Therapy in Nephrology
& Hypertension

Therapy in Nephrology & Hypertension

A Companion to Brenner & Rector's The Kidney

Third Edition

Christopher S. Wilcox, MD, PhD, FRCP(c), FACP

George E. Schreiner Professor of Nephrology and
Director, Georgetown University Hypertension,
   Kidney and Vascular Disorders Center
Department of Medicine
Co-Director of Angiogenesis Program
Lombardi Cancer Institute
Georgetown University
Chief of Division of Nephrology and Hypertension
Department of Medicine
Georgetown University Hospital
Washington, DC

SECTION EDITORS

Tomas Berl
Jonathan Himmelfarb
William E. Mitch
Barbara Murphy
David J. Salant
Alan S.L. Yu

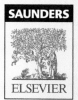

SAUNDERS

ELSEVIER

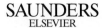

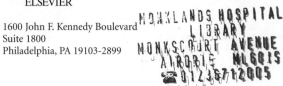

SAUNDERS
ELSEVIER

1600 John F. Kennedy Boulevard
Suite 1800
Philadelphia, PA 19103-2899

THERAPY IN NEPHROLOGY & HYPERTENSION: A COMPANION TO
BRENNER & RECTOR'S THE KIDNEY, THIRD EDITION ISBN: 978-1-4160-5484-9

Copyright © 2008 by Saunders, an imprint of Elsevier Inc.

Notice

Knowledge and best practice in this field are constantly changing. As new research and experience broaden our knowledge, changes in practice, treatment and drug therapy may become necessary or appropriate. Readers are advised to check the most current information provided (i) on procedures featured or (ii) by the manufacturer of each product to be administered, to verify the recommended dose or formula, the method and duration of administration, and contraindications. It is the responsibility of the practitioner, relying on their own experience and knowledge of the patient, to make diagnoses, to determine dosages and the best treatment for each individual patient, and to take all appropriate safety precautions. To the fullest extent of the law, neither the Publisher nor the Editors assume any liability for any injury and/or damage to persons or property arising out or related to any use of the material contained in this book.

The Publisher

Previous editions copyrighted 2003, 1999

Library of Congress Cataloging-in-Publication Data
Therapy in nephrology & hypertension : a companion to Brenner & Rector's
The kidney / [edited by] Christopher S. Wilcox. — 3rd ed.
    p. ; cm.
Includes bibliographical references and index.
ISBN 978-1-4160-5484-9
1. Kidneys—Diseases—Treatment. 2. Hypertension—Treatment. 3. Renal hypertension—Treatment. I. Wilcox, Christopher S. II. Brenner & Rector's the kidney. III. Title: Therapy in nephrology and hypertension. IV. Title: Brenner and Rector's the kidney.
[DNLM: 1. Kidney Diseases—therapy. 2. Female Urogenital Diseases—therapy. 3. Hypertension—therapy. 4. Kidney Diseases—complications. 5. Male Urogenital Diseases—therapy. 6. Nephrology—methods. WJ 300 T397 2008]

RC902.T487 2008
616.6′106—dc22

2008018832

Acquisitions Editor: Adrianne Brigido
Developmental Editor: Pamela Heatherington
Project Manager: David Saltzberg
Design Direction: Steven Stave

Printed in Canada

Last digit is the print number: 9 8 7 6 5 4 3 2 1

Salus servandra per scientiam doctrinamque
(Let us provide healing through science and learning)
I acknowledge my great fortune to have learnt the science of nephrology and hypertension
from the best in the field: Faisel S. Nashat, MD; Sir Stanley Peart, FRS; Gerhard Giebish, MD; and
Barry M. Brenner, MD, and to have had the strong support for my work from George E.
Schreiner, MD, who endowed the chair that I hold and Ms. Alma L. Gildenhorn, who chairs the board of the Cardiovascular
Kidney Hypertension Institute that I direct.

Aureus et carus umor fluat abunde
(O precious golden fluid, may it flow in abundance)

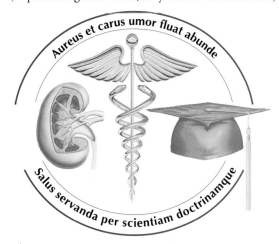

I express my deepest gratitude to those most influential in teaching me the practice of nephrology
and hypertension and the skills needed to develop a clinical and research program: William Slater, MD; William E. Mitch,
MD; and Craig C. Tisher, MD.

"During my years of teaching literature at Cornell and elsewhere I demanded of my students the passion of science and the patience of poetry."
Vladimir Nabokov
(***Strong Opinions**, Interviews, 1962*)

"Sell your cleverness and buy bewilderment;
Cleverness is mere opinion, bewilderment intuition."
Jalal al-Din Rumi
Persian poet and mystic, 1207–1273
(***Masnavi**, Book IV, Story II, as translated by E. H. Whinfield, 2000*)

The ideas and stimulating discussions that I have received from many colleagues, fellows, and students at the Universities of
Oxford, Cambridge, and London in the UK and Harvard, Florida, and Georgetown in the U.S.A. have been an inspiration for
me.

"Though I have all faith, so that I could remove mountains,
and have not love, I am nothing."
First Letter of St. Paul to the Corinthians, Chapter XIII
Holy Bible

Most important has been the sense of purpose and strength that accrues to my life and achievements from the love, understanding, and support of my dear wife, Linda; our beloved children, Mark, Juliette, Stuart, and Philip; and grandchildren
Henry, Isabelle, Anna, and Lauren; and from my dear brother, Frank, and his family.

In Memoriam
Stuart and Imogen Wilcox
and
Alex and Petra Wilcox

Contents

Preface

Therapy in Nephrology & Hypertension is a companion to *Brenner & Rector's The Kidney*. It provides comprehensive information and detailed discussion on the most critical areas relating to therapy. The aim is to provide a thoughtful overview of the rationale, specifics, efficacy, toxicity, and limitations of current therapeutics in renal disease and hypertension. A world-leading panel of expert contributors has been challenged to summarize and critique current clinical trials and to make their own treatment recommendations based on the results of these trials or, when these are not available, their own best clinical practice. They provide the background to these decisions and the details of the drugs used. Where possible, they have included an algorithm to summarize the steps involved in selection and monitoring of drug treatment.

The first two editions were coauthored with Hugh R. Brady. Sadly, his new responsibilities as President of University College, Dublin, Ireland, have precluded his involvement in this third edition. He has been hard indeed to replace. Rather than select another co-editor, I have chosen to distribute the editorial duties amongst a group of seven section editors. Each is a world expert in the fields that he or she covers. This ensures that the best current authors in the field have been selected to write the chapters and that the material has been critiqued by another true expert. I have been delighted with the results. This injection of new ideas and directions has led to the inclusion of many new chapters. Thirty of the 93 chapters have new primary authors.

Every chapter in this edition has been thoroughly revised and updated. Where new treatment modalities have been discovered and released, or new trials are available, these are included in the updated chapters.

It is you, the readers, who will evaluate the success of this textbook. Your comments, criticisms, and suggestions following its publication are greatly appreciated. They will be incorporated into the planning of the next edition. Please write to me to express comments on specific chapters, whether encouraging or otherwise, and any specific information or topics that you consider are either missing or inadequately or incorrectly covered. It is my aim to provide a comprehensive and up-to-date, fully referenced, and authoritative review of all the major areas of treatment in nephrology and hypertension by acknowledged experts in the field. I have retained the original concept of many short chapters since I believe this makes a large book, such as this, more accessible and readable and allows me to draw on a large expert authorship.

I wish to thank Barry Brenner for his continuing encouragement and trust in me to edit this important companion to his authoritative book; the many individuals at Saunders and Elsevier Science Publishing who have helped me pilot this project from inception to completion, most notably Ms. Pamela Hetherington, Ms. Adrianne Brigido, and Ms. Susan Pioli, who have undertaken the lead roles in preparing this new edition for publication; Ms. Emily Wing Kam Chan, who so diligently kept authors and section editors apprised of the progress of chapters and collated the entire book as chapters were passed on from section editors; and my wife for her understanding and support for this, yet another major academic project that necessarily takes time away from what we would otherwise spend together. Most important, I thank the section editors for the extraordinary dedication that they have shown to this project. Not only did I entrust them to recommend the selection of topics and authors, but also to read and correct the first proofs and to be the primary contacts for the authors as their chapters made their way through the process of submission, selection, correction, and final printing. Finally, I thank with great sincerity the many authors who have devoted their time and effort in busy academic lives to provide detailed, comprehensive, and fully referenced new chapters for this book.

Contributors

Enver Akalin, MD
Associate Professor of Medicine
Medical Director, Kidney and Pancreas Transplantation
Mount Sinai School of Medicine
New York, New York
Transplant Immunology and Immunosuppresssion

Alice Sue Appel, PhD
Research Associate
Columbia University College of Physicians and Surgeons
Research Associate
Division of Nephrology
Columbia Medical Center
New York, New York
Immunosuppressive Agents for the Therapy of Glomerular and Tubulointerstitial Disease

Gerald B. Appel, MD
Professor of Clinical Medicine
Columbia University College of Physicians and Surgeons
Director, Clinical Nephrology
Columbia University Medical Center
New York, New York
Immunosuppressive Agents for the Therapy of Glomerular and Tubulointerstitial Disease

Shakil Aslam, MD
Assistant Professor
Georgetown University School of Medicine
Assistant Professor
Georgetown University Hospital
Washington, DC
Antioxidant Therapy in Chronic Kidney Disease

Robert C. Atkins, MB BS, MSc, DSc, FRACP
School of Epidemiology and Preventive Medicine
Monash University
Victoria, Australia
Management of Infection-Associated Glomerulonephritis

Howard A. Austin III, MD
Adjunct Professor of Medicine
Uniformed Services University
Senior Clinical Investigator
National Institute of Diabetes and Digestive and Kidney Diseases
National Institutes of Health
Bethesda, Maryland
Lupus Nephritis; Idiopathic Membranous Nephropathy

James E. Balow, MD
Professor of Medicine
Uniformed Services University
Clinical Director and Chief
Kidney Disease Section
National Institute of Diabetes and Digestive and Kidney Diseases, National Institutes of Health
Bethesda, Maryland
Lupus Nephritis

Jonathan Barratt, MB ChB (Hons), PhD, MRCP
Senior Lecturer in Nephrology
Department of Infection, Immunity and Inflammation
University of Leicester
Honorary Consultant Nephrologist
John Walls Renal Unit
Leciester General Hospital
Leicester, United Kingdom
IgA Nephropathy and Henoch-Schönlein Purpura

Brendan J. Barrett, MB, MSc
Professor of Medicine (Nephrology and Clinical Epidemiology)
Memorial University of Newfoundland
Active Staff
Nephrology and Internal Medicine
Eastern Health
St. John's, Newfoundland and Labrador, Canada
Contrast Nephropathy

Bryan N. Becker, MD
Professor of Medicine
University of Wisconsin School of Medicine and Public Health
Madison, Wisconsin
Technical Aspects of Hemodialysis

Tomas Berl, MD
Professor of Medicine
Head, Division of Renal Diseases and Hypertension
University of Colorado Denver
Professor of Medicine
University of Colorado Hospital
Denver, Colorado
Therapy of Dysnatremic Disorders; Part III Editor; Part IV Editor

Catherine Blake, PhD, MMedSci
Senior Lecturer
School of Physiotherapy and Performance Science
University College Dublin
Dublin, Ireland
Measures to Improve Quality of Life in End-Stage Renal Disease Patients

Peter G. Blake, MB, FRCPC, FRCPI
Professor of Medicine
University of Western Ontario
Chief of Nephrology
London Health Sciences Centre
London, Ontario, Canada
Adequacy of Peritoneal Dialysis

Emily A. Blumberg, MD
Associate Professor of Medicine
Program Director, Infectious Diseases Fellowship
University of Pennsylvania
Director, Transplant Infectious Diseases
Hospital of the University of Pennsylvania
Philadelphia, Pennsylvania
Prevention and Treatment of Infection in Kidney Transplant Recipients

Joseph V. Bonventre, MD, PhD
Robert H. Ebert Professor of Molecular Medicine
Harvard Medical School
Chief, Renal Division
Brigham and Women's Hospital
Boston, Massachusetts
Experimental Strategies for Acute Kidney Injury

D. Craig Brater, MD
Professor of Medicine
Indiana University School of Medicine
Indianapolis, Indiana
Drug Dosing in Renal Failure

William E. Braun, MD
Staff
Department of Nephrology and Hypertension
Consultant in Organ Transplantation
Cleveland Clinic Foundation
Cleveland, Ohio
Cardiovascular and Other Noninfectious Complications after Renal Transplantation in Adults

Emmanuel L. Bravo, MD
Consultant
Department of Nephrology and Hypertension
Urological and Kidney Institute
Cleveland Clinic Foundation
Cleveland, Ohio
Adrenal Disorders

Zachary Z. Brener, MD
Assistant Professor of Clinical Medicine
Albert Einstein College of Medicine
Attending Nephrologist
Beth Israel Medical Center
New York, New York
Dialysis and Hemoperfusion in the Treatment of Poisoning and Drug Overdose

David M. Briscoe, MD
Associate Professor of Pediatrics
Harvard Medical School
Harvard University
Associate Professor
Childrens Hospital Boston
Boston, Massachusetts
Management of End-Stage Renal Disease in Childhood and Adolescence

Jonathan Bromberg, MD
Professor of Surgery, Immunology, and Gene and Cell Medicine
Chief, Transplantation Institute
Mount Sinai School of Medicine
New York, New York
Technical Aspects of Renal Transplantation and Surgical Complications

John Burkart, MD
Professor
Section of Nephrology
Corporate Director, Dialysis Program
Department of Internal Medicine
Wake Forest University
Winston-Salem, North Carolina
Techniques in Peritoneal Dialysis

Giovambattista Capasso, MD
Full Professor
Chair of Nephrology
Department of Internal Medicine
Second University
Director of Nephrology
Dialysis and Transplantation Unit
University General Hospital
Napoli, Italy
Diuretics and β-Blockers

Francesco P. Cappuccio, MD, MSc, FRCP, FFPH, FAHA
Cephalon Chair of Cardiovascular Medicine & Epidemiology
Cardiovascular & Epidemiology Research Group
Clinical Sciences Research Institute
University of Warwick Medical School
Honorary Consultant Physician
University Hospitals Conventry & Warwickshire NHS Trust
Coventry, United Kingdom
Dietary Salt Reduction

Culley C. Carson III, MD
Professor and Chief
Department of Surgery
Division of Urology
University of North Carolina School of Medicine
University of North Carolina Hospitals
Chapel Hill, North Carolina
Treatment of Erectile Dysfunction in Chronic Kidney Disease

Steven J. Chadban, BMed, PhD, FRACP
Associate Professor, Renal Medicine
University of Sydney
Senior Staff Sepcialist
Director of Kidney Transplantation
Royal Prince Alfred Hospital
Sydney, Australia
Management of Infection-Associated Glomerulonephritis

Arlene B. Chapman, MD
Professor of Medicine
Department of Medicine
Renal Division
Emory University School of Medicine
Atlanta, Georgia
Renal Cystic Disorders

Joline L.T. Chen, MD, MS
Assistant Professor
Boston University
Attending Nephrologist
Boston Medical Center
Boston, Massachusetts
Amyloidosis and Other Fibrillary and Monoclonal Immunoglobulin-Associated Kidney Diseases

Russell W. Chesney, MD
University of Tennessee Health Science Center
Vice President, Academic Affairs
Le Bonheur Children's Medical Center
Memphis, Tennessee
Noncystic Hereditary Diseases of the Kidney

Alfred K. Cheung, MD
Professor of Medicine
University of Utah
Staff Physician
Veterans Affairs Salt Lake City Healthcare System
Salt Lake City, Utah
Complications Associated with Hemodialysis

Monique E. Cho, MD
Staff Clinician
Kidney Disease Section
National Institute of Diabetes and Digestive and Kidney Diseases
National Institutes of Health
Bethesda, Maryland
Focal Segmental Glomerulosclerosis and Collapsing Glomerulopathy

Lewis M. Cohen, MD
Professor of Psychiatry
Tufts University
Baystate Medical Center
Springfield, Massachusetts
Neuropsychiatric Complications and Psychopharmacology of End-Stage Renal Disease; Palliative and Supportive Care

Paul R. Conlin, MD
Associate Professor of Medicine
Harvard Medical School
Interim Chief, Medical Service
VA Boston Healthcare System
Boston, Massachusetts
Nonpharmacologic Treatment

Dinna Cruz, MD, MPH
Nephrologist
Ospedale San Bortolo
Vicenza, Italy
Continuous Renal Replacement Therapies

Brett Cullis, MBChB
Specialist Registrar in Nephrology and Intensive Care Medicine
Derriford Hospital
Plymouth, United Kingdom
Dopaminergic and Pressor Agents in Acute Renal Failure

Gary C. Curhan, MD, ScD
Associate Professor of Medicine
Harvard Medical School
Associate Professor of Epidemiology
Harvard School of Public Health
Physician
Brigham and Women's Hospital
Boston, Massachusetts
Evaluation and Management of Kidney Stone Disease

John J. Curtis, MD
Professor of Medicine
Professor of Surgery
Division of Nephrology
University of Alabama at Birmingham
Birmingham, Alabama
Hypertension in Renal Transplant Recipients

Christopher J. Cutie, MD
Resident in Urology
Harvard Medical School
Massachusetts General Hospital
Boston, Massachusetts
Obstructive Uropathy

Giuseppe D'Amico, MD, FRCP
Emeritus Head
Division of Nephrology
S. Carlo Borromeo Hospital
Milano, Italy
Cryoglobulinemia and Hepatitis C–Associated Membranoproliferative Glomerulonephritis

Simon J. Davies, MD, FRCP
Professor of Nephrology and Dialysis Medicine
Institute for Science and Technology in Medicine
Faculty of Health
Keele University
Keele, United Kingdom
Consultant Nephrologist
University Hospital of North Staffordshire
Stoke-on-Trent, Staffordshire, United Kingdom
Complications of Peritoneal Dialysis

Connie L. Davis, MD
Professor of Medicine
University of Washington School of Medicine
Medical Director and Co Program Director
Kidney and Pancreas Transplant
University Hospital Medical Center
Seattle, Washington
*Evaluation of the Kidney Transplant Recipient and Living
   Kidney Donor*

Sara N. Davison, MD, MHSc
Associate Professor
University of Alberta
Nephrologist
University of Alberta Hospital
Edmonton, Alberta, Canada
Palliative and Supportive Care

Raffaele De Caterina, MD, PhD
Professor of Cardiology
Director, Institute of Cardiology
G. d'Annunzio University
Chief, University Cardiology Division
Ospedale Clinicizzato S.S. Annunziata
Chieti, Italy
Director, Laboratory for Thrombosis and Atherosclerosis
   Research
CNR Institute of Clinical Physiology
Pisa, Italy
Dietary Modulation of the Inflammatory Response

Laura M. Dember, MD
Associate Professor of Medicine
Boston University School of Medicine
Boston, Massachusetts
*Minimal Change Disease; Amyloidosis and Other Fibrillary and
   Monoclonal Immunoglobulin-Associated Kidney Diseases*

Mark Denton, MD, PhD
Consultant Nephrologist
Derriford Hospital
Honorary Senior Lecturer
Peninsula Medical School
Plymouth, United Kingdom
Dopaminergic and Pressor Agents in Acute Renal Failure

Thomas A. Depner, MD
Professor of Medicine
University of California, Davis, Medical Center
Director of Dialysis Services
University of California, Davis, Health System
Sacramento, California
Hemodialysis Adequacy

J. Eric Derksen, MD
Urology Section Chief
Penrose Hospital
Colorado Springs, Colorado
Treatment of Erectile Dysfunction in Chronic Kidney Disease

Vikas R. Dharnidharka, MD, MPH
Associate Professor
Chief, Division of Pediatric Nephrology
Fellowship Program Director
University of Florida College of Medicine
Medical Director, Pediatric Kidney Transplantation
Shands Hospital at the University of Florida
Gainesville, Florida
*Management of End-Stage Renal Disease in Childhood and
   Adolescence*

Bradley S. Dixon, MD
Associate Professor of Medicine
University of Iowa
Staff Physician
Veterans Affairs Medical Center
Iowa City, Iowa
Choice and Maintenance of Vascular Access

Hamish Dobbie, MB
Centre for Nephrology
University College London
London, United Kingdom
Diuretics and β-Blockers

Wilfred Druml, MD
Third Department of Medicine
Division of Nephrology
Vienna General Hospital
Medical University of Vienna
Vienna, Austria
Division of Nephrology
Baylor College of Medicine
Houston, Texas
Nutritional Management of Acute Renal Failure

Thomas D. DuBose, Jr., MD
Tinsley R. Harrison Professor and Chair of Internal Medicine
Professor of Physiology and Pharmacology
Wake Forest University School of Medicine
Chief of Internal Medicine Service
North Carolina Baptist Hospital
Winston-Salem, North Carolina
Metabolic and Respiratory Acidosis

Lance D. Dworkin, MD
Professor of Medicine
Vice Chairman for Research & Academic Affairs
The Warren Alpert Medical School of Brown University
Director, Division of Kidney Disease & Hypertension
Rhode Island Hospital
The Miriam Hospital
Providence, Rhode Island
Calcium Channel Blockers; Medical Management of Patients with Renal Artery Stenosis

David H. Ellison, MD
Head, Division of Nephrology and Hypertension
Professor of Medicine and Physiology and Pharmacology
Oregon Health & Science University
Staff Physician
Veterans Affairs Medical Center
Partland, Oregon
Diuretic Use in Edema and the Problem of Resistance

Stephen Z. Fadem, MD, FACP, FASN
Clinical Professor
Division of Nephrology
Baylor College of Medicine
Staff
The Methodist Hospital
Houston, Texas
Internet Resources for Nephrologists

John Feehally, MA, DM, FRCP
Professor of Renal Medicine
Department of Infection, Immunity and Inflammation
University of Leicester
Consultant Nephrologist
University Hospitals of Leicester
Leicester, United Kingdom
IgA Nephropathy and Henoch-Schönlein Purpura

Donald A. Feinfeld, MD
Professor of Clinical Medicine
Albert Einstein College of Clinical Medicine
Nephrology Fellowship Program Director
Beth Israel Medical Center
New York, New York
Dialysis and Hemoperfusion in the Treatment of Poisoning and Drug Overdose

Steven Fishbane, MD
Professor of Medicine
SUNY Stony Brook School of Medicine
Chief of Nephrology
Winthrop University Hospital
Mineola, New York
Iron and Erythropoietin-Related Therapies

John M. Fitzpatrick, MCh, FRSCI, FCUROL (SA), FRCS, FRCS(Glas)
Professor and Chairman
Department of Surgery
University College Dublin
Consultant Urologist
Mater Misericordiae University Hospital
Dublin, Ireland
Nephrolithiasis: Lithotripsy and Surgery

Daniel J. Ford, MB BCh, MRCP(UK)
Specialist Registrar in Renal Medicine
Southmead Hospital
Bristol, United Kingdom
Dopaminergic and Pressor Agents in Acute Renal Failure

Alessandro Fornasieri, MD
Consultant
Division of Nephrology
San Carlo Hospital
Milano, Italy
Cryoglobulinemia and Hepatitis C–Associated Membranoproliferative Glomerulonephritis

Marc B. Garnick, MD
Professor of Medicine
Harvard Medical School
Professor of Medicine
Beth Israel-Deaconess Medical Center
Boston, Massachusetts
Primary Neoplasms of the Kidney

Robert S. Gaston, MD
Professor of Medicine and Surgery
University of Alabama at Birmingham
Medical Director, Kidney and Pancreas Transplantation
University Hospital
Birmingham, Alabama
Hypertension in Renal Transplant Recipients

Michael J. Germain, MD
Professor of Medicine
Tufts University
Baystate Medical Center
Springfield, Massachusetts
Neuropsychiatric Complications and Psychopharmacology of End-Stage Renal Disease; Palliative and Supportive Care

Pere Ginès, MD, PhD
Professor of Medicine
University of Barcelona School of Medicine
Chairman, Liver Unit
Hospital Clínic
Barcelona, Catalonia, Spain
Management of Hepatorenal Syndrome

Joyce M. Gonin, MD
Associate Professor of Medicine
Georgetown University
Associate Professor of Medicine
Georgetown University Hospital
Washington, DC
Hyperhomocysteinemia

Eddie L. Greene, MD
Associate Professor of Medicine
Mayo Clinic College of Medicine
Mayo Clinic
Rochester, Minnesota
*Treatment of Sleep Disorders in Patients with Renal
    Dysfunction*

Scott M. Grundy, MD
Professor of Internal Medicine
University of Texas Southwestern Medical Center
Dallas, Texas
*Cholesterol Management in Patients with Chronic Kidney
    Disease*

Mounira Habli, MD
Fellow and Clinical Instructor
Division of Maternal Fetal Medicine
Department of Obstetrics and Gynecology
University of Cincinnati
Cincinnati, Ohio
Hypertension in Pregnancy; Renal Disease in Pregnancy

Andrew Hall, MA, MB, MRCP(UK)
Clinical Research Fellow
University College London
London, United Kingdom
Diuretics and β-Blockers

Mitchell L. Halperin, MD, FRCPC, FRS
Emeritus Professor of Medicine
University of Toronto
Attending Staff
Division of Nephrology
St. Michael's Hospital
Toronto, Ontario, Canada
Treatment of Hypokalemia and Hyperkalemia

Nikolas B. Harbord, MD
Attending
Department of Nephrology and Hypertension
Beth Israel Medical Center
New York, New York
*Dialysis and Hemoperfusion in the Treatment of Poisoning and
    Drug Overdose*

Peter Hewins, PhD, MRCP
Wellcome Trust Intermediate Clinical Fellow
University of Birmingham
Honorary Consultant Nephrologist
University Hospital Birmingham NHS Foundation Trust
Edgbaston, Birmingham, United Kingdom
Idiopathic Membranoproliferative Glomerulonephritis

Jonathan Himmelfarb, MD
Professor of Medicine
Director, Kidney Research Institute
Joseph Eschbach Endowed Chair for Kidney Research
Department of Medicine
Division of Nephrology
University of Washington
Seattle, Washington
Part VI Editor; Part XIII Editor

Norman K. Hollenberg, MD, PhD
Professor of Medicine
Harvard Medical School
Director of Physiologic Research Division
Brigham and Women's Hospital
Boston, Massachusetts
*ACE Inhibitors, Angiotensin Receptor Blockers,
    Mineralocortcoid Receptor Antigonists,
    and Renin Antagonists*

Enyu Imai, MD, PhD
Nephrology
Osaka University Graduate School of Medicine
Clinical Professor of Nephrology
Osaka University Hospital
Osaka, Japan
Prospects for Gene Therapy

Yoshitaka Isaka, MD, PhD
Advanced Technology for Transplantation
Osaka University Graduate School of Medicine
Osaka, Japan
Prospects for Gene Therapy

Hye Ryoun Jang, MD, PhD
Postdoctoral Fellow
Division of Nephrology
Department of Medicine
Johns Hopkins University School of Medicine
Baltimore, Maryland
Experimental Strategies for Acute Kidney Injury

David Jayne, MD, FRCP
Consultant in Nephrology
Addenbrooke's Hospital
Cambridge, United Kingdom
Plasmapheresis in Renal Diseases

Jay R. Kaluvapalle, MD
Fellow
University of Utah
Fellow
University of Utah Health Sciences Center
Salt Lake City, Utah
Complications Associated with Hemodialysis

Kamel S. Kamel, MD, FRCPC
Professor of Medicine
University of Toronto
Head, Division of Nephrology
St. Michael's Hospital
Toronto, Ontario, Canada
Treatment of Hypokalemia and Hyperkalemia

Suraj Kapa, MD
Resident, Internal Medicine
Mayo Clinic
Rochester, Minnesota
Treatment of Sleep Disorders in Patients with Renal Dysfunction

Norman M. Kaplan, MD
Clinical Professor of Internal Medicine
University of Texas Southwestern Medical School
Dallas, Texas
Individualization of Pharmacologic Therapy

Joana E. Kist-van Holthe, MD, PhD
Leiden University Medical Centre
Leiden, The Netherlands
Management of End-Stage Renal Disease in Childhood and Adolescence

Mary E. Klotman, MD
Murray Rosenberg Professor of Medicine
Chief, Division of Infectious Diseases
Mount Sinai School of Medicine
New York, New York
Hepatitis B– and HIV-Related Renal Diseases

Paul E. Klotman, MD
Mount Sinai School of Medicine
New York, New York
Hepatitis B– and HIV-Related Renal Diseases

Jeffrey B. Kopp, MD
Adjunct Professor
Uniformed Services University of the Health Sciences
Staff Clinician
Kidney Disease Section
National Institute of Diabetes and Digestive and Kidney Diseases
National Institutes of Health
Bethesda, Maryland
Focal Segmental Glomerulosclerosis and Collapsing Glomerulopathy

Lawrence R. Krakoff, MD
Professor of Medicine
Mount Sinai School of Medicine
New York, New York
Chief of Medicine
Englewood Hospital & Medical Center
Englewood, New Jersey
Decisions for Management of High Blood Pressure: A Perspective

Aaron C. Lentz, MD
Resident Physician
Department of Surgery
Division of Urology
University of North Carolina Hospitals
Chapel Hill, North Carolina
Treatment of Erectile Dysfunction in Chronic Kidney Disease

Susan M. Lerner, MD
Assistant Professor of Surgery
Mount Sinai School of Medicine
New York, New York
Technical Aspects of Renal Transplantation and Surgical Complications

Jerrold S. Levine, MD
Associate Professor of Medicine
Department of Medicine
Section of Nephrology
Adjunct Associate Professor
Department of Microbiology and Immunology
Medical Staff
University of Illinois at Chicago
Chief, Section of Nephrology
Medical Staff
Jesse Brown Veterans Affairs Medical Center
Chicago, Illinois
Management of Complications of Nephrotic Syndrome

Jeremy B. Levy, PhD, FRCP
Senior Lecturer
Imperial College London
Consultant Nephrologist
Imperial College Healthcare NHS Trust
Hammersmith Hospital
London, United Kingdom
Systemic Vasculitis and Pauci-Immune Glomerulonephritis

Edmund J. Lewis, MD
Professor of Medicine
Rush Medical College
Director, Section of Nephrology
Rush University Medical Center
Chicago, Illinois
Therapy for Diabetic Nephropathy

Julia B. Lewis, MD
Professor of Medicine
Director of Nephrology Fellowship Program
Vanderbilt University Medical Center
Nashville, Tennessee
Therapy for Diabetic Nephropathy

Shih-Hua Lin, MD
Professor of Medicine
Division of Nephrology
Department of Medicine
Director of Hemodialysis
Tri-Service General Hospital
National Defense Medical Center
Taipei, Taiwan, Republic of China
Treatment of Hypokalemia and Hyperkalemia

Francisco Llach, MD, FACP
Professor of Medicine
Director of Clinical Nephrology
Division of Nephrology and Hypertension
Georgetown University
Washington, DC
Hypercalcemia, Hypocalcemia, and Other Divalent Cation
 Disorders

Friedrich C. Luft, MD
Professor of Medicine
Medical Faculty of the Charité
Berlin, Germany
Helen C. Levitt Visiting Professor
Roy J. and Lucille A. Carver College of Medicine
University of Iowa
Iowa City, Iowa
Chief, Division of Nephrology and Hypertension
HELIOS-Klinikum-Berlin
Director, Experimental and Clinical Research Center,
 Max-Delbrück Center for Molecular Medicine
Berlin, Germany
Management of Volume Depletion and Established Acute Renal
 Failure

Samuel J. Mann, MD
Professor of Clinical Medicine
Division of Nephrology and Hypertension
Weill/Cornell Medical School
Attending
New York Presbyterian–Weill/Cornell Medical Center
New York, New York
Hypertensive Emergencies

Kevin J. Martin, MD
Professor of Internal Medicine
Director, Division of Nephrology
Saint Louis University
St. Louis, Missouri
Calcium, Phosphorus, Renal Bone Disease, and Calciphylaxis

Tahsin Masud, MD
Associate Professor of Medicine
Emory University School of Medicine
Atlanta, Georgia
Nutritional Therapy of Patients with Chronic Kidney Disease
 and Its Impact on Progressive Renal Insufficiency

Roy O. Mathew, MD
Fellow
University of California at San Diego
San Diego, California
Acute Dialysis Principles and Practice

W. Scott McDougal, AB, MD, AM (Hon)
Professor of Urology
Harvard Medical School
Chief of Urology
Massachusetts General Hospital
Boston, Massachusetts
Obstructive Uropathy

Michael McKusick, MD
Assistant Professor of Radiology
Mayo Medical School
Consultant, Vascular and Interventional Radiology and
 Vascular Surgery
Mayo Clinic
Rochester, Minnesota
Renovascular Hypertension and Ischemic Nephropathy:
 Angioplasty and Stenting

Ravindra L. Mehta, MD
Professor of Clinical Medicine
Associate Chair, Clinical Affairs, Department of Medicine
Division of Nephrology
University of California at San Diego
UCSD Medical Center
San Diego, California
Acute Dialysis Principles and Practice

Luigi Minetti, MD
Clinical Research Center for Rare Diseases Aldo e Cele Daccò
Villa Camozza
Ranica, Italy
Mario Negri Institute for Pharmacological Research
Negri Bergamo Laboratories
Bergamo, Italy
Treatment of Anemia and Bleeding in Chronic Kidney Disease

Adam M. Mirot, MD
Assistant Professor of Psychiatry
Tufts University School of Medicine
Boston, Massachusetts
Staff Psychiatrist
Psychiatric Consultation Service
Baystate Medical Center
Springfield, Massachusetts
Neuropsychiatric Complications and Psychopharmacology of
 End-Stage Renal Disease

William E. Mitch, MD
Gordon A. Cain Chair in Nephrology
Director, Division of Nephrology
Baylor College of Medicine
Houston, Texas
Nutritional Management of Acute Renal Failure; Nutritional
 Therapy of Patients with Chronic Kidney Disease and Its
 Impact on Progressive Renal Insufficiency; Part XII Editor;
 Part XVI Editor

Alvin H. Moss, MD
Professor of Medicine
Section of Nephrology
West Virginia University School of Medicine
Director, Center for Health Ethics and Law
Medical Director, Palliative Care Service
West Virginia University Hospital
Morgantown, West Virginia
Patient Selection for Dialysis and the Decision to Withhold or Withdraw Dialysis

Barbara Murphy, MB, BAO, BCH
Chief, Division of Nephrology
Department of Medicine
Mount Sinai School of Medicine
New York, New York
Part VII Editor; Part VIII Editor; Part XIV Editor

Mitra K. Nadim, MD
Assistant Professor of Clinical Medicine
University of Southern California Keck School of Medicine
Attending Nephrologist
USC University Hospital
Los Angeles, California
Diuretics in Acute Kidney Injury

Eric G. Neilson, MD
Hugh Jackson Morgan Professor of Medicine
Chariman, Department of Medicine
Vanderbilt University School of Medicine
Physician-in-Chief
Vanderbilt University Hospital
Nashville, Tennessee
Treatment of Acute Interstitial Nephritis

Elizabeth H. Nora, MD, PhD
Endocrinology and Internal Medicine
The Aurora Sheboygan Clinic
Sheboygan, Wisconsin
Treatment of Sleep Disorders in Patients with Renal Dysfunction

Marina Noris, PhD
Mario Negri Institute for Pharmacological Research
Clinical Research Center for Rare Diseases Aldo e Cele Daccò
Ranica, Bergamo, Italy
Thrombotic Microangiopathies

Pouneh Nouri, MD
Georgetown University
Assistant Professor of Medicine
Georgetown University Hospital
Washington, DC
Hypercalcemia, Hypocalcemia, and Other Divalent Cation Disorders; Management of Hypertension in Patients Receiving Dialysis

Man S. Oh, MD
Professor of Medicine
State University of New York
Downstate Medical Center
Brooklyn, New York
Treatment of Hypokalemia and Hyperkalemia

Yvonne M. O'Meara, MD, FRCPI
Senior Lecturer in Medicine
School of Medicine and Medical Sciences
University College Dublin
Consultant Nephrologist
Mater Misericordia University Hospital
Dublin, Ireland
Management of Complications of Nephrotic Syndrome

Biff F. Palmer, MD
Professor of Internal Medicine
Renal Fellowship Director
University of Texas Southwestern Medical Center
Dallas, Texas
Treatment of Metabolic and Respiratory Alkalosis

Vasilios Papademetriou, MD
Professor of Medicine
Georgetown University
Director, Hypertension and Cardiovascular Research
Department of Veterans Affairs Medical Center
Management of Associated Cardiovascular Risk in Essential Hypertension

Patrick S. Parfrey, MD, FRCPC
University Research Professor (Medicine)
Memorial University
Staff Nephrologist
Eastern Health
St. John's, Newfoundland and Labrador, Canada
Contrast Nephropathy

Manish P. Patel, MD
Division of Urology
School of Medicine
University of North Carolina at Chapel Hill
Chapel Hill, North Carolina
Treatment of Erectile Dysfunction in Chronic Kidney Disease

Marie-Noëlle Pépin, MD, FRCPC
Nephrologist
Associate Professor
Centre Hospitalier de l'Université de Montréal
Montreal, Quebec, Canada
Management of Hepatorenal Syndrome

William D. Plant, BSC, MB, MRCPI, FRCPE
Clinical Senior Lecturer in Nephrology
School of Medicine
University College Cork
Consultant Renal Physician
Cork University Hospital
Cork, Ireland
Measures to Improve Quality of Life in End-Stage Renal Disease Patients

Charles D. Pusey, DSc, FRCP, FRCPath
Professor of Medicine
Imperial College London
Honorary Consultant Physician
Imperial College Healthcare NHS Trust
London, United Kingdom
Systematic Vasculitis and Pauci-Immune Glomerulonephritis

Rizwan A. Qazi, MD
Assistant Professor of Internal Medicine
Saint Louis University School of Medicine
St. Louis, Missouri
Calcium, Phosphorus, Renal Bone Disease and Calciphylaxis

Hamid Rabb, MD
Professor of Medicine
Johns Hopkins University School of Medicine
Physician Director, Kidney & Pancreas Transplant
The Johns Hopkins Hospital
Baltimore, Maryland
Experimental Strategies for Acute Kidney Injury

Brian D. Radbill, MD
Assistant Professor
Department of Medicine
Clinical Director, Renal Division
Medical Director
Adult Hemodialysis
Mount Sinai School Medicine
New York, New York
Hepatitis B– and HIV-Related Renal Diseases

Frederic F. Rahbari-Oskoui, MD
Assistant Professor of Medicine
Emory University School of Medicine
Atlanta, Georgia
Renal Cystic Disorders

Andrew J. Rees, MB, MSc, FRCP, FMedSci
Marie Curie Excellence Chair
Institute of Pathology
Medical University of Vienna
Vienna, Austria
Antiglomerular Basement Membrane Antibody Disease

Giuseppe Remuzzi, MD
Professor of Nephrology
Director, Division of Nephrology and Dialysis
Ospedale Riuniti di Bergamo and Negri Bergamo
    Laboratories
Mario Negri Institute for Pharmacological Research
Bergamo, Italy
*Thrombotic Microangiopathies; Treatment of Anemia and
    Bleeding in Chronic Kidney Disease*

Zaccaria Ricci, MD
Medical Doctor
Bambino Gesù Hospital
Rome, Italy
Continuous Renal Replacement Therapies

Eberhard Ritz, MD
Professor of Medicine
Section of Nephrology
Department of Internal Medicine
University of Heidelberg
Heidelberg, Germany
Cardiovascular Complications of End-Stage Renal Disease

Nancy M. Rodig, MD
Instructor in Pediatrics
Harvard Medical School
Attending Physician in Nephrology
Children's Hospital Boston
Boston, Massachusetts
Management of Pediatric Kidney Disease

Claudio Ronco, MD
Professor of Nephrology
University of Padova
Padova, Italy
Professor of Nephrology
University of Bologna
Bologna, Italy
Director
Department of Nephrology Dialysis and Transplantation
San Bortolo Hospital
Vicenza, Italy
Continuous Renal Replacement Therapies

Robert H. Rubin, MD
Osborne Professor of Health Sciences and Technology
Professor of Medicine
Harvard Medical School
Director, Center for Experimental Pharmacology and
    Therapeutics
Massachusetts Institute of Technology
Associate Director
Division of Infectious Disease
Brigham and Women's Hospital
Boston, Massachusetts
Therapy of Urinary Tract Infection

Robert J. Rubin, MD
Clinical Professor of Medicine
Georgetown University
Attending Physician
Georgetown University Hospital
Washington, DC
Health Economics of End-Stage Renal Disease Treatment

Piero Ruggenenti, MD
Division of Nephrology and Dialysis
Azienda Ospedaliera Ospedali Riuniti di Bergamo and Mario
    Negri Institute for Pharmacological Research
Negri Bergamo Laboratories
Ranica, Bergamo, Italy
Thrombotic Microangiopathies

David J. Salant, MD
Professor of Medicine
Boston University School of Medicine
Chief, Renal Section
Boston Medical Center
Boston, Massachusetts
Minimal Change Disease; Part II Editor

Paul W. Sanders, MD
Professor of Medicine and Physiology & Biophysics
University of Alabama at Birmingham
Department of Veterans Affairs Medical Center
Birmingham, Alabama
Myeloma and Secondary Involvement of the Kidney in Dysproteinemias

Caroline O.S. Savage, PhD, FRCP
Professor of Nephrology
University of Birmingham
Professor of Nephrology
University Hospital Birmingham NHS Foundation Trust
Edgbaston, Birmingham, United Kingdom
Idiopathic Membranoproliferative Glomerulonephritis

Mohamed H. Sayegh, MD, FAHA, FASN
Warren E. Grupe and John P. Merrill Chair in Transplantation Medicine
Professor of Medicine and Pediatrics
Harvard Medical School
Director, Transplantation Research Center, Renal Division
Brigham and Women's Hospital
Children's Hospital Boston
Boston, Massachusetts
Diagnosis and Management of Renal Allograft Dysfunction

Arrigo Schieppati, MD
Mario Negri Institute for Pharmacological Research
Division of Nephrology and Dialysis
Azienda Ospedaliera
Ospedali Riuniti di Bergamo
Mario Negri Institute for Pharmacological Research
Negri Bergamo Laboratories
Bergamo, Italy
Treatment of Anemia and Bleeding in Chronic Kidney Disease

Bernd Schröppel, MD
Assistant Professor
Division of Nephrology
Mount Sinai School of Medicine
New York, New York
Transplant Immunology and Immunosuppresssion

Gerald Schulman, MD, FASN
Professor of Medicine
Vanderbilt University School of Medicine
Vanderbilt University Medical Center
Nashville, Tennessee
Technical Aspects of Hemodialysis

Douglas G. Shemin, MD
Associate Professor of Medicine
Warren Alpert Medical School of Brown University
Director, Hemodialysis Unit
Rhode Island Hospital
Providence, Rhode Island
Calcium Channel Blockers

Baha M. Sibai, MD
Professor
University of Cincinnati
Cincinnati, Ohio
Hypertension in Pregnancy; Renal Disease in Pregnancy

Sandra Silva, MD
International Fellow
Ospedale San Bortolo
Vicenza, Italy
Continuous Renal Replacement Therapies

Karen D. Sims, MD, PhD
Fellow
Infectious Diseases Division
Department of Medicine
University of Pennsylvania School of Medicine
Hospital of the University of Pennsylvania
Philadelphia, Pennsylvania
Prevention and Treatment of Infection in Kidney Transplant Recipients

James P. Smith, MD
Fellow, Division of Nephrology
Department of Medicine
Vanderbilt University Medical Center
Nashville, Tennessee
Treatment of Acute Interstitial Nephritis

Richard J.H. Smith, MD
Professor of Internal Medicine
Division of Nephrology, Otolaryngology and Pediatrics
Sterba Hearing Research Professor
Director, Molecular Otolaryngology Research Laboratories
Carver College of Medicine
University of Iowa
Iowa City, Iowa
Idiopathic Membranoproliferative Glomerulonephritis

Michael J.G. Somers, MD
Assistant Professor of Pediatrics
Harvard Medical School
Director of Clinical Services
Division of Nephrology
Children's Hospital Boston
Boston, Massachusetts
Management of Pediatric Kidney Disease

Virend K. Somers, MD, PhD
Professor of Medicine
Mayo Clinic
Rochester, Minnesota
Treatment of Sleep Disorders in Patients with Renal Dysfunction

Maarten W. Taal, MBChB, MMed, MD, FCP(SA), FRCP
Senior Lecturer
University of Nottingham Medical School at Derby
Consultant Renal Physician
Derby City General Hospital
Derby, United Kingdom
Prevention of Progressive Renal Failure

Yoshitsugu Takabatake, MD, PhD
Assistant Professor
Department of Nephrology
Osaka University School of Graduate Medicine
Osaka, Japan
Prospects for Gene Therapy

Eric N. Taylor, MD, MSc
Instructor in Medicine
Harvard Medical School
Associate Physician
Renal Division
Brigham and Women's Hospital
Boston, Massachusetts
Evaluation and Management of Kidney Stone Disease

Edward G. Tessier, PharmD, MPH, BCPS
Adjunct Assistant Professor
University of Massachusetts, Amherst School of Nursing
Clinical Pharmacist
Baystate Franklin Medical Center
Greenfield, Massachusetts
*Neuropsychiatric Complications and Psychopharmacology of
   End-Stage Renal Disease*

Stephen C. Textor, MD
Professor of Medicine
Mayo Clinic College of Medicine
Professor of Medicine
Vice-Chair, Division of Nephrology and Hypertension
Mayo Clinic
Rochester, Minnesota
*Renovascular Hypertension and Ischemic Nephropathy:
   Angioplasty and Stenting*

Joshua M. Thurman, MD
Assistant Professor of Medicine
University of Colorado Health Sciences Center
University of Colorado
Aurora, Colorado
Therapy of Dysnatremic Disorders

Nina E. Tolkoff-Rubin, MD
Professor of Medicine
Harvard Medical School
Medical Director, Dialysis and Renal Transplant
Massachusetts General Hospital
Boston, Massachussetts
Therapy of Urinary Tract Infection

Robert D. Toto, MD
Mary M. Conroy Professor of Kidney Diseases
Distinguished Teaching Professor
University of Texas Southwestern Medical Center
Dallas, Texas
*Cholesterol Management in Patients with Chronic Kidney
   Disease*

A. Neil Turner, PhD, FRCP
Professor of Nephrology
University of Edinburgh
Consultant Nephrologist
Edinburgh Royal Infirmary
Edinburgh, United Kingdom
Antiglomerular Basement Membrane Antibody Disease

Robert Unwin, BM, PhD, FRCP
Professor of Nephrology and Physiology
Centre for Nephrology
University College Medical School
Royal Free Campus
University College London
Honorary Consultant Nephrologist
Department of Nephrology and Transplantation
Royal Free Hospital
London, United Kingdom
Diuretics and β-Blockers

Joseph A. Vassalotti, MD
Clinical Assistant Professor of Medicine
Mount Sinai School of Medicine
New York, New York
Hepatitis B– and HIV-Related Renal Diseases

Gloria Lena Vega, PhD
Professor of Clinical Nutrition
Center for Human Nutrition
University of Texas Southwestern Medical Center
Dallas, Texas
*Cholesterol Management in Patients with Chronic Kidney
   Disease*

John P. Vella, MD, FACP, FRCP
Associate Professor of Medicine
University of Vermont School of Medicine
Burlington, Vermont
Director of Transplantation
Maine Medical Center
Portland, Maine
Diagnosis and Management of Renal Allograft Dysfunction

Meryl Waldman, MD
Nephrologist
Clinical Researcher
National Institutes of Health
Kidney Disease Section
Bethesda, Maryland
Lupus Nephritis

Ravinder K. Wali, MBBS, MD, MRCP
Associate Professor of Medicine and Nephrology
University of Maryland School of Medicine
Attending Physician
University of Maryland Hospital
Baltimore, Maryland
Complications Associated with Hemodialysis

Christoph Wanner, MD
Professor of Medicine
University of Wuerzburg
Chief, Division of Nephrology
Department of Medicine
University Hospital
Wuerzburg, Germany
Cardiovascular Complications of End-Stage Renal Disease

William L. Whittier, MD
Assistant Professor of Medicine
Section of Nephrology
Rush University Medical School
Assistant Professor of Medicine
Section of Nephrology
Rush University Medical Center
Chicago, Illinois
Therapy for Diabetic Nephropathy

Christopher S. Wilcox, MD, PhD, FRCP (UK), FACP
George E. Schreiner Professor of Nephrology and
Director, Georgetown University Hypertension,
    Kidney and Vascular Disorders Center
Department of Medicine
Co-Director of Angiogenesis Program
Lombardi Cancer Institute
Georgetown University
Chief of Division of Nephrology and Hypertension
Department of Medicine
Georgetown University Hospital
Washington, DC
Diuretic Use in Edema and the Problem of Resistance; Medical
    Management of Patients with Renal Artery Stenosis;
    Management of Hypertension in Patients Receiving Dialysis;
    Hyperhomocysteinemia

John D. Williams, MD, FRCP
Professor of Medicine
Cardiff University
University Hospital of Wales
Heath Park
Cardiff, United Kingdom
Complications of Peritoneal Dialysis

James F. Winchester, MD, FRCP(Glas), FACP
Professor of Clinical Medicine
Albert Einstein College of Medicine
Chief, Division of Nephrology and Hypertension
Vice-Chair, Department of Medicine
Beth Israel Medical Center
New York, New York
Dialysis and Hemoperfusion in the Treatment of Poisoning and
    Drug Overdose

Christina M. Wyatt, MD
Assistant Professor
Division of Nephrology
Mount Sinai School of Medicine
New York, New York
Hepatitis B– and HIV-Related Renal Diseases

Jane Y. Yeun, MD
Professor of Clinical Medicine
Director, Nephrology Fellowship Program
University of California, Davis, Medical Center
Sacramento, California
Nephrology Staff
Sacramento Veterans Affairs Medical Center
Mather, California
Hemodialysis Adequacy

Alan S.L. Yu, MB, BChir
Associate Professor of Medicine and Physiology
University of Southern California Keck School of Medicine
Attending Physician
Division of Nephrology
Los Angeles County-USC Medical Center
Los Angeles, California
Diuretics in Acute Kidney Injury; Part I Editor; Part V Editor;
    Part IX Editor

Carmine Zoccali, MD, PhD
Chief, Nephrology, Hypertension and Renal Transplantation
CNR-IBIM Clinical Epidemiology of Renal Diseases and
    Hypertension
Ospedali Riuniti
Reggio Calabria, Italy
Dietary Modulation of the Inflammatory Response

Acute Renal Failure

CONTENTS

Chapter 1

Management of Volume Depletion and Established Acute Renal Failure

Friedrich C. Luft

CHAPTER CONTENTS

ESTABLISHING ACUTE RENAL FAILURE

Acute Kidney Injury and the RIFLE Criteria

The introduction of a clear-cut clinical definition of acute renal failure with diagnostic criteria is an important advance in our thinking about patients with acute renal failure. The need was obvious because a doubling in serum creatinine in acutely hospitalized patients increases the mortality to 30%. Another doubling in serum creatinine increases this mortality to 60%.[1] A group of nephrologists and critical care specialists (since expanded to the Acute Kidney Injury Network) formulated the RIFLE criteria (www.ccm.upmc.edu/adqui/ADQI2/ADQI2g1.pdf).[2] The acronym RIFLE stands for the increasing severity classes Risk, Injury, and Failure and the two outcome classes Loss and End-stage kidney disease (Fig. 1-1). The three severity grades are defined based on the changes in serum creatinine or urine output, where the worst of each criterion is used. R, I, and F represent a 25%, 50%, or 75% decrease in glomerular filtration rate (GFR) (or corresponding increase in serum creatinine) and/or oliguria (<0.5 mL/kg/hr) for 6, 12, or 24 hours, respectively. These criteria are easily remembered; most clinical laboratories in the United States and Europe now calculate the GFR by means of the Modification of Diet in Renal Disease study formula. The appearance of R, I, or F in any patient is, of course, good grounds to rule out urinary tract obstruction with diagnostic ultrasonography to preclude postrenal causes of acute renal failure. The two outcome criteria, loss and end-stage kidney disease, are defined by the duration of renal function loss.

Urinary Indices

Although earlier clinicians seem to have had few problems in recognizing established acute renal failure, we have greater difficulties today. Prerenal azotemia is said to account for 40% of cases in hospitalized acute renal failure patients and 60% of community-acquired cases.[3,4] However, how do we distinguish between established acute renal failure and prerenal azotemia? The authors of the two cited reports were not precise in their estimates but espoused renal indices in making this distinction (Box 1-1). Some early investigators relied on specific gravity to reflect tubular function. All performed microscopy and were impressed by muddy brown urinary sediments. Urinary sodium, fractional excretion of sodium, urine-to-plasma creatinine ratio, urinary osmolarity, urine-to-plasma osmolality ratio, serum urea-to-creatinine ratio, and fractional excretion of urea appear to give variable and inconsistent results.[5] Bagshaw and colleagues[6] reviewed 27 papers on the subject that included approximately 1500 assessed patients. About half the patients were septic. Inadequate timing, lack of adequate controls, failure to perform all the tests, and lack of documented established acute renal failure or prerenal azotemia criteria were among the confounders. The authors concluded that the scientific basis for urinary indices and microscopy, particularly in septic acute renal failure patients, is weak. In his critique and commentary, Schrier[7] observed that fractional excretion of sodium or a renal failure index (urine sodium/urine-to-plasma creatinine ratio) less than 1.0 occurs in 85% to 94% of patients with prerenal azotemia and only in less than 4% of patients with oliguric established acute renal failure. These figures should inspire confidence. Nevertheless, in a sheep model of sepsis, renal blood flow increased remarkably (contrary to what was expected), while GFR and urinary output decreased.[8] Moreover, urinary sodium, fractional excretion of sodium, and fractional excretion of urea all decreased, suggesting that these indices are not reliable markers of a prerenal reduced renal blood flow state.[9]

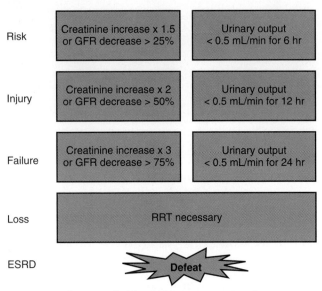

Risk	Creatinine increase x 1.5 or GFR decrease > 25%	Urinary output < 0.5 mL/min for 6 hr
Injury	Creatinine increase x 2 or GFR decrease > 50%	Urinary output < 0.5 mL/min for 12 hr
Failure	Creatinine increase x 3 or GFR decrease > 75%	Urinary output < 0.5 mL/min for 24 hr
Loss	RRT necessary	
ESRD	Defeat	

Figure 1-1 The remarkable RIFLE criteria to classify acute renal failure are shown. On the left are GFR (serum creatinine or cystatin C increases). On the right, even easier, are the urinary output criteria. Remarkably, this simple system exhibits high sensitivity on steps 1 to 3 and high specificity on steps 3 to 5. The breakdown variable is renal replacement therapy (RRT) and end-stage renal disease (ESRD). All consulting nephrologists should use the RIFLE criteria to facilitate patient care and to educate the non-nephrologic community. GFR, glomerular filtration rate.

Box 1-1 Common Renal Indices Assessing Tubular Function*

Urinary Concentration
Specific gravity (>1.020)
Urine osmolality (UOsm > 500 mOsm/kg H_2O)
Urine/plasma osmolality ratio (>1.5)
Urine/plasma creatinine ratio (>20:1)

Urine Sodium
UNa (<20 mmol/L)
$FE_{Na} = (U_{Na}/S_{Na}) \div (U_{Cr}/S_{Cr}) \times 100$ (<1%)

Urea Based
Serum urea-to-serum creatinine ratio (>10:1) when urea is expressed as blood urea nitrogen (BUN mg/dL)
$FE_{Un} = (U_{Urea}/S_{Urea}) \div (U_{Cr}/S_{Cr}) \times 100$ (<35%)

*Renal indices to separate established acute renal failure from prerenal azotemia has a time-honored role in acute nephrology. However, the value of renal indices is questionable. FE_{Na} and FE_{Urea} are probably the most discriminatory; the latter is of value in patients given loop diuretics. The RIFLE criteria are probably superior in terms of sensitivity (lower values) and specificity (higher values), respectively.
FE_{Na}, fractional excretion of sodium; FE_{Un}, fractional excretion of urea; S_{Cr}, serum creatinine; S_{Na}, serum sodium; S_{Urea}, serum urea; U_{Cr}, urinary creatinine; U_{Na}, urinary sodium; U_{Urea}, urinary urea.

Fractional excretion of urea warrants a special mention. In Europe, where loop diuretics are considered a vitamin—or a food—rather than a drug, nephrologists are faced with the problem that all patients have been subjected to loop diuretics before they are called. This state of affairs makes urinary sodium values and fractional excretion of sodium worthless as indicators. Carvounis and colleagues[10] tested 50 patients with prerenal azotemia, 27 of whom had been treated with diuretics and 25 of whom were shown to have established acute renal failure. They reported that a low (<35%) fractional excretion of urea was more sensitive and specific than fractional excretion of sodium for differentiating prerenal azotemia from established acute renal failure.

To summarize, renal indices will remain valuable exercises for residents and fellows on every nephrology service. They are also a valuable activity in terms of teaching renal physiology. Nevertheless, their value in diagnosing established acute renal failure, particularly in septic patients, remains unconvincing. Thus, *caveat emptor!*

VOLUME REPLACEMENT

Assessing the State of Hydration

A prospective, randomized trial has amply demonstrated that early goal-directed therapy provides significant benefits with respect to outcome in patients with severe sepsis and septic shock.[11] Volume expansion is a major part of the goal-directed therapy. All nephrologists would agree that volume expansion should be conducted in any hypovolemic patient to ameliorate prerenal azotemia and to avoid prerenal azotemia from developing into established acute renal failure. However, how good are we at determining whether a patient is hypovolemic? McGee and colleagues[12] reviewed this issue systematically. They searched Medline, personal files, and bibliographies of textbooks on physical diagnosis and identified 10 studies investigating postural vital signs or the capillary refill time of healthy volunteers, some of whom underwent phlebotomy of up to 1150 mL of blood, and four studies of patients presenting to emergency departments with suspected hypovolemia, usually due to vomiting, diarrhea, or decreased oral intake. McGee and colleagues[12] found that when clinicians evaluate adults with suspected blood loss, the most helpful physical findings are either severe postural dizziness (preventing measurement of upright vital signs) or a postural pulse increment of 30 beats per minute or more. The presence of either finding had a sensitivity for moderate blood loss of only 22%; however, the corresponding specificity was 98%. Supine hypotension and tachycardia were frequently absent, even after up to 1150 mL of blood loss. Surgeons in both world wars reported that soldiers with hemorrhagic shock actually had bradycardia approximately one third of the time. The finding of mild postural dizziness had no proven value. In patients with vomiting, diarrhea, or decreased oral intake, the presence of a dry axilla supports the diagnosis of hypovolemia, and moist mucous membranes and a tongue without furrows argue against it. McGee colleagues[12] also found that in adults, the capillary refill time and poor skin turgor had no diagnostic value. Thus, in patients with vomiting, diarrhea, or decreased oral intake, few findings have proven utility. Clinicians are left to measuring serum electrolytes, serum blood urea nitrogen, and creatinine levels when diagnostic certainty is required, provided they are confident in the renal indices described above. The clinical assessment of hypovolemia, although we all cling to our tests and firm beliefs in assessing whether a patient is "dry" (clinically, a meaningless term), would appear to be of little value.

In terms of volume expansion, we are not much better. Observing neck veins, listening for rales, poking for edema are all time-honored hallmarks to establish volume expansion or at least adequate filling pressures. Commonly, radiographs are obtained to assess volume status. Ely and colleagues[13] performed a prospective evaluation of 100 patients who had pulmonary artery occlusion pressure measured. Patients were divided into those who had a pulmonary artery occlusion pressure less than 18 mm Hg or more than 18 mm Hg. Objective (measured) vascular pedicle width and cardiothoracic ratio were better than any subjective interpretation of the radiographs. The authors found that the classic clinical signs of jugular venous distention, crackles on auscultation, and peripheral edema were poor indicators of volume status in these patients and were commonly frankly misleading. Furthermore, the pulmonary artery catheter itself is commonly misleading. Marik[14] termed the intravascular volume assessment, even with a pulmonary artery catheter, "a comedy of errors." Befuddled clinicians should not believe that the pulmonary artery catheter is a "dipstick" to assess "fullness of the tank." The pulmonary artery occlusion pressure cannot be a measure of ventricular preload because preload is a function of muscle fiber length (end-diastolic volume) and not end-diastolic pressure. Several randomized trials have questioned the value of pulmonary artery catheters in supplementing intensive care management; however, that topic is beyond the scope of this chapter.

Nonetheless, clinicians must make decisions about volume status and act accordingly. Most patients in the intensive care unit will have at least a central venous catheter. These catheters permit two measurements that are helpful in assessing oliguria. The first is the measurement of the central venous pressure itself and the second is its change in response to volume challenge. Here, care must be taken with patients receiving mechanical ventilation. In such patients, a central venous pressure greater than 10 mm Hg may still represent volume depletion. In ventilator-dependent patients, if the systolic blood pressure decreases after each lung inflation, cardiac filling pressures may very well be inadequate. Also helpful is the measurement of the central venous oxygen saturation. The value is generally approximately 70% (P-central-venous O_2 40 mm Hg). If the value is less than 50% (P-central-venous O_2 < 28 mm Hg), low cardiac output could be present. In patients with pulmonary artery catheters (or equivalent systems), oxygen delivery and oxygen use should be measured. Determining oxygen use is the primary utility of the pulmonary artery catheter.

Picking the "Right" Volume Expander

In 1861, Thomas Graham investigated the diffusion phenomenon and found that some substances could traverse a parchment membrane and others could not. He classified the substances as crystalloids or colloids accordingly. Crystalloid fluids are electrolyte solutions with small molecules that disperse freely throughout the extracellular space. The principal components are sodium and chloride. As a result, crystalloid volume resuscitation will expand the interstitial volume rather than the plasma volume. Infusion of 1 L of 0.9% sodium chloride (commonly and mistakenly called *physiologic saline*) adds 275 mL to the plasma volume and 825 mL to the interstitial volume. The total volume expansion is 1100 mL because the solution (154 mmol Na and 154 mmol Cl) is sufficiently hypertonic to shift fluid from the intracellular to the extracellular space. So much for isotonic physiologic sodium chloride! Furthermore, 0.9% sodium chloride contributes to hyperchloremic metabolic acidosis (Cl 154 mmol/L). Four liters of sodium chloride administered over a short period (not an uncommon practice in our intensive care unit) will reduce pH from 7.4 to 7.3.

Sidney Ringer and Alexis Hartmann provided us with an alternative to 0.9% saline that has been in use since the 1930s. Lactated Ringer's solution has the advantage of being more physiologic; however, the solution may bind certain drugs, including aminocaproic acid, amphotericin, ampicillin, and thiopental. Lactated Ringer's solution is also contraindicated when diluting red blood cell transfusions, since the solution can bind citrated anticoagulants in blood products. Contrary to popular belief, lactated Ringer's solution will not raise serum lactate levels significantly.

Dextrose solutions (50 g in 1000 mL or 5%) will not increase the plasma volume appreciably and are therefore useless in patients with volume depletion. Routine or aggressive infusion of dextrose-containing solutions can be harmful. When circulatory flow is compromised (shock), 5% dextrose can contribute to metabolic acid production. A 5% dextrose infusion promotes cell swelling. When dextrose is added to isotonic saline (D5 normal saline), the infusion fluid is hypertonic to plasma (560 mOsm/L). If glucose use is impaired (not unheard of in very ill patients), the hypertonic infusion creates an undesirable osmotic force that can promote cell contraction. Finally, hyperglycemia, resulting from dextrose infusions, has numerous deleterious effects including immunosuppression, increased risk of infection, brain injury aggravation, and increased mortality. The fact that more than 10% of intensive care unit patients are diabetic does not inspire confidence. The deleterious effects of hyperglycemia and the benefits of lowering blood sugar in critically ill patients have been convincingly shown in both surgical and medical intensive care unit patients.[15,16]

Are colloid-containing fluids better? Colloid fluids are more effective than crystalloids in expanding the plasma volume because they contain large, poorly diffusible, solute molecules that create an oncotic pressure to keep water in the vascular space. In healthy subjects, the colloid oncotic pressure of plasma is approximately 25 mm Hg while lying down; when standing, the value decreases to 20 mm Hg. A 1-L 5% albumin solution results in a 700-mL increment in the plasma volume and in only a 300-mL increase in the interstitial volume. Thus, 70% of this infusion remains in the intravascular space. Colloid fluids are threefold more effective in increasing intravascular volume than crystalloid solutions.

Albumin is expensive. Thus, alternatives are popular. Hydroxyethyl starch (hetastarch) is a chemically modified starch polymer that is available as a 6% solution in isotonic saline. There are three types of hetastarch solutions based on the average molecular weight, 450, 200, and 70 kd for high, medium, and lightweight hetastarch, respectively. In the United States, the heavy weight is favored. Hetastarch undergoes hydrolysis by amylases in the blood. The products less than 50 kd are eliminated by the kidneys (if these are working). Hetastarch can interfere with tissue factor and von Willebrand factor. Overt bleeding is uncommon but can complicate bypass operations. Hetastarch may increase serum amylase levels as a form of macroamylasemia, which is not a toxic effect. Anaphylactic reactions can occur with hetastarch but are rare. Dextrans are similar in kind and in substance to hetastarch solutions.

The colloid-crystalloid debate (warfare) continues, and no end is in sight. The fact that an acute blood loss is accompanied by a dramatic interstitial fluid volume deficit raised hopes for the crystalloid camp. However, clinicians prefer blood pressure to be measurable and to be maintained. What should we do? To help us, outcomes experts conducted a systematic review of randomized, controlled trials of resuscitation with colloids compared with crystalloids for volume replacement of critically ill patients.[17] The analysis was stratified according to patient type and quality of allocation concealment. Despite the inclusion of 37 randomized trials, resuscitation with colloids was associated with an increased absolute risk of 4% mortality, or four extra deaths for every 100 patients resuscitated. There was no evidence of differences in effect among patients with different types of injury that required fluid resuscitation. Suffice it to say, this meta-analysis generated much controversy.

The last word should have been the SAFE study.[18] In this study, 6997 patients requiring fluid resuscitation were randomized to 4% albumin or normal saline. The primary endpoint was death from any cause. The outcomes in the two groups were similar. However, the patients died of various causes, and there is no way to determine whether an intravenous fluid was somehow directly related to death. Subsequently, other studies have been published, including a recent study investigating three fluids in 129 children with dengue shock syndrome.[19] Ringer's lactate, 6% hydroxyethyl starch, and 6% dextran 70 were compared in the study. First, as a tribute to the investigators, only one patient died in the study. The treatments did not differ in outcomes. The authors concluded that initial resuscitation with Ringer's lactate is indicated for children with moderately severe dengue shock syndrome. Dextran 70 and 6% hydroxyethyl starch performed similarly in children with severe shock; however, dextran had more side effects.

Could hypertonic saline (hypertonic resuscitation) provide an answer?[20,21] A 7.5% sodium chloride solution has an osmolality 8.5 times that of plasma. The additional volume would come from the intracellular space. Preliminary data exist that suggest a role for such an approach. However, currently no controlled data exist. In case the notion results in discomfort, the idea that Na and Cl determine extracellular fluid volume (aside from the amount sequestered in bone) may require revision. An additional storage space for sodium influencing volume regulation may exist in proteoglycan-containing connective tissue.[22]

The resuscitation fluid should be selected based on the need of a specific problem in any given patient. For example, crystalloid fluids are designed to fill the extracellular space. They are particularly indicated when the interstitial space is compromised and would be appropriate for use in patients with loss of both interstitial and intravascular volume. Colloid fluids are designed to expand the plasma volume and are appropriate for patients with hypovolemia related to acute blood loss. Albumin-containing colloid fluids are appropriate for patients with hypovolemia associated with hypoalbuminemia. Tailoring fluid therapy to specific problems of fluid imbalance is the best approach to volume resuscitation in the intensive care unit. Most patients with acute kidney injury (AKI) can probably be managed with crystalloid volume replacement.

Monitoring and Administration

Blood loss is classified by the American College of Surgeons in terms of amount.[23] Class I is approximately 15%, class II is 15% to 30%, class III is 30% to 40%, class IV is more than 40%. The latter two classes generally would be picked up as AKI, at least according to the RIFLE criteria based on oliguria. Tachycardia is generally absent in the supine position; indeed, bradycardia may be present. Blood pressure is an insensitive marker of blood loss. The use of the hematocrit to estimate blood loss is naive and inappropriate.[24] Central venous and pulmonary artery catheters are commonly inserted into hypovolemic patients. Cardiac filling pressures will generally overestimate the intravascular volume status in hypovolemic patients.[25] Oxygen transport parameters may be very helpful as discussed earlier. If a pulmonary artery catheter is in place, its value lies in measuring Do_2 and Vo_2. Compensated hypovolemia is identified by a normal Vo_2 (>100 mL/min/m^2) and an O_2 extraction less than 50%. Hypovolemic shock is identified by an abnormally low Vo_2 (<100 mL/min/m^2) and an extraction rate greater than 50%. Lactate, $Paco_2$, and HCO_3 values can be obtained and are valuable monitoring parameters.

The Trendelenburg position (legs elevated and head below the horizontal plane) does *not* promote venous return to the heart and, according to careful study, is a worthless maneuver for this purpose. Friedrich Trendelenburg (1844–1924), an innovative surgeon, developed the position to perform perineal operations and *not* to treat shock. Generally, the central veins are cannulated in patients for volume resuscitation because larger veins permit more rapid fluid infusions, or so most clinicians believe. However, the rate of volume infusion is determined by the dimensions of the vascular catheter and not by the size of the vein. Hagen and Poisseuille showed clearly that wider bore (radius) and shorter length determine how fast infusions can run. The relationship they defined is $Q = \Delta P(\pi r^4/8 \mu L)$, where r is radius and L is length. Thus, short peripheral 14- or 16-gauge 5-cm catheters will allow a gravity crystalloid flow rate of 200 and 150 mL/min, respectively. The Hagen-Poiseuille relationship also predicts how fast whole blood and packed erythrocytes will flow. The μ value refers to viscosity. Whole blood flows approximately half as fast as crystalloid, whereas packed erythrocytes flow approximately one fourth as fast. A short, large catheter in a peripheral vein is of far greater value in treating shock than a small-bore, long central catheter.

The first priority in the volume-depleted patient is to support cardiac output. Worthwhile points to remember are that (1) colloid fluids are more effective than whole blood, packed cells, or crystalloids for increasing cardiac output; (2) erythrocyte concentrates are relatively ineffective in promoting cardiac output and flow slowly; (3) colloids add to the plasma volume, whereas crystalloid fluids primarily add to the interstitial volume; and (4) for a given effect on cardiac output, the volume of crystalloids must exceed that of colloids by approximately a factor of 3.

Role of the Fluid Challenge

What to do when we have little idea of what we are doing (Fig. 1-2)? This situation is common in critical care medicine,

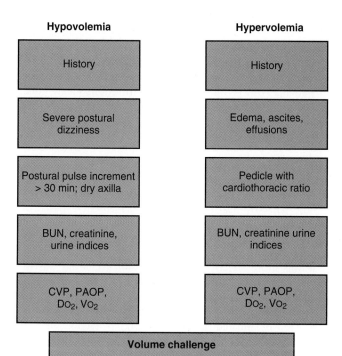

Hypovolemia

- History
- Severe postural dizziness
- Postural pulse increment > 30 min; dry axilla
- BUN, creatinine, urine indices
- CVP, PAOP, DO_2, VO_2

Hypervolemia

- History
- Edema, ascites, effusions
- Pedicle with cardiothoracic ratio
- BUN, creatinine urine indices
- CVP, PAOP, DO_2, VO_2

Volume challenge

Figure 1-2 The first step in assessing volume status in the critically ill is to keep in mind that all our clinical assessments, laboratory tests, and modes of patient monitoring are fallible and fraught with error. Severe postural dizziness is defined as the inability to stand upright. Postural pulse increment greater than 30 per minute may be absent with acute hemorrhage. Systolic blood pressure decreases (>20 mm Hg), although popular, have a sensitivity and specificity of approximately 10%. Serum and urine chemistries may also be misleading. Edema and ascites speak to the extracellular fluid volume, not to the circulating fluid volume. A chest radiograph may be helpful. Central catheters are not infallible "dipsticks" and commonly mislead. Careful clinical longitudinal assessment, measurement, and documentation are warranted. (Adapted from McGee S, Abernethy WB 3rd, Simel DL: The rational clinical examination. Is this patient hypovolemic? JAMA 1999;281:1022–1029; Ely WE, Smith AC, Chiles C, et al: Radiologic determination of intravascular volume status using portable, digital chest radiography: A prospective investigation in 100 patients. Crit Care Med 2001;29:1502–1512; and Marik PE: Assessment of intravascular volume: A comedy of errors. Crit Care Med 2001:29:1635–1636.)

and the fluid challenge strategy commonly helps and, if carefully done, should do no harm. Volume challenges of 500 to 1000 mL for crystalloids or 300 to 500 mL for colloids over the course of approximately an hour have been suggested for patients suspected of having sepsis, septic shock, or volume depletion due to other causes.[26] There is no evidence to favor crystalloid or colloid fluids in this regard. In patients with hypoalbuminemia (<3 g/dL), 5% albumin should be seriously considered for volume resuscitation.

Flushing the Kidneys: Role of Diuretics

Furosemide in the AKI setting is particularly deserving of a few comments. Furosemide is probably the most frequently administered drug in patients meeting the RIFLE criteria. In fact, the most common reason for nephrologic consultation in our hospital is, "This patient refuses to respond to furosemide." Mehta and colleagues[27] have investigated this issue. They determined whether the use of diuretics (mostly furosemide) was associated with adverse or favorable outcomes in critically ill patients with acute renal failure. Mehta and colleagues conducted a cohort study of 552 patients with acute renal failure in intensive care units at four academic medical centers. Patients were categorized by the use of diuretics on the day of nephrology consultation and, in companion analyses, by diuretic use at any time during the first week after consultation. They found that diuretics were used in 59% of patients at the time of nephrology consultation. This author is certain that in Europe the figure would be much closer to 100%. The patients treated with diuretics on or before the day of consultation were older and more likely to have a history of congestive heart failure, nephrotoxic (rather than ischemic or multifactorial) origin of acute renal failure, acute respiratory failure, and lower serum urea nitrogen concentrations. Mehta and colleagues[27] found that diuretic use was associated with a significant increase in the risk of death or nonrecovery of renal function. The increased risk was borne largely by patients who were relatively unresponsive to diuretics. Mehta and colleagues concluded that diuretics in critically ill patients with acute renal failure were associated with an increased risk of death and nonrecovery of renal function. The data were observational. The frustrated physicians probably gave the sicker, more oliguric patients more diuretics than the healthier patients. Numerous trials have been conducted on furosemide in the acute renal failure setting in the hope that the drug might decrease oxygen consumption or provide some other advantage for recovery. All controlled trials in this regard were negative. A recent meta-analysis underscored this point.[28] Nevertheless, the practice of administering furosemide to all persons with oliguria of any degree persists. Mehta and colleagues stated that in the absence of compelling contradictory data from a randomized, blinded clinical trial, the widespread use of diuretics in critically ill patients with acute renal failure should be discouraged.[27] The findings of Mehta and colleagues have had no effect on medical practice thus far, but should have. What do physicians seek to achieve with furosemide—a lower RIFLE score?

Management of Myoglobinuria

Myoglobinuria is a regular feature in trauma patients, but is also observed in any case of muscle injury. The presence of urinary myoglobin does not necessarily denote AKI; however, its absence indicates a substantial decrease in risk.[29] Muscle necrosis releases particularly large amounts of potassium and phosphorus. Myoglobin, when resorbed by the tubular cells, promotes substantial oxidative stress when the iron is released. Aggressive volume resuscitation to prevent hypovolemia and maintain renal blood flow is indicated. Alkalinization of the urine may help limit the renal injury. Trauma teams managing disaster or combat victims regularly begin aggressive volume expansion as soon as an extremity avails itself to allow vessel cannulation. This approach appears prudent. Israeli military physicians report that managing crush injuries with aggressive volume expansion and urine alkalinization protects from AKI.[30] However, the authors addressed the issue of trauma victims who, in all likelihood, have severe blood loss necessitating goal-directed therapy. Older patients with heart disease and other concomitant medical problems, such as developing myoglobinuria complicating statin therapy, should not necessarily be treated in the same fashion merely because they have an elevated creatine kinase level or urine that contains myoglobin.

ELECTROLYTE DISTURBANCES

Hypernatremia

Hypernatremia (Na > 150 mmol/L) associated with AKI is common and occurs in both children and adults. Here, volume assessment and the osmolar disturbance must be considered separately. Generally, hypernatremia coexists with volume contraction. However, the intensive care unit is an exception. The coexistence of hypernatremia and edema that develops in an intensive care unit invariably points to physician-induced therapeutic misadventures.[31] Conscious patients are generally able to protect themselves from this dilemma. When the constellation of volume expansion and edema develops on an outpatient basis, the physician should suspect (salt poisoning) abuse.[32]

In a recent review of 105 children admitted to a general pediatrics department, hypernatremic dehydration (volume contraction) represented 12% of all dehydration forms.[33] Half of the children were in shock. Severe dehydration was present in 90% of patients, and neurological signs were observed in 77%. The initial mean serum sodium concentration was 159 mmol/L. Acidosis and AKI were present in 97% and 77% of patients, respectively. The predominant cause of hypernatremic dehydration in these children was diarrhea (94%). The children were given intravenous rehydration with 5% glucose solution at an average of 147 mL/kg/day and containing a mean sodium level of 42 mmol/L. Serum sodium was normalized within the first 72 hours. The mortality rate was 11%. Another hypernatremia in infants relevant to nephrologists is that associated with breast-feeding.[34] This serious complication occurs when breast-feeding is insufficient and is often associated with hyperbilirubinemia. Neonatal hypernatremic dehydration results from inadequate transfer of breast milk from mother to infant. Furthermore, poor milk drainage from the breasts can result in persistence of high milk sodium concentrations. Breast-feeding–associated hypernatremia results only when breast-feeding is not properly established. The failure to diagnose hypernatremic dehydration can have serious consequences, including AKI, seizures, intracranial hemorrhage, vascular thrombosis, and death. Most breast-feeding–associated hypernatremia could be prevented if infants with excessive weight loss or inadequate breast milk transfer were judiciously given expressed breast milk if available and formula if necessary until breast milk production increases and breast-feeding difficulties are addressed by a health care provider well trained in lactation support.

Hypernatremia with AKI is a frequent problem in elderly individuals.[35] Changes in the physiologic responses to water deprivation are of particular interest in understanding the pathogenesis of hypernatremia in the elderly. In older persons, there are deficits in both the intensity and threshold of the thirst response. The ability to concentrate the urine also declines with age. There are both a decline in the GFR and an increased incidence of renal disease with advancing age, which may contribute to impaired ability to conserve water. Because of a decrease in the percentage of total body water with age, equal volumes of fluid loss in young and old individuals may represent more severe dehydration in the elderly. The correction of hypernatremia in the elderly requires particular care in terms of administering glucose-containing solutions. Hyperglycemia, coupled with hypernatremia, is particularly undesirable. Continuous venovenous hemofiltration has been used in patients with serum sodium concentrations greater than 200 mmol/L to lower the serum sodium concentration in a controlled fashion.[36]

Hyperkalemia

The most celebrated life-threatening electrolyte disturbance in patients with acute renal failure is hyperkalemia. The Cochrane database has reported on management.[37] Based on small studies, inhaled β-agonists, nebulized β-agonists, and intravenous insulin and glucose were all effective, and the combination of nebulized β-agonists and insulin and glucose was more effective than either alone. Dialysis was invariably effective. The results were equivocal for intravenous bicarbonate. Potassium-absorbing resin was not effective after 4 hours. The Cochrane authorities concluded that nebulized or inhaled salbutamol and intravenous insulin and glucose are the first-line therapies for the management of emergency hyperkalemia that are best supported by the evidence. Their combination may be more effective than either alone and should be considered when hyperkalemia is severe. In adult patients with coronary heart disease, nebulized or inhaled salbutamol would not appear to be a good idea. The experts concluded that further studies of the optimal use of combination treatments and of the adverse effects of treatments are needed.

Kamel and Wei[38] recently reviewed controversies in treating hyperkalemia. They concluded that insulin and glucose were frontline and that β-agonists were ineffective in a significant number of patients. Sodium bicarbonate should be reserved for patients who concomitantly have severe metabolic acidosis. Kamel and Wei[38] were also reluctant to use exchange resins in patients with acute hyperkalemia. The intravenous administration of calcium salts for hyperkalemia is commonly recommended.[39] Intermittent injections of 10 mL of 10% calcium gluconate and/or calcium chloride are given according to guidelines (www.clinicalschool.swan.ac.uk/wics/itugl/hik.him). Calcium salts do not alter the serum potassium concentration, although reversal of electrocardiographic findings is immediate and dramatic. The role of calcium remains unclear because the effect is only transient; calcium works in a minute, but the effect is also gone in minutes. Therefore, concomitant therapies (insulin and glucose) must be given. Furthermore, calcium should obviously not be given together with sodium bicarbonate because of precipitation. Nonetheless, the successful management of 46 cases of battlefield acute renal failure in Korea by the U.S. Army employed a continuous infusion containing calcium gluconate, sodium bicarbonate, insulin, and glucose.[40] Presumably, the amounts of sodium bicarbonate and calcium were low or the two were not given concomitantly.

Final words about the electrocardiogram are worthy of mention. Life-threatening hyperkalemia can occur with a relatively normal electrocardiogram, albeit it is unusual. Flat P waves, widened QRS complex, and tented T waves are welcome hyperkalemia signs that are taught to every medical student and illustrated in every textbook. However, these classic signs may be absent and instead there may be merely peculiar QRS conduction delays and more nonspecific signs. The wary clinician is duly suspicious.

Metabolic Acidosis

This topic and its treatment are discussed elsewhere. For intensivist nephrologists, type B lactic acidosis induced by metformin deserves a comment. The drug, which is indicated in almost all overweight patients with the metabolic syndrome, polycystic ovarian syndrome, and type 2 diabetes mellitus, has a mode of action that is now quite well understood.[41] Unfortunately, the drug can induce type B (without shock) lactic acidosis, and the risk is actually only relevant when renal function is impaired. Metformin should not be given to persons with a GFR less than 60 mL/min. In an earlier review, this author handled this topic fairly lightly,[42] but has since seen several patients with profound lactic acidosis that could only be attributed to metformin. In all cases, physicians had failed to discontinue the drug, despite an obvious decrease in renal function. Discontinuing metformin is the cornerstone of treatment.

MANAGING OTHER UREMIC COMPLICATIONS

Uremic Bleeding and Thrombosis

Uremic platelets function less well than platelets in a normal environment. Early studies proposed a role for guanidinosuccinic acid that accumulates when renal function falls to low levels. This idea was probably not a bad one because we now know that guanidinosuccinic acid in uremic blood depends on amidine being transferred to aspartic acid from L-arginine. L-Arginine is the major substrate of nitric oxide (NO) synthase. NO is the major modulator of vascular tone (endothelial function) that limits platelet adhesion to endothelium and platelet-platelet interaction, increasing the formation of cell cyclic guanosine monophosphate. Guanidinosuccinic acid causes cultured endothelial cells to produce NO. An increase in NO may also decrease fibrinogen binding to the platelet GP IIb/IIIa receptor. Noris and Remuzzi[43] point out that uremia is a high NO state, at least as far as the platelet is concerned. Platelets from uremic patients produce more NO. N^G-monomethyl-L-arginine restores platelet stickiness

and responses to adenosinediphosphate in uremic platelets. Noris and Remuzzi[43] argue that uremic bleeding is largely due to an exuberant formation of NO by uremic vessels, a process that is guanidinosuccinic acid dependent.

Nevertheless, treating uremic patients with N^G-monomethyl-L-arginine seems premature. NO synthase is already inhibited by asymmetrical dimethyl arginine that accumulates in patients with decreased renal function. Brunini and colleagues[44] suggest that reduced plasma L-arginine and NO production as well as increased tumor necrosis factor α, fibrinogen, and C-reactive protein levels in uremic patients cause increased aggregability of platelets, which could conceivably occur when uremic patients are poorly nourished and poorly dialyzed.

Treatment options center on recombinant erythropoietin or darbepoietin-α, adequate dialysis, desmopressin, tranexamic acid, or conjugated estrogens.[45] Thrombotic complications in uremia are caused by increased platelet aggregation and hypercoagulability. Erythrocyte-platelet aggregates, leukocyte-platelet aggregates, and platelet microparticles are found to a greater degree in uremic patients compared with healthy individuals. Increased platelet phosphatidylserine expression initiates phagocytosis and coagulation. Therapy with antiplatelet drugs does not reduce vascular access thrombosis but instead increases bleeding complications. Heparin-induced thrombocytopenia (type II) may develop in hemodialyzed patients, but is fortunately relatively uncommon. Furthermore, heparin-induced thrombocytopenia antibody-positive uremic patients generally develop only mild thrombocytopenia and only very few thrombotic complications. Substitution of heparin by hirudin, danaparoid, or regional citrate anticoagulation is an option in individual cases.

Drug-Dosing Principles

A scholarly chapter on this complicated issue follows, allowing only a few general comments here. Critical illness has a great impact on many pharmacokinetic parameters. An increased volume of distribution often results in drug underdosing, whereas organ impairment may lead to drug accumulation and overdosing. Renal replacement therapy (RRT) in critically ill patients with renal failure may significantly increase drug clearance, requiring drug-dosing adjustments. Drugs significantly eliminated by the kidney are likely to experience substantial removal during RRT, and a supplemental dose that corresponds to the amount of drug removed by RRT should be administered. Mechanisms of drug removal during RRT have been investigated in detail, along with methods for measuring or estimating RRT drug clearances. Numerous investigators have outlined approaches for drug-dosing adjustments, and the pharmacologic principles, particularly for antibiotic prescription, are readily available elsewhere.

Renal Replacement Therapy

Approximately 70% of patients with established acute renal failure require RRT. The primary indications remain volume expansion, electrolyte disturbances (primarily hyperkalemia), acid-base disorders (usually metabolic acidosis), and encephalopathy (uremic symptoms). The eponym A-E-I-O-U still serves a purpose in terms of student instruction (acidosis, electrolytes, intoxication, [volume] overload, and uremia).

However, the indications have been modified and made less restrictive, particularly as innovative therapies have become available. Uremic encephalopathy is an unusual indication nowadays. There are no creatinine or GFR values that absolutely indicate dialysis; the decision remains a clinical judgment. For hemodialysis and hemofiltration, appropriate blood access is required. Large-bore, double-lumen vascular catheters are used for this purpose. The catheters are introduced into the internal jugular or femoral veins. Subclavian vein access is relatively contraindicated because injury to this vessel is common. Subclavian vein thrombosis makes the peripheral veins of the corresponding extremity useless in terms of long-term hemodialysis blood access.[46] Should AKI patients with central access catheters receive thrombosis prophylaxis? They probably should.[47]

The dialysis care of AKI patients requiring it is outlined in detail elsewhere, and state-of-the-art recommendations are made. However, many patients requiring RRT receive much less than they deserve or what their physicians have prescribed. Venkataraman and colleagues[48] reviewed the records of AKI patients undergoing intermittent dialysis and found that they were prescribed 25 mL/kg/hr (too little in this author's view). However, they received only 16.5 mL/kg/hr. The logistics of dialysis in intensive care units is difficult; competing machinery, diagnostic test scheduling, multiple care teams, and other confounders all contribute to the dilemma.

Recovery and Prognosis

In the past, failure to recover from acute renal failure was associated with renal cortical necrosis, commonly after postpartum hemorrhage. Today, in younger individuals, non–Shiga's toxin–mediated hemolytic uremic syndrome is a prominent cause. Not appreciated particularly by non-nephrologist clinicians is the role of cholesterol emboli as a cause for nonreversible acute renal failure.[49] Few studies have addressed the issue of long-term outcome in established acute renal failure patients. Bagshaw[50] focused on this issue. He found that the survival rates were variable and ranged from 46% to 74%, 55% to 73%, 57% to 65%, and 65% to 70% at 90 days, 6 months, 1 year, and 5 years, respectively. Older age, comorbid illness, illness severity, septic shock, and RRT after cardiac surgery were associated with reduced survival. Recovery to independence from RRT occurred in 60% to 70% of survivors by 90 days. Health-related quality of life was generally good and perceived as acceptable. Acute renal failure survivors often experienced difficulty with mobility and limitations in activities of daily living. RRT was costly and achieved marginal cost-effectiveness in terms of quality-adjusted survival for those with a higher probability of survival. Bagshaw concluded that the long-term survival after acute renal failure was poor. Yet, most survivors recover sufficient function to become no longer dependent on RRT.

In the past, post–acute renal failure/post–obstructive diuresis were commonly observed during the recovery from acute renal failure, particularly when dialysis was not often used. One reason for this phenomenon was probably related to volume expansion. However, tubular dysfunction, particularly after obstruction, can occur. A patient with Burkitt's lymphoma and obstructing lymph nodes may claim the world's record. The patient developed anuria after aggressive chemotherapy and bowel surgery.[51] During recovery, as the patient's creatinine

concentration decreased from 7 to 1.5 mg/dL over a 5-day period, his urinary output increased from 0 to more than 80 L/day. The volume replacement given the patient was always close to, but less than, his output, suggesting that the clinicians were not contributing to the situation. Furthermore, daily weights did not suggest that volume expansion was responsible. The dramatic situation subsequently resolved. Clinicians must be aware that postoperative intra-abdominal hypertension is associated with acute renal failure as well as with subsequent post–obstructive diuresis. Abdominal pressures can be monitored via the bladder. Because acute renal failure is commonly elicited by shock, checking posterior pituitary function and renal concentrating ability is worthwhile in patients who are polyuric during recovery. Central diabetes insipidus after shock syndromes is well-known but less appreciated outside of the obstetrical service. Severe ischemic injury may also result in permanent alteration of renal capillary density and the predisposition to the development of renal fibrosis, with subsequent nephrogenic diabetes insipidus.

Management of the recovery phase of acute renal failure focuses on attention to details. Intake and output are routinely measured in every intensive care unit, whereas a general resistance to obtaining daily weights seems to be an international phenomenon. Strict and specialized hemodynamic monitoring is warranted. Medical management must be designed to avoid serious hemodynamic and metabolic disorders.

Established acute renal failure is similar to acute respiratory distress syndrome in that it is not a primary disease, but a complication of other disease processes, particularly septic shock.[52,53] Consequently, the mortality rate of acute renal failure mirrors the mortality rate of the primary diseases responsible for its development. Because these primary diseases have a high mortality rate, the fact that the mortality rate of acute renal failure has remained unchanged in the past 60 years is not surprising.[52–54] Furthermore, the fact that hemodialysis and other RRTs have not altered mortality also comes as no surprise. Unfortunately, this state of affairs has escaped the evidence-based medicine crowd that preaches discarding those interventions that have not been shown to improve mortality.

References

1. Kellum JA, Levin N, Bouman C, Lameire N: Developing a consensus classification system for acute renal failure. Curr Opin Crit Care 2002;8:509–514.
2. Hoste EAJ, Kellum JA: Acute kidney injury: Epidemiology and diagnostic criteria. Curr Opin Crit Care 2006;12:531–537.
3. Nolan CR, Anderson RJ: Hospital-acquired acute renal failure. J Am Soc Nephrol 1998;9:710–718.
4. Liano F, Pascual J: Epidemiology of acute renal failure: A prospective multicenter, community-based study. Madrid Acute Renal Failure Study Group. Kidney Int 1996;50:811–818.
5. Bellomo R: Defining, quantifying, and classifying acute renal failure. Crit Care Clin 2005;21:223–237.
6. Bagshaw SM, Langenberg C, Bellomo R: Urinary biochemistry and microscopy in septic acute renal failure: A systematic review. Am J Kidney Dis 2006;48:695–705.
7. Schrier RW: Urinary indices and microscopy in sepsis-related acute renal failure. Am J Kidney Dis 2006;48:838–841.

8. Langenberg C, Wan L, Egi M, et al: Renal blood flow in experimental septic acute renal failure. Kidney Int 2006;69:1996–2002.
9. Langenberg C, Wan L, Bagshaw SM, et al: Urinary biochemistry in experimental septic acute renal failure. Nephrol Dial Transplant 2006;21:3389–3397.
10. Carvounis CP, Nisar S, Guro-Razuman S. Significance of the fractional excretion of urea in the differential diagnosis of acute renal failure. Kidney Int 2002;62:2223–2229.
11. Rivers E, Nguyen B, Havstad S, et al: Early Goal-Directed Therapy Collaborative Group. Early goal-directed therapy in the treatment of severe sepsis and septic shock. N Engl J Med 2001;345:1368–1377.
12. McGee S, Abernethy WB 3rd, Simel DL: The rational clinical examination: Is this patient hypovolemic? JAMA 1999;281:1022–1029.
13. Ely WE, Smith AC, Chiles C, et al: Radiologic determination of intravascular volume status using portable, digital chest radiography: A prospective investigation in 100 patients. Crit Care Med 2001;29:1502–1512.
14. Marik PE: Assessment of intravascular volume: A comedy of errors. Crit Care Med 2001;29:1635–1636.
15. van den Berghe G, Wouters P, Weekers F, et al: Intensive insulin therapy in the critically ill patients. N Engl J Med 2001;345:1359–1367.
16. Van den Berghe G, Wilmer A, Hermans G, et al: Intensive insulin therapy in the medical ICU. N Engl J Med 2006;354:449–461.
17. Schierhout G, Roberts I: Fluid resuscitation with colloid or crystalloid solutions in critically ill patients: A systematic review of randomised trials. Br Med J 1998;316:961–964.
18. The SAFE Study Investigators: A comparison of albumin and saline for fluid resuscitation in the intensive care unit. N Engl J Med 2004;350:2247–2256.
19. Wills BA, Dung NM, Loan HT, et al: Comparison of three fluid solutions for resuscitation in dengue shock syndrome. N Engl J Med 2005;353:877–889.
20. Chiara O, Pelosi P, Brazzi L, et al: Resuscitation from hemorrhagic shock: Experimental model comparing normal saline, dextran, and hypertonic saline solutions. Crit Care Med 2003;31:1915–1922.
21. Cooper DJ, Myles PS, McDermott FT, et al: Prehospital hypertonic saline resuscitation of patients with hypotension and severe traumatic brain injury. JAMA 2004;291:1350–1357.
22. Titze J, Shakibaei M, Schafflhuber M, et al: Glycosaminoglycan polymerization may enable osmotically inactive Na+ storage in the skin. Am J Physiol Heart Circ Physiol 2004;22:803–810.
23. Committee on Trauma: Advanced Trauma Life Support Student Manual. Chicago: American College of Surgeons, 1989.
24. Cordts PR, LaMorte WW, Fisher JB, et al: Poor predictive value of hematocrit and hemodynamic parameters for erythrocyte deficits after extensive vascular operations. Surg Gynecol Obstet 1992;175:243–248.
25. Kumar A, Anel R, Bunnell E, et al: Pulmonary artery occlusion pressure and central venous pressure fail to predict ventricular filling volumes, cardiac performance, or the response to volume infusion in normal subjects. Crit Care Med 2004;32:691–699.
26. Vincent J-L, Gerlach H: Fluid resuscitation in severe sepsis and septic shock: An evidence-based review. Crit Care Med 2004;32(Suppl):S451–S454.
27. Mehta RL, Pascual MT, Soroko S, Chertow GM; PICARD Study Group. Diuretics, mortality, and nonrecovery of renal function in acute renal failure. JAMA 2002;288:2547–2553.
28. Ho KM, Sheridan DJ: Meta-analysis of frusemide to prevent or treat acute renal failure. Br Med J 2006;333:420.
29. Sharp LS, Orzycki GS, Feliciano DV: Rhabdomyolysis and secondary renal failure in critically ill patients. Am J Surg 2004;188:801–806.
30. Ashkenazi I, Isakovich B, Kluger Y, et al: Prehospital management of earthquake casualties buried under rubble. Prehospital Disaster Med 2005;20:122–133.
31. Kahn T: Hypernatremia with edema. Arch Intern Med 1999;159:93–98.
32. Raya A, Giner P, Aranegui P, et al: Fatal acute hypernatremia caused by massive intake of salt. Arch Intern Med 1992;152:640–646.
33. Chouchane S, Fehri H, Chouchane C, et al: Hypernatremic dehydration in children: Retrospective study of 105 cases. Arch Pediatr 2005;12:1697–1702.
34. Moritz ML, Manole MD, Bogen DL, Ayus JC: Breastfeeding-associated hypernatremia: Are we missing the diagnosis? Pediatrics 2005;116:e343–e347.
35. Ayus JC, Arieff AI: Abnormalities of water metabolism in the elderly. Semin Nephrol 1996;16:277–288.
36. Yang YF, Wu VC, Huang CC: Successful management of extreme hypernatraemia by haemofiltration in a patient with severe metabolic acidosis and renal failure. Nephrol Dial Transplant 2005;20:2013–2014.
37. Mahoney BA, Smith WA, Lo DS, et al: Emergency interventions for hyperkalaemia. Cochrane Database Syst Rev 2005;2:D003235.
38. Kamel KS, Wei C: Controversial issues in the treatment of hyperkalemia. Nephrol Dial Transplant 2003;18:2215–2218.
39. De Takats D: Using calcium salts for hyperkalemia. Nephrol Dial Transplant 2004;19:1333–1334.
40. Merony WH, Herndon RF: The management of acute renal insufficiency. JAMA 1954;155:877–892.
41. Zhou G, Myers R, Li Y, et al: Role of AMP-activated protein kinase in mechanism of metformin action. J Clin Invest 2001;108:1167–1174.
42. Luft FC: Lactic acidosis update for critical care clinicians. J Am Soc Nephrol 2001;12(Suppl 17):S15–S19.
43. Noris M, Remuzzi G: Uremic bleeding: Closing the circle after 30 years of controversies? Blood 1999;94:2569–2574.
44. Brunini TM, Mendes-Ribeiro AC, Ellory JC, Mann GE: Platelet nitric oxide synthesis in uremia and malnutrition: A role for L-arginine supplementation in vascular protection? Cardiovasc Res 2007;73:359–367.
45. Horl WH: Thrombocytopathy and blood complications in uremia. Wien Klin Wochenschr 2006;118:134–150.
46. Hernandez D, Diaz F, Fuino M, et al: Subclavian vascular access stenosis in dialysis patients: Natural history and risk factors. J Am Soc Nephrol 1998;9:1507–1510.
47. Francis CW: Clinical practice. Prophylaxis for thromboembolism in hospitalized medical patients. N Engl J Med 2007;356:1438–1444.
48. Venkataraman R, Kellum JA, Palevsky P: Dosing patterns for continuous renal replacement therapy at a large academic medical center in the United States. J Crit Care 2002;17:246–250.
49. Scolari F, Ravani P, Pola A, et al: Predictors of renal and patient outcomes in atheroembolic renal disease: A prospective study. J Am Soc Nephrol 2003;14:1584–1590.
50. Bagshaw SM: The long-term outcome after acute renal failure. Curr Opin Crit Care 2006;12:561–566.
51. Atamer T, Artim-Esen B, Yavuz S, Ecder T: Massive postobstructive diuresis in a patient with Burkitt's lymphoma. Nephrol Dial Transplant 2005;20:1991–1993.
52. Uchino S, Kellum JA, Bellomo R, et al: Acute renal failure in critically ill patients: A multinational, multicenter study. JAMA 2005;294:813–818.
53. Abernathy VE, Lieberthal W: Acute renal failure in the critically ill patient. Crit Care Clin 2002;18:203–212.
54. Singri N, Ahya SN, Levin ML: Acute renal failure. JAMA 2003;289:747–751.

Further Reading

Bagshaw SM: The long-term outcome after acute renal failure. Curr Opin Crit Care 2006;12:561–566.

Hoste EAJ, Kellum JA: Acute kidney injury: Epidemiology and diagnostic criteria. Curr Opin Crit Care 2006;12:531–537.

Mahoney BA, Smith WA, Lo DS, et al: Emergency interventions for hyperkalaemia. Cochrane Database Syst Rev 2005;(2):D003235.

Rivers E, Nguyen B, Havstad S, et al: Early Goal-Directed Therapy Collaborative Group. Early goal-directed therapy in the treatment of severe sepsis and septic shock. N Engl J Med 2001;345:1368–1377.

The SAFE Study Investigators: A comparison of albumin and saline for fluid resuscitation in the intensive care unit. N Engl J Med 2004;350:2247–2256.

Chapter 2

Dopaminergic and Pressor Agents in Acute Renal Failure

Daniel J. Ford, Brett Cullis, and Mark Denton

CHAPTER CONTENTS

DOPAMINERGIC AGENTS IN ACUTE RENAL FAILURE

Dopamine was first described by Barger and Dale[1] in 1910 and has been used in clinical practice since the 1960s. Its popularity stems from early work suggesting that at low doses, it had the ability to increase renal blood flow (RBF), diuresis, and natriuresis in both animal studies[2] and studies with healthy human volunteers.[3,4] It remained the mainstay of both treatment and prevention of acute renal failure (ARF) for three decades. However, since the 1990s, the evidence base for low-dose dopamine has been called into question and during the 2000s, the evidence against it being beneficial has become substantial.

Fenoldopam mesylate is a selective DA_1 receptor agonist. It is currently being used for treatment of hypertensive crises.[5] It has been hypothesized that fenoldopam may be beneficial in the treatment or prevention of ARF because of its DA_1 receptor selectivity.[6]

The following section looks at the physiology of dopamine and fenoldopam in both health and critical illness, and the reasons why dopamine was initially thought to be beneficial. It also covers the evidence for and against both dopamine and fenoldopam in the prevention of ARF in high-risk patients and in the treatment of ARF in the critically ill.

Dopamine

Physiology of Intrarenal Dopamine

Dopamine is synthesized by the kidney and is a critical regulator of sodium excretion.[7,8] It achieves this by directly inhibiting sodium reabsorption via inhibition of sodium transporters along almost the entire length of the nephron and by interacting with other regulators of sodium excretion, including atrial natriuretic peptide, catecholamines, vasopressin, angiotensin, and prostaglandins.[8] This physiologic role of dopamine is important to the understanding of the effects of exogenous dopamine and is therefore discussed briefly in this section.

Proximal tubule epithelial cells synthesize dopamine from the substrate L-dopa using the enzyme L-amino acid decarboxylase. L-Dopa enters the cell from the tubular lumen by a sodium-coupled transport mechanism. Dietary sodium load is the major factor controlling intrarenal dopamine synthesis; the exact mechanism linking increased salt intake to increased renal dopamine synthesis is not understood. Upon synthesis, intrarenal dopamine may act in an autocrine fashion by binding dopamine receptors on the proximal tubule cell or pass along the urinary space to bind to specific receptors on distal portions of the nephron. Importantly, the natriuretic effect of dopamine is prominent in states of sodium loading and is weak or negligible in salt-depleted states.[9,10]

Dopamine inhibits the activity of the Na/K ATPase in the proximal tubule, the thick ascending limb of Henle, the distal tubule, and the collecting duct. Dopamine also has profound effects on sodium entry into tubule cells via inhibition of the Na/H exchanger and Na/PO_4 exchanger in the proximal tubule. Dopamine also inhibits the Na/Cl cotransporter in the thick ascending limb and the vasopressin-stimulated sodium transporter in the collecting duct.

Intrarenal dopamine interacts with other hormonal regulators of sodium excretion. For example, the natriuretic effect of atrial natriuretic peptide is dependent on renal dopamine receptors. Conversely, the inhibitory effect of dopamine on the proximal tubule Na/H exchanger is potentiated by atrial natriuretic peptide. Dopamine and α-adrenergic agonists counteract each other's effect on basolateral Na/K ATPase. In addition, dopamine inhibits the stimulatory effect of angiotensin on Na/K ATPase in part by inhibition of angiotensin I receptor expression. Vasopressin-dependent sodium and water transport in the cortical collecting duct is inhibited by stimulation of dopamine receptors at these sites. Finally, dopamine enhances the synthesis of other locally acting natriuretic compounds, such as prostaglandin E_2.

Dopamine receptors are expressed on the renal vasculature.[11] DA_1 receptors are localized within the vessel wall media, whereas DA_2 receptors are present in the adventitia and are probably localized presynaptically on sympathetic nerve terminals. The vascular effects of dopamine in the kidney are mediated by dopamine released by dopaminergic nerves and circulating dopamine but not dopamine synthesized by the proximal tubules.[8]

Recent studies have examined the activity of renally synthesized dopamine in disease. In patients with both acute and chronic heart failure, proximal tubular uptake of the precursor L-dopa is enhanced perhaps to preserve renal dopamine production.[12] Patients with renal parenchymal disease have reduced activity of their renal dopaminergic system.[13]

Effects of Exogenous Dopamine on Renal Function in Healthy Persons

Dopamine can bind to at least three types of receptor: the dopamine receptor, the β-adrenoreceptor, and the α-adrenoreceptor.[14] There are differences in the affinity of these receptors for dopamine, and this accounts for the dose-response profile observed with infusion. In general, selective dopamine receptor stimulation occurs within an infusion rate range of 0.5 to 3.0 μg/kg/min. Further increases in infusion rate between 3 and 10 μg/kg/min result in increasing β-adrenoreceptor stimulation, and increased α-adrenoreceptor stimulation occurs at a rate between 5 and 20 μg/kg/min. These dose ranges are only approximate and must be interpreted with caution because they were derived from small studies using healthy patients.[14] In general, studies have shown a poor correlation between infusion rates and plasma dopamine levels in critically ill patients.[15] There is a high interpatient and intrapatient variability in the effects of any given dopamine infusion rate.[16] Thus, low-dose dopamine should not be referred to as renal dose dopamine because at this infusion rate (0.5–3 μg/kg/min) it is possible that all three receptor types are stimulated. Consistent with this, tachycardia is frequently seen in patients receiving low-dose dopamine.[17] Dopamine clearance is reduced in critically ill patients and in patients with renal impairment.[15]

In healthy adults, dopamine infusion increases RBF; the mechanism for this effect is dependent on the infusion rate.[3,18,19] At low infusion rates, dopamine induces renal vasodilation and increases RBF and can do this without any change in systemic hemodynamics—an effect mediated by dopaminergic receptors on the intrarenal vasculature.[20,21] This effect can be mimicked by selective DA_1 receptor agonists such as fenoldopam.[6] Stimulation of presynaptic DA_2 receptors on sympathetic nerve terminals with inhibition of norepinephrine release may further augment renal vasodilation and RBF.[22] With higher infusion rates, RBF is increased as a consequence of increases in cardiac output, mediated by β-adrenoreceptor stimulation.[23] In healthy humans, low-dose dopamine counteracts the reduction in RBF observed with norepinephrine infusion.[24,25]

Knowledge of how low-dose dopamine affects the intrarenal distribution of blood flow is important because specific areas of the kidney are more susceptible to ischemic injury than others. Most animal models have shown a preferential increase in cortical flow with dopamine.[7] This was confirmed in humans by Hoogenberg and colleagues[24] using a xenon washout technique. Dopamine-induced prostaglandin E_2 production may also enhance inner medullary blood flow.[26] Thus, dopamine may shunt blood away from the outer medulla, which would be detrimental in states of renal hypoperfusion given that the outer medulla contains the pars recta of the proximal tubule and the medullary thick ascending limb, two highly metabolically active portions of the nephron. In a study of patients with severe sepsis, low-dose dopamine increased RBF, but this was accompanied by a reduction in the renal oxygen extraction ratio, which led to no net change in renal oxygen consumption.[27]

Low-dose dopamine has minimal effects on the glomerular filtration rate (GFR) in healthy subjects.[16,19] Most studies report a mild increase in the GFR of approximately 10% to 20%, whereas others report no change as assessed by creatinine clearance or iothalamate clearance. Increases in the GFR are mediated by preferential afferent arteriolar vasodilation and an increase in intraglomerular pressure, as demonstrated in single-nephron studies.[28] The ultrafiltration coefficient remains unchanged with dopamine infusion.[7] The selective DA_1 receptor agonist fenoldopam did not change the GFR in healthy adults.[6]

The hemodynamic effects of low-dose dopamine infusion on healthy subjects differ with age, race, extracellular fluid volume status,[29] and duration of infusion.[30] In neonates, activation of α-adrenoreceptors occurs at much lower infusion rates.[31] In general, the selective vasodilatory effects of dopamine are not seen in young children.[32] With increasing age, the effects of dopamine on RBF and GFR are attenuated, perhaps because of impaired renal prostaglandin production.[33,34] Blacks are more likely to exhibit pressor responses to low-dose dopamine than whites.[35] Blacks also appear to be more resistant to the natriuretic effects of dopamine.[35]

A natriuresis is the most consistent physiologic response to low-dose dopamine in healthy humans.[19] This effect is rapid in onset and may be profound. It is abrogated by extracellular fluid volume depletion[29] and typically wanes after 24 hours of infusion, perhaps as a result of counteractive antinatriuretic factors or perhaps dopamine receptor down-regulation.[3,30,36,37] Oral dopamine receptor antagonists commonly used as antiemetic agents or to enhance gastric motility may or may not counteract the hemodynamic and natriuretic effects of dopamine.[38,39] In addition to the direct tubular effects of dopamine, dopamine infusion may induce natriuresis by inhibiting adrenal aldosterone production.[40,41]

Effects of Exogenous Dopamine on Renal Function in Disease States

Whereas low-dose dopamine consistently causes renal vasodilation in healthy adults, this effect is often attenuated or absent in critically ill patients (Table 2-1). Several factors may account for this, such as abnormal vasculature (e.g., atherosclerosis), hypertensive arteriopathy and renal artery stenosis, and counterregulatory effects of other vasoactive hormones, including increased activity of the renin-angiotensin-aldosterone system and the sympathetic nervous system.

Both extracellular volume depletion and hypoxemia have been shown to abrogate the renal effects of dopamine.[29,42] Some clinical settings in which studies have reported diminished effects of dopamine include chronic kidney disease,[43]

Table 2-1   Effects of Dopamine on Renal Hemodynamics and Sodium Excretion in Disease States

Disease State	Reference	RBF	GFR	UNa
Hypertension	Bhugi et al, 1989[45]	↔	NR	↑
Cardiac failure	McDonald et al, 1964[3]	↔	↔	↑
Septic shock on NE	Lherm et al, 1996[44]	NR	↔	↔
After vascular surgery	de Lasson et al, 1995[47]	↑	↔	↑
After vascular surgery	Girbes et al, 1996[40]	↑	↔	↑
Critically ill	Duke et al, 1994[17]	NR	↔	↑
Critically ill	Parker et al, 1981[46]	NR	↔	↑
Hypoxemia	Olsen et al, 1993[42]	↔	↔	↑
Chronic renal impairment	ter Wee et al, 1986[43]	↔	↔	↑
Acute renal failure	Lauschke et al, 2006[48]	NR	NR	↔

GFR, glomerular filtration rate; NE, norepinephrine; NR, not reported; RBF, renal blood flow; U_{Na}, urine sodium excretion.

cardiac failure,[3] septic shock treated with norepinephrine,[44] hypertension,[45] critically ill patients in intensive care units (ICUs),[17,46] and after vascular surgery.[40,47]

ter Wee and colleagues[43] found patients with chronic kidney disease to be less responsive than normal individuals to the renal vasodilatory action of dopamine. The increase in RBF and GFR observed with low-dose dopamine correlated with the baseline GFR. Patients with a baseline GFR of less than 50 mL/min showed no change in RBF or GFR with dopamine infusion.[43] McDonald and colleagues[3] showed that low-dose dopamine does not increase RBF in patients with clinical and radiologic heart failure.

Girbes and colleagues[40] looked at patients undergoing infrarenal aortic surgery. They found that low-dose dopamine did increase RBF, but this was accounted for by an increase in cardiac output rather than selective renal vasodilation. In a prospective crossover study comparing dobutamine and dopamine in critically ill patients, dopamine acted primarily as a diuretic and had no effect on creatinine clearance, whereas dobutamine, which had a greater effect on cardiac index, increased creatinine clearance. Lauschke and colleagues[48] looked at low-dose dopamine in patients with and without ARF. Dopamine was found to reduce renal resistive indices in patients without ARF, but increased resistive indices in patients with ARF. This suggests that dopamine can worsen renal perfusion in patients with ARF.

A study that did find an initial increase in creatinine clearance in critically ill patients treated with low-dose dopamine showed that this effect had disappeared after 48 hours, suggesting a tolerance to the effects of dopamine over time.[36] Marik[49] found that high levels of renin in critically ill patients may counteract the effects of dopamine.

In addition to these studies showing the reduction of the hemodynamic effects of dopamine in disease states as compared with healthy adults, it has been demonstrated that there is a poor correlation between dopamine infusion dose and dopamine plasma level,[15] calling into doubt the concept of low-dose dopamine.

In summary, the hemodynamic effects of dopamine that have been demonstrated in healthy adults are reduced in a number of disease states. The only effects that persist are increased diuresis and natriuresis.[50]

Value of Low-Dose Dopamine in Preventing Acute Renal Failure in High-Risk Patients

A limitation of the efficacy of any treatment designed to prevent ARF is the difficulty in predicting its occurrence and hence the correct timing of treatment. However, when patients are about to undergo a high-risk procedure, prophylactic administration of renoprotective agents can be timed appropriately. In these circumstances, judgment is required as to whether it is appropriate to expose all patients to the potential side effects of a given drug when the potential benefit may be gained by only a few patients. Several well-defined clinical situations are associated with renal hypoperfusion and a high risk of developing ARF. These include cardiac, vascular, and biliary surgery, renal and liver transplantation, and exposure to radiocontrast agents or vasoactive drugs. The prophylactic administration of low-dose dopamine in an attempt to prevent renal hypoperfusion and injury has been evaluated in these settings. Some of the studies looking at these individual populations are discussed and the larger meta-analyses that look at all these groups as a whole are reviewed. The major trials are summarized in Table 2-2.

Cardiovascular Surgery

Five studies have examined the efficacy of low-dose dopamine infusion in the prevention of ARF during cardiac surgery.[51–55] Three studies have examined the efficacy of low-dose dopamine infusion in the prevention of ARF during peripheral vascular surgery.[47,56,57] All studies failed to demonstrate a beneficial effect of dopamine on renal function, as assessed by urea (blood urea nitrogen [BUN]), creatinine, or creatinine clearance. However, the incidence of ARF in the control groups of some of these studies was low (perhaps a result of study participation), making it difficult to detect a benefit of dopamine. Three studies examined evidence of more subtle ischemic renal damage by measuring markers of tubule injury such as urinary retinal binding protein and β_2-microglobulin.[51–55] Overall, prophylactic low-dose dopamine infusion appeared to be

Table 2-2 Prospective, Randomized, Controlled Trials Examining the Ability of Low-Dose Dopamine to Prevent Acute Renal Failure in Patients at High Risk of Acute Kidney Injury

Study	Clinical Setting	Dopamine Regimen	Parameter	RENAL CONTROL	
				Preop	Postop
Lassnigg et al[51] (N = 82)	Cardiac surgery	2 μg/kg/min pre-surgery and 48 hr post-surgery	BUN	17.3 ± 5.9	23.7 ± 10.7
			Creat	0.96 ± 0.23	1.1 ± 0.36
			CrCl	99 ± 47	95 ± 54
			ARF	—	1 (2.3%)
Myles et al[52] (N = 52)	Elective CABG	3 μg/kg/min pre-surgery and 24 hr post-surgery	BUN	NR	NR
			Creat	1.02 ± 0.05	1.03 ± 0.05
			CrCl	127 ± 12	107 ± 15
			UO	NR	342 ± 130
Tang et al[53] (N = 42)	Cardiac surgery	3 μg/kg/min pre-surgery and 48 hr post-surgery	BUN*	5.2 ± 0.4	6.5 ± 1.5
			Creat	120 ± 5	113 ± 4
			UO*	27 ± 7	21 ± 4
Sumeray et al[54] (N = 48)	Cardiac surgery	2.5 μg/kg/min pre-surgery and 48 hr post-surgery	CrCl	68.2	70.0
			GFR	75.4	81.4
			UO	—	2050
Yavuz et al[55] (N = 22)	Cardiac surgery	2 μg/kg/min pre-surgery and for 48 hr post-surgery	CrCl	75.2	55.6
Baldwin et al[56] (N = 37)	Elective abdominal aortic surgery	3 μg/kg/min post-surgery for 24 hr	BUN	6.8	5.8
			Creat	1.3	1.2
			CrCl	72	83
			UO	NR	NR
Paul et al[57] (N = 27)	Elective infrarenal aortic clamping	3 μg/kg/min post-surgery for 24 hr mannitol	BUN	NR	NR
			Creat	NR	NR
			CrCl	96 ± 10	92 ± 7
			UO	150 ± 30	115 ± 30
Swygert et al[60] (N = 48)	Liver transplantation	3 μg/kg/min pre-surgery and 24 hr post-surgery	BUN	14 ± 1.7	33.5 ± 4.5
			SCr	1.0 ± 0.1	1.4 ± 0.1
			CrCl	82	58 ± 10

FUNCTION			
DOPAMINE			
Preop	Postop	Significant Difference?	Comment
16.2 ± 6.1	25.7 ± 8.1	No	ARF defined by increase in Creat > 0.5; statistically more ARF in third group receiving furosemide alone
0.98 ± 0.23	1.21 ± 0.45	No	
101 ± 35	72 ± 35	No	
–	0 (0%)	No	
NR	NR	–	CrCl Creat and UO assessed at day 7 postoperatively; no ARF in control group
1.05 ± 0.05	1.13 ± 0.14	No	
104 ± 16	91 ± 16	No	
NR	305 ± 160	No	
4.5 ± 0.3	6.4 ± 1.0	No	Parameters assessed at day 5; dopamine use associated with worse tubular injury (assessed by urine retinol-binding protein) (UO = mL/hr)
110 ± 6	1.13 ± 0.14	No	
28 ± 5	23 ± 4	No	
67.7	68.4	No	Parameters measured at day 5; urine markers of tubular injury were more preserved in dopamine group
74.4	73.7	No	
–	2229	No	
66.3	72.2	No	Creatinine clearance measured at day 7; significantly higher level of β_2-microglobulin in dopamine group
6.8	5.8	No	Parameters assessed at day 5; no ARF in control group; trend toward increased UO in control group
1.2	1.2	No	
89	85	No	
NR	NR	–	
NR	NR	–	Parameters assessed at day 1 postoperatively; CrCl decreased in both groups by 50% during clamp period (UO = mL/day)
NR	NR	–	
92 ± 7	92 ± 7	No	
130 ± 30	100 ± 30	No	
19.4 ± 3.7	31.6 ± 5.3	No	BUN/SCr assessed at day 7 and GFR at 1 mo postop (after 30 days of cyclosporine); incidence of postop ARF was 4% in both groups
1.3 ± 0.2	1.4 ± 0.2	No	
84	59 ± 6	No	

Continued

Table 2-2 Prospective, Randomized, Controlled Trials Examining the Ability of Low-Dose Dopamine to Prevent Acute Renal Failure in Patients at High Risk of Acute Kidney Injury—cont'd

| | | | | | RENAL | |
| | | | | | CONTROL | |
Study	Clinical Setting	Dopamine Regimen		Parameter	Preop	Postop
Parks et al[62] (N = 23)	Elective biliary surgery	3 μg/kg/min pre-surgery and 24 hr post-surgery		BUN	5.1 ± 0.6	4.8 ± 0.6
				SCr	72 ± 6	70 ± 7
				CrCl	70 ± 17	75 ± 10
				UO	46 ± 10	60 ± 20
Gare et al[67] (N = 66)	Coronary angiography in patients with DM and/or CRF	2 μg/kg/min and saline infusion for 48 hr	Saline	BUN*	7.3 ± 0.5	7.9 ± 0.8
				Creat*	100.6 ± 5.2	112.3 ± 8.0
Hans et al[68] (N = 55)	CRF (Creat 1.4–3.5); abdominal angiography	2.5 μg/kg/min 1 hr pre/ 12 hr post-procedure	Saline	ARF	—	44%
Kapoor et al[69] (N = 40)	Coronary angiography	5 μg/kg/min 30 min pre- and 6 hr post-procedure	Saline	BUN	20 ± 13	23 ± 8
				Creat	1.5 ± 7	2.0 ± 1.0
				ARF	—	50%
Stevens et al[70] (N = 77)	High-risk patients; DM, CRF, PVD; coronary angiography	2 μg/kg/min and saline infusion, furosemide, and mannitol	Saline	Creat	2.6 ± 0.9	3.1 ± 1.2
				UO	—	122 ± 54
				ARF	—	14.50%
				RRT	—	9.10%
Weisberg et al[71] (N = 50)	CRF (Creat >1.8); coronary angiography	2.5 μg/kg/min during and 2 hr post-procedure	Saline	RBF	247 ± 55	NR
				Creat	>1.8	NR
				ARF	—	40%
Abizaid et al[72] (N = 40)	CRF (Creat >1.5); coronary angiography	2.5 μg/kg/min 2 hr pre-procedure and saline infusion (1 mg/kg/hr); 12 hr pre-procedure	Saline	Creat	2.3 ± 0.8	2.8 ± 1.1
				ARF	—	6 (30%)

ARF, acute renal failure; BUN, blood urea nitrogen; CABG, coronary artery bypass grafting; Creat, serum creatinine; CRF, chronic renal failure; CrCl, creatinine clearance (mL/min); DM, diabetes mellitus; GFR, glomerular filtration rate; NR, not reported; PVD, peripheral vascular disease; RBF, renal blood flow; RRT, renal replacement therapy; U_{Na}, urine sodium excretion; UO, urine output.
BUN and Creat expressed as mg/dL unless marked by an asterisk, which indicates SI units.

FUNCTION			
DOPAMINE			
Preop	Postop	Significant Difference?	Comment
4.9 ± 0.6	6.0 ± 1.0	No	BUN in mmol/L; parameters assessed at day 5; no ARF in control group; all patients received a bolus of saline and furosemide postop
72 ± 6	68 ± 8	No	
90 ± 10	78 ± 12	No	
62 ± 10	55 ± 15	No	
6.9 ± 0.5	7.6 ± 0.6	No	Peak Creat within 5 days post-contrast; subgroup of patients with peripheral vascular disease did worse with dopamine
100.3 ± 5.4	117.5 ± 8.8	No	
—	18%	Yes	ARF defined by increase in Creat > 0.5 mg/dL by day 4 post-procedure; no RRT required
16 ± 8	15 ± 6	No	ARF defined by Creat > 25% above baseline; in all cases, ARF mild and reversible
1.5 ± 0.3	1.4 ± 0.3	Yes	
—	0%	Yes	
2.2 ± 0.4	2.7 ± 1.2	No	Parameters assessed at 24 and 48 hr; ARF defined by increase in Creat > 0.5 mg/dL
—	167 ± 58	Yes	
—	13.60%	No	
—	4.50%	No	
171 ± 23	NR	Yes	ARF defined by Creat > 25% above baseline RBF: thermodilution (mL/min per kidney)
> 1.8	NR	—	
—	30%	No	
1.9 ± 0.3	2.5 ± 0.6	No	Creat is peak value post-procedure; ARF defined by Creat > 25% above baseline
—	10 (50%)	No	

associated with increased renal tubular injury. A second study by Yavuz and colleagues[58] in patients undergoing coronary artery grafting showed a higher creatinine clearance in patients treated with both dopamine and diltiazem than those treated with either drug alone or placebo. However, it was a small study, with each of the four groups containing only 15 patients. The other studies looking at cardiac surgery were also relatively small (between 22 and 82 patients). Jones and colleagues[59] recruited 1100 patients undergoing cardiopulmonary bypass, to be prospectively randomized to dopamine, furosemide, mannitol, or control (ISRCTN 98672577, www. controlled-trials.com). This will perhaps provide more evidence in this particular subgroup of at-risk patients.

Liver Transplantation and Hepatobiliary Surgery

Liver transplantation is associated with a high incidence of renal failure, in part from the chronic renal hypoperfusion that complicates liver failure and the nephrotoxicity of hyperbilirubinemia and calcineurin inhibitors. In a large prospective, controlled trial involving 48 patients, perioperative infusion of dopamine was not associated with lower BUN or an improved creatinine clearance at 24 hours after surgery or with isotope GFR measured at 1 month.[60] The incidence of ARF was similar in both groups, but was very low at 4% compared with 40% to 60% in some series.

Two trials have looked at the effect of dopamine on patients with obstructive jaundice and hyperbilirubinemia who were undergoing surgery. In a prospective, randomized, controlled trial involving 40 patients, Wahbah and colleagues[61] concluded that administration of low-dose dopamine conferred no additional benefit over adequate hydration. Similarly, Parks and colleagues[62] randomized 23 patients to dopamine or saline infusion during surgery for obstructive jaundice and found no benefit of dopamine infusion on creatinine clearance 5 days after surgery.

Renal Transplantation

Four studies have examined the role of perioperative low-dose dopamine infusion during renal transplantation, including three prospective studies[63-65] and one retrospective study.[66] Endpoints measured included incidence of posttransplantation ARF, delayed graft function, requirements for dialysis, and allograft GFR at various points after transplantation. Three studies indicated no beneficial effects of perioperative dopamine infusion on allograft function. Indeed, dopamine-induced natriuresis and diuresis were often associated with fluid and electrolyte management problems in these patients. Carmellini and colleagues[64] reported a small but significantly higher GFR at 1 month in the dopamine-treated transplantation group. However, there were no significant differences in the rate of delayed graft function or in the requirement for dialysis between groups in this study.

Radiocontrast-Induced Nephropathy

Radiocontrast agents are a major cause of hospital-acquired ARF. Patients with diabetes, patients with preexisting renal impairment, and patients with intravascular volume depletion are most at risk of radiocontrast-induced nephropathy. In the majority of cases, radiocontrast-induced nephropathy is mild and reversible; however, contrast exposure may precipitate the need for permanent dialysis in patients with baseline chronic renal failure. The mechanism for this effect is contrast-induced intrarenal vasoconstriction. The role of prophylactic dopamine to prevent radiocontrast-induced nephropathy has been assessed in six trials.[67-72] Hans and colleagues[68] reported a significant reduction in ARF episodes (increase in creatinine >0.5 mg/dL) from 44% to 18% with dopamine infusion. Kapoor and colleagues[69] found similar results, although all cases of ARF were transient and not requiring acute dialysis. Four studies found no difference in the rate of ARF.[67-72] It is difficult to justify the use of prophylactic dopamine, considering its potential significant side effects (see "Potentially Deleterious Effects of Dopamine") including the need for central venous access, based on these studies.

Influence of Low-Dose Dopamine on Established Acute Renal Failure

Established acute tubular necrosis (ATN) is associated with a reduced GFR owing to several mechanisms, including (1) impaired glomerular perfusion secondary to preglomerular vasoconstriction, (2) back-leakage of glomerular filtrate through injured tubular epithelium, and (3) obstruction of the renal tubules by cellular debris.

Proponents of low-dose dopamine infusion argue that dopamine may improve the outcome of ATN by (1) improving renal perfusion, (2) inhibiting tubular transport processes and therefore improving the oxygen supply/demand relationship, and (3) "flushing out" renal tubules by inducing diuresis.

This presumption was strengthened by a small ($N = 23$) prospective, randomized, controlled trial (RCT) that looked at ARF in patients with falciparum malaria.[73] This study found that in patients with ARF, but with serum creatinine less than 400 μmol/L, dopamine reduced the recovery time from 17 days to 9 days.

Questions about the evidence base for dopamine began to be raised in a number of editorials and commentaries in the mid-1990s,[74-76] but despite this, there remained a strong tradition of dopamine use for the treatment of ARF. For example, a survey in 2001 found that 17 of 24 ICUs in New Zealand were still using dopamine for the treatment of ARF or oliguria. There is now considerable evidence to suggest that dopamine is, at best, ineffective at reducing mortality or the need for renal replacement therapy in ARF. Recently, three systematic reviews[77-79] and a large multicenter RCT[78] looked at the benefits of dopamine versus placebo in the treatment of ARF or the prevention of ARF in high-risk groups. The RCT from the Australian and New Zealand Intensive Care Society Clinical Trials Group looked at 328 patients in 23 ICUs. The inclusion criteria were two or more criteria for the systemic inflammatory response syndrome and one indicator of early renal dysfunction (urine output < 0.5 mL/kg/hr, serum creatinine > 150 μmol/L in the absence of premorbid renal dysfunction, or an increase in creatinine > 80 μmol/L within 24 hours). The patients were randomized to dopamine or placebo in a double-blind manner. The authors found no significant difference in primary outcome (peak serum creatinine) between the two groups, nor was there a difference in the increase in creatinine from baseline, the number of patients whose creatinine exceeded 300 μmol/L, the need for renal replacement therapy, the length of ICU stay, the length of hospital stay, or the number of deaths.[78]

In an observational study, Chertow and colleagues[80] analyzed a subgroup of patients who received low-dose dopamine in the placebo arm of a multicenter intervention trial. All patients in the placebo arm were adults with ARF (defined as an increase in the serum creatinine concentration of at least 1 mg/dL during 24–49 hours) and had a clinical history consistent with ATN. Dopamine had been administered to a portion of these patients at the discretion of the physician. A total of 86 patients received dopamine (<3 μg/kg/min) and 79 did not. Despite complex adjustment for treatment bias, low-dose dopamine treatment was not associated with a reduced risk of death or dialysis in patients with ATN.

Meta-analysis of Trials

Kellum and Decker[79] looked at 58 studies of 2149 patients, including 17 RCTs (854 patients). They included all studies looking at either the treatment or prevention of ARF and found no significant difference between dopamine and placebo in mortality or the need for renal replacement therapy. Marik[81] looked at 15 RCTs of 970 patients that included studies looking at either the prevention or treatment of early renal dysfunction. It demonstrated no significant difference between the absolute change in serum creatinine or the incidence of ARF between those patients receiving low-dose dopamine and those receiving placebo. Friedrich and colleagues[77] looked at 61 trials with 3359 patients; they included patients with or at risk for ARF and who were patients having cardiac, vascular, and other surgery; receiving radiologic contrast or other nephrotoxins; or had miscellaneous indications. Their review included the Australian and New Zealand Intensive Care Society study, which was the second largest study and dominated the clinical outcomes data (with a weighting of 68.1% for mortality and 27.4% for renal replacement therapy). As well as looking at mortality and the need for renal replacement therapy, the authors of this review also looked at a variety of renal physiologic indices. Their findings mirrored those of the previous reviews, showing no evidence that dopamine offers any clinically important benefits to patients with or at risk for ARF. These results were similar when the Australian and New Zealand Intensive Care Society study was excluded from the analysis (to ensure that one large study did not skew the results extraordinarily). The physiologic analysis showed an increased urine output of 24% with dopamine therapy on day 1. This effect decreased and was no longer significant beyond the first day. The authors concede that the inevitable heterogeneity of the systematic review meant that the analysis might have been underpowered to detect any subgroup effects.

Summary

The conclusion that we draw from these studies is that there is no evidence that dopamine is of any benefit over placebo in reduction of mortality or the need for renal replacement therapy in patients with or at risk of ARF. These disappointing results may be due to several factors: (1) the renal hemodynamic effects of dopamine appear to be attenuated in critically ill patients, (2) dopamine may have a detrimental effect on the intrarenal distribution of blood flow, and (3) inhibition of proximal tubule solute reabsorption may enhance distal delivery of solute and increase the workload of distal nephron segments.

The three recent meta-analyses all included studies looking at the benefit of dopamine in the prevention of ARF in high-risk groups. These failed to show any benefit of dopamine over placebo, and the authors concluded that low-dose dopamine should no longer be used for these indications. It could be argued that the obvious limitations of meta-analyses (i.e., the heterogeneous nature of the population studied) preclude extrapolation to individual subgroups. While there is a theoretical possibility that low-dose dopamine may be of benefit to one subgroup, this has not been indicated convincingly in any of a number of smaller trials. If this were to be the case, it would require a large prospective, randomized, controlled trial in one of the specific subgroups (for example, the study cited earlier that recruited 1100 patients undergoing coronary artery bypass grafting)[59] (ISRCTN 98672577, www.controlled-trials.com). Unless a future trial shows convincing evidence of benefit in a particular population, there should currently be no place for low-dose dopamine in the prevention of ARF in high-risk patients.

Potentially Deleterious Effects of Dopamine

Although proponents advocate the use of low-dose dopamine in ARF on the grounds that it may improve renal function and is unlikely to harm the patient, evidence is accumulating that the latter is a misconception. Table 2-3 outlines common adverse effects of low-dose dopamine. Administration of dopamine requires a central venous catheter. While this may be a routine procedure for patients undergoing cardiac surgery, for example, the additional risks of a central line for routine radiologic contrast procedures must be strongly considered. Local extravasation of dopamine adjacent to an artery may provoke distal ischemia and gangrene. Even at low doses, dopamine can, through β-receptor agonism, increase myocardial oxygen demand and precipitate tachyarrhythmias and myocardial ischemia.[82-84] There is evidence to suggest that in patients undergoing cardiac surgery, dopamine may increase the risk of postoperative atrial fibrillation or flutter by 74%.[84]

Neural dopamine is an inhibitory neurotransmitter in the carotid bodies, and dopamine infusion can suppress the respiratory drive induced by hypoxemia.[85] Dopamine can also lower blood Pao_2 by altering ventilation-perfusion matching within the lung, an effect arising from a shunt of blood away

Table 2-3 Deleterious Effects of Low-Dose Dopamine

Effect	Cause
Distal gangrene	Local extravasation of dopamine
Fluid and electrolyte imbalance	Inhibition of salt and water reabsorption
Tachyarrhythmias and myocardial ischemia	β-adrenoreceptor stimulation
Hypoxemia	Reduced respiratory drive; pulmonary shunting
Gut ischemia and bacterial translocation	Shunting of blood away from mucosal capillary bed
Catabolic	Inhibition of growth hormone release
Immunosuppression	Inhibition of prolactin release

from alveolar capillaries.[18,82] Hypoxemia may worsen myocardial ischemia in susceptible patients and delay recovery from ischemic ATN.

Fluid and electrolyte imbalance is common and has been reported in several studies using dopamine, especially after renal transplantation. The natriuresis and diuresis induced by inhibition of tubular sodium reabsorption and antidiuretic hormone release can cause severe volume depletion unless close monitoring of the patient permits sufficient fluid replacement. Potassium depletion is also a common result of the increased delivery of sodium to the distal tubule. Hypophosphatemia and hypomagnesemia have also been reported.

Low-dose dopamine suppresses pituitary function and inhibits prolactin and growth hormone secretion and hence may exacerbate the catabolic state in critically ill patients.[86] Hypoprolactinemia suppresses T-cell proliferation.[87]

Although low-dose dopamine increases total splanchnic blood flow, animal studies have shown that absolute intestinal mucosal flow is decreased as a result of dopamine-induced shunting of blood away from the mucosa.[88] This complication is of some concern, particularly in the critically ill patient in whom critical intestinal mucosal ischemia may lead to bacterial translocation and sepsis. When high-dose dopamine was compared with norepinephrine in patients with septic shock, dopamine was associated with a drop in gastric mucosal pH (an indicator of mucosal ischemia) compared with norepinephrine.[89]

Finally, low-dose dopamine hastened the onset of gut ischemia in a porcine model of hemorrhagic shock as a result of shunting blood away from the bowel mucosa rather than an absolute reduction in mesenteric blood flow.[90]

Fenoldopam

Fenoldopam mesylate is a selective DA_1 receptor agonist. It is currently being used for the treatment of hypertensive crises.[5] It has been hypothesized that fenoldopam may be beneficial in the treatment or prevention of ARF.[91] The reasons for this hypothesis, along with the evidence of its efficacy, are discussed in the following sections.

Rationale for Use of Fenoldopam

Dopamine receptors are expressed on the renal vasculature. DA_1 receptors are localized to the smooth muscle of the arterial beds, whereas DA_2 receptors are localized on the adventitia and probably on the sympathetic nerve terminals. It is the DA_1 receptor that mediates renal arterial vasodilation and natriuresis. DA_2 receptors cause vasoconstriction.[92]

Fenoldopam mesylate is a benzapine derivative that is a potent short-acting DA_1 receptor agonist. It is slightly more active than dopamine on the DA_1 receptor, but has no action on DA_2 or β- or α-adrenoreceptors. This action means that fenoldopam has none of the adrenergic effects of dopamine and may cause more vasodilation in the outer renal medulla than in the cortex.[93] This may be important given that the outer medulla contains the pars recta of the proximal tubule and the medullary thick ascending limb, two highly metabolically active portions of the nephron. Therefore, at lower doses (0.03–0.1 μg/kg/min) it increases RBF without affecting systemic hemodynamics. At higher doses (>1 μg/kg/min) it causes dose-related hypotension, and it is at these doses that it is used in the treatment of accelerated hypertension. There is

a suggestion that fenoldopam may improve renal function in patients with severe hypertension.[94]

Fenoldopam in the Prevention or Treatment of Acute Renal Failure

In the same way that the effects of dopamine have been studied in attempts to prevent ARF in high-risk populations, the same populations have been studied with respect to fenoldopam, although there is not yet the same volume of data as there is for dopamine. There is, however, at least one prospective RCT for most of the high-risk subgroups, as well as a large meta-analysis of all groups.

The meta-analysis reviewed 1290 patients in 16 RCTs.[95] The patients studied were all postoperative or in ICUs and were at risk of or had established ARF. They did not include patients at risk of contrast nephropathy. The authors of the meta-analysis found that the use of fenoldopam (versus placebo or usual care, including dopamine) significantly reduced the risk of acute kidney injury, the need for renal replacement therapy, and hospital mortality. In addition, the use of fenoldopam reduced the length of both ICU stay and total hospital stay. The authors did not find a significant incidence of hypotension or need for vasopressor use.

These findings are very promising in the search for a tool to help prevent or treat ARF. However, these findings should be interpreted with the caution that should accompany any meta-analysis. The limitations of this type of study include the heterogeneity of the population studied and the variation in definitive endpoints (for example, definition of acute kidney injury or parameters for commencing renal replacement therapy—only one study in the meta-analysis had predefined criteria indicating when a patient had reached a dialytic endpoint). These points are made by the authors as well as the acknowledgment that several of the studies were of suboptimal quality, increasing the risk of bias. They therefore conclude that their study supports the hypothesis that fenoldopam has renal protective effects, but given the limitations of meta-analyses, a larger multicenter RCT is required to confirm these results.

The benefits of fenoldopam in high-risk subgroups have, as with dopamine, been studied in a number of RCTs, some of which are listed in Table 2-4 (p. 24). Two studies have looked at fenoldopam in vascular surgery. Oliver and colleagues[96] compared fenoldopam with dopamine and nitroprusside in 60 patients undergoing elective aortic cross-clamping. They found no difference in urine output, serum creatinine, or creatinine clearance between the two groups. Halpenny and colleagues[97] also reviewed patients undergoing elective infrarenal cross-clamping, comparing fenoldopam with placebo in 28 patients. They found a decrease in creatinine clearance and an increase in serum creatinine in the control group compared with no change in the fenoldopam group. The relevance of this endpoint is unclear.

Three RCTs have looked at patients undergoing cardiac surgery. Bove and colleagues[98] randomized 80 patients to fenoldopam or dopamine. They found no difference in ARF, mortality, or length of ICU stay. The other two studies found an improvement in either creatinine clearance or serum creatinine.[99,100] Two studies have looked at fenoldopam in liver transplantation. Della Rocca and colleagues[101] compared fenoldopam with dopamine in 43 patients and found an improvement in serum creatinine and urea. Biancofiore and colleagues[102] compared fenoldopam, dopamine, and placebo groups ($N = 140$) and found a similar improvement in creatinine clearance. Neither study found a significant mortality benefit.

Four studies have reviewed fenoldopam in the prevention of contrast nephropathy. The first was a pilot study of 51 patients randomized to fenoldopam or placebo.[103] This study found an improvement in renal plasma flow, thus recommending further studies in this population. However, two of the other three trials showed no benefit of fenoldopam compared with either placebo or N-acetylcysteine,[104,105] whereas the third found fenoldopam to be less effective than N-acetylcysteine in preventing contrast nephropathy.[106]

There have been three RCTs of critically ill or septic patients with ARF. All three show promising trends in favor of fenoldopam, although none was able to confidently prove its value. In the largest of the three, 300 patients in ICUs with evidence of sepsis were randomized to fenoldopam or placebo.[107] The incidence of ARF (defined as an increase in serum creatinine > 150 μmol/L) was significantly lower in the fenoldopam group, although the incidence of severe ARF (creatinine > 300 μmol/L) failed to reach significance (10 in fenoldopam group versus 21 in control group; $P = .056$). Length of ICU stay was lower in the fenoldopam group, but mortality was not significantly different. The authors concluded that, although promising, their findings do not provide an adequate level of evidence to fully support the use of fenoldopam in this setting and they called for larger studies, adequately powered to assess endpoints such as mortality or the need for renal replacement therapy. Tumlin and colleagues[108] randomized 155 patients with early ATN to fenoldopam or placebo. There was a trend toward a benefit with fenoldopam, but it was not statistically significant. Certain subgroups reached statistical significance (nondiabetics and patients after cardiac surgery), but larger studies are required to confirm this. Brienza and colleagues[109] compared fenoldopam with dopamine in 100 patients in ICUs with early renal dysfunction. There was an improvement in serum creatinine levels at days 2, 3, and 4 in the fenoldopam group, although again the clinical significance of this finding is still not established.

Summary

Since its introduction into clinical use in the 1960s, low-dose dopamine became standard therapy for the treatment or prevention of ARF for three decades. Its use has diminished over the past 10 years as evidence suggesting a lack of benefit has grown. More recently, there have been three systemic reviews and one large, multicenter, randomized, controlled trial that have strengthened the argument against low-dose dopamine. Proponents of low-dose dopamine may argue that there remains a possibility of a subgroup of at-risk patients who may benefit from this therapy, although there are very few data to suggest that this is the case. Therefore, future use of dopamine for this purpose cannot be justified outside the confines of prospective RCTs, if at all. These recommendations should not preclude the use of dopamine for its systemic effects in heart failure or septic shock, when dopamine, like other inotropes or vasopressors, may afford a valuable increase in cardiac output and tissue perfusion.

Some of the properties of dopamine, which may contribute to its apparent lack of overall benefit, include DA_2 receptor agonism and β- and α-adrenoreceptor agonism. Fenoldopam is a selective DA_1 receptor agonist that does not share these other properties. It has therefore been suggested that low-dose

fenoldopam may be beneficial in the prevention or treatment of ARF. At present, the studies on fenoldopam, including one meta-analysis, have mostly been encouraging, although there is less evidence to support its protective properties against radiocontrast-induced nephropathy. However, while in previous years, a very promising meta-analysis would have been enough to provoke widespread use of this treatment, the legacy of three decades of dopamine use with no evidence base remains very prominent in our memories.[110] Therefore, although fenoldopam remains a very encouraging prospect, the authors of these studies as well as other editorials have all been quite restrained in their conclusions and have called for further large, multicenter, randomized, controlled trials to support these promising findings.

VASOPRESSOR AGENTS IN ACUTE RENAL FAILURE

Volume depletion is by far the most common cause of renal hypoperfusion; if adequate fluid resuscitation has failed to improve arterial pressure, renal perfusion, and kidney function, it then becomes necessary to consider cardiogenic or distributive shock. Distributive shock is most likely to occur in the setting of severe sepsis, and in this case, one needs to consider the use of vasopressors. The vasopressors available for clinical use include norepinephrine, epinephrine, phenylephrine, dopamine, and vasopressin. Dopamine was covered in the previous section and is therefore not mentioned here. This section reviews the utility of vasopressors in improving renal perfusion and function in patients with sepsis-induced ARF.

Vasopressors promote vasculature smooth muscle contraction, increase systemic vascular resistance, and augment blood pressure in septic patients. By augmenting systemic blood pressure and renal perfusion pressure, they may improve renal function. However, renal failure in the setting of septic shock is not simply a consequence of systemic hypotension. Hypoperfusion of the kidney in sepsis may be exacerbated by concomitant renal vasoconstriction, and improving systemic blood pressure alone may not necessarily improve renal perfusion. Animal studies show variable changes in renal vascular resistance in sepsis-induced ARF.[111–114] A recent review by Langeberg and colleagues[115] showed that of 137 studies published, 69 showed increased renal vascular resistance, 16 showed no change, and 52 showed a decrease. This has never been studied in humans.

Very few studies have been done to specifically assess the appropriate target blood pressure sought with vasopressors in patients with sepsis-induced ARF. There have been numerous trials in ICU patients comparing various blood pressure targets on outcome, but they have not looked at renal function as a primary endpoint. Hayes and colleagues[116] chose a mean arterial pressure (MAP) target of 80 mm Hg when attempting to improve oxygen delivery, but showed no improvement in predicted outcomes. The early goal-directed therapy trial on which many guidelines of the surviving sepsis campaign are based used a target MAP of 65 mm Hg.[117,118] Bougoin and colleagues[119] randomized 40 patients with septic shock to a norepinephrine infusion to achieve a MAP of either 65 or 85 mm Hg. Endpoints were spot creatinine clearance, urine flow, and serum creatinine. They found no difference in any of these endpoints and therefore suggested that there was no

Table 2-4 Prospective Randomized, Controlled Trials Examining the Ability of Fenoldopam to Prevent Acute Renal Failure in High-Risk Patients

Study	Clinical Setting	Fenoldopam Regimen	Parameter	RENAL CONTROL	
				Preop	Postop
Oliver et al[95] (N = 60)	Elective AAA repair	0.05 µg/kg/min start dose	UO (first 24 hr)	1.3 ± 0.2	2755 mL
			Creat (mg/dL)		1.2 ± 0.4
			CrCl		68.3
Bove et al[97] (N = 80)	Cardiac surgery	0.05 µg/kg/min	Creat	1.54 ± 0.59	1.6 ± 0.69
			Death (%)		7.5
			ARF (%)		40
Halpenny et al[99] (N = 31)	Cardiac surgery	0.1 µg/kg/min	UO (mL/min)	1.5	3.8
			Creat	96	78
			CrCl	107	71
Della Rocca et al[100] (N = 43)	Liver transplant	0.1 µg/kg/min	Creat	0.98	1.66
			Urea (mg/dL)	21	29
			CrCl	87	68
			ICU stay (hr)		48
			Hosp stay (days)		16.5
Biancofiore et al[101] (N = 140)	Liver transplant	0.1 µg/kg/min		Dop/placebo	Dop/placebo
			Creat	0.85/0.88	0.9/0.9
			CrCl	102.5/110.7	−12.3%/−39%
Tumlin et al[102] (N = 45)	Contrast	0.1 µg/kg/min	Renal plasma flow		−33.2%
			Contrast nephropathy		40%
			Peak Creat (mg/dL)		3.6
Ng et al[103] (N = 84)	Contrast	0.1 µg/kg/min	Change in Creat (72 hr)		0.2
Stone et al[104] (N = 315)	Contrast	0.05–0.1 µg/kg/min	Creat increase > 25%		30.1%
			Creat increase > 0.5 mg/dL		24.0%
Briguori et al[105] (N = 192)	Contrast	0.1 µg/kg/min	Creat		1.72
			Creat increase > 0.5 mg/dL		4.1%
Morelli et al[106] (N = 300)	Sepsis on ICU	0.09 µg/kg/min	Creat (µmol/l)	102.9 ± 88	176 ± 150.4
			Creat increase (%)		71 ± 101
			Mortality (%)		44
			Cases of ARF (Cr >150)		34%
			Cases of severe ARF (Cr > 300)		14%
			Length of ICU stay (days)		13

FUNCTION				
DOPAMINE				
Preop	Postop	Significant Difference?	Comment	
1.2 ± 0.3	2939 mL	No	Control = dopamine	
	1.1 ± 0.5	No	2 μg/kg/min and nitroprusside	
	78.6	No	Creat and CrCl measured at 72 hr	
1.56 ± 0.78	1.7 ± 0.86	No	ARF defined as 25% increase Creat	
	10	No		
	42.5	No	Control = dopamine 2.5 μg	
1.5	4.4	$P < .01$	UO measured 0–4 hr postop; not significant at later stages	
93	76			
93	93	$P < .01$		
1.00	1.18	$P = .004$	Control = dopamine 2 μg/kg/min; post = postop day 3	
20	23	$P = .01$		
85	76	NS		
	48	NS		
	16.0	NS		
			Control = dopamine 3 μg/kg/min or placebo	
0.81	1.0	NS		
110	+ 3%	$P < .001$		
	±15.8%	$P < .05$	Control = saline	
	21%	NS		
	2.8	$P < .05$		
	0.08	$P = .4$	Control = N-acetylcysteine	
	33.6%	NS	Control = placebo	
	28.5%	NS		
	1.75		Control = N-acetylcysteine	
	13.7%	$P = .019$		
89.8 ± 26.4	132 ± 88	$P = .003$	Control = placebo	
	46 ± 78	$P = .22$		
	34.7	No		
	19.3%	$P = .006$		
	6.7%	No		
	8	$P < .001$		

Continued

Table 2-4 Prospective Randomized, Controlled Trials Examining the Ability of Fenoldopam to Prevent Acute Renal Failure in High-Risk Patients—cont'd

Study	Clinical Setting	Fenoldopam Regimen	Parameter	RENAL CONTROL	
				Preop	Postop
Tumlin et al[07] (N = 155)	Critically ill	0.05–0.2 µg/kg/min	Creat	1.25	2.24
			Creat > 1.5		31%
			Death and dialysis		37.0%
			Dialysis		25.3%
Brienza et al[108] (N = 100)	Critically ill	0.1 µg/kg/min	Mean Creat increase		0.09
			Patients with > 10% Creat increase		38%
			Creat (at day 3) 1.91		1.86

AAA, abdominal aortic aneurysm; ARF, acute renal failure; CrCl, creatinine clearance; Creat, creatinine; Hosp, hospital; ICU, intensive care unit; NS, not significant; UO, urine output.

point in targeting a higher pressure. The study was limited in that it continued for only 8 hours, during which creatinine and, potentially, creatinine clearance would not normally change significantly. There was a significant reduction in the oxygen extraction ratio and serum lactate in the higher pressure group, suggesting that there may be some overall benefit. The problem with setting a specific target blood pressure is that higher doses of vasopressors can induce unwanted tissue vasoconstriction, and therefore the lowest dose possible that achieves adequate urine output is the optimum.

Norepinephrine

Norepinephrine is one of the most commonly used vasopressors and has by far the most evidence supporting its use in renal failure. It acts primarily on α-adrenergic receptors, although there is some β-adrenergic effect. This means that it is able to increase the MAP by vasoconstriction with little increase in cardiac output and myocardial oxygen demand. It is clinically proven to increase the MAP effectively, and in randomized, controlled trials comparing it with dopamine, it was more effective at increasing the blood pressure and had better effect on oxygen extraction ratios and splanchnic blood flow.[120–123] Martin and colleagues[122] compared 32 patients with vasoplegic shock who were treated with dopamine or norepinephrine and showed that there was adequate restoration of blood pressure or systemic vascular resistance in 31% and 98%, respectively.

There has long been concern over the use of norepinephrine in the setting of ARF because it was shown to cause renal vasoconstriction and ARF. This concern was raised by an animal model of ARF in which high doses of norepinephrine were infused directly into the renal artery. These animals were normotensive and not septic and therefore far removed from the clinical situation.[124] In the face of hypovolemia, norepinephrine does worsen renal function and hence fluid resuscitation is imperative.[124,125]

In septic animals and humans, there is evidence that norepinephrine infusion improves renal function. The proposed mechanisms are (1) an increased MAP and therefore perfusion pressure, (2) relatively greater efferent than afferent arteriolar vasoconstriction with consequent increased intraglomerular pressure, and (3) better regional blood flow.[111,126,127] The details of these studies are outlined in the following.

Animal Studies

Table 2-5 (p. 28) summarizes some of the animal studies performed to determine the effects of norepinephrine infusion on renal hemodynamics and function in experimental models of sepsis induced ARF.[112,127–130] Bellomo and colleagues[113] looked at RBF with norepinephrine before and after treatment with lipopolysaccharide (LPS) in dogs. RBF was unchanged when norepinephrine was infused in nonseptic animals; however, once they had been given LPS, norepinephrine induced a marked increase in RBF from baseline. Similarly, in dogs injected with *Escherichia coli*, there was almost complete restoration of RBF to presepsis levels in those treated with norepinephrine.[130] Boffa and colleagues[111] injected LPS into mice and at 14 hours measured the MAP, RBF, renal vascular resistance, GFR, and urine flow. The animals were exposed to vasoconstrictors norepinephrine, angiotensin II, and N-nitro-L-arginine methyl ester both before LPS injection and then again 14 hours after LPS. They showed that norepinephrine did not decrease the GFR in control animals. In the animals with septic shock, all the agents increased the MAP to a similar degree, but there was a

FUNCTION			
DOPAMINE			
Preop	Postop	Significant Difference?	Comment
1.17	2.02	NS	Control = placebo
	29%	NS	
	27.5%	NS	
	16.3%	NS	
	−0.29	$P < 0.05$	Control = dopamine 2 μg/kg/min
	16%	$P < 0.05$	
1.93	1.54		

45% increase in the GFR in the norepinephrine group, which was not seen with the other agents. Di Giantomasso and colleagues[131,132] showed in sheep treated with *E. coli* that norepinephrine was able to significantly increase creatinine clearance and urine flow 2 hours after the onset of sepsis.

Human Studies

There is a paucity of good studies assessing the benefit of norepinephrine in patients with septic shock. One concern with the use of norepinephrine is that it may worsen perfusion to some tissues due to its vasoconstrictive effect. However, these concerns have not been supported by most studies: Martin and colleagues[122] compared norepinephrine and dopamine in septic shock and were able to show a significant reduction from baseline of serum lactate concentration with norepinephrine, suggesting improvement rather than worsening of tissue ischemia and that reduction of lactate correlates closely with survival in acute sepsis. Splanchnic blood flow is also improved or maintained in septic shock with norepinephrine.[133]

Bourgoin and colleagues[119] showed that in 28 patients randomized to receive norepinephrine to maintain an MAP of 65 or 85 mm Hg, there was improvement from baseline of both creatinine clearance and urine flow rate. There was no difference between the two groups, however. Desjars and colleagues[134] measured creatinine clearance and urine flow rates in septic patients before and 24 hours after starting norepinephrine. They showed an increase in both variables in all patients. Marin and colleagues[126] looked at 25 patients with septic shock who were treated with norepinephrine and showed improvements in urine flow, creatinine, and creatinine clearance in 20 patients. Redl-Wenzel and colleagues[135] looked at 56 patients who remained hypotensive despite dopamine and dobutamine. They were then started on norepinephrine with a target blood pressure of 60 mm Hg. There was a significant improvement in creatinine clearance at 48 hours from 73 mL/min to 102 mL/min. Albanese and colleagues[136] performed a prospective, randomized, controlled trial in septic patients comparing norepinephrine and terlipressin. The renal parameters assessed were urine flow and creatinine clearance. Twenty patients were enrolled in this open-label study. There was no statistical difference between the two groups in both parameters; however, both groups did improve significantly from baseline.

Albanese and colleagues[137] also looked at two groups of ICU patients receiving norepinephrine. There were 14 patients with septic shock and 12 patients with head injuries. In the septic patients, there was an increase in urine flow rate from 14 mL/hr to 102 mL/hr. There was also a statistically significant increase in creatinine clearance. This is in contrast to those patients with head injuries who had no change in urine flow rate or creatinine clearance.

On the grounds of the above information, norepinephrine may well confer benefit in ARF in patients with distributive shock and can be recommended for this purpose. The recommended dose is 0.1 to 2 μg/kg/min.

Epinephrine

Epinephrine has both α- and β-adrenergic properties, with the former becoming more predominant at higher doses. It is able to increase the systemic arterial pressure by both increasing systemic vascular resistance and increasing cardiac output. This would appear at the outset to be the optimal way to treat patients with septic shock as they have both severe vasoplegia and myocardial dysfunction. Although it has been shown to improve blood pressure in a number of trials,[138–141] the major concern with its use has been that at clinically

Table 2-5 Effects of Norepinephrine Infusion on Renal Hemodynamics and Renal Function in Experimental Models of Sepsis

Study	Study Type	Animal Model	Norepinephrine Infusion Rate
Anderson et al[128]	Controlled trial of intravenous and renal-arterial norepinephrine infusion in nonseptic animals	Dog	0.1–0.4 μg/kg/min
Di Giantomasso et al[130]	Randomized, placebo-controlled animal trial using norepinpehrine in experimental sepsis	Merino sheep	0.4 μg/kg/min
Peng et al[129]	Controlled trial of increasing doses of norepinephrine in experimental bacteremia	Dog	0.1–0.5 μg/kg/min
Bellomo et al[112]	Controlled trial comparing response to norepinephrine before and after the induction of sepsis	Dog	0.3 μg/kg/min
Di Giantomasso et al[131]	Randomized, placebo-controlled trial comparing renal response to norepinephrine and low-dose dopamine in experimental sepsis	Merino sheep	0.4 μg/kg/min
Boffa and Arendshorst[110]	Placebo-controlled trial of norepinephrine versus placebo, then norepinephrine versus nitric oxide synthase inhibition or angiotensin II	Balb C mice	6 μg/kg/min
Di Giantomasso et al[113]	Controlled trial assessing the effect of norepinephrine versus placebo on regional renal blood flow in sepsis	Merino sheep	0.4 μg/kg/min

*$P < .01$.
†$P < .05$.
‡$P = .018$.
N/T, not tested.

relevant doses, it impairs splanchnic perfusion and increases systemic lactate.[138–140,142–144] The hyperlactatemia may not necessarily be due to tissue ischemia because in studies that looked over a longer period, the lactate increased transiently and then decreased progressively in survivors.[138]

There is a paucity of experimental and clinical trials looking specifically at the use of epinephrine in renal failure. Di Giantomasso and colleagues,[139] using their septic sheep model, looked at renal hemodynamics with the use of epinephrine. It reduced RBF and increased renal vascular resistance in a manner similar to that seen previously with the use of norepinephrine. In contrast to norepinephrine, creatinine clearance actually decreased slightly. Krejci and colleagues[142] showed an increase in RBF associated with epinephrine infusion that was greater than that seen with norepinephrine; however, there was no measurement of urine output or other renal function variables. Day and colleagues[140] performed an elaborate study using thermodilution catheters placed in the renal veins vof patients with severe sepsis or malaria to measure RBF, lactate concentrations, and renal vascular resistance indices. Patients then received either dopamine or epinephrine in a crossover manner. The trial was stopped early due to significant hyperlactatemia in the epinephrine group. Epinephrine did, however, result in an increase in renal vascular resistance and renal oxygen extraction ratios. There are, however, several limitations to the study. Only eight patients received epinephrine and only four received the full dose. There were a number of patients with malaria, which may respond differently due to different pathologic mechanisms in the kidney. These few studies are the main clinical trials looking specifically at epinephrine in sepsis-induced renal failure. Based on current evidence, epinephrine cannot be recommended for the initial management of patients with renal failure in the intensive care setting.

Phenylephrine

Phenylephrine is a specific α-adrenoreceptor agonist that is used in some ICUs to treat hypotension associated with septic shock. There is currently very little evidence of its use in patients with renal failure. Krejci and colleagues[142] showed that phenylephrine increases RBF more than norepinephrine in septic pigs and the increase in RBF correlated with the in-

Effect of Norepinephrine on Renal Blood Flow	Effect of Norepinephrine on Renal Vascular Resistance	Effect of Norepinephrine on Urine Output	Effect of Norepinephrine on Glomerular Filtration Rate	Effect of Norepinephrine on Regional Blood Flow
Increased 61%*	Decreased	N/T	Increased linearly up to 20%[†]	N/T
No change	Nonsignificant decrease	117 mL/hr versus 51 mL/hr (placebo)[†]	83 mL/min versus 41 mL/min (placebo)[†]	N/T
Increased in bacteremia at doses ≥ 0.3 μg/kg/min but decreased in normal animals	N/T	N/T	N/T	N/T
Increase not significant	No significant difference from control	N/T	N/T	N/T
Increased 29%[‡]	Decreased 8%[‡]	228 mL/hr versus 49 mL/hr (placebo)	N/T	N/T
No change	No change	44% increase*	45% increase*	N/T
N/T	N/T	57% increase*	N/T	54% increase in medullary blood flow[†]; 34% increase in cortical blood flow (not significant)

crease in systemic pressure. It was postulated that, because phenylephrine constricts larger arterioles and not terminal ones, there may be better microvascular perfusion compared with norepinephrine. There was, however, no difference in splanchnic metabolic variables between the two agents. In the only study in humans to assess the effect of phenylephrine in septic shock, Gregory and colleagues[145] looked retrospectively at 13 patients and assessed response. Phenylephrine resulted in a marked increase in the MAP, systemic vascular resistance, and cardiac index. There was a significant increase in urine flow, but no change in creatinine.

Vasopressin

Vasopressin is a potent vasoconstrictive agent released by the posterior pituitary in response to baroreceptor stimulation caused by hypotension.[146] In septic shock, it has been shown that in the first 24 hours there is a significant (as much as 10-fold) increase in plasma levels; however, these then rapidly decrease to baseline levels. Exogenous administration of low-dose vasopressin in patients with septic

shock improves blood pressure significantly, and this effect is further augmented by catecholamines. Vasopressin 1 (V_1) receptors are present on vascular smooth muscle cells and through phospholipase C are able to increase intracellular calcium and sensitize the contractile apparatus to the calcium, thereby causing contraction. It therefore is able to overcome the mechanisms through which catecholamine resistance occurs.[146–148]

The effects of vasopressin on the kidney in septic shock is becoming better understood. Vasopressin is able to elevate the MAP and therefore will increase renal perfusion pressure.[149–154] Vasopressin may result in selective efferent arteriolar vasoconstriction. This was first suggested in 1956 by Wagener and Braunwald,[155] who looked at three patients with autonomic failure and showed that vasopressin caused a decrease in renal plasma flow using para-aminohippurate clearance; however, GFR remained constant (inulin clearance) suggesting that there was selective efferent arteriolar vasoconstriction. Using an in vitro model, Edwards and colleagues[156] showed that selective efferent arteriolar constriction was reversed by a V_1 receptor antagonist.

Animal Studies

Albert and colleagues[157] showed that vasopressin selectively enhanced renal cortical blood flow in endotoxin-treated animals. In rodents, Levy and colleagues[158] showed that vasopressin did not change RBF in endotoxin-treated animals, but it did significantly increase urine output and inulin-measured GFR. In contrast to these findings, two studies by Malay and colleagues[153] and Lefaivre and colleagues[159] showed there was a decrease in RBF in endotoxemic pigs and rabbits, respectively.

Human Studies

Landry and colleagues[160] described the response to vasopressin in five patients with refractory shock unresponsive to standard vasopressors. In all the patients, there was a significant increase in the MAP. In three of the five patients, there was a marked increase in urine output. Another study randomized 48 patients with septic shock to receive either vasopressin (4 U/hr) with norepinephrine or norepinephrine alone. In the group randomized to vasopressin with norepinephrine, there were a significantly higher MAP and cardiac index. There was improved gastric pH in the vasopressin group, but also increased bilirubin and reduced platelets. Urine output was not reported; however, there was no change in creatinine after 48 hours.[150] Tsuneyoshi and colleagues[151] also reported a prospective, case-controlled study on patients with septic shock treated with norepinephrine. Vasopressin was added to norepinephrine at a rate of 0.04 U/min in 16 patients. There was a significant improvement in blood pressure and a decrease in norepinephrine requirements. Urine output had significantly increased by 16 hours in the 10 patients who were oliguric but not anuric. Those patients who were anuric did not improve; however, this could be expected if ATN has already occurred.

Retrospective studies in larger numbers of patients have also been reported. These studies show that vasopressin decreases norepinephrine requirements[161] and increases urine output.[152] Albanese and colleagues[136] performed a randomized, open-label study of terlipressin (a synthetic vasopressin analogue) compared with norepinephrine. Twenty patients with septic shock and two with organ failure were randomized to receive either norepinephrine in incremental doses or terlipressin in a 1-mg bolus every 6 hours (equivalent to 0.03–0.04 U/min vasopressin). All patients achieved the target MAP of 60 to 70 mm Hg. Measurements at 6 hours showed significant reduction in lactate in both groups. Urine output and creatinine clearance significantly increased in both groups, and there was no difference between the two agents. Another randomized, controlled trial by Patel and colleagues[154] looked at 24 patients with septic shock and randomized them to a blinded infusion of either norepinephrine or vasopressin. All patients were on high-dose norepinephrine at the start of the study. The observation time was only 4 hours. During this time, there was no difference in blood pressure or cardiac index. Those patients in the norepinephrine group showed no change in urine output (25 to 15 mL/min) or creatinine clearance. In the vasopressin group, there was an increase in urine output from 32.5 to 65 mL/hr and a 75% increase in creatinine clearance. There was no difference in indirect markers of splanchnic blood flow, nor were there electrocardiographic changes consistent with ischemia. This study is of great interest; however, it has the obvious limitation of being conducted over only a very short period of time.

Vasopressin and its analogue terlipressin appear to have a beneficial effect on renal function and are effective at increasing blood pressure in septic shock. The VASST study, a multicenter double-blind randomized controlled trial, randomized patients with septic shock to receive either vasopressin ($N = 397$) or norepinephrine ($N = 382$) in addition to open-label vasopressors. There was no difference in 28- or 90-day mortality between the two groups, but there was significantly reduced mortality in the vasopressin group, with less severe septic shock.[162] A planned post-hoc analysis presented in abstract form looked at patients stratified by the RIFLE criteria for acute kidney injury.[163] The risk group treated with vasopressin had a significantly lower incidence of renal failure compared to the norepinephrine group (21.2% vs. 41.2%, $P = .02$), and this was associated with reduced mortality. There was no difference in renal outcomes between the injury and failure groups. When all patients in the study were included, there was a trend toward lower creatinine and increased urine output in the vasopressin group (personal correspondence). It is therefore recommended that vasopressin be added to norepinephrine in oliguric sepsis. The recommended dose of vasopressin is 0.01 to 0.04 U/min, and terlipressin is 1 to 2 mg every 6 hours. This should be titrated against blood pressure and not serum vasopressin levels.[146,148]

There have been a number of concerns raised about the use of vasopressin. First is a hepatotoxic effect due to reduced hepatic blood flow and manifest by increased liver transaminases and bilirubin.[150,164] Second is a detrimental effect on coronary blood flow highlighted by animal studies. In clinical studies, vasopressin use has not caused ischemic electrocardiographic changes or increased troponin I levels.[150] Third is a procoagulant side effect due to the presence of V_1 receptors on platelets resulting in platelet aggregation. This is of specific concern in patients who already have poor microvascular blood flow. Patients often become thrombocytopenic when treated with vasopressin.[150]

SUMMARY

In shock states, fluid resuscitation is of prime importance. When fluid resuscitation does not adequately improve blood pressure and distributive shock has been confirmed, vasopressors should be used. In patients with ARF, current evidence suggests the use of norepinephrine at a dose of 0.01 to 2.0 µg/kg/min in the first instance. This has been shown in both animal and human trials of sepsis to improve RBF and function. The aim is to increase the MAP to more than 60 mm Hg and potentially higher if there is significant underlying premorbid hypertension. Aiming for higher targets may in fact be detrimental due to vasoconstriction of both renal and splanchnic vascular beds, and therefore one must target the lowest MAP that achieves the endpoint of regional perfusion and improvement in renal function. The addition of vasopressin to norepinephrine is recommended in oliguric sepsis. High-dose dopamine, phenylephrine, and epinephrine are able to improve blood pressure in sepsis and do not appear to cause harm to renal function, but, due to a lack of evidence, their use cannot be recommended as first-line therapy to treat ARF associated with sepsis.

References

1. Barger G, Dale HH: Chemical structure and sympathomimetic action of amines. J Physiol 1910;41:19–59.
2. McNay JL, McDonald RH Jr, Goldberg LI: Direct renal vasodilatation produced by dopamine in the dog. Circ Res 1965;16: 510–517.
3. McDonald RH Jr, Goldberg LI, McNay JL, Tuttle EP Jr: Effect of dopamine in man: Augmentation of sodium excretion, glomerular filtration rate, and renal plasma flow. J Clin Invest 1964;43: 1116–1124.
4. Goldberg LI: Cardiovascular and renal actions of dopamine: Potential clinical applications. Pharmacol Rev 1972;24:1–29.
5. Tumlin JA, Dunbar LM, Oparil S, et al: Fenoldopam, a dopamine agonist, for hypertensive emergency: A multicenter randomized trial. Fenoldopam Study Group. Acad Emerg Med 2000;7:653–662.
6. Mathur VS, Swan SK, Lambrecht LJ, et al: The effects of fenoldopam, a selective dopamine receptor agonist, on systemic and renal hemodynamics in normotensive subjects. Crit Care Med 1999;27:1832–1837.
7. Lee MR: Dopamine and the kidney: Ten years on. Clin Sci (Lond) 1993;84:357–375.
8. Aperia AC: Intrarenal dopamine: A key signal in the interactive regulation of sodium metabolism. Annu Rev Physiol 2000;62: 621–647.
9. Hansell P, Fasching A: The effect of dopamine receptor blockade on natriuresis is dependent on the degree of hypervolemia. Kidney Int 1991;39:253–258.
10. Bryan AG, Bolsin SN, Vianna PT, Haloush H: Modification of the diuretic and natriuretic effects of a dopamine infusion by fluid loading in preoperative cardiac surgical patients. J Cardiothorac Vasc Anesth 1995;9:158–163.
11. Carey RM, Siragy HM, Felder RA: Physiological modulation of renal function by the renal dopaminergic system. J Auton Pharmacol 1990;10(Suppl 1):s47–s51.
12. Ferreira A, Bettencourt P, Pestana M, et al: Heart failure, aging, and renal synthesis of dopamine. Am J Kidney Dis 2001;38:502–509.
13. Pestana M, Jardim H, Correia F, et al: Renal dopaminergic mechanisms in renal parenchymal diseases and hypertension. Nephrol Dial Transplant 2001;16(Suppl 1):53–59.
14. D'Orio V, el Allaf D, Juchmes J, Marcelle R: The use of low doses of dopamine in intensive care medicine. Arch Int Physiol Biochim 1984;92:S11–S20.
15. Juste RN, Moran L, Hooper J, Soni N: Dopamine clearance in critically ill patients. Intensive Care Med 1998;24:1217–1220.
16. MacGregor DA, Butterworth JF, Zaloga CP, et al: Hemodynamic and renal effects of dopexamine and dobutamine in patients with reduced cardiac output following coronary artery bypass grafting. Chest 1994;106:835–841.
17. Duke GJ, Briedis JH, Weaver RA: Renal support in critically ill patients: Low-dose dopamine or low-dose dobutamine? Crit Care Med 1994;22:1919–1925.
18. Goldberg LI: Dopamine—clinical uses of an endogenous catecholamine. N Engl J Med 1974;291:707–710.
19. Olsen NV: Effects of dopamine on renal haemodynamics tubular function and sodium excretion in normal humans. Dan Med Bull 1998;45:282–297.
20. Hughes JM, Beck TR, Rose CE Jr, Carey RM: The effect of selective dopamine-1 receptor stimulation on renal and adrenal function in man. J Clin Endocrinol Metab 1988;66:518–525.
21. Yura T, Yuasa S, Fukunaga M, et al: Role for Doppler ultrasound in the assessment of renal circulation: Effects of dopamine and dobutamine on renal hemodynamics in humans. Nephron 1995;71:168–175.
22. Bughi S, Jost-Vu E, Antonipillai I, et al: Effect of dopamine2 blockade on renal function under varied sodium intake. J Clin Endocrinol Metab 1994;78:1079–1084.
23. Olsen NV, Lang-Jensen T, Hansen JM, et al: Effects of acute beta-adrenoceptor blockade with metoprolol on the renal response to dopamine in normal humans. Br J Clin Pharmacol 1994;37:347–353.
24. Hoogenberg K, Smit AJ, Girbes AR: Effects of low-dose dopamine on renal and systemic hemodynamics during incremental norepinephrine infusion in healthy volunteers. Crit Care Med 1998;26: 260–265.
25. Richer M, Robert S, Lebel M: Renal hemodynamics during norepinephrine and low-dose dopamine infusions in man. Crit Care Med 1996;24:1150–1156.
26. Hubbard PC, Henderson IW: Renal dopamine and the tubular handling of sodium. J Mol Endocrinol 1995;14:139–155.
27. Day NP, Phu NH, Mai NT, et al: Effects of dopamine and epinephrine infusions on renal hemodynamics in severe malaria and severe sepsis. Crit Care Med 2000;28:1353–1362.
28. Seri I, Aperia A: Contribution of dopamine 2 receptors to dopamine-induced increase in glomerular filtration rate. Am J Physiol 1988;254:F196–F201.
29. Agnoli GC, Cacciari M, Garutti C, et al: Effects of extracellular fluid volume changes on renal response to low-dose dopamine infusion in normal women. Clin Physiol 1987;7:465–479.
30. Orme ML, Breckenridge A, Dollery CT: The effects of long term administration of dopamine on renal function in hypertensive patients. Eur J Clin Pharmacol 1973;6:150–155.
31. Seri I, Rudas G, Bors Z, et al: Effects of low-dose dopamine infusion on cardiovascular and renal functions, cerebral blood flow, and plasma catecholamine levels in sick preterm neonates. Pediatr Res 1993;34:742–749.
32. Prins I, Plotz FB, Uiterwaal CS, van Vught HJ: Low-dose dopamine in neonatal and pediatric intensive care: A systematic review. Intensive Care Med 2001;27:206–210.
33. Mulkerrin E, Epstein FH, Clark BA: Reduced renal response to low-dose dopamine infusion in the elderly. J Gerontol A Biol Sci Med Sci 1995;50:M271–M275.
34. Fuiano G, Sund S, Mazza G, et al: Renal hemodynamic response to maximal vasodilating stimulus in healthy older subjects. Kidney Int 2001;59:1052–1058.
35. Marinac JS, Willsie SK, Dew M, et al: Pharmacodynamic effects of dopamine stratified by race. Am J Ther 2001;8:27–34.
36. Ichai C, Passeron C, Carles M, et al: Prolonged low-dose dopamine infusion induces a transient improvement in renal function in hemodynamically stable, critically ill patients: A single-blind, prospective, controlled study. Crit Care Med 2000;28:1329–1335.
37. Braun GG, Bahlmann F, Brandl M, Knoll R: Long term administration of dopamine: Is there a development of tolerance? Prog Clin Biol Res 1989;308:1097–1099.
38. MacDonald TM: Metoclopramide, domperidone and dopamine in man: Actions and interactions. Eur J Clin Pharmacol 1991; 40:225–230.
39. Munn J, Tooley M, Bolsin S, et al: Effect of metoclopramide on renal vascular resistance index and renal function in patients receiving a low-dose infusion of dopamine. Br J Anaesth 1993;71:379–382.
40. Girbes AR, Lieverse AG, Smit AJ, et al: Lack of specific renal haemodynamic effects of different doses of dopamine after infrarenal aortic surgery. Br J Anaesth 1996;77:753–757.
41. Smit AJ, Meijer S, Wesseling H, et al: Effect of metoclopramide on dopamine-induced changes in renal function in healthy controls and in patients with renal disease. Clin Sci (Lond) 1988;75:421–428.
42. Olsen NV, Hansen JM, Kanstrup IL, et al: Renal hemodynamics, tubular function, and response to low-dose dopamine during acute hypoxia in humans. J Appl Physiol 1993;74:2166–2173.
43. ter Wee PM, Rosman JB, van der Geest S, et al: Renal hemodynamics during separate and combined infusion of amino acids and dopamine. Kidney Int 1986;29:870–874.

44. Lherm T, Troche G, Rossignol M, et al: Renal effects of low-dose dopamine in patients with sepsis syndrome or septic shock treated with catecholamines. Intensive Care Med 1996;22:213–219.

45. Bughi S, Horton R, Antonipillai I, et al: Comparison of dopamine and fenoldopam effects on RBF and prostacyclin excretion in normal and essential hypertensive subjects. J Clin Endocrinol Metab 1989;69:1116–1121.

46. Parker S, Carlon GC, Isaacs M, et al: Dopamine administration in oliguria and oliguric renal failure. Crit Care Med 1981;9: 630–632.

47. de Lasson L, Hansen HE, Juhl B, et al: A randomised, clinical study of the effect of low-dose dopamine on central and renal haemodynamics in infrarenal aortic surgery. Eur J Vasc Endovasc Surg 1995;10:82–90.

48. Lauschke A, Teichgraber UK, Frei U, Eckardt KU: 'Low-dose' dopamine worsens renal perfusion in patients with acute renal failure. Kidney Int 2006;69:1669–1674.

49. Marik PE: Low-dose dopamine in critically ill oliguric patients: The influence of the renin-angiotensin system. Heart Lung 1993;22:171–175.

50. Pavoni V, Verri M, Ferraro L, et al: Plasma dopamine concentration and effects of low dopamine doses on urinary output after major vascular surgery. Kidney Int Suppl 1998;66: S75–S80.

51. Lassnigg A, Donner E, Grubhofer G, et al: Lack of renoprotective effects of dopamine and furosemide during cardiac surgery. J Am Soc Nephrol 2000;11:97–104.

52. Myles PS, Buckland MR, Schenk NJ, et al: Effect of "renal-dose" dopamine on renal function following cardiac surgery. Anaesth Intensive Care 1993;21:56–61.

53. Tang AT, El-Gamel A, Keevil B, et al: The effect of 'renal-dose' dopamine on renal tubular function following cardiac surgery: Assessed by measuring retinol binding protein (RBP). Eur J Cardiothorac Surg 1999;15:717–722.

54. Sumeray M, Robertson C, Lapsley M, et al: Low dose dopamine infusion reduces renal tubular injury following cardiopulmonary bypass surgery. J Nephrol 2001;14:397–402.

55. Yavuz S, Ayabakan N, Dilek K, Ozdemir A: Renal dose dopamine in open heart surgery: Does it protect renal tubular function? J Cardiovasc Surg (Torino) 2002;43:25–30.

56. Baldwin L, Henderson A, Hickman P: Effect of postoperative low-dose dopamine on renal function after elective major vascular surgery. Ann Intern Med 1994;120:744–747.

57. Paul MD, Mazer CD, Byrick RJ, et al: Influence of mannitol and dopamine on renal function during elective infrarenal aortic clamping in man. Am J Nephrol 1986;6:427–434.

58. Yavuz S, Ayabakan N, Goncu MT, Ozdemir IA: Effect of combined dopamine and diltiazem on renal function after cardiac surgery. Med Sci Monit 2002;8:PI45–PI50.

59. Jones D, Bellomo R: Renal-dose dopamine: From hypothesis to paradigm to dogma to myth and, finally, superstition? J Intensive Care Med 2005;20:199–211.

60. Swygert TH, Roberts LC, Valek TR, et al: Effect of intraoperative low-dose dopamine on renal function in liver transplant recipients. Anesthesiology 1991;75:571–576.

61. Wahbah AM, el-Hefny MO, Wafa EM, et al: Perioperative renal protection in patients with obstructive jaundice using drug combinations. Hepatogastroenterology 2000;47:1691–1694.

62. Parks RW, Diamond T, McCrory DC, et al: Prospective study of postoperative renal function in obstructive jaundice and the effect of perioperative dopamine. Br J Surg 1994;81:437–439.

63. Grundmann R, Kindler J, Meider G, et al: Dopamine treatment of human cadaver kidney graft recipients: A prospectively randomized trial. Klin Wochenschr 1982;60:193–197.

64. Carmellini M, Romagnoli J, Giulianotti PC, et al: Dopamine lowers the incidence of delayed graft function in transplanted kidney patients treated with cyclosporine A. Transplant Proc 1994;26:2626–2629.

65. Kadieva VS, Friedman L, Margolius LP, et al: The effect of dopamine on graft function in patients undergoing renal transplantation. Anesth Analg 1993;76:362–365.

66. Sandberg J, Tyden G, Groth CG: Low-dose dopamine infusion following cadaveric renal transplantation: No effect on the incidence of ATN. Transplant Proc 1992;24:357.

67. Gare M, Haviv YS, Ben-Yehuda A, et al: The renal effect of low-dose dopamine in high-risk patients undergoing coronary angiography. J Am Coll Cardiol 1999;34:1682–1688.

68. Hans SS, Hans BA, Dhillon R, et al: Effect of dopamine on renal function after arteriography in patients with pre-existing renal insufficiency. Am Surg 1998;64:432–436.

69. Kapoor A, Sinha N, Sharma RK, et al: Use of dopamine in prevention of contrast induced acute renal failure—a randomised study. Int J Cardiol 1996;53:233–236.

70. Stevens MA, McCullough PA, Tobin KJ, et al: A prospective randomized trial of prevention measures in patients at high risk for contrast nephropathy: Results of the P.R.I.N.C.E. Study. Prevention of Radiocontrast Induced Nephropathy Clinical Evaluation. J Am Coll Cardiol 1999;33:403–411.

71. Weisberg LS, Kurnik PB, Kurnik BR: Risk of radiocontrast nephropathy in patients with and without diabetes mellitus. Kidney Int 1994;45:259–265.

72. Abizaid AS, Clark CE, Mintz GS, et al: Effects of dopamine and aminophylline on contrast-induced acute renal failure after coronary angioplasty in patients with preexisting renal insufficiency. Am J Cardiol 1999;83:260–263.

73. Lumlertgul D, Keoplung M, Sitprija V, et al: Furosemide and dopamine in malarial acute renal failure. Nephron 1989;52:40–44.

74. Denton MD, Chertow GM, Brady HR: "Renal-dose" dopamine for the treatment of acute renal failure: Scientific rationale, experimental studies and clinical trials. Kidney Int 1996;50:4–14.

75. Cottee DB, Saul WP: Is renal dose dopamine protective or therapeutic? No. Crit Care Clin 1996;12:687–695.

76. Burton CJ, Tomson CR. Can the use of low-dose dopamine for treatment of acute renal failure be justified? Postgrad Med J 1999;75:269–274.

77. Friedrich JO, Adhikari N, Herridge MS, Beyene J: Meta-analysis: Low-dose dopamine increases urine output but does not prevent renal dysfunction or death. Ann Intern Med 2005;142: 510–524.

78. Bellomo R, Chapman M, Finfer S, et al: Low-dose dopamine in patients with early renal dysfunction: A placebo-controlled randomised trial. Australian and New Zealand Intensive Care Society (ANZICS) Clinical Trials Group. Lancet 2000;356: 2139–2143.

79. Kellum JA, Decker JM: Use of dopamine in acute renal failure: A meta-analysis. Crit Care Med 2001;29:1526–1531.

80. Chertow GM, Sayegh MH, Allgren RL, Lazarus JM: Is the administration of dopamine associated with adverse or favorable outcomes in acute renal failure? Auriculin Anaritide Acute Renal Failure Study Group. Am J Med 1996;101:49–53.

81. Marik PE: Low-dose dopamine: A systematic review. Intensive care Med 2002;28:877–883.

82. Duke GJ, Bersten AD: Dopamine and renal salvage in the critically ill patient. Anaesth Intensive Care 1992;20:277–287.

83. Chiolero R, Borgeat A, Fisher A: Postoperative arrhythmias and risk factors after open heart surgery. Thorac Cardiovasc Surg 1991;39:81–84.

84. Argalious M, Motta P, Khandwala F, et al: "Renal dose" dopamine is associated with the risk of new-onset atrial fibrillation after cardiac surgery. Crit Care Med 2005;33:1327–1332.

85. Van De Borne P, Somers VK: Dopamine and congestive heart failure: Pharmacology, clinical use, and precautions. Congest Heart Fail 1999;5:216–221.

86. Van den Berghe G, de Zegher F: Anterior pituitary function during critical illness and dopamine treatment. Crit Care Med 1996;24:1580–1590.

87. Devins SS, Miller A, Herndon BL, et al: Effects of dopamine on T-lymphocyte proliferative responses and serum prolactin concentrations in critically ill patients. Crit Care Med 1992;20: 1644–1649.

88. Giraud GD, MacCannell KL: Decreased nutrient blood flow during dopamine- and epinephrine-induced intestinal vasodilation. J Pharmacol Exp Ther 1984;230:214–220.

89. Marik PE, Mohedin M: The contrasting effects of dopamine and norepinephrine on systemic and splanchnic oxygen utilization in hyperdynamic sepsis. JAMA 1994;272:1354–1357.

90. Segal JM, Phang PT, Walley KR: Low-dose dopamine hastens onset of gut ischemia in a porcine model of hemorrhagic shock. J Appl Physiol 1992;73:1159–1164.

91. Singer I, Epstein M: Potential of dopamine A-1 agonists in the management of acute renal failure. Am J Kidney Dis 1998;31: 743–755.

92. Siragy HM, Felder RA, Peach MJ, Carey RM: Intrarenal DA2 dopamine receptor stimulation in the conscious dog. Am J Physiol 1992;262:F932–F938.

93. Kien ND, Moore PG, Jaffe RS: Cardiovascular function during induced hypotension by fenoldopam or sodium nitroprusside in anesthetized dogs. Anesth Analg 1992;74:72–78.

94. Shusterman NH, Elliott WJ, White WB: Fenoldopam, but not nitroprusside, improves renal function in severely hypertensive patients with impaired renal function. Am J Med 1993;95:161–168.

95. Landoni G, Biondi-Zoccai GG, Tumlin JA, et al: Beneficial impact of fenoldopam in critically ill patients with or at risk for acute renal failure: A meta-analysis of randomized clinical trials. Am J Kidney Dis 2007;49:56–68.

96. Oliver WC Jr, Nuttall GA, Cherry KJ, et al: A comparison of fenoldopam with dopamine and sodium nitroprusside in patients undergoing cross-clamping of the abdominal aorta. Anesth Analg 2006;103:833–840.

97. Halpenny M, Rushe C, Breen P, et al: The effects of fenoldopam on renal function in patients undergoing elective aortic surgery. Eur J Anaesthesiol 2002;19:92–99.

98. Bove T, Landoni G, Calabro MG, et al: Renoprotective action of fenoldopam in high-risk patients undergoing cardiac surgery: A prospective, double-blind, randomized clinical trial. Circulation 2005;111:3230–3235.

99. Caimmi PP, Pagani L, Micalizzi E, et al: Fenoldopam for renal protection in patients undergoing cardiopulmonary bypass. J Cardiothorac Vasc Anesth 2003;17:491–494.

100. Halpenny M, Lakshmi S, O'Donnell A, et al: Fenoldopam: Renal and splanchnic effects in patients undergoing coronary artery bypass grafting. Anaesthesia 2001;56:953–960.

101. Della Rocca G, Pompei L, Costa MG, et al: Fenoldopam mesylate and renal function in patients undergoing liver transplantation: A randomized, controlled pilot trial. Anesth Analg 2004;99:1604–1609.

102. Biancofiore G, Della Rocca G, Bindi L, et al: Use of fenoldopam to control renal dysfunction early after liver transplantation. Liver Transpl 2004;10:986–992.

103. Tumlin JA, Wang A, Murray PT, Mathur VS: Fenoldopam mesylate blocks reductions in renal plasma flow after radiocontrast dye infusion: A pilot trial in the prevention of contrast nephropathy. Am Heart J 2002;143:894–903.

104. Ng TM, Shurmur SW, Silver M, et al: Comparison of N-acetylcysteine and fenoldopam for preventing contrast-induced nephropathy (CAFCIN). Int J Cardiol 2006;109:322–328.

105. Stone GW, McCullough PA, Tumlin JA, et al: Fenoldopam mesylate for the prevention of contrast-induced nephropathy: A randomized controlled trial. JAMA 2003;290:2284–2291.

106. Briguori C, Marenzi G: Contrast-induced nephropathy: Pharmacological prophylaxis. Kidney Int Suppl 2006:S30–S38.

107. Morelli A, Ricci Z, Bellomo R, et al: Prophylactic fenoldopam for renal protection in sepsis: A randomized, double-blind, placebo-controlled pilot trial. Crit Care Med 2005;33:2451–2456.

108. Tumlin JA, Finkel KW, Murray PT, et al: Fenoldopam mesylate in early acute tubular necrosis: A randomized, double-blind, placebo-controlled clinical trial. Am J Kidney Dis 2005;46:26–34.

109. Brienza N, Malcangi V, Dalfino L, et al: A comparison between fenoldopam and low-dose dopamine in early renal dysfunction of critically ill patients. Crit Care Med 2006;34:707–714.

110. Kellum JA: Prophylactic fenoldopam for renal protection? No, thank you, not for me–not yet at least. Crit Care Med 2005;33: 2681–2683.

111. Boffa JJ, Arendshorst WJ: Maintenance of renal vascular reactivity contributes to acute renal failure during endotoxemic shock. J Am Soc Nephrol 2005;16:117–124.

112. Treggiari MM, Romand JA, Burgener D, et al: Effect of increasing norepinephrine dosage on regional blood flow in a porcine model of endotoxin shock. Crit Care Med 2002;30: 1334–1339.

113. Bellomo R, Kellum JA, Wisniewski SR, Pinsky MR: Effects of norepinephrine on the renal vasculature in normal and endotoxemic dogs. Am J Respir Crit Care Med 1999;159:1186–1192.

114. Di Giantomasso D, Morimatsu H, May CN, Bellomo R: IntraRBF distribution in hyperdynamic septic shock: Effect of norepinephrine. Crit Care Med 2003;31:2509–2513.

115. Langenberg C, Bellomo R, May CN, et al: Renal vascular resistance in sepsis. Nephron Physiol 2006;104:1–11.

116. Hayes MA, Timmins AC, Yau EH, et al: Elevation of systemic oxygen delivery in the treatment of critically ill patients. N Engl J Med 1994;330:1717–1722.

117. Rivers E, Nguyen B, Havstad S, et al: Early goal-directed therapy in the treatment of severe sepsis and septic shock. N Engl J Med 2001;345:1368–1377.

118. Dellinger RP, Carlet JM, Masur H, et al: Surviving Sepsis Campaign guidelines for management of severe sepsis and septic shock. Intensive Care Med 2004;30:536–555.

119. Bourgoin A, Leone M, Delmas A, et al: Increasing mean arterial pressure in patients with septic shock: Effects on oxygen variables and renal function. Crit Care Med 2005;33:780–786.

120. Zhou SX, Qiu HB, Huang YZ, et al: Effects of norepinephrine, epinephrine, and norepinephrine-dobutamine on systemic and gastric mucosal oxygenation in septic shock. Acta Pharmacol Sin 2002;23:654–658.

121. De Backer D, Creteur J, Silva E, Vincent JL: Effects of dopamine, norepinephrine, and epinephrine on the splanchnic circulation in septic shock: Which is best? Crit Care Med 2003; 31:1659–1667.

122. Martin C, Papazian L, Perrin G, Saux P, Gouin F. Norepinephrine or dopamine for the treatment of hyperdynamic septic shock? Chest 1993;103:1826–1831.

123. Guerin JP, Levraut J, Samat-Long C, et al. Effects of dopamine and norepinephrine on systemic and hepatosplanchnic hemodynamics, oxygen exchange, and energy balance in vasoplegic septic patients. Shock 2005;23:18–24.

124. Cronin RE, de Torrente A, Miller PD, et al: Pathogenic mechanisms in early norepinephrine-induced acute renal failure: Functional and histological correlates of protection. Kidney Int 1978;14:115–125.

125. Murakawa K, Kobayashi A: Effects of vasopressors on renal tissue gas tensions during hemorrhagic shock in dogs. Crit Care Med 1988;16:789–792.

126. Marin C, Eon B, Saux P, et al: Renal effects of norepinephrine used to treat septic shock patients. Crit Care Med 1990;18: 282–285.

127. Llinas MT, Lopez R, Rodriguez F, et al: Role of COX-2-derived metabolites in regulation of the renal hemodynamic response to norepinephrine. Am J Physiol Renal Physiol 2001;281: F975–F982.

128. Inscho EW, Carmines PK, Navar LG: Prostaglandin influences on afferent arteriolar responses to vasoconstrictor agonists. Am J Physiol 1990;259:F157–F163.

129. Anderson WP, Korner PI, Selig SE: Mechanisms involved in the renal responses to intravenous and renal artery infusions of noradrenaline in conscious dogs. J Physiol 1981;321: 21–30.

130. Peng ZY, Critchley LA, Fok BS: The effects of increasing doses of noradrenaline on systemic and renal circulations in acute bacteraemic dogs. Intensive Care Med 2005;31:1558–1163.

131. Di Giantomasso D, May CN, Bellomo R: Norepinephrine and vital organ blood flow during experimental hyperdynamic sepsis. Intensive Care Med 2003;29:1774–2781.

132. Di Giantomasso D, Morimatsu H, May CN, Bellomo R: Increasing RBF: Low-dose dopamine or medium-dose norepinephrine. Chest 2004;125:2260–2267.

133. Hollenberg SM, Ahrens TS, Annane D, et al: Practice parameters for hemodynamic support of sepsis in adult patients: 2004 update. Crit Care Med 2004;32:1928–1948.

134. Desjars P, Pinaud M, Bugnon D, Tasseau F: Norepinephrine therapy has no deleterious renal effects in human septic shock. Crit Care Med 1989;17:426–429.

135. Redl-Wenzl EM, Armbruster C, Edelmann G, et al: The effects of norepinephrine on hemodynamics and renal function in severe septic shock states. Intensive Care Med 1993;19:151–154.

136. Albanese J, Leone M, Delmas A, Martin C: Terlipressin or norepinephrine in hyperdynamic septic shock: A prospective, randomized study. Crit Care Med 2005;33:1897–1902.

137. Albanese J, Leone M, Garnier F, et al: Renal effects of norepinephrine in septic and nonseptic patients. Chest 2004;126:534–539.

138. Bollaert PE, Bauer P, Audibert G, et al: Effects of epinephrine on hemodynamics and oxygen metabolism in dopamine-resistant septic shock. Chest 1990;98:949–953.

139. Di Giantomasso D, Bellomo R, May CN: The hemodynamic and metabolic effects of epinephrine in experimental hyperdynamic septic shock. Intensive Care Med 2005;31:454–462.

140. Day NP, Phu NH, Bethell DP, et al: The effects of dopamine and adrenaline infusions on acid-base balance and systemic haemodynamics in severe infection. Lancet 1996;348:219–223.

141. Smythe CM, Nickel JF, Bradley SE: The effect of epinephrine (USP), l-epinephrine, and l-norepinephrine on glomerular filtration rate, renal plasma flow, and the urinary excretion of sodium, potassium, and water in normal man. J Clin Invest 1952;31:499–506.

142. Krejci V, Hiltebrand LB, Sigurdsson GH: Effects of epinephrine, norepinephrine, and phenylephrine on microcirculatory blood flow in the gastrointestinal tract in sepsis. Crit Care Med 2006;34:1456–1463.

143. Mackenzie SJ, Kapadia F, Nimmo GR, et al: Adrenaline in treatment of septic shock: Effects on hemodynamics and oxygen transport. Intensive Care Med 1991;17:36–39.

144. Seguin P, Bellissant E, Le Tulzo Y, et al: Effects of epinephrine compared with the combination of dobutamine and norepinephrine on gastric perfusion in septic shock. Clin Pharmacol Ther 2002;71:381–388.

145. Gregory JS, Bonfiglio MF, Dasta JF, et al: Experience with phenylephrine as a component of the pharmacologic support of septic shock. Crit Care Med 1991;19:1395–1400.

146. Delmas A, Leone M, Rousseau S, et al: Clinical review: Vasopressin and terlipressin in septic shock patients. Crit Care 2005;9:212–222.

147. Schrier RW, Wang W: Acute renal failure and sepsis. N Engl J Med 2004;351:159–169.

148. Barrett LK, Singer M, Clapp LH: Vasopressin: Mechanisms of action on the vasculature in health and in septic shock. Crit Care Med 2007;35:33–40.

149. Landry DW, Levin HR, Gallant EM, et al: Vasopressin deficiency contributes to the vasodilation of septic shock. Circulation 1997;95:1122–1125.

150. Dunser MW, Mayr AJ, Ulmer H, et al: Arginine vasopressin in advanced vasodilatory shock: A prospective, randomized, controlled study. Circulation 2003;107:2313–2319.

151. Tsuneyoshi I, Yamada H, Kakihana Y, et al: Hemodynamic and metabolic effects of low-dose vasopressin infusions in vasodilatory septic shock. Crit Care Med 2001;29:487–493.

152. Holmes CL, Walley KR, Chittock DR, et al: The effects of vasopressin on hemodynamics and renal function in severe septic shock: A case series. Intensive Care Med 2001;27:1416–1421.

153. Malay MB, Ashton RC Jr, Landry DW, Townsend RN: Low-dose vasopressin in the treatment of vasodilatory septic shock. J Trauma 1999;47:699–705.

154. Patel BM, Chittock DR, Russell JA, Walley KR: Beneficial effects of short-term vasopressin infusion during severe septic shock. Anesthesiology 2002;96:576–582.

155. Braunwald E, Wagner HN Jr: The pressor effect of the antidiuretic principle of the posterior pituitary in orthostatic hypotension. J Clin Invest 1956;35:1412–1418.

156. Edwards RM, Trizna W, Kinter LB: Renal microvascular effects of vasopressin and vasopressin antagonists. Am J Physiol 1989;256:F274–F278.

157. Albert M, Losser MR, Hayon D, et al: Systemic and renal macro- and microcirculatory responses to arginine vasopressin in endotoxic rabbits. Crit Care Med 2004;32:1891–1898.

158. Levy B, Vallee C, Lauzier F, et al: Comparative effects of vasopressin, norepinephrine, and L-canavanine, a selective inhibitor of inducible nitric oxide synthase, in endotoxic shock. Am J Physiol Heart Circ Physiol 2004;287:H209–H215.

159. Faivre V, Kaskos H, Callebert J, et al: Cardiac and renal effects of levosimendan, arginine vasopressin, and norepinephrine in lipopolysaccharide-treated rabbits. Anesthesiology 2005;103: 514–521.

160. Landry DW, Levin HR, Gallant EM, et al: Vasopressin pressor hypersensitivity in vasodilatory septic shock. Crit Care Med 1997;25:1279–1282.

161. Durairaj SK, Haywood LJ: Hemodynamic effects of dopamine in patients with resistant congestive heart failure. Clin Pharmacol Ther 1978;24:175–185.

162. Russell JA, Walley KR, Singer J, et al: Vasopressin versus norepinephrine infusion in patients with septic shock. N Engl J Med 2008;28;358:877–887.

163. Gordon A, Russell J, Holmes Boulton C, et al: The effect of vasopressin on renal function in septic shock. Am J Respir Crit Care Med 2007;175:A596.

164. Dunser MW, Mayr AJ, Ulmer H, et al: The effects of vasopressin on systemic hemodynamics in catecholamine-resistant septic and postcardiotomy shock: A retrospective analysis. Anesth Analg 2001;93:7–13.

Further Reading

Bourgoin A, Leone M, Delmas A, et al: Increasing mean arterial pressure in patients with septic shock: Effects on oxygen variables and renal function. Crit Care Med 2005;33:780–786.

Delmas A, Leone M, Rousseau S, et al: Clinical review: Vasopressin and terlipressin in septic shock patients. Crit Care 2005;9:212–222.

Hollenberg S, Ahrens T, Annane D, et al: Practice parameters for hemodynamic support of sepsis in adult patients: 2004 update. Crit Care Med 2004;32:1928–1948.

Holmes CL, Walley KR: Bad medicine: Low-dose dopamine in the ICU. Chest 2003;123:1266–1275.

Kellum JA: Prophylactic fenoldopam for renal protection? No, thank you, not for me—not yet at least. Crit Care Med 2005;33:2681–2683.

Rivers E, Nguyen B, Havstad S, et al: Early goal-directed therapy in the treatment of severe sepsis and septic shock. N Engl J Med 2001;345:1368–1377.

Venkataraman R, Kellum JA: Prevention of acute renal failure. Chest 2007;131:100–108.

Chapter 3

Diuretics in Acute Kidney Injury

Mitra K. Nadim and Alan S.L. Yu

BACKGROUND

Acute kidney injury (AKI) remains a common problem with a prevalence of 5% in patients admitted to the hospital and 30% to 50% in those admitted to an intensive care unit. Despite significant advances in supportive care, the morbidity and mortality associated with AKI remain high. Multiple pathophysiologic factors contribute to renal injury in AKI, including vasoconstriction, reduced glomerular capillary permeability, tubular obstruction by casts and swollen epithelial cells, and back-leakage of filtrate through an altered epithelium.[1,2] Over the past two decades, a variety of approaches have been explored by investigators to prevent or ameliorate AKI or accelerate the recovery of patients with AKI, of which the use of diuretics remains one of the most frequently used for this purpose. However, outcome data to support the use of diuretics remain sparse. Extensive data from animal studies suggest that diuretics given prophylactically before renal injury, or very early in so-called incipient AKI, may ameliorate the subsequent course of AKI, whereas their administration once AKI is established has generally been ineffective (see Conger[3] for review). However, the data supporting a beneficial role for diuretics in human AKI are inconsistent. Evaluation of the available human studies is further complicated by the heterogeneity of AKI and varies widely in the definition of AKI, the underlying etiology of renal injury, the severity of disease, and the phase of AKI at which the diuretics were administered.

This chapter discusses the clinical data for the use of mannitol, loop diuretics, and natriuretic peptides in patients with AKI. Complications of diuretic therapy are considered, and recommendations are given for the use and dosing of diuretics. With the exception of a few small randomized, controlled trials, most of the data are from retrospective or case-control studies that are confounded by multiple factors. We focus on the recent prospective clinical trials and refer the reader to several excellent reviews[4–8] for a summary of the earlier work.

USE OF DIURETICS IN THE PREVENTION OF ACUTE KIDNEY INJURY

Mannitol

The prophylactic use of mannitol began in the 1960s when it was introduced for use in patients undergoing cardiovascular surgery to maintain intraoperative urine flow.[9] Since then, prophylactic mannitol has also been recommended for patients considered to be at high risk of AKI, such as those undergoing vascular (aortic aneurysm) surgery or cardiac surgery or patients developing obstructive jaundice; yet several small randomized, controlled trials have found no reduction in the incidence of AKI with mannitol administration.[10–13] Over the past few decades, there have been several theoretical arguments favoring the use of mannitol. First, mannitol increases renal blood flow in both the renal cortex and medulla by reducing renal vascular resistance.[14] Second, by increasing urine flow, mannitol could lead to relief of tubular obstruction by casts and cellular debris and to a reduction in the concentration of tubular toxins such as myoglobin or hemoglobin.[15] Finally, mannitol may reduce epithelial cell swelling[16] as well as scavenge harmful free radicals,[17] thereby ameliorating hypoxic reperfusion injury. Although studies in animals have shown that mannitol helps to protect the kidney against ischemic injury, human studies fail to demonstrate the efficacy of mannitol in preventing AKI.[5,18]

There are compelling data that mannitol causes a higher incidence of radiocontrast-induced nephrotoxicity as compared with saline plasma volume expansion alone in either diabetic or nondiabetic patients.[19,20] Solomon and colleagues[19] found that 25 g of mannitol before contrast administration plus plasma volume expansion with saline was not associated with any reduction in risk compared with saline alone; instead, there was a trend toward harm. A forced diuresis regimen that included intravenous crystalloid, mannitol, furosemide, and low-dose dopamine similarly exerted no effect on the overall incidence of contrast-induced nephropathy.[20] The trial design allowed independent evaluation of the effects of mannitol, and the results demonstrated no additive benefit. In patients with both diabetes and chronic kidney disease receiving a radiocontrast agent, mannitol increased the incidence of nephrotoxicity.[21,22]

Forced alkaline diuresis with intravenous fluids and mannitol has been advocated in the setting of rhabdomyolysis to create an osmotic diuresis,[23,24] vasodilation of renal vasculature,[25] and free-radical scavenging.[26,27] However, available evidence suggests that mannitol offers no benefit over and above aggressive fluid resuscitation.[28–30] Furthermore, mannitol can be harmful if urine output cannot be maintained.

Mannitol may have a beneficial role in the prevention of AKI after renal transplantation. In small studies of patients undergoing kidney transplantation, mannitol administration appears to have salutary effects with regard to AKI. In these studies, 250 mL of 20% mannitol given immediately before vessel unclamping reduced the incidence of AKI, as determined by a decreased need for posttransplantation dialysis.[31–38] However, no durable outcome difference at 3 months was found compared with patients who did not receive mannitol.[38] The practice of using mannitol in renal transplantation varies by center, and its potential benefit remains to be confirmed by larger multicenter trials.

Loop Diuretics

Loop diuretics have vasodilatory properties and, like mannitol, increase urine flow and could relieve tubular obstruction and reduce the concentration of tubular toxins.[15] However, it has been postulated that the increased renal blood flow induced by loop diuretics may be maldistributed and potentially harmful.[39,40] Furthermore, by inhibiting active solute transport, loop diuretics reduce the oxygen and adenosine triphosphate requirements of the tubular epithelium, thereby possibly improving tolerance of hypoxia.[41] A systematic review of seven randomized, controlled trials comparing fluids alone with diuretics in patients at risk of AKI from various causes found no evidence of improved survival, decreased incidence of AKI, or need for dialysis associated with diuretics.[42]

Furosemide is widely used to prevent the development of AKI despite a lack of evidence of its efficacy in humans. In a double-blind, randomized, controlled trial ($N = 126$) examining the effectiveness of furosemide and dopamine in preventing AKI in patients with normal renal function after cardiac surgery, Lassnigg and colleagues[43] found that compared with 0.9% saline, furosemide was associated with an increased risk of the development of AKI. As the increased sodium and water excretion in the furosemide group was not fully replaced, these results could potentially be due to relative hypovolemia, although objective indices such as pulmonary capillary wedge pressures were not significantly different between the two groups.

Three prospective controlled studies have evaluated the role of furosemide in preventing AKI induced by radiocontrast material and found no benefit.[39,44,45] In two of the studies, administration of furosemide before radiocontrast resulted in worsening of the decline in renal function that was associated with net loss of body weight,[39,44] again suggesting that it had caused hypovolemia (Table 3-1).

USE OF DIURETICS IN ESTABLISHED ACUTE KIDNEY INJURY

Mannitol

There have been no controlled studies of the use of mannitol in early or established AKI. Although several uncontrolled studies performed before 1970 demonstrate that mannitol can restore urine flow when administered early in the course of

Table 3-1 Summary of Randomized, Controlled Clinical Trials of Diuretics in the Prevention of Acute Kidney Injury

Study	Patients	Control	Intervention	Effect of Intervention on Renal Recovery
Solomon et al[39]	78 patients with chronic kidney disease who underwent cardiac angiography	Saline	Mannitol and saline Furosemide and saline	Worse
Weisberg et al[75]	50 patients undergoing radiocontrast study	Saline	Mannitol and saline	None
Stevens et al[45]	98 patients undergoing radiocontrast study	Saline	Mannitol, furosemide, dopamine, and saline	None
Weinstein et al[44]	18 patients undergoing radiocontrast study	Saline	Furosemide	Worse
Van Valenberg et al[31]	131 patients undergoing cadaveric renal transplantation	Saline	Mannitol and saline	Better
Lassnigg et al[43]	126 patients undergoing elective cardiac surgery	Saline	Furosemide and saline	Worse
Nicholson et al[18]	28 patients undergoing abdominal aortic surgery	Saline	Mannitol	None

oliguric AKI, there is no evidence that it improves outcome in terms of renal function.[46–49]

Loop Diuretics

Several retrospective studies, reviewed by Conger,[5] have found no effect of furosemide on renal function or mortality in patients with AKI of various etiologies. A recent prospective observational study by Mehta and colleagues[50] found that diuretic use was associated with an increased risk of death and failure of renal function to recover in critically ill patients with established AKI. However, the increased risk was mainly in patients who were relatively unresponsive to diuretics. This suggests that the use of diuretics may be a marker of a sicker patient population (i.e., there was residual confounding by unobserved factors) rather than a direct cause of the poor outcome. This conclusion is supported by the recently reported results of an even larger, prospective, multinational, observational cohort study that found no association between the use of diuretics and mortality rate in critically ill patients with AKI.[51] There have now been six randomized, controlled trials of loop diuretics in established AKI[52–57] of which three were placebo-controlled trials,[53,55,56] and in five of these studies,[52–56] the use of loop diuretics failed to have a significant impact on renal function recovery or patient survival (Table 3-2). The recent study by Cantarovich and colleagues[56] is the largest prospective, randomized, double-blind, placebo-controlled study to date and the only one to be performed in the modern era. It was designed to have an 80% power to detect a 15% difference in the primary endpoint, which was 1-month survival. Despite this, they found that furosemide had no effect on patient survival or renal recovery rate.

Natriuretic Peptides

Despite encouraging experimental data with the use of the atrial natriuretic peptide anaritide on ischemic AKI,[58,59] results have been disappointing in humans. In two large, multicenter, prospective, randomized, placebo-controlled trials in patients with AKI due to acute tubular necrosis of various etiologies, atrial natriuretic peptide infusion for 24 hours had no effect on the need for dialysis, the rate of dialysis-free survival, and overall mortality rate.[60,61] In both studies, however, approximately 90% of the patients in the anaritide group became hypotensive (systolic blood pressure < 90 mm Hg), which could have resulted in reduced renal perfusion.[60,61] In a more recent single-center trial of patients ($N = 61$) with heart failure, recombinant atrial natriuretic peptide given for a longer period of time after cardiac surgery decreased the probability of dialysis and improved dialysis-free survival[62] (see Table 3-2).

USE OF DIURETICS IN THE MANAGEMENT OF COMPLICATIONS OF ACUTE KIDNEY INJURY

Although there is no evidence that diuretics are effective at preventing or altering the course of AKI, they are very useful in the management of oliguria and volume overload in this setting.

Table 3-2 Summary of Randomized, Controlled Clinical Trials of Diuretics in the Setting of Established Acute Kidney Injury

Study	Patients	Control	Intervention	Effect of Intervention on Renal Recovery
Brown et al[54]	58 patients with postoperative AKI	Furosemide infusion × 4 hr	Furosemide infusion × 4 hr followed by IV bolus or oral furosemide 1 g tid	None
Shilliday et al[55]	92 patients with AKI of various etiologies	Placebo IV infusion, mannitol, and dopamine	Furosemide or torsemide, mannitol, and dopamine	None
Sirivella et al[57]	100 patients with postoperative oliguric or anuric AKI	Furosemide, bumetanide, or ethacrynic acid intermittent bolus	Furosemide, mannitol, and dopamine continuous infusion	Better
Kleinknecht et al[53]	66 with oliguric AKI	Placebo	Intervention: furosemide bolus every 4 hr	None
Cantarovich et al[56]	330 patients with AKI requiring renal replacement therapy	Placebo	Furosemide infusion or oral given after dialysis	None
Allgren et al[61]	504 patients with oliguric and nonoliguric AKI	Placebo	ANP	None
Lewis et al[60]	222 patients with oliguric AKI	Placebo	ANP	None
Sward et al[62]	61 patients with postoperative AKI	Saline	ANP	Better

AKI, acute kidney injury; ANP, atrial natriuretic peptide.

Several studies have shown that diuretics administered early in the course of oliguric AKI, usually within 24 to 48 hours of onset,[48,49,63] can induce a sustained diuresis in some patients, in some cases even after a single bolus dose. Although individuals who are successfully converted in this manner from oliguric to nonoliguric AKI have a better prognosis than those who are diuretic resistant,[49] this likely reflects the milder severity of their underlying renal injury and not any effect of the diuretic to alter the natural history of the disease. Thus, patients who are diuretic responsive had not only a shorter duration of oliguria, but also higher urine output and better urinary concentrating ability than diuretic-resistant patients.[47,49,64] Successful reversal of oliguria, even in the initial absence of overt hypervolemia, might be expected to reduce the subsequent need for dialysis or ultrafiltration. Indeed this has been shown in some studies,[57] although not in others.[54] Our approach is to administer a single bolus of a diuretic within 24 hours of the onset of oliguria, once established AKI has been confirmed, to attempt to convert to nonoliguric AKI only after careful correction of the volume status and for a very limited time. We favor loop diuretics over mannitol because they appear to be safer and may also be more effective.[63] If there is no diuretic response to a maximally effective dose (see later), further doses should not be given as there is a significant risk of ototoxicity.[53–56] If there is a diuretic response, but it is transient and not sustained, further doses of diuretic, given either as repeated boluses or as a continuous infusion, should be given only if required in a hypervolemic patient to maintain appropriate fluid balance.

PHARMACOLOGY AND DOSE RECOMMENDATIONS

Mannitol may be given in boluses of 12.5 to 25 g or as a continuous infusion of up to 200 g per 24 hours. It is rapidly distributed in the extracellular space, results in the onset of diuresis within 15 to 30 minutes, and has a half-life of 70 to 100 minutes in the setting of normal renal function. In the setting of renal dysfunction, mannitol may accumulate and cause plasma volume expansion as well as itself causing AKI.[65,66] It should therefore be administered with caution, if at all, to anuric patients. Moreover, as with all diuretics, mannitol may induce AKI due to excessive osmotic diuresis in patients with hypovolemia, thereby exacerbating the renal injury.

The effectiveness of loop diuretics in patients with AKI is reduced due to decreased urinary excretion. This may be overcome by administering doses that achieve high enough serum concentrations to provide entry of sufficient amounts of diuretic into the urine. Treatment should be initiated with an intravenous bolus dose. A reasonable starting dose is 40 mg furosemide, 1 mg bumetanide, or 25 mg torsemide. If there is no response within 30 to 60 minutes, the dose should be increased by repeatedly doubling the dose until either diuresis is achieved or the maximum safe dose is reached. We consider a maximum single dose of 160 mg IV furosemide with a maximum total daily dose of 1 g to be safe or 6 to 8 mg IV bumetanide to be safe, and these will produce the upper plateau of the dose-response curve.[67] Higher doses may incur an unacceptable risk of ototoxicity.[54] In a recent meta-analysis, high-dose furosemide (1.0–3.4 g/day) was associated with an increased risk of temporary deafness and tinnitus, which resolved after treatment was stopped.[68]

Some advocate maintaining a continuous infusion of intravenous loop diuretics in order to maintain a safe and constant plasma level. In two of these trials, continuous infusion was more effective at reversing oliguria.[54,57] In the study by Sirivella and colleagues,[57] 90% of the patients receiving intermittent bolus diuretics required dialysis compared with only 6.7% of the patients receiving the continuous infusion of furosemide, dopamine, and saline. However, this study was flawed because there was no true control group. A recent meta-analysis (Cochrane review) comparing continuous infusion versus bolus injection of loop diuretics in patients with congestive heart failure showed greater diuresis and better safety profile when given as a continuous infusion.[69] In a small crossover, randomized study of eight patients with chronic kidney disease (mean creatinine clearance = 17 mL/min), continuous IV infusion of bumetanide was more effective (i.e., greater net sodium excretion) and less toxic when compared with conventional intermittent bolus.[70] Brown and colleagues[54] randomized 58 patients with established acute renal failure to receive either a one-time bolus of furosemide or a bolus followed by a continuous infusion. Although the continuous infusion was more effective at reversing oliguria, there was no difference in the need for dialysis, duration of renal failure, or mortality between the two groups. An infusion of furosemide may be given at 5 to 40 mg/hr after a bolus dose.[71] The half-life of furosemide is intermediate, with bumetanide having a shorter half-life and torsemide having a longer half-life. Therefore, the benefits of continuous infusion may be greater for bumetanide and furosemide than for torsemide.

If the loop diuretic alone is ineffective, a thiazide diuretic may also be added (e.g., 250 or 500 mg IV chlorothiazide, given 30 minutes before a 200-mg IV bolus of furosemide). This combination has been studied in patients with chronic kidney disease,[72] but can also be effective in patients with AKI. Thiazide diuretics alone are ineffective when the glomerular filtration rate is less than 30 mL/min, but may retain benefit when added to a regimen containing a loop diuretic. If no increase in urine output occurs in response to 200 mg furosemide given in combination with a thiazide diuretic, additional doses should not be administered until recovery of renal function is evident.

Several studies have looked into the use of albumin in conjunction with furosemide in hypoalbuminemic patients. In patients with severe hypoalbuminemia, the volume of distribution of furosemide, which in plasma is normally tightly protein bound, is markedly increased; thus, coadministration of furosemide with IV albumin could theoretically improve delivery of furosemide to the tubular lumen and thus improve the natriuretic effect of furosemide. One crossover, randomized, controlled trial (nine patients with nephrotic syndrome with a mean albumin of 2.9 g/dL) compared three interventions: furosemide alone, furosemide plus albumin, and albumin alone.[72] It found that furosemide was superior to albumin alone, and furosemide plus albumin resulted in the greatest urinary sodium and volume excretion. The glomerular filtration rate was not significantly affected by either intervention. The clinical significance of this finding is unclear. In a randomized trial of 1126 cirrhotic patients with ascites not responding to bed rest or low-sodium diet,[73] patients assigned to receive diuretics plus albumin (12.5 g/day as inpatients or 25 g/wk as outpatients) had a shorter hospital stay, decreased recurrence of ascites during a 3-year follow-up period, and a decreased number of hospital readmissions. There was no difference in the two groups with respect to survival and incidence of other complications. Mean albumin level was 3.1 g/dL. However, a more recent trial failed to show any convincing advantage to this approach.[74]

CONCLUSION

In summary, although we would not discourage the use of diuretics in patients with AKI, we find insufficient evidence to support their use for prevention or treatment of AKI, and some evidence to suggest that they may be harmful if given intercurrently with an acute renal insult. Diuretics may safely be used to treat the complications of AKI and probably do not affect patient mortality or the rate of renal recovery.

References

1. Thadhani R, Pascual M, Bonventre JV: Acute renal failure. N Engl J Med 1996;334:1448–1460.
2. Kellum JA: Use of diuretics in the acute care setting. Kidney Int 1998;66(Suppl):S67–S70.
3. Conger JD: Drug therapy in acute renal failure. In Lazarus JM, Brenner BM (eds): Acute Renal Failure, 3rd ed. New York: Churchill Livingstone, 1993, pp 527–552.
4. Fink M: Are diuretics useful in the treatment or prevention of acute renal failure? South Med J 1982;75:329–334.
5. Conger JD: Interventions in clinical acute renal failure: What are the data? Am J Kidney Dis 1995;26:565–576.
6. Shilliday I, Allison MEM: Diuretics in acute renal failure. Ren Fail 1994;16:3–17.
7. Better OS, Rubinstein I, Winaver JM, Knochel JP: Mannitol therapy revisited, 1940–1997. Kidney Int 1997;51:886–894.
8. Lameire AL, Vanholder R: Pathophysiologic features and prevention of human and experimental acute tubular necrosis. J Am Soc Nephrol 2001;12:S20–S32.
9. Barry KC, Cohen A, Knochel JP, et al: Mannitol infusion II. The prevention of acute functional renal failure during resection of an aneurysm of the abdominal aorta. N Engl J Med 1961; 264:967–971.
10. Ip-Yam PC, Murphy S, Baines M, et al: Renal function and proteinuria after cardiopulmonary bypass: The effects of temperature and mannitol. Anesth Analg 1994;78:542–547.
11. Beall AC Jr, Hall CW, Morris GC Jr, Debakey ME: Mannitol-induced osmotic diuresis during renal artery occlusion. Ann Surg 1965;161:46–52.
12. Gubern JM, Sancho JJ, Simo J, Sitges-Serra A: A randomized trial on the effect of mannitol on postoperative renal function in patients with obstructive jaundice. Surgery 1988;103:19–44.
13. Gubern JM, Martinez-Rodenas F, Sitges-Serra A. Use of mannitol as a measure to prevent postoperative renal failure in patients with obstructive jaundice. Am J Surg 1990;159:444–445.
14. Velasquez MT, Notargiacomo AV, Cohn JN: Comparative effects of saline and mannitol on renal cortical blood flow and volume in the dog. Am J Physiol 1973;224:322–327.
15. Star RA: Treatment of acute renal failure. Kidney Int 1998;54: 1817–1831.
16. Mason J, Joeris B, Welsch J, Kriz W: Vascular congestion in ischemic renal failure: The role of cell swelling. Miner Electrolyte Metab 1989;15:114–124.
17. Magovern GJ, Bolling SF, Casale AS, et al: The mechanisms of mannitol in reducing ischemic injury: Hyperosmolarity or hydroxyl scavenger? Circulation 1984;70(Suppl 1):91–95.
18. Nicholson ML, Baker DM, Hopkinson BR, Wenham PW: Randomized controlled trial of the effect of mannitol on renal reperfusion injury during aortic aneurysm surgery. Br J Surg 1996;83:1230–1233.
19. Solomon R, Werner C, Mann D, et al: Effects of saline, mannitol, and furosemide to prevent acute decreases in renal function induced by radiocontrast agents. N Engl J Med 1994;331:416–420.
20. Stevens MA, McCullough PA, Tobin KJ, et al: A prospective randomized trial of prevention measures in patients at high risk for contrast nephropathy: Results of the P.R.I.N.C.E. Study. Prevention of Radiocontrast Induced Nephropathy Clinical Evaluation. J Am Coll Cardiol 1999;33:203–211.
21. Anto HR, Chou SY, Porush JG, Shapiro WB: Infusion intravenous pyelography and renal function. Effect of hypertonic mannitol in patients with chronic renal insufficiency. Arch Intern Med 1981; 141:652–656.
22. Weisberg LS, Kurnik PB, Kurnik BR: Risk of radiocontrast nephropathy in patients with and without diabetes mellitus. Kidney Int 1994;45:159–165.
23. Abassi ZA, Hoffman A, Better OS: Acute renal failure complicating muscle crush injury. Semin Nephrol 1998;18:558–565.
24. Malinoski DJ, Slater MS, Mullins RJ: Crush injury and rhabdomyolysis. Crit Care Clin 2004;20:171–192.
25. Johnston PA, Bernard DB, Perrin NS, Levinsky NG: Prostaglandins mediate the vasodilatory effect of mannitol in the hypoperfused rat kidney. J Clin Invest 1981;68:127–133.
26. Tay M, Comper WD, Vassiliou P, et al: The inhibitory action of oxygen radical scavengers on proteinuria and glomerular heparan sulphate loss in the isolated perfused kidney. Biochem Int 1990;20:467–478.
27. Bratell S, Folmerz P, Hansson R, et al: Effects of oxygen free radical scavengers, xanthine oxidase inhibition and calcium entry-blockers on leakage of albumin after ischaemia: An experimental study in rabbit kidneys. Acta Physiol Scand 1988;134: 15–41.
28. Brown CV, Rhee P, Chan L, et al: Preventing renal failure in patients with rhabdomyolysis: Do bicarbonate and mannitol make a difference? J Trauma 2004;56:6191–6196.
29. Homsi E, Barreiro MF, Orlando JM, Higa EM: Prophylaxis of acute renal failure in patients with rhabdomyolysis. Ren Fail 1997;19:283–288.
30. Girbes AR: Prevention of acute renal failure: Role of vaso-active drugs, mannitol and diuretics. Int J Artif Organs 2004;27: 1049–1053.
31. van Valenberg PL, Hoitsma AJ, Tiggeler RG, et al: Mannitol as an indispensable constituent of an intraoperative hydration protocol for the prevention of acute renal failure after renal cadaveric transplantation. Transplantation 1987;44:784–788.
32. Tiggeler RG, Berden JH, Hoitsma AJ, Koene RA: Prevention of acute tubular necrosis in cadaveric kidney transplantation by the combined use of mannitol and moderate hydration. Ann Surg 1985;201:246–251.
33. Porras I, Gonzalez-Posada JM, Losada M, et al: A multivariate analysis of the risk factors for posttransplant renal failure: Beneficial effect of a flush solution with mannitol. Transplant Proc 1992;24:12–13.
34. Richards KF, Belnap LP, Rees WV, Stevens LE: Mannitol reduces ATN in cadaveric allografts. Transplant Proc 1989;21:1228–1229.
35. Grino JM, Miravitlles R, Castelao AM, et al: Flush solution with mannitol in the prevention of post-transplant renal failure. Transplant Proc 1987;19:5140–5142.
36. Hoitsma AJ, Groenewoud AF, Berden JH, et al: Important role for mannitol in the prevention of acute renal failure after cadaveric kidney transplantation. Transplant Proc 1987;19: 2063–2064.
37. Lauzurica R, Teixido J, Serra A, et al: Hydration and mannitol reduce the need for dialysis in cadaveric kidney transplant recipients treated with CyA. Transplant Proc 1992;24:16–17.

38. Weimar W, Geerlings W, Bijnen AB, et al: A controlled study on the effect of mannitol on immediate renal function after cadaver donor kidney transplantation. Transplantation 1983;35:19–101.

39. Solomon R, Werner C, Mann D, et al: Effects of saline, mannitol, and furosemide to prevent acute decreases in renal function induced by radiocontrast agents. N Engl J Med 1994;331:1416–1420.

40. Brezis M, Rosen S: Hypoxia of the renal medulla: Its implications for disease. N Engl J Med 1995;332:647–655.

41. Brezis M, Rosen S, Silva P, Epstein FH: Transport activity modified thick ascending limb damage in the isolated perfused kidney. Kidney Int 1984;25:65–72.

42. Kellum JA: The use of diuretics and dopamine in acute renal failure: A systematic review of the evidence. Crit Care 1997;1:23–59.

43. Lassnigg A, Donner E, Grubhofer G, et al: Lack of renoprotective effects of dopamine and furosemide during cardiac surgery. J Am Soc Nephrol 2000;11:97–104.

44. Weinstein JM, Heyman S, Brezis M: Potential deleterious effect of furosemide in radiocontrast nephropathy. Nephron 1992;62:413–415.

45. Stevens NA, McCullough PA, Tobin KJ, et al: A prospective randomized trial of prevention measures in patients at high risk for contrast nephropathy: Results of the PRINCE study. J Am Coll Cardiol 1999;33:403–411.

46. Barry K, Malloy J: Oliguric renal failure: Evaluation and therapy by the intravenous infusion of mannitol. JAMA 1962;179:510–562.

47. Eliahou H: Mannitol therapy in oliguria of acute onset. Br Med J 1964;1:807–811.

48. Luke R, Linton A, Briggs J, Kennedy A: Mannitol therapy in acute renal failure. Lancet 1965;1:980–984.

49. Luke R, Briggs J, Allison M, Kennedy A: Factors determining response to mannitol in acute renal failure. Am J Med Sci 1970;259:168–173.

50. Mehta RL, Pascual MT, Soroko S, Chertow GM: Diuretics, mortality, and nonrecovery of renal function in acute renal failure. JAMA 2002;288:2547–2553.

51. Uchino S, Doig GS, Bellomo R, et al: Diuretics and mortality in acute renal failure. Crit Care Med 2004;32:1669–1677.

52. Cantarovich F, Locatelli A, Fernandez JC: Frusemide in high doses in the treatment of acute renal failure. Postgrad Med J 1971;47:13–19.

53. Kleinknecht D, Ganeval D, Gonzalez-Duque LA, Fermanian J: Furosemide in acute oliguric renal failure. A controlled trial. Nephron 1976;17:51–58.

54. Brown CB, Ogg CS, Cameron JS: High dose furosemide in acute renal failure: A controlled trial. Clin Nephrol 1981;15:90–96.

55. Shilliday IR, Quinn KJ, Allison ME: Loop diuretics in the management of acute renal failure: A prospective, double-blind, placebo-controlled, randomized study. Nephrol Dial Transplant 1997;12:2592–2596.

56. Cantarovich F, Rangoonwala B, Lorenz H, et al: High-dose furosemide for established ARF: A prospective, randomized, double-blind, placebo-controlled, multicenter trial. Am J Kidney Dis 2004;44:302–309.

57. Sirivella S, Gielchinsky I, Parsonnet V: Mannitol, furosemide, and dopamine infusion in postoperative renal failure complicating cardiac surgery. Ann Thorac Surg 2000;69:501–506.

58. Conger JD, Falk SA, Yuan BH, Schrier RW: Atrial natriuretic peptide and dopamine in a rat model of ischemic acute renal failure. Kidney Int 1989;35:5126–32.

59. Nakamoto M, Shapiro JI, Shanley PF, et al: In vitro and in vivo protective effect of atriopeptin III on ischemic acute renal failure. J Clin Invest 1987;80:398–705.

60. Lewis J, Salem MM, Chertow GM, et al: Atrial natriuretic factor in oliguric acute renal failure. Anaritide Acute Renal Failure Study Group. Am J Kidney Dis 2000;36:467–474.

61. Allgren RL, Marbury TC, Rahman SN, et al: Anaritide in acute tubular necrosis. Auriculin Anaritide Acute Renal Failure Study Group. N Engl J Med 1997;336:1228–1234.

62. Sward K, Valsson F, Odencrants P, et al: Recombinant human atrial natriuretic peptide in ischemic acute renal failure: A randomized placebo-controlled trial. Crit Care Med 2004;32:6310–6315.

63. Kjellstrand C: Ethacrynic acid in acute tubular necrosis. Indications and effect on the natural course. Nephron 1972;9:337–348.

64. Scheer RL: The effects of hypertonic mannitol on oliguric patients. Am J Med Sci 1965;250:35–43.

65. van Hengel P, Nikken JJ, de Jong GM, et al: Mannitol-induced acute renal failure. Neth J Med 1997;50:11–24.

66. Visweswaran P, Massin EK, Dubose TD: Mannitol-induced acute renal failure. J Am Soc Nephrol 1997;8:1028–1033.

67. Voelker JR, Cartwright-Brown D, Anderson S, et al: Comparison of loop diuretics in patients with chronic renal insufficiency. Kidney Int 1987;32:472–478.

68. Ho KM, Sheridan DJ: Meta-analysis of furosemide to prevent or treat acute renal failure. Br Med J 2006;333:420.

69. Salvador DR, Rey NR, Ramos GC, Punzalan FE: Continuous infusion versus bolus injection of loop diuretics in congestive heart failure. Cochrane Database Syst Rev 2005;3:D003178.

70. Rudy DW, Voelker JR, Greene PK, et al: Loop diuretics for chronic renal insufficiency: A continuous infusion is more efficacious than bolus therapy. Ann Intern Med 1991;115:560–566.

71. Martin SJ, Danzinger LH: Continuous infusion of loop diuretics in the critically ill: A review of the literature. Crit Care Med 1994;22:1323–1329.

72. Fliser D: Loop diuretics and thiazides—the case for their combination in chronic renal failure. Nephrol Dial Transplant 1996;11:408–423.

73. Gentilini P, Casini-Raggi V, Di Fiore G, et al: Albumin improves the response to diuretics in patients with cirrhosis and ascites: Results of a randomized, controlled trial. J Hepatol 1999;30:439–445.

74. Chalasani N, Gorski JC, Horlander JC Sr, et al: Effects of albumin/furosemide mixtures on responses to furosemide in hypoalbuminemic patients. J Am Soc Nephrol 2001;12:1010–1016.

75. Weisberg LS, Kurnik PB, Kurnik BRC: Risk of radiocontrast nephropathy in patients with and without diabetes mellitus. Kidney Int 1994;45:259–265.

Further Reading

Cantarovich F, Rangoonwala B, Lorenz H, et al: High-dose furosemide for established ARF: A prospective, randomized, double-blind, placebo-controlled, multicenter trial. Am J Kidney Dis 2004;44:302–309.

Ho KM, Sheridan DJ: Meta-analysis of frusemide to prevent or treat acute renal failure. Br Med J 2006;333:420.

Mehta RL, Pascual MT, Soroko S, Chertow GM: Diuretics, mortality, and nonrecovery of renal function in acute renal failure. JAMA 2002;288:2547–2553.

Uchino S, Doig GS, Bellomo R, et al: Diuretics and mortality in acute renal failure. Crit Care Med 2004;32:1669–1677.

Chapter 4

Contrast Nephropathy

Brendan J. Barrett and Patrick S. Parfrey

Iodinated contrast media are commonly injected intravascularly, into either an artery or vein, to enhance images during diagnostic or interventional radiologic procedures. Most of the recent literature on contrast-induced nephropathy (CIN) has been in the setting of cardiac angiography and percutaneous coronary intervention. Estimates of risk, the mechanism of kidney injury, and the impact of preventive therapies may differ according to the population studied. There is no specific therapy for CIN once it occurs, with supportive measures applied as usual for acute kidney injury.

EPIDEMIOLOGY

Sensitive tests of kidney function commonly identify mild, transient reduction after contrast injection.[1] CIN has been reported to be the third most common cause of acute renal failure in hospitalized patients.[2] The reported incidence of CIN varies among studies due to differences in definition, background risk, type and dose of contrast, imaging procedure, and the frequency of other potential causes of acute renal failure. There is no specific diagnostic marker for CIN in humans, and contrast may be a contributory cause rather than a sole cause of acute kidney injury. Concomitant insults may include low blood volume, surgery, atheroembolic disease, and other nephrotoxins. In one study of patients having coronary angiography, serum creatinine increased by more than 25% in 14.5% (95% confidence interval: 12.9%–16.1%) of cases, whereas 0.77% required dialysis.[3] The literature on risk after intravenous injection of modern contrast agents is sparse. The frequency of minor changes in serum creatinine after intravenous contrast appear to be many-fold less common than after cardiac angiography, and the importance of considering the background rate of acute change in kidney function has recently been re-emphasized.[4,5] The presence or absence of risk factors and the type of imaging procedure are most relevant. Preexisting renal function is a major determinant of the risk of CIN.[3] Although minor, usually transient changes in serum creatinine after contrast have been associated with prolonged hospital stay, adverse cardiac events, and higher mortality both in hospital and in the long term.[3,6–10] These associations may be explained at least in part by comorbidities, acuity of illness, or alternate causes of acute kidney injury such as atheroembolism.

PATHOGENETIC BASIS FOR PREVENTION

CIN likely results from both ischemic injury and direct tubular cell toxicity.[11] A reduction in medullary perfusion, possibly mediated by increased endothelin and adenosine together with reduced nitric oxide and prostacyclin, has been considered important.[12] The nature of the contrast including its physical properties such as viscosity and osmolality, associated ions, concentration, concomitant hypoxia, and oxygen free radical generation may each be related to the degree of cellular damage.[11,13] Although controversy remains about the exact pathogenesis in humans and the relevance of animal models, pathogenetic considerations underlie most efforts to reduce contrast nephrotoxicity.

ASSESSMENT OF RISK

The first steps in preventing CIN are to identify risk factors and review the need for contrast. The most important risk factors are preexisting kidney disease, diabetes, poor cardiac function, hypotension, anemia, and older age. Most risk factors can be detected with a routine history and physical examination. It is not necessary to measure serum creatinine on every patient, but this should be done before intra-arterial contrast and in patients with a history of kidney disease, proteinuria, kidney surgery, diabetes, hypertension, or gout.[14] Patients with reduced kidney function may be more accurately recognized if creatinine clearance or the glomerular filtration rate are estimated from the serum creatinine. Some risk factors such as volume depletion may be corrected before contrast. The risk of CIN increases exponentially with the number of risk factors present.[7,9,15] Validated risk prediction models have been developed for those having percutaneous coronary intervention.[16]

Alternate imaging modalities not requiring contrast should be considered in those with any risk factors. High-dose gadolinium chelates should not be substituted for iodinated radiocontrast media in those patients at risk of CIN, as they have been shown to be at least as nephrotoxic as the latter media when used in this fashion.[17] Serum creatinine should be measured again at 24 to 72 hours post-contrast in patients at risk of CIN.

SPECIFIC PROPHYLACTIC THERAPIES

Table 4-1 summarizes the most commonly used prophylactic measures supported by at least some evidence.

Fluid Administration

Administration of fluids is recommended to reduce the risk of CIN. However, data to support a specific fluid regimen are lacking and the optimal fluid regimen remains unclear. The trials evaluating prophylactic fluid therapy generally lack power. In two trials, prolonged IV saline was superior to an oral fluid regimen with or without a brief IV fluid bolus.[18,19] No difference between fluid regimens was found in two other trials comparing IV saline with either oral salt and water or oral water and brief IV fluid.[20,21] A final small trial, marred by excessive dropouts, showed a trend to less CIN with more prolonged precontrast IV fluid.[22] Isotonic saline was slightly better than 0.45% saline in a large trial of patients with good kidney function.[23] Almost all participants in these trials received intra-arterial contrast. Based on this evidence, the recommendations for the present are to ensure that patients receiving contrast are in a state of optimal hydration as determined by clinical assessment. Fluid restriction before injection of contrast should be limited to when truly necessary. For those at risk of CIN, particularly those undergoing cardiac angiography, it is recommended that consideration be given to infusing 0.9% saline intravenously for at least 6 hours before and after contrast, in the absence of data showing that shorter duration or oral fluid supplementation is comparable.

Bicarbonate

Alkalinization of tubular fluid has been proposed to reduce the rate of CIN. The mechanism of any benefit might include reduction in pH-dependent free radical generation in the kidney. In the only reported trial to date involving 119 patients, 81% of whom were undergoing cardiac angiography, isotonic sodium bicarbonate resulted in a lower frequency of CIN (defined as a 25% increase in serum creatinine within 2 days) compared with 0.9% saline infusion.[24] However, the trial was terminated early due to a lower than expected rate of events in the bicarbonate group, but the timing of the interim analysis and the stopping rules were not prespecified and the P value for the difference in event rates was higher than generally used to prematurely terminate a trial. It is also unclear whether any benefit from bicarbonate would be seen if patients were also treated with N-acetylcysteine (NAC). This question has not been properly addressed, but no additional benefit was seen in a retrospective analysis at one center.[25] Although it is reasonable to use bicarbonate infusion in an effort to reduce the rate of CIN, the results of this trial require replication before this can be recommended as the fluid of choice.

N-Acetylcysteine

NAC might reduce the nephrotoxicity of contrast through antioxidant and vasodilatory effects.[26] The results of an initial trial were dramatic, but the event rate in the controls was unexpectedly high for patients given low-dose IV low-osmolality contrast.[27] Subsequent trials have largely involved patients with reduced kidney function having cardiac angiography. Some have shown benefit and others not; many are limited by low power and a lack of blinding. The dose of NAC employed in most trials has not been chosen based on pharmacologic principles. Two trials comparing doses of NAC have suggested

Table 4-1   Therapies Commonly Used to Reduce the Risk of Contrast-Induced Nephropathy

Therapy	Dose	Route	Frequency	Comments
Fluid therapy	Varies from unrestricted PO fluids to 1 mL/kg/hr	IV or PO	Usually continuous from pre- to postcontrast. Some use bolus therapy pre-contrast	No one regimen proven best. IV 0.9% saline at 1 mL/kg/hr from 12 hr pre to 12 hr post most established. May increase risk of pulmonary edema
Isotonic sodium bicarbonate	3 mL/kg/hr × 1 hr, then 1 mL/kg/hr × 6 hr	IV	Infusion from 1 hr pre- and for 6 hr postcontrast	Only one supporting trial with caveats. May increase risk of pulmonary edema
N-acetylcysteine	Varies from 600–1200 mg bid PO to 150 mg/kg IV bolus	PO or IV	Varies, q12h for 4 doses beginning precontrast most common	Supporting study results heterogeneous
Theophylline and related	Varies 125–200 mg PO or 4–5 mg/kg IV bolus ± 0.4 mg/kg IV infusion	PO or IV	Varies from q12h PO to single IV bolus ± infusion for 24–72 hr	Limited evidence of efficacy, concern about potential cardiotoxicity

that higher doses may be required, especially if higher doses of contrast are being employed.[28,29] Several meta-analyses of trials of NAC have been reported. The trials included in these analyses vary, but more recent and comprehensive meta-analyses suggest some benefit to NAC (pooled odds ratio ranged from 0.54 to 0.73 for contrast nephropathy defined variably as increases in serum creatinine).[30–34] However, this estimate must be interpreted with caution, given the heterogeneous results of the individual trials and the possibility of publication bias, with small negative studies underrepresented. Also, the effect of NAC on outcomes other than minor changes in serum creatinine is largely unknown. Indeed, studies in healthy volunteers have suggested that NAC might have an effect on creatinine levels unrelated to an effect on the glomerular filtration rate.[35] However, in a recent trial involving patients undergoing primary angioplasty after myocardial infarction, NAC showed a dose-related improvement in CIN (defined as a serum creatinine increase), and there was a parallel beneficial effect on in-hospital death.[29]

Theophylline

Theophylline and aminophylline have the potential to reduce CIN through antagonizing adenosine-mediated vasoconstriction. These drugs have been tested in several small trials. Recent meta-analyses found that the mean increase in serum creatinine was significantly, but only slightly, lower at 48 hours after contrast among those receiving active therapy compared with placebo. The clinical importance of this finding is not clear.[36,37] There was heterogeneity among studies with regard to changes in serum creatinine. There is potential for adverse effects with theophylline. The optimal dose for prevention of CIN has not been established. Further studies are warranted.

Other Pharmacologic Agents

Several other interventions have been proposed to reduce the risk of CIN, but data are limited to support them. Forced diuresis with furosemide, mannitol, dopamine, or a combination of these given at the time of the contrast exposure has been associated with similar or higher rates of CIN when compared with prophylactic fluids alone.[38–41] Negative fluid balance might underlie some of the detrimental effects.

Generally small randomized trials of vasodilation with dopamine, fenoldopam, atrial natriuretic peptide, calcium channel blockers, prostaglandin E_1, or a nonselective endothelin receptor antagonist failed to show a reduction in the rate of CIN compared with fluid therapy.[41–46]

Two studies of captopril as a prophylactic agent yielded divergent results. In the first trial, serum creatinine increased by more than 0.5 mg/dL (44 μmol/L) in two (6%) patients given captopril for 3 days versus 10 (29%) given placebo ($P < .02$).[47] In the second study, CIN was reported as occurring in five (8.3%) patients given captopril versus one (3.1%) given placebo ($P = .02$).[48]

Ascorbic acid as an antioxidant has been tested in a single randomized trial with patients undergoing cardiac angiography.[49] Serum creatinine increased by 25% or more than 0.5 mg/dL (44 μmol/L) within 2 to 5 days in 11 (9%) patients given ascorbic acid versus 23 (20%) given placebo ($P = .02$).[49] However, these results are difficult to interpret as the baseline serum creatinine level was lower in the placebo group and both groups reached a similar level post-contrast.

Prophylactic Renal Replacement Therapy

Hemodialysis during or shortly after contrast has not been shown to prevent CIN.[50–52] In a trial of prophylactic hemofiltration in an intensive care unit before and after contrast involving patients with a mean creatinine clearance of 26 mL/min undergoing cardiac procedures, a 25% increase in serum creatinine was seen in three (5%) patients undergoing hemofiltration versus 28 (50%) given fluid alone ($P < .001$).[53] These results were replicated in a further trial by the same investigators, in which they also showed that hemofiltration limited to the post-contrast period was not significantly different from saline alone.[54] However, as changes in serum creatinine during and soon after hemofiltration are affected by creatinine removal, such changes in serum creatinine do not reliably reflect changes in kidney function. The mechanism of benefit, if any, to the kidney remains speculative. Marenzi and colleagues[54] suggest controlled high-volume administration as one possibility, but their hemofiltration protocol should lead to a neutral, not positive, fluid balance. In both trials, hemofiltration, especially pre- and post-contrast, was associated with reduced in-hospital cardiovascular mortality, but the mechanism by which this might occur is unclear. Given the resource implications and the problems with interpreting the true effect on kidney function, hemofiltration is not recommended at this time as a means to prevent CIN.

CONSIDERATIONS RELATED TO CONTRAST MEDIA

Contrast media can be classified in a number of ways including by osmolality, viscosity, and ionicity. High-osmolality agents such as sodium diatrizoate have been largely abandoned because of their greater general toxicities. In a meta-analysis of comparative trials, an increase in serum creatinine more than 0.5 mg/dL (44 μmol/L) after contrast in patients with reduced kidney function was less frequent with low- as opposed to high-osmolal media (odds ratio = 0.61, 95% confidence interval: 0.48–0.77).[55] Results in subgroups of trials were qualitatively similar, but statistical significance could only be shown for intra-arterial injection and in those with preexisting renal impairment. Due to the small number of events, no conclusion could be reached about the need for dialysis.

More recent trials have compared the nephrotoxicity of low-osmolal media such as iohexol or iopamidol with the iso-osmolal agent iodixanol. The results have not been totally consistent. A patient level meta-analysis of data from 16 trials in the database of GE Healthcare found that CIN defined as a 0.5-mg/dL increase in creatinine by 3 days post-contrast occurred in 1.4% after intra-arterial iodixanol versus 3.5% after low-osmolality agents.[56] The difference was more pronounced in those with existing kidney disease with or without diabetes. A further trial comparing iodixanol with iopamidol in 414 patients having cardiac angiography did not find any difference in the rate of CIN.[57] Similarly, comparative trials after intravenous injection of iodixanol versus low-osmolality agents have all shown similar rates of CIN with either agent.[58,59] An analysis of the frequency of CIN before and after hospitals in Sweden switched to iodixanol suggested a higher rate of CIN with iodixanol.[60] Given the disparity in

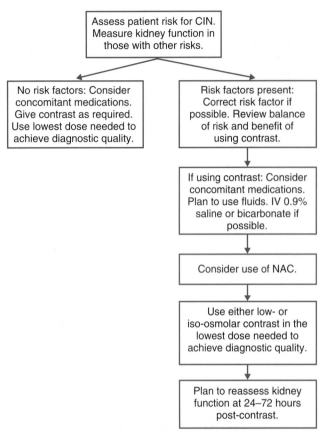

Figure 4-1 Algorithm for managing the risk of contrast-induced nephropathy (CIN). NAC, N-acetylcysteine.

the results, either low- or iso-osmolal media are acceptable at this time for patients at risk of CIN.

The nephrotoxicity of radiocontrast agents seems to be dose related. This has not always been clear when exposure to contrast has been measured as the volume injected (in milliliters). However, different contrast agents have varying concentrations of iodine and iodinated media are largely excreted through the kidney. It has been shown that the area under the curve as a measure of contrast exposure is closely estimated by dividing the grams of iodine injected by creatinine clearance.[61] The related measure contrast volume (mL) × kg body weight ÷ serum creatinine in mg/dL has been associated with risk of CIN.[62,63] Exceeding a value of 5 mL × kg body weight ÷ serum creatinine in mg/dL strongly predicts nephropathy requiring dialysis.[63] Therefore, the volume of contrast injected should be limited to the minimum required to complete the diagnostic or therapeutic procedure.

MANAGING CONCOMITANT MEDICATIONS

Because of the risk of lactic acidosis when CIN occurs in a patient with diabetes receiving metformin, it is recommended that this drug be stopped at least from the time of contrast injection and held until CIN has been excluded.[5,64] The balance of risks and benefits associated with interrupting therapy with diuretics, angiotensin-converting enzyme inhibitors, and angiotensin receptor blockers in cases at risk of CIN has not been thoroughly studied to date.[65] It is generally recommended that NSAID therapy be interrupted, but empirical data on which to base this are lacking.

RECOMMENDED OVERALL RISK MINIMIZATION STRATEGY

Figure 4-1 outlines an overall approach to minimizing the risk of CIN. The steps involved include an assessment of risk, review of the balance of risks and benefits associated with the use of contrast for the particular case, use of fluid prophylaxis, consideration of specific prophylactic drug therapy, management of concomitant drug therapy, choice of type and dose of contrast, and postcontrast follow-up.

References

1. Katholi RE, Taylor GJ, McCann WP, et al: Nephrotoxicity from contrast media: Attenuation with theophylline. Radiology 1995;195:17–22.
2. Nash K, Hafeez A, Hou S: Hospital-acquired renal insufficiency. Am J Kidney Dis 2002;39:930–936.
3. McCullough PA, Wolyn R, Rocher LL, et al: Acute renal failure after coronary intervention: Incidence, risk factors, and relationship to mortality. Am J Med 1997;103:368–375.
4. Katzberg R, Barrett B: Risk of iodinated contrast material—induced nephropathy with intravenous administration. Radiology 2007;243:622–628.
5. Rao QA, Newhouse JH: Risk of nephropathy after intravenous administration of contrast material: A critical literature analysis. Radiology 2006;239:392–397.
6. Abizaid AS, Clark CE, Mintz GS, et al: Effects of dopamine and aminophylline on contrast-induced acute renal failure after coronary angioplasty in patients with preexisting renal insufficiency. Am J Cardiol 1999;83:260–263.
7. Bartholomew BA, Harjai KJ, Dukkipati S, et al: Impact of nephropathy after percutaneous coronary intervention and a method for risk stratification. Am J Cardiol 2004;93:1515–1519.
8. Dangas G, Iakovou I, Nikolsky E, et al: Contrast-induced nephropathy after percutaneous coronary interventions in relation to chronic kidney disease and hemodynamic variables. Am J Cardiol 2005;95:13–19.
9. Marenzi G, Lauri G, Assanelli E, et al: Contrast-induced nephropathy in patients undergoing primary angioplasty for acute myocardial infarction. J Am Coll Cardiol 2004;44:1780–1785.
10. Rihal CS, Textor SC, Grill DE, et al: Incidence and prognostic importance of acute renal failure after percutaneous coronary intervention. Circulation 2002;105:2259–2264.
11. Persson PB, Hansell P, Liss P: Pathophysiology of contrast medium-induced nephropathy. Kidney Int 2005;68:14–22.
12. Heyman SN, Brezis M, Epstein FH, et al: Early renal medullary hypoxic injury from radiocontrast and indomethacin. Kidney Int 1991;40:632–642.
13. Katholi RE, Woods WT, Taylor GJ, et al: Oxygen free radicals and contrast nephropathy. Am J Kidney Dis 1998;32:64–71.
14. Thomsen HS, Morcos SK, Members of the Contrast Media Safety Committee of European Society of Urogenital Radiology (ESUR): In which patients should serum creatinine be measured before iodinated contrast medium injection? Eur Radiol 2005;15:749–754.
15. Rich MW, Crecelius CA: Incidence, risk factors, and clinical course of acute renal insufficiency after cardiac catheterization in patients 70 years of age or older. Arch Intern Med 1995; 150:1237–1242.

16. Mehran R, Aymong ED, Nikolsky E, et al: A simple risk score for prediction of contrast-induced nephropathy after percutaneous coronary intervention. J Am Coll Cardiol 2004;44:1393–1399.

17. Thomsen HS, Almen T, Morcos SK, Contrast Media Safety Committee of the European Society of Urogenital Radiology (ESUR): Gadolinium-containing contrast media for radiographic examinations: A position paper. Eur Radiol 2002;12:2600–2605.

18. Bader BD, Berger ED, Heede MB, et al: What is the best hydration regimen to prevent contrast media-induced nephrotoxicity? Clin Nephrol 2004;62:1–7.

19. Trivedi HS, Moore H, Nasr S, et al: A randomized prospective trial to assess the role of saline hydration on the development of contrast nephrotoxicity. Nephron Clin Pract 2003;93:c29–c34.

20. Dussol B, Morange S, Loundoun A, et al: A randomized trial of saline hydration to prevent contrast nephropathy in chronic renal failure patients. Nephrol Dial Transplant 2006;21:2120–2126.

21. Taylor AJ, Hotchkiss D, Morse RW, et al: PREPARED: PREParation for Angiography in Renal Dysfunction. Chest 1998;114:1570–1574.

22. Krasuski RA, Beard BM, Geoghagan JD, et al: Optimal timing of hydration to erase contrast-associated nephropathy: The OTHER CAN study. J Invasive Cardiol 2003;15:699–702.

23. Mueller C, Buettner HJ, Petersen J, et al: Prevention of contrast media-associated nephropathy. Randomized comparison of 2 hydration regimens in 1620 patients undergoing coronary angioplasty. Arch Intern Med 2002;162:329–336.

24. Merten GJ, Burgess WP, Gray LV, et al: Prevention of contrast-induced nephropathy with sodium bicarbonate: A randomized controlled trial. JAMA 2004;291:2328–2334.

25. Schmidt P, Pang D, Nykamp D, et al: N-acetylcysteine and sodium bicarbonate versus N-acetylcysteine and standard hydration for the prevention of radiocontrast-induced nephropathy following coronary angiography. Ann Pharmacother 2007;41:46–50.

26. Fishbane S, Durham JH, Marzo K, Rudnick M: N-acetylcysteine in the prevention of radiocontrast-induced nephropathy. J Am Soc Nephrol 2004;15:251–260.

27. Tepel M, van der Giet M, Schwarzfeld C, et al: Prevention of radiographic contrast-agent-induced reductions in renal function by acetylcysteine. N Engl J Med 2000;343:180–184.

28. Briguori C, Colombo A, Violante A, et al: Standard vs double dose of N-acetylcysteine to prevent contrast agent associated nephrotoxicity. Eur Heart J 2004;25:206–211.

29. Marenzi G, Assanelli E, Marana I, et al: N-acetylcysteine and contrast-induced nephropathy in primary angioplasty. N Engl J Med 2006;354:2773–2782.

30. Bagshaw SM, Ghali WA: Acetylcysteine for prevention of contrast-induced nephropathy after intravascular angiography: A systematic review and meta-analysis. BMC Med 2004;2:38. Available at: www.biomedcentral.com/1741-7015/2/38 (accessed January 14, 2005).

31. Duong MH, MacKenzie TA, Malenka DJ: N-acetylcysteine prophylaxis significantly reduces the risk of radiocontrast-induced nephropathy: Comprehensive meta-analysis. Catheter Cardiovasc Interv 2005;64:471–479.

32. Kshirsagar AV, Poole C, Mottl A, et al: N-acetylcysteine for the prevention of radiocontrast induced nephropathy: A meta-analysis of prospective controlled trials. J Am Soc Nephrol 2004;15:761–769.

33. Nallamothu BK, Shojania KG, Saint S, et al: Is acetylcysteine effective in preventing contrast-related nephropathy? A meta-analysis. Am J Med 2004;117:938–947.

34. Pannu N, Manns B, Lee H, Tonelli M. Systematic review of the impact of N-acetylcysteine on contrast nephropathy. Kidney Int 2004;65:1266–1274.

35. Hoffmann U, Fischereder M, Kruger B, et al: The value of N-acetylcysteine in the prevention of radiocontrast agent-induced nephropathy seems questionable. J Am Soc Nephrol 2004;15:407–410.

36. Bagshaw SM, Ghali WA: Theophylline for prevention of contrast-induced nephropathy. Arch Intern Med 2005;165:1087–1093.

37. Ix JH, McCulloch CE, Chertow GM: Theophylline for the prevention of radiocontrast nephropathy: A meta-analysis. Nephrol Dial Transplant 2004;19:2747–2753.

38. Solomon R, Werner C, Mann D, et al: Effects of saline, mannitol, and furosemide on acute decreases in renal function induced by radiocontrast agents. N Engl J Med 1994;331:1416–1420.

39. Stevens MA, McCullough PA, Tobin KJ, et al: A prospective randomized trial of prevention measures in patients at high risk for contrast nephropathy. J Am Coll Cardiol 1999;33:403–411.

40. Weinstein J-M, Heyman S, Brezis M: Potential deleterious effect of furosemide in radiocontrast nephropathy. Nephron 1992;62:413–415.

41. Weisberg LS, Kurnik PB, Kurnik BRC: Risk of radiocontrast nephropathy in patients with and without diabetes mellitus. Kidney Int 1994;45:259–265.

42. Khoury Z, Schlicht JR, Como J, et al: The effect of prophylactic nifedipine on renal function in patients administered contrast media. Pharmacotherapy 1995;15:59–65.

43. Kurnik BR, Allgren RL, Genter FC, et al: Prospective study of atrial natriuretic peptide for the prevention of radiocontrast-induced nephropathy. Am J Kidney Dis 1998;31:674–680.

44. Sketch MH, Whelton A, Schollmayer E, et al: Prevention of contrast media-induced renal dysfunction with prostaglandin E$_1$: A randomized, double-blind, placebo-controlled study. Am J Ther 2001;8:155–162.

45. Stone GW, McCullough PA, Tumlin JA, et al: Fenoldopam mesylate for the prevention of contrast-induced nephropathy: A randomized controlled trial. JAMA 2003;290:2284–2291.

46. Wang A, Holcslaw T, Bashore TM, et al: Exacerbation of radiocontrast nephrotoxicity by endothelin receptor antagonism. Kidney Int 2000;57:1675–1680.

47. Gupta RK, Kapoor A, Tewari S, et al: Captopril for prevention of contrast-induced nephropathy in diabetic patients: A randomised study. Indian Heart J 1999;51:521–526.

48. Toprak O, Cirit M, Bayata S, et al: [The effect of pre-procedural captopril on contrast-induced nephropathy in patients who underwent coronary angiography] [in Turkish] Anadolu Kardiyol Derg 2003;3:98–103.

49. Spargias K, Alexopoulos E, Kyrzopoulos S, et al: Ascorbic acid prevents contrast-mediated nephropathy in patients with renal dysfunction undergoing coronary angiography or intervention. Circulation 2004;110:2837–2842.

50. Frank H, Werner D, Lorusso V, et al: Simultaneous hemodialysis during coronary angiography fails to prevent radiocontrast-induced nephropathy in chronic renal failure. Clin Nephrol 2003;60:176–182.

51. Sterner G, Frennby B, Kurkus J, Nyman U: Does post-angiographic hemodialysis reduce the risk of contrast-medium nephropathy? Scand J Urol Nephrol 2000;34:323–326.

52. Vogt B, Ferrari P, Schonholzer C, et al: Prophylactic hemodialysis after radiocontrast media in patients with renal insufficiency is potentially harmful. Am J Med 2001;111:692–698.

53. Marenzi G, Marana I, Lauri G, et al: The prevention of radiocontrast-agent-induced nephropathy by hemofiltration. N Engl J Med 2003;349:1333–1340.

54. Marenzi G, Lauri G, Campodonico J, et al: Comparison of two hemofiltration protocols for prevention of contrast-induced nephropathy in high-risk patients. Am J Med 2006;119:155–162.

55. Barrett BJ, Carlisle EJ: Metaanalysis of the relative nephrotoxicity of high- and low-osmolality iodinated contrast media. Radiology 1993;188:171–178.

56. McCullough PA, Bertrand ME, Brinker JA, Stacul F: A meta-analysis of the renal safety of isosmolar iodixanol compared with low-osmolar contrast media. J Am Coll Cardiol 2006;48:692–699.

57. Solomon RJ, Natarajan MK, Doucet S, et al, Investigators of the CARE Study: Cardiac Angiography in Renally Impaired Patients

(CARE) study: A randomized double-blind trial of contrast-induced nephropathy in patients with chronic kidney disease. Circulation 2007;115:3189–3196.

58. Barrett BJ, Katzberg RW, Thomsen HS, et al, for the IMPACT Study Investigators: Contrast-induced nephropathy in patients with chronic kidney disease undergoing computed tomography: A double blind comparison of iodixanol and iopamidol. Invest Radiol 2006;41:815–821.

59. Carraro M, Malalan F, Antonione R, et al: Effects of a dimeric vs a monomeric non-ionic contrast medium on renal function in patients with mild to moderate renal insufficiency: A double-blind, randomized clinical trial. Eur Radiol 1998;8:144–147.

60. Liss P, Persson PB, Hansell P, Lagerqvist B: Renal failure in 57 925 patients undergoing coronary procedures using iso-osmolar or low-osmolar contrast media. Kidney Int 2006;70:1811–1817.

61. Sherwin PF, Cambron R, Johnson JA, Pierro JA: Contrast dose-to-creatinine clearance ratio as a potential indicator of risk for radiocontrast-induced nephropathy: Correlation of D/CrCL with area under the contrast concentration-time curve using iodixanol. Invest Radiol 2005;40:598–603.

62. Cigarroa RG, Lange RA, Williams RH, Hillis LD: Dosing of contrast material to prevent contrast nephropathy in patients with renal disease. Am J Med 1989;86:649–652.

63. Freeman RV, O'Donnell MO, Share D, et al, for the Blue Cross Blue Shield of Michigan Cardiovascular Consortium: Nephropathy requiring dialysis after percutaneous coronary intervention and the critical role of an adjusted contrast dose. Am J Cardiol 2002;90:1068–1073.

64. Thomsen HS: Guidelines for contrast media from the European Society of Urogenital Radiology. AJR Am J Roentgenol 2003;181:1463–1471.

65. Erley C: Concomitant drugs with exposure to contrast media. Kidney Int Suppl 2006;100:S20–S24.

Further Reading

Pannu N, Wiebe N, Tonelli M; Alberta Kidney Disease Network: Prophylaxis strategies for contrast-induced nephropathy. JAMA 2006;295:2765–2779.

Solomon R, Deray G, on behalf of the consensus panel for CIN. How to prevent contrast-induced nephropathy and manage risk patients: Practical recommendations. Kidney Int 2006;69:551–553.

Thomsen HS: How to avoid CIN: Guidelines from the European Society for Urogenital Radiology. Nephrol Dial Transplant 2005;20(Suppl 1):i18–i22.

Chapter 5

Management of Hepatorenal Syndrome

Marie-Noëlle Pépin and Pere Ginès

Hepatorenal syndrome (HRS) is a systemic condition that usually occurs in patients with advanced liver disease and combines cardiovascular and kidney disturbances.[1–5] Severe reduction in the glomerular filtration rate develops in the absence of significant renal lesions as a final consequence of an extreme splanchnic arterial vasodilation secondary to portal hypertension.[6–11] Bacterial translocation probably plays a major role in the induction of the splanchnic arterial vasodilation responsible for decrease in systemic vascular resistances and arterial underfilling.[12–20] The kidney perceives this decreased blood flow and initiates afferent arterial vasoconstriction and activation of the renin-angiotensin system.[21,22] It also responds to sympathetic nervous system activation by increasing sodium retention and vasoconstriction in an attempt to improve kidney perfusion.[23,24] Although initially compensated by the secretion of vasodilators within the renal circulation, vasoconstriction can progress to a severe reduction in the glomerular filtration rate, the so-called HRS. At this stage, patients constantly have alterations of renal solute-free water excretion as a consequence of increased vasopressin release and usually have a serum sodium lower than 130 mEq/L.[25–29] Among patients with cirrhosis and ascites without renal failure, marked renal sodium retention and presence of hyponatremia have been identified as risk factors for the development of HRS.[30] Some triggering events can precipitate HRS, among them bacterial infections, particularly spontaneous bacterial peritonitis (i.e., the spontaneous infection of the ascitic fluid in the absence of an intra-abdominal source of infection).[17] However, in other patients, HRS develops spontaneously without any apparent triggering event.

Besides vasoconstriction in the renal circulation, patients with HRS also have vasoconstriction in other nonsplanchnic vascular beds, including the lower and upper extremities, brain, and liver.[17,31,32] Reduced blood flow in the latter two territories may play a role in some of the clinical features seen in patients with HRS, such as encephalopathy and worsening of liver function, respectively. A decrease in cardiac function may also contribute to arterial underfilling in patients with HRS. The cardiac dysfunction is likely due to cirrhotic cardiomyopathy, the origin of which is still under investigation.[17,33–38]

Two different patterns of renal failure (steady and progressive) define two different clinical types of HRS: type 1 and type 2 HRS.[39,40] The rate of progression used to define type 1 HRS has been arbitrarily set as a 100% increase in serum creatinine reaching a value greater than 2.5 mg/dL (221 μmol/L) in less than 2 weeks. Patients not meeting these criteria of progression are considered to have type 2 HRS. There is consensus to establish the diagnosis of HRS when serum creatinine is greater than 1.5 mg/dL (133 μmol/L),[40,41] which corresponds approximately to a glomerular filtration rate lower than 30 mL/min.[42] Because of the lack of specific diagnostic procedures for HRS, the diagnosis of HRS relies on the exclusion of other conditions that may cause renal failure in cirrhosis, particularly volume depletion, shock, treatment with nephrotoxic drugs, and parenchymal kidney diseases.[40,43–45] Box 5-1 shows the diagnostic criteria of HRS proposed in a recent consensus workshop of the International Ascites Club.[41] Reflecting the systemic nature of the disease, patients with type 1 HRS usually present signs of multiorgan failure. By contrast, in patients with type 2 HRS renal failure almost goes unnoticed, as the main clinical problem is refractory ascites and frequent need for repeated large-volume paracentesis due to poor response to diuretic therapy.[40,41] Some patients with type 2 HRS eventually progress to type 1 HRS, often as a consequence of an acute event such as bacterial infections. Outcome is different for the two types of HRS, as patients with type 1 HRS have a median survival of only 1 month, whereas the median survival is 7 months for patients with type 2 HRS.[39,46]

In recent years, major advances have been made in the field of HRS, particularly in its pathogenesis and management. The aim of the current chapter is to review the management of HRS in patients with cirrhosis, with particular emphasis on type 1 HRS. An update on the pathogenesis of HRS may be found in several recent reviews.[4,47–49]

MANAGEMENT OF TYPE 1 HEPATORENAL SYNDROME

General Measures

Diuretics should be withdrawn in all patients with cirrhosis and renal failure, regardless of whether there is suspicion of HRS, and patients should be placed on a low-salt diet (<2 g/day). If

Box 5-1 Diagnostic Criteria for Hepatorenal Syndrome in Cirrhosis

1. Cirrhosis with ascites
2. Serum creatinine > 1.5 mg/dL (133 μmol/L)
3. No improvement in serum creatinine (decrease to a level <1.5 mg/dL after at least 2 days off diuretics and volume expansion with albumin 1 g/kg body weight up to a maximum of 100 g/day)
4. Absence of shock
5. No current or recent treatment with nephrotoxic drugs
6. Absence of signs of parenchymal renal disease, as suggested by proteinuria (>500 mg/day) or hematuria (>50 red blood cells per high-power field), and/or abnormal renal ultrasound scan

From Salerno F, Gerbes A, Ginès P, et al: Diagnosis, prevention and treatment of the hepatorenal syndrome in cirrhosis. A consensus workshop of the International Ascites Club. Gut 2007;56: 1310–1318.

Table 5-1 Treatment Options for Hepatorenal Syndrome and Mechanism of Action

Therapy	Mechanism of Action
Liver transplantation	Improvement in liver function and normalization of circulatory disturbances in the portal and systemic circulations
Transjugular intrahepatic portosystemic shunt	Reduction in portal pressure and suppression of the activity of vasoconstrictor systems
Vasoconstrictors (terlipressin, α-adrenergic agonists)	Vasoconstriction of the splanchnic circulation and suppression of the activity of vasoconstrictor systems
Albumin	Improvement in effective arterial blood volume? Improvement of endothelial function? Antioxidant activity?
Renal replacement therapy	Supplies renal detoxification functions
Albumin dialysis (MARS, Prometheus)*	Supplies liver detoxification functions. Improvement of circulatory function?

*Currently under clinical investigation.

the patient presents with hyponatremia, which is usually the case, fluid intake should be restricted to 1.0 to 1.5 L/day to avoid a positive fluid balance and further decrease in serum sodium concentration. The administration of saline solutions may markedly increase ascites and edema due to the presence of severe renal sodium retention and therefore is not recommended. For this same reason and the lack of severe metabolic acidosis in most patients, the routine administration of sodium bicarbonate is not advisable. Early identification of infections and treatment with broad-spectrum antibiotics is fundamental because severe infections are very common and contribute to death in many of these patients. Considering that antibiotic prophylaxis is effective in the prevention of bacterial infections in other high-risk groups, such as patients with advanced cirrhosis and gastrointestinal bleeding,[50] it is possible that antibiotic prophylaxis is also effective in preventing bacterial infections in patients with type 1 HRS, but this has not been specifically investigated.

Specific Therapies

Several therapeutic approaches, which are discussed in the following sections, can be used in the management of type 1 HRS (Table 5-1).

Liver Transplantation

Liver transplantation is the treatment of choice for patients with cirrhosis and type 1 HRS without contraindications to transplantation because it allows the cure of both liver disease and associated renal failure.[51–53] It is now well established that patients with HRS have a satisfactory long-term survival with liver transplantation alone (approximately 70% at 3 years after transplantation in most transplantation centers), yet slightly lower than that of transplant recipients without HRS.[52,54–57] The main issue in liver transplantation for patients with type 1 HRS is the high mortality rate in the waiting list due to short survival expectancy in the setting of prolonged waiting times in most transplantation centers. This can be improved by assigning patients with type 1 HRS a high priority for transplantation, which can be accomplished by using the MELD (Model for End-stage Liver Disease) score.[58,59] This is a score of severity of cirrhosis used in many countries to allocate organs for liver transplantation, which includes three variables: two of liver function, serum bilirubin, and international normalization ratio (a standardized unit for Quick time) and one of renal function and serum creatinine (for calculation, please visit www.mayoclinic.org/meld/mayomodel6.html or www.unos.org). For the same degree of liver failure, MELD score values increase progressively as serum creatinine values increase (minimum value 6 points; maximum value 40 points). The maximum value of serum creatinine to be used in the calculation of MELD is 4 mg/dL. This value is also used for patients on renal replacement therapy. Patients with type 1 HRS usually have higher MELD scores than those of patients with type 2 HRS due to a greater impairment of liver and renal function. In patients with HRS, the MELD score is an excellent predictive factor of survival. Because patients with type 1 HRS have very high MELD score values, the use of this score as a system for organ allocation in liver transplantation may likely increase the applicability of liver transplantation in this patient population and help reduce waiting list mortality.

In addition to using the MELD score for organ allocation, patients with type 1 HRS awaiting liver transplantation may possibly benefit from treatment of HRS aimed at improving renal function before transplantation. Although not assessed yet in prospective studies, the reversal of HRS before transplantation may help patients reach transplantation and improve posttransplantation outcome, and, in particular, reduce the frequent occurrence of chronic renal failure.[52,55,60] A retrospective study including a small number of patients with HRS treated with vasoconstrictors before transplantation (see later) showed that patients with HRS who responded to therapy with an improvement in renal function had an outcome after transplantation that was not different from that of a control group of transplant recipients without HRS matched by age and severity of cirrhosis.[61]

The use of combined liver-kidney transplantation (CLKT) has also been suggested as an approach to therapy of HRS, but it is still a matter of debate. A clear benefit of CLKT on the evolution of renal function and patient survival compared with liver transplantation alone has not been demonstrated.[54,56] Conversely, CLKT increases the use of kidneys for a group of patients in whom native kidney function may recover spontaneously after liver transplantation alone.[51–53] Therefore, the use of CLKT in a scenario of growing lists for kidney transplantation in patients with permanent end-stage kidney disease remains very contentious. As a result, it appears that CLKT should not be recommended currently as standard therapy for patients with HRS. There remain doubts in the specific circumstance of patients with HRS who have been on dialysis for a prolonged period before liver transplantation and therefore have poor chances of regaining renal function after transplantation.[56,62,63] It is currently unknown how much time on dialysis before liver transplantation prevents recovery from HRS in the posttransplantation period. A panel recently proposed guidelines to help select between liver transplantation alone or CLKT.[64] They recommended that patients with HRS requiring more than 6 weeks of dialysis should be evaluated for CLKT. For patients with HRS not on dialysis or with shorter duration of dialysis, prognosis was estimated to be good and liver transplantation alone was considered to be sufficient. Obviously, more studies are needed in this area.

Finally, kidney transplantation after liver transplantation was recently proposed as an alternative to CLKT for patients with HRS who needed dialysis for more than 30 days after liver transplantation.[57] This suggestion was based on findings of a 1-year survival rate 40% lower in patients who required dialysis for more than 30 days compared with patients who required dialysis for less than 30 days. Although kidney after liver transplantation may be a reasonable approach in some patients, the information is still very limited.

Pharmacologic Therapy

Early studies assessed the use of vasodilators, such as dopamine and prostaglandins, with the aim of reversing the intense renal vasoconstriction characteristic of HRS. However, in addition to not improving renal function, these drugs may further impair systemic hemodynamics, which is already markedly altered in patients with advanced cirrhosis.[65–68] Recent research on management of HRS has been directed toward reversal of major pathogenic events such as arterial splanchnic vasodilation and portal hypertension. This may be achieved by the administration of vasoconstrictor drugs or maneuvers aimed at reducing portal pressure. Several recent studies have shown that the administration of vasoconstrictor drugs is associated with an improvement in renal function in a significant number of patients with HRS (Table 5-2). The rationale of vasoconstrictor therapy is to improve circulatory function by causing vasoconstriction of the extremely dilated splanchnic arterial bed, which subsequently improves arterial underfilling, reduces the activity of the endogenous vasoconstrictor systems, and increases renal perfusion.[69–71] Two types of drugs have been used: vasopressin analogues (mainly terlipressin) and α-adrenergic agonists (norepinephrine and midodrine), which act on V1 vasopressin receptors and α_1-adrenergic receptors, respectively, present in vascular smooth muscle cells.

Vasopressin Analogues

The first analogue of vasopressin investigated was ornipressin (8-ornithin vasopressin), an agent with a predominant affinity for V1 receptors located in the vascular smooth muscle cells, particularly abundant in the splanchnic vessels. Ornipressin was initially given in studies of small numbers of patients as an IV infusion of 6 U/hr over 4 hours.[69,72] During the infusion, the mean arterial pressure increased, cardiac output decreased, and renal blood flow and glomerular filtration rate improved as did sodium excretion. Following these positive findings, the effects of a more prolonged administration of ornipressin were investigated. Guevara and colleagues[73] treated eight patients for 3 days with a stepped-dose infusion of ornipressin (2–6 U/hr) plus albumin without observing any side effects but with only a slight improvement in the glomerular filtration rate. They subsequently treated eight additional patients for a longer period

Table 5-2 Vasoconstrictor Drugs Used in the Treatment of Hepatorenal Syndrome

Drug	Dose Range	Median Duration of Therapy	Response to Therapy (%)*	Severe Side Effects (%)†
Terlipressin	1–2 mg/4–12 hr IV bolus	15 days	52‡	13
Norepinephrine	0.1–3 mg/hr IV perfusion	15 days	77§	5
Midodrine	7.5–12.5 mg/8 hr PO	—	43‖	1

*Response to therapy as defined by complete reversal of hepatorenal syndrome (serum creatinine < 1.5 mg/dL (133 μmol/L) in most studies.
†Severe side effects include cardiac arrhythmia or ischemia, other ischemic events, dyspnea, and circulatory overload.
‡From references 77–81, 83–85, and 90. Total number of patients included is 255.
§From references 87 and 90. Total number of patients included is 22.
‖From references 86, 88, and 89. Midodrine was given in association with octreotide. Total number of patients included is 79.

(15 days) with the same regimen. Treatment was associated with a marked improvement in the glomerular filtration rate in four of seven patients treated. Ornipressin had to be discontinued in the remaining three patients because of severe ischemic complications (ischemic colitis and tongue ischemia). A good response rate (four of seven patients) with ornipressin (6 U/hr) plus low-dose dopamine, but without albumin, was also reported in a subsequent study performed by Gülberg and colleagues.[74] One of the patients developed severe intestinal ischemia. These studies confirmed the reversibility of HRS under pharmacologic therapy with a vasoconstrictor drug. However, due to the high incidence of adverse events related to ornipressin, the research was then focused on terlipressin, an analogue of vasopressin approved for the treatment of gastrointestinal bleeding caused by esophageal varices.[75,76]

Terlipressin, a product of the cleavage of triglycil-lysine-vasopressin, is the vasoconstrictor drug that has been used more frequently in HRS and thus far does not seem to share the high rate of ischemic complications observed with ornipressin. Moreover, its slow metabolism results in a prolonged half-life, which allows intermittent IV dosing. A preliminary crossover study demonstrated that terlipressin treatment for 2 days was more effective than placebo in improving renal function in patients with HRS without causing adverse effects.[70] However, improvement was very mild due to the short duration of treatment. A number of nonrandomized phase 2 studies using combined therapy of terlipressin (0.5–2 mg/4 hr for 15 days) plus albumin (1 g/kg of body weight on the first day and 20–40 g/day thereafter) including a total of 152 patients (87% with type 1 HRS) have shown a high response rate, ranging from 44% to 77%.[77–81] In most studies, the definition used for response to therapy was a decrease in serum creatinine to less than 1.5 mg/dL (133 μmol/L), although in some studies a decrease of 20% to 30% of serum creatinine from baseline was considered a response to therapy. The average survival rate of patients included in these phase 2 studies was 60% at 1 month. Recurrence of HRS after terlipressin withdrawal may occur in as many as 20% of patients, although some studies reported a higher rate, and treatment of recurrence is usually effective.[77–79,81,82]

So far, only three randomized, comparative studies have been reported assessing the effects of terlipressin on renal function and survival in patients with HRS.[83–85] One small trial from Solanki and colleagues[83] randomized 24 patients to either low-dose terlipressin (1 mg/12 hr) or placebo for 15 days in combination with albumin and fresh frozen plasma. Complete reversal of HRS was observed in 42% of patients treated with terlipressin. Survival was longer in patients treated with terlipressin compared with those treated with placebo, and transient cardiac arrhythmia was seen in three patients treated with terlipressin. The results of two larger randomized, controlled studies were reported recently.[84,85] The Spanish trial[85] included 46 patients with HRS, 74% of them with type 1 HRS, and the American trial[84] included 112 patients, all with type 1 HRS. The two studies used very similar treatment regimens of terlipressin plus albumin for 2 weeks. The starting dose of terlipressin was 1 mg/4 to 6 hr IV and was increased to a maximum of 2 mg/4 to 6 hr after 2 to 3 days if there was no response to therapy as defined by a reduction in serum creatinine of greater than 25% to 30% of pretreatment values. Reversal of HRS, as defined by a decrease in serum creatinine to less than 1.5 mg/dL, was observed in 39% of patients in the Spanish study and 34% of patients in the American study. In addition to a marked decrease in the high serum creatinine levels, response to therapy was characterized by an increase in arterial pressure, high urine output, and a marked increase in the low serum sodium concentration.[85] The latter could be due to improved glomerular filtration rate and/or suppression of antidiuretic hormone after improvement in effective arterial blood volume and is consistent with a predominant action of terlipressin on V1 over V2 antidiuretic hormone receptors. The frequency of ischemic side effects requiring the discontinuation of treatment was approximately 10%. Some patients developed transient pulmonary edema during the first few days of therapy, even with close monitoring of central venous pressure. In none of the studies was treatment with terlipressin and albumin associated with an improved survival compared with the control group of patients treated with albumin alone. However, both studies showed that responders in terms of improvement in renal function after therapy had a significant, albeit moderate, increase in survival compared with nonresponders (median survival > 90 days versus 13 days, respectively, in one of the studies).[85] Nevertheless, it is important to emphasize that despite the improved survival, responders still have a high risk of death in the short term, which is particularly important in patients awaiting liver transplantation. Further studies in larger patient populations are needed to definitively assess the effect of treatment with terlipressin on survival of patients with type 1 HRS.

There are two major shortcomings of the treatment with terlipressin: lack of availability in some countries and high cost, the latter being a major limiting factor for its use in some areas of the world. These two drawbacks have prompted the investigation of other vasoconstrictor drugs.

α-Adrenergic Agonists

α-Adrenergic agonists (norepinephrine, midodrine) represent an attractive alternative to terlipressin because of the low cost and wide availability compared with terlipressin.[86–90] However, the information on the efficacy and side effects of α-adrenergic agonists in patients with type 1 HRS is still very limited. A small study from Angeli and colleagues[86] looked at the efficacy of midodrine in combination with octreotide, a somatostatin analogue used for gastrointestinal bleeding, and compared it with nonpressor doses of dopamine (both groups also received albumin 20–40 g/day). The rationale for the use of a somatostatin analogue is to suppress glucagon as well as other splanchnic vasodilator peptides. In the five patients treated with octreotide and midodrine, the authors observed an improvement in serum creatinine and glomerular filtration rate, as well as sodium excretion, and suppression of renin and aldosterone with a decrease in glucagon and nitric oxide levels. No changes or even a worsening of renal parameters were observed in a small control group of nonrandomized patients. In a retrospective study, patients treated with octreotide and midodrine had a higher rate of sustained response (40%) and a lower mortality rate (43%) compared with contemporaneous patients not treated (10% and 71%, respectively), although the study is limited by the retrospective design.[89] It appears that octreotide alone without the simultaneous use of vasoconstrictors does not improve renal function. In fact, a small placebo-controlled, crossover trial showed that octreotide plus albumin was not effective for the treatment of HRS.[91]

Norepinephrine in combination with albumin has been assessed because of its potent vasoconstrictor effect on both arterial and venous circulation and its wide availability. Infusion of norepinephrine (0.5–3 mg/hr) together with administration of albumin and furosemide to keep central venous pressure in the range of 4 to 10 cm of water was shown to reverse type 1 HRS in 10 of 12 patients after a median of 7 days.[87] In addition to an increase in mean arterial pressure and a marked decrease in the activity of the renin-aldosterone system, sodium excretion also increased. The only adverse event reported was an episode of reversible myocardial hypokinesia probably related to cardiac ischemia. Three patients could undergo liver transplantation with a normal serum creatinine. A recent randomized study compared norepinephrine plus albumin with terlipressin plus albumin until reversal of HRS or 15 days of therapy.[90] The study randomized 22 patients with HRS (either type 1 or 2) and observed a reversal rate of 70% with norepinephrine and 83% (not significant) with terlipressin. Both groups had a significant improvement in circulatory function. The results of these two studies suggest that norepinephrine may be a good alternative to terlipressin. Nevertheless, larger studies are needed to confirm that α-adrenergic agonists are equally effective as terlipressin in the management of HRS.

Adjunctive Therapy to Vasoconstrictors

In most studies, vasoconstrictors have been given in combination with IV albumin with the aim of further improving the arterial underfilling. The rationale of the concomitant use of albumin is in part based on studies of head-of-water immersion in patients with ascites without HRS that showed that expansion of central blood volume (together with a vasoconstrictor) is necessary to overcome sodium avidity and achieve a negative sodium balance.[92] In addition to its effects as plasma expander, albumin administration may also have beneficial effects related to its antioxidant properties or its ability to improve endothelial function, although this clearly needs further studies.[93] The possible role of albumin in improving response to vasoconstrictors for patients with HRS was investigated in two studies, the designs of which unfortunately limit their conclusions. Ortega and colleagues[81] undertook a sequential observational study, in which the first 13 patients were given terlipressin (0.5 up to 2 mg/4 hr) plus albumin (1 g/kg of body weight for the first day followed by 20–40 g/day thereafter) and the subsequent eight patients received terlipressin alone. In the group receiving the combined therapy, 77% achieved a complete reversal of HRS (decrease in serum creatinine value to < 1.5 mg/dL) compared with significantly lower percentage (25%) in the group receiving terlipressin alone. The second study was a retrospective evaluation of a group of patients treated with terlipressin.[80] In the 68 patients who received terlipressin in combination with albumin, the response rate (decrease in serum creatinine > 20%) was 62% compared with 48% in the 23 patients who were given terlipressin alone. This difference in response rate was not significant. Until further studies assessing the role of simultaneous albumin administration are done, the specific properties of albumin and its beneficial effect in combination with vasoconstrictor drugs on reversal of HRS remain controversial. However, as the majority of studies showing reversal of HRS have used albumin, its use as an adjunctive therapy to vasoconstrictors is currently recommended.[41,77,81,83–85,93] Whether plasma expansion could be done with synthetic agents such as hydroxyethyl starch instead of albumin remains to be assessed.[94] Nevertheless, accumulation of these agents and osmotic tubular damage reported in renal failure could be problematic.[95,96]

Transjugular Intrahepatic Portosystemic Shunts

Only a few studies have reported on the effects of a transjugular intrahepatic portosystemic shunt (TIPS) in patients with type 1 HRS.[97,98] A TIPS is a stent placed via the jugular vein in the liver parenchyma to create a direct communication between portal vein and hepatic veins aimed at reducing the increased portal pressure characteristic of advanced cirrhosis and HRS. In patients with type 1 HRS, a TIPS improves circulatory function and reduces the activity of vasoconstrictor systems. This is associated with a slow decrease in serum creatinine levels in approximately 60% of patients. Median survival after insertion of a TIPS in patients with type 1 HRS ranges between 2 and 4 months. The utility of a TIPS in patients with type 1 HRS is low because a TIPS is contraindicated in patients with severe liver failure, manifested by high serum bilirubin levels and/or high MELD scores and/or hepatic encephalopathy, which are common findings in the setting of type 1 HRS. Hepatic encephalopathy is particularly common after TIPS placement and is directly related to the shunting of the blood to the systemic circulation. In two studies including a small number of patients, TIPSs have been used as a sequential therapy in selected patients with HRS in whom renal function improved after treatment with vasoconstrictors (either terlipressin or midodrine plus octreotide).[79,88] In both studies, a TIPS further improved renal function. In one of the studies, sodium excretion also improved, and there was a marked decrease in renin and aldosterone at 1 month post–TIPS insertion.[88] Although this approach (vasoconstrictors followed by TIPS insertion) appears promising, more information is needed before it can be generalized in clinical practice.

Other Therapeutic Methods

Renal replacement therapy (hemodialysis or continuous venovenous hemodiafiltration) has been used in the management of patients with type 1 HRS, especially in patients who are candidates for liver transplantation, in an attempt to keep patients alive until liver transplantation is performed or a spontaneous improvement in renal function occurs.[99–103] Unfortunately, the potential beneficial effect of this approach has not been unequivocally demonstrated.[104] The clinical experience is that most patients do not tolerate hemodialysis well and develop major side effects, including severe arterial hypotension, bleeding, and infections, that may contribute to death during treatment. Some authors have suggested a better tolerance for continuous venovenous hemodiafiltration, but no study compared both therapies in patients with the same degree of liver impairment and studies done in the general intensive care unit population failed to demonstrate any superiority of one over the other.[104–108] Conversely, findings that indicate the need for renal replacement therapy (severe fluid overload, acidosis, or hyperkalemia) are uncommon in type 1 HRS, at least in early stages. Therefore, the initial therapy for these patients should probably include measures aimed at improving circulatory function (particularly vasoconstrictors) before renal replacement therapy is started.

Extracorporeal albumin dialysis, such as the molecular adsorbents recirculation system, is a system that uses an albumin-containing dialysate that is recirculated and perfused through a charcoal and anion-exchanger column, combined with a hemodialysis filter. It has been reported that the molecular adsorbents recirculation system improves renal function and survival in a small series of patients with HRS, but these results require confirmation in larger series of patients.[109] A multicenter European study (the Helios study) using a new extracorporeal adsorbent dialysis system, called Prometheus and based on recycling of patients' own albumin, is actually under way to specifically assess the efficacy of this device in patients with HRS. The use of albumin dialysis in the treatment of HRS should currently be restricted to investigational purposes.

Recommendations for Therapy of Type 1 Hepatorenal Syndrome

Given the limited information, particularly the low number of randomized, controlled studies on treatments of HRS, the following recommendations are based both on existing data and on the authors' experience (Fig. 5-1).

In patients who are candidates for liver transplantation, every effort should be made to include patients on the waiting list as soon as possible. Most patients with type 1 HRS will die while awaiting transplantation due to their extremely poor prognosis unless a system of prioritization of patients exists. In this regard, the use of MELD score as a system for organ allocation may increase the applicability of transplantation in patients with type 1 HRS by reducing waiting list mortality. Considering the relatively high morbidity and

mortality after liver transplantation in patients with type 1 HRS, patients should ideally be treated while awaiting transplantation in an attempt to improve renal function before transplantation. Among the different treatments available, the administration of vasoconstrictors plus albumin appears to be the method of choice because of its efficacy and easy applicability. Treatment with vasoconstrictors improves survival in responder patients and may also improve outcome after transplantation. However, given the limited survival effect, patients responding to therapy should probably be maintained on the waitlist with their pretreatment MELD score to avoid reducing their access to transplantation. Among the different vasoconstrictors available, terlipressin has been the drug most commonly used and should be considered the first choice of treatment. Norepinephrine or midodrine appear to be suitable alternatives if terlipressin is not available. Midodrine should be given in association with octreotide. Patients treated with vasoconstrictors should be hospitalized and closely monitored for adverse events, particularly ischemic complications and circulatory overload. Renal replacement therapy or insertion of a TIPS should be reserved for patients not responding to vasoconstrictors. Methods of albumin dialysis should be used only in the setting of prospective studies.

Recommendations for patients with type 1 HRS who are not candidates for liver transplantation are difficult to propose with the limited available information. In these patients,

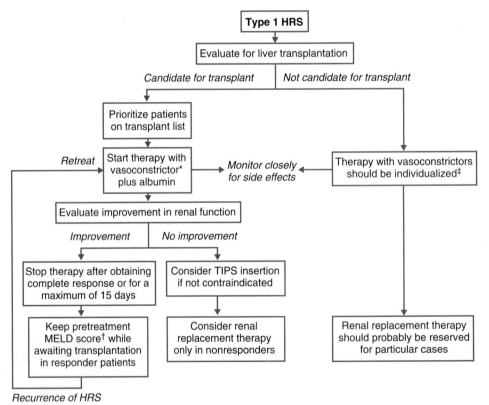

Figure 5-1 Proposed algorithm for the management of type 1 hepatorenal syndrome (HRS). *Either terlipressin, if available, or norepinephrine; therapy with a combination of midodrine and octreotide could also be an option. †MELD (Model for End-Stage Liver Disease) score (see text for details). ‡Patients for whom a limited survival advantage (in case of response) could be beneficial (e.g., alcoholic patients who could reach abstinence period sufficient to be placed on transplant list). TIPS, transjugular intrahepatic portosystemic shunt.

the appropriateness of a specific therapy for HRS should be evaluated in the context of the clinical characteristics of patients (e.g., age, severity of liver failure, possible improvement in liver disease). If treatment is considered appropriate, vasoconstrictors are probably the best option. A TIPS has a low utility and a high cost and is not available in many centers. Methods of renal replacement therapy should probably be used only in very specific cases, whereas albumin dialysis should be used only in the setting of prospective controlled studies.

MANAGEMENT OF TYPE 2 HEPATORENAL SYNDROME

General Measures

Unlike patients with type 1 HRS, patients with type 2 HRS can be managed as outpatients unless they develop complications that require hospitalization. The most frequent clinical finding of these patients is refractory ascites. Diuretics should be given only if they cause a significant natriuresis (i.e., urine sodium > 30 mEq/day).[110] Care should be taken with the use of spironolactone and other potassium-sparing diuretics in these patients because of the risk of developing hyperkalemia. Repeated paracentesis with IV albumin is likely the method of choice for the treatment of large ascites in these patients.[110] If hyponatremia is present, total fluid intake should be restricted to approximately 1000 to 1500 mL/day. Bacterial infections should be diagnosed and treated early due to the risk of precipitating type 1 HRS. Patients with low protein concentration in the ascitic fluid (<15 g/L) should receive prophylactic treatment with norfloxacin (400 mg/day) to prevent the development of

spontaneous bacterial peritonitis and reduce the risk of type 1 HRS (see later).[111]

Specific Therapies

Liver transplantation is the treatment of choice for candidate patients. As for patients with type 1 HRS, the use of MELD score for organ allocation in liver transplantation is probably the best method to reduce mortality of those on the waitlist. Results from small studies suggest that the administration of vasoconstrictors improves renal function in these patients.[79,81,85,90] Because of the paucity of data in patients with type 2 HRS, it is currently unknown whether all patients should be treated with vasoconstrictors. Candidates for liver transplantation should probably be treated to improve renal function before transplantation. The use of a TIPS in patients with type 2 HRS is associated with an improvement in renal function, better control of ascites, and decreased risk of progression from type 2 to type 1 HRS.[112] However, a TIPS does not improve survival in these patients compared with treatment with repeated paracentesis and IV albumin.[112,113] Therefore, the beneficial effects of a TIPS in reducing ascites recurrence rate and progression to type 1 HRS in patients with type 2 HRS should be weighed against the lack of improvement in survival rate, increased risk of encephalopathy, and high costs. Recommendations for the management of patients with type 2 HRS are outlined in Figure 5-2.

PREVENTION

There is limited, yet important, information on the prevention of HRS. Two strategies are used to prevent the development of HRS in patients with cirrhosis. The first strategy is to use

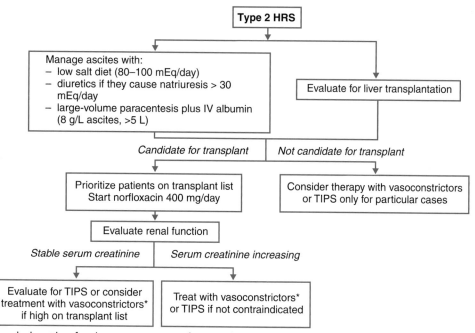

Figure 5-2 Proposed algorithm for the management of type 2 hepatorenal syndrome (HRS). *Terlipressin should be the preferred choice as information for norepinephrine and midodrine is lacking or limited. TIPS, transjugular intrahepatic portosystemic shunt.

Box 5-2 Key Concepts

1. HRS is a relatively common complication of cirrhosis and is characterized by a marked splanchnic arterial vasodilation leading to an extreme underfilling of the arterial circulation resulting in a marked renal vasoconstriction and reduction in glomerular filtration rate.
2. Liver transplantation is the definitive treatment for selected patients. However, waitlist mortality is high and posttransplantation outcome impaired in patients with HRS, particularly in those with type 1 HRS. Treatment of HRS before transplantation may help reduce waitlist mortality and improve posttransplantation outcome.
3. Specific treatments for HRS are aimed at improving the underfilling of the arterial circulation and include vasoconstrictors plus albumin and insertion of a TIPS. Both restoring effective plasma volume and improving vasodilation seem essential for the reversal of HRS.
4. The best treatment option for patients with type 1 HRS is terlipressin plus albumin because they improve renal function in as many as 40% of patients. Alternative drugs are norepinephrine and midodrine, but information is limited. A TIPS may be effective but has low applicability because it is contraindicated in patients with poor liver function.
5. Response to therapy (i.e., improvement in renal function) with vasoconstrictors is associated with an increased survival rate.
6. Hemodialysis should probably be used only in candidates for transplantation not responding to pharmacologic treatment. Extracorporeal albumin dialysis is promising, but requires further evaluation. CKLT should not be used in patients with type 1 HRS unless prolonged hemodialysis makes reversal of HRS unlikely.
7. Treatment of type 2 HRS with vasoconstrictors plus albumin is effective, but information is very limited. A TIPS improves renal function and management of ascites in these patients, but does not seem to improve survival, although more studies are needed.
8. Effective prevention of HRS in patients with spontaneous bacterial peritonitis is achieved by the administration of albumin together with antibiotics. The long-term administration of norfloxacin to patients with cirrhosis and ascites is associated with a reduced risk of developing HRS. Pentoxifylline reduces the risk of HRS in patients with alcoholic hepatitis.

albumin to prevent the deterioration of circulatory function that frequently occurs in patients with cirrhosis and spontaneous bacterial peritonitis.[114] In patients with spontaneous bacterial peritonitis, the administration of albumin (1.5 g/kg IV at the diagnosis of the infection and 1 g/kg IV 48 hours later) together with antibiotics improves circulatory function and reduces markedly the occurrence of HRS compared with the standard treatment with antibiotics alone (10% in the albumin group versus 33% in the nonalbumin group).[114] This effective prevention of HRS results in an improvement in survival.

The second strategy used for the prevention of HRS is either the inhibition of cytokines related to bacterial products, particularly tumor necrosis factor α, or selective intestinal decontamination to suppress the deleterious effects of bacterial translocation on cardiovascular function.[20,115] In patients with alcoholic hepatitis, the administration of pentoxifylline (400 mg three times daily), a drug that inhibits tumor necrosis factor α, was shown to reduce the occurrence of HRS and mortality (8% and 24%, respectively) compared with a control group (35% and 46%, respectively).[116] Finally, a recent study showed that long-term treatment with norfloxacin (400 mg/day) in patients with advanced cirrhosis and ascites was associated with a lower risk of developing HRS compared with a control group of patients receiving placebo.[111] In this study, the beneficial effect of norfloxacin in the prevention of HRS was not related to the effect of the drug in preventing the development of spontaneous bacterial peritonitis. More studies are needed to further evaluate these and other strategies for the prevention of HRS in cirrhosis.

Box 5-2 reviews key concepts in this chapter.

References

1. Moreau R, Lebrec D: Review article: Hepatorenal syndrome—definitions and diagnosis. Aliment Pharmacol Ther 2004; 20(Suppl 3):24–28.
2. Arroyo V, Terra C, Torre A, Ginès P: Hepatorenal syndrome in cirrhosis: Clinical features, diagnosis, and management. In Ginès P, Arroyo V, Rodés J, Schrier RW (eds): Ascites and Renal Dysfunction in Liver Disease. Malden, MA: Blackwell Publishing, 2005, pp 341–359.
3. Cárdenas A, Ginès P: Therapy insight: Management of hepatorenal syndrome. Nat Clin Pract Gastroenterol Hepatol 2006;3:338–348.
4. Wadei H, Mai ML, Ahsan N, Gonwa TA: Hepatorenal syndrome: Pathophysiology and management. Clin J Am Soc Nephrol 2006;1:1066–1079.
5. Arroyo V, Terra C, Ginès P: Advances in the pathogenesis and treatment of type-1 and type-2 hepatorenal syndrome. J Hepatol 2007;46:535–546.
6. Flint A: Clinical report on hydro-peritoneum based on an analysis of forty-six cases. Am J Med Sci 1863;45:306–339.
7. Ring-Larsen H: Renal blood flow in cirrhosis: Relation to systemic and portal haemodynamics and liver function. Scand J Clin Lab Invest 1977;37:635–642.
8. Vorobioff J, Bredfeldt J, Groszmann R: Hyperdynamic circulation in portal-hypertensive rat model: A primary factor for maintenance of chronic portal hypertension. Am J Physiol 1983;244: G52–G57.
9. Schrier RW, Arroyo V, Bernardi M, et al: Peripheral arterial vasodilation hypothesis: A proposal for the initiation of renal sodium and water retention in cirrhosis. Hepatology 1988;8: 1151–1157.
10. Martin PY, Ginès P, Schrier RW: Mechanisms of disease—nitric oxide as a mediator of hemodynamic abnormalities and sodium and water retention in cirrhosis. N Engl J Med 1998;339:533–541.

11. Arroyo V, Colmenero J: Ascites and hepatorenal syndrome in cirrhosis: Pathophysiological basis of therapy and current management. J Hepatol 2003;38(Suppl 1):S69–S89.

12. Hamilton G, Phing R, Hutton R, et al: The relationship between prostacyclin activity and pressure in the portal vein. Hepatology 1982;2:236–242.

13. Guarner C, Soriano G, Tomas A, et al: Increased serum nitrite and nitrate levels in patients with cirrhosis: Relationship to endotoxemia. Hepatology 1993;18:1139–1143.

14. Battista S, Bar F, Mengozzi G, et al: Hyperdynamic circulation in patients with cirrhosis: direct measurement of nitric oxide levels in hepatic and portal veins. J Hepatol 1997;26:75–80.

15. Sarela A, Mihaimeed F, Batten J, et al: Hepatic and splanchnic nitric oxide activity in patients with cirrhosis. Gut 1999;44:749–753.

16. Wiest R, Groszmann R: Nitric oxide and portal hypertension: Its role in the regulation of intrahepatic and splanchnic vascular resistance. Semin Liver Dis 1999;19:411–426.

17. Ruiz-Del-Arbol L, Urman J, Fernandez J, et al: Systemic, renal, and hepatic hemodynamic derangement in cirrhotic patients with spontaneous bacterial peritonitis. Hepatology 2003;38:1210–1218.

18. Grange JD, Amiot X: Nitric oxide and renal function in cirrhotic patients with ascites: From physiopathology to practice. Eur J Gastroenterol Hepatol 2004;16:567–570.

19. Blendis L, Wong F: SBP and the pathogenesis of renal failure: The hidden triangle. Gastroenterology 2004;127:352–354.

20. Wiest R, Garcia-Tsao G: Bacterial translocation (BT) in cirrhosis. Hepatology 2005;41:422–433.

21. Schroeder E, Anderson G, Goldman S, Streeten D: Effect of blockade of angiotensin II on blood pressure, renin and aldosterone in cirrhosis. Kidney Int 1976;9:511–519.

22. Arroyo V, Planas R, Gaya J, et al: Sympathetic nervous activity, renin-angiotensin system and renal excretion of prostaglandin E2 in cirrhosis. Relationship to functional renal failure and sodium and water excretion. Eur J Clin Invest 1983;13:271–278.

23. Henriksen J, Ring-Larsen H, Christensen NJ: Autonomic nervous function in liver disease. In Bomzom A, Blendis L (eds): Cardiovascular Complications of Liver Disease. Boca Raton, FL: CRC Press, 1990, pp 63–79.

24. Dudley FJ, Esler M: The sympathetic nervous system in cirrhosis. In Ginès P, Arroyo V, Rodés J, Schrier RW (eds): Ascites and Renal Dysfunction in Liver Disease. Malden, MA: Blackwell Publishing, 2005, pp 54–72.

25. Arroyo V, Rodés J, Gutierrez-Lizarraga MA, Revert L: Prognostic value of spontaneous hyponatremia in cirrhosis with ascites. Am J Dig Dis 1976;21:249–256.

26. Anderson R, Cronin R, McDonald K, Schrier R: Mechanisms of portal hypertension-induced alterations in renal hemodynamics, renal water excretion and renin secretion. J Clin Invest 1976;58:964–970.

27. Schrier RW: Pathogenesis of sodium and water retention in high-output and low-output cardiac failure, nephrotic syndrome, cirrhosis, and pregnancy. N Engl J Med 1988;319:1065–1072.

28. Ginès P, Berl T, Bernardi M, et al: Hyponatremia in cirrhosis: From pathogenesis to treatment. Hepatology 1998;28:851–864.

29. Porcel A, Diaz F, Rendon P: Dilutional hyponatremia in patients with cirrhosis and ascites. Arch Intern Med 2002;162:323–328.

30. Ginès A, Escorsell A, Ginès P, et al: Incidence, predictive factors, and prognosis of the hepatorenal syndrome in cirrhosis with ascites. Gastroenterology 1993;105:229–236.

31. Maroto A, Ginès P, Arroyo V, et al: Brachial and femoral artery blood flow in cirrhosis: Relationship to kidney dysfunction. Hepatology 1993;17:788–793.

32. Lagi A, La Villa G, Barletta G: Cerebral autoregulation in patients with cirrhosis and ascites. A transcranial study. J Hepatol 1997;27:114–120.

33. Bernardi M, Rubboli A, Trevisani F, et al: Reduced cardiovascular responsiveness to exercise-induced sympathoadrenergic stimulation in patients with cirrhosis. J Hepatol 1991;12:207–216.

34. Pozzi M, Carugo S, Boari G, et al: Evidence of functional and structural cardiac abnormalities in cirrhotic patients with and without ascites. Hepatology 1997;26:1131–1137.

35. Wong F, Liu P, Lilly L, et al: Role of cardiac structural and functional abnormalities in the pathogenesis of hyperdynamic circulation and renal sodium retention in cirrhosis. Clin Sci (Lond) 1999;97:259–267.

36. Torregrosa M, Aguade S, Dos L, et al: Cardiac alterations in cirrhosis: Reversibility after liver transplantation. J Hepatol 2005;42:68–74.

37. Liu H, Lee SS: The heart in cirrhosis. In Ginès P, Arroyo V, Rodés J, Schrier RW (eds): Ascites and Renal Dysfunction in Liver Disease. Malden, MA: Blackwell Publishing, 2005, pp 186–197.

38. Ruiz-Del-Arbol L, Monescillo A, Arocena C, et al: Circulatory function and hepatorenal syndrome in cirrhosis. Hepatology 2005;42:239–240.

39. Alessandria C, Ozdogan O, Guevara M, et al: MELD score and clinical type predict prognosis in hepatorenal syndrome: Relevance to liver transplantation. Hepatology 2005;41:1282–1289.

40. Arroyo V, Ginès P, Gerbes AL, et al: Definition and diagnostic criteria of refractory ascites and hepatorenal syndrome in cirrhosis. International Ascites Club. Hepatology 1996;23:164–176.

41. Salerno F, Gerbes A, Ginès P, et al: Diagnosis, prevention and treatment of the hepatorenal syndrome in cirrhosis. A consensus workshop of the International Ascites Club. Gut 2007;56:1310–1318.

42. Bataller R, Ginès P, Guevara M, Arroyo V: Hepatorenal syndrome. Semin Liver Dis 1997;17:233–247.

43. Lhotta K: Beyond hepatorenal syndrome: Glomerulonephritis in patients with liver disease. Semin Nephrol 2002;22:302–308.

44. Poole B, Schrier RW, Jani A: Glomerular disease in cirrhosis. In Ginès P, Arroyo V, Rodés J, Schrier RW (eds): Ascites and Renal Dysfunction in Liver Disease. Malden, MA: Blackwell Publishing, 2005, pp 360–370.

45. Salerno F, Badalamenti S: Drug-induced renal failure in cirrhosis. In Ginès P, Arroyo V, Rodés J, Schrier R (eds): Ascites and Renal Dysfunction in Liver Disease. Malden, MA: Blackwell Publishing, 2005, pp 372–382.

46. Watt K, Uhanova J, Minuk G: Hepatorenal syndrome: Diagnostic accuracy, clinical features, and outcome in a tertiary care center. Am J Gastroenterol 2002;97:2046–2050.

47. Blendis L, Wong F: The natural history and management of hepatorenal disorders: From pre-ascites to hepatorenal syndrome. Clin Med 2003;3:154–159.

48. Moller S, Henriksen JH: Review article: Pathogenesis and pathophysiology of hepatorenal syndrome—is there a scope for prevention? Aliment Pharmacol Ther 2004;20(Suppl 3):31–41.

49. Guevara M, Ortega R, Ginès P, Rodés J: Pathogenesis of renal vasoconstriction in cirrhosis. In Ginès P, Arroyo V, Rodés J, Schrier RW (eds): Ascites and Renal Dysfunction in Liver Disease. Malden, MA: Blackwell Publishing, 2005, pp 329–340.

50. Fernandez J, Ruiz-Del-Arbol L, Gomez C, et al: Norfloxacin versus ceftriaxone in the prophylaxis of infections in patients with advanced cirrhosis and hemorrhage. Gastroenterology 2006;131:1049–1056.

51. Iwatsuki S, Popovtzer MM, Corman JL, et al: Recovery from "hepatorenal syndrome" after orthotopic liver transplantation. N Engl J Med 1973;289:1155–1159.

52. Gonwa TA, Morris CA, Goldstein RM, et al: Long-term survival and renal function following liver transplantation in patients with and without hepatorenal syndrome—experience in 300 patients. Transplantation 1991;51:428–430.

53. Rimola A, Navasa M, Grande L, Garcia-Valdecasas JC: Liver transplantation for patients with cirrhosis and ascites. In Ginès P, Arroyo V, Rodés J, Schrier RW (eds): Ascites and Renal Dysfunction in Liver Disease. Malden, MA: Blackwell Publishing, 2005, pp 271–285.

54. Jeyarajah D, Gonwa TA, McBride MA, et al: Hepatorenal syndrome: Combined liver kidney transplants versus isolated liver transplant. Transplantation 1997;64:1760–1765.

55. Nair S, Verma S, Thuluvath PJ: Pretransplant renal function predicts survival in patients undergoing orthotopic liver transplantation. Hepatology 2002;35:1179–1185.

56. Ruiz R, Kunitake H, Wilkinson AH, et al: Long-term analysis of combined liver and kidney transplantation at a single center. Arch Surg 2006;141:735–741.

57. Ruiz R, Barri YM, Jennings LW, et al: Hepatorenal syndrome: A proposal for kidney after liver transplantation (KALT). Liver Transplant 2007;13:838–843.

58. Malinchoc M, Kamath PS, Gordon FD, et al: A model to predict poor survival in patients undergoing transjugular intrahepatic portosystemic shunts. Hepatology 2000;31:864–871.

59. Wiesner R, Edwards E, Freeman R, et al: Model for End-Stage Liver Disease (MELD) and allocation of donor livers. Gastroenterology 2003;124:91–96.

60. O'Riordan A, Wong V, McQuillan R, et al: Acute renal failure, as defined by the RIFLE criteria, post-liver transplantation. Am J Transplant 2007;7:168–176.

61. Restuccia T, Ortega R, Guevara M, et al: Effects of treatment of hepatorenal syndrome before transplantation on posttransplantation outcome. A case-control study. J Hepatol 2004;40:140–146.

62. Jeyarajah D, Gonwa TA, McBride MA, et al: Hepatorenal syndrome. Transplantation 1997;64:1760–1765.

63. O'Mahony C, Barshes N, Vierling J, et al: Combined liver and kidney transplantation should be considered in patients with hepatorenal syndrome requiring renal replacement therapy greater than 1 week [abstract 783]. Transplantation 2006; 82(Suppl 3 WTC):331.

64. Davis CL, Feng S, Sung R, et al: Simultaneous liver-kidney transplantation: Evaluation to decision making. Am J Transplant 2007;7:1702–1709.

65. Bennet W, Keefe E, Melnyk C, et al: Response to dopamine hydrochloride in the hepatorenal syndrome. Arch Intern Med 1975;135:964–971.

66. Wilson J. Dopamine in the hepatorenal syndrome. JAMA 1977;238:2719–2720.

67. Ginès A, Salmeron JM, Ginès P: Oral misoprostol or intravenous prostaglandin E2 do not improve renal function in patients with cirrhosis and ascites with hyponatremia or renal failure. J Hepatol 1993;17:220–226.

68. Clewell J, Walker-Renard P: Prostaglandins for the treatment of hepatorenal syndrome. Ann Pharmacother 1994;28:54–55.

69. Lenz K, Hortnagl H, Druml W, et al: Ornipressin in the treatment of functional renal failure in decompensated liver cirrhosis. Effects on renal hemodynamics and atrial natriuretic factor. Gastroenterology 1991;101:1060–1067.

70. Hadengue A, Gadano A, Moreau R, et al: Beneficial effects of the 2-day administration of terlipressin in patients with cirrhosis and hepatorenal syndrome. J Hepatol 1998;29:565–570.

71. Therapondos G, Stanley A, Hayes P: Systemic, portal and renal effects of terlipressin in patients with cirrhotic ascites: Pilot study. J Gastroenterol Hepatol 2004;19:73–77.

72. Lenz K, Hortnagl H, Druml W, et al: Beneficial effect of 8-ornithin vasopressin on renal dysfunction in decompensated cirrhosis. Gut 1989;30:90–96.

73. Guevara M, Ginès P, Fernandez-Esparrach G, et al: Reversibility of hepatorenal syndrome by prolonged administration of ornipressin and plasma volume expansion. Hepatology 1998;27:35–41.

74. Gülberg V, Bilzer M, Gerbes AL: Long-term therapy and retreatment of hepatorenal syndrome type 1 with ornipressin and dopamine. Hepatology 1999;30:870–875.

75. Feu F, Del Arbol LR, Banares R, et al: Double-blind randomized controlled trial comparing terlipressin and somatostatin for acute variceal hemorrhage. Gastroenterology 1996;111:1291–1299.

76. Escorsell A, Del Arbol LR, Planas R, et al: Multicenter randomized controlled trial of terlipressin versus sclerotherapy in the treatment of acute variceal bleeding: The TEST study. Hepatology 2000;32:471–476.

77. Uriz J, Ginès P, Cárdenas A, et al: Terlipressin plus albumin infusion: An effective and safe therapy of hepatorenal syndrome. J Hepatol 2000;33:43–48.

78. Mulkay JP, Louis H, Donckier V, et al: Long-term terlipressin administration improves renal function in cirrhotic patients with type 1 hepatorenal syndrome: A pilot study. Acta Gastroenterol Belg 2001;64:15–19.

79. Alessandria C, Venon W, Marzano A: Renal failure in cirrhotic patients: Role of terlipressin in clinical approach to hepatorenal syndrome type 2. Eur J Gastroenterol Hepatol 2002;14:1363–1368.

80. Moreau R, Durand F, Poynard T, et al: Terlipressin in patients with cirrhosis and type 1 hepatorenal syndrome: A retrospective multicenter study. Gastroenterology 2002;122:923–930.

81. Ortega R, Ginès P, Uriz J, et al: Terlipressin therapy with and without albumin for patients with hepatorenal syndrome: Results of a prospective, nonrandomized study. Hepatology 2002;36:941–948.

82. Colle I, Durand F, Pessione F, et al: Clinical course, predictive factors and prognosis in patients with cirrhosis and type 1 hepatorenal syndrome treated with terlipressin: A retrospective analysis. J Gastroenterol Hepatol 2002;17:882–888.

83. Solanki P, Chawla A, Garg R, et al: Beneficial effects of terlipressin in hepatorenal syndrome: A prospective, randomized placebo-controlled clinical trial. J Gastroenterol Hepatol 2003;18:152–156.

84. Sanyal AJ, Boyer T, Garcia-Tsao G, et al: A randomized prospective, double blind placebo controlled trial of terlipressin for type 1 hepatorenal syndrome. Gastroenterology 2008, in press.

85. Martín-Llahí M, Pépin MN, Guevara M, et al: Terlipressin and albumin vs albumin in patients with cirrhosis and hepatorenal syndrome: A randomized study. Gastroenterology 2008, in press.

86. Angeli P, Volpin R, Gerunda G, et al: Reversal of type 1 hepatorenal syndrome with the administration of midodrine and octreotide. Hepatology 1999;29:1690–1697.

87. Duvoux C, Zanditenas D, Hezode C, et al: Effects of noradrenalin and albumin in patients with type I hepatorenal syndrome: A pilot study. Hepatology 2002;36:374–380.

88. Wong F, Pantea L, Sniderman K: Midodrine, octreotide, albumin, and TIPS in selected patients with cirrhosis and type 1 hepatorenal syndrome. Hepatology 2004;40:55–64.

89. Esrailian E, Pantangco E, Kyulo N, et al: Octreotide/midodrine therapy significantly improves renal function and 30-day survival in patients with type 1 hepatorenal syndrome. Dig Dis Sci 2007;52:742–748.

90. Alessandria C, Ottobrelli A, Debernardi-Venon W, et al: Noradrenalin vs terlipressin in patients with hepatorenal syndrome: A prospective, randomized, unblinded, pilot study. J Hepatol 2007;47:499–505.

91. Pomier-Layrargues G, Paquin SC, Hassoun Z, et al: Octreotide in hepatorenal syndrome: A randomized, double-blind, placebo-controlled, crossover study. Hepatology 2003;38:238–243.

92. Nicholls KM, Shapiro MD, Kluge R, et al: Sodium excretion in advanced cirrhosis: Effect of expansion of central blood volume and suppression of plasma aldosterone. Hepatology 1986;6:235–238.

93. Wong F: Drug insight: The role of albumin in the management of chronic liver disease. Nat Clin Pract Gastroenterol Hepatol 2007;4:43–51.

94. Saner F, Kavuk I, Lang H, et al: Terlipressin and gelafundin: Safe therapy of hepatorenal syndrome. Eur J Med Res 2004;9:78–82.

95. Davidson I: Renal impact of fluid management with colloids: A comparative review. Eur J Anaesthesiol 2006;23:721–738.

96. Vincent J: The pros and cons of hydroxyethyl starch solutions. Anesth Analg 2007;104:484–486.

97. Guevara M, Ginès P, Bandi JC, et al: Transjugular intrahepatic portosystemic shunt in hepatorenal syndrome: Effects on renal function and vasoactive systems. Hepatology 1998;28:416–422.

98. Brensing KA, Textor J, Perz J, et al: Long term outcome after transjugular intrahepatic portosystemic stent-shunt in non-transplant cirrhotics with hepatorenal syndrome: A phase II study. Gut 2000;47:288–295.

99. Keller F, Heinze H, Jochimsen F, et al: Risk factors and outcome of 107 patients with decompensated liver disease and acute renal failure (including 26 patients with hepatorenal syndrome): The role of hemodialysis. Ren Fail 1995;17:135–146.

100. Richardson D, Stoves J, Davies M, Davison A: Liver transplantation for dialysis dependent hepatorenal failure. Nephrol Dial Transplant 1999;14:2742–2745.

101. Eckardt K, Frei U: Reversibility of hepatorenal syndrome in an anuric patient with Child C cirrhosis requiring haemodialysis for 7 weeks. Nephrol Dial Transplant 2000;15:1063–1065.

102. Capling R, Bastani B: The clinical course of patients with type 1 hepatorenal syndrome maintained on hemodialysis. Ren Fail 2004;26:563–568.

103. Storm C, Bernhardt W, Schaeffner E, et al: Immediate recovery of renal function after orthotopic liver transplantation in a patient with hepatorenal syndrome requiring hemodialysis for more than 8 months. Transplant Proc 2007;39:544–546.

104. Witzke O, Baumann M, Patschan D, et al: Which patients benefit from hemodialysis therapy in hepatorenal syndrome? J Gastroenterol Hepatol 2004;19:1369–1373.

105. Mehta RL, McDonald B, Gabbai FB, et al: A randomized clinical trial of continuous versus intermittent dialysis for acute renal failure. Kidney Int 2001;60:1154–1163.

106. Augustine JJ, Sandy D, Seifert TH, Paganini EP: A randomized controlled trial comparing intermittent with continuous dialysis in patients with ARF. Am J Kidney Dis 2004;44:1000–1007.

107. Uehlinger DE, Jakob SM, Ferrari P, et al: Comparison of continuous and intermittent renal replacement therapy for acute renal failure. Nephrol Dial Transplant 2005;20:1630–1637.

108. Vinsonneau C, Camus C, Combes A, et al: Continuous venovenous haemodiafiltration versus intermittent haemodialysis for acute renal failure in patients with multiple-organ dysfunction syndrome: A multicentre randomised trial. Lancet 2006;368:379–385.

109. Mitzner SR, Stange J, Klammt S, et al: Improvement of hepatorenal syndrome with extracorporeal albumin dialysis MARS: Results of a prospective, randomized, controlled clinical trial. Liver Transplant 2000;6:277–286.

110. Moore KP, Wong F, Ginès P, et al: The management of ascites in cirrhosis: Report on the consensus conference of the International Ascites Club. Hepatology 2003;38:258–266.

111. Fernández J, Navasa M, Planas R, et al: Primary prophylaxis of spontaneous bacterial peritonitis delays hepatorenal syndrome and improves survival in cirrhosis. Gastroenterology 2007;133:818–824.

112. Ginès P, Uriz J, Calahorra B, et al: Transjugular intrahepatic portosystemic shunting versus paracentesis plus albumin for refractory ascites in cirrhosis. Gastroenterology 2002;123:1839–1847.

113. Albillos A, Bañares R, Gonzalez M, et al: A meta-analysis of transjugular intrahepatic portosystemic shunt versus paracentesis for refractory ascites. J Hepatol 2005;43:990–996.

114. Sort P, Navasa M, Arroyo V, et al: Effect of intravenous albumin on renal impairment and mortality in patients with cirrhosis and spontaneous bacterial peritonitis. N Engl J Med 1999;341:403–409.

115. Rasaratnam B, Kaye D, Jennings G, et al: The effect of selective intestinal decontamination on the hyperdynamic circulatory state in cirrhosis—a randomized trial. Ann Intern Med 2003;139:186–193.

116. Akriviadis E, Botla R, Briggs W, et al: Pentoxifylline improves short-term survival in severe acute alcoholic hepatitis: A double-blind, placebo-controlled trial. Gastroenterology 2000;119:1637–1648.

Further Reading

Arroyo V, Terra C, Ginès P: Advances in the pathogenesis and treatment of type-1 and type-2 hepatorenal syndrome. J Hepatol 2007;46:935–946.

Arroyo V, Terra C, Torre A, Ginès P: Hepatorenal syndrome in cirrhosis: Clinical features, diagnosis, and management. In Ginès P, Arroyo V, Rodés J, Schrier RW (eds): Ascites and Renal Dysfunction in Liver Disease. Malden, MA: Blackwell Publishing, 2005, pp 341–359.

Cárdenas A, Ginès P: Therapy insight: Management of hepatorenal syndrome. Nat Clin Pract Gastroenterol 2006;3:338–348.

Dagher L, Moore K: The hepatorenal syndrome. Gut 2001;49:729–737.

Ginès P, Cárdenas A, Arroyo V, Rodés J: Management of cirrhosis and ascites. N Engl J Med 2004;350:1646–1654.

Gonwa TA, Morris CA, Goldstein RM, et al: Long-term survival and renal function following liver transplantation in patients with and without hepatorenal syndrome—experience in 300 patients. Transplantation 1991;51:428–430.

Moreau R, Lebrec D: The use of vasoconstrictors in patients with cirrhosis: Type 1 HRS and beyond. Hepatology 2006;43:385–394.

Salerno F, Gerbes A, Ginès P, et al: Diagnosis, prevention and treatment of the hepatorenal syndrome in cirrhosis. A consensus workshop of the international ascites club. Gut 2007;56:1310–1318.

Wadei HM, Mai ML, Ahsan N, Gonwa TA: Hepatorenal syndrome: Pathophysiology and management. Clin J Am Soc Nephrol 2006;1:1066–1079.

Chapter 6

Acute Dialysis Principles and Practice

Roy O. Mathew and Ravindra L. Mehta

The traditional concept of acute renal failure (ARF) has been recently redefined as acute kidney injury (AKI).[1] A collaboration of several societies has led to the creation of the Acute Kidney Injury Network (AKIN), which has proposed diagnostic and staging criteria for AKI based on the RIFLE criteria (Risk, Injury, Failure, Loss, End stage).[2] As is evident by these criteria, patients who suffer AKI may progress through various stages that correlate with outcomes. When renal replacement therapy (RRT)/support is required, there is a far worse prognosis than with lesser degrees of renal injury.[3–5] Several dialysis techniques are now available for RRT to manage AKI. Acute intermittent hemodialysis (IHD), peritoneal dialysis, and continuous techniques are the mainstays of treatment modalities. This chapter reviews the indications, modalities, and administration guidelines for acute hemo- and peritoneal dialysis.

TECHNIQUE PRINCIPLES

Modalities

Dialysis modalities can be segregated by the type of clearance and duration of therapy. Variations in clearance technique include hemodialysis, hemofiltration, and hemodiafiltration (combining the former two). Therapy may be administered continuously, intermittently, or some combination of the two. Continuous modalities are discussed further in Chapter 7. Intermittent therapies all depend on diffusion-based transfer of solutes and use convection predominantly for fluid removal. The duration of therapy usually is short (3–6 hours) with sessions provided on a daily, alternate-day, or three times per week frequency. Alternatively, the duration can be prolonged (6–16 hours) with adjustments in the blood and dialysate flow rates. These hybrid modalities are termed slow low-efficiency dialysis (SLED), slow continuous dialysis, or extended daily dialysis (EDD).

Intermittent hemodialysis (IHD) is the procedure that has been widely used over the past four decades in patients with end-stage renal disease and those with ARF. The vast majority of IHD is performed using a single-pass of dialysate at flow rates greater than that of blood. Several important technological advances have made the procedure safer and more suited for the ARF patient. The availability of variable sodium concentrations in the dialysate, biocompatible membranes, bicarbonate-based dialysate, and volumetrically controlled ultrafiltration offer certain advantages that are particularly well suited to the ARF patient.[6,7] Nevertheless, most centers use a fairly standard regimen for administration of the therapy. Because of limitations imposed by the use of dual-lumen catheters for vascular access, only moderate blood flow rates (200–250 mL/min) can be achieved. The standard dialysate flow rates used are 500 mL/min. IHD offers the advantage of providing for rapid correction of electrolyte and acid-base disturbances. A major disadvantage of IHD is the limited time (usually 3–4 hours) of total therapy per day. As a result, the patient will remain without renal support for the majority of the day during which fluid regulation, acid-base balance, and electrolyte homeostasis are not possible. Another important disadvantage of IHD is that patients with hemodynamic instability may not tolerate the higher blood flow rates needed to achieve an adequate level of diffusive clearance in the limited duration of the treatment. More important is the demonstration that intradialytic hypotension may contribute to delayed renal recovery.[8,9] Of interest is the demonstration by Schortgen and colleagues[10] that implementation of strict guidelines for the management and prevention of intradialytic hypotension helped reduce the incidence of such episodes, but did not affect overall mortality.

Sorbent system IHD is a system that regenerates dialysate by passing it through a sorbent cartridge that contains five distinct layers.[11,12] The first layer contains activated carbon, the second contains urease, which converts urea to ammonium carbonate, and the third layer contains zirconium phosphate in which cations such as potassium, calcium, and magnesium are adsorbed and exchanged for hydrogen and sodium ions. The fourth layer of the cartridge contains hydrated zirconium oxide to which phosphate and fluoride are adsorbed and exchanged for acetate. The fifth layer contains activated carbon, which removes creatinine and other waste products. Although this system is used only infrequently, it provides the advantage of eliminating the need for a source of pure water and providing a system that is highly portable. In addition, because of the unique characteristics of the regenerating system, sorbent IHD allows for greater flexibility in custom tailoring the dialysate. The greatest disadvantage of the sorbent system is that it is less efficient than single-pass IHD. The slower flow rate of dialysate and the overall adsorptive capacity of the sorbent cartridge impose the main limitations on efficiency of diffusive clearance. Previous sorbent-based systems (REDY) are also seeing a reemergence with the development of the Alliant System.[13]

Intermittent hemodiafiltration (IHF) uses convective clearance for solute removal. The main disadvantage of IHD is the need for large volumes of sterile replacement fluid. Therefore, the expense associated with IHD has limited its use in the United States. Proponents of the therapy claim that it offers greater hemodynamic stability and improved middle molecule clearance. Because of these advantages, IHD has been used extensively in Europe.[14]

Intermittent ultrafiltration uses the same device as with IHD, but differs in that the main use of IHD is in fluid removal. Typically, the procedure is used for treatment of pulmonary edema or severe cardiomyopathy with resistant fluid overload. Because the same machine used for IHD is also used for IUF, some centers use a combination of IUF and IHD in series. Such an approach provides greater hemodynamic stability and the ability to quickly treat volume overload. A major disadvantage is the loss of time available for diffusive solute clearance.

In 1999, Schlaeper and colleagues[15] reported the use of slow continuous dialysis in which blood flow rates were 100 to 200 mL/min and dialysate flow rates were 100 to 300 mL/min. Patients were treated for 12 hours during the day or evening. The procedure was thought to be safe, efficient, and relatively simple. Extended daily dialysis (EDD) was initially described by Kumar and colleagues.[16] EDD or SLED differs from IHD in that blood flow (QB) and dialysate flow (QD) are intentionally kept low but the duration is extended to maintain the strength or intensity. Typical QB is 125 to 250 mL/min and QD is 200 to 400 mL/min. Typical run times are 8 to 12 hours. Furthermore, dialysis may be performed at night to avoid scheduling conflicts.[17–24] Hybrid modalities have been run at night for 8 to 12 hours using intensive care unit (ICU) staff, thereby eliminating interruption of therapy and reducing staff requirements. Studies comparing hybrid modalities to continuous RRT (CRRT) have revealed favorable hemodynamic tolerance in critically ill patients while achieving dialysis adequacy and ultrafiltration targets.[17,22,23,25] The use of standard IHD machines allows some cost savings by eliminating the need for specialized dialysate or replacement fluid. Anticoagulation use has also been shown to be less in SLED as compared with CRRT because SLED may be run without anticoagulation (saline flushes). Recently, a new system has been designed specifically for the hybrid modality. This system is called the Genius single-pass dialysis system (Fresenius).

Peritoneal dialysis was the first "continuous" form of dialysis therapy used in the acute setting. In peritoneal dialysis, the patient's peritoneum acts as the semipermeable dialysis membrane. Dialysate consists of a sterile, lactate-based solution inserted via a peritoneal catheter into the abdominal cavity. Diffusion occurs from the blood perfusing the peritoneum to the fluid in the abdominal cavity across the peritoneum. Once the dialysate becomes saturated (3–4 hours), it is removed and fresh dialysate is instilled. Fluid removal is achieved by using an osmotic pressure mechanism in which varying dextrose concentrations in the dialysate provide an osmotic gradient for water flow from the patient's blood to the peritoneum. The process of dialysate instillation and removal can be automated with cyclers. The main advantages of peritoneal dialysis are that it is less labor intensive than hemodialysis and does not require anticoagulation. The major disadvantage is that dialysis is relatively inefficient because total solute removal is limited by total peritoneal effluent. Moreover, transfer across the peritoneum is highly influenced by both the anatomy of the peritoneum and the underlying hemodynamic status of the patient. Another major disadvantage is that the procedure requires the placement of a peritoneal catheter into the abdominal cavity, which may add to the morbidity of the already compromised ICU patient.

Considerable debate has ensued over the choice of modality in the acute setting, especially for the critically ill. Over the years, continuous modes of renal replacement have become the preferred modality of treating physicians. In 1999, Mehta and Letteri[26] reported on a survey performed among U.S. nephrologists that revealed 70% of those responding used IHD as the acute renal replacement modality. A recent survey during the Third International Critical Care Nephrology Conference in Vicenza, Italy, revealed several changing trends. First, the care of patients with ARF has been accepted by multiple specialties. Thirty-six percent of respondents were intensivists; nephrologists represented 52% of the attendees. Second, the overwhelming majority of respondents preferred to use continuous modes of renal replacement. Intensivists preferred CRRT more than nephrologists, who preferred IHD. Acute peritoneal dialysis (PD) was listed as an option by approximately 20% of participants, although actual use was not addressed. If used, PD was considered solely by nephrologists.[27] The DOse REsponse Multicentre collaborative Initiative (DO RE MI) study is an ongoing multicenter study to examine current use and dosing patterns of renal replacement in the acute setting.[28] Preliminary data suggest that CRRT has become the preferred modality, especially for those patients who are hemodynamically unstable. A few, small randomized clinical trials have been unable to demonstrate a consistent overall survival benefit of CRRT over IHD; however, differences in renal recovery tend to favor continuous modalities over intermittent.[29–34] At present, all the available modalities are viable options for managing patients with AKI; however, the choice of modality needs to be tailored to the clinical need.

Indications and Timing of Initiation for Dialysis

Hyperkalemia, severe hyperphosphatemia, severe hyperuricemia, severe acidemia, and uremia-related complications (coma, pericarditis, and seizures) are all accepted indications for starting dialysis. However, there is wide variability on the timing of initiation of dialysis even when these indications are present. Aside from situations in which there are severe derangements, most nephrologists have a tendency to avoid dialysis for as long as possible. Two major factors contribute to the decision to delay dialysis. First, the dialysis procedure itself is not without risk. Hypotension, arrhythmias, and complications of vascular access placement are not uncommon.[35] Second is the concern that dialysis may delay recovery of renal function.[9,36] Therefore, in general, dialysis in current practice is initiated when clinical features of significant volume overload and solute imbalance dictate a need for intervention. Common parameters used for defining the indications and timing of dialysis for AKI include the level of blood urea nitrogen and creatinine, presence of oliguria, evidence of heart failure and pulmonary edema, and an estimate of the catabolic state.[37,38]

Continued debate ensues over the appropriate level of BUN above which one should always start dialysis. Underlying is the multitude of reasons that BUN may be elevated, as well as variability in the level at which complications arise. Liu and colleagues[39] examined the mortality associated with a high versus low starting BUN. In this prospective cohort analysis, patients with BUN less than 76 mg/dL (mean BUN, 46 mg/dL) had a trend toward higher mortality (14- and 28-day mortality: 0.80 and 0.69 in low BUN versus 0.75 and 0.54 for high BUN, respectively). In contrast, a randomized, controlled trial conducted in oliguric critically ill patients in the Netherlands revealed no significant difference in hospital mortality with early (mean BUN, 46 mg/dL) versus late (mean BUN, 105 mg/dL) hemofiltration initiation.[40]

Oliguria and its associated complications are a serious contributor to morbidity of AKI. The use of diuretics to support urine flow has been debated in the literature with no clear indication that it either hurts or helps in oliguria.[41–43] Given the added comfort of volume control, maintenance of urine volume with or without diuretics may unnecessarily delay the onset of dialysis in select individuals. Liangos and colleagues[44] examined the relationship of urine volume to timing of initiation of dialysis and overall mortality. Nonsurvivors had significantly higher urine volumes and severity of illness than survivors (1.5 L/day versus 0.7 L/day). Nonsurvivors also had lower BUN at start of nephrology consult (42 versus 76 mg/dL, $P = .01$). What this study had demonstrated was the increasing complexity of the natural history of AKI. Seemingly mild clinical deterioration (as evidenced by lower APACHE [Acute Physiology, Age, and Chronic Health Evaluation] II score at consult) resulted in delayed initiation of therapy and ultimately poor outcomes. Neither laboratory nor clinical data alone seem to predict when dialysis should be initiated. The combination provides the basis for the decision-making process in initiating therapy with dialysis.

A key issue is the timing of involvement of the nephrologist in the care of individuals with AKI. Late consultation with a nephrologist was associated with lower BUN (mean 47 mg/dL versus 77 mg/dL in late versus early groups, respectively) and higher urine output (mean 1180 versus 608 mL in late versus early groups) was reported in a prospective observation trial conducted among ICU patients requiring a nephrology consultation.[45] Late nephrology consultation was also associated with higher in-hospital mortality and lower recovery of renal function in survivors (adjusted odds ratio = 1.5, although not statistically significant). AKI involves a complex physiologic milieu that requires early aggressive collaborative management to provide appropriate therapy in a timely manner.

Despite the absence of standards for initiation of dialysis in the ICU, several important factors need to be considered when making the decision to provide RRT. An important distinction in the ICU patient is the recognition that ARF does not occur in isolation from other organ-system dysfunction. Consequently, providing dialysis can be viewed as a form of renal support rather than mere replacement.[46] For example, in the presence of oliguric renal failure, administration of large volumes of fluid to patients with multiple organ failure may lead to impaired oxygenation. In such a setting, early intervention with extracorporeal therapies for management of fluid balance may significantly affect the function of other organs irrespective of more traditional indices of renal failure, such as BUN. Several pieces of evidence point to the importance of fluid overload in determining outcomes of AKI. We showed in a randomized, controlled trial comparing intermittent therapies with continuous therapies that patients dialyzed for solute control had a better outcome than those dialyzed for volume control.[32] Moreover, patients dialyzed for both solute and volume control had the worst outcome. Mukau and Latimer[47] showed that 95% of their patients with postoperative ARF had fluid excesses of more than 10 L at initiation of dialysis. Recent studies have suggested that achieving a negative fluid balance in the first 3 days of admission for septic shock was a predictor of better survival.[48] Foland and colleagues[49] have shown that pediatric patients receiving continuous venovenous hemofiltration (CVVH) with more than 10% fluid overload before initiation of CVVH have a poor prognosis. Consequently, fluid regulation seems to be an important consideration when deciding to initiate dialysis in the ICU patient with ARF. Moreover, such renal support provides volume "space," which permits for the administration of nutritional support without limitations.[50] Although there are currently no trials exploring the timing of intervention for acute dialysis, the availability of the Acute Kidney Injury Network staging system should permit an improved characterization of AKI. Ongoing analyses are being performed on the utility of RIFLE criteria as predictors of mortality as well as indicators for therapy initiation.[4,51–53]

Prescription for Acute Dialysis

Acute Kidney Injury Patients

The acute dialysis prescription includes dialysis operational characteristics, duration, and frequency as the main parameters defining the dose of therapy. The operational characteristics are determined by the type of dialyzer, QB, and QD. QB is dependent on access type, with fistulas and grafts providing the highest flows and temporary polyurethane catheters providing the lowest flows before recirculation becomes an issue. The QD should be adjusted based on the QB to facilitate a maximal gradient with single-pass systems. In acute IHD, especially at high starting BUN, dialysis is initiated at half the target QB and QD. This is to prevent dialysis disequilibrium (DD) syndrome, which has been linked to rapid decreases in BUN in dialysis-naive patients. The duration of each dialysis session determines the delivered dose per unit of time. Dialysis sessions of 4 to 5 hours are often required to achieve adequate solute and fluid removal without significant hemodynamic disturbance.[33] Shorter sessions are typically used in dialysis initiation and then longer sessions are introduced gradually to meet adequacy goals. Daily hemodialysis has been proven to provide improved survival benefit in critically ill patients.[54] To address the need for prolonged therapy and accommodate the hectic schedule of the hospitalized patient requiring RRT, hybrid therapies have been designed. Table 6-1 compares IHD with different hybrid therapies.

Long-Term Dialysis Patients

Traditional guidelines for outpatient management of end-stage renal disease (ESRD) patients involve three times weekly dosing frequency of IHD. When these patients are hospitalized, the utility of continuing this regimen versus intensive therapy delivery has not been extensively studied. One recent observational study compared the mortality of patients who suffered AKI requiring RRT and had no history of renal insufficiency with ESRD patients requiring ICU admission.[55] This study demonstrated significantly higher hospital mortality among de novo AKI patients compared with ESRD patients (34% and 14%, respectively). Dialysis delivered to the ESRD population was every other day dosing (mean, every 1.95 ± 0.3 days). No comparison with less or more dosing was performed. A recent observational trial described the clinical characteristics of long-term hemodialysis patients admitted to the ICU.[56] This trial highlighted the influence of long-term phosphate management on ICU mortality in this population. No mention of dialysis dosing was given in this study. Until larger prospective cohort or randomized, controlled trials are conducted regarding dosing frequency in hospitalized ESRD patients, no specific recommendations can be made. Nevertheless, a thorough evaluation of the severity of illness and metabolic needs of the patient should serve as a general guide to dosing frequency.

Toxin/Drug Removal

Certain drug or toxin overdoses may be regulated by dialytic or adsorbent removal of the compound from circulation. This depends on the size and degree of albumin binding of the compound of interest. Charcoal hemoperfusion techniques for toxin removal are rarely, if ever, used. The cartridges are expensive to purchase and have a very short shelf life, and hemodialysis or hemodiafiltration (intermittent or continuous) techniques provide adequate removal of toxins. A recent survey in New York City found that, of 34 hospitals that responded to a survey about charcoal hemoperfusion use, only 3 centers actually used the technique; the conditions for which it was used were theophylline toxicity and aluminum overdose.[57] The intensity and frequency of dialysis required for toxin removal depend largely on the individual drug/toxin pharmacokinetics. Table 6-2 lists common toxicities, indications, and prescriptions for hemodialysis.[58,59]

Isolated Fluid Removal

Ultrafiltration has become a therapeutic maneuver in managing decompensated congestive heart failure with refractory volume overload. The UNLOAD trial group recently reported results from a randomized trial of ultrafiltration (using the Aquadex machine) compared with diuretics for acute decompensated heart failure. In this manufacturer-sponsored trial, patients with clinically determined heart failure decompensation (no EF in eligibility criteria) with no or only moderate renal disease (creatinine < 3 mg/dL) who received early ultrafiltration achieved greater volume removal and improved dyspnea score after 48 hours of treatment.[60] The Aquadex system is specifically designed to provide slow ultrafiltration using slow QB (10–50 mL/min). Traditional CRRT machines have also been used to provide IHD in congestive heart failure.[61]

Factors Influencing Acute Dialysis Delivery

Access

Acute hemodialysis access is a major factor in the delivery of an adequate dialysis dose. Modern dialysis catheters are composed of polyurethane, which is stiff at room temperature and then softens at body temperature; this facilitates access placement. Catheter length should be appropriate for the location of placement. Femoral catheters should be no shorter than

Table 6-1 Comparison of Intermittent Hemodialysis with Hybrid Therapies

| | ACUTE IHD | | SLED/EDD | |
	Initiation	Maintenance	Initiation	Maintenance
Duration	2–2.5 hr	4–5 hr	8–12 hr	8–12 hr
Frequency	Daily for 2–3 days	Alternate day to daily depending on severity of illness	Daily	Daily
Filter	Synthetic or modified cellulose/small	Synthetic or modified cellulose/large	Synthetic or modified cellulose/small or large	Synthetic or modified cellulose/small or large
Q_B (mL/min)	200–250	250–350	150–250	150–250
Q_D (mL/min)/flow	400–500/counter- or syncurrent	500–800/countercurrent	16–20/countercurrent	16–20/countercurrent

EDD, extended daily dialysis; IHD, intermittent hemodialysis; QB, blood flow; QD, dialysate flow; SLED, slow-efficiency dialysis.

Table 6-2   Common Toxicities, Indications, and Prescription for Hemodialysis

Toxicity	Indications for HD	Dialysis Prescription[130]
Acetaminophen	Acute HD if concomitant renal failure (RIFLE criteria) requiring RRT; not for drug removal; N-acetylcysteine is still treatment of choice	Per general acute prescription section
Alcohols (ethylene glycol/methanol)	Refractory acidosis, visual impairments, renal failure, and pulmonary edema	Duration: typically long duration (6–8 hr); frequency: daily until serum levels undetectable; dialysate: high bicarbonate (e. g., 40 mEq/L) in the face of severe acidosis; QB/QD: high flows to maximize clearance; caution: hypophosphatemia with extended dialysis
Cyclic antidepressants (classic: carbamazepime)	Helpful in drug removal; no studies documenting aid in high bicarbonate dialysate to aid with blood alkalinization for management of toxicity	Duration: typically shorter sessions given the high Vd, especially of TCA; frequency: daily until symptoms resolve or levels therapeutic or undetectable; dialysate: no specific recommendations; QB/QD: low initial flows and increase as needed/tolerated
Lithium	If levels > 4 mmol/L after acute ingestion or ≥ 2.5 mmol/L after long-term ingestion, renal failure, severe neurologic dysfunction; treatment may be needed daily and over extended periods of time (4–6 hr) as rebound levels are frequent problem	Duration: initially 6–8 hr and then subsequent sessions 3–4 hr; frequency: typically daily until lithium levels do not rebound to supratherapeutic levels; dialysate: bicarbonate based dialysate; QB/QD: high flows to maximize clearance
Salicylates	HD if levels > 100 mg/dL in acute ingestion, seizures, persistent electrolyte abnormalities, presistent altered level of consciousness, or refractory acidosis	Duration: initially 6–8 hr and then shorter as symptoms/levels permit; frequency: daily to alternate day; dialysate: bicarbonate based; QB/QD: high flows if severe acidosis present
Metformin	HD for severe lactic acidosis; may require prolonged daily therapy	Duration: longer sessions initially (some reports suggest 21–24 hr[138]; frequency: daily until acidosis resolves; dialysate: bicarbonate based (may need high levels, i.e., 40 mEq/L); QB/QD: high flows to maximize clearance of lactate

HD, hemodialysis; QB, blood flow; QD, dialysate flow; RRT, renal replacement therapy; TCA, tricyclic antidepressant; Vd, volume of distribution.

20 cm; right internal jugular placement requires anywhere between 13.5 and 16 cm depending on the size of the patient, and left internal jugular catheters necessitate approximately 16 to 20 cm catheters. Leblanc and colleagues[62] showed that recirculation rates varied based on the site and length of the catheters. Subclavian catheters (13.5–19.5 cm) had recirculation rates of 4.1%, whereas femoral catheters had recirculation rates of more than 20% (13.5 cm) and 12.1% (19.5 cm). Subclavian vein insertion has been discouraged due to the finding of stenosis as a late complication. This is especially important in patients who will potentially require long-term hemodialysis access in the future.[63,64] For these patients, subclavian catheters are contraindicated unless no other site is available.[65] Furthermore, unless done by trained individuals, subclavian catheter placement has high rates of complications including hemothorax and pneumothorax.[66] Femoral and right internal jugular arteries are the most common sites of insertion. Use of femoral catheters is associated with higher rates of recirculation and infection and less efficient dialysis delivery.[62,63,67] A recent study from France demonstrated the possibility of using tunneled silicone femoral catheters for acute hemodialysis.[67] Decreased recirculation, improved delivered Kt/V to prescribed Kt/V (where K = dialyzer urea clearance, t = dialysis time, V = urea volume of distribution) ratios, and decreased rates of infection were found compared with nontunneled femoral catheters. No comparisons with internal jugular catheters were made. This, along with the fact that few institutions have trained individuals available for placement of such catheters in the acute setting, limits the general applicability of this study.

A considerable amount of catheter hours are spent in nonuse. During these times, adequate patency must be ensured to prevent local complications (i.e., thrombosis) and obviate risks of reinsertion. Catheter lock solutions have traditionally been composed of heparin-containing saline solutions. Heparin carries the risk of hemorrhage if accidentally instilled into the patient and is contraindicated in those with heparin-induced thrombocytopenia (HIT).

Citrate (trisodium citrate) catheter locks compared with heparin locks have been studied with regard to catheter patency and complications. Catheter patency is equivalent, if not superior, to heparin.[69,70] Furthermore, in vitro studies demonstrate protection against biofilm formation with citrate solutions compared with heparin solutions, although reduction in catheter-related bacteremia has been inconsistently shown in studies.[69–72] Catheter lock solutions containing citrate are typically 4% to 49% citrate solutions.

Anticoagulation

Adequate system anticoagulation is paramount to achieving an optimally delivered dialysis dose. Heparin has been the mainstay of long-term and acute hemodialysis protocols. This is due to its ready availability, ease of administration, comfort among users with the agent, its monitoring, and its safety profile. There are several methods for administering heparin during dialysis. The standard method involves administering heparin systemically either as a continuous infusion or as repeated bolus units. The continuous infusion method is begun by giving a bolus, typically approximately 2000 U, waiting 3 to 4 minutes, and then continuous administration of 1200 U/hr. The therapeutic goal is to prolong the activated clotting time (ACT) to baseline plus 80%. Prolongation of ACT is directly proportional to the amount of heparin given. If the ACT is not prolonged to 180% of baseline after the initial bolus, then an additional amount should be given to reach the goal before the continuous amount is started. The repeated-bolus method involves administering approximately 4000 U of heparin as an initial bolus to prolong the ACT to well above the 180% target. This is repeated an hour later with a 2000-U bolus and then another hour later with 1000 U. The anticoagulation should be stopped approximately 1 hour before completion of therapy to prevent excessive residual anticoagulation.[73]

In those patients at increased risk of hemorrhagic complications but not actively bleeding or immediately postoperative, a protocol of "tight" heparin or no anticoagulation may be followed. Tight heparin protocols are typically only given as single-bolus plus continuous-infusion administration. This is to prevent the large swings in ACT as seen by the repeated-bolus technique. The therapeutic goal for the tight heparin protocol is to prolong the ACT to no longer than 130% of baseline. This is typically achieved by giving 750 U as an initial bolus and then administering a continuous infusion of 600 U/hr. Again, adjustments should be made based on target ACT prolongation of 130%. This is the typical anticoagulation protocol followed for AKI patients. A no-anticoagulation protocol may also be followed, but is generally reserved for those who are at high risk of bleeding—notably, those who are actively bleeding, those who are immediately postoperative, or those in whom heparin is contraindicated (i.e., HIT patients). The system is primed with heparinized saline (1000 U/mL), unless HIT is present, in which case, normal saline alone is used. Once blood is circulating, rapid saline boluses administered prefilter every 30 minutes should provide adequate filter life in approximately 95% of cases. More frequent rinsing may be performed based on clinical inspection.

Citrate has been used as an anticoagulant for extracorporeal circuits for many years now. Its safety and efficacy have been demonstrated in numerous trials, but predominantly in the CRRT literature. Regional citrate anticoagulation may also be used during IHD. Administration has traditionally been given in the presence of a calcium-free dialysate. Recent studies, however, have demonstrated the possibility of using low calcium dialysate with regional citrate anticoagulation and still achieving adequate dialysis with adequate filter life.[74] A summary of available anticoagulants and dosing strategies in IHD and SLED/EDD is given in Table 6-3.

Dialyzer

Several studies have examined the role of the dialyzer membrane itself in renal recovery after AKI. Biocompatibility refers to the degree to which complement is activated by blood-dialyzer contact. The traditional unsubstituted cellulose membranes (i.e., cuprophane) are considered bioincompatible due to the high degree of complement activation and leukodepletion. The new synthetic brands (polysulfone, acrylonitrile, polymethylmethacrylate) are considered biocompatible. Modified cellulose membranes have intermediate characteristics (i.e., meltspun cellulose diacetate). Dialyzer membranes have been further segregated based on the ability to remove mid- to large-size molecules (high versus low flux). Flux is measured based on the clearance of β_2-microglobulin (>20 mL/min being high flux). In the long-term hemodialysis setting, high-flux synthetic or substituted cellulose membranes have become the norm due to decreased dialyzer reactions and improvements in clinical outcomes. In the acute setting, however, studies have not demonstrated a consistent benefit of synthetic high-flux membranes in terms of renal recovery or mortality. One meta-analysis did reveal that synthetic membranes conferred improved overall survival compared with cellulose acetate membranes, but there were no differences in renal survival.[75] As mentioned in this meta-analysis, the survival advantage may not persist when compared with modified cellulose membranes. In a randomized trial comparing synthetic with modified cellulose (meltspun cellulose diacetate) membranes, no differences in renal or patient survival were demonstrated.[76] Furthermore, there was no improvement in survival based on high- versus low-flux synthetic membranes. No definitive recommendations can be made regarding modified cellulose versus synthetic membranes for ARF at this time. Cellulose acetate membranes should be avoided as there is evidence of decreased survival with their use.

Dialysate (Bicarbonate/Acetate)

Bicarbonate-buffered dialysate solutions are the current standard in acute or long-term renal replacement. Lactate is the buffer base for PD solutions given its stability and conversion of lactate to bicarbonate by the liver. Thus, lactate-based dialysate is particularly avoided in those with decreased ability to metabolize lactate, such as those with liver failure or immediately after liver transplantation. If dialysis is emergently needed and lactate-based PD fluid is readily available, it may be used in acutely ill patients with preserved liver function.[77,78] Acetate-based dialysate has also been used but has a tendency to exacerbate dialysis-induced hypoxemia (see later).

Sodium may be varied based on patient natremia or on the need to buffer intradialytic hypotension in susceptible patients (see "Preventing and Managing Complications of Acute Dialysis"). Potassium and calcium may likewise be altered based on patient needs.

Table 6-3 Summary of Available Anticoagulants and Dosing Strategies in Intermittent Hemodialysis and Slow-Efficiency Dialysis/Extended Daily Dialysis

Method	Filter Priming	Initial Dose	Maintenance Dose	Monitoring	Pro	Con	Overanticoagulation
No anticoagulation	None or with heparinized saline (5–8 IU/mL)	N/A	N/A	Filter thrombosis, filter pressure	No monitoring or risks associated with other anticoagulation regimens; adequate filter patency in high-risk patients (active bleeding or immediately postoperative)	Inadequate filter patency or dialysis adequacy due to decreased dialyzer performance over time	N/A
Heparin	Heparinized saline (5–8 IU/mL)	2000–5000 IU prefilter	3–15 IU/kg/hr prefilter	aPTT/ACT 1.5–2 times the upper limit of normal	Familiarity, effective anticoagulation, ease of monitoring in catheterized patient	Increased risk of hemorrhagic complications, HIT, adrenal insufficiency	Protamine administered 10 mg: 100 U heparin (dose should be sum of previous 2–3 hr of heparin administration)
Tight heparin	Heparinized saline	750–1000 IU prefilter	None, periodic bolus administration of 400–600 IU	Target ACT to 1.3–1.4 times the upper limit of normal	Same as above, may provide low bleeding risk in high-risk patients	Same as above	Same as above
LMWH (dalteparin)	Heparinized saline or 1.5–2.5 UmL dalteparin	20-U/kg bolus	Prefilter administration at 10 IU/kg/hr	Recommendations are to monitor anti-Xa activity of 0.25–0.35 IU/mL	Similar patency rates as with heparin	More costly and pitfalls of heparin persist	Protamine may be tried as above; blood products may be required
LMWH (enoxaparin)		750 U	0.05 mg/kg/hr	Anti-Xa activity 0.25–0.35 IU/mL	Same as above	Same as above	Same as above

Argatroban	None or with heparinized saline if no HIT present	250 μg/kg	0.5–2 μg/kg/min	aPTT aiming for 1–1.4 times the upper limit of normal	Safe in renal failure; established as treatment for HIT	No antidote for bleeding and aPTT may not absolutely correlate with anticoagulation	No antidote available; blood products may be required
Citrate (TSC or ACD-A administered alone prefilter)		140–160 mL/hr of 4% TSC given prefilter (3%–8% of the blood flow rates) or ACD-A at 250 mL/hr	Vary rate of citrate in 5–10-mL/hr increments to maintain desired postfilter ionized calcium rates	Maintain postfilter ionized calcium, at 0.2–0.3 mmol/L; use systemically administered calcium to maintain systemic ionized calcium within the normal laboratory range (1.0–1.2 mmol/L)	Ease of administration, ease of monitoring, low incidence of adverse events, ease of discontinuation if complications arise; there may be improved biocompatibility with citrate[139,140]	Difficulty in obtaining appropriate dialysate and citrate solution (depends on pharmacy availability); potential for metabolic alkalosis, hypernatremia, hyper-/hypocalcemia, or citrate toxicity	Rarely, if ever occurs; if total calcium-to-ionized-calcium ratio > 2.1, then lower citrate rate or turn off citrate anticoagulation

ACD-A, acid citrate dextrose-A solution; ACT, activated clotting time; aPTT, activated partial thromboplastin time; HIT, heparin-induced thrombocytopenia; LMWH, low molecular weight heparin; N/A, not applicable; TSC, trisodium citrate.

Preventing and Managing Complications of Acute Dialysis

Hypotension

Intradialytic hypotension is a significant problem in both the long-term and acute dialysis setting. This is more of a problem in ARF as renal recovery has to be one of the goals of overall treatment. Manns and colleagues[36] showed that IHD was associated with a decrease in the glomerular filtration rate during and after the procedure compared with the preprocedure glomerular filtration rate. Conversely, a study by John and colleagues[79] examined the effects of intradialytic hypotension on splanchnic perfusion as represented by gastric intramucosal pH and P_{CO_2}. Despite decreases in mean arterial pressure of more than 20% from baseline in IHD compared with CVVH, there was no significant impact on intramucosal acid-base status, nor was there a sustained impact on systemic hemodynamics. These findings were limited to a 24-hour period, and thus it is difficult to say whether repeated hypotensive insults would ultimately result in subtle organ damage. Two studies comparing the renal survival of patients undergoing CRRT versus IHD have demonstrated that there is a trend toward improved renal recovery in CRRT.[29,30] Improvements in hemodialysis techniques have been put forth that aim to reduce the hemodynamic challenges of traditional IHD. Paganini and colleagues[80] have compared variable sodium and ultrafiltration modeling with a fixed scenario in critically ill patients with ARF requiring RRT. Variable sodium modeling (160 mEq/L to 140 mEq/L over the course of dialysis) and ultrafiltration (50% ultrafiltration in the first hour and 50% over the remainder of the dialysis session) afforded improved hemodynamic stability compared with fixed sodium and ultrafiltration. Furthermore, a randomized, controlled trial comparing IHD with continuous venovenous hemodiafiltration (CVVHDF) demonstrated significant adherence and hemodynamic tolerance in the IHD arm when a strict protocol for IHD administration was followed.[33] In this study, IHD was administered for 4 hours or longer, with high fixed sodium (150 mmol/L), low dialysate temperature (35°C), QB of 250 mL/min, and QD of 500 mL/min. Hypotension occurred no more frequently in the IHD arm than in the CVVHDF arm. Despite similar survival rates, no mention was made regarding renal survival. Dheenan and Henrich[81] examined various techniques for hemodynamic buffering in ESRD patients and also demonstrated beneficial effects of high sodium, sodium modeling, and cool dialysate. They caution that fixed high sodium may result in net sodium gain and resultant intradialytic weight gains. The impact on AKI patients is not well described.

Hypoxia

Alveolar hypoventilation with resultant reductions in arterial oxygen tension during hemodialysis had been described during the use of acetate-buffered dialysate.[82,83] Early comparison trials of bicarbonate-buffered dialysate had not demonstrated a significant difference in rates of intra- and postdialysis hypoxemia.[84] It is now recognized that a relative alkalosis, either by utilization of CO_2 in the conversion of acetate to bicarbonate or by diffusion from high bicarbonate dialysate, induces hypoventilation.[85,86] Mildly elevated bicarbonate in the dialysate (~30 mEq/L) does not induce significant hypoventilation and resultant hypoxemia.[85] It is not clear, however, what, if any,

are the clinical consequences of dialysis-induced hypoxemia. Studies of long-term hemodialysis patients have revealed mild silent cardiac ischemic events and decreases in transcutaneous oxygen tension in patients with peripheral vascular disease.[87,88] This would be expected to be pronounced in those with underlying lung pathology, although a study by Pitcher and colleagues[86] did not demonstrate significant differences in arterial O_2 changes in normals and those with chronic obstructive pulmonary disorder after hemodialysis. With the more commonplace use of bicarbonate-based dialysate, dialysis-induced hypoxemia has become a minor problem and one not likely to have significant clinical consequences for the majority of AKI patients requiring IHD.

Dialysis Disequilibrium Syndrome

DD syndrome occurs due to rapid urea removal and resultant brain edema. Urea is not an effective osmolar agent and thus should not result in significant fluid shifts regardless of the degree of urea gradient change. Biochemical profiles of urea transporters in the brain of chronic uremia have elucidated the mechanisms underlying this syndrome. Down-regulation of brain urea transporters and increased aquaporins (AQ4 and AQ9) in the brain have been demonstrated in chronic uremia in five of six nephrectomized rats.[89] This is more commonly seen in chronic kidney disease patients who are started on hemodialysis but has been reported in AKI as well.[90,91] Patients with previous brain trauma or cerebrovascular events seem to be most susceptible to developing DD syndrome.[90] Symptoms may be mild such as headaches, dizziness, and blurry vision or more severe such as acute delirium and, in rare cases, brain death.[90] The ideal therapy for DD syndrome is prevention. As mentioned previously, reduced intensity of initial dialysis sessions affords more gradual removal of urea and time for osmotic gradient adjustment in the brain. SLED/EDD is administered in such a fashion as to eliminate the traditional difficulties of IHD with regard to DD. Slow QB and QD are the norm for the hybrid procedures and may confer protection against the development of DD syndrome. Mannitol may also be administered with initiating dialysis sessions to facilitate water egress from the brain.[91]

Bacterial Endotoxin–Related Pyrogenic Reactions

Dialysate provided for long-term hemodialysis is allowed 100 to 200 cfu/mL of bacteria or 0.25 to 2 EU/mL of endotoxin. This is based on decreased pyrogen response at these levels. However, evidence of chronic inflammation and downstream effects (malnutrition, decreased erythropoietin response, β_2-microglobulin levels) related to systemic responses to these low levels of endotoxin has been mounting.[92–94] Similar trials have not been conducted in the acute population.

Quality Assurance

Dose Monitoring and Goals

The simplest measure of dialysis adequacy is the urea reduction ratio. According to measured kinetics in the long-term hemodialysis setting, a delivered Kt/V of 1.0 corresponds to a urea reduction ratio of 60%.[73] Outcome studies in the ESRD population, most notably HEMO and the National Cooperative Dialysis Study (NCDS), have demonstrated correlations between delivered single pool (sp) Kt/V and morbidity and mortaility.[95,96] The NCDS revealed that mortality was increased if delivered spKt/V was less than 1. The HEMO study, utilizing spKt/V of 1.2 as the standard arm, established that delivering higher doses in the conventional three times per week model conferred no additional survival benefit.[96] As such, the hemodialysis adequacy work group for the National Kidney Foundation (NKF) has recommended that the target for minimal dialysis adequacy, for ESRD managment, be an spKt/V of 1.2.[97] Similar guidelines are lacking in acute hemodialysis, and thus considerable attention is being given to determining dose-outcome associations as well as appropriate dose delivery and quantification in recent years.

How does the dose of dialysis predict clinical outcomes in acute hemodialysis? A retrospective cohort analysis of acute hemodialysis and CRRT patients revealed little effect of Kt/V on mortality in patients with either high- or low-severity scores (Cleveland Clinic Foundation intensive care unit acute renal failure scores).[98] The severity score assessed critically ill patients requiring acute RRT on a 20-point scale based on select clinical variables (gender, mechanical ventilation, platelet count, surgical status, change in blood urea nitrogen, and serum creatinine). Those with scores less than 5 had the best survival rate and those with scores higher than 14 had the worst survival, regardless of the delivered dose of dialysis. The intermediate range was defined by a score between 5 and 14. Patients in this serverity range who received a higher dose of dialysis (Kt/V > 1) demonstrated lower mortality than those patients who received a lower dose (Kt/V ≤ 1).[99] A prospective analysis of alternate-day versus daily hemodialysis in ARF revealed that higher delivered Kt/V correlated with improved survival.[54] Higher Kt/V was accomplished by daily, rather than alternate-day, dialysis. The dependence of survival on dose appears to be a direct relationship up to a point, and a function of overall disease severity. Ronco and colleagues[100] describe this elegantly in a recent review regarding the dose of RRT in AKI.

The appropriate target of dose for acute IHD has not been clearly established. In CRRT, a high dose or the dose at which survival is affected has been demonstrated at 35 mL/kg/hr of ultrafiltration or effluent volume.[101] This corresponds to a delivered Kt/V of 1.4 in a 70-kg man dialyzed for 24 hours.[102] Prescribing acute dialysis sessions with the goal of 1.4 would deliver a Kt/V of approximately 1.2.[103] Reasons for the discrepancy between the prescribed and delivered dose of dialysis have been explored in several prospective studies.[99,103,104] Reasons stated for this discrepancy include lack of a steady state of urea nitrogen appearance, variable function, and high recirculation with temporary catheters, decreased QB, multiple interruptions, and decreased dialyzer clearance, especially in anticoagulation-free dialysis.[105] Studies have examined alternate methodologies to calculate dose in acute hemodialysis. The concept of using only K × t has been put forth as an accurate measure of dialysis delivery in long-term hemodialysis patients.[106] Ridel and colleagues[107] studied Kt as measured by ionic dialysance compared with dialysate sampling. Kt ionic dialysance revealed acceptable correlation with Kt from dialysate sampling. No corresponding studies of outcome measures using Kt ionic dialysance as the therapeutic goal in AKI have been carried out to date.

The concept of equivalent renal urea clearance (EKRjc) has been suggested as an accurate and simple means of expressing dialysis dose in AKI.[108] Casino and Marshall[108] note that the EKRjc meets several important criteria for acute dose quantification: independence from steady-state urea concentration, ease of calculation in the clinical setting that is applicable regardless of schedule (e.g., three times per week, alternate day, continuous), incorporating appropriate estimate of urea Vd in the acute setting, and allowing comparison with residual renal urea clearance. The first and third requirements are met in that urea removal (j) is used instead of urea generation and that minimal interdialytic periods are required to calculate interdialytic urea changes. With regard to inaccuracies in determinations of V in the acute setting, EKRjc as presented in their analysis is accurate within approximately 5% of their theoretical standard (dpEKRjc) when the estimated Vd is within 25% of the true Vd. EKRjc is proposed as a fair comparison of clearance across modalities. Studies have looked at EKRjc in SLEDD and CRRT.[17,108–110] Further comparative studies will be required to determine the strength of EKRjc to predict outcomes in AKI.

In dose delivery, more seems to be better in much of medicine. However, this has not proven true in many well-designed randomized studies examining dose delivery in dialysis.[96] In the landmark study of Ronco and colleagues,[101] no significant difference was noted between the 35- and 45-mL/kg/hr dose groups. One possible explanation for the potential for harm at higher doses of dialysis is that, in the critically ill patient, pro- and anti-inflammatory markers coexist in a delicate balance of activity.[102] If the dose of dialysis is high enough, anti-inflammatory mediators may be removed at similar or greater rates as those of proinflammatory mediators. Caution needs to be taken in blanket prescriptions of high Kt/V (>1.2) until well-designed trials have indicated a clear benefit for AKI patients.

ACUTE PERITONEAL DIALYSIS

PD was first attempted in the acute setting in 1923, albeit unsuccessfully; it was not until the 1950s that the procedure became standardized and more commonplace.[111] Today, the use of acute PD has been limited to pediatric populations and in developing countries where access to blood purification techniques are severely limited. Given the higher clearances achieved with hemodialysis techniques when the technologies are available, these have been the preferred modalities for AKI requiring RRT. General indications for acute PD are similar to those for acute HD. Acute PD may be particularly useful in two clinical settings: cirrhosis and decompensated heart failure. Recent reports have suggested beneficial uses in cirrhotic patients with ascites requiring RRT, though this is better tolerated in the chronic population and less so in the acute population.[112] Heart failure, conversely, may benefit from less aggressive fluid removal that is afforded by PD.[113] Additional indications include control of hyperthermia and treatment of necrotizing/hemorrhagic pancreatitis with concomitant renal failure when abdominal cavity washing is beneficial.[73] Contraindications to PD include recent abdominal surgery (especially when accompanied by drain placement), adynamic ileus, peritoneal fibrosis/adhesions, and emergency situations (i.e., flash pulmonary edema, poisoning, or drug intoxication).[73,114] Although not proven, fears of uncontrolled fluid shifts have led people away from acute PD in acute brain injury individuals requiring RRT.[115]

Acute PD, although easy to perform in the acute setting, does not achieve clearances that approximate those with IHD or CRRT. The issue of adequacy of PD in the severely hypercatabolic patient has not been extensively studied, although small trials have looked at various PD modalities in hypercatabolic patients. Chitalia and colleagues[116] examined two different types of PD (tidal PD and continuous exchange/equilibrium PD [CEPD]). In this randomized, controlled trial, tidal PD provided better clearances than CEPD. Using K/DOQI standards for long-term PD, tidal PD provided weekly creatinine clearance of 68.54 L/1.73 m² and weekly KtT/V of 2.43 versus 58.85 L/1.73 m² and 1.8 KtT/V for CEPD.[116] In another recent trial of CEPD using a flexible Tenckhoff catheter and automated cycler, adequate metabolic control was achieved after 3 days.[117] These patients had a mean APACHE II score of 32%, and 76.6% required ICU admission. Although both trials suggested adequate clearances for patients with AKI requiring RRT, no comparisons with blood purification modalities were carried out. This is especially important in that in the long-term setting PD, although providing lower clearances than IHD, affords adequate management of end-stage renal disease. This has not been officially compared in the acute setting.

Peritoneal access had been the limiting factor for therapy during the early years. Early access included such makeshift items as thermometer casing with a piece of tape attached to pull it out of the peritoneal cavity.[118] It was not until the introduction of the flexible Tenckhoff catheter in the 1960s that PD became a more generally applicable process.[119] Surgically inserted Tenckhoff catheters remain the most commonly used. Others such as the Cook Tenckhoff and Cook Mac-Lock multipurpose drainage catheter have been used without much proven benefit over the traditional Tenckhoff.[119,120] There are acute peritoneal catheters that may be inserted at the bedside by trained individuals. Access is typically obtained in one of three locations on the abdominal wall: infraumbilical, right lower quadrant, or left lower quadrant. The left lower quadrant is generally preferred to avoid the cecum and the bladder. Rigid catheters that are used for acute PD tend to be more prone to kinking. This leads to increased alarms with the automated cyclers. Acute catheters should not remain in place for longer than 3 days as infection rates increase considerably after this time.

Dose calculation in PD involves consideration of dialysate composition and volume, session duration, and mode of exchange. Current PD fluids use lactate as the bicarbonate source. PD tends to remove significant amounts of calcium and magnesium, so replacement is typically added to the dialysate. Bicarbonate solutions cause precipitation of calcium and magnesium and are thus avoided in long-term PD. The obvious difficulty is that ARF patients may also be unable to adequately convert lactate to bicarbonate. Furthermore, patients with any form of shock may have worsening acidosis with lactate solutions. A randomized trial comparing bicarbonate with lactate-buffered dialysate in critically ill patients requiring RRT revealed excellent metabolic control with bicarbonate compared with lactate.[121] Lactate-buffered solutions tended to correct acidosis more slowly and bicarbonate-buffered solutions tended to have lower calcium and magnesium levels; neither resulted in significant clinical consequences. If bicarbonate-based dialysate is to be used, it should be devoid of calcium and magnesium. A two-bag system designed to introduce bicarbonate at the time of fill is preferable.

Dextrose is used as an osmotic agent in PD fluids. Dextrose concentration is varied depending on the degree of fluid removal desired. Standard concentrations are 1.5%, 2.5%, and 4.25% dextrose. Icodextrins are alternative osmotic agents used in PD fluids in the long-term setting. These substances are polyglucose agents that have much lower transmission across peritoneal membranes (high reflection coefficient) and thus retain osmotic capability longer.[122] Hyperglycemia may also be prevented with the polyglucose agents.[123,124] Despite these potential benefits, the use of icodextrin in the acute setting has not been studied. Furthermore, icodextrins are associated with sterile hypersensitivity peritonitis.[125,126] These may lead to unnecessary antibiotic exposure in the acutely ill patient. In the adult, average peritoneal capacity is approximately 2 L of dialysate. Smaller volumes should be used in smaller individuals and those with pulmonary disease or abdominal wall/inguinal hernias. In addition, smaller volumes (500–1000 mL) are very often used when PD is started to prevent leakage around the newly placed catheter. In pediatric populations, the issue of high-volume (20 mL/kg per exchange) versus low-volume (10 mL/kg per exchange) exchanges has been addressed in the literature.[127,128] These trials suggest that low-volume exchanges provide adequate clearance without respiratory compromise or complications related to dialysate leakage. Low sodium dialysate (129 mmol/L) in association with high dextrose concentration (2.86%) has been studied in the pediatric AKI population with resultant enhanced sodium removal without sacrifice of ultrafiltration capacity.[129]

Choice of modality (manual/autocycled) will depend on the patient's needs. Manual modalities may be chosen for those who are more stable with fewer volume management needs. Hypercatabolic patients with significant volume overload will need nearly continuous exchange that cannot be maintained via a manual modality. Such patients will be better served with an automated cycler. The dose of delivery should be individualized to the patient's needs. In CEPD, each fill lasts approximately 10 minutes (200 mL/min). The fluid should dwell for 30 minutes and then be drained for 20 minutes. Exchanges are performed every hour, giving the patients 48 L of dialysate exchanged on a daily basis.[121] As the patient stabilizes, the dwells may be extended to 3 to 4 hours. Variations in dialysate flow have been introduced. Tidal PD is a modality in which a fraction of the dialysate cycles continuously throughout the dialysis period. Continuous-flow PD is a modality in which the entire volume of dialysate cycles through the abdomen in a continuous manner over several hours. This is facilitated by new techniques by which the dialysate is recycled and reinfused into the abdomen.[130]

Aside from the trial by Chitalia and colleagues,[116] few studies have examined the utility of adequacy guidelines for acute PD. Current long-term PD patient guidelines suggest a minimum weekly Kt/V of 1.7 for adequate delivery in anuric patients; however, there is considerable debate as to the appropriate level for the majority of patients.[114,131] The dose in PD is determined by the 24-hour drain volume multiplied by the number of days per week of dialysis adjusted for urea Vd.[114] Anthropometric formulas (i.e., Watson formulas) are typically used to determine urea Vd.[132] Solute reduction index ([24-hour urea removed (grams)]/[predialysis BUN × total body weight] × 100) may also be used to determine PD adequacy in AKI.[116] Goals for this have not been stringently established; Chitalia and colleagues[116] put forth a solute reduction index of more than 20% comparable with weekly Kt/V of more than 2.[114] Studies are required to evaluate the efficacy of these models in acute patients, especially given the lack of urea generation and urea Vd steady state in acute patients as mentioned previously.

Complications related to acute PD are bowel perforations during catheter insertion, fluid leak around the catheter site, exit site infection, peritonitis, hemothorax, or hyperglycemia. A potentially life-threatening complication related to acute PD catheters relates to bowel incarceration after removal of the catheter.[133] This complication may be prevented by proper closure of the laparotomy incision after catheter removal. Pulmonary compromise has been one of the prime fears of using PD in critically ill patients. Patients on long-term PD have revealed minor alterations in pulmonary function without effects on acid-base status or oxygenation.[134] Significant complications (hydro-/hemothorax) are rare and typically managed with conservative measures.[135,136] PD results in large protein and amino acid losses in the dialysate. Studies in critically ill patients receiving acute PD have demonstrated this as well; however, serum albumin levels were not altered significantly.[117,121] Amino acid–supplemented dialysate has been shown to allow uptake and reduce losses in the dialysate in acutely ill children; however, serum albumin levels were not significantly altered from baseline.[137]

References

1. Mehta RL, Kellum JA, Shah SV, et al: Acute Kidney Injury Network: Report of an initiative to improve outcomes in acute kidney injury. Crit Care 2007;11:R31.
2. Bellomo R, Ronco C, Kellum JA, et al: Acute renal failure—definition, outcome measures, animal models, fluid therapy and information technology needs: The Second International Consensus Conference of the Acute Dialysis Quality Initiative (ADQI) Group. Crit Care 2004;8:204–212.
3. Chertow GM, Burdick E, Honour M, et al: Acute kidney injury, mortality, length of stay, and costs in hospitalized patients. J Am Soc Nephrol 2005;16:365–370.
4. Abosaif NY, Tolba YA, Heap M, et al: The outcome of acute renal failure in the intensive care unit according to RIFLE: Model application, sensitivity, and predictability. Am J Kidney Dis 2005;46:1038–1048.
5. Cruz DN, Bolgan I, Perazella MA, et al: North East Italian Prospective Hospital Renal Outcome Survey on Acute Kidney Injury (NEiPHROS-AKI): Targeting the problem with the RIFLE criteria. Clin J Am Soc Nephrol 2007;2:418–425.
6. de Vries PM, Olthof CG, Solf A, et al: Fluid balance during haemodialysis and haemofiltration: The effect of dialysate sodium and a variable ultrafiltration rate. Nephrol Dial Transplant 1991;6:257–263.
7. Karsou SA, Jaber BL, Pereira BJ: Impact of intermittent hemodialysis variables on clinical outcomes in acute renal failure. Am J Kidney Dis 2000;35:980–991.
8. Solez K, Morel-Maroger L, Sraer JD: The morphology of "acute tubular necrosis" in man: Analysis of 57 renal biopsies and a comparison with the glycerol model. Medicine 1979;58:362–376.
9. Conger J: Does hemodialysis delay recovery from acute renal failure? Semin Dial 1990;3:146–150.
10. Schortgen F, Soubrier N, Delclaux C, et al: Hemodynamic tolerance of intermittent hemodialysis in critically ill patients. Usefulness of practice guidelines. Am J Respir Crit Care Med 2000;162:197–202.
11. Solutions R: Available at: http://www.renalsolutionsinc.com/home/documents/thehistoryofsorbentdialysisforpdf.pdf. Accessed July 30, 2007.
12. Nissenson A, Fine R (eds): Clinical Dialysis, 4th ed. New York: McGraw-Hill, 2005.
13. Ash SR: The Allient dialysis system. Semin Dial 2004;17:164–166.
14. Botella J, Ghezzi PM, Sanz-Moreno C: Adsorption in hemodialysis. Kidney Int 2000;76:S60–S65.
15. Schlaeper C, Amerling R, Manns M, Levin NW: High clearance continuous renal replacement therapy with a modified dialysis machine. Kidney Int 1999;72:S20–S23.
16. Kumar VA, Craig M, Depner TA, Yeun JY: Extended daily dialysis: A new approach to renal replacement for acute renal failure in the intensive care unit. Am J Kidney Dis 2000;36:294–300.
17. Berbece AN, Richardson RM: Sustained low-efficiency dialysis in the ICU: Cost, anticoagulation, and solute removal. Kidney Int 2006;70:963–968.
18. Finkel KW, Foringer JR: Safety of regional citrate anticoagulation for continuous sustained low efficiency dialysis (C-SLED) in critically ill patients. Ren Fail 2005;27:541–545.
19. Fliser D, Kielstein JT: Technology insight: treatment of renal failure in the intensive care unit with extended dialysis. Nat Clin Pract Nephrol 2006;2:32–39.
20. Kielstein JT, Kretschmer U, Ernst T, et al: Efficacy and cardiovascular tolerability of extended dialysis in critically ill patients: A randomized controlled study. Am J Kidney Dis 2004;43:342–349.
21. Kumar VA, Yeun JY, Depner TA, Don BR: Extended daily dialysis vs. continuous hemodialysis for ICU patients with acute renal failure: A two-year single center report. Int J Artif Organs 2004;27:371–379.
22. Lonnemann G, Floege J, Kliem V, et al: Extended daily veno-venous high-flux haemodialysis in patients with acute renal failure and multiple organ dysfunction syndrome using a single path batch dialysis system. Nephrol Dial Transplant 2000;15:1189–1193.
23. Marshall MR, Golper TA, Shaver MJ, et al: Sustained low-efficiency dialysis for critically ill patients requiring renal replacement therapy. Kidney Int 2001;60:777–785.
24. Marshall MR, Golper TA, Shaver MJ, et al: Urea kinetics during sustained low-efficiency dialysis in critically ill patients requiring renal replacement therapy. Am J Kidney Dis 2002;39:556–570.
25. Liao Z, Zhang W, Hardy PA, et al: Kinetic comparison of different acute dialysis therapies. Artif Organs 2003;27:802–807.
26. Mehta RL, Letteri JM: Current status of renal replacement therapy for acute renal failure. Am J Nephrol 1999;19:377–382.
27. Ricci Z, Ronco C, D'Amico G, et al: Practice patterns in the management of acute renal failure in the critically ill patient: An international survey. 2006;21:690–696.
28. Monti G, Herrera M, Kindgen-Milles D, et al: The DOse REsponse Multicentre International Collaborative Initiative (DO-RE-MI)1. Contrib Nephrol 2007;156:434–443.
29. Bell M, SWING, Granath F, et al: Continuous renal replacement therapy is associated with less chronic renal failure than intermittent haemodialysis after acute renal failure. Intensive Care Med 2007;33:773–780.
30. Jacka MJ, Ivancinova X, Gibney RT: Continuous renal replacement therapy improves renal recovery from acute renal failure. Can J Anaesth 2005;52:327–332.
31. Cho KC, Himmelfarb J, Paganini E, et al: Survival by dialysis modality in critically ill patients with acute kidney injury. J Am Soc Nephrol 2006;17:3132–3138.
32. Mehta RL, McDonald B, Gabbai FB, et al: A randomized clinical trial of continuous versus intermittent dialysis for acute renal failure. Kidney Int 2001;60:1154–1163.
33. Vinsonneau C, Camus C, Combes A, et al: Continuous venovenous haemodiafiltration versus intermittent haemodialysis for acute renal failure in patients with multiple-organ dysfunction syndrome: A multicentre randomised trial. Lancet 2006;368:379–385.
34. Misset B, Timsit JF, Chevret S, et al: A randomized cross-over comparison of the hemodynamic response to intermittent hemodialysis and continuous hemofiltration in ICU patients with acute renal failure. Intensive Care Med 1996;22:742–746.

35. Fiaccadori E, Gonzi G, Zambrelli P, Tortorella G: Cardiac arrhythmias during central venous catheter procedures in acute renal failure: A prospective study. J Am Soc Nephrol 1996;7:1079–1084.

36. Manns M, Sigler MH, Teehan BP: Intradialytic renal haemodynamics—potential consequences for the management of the patient with acute renal failure. Nephrol Dial Transplant 1997;12:870–872.

37. Mehta R: Renal replacement therapy for ARF: Matching the method to the patient. Semin Dial 1993;6:253–259.

38. Mehta RL, Letteri JM: Current status of renal replacement therapy for acute renal failure. A survey of US nephrologists. The National Kidney Foundation Council on Dialysis. Am J Nephrol 1999;19:377–382.

39. Liu KD, Himmelfarb J, Paganini E, et al: Timing of initiation of dialysis in critically ill patients with acute kidney injury. Clin J Am Soc Nephrol 2006;1:915–919.

40. Bouman CS, Oudemans-Van Straaten HM, Tijssen JG, et al: Effects of early high-volume continuous venovenous hemofiltration on survival and recovery of renal function in intensive care patients with acute renal failure: A prospective, randomized trial. Crit Care Med 2002;30:2205–2211.

41. Cantarovich F, Rangoonwala B, Lorenz H, et al: High-dose furosemide for established ARF: A prospective, randomized, double-blind, placebo-controlled, multicenter trial. Am J Kidney Dis 2004;44:402–409.

42. Mehta RL, Pascual MT, Soroko S, Chertow GM: Diuretics, mortality, and nonrecovery of renal function in acute renal failure. JAMA 2002;288:2547–2553.

43. Uchino S, Doig GS, Bellomo R, et al: Diuretics and mortality in acute renal failure. Crit Care Med 2004;32:2669–2677.

44. Liangos O, Rao M, Balakrishnan VS, et al: Relationship of urine output to dialysis initiation and mortality in acute renal failure. Nephro. Clin Pract 2005;99:c56–c60.

45. Mehta RL, McDonald B, Gabbai F, et al: Nephrology consultation in acute renal failure: Does timing matter? Am J Med 2002;113:456–461.

46. Mehta RL: Indications for dialysis in the ICU: Renal replacement vs. renal support. Blood Purif 2001;19:227–232.

47. Mukau L, Latimer RG: Acute hemodialysis in the surgical intensive care unit. Am Surg 1988;54:548–552.

48. Alsous F, Khamiees M, DeGirolamo A, et al: Negative fluid balance predicts survival in patients with septic shock: A retrospective pilot study. Chest 2000;117:1749–1754.

49. Foland JA, Fortenberry JD, Warshaw BL, et al: Fluid overload before continuous hemofiltration and survival in critically ill children: A retrospective analysis. Crit Care Med 2004;32:1771–1776.

50. Weiss L, Danielson BG, Wikstrom B, et al: Continuous arteriovenous hemofiltration in the treatment of 100 critically ill patients with acute renal failure: Report on clinical outcome and nutritional aspects. Clin Nephrol 1989;31:184–189.

51. Lopes JA, Jorge S, Resina C, et al: Prognostic utility of RIFLE for acute renal failure in patients with sepsis. Crit Care 2007;11:408.

52. Uchino S, Bellomo R, Goldsmith D, et al: An assessment of the RIFLE criteria for acute renal failure in hospitalized patients. Crit Care Med 2006;34:1913–1917.

53. Honoré PM, Joannes-Boyau O, Gressens B: Blood and plasma treatments: High-volume hemofiltration—a global view. Contrib Nephrol 2007;156:371–386.

54. Schiffl H, Lang SM, Fischer R: Daily hemodialysis and the outcome of acute renal failure. N Engl J Med 2002;346:305–310.

55. Clermont G, Acker CG, Angus DC, et al: Renal failure in the ICU: Comparison of the impact of acute renal failure and end-stage renal disease on ICU outcomes. Kidney Int 2002;62:986–996.

56. Manhes G, Heng AE, Aublet-Cuvelier B, et al: Clinical features and outcome of chronic dialysis patients admitted to an intensive care unit. Nephrol Dial Transplant 2005;20:1127–1133.

57. Shalkham AS, Kirrane BM, Hoffman RS, et al: The availability and use of charcoal hemoperfusion in the treatment of poisoned patients. Am J Kidney Dis 2006;48:239–241.

58. Zimmerman JL: Poisonings and overdoses in the intensive care unit: General and specific management issues. Crit Care Med 2003;31:2794–2801.

59. Guo PY, Storsley LJ, Finkle SN: Severe lactic acidosis treated with prolonged hemodialysis: Recovery after massive overdoses of metformin. Semin Dial 2006;19:80–83.

60. Costanzo MR, Guglin ME, Saltzberg MT, et al: Ultrafiltration versus intravenous diuretics for patients hospitalized for acute decompensated heart failure. J Am Coll Cardiol 2007;49:675–683.

61. Libetta C, Sepe V, Zucchi M, et al: Intermittent haemodiafiltration in refractory congestive heart failure: BNP and balance of inflammatory cytokines. Nephrol Dial Transplant 2007;22:2013–2019.

62. Leblanc M, Fedak S, Mokris G, Paganini EP: Blood recirculation in temporary central catheters for acute hemodialysis. Clin Nephrol 1996;45:315–319.

63. Canaud B, Desmeules S, Klouche K, et al: Vascular access for dialysis in the intensive care unit. Best Pract Res Clin Anaesthesiol 2004;18:159–174.

64. Clark DD, Albina JE, Chazan JA: Subclavian vein stenosis and thrombosis: A potential serious complication in chronic hemodialysis patients. Am J Kidney Dis 1990;15:265–268.

65. Oliver MJL: Acute dialysis catheters. Semin Dial 2001;14:432–435.

66. Kamran T, Zaheer K, Khan AA, et al: Applications and complications of subclavian vein catheterization for hemodialysis. J Coll Physicians Surg Pak 2003;13:40–43.

67. Liangos O, Rao M, Ruthazer R, et al: Factors associated with urea reduction ratio in acute renal failure. Artif Organs 2004;28:1076–1081.

68. Klouche K, Amigues L, Deleuze S, et al: Complications, effects on dialysis dose, and survival of tunneled femoral dialysis catheters in acute renal failure. Am J Kidney Dis 2007;49:99–108.

69. Grudzinski L, Quinan P, Kwok S, Pierratos A: Sodium citrate 4% locking solution for central venous dialysis catheters—an effective, more cost-efficient alternative to heparin. Nephrol Dial Transplant 2007;22:471–476.

70. Weijmer MC, van den Dorpel MA, Van de Ven PJ, et al: Randomized, clinical trial comparison of trisodium citrate 30% and heparin as catheter-locking solution in hemodialysis patients. J Am Soc Nephrol 2005;16:2769–2777.

71. Shanks RM, Sargent JL, Martinez RM, et al: Catheter lock solutions influence staphylococcal biofilm formation on abiotic surfaces. Nephrol Dial Transplant 2006;21:2247–2255.

72. Weijmer MC, Debets-Ossenkopp YJ, Van De Vondervoort FJ, ter Wee PM: Superior antimicrobial activity of trisodium citrate over heparin for catheter locking. Nephrol Dial Transplant 2002;17:2189–2195.

73. Daugirdas J, Blake P, Ing T (eds): Handbook of Dialysis, 3rd ed. Philadelphia: Lippincott Williams & Wilkins, 2001.

74. Cointault O, Kamar N, Bories P, et al: Regional citrate anticoagulation in continuous venovenous haemodiafiltration using commercial solutions. Nephrol Dial Transplant 2004;19:171–178.

75. Subramanian S, Venkataraman R, Kellum JA: Influence of dialysis membranes on outcomes in acute renal failure: A meta-analysis. Kidney Int 2002;62:1819–1823.

76. Gastaldello K, Melot C, Kahn R-J, et al: Comparison of cellulose diacetate and polysulfone membranes in the outcome of acute renal failure. A prospective randomized study. Nephrol Dial Transplant 2000;15:224–230.

77. Zimmerman D, Cotman P, Ting R, et al: Continuous veno-venous haemodialysis with a novel bicarbonate dialysis solution: Prospective cross-over comparison with a lactate buffered solution. Nephrol Dial Transplant 1999;14:2387–2391.

78. Kierdorf HP, Leue C, Arns S: Lactate- or bicarbonate-buffered solutions in continuous extracorporeal renal replacement therapies. Kidney Int 1999:S32–S36.

79. John S, Griesbach D, Baumgartel M, et al: Effects of continuous haemofiltration vs intermittent haemodialysis on systemic haemodynamics and splanchnic regional perfusion in septic shock patients: A prospective, randomized clinical trial. Nephrol Dial Transplant 2001;16:320–327.

80. Paganini EP, Sandy D, Moreno L, et al: The effect of sodium and ultrafiltration modelling on plasma volume changes and haemodynamic stability in intensive care patients receiving haemodialysis for acute renal failure: A prospective, stratified, randomized, crossover study. Nephrol Dial Transplant 1996;11(Suppl 8):32–37.

81. Dheenan S, Henrich WL: Preventing dialysis hypotension: A comparison of usual protective maneuvers. Kidney Int 2001;59:1175–1181.

82. Carlon GC, Campfield PB, Goldiner PL, Turnbull AD: Hypoxemia during hemodialysis. Crit Care Med 1979;7:497–499.

83. Patterson RW, Nissenson AR, Miller J, et al: Hypoxemia and pulmonary gas exchange during hemodialysis. J Appl Physiol 1981;50:259–264.

84. Hunt JM, Chappell TR, Henrich WL, Rubin LJ: Gas exchange during dialysis. Contrasting mechanisms contributing to comparable alterations with acetate and bicarbonate buffers. Am J Med 1984;77:255–260.

85. Ganss R, Aarseth HP, Nordby G: Prevention of hemodialysis associated hypoxemia by use of low-concentration bicarbonate dialysate. Asaio J 1992;38:820–822.

86. Pitcher WD, Diamond SM, Henrich WL: Pulmonary gas exchange during dialysis in patients with obstructive lung disease. Chest 1989;96:1136–1141.

87. Hinchliffe RJ, Kirk B, Bhattacharjee D, et al: The effect of haemodialysis on transcutaneous oxygen tension in patients with diabetes—a pilot study. Nephrol Dial Transplant 2006;21:1981–1983.

88. Munger MA, Ateshkadi A, Cheung AK, et al: Cardiopulmonary events during hemodialysis: Effects of dialysis membranes and dialysate buffers. Am J Kidney Dis 2000;36:130–139.

89. Trinh-Trang-Tan MM, Cartron JP, Bankir L: Molecular basis for the dialysis disequilibrium syndrome: Altered aquaporin and urea transporter expression in the brain. Nephrol Dial Transplant 2005;20:1984–1988.

90. Bagshaw S, Peets A, Hameed M, et al: Dialysis disequilibrium syndrome: Brain death following hemodialysis for metabolic acidosis and acute renal failure—a case report. BMC Nephrol 2004;5:9.

91. DiFresco V, Landman M, Jaber BL, White AC: Dialysis disequilibrium syndrome: An unusual cause of respiratory failure in the medical intensive care unit. Intensive Care Med 2000;26:628–630.

92. Lonnemann G: Chronic inflammation in hemodialysis: The role of contaminated dialysate. Blood Purif 2000;18:214–223.

93. Ward RA: Ultrapure dialysate. Semin Dial 2004;17:489–497.

94. Arizono K, Nomura K, Motoyama T, et al: Use of ultrapure dialysate in reduction of chronic inflammation during hemodialysis. Blood Purif 2004;22(Suppl 2):26–29.

95. Eknoyan G, Beck GJ, Cheung AK, et al: Effect of dialysis dose and membrane flux in maintenance hemodialysis. N Engl J Med 2002;347:2010–2019.

96. Saran R, Canaud BJ, Depner TA, et al: Dose of dialysis: Key lessons from major observational studies and clinical trials. Am J Kidney Dis 2004;44(5 Suppl 2):47–53.

97. Hemodialysis Adequacy 2006 Work Group: Clinical practice guidelines for hemodialysis adequacy, update 2006. Am J Kidney Dis 2006;48:S2–S90.

98. Paganini E, Tapolyai M, Goormastic M, et al: Establishing a dialysis therapy/patient outcome link in intensive care unit acute dialysis for patients with acute renal failure. Am J Kid Dis 1996;28:S81–S89.

99. Paganini EP, Kanagasundaram NS, Larive B, Greene T: Prescription of adequate renal replacement in critically ill patients. Blood Purif 2001;19:238–244.

100. Ronco C, Ricci Z, Bellomo R: Current worldwide practice of dialysis dose prescription in acute renal failure. Curr Opin Crit Care 2006;12:551–556.

101. Ronco C, Bellomo R, Homel P, et al: Effects of different doses in continuous veno-venous haemofiltration on outcomes of acute renal failure: A prospective randomised trial. Lancet 2000;356:26–30.

102. Ricci Z, Ronco C: Renal replacement. II: Dialysis dose. Crit Care Clin 2005;21:357–366.

103. Evanson JA, Himmelfarb J, Wingard R, et al: Prescribed versus delivered dialysis in acute renal failure patients. Am J Kidney Dis 1998;32:731–738.

104. Evanson JA, Ikizler TA, Wingard R, et al: Measurement of the delivery of dialysis in acute renal failure. Kidney Int 1999;55:1501–1508.

105. Leblanc M, Tapolyai M, Paganini EP: What dialysis dose should be provided in acute renal failure? A review. Adv Renal Replace Ther 1995;2:255–264.

106. Lowrie EG, Chertow GM, Lew NL, et al: The urea [clearance × dialysis time] product (Kt) as an outcome-based measure of hemodialysis dose. Kidney Int 1999;56:729–737.

107. Ridel C, Osman D, Mercadal L, et al: Ionic dialysance: A new valid parameter for quantification of dialysis efficiency in acute renal failure? Intensive Care Med 2007;33:460–465.

108. Casino FG, Marshall MR: Simple and accurate quantification of dialysis in acute renal failure patients during either urea non-steady state or treatment with irregular or continuous schedules. Nephrol Dial Transplant 2004;19:1454–1466.

109. Marshall MR, Ma T, Galler D, et al: Sustained low-efficiency daily diafiltration (SLEDD-f) for critically ill patients requiring renal replacement therapy: Towards an adequate therapy. Nephrol Dial Transplant 2004;19:877–884.

110. Marshall MR, Golper TA, Shaver MJ, et al: Urea kinetics during sustained low-efficiency dialysis in critically ill patients requiring renal replacement therapy. Am J Kidney Dis 2002;39:556–570.

111. Cleve E, Smith F, Hensler N: Peritoneal dialysis in renal failure. Am J Med Sci 1960;240:319–326.

112. Howard CS, Teitelbaum I: Renal replacement therapy in patients with chronic liver disease. 2005;18:212–216.

113. Gabriel DP, Fernandez-Cean J, Balbi AL: Utilization of peritoneal dialysis in the acute setting. 2007;27:328–331.

114. Gabriel DP, Nascimento GVR, Caramori JT, et al: Peritoneal dialysis in acute renal failure. Ren Fail 2006;28:451–456.

115. Davenport A: Renal replacement therapy in the patient with acute brain injury. Am J Kidney Dis 2001;37:457–466.

116. Chitalia VC, Almeida AF, Rai H, et al: Is peritoneal dialysis adequate for hypercatabolic acute renal failure in developing countries? Kidney Int 2002;61:747–757.

117. Gabriel DP, do Nascimento GV, Caramori JT, et al: High volume peritoneal dialysis for acute renal failure. Perit Dial Int 2007;27:277–282.

118. Bracey D: Acute renal failure: Two cases treated with decapsulation and peritoneal dialysis. Br J Surg 1951;38:482–488.

119. Twardowski ZJ: History of peritoneal access development. Int J Artif Organs 2006;29:2–40.

120. Auron A, Warady BA, Simon S, et al: Use of the multipurpose drainage catheter for the provision of acute peritoneal dialysis in infants and children. Am J Kidney Dis 2007;49:650–655.

121. Thongboonkerd V, Lumlertgul D, Supajatura V: Better correction of metabolic acidosis, blood pressure control, and phagocytosis with bicarbonate compared to lactate solution in acute peritoneal dialysis. Artif Organs 2001;25:99–108.

122. Heimburger O: Peritoneal transport with icodextrin solution. Contrib Nephrol 2006;150:97–103.

123. Gursu EM, Ozdemir A, Yalinbas B, et al: The effect of icodextrin and glucose-containing solutions on insulin resistance in CAPD patients. Clin Nephrol 2006;66:263–268.

124. Amici G, Orrasch M, Da Rin G, Bocci C: Hyperinsulinism reduction associated with icodextrin treatment in continuous ambulatory peritoneal dialysis patients. Adv Perit Dial 2001;17:80–83.

125. Boer WH, Vos PF, Fieren MW: Culture-negative peritonitis associated with the use of icodextrin-containing dialysate in twelve patients treated with peritoneal dialysis. Perit Dial Int 2003;23:33–38.

126. MacGinley R, Cooney K, Alexander G, et al: Relapsing culture-negative peritonitis in peritoneal dialysis patients exposed to icodextrin solution. Am J Kidney Dis 2002;40:1030–1035.

127. Golej J, Kitzmueller E, Hermon M, et al: Low-volume peritoneal dialysis in 116 neonatal and paediatric critical care patients. Eur J Pediatr 2002;161:385–389.

128. Wood EG, Lynch RE, Fleming SS, Bunchman TE: Ultrafiltration using low volume peritoneal dialysis in critically ill infants and children. Adv Perit Dial 1991;7:266–268.

129. Vande Walle JG, Raes AM, De Hoorne J, Mauel R: Need for low sodium concentration and frequent cycles of 3.86% glucose solution in children treated with acute peritoneal dialysis. Adv Perit Dial 2005;21:204–208.

130. Ronco C, Amerling R: Continuous flow peritoneal dialysis: Current state-of-the-art and obstacles to further development. Contrib Nephrol 2006;150:310–320.

131. Winchester JF, Harbord N, Audia P, et al: The 2006 K/DOQI guidelines for peritoneal dialysis adequacy are not adequate. Blood Purif 2007;25:103–105.

132. Henrich WL (ed): Principles and Practice of Dialysis, 3rd ed. Philadelphia: Lippincott Williams & Wilkins, 2004.

133. Wong K, Lan LC, Lin SC, Tam P: Small bowel herniation and gangrene from peritoneal dialysis catheter exit site. Pediatr Nephrol 2003;18:301–302.

134. Ahluwalia M, Ishikawa S, Gellman M, et al: Pulmonary functions during peritoneal dialysis. Clin Nephrol 1982;18:251–256.

135. Cruces RP, Roque EJ, Ronco MR, et al: [Massive acute hydrothorax secondary to peritoneal dialysis in a hemolytic uremic syndrome. Report of one case]. Rev Med Chil 2006;134:91–94.

136. Chow KM, Szeto CC, Li PK-T: Management options for hydrothorax complicating peritoneal dialysis. Semin Dial 2003;16:389–394.

137. Vande Walle J, Raes A, Dehoorne J, et al: Combined amino-acid and glucose peritoneal dialysis solution for children with acute renal failure. Adv Perit Dial 2004;20:226–230.

138. Guo PYF, Storsley LJ, Finkle SN: Severe lactic acidosis treated with prolonged hemodialysis: Recovery after massive overdoses of metformin. Semin Dial 2006;19:80–83.

139. Gabutti L, Ferrari N, Mombelli G, et al: The favorable effect of regional citrate anticoagulation on interleukin-1beta release is dissociated from both coagulation and complement activation. J Nephrol 2004;17:819–825.

140. Hofbauer R, Moser D, Frass M, et al: Effect of anticoagulation on blood membrane interactions during hemodialysis. Kidney Int 1999;56:1578–1583.

Further Reading

Bellomo R: Do we know the optimal dose for renal replacement therapy in the intensive care unit? Kidney Int 2006;70:1202–1204.

Fliser D, Kielstein JT: Technology insight: Treatment of renal failure in the intensive care unit with extended dialysis. Nat Clin Pract Nephrol 2006;2:32–39.

Gabriel DP, Nascimento GVR, Caramori JT, et al: Peritoneal dialysis in acute renal failure. Ren Fail 2006;28:451–456.

John S, Eckardt KU: Renal replacement therapy in the treatment of acute renal failure—intermittent and continuous. Semin Dial 2006;19:455–464.

Ronco C, Ricci Z, Bellomo R: Current worldwide practice of dialysis dose prescription in acute renal failure. Curr Opin Crit Care 2006;12:551–556.

Chapter 7

Continuous Renal Replacement Therapies

Dinna Cruz, Zaccaria Ricci, Sandra Silva, and Claudio Ronco

In the past decade, the change in the epidemiology of acute renal failure has made critical care nephrology an emerging subspecialty of intensive care medicine. Dedicated literature and a series of physicians and nurses have made an effort to bridge the knowledge and experience from nephrology and critical care medicine in response to an increased incidence of acute kidney injury (AKI) in intensive care unit (ICU) patients.[1] The use of continuous renal replacement therapies (CRRTs) is constantly increasing, especially in the setting of intensive care and critically ill patients, as originally advocated by Kramer and colleagues.[2]

The kidneys remove water, various solutes, and nonvolatile acids, thereby maintaining homeostasis; they also metabolize inflammatory mediators and excrete administered drugs or their metabolites. Thus, the optimal treatment of acute renal failure should closely mimic the functions of the kidney. Different renal replacement therapy (RRT) strategies present advantages and disadvantages, and the application of a given technique should be decided based on specific indications and careful evaluation of patient's clinical conditions. In this setting, CRRTs are generally chosen for sicker patients for whom hemodialysis or peritoneal dialysis is contraindicated or even precluded.

EVOLUTION OF CONTINUOUS THERAPIES

The Birth of Continuous Renal Replacement Therapies

The origin of the new era of extracorporeal treatment of acute renal failure can definitely be found in the mid-1970s, when continuous arteriovenous hemofiltration (CAVH) appeared on the scene. Up to that point, AKI was treated with conservative measures: peritoneal dialysis or intermittent hemodialysis (IHD). All techniques had the limitations of low clearance rates, poor fluid management control, and many complications. CAVH was developed by Peter Kramer in 1977, and it immediately became an important alternative treatment for

AKI in those patients in whom peritoneal dialysis or IHD was clinically or technically precluded.[3] This opened the doors of ICUs to a dedicated dialysis technology that experienced a flourishing evolution in subsequent years. In the mid-1980s, the technology of CAVH was extended to infants and children, and newly designed hemofilters permitted the application of the technique even to newborns. CAVH presented important advantages over IHD. These were particularly apparent in the areas of hemodynamic stability, control of circulating volume, and nutritional support. However, CAVH also had serious shortcomings that included the need for arterial cannulation (or construction of a Scribner arteriovenous shunt) and the limited solute clearance that could be achieved even under optimal operating circumstances (10 ± 12 mL/min for small solutes such as urea). Initial technical modifications, such as predilution (i.e., the infusion of the replacement solution before the filter instead of after it), did improve creatinine clearance, but the next major technical advance was the creation of an additional side port to the hemofilter. Through this port countercurrent dialysate could be infused at slow flow rates (i.e., 1 L/hr) to achieve additional diffusive solute clearance: this modified technique was named continuous arteriovenous hemodiafiltration or hemodialysis (CAVHDF or CAVHD). With the arrival of CAVHDF-CAVHD, IHD was used even less because uremic control could be achieved in all patients irrespective of their weight or catabolic state simply by increasing the countercurrent dialysate flow rates to 1.5 or 2 L/hr as necessary.

Venovenous Pumped Techniques

Arteriovenous therapies were simple because they did not require a peristaltic blood pump, but the morbidity associated with arterial cannulation was substantial. For this reason, venovenous techniques using a double-lumen central venous catheter for vascular access were considered preferable and safer. Thus, within a few years, continuous venovenous hemofiltration (CVVH) replaced CAVH because of its improved performance and safety. The advance was made possible by the use of blood pumps, calibrated ultrafiltration control systems, and double-lumen venous catheters. In this setting, improved safety and reliability were then offered by CVVH or continuous venovenous hemodiafiltration or continuous venovenous hemodialysis. These treatments started to be widely used at the end of the 1980s and achieved excellent uremic control using high blood flows ($\geq$150 mL/min) and large membrane surface areas ($\geq$0.8 m^2). To facilitate nursing care, ultrafiltration was soon controlled by devices with reasonable precision. Thus, for clinical purposes, ultrafiltration and reinfusion could be fully regulated to achieve the desired therapeutic goals. In the late 1980s, specific machines for CRRTs were designed and a new era of renal replacement in the critically ill patient began.[4] The therapy started to be standardized and clear indications began to be defined. The evolution of technology did not stop, however, and the recent demand for higher efficiency and exchange volumes has spurred new interest in a further generation of machines with better performance, integrated information technology, and easy-to-use operator interfaces.

Recent Advances in Continuous Renal Replacement Therapies

The latest generation of machines available on the market today, representing the evolution of the past decade of research and development, is shown in Figure 7-1. Specific machines have now been designed to permit safe and reliable performance of the therapy. These new devices are equipped with a user friendly interface that allows for easy performance and monitoring. The apparent complexity of the circuit is made simple by a self-loading circuit or a cartridge that includes the filter and the blood and dialysate lines. Priming is performed automatically by the machine and pre- or postdilution (reinfusion of substitution fluid

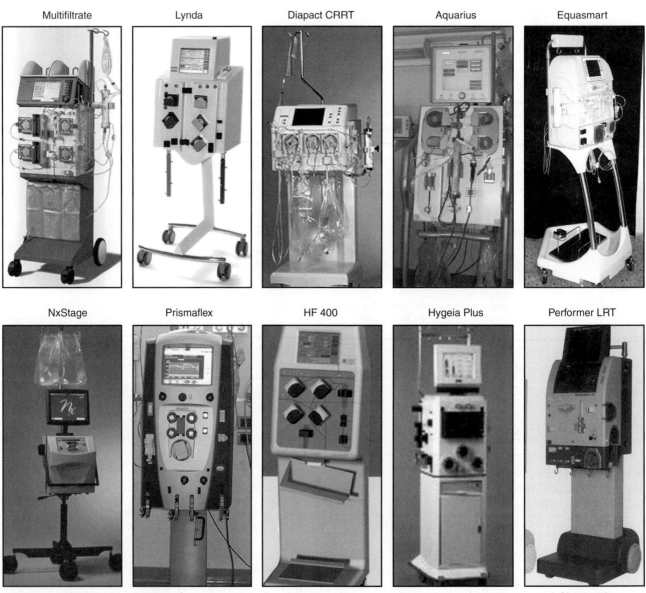

Figure 7-1 The latest generation of continuous renal replacement therapy machines. **Top,** The Fresenius Multifiltrate, The Bellco Lynda, The B. Braun Diapact CRRT, The Edwards Aquarius, The Medica Equasmart. **Bottom,** The NxStage, The Gambro Prosmaflex, The Infomed HF 400, The Hygeia Plus, The RAND Performer LRT.

before or after the filter) can easily be performed by changing the position of the reinfusion line. These new machines permit all CRRTs to be performed by programming the flows and the total amounts of fluid to be exchanged or circulated as a countercurrent dialysate at the beginning of the session.

A schematic drawing of different techniques available today for the therapy of the critically ill patient with renal and other organ dysfunction is given in Figure 7-2. An important advance in the past decade has been the use of either increased exchange volumes in hemofiltration or the combined use of adsorbent techniques.[5] Early data suggest that high-volume hemofiltration (HVHF) and continuous plasma filtration coupled with adsorption may have a beneficial effect on clinical outcome in patients with severe sepsis and septic shock (see following discussion).

The effect of different modalities of CRRT on length of stay and recovery of renal function in the general population is still under evaluation, since the case mix is changing in every study and the populations treated are not homogeneous. In this field, further research is needed. Adequate technical support becomes mandatory, therefore, to fulfill all these expectations. The evolution of understanding of the above-mentioned concepts has led to the improvement of technology and the generation of new machines and devices compatible with the demand for increased efficiency, accuracy, safety, performance, and cost/benefit ratio. At present, almost all CRRTs can be delivered in a safe, adequate, and flexible way, thanks to devices specifically designed for critically ill patients, to a point that multiple organ support therapy is envisaged as a possible therapeutic approach in the critical care setting.[6] Nevertheless, CRRTs cannot be considered simple therapies that can be prescribed and administered by everybody. Thorough education and training are quintessential for the personnel dealing with these techniques. Dedicated nurses and knowledgeable specialists are required to administer a therapy with optimal features of safety and efficacy.

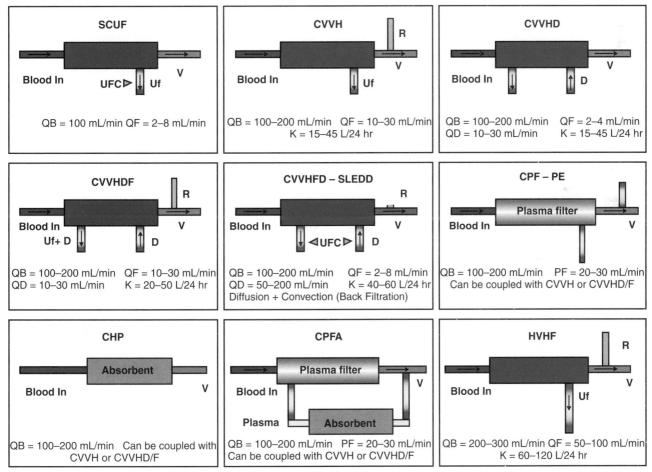

Figure 7-2 Techniques available today for renal replacement in the intensive care unit. CAVH, continuous arteriovenous hemofiltration; CHP, continuous hemoperfusion; CPFA, continuous plasmafiltration coupled with adsorption; CPF-PE, continuous plasmafiltration–plasma exchange; CVVH, continuous venovenous hemofiltration; CVVHD, continuous venovenous hemodialysis; CVVHDF, continuous venovenous hemodiafiltration; CVVHFD, continuous venovenous high-flux dialysis; D, dialysate; HVHF, high-volume hemofiltration; K, clearance; PF, plasma filtrate flow; QB, blood flow; QD, dialysate flow; QF, ultrafiltration rate; R, replacement; SCUF, slow continuous ultrafiltration; SLEDD, sustained low efficiency daily dialysis; UFC, ultrafiltration control system; V, venous return.

CLINICAL ASPECTS OF CONTINUOUS RENAL REPLACEMENT THERAPIES

Fluid Removal

CRRT slowly and continuously removes fluid, mimicking the urine output, whereas IHD must extract up to 2 days worth of administered fluid plus excess body water, which may be pathologically present in the anuric patient. The intravascular volume depletion associated with IHD is due to both the high rate of fluid removal required and the transcellular and interstitial fluid shifts caused by the rapid dialytic loss of solute.[7] The major consequence of rapid fluid removal is hemodynamic instability. Critically ill patients need continuous volume infusions: blood and fresh frozen plasma, vasopressors and other continuous infusions, and parenteral and enteral nutrition, which must be delivered without restriction or interruption even in hypercatabolic patients. In the clinical picture of an anuric patient, this means a constant risk of fluid overload and high daily ultrafiltration requirements. The extreme example of the patient who cannot afford intravascular volume shifts is the patient with acute respiratory distress syndrome, the septic patient who is becoming refractory to vasopressors, or the patient with cerebral edema. Furthermore, all critically ill patients tolerate hypotension poorly, with a definite risk of cardiac arrest, particularly if they are already inotrope dependent. Indeed, the damaged kidneys, which have temporarily lost pressure-flow autoregulation, may also be threatened with fresh ischemic lesions occurring with each episode of IHD,[8] leading to a delay in renal recovery. Interestingly, recent reports have suggested a benefit of CRRTs with respect to recovery of renal function (see following discussion).

The importance of fluid balance management is enhanced in the specific category of patients with decompensated heart failure. In fact, it is just such patients who may well respond positively to continuous ultrafiltration with an increase in cardiac index, while avoiding a decrease in arterial pressure, due to a change in the preload optimizing myocardial contractility on the Starling curve.[7] Many patients with congestive cardiac failure nonresponsive to conventional therapy are now successfully treated in this way.[9]

In critically ill children, the correction of water overload is considered a priority: it has been shown that restoring an adequate water content in small children is the main independent variable for outcome prediction.[10,11] This concept is even more important in critically ill neonates in whom a relatively larger amount of fluid must be administered to deliver an adequate amount of drug infusion, parenteral/enteral nutrition, and blood derivates.

Solute Removal and Electrolyte Balance

An attribute of IHD often quoted by proponents is that it is highly efficient at clearing solutes such as urea. In fact, this is both a false argument and a disadvantage. The primary rationale of using continuous therapy is to maintain a more physiologic constant removal of fluid and solute, among other things. In the process, the cumulative clearance of urea and creatinine by a continuous method is significantly superior to that achieved by IHD administered as often as four times per week, even in septic patients. Indeed, IHD six times per week would be required to achieve the same uremic control.[12]

The detailed physiologic impact of better uremic control has not been fully elucidated. Uremia causes immunosuppression with impaired phagocytosis and defective lymphocyte and monocyte function, which could well be important in the ICU setting. Extrapolating from data established in patients with end-stage renal disease, better uremic control is clearly advantageous. In the National Cooperative Dialysis Study, there was a higher morbidity, including cardiovascular events and hospitalization rate, in patients with end-stage renal disease hemodialyzed to a target average urea concentration of 100 mg/dL (36 mmol/L) compared to the group whose target was 50 mg/dL (18 mmol/L).[13] There is, however, uncertainty regarding the relative contributions of uremia, malnutrition, and bioincompatible membranes in these older studies.[14] Furthermore, work needs to be done specifically on patients with AKI.

A landmark study by Ronco and co-workers[15] is at present the only randomized trial in AKI that showed that a high (adequate) dialytic dose (metabolic control) improved survival: in this study, continuous venovenous postdilution hemofiltration at 35 mL/kg/hr or 45 mL/kg/hr was associated with improved survival when compared with 20 mL/kg/hr in 425 critically ill patients with AKI.[15] This suggests that 35 mL/kg/hr should be considered the minimum adequate CRRT dose in patients with AKI.

One specific comment must be made concerning the difference between CVVH and all other techniques, including dialysis and the use of diuretics. In all pharmacologic and dialytic techniques, the removal of sodium and water cannot be dissociated and the mechanisms are strictly correlated. In particular, the diuretic effect is based on natriuresis, while ultrafiltration during dialysis may result in hypo- or hypertonia, depending on the interference with diffusion and removal of other molecules such as urea and other electrolytes. In such circumstances, water removal is linked to other solutes in proportions that are dependent on the technique used. In CVVH, the mechanism of ultrafiltration produces a fluid that is substantially similar to plasma water except for a minimal interference due to Donnan effects. In such a technique, ultrafiltration is basically iso-osmotic and isonatremic and water and sodium removal cannot be dissociated, with sodium elimination linked to the sodium plasma water concentration. However, the sodium balance can be significantly affected by the sodium concentration in the replacement solution. Sodium removal can be dissociated from water removal in CVVH, thus obtaining a real manipulation of the sodium pool in the body. This effect cannot be achieved with any other technique. The advantage is that one can normalize not only plasma concentrations but also the electrolyte content in the extracellular and possibly intracellular volume.[16]

Immunomodulatory Effects

One of the most active areas of research in intensive care in recent years involves the modulation of the septic response to reduce the persistently high mortality in sepsis syndrome and the potential benefit of CRRT. Although there is skepticism that any improvement might be due to nonspecific changes such as fluid removal or lowering the core temperature in febrile patients, there is evidence that cytokines and complement, among other mediators, are cleared from the blood by convection and/or adsorption onto high-flux synthetic hemofilter membranes. There is little doubt that it is important to use biocompatible membranes, and if mediator removal is to be effective, it needs to be continuous and convective, not intermittent and diffusive.[17]

HVHF or continuous plasma filtration coupled with adsorption (CPFA) has been investigated as potent immunomodulatory treatments in sepsis. Since sepsis and systemic inflammatory response syndrome are characterized by a cytokine network that is synergistic, redundant, autocatalytic, and self-augmenting, the control of such a nonlinear system cannot be approached by simple blockade or elimination of some specific mediators. Therefore, nonspecific removal of a broad range of inflammatory mediators by HVHF and CPFA may be beneficial, as recently suggested based on the peak concentration hypothesis.[18] The high dose that characterizes HVHF can be delivered by using either a constantly high exchange rate or delivering a pulse (for 6–8 hours) of very high-volume hemofiltration (85–100 mL/kg/hr) followed by standard doses.[19] In both cases, cytokine half-lives and concentrations are affected, the first by the continuous modality and the second by the nonspecific decapitation of peaks. Therefore, rather than a detailed analysis of each molecule involved, we envisage as much more interesting and useful a teleologic analysis of the impact of HVHF on more integrated events such as monocyte cell responsiveness, including apoptosis, neutrophil-priming activity, and oxidative burst.[18,20] Whether these effects translate into significant changes in end-organ damage by inflammatory mediators or result in a reproducible reduction in mortality and/or morbidity is still being elucidated.

Side Effects of Continuous Renal Replacement Therapies

Although considerable attention has focused on the perceived benefits of CRRTs, there has been less emphasis on the possibility that CRRT might confer increased risk. As a continuous extracorporeal therapy, CRRT often requires continuous anticoagulation, which can increase bleeding risk. Conversely, clotting of the extracorporeal circuit also occurs frequently with CRRTs, which might contribute to blood loss and could exacerbate anemia in critically ill patients. The increased solute transfer associated with the use of CRRTs might enhance removal of amino acids, vitamins, catecholamines, and other solutes with a beneficial function in critically ill patients. Continuous therapies must be continuous to work: how many treatments really last more than 18 to 20 hours per day? Downtime due to filter-circuit-catheter clotting, circuit change, frequent replacement solution bag substitution, and patient mobility (surgery, diagnostics) should be carefully monitored and might significantly affect dialysis dose.[21] Also of concern are recent reports that technical problems with the delivery of CRRTs, including machine malfunction, medication errors, and compounding errors, might contribute to increased patient morbidity and mortality. Detection of safety problems and/or adverse events is particularly difficult when there are high rates of expected morbidity and mortality in the population undergoing a procedure, as is the case with CRRTs in critically ill patients with AKI. Currently, few available studies in the nephrology literature provide substantive information on the safety or adverse effects of CRRTs or IHD in the critically ill population. After the introduction of new technology and devices into medical practice, there is a natural tendency to assume that the novel therapeutic approach is providing benefit. This is especially the case when a therapy is administered to a critically ill patient 24 hours per day and becomes part of the typical equipment of an ICU bed: the level of attention is probably superior when a dedicated dialysis nurse administers the treatment for few hours during a day shift. Nonetheless, a new generation of dedicated CRRT machines has been recently released with strict safety features and the possibility of a high range of prescriptions. In any case, the ideal therapy still does not exist and specific ICU staff training is mandatory before the routine use of such modern monitors: there will never be a solution to the unwise use of a perfect system.[22]

Clinical Trials Focusing on Mortality

Four recently published randomized clinical trials and one multicenter observational study tested the hypothesis that outcomes with CRRTs are superior to those with IHD.[23–27] None of these studies showed a superior outcome for CRRTs compared with IHD. The results of these studies are surprising and, in some cases, strongly criticized for methodology and group randomization.[28] Nevertheless, they certainly do not support the belief that CRRTs provide better outcomes than IHD. One of the common key points of these recent trials can be that IHD has become safer and more efficacious with contemporary dialytic techniques. Furthermore, a liberal and extended use of CRRTs might have become less safe and/or efficacious than previously considered or expected. The concept that CRRTs can provide more hemodynamic stability, more effective volume homeostasis, and better blood pressure support than IHD has been the basis for the assumption that CRRTs are superior therapies. Over the past two decades, however, technical advances in the delivery of IHD have dramatically decreased the propensity of IHD to cause intradialytic hypotension. These advances include the introduction of volume-controlled dialysis machines, the routine use of biocompatible synthetic dialysis membranes, the use of bicarbonate-based dialysate, and the delivery of higher doses of dialysis. In an important study, Schortgen[29] demonstrated that there were a lower rate of hemodynamic instability and better outcomes after implementation of a clinical practice algorithm designed to improve hemodynamic tolerance to IHD. Recommendations included priming the dialysis circuit with isotonic saline, setting dialysate sodium concentration at more than 145 mmol/L, discontinuing vasodilator therapy, and setting dialysate temperature to below 37°C. Thus, the original rationale for the widely held assumption that CRRTs are superior therapies may have dissipated over time. Examining the results of recently published observational studies and randomized trials reveals no convincing evidence to support superiority of CRRTs over IHD in terms of mortality in the management of most critically ill patients with AKI.[30]

Clinical Studies and Renal Recovery

However, is mortality the only relevant endpoint to examine? There is a certain tendency to neglect the kidney once it has failed, based on the misconception that one can do no further harm to an organ that has already failed. However, renal recovery is an equally important clinical endpoint. Long-term dialysis is not only associated with significant impairment in health-related quality of life,[31] it is also an expensive therapy, costing on average U.S. $69,751 per year.[32] Moreover, chronic kidney disease of milder severity (stage 2 or 3) is likewise associated with adverse patient outcomes and high health care costs, suggesting that the presence of any sustained renal impairment is potentially significant.[33] Therefore, treatment of all patients with intermittent hemodialysis on the presumption of equipoise based on mortality outcomes may be inappropriate from both clinical and economic standpoints because it disregards potential downstream effects. Better rates of renal recovery might save significant resources and affect long-term well-being among survivors.

Three observational studies and one randomized, controlled study reported renal-related outcomes.[23,34-36] In a single-center observational study, dialysis independence was significantly higher among patients initially treated with CRRTs (87%) versus IHD (36%).[35] Similar results were seen in a Swedish multicenter study in which 91.7% of patients treated with CRRTs were dialysis independent at 3 months compared with 83.5% of IHD patients.[34] A large international multicenter database confirmed these findings.[36] Unadjusted dialysis dependence at hospital discharge was higher after CRRTs (85.5%) than after IHD (66.2%). Last, the randomized, controlled trial by Mehta and colleagues,[23] often quoted as a "negative" trial, found CRRTs to be beneficial regarding renal recovery. Chronic renal insufficiency at death or hospital discharge was diagnosed in 17% of patients whose therapy was IHD versus only 4% of those whose initial therapy was CRRTs ($P = .01$). For patients receiving an adequate trial of monotherapy, recovery of renal function was 92% for CRRTs versus 59% for IHD ($P < .01$). A pathophysiologic explanation for this observation can be easily found. In at least one study, a significantly higher incidence of hypotension was seen among patients treated with IHD as opposed to CRRTs.[37] The gentle but effective correction of metabolic and fluid derangements and the maintenance of a steady correction of homeostasis by CRRTs may influence the process of recovery of the kidney during and after the acute injury has occurred. When seen in this light, CRRT is a potentially valuable tool to aid renal recovery.

Clinical Effects of Hybrid Techniques

Hybrid techniques have been given a variety of names, such as sustained low efficiency daily dialysis (SLEDD), prolonged intermittent daily RRT, extended daily dialysis (EDD), or simply extended dialysis,[38-41] depending on variations in schedule and type of solute removal (convective or diffusive). Theoretically speaking, the purpose of such therapy would be the optimization of the advantages offered by either CRRTs or IHD, including efficient solute removal with minimum solute disequilibrium, reduced ultrafiltration rate with hemodynamic stability, optimized delivered-to-prescribed ratio, low anticoagulant needs, decreased cost of therapy delivery, efficiency of resource use, and improved patient mobility. Initial case series have shown the feasibility and high clearances that potentially are associated with such approaches. The arrival of technology that can be used in the ICU by ICU nurses to deliver SLEDD with convective components offers further options from a therapeutic point of view. One can now easily use technology in the ICU to generate ultrapure replacement fluid and administer it as in CRRTs, but at lower cost, in greater amounts, and for shorter periods of time, or combine such hemofiltration with diffusion, or use pure diffusion at any chosen clearance for a period of time that can encompass a given nursing shift, the 9 to 5 maximum staff availability period, or the nighttime period.

A recent randomized trial comparing CVVH and EDD with filtration (EDDf) found that both techniques achieved correction of several electrolyte abnormalities present before intervention.[42] The potential risk of hypophosphatemia in CVVH patients suggests the need for vigilance and frequent serum phosphate monitoring. Importantly, in all patients, hypo- or hyperkalemia/-magnesemia were avoided with the prescriptions used. Although the serum sodium was maintained within the normal range and was similar in both groups, there were significant differences in the chloride concentration. The relative hyperchloremia in the EDDf patients was almost certainly due to the greater concentration of chloride in the fluids used for EDDf (111.8 mmol/L) than in the fluids used for CVVH (100.75 mmol/L). The authors found that the two therapies affected metabolic acid-base variables differently. First, the concentration of lactate was lower with EDDf throughout the study period. This difference was likely explained by the use of lactate as buffer during CVVH, compared with bicarbonate during EDDf. Second, despite the increase in lactate with CVVH, median pH, bicarbonate, and base excess values were all less acidotic with continuous treatment. These findings are consistent with both the lower amount of buffer in EDDf fluids (26 mEq/L) than in CVVH (45 mEq/L) and the relative hyperchloremia of these fluids. The effect of hyperchloremia is also likely to explain the difference in mean apparent strong ion difference between the two groups. A decrease in CO_2 in response to this metabolic acidosis accounted for the lower effective strong ion difference values observed during EDDf. Conversely, the strong ion gap was similar for both treatments, in keeping with likely equivalent clearance of unmeasured acids. Although the clinical significance of these differences is uncertain, a higher bicarbonate concentration in EDDf fluids may be desirable.

CONCLUSIONS

Comparing intermittent and continuous therapies can be misleading. Besides the difficulty of conducting a well-designed, adequately powered, randomized trial (requiring at least 1200 patients), continuous and intermittent therapies represent a continuum in the management of AKI; thus, sicker patients would derive greater benefit from CRRTs, whereas less severely ill patients might take advantage of daily extended or intermittent treatments.

The choices today are almost limitless: Should the therapy be 3 or 4 hours of IHD with standard settings? Or should it be CRRT at 35 mL/kg/hr effluent flow rate? Or should it be SLEDD at blood and dialysate flow rates of 150 mL/min for 8 hours during the day? Or should we apply SLEDD for 12 hours overnight? Or should we add a convective component to SLEDD and make it SLEDD with filtration? Or should we combine CRRT for the first 2 or 3 days when the patient is in the hyperacute phase, with SLEDD thereafter as recovery takes place? Indeed, from the point of view of the intensivist, the modes of RRT are beginning to resemble the modes of mechanical ventilation, with ventilator settings seamlessly being changed to fit into the therapeutic goals and patient needs and phases of illness. Just as stereotyped approaches to ventilation are anachronistic and inappropriately try to fit the patient into a fixed therapy rather than tailoring the therapy to the patient, so should RRT be adjusted to fulfill the needs of the individual and his or her illness. Just as the concept of showing that one mode of ventilation is better than another seems a lost cause, the same might happen with RRT. In the light of current knowledge, it is prudent to say that the best RRT for a patient is the safest, the simplest, and the more efficient that the center can provide. Until definitive data become available, be it about mortality or renal recovery, personal experience and local circumstances remain major determinants in the selection of a given RRT mortality.

References

1. Ronco C: Critical care nephrology: The journey has begun. Int J Artif Organs 2004;27:349–351.
2. Kramer P, Wigger W, Rieger J, et al: Arteriovenous haemofiltration: A new and simple method for treatment of over-hydrated patients resistant to diuretics. Klin Wochenschr 1977;55:1121–1122.
3. Lauer A, Saccaggi A, Ronco C, et al: Continuous arterio-venous hemofiltration in the critically ill patient. Ann Intern Med 1983;99:455–460.
4. Ronco C, Bellomo R: The evolving technology for continuous renal replacement therapy from current standards to high volume hemofiltration. Curr Opin Crit Care 1997;3:426–433.
5. Reiter K, Bellomo R, Ronco C, Kellum J: Pro/con clinical debate: Is high-volume hemofiltration beneficial in the treatment of septic shock? Crit Care 2002;6:18–21.
6. Ronco C, Bellomo R: Acute renal failure and multiple organ dysfunction in the ICU: From renal replacement therapy (RRT) to multiple organ support therapy (MOST). Int J Artif Organs 2002;25:733–747.
7. Lauer A, Alvis R, Avram M: Hemodynamic consequences of continuous arteriovenous hemofiltration. Am J Kidney Dis 1988;12:110–115.
8. Conger JD, Robinette JB, Hammond WS: Differences in vascular reactivity in models of ischemic acute renal failure. Kidney Int 1991;39:1087–1097.
9. Costanzo MR, Guglin ME, Saltzberg MT, et al, for the UNLOAD Trial Investigators: Ultrafiltration versus intravenous diuretics for patients hospitalized for acute decompensated heart failure. J Am Coll Cardiol 2007;49:675–683.
10. Goldstein SL, Currier H, Graf C, et al: Outcome in children receiving continuous veno-venous hemofiltration. Pediatrics 2001;107:1309–1312.
11. Foland JA, Fortenberry JD, Warshaw BL, et al: Fluid overload before continuous hemofiltration and survival in critically ill children: A retrospective analysis. Crit Care Med 2004;32:1771–1776.
12. Clark WR, Mueller BA, Alaka KJ, Macias VL: A comparison of metabolic control by continuous and intermittent therapies in acute renal failure. J Am Soc Nephrol 1994;4:1113–1120.
13. Lowrie EG, Laird NM, Parker TF, Sargent JA: Effect of the hemodialysis prescription on patient morbidity: Report from the National Cooperative Dialysis Study. N Engl J Med 1981;305:1176–1181.
14. Hammerschmid DE, Goldberg R, Raij L, Kay NE: Leukocyte abnormalities in renal failure and hemodialysis. Semin Nephrol 1985;5:91–103.
15. Ronco C, Bellomo R, Homel P, et al: Effects of different doses in continuous veno-venous haemofiltration on outcomes of acute renal failure: A prospective randomised trial. Lancet 2000;356:26–30.
16. Ronco C, Ricci Z, Bellomo R, Bedogni F: Extracorporeal ultrafiltration for the treatment of overhydration and congestive heart failure. Cardiology 2001;96:155–168.
17. Venkataraman R, Subramanian S, Kellum JA: Clinical review: Extracorporeal blood purification in severe sepsis. Crit Care 2003;7:139–145.
18. D'Intini V, Bordoni V, Bolgan I, et al: Monocyte apoptosis in uremia is normalized with continuous blood purification modalities. Blood Purif 2004;22:9–12.
19. Brendolan A, D'Intini V, Ricci Z, et al: Pulse high volume hemofiltration. Int J Artif Organs 2004;27:398–403.
20. Mariano F, Tetta C, Guida G, et al: Hemofiltration reduces the serum priming activity on neutrophils chemiluminescence in septic patients. Kidney Int 2001;60:1598–1605.
21. Uchino S, Fealy N, Baldwin I, et al: Continuous is not continuous: The incidence and impact of circuit "down-time" on uraemic control during continuous veno-venous haemofiltration. Intensive Care Med 2003;29:575–578.
22. Ronco C, Ricci Z, Bellomo R, et al: Management of fluid balance in CRRT: A technical approach. Int J Artif Organs 2005;28:765–776.
23. Mehta RL, McDonald B, Gabbai F, et al: A randomized clinical trial of continuous vs intermittent dialysis for acute renal failure. Kidney Int 2001;60:1154–1163.
24. Uehlinger DE, Jakob SM, Ferrari P, et al: Comparison of continuous and intermittent renal replacement therapy for acute renal failure. Nephrol Dial Transplant 2005;20:1630–1637.
25. Augustine JJ, Sandy D, Seifert TH, Paganini EP: A randomized controlled trial comparing intermittent with continuous dialysis in patients with ARF. Am J Kidney Dis 2004;44:1000–1007.
26. Vinsonneau C, Camus C, Combes A, et al, for the Hemodiafe Study Group: Continuous venovenous haemodiafiltration versus intermittent haemodialysis for acute renal failure in patients with multiple-organ dysfunction syndrome: A multicentre randomised trial. Lancet 2006;368:379–385.
27. Cho KC: Survival by dialysis modality in critically ill patients with acute kidney injury. J Am Soc Nephrol 2006;17:3132–3138.
28. Kellum J, Palevsky P: Renal support in acute kidney injury. Lancet 2006;368:344–345.
29. Schortgen F: Hemodynamic tolerance of intermittent hemodialysis in critically ill patients: Usefulness of practice guidelines. Am J Respir Crit Care Med 2000;162:197–202.
30. Himmelfarb J: Continuous dialysis is not superior to intermittent dialysis in acute kidney injury of the critically ill patient. Nat Clin Pract Nephrol 2007;3:120–121.
31. Gokal R: Quality of life in patients undergoing renal replacement therapy. Kidney Int 1993;40:S23–S27.
32. Manns BJ, Taub KJ, Donaldson C: Economic evaluation and end-stage renal disease: From basics to bedside. Am J Kidney Dis 2000;36:12–28.
33. Culleton BF, Larson MG, Wilson PW, et al: Cardiovascular disease and mortality in a community-based cohort with mild renal insufficiency. Kidney Int 1999;56:2214–2219.
34. Bell M, SWING, Granath F, et al: Continuous renal replacement therapy is associated with less chronic renal failure than intermittent haemodialysis after acute renal failure. Intensive Care Med 2007;33:773–780.
35. Jacka MJ, Ivancinova X, Gibney RTN: Continuous renal replacement therapy improves renal recovery from acute renal failure. Can J Anaesth 2005;52:327–332.
36. Uchino S, Bellomo R, Kellum JA, et al, for The Beginning and Ending Supportive Therapy for the Kidney (B.E.S.T. Kidney) Investigators Writing Committee. Patient and kidney survival by dialysis modality in critically ill patients with acute kidney injury. Int J Artif Organs 2007;30:281–292.
37. Uchino S, Kellum JA, Bellomo R, et al: Acute renal failure in critically ill patients. A multinational, multicenter study. JAMA 2005;294:813–818.
38. Marshall MR, Golper TA, Shaver MJ, et al: Urea kinetics during sustained low efficiency dialysis in critically ill patients requiring renal replacement therapy. Am J Kidney Dis 2002;39:556–570.

39. Naka T, Baldwin I, Bellomo R, et al: Prolonged daily intermittent renal replacement therapy in ICU patients by ICU nurses and ICU physicians. Int J Artif Organs 2004;27:380–387.

40. Kumar VA, Craig M, Depner T, Yeun JY: Extended daily dialysis: A new approach to renal replacement for acute renal failure in the intensive care unit. Am J Kidney Dis 2000;36:294–300.

41. Kielstein JT, Kretschmer U, Ernst T, et al: Efficacy and cardiovascular tolerability of extended dialysis in critically ill patients: A randomized controlled study. Am J Kidney Dis 2004;43: 342–349.

42. Baldwin I, Naka T, Koch B, et al: A pilot randomised controlled comparison of continuous veno-venous haemofiltration and extended daily dialysis with filtration: Effect on small solutes and acid-base balance. Intensive Care Med 2007;33:830–835.

Further Reading

Augustine JJ, Sandy D, Seifert TH, Paganini EP: A randomized controlled trial comparing intermittent with continuous dialysis in patients with ARF. Am J Kidney Dis 2004;44:1000–1007.

Bell M, SWING, Granath F, et al: Continuous renal replacement therapy is associated with less chronic renal failure than intermittent haemodialysis after acute renal failure. Intensive Care Med 2007;33:773–780.

Cho KC, Himmelfarb J, Paganini E, et al: Survival by dialysis modality in critically ill patients with acute kidney injury. J Am Soc Nephrol 2006;17:3132–3138.

Clark WR, Letteri JJ, Uchino S, et al: Recent clinical advances in the management of critically ill patients with acute renal failure. Blood Purif 2006;24:487–498.

Hoste EA, Kellum JA: Acute kidney dysfunction and the critically ill. Minerva Anesthesiol 2006;72:133–143.

Mehta RL, McDonald B, Gabbai F, et al: A randomized clinical trial of continuous vs. intermittent dialysis for acute renal failure. Kidney Int 2001;60:1154–1163.

Vinsonneau C, Camus C, Combes A, et al, for the Hemodiafe Study Group. Continuous venovenous haemodiafiltration versus intermittent haemodialysis for acute renal failure in patients with multiple-organ dysfunction syndrome: A multicentre randomised trial. Lancet 2006;368:379–385.

Uchino S, Bellomo R, Kellum JA, et al, for The Beginning and Ending Supportive Therapy for the Kidney (B.E.S.T. Kidney) Investigators Writing Committee: Patient and kidney survival by dialysis modality in critically ill patients with acute kidney injury. Int J Artif Organs 2007;30:281–292.

Chapter 8

Nutritional Management of Acute Renal Failure

Wilfred Druml and William E. Mitch

CHAPTER CONTENTS

Nutritional support is a cornerstone in the complex therapeutic strategies designed to care for the patient with acute renal failure (ARF). ARF is a hypermetabolic, proinflammatory, and pro-oxidative clinical syndrome.[1] Metabolism and nutrient requirements for ARF patients are affected not only by the acutely uremic state per se, but also by the type and intensity of renal replacement therapy and by the underlying disease process and associated complications. Any nutritional program for an ARF patient must take into consideration this complex metabolic environment and must be coordinated with renal replacement therapy.

ARF is associated with an excess attributable mortality being interrelated with the systemic immunologic and metabolic consequences of ARF, and these factors are aggravated by malnutrition.[1,2] The objectives of nutritional therapy are to maintain lean body mass and to stimulate immunocompetence and repair functions and are aimed at mitigating the inflammatory state while improving oxygen radical scavenging system and endothelial functions. Despite the difficulty of demonstrating clear-cut benefits of nutritional interventions in the prognosis of critically ill patients, an increasing number of investigations have led to the conclusion that nutrition improves the course of disease and prognosis.[3]

The principles of nutritional support for ARF differ fundamentally from those for patients with chronic kidney disease (CKD) because diets or infusions that satisfy minimal requirements in CKD will not necessarily be sufficient for acutely ill ARF patients. Specifically, it is not renal dysfunction that principally determines nutrient needs. Instead, the severity of diseases/conditions associated with hypercatabolism, the nutritional state, and the type and frequency of renal replacement therapy determine nutrient requirements.

For many years, parenteral nutrition was the preferred route of nutritional support in patients with ARF. During the past decade, enteral nutrition has become the primary type of nutritional support for ARF patients who can tolerate enteral/oral feeding.[4] It is an unfortunate fact that few systematic studies have been conducted of nutritional support in ARF; most recommendations thus are necessarily based on expert opinion rather then on controlled studies.

METABOLIC ALTERATIONS AND NUTRIENT REQUIREMENTS IN ACUTE RENAL FAILURE

ARF is associated with a broad pattern of disturbances of physiologic functions that exert a pronounced impact on morbidity and mortality. In many cases, ARF is not an isolated event but a complication of sepsis, trauma, or multiple organ failure so metabolic changes in such patients will be determined by the acute uremic state plus the underlying disease process and/or complications (severe infections and organ dysfunction) and by the type and intensity of renal replacement therapy. The acute loss of excretory renal function affects water, electrolyte, and acid-base metabolism and has a profound effect on the *milieu interieur*. There are specific alterations in protein, amino acid, carbohydrate, and lipid metabolism.[5]

As noted, the optimal intake of nutrients in ARF patients is influenced more by the nature of the illness causing ARF, the extent of catabolism, and type and frequency of dialysis rather than renal dysfunction per se.[6] ARF patients present as a heterogeneous group of subjects with widely differing nutrient requirements, and in individual patients, requirements can vary considerably (Box 8-1).

Energy Metabolism and Energy Requirements

In contrast to experimental animals, in which ARF is associated with decreased oxygen consumption (uremic hypometabolism), energy expenditure is normal in patients with uncomplicated ARF. However, sepsis or multiple organ failure will increase oxygen consumption by 30% on average,[7] so energy metabolism is determined more by the underlying disease process than by ARF. There are well-defined complications of administering excessive energy substrates; thus, feeding should not exceed actual rates of energy expenditure. Complications, if any, from slightly underfeeding are less deleterious than those arising from overfeeding. For example, increasing energy intake from 30 to 40 kcal/kg body weight (BW)/day in ARF patients was shown to increase metabolic complications, such as hyperglycemia and hypertriglyceridemia, and had no beneficial effects.[8] Since basal energy expenditure cannot be measured easily, it should be estimated from standard formulas such as the Harris-Benedict equation plus corrections for the degree of hypermetabolism (i.e., a stress factor). Please note that in most clinical situations, energy requirements are 20 to 25 kcal/kg BW/day and rarely higher than 130% of basal energy expenditure.

Amino Acid/Protein Metabolism

A hallmark of ARF is excessive protein catabolism and sustained negative nitrogen balance. It is impossible to block or compensate for protein losses by nutritional strategies. Hyper-catabolism causes excessive release of amino acids from skeletal muscle, and there is also defective utilization of amino acids in the synthesis of muscle protein.[9,10] Hepatic gluconeogenesis (and ureagenesis) and synthesis of a number of proteins including acute phase proteins are all increased. ARF also causes an imbalance in amino acid pools in plasma and in the intracellular compartment; the utilization of amino acids after intravenous infusion is also defective.[11]

Release of inflammatory mediators (e.g., tumor necrosis factor α, interleukins), endocrine factors (catabolic hormones, hyperparathyroidism), circulating proteases, and catabolism stimulated by renal replacement therapy each contribute to accelerated protein breakdown in ARF (Box 8-2). A major catabolic factor is insulin resistance, which interrupts the control of protein turnover.[12] In muscle, both insulin-mediated stimulation of protein synthesis and inhibition of protein degradation are depressed in ARF. Metabolic acidosis has been identified as one important factor that stimulates protein breakdown.[13] Nitrogen losses in ARF patients are augmented if stressful factors such as inadequate nutrition, infection, trauma, sepsis, and thermal injury are present.

Protein and amino acid metabolism is also impaired by the loss of renal tissue since several amino acids are synthesized and/or metabolized by the kidney.[14] Indeed, the loss of kidney function can make several amino acids (e.g., tyrosine, arginine, serine, cysteine) conditionally indispensable. Moreover, the renal degradation of peptides is retarded in ARF, so catabolism of peptide hormones and inflammatory cytokines is retarded, a mechanism by which the inflammatory response in ARF is augmented.[15]

Anticatabolic Strategies in Acute Renal Failure

Anticatabolic strategies can be aimed at various targets (see Box 8-2). Nutrition is of paramount importance in mitigating catabolism. However, hypercatabolism in ARF can only be reduced and is not completely suppressed by conventional nutritional substrates (including branched-chain

---

Box 8-1 Important Metabolic Abnormalities Induced by Acute Renal Failure

Activation of amino acid and protein catabolism (especially in muscle)
Peripheral glucose intolerance/increased gluconeogenesis
Inhibition of lipolysis and altered fat clearance
Depletion of the antioxidant system
Induction of a proinflammatory state
Impairment of immunocompetence
Complex endocrine abnormalities: hyperparathyroidism, insulin resistance, erythropoietin resistance, resistance to growth factors, etc.

Box 8-2 Protein Catabolism in Acute Renal Failure: Contributing Factors

Impaired metabolic functions caused by accumulating uremic toxins
Endocrine factors
    Insulin resistance
    Increased secretion of catabolic hormones (catecholamines, glucagon, glucocorticoids)
    Hyperparathyroidism
    Suppression of release/resistance to growth factors
Acidosis stimulation of amino acid and protein catabolism
Acute phase reaction: systemic inflammatory response syndrome (activation of cytokine network)
Release of proteases
Inadequate supply of nutritional substrates
Renal replacement therapy
    Loss of nutritional substrates
    Activation of protein catabolism

amino acids). Whether specific nutrients such as glutamine or lipids can exert a more pronounced benefit for protein balance remains to be shown. Further therapeutic targets include hormones (especially the use of insulin and growth factors) and mediators (anti-inflammatory strategies) (see later). Finally, the enzyme systems that catalyze protein breakdown (e.g., the ubiquitin-proteasome system) potentially can be blocked. Obviously, inhibiting protein catabolism systems should not present a primary target of therapy because many metabolic pathways would be impaired. It appears that more upstream therapeutic interventions aimed at mitigating the underlying inflammatory process will be required.

Anti-inflammatory strategies using anticytokines have been reported to limit the release or action of inflammatory mediators in animal experiments. Unfortunately, they have not been successful in clinical trials of patients with critical illnesses. However, it should be recognized that several nutritional factors such as amino acids (glutamine, glycine, arginine), ω-3 fatty acids and selenium can modify inflammatory responses and the release of mediators and can mitigate oxidative injury, presenting a promising field in nutritional intervention in patients with ARF.

There is hope that the use of growth factors in ARF patients (e.g., recombinant human growth hormone or insulin-like growth factor I) would be beneficial. In sharp contrast to findings from animal experiments, available clinical results from treating acutely ill patients have been disappointing: a multicenter study of insulin-like growth factor I administration to ARF patients was prematurely terminated because of a lack of benefit; recombinant human growth hormone was even associated with increased mortality in critically ill patients, many of whom had ARF.[16,17]

Protein/Amino Acid Requirements

The most controversial question in nutritional support of patients with ARF concerns the optimal intake of amino acids/protein. Unfortunately, few studies have attempted to define requirements. The optimal daily protein or amino acid requirement seems to be above the minimum level of 0.6 g of protein/kg BW/day recommended for CKD patients or the recommended allowance (RDA) of 0.8 g/kg BW/day for normal subjects. Even for noncatabolic patients during polyuric recovery phase of ARF, an amino acid intake of 1 g/kg BW/day was found to be necessary to achieve a neutral nitrogen balance.[18] Some studies have tried to evaluate protein/amino acids requirements in critically ill patients with ARF on continuous renal replacement therapy (CRRT). In these patients, a protein catabolic rate of 1.4 to 1.7 g/kg BW/day was observed,[6,19,20] and there was an inverse relationship between protein and energy provision and protein catabolic rate. Overall, the nitrogen deficit was less in patients receiving nutritional support. A protein intake of about 1.5 g/kg BW/day was recommended.

Thus, unless renal insufficiency will be brief and there is no associated catabolic illness, the intake of protein or amino acids should not be lower than 1.0 g/kg BW/day. It should be emphasized that hypercatabolism cannot be overcome by increasing protein or protein/amino acid intake to more than 1.5 g. This level is in accordance with general recommendations for critically ill patients. Any exaggerated protein intake,

as recently suggested by some authors,[21,22] has not proven to be beneficial and simply stimulates the formation of urea and other nitrogenous waste products, can induce hyperammonemia, and may aggravate uremic complications. For patients treated by hemodialysis/continuous hemofiltration/peritoneal dialysis, extra protein/amino acid intake of 0.2 g/kg BW/day (again to a maximum of 1.5–1.7 g/kg BW/day) should be provided to compensate for losses occurring during therapy.

Carbohydrate Metabolism in Acute Renal Failure

ARF is characterized by an insulin-resistant state that is closely related to the prognosis of the patients.[23] Maximal insulin-stimulated glucose uptake by skeletal muscle is lower, whereas the insulin concentration causing half-maximal uptake is normal, indicating the presence of a postreceptor defect rather than impaired sensitivity.[24] A second feature of abnormal glucose metabolism in ARF is accelerated hepatic gluconeogenesis from the amino acids released during catabolism. Hepatic extraction of amino acids and their conversion to glucose and urea production all are increased by ARF. In contrast to healthy adults, hepatic gluconeogenesis from amino acids and thus protein catabolism cannot be completely suppressed by exogenous infusions of glucose.[25]

The metabolism of insulin is grossly abnormal in ARF; endogenous insulin secretion is decreased in the basal state and during a glucose infusion. Renal insulin catabolism is blunted and, surprisingly, insulin catabolism by the liver is consistently decreased in ARF.[26] As a consequence, many ARF patients express hyperglycemia. This is relevant because hyperglycemia in critically ill patients is recognized as an important determinant of the evolution of complications such as infections (but also of kidney injury) and prognosis.[27] Normoglycemia must be strictly maintained during nutritional support in ARF patients.

Lipid Metabolism in Acute Renal Failure

Profound alterations in lipid metabolism occur in patients with ARF; the triglyceride content of plasma lipoproteins is increased, whereas total cholesterol and, in particular, high-density lipoprotein cholesterol are decreased.[28] The major cause of lipid abnormalities is impaired lipolysis. The activities of both lipolytic systems, lipoprotein lipase and hepatic triglyceride lipase, are decreased to less than 50% of normal.[29] Whether increased hepatic synthesis contributes to hypertriglyceridemia in ARF remains unsettled. In contrast to CKD, carnitine deficiency does not participate in the development of lipid abnormalities in ARF. Plasma carnitine levels in ARF patients are increased due to both increased release from muscle tissue and activated hepatic synthesis.[30] The nutritional relevance of abnormal lipid metabolism is that lipid particles of artificial fat emulsions are metabolized like very low density lipoprotein lipids; their elimination is delayed in ARF. The delayed lipolysis in ARF contrasts with other acute illnesses such as surgery, trauma, and sepsis, in which fat elimination and utilization are enhanced to cover increased energy requirements via the oxidation of free fatty acids.[31] Moreover, intestinal absorption of lipids is retarded in renal failure.

Micronutrients

Requirements for water-soluble vitamins in patients with ARF are increased, mainly because of losses induced by renal replacement therapies. Caution should be used in prescribing vitamin C because it is a precursor of oxalic acid and an excess (>250 mg/day) can result in secondary oxalosis.[32] In contrast to CKD, the requirements of vitamins A, E, and D (but not vitamin K) are increased in patients with ARF, and a daily supplement should be provided.[33] This is possible because most multivitamin preparations for parenteral infusions contain the RDA of vitamins.

Requirements of trace elements are poorly defined for ARF patients. Parenteral infusions carry the risk of inducing toxic effects because the regulation of trace element homeostasis, including gastrointestinal absorption and impaired renal excretion is impaired in ARF. Nevertheless, selenium concentrations in plasma and erythrocytes are consistently decreased in patients with ARF and CKD. Selenium supplementation can reduce the evolution of organ dysfunctions and ARF and potentially improve prognosis in critically ill patients with sepsis.[34] Several micronutrients are part of the organism's defense mechanisms against oxygen free radical–induced injury. This is relevant because ARF is a pro-oxidative state and profound depression in antioxidant-status has been documented in patients with ARF.[35,36] Repletion of the antioxidative system is an important aim in nutritional support of renal failure patients.

Electrolytes

Derangements in electrolyte balance in patients with ARF are extremely variable, so no standard recommendations can be given. Electrolyte requirements not only vary considerably among patients, but it must be noted that abnormalities can fundamentally change during the course of the disease.[37] Notably, hypokalemia, hypophosphatemia, and hypomagnesemia are frequently present in ARF patients, especially those with nonoliguric ARF and the patients treated by CRRT. Nutrition support, especially parenteral nutrition with a low electrolyte content, can induce hypophosphatemia and hypokalemia, respectively (the refeeding syndrome).[38] Thus, electrolyte requirements have to be evaluated in patients with ARF on a day-to-day basis.

METABOLIC IMPACT OF EXTRACORPOREAL THERAPY

The impact of renal replacement therapies on metabolism is manifold. Protein catabolism is caused not only by substrate losses, but also by activation of protein breakdown mediated by release of leukocyte-derived proteases and inflammatory mediators.[39] Potentially, dialysis induces also an inhibition of muscular protein synthesis.[40] Several water-soluble substances, such as vitamins and carnitine, are lost during hemodialysis, and it has been suggested that generation of reactive oxygen species is augmented during dialysis treatment (Box 8-3).

Recently, CRRT (continuous hemofiltration and/or continuous hemodialysis) have been widely used to manage critically ill patients with ARF. The metabolic consequences of these modalities reflect the continuous mode of therapy and the recommended high fluid turnover.[41]

One major effect of CRRT is the elimination of small- and medium-sized molecules. Amino acid losses can be estimated from the volume of the filtrate and the average plasma concentrations. Usually, amino acid loss accounts for 5 to 15 g of amino acid per day, representing approximately 10% to 15% of amino acid intake.[42] Water-soluble vitamins, such as folic acid and vitamins B_1, B_6, and C are also eliminated during CRRT, so their intake should be higher than the RDA to maintain plasma concentrations.[43] There are also relevant losses of selenium during CRRT accounting for as much as twice the daily RDA.[44]

CLINICAL EXPERIENCES WITH NUTRITIONAL SUPPORT IN ACUTE RENAL FAILURE

Unfortunately, only a limited number of controlled trials on nutritional support in ARF have been done. Few are prospective and fulfill minimal requirements in study design with respect to patient numbers, definition of endpoints, and stratification of groups. Early investigations compared nutritional support with amino acids plus glucose versus glucose alone.[45] Pooled results of the four best studies reveal a mortality rate of 64% with glucose infusion only compared with a 42% mortality rate when a more complete parenteral nutrition solution was provided.[6] Combining these results with other retrospective investigations, the data are consistent with the conclusion that nutritional support is effective and that sicker patients with more complications will derive benefit from nutritional therapy. Other investigations have evaluated the optimal type of amino acid solution and the quantity of amino acids/protein to be used. These studies have not generated conclusive results with regard to an improved survival rate or an improvement in

---

Box 8-3 Metabolic Effects of Renal Replacement Therapy in Acute Renal Failure

Intermittent Hemodialysis
Loss of water-soluble molecules
  Amino acids
  Water-soluble vitamins
  L-carnitine, etc.
Activation of protein catabolism
  Loss of amino acids
  Loss of proteins
  Cytokine release (tumor necrosis factor α, etc.)
Inhibition of protein synthesis
Increase in eactive oxygen species production

Continuous Renal Replacement Therapy
Heat loss
Excessive load of substrates (lactate, citrate, glucose, etc.)
Loss of nutrients (amino acids, vitamins, selenium, etc.)
Loss of electrolytes (phosphate, magnesium)
Elimination of (short-chain) proteins (hormones, potential inflammatory mediators but also albumin)
Metabolic consequences of bioincompatibility (induction/activation of mediator cascades, of an inflammatory reaction, stimulation of protein catabolism)

nitrogen balance, but the numbers of patients studied is small or no matched control group or patients were not hypercatabolic.[37,46] This includes some recent investigations using high amounts of protein/amino acids in nutritional support in patients with ARF on CRRT (see previously).[22] Most of these studies have evaluated parenteral nutrition in patients with ARF, but enteral nutrition is now the first line of nutritional support. Unfortunately, few systematic studies of the potential benefits of enteral nutrition in ARF patients are available.[4,47,48]

In some ways, the ongoing controversy over the efficiency of nutritional support in ARF reflects a basic misunderstanding of the objectives of nutritional therapy. Nutritional support presents just one element of a complex pattern of therapeutic interventions, so it can be argued that patient survival should not be the sole endpoint of a nutritional evaluation. Nevertheless, there are reports demonstrating a beneficial effect of timely instituted and qualitatively/quantitatively adapted nutritional support on the course of acute disease states and patient survival.[3]

IMPACT OF NUTRITIONAL INTERVENTIONS ON RENAL FUNCTION AND/OR RECOVERY FROM ACUTE RENAL FAILURE

Starvation accelerates protein breakdown and impairs protein synthesis in the kidney, whereas refeeding exerts the opposite effects. In the experimental animal model, provision of amino acids or total parenteral nutrition accelerates tissue repair and recovery of renal function. In patients, however, this has been much more difficult to prove; only one study has reported a positive effect of nutrition on the resolution of ARF.[45] Available evidence, however, suggests that the provision of substrates may enhance tissue regeneration and, potentially, renal tubular repair. Conversely, high doses of amino acids can induce toxic damage to renal tubules subjected to ischemic or nephrotoxic insults.[49] In part, this "therapeutic paradox" in ARF is related to an increase in metabolic work occurring when oxygen is limited (similar observations have been made with glucose infusions during renal ischemia). In summary, during the insult phase of ARF (similar to the ebb phase after trauma, major operations, etc.), exaggerated amounts of nutritional intake can aggravate tissue injury and must be avoided. In contrast, certain amino acids may be renoprotective. Glycine and, to a lesser degree, alanine have been shown to limit tubular injury in ischemic and nephrotoxic experimental models of ARF. Arginine (possibly by producing nitric oxide) also is reported to preserve renal function (but may also accentuate tubular injury) in experimental models of ARF.[50] In a nephrotoxic model, protein-rich nutrition was shown to limit tubular injury.[51] Clinically, high amino acid intake was shown to preserve water balance while increasing diuresis and reducing the need for diuretic therapy in patients with nonoliguric ARF.[52]

Various other endocrine-metabolic interventions (e.g., thyroxine, human growth hormone, epidermal growth factor, insulin-like growth factor I) can accelerate regeneration in experimental ARF. In the rat, insulin-like growth factor I accelerates recovery from ischemic ARF and improves nitrogen balance. Unfortunately, these approaches have not been effective in clinical studies of ARF patients (see previously). Nevertheless, a prominent goal in studies of ARF is to stimulate renal regeneration by several mechanisms, including growth factors, stem cells, and erythropoietin.

PATIENT CLASSIFICATION

Ideally, a nutritional program should be designed for each ARF patient because these patients are extremely heterogeneous. In practice, it is advisable to distinguish at least three levels of dietary requirements according to the severity of disease and the extent of protein catabolism associated with the underlying disease (Table 8-1). The first group includes patients without excess catabolism; they will have a urea appearance rate of less than 5 g of nitrogen more than nitrogen intake. ARF is usually caused by nephrotoxins (e.g., aminoglycosides, contrast media, mismatched blood transfusions). In most cases, these patients can be fed orally, and the prognosis for recovery of renal function and for survival is excellent. A second group includes patients with moderate hypercatabolism as signified by a urea appearance rate exceeding nitrogen intake by 5 to 10 g of nitrogen per day. These patients frequently suffer from complicating infections, peritonitis, or moderate traumatic injuries associated with ARF. Nutritional support and dialysis are often required. In the third category of patients, ARF occurs in association with severe trauma, burns, or overwhelming sepsis. Urea appearance is markedly elevated (>10 g/day above nitrogen intake). Treatment strategies are complex and include enteral/parenteral nutrition, hemodialysis, and blood pressure or ventilatory support (see Table 8-1). Insulin is often required to maintain blood glucose concentrations within acceptable levels. Dialysis/continuous hemofiltration is recommended as necessary to maintain fluid balance and a blood urea nitrogen less than 80 mg/dL. The mortality rate in this group exceeds 60% to 80%, and in addition to the severity of the underlying illness, ARF is a major independent contributor to poor prognosis.[2,53]

NUTRIENT ADMINISTRATION

Important questions are which patients require nutritional support and when should it be initiated? Both decisions are influenced by the nutritional state of the patient as well as the type and degree of hypercatabolism associated with the underlying illness. During the acute phase of ARF (i.e., within the first 24 hours after trauma, surgery, etc.), nutritional support should be avoided because infusion of large quantities of amino acids or glucose during this ebb phase will increase oxygen requirements and aggravate tubular injury and the degree of renal function loss. If the nutritional status of the patient is normal (e.g., based on plasma protein concentrations, anthropometric measurements, and, most importantly, clinical judgment) and if the patient will resume a normal diet within 5 days, no specific nutritional support is necessary. However, if there is evidence of lost protein and energy stores, nutritional therapy should be initiated regardless of whether the patient is likely to eat within 5 days.

For all patients, some estimate of the type and severity of complicating diseases should be made. For patients with evidence of protein catabolism (see Table 8-1, groups 2 and 3), nutritional support should be instituted early and dialysis used to keep the blood urea nitrogen less than 80 mg/dL. Since metabolic

Table 8-1 Patient Classification and Nutrient Requirements in Patients with Acute Renal Failure

	EXTENT OF CATABOLISM		
	Mild	Moderate	Severe
Excess urea appearance (above N intake)	<5g	5–10 g	>10 g
Examples of clinical settings	Drug toxicity	Elective surgery ± infection	Severe injury or sepsis
Mortality	20%	60%	60%–80%
Dialysis/hemofiltration frequency	Rare	As needed	Frequent
Route of nutrient administration	Oral	Enteral and/or parenteral	Enteral and/or parenteral
Energy recommendations (kcal/kg BW/day)	20–25	20–30	25–30 (35)
Energy substrates: Glucose/fat (g/kg BW/day)	Glucose 3.0–5.0	Glucose + fat (3.0–5.0 glucose, 0.5–1.0 fat)	Glucose + fat (3.0–5.0 glucose, 0.8–1.2 fat)
Amino acids/protein (g/kg/day)	0.6–1.0 EAA (+ NEAA)	1.0–1.4 EAA + NEAA	1.2–1.5 (1.7) EAA + NEAA
Nutrients used Oral/enteral Parenteral	Food	Enteral formulas	Enteral formulas
		EAAs + specific NEAAs (general or "nephro" solutions)	
		Glucose 50%–70% + fat emulsions 10% or 20%	
		Glucose 50%–70%	
		Multivitamin and multitrace element preparations*	

*Consider increased micronutrient requirements
BW, body weight; EAAs, essential amino acids; NEAAs, nonessential amino acids.

abnormalities associated with ARF generally occur when creatinine clearance decreases to less than 50 mL/min, nutritional regimens should be designed to counteract specific metabolic abnormalities if renal function is below this threshold. Therapeutic attention must focus on methods that provide an optimal nutritional regimen to prevent both the loss of lean body mass and hospital-acquired malnutrition and to stimulate immunocompetence while supporting patients to survive the acute illness. Nutritional support should be started early and must be both quantitatively and qualitatively sufficient (Fig. 8-1).

Oral Feedings

Oral feedings should be encouraged in all patients who can tolerate them. This is required because of the beneficial effects of food on the function of the intestine (see later). Initially, 40 g/day of high-quality protein (e.g., egg protein) should be given to provide a daily protein requirement of approximately 0.6 g/kg BW/day. Protein intake should be increased to 0.8 to 1.0 g protein/kg BW/day if the BUN is maintained at less than 100 mg/dL, but patients treated by hemodialysis will require a protein intake of 1 to 1.2 g/kg BW/day, whereas those treated by peritoneal dialysis will need 1.4 g/kg BW/day of protein to counteract losses of both amino acids and protein during peritoneal dialysis. Because water-soluble vitamins in such diets might be insufficient, a supplement is recommended.

Enteral Nutrition

Whenever possible, enteral feeding, providing at least a portion of nutritional needs, should be performed.[4,47] Even small amounts of nutrients serve to maintain normal intestinal structure and function and limit bacterial translocation from the gut. Enteral feeding also may help prevent the development of infections. It also may exert beneficial effect on kidney function; in experimental ARF, enteral compared with parenteral nutrient administration was found to improve renal function.[54] In two clinical studies, enteral nutrition was a factor associated with an improved prognosis in ARF patients.[22,53] Despite the fact that this practice is used in most critical care units, there are few systematic studies on enteral nutrition in ARF patients.[48]

Enteral diets are given through a small (8–10 French) soft feeding tube positioned with the tip in the stomach or jejunum, and nutrients are administered by pump either intermittently or continuously. The gastric contents should be aspirated every 2 to 3 hours until adequate gastric emptying and intestinal peristalsis are established. This will prevent vomiting and bronchopulmonary aspiration and is required because ARF is associated with a profound impairment of gastric and intestinal motility. Enteral nutrition should be started slowly, and the infusion gradually increased over several days until nutritional requirements are satisfied. Potentially treatable side effects include nausea, vomiting, diarrhea, abdominal distention, and cramping.

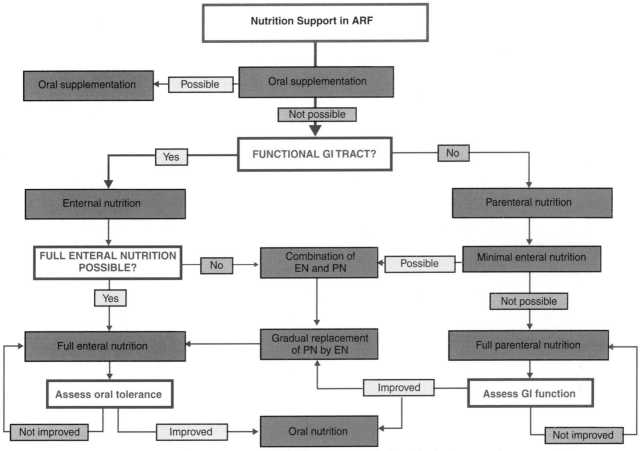

Figure 8-1 Flow chart for nutritional support in patients with acute renal failure (ARF). EN, enteral nutrition; GI, gastrointestinal; PN, parenteral nutrition. (Adapted from Druml W, Jadrna K, for the AKE. Recommendations for enteral and parenteral nutrition in the adult. Vienna: Austrian Society for Clinical Nutrition, 2008, p 14).

Enteral Feeding Formulas

No commercially available enteral diets have been specifically developed for patients with ARF. The use of conventional tube feeding formulas designed for subjects with normal renal function can be limited by the fixed composition of nutrients and high content of protein and electrolytes (especially potassium and phosphates). Specialized ready-to-use liquid diets developed for CKD patients or for hemodialysis patients can be used for ARF patients. In those patients who do not require extracorporal therapy, preparations with a reduced protein content (high-quality proteins provided in part as oligopeptides or free amino acids) but with a restricted electrolyte concentration can be given. For catabolic ARF patients, preparations with a moderate protein content and a reduced electrolyte content present the optimal diet currently. Whether enteral diets containing specific nutrients such as glutamine, arginine, ω-3 fatty acids, and nucleotides (immunonutrition) will exert advantages in patients with ARF remains to be shown.

Parenteral Nutrition

Parenteral nutrition should not be viewed as alternative but rather complementary nutritional support because many ARF patients are not able to meet their nutritional requirements by enteral infusions alone. Moreover, ARF frequently occurs in patients with gastrointestinal dysfunction (e.g., pancreatitis) or in hypercatabolic patients with multiple organ dysfunction; thus, a total or supplementary parenteral nutrient supply may become necessary.[55]

Substrates for Parenteral Nutrition in Acute Renal Failure

Amino Acid Solutions

Amino acid solutions containing exclusively essential amino acids should no longer be used. There is controversy whether parenteral nutrition for ARF patients should consist of general amino acid solutions containing essential amino acids plus nonessential amino acids in standard proportions or should be limited to nephro solutions that contain essential amino acids in modified proportions and specific nonessential amino acids that might be conditionally essential. For example, tyrosine is regarded as a conditionally essential amino acid in ARF patients, but tyrosine has a low water-solubility index. Consequently, tyrosine is supplied as tyrosine dipeptides such as glycyl tyrosine in modern nephro solutions because the conjugates increase tyrosine solubility. Glutamine has been termed a conditionally essential amino acid in catabolic illness because it may exert beneficial effects on renal function and can improve survival in critically ill patients. These benefits were found to be most pronounced in ARF patients (4 of 24 survivors without, 14 of 23 with glutamine, $P < .02$).[56] Since free glutamine is not stable in aqueous solutions, glutamine-containing dipeptides can be given as a glutamine source for parenteral nutrition. Despite considerable investigation, there is no persuasive evidence that mixtures enriched with branched-chain amino acids exert significant blunting of protein catabolism and loss of muscle mass.

Energy Substrates: Carbohydrates

Glucose is the main energy substrate in total parenteral nutrition. However, when glucose intake is increased to more than 3 to 5 g/kg BW/day, the extra glucose is not oxidized but instead increases lipogenesis.[57] This is undesirable because it induces fatty infiltration of the liver and excessive carbon dioxide production, yielding hypercarbia. The amount of glucose that can be infused is also often limited by impaired glucose utilization, a complication of ARF. In this case, insulin is needed to maintain normoglycemia. Consequently, energy requirements cannot be met by glucose alone unless excessive amounts of insulin are infused; thus, a portion of the energy requirement should be covered by lipid emulsions. The most suitable means of providing energy substrates to critically ill patients is not with glucose or lipids, but with glucose plus lipids. Other carbohydrates including fructose, sorbitol, and xylitol are available in some countries (but not in the United States). They should not be used in patients with ARF because they exert adverse metabolic effects.

Fat Emulsions

The advantages of intravenous lipids include their high energy content per gram of lipids and low osmolality, being a source of essential fatty acids, and having a low frequency of hepatic side effects compared with glucose (i.e., less fatty infiltration of the liver and hyperbilirubinemia) and less carbon dioxide production (especially important for patients with compromised respiratory function). Altered lipid metabolism caused by ARF should not prevent lipid emulsion use; the amount infused should be adjusted to the patient's capacity to use lipids. Usually, 1 g of fat/kg BW/day will not increase plasma triglycerides substantially, so approximately 20% to 30% of energy requirements can be met by lipid infusion. Lipid emulsions are not hyperosmolar and can be infused into a peripheral vein.

Conventional lipid emulsions contain large amounts of triglycerides with polyunsaturated fatty acids (mainly from soy oil). Because of the potential generation of proinflammatory and vasoconstrictor eicosanoids from polyunsaturated fatty acids, these lipid preparations are increasingly exchanged for emulsions in which soy oil is replaced by coconut oil (containing medium triglycerides) and/or olive oil or fish oil (containing ω-3-fatty acids). For critically ill patients, these novel formulas have been associated with a mitigation of the inflammatory state, a reduction in the length of hospital stay, and potentially an improved prognosis.[58,59] This is speculative because systematic investigations of these newer emulsions in patients with ARF are not available. For medium triglyceride–containing emulsions, metabolic advantages include a faster elimination from plasma, complete carnitine-independent metabolism, and a triglyceride-lowering effect. Unfortunately, the defect in lipolysis characteristic of ARF cannot be circumvented by using medium triglycerides.[31] Lipids should not be administered in the presence of hyperlipidemia (e.g., plasma triglycerides > 350 mg/dL) or when there is activated intravascular coagulation, acidosis (pH < 7.25), or impaired macro-/microcirculation.

Parenteral Solutions

Standard solutions are composed of amino acids, glucose, and lipids with vitamins, trace elements, and electrolytes added as required (see Table 8-2). Recently, all-in-one solutions (in three-chamber bags) in which all nutrients are present have proven efficacious and gained wider acceptance. If hyperglycemia is present, insulin can be added or administered separately. To ensure optimal nutrient utilization and to avoid creating metabolic derangements (such as hyperglycemia, hypertriglyceridemia, an excessive increase in the blood urea nitrogen, and a mineral unbalance), the infusion should be started at a low

Table 8-2 Parenteral Nutrition in Acute Renal Failure: Renal Failure Fluid (All-in-One Solution)*

Component	Quantity	Remarks
Glucose 30%–70%	500 mL	In the presence of severe insulin resistance, use glucose 30%
Fat emulsion 10%–20%	500 mL	Start with 10%, switch to 20% if triglycerides are <350 mg/dL
Amino acids 6.5%–10%	500 mL	General or special nephro amino acid solutions including EAAs and NEAAs
Water-soluble vitamins†	2 × RDA	Limit vitamin C intake to <250 mg/day
Fat-soluble vitamins†	RDA	Increased requirements of vitamin E
Trace elements†	RDA	Plus selenium 100–300 μg/day
Electrolytes	As required	Caution: hypophosphatemia or hypokalemia after initiation of TPN
Insulin	As required	Added directly to the solution or given separately

*"All-in-one solution" with all components contained in a single bag, infusion rate initially 50% of requirements, to be increased over a period of 3 days to satisfy requirements
†Combination products containing the recommended daily allowances (RDA)
EAAs, essential amino acids; NEAAs, nonessential amino acids; TPN, total parenteral nutrition.

Table 8-3   A Minimal Suggested Schedule for Monitoring of Nutritional Support

	PATIENT METABOLICALLY	
Variables	Unstable	Stable
Blood glucose, potassium	4–6 times/day	Daily
Osmolality	Daily	Once weekly
Electrolytes (sodium, chloride)	Daily	Three times per week
Calcium, phosphate, magnesium	Daily	Three times per week
BUN/BUN increase/day	Daily	Daily
UNA	Daily	Once weekly
Triglycerides	Daily	Twice weekly
Blood gas analysis/pH	Daily	Once weekly
Ammonia	Twice weekly	Once weekly
Transaminases + bilirubin	Twice weekly	Once weekly

BUN, blood urea nitrogen; UNA, urea nitrogen appearance rate.

rate (providing approximately 50% of requirements) and gradually increased over several days. Optimally, the solution should be infused continuously over 24 hours to avoid marked changes in substrate concentrations and to achieve maximal utilization for anabolism. Because fluids are restricted in ARF patients, the parenteral nutrition solutions are hyperosmolar and hence must be infused through a central venous catheter to avoid damage to peripheral veins. The use of special venous catheters both as infusion ports and for temporary dialysis access is possible, but they carry a significant risk of infection.

COMPLICATIONS AND MONITORING OF NUTRITIONAL SUPPORT

Complications and side effects of nutritional support in ARF patients do not differ fundamentally from those observed in other patient groups. Hypervolemia and electrolyte imbalances, however, can develop rapidly, and altered utilization of several nutrients make it unwise to give an exaggerated intake of protein or glucose (see previously). If an excess is given, metabolic derangements and waste product accumulation will occur. Most complications of nutritional support are related to an excess intake of substrates (e.g., hyperglycemia, hypertriglyceridemia, hyperkalemia, an accelerated increase in BUN or in carbon dioxide production). More rare is the development of deficiencies (e.g., minerals, vitamins, essential fatty acids). Thus, nutritional therapy in ARF patients requires more frequent monitoring than in other patient groups (Table 8-3).

SUMMARY

Acute loss of renal function causes complex metabolic abnormalities affecting not only water, electrolyte, and acid-base balance but also amino acid, carbohydrate, and lipid metabolism. Moreover, the critically ill ARF patient presents a hypercatabolic, proinflammatory, and pro-oxidative state. The excess attribut-

able mortality of ARF is tightly interrelated with the systemic immunologic and metabolic consequences of ARF, factors that are aggravated by malnutrition. Knowledge about the pathophysiology of these metabolic changes, understanding the metabolic side effects of renal replacement therapies, and improved definitions of nutritional requirements plus advancements in nutritional techniques have improved the success of nutritional therapy in ARF. Dietary restrictions based on the principles of treating CKD patients have been largely abandoned in favor of an approach that is directed at meeting nutrient requirements. There is no longer doubt that enteral nutrition is the preferred route of meeting nutritional requirements in ARF patients. Even small amounts of food can help support intestinal functions (and potentially improve renal function). Nevertheless, many ARF patients have severe limitations to enteral nutrition and require supplementary or even total parenteral nutrition.

Unfortunately, nutritional support has not convincingly reduced the morbidity and mortality associated with ARF. We believe that future advances in nutritional therapy will not be based on a quantitative approach to provide nitrogen and energy requirements. Instead, the developments will move toward a more qualitative type of metabolic support taking advantage of specific pharmacologic effects of nutrients.

References

1. Kelly KJ: Acute renal failure: Much more than a kidney disease. Semin Nephrol 2006;26:105–113.
2. Druml W: Acute renal failure is not a "cute" renal failure! Intensive Care Med 2004;30:1886–1890.
3. Artinian V, Krayem H, DiGiovine B: Effects of early enteral feeding on the outcome of critically ill mechanically ventilated medical patients. Chest 2006;129:960–967.
4. Cano N, Fiaccadori E, Tesinsky P, et al: ESPEN Guidelines on Enteral Nutrition: Adult renal failure. Clin Nutr 2006;25:295–310.
5. Druml W, Mitch W: Metabolic abnormalities in acute renal failure. Semin Dial 2006;9:484–490.
6. Druml W: Nutritional support in acute renal failure. In Mitch W, Saulo K (eds): Handbook of Nutrition and the Kidney. Philadelphia: Lippincott Williams & Wilkins, 2005, pp 95–114.

7. Schneeweiss B, Graninger W, Stockenhuber F, et al: Energy metabolism in acute and chronic renal failure. Am J Clin Nutr 1990;52:596–601.
8. Fiaccadori E, Maggiore U, Rotelli C, et al: Effects of different energy intakes on nitrogen balance in patients with acute renal failure: A pilot study. Nephrol Dial Transplant 2005;20:1976–1980.
9. Druml W: Protein metabolism in acute renal failure. Miner Electrolyte Metab 1998;24:47–54.
10. Price SR, Reaich D, Marinovic AC, et al: Mechanisms contributing to muscle-wasting in acute uremia: Activation of amino acid catabolism. J Am Soc Nephrol 1998;9:439–443.
11. Druml W, Fischer M, Liebisch B, et al: Elimination of amino acids in renal failure. Am J Clin Nutr 1994;60:418–423.
12. Wang X, Hu Z, Hu J, et al: Insulin resistance accelerates muscle protein degradation: Activation of the ubiquitin-proteasome pathway by defects in muscle cell signaling. Endocrinology 2006;147:4160–4168.
13. Mitch WE: Robert H. Herman Memorial Award in Clinical Nutrition Lecture, 1997. Mechanisms causing loss of lean body mass in kidney disease. Am J Clin Nutr 1998;67:359–366.
14. van de Poll MC, Soeters PB, Deutz NE, et al: Renal metabolism of amino acids: Its role in interorgan amino acid exchange. Am J Clin Nutr 2004;79:185–197.
15. Zager RA, Johnson AC, Lund S, Hanson S: Acute renal failure: Determinants and characteristics of the injury-induced hyperinflammatory response. Am J Physiol Renal Physiol 2006;291: F546–F556.
16. Hirschberg R, Kopple J, Lipsett P, et al: Multicenter clinical trial of recombinant human insulin-like growth factor I in patients with acute renal failure. Kidney Int 1999;55:2423–2432.
17. Takala J, Ruokonen E, Webster NR, et al: Increased mortality associated with growth hormone treatment in critically ill adults. N Engl J Med 1999;341:785–792.
18. Druml W: Nutritional management of acute renal failure. J Ren Nutr 2005;15:63–70.
19. Chima CS, Meyer L, Hummell AC, et al: Protein catabolic rate in patients with acute renal failure on continuous arteriovenous hemofiltration and total parenteral nutrition. J Am Soc Nephrol 1993;3:1516–1521.
20. Leblanc M, Garred LJ, Cardinal J, et al: Catabolism in critical illness: Estimation from urea nitrogen appearance and creatinine production during continuous renal replacement therapy. Am J Kidney Dis 1998;32:444–453.
21. Bellomo R, Tan HK, Bhonagiri S, et al: High protein intake during continuous hemodiafiltration: Impact on amino acids and nitrogen balance. Int J Artif Organs 2002;25:261–268.
22. Scheinkestel CD, Kar L, Marshall K, et al: Prospective randomized trial to assess caloric and protein needs of critically ill, anuric, ventilated patients requiring continuous renal replacement therapy. Nutrition 2003;19:909–916.
23. Basi S, Pupim LB, Simmons EM, et al: Insulin resistance in critically ill patients with acute renal failure. Am J Physiol Renal Physiol 2005;289:F259–F264.
24. May RC, Clark AS, Goheer MA, Mitch WE: Specific defects in insulin-mediated muscle metabolism in acute uremia. Kidney Int 1985;28:490–497.
25. Cianciaruso B, Bellizzi V, Napoli R, et al: Hepatic uptake and release of glucose, lactate, and amino acids in acutely uremic dogs. Metabolism 1991;40:261–269.
26. Cianciaruso B, Sacca L, Terracciano V, et al: Insulin metabolism in acute renal failure. Kidney Int Suppl 1987;22:S109–S112.
27. Van den Berghe G, Wilmer A, Hermans G, et al: Intensive insulin therapy in the medical ICU. N Engl J Med 2006;354:449–461.
28. Druml W, Laggner A, Widhalm K, et al: Lipid metabolism in acute renal failure. Kidney Int Suppl 1983;16:S139–S142.
29. Druml W, Zechner R, Magometschnigg D, et al: Post-heparin lipolytic activity in acute renal failure. Clin Nephrol 1985;23: 289–293.
30. Wanner C, Riegel W, Schaefer RM, Horl WH: Carnitine and carnitine esters in acute renal failure. Nephrol Dial Transplant 1989;4:951–956.
31. Druml W, Fischer M, Sertl S, et al: Fat elimination in acute renal failure: Long-chain vs medium-chain triglycerides. Am J Clin Nutr 1992;55:468–472.
32. Canavese C, Salomone M, Massara C, et al: Primary oxalosis mimicking hyperparathyroidism diagnosed after long-term hemodialysis. Am J Nephrol 1990;10:344–349.
33. Druml W, Schwarzenhofer M, Apsner R, Horl WH: Fat-soluble vitamins in patients with acute renal failure. Miner Electrolyte Metab 1998;24:220–226.
34. Angstwurm MW, Engelmann L, Zimmermann T, et al: Selenium in Intensive Care (SIC): Results of a prospective randomized, placebo-controlled, multiple-center study in patients with severe systemic inflammatory response syndrome, sepsis, and septic shock. Crit Care Med 2007;35:118–126.
35. Metnitz GH, Fischer M, Bartens C, et al: Impact of acute renal failure on antioxidant status in multiple organ failure. Acta Anaesthesiol Scand 2000;44:236–240.
36. Himmelfarb J, McMonagle E, Freedman S, et al: Oxidative stress is increased in critically ill patients with acute renal failure. J Am Soc Nephrol 2004;15:2449–2456.
37. Druml W: Nutritional support in patients with acute renal failure. In Molitoris B, Finn W (eds): Acute Renal Failure. A Companion to Brenner & Rector's The Kidney. Philadelphia: WB Saunders, 2001, pp 465–489.
38. Kurtin P, Kouba J: Profound hypophosphatemia in the course of acute renal failure. Am J Kidney Dis 1987;10:346–349.
39. Veeneman JM, Kingma HA, Boer TS, et al: Protein intake during hemodialysis maintains a positive whole body protein balance in chronic hemodialysis patients. Am J Physiol Endocrinol Metab 2003;284:E954–E965.
40. Pupim LB, Flakoll PJ, Brouillette JR, et al: Intradialytic parenteral nutrition improves protein and energy homeostasis in chronic hemodialysis patients. J Clin Invest 2002;110:483–492.
41. Druml W: Metabolic aspects of continuous renal replacement therapies. Kidney Int Suppl 1999;72:S56–S61.
42. Frankenfield DC, Badellino MM, Reynolds HN, et al: Amino acid loss and plasma concentration during continuous hemodiafiltration. JPEN J Parenter Enteral Nutr 1993;17:551–561.
43. Fortin MC, Amyot SL, Geadah D, Leblanc M: Serum concentrations and clearances of folic acid and pyridoxal-5-phosphate during venovenous continuous renal replacement therapy. Intensive Care Med 1999;25:594–598.
44. Berger MM, Shenkin A, Revelly JP, et al: Copper, selenium, zinc, and thiamine balances during continuous venovenous hemodiafiltration in critically ill patients. Am J Clin Nutr 2004;80: 410–416.
45. Abel RM, Beck CH Jr, Abbott WM, et al: Improved survival from acute renal failure after treatment with intravenous essential L-amino acids and glucose. Results of a prospective, double-blind study. N Engl J Med 1973;288:695–699.
46. Feinstein EI, Kopple JD, Silberman H, Massry SG: Total parenteral nutrition with high or low nitrogen intakes in patients with acute renal failure. Kidney Int Suppl 1983;16:S319–S323.
47. Druml W, Mitch W: Enteral nutrition in renal disease. In Rolandelli RH, Bankhead R, Boullata JI, Compher CW (eds): Clinical Nutrition: Enteral and Tube Feeding, 4th ed. Philadelphia: WB Saunders, 2005, pp 471–485.
48. Fiaccadori E, Maggiore U, Giacosa R, et al: Enteral nutrition in patients with acute renal failure. Kidney Int 2004;65:999–1008.
49. Zager RA: Amino acid hyperalimentation in acute renal failure: A potential therapeutic paradox. Kidney Int Suppl 1987;22: S72–S75.
50. Schramm L, Weierich T, Heldbreder E, et al: Endotoxin-induced acute renal failure in rats: Effects of L-arginine and nitric oxide synthase inhibition on renal function. J Nephrol 2005;18:374–381.

51. Pons M, Plante I, LeBrun M, et al: Protein-rich diet attenuates cyclosporin A-induced renal tubular damage in rats. J Ren Nutr 2003;13:84–92.
52. Singer P: High-dose amino acid infusion preserves diuresis and improves nitrogen balance in non-oliguric acute renal failure. Wien Klin Wochenschr 2007:119:218–222.
53. Metnitz PG, Krenn CG, Steltzer H, et al: Effect of acute renal failure requiring renal replacement therapy on outcome in critically ill patients. Crit Care Med 2002;30:2051–2058.
54. Mouser JF, Hak EB, Kuhl DA, et al: Recovery from ischemic acute renal failure is improved with enteral compared with parenteral nutrition. Crit Care Med 1997;25:1748–1754.
55. Heidegger CP, Romand JA, Treggiari MM, Pichard C: Is it now time to promote mixed enteral and parenteral nutrition for the critically ill patient? Intensive Care Med 2007;33:963–969.
56. Griffiths RD, Jones C, Palmer TE: Six-month outcome of critically ill patients given glutamine-supplemented parenteral nutrition. Nutrition 1997;13:295–302.
57. Tappy L, Schwarz JM, Schneiter P, et al: Effects of isoenergetic glucose-based or lipid-based parenteral nutrition on glucose metabolism, de novo lipogenesis, and respiratory gas exchanges in critically ill patients. Crit Care Med 1998;26:860–867.
58. Huschak G, Zur Nieden K, Hoell T, et al: Olive oil based nutrition in multiple trauma patients: A pilot study. Intensive Care Med 2005;31:1202–1208.
59. Heller AR, Rossler S, Litz RJ, et al: Omega-3 fatty acids improve the diagnosis-related clinical outcome. Crit Care Med 2006;34:972–979.

Further Reading

Cano N, Fiaccadori E, Tesinsky P, et al: ESPEN Guidelines on Enteral Nutrition: Adult renal failure. Clin Nutr 2006;25:295–310.
Druml W: Nutritional management of acute renal failure. J Renal Nutr 2005;15:63–70.
Druml W, Mitch WE: Metabolic abnormalities in acute renal failure. Semin Dial 1996;9:484–490.
Druml W, Mitch WE: Enteral nutrition in renal disease. In Rolandelli RH, Bankhead R, Boullata JI, Compher CW (eds): Clinical Nutrition: Enteral and Tube Feeding, 4th ed. Philadelphia: WB Saunders, 2005, pp 471–485.

Chapter 9

Experimental Strategies for Acute Kidney Injury

Hye Ryoun Jang, Joseph V. Bonventre, and Hamid Rabb

The high incidence and lack of specific early diagnostic tools and effective therapeutic approaches to acute kidney injury (AKI)/acute renal failure underlie the importance of exploration of novel experimental strategies to make advances in the care of patients with this syndrome. This overview is divided into four sections. The first section reviews experimental models of AKI. The second section discusses general advances in the pathophysiology of AKI using current experiment models. The third focuses on novel diagnostics and the fourth on experimental therapeutics that are promising for clinical translation. Owing to space limitations, we have had to be selective and focus on recent advances. For more in-depth review, we refer the reader to previous editions of this chapter as well as to the updated comprehensive AKI chapter in the parent textbook.[1-3]

EXPERIMENTAL MODELS OF ACUTE KIDNEY INJURY

Experimental models of AKI can be divided into two categories: in vivo and in vitro. Studies can be further subdivided according to how AKI is simulated: ischemia-reperfusion injury (IRI), sepsis, or nephrotoxic agents.

In Vivo

A large number of studies of AKI have been conducted in rodents, especially rats. More recently, because of the opportunity to apply genetic approaches to change the expression of proteins in mice, this species has increased in popularity as a model. IRI models have been established in mice.[4] Mice can be genetically engineered with specific deficiencies in cytokines, surface markers, or certain cell populations. When dealing with mice, however, it is important to recognize that different background strains have strain-specific responses to

AKI, highlighting the importance of using appropriate strain controls.[5] Age and sex of the animal used also have to be considered because the susceptibility to AKI can vary according to age or sex.[6] Female mice are known to be resistant to IRI-induced AKI but more sensitive to cisplatin-induced AKI.[7] The weaknesses of rodent models include unique physiology, size difference from humans, and key immunologic differences that limit applicability to humans. Large mammals such as dogs,[8,9] pigs, and sheep[10] have been used, but less commonly than rodents. The pig kidney has many similarities to the human kidney, both anatomically and physiologically,[11] and may be well suited to simulate the hemodynamic changes encountered during AKI. However, the high costs involved in developing and maintaining large mammalian models and also ethical issues have limited their use. A few newer animal models, such as zebrafish[12] for nephrotoxic drug–induced AKI or Caenorhabditis elegans[13-15] for understanding cellular response to hypoxia are promising. Hentschel and Bonventre[16] recently reviewed novel nonrodent models of AKI.

IRI-induced AKI models are widely used to simulate both native kidney and transplant injury. In mice, IRI is usually performed using microvascular clamps on renal pedicles, occluding the artery and vein while sparing the ureter. Clamping the renal artery alone followed by reperfusion is more often used in larger animals. Unilateral renal pedicle clamp followed by contralateral nephrectomy is also widely used as a variant of this model to study IRI-induced AKI to simulate transplant injury more closely. Strict attention to temperature during ischemia and surgical technique are required for reproducibility in the clamp model. A major limitation is that most patients with native kidney AKI do not undergo IRI in the same manner; the period of ischemia is usually not accompanied by abdominal surgery, and it is usually in the context of whole-body ischemia. Sepsis-induced AKI models are usually induced by administration of lipopolysaccharide or cecal ligation and puncture (CLP). Although the CLP model may be closer to the clinical situation, some laboratories have had difficulty achieving a reliable and reproducible increase in serum creatinine with this model. Star and colleagues[17] recently refined this model in aged mice and found that ethyl pyruvate inhibited renal and multiple organ damage, even when the ethyl pyruvate was administered 12 hours after CLP. Key to this model was employing a fluid resuscitation and antibiotic strategy after CLP. The model results in a two- to threefold increase in serum creatinine concentration, which is less than the increases frequently seen in patients with sepsis, but it does embody many components of similarity to the multiorgan disease state of patients with sepsis and AKI. The same group subsequently reported a CLP model in aged rats,[18] demonstrating that this rat model has more inconsistency with development of AKI, defined as a doubling of serum creatinine. The heterogeneity of response was taken advantage of by the authors as they performed proteomic analysis on collected urine from rats that developed AKI and compared patterns with those obtained on urine from rats that did not develop AKI.

Many nephrotoxicants pertinent to human disease can be reproduced in rodent models. Cisplatin, a common chemotherapeutic agent, has many pathophysiologic features that overlap with IRI. Other nephrotoxicants such as gentamicin have been studied for many years, whereas recently much more attention is being devoted to environmental nephrotoxicants such as cadmium.[19] Dosing with various nephrotoxicants in animals may differ considerably from what it takes to produce toxicity in humans. Although some models exist for radiocontrast nephropathy, these models are generally multicomponent and difficult to reliably reproduce as well as difficult to translate from one species to another.[20] Thus, given its importance to human exposure, this represents an important opportunity to develop more clinically oriented disease models in vivo. The recently recognized strong association between gadolinium and nephrogenic systemic fibrosis during CKD and during AKI represents a new opportunity for development of models to study gadolinium effects during AKI.

In Vitro

Most in vitro studies of AKI have been performed with cell culture methods. Hypoxic chambers or chemical anoxia are commonly used. Strengths of in vitro approaches are the ability to tightly control the environment and evaluate the specific cellular response. However, in vitro conditions are quite different from in vivo conditions, and single cells in isolation do not represent the true complex milieu in which a kidney cell population responds to injury and repair. Use of immortalized cells in culture, which increases the ease of obtaining cells, further distances the cell of study from the human kidney. It is important to recognize that cells placed in culture change their metabolic characteristics quite dramatically; to the extent that metabolism is linked to function, many functional characteristics would also be expected to change. There are, however, situations in which in vitro approaches nicely complement in vivo ones, because the mechanism at the cellular level can often be dissected more effectively in vitro. As an example, cell culture methods have been very useful in revealing the molecular mechanisms of apoptosis or regeneration of tubular epithelial cells.

ADVANCES IN PATHOPHYSIOLOGY OF ACUTE KIDNEY INJURY

In AKI models, there have been at least six main pathophysiologic themes: (1) imbalance between vasoconstrictive and vasodilatory factors, (2) inflammation, (3) tubular dysfunction and intratubular obstruction, (4) cell death by necrosis or apoptosis, (5) preconditioning, and (6) organ cross talk.

Imbalance between Vasoconstrictive and Vasodilatory Influences

Although total renal blood flow reaches 25% of cardiac output, the majority of that flow is directed to the renal cortex[21] and the distribution of renal blood flow may be abnormal after ischemia even though total renal blood flow after ischemia may be close to normal.[22] The outer medulla is hypoxic under normal conditions and is particularly sensitive to further decrements in blood flow.[23] There have been a number of studies exploring the balance between renal vasoconstrictive and vasodilatory influences in AKI and many therapeutic attempts to increase renal blood flow and ameliorate abnormal redistribution. Nitric oxide, endothelin, atrial natriuretic peptide, angiotensin II, dopamine, eicosanoids, and platelet-activating factors are candidate mediators of the intrarenal balance between vasoconstriction and vasodilation in postischemic kidneys.[1] Recently, renal endothelial dysfunction and impaired autoregulation during AKI from excess nitric oxide were reported.[24] Although atrial natriuretic peptide, dopamine, calcium channel blockers, and eicosanoid products of phospholipase A_2 enzymes, including prostaglandins, have been reported to be implicated in the pathophysiology of AKI, there is no convincing evidence of protective effects in humans.[2]

Inflammation

Inflammation is thought to be of greatest importance for AKI at the level of the microvasculature. The flow of leukocytes through capillaries and small venules can be adversely affected by cell-cell interactions, such as platelet plugging, or blood cell–endothelium interactions resulting in leukocyte adhesion and transmigration through the endothelial layer. The important role of leukocyte-endothelium adhesion molecules, particularly CD11/CD18, intercellular adhesion molecule (ICAM)-1, E-selectin, P-selectin, and tissue-type plasminogen activator in IRI-induced AKI, has already been demonstrated.[4,25–30] However, clinical trials with a CD11a/CD18 or ICAM-1 monoclonal antibody did not demonstrate any protective effect.[31,32] Several studies have elucidated significant pathophysiologic roles for T cells during the initiation phase of IRI-induced AKI.[33–37] A "hit-and-run" hypothesis regarding T cells was proposed to explain that few T cells were detected in the kidneys during the insult phase of IRI-induced AKI.[38] Isolation and assessing phenotypes of lymphocytes from the postischemic kidneys[36] and confirmation of the existence of T cells in the kidneys within 1 hour of IRI[39] directly support the "hit-and-run" hypothesis. It was demonstrated that the CD4$^+$ T cells have an important pathophysiologic role in IRI-induced AKI,[34] that CD4 cells of the Th1 phenotype are pathogenic, and that the Th2 phenotype can be protective.[40] The role of T cells, however, is more complex than initially expected. Although T-cell depletion with thymectomy followed by T cell–depleting antibody administration improved the course of experimental IRI,[41] mice deficient in both T and B cells were not protected from IRI.[42] The role of T-cell receptor in IRI is another important question to be solved. The T-cell receptor appears to play a role in the full injury response to IRI, although alloantigen-independent activation in IRI could also participate.[36] The role of B cells in AKI has had limited study, but there may be a role for these cells.[43] Natural killer T (NKT) cells are another lymphocyte population that can respond to nonprotein antigens and have been implicated in experimental AKI.[44] Macrophages are well established to migrate to the kidney during AKI and likely play an important role in the cellular inflammatory cascade.[45] Interleukin-1–dependent inflammatory cascades[46] and alternative complement pathway[47] were also implicated to have some role in pathogenesis of IRI.

The severity of tubular damage in the outer medulla could increase with increasing distance from vascular bundles, which is also consistent with the important role of local oxygen gradients.[48,49] In experimental AKI models in which vascular changes are induced by inactivation of prostaglandin and nitric oxide synthesis in the setting of contrast medium administration, medullary thick ascending limb of the loop of Henle oxygen consumption appears to correlate with tubular damage since furosemide, which inhibits NKCC2 in the medullary thick ascending limb of the loop of Henle, confers structural and functional protection.[50]

Tubular Cell Dysfunction and Intratubular Obstruction

Coexistence of renal tubular dysfunction and down-regulation of tubular sodium transporters, especially NHE3, Na$^+$/K$^+$-ATPase, and NKCC2 after IRI, has been reported.[51–54] More recently, NHE activation, followed by renal endothelin-1 overproduction, seems to play an important role in the pathogenesis of IRI-induced AKI, as demonstrated by administering pre- and post-treatment of 5-N-ethyl-N-isopropyl amiloride in mice IRI model.[55] Renal tubular dysfunction in sepsis-associated AKI is associated with a marked down-regulation of ROMK, NKCC2, ENaC, Na$^+$/K$^+$-ATPase, and NHE3, with attenuation of these effects by glucocorticoid treatment.[56] Peritubular capillary dysfunction and renal tubular epithelial cell stress were also found after lipopolysaccharide administration in mice using intravital video microscopy.[57] Reactive nitrogen species were implicated as an important mediator in sepsis-induced peritubular dysfunction.[58] Protein C may play a role in sepsis-associated AKI: a rapid decrease in protein C after sepsis was reported with an increase in blood urea nitrogen and expression of known markers of renal injury, including neutrophil gelatinase–associated lipocalin, CXCL1, and CXCL2 in a CLP model of sepsis.[59] In experimental settings mimicking hyperdynamic sepsis, a marked increase in renal blood flow with severe renal vasodilatation was observed in a sheep model.[10] Caspase-1,[60–62] Toll-like receptor 4,[63] myeloid differentiation factor 88,[64] heme oxygenase-1,[65] thromboxane

receptor,[66] and T-cell modulation of neutrophils via the CD28 pathway[67] have been implicated in the pathogenesis of sepsis-induced AKI.

Cell Necrosis and Apoptosis

Proteins such as prostate apoptosis response-4,[68] a leucine zipper protein linked to apoptotic cell death in prostate cancer and neuronal tissues, and calpain,[69] an intracellular Ca^{2+}-dependent cysteine protease that is released in the extracellular milieu by tubular epithelial cells, were also recently proposed as novel and early mediators of renal tubule cell injury following IRI. Various mediators have been shown to be involved in cisplatin-induced AKI: T cells,[70] Fas and tumor necrosis factor (TNF) receptor 1,[71] TNF receptor 2,[72] caspase-1,[73] p53,[74] and p21,[75] a cell cycle–inhibitory protein. Prostaglandin E$_2$ has been implicated in mercury chloride–induced AKI,[76] caspases in glycerol-induced AKI,[77] and A$_1$ adenosine receptor in acute radiocontrast nephropathy.[78] Fas-associated death domain, an adaptor protein required for the transmission of the death signal from lethal receptors of the TNF superfamily, and TNF-like weak inducer of apoptosis (TWEAK), a member of the TNF superfamily, were found to play an important role in apoptosis of renal tubular cells in culture.[79,80] Extracellular signal–regulated kinase can elicit apoptosis in epithelial cells by activating caspase-3 and inhibiting Akt pathways, leading to nuclear condensation through caspase-3 and histone H$_2$B phosphorylation in H$_2$O$_2$-induced renal proximal tubular cell apoptosis during IRI.[81] Although Bid, a proapoptotic Bcl-2 family protein, was shown to be involved in the pathogenesis of ischemic injury,[82] apoptosis-antagonizing transcription factor, a leucine zipper domain–containing protein, was reported to protect renal tubule cells against apoptosis induced by IRI.[83]

Preconditioning

Over a number of years, it has been appreciated that the kidney can be preconditioned by previous toxin or ischemic exposure so that it is more resistant to subsequent toxins or ischemia.[84] The mechanisms of this protection are not completely understood. Inducible nitric oxide synthase is an important contributor but does not account for all the protection.[85] A complex pattern of hypoxia-inducible transcription factor activation appears to play an important role in tissue preservation in response to regional renal hypoxia,[86] and preconditioning activation of hypoxia-inducible transcription factor ameliorates ischemic injury.[87] A recent study demonstrated that activation of heat shock protein-70 by heat preconditioning also attenuated ischemic renal injury via inhibition of NF-κB–mediated inflammation.[88]

Organ Cross Talk

Given that many patients die during AKI of distant organ effects, a new area of investigation has been the mechanisms of distant organ effects of AKI. A major inflammatory and proapoptotic response occurs in the lung, heart, and brain during AKI.[89–91] An increase in lung vascular permeability occurs during AKI, more severe than the change associated with the same increase in serum creatinine caused by an acute removal of kidneys, implicating reperfusion products in addition to uremia as the cause. The time after AKI can have an important influence on the type of extrarenal response because lung responses can be proinjurious or protective.[89] It is also important to recognize that pathophysiologic processes in distant organs can also influence kidney function.[92] Further specific pathophysiologic targets for therapy are discussed later in the section on future preventive and therapeutic strategies.

EXPERIMENTAL APPROACHES FOR EARLY DIAGNOSIS OF ACUTE KIDNEY INJURY

The increase in serum creatinine or decrease in urine output is not sensitive enough to reveal early injury events in the kidney. There is an important need for novel biomarkers of AKI, much like serum troponin can be used to detect early acute myocardial injury. Many novel biomarkers such as urinary Toll-like receptor 4,[93] malondialdehyde,[94] keratinocyte-derived chemokine,[95] neutrophil gelatinase–associated lipocalin,[96] spermidine/spermine (N_1-acetyltransferase),[97] and kidney injury molecule-1,[98] a type 1 membrane protein with extracellular immunoglobulin and mucin domains, can increase well before an increase in serum creatinine occurs in AKI models (Box 9-1). The cyclin-dependent kinase inhibitor p21, a kind of stress-induced gene, and mouse telomerase reverse transcriptase could serve as a novel marker for estimating the ischemic period.[99] However, the jury is still out on the best approach to use one or several urinary or serum tests in diagnosing or classifying AKI.[100] This topic is covered in much greater detail in a review.[101]

Newer technologies have been embraced to detect novel biomarkers: proteomics using special techniques such as difference in-gel electrophoresis[18] and 1H-nuclear magnetic resonance spectroscopy.[102] Novel imaging approaches are also promising for the detection and staging of AKI. A new radiometric measurement technique has been developed based on intravital fluorescence microscopy that allows rapid evaluations of renal function in rodent models.[103] By using this technique, plasma clearance rates of a fluorescent glomerular filtration rate marker can be measured in less than 5 minutes following a bolus infusion of a fluorescent dye mixture into the bloodstream. Ultrasmall superparamagnetic iron oxide–enhanced magnetic resonance imaging,[104] magnetic resonance imaging with dendrimer-based contrast,[105,106] and Apo-Sense,[107] a family of small-molecule compounds capable of selectively targeting and accumulating within apoptotic/necrotic cells, have been proposed as imaging techniques for diagnosing early renal injury before azotemia develops.

EXPERIMENTAL STRATEGIES FOR PREVENTION OR TREATMENT OF ACUTE KIDNEY INJURY

The major experimental approach in this field involves the application of novel pharmacologic and cell-based therapy (Box 9-2). Another approach, although performed by limited groups but with great promise, is to use novel devices or innovative use of existing approaches, taking advantage of advances in bioengineering and tissue engineering.

Growth factors have shown great promise in experimental models, but a small study in humans with insulin-like growth factor I was not protective.[108] That does not exclude, however, the possibility for other growth factors to have therapeutic potential. There has been recent interest in applying agents that prevent lymphocyte infiltration into the kidney, such as the sphingosine-1-phosphate type 1 receptor agonists FTY720[109] and SEW2871,[39] which were successful in mice IRI models. Although FTY720 will likely not be used in human transplantation, similar agents with better side effect profiles have promise. Erythropoietin (EPO) and similar agents could have potential for human AKI. EPO has been shown to decrease mortality in experimental AKI[110] and can also provide renoprotection at a

---

Box 9-1 Some Novel Biomarkers and Imaging Techniques That Deserve Increased Evaluation for Early Diagnosis of Acute Kidney Injury

Novel Biomarkers
Urine
 Kidney injury molecule-1
 Neutrophil gelatinase–associated lipocalin
 Toll-like receptor 4
 Malondialdehyde
 Keratinocyte-derived chemokine (Gro-α)
 Cytokines and chemokines
 Urine epigenetics/DNA methylation
Gene
 Cyclin-dependent kinase inhibitor p21
 Spermidine/spermine (N_1-acetyltransferase)
 Mouse telomerase reverse transcriptase

Novel Imaging Techniques
 Ultrasmall superparamagnetic iron oxide–enhanced MRI
 MRI with dendrimer-based contrast
 ApoSense technique

MRI, magnetic resonance imaging.

Box 9-2 Experimental Preventive or Therapeutic Agents for Acute Kidney Injury

Stem cell therapy
Renal tubule assist device or bioartificial kidneys

In IRI Models
Sphingosine-1-phosphate type 1 receptor agonists
Erythropoietin
Trimetazidine
Caspase inhibitors
Selectin ligand inhibitors
Antiapoptotic agents
CD4+ T cells of the Th2 phenotype
New molecules identified by subtraction/array/
 proteomic techniques

In Sepsis-induced AKI Models
Activated protein C
Levosimendan
Ethyl pyruvate

AKI, acute kidney injury; IRI, ischemia-reperfusion injury.

high dose,[111] a low dose,[112] and after pretreatment with EPO.[113] Endothelial cells are a potential target of the cytoprotective effects of EPO.[114,115] However no significant change in renal outcome was observed in human studies in which EPO was administered to acutely ill patients.[116] Darbepoetin, a clinically used variant of EPO, was reported to have a renoprotective effect in IRI-induced AKI.[117]

Using current immunosuppressive drugs for AKI has been limited to date by their nonimmune side effect profile. Cyclosporine or rapamycin were reported to aggravate damage in ischemic organs, negatively affecting posttransplantation recovery in a concentration-dependent fashion.[118]

Cyclosporine also delayed tubular regeneration after IRI. Rapamycin delayed but did not prevent renal recovery after AKI in rats undergoing renal artery occlusion likely due to acquired tubular cell resistance to rapamycin.[119] By contrast, pretreatment with mycophenolate mofetil led to reduced IRI in rats by decreasing the expression of ICAM-1 and infiltration of macrophages and lymphocytes, and this is a relatively well-understood agent with an acceptable toxicity profile in humans.[120]

Trimetazidine, an anti-ischemic metabolic agent that inhibits fatty acid metabolism, enhanced hypoxia-inducible transcription-1α expression and reduced tubulointerstitial fibrosis in a pig IRI model.[121] Other novel potential therapeutic agents include olprinone,[122] L-carnosine,[123] inhibitory monoclonal antibody to mouse factor B[124] and CD55/CD59[125] for targeting complement system, fructose-1,6-diphosphate,[126] ghrelin,[127] peroxisome proliferator–activated receptor β/δ,[128] geranylgeranylacetone,[129] the oxygen radical scavenger edaravone,[130] apotransferrin,[131] nitric oxide precursor L-arginine,[132] α_1-acid glycoprotein,[133] and the tyrosine kinase inhibitor tyrphostin AG126.[134] For each of these agents, a rationale can be developed for why they might be effective.

Granulocyte colony–stimulating factor was reported to attenuate renal injury in IRI-induced AKI,[135,136] cisplatin-induced AKI,[137] and folic acid–induced AKI,[138] but to worsen renal injury in another setting of IRI-induced AKI.[139] Activated protein C,[140] levosimendan,[141] and ethyl pyruvate[17] hold promise for sepsis-induced AKI. Several conventional agents such as 3-hydroxy-3-methylglutaryl coenzyme A reductase inhibitor,[142–144] mineralocorticoid receptor blocker,[145,146] minocycline,[147] docosahexaenoic acid (all cis 4,7,10,13,16,19 docosahexaenoic acid C22: n-3),[148] and magnesium supplementation combined with N-acetylcysteine[149] have had beneficial effects in animal models and are candidates to test in humans.

Fibrate,[150,151] MEK inhibitor,[152] peroxisome proliferator–activated receptor α ligand,[153] and antioxidants[154] can ameliorate renal injury in experimental cisplatin-induced AKI. Kallikrein/kinin was reported to have renoprotective effects by inhibiting inflammatory cell recruitment and apoptosis through suppression of oxidative stress–mediated signaling pathways in gentamicin-induced nephrotoxicity.[155]

It is important to consider why many pharmacologic agents have demonstrated renoprotective effects or therapeutic potentials in animal models, but have failed in human clinical trials. Dose and timing of pharmacologic agents could be an important factor. In most animal studies, supraphysiologic doses, not tolerated by patients, were usually administered prior to or very early during the renal insult, whereas much smaller doses were administered, usually after established AKI, in clinical trials. The difference in physiologic and immunologic characteristics and responses between humans and animals also has to be considered.

Stem-cell therapy is a novel and promising approach for mitigating tissue damage or hastening the healing process after AKI. Hematopoietic stem cells and mesenchymal stem cells were beneficial in experimental AKI, and the mode of actions was initially thought to be from directly repopulating and repairing renal tubules.[135,156–158] However, more recent reports have proposed that the restoration of tubular epithelial cells relies on replication of intrinsic tubular cells more than exogenous cells.[159–161] Recent reports have demonstrated that mesenchymal stem cells ameliorated tissue damage after IRI in mice,[162] and exogenous mesenchymal stem cells trafficked into the kidneys injured by glycerol.[163] It is very likely that paracrine mechanisms play a key role in the healing effect of exogenously administered stem cells. This topic has recently been reviewed much more extensively.[164]

The bioartificial renal tubule assist device (RAD) was introduced as a therapeutic approach that combined cell therapy and hemodialysis or hemofiltration.[165] The RAD is a cartridge containing living renal proximal tubule cells isolated from deceased donor kidneys, grown in confluent monolayers along the inner surface of the hollow fibers in a conventional hemofiltration cartridge.[166,167] The bioartificial kidney, consisting of a filtration device (a conventional high-flux hemofilter) followed in series by the RAD, showed promise in acutely uremic dogs after bilateral nephrectomies[168,169] and also in septic shock models using dogs and pigs.[170,171] Continuous bioartificial kidney therapy was recently tested on a porcine multiple organ dysfunction syndrome with AKI model, with measured decrements in serum TNF-α, increment of serum interleukin-10, and consequently prolonged survival.[172] Although controlled trials with a small number of patients failed to demonstrate that the RAD could confer a survival advantage in sepsis-induced AKI, recent phase I/II clinical trials were promising.[173,174]

In summary, there have been many advances in our understanding of AKI over the past few years. The current focus is to translate findings from the laboratory into improved diagnosis, prevention, and treatment for our patients. There is a great need and many candidates to evaluate more completely.

References

1. Rabb H, Bonventre JV: Experimental strategies for acute renal failure—the future. In Brady HR, Wilcox CS (eds): Therapy in Nephrology and Hypertension: A Companion to Brenner and Rector's The Kidney. Philadelphia: WB Saunders, 1999, pp 72–80.
2. Rabb H, Bonventre JV: Experimental strategies for acute renal failure: The future. In Brady HR, Wilcox CS (eds): Therapy in Nephrology and Hypertension: A Companion to Brenner and Rector's The Kidney, 2nd ed. Philadelphia: WB Saunders, 2003, pp 87–91.
3. Clarkson M, Friedewald J, Eustace J, et al: Acute renal failure/acute kidney injury. In Brenner BM (ed): Brenner and Rector's The Kidney, 8th ed. Philadelphia: WB Saunders, 2007, pp 943–986.
4. Kelly KJ, Williams WW Jr, Colvin RB, et al: Antibody to intercellular adhesion molecule 1 protects the kidney against ischemic injury. Proc Natl Acad Sci U S A 1994;91:812–816.
5. Burne MJ, Haq M, Matsuse H, et al: Genetic susceptibility to renal ischemia reperfusion injury revealed in a murine model. Transplantation 2000;69:1023–1025.

6. Park KM, Kim JI, Ahn Y, et al: Testosterone is responsible for enhanced susceptibility of males to ischemic renal injury. J Biol Chem 2004;279:52282–52292.

7. Wei Q, Wang MH, Dong Z: Differential gender differences in ischemic and nephrotoxic acute renal failure. Am J Nephrol 2005;25:491–499.

8. Lewis RM, Rice JH, Patton MK, et al: Renal ischemic injury in the dog: Characterization and effect of various pharmacologic agents. J Lab Clin Med 1984;104:470–479.

9. Riley AL, Alexander EA, Migdal S, et al: The effect of ischemia on renal blood flow in the dog. Kidney Int 1975;7:27–34.

10. Langenberg C, Wan L, Egi M, et al: Renal blood flow in experimental septic acute renal failure. Kidney Int 2006;69:1996–2002.

11. Killion D, Canfield C, Norman J, et al: Exogenous epidermal growth factor fails to accelerate functional recovery in the auto-transplanted ischemic pig kidney. J Urol 1993;150:1551–1556.

12. Hentschel DM, Park KM, Cilenti L, et al: Acute renal failure in zebrafish: A novel system to study a complex disease. Am J Physiol Renal Physiol 2005;288:F923–F929.

13. Padilla PA, Nystul TG, Zager RA, et al: Dephosphorylation of cell cycle-regulated proteins correlates with anoxia-induced suspended animation in Caenorhabditis elegans. Mol Biol Cell 2002;13:1473–1483.

14. Shen C, Nettleton D, Jiang M, et al: Roles of the HIF-1 hypoxia-inducible factor during hypoxia response in Caenorhabditis elegans. J Biol Chem 2005;280:20580–20588.

15. Shen C, Shao Z, Powell-Coffman JA: The Caenorhabditis elegans rhy-1 gene inhibits HIF-1 hypoxia-inducible factor activity in a negative feedback loop that does not include vhl-1. Genetics 2006;174:1205–1214.

16. Hentschel DM, Bonventre JV: Novel non-rodent models of kidney disease. Curr Mol Med 2005;5:537–546.

17. Miyaji T, Hu X, Yuen PS, et al: Ethyl pyruvate decreases sepsis-induced acute renal failure and multiple organ damage in aged mice. Kidney Int 2003;64:1620–1631.

18. Holly MK, Dear JW, Hu X, et al: Biomarker and drug-target discovery using proteomics in a new rat model of sepsis-induced acute renal failure. Kidney Int 2006;70:496–506.

19. Prozialeck WC, Vaidya VS, Liu J, et al: Kidney injury molecule-1 is an early biomarker of cadmium nephrotoxicity. Kidney Int 2007;72:985–993.

20. Heyman SN, Lieberthal W, Rogiers P, et al: Animal models of acute tubular necrosis. Curr Opin Crit Care 2002;8:526–534.

21. Chou SY, Porush JG, Faubert PF: Renal medullary circulation: Hormonal control. Kidney Int 1990;37:1–13.

22. Thadhani R, Pascual M, Bonventre JV: Acute renal failure. N Engl J Med 1996;334:1448–1460.

23. Brezis M, Rosen S: Hypoxia of the renal medulla—its implications for disease. N Engl J Med 1995;332:647–655.

24. Guan Z, Gobe G, Willgoss D, et al: Renal endothelial dysfunction and impaired autoregulation after ischemia-reperfusion injury result from excess nitric oxide. Am J Physiol Renal Physiol 2006;291:F619–F628.

25. Rabb H, Mendiola CC, Dietz J, et al: Role of CD11a and CD11b in ischemic acute renal failure in rats. Am J Physiol 1994;267: F1052–F1058.

26. Kelly KJ, Williams WW Jr, Colvin RB, et al: Intercellular adhesion molecule-1-deficient mice are protected against ischemic renal injury. J Clin Invest 1996;97:1056–1063.

27. Haller H, Dragun D, Miethke A, et al: Antisense oligonucleotides for ICAM-1 attenuate reperfusion injury and renal failure in the rat. Kidney Int 1996;50:473–480.

28. Singbartl K, Ley K: Protection from ischemia-reperfusion induced severe acute renal failure by blocking E-selectin. Crit Care Med 2000;28:2507–2514.

29. Singbartl K, Green SA, Ley K: Blocking P-selectin protects from ischemia/reperfusion-induced acute renal failure. FASEB J 2000;14:48–54.

30. Roelofs JJ, Rouschop KM, Leemans JC, et al: Tissue-type plasminogen activator modulates inflammatory responses and renal function in ischemia reperfusion injury. J Am Soc Nephrol 2006;17:131–140.

31. Salmela K, Wramner L, Ekberg H, et al: A randomized multicenter trial of the anti-ICAM-1 monoclonal antibody (enlimomab) for the prevention of acute rejection and delayed onset of graft function in cadaveric renal transplantation: A report of the European Anti-ICAM-1 Renal Transplant Study Group. Transplantation 1999;67:729–736.

32. Vincenti F, Mendez R, Pescovitz M, et al: A phase I/II randomized open-label multicenter trial of efalizumab, a humanized anti-CD11a, anti-LFA-1 in renal transplantation. Am J Transplant 2007;7:1770–1777.

33. Rabb H, Daniels F, O'Donnell M, et al: Pathophysiological role of T lymphocytes in renal ischemia-reperfusion injury in mice. Am J Physiol Renal Physiol 2000;279:F525–F531.

34. Burne MJ, Daniels F, El Ghandour A, et al: Identification of the CD4+ T cell as a major pathogenic factor in ischemic acute renal failure. J Clin Invest 2001;108:1283–1290.

35. De Greef KE, Ysebaert DK, Dauwe S, et al: Anti-B7-1 blocks mononuclear cell adherence in vasa recta after ischemia. Kidney Int 2001;60:1415–1427.

36. Ascon DB, Lopez-Briones S, Liu M, et al: Phenotypic and functional characterization of kidney-infiltrating lymphocytes in renal ischemia reperfusion injury. J Immunol 2006;177:3380–3387.

37. Day YJ, Huang L, Ye H, et al: Renal ischemia-reperfusion injury and adenosine 2A receptor-mediated tissue protection: The role of CD4+ T cells and IFN-gamma. J Immunol 2006;176: 3108–3114.

38. Friedewald JJ, Rabb H: Inflammatory cells in ischemic acute renal failure. Kidney Int 2004;66:486–491.

39. Lai LW, Yong KC, Igarashi S, et al: A sphingosine-1-phosphate type 1 receptor agonist inhibits the early T-cell transient following renal ischemia-reperfusion injury. Kidney Int 2007;71: 1223–1231.

40. Yokota N, Burne-Taney M, Racusen L, et al: Contrasting roles for STAT4 and STAT6 signal transduction pathways in murine renal ischemia-reperfusion injury. Am J Physiol Renal Physiol 2003;285:F319–F325.

41. Yokota N, Daniels F, Crosson J, et al: Protective effect of T cell depletion in murine renal ischemia-reperfusion injury. Transplantation 2002;74:759–763.

42. Park P, Haas M, Cunningham PN, et al: Injury in renal ischemia-reperfusion is independent from immunoglobulins and T lymphocytes. Am J Physiol Renal Physiol 2002;282:F352–F357.

43. Burne-Taney MJ, Ascon DB, Daniels F, et al: B cell deficiency confers protection from renal ischemia reperfusion injury. J Immunol 2003;171:3210–3215.

44. Li L, Huang L, Sung SS, et al: NKT cell activation mediates neutrophil IFN-gamma production and renal ischemia-reperfusion injury. J Immunol 2007;178:5899–5911.

45. Day YJ, Huang L, Ye H, et al: Renal ischemia-reperfusion injury and adenosine 2A receptor-mediated tissue protection: Role of macrophages. Am J Physiol Renal Physiol 2005;288:F722–F731.

46. Furuichi K, Wada T, Iwata Y, et al: Interleukin-1-dependent sequential chemokine expression and inflammatory cell infiltration in ischemia-reperfusion injury. Crit Care Med 2006;34: 2447–2455.

47. Thurman JM, Ljubanovic D, Edelstein CL, et al: Lack of a functional alternative complement pathway ameliorates ischemic acute renal failure in mice. J Immunol 2003;170:1517–1523.

48. Agmon Y, Peleg H, Greenfeld Z, et al: Nitric oxide and prostanoids protect the renal outer medulla from radiocontrast toxicity in the rat. J Clin Invest 1994;94:1069–1075.

49. Heyman SN, Brezis M, Epstein FH, et al: Early renal medullary hypoxic injury from radiocontrast and indomethacin. Kidney Int 1991;40:632–642.

50. Heyman SN, Brezis M, Greenfeld Z, et al: Protective role of furosemide and saline in radiocontrast-induced acute renal failure in the rat. Am J Kidney Dis 1989;14:377–385.

51. Fernandez-Llama P, Andrews P, Turner R, et al: Decreased abundance of collecting duct aquaporins in post-ischemic renal failure in rats. J Am Soc Nephrol 1999;10:1658–1668.

52. Kwon TH, Frokiaer J, Han JS, et al: Decreased abundance of major Na+ transporters in kidneys of rats with ischemia-induced acute renal failure. Am J Physiol Renal Physiol 2000;278:F925–F939.

53. Van Why SK, Mann AS, Ardito T, et al: Expression and molecular regulation of (Na+K+ATPase) after renal ischemia. Am J Physiol 1994;267:F75–F85.

54. Wang Z, Rabb H, Haq M, et al: A possible molecular basis of natriuresis during ischemic-reperfusion injury in the kidney. J Am Soc Nephrol 1998;9:605–613.

55. Yamashita J, Ohkita M, Takaoka M, et al: Role of Na+/H+ exchanger in the pathogenesis of ischemic acute renal failure in mice. J Cardiovasc Pharmacol 2007;49:154–160.

56. Schmidt C, Hocherl K, Schweda F, et al: Regulation of renal sodium transporters during severe inflammation. J Am Soc Nephrol 2007;18:1072–1083.

57. Wu L, Tiwari MM, Messer KJ, et al: Peritubular capillary dysfunction and renal tubular epithelial cell stress following lipopolysaccharide administration in mice. Am J Physiol Renal Physiol 2007;292:F261–F268.

58. Wu L, Gokden N, Mayeux PR: Evidence for the role of reactive nitrogen species in polymicrobial sepsis-induced renal peritubular capillary dysfunction and tubular injury. J Am Soc Nephrol 2007;18:1807–1815.

59. Gupta A, Berg DT, Gerlitz B, et al: Role of protein C in renal dysfunction after polymicrobial sepsis. J Am Soc Nephrol 2007;18:860–867.

60. Wang W, Faubel S, Ljubanovic D, et al: Endotoxemic acute renal failure is attenuated in caspase-1-deficient mice. Am J Physiol Renal Physiol 2005;288:F997–F1004.

61. Tiwari MM, Brock RW, Megyesi JK, et al: Disruption of renal peritubular blood flow in lipopolysaccharide-induced renal failure: Role of nitric oxide and caspases. Am J Physiol Renal Physiol 2005;289:F1324–F1332.

62. Guo R, Wang Y, Minto AW, et al: Acute renal failure in endotoxemia is dependent on caspase activation. J Am Soc Nephrol 2004;15:3093–3102.

63. Cunningham PN, Wang Y, Guo R, et al: Role of Toll-like receptor 4 in endotoxin-induced acute renal failure. J Immunol 2004;172:2629–2635.

64. Dear JW, Yasuda H, Hu X, et al: Sepsis-induced organ failure is mediated by different pathways in the kidney and liver: Acute renal failure is dependent on MyD88 but not renal cell Apoptosis. Kidney Int 2006;69:832–836.

65. Poole B, Wang W, Chen YC, et al: Role of heme oxygenase-1 in endotoxemic acute renal failure. Am J Physiol Renal Physiol 2005;289:F1382–F1385.

66. Boffa JJ, Just A, Coffman TM, et al: Thromboxane receptor mediates renal vasoconstriction and contributes to acute renal failure in endotoxemic mice. J Am Soc Nephrol 2004;15:2358–2365.

67. Singbartl K, Bockhorn SG, Zarbock A, et al: T cells modulate neutrophil-dependent acute renal failure during endotoxemia: Critical role for CD28. J Am Soc Nephrol 2005;16:720–728.

68. Xie J, Guo Q: Par-4 is a novel mediator of renal tubule cell death in models of ischemia-reperfusion injury. Am J Physiol Renal Physiol 2007;292:F107–F115.

69. Frangie C, Zhang W, Perez J, et al: Extracellular calpains increase tubular epithelial cell mobility. Implications for kidney repair after ischemia. J Biol Chem 2006;281:26624–26632.

70. Liu M, Chien CC, Burne-Taney M, et al: A pathophysiologic role for T lymphocytes in murine acute cisplatin nephrotoxicity. J Am Soc Nephrol 2006;17:765–774.

71. Tsuruya K, Ninomiya T, Tokumoto M, et al: Direct involvement of the receptor-mediated apoptotic pathways in cisplatin-induced renal tubular cell death. Kidney Int 2003;63:72–82.

72. Ramesh G, Reeves WB: TNFR2-mediated apoptosis and necrosis in cisplatin-induced acute renal failure. Am J Physiol Renal Physiol 2003;285:F610–F618.

73. Faubel S, Ljubanovic D, Reznikov L, et al: Caspase-1-deficient mice are protected against cisplatin-induced apoptosis and acute tubular necrosis. Kidney Int 2004;66:2202–2213.

74. Jiang M, Yi X, Hsu S, et al: Role of p53 in cisplatin-induced tubular cell apoptosis: Dependence on p53 transcriptional activity. Am J Physiol Renal Physiol 2004;287:F1140–F1147.

75. Zhou H, Fujigaki Y, Kato A, et al: Inhibition of p21 modifies the response of cortical proximal tubules to cisplatin in rats. Am J Physiol Renal Physiol 2006;291:F225–F235.

76. Vukicevic S, Simic P, Borovecki F, et al: Role of EP2 and EP4 receptor-selective agonists of prostaglandin E2 in acute and chronic kidney failure. Kidney Int 2006;70:1099–1106.

77. Homsi E, Janino P, de Faria JB: Role of caspases on cell death, inflammation, and cell cycle in glycerol-induced acute renal failure. Kidney Int 2006;69:1385–1392.

78. Lee HT, Jan M, Bae SC, et al: A1 adenosine receptor knockout mice are protected against acute radiocontrast nephropathy in vivo. Am J Physiol Renal Physiol 2006;290:F1367–F1375.

79. Justo P, Sanz AB, Lorz C, et al: Lethal activity of FADD death domain in renal tubular epithelial cells. Kidney Int 2006;69:2205–2211.

80. Justo P, Sanz AB, Sanchez-Nino MD, et al: Cytokine cooperation in renal tubular cell injury: The role of TWEAK. Kidney Int 2006;70:1750–1758.

81. Zhuang S, Yan Y, Daubert RA, et al: ERK promotes hydrogen peroxide-induced apoptosis through caspase-3 activation and inhibition of Akt in renal epithelial cells. Am J Physiol Renal Physiol 2007;292:F440–F447.

82. Wei Q, Yin XM, Wang MH, et al: Bid deficiency ameliorates ischemic renal failure and delays animal death in C57BL/6 mice. Am J Physiol Renal Physiol 2006;290:F35–F42.

83. Xie J, Guo Q: Apoptosis antagonizing transcription factor protects renal tubule cells against oxidative damage and apoptosis induced by ischemia-reperfusion. J Am Soc Nephrol 2006;17:3336–3346.

84. Bonventre JV: Kidney ischemic preconditioning. Curr Opin Nephrol Hypertens 2002;11:43–48.

85. Park KM, Byun JY, Kramers C, et al: Inducible nitric-oxide synthase is an important contributor to prolonged protective effects of ischemic preconditioning in the mouse kidney. J Biol Chem 2003;278:27256–27266.

86. Rosenberger C, Heyman SN, Rosen S, et al: Up-regulation of HIF in experimental acute renal failure: Evidence for a protective transcriptional response to hypoxia. Kidney Int 2005;67:531–542.

87. Bernhardt WM, Campean V, Kany S, et al: Preconditional activation of hypoxia-inducible factors ameliorates ischemic acute renal failure. J Am Soc Nephrol 2006;17:1970–1978.

88. Jo SK, Ko GJ, Boo CS, et al: Heat preconditioning attenuates renal injury in ischemic ARF in rats: Role of heat-shock protein 70 on NF-kappaB-mediated inflammation and on tubular cell injury. J Am Soc Nephrol 2006;17:3082–3092.

89. Zarbock A, Schmolke M, Spieker T, et al: Acute uremia but not renal inflammation attenuates aseptic acute lung injury: A critical role for uremic neutrophils. J Am Soc Nephrol 2006;17:3124–3131.

90. Hoke TS, Douglas IS, Klein CL, et al: Acute renal failure after bilateral nephrectomy is associated with cytokine-mediated pulmonary injury. J Am Soc Nephrol 2007;18:155–164.

91. Kingma JG Jr, Vincent C, Rouleau JR, et al: Influence of acute renal failure on coronary vasoregulation in dogs. J Am Soc Nephrol 2006;17:1316–1324.

92. Choi WI, Quinn DA, Park KM, et al: Systemic microvascular leak in an in vivo rat model of ventilator-induced lung injury. Am J Respir Crit Care Med 2003;167:1627–1632.

93. Zager RA, Johnson AC, Lund S, et al: Toll-like receptor (TLR4) shedding and depletion: Acute proximal tubular cell responses to hypoxic and toxic injury. Am J Physiol Renal Physiol 2007;292:F304–F312.

94. Zhou H, Kato A, Miyaji T, et al: Urinary marker for oxidative stress in kidneys in cisplatin-induced acute renal failure in rats. Nephrol Dial Transplant 2006;21:616–-623.

95. Molls RR, Savransky V, Liu M, et al: Keratinocyte-derived chemokine is an early biomarker of ischemic acute kidney injury. Am J Physiol Renal Physiol 2006;290:F1187–F1193.

96. Mishra J, Ma Q, Prada A, et al: Identification of neutrophil gelatinase-associated lipocalin as a novel early urinary biomarker for ischemic renal injury. J Am Soc Nephrol 2003;14:2534–2543.

97. Zahedi K, Wang Z, Barone S, et al: Expression of SSAT, a novel biomarker of tubular cell damage, increases in kidney ischemia-reperfusion injury. Am J Physiol Renal Physiol 2003;284:F1046–F1055.

98. Ichimura T, Hung CC, Yang SA, et al: Kidney injury molecule-1: a tissue and urinary biomarker for nephrotoxicant-induced renal injury. Am J Physiol Renal Physiol 2004;286:F552–F563.

99. Hochegger K, Koppelstaetter C, Tagwerker A, et al: p21 and mTERT are novel markers for determining different ischemic time periods in renal ischemia-reperfusion injury. Am J Physiol Renal Physiol 2007;292:F762–F768.

100. Bagshaw SM, Langenberg C, Wan L, et al: A systematic review of urinary findings in experimental septic acute renal failure. Crit Care Med 2007;35:1592–1598.

101. Waikar SS, Bonventre JV: Biomarkers for the diagnosis of acute kidney injury. Curr Opin Nephrol Hypertens 2007;16:557–564.

102. Portilla D, Li S, Nagothu KK, et al: Metabolomic study of cisplatin-induced nephrotoxicity. Kidney Int 2006;69:2194–2204.

103. Yu W, Sandoval RM, Molitoris BA: Rapid determination of renal filtration function using an optical ratiometric imaging approach. Am J Physiol Renal Physiol 2007;292:F1873–F1880.

104. Jo SK, Hu X, Kobayashi H, et al: Detection of inflammation following renal ischemia by magnetic resonance imaging. Kidney Int 2003;64:43–51.

105. Dear JW, Kobayashi H, Brechbiel MW, et al: Imaging acute renal failure with polyamine dendrimer-based MRI contrast agents. Nephron Clin Pract 2006;103:c45–c49.

106. Dear JW, Kobayashi H, Jo SK, et al: Dendrimer-enhanced MRI as a diagnostic and prognostic biomarker of sepsis-induced acute renal failure in aged mice. Kidney Int 2005;67:2159–2167.

107. Damianovich M, Ziv I, Heyman SN, et al: ApoSense: A novel technology for functional molecular imaging of cell death in models of acute renal tubular necrosis. Eur J Nucl Med Mol Imaging 2006;33:281–291.

108. Hirschberg R, Kopple J, Lipsett P, et al: Multicenter clinical trial of recombinant human insulin-like growth factor I in patients with acute renal failure. Kidney Int 1999;55:2423–2432.

109. Awad AS, Ye H, Huang L, et al: Selective sphingosine 1-phosphate 1 receptor activation reduces ischemia-reperfusion injury in mouse kidney. Am J Physiol Renal Physiol 2006;290:F1516–F1524.

110. Nemoto T, Yokota N, Keane WF, et al: Recombinant erythropoietin rapidly treats anemia in ischemic acute renal failure. Kidney Int 2001;59:246–251.

111. Yang CW, Li C, Jung JY, et al: Preconditioning with erythropoietin protects against subsequent ischemia-reperfusion injury in rat kidney. FASEB J 2003;17:1754–1755.

112. Sharples EJ, Patel N, Brown P, et al: Erythropoietin protects the kidney against the injury and dysfunction caused by ischemia-reperfusion. J Am Soc Nephrol 2004;15:2115–2124.

113. Patel NS, Sharples EJ, Cuzzocrea S, et al: Pretreatment with EPO reduces the injury and dysfunction caused by ischemia/

reperfusion in the mouse kidney in vivo. Kidney Int 2004;66:983–989.

114. Bahlmann FH, De Groot K, Spandau JM, et al: Erythropoietin regulates endothelial progenitor cells. Blood 2004;103:921–926.

115. Scalera F, Kielstein JT, Martens-Lobenhoffer J, et al: Erythropoietin increases asymmetric dimethylarginine in endothelial cells: Role of dimethylarginine dimethylaminohydrolase. J Am Soc Nephrol 2005;16:892–898.

116. Silver M, Corwin MJ, Bazan A, et al: Efficacy of recombinant human erythropoietin in critically ill patients admitted to a long-term acute care facility: A randomized, double-blind, placebo-controlled trial. Crit Care Med 2006;34:2310–2316.

117. Johnson DW, Pat B, Vesey DA, et al: Delayed administration of darbepoetin or erythropoietin protects against ischemic acute renal injury and failure. Kidney Int 2006;69:1806–1813.

118. Goncalves GM, Cenedeze MA, Feitoza CQ, et al: The role of immunosuppressive drugs in aggravating renal ischemia and reperfusion injury. Transplant Proc 2007;39:417–420.

119. Lieberthal W, Fuhro R, Andry C, et al: Rapamycin delays but does not prevent recovery from acute renal failure: Role of acquired tubular resistance. Transplantation 2006;82:17–22.

120. Ventura CG, Coimbra TM, de Campos SB, et al: Mycophenolate mofetil attenuates renal ischemia/reperfusion injury. J Am Soc Nephrol 2002;13:2524–2533.

121. Jayle C, Favreau F, Zhang K, et al: Comparison of protective effects of trimetazidine against experimental warm ischemia of different durations: Early and long-term effects in a pig kidney model. Am J Physiol Renal Physiol 2007;292:F1082–F1093.

122. Anas C, Ozaki T, Maruyama S, et al: Effects of olprinone, a phosphodiesterase III inhibitor, on ischemic acute renal failure. Int J Urol 2007;14:219–225.

123. Kurata H, Fujii T, Tsutsui H, et al: Renoprotective effects of l-carnosine on ischemia/reperfusion-induced renal injury in rats. J Pharmacol Exp Ther 2006;319:640–647.

124. Thurman JM, Royer PA, Ljubanovic D, et al: Treatment with an inhibitory monoclonal antibody to mouse factor B protects mice from induction of apoptosis and renal ischemia/reperfusion injury. J Am Soc Nephrol 2006;17:707–715.

125. Yamada K, Miwa T, Liu J, et al: Critical protection from renal ischemia reperfusion injury by CD55 and CD59. J Immunol 2004;172:3869–3875.

126. Antunes N, Martinusso CA, Takiya CM, et al: Fructose-1,6 diphosphate as a protective agent for experimental ischemic acute renal failure. Kidney Int 2006;69:68–72.

127. Takeda R, Nishimatsu H, Suzuki E, et al: Ghrelin improves renal function in mice with ischemic acute renal failure. J Am Soc Nephrol 2006;17:113–121.

128. Letavernier E, Perez J, Joye E, et al: Peroxisome proliferator-activated receptor beta/delta exerts a strong protection from ischemic acute renal failure. J Am Soc Nephrol 2005;16:2395–2402.

129. Suzuki S, Maruyama S, Sato W, et al: Geranylgeranylacetone ameliorates ischemic acute renal failure via induction of Hsp70. Kidney Int 2005;67:2210–2220.

130. Doi K, Suzuki Y, Nakao A, et al: Radical scavenger edaravone developed for clinical use ameliorates ischemia/reperfusion injury in rat kidney. Kidney Int 2004;65:1714–1723.

131. de Vries B, Walter SJ, von Bonsdorff L, et al: Reduction of circulating redox-active iron by apotransferrin protects against renal ischemia-reperfusion injury. Transplantation 2004;77:669–675.

132. Schneider R, Raff U, Vornberger N, et al: L-Arginine counteracts nitric oxide deficiency and improves the recovery phase of ischemic acute renal failure in rats. Kidney Int 2003;64:216–225.

133. de Vries B, Walter SJ, Wolfs TG, et al: Exogenous alpha-1-acid glycoprotein protects against renal ischemia-reperfusion injury by inhibition of inflammation and apoptosis. Transplantation 2004;78:1116–1124.

134. Chatterjee PK, Patel NS, Kvale EO, et al: The tyrosine kinase inhibitor tyrphostin AG126 reduces renal ischemia/reperfusion injury in the rat. Kidney Int 2003;64:1605–1619.

135. Lin F, Cordes K, Li L, et al: Hematopoietic stem cells contribute to the regeneration of renal tubules after renal ischemia-reperfusion injury in mice. J Am Soc Nephrol 2003;14:1188–1199.

136. Stokman G, Leemans JC, Claessen N, et al: Hematopoietic stem cell mobilization therapy accelerates recovery of renal function independent of stem cell contribution. J Am Soc Nephrol 2005;16:1684–1692.

137. Iwasaki M, Adachi Y, Minamino K, et al: Mobilization of bone marrow cells by G-CSF rescues mice from cisplatin-induced renal failure, and M-CSF enhances the effects of G-CSF. J Am Soc Nephrol 2005;16:658–666.

138. Fang TC, Alison MR, Cook HT, et al: Proliferation of bone marrow-derived cells contributes to regeneration after folic acid-induced acute tubular injury. J Am Soc Nephrol 2005;16:1723–1732.

139. Togel F, Isaac J, Westenfelder C: Hematopoietic stem cell mobilization-associated granulocytosis severely worsens acute renal failure. J Am Soc Nephrol 2004;15:1261–1267.

140. Gupta A, Rhodes GJ, Berg DT, et al: Activated protein C ameliorates LPS-induced acute kidney injury and downregulates renal INOS and angiotensin 2. Am J Physiol Renal Physiol 2007;293:F245–F254.

141. Zager RA, Johnson AC, Lund S, et al: Levosimendan protects against experimental endotoxemic acute renal failure. Am J Physiol Renal Physiol 2006;290:F1453–F1462.

142. Yokota N, O'Donnell M, Daniels F, et al: Protective effect of HMG-CoA reductase inhibitor on experimental renal ischemia-reperfusion injury. Am J Nephrol 2003;23:13–17.

143. Yasuda H, Yuen PS, Hu X, et al: Simvastatin improves sepsis-induced mortality and acute kidney injury via renal vascular effects. Kidney Int 2006;69:1535–1542.

144. Sabbatini M, Pisani A, Uccello F, et al: Atorvastatin improves the course of ischemic acute renal failure in aging rats. J Am Soc Nephrol 2004;15:901–909.

145. Mejia-Vilet JM, Ramirez V, Cruz C, et al: Renal ischemia-reperfusion injury is prevented by the mineralocorticoid receptor blocker spironolactone. Am J Physiol Renal Physiol 2007;293:F78–F86.

146. Feria I, Pichardo I, Juarez P, et al: Therapeutic benefit of spironolactone in experimental chronic cyclosporine A nephrotoxicity. Kidney Int 2003;63:43–52.

147. Kelly KJ, Sutton TA, Weathered N, et al: Minocycline inhibits apoptosis and inflammation in a rat model of ischemic renal injury. Am J Physiol Renal Physiol 2004;287:F760–F766.

148. Kielar ML, Jeyarajah DR, Zhou XJ, et al: Docosahexaenoic acid ameliorates murine ischemic acute renal failure and prevents increases in mRNA abundance for both TNF-alpha and inducible nitric oxide synthase. J Am Soc Nephrol 2003;14:389–396.

149. de Araujo M, Andrade L, Coimbra TM, et al: Magnesium supplementation combined with N-acetylcysteine protects against postischemic acute renal failure. J Am Soc Nephrol 2005;16:3339–3349.

150. Nagothu KK, Bhatt R, Kaushal GP, et al: Fibrate prevents cisplatin-induced proximal tubule cell death. Kidney Int 2005;68:2680–2693.

151. Li S, Gokden N, Okusa MD, et al: Anti-inflammatory effect of fibrate protects from cisplatin-induced ARF. Am J Physiol Renal Physiol 2005;289:F469–F480.

152. Jo SK, Cho WY, Sung SA, et al: MEK inhibitor, U0126, attenuates cisplatin-induced renal injury by decreasing inflammation and apoptosis. Kidney Int 2005;67:458–466.

153. Li S, Basnakian A, Bhatt R, et al: PPAR-alpha ligand ameliorates acute renal failure by reducing cisplatin-induced increased expression of renal endonuclease G. Am J Physiol Renal Physiol 2004;287:F990–F998.

154. Tsuruya K, Tokumoto M, Ninomiya T, et al: Antioxidant ameliorates cisplatin-induced renal tubular cell death through inhibition of death receptor-mediated pathways. Am J Physiol Renal Physiol 2003;285:F208–F218.

155. Bledsoe G, Crickman S, Mao J, et al: Kallikrein/kinin protects against gentamicin-induced nephrotoxicity by inhibition of inflammation and apoptosis. Nephrol Dial Transplant 2006;21:624–633.

156. Morigi M, Imberti B, Zoja C, et al: Mesenchymal stem cells are renotropic, helping to repair the kidney and improve function in acute renal failure. J Am Soc Nephrol 2004;15:1794–1804.

157. Lange C, Togel F, Ittrich H, et al: Administered mesenchymal stem cells enhance recovery from ischemia/reperfusion-induced acute renal failure in rats. Kidney Int 2005;68:1613–1617.

158. Kale S, Karihaloo A, Clark PR, et al: Bone marrow stem cells contribute to repair of the ischemically injured renal tubule. J Clin Invest 2003;112:42–49.

159. Duffield JS, Bonventre JV: Kidney tubular epithelium is restored without replacement with bone marrow-derived cells during repair after ischemic injury. Kidney Int 2005;68:1956–1961.

160. Duffield JS, Park KM, Hsiao LL, et al: Restoration of tubular epithelial cells during repair of the postischemic kidney occurs independently of bone marrow-derived stem cells. J Clin Invest 2005;115:1743–1755.

161. Lin F, Moran A, Igarashi P: Intrarenal cells, not bone marrow-derived cells, are the major source for regeneration in postischemic kidney. J Clin Invest 2005;115:1756–1764.

162. Semedo P, Wang PM, Andreucci TH, et al: Mesenchymal stem cells ameliorate tissue damages triggered by renal ischemia and reperfusion injury. Transplant Proc 2007;39:421–423.

163. Herrera MB, Bussolati B, Bruno S, et al: Exogenous mesenchymal stem cells localize to the kidney by means of CD44 following acute tubular injury. Kidney Int 2007;72:430–441.

164. Humphreys BD, Bonventre JV: Mesenchymal stem cells in acute kidney injury. Annu Rev Med 2008;59:311–325.

165. Fissell WH, Kimball J, MacKay SM, et al: The role of a bioengineered artificial kidney in renal failure. Ann N Y Acad Sci 2001;944:284–295.

166. Humes HD, Cieslinski DA: Interaction between growth factors and retinoic acid in the induction of kidney tubulogenesis in tissue culture. Exp Cell Res 1992;201:8–15.

167. Humes HD, Krauss JC, Cieslinski DA, et al: Tubulogenesis from isolated single cells of adult mammalian kidney: Clonal analysis with a recombinant retrovirus. Am J Physiol 1996;271:F42–F49.

168. Humes HD, Buffington DA, MacKay SM, et al: Replacement of renal function in uremic animals with a tissue-engineered kidney. Nat Biotechnol 1999;17:451–455.

169. Humes HD, Fissell WH, Weitzel WF, et al: Metabolic replacement of kidney function in uremic animals with a bioartificial kidney containing human cells. Am J Kidney Dis 2002;39:1078–1087.

170. Fissell WH, Lou L, Abrishami S, et al: Bioartificial kidney ameliorates gram-negative bacteria-induced septic shock in uremic animals. J Am Soc Nephrol 2003;14:454–461.

171. Humes HD, Buffington DA, Lou L, et al: Cell therapy with a tissue-engineered kidney reduces the multiple-organ consequences of septic shock. Crit Care Med 2003;31:2421–2428.

172. Huijuan M, Xiaoyun W, Xumin Y, et al: Effect of continuous bio-artificial kidney therapy on porcine multiple organ dysfunction syndrome with acute renal failure. ASAIO J 2007;53:329–334.

173. Humes HD, Weitzel WF, Bartlett RH, et al: Initial clinical results of the bioartificial kidney containing human cells in ICU patients with acute renal failure. Kidney Int 2004;66:1578–1588.

174. Williams W, Tumlin J, Murray P, et al: Renal bioreplacement therapy (RBT) reduces mortality in ICU patients with acute renal failure (ARF). In Renal Week 2006, San Diego, 2006.

Further Reading

Clarkson M, Friedewald J, Eustace J, et al: Acute renal failure/acute kidney injury. In Brenner BM (ed): Brenner and Rector's The Kidney, 8th ed. Philadelphia: WB Saunders, 2007, pp 943–986.

Dear JW, Yasuda H, Hu X, et al: Sepsis-induced organ failure is mediated by different pathways in the kidney and liver: Acute renal failure is dependent on MyD88 but not renal cell apoptosis. Kidney Int 2006;69:832–836.

Hentschel DM, Bonventre JV: Novel non-rodent models of kidney disease. Curr Mol Med 2005;5:537–546.

Lai LW, Yong KC, Igarashi S, et al: A sphingosine-1-phosphate type 1 receptor agonist inhibits the early T-cell transient following renal ischemia-reperfusion injury. Kidney Int 2007;71:1223–1231.

Singbartl K, Bockhorn SG, Zarbock A, et al: T cells modulate neutrophil-dependent acute renal failure during endotoxemia: Critical role for CD28. J Am Soc Nephrol 2005;16:720–728.

PART II

Diseases of Glomeruli, Microvasculature, and Tubulointerstitium

CONTENTS

Chapter 10

Immunosuppressive Agents for the Therapy of Glomerular and Tubulointerstitial Disease

Alice Sue Appel and Gerald B. Appel

CHAPTER CONTENTS

Many glomerular and a number of tubulointerstitial diseases are the result of immunologic processes that damage the kidney. A variety of immunosuppressive agents have been used in the treatment of these diseases and many more are currently undergoing study. Only a few of these agents have been studied in controlled, randomized trials in any parenchymal renal disease and virtually none of them are approved by the U.S. Food and Drug Administration for the treatment of glomerular diseases. Many medications have been adopted after proving effective as immunosuppressives in transplantation. Others have been studied in rheumatologic and other immunologic disorders. Most have been used in combinations with other drugs blocking the immune system, thus making the specific role of any one agent less clear. Since many are broad-spectrum blockers of the immune response, attributing efficacy in reducing proteinuria or prolonging renal survival to one specific blocking action in the immune cascade is often impossible. In this chapter, we present a brief overview of the mechanism of the immune responses and then discuss the current and potential future medications used for immunosuppressive therapy for glomerular and tubulointerstitial diseases.

OVERVIEW OF THE IMMUNE RESPONSE AND IMMUNOSUPPRESSIVES

Self-tolerance refers to a lack of immune responsiveness to the tissues of one's own body. Two main mechanisms explaining self-tolerance deal with central tolerance and peripheral tolerance.[1] Central tolerance is the process of the deletion of self-reactive lymphocytes (B and T cells) during their maturation process in bone marrow for the former and thymus for the latter. Peripheral tolerance is the process of backup tolerance in peripheral tissues to self-reactive T cells that have escaped deletion in the thymus.

Autoimmune disease is believed to result from the bypass of at least one of the mechanisms of self-tolerance, and the mechanism differs from disease to disease. Often there is an interaction among immunologic, genetic, and even microbial factors. Classically, the immune system has been divided into two classes: humoral, mediated by soluble antibody proteins, and cellular, mediated by lymphocytes. Immune complex–mediated glomerulonephritis is a classic humoral response, whereas alterations in T-cell function may underlie the pathogenetic defects in minimal change disease. However, in some glomerular diseases such as antineutrophilic cytoplasmic antibody (ANCA)–positive glomerulonephritis, there is evidence of involvement of both humoral and cell-mediated limbs of the immune system. This chapter deals with current and possibly future immunosuppressive treatments for glomerular disease in terms of their mechanisms, efficacy, and toxicities. Although much is known about the mechanisms of actions of many immunosuppressive drugs, it is clear that most have multiple effects in blockade of the immune response. Even monoclonal antibodies may have pleiotropic effects. Thus, understanding synergistic immunomodulation requires adequate study in animal models and in humans with glomerular disease.

Moreover, there is no immunosuppressive agent that does not have the potential to produce serious side effects. Some adverse reactions are relatively specific to a given drug such as hair growth and gum hyperplasia with cyclosporine or alopecia and hemorrhagic cystitis with cyclophosphamide. However, it is important to note that along with use of virtually all immunosuppressive agents there exists the potential for a marked increase in both infection and neoplasia. These factors must always be taken into account when one is treating with immunosuppressive agents. In treating any individual patient, the risks versus benefits of the immunosuppressives must be weighed.

IMMUNOSUPPRESSIVE AGENTS

Glucocorticoids

Glucocorticoids (e.g., prednisone, methylprednisolone) have been used for many decades as both immunosuppressive and anti-inflammatory agents. They suppress both cell-mediated immunity, by inhibiting genes that code for important cytokines including interleukins 1 through 6 and 8 and interferon-γ, and humoral immunity, by diminishing B-cell clonal expansion and antibody synthesis. At high doses, they also directly kill T and B cells, which could account for the powerful immunosuppressive effects of pulse steroids.

As long ago as the 1950s, they were used for the treatment of idiopathic nephrotic syndrome and lupus nephritis. Currently, they are commonly used in numerous glomerular diseases including minimal change disease, focal glomerulosclerosis, membranous nephropathy, lupus nephritis, and rapidly progressive glomerulonephritides, as well as in acute interstitial nephritis. They may be used alone or in conjunction with other immunosuppressants.[2]

Unfortunately, these agents are associated with many potential adverse effects, and close monitoring for side effects is crucial. Toxicities include an increased susceptibility to infection, impaired glucose metabolism, sodium retention and hypertension, accelerated bone loss with accompanying osteoporosis (which may be diminished by the use of calcium, vitamin D supplements, and bisphosphonates),[3] cataracts, and cushingoid appearance and other cosmetic effects. The latter complication must be strongly considered when treating young people and others who are especially concerned about their appearance since these patients often discontinue the use of these drugs rather than tolerate the social consequences of cosmetic changes.

Azathioprine

Azathioprine has been used in humans as an immunosuppressant since the early 1960s. It is actually a prodrug, which is converted in the body to its active metabolite 6-mercaptopurine, which acts by inhibiting the formation of phosphoribosyl pyrophosphate, an intermediate in purine formation.

Azathioprine has been used to treat many immunologic glomerular diseases including lupus, IgA nephropathy, and vasculitis. It is the focus of many ongoing studies dealing with maintenance of remission in severe proliferative glomerulonephritides such as lupus nephritis and ANCA-positive disease.[4]

Acute myelosuppression with resulting leukopenia, megaloblastic anemia, and thrombocytopenia can be caused by azathioprine therapy due to the incorporation of azathioprine-derived 6-thioguanine nucleotides into DNA.[5] The metabolite of azathioprine, 6-mercaptopurine, is deactivated by the enzyme thiopurine S-methyltransferase, and those with a genetic polymorphism for thiopurine S-methyltransferase are particularly susceptible to such toxicity.[5] This genetic abnormality occurs in approximately 1 per 220 individuals, and screening for it before starting azathioprine therapy has been recommended, although rarely practiced clinically.[6] Other side effects include nausea, vomiting, diarrhea, and hepatotoxicity, although liver function tests usually return to normal after discontinuation of the drug. Another concern is the interaction between azathioprine and allopurinol,[7] which results in potentiating the bone marrow suppression caused by the azathioprine. This results because allopurinol impairs the metabolism of the azathioprine. Both drugs should not be used together unless absolutely necessary and then only with very great caution. Although it was previously believed that there was no significant teratogenicity attributable to azathioprine,[8] leukopenia and/or thrombocytopenia have been reported in neonates whose mothers had taken azathioprine throughout pregnancy.[9]

ALKYLATING AGENTS

Cyclophosphamide

Drugs of the nitrogen mustard alkylating agent class of which cyclophosphamide is the most commonly used have been known to be immunosuppressants since the 1950s.[10] Cyclophosphamide is actually a prodrug, converted in the liver by mixed-function oxidase enzymes to the active metabolites 4-hydroxy-cyclophosphamide and phosphoramide mustard. The result is the binding of these agents to and the cross-linking of DNA, thus inhibiting cell proliferation and function. This frequently results in dose-dependent neutropenia and lymphopenia with reductions of both B cells and $CD4^+$ and $CD8^+$ T cells.[11]

Cyclophosphamide has been used to treat autoimmune glomerular diseases, both as intravenous pulses and in an oral form. For many years, it was the first-line therapy for severe lupus nephritis, and it remains the drug of choice for most patients with severe crescentic rapidly progressive glomerulonephritis whether related to ANCA-positive disease or antiglomerular basement membrane disease.[4,12–14] Cyclophosphamide has also been used to treat steroid-resistant minimal change disease and focal glomerulosclerosis, IgA nephropathy, and membranous nephropathy.[15,16] Because of its toxicity (see "Mycophenolate Mofetil"), newer immunosuppressants with fewer adverse side effects, such as mycophenolate mofetil, are now becoming the alternate treatments.

The adverse effects of cyclophosphamide can be severe. There is significant dose-dependent bone marrow depression with granulocytes, lymphocytes, erythrocytes, and platelets all affected. The effect on leukocytes is most pronounced, and the aim should be to keep the total white blood cell count greater than $3000/mm^3$. Infections are especially common in those who are neutropenic, but major bacterial and fungal infections can also occur without neutropenia, especially in the presence of concomitant treatment with glucocorticoids.

Another important adverse effect of oral cyclophosphamide, although rare with intravenous dosing, is hemorrhagic cystitis with the increased risk of developing bladder cancer.[17] A small percentage of the cyclophosphamide metabolite aldophosphamide is converted to acrolein, which is toxic to bladder epithelium. Aggressive hydration should be encouraged to prevent this complication. Infertility in both males and females may also occur with the use of cyclophosphamide. Clearly, the patient's age and desire to have children must be taken into consideration before using this agent. If cyclophosphamide remains the drug of choice, a suggestion would be to have the patient's ova or sperm banked before initiation of therapy. Also, pregnant women should not be given cyclophosphamide unless absolutely necessary because of teratogenicity. Other common adverse effects include nausea, hair loss, mouth sores, and hyponatremia due to increased secretion of antidiuretic hormone.

Because of the major toxicities of the alkylating agents, a strategy that should be strongly considered is induction therapy with cyclophosphamide and then maintenance therapy with a less toxic drug such as mycophenolate mofetil and azathioprine. Studies are now under way to determine the effectiveness of this strategy.[4,18]

Chlorambucil

Like cyclophosphamide, chlorambucil is a nitrogen mustard alkylating agent. It has been used to treat steroid-resistant minimal change disease and focal glomerulosclerosis, as part of an alternating monthly regimen with corticosteroids to treat membranous nephropathy, and for several other immune renal diseases.[19] Its mechanism of action is primarily binding to and cross-linking of DNA, resulting in apoptosis or defective cellular function with reductions in both B and T cells (CD4$^+$ and CD8$^+$).

The major adverse side effect of chlorambucil is bone marrow suppression, causing anemia, neutropenia, and thrombocytopenia. Other toxicities include gastrointestinal disturbances, central nervous system side effects including seizures and tremors, hepatotoxicity, and infertility. In some studies, it was found to have greater toxicity than cyclophosphamide and hence it is used infrequently in clinical nephrology at this time.[20] Chlorambucil should never be used during pregnancy due to its strong teratogenic potential.

CALCINEURIN INHIBITORS

This class of immunosuppressive drugs includes cyclosporine and tacrolimus (previously known as FK506). The immunosuppressive activity of cyclosporine was first noted in 1972, and tacrolimus was discovered in 1984.[21]

Originally used to prevent transplant rejection, the use of both drugs as immunosuppressive agents has widely expanded. Both cyclosporine and tacrolimus have been used to treat minimal change disease, focal glomerulosclerosis, membranous nephropathy, and as an adjunct to treatment of many proliferative glomerulonephritides.[22,23]

Cyclosporine is a cyclic polypeptide consisting of 11 amino acids and tacrolimus is a macrolide lactone. Both exhibit similar immunosuppressant mechanisms in their effects on both humoral and cell-mediated responses. They act chiefly by inhibiting calcineurin. Cyclosporine first binds to the cytoplasmic protein cyclophilin; the cyclosporine-cyclophilin complex then binds to and competitively inhibits the calcium-sensitive phosphatase calcineurin,[24–26] an enzyme that normally dephosphorylates the nuclear factor of activated T cells. T cells are especially sensitive to calcineurin inhibition because of their low calcineurin content. Tacrolimus binds to FK binding protein, an immunophilin, and forms a new complex (FK binding protein-12–FK506) that interacts with and inhibits calcineurin.[24,25] The result of both agents is the inhibition of a number of transcription factors, leading to decreased production of various cytokines, especially interleukin-2. In addition, both cyclosporine and tacrolimus inhibit the activation of the T-cell transcription factors AP-1 and NK-κB.[26] Fortunately, unlike many other immunosuppressive drugs, neither cyclosporine nor tacrolimus is myelosuppressive.[26]

Both cyclosporine and tacrolimus exhibit similar adverse side effects. First, both drugs are nephrotoxic and may cause acute renal insufficiency (usually reversible after lowering or discontinuing the medication) or chronic renal insufficiency (often irreversible).[27,28] The acute manifestations may result from both renal vasoconstriction (affecting both afferent and efferent glomerular arterioles) and tubular toxicity. Rarely, hemolytic uremic syndrome may also occur. Hypertension is also a common side effect of both drugs, usually appearing within weeks of beginning treatment. Reduction in the dose often ameliorates the hypertension, but antihypertensive therapy is often required.

Neurological toxicity, particularly with tremor, is also not uncommon, especially with tacrolimus at high doses.[29–31] Gastrointestinal side effects, including loss of appetite, nausea and vomiting, and diarrhea, occur and are also more frequently noted with tacrolimus.[32] On the other hand, both gingival hyperplasia and hirsutism occur with cyclosporine but not with tacrolimus.[33] Tacrolimus may cause alopecia.[34,35] Both the cosmetic effects of hirsutism and alopecia should be taken into account when treating patients who are highly concerned with their appearance. Both tacrolimus and cyclosporine are associated with an increased risk of developing diabetes. Although the data are somewhat conflicting, in general, this is more common with tacrolimus than cyclosporine.[36–38] Hyperkalemia and hypomagnesemia are associated with the use of both medications due to renal tubular malfunction. Hyperuricemia with resulting gout also may occur with both drugs.

Cyclosporine and tacrolimus are both metabolized by the cytochrome P-450 3A enzymes in the liver. Therefore, one must be aware that other drugs metabolized by the same system, including diltiazem, verapamil, ketoconazole, allopurinol, erythromycin, and numerous others, can result in an elevation of cyclosporine and tacrolimus blood levels. Patients should also be informed that they should not drink grapefruit juice while they are taking cyclosporine or tacrolimus for the same reason.[39,40] Conversely, certain medications, such as rifampin and phenobarbital, may reduce the level of cyclosporine or tacrolimus by induction of cytochrome P-450. Certain statins (simvastatin, lovastatin, and atorvastatin) are metabolized by the cytochrome P-450 3A4 system. Concomitant use of these lipid-lowering agents with cyclosporine may increase their plasma concentrations and increases the risk of myopathy with possible accompanying rhabdomyolysis.[41] (Note that rosuvastatin and pravastatin are excreted mainly unchanged so that cytochrome P-450 3A inhibitors do not significantly increase their plasma concentrations.[41]) However, because of the major cardioprotective effects of the statins, many believe that the benefits of statin therapy for patients on cyclosporine far outweigh the risk of rhabdomyolysis as long as the patients are carefully monitored.[42–44]

To avoid nephrotoxicity and other side effects, serial levels of cyclosporine and tacrolimus should be obtained. Trough levels are commonly measured just before the next dose of the drug.

SIROLIMUS

Sirolimus (rapamycin) is produced from the bacteria *Streptomyces hygroscopicus*. It was first discovered in a soil sample from Easter Island (or Rapa Nui Island, hence the name rapamycin).[45]

It is a lipophilic macrolide like tacrolimus but is not a calcineurin inhibitor. Like tacrolimus, it first binds to the immunophilin FK binding protein-12. However, the sirolimus–FK binding protein-12 complex then binds directly in mammals to cytosolic protein kinases known as mammalian targets of rapamycin or mTOR, resulting in the inhibition of the growth of hematopoietic and lymphoid cells. The mechanism by which it does this is thought to be regulation of the cell cycle through inhibition of growth factor–related signal transduction,[46,47] which results in blockade of the G1 to S phase transition. Thus, the major immunosuppressive activity of sirolimus is to inhibit proliferation of T cells. Therefore, sirolimus acts at a later stage in the immune response than the calcineurin inhibitors and may act synergistically with the latter.

Initial enthusiasm for the use of sirolimus in the treatment of glomerular diseases has been tempered by reports of acute renal failure in such patients as well as the potential induction of focal glomerulosclerosis in patients with renal allografts.[48–50] Nevertheless, there are reports of successful use of this agent in steroid-resistant focal glomerulosclerosis.[51]

Unlike cyclosporine and tacrolimus, sirolimus does not appear to be nephrotoxic. The drug, however, is certainly not benign in terms of other side effects. These include hyperlipidemia and especially hypertriglyceridemia, nausea and diarrhea, elevated liver function tests, and myelosuppression. Sirolimus may also impair wound healing so that some prefer to avoid its use in the immediate postoperative period.

MYCOPHENOLATE MOFETIL

Mycophenolate mofetil (MMF), derived from the fungus *Penicillium stoloniferum*, is metabolized to its active form mycophenolic acid in the liver. Its mechanism of action is to inhibit the enzyme inosine monophosphate dehydrogenase, crucial for the de novo synthesis of guanosine nucleotides.[52,53] Since lymphocytes do not have a salvage pathway for purine synthesis but rely entirely on de novo synthesis, MMF selectively blocks T- and B-cell proliferation. Unlike alkylating agents such as cyclophosphamide, mycophenolic acid has little impact on tissues with high proliferative activity that possess a salvage pathway for nucleotide synthesis (e.g., skin, intestine, bone marrow). This provides a more favorable tolerability and toxicity profile than many other commonly used immunosuppressants. MMF may also limit glomerular injury and prevent progressive renal scarring and fibrosis by inhibiting proliferation of mesangial cells and by decreasing lymphocyte migration into renal tissue by altering adhesion molecule function with impaired glycosylation.[52–57] Moreover mycophenolic acid seems to lessen the expression of the inducible form of nitric acid synthase in the renal cortex[58] and may slow the development of atherosclerosis.

MMF has been used as a standard component of modern immunosuppressive regimens for transplantation. It has been shown to be effective in several induction and maintenance studies of severe lupus nephritis and is currently being studied in focal glomerulosclerosis, IgA nephropathy, membranous nephropathy, and as maintenance therapy for ANCA-positive glomerulonephritides.[18,59–61] It has also proven successful in the therapy of steroid-resistant or intolerant acute interstitial nephritis.[62]

The most common adverse effect of MMF is gastrointestinal upset including nausea, abdominal cramps, and diarrhea. This can often be ameliorated by dividing the daily amount of the drug into three or four doses. Leukopenia, which is often responsive to dose reduction, may be seen. As with all other immunosuppressant medications, there is an increased risk of infectious complications.

RITUXIMAB

Rituximab was first approved in 1997 for the treatment of B-cell lymphoma. It is a chimeric (mouse-human) antibody, 60% to 65% human, that binds to the CD20 antigen, a phosphoprotein found commonly on B cells but not on stem cells or mature plasma cells. Rituximab is composed of the variable region of a murine anti-human CD20 monoclonal antibody fused to the human IgG1κ constant region. Rituximab binds to a conformational epitope on CD20 and deletes CD20$^+$ B cells, by a combination of mechanisms, including direct complement-mediated cytolysis, antibody-dependent, cell-mediated cytotoxicity via binding to the Fcγ receptor on cytotoxic cells, and deregulation of survival pathways with resulting apoptosis.[63–65] Among the B cells deleted are those responsible for the production of self-reactive antibodies.[66]

Although originally used for the treatment of B-cell lymphoma, the use of rituximab has spread as a possible treatment choice for numerous autoimmune diseases. In nephrology, it is being actively studied as an immunomodulator in lupus and lupus nephritis, Wegener's granulomatosis, and other ANCA-positive rapidly progressive glomerulonephritides.[67] It has also been used in membranous nephropathy and isolated cases of minimal change disease and focal glomerulosclerosis (see Chapters 19 and 21 for details).

As with other immunosuppressive drugs, rituximab is not without adverse side effects. Rituximab is given weekly for four consecutive doses of 375 mg/m^2 or two doses of 1000 mg given 2 weeks apart. Infusion more rapidly than over 4 hours or without concomitant methylprednisolone can result in allergic phenomena with wheezing, shortness of breath, pulmonary reactions, and hypotension. Other side effects include reactivation of hepatitis B and other viral infections. In several lupus patients, immune toxicity resulting from the loss of B cells has led to activation of JC virus and fatal progressive multifocal leukoencephalopathy.[68] The efficacy of rituximab may be abrogated by the development of antichimeric antibodies. It is still unclear how commonly such antibodies will develop in response to this chimeric, partially murine antibody. The development of fully humanized anti–B cell monoclonal antibodies is already under way.

OTHER POTENTIAL IMMUNOSUPPRESSIVE AGENTS

T lymphocytes require two signals for activation. The first signal occurs with presentation of antigen to the T-cell receptor, while the second signal is an interaction of costimulatory molecules on T lymphocytes and antigen-presenting cells. Blockade of this second costimulatory signal interrupts the immune response. A number of agents have been developed to modulate the immune system based on this mechanism.

CD40, a member of the tumor necrosis factor receptor family, is expressed on antigen-presenting cells including B cells and macrophages.[69] The ligand of CD40 is CD154 (CD40 ligand), which is expressed on activated CD4[+] T cells and some CD8[+] T cells. Although a murine anti-CD154 analogue was successful in murine lupus, results with two different humanized anti-CD40 monoclonal antibodies (BG9588 and IDEC-131) have not been successful in human lupus nephritis.[70,71] BG9588 (riplizumab) was associated with unacceptable thromboembolic phenomena, and IDEC-131 was ineffective in reaching stated endpoints of therapy.

Another costimulatory pathway involves CD28 and CD80/86. CD28 is present on T cells and binds to CD80 (B7-1) and CD86 (B7-2) on antigen-presenting cells. CTLA-4 competes with CD28 for the same B7 ligands and antagonizes CD28-dependent costimulation.[69] CTLA4-Ig is a recombinant fusion molecule that combines the extracellular domain of human CTLA4 with the constant region (Fc) of the human IgG1 heavy chain. Two preparations of CTLA4Ig have been used clinically to modulate costimulation.[72] Abatacept binds CD80 more avidly than CD86 while belatacept (LEA29Y) binds even more avidly to both CD80 and CD86 and provides more potent inhibition of T-cell activation. Both agents have been studied in transplantation, and trials are ongoing in lupus nephritis. Similar costimulatory blockade could prove useful in a number of other immune-mediated glomerulonephritides.

Mizoribine

Mizoribine, an immunosuppressant agent not approved yet in the United States, has been used in Japan for the treatment of lupus nephritis and glomerulonephritis. Its active form, mizoribine-5-P, selectively inhibits inosine monophosphate synthetase and guanosine monophosphate synthetase, resulting in blocking synthesis of guanine nucleotides. There is inhibition of T-cell activation and proliferation associated with a decease in intracellular guanosine triphosphate.[73] In Japan, mizoribine, in addition to preventing transplant rejection, has been used in the treatment of rheumatoid arthritis, steroid-resistant nephrotic syndrome, and systemic lupus nephritis.[74–76]

The safety profile of mizoribine has been reported to be as safe or safer than that of other immunosuppressant agents. Adverse effects have been reportedly less severe with mizoribine than with other such drugs, especially azathioprine.[73] There is one report of rhabdomyolysis in a patient also treated with a fibrate, and there is warning against the use of both drugs together.[77] Also, at the highest doses, mizoribine has been reported to increase uric acid levels.[78]

INTRAVENOUS IMMUNOGLOBULIN

Intravenous immunoglobulin (IVIG) has been used to treat lupus nephritis, Henoch-Schönlein purpura, and a number of other glomerulonephritides.[79–81] Almost all studies have been small in size, and most have been uncontrolled and combined with other therapies. IVIG has a variety of immune-modulating actions including acceleration of IgG catabolism. Thus, the role of IVIG remains unclear in any glomerular disease. Since these agents possess a number of potential adverse side effects including acute renal failure,

especially seen with sucrose-based IVIG, they should be used cautiously until their precise role has been clarified.

OTHER MODULATORS OF THE IMMUNE RESPONSE

Another area of potential interest is in designer molecules that modulate a specific element of the immune response. For example, LPJ 394, a complex of four oligonucleotides, was designed to induce B-cell anergy by binding surface immunoglobulin without T-cell help.[82] Despite effectively reducing anti–double-stranded DNA antibody levels in murine and human lupus, this agent has not yet been established as clinically effective in humans. Antagonists of tumor necrosis factor α are clinically available for the treatment of rheumatoid arthritis. They have been associated with severe infections including activation of tuberculosis in some patients and the induction of systemic lupus in some rheumatoid patients. They have not proven effective in maintaining remissions in ANCA-positive vasculitis.[83] As the effector limb of the immune system becomes better studied, there will clearly be a variety of new targets for the prevention of glomerular damage. Potential therapeutic targets include cytokines (i.e., interleukin-6, interleukin-10,[84] IL-18) B-lymphocyte stimulator,[85–87] interferons (i.e., type I)[88–90], Toll-like receptor (TLR9 blockade),[91,92] adhesion molecules, and complement components. Agents to modulate these factors will probably be combined with conventional therapy to induce remission in glomerular diseases as well as to maintain patients in remission. A major challenge will be understanding the interactions between newer immunomodulator drugs and currently used immunosuppressives.

References

1. Kumar V, Cotran RS, Robbins SL (eds): Robbins Basic Pathology, 7 ed. Philadelphia: Elsevier, 2003, pp 126–132.
2. Austin HA III, Klippel JH, Balow JE, et al: Therapy of lupus nephritis. Controlled trial of prednisone and cytotoxic drugs. N Engl J Med 1986;314:614–619.
3. Curtis JR, Saag KG: Prevention and treatment of glucocorticoid osteoporosis. Curr Osteoporos Rep 2007;5:14–21.
4. Hossiau FA, Vasconcelos C, D'Cruz D, et al: Immunosuppressive therapy in lupus nephritis: The Euro-Lupus Nephritis Trial, a randomized trial of low-dose versus high-dose intravenous cyclophosphamide. Arthritis Rheum 2002;46:2121–2131.
5. Lennard I, Van Loon JA, Weinshilboum RM: Pharmacogenetics of acute azathioprine toxicity: Relationship to thiopurine methyltransferase genetic polymorphism. Clin Pharmacol Ther 1989;46:149–154.
6. Holme SA, Duley JA, Sanderson J, et al: Erythrolytic thiopurine methyltransferase assessment prior to azathioprine use in the UK. Q J Med 2002;95:439–444.
7. Stamp L, Searle M, O'Donnell J, Chapman P: Gout in solid organ transplantation: A challenging clinical problem. Drugs 2005;65:2593–2611.
8. Lu CY, Sicher SC, Vasquez MA: Prevention and treatment of renal allograft rejection: New therapeutic approaches and new insights into established therapies. J Am Soc Nephrol 1993;4:1239–1256.
9. GlaxoSmithKline, Inc.: Monograph "Imuran," 2005.
10. Brock N: The history of the oxazaphosphorine cytostatics. Cancer 1996;78:542–547.

11. Varkila K, Hurme M: The effect of cyclophosphamide on cytotoxic T-lymphocyte responses. Immunology 1983;48:433–438.

12. Illei GG, Austin HA, Crane M, et al: Combination therapy with pulse cyclophosphamide plus pulse methylprednisolone improves long-term renal outcome without adding toxicity in patients with lupus nephritis. Ann Intern Med 2001;135:248–257.

13. Jayne D, Rasmussen N, Andrassy K, et al: A randomized trial of maintenance therapy for vasculitis associated with ANCA. N Engl J Med 2003;349:36–44.

14. Pusey CD: Anti-glomerular basement membrane disease. Kidney Int 2003;64:1535–1550.

15. Ballardie FW, Roberts IS: Controlled prospective trial of prednisolone and cytotoxics in progressive IgA nephropathy. J Am Soc Nephrol 2002;13:142–148.

16. Appel GB: Glomerular diseases and the nephrotic syndrome. In Goldman L, Ausiello D (eds): Cecil Textbook of Medicine, 23rd ed. Philadelphia, Elsevier, 2008, pp 866–877.

17. Talar-Williams C, Hijazi YM, Walther MM, et al: Cyclophosphamide-induced cystitis and bladder cancer in patients with Wegener's granulomatosis. Ann Intern Med 1996;124:477–484.

18. Contreras G, Pardo V, Leclercq B, et al: Sequential therapies for proliferative lupus nephritis. N Engl J Med 2004;350:971–980.

19. Ponticelli C, Zucchelli P, Passerini P, et al: A 10-year follow-up of a randomized study with methylprednisolone and chlorambucil in membranous nephropathy. Kidney Int 1995;48:1600–1604.

20. Ponticelli C, Altieri P, Scolari F, et al: A randomized study comparing methylprednisolone plus chlorambucil versus methylprednisolone plus cyclophosphamide in idiopathic membranous nephropathy. J Am Soc Nephrol 1998;9:444–450.

21. Borel JF: History of the discovery of cyclosporine and of its early pharmacological development. Wien Klin Wochenschr 2002;114:433–437.

22. Cattran DC, Appel GB, Hebert L, et al: A multicenter trial of cyclosporine in patients with steroid resistant focal and segmental glomerulosclerosis. Kidney Int 1999;56:2220–2226.

23. Cattran DC, Appel GB, Hebert LA, et al, for the North American Nephrotic Syndrome Study Group: Cyclosporine in steroid resistant membranous nephropathy: A randomized trial. Kidney Int 2001;59:1484–1490.

24. Weiderrecht G, Lam E, Hung S, et al: The mechanism of action of FK506 and cyclosporine A. Ann N Y Acad Sci 1993;696:9–19.

25. Clipstone NA, Crabtree GR: Calcineurin is a key signaling enzyme in T lymphocyte activation and the target of the immunosuppressive drugs cyclosporine A and FK506. Ann N Y Acad Sci 1993;696:20–30.

26. Matsuda S, Koyasu S: Mechanisms of action of cyclosporine. Immunopharmacology 2000;47:119–125.

27. Remuzzi G, Piereco N: Cyclosporine-induced renal dysfunction in experimental animals and humans. Kidney Int 1995;52:S70–S74.

28. Porayko MK, Textor SC, Krom RA: Nephrotoxicity of FK506 and cyclosporine when used as primary immunosuppression in liver transplant recipients. Transplant Proc 1993;25:665–668.

29. Schwartz RB, Bravo SM, First MR, et al: Cyclosporine neurotoxicity and its relationship to hypertensive encephalopathy: CT and MR findings in 16 cases. AJR Am J Roentgenol 1995;165:627–631.

30. Eidelman BH, Abu-Elmagd K, Wilson J, et al: Neurologic complications of FK506. Transplant Proc 1991;23:3175–3178.

31. Wijdicks EF, Wiesner RH, Krom RA: Neurotoxicity in liver transplant recipients with cyclosporine immunosuppression. Neurology 1995;45:1962–1964.

32. Mor E, Sheiner PA, Schwartz ME, et al: Reversal of severe FK506 side effects by conversion to cyclosporine-based immunosuppression. Transplantation 1994;58:380–383.

33. Thorp M, DeMattos A, Bennet W, et al: The effect of conversion from cyclosporine to tacrolimus on gingival hyperplasia, hirsutism, and cholesterol. Transplantation 2000;69:1218–1220.

34. Tricot L, Lebbe C, Pillebout E, et al: Tacrolimus-induced alopecia in female kidney-pancreas transplant recipients. Transplantation 2000;80:1546–1549.

35. Shapiro J, Jordan ML, Scantlebury VP, et al: Alopecia as a consequence of tacrolimus therapy. Transplantation 1998;65:1284.

36. First MR, Gerber DA, Hariharan S, et al: Posttransplant diabetes mellitus in kidney allograft recipients: Incidence, risk factors, and management. Transplantation 2002;73:379–386.

37. Johnson C, Ahsan N, Gonwa T, et al: Randomized trial of tacrolimus (Prograf) in combination with azathioprine or mycophenolate mofetil versus cyclosporine (Neoral) with mycophenolate mofetil after cadaveric kidney transplantation. Transplantation 2000;69:534–841.

38. Neylan JF, for the FK506 Kidney Transplant Study Group: Racial differences in renal transplantation after immunosuppression with tacrolimus versus cyclosporine. Transplantation 1998;65:515–523.

39. Fujita K: Food-drug interactions via human cytochrome P450 3. Drug Metab Drug Interact 2004;20:195–217.

40. Dahan A, Altman H: Food-drug interaction: Grapefruit juice augments drug bioavailability—mechanism, extent and relevance. Eur J Clin Nutr 2004;58:1–9.

41. Neuvonen PJ, Niemi M, Backman JT: Drug interactions with lipid-lowering drugs; mechanisms and clinical relevance. Clin Pharmacol Ther 2006;80:565–581.

42. Vanhaecke J, Van Cleemput J, Van Lierde J, et al: Safety and efficacy of low dose simvastatin in cardiac transplant recipients treated with cyclosporine. Transplantation 1994;15:582–585.

43. Arnadottir M, Eriksson LO, Germershausen JI, Thysell H: Low-dose simvastatin is a well-tolerated and efficacious cholesterol-lowering agent in cyclosporin-treated kidney transplant recipients: Double-blind, randomized, placebo-controlled study in 40 patients. Nephron 1994;68:57–62.

44. Panici V, Manca-Rizza G, Paoletti S, et al: Safety and effects on the lipid and C-reactive protein plasma concentration of the association of ezetimib plus atorvastatin in renal transplant patients treated by cyclosporine-A: A pilot study. Biomed Pharmacother 2006;60:549–552.

45. Pritchard DI: Sourcing a chemical succession for cyclosporine from parasites and human pathogens. Drug Discovery Today 2005;19:688–691.

46. Chung J, Kao CJ, Crabtree GR, et al: Rapamycin-FKBP specifically blocks growth-dependent activation of and signaling by the 70 kd S6 protein kinases. Cell 1992;69:1227–1236.

47. Morice WG, Brunn GJ, Wiederrecht G, et al: Rapamycin-induced inhibition of p34cdc2 kinase activation is associated with G1/S-phase growth arrest in t lymphocytes. J Biol Chem 1993;268:3734–3738.

48. Cho ME, Hurle JK, Kopp JB: Sirolimus therapy of focal segmental glomerulosclerosis is associated with nephrotoxicity. Am J Kidney Dis 2007;49:210–217.

49. Fervenza FC, Fitzpatrick PM, Mertz J, et al: Acute rapamycin nephrotoxicity in native kidneys of patients with chronic glomerulopathies. Nephrol Dial Transplant 2004;19:1288–1292.

50. Izzedine H, Brochieriou I, Frances C: Post-transplantation proteinuria and sirolimus. N Engl J Med 2005;353:288–289.

51. Tumlin JA, Miller D, Near M, et al: A prospective, open-label trial of sirolimus in the treatment of focal segmental glomerulosclerosis. Clin J Am Soc Nephrol 2006;1:109–116.

52. Allison AC, Eugui EM: Mycophenolate mofetil and its mechanisms of action. Immunopharmacology 2000;47:85–116.

53. Appel GB, Radhakrishnan J, Ginzler E: Use of mycophenolate mofetil in autoimmune and renal diseases. Transplantation 2005;80(2 Suppl):S265–S271.

54. Hauser IA, Renders L, Radeke HH, et al: Mycophenolate mofetil inhibits rat and human mesangial proliferation by guanosine depletion. Nephrol Dial Transplant 1999;14:58–63.

55. Badid C, Vincent M, McGregor B, et al: Mycophenolate mofetil reduces myofibroblast infiltration and collagen III deposition in rat remnant kidney. Kidney Int 1999;58:51–61.

56. Allison AC, Eugui EM: Immunosuppressive and other effects of mycophenolic acid and an ester prodrug mycophenolate mofetil. Immunol Rev 1993;136:5–28.

57. Blaheta RA, Lechel K, Wittig B, et al. Mycophenolate mofetil impairs transendothelial migration of allogenic CD4 and CD8 T-cells. Transplant Proc 1999;31:1250–1252.

58. Lui SL, Tsang R, Wong D, et al: Effect of mycophenolate mofetil on severity of nephritis and nitric acid production in lupus-prone MPR/lpr mice. Lupus 2002;11:411–418.

59. Ginzler EM, Dooley MA, Aranow C, et al: Mycophenolate mofetil or intravenous cyclophosphamide for lupus nephritis. N Engl J Med 2005;353:2219–2228.

60. Cattran DC, Wang MM, Appel GB, et al: Mycophenolate mofetil in the treatment of focal segmental glomerulosclerosis. Clin Nephrol 2004;62:605–611.

61. Branten AJ, du Buf-Vereijken PW, Vervloet M, Wetzels JF: Mycophenolate mofetil in idiopathic membranous nephropathy: A clinical trial with comparison to a historic control group treated with cyclophosphamide. Am J Kidney Dis 2007;50: 248–256.

62. Preddie D, Nickolas T, Radhakrishnan J, et al: Use of MMF in refractory acute interstitial nephritis. Clin J Am Soc Nephrol 2006;1:718–721.

63. Binder M, Otto F, Mertelsmann R, et al: The epitope recognized by rituximab. Blood 2006;108:1975–1978.

64. Maloney DG: Mechanism of action of rituximab. Anticancer Drugs 2001;12(Suppl 2):S1–S4.

65. Liu Y, Zheng M, Lai Z, et al: Inhibition of human B-cell lymphoma by an anti-CD20 antibody and its chimeric F(ab')2fragment via induction of apoptosis. Cancer Lett 2004;205:243–253.

66. Anolik JH, Barnard J, Cappione A, et al: Rituximab improves peripheral B cell abnormalities in human systemic lupus erythematosus. Arthritis Rheum 2004;50:3580–3590.

67. Appel GB, Looney J, Eisenberg RA, et al: Protocol for the lupus nephritis assessment with rituximab (LUNAR) study. ASN Abstract, 2006.

68. FDA Alert: Progressive multifocal leukoencephalopathy, December 2006. Available at: www.fda.gov/cder/drug/InfoSheets/HCP/rituximab.pdf.

69. Appel GB, Waldman M: Update on the treatment of lupus nephritis. Kidney Int 2006;70:1403–1412.

70. Biancone L, Deambrosis I, Camussi G: Lymphocyte costimulatory receptors in renal disease and transplantation. J Nephrol 2002;15:7–16.

71. Kalunian KC, Davis JC Jr, Merrill JT, et al: Treatment of systemic lupus erythematosus by inhibition of T cell costimulation with anti-CD154: A randomized, double-blind, placebo-controlled trial. Arthritis Rheum 2002;46:3251–3258.

72. Davis JC Jr, Totoritis MC, Rosenberg J, et al: Phase I clinical trial of a monoclonal antibody against CD40-ligand (IDEC-131) in patients with systemic lupus erythematosus. J Rheumatol 2001;28:95–101.

73. Yokota S: Mizoribine: Mode of action and effects in clinical use. Pediatr Int 2002;44:196–198.

74. Yumura W, Suganuma S, Uchida K, et al: Effects of long-term treatment with mizoribine in patients with proliferative lupus nephritis. Clin Nephrol 2005;64:28–34.

75. Kuroda T, Hirose S, Tanabe et al: Mizoribine therapy for patients with lupus nephritis: The association between peak mizoribine concentration and clinical efficacy. Mod Rheumatol 2007;17:206–212.

76. Hirayama K, Kobayashi AM, Hashimoto Y, et al: Treatment with the purine synthesis inhibitor mizoribine for ANCA-associated renal vasculitis. Am J Kidney Dis 2004;44:57–63.

77. Morimoto S, Fujoka Y, Tsusumi C, et al: Mizoribine-induced rhabdomyolysis in a rheumatoid arthritis patient receiving benzafibrate treatment. Am J Med 2005;329:211–213.

78. Stypinski D, Obaidi M, Combs M, et al: Safety, tolerability and pharmacokinetics of higher dose mizoribine in healthy male volunteers. Br J Clin Pharmacol 2007;63:459–468.

79. Yu Z, Lennon VA: Mechanism of intravenous immunoglobulin therapy in antibody-mediated autoimmune disease. N Engl J Med 1999;340:227–228.

80. Toubi E, Kessel A, Shoenfeld Y: High dose intravenous immunoglobulin: An option in the treatment of SLE. Hum Immunol 2005:66:395–402.

81. Orbach H, Tishler M, Shoenfeld Y: Intravenous immunoglobulin and the kidney—a two-edged sword. Semin Arthritis Rheum 2004;34:593–601.

82. Abetimus: Abetimus sodium, LJP 394. BioDrugs 2003;17:212–215.

83. Huugen D, Tervaert JWC, Heeringa P: TNF-alpha bioactivity-inhibiting therapy in ANCA-associated vasculitis: Clinical and experimental considerations. Clin J Am Soc Nephrol 2006; 1:1100–1107.

84. Llorente L, Richaud-Patin Y, Garcia-Padilla C, et al: Clinical and biologic effects of anti-interleukin-10 monoclonal antibody administration in systemic lupus erythematosus. Arthritis Rheum 2000;43:1790–1800.

85. Stohl W, Metyas S, Tan SM, et al: B lymphocyte stimulator overexpression in patients with systemic lupus erythematosus: Longitudinal observations. Arthritis Rheum 2003;48:3475–3486.

86. Stohl W: Targeting B lymphocyte stimulator in systemic lupus erythematosus and other autoimmune rheumatic disorders. Expert Opin Ther Targets 2004;8:177–189.

87. Zhang J, Roschke V, Baker KP, et al: Cutting edge: A role for B lymphocyte stimulator in systemic lupus erythematosus. J Immunol 2001;166:6–10.

88. Crow MK: Interferon-alpha: A new target for therapy in systemic lupus erythematosus? Arthritis Rheum 2003;48:2396–2401.

89. Baechler EC, Gregersen PK, Behrens TW: The emerging role of interferon in human systemic lupus erythematosus. Curr Opin Immunol 2004;16:801–807.

90. Schwarting A, Paul K, Tschirner S, et al: Interferon-beta: A therapeutic for autoimmune lupus in MRL-Faslpr mice. J Am Soc Nephrol 2005;16:3264–3272.

91. Leadbetter EA, Rifkin IR, Hohlbaum AM, et al: Chromatin-IgG complexes activate B cells by dual engagement of IgM and Toll-like receptors. Nature 2002;416:603–607.

92. Anders HJ, Vielhauer V, Eis V, et al: Activation of Toll-like receptor-9 induces progression of renal disease in MRL-Fas(lpr) mice. FASEB J 2004;18:534–536.

Further Reading

Appel GB: Glomerular disease and the nephrotic syndrome. In Goldman L, Ausiello D (eds): Cecil Textbook of Medicine, 23rd ed. Philadelphia, Elsevier, 2008, pp 866–877.

Appel GB, Radhakrishnan J, Ginzler E: Use of mycophenolate mofetil in autoimmune and renal diseases. Transplantation. 2005;80(2 Suppl):S265–S271.

Appel GB, Waldman M: Update on the treatment of lupus nephritis. Kidney Int 2006;70:1403–1412.

Biancone L, Deambrosis I, Camussi G: Lymphocyte costimulatory receptors in renal disease and transplantation. J Nephrol 2002;15:7–16.

Matsuda S, Koyasu S: Mechanisms of action of cyclosporine. Immunopharmacology 2000;47:119–125.

Maloney DG: Mechanism of action of rituximab. Anticancer Drugs 2001;12(Suppl 2):S1–S4.

Markowitz G, Appel GB: Use of MMF in refractory acute interstitial nephritis. Clin J Am Soc Nephrol 2006;1:718–721.

Orbach H, Tishler M, Shoenfeld Y: Intravenous immunoglobulin and the kidney—a two-edged sword. Semin Arthritis Rheum 2004;34:593–601.

Preddie D, Nickolas T, Radhakrishnan J, et al: Use of MMF in refractory acute interstitial nephritis. Clin J Am Soc Nephrol 2006;1:718–721.

Chapter 11

Dietary Modulation of the Inflammatory Response

Raffaele De Caterina and Carmine Zoccali

INFLAMMATION AND POINTS OF ATTACK FOR ITS MODULATION

Inflammation can be classically defined as the reaction of a living vascularized tissue to localized damage,[1] and it plays a role in both normal repair reactions and the pathogenesis of disease. The inflammatory reactions are usually defined as acute or chronic based on both their temporal duration and the prevailing phenomena occurring. Acute inflammation, lasting minutes to hours, has its main features in fluid and plasma protein exudation (edema) and leukocyte (mainly neutrophil) migration.[2] Chronic inflammation lasts longer, is less stereotyped, and is associated histologically with the presence of lymphocytes and macrophages as well as with the proliferation of small blood vessels and of connective tissue.[3] Inflammatory phenomena are at the basis of a number of disease processes of either systemic or organ-specific nature, ranging from classic rheumatic diseases to bronchial airway hyperresponsiveness, inflammatory bowel disease, kidney diseases, psoriasis, and atopic eczema. Tissue phenomena occurring in inflammation include modification of blood flow and vessel diameter, changes in vascular permeability, leukocyte exudation and phagocytosis, remodeling of the extracellular matrix, and cell proliferation. Each phase of the inflammatory reaction is sustained by the local production of mediators, including vasoactive amines, plasma and tissue proteases, arachidonic acid metabolites, cytokines, chemokines and growth factors, lysosomal components, and reactive oxygen species, each of which may be a theoretical target for drugs or therapeutic interventions. It has recently been appreciated that many of these phases may be modulated by diet. Dietary modulation of the inflammatory reaction is thus now achievable as a therapeutic option in the treatment of a variety of human diseases. Selected dietary components can also be supplemented in amounts not easily achieved through the diet, thus configuring truly pharmacologic modalities based on dietary components. This chapter reviews the main options currently available for these interventions, their proposed rationale and mechanism of action, clinical results, and some current therapeutic recommendations. Most of these are currently based on manipulation of fatty acid (FA) intake, but important new notions in this area deal with the link of obesity and inflammation with the consequent target of weight loss through restriction of dietary calorie intake and the link with salt sensitivity, inflammation, and hypertension.

HIGHLY UNSATURATED AND N-3 FATTY ACIDS

Present mainly in seafood, and therefore better known as fish oils, highly unsaturated FAs of the n-3 series (ω-3 FAs) are probably the best example of how diet may affect inflammation. These compounds exert a remarkable variety of biologic effects[4,5]; because of this, they are currently being tested in a variety of clinical situations as disparate as coronary artery disease,[6,7] hypertension,[8,9] some dyslipidemias,[10] cancer,[11–13] diabetes,[14] renal diseases,[15] and a number of inflammatory states.[16] The reader is referred to the cited reviews covering their use in these conditions, whereas this section focuses on their use in inflammatory states and renal disease.

Biologic Properties and Effects of N-3 Fatty Acids and Their Potential Relevance to Inflammation

Current medical interest in n-3 fatty acids stems from observations of the different prevalence of some chronic diseases in the Greenland (Eskimo) population relative to Western populations.[17] Diseases with lower prevalence in Inuit compared with control Danes include myocardial infarction, from which the main source of interest for these compounds as preventive agents in coronary artery disease has derived, but also conditions such as psoriasis, bronchial asthma, diabetes mellitus, and thyrotoxicosis,[17] which share a background of inflammation or a derangement of immunity. Increased nutritional intake of fish and marine mammals, providing an increased supply of n-3 FAs, was pointed out as the main factor responsible for such differences.[18,19] Mammals in general cannot synthesize FAs with double bonds distal to the ninth carbon atom (starting counts from the methyl end of the carbon chain), although they are able, to some extent, to elongate (increase carbon chain length) and further desaturate (increase the number of double bonds) the aliphatic chain. Two main families of long-chain polyunsaturated FAs exist, biologically derived from the shortest nonsynthesizable precursors linoleic acid (C18:2 n-6)

and α-linolenic acid (C18:3) (Fig. 11-1). Linoleic acid is abundant in oils from most vegetable seeds such as corn and safflower. α-Linolenic acid is found in the chloroplasts of green leafy vegetables. Humans can desaturate and elongate α-linolenic acid to eicosapentaenoic acid (EPA) and, further, to docosahexaenoic acid (DHA). However, the elongation and desaturation processes are likely to be slow and possibly further limited by aging[20] and disease conditions.[21] For these reasons, EPA and DHA are considered, to a large extent, nutritionally essential and nearly exclusively derived from fish. Fish increase their membrane content by eating the phytoplankton rich in either the precursor α-linolenic acid or the more elongated compounds EPA and DHA. Fatty fish living in cold seas (e.g., mackerel, salmon, herring) are particularly rich in these compounds, which may give them a selective advantage in preventing low temperature–related loss in membrane fluidity in cell membranes.[20] Concentrated formulations of EPA and DHA are now available from industrial processing of the body fat from fish and are undergoing clinical trials as dietary supplements or pharmacologic agents.

The n-3 FAs exert a remarkable variety of biologic effects, many of which may affect inflammation and clinical conditions related to their presence (Fig. 11-2). The most important of these are now discussed in greater detail.

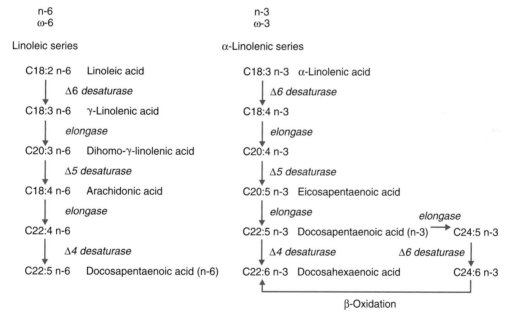

Figure 11-1   Metabolism and nomenclature of the main polyunsaturated fatty acid (FA) of the linoleic series *(left)* and the α-linolenic series *(right)*. The two metabolic pathways, although largely using the same enzymes without appreciable substrate specificity, are entirely distinct and not interconvertible in animals and humans. Regulation of elongase and desaturates is largely unknown. Both pathways use the same enzymes for chain elongation and desaturation. Recent findings, however, have indicated that formation of docosahexaenoic acid (DHA) from 22:5 n-3 occurs through an initial chain elongation to 24:5 n-3 (in either mitochondria or peroxisomes), which is in turn desaturated in microsomes at position 6 to yield 24:6 n-3. The chain is then shortened via b-oxidation to yield DHA. This novel biosynthetic pathway is commonly referred to as Sprecher's shunt.[122] Dihomo-g-linolenic acid is the precursor of prostaglandins of the 1 series. Arachidonic acid is the most common eicosanoid precursor; eicosapentaenoic acid is the most common precursor of the prostaglandins of the 3 series and of leukotrienes of the 5 series, and the most abundant polyunsaturated FA present in fish oil concentrates; DHA is the most abundant n-3 FA accumulated in tissues (especially in the central nervous system) and in fish, and can exert its effects partially by retroconversion to eicosapentaenoic acid and partially by itself. See text for further details. (Modified from De Caterina R, Endres S, Kristensen S, Schmidt E: n-3 Fatty acids and renal diseases. Am J Kidney Dis 1994;24:397–415.)

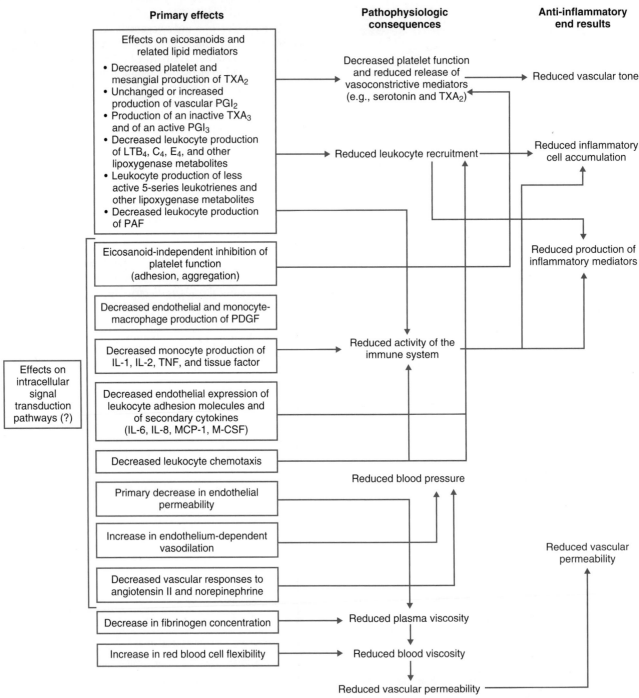

Figure 11-2 Biologic effects of n-3 fatty acids (FAs) and the rationale for their anti-inflammatory use. IL, interleukin; LT, leukotriene; MCP-1, monocyte chemoattractant protein-1; M-CSF, macrophage colony–stimulating factor; PAF, platelet-activating factor; PDGF, platelet-derived growth factor; PG, prostaglandin; TNF, tumor necrosis factor; TX, thromboxane. See text for details and references.

Production of Eicosanoids and Related Lipid Mediators

Until recently, the prevailing hypothesis to explain the protean effects of n-3 FAs was that their action could be related to the different profile of activities of neosynthesized, soluble lipid mediators derived from EPA as opposed to those derived from the normally more abundant arachidonic acid (AA) (Fig. 11-3).

Both AA and EPA are FAs with 20 (in Greek, *eicosa*) carbon atoms and four or five *cis* double bonds, each one inducing a bending of the otherwise linear aliphatic chain. These bendings allow the occurrence of a hairpin configuration and the subsequent enzymatic transformation of the FA precursor in a variety of compounds commonly designated eicosanoids. This term now encompasses a number of classes of related compounds, named prostaglandins, thromboxanes (TXs), leukotrienes (LTs), hydroxy- and epoxy-FAs, lipoxins, and isoprostanes.

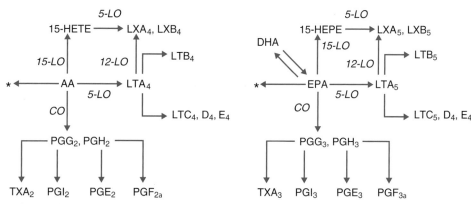

Figure 11-3 An updated schema for the origin of the main eicosanoids deriving from the linoleic series (metabolites of arachidonic acid [AA]) and of the α-linolenic series (metabolites of eicosapentaenoic acid [EPA]) with relevance to inflammation physiology and pathophysiology. The best characterized metabolic pathway, catalyzed by the enzyme prostaglandin (PG) H synthase (cyclooxygenase [CO], of which a constitutive form and an inducible form are now known), leads to the formation of prostanoids (PGs[82]) and thromboxanes (TXs) of the 2 series from AA and of the 3 series from EPA. AA and EPA also can be metabolized in leukocytes and some connective tissue cells via the enzyme 5-lipoxygenase (5-LO) to leukotrienes (LTs) A4 and A5, respectively. These labile intermediates can be converted to the more stable LTB (endowed with potent chemotactic properties) or by the addition of a peptide residue to the sulfidopeptide LTs (LTC, LTD, LTE), which are powerful vasoconstrictors and able to increase vascular permeability. The schema also outlines the possible complex metabolization of both AA and EPA toward lipoxins (LXs), which are also endowed with vasoactive properties. Lipoxins arise through the combined action of 5-LO and other LOs (15-LO and 12-LO). Cell-cell interactions, including exchanges of substrates and of intermediate metabolites, are thought to be particularly relevant to the generation of LO metabolites. On the average, metabolites derived from EPA are less active than the corresponding species derived from AA, potentially explaining the reduction in many cellular responses occurring when n-3 fatty acids are added to the diet. More importantly, EPA is a worse substrate for the metabolizing enzymes than AA, leading to a net absolute reduction in the amount of metabolites generated. The schema also outlines the bidirectional relationship of EPA and DHA, by which the latter compound may serve as a storage compartment for EPA. The asterisk denotes other potential metabolic conversions of AA and EPA to bioactive compounds, which have been recently appreciated in particular organ systems. These include the generation of isoprostanes, ω-3 hydroxylation, epioxygenase, and cytochrome P-450/allylic oxidation products. 15-HEPE, 15-hydroxypentaenoic acid; 15-HETE, 15-hydroxytetraenoic acid. (Modified and updated from De Caterina R, Endres S, Kristensen S, Schmidt E: n-3 Fatty acids and renal diseases. Am J Kidney Dis 1994;24:397–415.)

The initial step in the biosynthesis of these compounds is thought to be a receptor- or physical perturbation–mediated influx of Ca^{2+} ions, causing translocation of a cytoplasmic phospholipase A_2 to the cell membrane.[22,23] The enzyme then catalyzes the hydrolysis of the esterified AA in the sn-2 position.[24,25] A variety of phospholipase A_2 have now been identified, differing in molecular weight, calcium sensitivity, and the specificity for AA.[26] The activity of these enzymes appears to be increased by a phospholipase A_2–activating protein, which is activated by cytokines such as interleukin (IL)-1 and tumor necrosis factor (TNF).[27] A secretory phospholipase A_2 present on the surface of mast cells and other cells may also be involved in the liberation of AA.[28,29]

Physical stimuli–or agonist-induced activation of cytoplasmic phospholipase A_2 leads to a liberation of free AA. When EPA partially replaces AA as the polyunsaturated FA in the sn-2 position of glycerophospholipids, free EPA is produced. AA or EPA then becomes available for a variety of enzymes able to drive their further metabolism in directions depending on the cell type where such activation processes occur (see Fig. 11-1). Thus, in platelets and a few other tissues (including the kidney), AA is metabolized to TXA_2, a powerful vasoconstrictor and inducer of platelet activation. The replacement of EPA leads to the production of a much weaker TXA_3. On the other hand, in endothelia, products of AA and EPA are the almost equally active prostaglandins I_2 and I_3, both vasodilators and inhibitors of platelet activation. In leukocytes, which are pivotal cells in inflammation, the main metabolism of AA is toward the production of LTs, endowed with chemotactic (LTB_4) or vaso- or bronchoconstrictive and endothelium-permeabilizing properties (LTC_4, LTD_4, and LTE_4). EPA also acts as a poor substrate for AA-metabolizing enzymes, leading to a decreased net production of derived compounds (reviewed in De Caterina and Zampolli[30]). Lipoxygenase products of EPA are the weaker corresponding LTs of the 5 series (LTB_5, C_5, D_5, E_5) (see Fig. 11-3), although, in this regard, the most relevant property of n-3 FA incorporation in membrane phospholipids appears to be the reduced production of such mediators.[31] As a result, a shift in the relative abundance of AA and EPA leads to a new balance of eicosanoids, favoring vasodilating, antiplatelet, and less proinflammatory compounds. Elevated TXA_2 (by urinary assays of metabolites of its hydrolytic product TXB_2) has been found in patients with systemic lupus erythematosus[32] and in a variety of renal diseases including chronic glomerular disease,[33] diabetic nephropathy,[34] renal damage caused by cyclosporine,[35] renal transplant rejection,[36] and proteinuric syndromes.[37–40] Substitution of EPA for AA reduces platelet[41–45] as well as renal production of TX.[40] In addition, n-3 FAs have been found to reduce the gene expression of cyclo-oxygenase-2,[46] leading to the net reduction in the output of proinflammatory prostanoids. In addition, some of the anti-inflammatory effects of n-3 FAs may derive from their conversion, mainly through a cytochrome P-450–mediated pathway, to oxygenated products that carry potent protective bioactions present in resolving inflammatory exudates and therefore termed resolvins.[47–49] Resolvin E_1 is biosynthesized in vivo from EPA via transcellular biosynthetic routes during cell-cell interactions, and thus resolvin E_1 is formed in vivo during multicellular responses such as inflammation and microbial infections. Resolvin E_1 protects tissues from leukocyte-mediated injury and counterregulates proinflammatory gene expression. These newly identified resolvins may underlie the beneficial actions of n-3 polyunsaturated FAs, especially in chronic disorders where unresolved inflammation is a key mechanism of pathogenesis.

Overall, these changes may be an explanation for some of the anti-inflammatory, antihypertensive, and renal effects of n-3 FAs.

Modulation of Cell Activation and Cytokine Production

In addition to changes in eicosanoid metabolism, increased attention is being now paid to n-3 FAs as possible modulators of cytokine production. When administered to healthy volunteers, n-3 FAs decrease bacterial lipopolysaccharide-induced production of the proinflammatory cytokines IL-1 and TNF-α from peripheral blood mononuclear cells.[50,51] In cultured human endothelial cells, the membrane enrichment of n-3 FAs, by supplementation of culture medium with DHA, reduces the ability of endothelial cells to respond to stimulation with bacterial lipopolysaccharide, IL-1, IL-4, or TNF in terms of surface expression of the leukocyte adhesion molecules vascular cell adhesion molecule-1, intercellular adhesion molecule-1, and E-selectin, as well as release of soluble mediators of endothelial activation, such as IL-6 and IL-8, which are able to provide positive feedback for the amplification of the inflammatory response.[52–55] Similarly, n-3 FAs also inhibit the gene expression of cyclooxygenase-2,[46] thereby providing another negative interference on inflammation. This provides a basis for a reduced responsiveness of cells to inflammatory stimuli, probably due to the ability of n-3 FAs to modulate the activation of transcription factors (nuclear factor κB),[46,52–55] which can coordinate the concerted activation of a variety of genes involved in acute inflammation, atherosclerosis, and the modulation of the immune response.[55–57] Other reported properties of n-3 FAs, including the ability to modulate the expression of tissue factor by stimulated monocytes,[58,59] or of platelet-derived growth factor–like proteins in endothelial cells[60] or monocytes[61] could be due to the same or a similar underlying mechanism of action.

Other Biologic Properties of N-3 Fatty Acids Related to Modulation of Inflammation

Other effects of n-3 FAs include reduction of monocyte and neutrophil chemotaxis[62–65] and leukocyte inflammatory potential,[66] possibly by modulating cytokine and chemokine production. Total blood viscosity is reduced by n-3 FAs,[67–69] most probably through a combined effect on red blood cell deformability[20] and plasma viscosity, the main determinant of which, concentration of fibrinogen, is favorably reduced by these compounds.[70–72] In addition, n-3 FAs have been reported to increase endothelium-dependent vasodilation[73,74]

and to decrease vasoconstrictive responses to angiotensin II.[75,76] At least some of these effects may be due to a modulation of intracellular signal transduction pathways, partly due to the function of FAs as intracellular second messengers themselves in cell activation[77] (see Fig. 11-2). In general, n-3 FAs have been found to reduce the increase in intracellular calcium in response to agonists. In particular, the enrichment of cellular phospholipids with DHA inhibits calcium transients.[78–80] In cardiac myocytes, this may occur through a modulation of the L-type calcium channel.[81] Alternatively, changes in agonist-induced increase in intracellular calcium may occur through an alteration of the agonist-receptor affinity[82] or cell membrane physicochemical characteristics.[83,84] Postreceptor signaling pathways and the formation of second messengers involved in the mobilization of intracellular calcium may be inhibited by reductions of the production of inositol trisphosphate[85,86] or by conversion of FAs to cytochrome P-450 epoxygenase metabolites.[87,88] By some of these mechanisms, fish oil has been reported protective against proteinuria in animal models[89] as well as in humans with glomerular kidney diseases.[40]

ESSENTIAL FATTY ACID DEFICIENCY

More than 25 years ago, it was established that essential FA (EFA) deficiency was able to prevent the lethal glomerulonephritis that occurs in the New Zealand black × New Zealand white model of murine lupus.[90] The original report was followed by others showing similar results for supplementation with n-3 FAs in both the New Zealand black × New Zealand white and MRL1pr models of murine lupus.[91–93] A proximal step in the pathogenesis of the glomerulonephritis in murine lupus is the formation of autoantibodies. Suppression of such an event did not appear to be involved in these protective effects. Dietary polyunsaturated FA manipulation was found to be effective even when started late in the disease, after a full-blown autoantibody response.[92] Also, investigations on the mechanism of action of EFA deficiency were not able to show clear results of suppression of lymphocyte responses.[94] Therefore, it was reasoned that FAs had to act distally to the deposition of immune complexes in glomeruli. The original hypothesis entertained at that time was that the efficacy of dietary polyunsaturated FA manipulation was through diminished levels of active cyclooxygenase metabolites.[93] However, several lines of evidence subsequently argued against such a simplistic explanation. These were mainly that (1) pharmacologic inhibition of cyclooxygenase in murine lupus did not reproduce the beneficial effects of FA manipulation[95] and that (2) EFA deprivation was not inevitably accompanied by a decrease in tissue AA or the production of cyclooxygenase metabolites.[96] Subsequent studies in normal glomeruli showed that EFA deficiency has the unique ability to modulate macrophage migration, dramatically depleting the resident population of glomerular and renal interstitial macrophages.[97] The specific deficiency of n-6 FAs was responsible for these effects because the administration of linoleic acid (18:2 n-6), but not that of α-linolenic acid (18:3 n-3), reversed the decrease in macrophage population.[97] These changes were interpreted as due to an attenuated ability of glomeruli from EFA-deficient animals to generate LTB_4.[98] More recently, it was observed that EFA deficiency attenuates the immunologic, metabolic, and functional alterations accompanying nephrotoxic nephritis, a model of immune-mediated glomerulonephritis.[99,100] In this model, multiple mechanisms appear operative in different phases, including an early role for neutrophil-platelet interactions, causing increased glomerular LTB$_4$ and TX synthesis and consequent proteinuria and involving complement and possibly fibrinogen, P-selectin, and eicosanoids.[101] EFA deficiency does not alter neutrophil influx in the glomeruli, but affects the acute increase in glomerular LTB$_4$ and TX[99] and other neutrophil functions, such as the generation of superoxide anion,[102] similarly to what occurs with n-3 FA supplementation.[62] A role for the generation of platelet-aggregating factor, the production of which is also impaired by EFA deficiency[103] as well as by n-3 FA supplementation,[104] has been postulated.[105] In later phases of nephrotoxic nephritis, the critical cellular effector system is the monocyte macrophage, which appears to mediate the increase in glomerular TX production, proteinuria, and the decline in renal function.[106,107] EFA deficiency dramatically inhibits the elicitation of monocyte macrophages into the glomerulus in this model of renal inflammatory disease, and this effect is not attributable to either platelet-aggregating factor or LTB$_5$ because it is not inhibited by platelet-aggregating factor receptor blockade or 5-lipoxygenase inhibition.[108] Because no defect in in vitro sensitivity to chemotactic agents in monocyte/macrophages from EFA-deficient animals is also demonstrable,[99] it is likely that glomerular production of a monocyte-specific chemoattractant or monocyte adherence is impaired, similar to what was demonstrated with n-3 FA supplementation.[52,54] FA manipulation with EFA deficiency has also been shown to be effective in decreasing the late glomerulosclerosis,[109,110] which is a consequence of glomerular injury and inflammation regardless of the initiating insult.[111]

STUDIES IN HUMANS WITH DIETARY MANIPULATION OF FATTY ACID INTAKE

Along with the elucidation of their many biologic properties, studies have been performed to explore the potential usefulness mostly of dietary supplementation with n-3 FAs in a number of pathologic conditions in which inflammation is either the most prominent or an essential component. Such conditions include rheumatoid arthritis,[112] systemic lupus erythematosus[113] and other rheumatic diseases,[114] ulcerative colitis,[115–117] Crohn's disease,[118–120] and bronchial asthma.[121] Results of the vast majority of these trials have been critically reviewed.[122,123] Several well-controlled, double-blind trials of the effects of n-3 FAs in rheumatoid arthritis have reported statistically significant beneficial effects, which were, however, of a small magnitude and modest clinical impact. Such studies were conducted with doses in the range of 5 to 6 g/day, with minimal side effects, justifying the hypothesis that larger doses might possibly have a greater clinical efficacy. Inconsistent results, possibly for similar reasons, have also been reported in inflammatory respiratory diseases (i.e., allergic asthma)[124,125] and inflammatory skin diseases.[126–128] Promising, yet not definitive, studies have been reported in systemic lupus erythematosus.[129] A double-blind, placebo-controlled clinical trial in patients with Crohn's disease at high risk of relapse showed

that 59% of patients kept on 2.7 g/day of n-3 FAs remained in remission compared with 26% in the placebo group.[120] This is the most promising result obtained so far in this disease category. Compared with previous less favorable results obtained by others,[118,119] the authors hypothesized a better compliance in the last study due to a special coating that enhances protection of the n-3 FA capsules against gastric acidity and the consequent occurrence of gastric side effects.[120] Also, four double-blind, placebo-controlled trials in ulcerative colitis, with doses of n-3 FAs ranging between 2.7 and 5.4 g/day, have documented moderate clinical improvements, mostly in remission induction.[115–118] The variable results obtained by dietary supplementation with n-3 FAs in different inflammatory conditions can possibly be explained by the variable nature of inflammation in these conditions. A unitary explanation of these discrepancies is, however, lacking at present.

Studies with Supplementation of N-3 Fatty Acids in Renal Disease

Against a background of older literature indicating promising effects in slowing down the progression of glomerular sclerosis and reducing proteinuria in various forms of renal diseases (reviewed by De Caterina and colleagues[15]), more recent human studies fall in the following two main categories: (1) studies with intermediate mechanistic endpoints showing that in patients on hemodialysis, n-3 FAs may ameliorate the lipid profile by reducing plasma levels of triglycerides, remnant lipoproteins, and, contrary to common expectations, lipid peroxidation[130]; increase high-density lipoprotein cholesterol[131]; synergize the lipid-lowering effects of statins[132]; reduce LT formation[133]; and increase heart rate variability, a prognostic marker of arrhythmic death in these patients,[134] and showing that in patients after renal transplantation, n-3 FAs may have, like in other clinical conditions,[8,44] favorable effects on blood pressure[135] and improvement in cyclosporine absorption and metabolism[136] and (2) studies with clinical endpoints, mostly confined to the setting of IgA nephropathy.[137] In this disease, a prospective, double-blind trial had originally shown beneficial effects of n-3 FAs.[138] This was confirmed in a follow-up of the original cohort of longer than 6 years.[139] A more recent study in IgA nephropathy has confirmed positive effects.[140] Possible differences between animal and human studies using fish oils are the larger doses generally used in animal studies and the different background diet, whereby in experimental studies the animals are usually placed on a n-3 enriched diet without exposure to competing n-6–containing food, whereas human studies have usually involved n-3 supplements, with patients usually eating a regular diet rich in competing n-6 FAs. Future studies in patients will have to address the issues of the background diet and of the achieved ratio of n-3/n-6 FAs.

VITAMINS AND OTHER NUTRIENTS

There are scanty and occasional reports in the literature of other nutrients able to modulate selected examples of inflammation. Thus, plasma levels of pyridoxal-5′-phosphate (vitamin B$_6$) have been found to be reduced in patients with rheumatoid arthritis, and this reduction is in some way correlated with an increased production of the inflammatory mediator TNF-α by peripheral blood monocytes.[141] Antioxidant vitamins, mostly vitamin E[142] and β-carotene (vitamin A),[143] have occasionally been reported to modulate the inflammatory response in a variety of experimental models and some clinical conditions. Their effects, although with a clear biologic rationale in interfering with redox-mediated intracellular signal transduction pathways activated by cytokines, are weak at best, and their clinical impact appears to be minor.

OBESITY AS AN INFLAMMATORY STATE

An effective immune response to infectious agents and the capability of repairing tissue damage and storing energy to be spent in situations of environmental food deprivation, such as during long famine periods, are fundamental functions of living organisms. In an evolutionary perspective, it is not unexpected that metabolic and immune pathways evolved in an interdependent manner and that the immune response and metabolic control systems in part share the same cellular mechanisms.[144] Cytokines, transcription factors, and some lipids represent regulatory signals both for the metabolic and the immune response to infection. Stimulation of the immune system activates metabolic pathways that mobilize stored body fuels and in parallel suppresses pathways conducive to energy storage, such as the insulin signaling pathway.[145] This adaptive response serves to provide the energy input required to mount and sustain the inflammatory response (Fig. 11-4). Starvation suppresses the immune system, whereas overfeeding and fat excess have an opposite influence on the immune response. For millennia, starvation and malnutrition have been recognized as major risk factors for infection and death. In this scenario, the integrated functioning of the inflammatory and the metabolic responses aimed at generating an appropriate response to infectious agents emerged as a trait advantageous for survival. Although famine still remains a problem of considerable dimensions in less economically developed countries, in most Western countries the major threat to human health is now represented by the epidemics of obesity-driven diseases such as diabetes, hypertension, and dyslipidemia and to related atherosclerotic complications,[146]

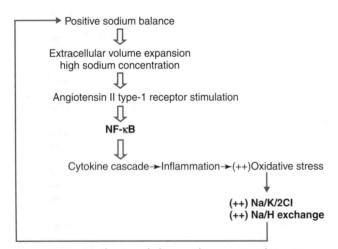

Figure 11-4   Mechanisms linking sodium-sensitive hypertension to inflammatory signals. See text for further explanations. NF-κB, nuclear factor κB.

that is, to a set of diseases and complications causally related to altered metabolic and immune mechanisms.

TNF-α was the first biochemical link discovered between the adipose tissue and immune mechanisms/inflammation. TNF-α alters insulin sensitivity, as shown by the observation that the obese TNF-α knockout mouse has better insulin sensitivity than the obese wild-type mouse.[147] Beyond TNF-α, fat cells are endowed with the ability to express a large series of inflammatory genes. These cells produce a series of compounds involved in adaptive and innate immunity. These include leptin, a hormone central to immunosuppression associated with starvation, and the large, continuously expanding repertoire of adipokines, now including, among others, adiponectin, resistin, and visfatin, all identified as fundamental factors in the regulation of insulin sensitivity as well as in the innate immune response.[148] The prototypical innate immunity cell, the macrophage, has similarities with the adipocyte because it expresses gene products typical of the adipocyte, such as the cytoplasmic FA-binding protein, adipocyte lipid-binding protein 2, and peroxisome proliferator activated receptor-γ.[149–152] Macrophages have lipid-storage capabilities, and the lipid-overloaded macrophage is a key factor in the processes leading to atherosclerotic plaque formation. Conversely, preadipocytes may differentiate into fully functional macrophages.[153] It is important to note that in obese patients, these two cell types, the macrophage and the adipocyte, colocalize in adipose tissue,[154] thus forming an integrated system participating in the innate immune response and in metabolic regulation.

Weight Loss and Inflammation in Obesity

There is substantial evidence that circulating levels of major cytokines such as TNF-α, IL-6, and IL-1β as well as C-reactive protein (the main inflammatory penthraxin synthesized in the liver) are associated with measures of adiposity, such as the waist circumference, the waist-to-hip ratio, and body mass index.[155] The causal nature of this link has been tested in a variety of intervention studies of weight loss in obese patients. Weight loss, no matter whether achieved through diet, exercise, or a surgical intervention, is accompanied by a decline in the level of C-reactive protein (CRP) and other circulating cytokines. The magnitude of the association between body fat and inflammation as well as the dose-response relationship between changes in weight loss and changes in CRP have been recently examined in a thorough meta-analysis encompassing the full series of medical and surgical interventions currently applied to induce weight loss.[156] Reduction in body weight was consistently associated with a decline in CRP level across a wide range of weight loss. In the combined analysis of the various interventions, the strength of the association was quite high because as much as 72% of the variance in CRP change was explained by concomitant weight loss, and each kg of weight loss corresponded to a decrease in CRP of 0.13 mg/L. The largest decreases in CRP level (by 5–10 mg/L) were observed in surgical intervention studies, which achieved the most pronounced weight changes (by 30–45 kg). The consistent association between decreases in inflammatory markers and weight loss, observed in diverse lifestyle-related interventions and in surgical studies, supports the hypothesis that inflammation represents one of the relevant mechanisms transducing the risk of vascular complications in obesity.

Collectively, these studies document that weight loss is probably the most effective intervention for reducing inflammation in obese patients.

INFLAMMATION AND HYPERTENSION

Although still overlooked, it is well demonstrated that hypertension per se (i.e., independent of excess weight, obesity, and other risk factors) is closely linked to inflammation. Plasma concentrations of IL-6 are significantly associated with blood pressure levels in apparently healthy men.[157] The propensity at mounting amplified inflammatory responses to hypertensive stimuli in hypertensive patients is epitomized by the observation that in vitro monocytes of these patients show an amplified synthesis of IL-1β in response to angiotensin II.[158]

Mechanistically, inflammation may be an integral part of the very same process leading to arterial damage in hypertensive patients. Activation of resident cells in the media or the adventitia may produce a variety of inflammatory compounds influencing the vascular tone. This hypothesis is supported by the consistent link between plasma CRP, IL-6, and TNF-α and indexes of arterial rigidity.[159] Of note, in the Women's Health Study cohort, CRP predicts the future development of hypertension.[160] CRP may play a direct role in arterial damage because it is associated with impaired endothelial function[161] and because it activates monocytes, vascular smooth muscle, and endothelial cells, thereby generating a proatherogenic milieu.

A major regulator of vascular tone, angiotensin II, has now also emerged as a major determinant of inflammation. Macrophages express high levels of angiotensin-converting enzyme (ACE). In addition, in experimental atherosclerosis, there is a close association between macrophages in the intima-media and angiotensin II.[162] Angiotensin II, through nuclear factor κB, activates the major cytokine cascade, including TNF-α, IL-6, and monocyte chemoattractant protein-1.[163,164] Increased vascular superoxide anion (O_2^-) production and altered vascular relaxation are hallmarks of angiotensin II–induced hypertension.[165] The association between inflammation and cardiovascular damage in experimental models and in humans seems to be causal in nature because a variety of studies with angiotensin-converting enzyme inhibitors or angiotensin II type 1 receptor blockers demonstrated that these drugs not only improve target organ damage and the clinical outcome,[166–169] but also reduce the plasma levels of a variety of inflammation markers.[170] Thus, inflammation is not only a hallmark of established hypertension, but also an alteration that may precede and predict the development of hypertension.

Sodium and Inflammation in Hypertension

It is now well established that sodium may induce hypertension by mechanism(s) beyond the expansion of extracellular volume. High sodium concentration induces cardiac myoblast and smooth muscle cell hypertrophy[171] and up-regulates the angiotensin II type 1 receptor,[172] that is, the receptor that triggers vasoconstrictive and also proinflammatory responses. In cells of the proximal tubule, high sodium concentrations per se activate nuclear factor κB, which is, as highlighted previously, a transcription factor for a variety of proinflammatory cytokines, chemokines, and adhesion molecules. This phenomenon is of relevance for intrarenal inflammation, a process now considered a fundamental pathogenetic step in salt-sensitive hypertension (see later). Conversely, sodium has a direct effect on the production of transforming growth factor-β in the kidney cortex of Dahl rats within just 1 day of increasing salt intake,[173] a phenomenon that may be implicated in the progression of renal disease in this model. Apart from its profibrotic effects, transforming growth factor-β may have a direct effect on blood pressure. Indeed, mice lacking emilin-1, an endogenous inhibitor of transforming growth factor-β, have reduced vessel diameter, increased peripheral vascular resistance, and hypertension.[174]

Inflammation appears to be a central mechanism in salt-sensitive hypertension. Activation of nuclear factor κB and up-regulation of TNF-α correlate with hypertension in the Dahl salt-sensitive rat,[175] and this effect seems to be causally implicated in salt-sensitive hypertension because immunosuppression by mycophenolic acid ameliorates blood pressure in this model.[176] Importantly, oxidative stress, a feature of inflammation, enhances the Na/K/2Cl cotransport and luminal Na/H exchange,[177] thus favoring salt retention. Furthermore, high salt intake triggers oxidative stress by stimulating a fundamental enzyme in the control of superoxide anion generation at the cellular level, reduced nicotinamide adenine dinucleotide phosphate oxidase.[178] Overall, there is therefore coherent, substantial evidence that, in experimental models, salt-induced hypertension is a process characterized by intrarenal inflammation and that inflammation is a key factor mediating the effect of salt on blood pressure and on renal damage in these models.

Salt Sensitivity and Inflammation in Human Hypertension

Salt sensitivity in humans is recognized as an independent driver of cardiovascular events.[179] Salt-sensitive patients frequently do not show the physiologic nocturnal blood pressure decrease[180] and exhibit a greater prevalence of left ventricular hypertrophy,[181] and clear-cut endothelial dysfunction.[182] The nondipping pattern of blood pressure[183] and left ventricular hypertrophy[184] are both well-known correlates of a systemic low-grade inflammatory state in essential hypertensive patients, and salt-induced endothelial dysfunction, a likely consequence of a salt-induced systemic and renal inflammation, is the most probable link between salt sensitivity and atherosclerotic complications in these patients. Soluble intercellular and vascular cell adhesion molecules and E-selectin are elevated in salt-sensitive hypertensive patients.[185] Recent observations indicate that levels of metalloproteinase-9, an enzyme involved in plaque stability, are lower in salt-sensitive than in salt-resistant patients, whereas type 1 tissue inhibitor of metalloproteinases shows an opposite pattern, suggesting that the balance between the two is skewed toward enhanced collagen deposition in the vascular wall in salt-sensitive patients.[186] Thus, findings in salt-sensitive forms of human hypertension appear consistent with data in experimental models. However, there is very little information on the effects of manipulating salt intake on inflammation in salt-sensitive patients. In the only study performed so far, no change in serum CRP, serum intercellular adhesion molecule-1, serum vascular adhesion molecule-1, or IL-6 was observed in either salt-sensitive or salt-resistant hypertensive patients 2 weeks after switching from a high (250 mmol/day) to a low (50 mmol/day) salt intake.[186] It should be noted, however, that 2 weeks may be too short a time to allow the effect of high salt intake on inflammation to dissipate. Indeed, studies exploring the effect of pharmacologic interventions on the main inflammatory biomarker CRP suggest that a substantially longer treatment period is needed for the effect of statins on CRP to be fully manifest in patients with primary and secondary forms of dyslipidemia, coronary heart disease, and renal diseases.[187]

CONCLUSIONS

Modulation of long-chain polyunsaturated FA intake, mostly by increasing the relative proportions of n-3 versus n-6 FAs, is probably the clearest example of how diet may modulate inflammation. It is possible that many of the epidemiologic differences in the incidence of inflammatory diseases among different populations can be tracked back to different nutritional intake of selected, quantitatively minor nutritional components such as n-3 FAs. An additional important notion in the past years has been the role of inflammation in explaining the link between obesity and cardiovascular risk, whereby dietary restriction of calorie intake exerts remarkable anti-inflammatory effects likely intervening in the pathogenetic events linking excess body weight to cardiovascular risk. Finally, the link between dietary sodium intake, salt sensitivity, and hypertension has been highlighted by recent research. The clarification of the mechanisms of action of these dietary components and a better documentation of the spectrum of clinical possibilities offered by dietary manipulation of the intake of such compounds, linking together classic nutritional science, molecular biology, epidemiology, and clinical medicine, are a frontier for nutritional research in the years to come and are likely to gain a place for these compounds in the therapy of inflammatory disorders.

References

1. Robbins S, Cotran R, Kumar V: Inflammation and repair processes. In Pathologic Basis of Disease, 3rd ed. Philadelphia: WB Saunders, 1984.
2. McIntyre TM, Modur V, Prescott SM, Zimmerman GA: Molecular mechanisms of early inflammation. Thromb Haemost 1997;78:302–305.
3. Majno G: Chronic inflammation: Links with angiogenesis and wound healing. Am J Pathol 1998;153:1035–1039.
4. Kang JX: The importance of omega-6/omega-3 fatty acid ratio in cell function. The gene transfer of omega-3 fatty acid desaturase. World Rev Nutr Diet 2003;92:23–36.
5. De Caterina R, Massaro M: Omega-3 fatty acids and the regulation of expression of endothelial pro-atherogenic and pro-inflammatory genes. J Membr Biol 2005;206:103–116.
6. GISSI-Prevenzione Investigators: Dietary supplementation with n-3 polyunsaturated fatty acids and vitamin E after myocardial infarction: Results of the GISSI-Prevenzione trial. Lancet 1999;354:447–455.
7. Yokoyama M, Origasa H, Matsuzaki M, et al: Effects of eicosapentaenoic acid on major coronary events in hypercholesterolaemic patients (JELIS): A randomised open-label, blinded endpoint analysis. Lancet 2007;369:1090–1098.
8. Holm T, Andreassen AK, Aukrust P, et al: Omega-3 fatty acids improve blood pressure control and preserve renal function in hypertensive heart transplant recipients. Eur Heart J 2001;22:428–436.
9. Mori TA: Omega-3 fatty acids and hypertension in humans. Clin Exp Pharmacol Physiol 2006;33:842–846.
10. Harris WS: Omega 3 fatty acids and human chylomicron metabolism. World Rev Nutr Diet 2001;88:163–167.
11. Reddy BS: Omega-3 fatty acids in colorectal cancer prevention. Int J Cancer 2004;112:1–7.
12. Tavani A, Franceschi S, Levi F, La Vecchia C: Fish, omega-3 polyunsaturated fat intake and cancer at selected sites. World Rev Nutr Diet 2005;94:166–175.
13. MacLean CH, Newberry SJ, Mojica WA, et al: Effects of omega-3 fatty acids on cancer risk: A systematic review. JAMA 2006;295:403–415.
14. De Caterina R, Madonna R, Bertolotto A, Schmidt EB: n-3 Fatty acids in the treatment of diabetic patients: Biological rationale and clinical data. Diabetes Care 2007;30:1012–1026.
15. De Caterina R, Endres S, Kristensen S, Schmidt E: n-3 Fatty acids and renal diseases. Am J Kidney Dis 1994;24:397–415.
16. Simopoulos AP: Omega-3 fatty acids in inflammation and autoimmune diseases. J Am Coll Nutr 2002;21:495–505.
17. Kromann N, Green A: Epidemiological studies in the Upernavik District, Greenland. Acta Med Scand 1980;208:401–406.
18. Dyerberg J, Bang H, Hjorne N: Fatty acid composition of the plasma lipids in Greenland Eskimos. Am J Clin Nutr 1975;28:958–966.
19. Bang H, Dyerberg J, Hjorne N: The composition of food consumed by Greenland Eskimos. Acta Med Scand 1976;200:69–73.
20. Popp-Snijders C, Schouten J, van der Meer J, van der Veen E: Fatty-fish induced changes in membrane lipid composition and viscosity of human erythrocyte suspensions. Scand J Clin Invest 1986;46:253–258.
21. Singer P, Jaeger W, Voigt S, Thiel H: Defective desaturation and elongation of n-6 and n-3 fatty acids in hypertensive patients. Prostaglandins Leukot Med 1984;15:159–165.
22. Sharp J, White D, Chious X, et al: Molecular cloning and expression of human (Ca2+ sensitive) cytosolic phospholipase A2. J Biol Chem 1991;266:14850–14853.
23. Clark J, Lin L, Kriz R, et al: A novel arachidonic acid-selective cytosolic PLA2 contains a (Ca2+ dependent) translocation domain with homology to PKC and GAP. Cell 1991;65:1043–1051.
24. Mayer R, Marshall L: New insights on mammalian phospholipase A2(s): Comparison of arachidonoyl-selective and -nonselective enzymes. FASEB J 1993;7:339–348.
25. Glaser K, Mobilio D, Chang J, Senko N: Phospholipase A2 enzymes: Regulation and inhibition. Trends Pharmacol Sci 1993;14:92–98.
26. Schaloske RH, Dennis EA: The phospholipase A2 superfamily and its group numbering system. Biochim Biophys Acta 2006;1761:1246–1259.
27. Clark M, Ögü L, Conway T, et al: Cloning of a phospholipase A2-activating protein. Proc Natl Acad Sci USA 1991;88:5418–5422.
28. Kramer R, Hession C, Johansen B, et al: Structure and properties of a human non-pancreatic phospholipase A2. J Biol Chem 1989;264:5768–5775.
29. Rosengren B, Jonsson-Rylander AC, Peilot H, et al: Distinctiveness of secretory phospholipase A2 group IIA and V suggesting unique roles in atherosclerosis. Biochim Biophys Acta 2006;1761:1301–1308.
30. De Caterina R, Zampolli A: From asthma to atherosclerosis—5-lipoxygenase, leukotrienes, and inflammation. N Engl J Med 2004;350:4–7.
31. Knapp H: Omega-3 fatty acids in respiratory diseases: A review. J Am Coll Nutr 1995;14:18–23.
32. Patrono C, Ciabattoni G, Remuzzi G, et al: Functional significance of renal prostacyclin and thromboxane A2 production in patients

with systemic lupus erythematosus. J Clin Invest 1985;76: 1011–1018.

33. Ciabattoni G, Cinotti G, Pierucci A, et al: Effect of sulindac and ibuprofen in patients with chronic glomerular disease. Evidence for the dependence of renal function on prostacyclin. N Engl J Med 1984;310:279–283.

34. Craven P, Melhem M, DeRubertis F: Thromboxane in the pathogenesis of glomerular injury in diabetes. Kidney Int 1992;42:937–946.

35. Perico N, Benigni A, Zoja C, et al: Functional significance of exaggerated renal thromboxane A2 synthesis induced by cyclosporin A. Am J Physiol 1986;251:F581–F587.

36. Foegh M, Lim K, Alijani M, et al: Thromboxane and inflammatory cell infiltration in the allograft of renal transplant patients. Transplant Proc 1987;19:3633–3636.

37. Remuzzi G, Imberti L, Rossini M, et al: Increased glomerular thromboxane synthesis as a possible cause of proteinuria in experimental nephrosis. J Clin Invest 1985;75:94–101.

38. Stahl R: Die Bedeutung von Eicosanoiden bei glomerulären Erkrankungen. Klin Wochenschr 1986;64:813–823.

39. Remuzzi G, FitzGerald G, Patrono C: Thromboxane synthesis and action within the kidney. Kidney Int 1992;41:1483–1493.

40. De Caterina R, Caprioli R, Giannessi D, et al: n-3 Polyunsaturated fatty acids reduce proteinuria in patients with chronic glomerular disease. Kidney Int 1993;44:843–850.

41. Dyerberg J, Bang H, Stofferson E, et al: Eicosapentaenoic acid and prevention of thrombosis and atherosclerosis. Lancet 1978;2:117–119.

42. von Schacky C, Fischer S, Weber P: Long-term effects of dietary marine ω-3 fatty acids upon plasma and cellular lipids, platelet function, and eicosanoids formation in humans. J Clin Invest 1985;76:1626–1631.

43. von Schacky C, Weber P: Metabolism and effects on platelet function of the purified eicosapentaenoic and docosahexaenoic acids in humans. J Clin Invest 1985;76:2446–2450.

44. Knapp H, FitzGerald G: Anti-hypertensive effects of fish oil. A controlled study of polyunsaturated fatty acid supplementation in essential hypertension. N Engl J Med 1989;320:1037–1043.

45. De Caterina R, Giannessi D, Mazzone A, et al: Vascular prostacyclin is increased in patients ingesting omega-3 polyunsaturated fatty acids before coronary artery bypass graft surgery. Circulation 1990;82:428–438.

46. Massaro M, Habib A, Lubrano L, et al: The omega-3 fatty acid docosahexaenoate attenuates endothelial cyclooxygenase-2 induction through both NADP(H) oxidase and PKC epsilon inhibition. Proc Natl Acad Sci U S A 2006;103:15184–15189.

47. Serhan CN, Hong S, Gronert K, et al: Resolvins: A family of bioactive products of omega-3 fatty acid transformation circuits initiated by aspirin treatment that counter proinflammation signals. J Exp Med 2002;196:1025–1037.

48. Serhan CN, Arita M, Hong S, Gotlinger K: Resolvins, docosatrienes, and neuroprotectins, novel omega-3-derived mediators, and their endogenous aspirin-triggered epimers. Lipids 2004; 39:1125–1132.

49. Arita M, Yoshida M, Hong S, et al: Resolvin E1, an endogenous lipid mediator derived from omega-3 eicosapentaenoic acid, protects against 2,4,6-trinitrobenzene sulfonic acid-induced colitis. Proc Natl Acad Sci U S A 2005;102:7671–7676.

50. Endres S, Ghorbany R, Kelley V, et al: The effect of dietary supplementation with n-3 polyunsaturated fatty acids on the synthesis of interleukin-1 and tumor necrosis factor by mononuclear cells. N Engl J Med 1989;320:265–271.

51. Meydani S, Endres S, Wood M, et al: Oral n-3 fatty acid supplementation suppresses cytokine production and lymphocyte proliferation: Comparison in young and older women. J Nutr 1991;121:547–555.

52. De Caterina R, Cybulsky MI, Clinton SK, et al: The omega-3 fatty acid docosahexaenoate reduces cytokine-induced expression of pro-atherogenic and pro-inflammatory proteins in human endothelial cells. Arterioscl Thromb 1994;14:1829–1836.

53. De Caterina R, Libby P: Control of endothelial leukocyte adhesion molecules by fatty acids. Lipids 1996;31(Suppl 1):557–563.

54. De Caterina R, Liao JK, Libby P: Fatty acid modulation of endothelial activation. Am J Clin Nutr 2000;71(1 Suppl):213S–223S.

55. De Caterina R: Endothelial dysfunctions: Common denominators in vascular disease. Curr Opin Lipidol 2000;11:9–23.

56. Bauerle P: The inducible transcription activator NF-kB: Regulation by distinct protein subunits. Biochim Biophys Acta 1991;1072:63–80.

57. Collins T, Cybulsky MI: NF-κB: Pivotal mediator or innocent bystander in atherogenesis? J Clin Invest 2001;107:255–264.

58. Hansen J, Olsen J, Wilsgard L, Osterud B: Effects of dietary supplementation with cod liver oil on monocyte thromboplastin synthesis, coagulation and fibrinolysis. J Intern Med Suppl 1989;225:133–139.

59. Tremoli E, Eligini S, Colli S, et al: Effects of omega 3 fatty acid ethyl esters on monocyte tissue factor expression. World Rev Nutr Diet 1994;76:55–59.

60. Fox P, DiCorleto P: Fish oils inhibit endothelial cell production of platelet-derived growth factor-like protein. Science 1988; 41:453–456.

61. Kaminski W, Jendraschak E, Kiefl R, von Schacky C: Dietary omega-3 fatty acids lower levels of platelet-derived growth factor mRNA in human mononuclear cells. Blood 1993;71: 1871–1879.

62. Lee T, Hoover R, Williams J, et al: Effect of dietary enrichment with eicosapentaenoic and docosahexaenoic acids on in vitro neutrophil and monocyte leukotriene generation and neutrophil function. N Engl J Med 1985;312:1217–1224.

63. Schmidt E, Dyerberg J: n-3 Fatty acids and leukocytes. J Intern Med 1989;225(Suppl 1):151–158.

64. Schmidt E, Pedersen J, Ekelund S, et al: Cod liver oil inhibits neutrophil and monocyte chemotaxis in healthy males. Atherosclerosis 1989;77:53-57.

65. Schmidt E, Pedersen J, Varming K, et al: n-3 Fatty acids and leukocyte chemotaxis. Effects in hyperlipidemia and dose-response studies in healthy men. Arteriosclerosis Thromb 1991;11: 429–435.

66. Fisher M, Upchurch K, Levine P, et al: Effects of dietary fish oil supplementation on polymorphonuclear leucocyte inflammatory potential. Inflammation 1986;10:387–392.

67. Terano T, Hirai A, Hamazaki T, et al: Effect of oral administration of highly purified eicosapentaenoic acid on platelet function, blood viscosity and red cell deformability in healthy human subjects. Atherosclerosis 1983;46:321–331.

68. Cartwright I, Pockley A, Galloway J, et al: The effects of dietary ω3 polyunsaturated fatty acids on erythrocyte membrane phospholipids, erythrocyte deformability and blood viscosity in healthy volunteers. Atherosclerosis 1985;55:267–281.

69. Ernst E: Effects of n-3 fatty acids on blood rheology. J Intern Med 1989;225(Suppl 731):129–133.

70. Hostmark A, Bjerkedal T, Kierulf P, et al: Fish oil and plasma fibrinogen. Br Med J 1988;297:180–181.

71. Radak K, Deck C, Huster G: Dietary supplementation with low-dose fish oils lowers fibrinogen levels: A randomized, double-blind controlled study. Ann Intern Med 1989;111:757–758.

72. Flaten H, Hostmark A, Kierulf P, et al: Fish-oil concentrate: Effects on variables related to cardiovascular disease. Am J Clin Nutr 1990;52:300–306.

73. Boulanger C, Schini V, Hendrickson H, Vanhoutte P: Chronic exposure of cultured endothelial cells to eicosapentaenoic acid potentiates the release of endothelium-dependent relaxing factor(s). Br J Pharmacol 1990;99:176–180.

74. Vanhoutte P, Shimokawa H, Boulanger C: Fish oil and the platelet-blood vessel wall interaction. World Rev Nutr Diet 1991;66:233–244.

75. Coddee J, Croft E, Barden A, et al: An inhibitory effect of dietary polyunsaturated fatty acids on renin secretion in the isolated perfused rat kidney. J Hypertens 1984;2:265–270.

76. Goodfriend T, Ball D: Fatty acids effects on angiotensin receptors. J Cardiovasc Pharmacol 1986;8:1276–1283.

77. Sellmayer A, Obermeier H, Weber C, Weber P: Modulation of cell activation by n-3 fatty acids. In De Caterina R, Endres S, Kristensen S, Schmidt E (eds): n-3 Fatty Acids and Vascular Disease. Berlin: Springer-Verlag, 1993, pp 21–30.

78. Hallaq H, Smith T, Leaf A: Protective effect of eicosapentaenoic acid on ouabain toxicity in neonatal rat cardiac myocytes. Proc Natl Acad Sci USA 1990;87:7834–7838.

79. Weber C, Aepfelbacher M, Lux I, et al: Docosahexaenoic acid inhibits PAF and LTD4-stimulated [Ca++ increase in differentiated monocytic U937 cells. Biochim Biophys Acta 1991;1133:38–45.

80. Locher R, Sachinidis A, Brunner C, Vetter W: Intracellular free calcium concentration and thromboxane A2 formation of vascular smooth muscle cells are influenced by fish oil and n-3 eicosapentaenoic acid. Scand J Lab Invest 1991;51:541–547.

81. Hallaq H, Smith T, Leaf A: Modulation of dihydropyridine-sensitive calcium channels in heart cells by fish oil fatty acids. Proc Natl Acad Sci USA 1992;89:1760–1764.

82. Swann P, Parent C, Croset M, et al: Enrichment of platelet phospholipids with eicosapentaenoic acid and docosahexaenoic acid inhibits thromboxane A2/prostaglandin H2 receptor binding and function. J Biol Chem 1990;265:21692–21697.

83. Salem N, Kim H, Yergey J: Docosahexaenoic acid: Membrane function and metabolism. In Simopoulos A, Kifer R, Martin R (eds): Health Effects of Polyunsaturated Fatty Acids in Seafoods. Orlando, FL: Academic Press, 1986, pp 263–318.

84. Ehringer W, Belcher D, Wassal S, Stillwell W: A comparison of the effects of linolenic (18:3 ω3) and docosahexaenoic (22:6 ω3) acids on phospholipid bilayers. Chem Phys Lipids 1990;54:79–88.

85. Locher R, Sachinidis A, Steiner A, et al: Fish oil affects phosphoinositide turnover and thromboxane A metabolism in cultured vascular smooth cells. Biochim Biophys Acta 1989;1012:279–283.

86. Medini L, Colli S, Mosconi C, et al: Diets rich in n-9, n-6 and n-3 fatty acids differentially affect the generation of inositol phosphates and of thromboxane by stimulated platelets in the rabbit. Biochem Pharmacol 1990;39:129–133.

87. Force T, Hyman G, Hajjar R, et al: Non cyclooxygenase metabolites of arachidonic acid amplify the vasopressin-induced Ca2+ signal in glomerular mesangial cells by releasing Ca2+ from intracellular stores. J Biol Chem 1991;266:4295–4302.

88. Oliw E, Sprecher H: Metabolism of polyunsaturated (n-3) fatty acids by monkey seminal vesicles: Isolation and biosynthesis of ω3 epoxides. Biochim Biophys Acta 1991;1086:287–294.

89. Weise WJ, Natori Y, Levine JS, et al: Fish oil has protective and therapeutic effects on proteinuria in passive Heymann nephritis. Kidney Int 1993;43:359–368.

90. Hurd E, Johnston J, Okita J, et al: Prevention of glomerulonephritis and prolonged survival in New Zealand Black/New Zealand White F1 hybrid mice fed an essential fatty acid-deficient diet. J Clin Invest 1981;67:476–485.

91. Prickett J, Robinson D, Steinberg A: Dietary enrichment with the polyunsaturated fatty acid eicosapentaenoic acid prevents proteinuria and prolongs survival in NZB × NZW F1 mice. J Clin Invest 1981;68:556–559.

92. Robinson D, Prickett J, Polisson R, et al: The protective effect of dietary fish oil in murine lupus. Prostaglandins 1985;30:51–75.

93. Kelley V, Ferretti A, Izui S, Strom T: A fish oil diet rich in eicosapentaenoic acid reduces cyclooxygenase metabolites, and suppresses lupus in MRL-1pr mice. J Immunol 1985;134:1914–1919.

94. Yamanaka W, Clemans G, Hutchinson M: Essential fatty acid deficiency in humans. Prog Lipid Res 1981;19:187–215.

95. Kelley V, Iaui S, Halushka P: Effect of ibuprofen, a fatty acid cyclooxygenase inhibitor on murine lupus. Clin Immunol Immunopathol 1982;25:223–231.

96. Lefkowith J, Filippo B, Sprecher H, Needleman P: Paradoxical conservation of cardiac and renal arachidonate content in essential fatty acid deficiency. J Biol Chem 1985;260:15736–15744.

97. Lefkowith J, Schreiner G: Essential fatty acid deficiency depletes rat glomeruli of resident mesangial macrophages and inhibits angiotensin II-stimulated eicosanoid synthesis. J Clin Invest 1987;80:947–956.

98. Lefkowith J, Morrison A, Schreiner G: Glomerular leukotriene B4 synthesis: Manipulation by (n-6) fatty acid deprivation and cellular origin. J Clin Invest 1988;82:1655–1660.

99. Schreiner G, Rovin B, Lefkowith J: The anti-inflammatory effects of essential fatty acid deficiency in experimental glomerulonephritis: The modulation of macrophage migration and eicosanoid metabolism. J Immunol 1989;143:3192–3199.

100. Takahashi K, Kato T, Schreiner G, et al: Essential fatty acid deficiency normalizes function and histology in rat nephrotoxic nephritis. Kidney Int 1992;41:1245–1253.

101. Wu X, Pippin J, Lefkowith JB: Platelets and neutrophils are critical to the enhanced glomerular arachidonate metabolism in acute nephrotoxic nephritis in rats. J Clin Invest 1993;91:766–773.

102. Gyllenhammar H, Palmblad J: Linoleic acid-deficient rat neutrophils show decreased bactericidal capacity, superoxide formation and membrane depolarization. Immunology 1989;66:616–620.

103. Ramesha C, Pickett W: Platelet-activating factor and leukotriene biosynthesis is inhibited in polymorphonuclear leukocytes depleted of arachidonic acid. J Biol Chem 1986;261:7592–7599.

104. Sperling R, Robin J, Kylander K, et al: The effects of n-3 polyunsaturated fatty acids on the generation of platelet-activating factor receptor by human monocytes. J Immunol 1987;139:4186–4191.

105. Baldi E, Emancipator S, Hassan M, Dunn M: Platelet activating factor receptor blockade ameliorates murine systemic lupus erythematosus. Kidney Int 1990;38:1030–1038.

106. Takahashi K, Schreiner G, Yamashita K, et al: Predominant functional roles for thromboxane A2 and prostaglandin E2 during late nephrotoxic serum glomerulonephritis in the rat. J Clin Invest 1990;85:1974–1982.

107. Lefkowith J, Nagamatsu T, Pippin J, Schreiner G: Role of leukocytes in metabolic and functional derangements of experimental glomerulonephritis. Am J Physiol 1991;261:F213–F220.

108. Rovin B, Lefkowith J, Schreiner G: Mechanisms underlying the anti-inflammatory effects of essential fatty acid deficiency in experimental glomerulonephritis: Inhibited release of a glomerular chemoattractant. J Immunol 1990;145:1238–1245.

109. Diamond J, Pesek I, Ruggieri S, Karnowsky M: Essential fatty acid deficiency during acute puromycin nephrosis ameliorates late renal injury. Am J Physiol 1989;257:F798–F807.

110. Diamond J, Ding G, Frye J, Diamond I: Glomerular macrophages and the mesangial proliferative response in the experimental nephrotic syndrome. Am J Pathol 1992;141:887–894.

111. El Nahas A: Growth factors and glomerular sclerosis. Kidney Int 1992;41:S15–S20.

112. Kremer J, Jubiz W, Michalek A, et al: Fish-oil fatty acid supplementation in active rheumatoid arthritis: A double-blinded, controlled, crossover study. Ann Intern Med 1987;106:497–503.

113. Westberg G, Tarkowski A: Effect of MaxEPA in patients with systemic lupus erythematosus. Scand J Rheumatol 1990;19:137–143.

114. Allen B: Fish oil in combination with other therapies in the treatment of psoriasis. Health effects of ω3 polyunsaturated fatty acids in seafoods. World Rev Nutr Diet 1991;66:436–445.

115. Hawthorne A, Daneshmend T, Hawkey C, et al: Treatment of ulcerative colitis with fish oil supplementation. Gut 1992;33:922–928.

116. Stenson W, Cort D, Rodgers J, et al: Dietary supplementation with fish oil in ulcerative colitis. Ann Intern Med 1992;116: 606–614.
117. Aslan A, Triadafilopoulos G: Fish oil fatty acid supplementation in active ulcerative colitis: A double-blind, placebo-controlled, crossover study. Am J Gastroenterol 1992;87:432–437.
118. Lorenz R, Weber P, Szinmau P, et al: Supplementation with n-3 fatty acids from fish oil in chronic inflammatory bowel disease— a randomized, placebo-controlled, double-blind cross-over trial. J Intern Med Suppl 1989;225:225–232.
119. Matè J, Castaños R, Garcia-Samaniego J, Pajares J: Does dietary fish oil maintain the remission of Crohn's disease (CD): A study case control [abstract]. Gastroenterology 1991;100 (Suppl):A228.
120. Belluzzi A, Brignola C, Campieri M, et al: Effect of an enteric-coated fish-oil preparation on relapses in Crohn's disease. N Engl J Med 1996;334:1557–1560.
121. Arm J, Horton C, Mencia-Huerta J, Lee T: The effects of dietary supplementation with fish oil lipids on the airway response to inhaled allergen in bronchial asthma. Am Rev Respir Dis 1989;139:1395–1402.
122. De Caterina R: Summary statement: Clinical trials with ω3 fatty acids. In Galli C, Simopoulos A, Tremoli E (eds): Effects of Fatty Acids and Lipids in Health and Disease. World Rev Nutr Diet. Basel: Karger, 1994, pp 130–132.
123. Sijben JW, Calder PC: Differential immunomodulation with long-chain n-3 PUFA in health and chronic disease. Proc Nutr Soc 2007;66:237-59.
124. Dry J, Vincent D: Effect of a fish oil diet on asthma: Results of a 1-year double-blind study. Int Arch Allergy Appl Immunol 1991;95:156–157.
125. Thien F, Mencia-Huerta J, Lee T: Dietary fish oil effects on seasonal hay fever and asthma in pollen-sensitive subjects. Am Rev Respir Dis 1993;147:1138–1143.
126. Gupta A, Ellis C, Tellner D, et al: Double-blind, placebo-controlled study to evaluate the efficacy of fish oil and low-dose UVB in the treatment of psoriasis. Br J Dermatol 1989;120:801–807.
127. Henneicke-von Zepelin H, Mrowietz U, Farber L, et al: Highly purified omega-3-polyunsaturated fatty acids for topical treatment of psoriasis. Results of a double-blind, placebo-controlled multicentre study. Br J Dermatol. 1993;129:713–717.
128. Soyland E, Funk J, Rajka G, et al: Effect of dietary supplementation with very-long-chain n-3 fatty acids in patients with psoriasis. N Engl J Med 1993;328:1812–1816.
129. Leiba A, Amital H, Gershwin ME, Shoenfeld Y: Diet and lupus. Lupus 2001;10:246–248.
130. Ando M, Sanaka T, Nihei H: Eicosapentaenoic acid reduces plasma levels of remnant lipoproteins and prevents in vivo peroxidation of LDL in dialysis patients. J Am Soc Nephrol 1999;10:2177–2184.
131. Khajehdehi P: Lipid-lowering effect of polyunsaturated fatty acids in hemodialysis patients. J Renal Nutr 2000;10:191–195.
132. Grekas D, Kassimatis E, Makedou A, et al: Combined treatment with low-dose pravastatin and fish oil in post-renal transplantation dislipidemia. Nephron 2000;88:329–333.
133. Løssl K, Skou HA, Christensen JH, Schmidt EB: The effect of n-3 fatty acids on leukotriene formation from neutrophils in patients on hemodialysis. Lipids 1999;34:S185.
134. Christensen JH, Aarøe J, Knudsen N, et al: Heart rate variability and n-3 fatty acids in patients with chronic renal failure—a pilot study. Clin Nephrol 1998;49:102–106.
135. Santos J, Queirós J, Silva F, et al: Effects of fish oil in cyclosporine-treated renal transplant recipients. Transplant Proc 2000;32: 2605–2608.
136. Busnach G, Stragliotto E, Minetti E, et al: Effect of n-3 polyunsaturated fatty acids on cyclosporine pharmacokinetics in kidney graft recipients: A randomized placebo-controlled study. J Nephrol 1998;11:87–93.
137. Donadio JV: The emerging role of omega-3 polyunsaturated fatty acids in the management of patients with IgA nephropathy. J Renal Nutr 2001;11:122–128.
138. Donadio JV, Bergstralh EJ, Offord KP, et al, for the Mayo Nephrology Collaborative Group: A controlled trial of fish oil in IgA nephropathy. N Engl J Med 1994;331:1194–1199.
139. Donadio JVJ, Grande JP, Bergstralh EJ, et al, for the Mayo Nephrology Collaborative Group: The long-term outcome of patients with IgA nephropathy treated with fish oil in a controlled trial. J Am Soc Nephrol 1999;10:1772–1777.
140. Sulikowska B, Nieweglowski T, Manitius J, et al: Effect of 12-month therapy with omega-3 polyunsaturated acids on glomerular filtration response to dopamine in IgA nephropathy. Am J Nephrol 2004;24:474–482.
141. Roubenoff R, Roubenoff R, Selhub J, et al: Abnormal vitamin B6 status in rheumatoid cachexia. Association with spontaneous tumor necrosis factor alpha production and markers of inflammation. Arthritis Rheum 1995;38:105–109.
142. Pringle K: Modulation of the inflammatory response by antioxidants. Dissert Abstr Int 1995;56:690.
143. Driscoll H, Chertow B, Jelic T, et al: Vitamin A status affects the development of diabetes and insulitis in BB rats. Metabolism 1996;45:248–253.
144. Zoccali C, Tripepi G, Cambareri F, et al: Adipose tissue cytokines, insulin sensitivity, inflammation, and cardiovascular outcomes in end-stage renal disease patients. J Ren Nutr 2005;15: 125–130.
145. Wellen KE, Hotamisligil GS: Inflammation, stress, and diabetes. J Clin Invest 2005;115:1111–1119.
146. Obesity: Preventing and managing the global epidemic. Report of a WHO consultation. World Health Organ Tech Rep Ser 2000;894:1–253.
147. Uysal KT, Wiesbrock SM, Marino MW, Hotamisligil GS: Protection from obesity-induced insulin resistance in mice lacking TNF-alpha function. Nature 1997;389:610–614.
148. Trayhurn P, Wood IS: Adipokines: Inflammation and the pleiotropic role of white adipose tissue. Br J Nutr 2004;92: 347–355.
149. Hotamisligil GS, Shargill NS, Spiegelman BM: Adipose expression of tumor necrosis factor-alpha: Direct role in obesity-linked insulin resistance. Science 1993;259:87–91.
150. Tontonoz P, Nagy L, Alvarez JG, et al: PPARgamma promotes monocyte/macrophage differentiation and uptake of oxidized LDL. Cell 1998;93:241–252.
151. Bouloumie A, Sengenes C, Portolan G, et al: Adipocyte produces matrix metalloproteinases 2 and 9: Involvement in adipose differentiation. Diabetes 2001;50:2080–2086.
152. Makowski L, Boord JB, Maeda K, et al: Lack of macrophage fatty-acid-binding protein aP2 protects mice deficient in apolipoprotein E against atherosclerosis. Nat Med 2001;7:699–705.
153. Charriere G, Cousin B, Arnaud E, et al: Preadipocyte conversion to macrophage. Evidence of plasticity. J Biol Chem 2003;278:9850–9855.
154. Weisberg SP, McCann D, Desai M, et al: Obesity is associated with macrophage accumulation in adipose tissue. J Clin Invest 2003;112:1796–1808.
155. Visser M, Bouter LM, McQuillan GM, et al: Elevated C-reactive protein levels in overweight and obese adults. JAMA 1999;282: 2131–2135.
156. Selvin E, Paynter NP, Erlinger TP: The effect of weight loss on C-reactive protein: A systematic review. Arch Intern Med 2007;167:31–39.
157. Chae CU, Lee RT, Rifai N, Ridker PM: Blood pressure and inflammation in apparently healthy men. Hypertension 2001;38: 399–403.
158. Dorffel Y, Latsch C, Stuhlmuller B, et al: Preactivated peripheral blood monocytes in patients with essential hypertension. Hypertension 1999;34:113–117.

159. Mahmud A, Feely J: Arterial stiffness is related to systemic inflammation in essential hypertension. Hypertension 2005;46:1118–1122.

160. Sesso HD, Buring JE, Rifai N, et al: C-reactive protein and the risk of developing hypertension. JAMA 2003;290:2945–2951.

161. Fichtlscherer S, Rosenberger G, Walter DH, et al: Elevated C-reactive protein levels and impaired endothelial vasoreactivity in patients with coronary artery disease. Circulation 2000;102:1000–1006.

162. Potter DD, Sobey CG, Tompkins PK, et al: Evidence that macrophages in atherosclerotic lesions contain angiotensin II. Circulation 1998;98:800–807.

163. Han Y, Runge MS, Brasier AR: Angiotensin II induces interleukin-6 transcription in vascular smooth muscle cells through pleiotropic activation of nuclear factor-kappa B transcription factors. Circ Res 1999;84:695–703.

164. Ruiz-Ortega M, Ruperez M, Lorenzo O, et al: Angiotensin II regulates the synthesis of proinflammatory cytokines and chemokines in the kidney. Kidney Int Suppl 2002:12–22.

165. Rajagopalan S, Kurz S, Munzel T, et al: Angiotensin II-mediated hypertension in the rat increases vascular superoxide production via membrane NADH/NADPH oxidase activation. Contribution to alterations of vasomotor tone. J Clin Invest 1996;97:1916–1923.

166. Casas JP, Chua W, Loukogeorgakis S, et al: Effect of inhibitors of the renin-angiotensin system and other antihypertensive drugs on renal outcomes: Systematic review and meta-analysis. Lancet 2005;366:2026–2033.

167. Remuzzi G, Macia M, Ruggenenti P: Prevention and treatment of diabetic renal disease in type 2 diabetes: The BENEDICT study. J Am Soc Nephrol 2006;17:S90–S97.

168. Ruster C, Wolf G: Renin-angiotensin-aldosterone system and progression of renal disease. J Am Soc Nephrol 2006;17:2985–2991.

169. Strippoli GF, Bonifati C, Craig M, et al: Angiotensin converting enzyme inhibitors and angiotensin II receptor antagonists for preventing the progression of diabetic kidney disease. Cochrane Database Syst Rev 2006:CD006257.

170. Schieffer B, Bunte C, Witte J, et al: Comparative effects of AT1-antagonism and angiotensin-converting enzyme inhibition on markers of inflammation and platelet aggregation in patients with coronary artery disease. J Am Coll Cardiol 2004;44:362–368.

171. Gu JW, Anand V, Shek EW, et al: Sodium induces hypertrophy of cultured myocardial myoblasts and vascular smooth muscle cells. Hypertension 1998;31:1083–1087.

172. Ruan X, Wagner C, Chatziantoniou C, et al: Regulation of angiotensin II receptor AT1 subtypes in renal afferent arterioles during chronic changes in sodium diet. J Clin Invest 1997;99:1072–1081.

173. Sanders PW: Salt intake, endothelial cell signaling, and progression of kidney disease. Hypertension 2004;43:142–146.

174. Zacchigna L, Vecchione C, Notte A, et al: Emilin1 links TGF-beta maturation to blood pressure homeostasis. Cell 2006;124:929–942.

175. Rodriguez-Iturbe B, Ferrebuz A, Vanegas V, et al: Early and sustained inhibition of nuclear factor-kappaB prevents hypertension in spontaneously hypertensive rats. J Pharmacol Exp Ther 2005;315:51–57.

176. Mattson DL, James L, Berdan EA, Meister CJ: Immune suppression attenuates hypertension and renal disease in the Dahl salt-sensitive rat. Hypertension 2006;48:149–156.

177. Juncos R, Hong NJ, Garvin JL: Differential effects of superoxide on luminal and basolateral Na+/H+ exchange in the thick ascending limb. Am J Physiol Regul Integr Comp Physiol 2006;290:R79–R83.

178. Kitiyakara C, Chabrashvili T, Chen Y, et al: Salt intake, oxidative stress, and renal expression of NADPH oxidase and superoxide dismutase. J Am Soc Nephrol 2003;14:2775–2782.

179. Morimoto A, Uzu T, Fujii T, et al: Sodium sensitivity and cardiovascular events in patients with essential hypertension. Lancet 1997;350:1734–1737.

180. de la Sierra A, Lluch MM, Coca A, et al: Assessment of salt sensitivity in essential hypertension by 24-h ambulatory blood pressure monitoring. Am J Hypertens 1995;8:970–977.

181. de la Sierra A, Lluch MM, Pare JC, et al: Increased left ventricular mass in salt-sensitive hypertensive patients. J Hum Hypertens 1996;10:795–799.

182. Bragulat E, de la Sierra A, Antonio MT, Coca A: Endothelial dysfunction in salt-sensitive essential hypertension. Hypertension 2001;37:444–448.

183. Bellelli G, Rozzini R, Battista Frisoni G, Trabucchi M: Is C-reactive protein an independent risk factor for essential hypertension? J Hypertens 2001;19:2107.

184. Mehta SK, Rame JE, Khera A, et al: Left ventricular hypertrophy, subclinical atherosclerosis, and inflammation. Hypertension 2007;49:1385–1391.

185. Ferri C, Bellini C, Desideri G, et al: Clustering of endothelial markers of vascular damage in human salt-sensitive hypertension: Influence of dietary sodium load and depletion. Hypertension 1998;32:862–868.

186. Larrousse M, Bragulat E, Segarra M, et al: Increased levels of atherosclerosis markers in salt-sensitive hypertension. Am J Hypertens 2006;19:87–93.

187. Ferns GA: Differential effects of statins on serum CRP levels: Implications of recent clinical trials. Atherosclerosis 2003;169:349–351.

Further Reading

Arita M, Yoshida M, Hong S, et al: Resolvin E1, an endogenous lipid mediator derived from omega-3 eicosapentaenoic acid, protects against 2,4,6-trinitrobenzene sulfonic acid-induced colitis. Proc Natl Acad Sci USA 2005;102:7671–7676.

De Caterina R, Massaro M: Omega-3 fatty acids and the regulation of expression of endothelial pro-atherogenic and pro-inflammatory genes. J Membr Biol 2005;206:103–116.

De Caterina R, Zampolli A: From asthma to atherosclerosis—5-lipoxygenase, leukotrienes, and inflammation. N Engl J Med 2004;350:4–7.

Endres S, Ghorbany R, Kelley V, et al: The effect of dietary supplementation with n-3 polyunsaturated fatty acids on the synthesis of interleukin-1 and tumor necrosis factor by mononuclear cells. N Engl J Med 1989;320:265–271.

GISSI-Prevenzione Investigators: Dietary supplementation with n-3 polyunsaturated fatty acids and vitamin E after myocardial infarction: Results of the GISSI-Prevenzione trial. Lancet 1999;354:447–455.

Massaro M, Habib A, Lubrano L, et al: The omega-3 fatty acid docosahexaenoate attenuates endothelial cyclooxygenase-2 induction through both NADP(H) oxidase and PKC epsilon inhibition. Proc Natl Acad Sci USA 2006;103:15184–15189.

Rodriguez-Iturbe B, Ferrebuz A, Vanegas V, et al: Early and sustained inhibition of nuclear factor-kappaB prevents hypertension in spontaneously hypertensive rats. J Pharmacol Exp Ther 2005;315:51–57.

Wellen KE, Hotamisligil GS: Inflammation, stress, and diabetes. J Clin Invest 2005;115:1111–1119.

Yokoyama M, Origasa H, Matsuzaki M, et al: Effects of eicosapentaenoic acid on major coronary events in hypercholesterolaemic patients (JELIS): A randomised open-label, blinded endpoint analysis. Lancet 2007;369:1090–1098.

Zoccali C, Tripepi G, Cambareri F, et al: Adipose tissue cytokines, insulin sensitivity, inflammation, and cardiovascular outcomes in end-stage renal disease patients. J Ren Nutr 2005;15:125–130.

Chapter 12

Plasmapheresis in Renal Diseases

David Jayne

CHAPTER CONTENTS

Plasma exchange is the removal of plasma from a patient and replacement with fresh frozen plasma or a substitute for plasma. The procedure is frequently termed *plasmapheresis* when solutions other than plasma (e.g., isotonic saline) are used as replacement fluid. *Pheresis* is derived from the Greek word for "to take away." The terms *plasma exchange* and *plasmapheresis* are interchangable, and current literature does not distinguish between them.

Plasmapheresis was first introduced to nephrology for the removal of cryoglobulins in 1967, of alloantibodies in transplantation in 1970, and of antiglomerular basement membrane (GBM) antibodies in anti-GBM disease in 1976.[1–3] It has become increasingly employed in renal diseases in which circulating factors, especially antibodies, are believed to contribute to disease pathophysiology. The strength of the theoretical rationale for plasmapheresis varies among indications and is complicated by the nonspecific nature of plasma exchange when potential unidentified pathogenic agents are also removed. Plasmapheresis is an invasive and expensive procedure that carries some risk to the patient. The evidence base for plasmapheresis remains relatively weak, with only a small number of randomized trials with more than 100 patients, and no trials in renal disease have been blinded.

MECHANISM OF ACTION

By removal of plasma, plasmapheresis removes any substance that exists in the plasma compartment. The rational use of plasmapheresis requires identification of the circulating factor to remove and the serial measurement of the factor to guide plasmapheresis dosing. Plasmapheresis is often combined with other treatments to control the target disease. For example, in anti-GBM disease, plasmapheresis rapidly reduces levels of circulating pathogenic anti-GBM antibodies; renal inflammation is reduced with steroids and cyclophosphamide suppresses further antibody production.[4] Other indications include the removal of components other than immunoglobulins, such as the removal of prothrombotic von Willebrand's factor (vWF) multimers by plasmapheresis in thrombotic thrombocytopenic purpura (TTP).[5] In this setting plasma infusion is also beneficial by replacing a deficient vWF cleaving metalloprotease. Thus, the nature of the replacement fluid may contribute to the therapeutic mechanism of the procedure (Table 12-1).

There are many other potential secondary mechanisms of plasma exchange that are less understood and will be of different relevance in different disease settings. For example, the pathology of small-vessel vasculitis includes inflammatory cytokines and chemokines and microthrombosis. The removal of these factors along with fibrinogen and other coagulation factors may be relevant to the therapeutic effect of plasma exchange. In autoimmune settings, prolonged immunoregulatory effects of plasmapheresis on lymphocyte activity and antibody production have been demonstrated, and plasmapheresis improves immune complex clearance.[6–8] Until these other mechanisms of plasmapheresis are better understood, they cannot be used to support its use in the absence of an identified circulating factor or secure clinical evidence.

TECHNICAL CONSIDERATIONS

Plasmapheresis involves withdrawal of venous blood, separation of plasma from blood cells, and reinfusion of cells plus donor plasma or another replacement solution. Plasma and blood cells may be separated by centrifugation or membrane filtration (Fig. 12-1).

Table 12-1   Possible Mechanisms of Action of Plasmapheresis

Mechanism	Example of Disease
Removal of Circulating Pathologic Factors	
Autoantibodies	Anti-GBM antibody disease, ANCA-associated vasculitis
Donor-specific antibodies	ABO-incompatible transplantation, HLA sensitization
IgA immune complexes	Crescentic IgA nephropathy, Henoch-Schönlein purpura
Cryoglobulin	Cryoglobulinemia
Myeloma protein	Myeloma cast nephropathy
Prothrombotic factors	Thrombotic microangiopathy
Replacement of Deficient Plasma Factors	
Antithrombotic or fibrinolytic factor	Thrombotic microangiopathy
Effects on the Immune System	
Removal of complement products	Lupus nephritis
	Transplantation
Effect on Immunoregulation	
Improvement in reticuloendothelial system function	SLE, cryoglobulinemia

ANCA, antineutrophil cytoplasmic antibody; GBM, glomerular basement membrane; HLA, human leukocyte antigen; IgA, immunoglobulin A; SLE, systemic lupus erythematosus.
Adapted from Madore F, Lazarus M, Brady H: Plasma exchange in renal diseases. J Am Soc Nephrol 1996;7: 367–386, with permission.

Centrifugation Technique

The use of centrifugal force causes whole blood to separate into various components according to their specific gravity, and the separation is monitored by sensors on the centrifuge or by computer algorithms.[9] Centrifugation can be intermittent or continuous. With intermittent centrifugation, blood is drawn in successive batches and separated. The cycle is repeated as often as necessary to remove the desired volume of plasma (usually, the equivalent of 1.0–1.5 plasma volumes or 2.5–4.0L during a session). The advantages of intermittent centrifugation include relative simplicity of operation, portability of the machines, and adequacy of a single-needle peripheral venipuncture. The disadvantages are slowness (typically > 4 hr) and the relatively large extracorporeal blood volume required (>225 mL). With continuous-flow equipment, blood is fed continuously into a rapidly rotating bowl in which red cells, leukocytes, platelets, and plasma separate into layers. Any layer or layers can be removed, and the remainder is returned to the patient with replacement fluid (see Fig. 12-1A). Continuous-flow centrifugation is faster and most operations (anticoagulation, collection procedures, fluid replacement) are automated. Disadvantages include higher cost, relative immobility of the equipment, and the requirement of either two venipunctures or insertion of a dual-lumen catheter.

Membrane Filtration Technique

Membrane filtration technology provides an alternative to centrifugation. The patient's blood is pumped through a parallel-plate or hollow-fiber filter at a continuous flow rate, typically 50 to 200 mL/min (see Fig. 12-1B). The membranes usually have pores of 0.2- to 0.6-μm diameter, sufficient to allow passage of plasma while retaining cells. Plasma is collected and weighed regularly, and the infusion rate of replacement fluid is adjusted manually or automatically to maintain intravascular volume. Membrane filtration can be performed using conventional hemodialysis equipment, but with increasing automation, specifically designed machines are safer and more convenient. Patients with acute renal failure can receive hemodialysis and plasmapheresis sequentially, using the same machine. In general, plasma can be removed at a rate of 30 to 50 mL/min (at a blood flow rate of 100 mL/min), and the average time required for a typical membrane filtration is less than 3 hours. The potential disadvantages of membrane filtration include activation of complement and leukocytes on the artificial membrane and the need for a large-vein catheter to obtain adequate blood flow rates.[10]

Membrane filtration is as safe and efficient as centrifugal plasmapheresis.[11] Automated continuous-flow centrifugal devices are more expensive than membrane-based filtration devices; however, the major costs of plasmapheresis relate to blood products, disposable blood lines, filters or centrifuge bowls, and staff time. In 2007, reimbursement rates for plasmapheresis in the United States were more than $1800 per procedure.

Selective Plasmapheresis Techniques

More sophisticated approaches achieve selective removal of immunoglobulins or other specific molecules. They have the joint aims of more efficient removal of the target factor and avoidance of the need for blood factor replacements and their associated cost and adverse reactions. In double-filtration apheresis following conventional plasmapheresis, separated

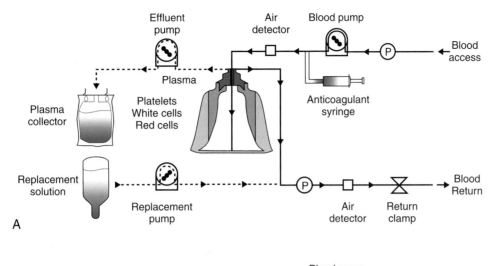

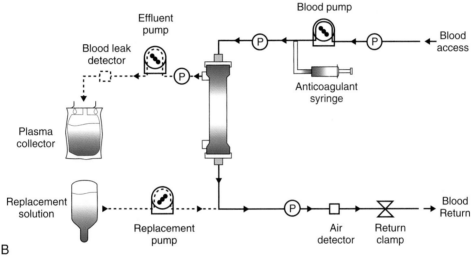

Figure 12-1 Centrifugal separator (**A**) and membrane filtration (**B**) systems for plasma exchange. **A,** Blood is pumped into the separator container. As the centrifuge revolves, different blood components are separated into discrete layers, which can be harvested separately. Plasma is pumped out of the centrifuge into a collection chamber. Red cells, leukocytes, and platelets are returned to the patient, along with replacement fluid. **B,** Blood is pumped into a biocompatible membrane that allows the filtration of plasma while retaining cellular elements. P, pressure monitor.

plasma is passed through a second filter for which the pore size can be selected according to the indication. The remaining plasma is then returned to the patient.[11] More than one plasma volume can be treated in one procedure, allowing more complete removal of the target factor. This is of potential use for the removal of donor-specific antibodies for immediate pretransplantation desensitization, for the removal of pathogenic antibodies in a seriously ill patient, for patients who cannot tolerate plasmapheresis, or for patients in whom conventional plasmapheresis provides inadequate target factor removal.

Modifications to the double-filtration process combine ligands for the target protein in the secondary column, so-called immunoabsorption. Examples include staphylococcal protein A to remove IgG antibodies, blood protein antigens A and B to remove anti-A and anti-B antibodies, and L-tryptophan or phenylalanine to remove autoantibodies.[12–15] These procedures have been used in case series in renal diseases; however, a prospective, randomized trial in 44 patients with rapidly progressive glomerulonephritis (RPGN) found no difference in outcome between plasmapheresis and protein A immunoabsorption.[16,17]

The high cost of secondary columns and complexity of double plasma treatment systems is currently limiting their availability, but with the increasing costs of blood products, they will become more attractive in the future.

Anticoagulation

Both centrifugation and membrane plasmapheresis require anticoagulation to prevent activation of the clotting mechanisms within the extracorporeal circuit. The most frequently used anticoagulant for centrifugation procedures is citrate. Acid-citrate dextrose is infused continuously at a rate adjusted according to the blood flow rate. Citrate chelates the divalent cations calcium and magnesium and may result in symptomatic hypocalcemia, especially with albumin replacement solutions that contain no calcium or magnesium. Standard unfractionated heparin is the most frequently used anticoagulant for membrane plasmapheresis. The required dose of heparin is approximately twice that needed for hemodialysis because a substantial amount of the infused heparin is removed along with the plasma.

Replacement Fluids

The typical replacement fluids are fresh frozen plasma, 5% albumin or other plasma derivatives (e.g., cryosupernatant), and crystalloids (e.g., 0.9% saline or Ringer's lactate). The choice of fluid has implications for the efficacy of the procedure, oncotic pressure, coagulation, and spectrum of adverse effects. Albumin is usually preferred to plasma because of the risk of hypersensitivity reactions and transmission of viral infections with the latter. When directly compared for the treatment of autoimmune disease, there was no difference in efficacy of plasmapheresis between albumin or plasma replacement.[18] Albumin (5%) is either used as 100% volume replacement or diluted 50:50 (volume/volume) with 0.9% saline. The exact composition of replacement fluids is tailored to the needs of the patient. For example, plasma is the replacement fluid of choice in patients with thrombotic microangiopathy (TMA) because the infusion of normal plasma may contribute to the replacement of a deficient plasma factor.[5] Plasma or a plasma derivative dosed at 6 to 12 mL/kg is used toward the end of the procedure in patients at risk of bleeding (e.g., after renal biopsy or those with liver disease or disseminated intravascular coagulation) or requiring intensive therapy (e.g., daily exchanges for several weeks). Alternatively fibrinogen levels can be monitored and plasma protein replacement dosed against fibrinogen levels. Albumin replacement and plasma replacement are equally effective at reducing plasma viscosity.[19]

EFFICACY OF PLASMAPHERESIS IN SPECIFIC RENAL DISEASES

General Comments

Clinical application of plasmapheresis was based initially on anecdotal or uncontrolled studies. The past two decades have witnessed a more rigorous reexamination of the efficacy of therapeutic plasma exchange.[20–23] However, for many disorders, there are few prospective, controlled clinical trials with adequate statistical power to allow definitive conclusions to be reached regarding the efficacy of plasmapheresis. In addition, other factors complicate the interpretation of published literature. First, the natural history of many diseases under investigation (e.g., lupus) is characterized by spontaneous exacerbations and remissions, making it difficult to evaluate whether any improvement is attributable to plasmapheresis. Second, treatment protocols vary widely between centers, making the comparison between

published studies hazardous. Finally, plasmapheresis is often combined with other therapies, making it harder to determine the value of the intervention. The therapeutic use of plasmapheresis in specific renal conditions is reviewed with reference to the pathogenesis when known, the strength of clinical trial evidence, and details of specific plasmapheresis regimens. Renal diseases in which plasmapheresis has been used include the various causes of RPGN, systemic lupus erythematosus, the TMAs, multiple myeloma, cryoglobulinemia, and renal transplantation.

Antiglomerular Basement Membrane Antibody Disease

Anti-GBM antibody disease (see also Chapter 18) typically presents as RPGN with or without pulmonary hemorrhage (Goodpasture's syndrome). Circulating anti-GBM antibodies are detected in more than 90% of patients, and, in general, disease activity correlates with the level of circulating anti-GBM antibodies.[24] Before 1975, anti-GBM–induced nephritis had a very poor prognosis, and more than 85% of patients treated with steroids and cytotoxic drugs progressed to end-stage renal disease (ESRD).[4] Against this background, the results of more than 20 uncontrolled studies including more than 250 patients, published over the past 20 years, suggest that survival rates greater than 80% and renal preservation rates greater than 45% may be obtained with therapeutic regimens combining plasmapheresis and immunosuppressive drugs.[4] These results compare favorably with historic data suggesting a patient survival rate of 45% and progression to ESRD in 85%. The largest published series involved 71 patients, and the outcome is detailed in Table 12-2. The chance of renal recovery was particularly poor for the most common subgroup, which is those presenting with a serum creatinine greater than 500 μmol/L and an immediate dialysis requirement due to oliguria or anuria. Less than 10% recovered renal function, and none of those in this subgroup who had 100% crescents on renal biopsy recovered. Several other centers have also reported that patients with a serum creatinine level greater than 500 μmol/L are unlikely to respond to therapy and regain renal function.

The specific role of plasmapheresis in anti-GBM disease has never been properly assessed by prospective, randomized, controlled trials. Only two controlled studies have evaluated the efficacy of plasmapheresis as an adjunct to conventional immunosuppressive therapy in this disease.[25,26] Although small (17 and 20 patients), both studies suggested a benefit as evidenced by faster decrease in anti-GBM antibody titers, lower serum creatinine after therapy, and fewer patients progressing

Table 12-2 Renal Outcome and Survival of 71 Patients with Anti-GBM Disease

Renal Function at Presentation	No. of Patients	PATIENT SURVIVAL		RENAL SURVIVAL	
		12 Mo	90 Mo	12 Mo	90 Mo
Creatinine < 500 μmol/L	19	19 (100%)	16 (84%)	18 (95%)	18 (95%)
Creatinine > 500 μmol/L	13	11 (83%)	8 (62%)	9 (82%)	4 (50%)
Dialysis dependent	39	26 (65%)	14 (36%)	2 (8%)	2 (5%)
Total	71	55 (77%)	38 (54%)	29 (53%)	25 (35%)

Data from Levy JB, Turner AN, Rees AJ, Pusey CD: Long-term outcome of anti-glomerular basement membrane antibody disease treated with plasma exchange and immunosuppression. Ann Intern Med 2001;134:1033–1042.

to renal failure. However, the authors were cautious about concluding that plasmapheresis had been responsible for the improved outcome because the groups receiving plasmapheresis had milder disease than the control groups.

Thus, there is good evidence based on an understanding of the pathogenesis and from nonrandomized trials with historic comparison that plasmapheresis in combination with steroids and immunosuppressive drugs improves renal outcome in patients with anti-GBM disease but without an immediate dialysis requirement. Plasmapheresis can accelerate disappearance of anti-GBM antibody and improve renal function if instituted promptly. Patients with oliguria/anuria and serum creatinine greater than 500 μmol/L (5.8 mg/dL) are unlikely to recover renal function, especially if the renal biopsy specimen demonstrates 100% crescents. Plasmapheresis is hard to justify in this setting unless lung hemorrhage is present. Lung hemorrhage is a life-threatening manifestation of anti-GBM disease and is more common in cigarette smokers. Urgent plasmapheresis is required to rapidly reduce anti-GBM levels with attention paid to replacement of coagulation factors, without which hemorrhage may be exacerbated.

Daily plasmapheresis involving 60 mL/kg phereses is usually continued for 10 to 12 days with measurement of anti-GBM levels. The target is to continue plasmapheresis until pretreatment levels fall into the normal range. Once this is achieved, plasmapheresis may be stopped but anti-GBM measurement should continue because an antibody rebound may occur in the days following its withdrawal. Late relapse of anti-GBM disease is rare.

One third of patients with RPGN and anti-GBM antibodies also have antineutrophil cytoplasm antibodies (ANCAs) and features of systemic vasculitis.[27] Such patients present with severe nephritis and are more likely to have pulmonary hemorrhage and are generally older than those with anti-GBM alone. The chances of renal recovery appear similar to those in patients with anti-GBM alone, and initial management is similar.[28] This subgroup differs from those with pure anti-GBM disease in that relapse may occur during long-term follow-up. Anti-GBM is negative at the time of relapse, but ANCA is usually positive.

Antineutrophil Cytoplasm Antibody–Associated Vasculitis

The renal lesion in Wegener's granulomatosis and microscopic polyangiitis is a focal, necrotizing glomerulonephritis in association with circulating ANCAs with specificity for proteinase 3 (proteinase 3–ANCA) or myeloperoxidase (myeloperoxidase-ANCA).[29] When disease is limited to the kidney, the term renal-limited vasculitis has been used. These syndromes are grouped under the term ANCA-associated vasculitis (AAV) (see also Chapter 17). The majority of cases have few or no immune deposits (pauci-immune), but 30% have appreciable immunoglobulin deposition. The pathogenicity of ANCA has been demonstrated in vitro and in experimental animals.[30] In human disease, ANCAs appear likely to contribute to the pathogenesis, but other mechanisms are important and ANCAs are not detectable in 5% of pauci-immune crescentic glomerulonephritis.[31] Plasmapheresis reduces levels of circulating ANCAs and adhesion molecules in vasculitis but has little effect on the high cytokine levels.[32] The typical clinical presentation is with RPGN, but an earlier phase with hematuria, proteinuria, and preserved renal function is often found when extrarenal manifestations dominate the presentation.

Conventional therapy employs the combination of high-dose corticosteroids and cyclophosphamide.[33]

Early randomized, controlled trials evaluated the efficacy of plasmapheresis as an adjunct to immunosuppressive therapy in patients with pauci-immune RPGN and varying degrees of renal failure, mostly before the availability of ANCA testing (Table 12-3).[22,34–40] Two studies randomly assigned patients to receive immunosuppressive agents with or without plasmapheresis and found no statistically significant difference between the two groups as judged by serum creatinine or dialysis dependence.[35,37] Three other studies demonstrated better renal outcomes in subgroup analyses of those presenting with severe disease.[36,38,39] Nonrandomized, controlled studies and other case series have indicated a recovery rate of 75% in those presenting in renal failure with a creatinine level greater than 5.8 mg/dL (500 μmol/L); this appears superior to that reported in series not using plasmapheresis in which recovery rates of 40% to 50% were seen.[41–43]

A recent study focused on 137 AAV patients presenting with a creatinine level greater than 5.8 mg/dL (500 μmol/L) who were randomized to either seven plasmapheresis sessions of 60 mL/kg within 14 days or three daily infusions of 1000 mg of methylprednisolone.[22] All patients received oral cyclophosphamide and the same oral corticosteroid regimen. Renal recovery occurred in 69% of the pheresis group and 49% of the control group. Risk of progression to ESRD was reduced by pheresis by 24%.[44] Thus, this study confirmed the benefit of pheresis seen earlier for the subgroup of patients presenting in renal failure, and plasmapheresis can now be routinely recommended for this indication. In a multivariate analysis studying predictive factors for renal recovery in this subgroup, the use of plasmapheresis remained associated with an improved outcome even in the presence of severe histologic features.[45]

Uncertainty remains regarding the role of plasmapheresis in AAV with RPGN and serum creatinine less than 500 μmol/L. Studies that have reported on this varied in the number of plasmapheresis sessions, and there is no established measure by which to judge how many sessions are needed. There also are no data to support or refute using ANCA levels in this setting; however, persistence of ANCA, lack of renal improvement as judged by urine output and serum creatinine, and activity of extrarenal vasculitis suggest that prolonged plasmapheresis may be required.

Pulmonary hemorrhage occurring with RPGN is termed pulmonary renal syndrome. AAV is the cause in 80% of cases, and it has been suggested that the pathogenesis of alveolar capillaritis is similar to that occurring in the glomeruli. Lung hemorrhage can be life threatening, and plasmapheresis is frequently used for this indication, but no randomized trials have addressed this presentation.[46,47] Whether plasmapheresis has a role for the treatment of other severe extrarenal manifestations of vasculitis is unknown, with inconclusive randomized trials providing conflicting evidence.[34,48]

Lupus Nephritis

Nephritis (see also Chapter 15) occurs in one third of patients with systemic lupus erythematosus and implies a poor prognosis with mortality rate of 12% and risk of progression to ESRD of 12% at 10 years with poorer outcomes in black populations.[49,50] The pathogenesis is complex with dysregulation of cellular, antibody, and cytokine/chemokine immune components. A belief in

Table 12-3 Randomized Controlled Trials Evaluating the Efficacy of Plasmapheresis in Treatment of Rapidly Progressive Glomerulonephritis and Antineutrophil Cytoplasm Antibody–Associated Vasculitis

Ref.	Disease Subgroup	No. of Patients	Initial Renal Function	No. of Phereses	Concomitant Therapy	Renal Outcome	Mortality
Glockner et al[37],*	RPGN[†]	26	46% dialysis	11	Steroids	*Improved GFR:*	
					AZA	Pheresis 69%	Pheresis 7%
					CYC	Controls 73%	Controls 8%
Cole et al[35],*	RPGN[†]	323	4% dialysis	10	Steroids	*Dialysis requirement:*	
					AZA	Pheresis 75%	Pheresis 13%
						Controls 71%	Controls 0%
Pusey et al[36]	RPGN[†]	48	39% dialysis	9	Steroids	No benefit for entire group	
					AZA	*Dialysis subgroup, recovery:*	
					CYC	Pheresis 91% (survivors)	Pheresis 48%
						Controls 37% (survivors)	Controls 35%
						$P < .05$	
Rifle and Dechelette[39],*	RPGN[†]		79% dialysis	9	Steroids	Benefit for entire group	
					CYC	*Dialysis subgroup, recovery:*	
					Heparin	Pheresis 75%	
						Controls 0%	
						$P < .05$	
Mauri et al[38]	RPGN[†]	22	50% serum creatinine > 800 μmol/L	6	Steroids	No benefit for entire group	
					CYC	*Creatinine >800 subgroup, follow-up creatinine:*	
						Pheresis 728 μmol/L	
						Controls 1163 μmol/L	
						$P < 0.05$	
Jayne et al[44]	AAV	137	Creatinine > 500 μmol/L	7	Steroids	*Renal recovery at 3 mo:*	*At 12 mo:*
					Controls, IV steroid	Pheresis 69%	Pheresis 27%
					CYC/AZA	Controls 49%	Controls 24%
						$P < 0.05$	

*Studies included patients with immune complex deposits.
†Studies included rapidly progressive glomerulonephritis (RPGN) with or without systemic vasculitis and excluded antiglomerular basement membrane disease.
AAV, antineutrophil cytoplasm antibody–associated vasculitis; AZA, azathioprine; CYC, cyclophosphamide.

the pathogenicity of circulating anti–double-stranded DNA antibodies or immune complexes developed from animal models inspired interest in plasmapheresis, and case reports and uncontrolled case series indicated a potential role in human disease.

The Lupus Nephritis Collaborative Study Group assessed the value of plasmapheresis as an adjunct to prednisone and cyclophosphamide in 86 patients with severe lupus nephritis.[51] Patients underwent plasmapheresis three times weekly for 4 weeks and were followed for an average of 136 weeks. Plasmapheresis caused a rapid reduction of serum anti–double-stranded DNA antibodies and cryoglobulins, but did not influence renal function or mortality. Importantly, patients receiving plasmapheresis tended to have a worse outcome. Four smaller randomized, controlled trials of plasmapheresis have been reported, although some patients included in these trials had mild disease (Table 12-4).[51–55] Plasmapheresis produced significant reduction in circulating immune complexes and anti-DNA antibodies, but the frequency and degree of partial or complete remission were the same in both plasmapheresis and control groups. Experimental evidence suggesting increased autoantibody production after plasmapheresis led to a theory that autoreactive lymphocytes might become more sensitive to cyclophosphamide in this setting.[56] Despite encouraging results in an uncontrolled study, a randomized, controlled trial found no additional benefit of sequential plasmapheresis and high-dose cyclophosphamide when compared with conventional cyclophosphamide dosing without plasmapheresis, and the sequential group had more severe adverse events.[56–58]

The results of the randomized trials do not exclude a beneficial role for plasmapheresis in defined subgroups, and no good studies have examined its role in lupus nephritis with RPGN, refractory lupus nephritis, or lupus nephritis with TMA. The evidence from TMA in other disease settings suggests an indication for plasmapheresis, and case series of catastrophic antiphospholipid syndrome also support its use.[59,60] Furthermore, there are uncommon extrarenal lupus manifestations associated with pathogenic autoantibodies, such as secondary diabetes with insulin receptor antibodies, in which plasmapheresis has been helpful.[61] Therefore, although plasmapheresis cannot be recommended for the routine treatment of severe lupus nephritis, it retains a potential role in certain subsets of patients.[62,63] Infection is the major cause of early mortality in SLE, and the possible increased infective risk of immunoglobulin removal by plasmapheresis in addition to high-dose corticosteroids and immunosuppression should be considered.

Cryoglobulinemia

Mixed (type II) cryoglobulinemia (see also Chapter 14), reflecting immune complexes containing monoclonal IgM rheumatoid factor and polyclonal IgG that precipitate within the glomerular

Table 12-4 Randomized, Controlled Trials Evaluating the Efficacy of Plasmapheresis in the Treatment of Lupus Nephritis

Ref	No. of Patients	Disease Severity	Initial Renal Function	No. of Phereses	Concomitant Therapy	Primary Endpoint	Mortality
Lewis et al[51]	86	Severe	Creatinine 180 µmol/L	12	Steroids	ESRD: Pheresis 20%	Pheresis 25%
					Cyclophosphamide	Controls 13%	Controls 17%
Wei et al[52]	20	Mild	GFR > 20 mL/min	6	Steroids Antimalarials	Remission: Pheresis 55% Controls 33%	
Dreksen et al[53]	20	Refractory	GFR mean 30 mL/min	9	Steroids	Remission: Pheresis 33% Control 18%	
French Group[54]	12		<50% crescents	23	Steroids	Remission: Pheresis 34% Controls 39%	
Clark et al[55]	39	Mild	GFR > 30 mL/min		Steroids	Serum creatinine: Pheresis 97 µmol/L	Pheresis 5%
					Azathioprine	Controls 124 µmol/L	Controls 0%

ESRD, end-stage renal disease; GFR, glomerular filtration rate.

capillary lumen, is often associated with a proliferative or membranoproliferative glomerulonephritis and a variable but sometimes rapidly progressive course. The majority of cases of type II cryoglobulinemia occur in association with chronic hepatitis C virus infection.[64] It may also be associated with non-Hodgkin's lymphoma or occur in isolation, that is, mixed essential cryoglobulinemia. Circulating cryoglobulins can be directly measured, and the level of monoclonal IgM, rheumatoid factor activity, and complement levels also reflect disease activity. Proteinuria is often of nephrotic range and extrarenal manifestations of systemic vasculitis are typically present.

Because cryoglobulins are restricted to the plasma compartment, their levels are rapidly and predictably reduced by plasmapheresis. Although case series have shown improved renal function in 55% to 87% of patients and improved survival (~25% mortality rate) compared with historic data (~55% mortality rate), the efficacy has never been subjected to a prospective, randomized, controlled clinical trial despite 30 years of experience.[65]

Management of cryoglobulinemia should address the underlying cause as well as the inflammatory manifestations. In hepatitis C–associated cryoglobulinemia, control of viral replication with interferon-α and ribavirin will abolish cryoglobulin production. Plasmapheresis increases the clearance of interferon-α and dosing may need to be adjusted.[66,67] Uremic patients tolerate interferon-α poorly and have a high frequency of *Staphylococcus aureus* sepsis. Plasmapheresis and corticosteroids may be required in the acute presentation or for the management of disease flare, but prolonged therapy is unnecessary if viral replication is controlled. In contrast, for mixed essential cryoglobulinemia, chronic intermittent plasma exchange may be required to control cryoglobulin levels, which are usually refractory to conventional immunosuppressives, including cyclophosphamide.[68] After an intensive course of three to five plasmaphereses, measurement of sequential cryoglobulin levels will allow the rate of synthesis to be assessed. A return of cryoglobulins does not necessarily imply return of glomerulonephritis or other inflammatory disease, and long-term therapy with corticosteroids and immunosuppression may dissociate cryoglobulin levels from disease activity. However, in those cases in which active inflammation persists, long-term intermittent plasmapheresis may be required.[67] Intravenous immunoglobulin may precipitate a cryoglobulinemic crisis but can be administered more safely immediately after plasma exchange. Rituximab and other therapeutic monoclonal antibodies are showing promise in a proportion of cryoglobulinemic patients but will be cleared by plasmapheresis, and their administration should also be planned to follow the procedure.[69]

The requirement for plasmapheresis should be determined by clinical severity. In subacute presentations with preserved renal function, corticosteroids with antiviral therapy in hepatitic C–associated disease or corticosteroids with an immunosuppressive in mixed essential disease may be sufficient. Plasmapheresis is indicated for persistent nephrotic syndrome, progressive renal failure, and severe extrarenal features, such as polyneuropathy. The frequency of plasmapheresis should be guided by the cryocrit, rheumatoid factor and complement levels, proteinuria, and serum creatinine. Volume should be replaced with albumin and saline and not plasma. Patients should be treated in a warm room with all infusions heated to 37°C to avoid cold precipitation of cryoglobulins. Despite optimal therapy in this subgroup of

patients, adverse events, including severe infection, are common and the risk of progression to ESRD is high.

IgA Nephropathy and Henoch-Schönlein Purpura

IgA nephropathy and Henoch-Schönlein purpura (HSP) (see also Chapter 16) represent a spectrum of manifestations of the same disease and are characterized by production of aberrantly glycosylated IgA1, circulating IgA rheumatoid factors, and IgA-containing immune complexes and mesangial deposition of IgA. Although serum total IgA concentration is elevated in 33% to 55% of patients, circulating IgA levels do not correlate with the severity or activity of disease. IgA nephropathy has a benign course in 50% to 70%, but those with proteinuria, hypertension, and glomerular or interstitial scarring follow a slowly progressive course with an appreciable risk of ESRD at 20 years. Less frequently, IgA nephropathy has a rapidly progressive course with glomerular necrosis, crescents, and deteriorating renal function. This also occurs in 24% of children and 31% of adults with HSP, accompanied by extrarenal features of systemic vasculitis.[70] Plasmapheresis has been employed in this setting in small case series.[71,72] Roccatello and colleagues[71] reported on their experience in treating six adults with crescentic IgA disease using plasmapheresis in addition to steroids and cyclophosphamide. All patients improved in the short term, but subsequent deterioration in renal function was observed in more than half of these patients. Sixteen children with HSP and severe renal involvement were treated with plasmapheresis alone; 15 recovered and one, referred late, developed ESRD.[73] Reversal of renal histologic activity and prevention of chronic changes was observed in six children who underwent biopsy before and after plasmapheresis plus immunosuppression.[74] Unfortunately, the uncontrolled nature of these observations does not permit definitive conclusions about the efficacy of plasmapheresis.

There is no consensus or randomized, controlled trials to guide either the use of corticosteroids or immunosuppressive drugs or plasmapheresis for the treatment of RPGN in IgA nephropathy or HSP. A rationale exists for the use of plasmapheresis to remove circulating IgA, and existing data are supportive but not conclusive.[75]

Focal Segmental Glomerulosclerosis and Relapsing Nephrotic Syndrome

A circulating pathogenic factor has been partly identified in focal segmental glomerulosclerosis (FSGS) that indicates plasmapheresis may be an effective treatment.[76] Small case series of patients with primary FSGS or relapsing nephrotic syndrome have reported benefit with prolonged plasmapheresis in a proportion of patients.[77–79] Reduction of proteinuria was used to determine the efficacy of plasmapheresis and the need for further treatment. The use of plasmapheresis for recurrent FSGS is discussed in the following section.

Thrombotic Microangiopathy

TMA (see also Chapter 26) is the renal lesion seen in hemolytic-uremic syndrome (HUS) and TTP and is found in conjunction with consumptive thrombocytopenia, microangiopathic hemolytic anemia, renal failure, and extrarenal organ involvement.[80] The pathogenesis may involve the accumulation of vWF multimers as a result of a deficiency of a vWF cleaving metalloprotease, ADAMTS 13, or the presence of an inhibitor to ADAMTS 13.[5] The vWF multimers cause endothelial cell and platelet activation and consequent microvascular thrombosis. An autoantibody blocking the activity of ADAMTS 13 is present in some spontaneous cases and when TMA occurs in association with systemic lupus erythematosus.[81] Infection-associated TMA results from a circulating toxin that causes direct endothelial injury and platelet activation. The rationale for therapy is the removal of pathogenic autoantibody, vWF multimers, or other pathogenic factors and the replacement of deficient antithrombotic and fibrinolytic factors with normal plasma. Plasmapheresis will also remove other circulating procoagulant and inflammatory factors. Therapeutic plasma exchange has been suggested mainly for adult HUS-TTP, although some studies have also included cases with childhood diarrhea-associated HUS.

Most of the evidence in favor of the role of plasmapheresis in HUS-TTP originates from uncontrolled or retrospective studies and from comparison with historical data.[80,82] Before the introduction of plasma infusion and plasmapheresis, TTP typically progressed rapidly and was almost uniformly fatal (93% fatality rate; 79% within 90 days). With plasmapheresis using fresh frozen plasma, remission rates of greater than 75% and survival rates greater than 85% have been consistently reported.[82] The underlying cause of TMA influences the outcome with idiopathic or autoimmunity-associated cases having a superior outcome when compared to those associated with malignancy or bone marrow transplantation.[83]

Two randomized, controlled trials compared plasma exchange with plasma infusion (Table 12-5).[84,85] Rock and colleagues[84] randomized patients with TTP to either plasma exchange or plasma infusion with fresh frozen plasma and observed that patients receiving plasma exchange had a better response rate and superior survival. Although the authors concluded that plasma exchange is superior to plasma infusion, interpretation should be guarded because patients undergoing plasma exchange received three times as much plasma as patients undergoing plasma infusion. Indeed, a smaller multicenter controlled trial did not observe a difference in outcome when patients were randomized to receive either daily infusions of 15 mL/kg of fresh frozen plasma or plasma exchange with a mixture of 15 mL/kg of fresh frozen

plasma and 45 mL/kg of 5% albumin as replacement fluid (see Table 12-5).[85] Thus, the exact role of plasma removal and plasma infusion in the beneficial effect of plasma exchange remains controversial. A retrospective analysis has found that mortality in TMA is related to low plasmapheresis dosing.[86] Predictive factors for mortality were age older than 40 years, hemoglobin less than 9 mg/dL, and fever; the authors suggested that those with a more severe prognosis should receive more plasmapheresis, but this has not been prospectively examined. A further retrospective review of idiopathic TTP found a mortality of 11%, a response to plasmapheresis rate of 80%, and an association of low hemoglobin with response to plasmapheresis; elevated lactate dehydrogenase levels after therapy predicted relapse.[83] Persistence of low ADAMTS 13 activity or high inhibitor levels after plasmapheresis is associated with a poor outcome, and these assays may be useful to titrate therapy.[81]

Plasmapheresis in combination with plasma infusion is now widely recommended for TMA regardless of its cause. Therapy aims to restore a platelet count to more than 150×10^9 L, with a low hemoglobin and elevated lactate dehydrogenase levels indicating a need for a longer treatment course. Typically, daily plasmapheresis of 60 mL/kg is required for 7 to 14 days with whole plasma or cryosupernatant plasma replacement.[82]

Renal Failure Associated with Multiple Myeloma

See also Chapters 23 and 40.

Renal failure complicates 3% to 9% of cases of multiple myeloma, of which 80% to 90% develop ESRD, and their survival is poor. Renal impairment can be caused by a variety of factors, including precipitation of free light chains within renal tubules and direct toxicity to tubule epithelium. Other factors frequently implicated include hypercalcemia, hyperuricemia, amyloidosis, hyperviscosity, infections, and chemotherapeutic agents. Measurement of circulating free light chains has shown that plasmapheresis is relatively inefficient at their removal, whereas hemodialysis with protein-leaking dialyzers is more effective.[87,88] Randomized, controlled trials have evaluated plasmapheresis in multiple myeloma but preceded the availability of free light chain assays (Table 12-6).[89,90] Johnson and colleagues[89] randomized patients to either chemotherapy and

Table 12-5 Randomized, Controlled Studies Comparing Plasmapheresis and Plasma Infusion in the Treatment of Thrombotic Microangiopathy

Ref	No. of Patients	Diagnosis	Mean Serum Creatinine at Presentation	No. of Phereses	Other Therapies	Remission Rate*	Mortality
Rock et al[84]	102 (adults)	TTP	138 μmol/L	3–36	Aspirin	Pheresis 78%	Pheresis 22%
					Dipyridamole	Controls 49%	Controls 37%
						(P < .05)	(P < .05)
Henon[85]	40 (adults)	TTP	278 μmol/L	3–35	Aspirin	Pheresis 80%	Pheresis 15%
					Dipyridamole	Controls 52%	Controls 3%
						(P = ns)	(P = ns)

*Remission defined as platelet count > 150,000 $\times$ 10⁹/L.
TTP, thrombotic thrombocytopenic purpura.

Table 12-6 Randomized, Controlled Trials Evaluating the Efficacy of Plasmapheresis in the Treatment of Acute Renal Failure Associated with Multiple Myeloma

Ref	No. of Patients	No. on Dialysis	No. of Phereses	Concomitant Therapy	Renal Recovery	Mortality
Johnson et al[89]	21	12 of 21	3–12	Forced diuresis	Pheresis 43%	Pheresis 25%*
				Steroids	Controls 0%	Controls 25%
				Melphalan	(P < .05)	
Zucchelli et al[90]	29	24 of 29	5	Forced diuresis	Pheresis 48%	Pheresis 34%
				Steroids	Controls 18%	Controls 72%
				Cyclophosphamide	(P < .05)	(P = ns)

*No significant difference for renal recovery or mortality.

forced diuresis with or without plasmapheresis and could detect only a small and nonsignificant benefit on renal function despite lowering of plasma concentration of myeloma protein. There was no difference in patient survival. In contrast, Zucchelli and colleagues[90] randomized patients to receive steroids and cyclophosphamide with or without plasmapheresis and observed significant improvements in renal outcome and patient survival. A similar trend was noted in at least three other nonrandomized studies and case series. The Canadian Apheresis Group study found no superior outcome of five to seven plasmaphereses in 104 patients with acute renal failure at the onset of myeloma.[23]

A decision to use plasmapheresis in multiple myeloma with renal failure should be preceded by attention to reversible factors including volume depletion and hypercalcemia. The role of plasmapheresis remains controversial, and the role of free light chain assays and their removal by hemodialysis requires further attention. While plasmapheresis dosing can be guided by renal recovery, existing data suggest that substantial free light chain removal requires prolonged therapy.

Renal Transplantation

Investigations of plasmapheresis in renal transplantation have focused on desensitization, treatment of rejection, and prevention and treatment of recurrent glomerular disease. Comparison of studies is complicated by different background immunosuppressive regimens and variable combination of plasmapheresis with therapeutic antibodies and intravenous immunoglobulin.

Plasmapheresis is increasingly employed to permit desensitization for ABO incompatibility or remove anti-HLA antibodies in sensitized patients. ABO incompatibility is a barrier to live kidney donation in 30% to 50% of cases, and removal of alloantibodies before and immediately after transplantation in combination with immunosuppression, rituximab, intravenous immunoglobulin, or splenectomy has led to graft survival rates similar to those of ABO-compatible transplants.[15] Procedures have involved conventional plasmapheresis or semiselective removal of immunoglobulin by double-filtration pheresis, staphylococcal protein A immunoabsorption, or selective removal of anti-A and anti-B antibodies using a blood group A and B antigen column. The dosing of plasmapheresis before

and after transplantation is titrated against circulating anti-A/B antibodies.

Approximately 20% of patients waiting for cadaveric transplantation have high titers of preformed cytotoxic antibodies that render them at high risk of hyperacute and acute allograft rejection. Plasmapheresis and immunoadsorption are also effective in the removal of cytotoxic anti-HLA antibodies before transplantation, permitting successful transplantation.[12] Prophylactic plasmapheresis of highly sensitized patients in the immediate postoperative period has not shown a major benefit over conventional antirejection prophylaxis.

Evidence supporting removal of donor-specific cytotoxic antibodies and inflammatory mediators in humoral rejection with prominent vascular injury by plasmapheresis in combination with other strategies has been controversial, with older studies reaching conflicting conclusions and more recent, uncontrolled studies reporting benefits on long-term graft function.[91,92] In a comparison with historic controls, the combination of plasmapheresis and intravenous immunoglobulin led to superior graft outcomes in humoral rejection than the additional use of intravenous immunoglobulin alone.[93] The recent identification of antibodies targeting the angiotensin II receptor type I in association with humoral rejection provides a further target for plasmapheresis.[94] Circulating antiendothelial antibodies have been identified in certain cases of humoral rejection associated with a high risk of graft failure; their removal by plasmapheresis is advocated according to the results of several small studies.[91,92] Where donor-specific or other pathogenetic antibodies are identified, dosing of plasmapheresis can be titrated against their levels.[94] Four randomized, controlled trials have been conducted on the efficacy of plasmapheresis in the treatment of established acute rejection (Table 12-7).[95–98] Blake and colleagues[95] randomized 85 patients to receive conventional antirejection therapy with or without plasmapheresis for treatment of all episodes of acute rejection occurring within the first 3 months after transplantation. There was no statistically significant difference in 5-year actuarial graft survival, although there was a trend toward superior graft survival in patients undergoing plasmapheresis. Two of these studies[96,97] did not observe a significant difference in graft survival, whereas the third study[98] suggested a benefit. Thus, all the data published to date do not support the use of therapeutic plasmapheresis for the prevention or

Table 12-7 Randomized, Controlled Trials Evaluating the Efficacy of Plasmapheresis in the Treatment of Acute Allograft Rejection

Ref	No. of Patients	Diagnosis	Graft Biopsy	No. of Phereses	Concomitant Therapy	Graft Survival
Blake et al[95]	85	Acute rejection	Vascular or cellular	5	Steroids (IV)	Pheresis 64% Controls 51%
Allen et al[97]	27	Steroid-resistant rejection	Vascular	6	Steroids (IV) Heparin (SC)	Pheresis 18% Controls 38%
Kirubakaran et al[96]	24	Acute rejection	Vascular	8	Steroids (IV)	Pheresis 33% Controls 75%
Bonomini et al[98]	44	Steroid-resistant rejection	Vascular	3–7	Steroids (IV) Cyclophosphamide	Pheresis 70%* Controls 19%

*Statistically significant benefit of plasmapheresis versus control group ($P < .5$).

treatment of acute rejection. The literature on therapeutic plasmapheresis in chronic allograft nephropathy is limited to a few uncontrolled series, and the results in general have been disappointing, with improvement in graft function being, at best, modest and usually transient.[99]

The presence of a circulating pathogenetic factor and the high rate of recurrent disease have provided a rationale for plasmapheresis in posttransplantation FSGS. Several small studies have reported success both in the prevention of recurrent disease by pre- and posttransplantation plasmapheresis or immunoabsorption and in its treatment, as judged by a reduction in proteinuria, after transplantation.[77,100–104] Further work is required to enable better prediction of the risk of recurrent disease, an understanding of plasmapheresis failure when it is ineffective, and a guide to plasmapheresis dosing in the absence of an accessible biomarker. TMA with or without associated HUS occurs de novo post-transplantation or as recurrent disease; plasmapheresis has been used in both its treatment and prevention.[82,105] The role of plasmapheresis in other glomerulopathies with a high risk of recurrence, such as dense deposit disease, is unclear.

Other Indications

Other indications included hepatitis B–associated polyarteritis, serum sickness, and toxin removal. Polyarteritis nodosa associated with hepatitis B infection has been effectively treated in an observational study by corticosteroids, plasma exchange, and lamivudine. All patients had remission of vasculitis and the majority lost hepatitis B early antigen and hepatitis B virus DNA from the circulation. Randomized trials have not shown a benefit in polyarteritis nodosa without hepatitis B infection.[48]

Serum sickness reactions after polyclonal or monoclonal antibodies, such as antithymocyte globulin, that fail to respond rapidly to corticosteroids, have improved after one or two plasmapheresis procedures.[106] With increasing use of therapeutic monoclonal antibodies, there is a need for a study of the role of plasmapheresis in the management of severe infusion reactions associated with an antiglobulin

response or unintended effects of the primary therapeutic antibody.

The removal of toxic substances by plasmapheresis is indicated when those substances are not readily removed by hemodialysis or charcoal hemoperfusion due to high levels of protein binding.[107] Examples include amanita toxin of *amanita phylloides*, digoxin in combination with antidigoxin antibodies, tricyclic antidepressants and heavy metals in combination with chelation agents.[108] Plasmapheresis dosing can be guided by guided by plasma levels, the volume of distribution of the toxin, and clinical parameters.

COMPLICATIONS OF PLASMAPHERESIS

Plasmapheresis is an invasive procedure with potential complications relating to vascular access, the extracorporeal procedure itself, the removal of coagulation factors and other plasma proteins, and the use of large volumes of pooled plasma products. Adverse events of the procedure occur in one third of patients, are usually mild, and rarely lead to discontinuation or hospital admission.[109] They comprise fever, urticaria, pruritus, hypocalcemic symptoms, and hypotension and are more common with fresh frozen plasma volume replacement than with albumin/saline. More severe reactions include anaphylaxis, thrombocytopenia, and hemorrhage and occur in 0.5% to 3.1% of treated patients.[110] The risk of hemorrhage after plasmapheresis is increased in the presence of uremia, coagulopathy, and thrombocytopenia or after a surgical procedure including renal biopsy. Complications of vascular access include hematomas, pneumothorax, thromboses, and catheter infections. Transmission of chronic viral infections through the use of blood products is now very rare, and there is a theoretical risk of other infections, including prions. Symptomatic hypocalcemia resulting from infusion of citrate (either as the treatment's anticoagulant or in fresh frozen plasma) complicates 1.5% to 9% of treatments. Hypotensive episodes occur in 4% to 7% of patients and can be triggered by vasovagal episodes, delayed or inadequate volume replacement, hypo-oncotic fluid replacement, or anaphylaxis. Repeated plasmapheresis depletes immunoglobulins and other immune reactants, which potentially increases the infective risk, especially in immunosuppressed or uremic patients. However, infection rates reported from randomized trials in the treatment of lupus nephritis and ANCA-associated vasculitis do not support this contention.[22,111,112] Intravenous immunoglobulin therapy has been used in the intensive care setting to reduce infective risk of immunosuppressed patients, including those treated with plasmapheresis, but there is no evidence that routine immunoglobulin replacement after a course of plasmapheresis is justified.

CONCLUSIONS

Use of plasmapheresis has changed in recent years reflecting the availability of evidence largely obtained from controlled, prospective studies. This evidence supports its use for anti-GBM disease, ANCA vasculitis with severe renal failure, refractory cryoglobulinemia, thrombotic microangiopathy, and desensitization before renal transplantation. In contrast, there is no role for plasmapheresis in the routine treatment of lupus nephritis or allograft rejection. More evidence is required to determine whether plasmapheresis is beneficial in other forms of ANCA vasculitis, certain severe lupus subgroups, crescentic IgA nephropathy and HSP, FSGS, multiple myeloma, and humoral transplant rejection. Plasmapheresis remains an expensive and nonspecific therapy in which side effects are common. Newer techniques, such as double filtration and immunoabsorption, offer the opportunity of equal or greater efficacy and reduced toxicity and merit further evaluation.

References

1. Lockwood CM, Rees AJ, Pearson TA, et al: Immunosuppression and plasma-exchange in the treatment of Goodpasture's syndrome. Lancet 1976;1:711–715.
2. Bastin R, Petrover M, Seligmann M, et al: [Fatal acute renal insufficiency complicating Waldenstrom's disease with cryoglobulinemia]. Bull Mem Soc Med Hop Paris 1967;118:259–272.
3. Merkel FK, Bier M, Beavers CD, et al: Delay of the heterograft reaction by selective plasmapheresis. Surg Forum 1970;21:261–263.
4. Levy JB, Turner AN, Rees AJ, Pusey CD: Long-term outcome of anti-glomerular basement membrane antibody disease treated with plasma exchange and immunosuppression. Ann Intern Med 2001;134:1033–1042.
5. Furlan M: Deficient activity of von Willebrand factor-cleaving protease in thrombotic thrombocytopenic purpura. Expert Rev Cardiovasc Ther 2003;1:243–255.
6. Lockwood CM, Worlledge S, Nicholas A, et al: Reversal of impaired splenic function in patients with nephritis or vasculitis (or both) by plasma exchange. N Engl J Med 1979;300:524–530.
7. Bystryn JC, Graf MW, Uhr JW: Regulation of antibody formation by serum antibody II. Removal of specific antibody by means of exchange transfusion. J Exp Med 1970;132:1279–1287.
8. Yokoyama H, Wada T, Furuichi K: Immunomodulation effects and clinical evidence of apheresis in renal diseases. Ther Apher Dial 2003;7:513–519.
9. Burgstaler EA, Pineda AA: Therapeutic plasma exchange: A paired comparison of Fresenius AS104 vs. COBE Spectra. J Clin Apher 2001;16:61–66.
10. Siami GA, Siami FS: Membrane plasmapheresis in the United States: A review over the last 20 years. Ther Apher 2001;5:315–320.
11. Siami FS, Siami GA: Plasmapheresis by using secondary membrane filters: Twelve years of experience. ASAIO J 2000;46:383–388.
12. Taube D, Palmer A, Welsh K, et al: Removal of anti-HLA antibodies prior to transplantation: An effective and successful strategy for highly sensitised renal allograft recipients. Transplant Proc 1989;21:694–695.
13. Elliott JD, Lockwood CM, Hale G, Waldmann H: Semi-specific immuno-absorption and monoclonal antibody therapy in ANCA positive vasculitis: Experience in four cases. Autoimmunity 1998;28:163–171.
14. Sugimoto K, Yamaji K, Yang KS, et al: Immunoadsorption plasmapheresis using a phenylalanine column as an effective treatment for lupus nephritis. Ther Apher Dial 2006;10:187–192.
15. Tyden G, Kumlien G, Fehrman I: Successful ABO-incompatible kidney transplantations without splenectomy using antigen-specific immunoadsorption and rituximab. Transplantation 2003;76:730–731.
16. Stegmayr BG, Almroth G, Berlin G, et al: Plasma exchange or immunoadsorption in patients with rapidly progressive crescentic glomerulonephritis. A Swedish multi-center study. Int J Artif Organs 1999;22:81–87.
17. Esnault VL, Testa A, Jayne DR, et al: Influence of immunoadsorption on the removal of immunoglobulin G autoantibodies in crescentic glomerulonephritis. Nephron 1993;65:180–184.
18. Bambauer R, Arnold A: Plasmapheresis with a substitution solution of human serum protein (5%) versus plasmapheresis with a substitution solution of human albumin (5%) in patients suffering from autoimmune diseases. Artif Organs 1999;23:1079–1087.
19. Arslan O, Tek I, Arat M, et al: Effects of replacement fluids on plasma viscosity used for therapeutic plasma exchange. Ther Apher Dial 2004;8:144–147.
20. Clark WF, Rock GA, Buskard N, et al: Therapeutic plasma exchange: An update from the Canadian Apheresis Group. Ann Intern Med 1999;131:453–462.
21. Rahman T, Harper L: Plasmapheresis in nephrology: An update. Curr Opin Nephrol Hypertens 2006;15:603–609.
22. Jayne DR, Gaskin G, Rasmussen N, et al: Randomized trial of plasma exchange or high-dosage methylprednisolone as adjunctive therapy for severe renal vasculitis. J Am Soc Nephrol 2007;20:2180–2188.
23. Clark WF, Stewart AK, Rock GA, et al: Plasma exchange when myeloma presents as acute renal failure: A randomized, controlled trial. Ann Intern Med 2005;143:777–784.
24. Wilson CB, Dixon FJ: Immunopathology and glomerulonephritis. Annu Rev Med 1974;25:83–98.
25. Simpson IJ, Doak PB, Williams LC, et al: Plasma exchange in Goodpasture's syndrome. Am J Nephrol 1982;2:301–311.
26. Johnson JP, Moore J Jr, Austin HA 3rd, et al: Therapy of anti-glomerular basement membrane antibody disease: Analysis of prognostic significance of clinical, pathologic and treatment factors. Medicine (Baltimore) 1985;64:219–227.
27. Jayne DR, Marshall PD, Jones SJ, Lockwood CM: Autoantibodies to GBM and neutrophil cytoplasm in rapidly progressive glomerulonephritis. Kidney Int 1990;37:965–970.
28. Levy JB, Hammad T, Coulthart A, et al: Clinical features and outcome of patients with both ANCA and anti-GBM antibodies. Kidney Int 2004;66:1535–1540.
29. Jennette JC, Falk RJ, Andrassy K, et al: Nomenclature of systemic vasculitides. Proposal of an international consensus conference. Arthritis Rheum 1994;37:187–192.
30. Xiao H, Heeringa P, Hu P, et al: Antineutrophil cytoplasmic autoantibodies specific for myeloperoxidase cause glomerulonephritis and vasculitis in mice. J Clin Invest 2002;110:955–963.

31. Morgan MD, Harper L, Williams J, Savage C: Anti-neutrophil cytoplasm-associated glomerulonephritis. J Am Soc Nephrol 2006;17:1224–1234.

32. Tesar V, Jelinkova E, Masek Z, et al: Influence of plasma exchange on serum levels of cytokines and adhesion molecules in ANCA-positive renal vasculitis. Blood Purif 1998;16:72–80.

33. Jayne D, Rasmussen N, Andrassy K, et al: A randomized trial of maintenance therapy for vasculitis associated with antineutrophil cytoplasmic autoantibodies. N Engl J Med 2003;349:36–44.

34. Szpirt WRN: Plasma exchange and cyclosporin A in Wegener's granulomatosis. Int J Artif Organs 1996;10:501–505.

35. Cole E, Cattran D, Magil A, et al: A prospective randomized trial of plasma exchange as additive therapy in idiopathic crescentic glomerulonephritis. The Canadian Apheresis Study Group. Am J Kidney Dis 1992;20:261–269.

36. Pusey CD, Rees AJ, Evans DJ, et al: Plasma exchange in focal necrotizing glomerulonephritis without anti-GBM antibodies. Kidney Int 1991;40:757–763.

37. Glockner WM, Sieberth HG, Wichmann HE, et al: Plasma exchange and immunosuppression in rapidly progressive glomerulonephritis: A controlled, multi-center study. Clin Nephrol 1988;29:1–8.

38. Mauri JM, Gonzalez MT, Poveda R, et al: Therapeutic plasma exchange in the treatment of rapidly progressive glomerulonephritis. Plasma Ther Transfus Technol 1985;6:587–591.

39. Rifle G, Dechelette E: Treatment of rapidly progressive glomerulonephritis by plasma exchange and methyl prednisolone pulses. Prog Clin Biol Res 1990;337:263–267.

40. Guillevin L, Cevallos R, Durand-Gasselin B, et al: Treatment of glomerulonephritis in microscopic polyangiitis and Churg-Strauss syndrome. Indications of plasma exchanges, meta-analysis of 2 randomized studies on 140 patients, 32 with glomerulonephritis. Ann Med Interne (Paris) 1997;148:198–204.

41. Aasarod K, Iversen BM, Hammerstrom J, et al: Clinical outcome of patients with Wegener's granulomatosis treated with plasma exchange. Blood Purif 2002;20:167–173.

42. Frasca GM, Soverini ML, Falaschini A, et al: Plasma exchange treatment improves prognosis of antineutrophil cytoplasmic antibody-associated crescentic glomerulonephritis: A case-control study in 26 patients from a single center. Ther Apher Dial 2003;7:540–546.

43. Bolton WK, Sturgill BC: Methylprednisolone therapy for acute crescentic rapidly progressive glomerulonephritis. Am J Nephrol 1989;9:368–375.

44. Jayne DR, Gaskin G, Rasmussen N, et al: Randomized trial of plasma exchange or high-dosage methylprednisolone as adjunctive therapy for severe renal vasculitis. J Am Soc Nephrol 2007;18:2180–2188.

45. de Lind van Wijngaarden RA, Hauer HA, Wolterbeek R, et al: Chances of renal recovery for dialysis-dependent ANCA-associated glomerulonephritis. J Am Soc Nephrol 2007;18:2189–2197.

46. Specks U: Diffuse alveolar hemorrhage syndromes. Curr Opin Rheumatol 2001;13:12–17.

47. Gallagher H, Kwan JT, Jayne DR: Pulmonary renal syndrome: A 4-year, single-center experience. Am J Kidney Dis 2002;39:42–47.

48. Guillevin L, Lhote F, Cohen P, et al: Corticosteroids plus pulse cyclophosphamide and plasma exchanges versus corticosteroids plus pulse cyclophosphamide alone in the treatment of polyarteritis nodosa and Churg-Strauss syndrome patients with factors predicting poor prognosis. A prospective, randomized trial in sixty-two patients. Arthritis Rheum 1995;38:1638–1645.

49. Korbet SM, Schwartz MM, Evans J, Lewis EJ: Severe lupus nephritis: Racial differences in presentation and outcome. J Am Soc Nephrol 2007;18:244–254.

50. Cervera R, Khamashta MA, Font J, et al: Morbidity and mortality in systemic lupus erythematosus during a 10-year period: A comparison of early and late manifestations in a cohort of 1,000 patients. Medicine (Baltimore) 2003;82:299–308.

51. Lewis EJ, Hunsicker LG, Lan SP, et al: A controlled trial of plasmapheresis therapy in severe lupus nephritis. The Lupus Nephritis Collaborative Study Group. N Engl J Med 1992;326:1373–1379.

52. Wei N, Klippel JH, Huston DP, et al: Randomised trial of plasma exchange in mild systemic lupus erythematosus. Lancet 1983;1:17–22.

53. Derksen RH, Hene RJ, Kallenberg CG, et al: Prospective multi-centre trial on the short-term effects of plasma exchange versus cytotoxic drugs in steroid-resistant lupus nephritis. Neth J Med 1988;33:168–177.

54. French Group: Randomised trial of plasma exchange in severe acute systemic lupus erythematosus. Plasma Ther Transfus Technol 1985;6:535–539.

55. Clark WF, Cattran DC, Balfe JW, et al: Chronic plasma exchange in systemic lupus erythematosus nephritis. Proc Eur Dial Transplant Assoc 1983;20:629–635.

56. Euler HH, Guillevin L: Plasmapheresis and subsequent pulse cyclophosphamide in severe systemic lupus erythematosus. An interim report of the Lupus Plasmapheresis Study Group. Ann Med Interne (Paris) 1994;145:296–302.

57. Wallace DJ, Goldfinger D, Pepkowitz SH, et al: Randomized controlled trial of pulse/synchronization cyclophosphamide/apheresis for proliferative lupus nephritis. J Clin Apher 1998;13:163–166.

58. Euler HH, Schroeder JO, Harten P, et al: Treatment-free remission in severe systemic lupus erythematosus following synchronization of plasmapheresis with subsequent pulse cyclophosphamide. Arthritis Rheum 1994;37:1784–1794.

59. Bucciarelli S, Espinosa G, Cervera R, et al: Mortality in the catastrophic antiphospholipid syndrome: Causes of death and prognostic factors in a series of 250 patients. Arthritis Rheum 2006;54:2568–2576.

60. Asherson RA, Cervera R, de Groot PG, et al: Catastrophic antiphospholipid syndrome: International consensus statement on classification criteria and treatment guidelines. Lupus 2003;12:530–534.

61. Coll AP, Morganstein D, Jayne D, et al: Successful treatment of Type B insulin resistance in a patient with otherwise quiescent systemic lupus erythematosus. Diabet Med 2005;22:814–815.

62. Stummvoll GH, Aringer M, Jansen M, et al: Immunoadsorption (IAS) as a rescue therapy in SLE: Considerations on safety and efficacy. Wien Klin Wochenschr 2004;116:716–724.

63. Pagnoux C, Korach JM, Guillevin L: Indications for plasma exchange in systemic lupus erythematosus in 2005. Lupus 2005;14:871–877.

64. Ferri C, Mascia MT: Cryoglobulinemic vasculitis. Curr Opin Rheumatol 2006;18:54–63.

65. Berkman EM, Orlin JB: Use of plasmapheresis and partial plasma exchange in the management of patients with cryoglobulinemia. Transfusion 1980;20:171–178.

66. Hausfater P, Cacoub P, Assogba U, et al: Plasma exchange and interferon-alpha pharmacokinetics in patients with hepatitis C virus-associated systemic vasculitis. Nephron 2002;91:627–630.

67. Garini G, Allegri L, Vaglio A, Buzio C: Hepatitis C virus-related cryoglobulinemia and glomerulonephritis: Pathogenesis and therapeutic strategies. Ann Ital Med Int 2005;20:71–80.

68. Beddhu S, Bastacky S, Johnson JP: The clinical and morphologic spectrum of renal cryoglobulinemia. Medicine (Baltimore) 2002;81:398–409.

69. Koukoulaki M, Abeygunasekara SC, Smith KG, Jayne DR: Remission of refractory hepatitis C-negative cryoglobulinaemic vasculitis after rituximab and infliximab. Nephrol Dial Transplant 2005;20:213–216.

70. Coppo R, Amore A, Gianoglio B: Clinical features of Henoch-Schönlein purpura. Italian Group of Renal Immunopathology. Ann Med Interne (Paris) 1999;150:143–150.

71. Roccatello D, Ferro M, Coppo R, et al: Report on intensive treatment of extracapillary glomerulonephritis with focus on crescentic IgA nephropathy. Nephrol Dial Transplant 1995;10:2054–2059.

72. Coppo R, Basolo B, Roccatello D, et al: Plasma exchange in progressive primary IgA nephropathy. Int J Artif Organs 1985;8:55–58.

73. Shenoy M, Ognjanovic MV, Coulthard MG: Treating severe Henoch-Schönlein and IgA nephritis with plasmapheresis alone. Pediatr Nephrol 2007;22:1167–1171.

74. Kawasaki Y, Suzuki J, Murai M, et al: Plasmapheresis therapy for rapidly progressive Henoch-Schönlein nephritis. Pediatr Nephrol 2004;19:920–923.

75. Zaffanello M, Brugnara M, Franchini M: Therapy for children with Henoch-Schonlein purpura nephritis: A systematic review. Sci World J 2007;7:20–30.

76. Savin VJ, Sharma R, Sharma M, et al: Circulating factor associated with increased glomerular permeability to albumin in recurrent focal segmental glomerulosclerosis. N Engl J Med 1996;334:878–883.

77. Bosch T, Wendler T: Extracorporeal plasma treatment in primary and recurrent focal segmental glomerular sclerosis: A review. Ther Apher 2001;5:155–160.

78. Stirling CM, Mathieson P, Boulton-Jones JM, et al: Treatment and outcome of adult patients with primary focal segmental glomerulosclerosis in five UK renal units. Q J Med 2005;98:443–449.

79. Ghiggeri GM, Musante L, Candiano G, et al: Protracted remission of proteinuria after combined therapy with plasmapheresis and anti-CD20 antibodies/cyclophosphamide in a child with oligoclonal IgM and glomerulosclerosis. Pediatr Nephrol 2007;22:1953–1956.

80. Nguyen TC, Stegmayr B, Busund R, et al: Plasma therapies in thrombotic syndromes. Int J Artif Organs 2005;28:459–465.

81. Zheng XL, Kaufman RM, Goodnough LT, Sadler JE: Effect of plasma exchange on plasma ADAMTS13 metalloprotease activity, inhibitor level, and clinical outcome in patients with idiopathic and nonidiopathic thrombotic thrombocytopenic purpura. Blood 2004;103:4043–4049.

82. Hwang WY, Chai LY, Ng HJ, et al: Therapeutic plasmapheresis for the treatment of the thrombotic thrombocytopenic purpura-haemolytic uraemic syndromes. Singapore Med J 2004;45:219–223.

83. Tuncer HH, Oster RA, Huang ST, Marques MB: Predictors of response and relapse in a cohort of adults with thrombotic thrombocytopenic purpura-hemolytic uremic syndrome: A single-institution experience. Transfusion 2007;47:107–114.

84. Rock GA, Shumak KH, Buskard NA, et al: Comparison of plasma exchange with plasma infusion in the treatment of thrombotic thrombocytopenic purpura. Canadian Apheresis Study Group. N Engl J Med 1991;325:393–397.

85. Henon P: [Treatment of thrombotic thrombopenic purpura. Results of a multicenter randomized clinical study]. Presse Med 1991;20:1761–1767.

86. Wyllie BF, Garg AX, Macnab J, et al: Thrombotic thrombocytopenic purpura/haemolytic uraemic syndrome: A new index predicting response to plasma exchange. Br J Haematol 2006;132:204–209.

87. Hutchison CA, Cockwell P, Reid S, et al: Efficient removal of immunoglobulin free light chains by hemodialysis for multiple myeloma: In vitro and in vivo studies. J Am Soc Nephrol 2007;18:886–895.

88. Cserti C, Haspel R, Stowell C, Dzik W: Light-chain removal by plasmapheresis in myeloma-associated renal failure. Transfusion 2007;47:511–514.

89. Johnson WJ, Kyle RA, Pineda AA, et al: Treatment of renal failure associated with multiple myeloma. Plasmapheresis, hemodialysis, and chemotherapy. Arch Intern Med 1990;150:863–869.

90. Zucchelli P, Pasquali S, Cagnoli L, Rovinetti C: Plasma exchange therapy in acute renal failure due to light chain myeloma. Trans Am Soc Artif Intern Organs 1984;30:36–39.

91. Shah A, Nadasdy T, Arend L, et al: Treatment of C4d-positive acute humoral rejection with plasmapheresis and rabbit polyclonal antithymocyte globulin. Transplantation 2004;77:1399–1405.

92. Ibernon M, Gil-Vernet S, Carrera M, et al: Therapy with plasmapheresis and intravenous immunoglobulin for acute humoral rejection in kidney transplantation. Transplant Proc 2005;37:3743–3745.

93. Lehrich RW, Rocha PN, Reinsmoen N, et al: Intravenous immunoglobulin and plasmapheresis in acute humoral rejection: Experience in renal allograft transplantation. Hum Immunol 2005;66:350–358.

94. Dragun D, Muller DN, Brasen JH, et al: Angiotensin II type 1-receptor activating antibodies in renal-allograft rejection. N Engl J Med 2005;352:558–569.

95. Blake P, Sutton D, Cardella CJ: Plasma exchange in acute renal transplant rejection. Prog Clin Biol Res 1990;337:249–252.

96. Kirubakaran MG, Disney AP, Norman J, et al: A controlled trial of plasmapheresis in the treatment of renal allograft rejection. Transplantation 1981;32:164–165.

97. Allen NH, Dyer P, Geoghegan T, et al: Plasma exchange in acute renal allograft rejection. A controlled trial. Transplantation 1983;35:425–428.

98. Bonomini V, Vangelista A, Frasca GM, et al: Effects of plasmapheresis in renal transplant rejection. A controlled study. Trans Am Soc Artif Intern Organs 1985;31:698–703.

99. Frasca GM, Martella D, Vangelista A, Bonomini V: Ten years experience with plasma exchange in renal transplantation. Int J Artif Organs 1991;14:51–55.

100. Valdivia P, Gonzalez Roncero F, Gentil MA, et al: Plasmapheresis for the prophylaxis and treatment of recurrent focal segmental glomerulosclerosis following renal transplant. Transplant Proc 2005;37:1473–1474.

101. Gohh RY, Yango AF, Morrissey PE, et al: Preemptive plasmapheresis and recurrence of FSGS in high-risk renal transplant recipients. Am J Transplant 2005;5:2907–2912.

102. Otsubo S, Tanabe K, Shinmura H, et al: Effect of post-transplant double filtration plasmapheresis on recurrent focal and segmental glomerulosclerosis in renal transplant recipients. Ther Apher Dial 2004;8:299–304.

103. Garcia CD, Bittencourt VB, Tumelero A, et al: Plasmapheresis for recurrent posttransplant focal segmental glomerulosclerosis. Transplant Proc 2006;38:1904–1905.

104. Dantal J, Bigot E, Bogers W, et al: Effect of plasma protein adsorption on protein excretion in kidney-transplant recipients with recurrent nephrotic syndrome. N Engl J Med 1994;330:7–14.

105. Ponticelli C: De novo thrombotic microangiopathy. An underrated complication of renal transplantation. Clin Nephrol 2007;67:335–340.

106. Tanriover B, Chuang P, Fishbach B, et al: Polyclonal antibody-induced serum sickness in renal transplant recipients: Treatment with therapeutic plasma exchange. Transplantation 2005;80:279–281.

107. Nenov VD, Marinov P, Sabeva J, Nenov DS: Current applications of plasmapheresis in clinical toxicology. Nephrol Dial Transplant 2003;18:56–58.

108. Santos-Araujo C, Campos M, Gavina C, et al: Combined use of plasmapheresis and antidigoxin antibodies in a patient with severe digoxin intoxication and acute renal failure. Nephrol Dial Transplant 2007;22:257–258.

109. Shemin D, Briggs D, Greenan M: Complications of therapeutic plasma exchange: A prospective study of 1,727 procedures. J Clin Apher 2007;22:270–276.

110. Mokrzycki MH, Kaplan AA: Therapeutic plasma exchange: Complications and management. Am J Kidney Dis 1994;23:817–827.

111. Bussel A, Jais JP: Side effects and mortality associated with plasma exchange: A three year experience with a regional register. Life Support Syst 1987;5:353–358.

112. Pohl MA, Lan SP, Berl T: Plasmapheresis does not increase the risk for infection in immunosuppressed patients with severe lupus nephritis. The Lupus Nephritis Collaborative Study Group. Ann Intern Med 1991;114:924–929.

Further Reading

Crosson JT: Focal segmental glomerulosclerosis and renal transplantation. Transplant Proc 2007;39:737–743.

ICON Health Publications: Plasmapheresis—A Medical Dictionary, Bibliography, and Annotated Research Guide to Internet References. San Diego: ICON Health Publications, 2004.

Nguyen TC, Stegmayr B, Busund R, et al: Plasma therapies in thrombotic syndromes. Int J Artif Organs 2005;28:459–465.

Pagnoux C: Plasma exchange for systemic lupus erythematosus. Transfus Apher Sci 2007;36:187–193.

Rahman T, Harper L: Plasmapheresis in nephrology: An update. Curr Opin Nephrol Hypertens 2006;15:603–609.

Siami GA, Siami FS: Membrane plasmapheresis in the United States: A review over the last 20 years. Ther Apher 2001;5:315–320.

Chapter 13

Management of Infection-Associated Glomerulonephritis

Steven J. Chadban and Robert C. Atkins

CHAPTER CONTENTS

An association between glomerulonephritis and infectious disease has long been recognized. Glomerular damage occurs in infection-associated glomerulonephritis as a result of three pathogenic pathways: the direct renal effects of the invading microorganism, the sepsis-induced dysregulation of systemic circulation and homeostasis, and, most importantly, the innate and adaptive host immune responses to microbial antigens. Current clinical therapies actively target the invading organism and provide support for host homeostasis, whereas the aberrant host immune response is not directly addressed.

The epidemiology of infectious disease and the problems in producing reliable and accurate animal models make infection-associated glomerulonephritis a difficult condition to study. Despite some advances in our understanding of the immunopathogenesis, little impact has been made on specific immunotherapy, and the treatment of infection-associated glomerulonephritis remains largely empirical rather than evidence based. With these limitations in mind, this chapter briefly reviews recent conceptual advances in the understanding of this form of glomerulonephritis and then discusses current therapeutic strategies associated with specific organisms and sites of infection. Approaches to management are provided and avenues amenable to future research highlighted. Renal diseases caused by infections

with human immunodeficiency virus (HIV) and hepatitis B virus are covered in Chapter 24 and hepatitis C virus in Chapter 14. Drug doses, including correction factors for renal dysfunction, are listed in Chapter 91.

RECENT DEVELOPMENTS IN INFECTION-ASSOCIATED GLOMERULONEPHRITIS

The epidemiology of infection-associated glomerulonephritis has changed. Classic poststreptococcal glomerulonephritis (PSGN) remains the most common cause of the nephritic syndrome in some communities.[1,2] Staphylococcal infection has, however, become a far more frequent precipitant of glomerulonephritis in developed countries.[3] Infective endocarditis is now the bacterial infection most frequently associated with glomerulonephritis in developed countries and is predominantly caused by staphylococci introduced via needles or surgery.[3,4] In Europe and North America, hepatitis C is a common cause of cryoglobulinemia and membranoproliferative glomerulonephritis, whereas on a worldwide scale, hepatitis B and malaria persist as dominant causes of the nephrotic syndrome.[5]

As the epidemiology has evolved, the classification of glomerulonephritis resulting from infection has broadened. As the incidence of PSGN in developed countries has decreased, infection with an increasing number of other microorganisms has been associated with glomerular disease. The glomerular lesions induced include classic postinfectious exudative endocapillary changes, but also mesangioproliferative, mesangiocapillary, crescentic, and membranous lesions. The time course varies such that clinical glomerulonephritis may become apparent during the acute or chronic infective phase or during convalescence. Accordingly, the term *postinfectious glomerulonephritis* is best used with specific reference to poststreptococcal disease, whereas the broader term *infection-associated glomerulonephritis* is the more appropriate nomenclature to apply to the entire spectrum of glomerulonephritis that results from infection.

The importance of host immune status is increasingly recognized as being central to the development of infection-associated glomerulonephritis and to the patient's prognosis. Alcoholism is prevalent throughout the world and is now well recognized as conferring both an increased susceptibility to infection-associated glomerulonephritis and a poor prognosis for this condition.[3,6] In addition, the immune dysregulation induced by chronic viral infections may enhance patient susceptibility to glomerulonephritis, particularly in the case of infections with hepatitis B, hepatitis C, and HIV.

Progress in molecular biologic technology has facilitated new insights into the pathogenesis of glomerulonephritis.[7] Infectious organisms may produce glomerular damage via several mechanisms:

1. Direct cytopathic effects, e.g., staphylococcal antigens may induce glomerular damage in the absence of immunoglobulin
2. Engagement of innate immune receptors by microorganisms, such as Toll-like receptor 4 engagement by bacterial lipopolysaccharide, causing activation of inflammatory cells and intrinsic kidney cells
3. Host cell–mediated damage due to the presence of the organism within renal cells, with subsequent cell surface antigen expression serving to attract cytotoxic T cells
4. Deposition of circulating immune complexes or cryoglobulins within the glomerulus
5. Formation of in situ immune complexes to planted infective antigens
6. Induction of autoimmunity via the development of cross-reactive antibodies
7. Indirect effects of infection mediated by cytokines and growth factors[8,9]

Various infections have been shown to induce glomerular damage via these mechanisms, although one major discrepancy exists. Humans incur infection many times a year during every year of their life, yet only a minority develop clinical nephritis. The reason that only some individuals develop glomerulonephritis in response to infection with particular organisms remains an enigma. Certainly some strains of organism are more nephrogenic than others (e.g., nephritogenic versus nonnephrogenic streptococci). Patient susceptibility factors have also been identified, such as complement deficiency, whereas others remain unidentified but inferred, such as familial susceptibility to PSGN. It appears likely that several infection-dependent and host-dependent factors must interact to produce infection-associated glomerulonephritis.

The diagnosis of infection-associated glomerulonephritis should be considered in three broad clinical settings. First, the patient who develops renal dysfunction or an abnormal urinary sediment in the context of an infectious illness may have infection-associated glomerulonephritis. This should be differentiated from renal tract infection, interstitial nephritis (due to infection or therapy), preexisting or concurrent renal disease, and the indirect effects of fever on urinary protein and red cell content. Second, infection-associated glomerulonephritis remains underdiagnosed as a cause of glomerulonephritis in the general community and should therefore be considered in all patients presenting with glomerular abnormalities.[10] Risk factors for infection with potentially nephritogenic organisms should be sought in the patient history. Examination for signs of infection such as skin rash, needle tracks, and stigmata of endocarditis should be performed. Specific serologic investigations, tailored to the epidemiology of infectious disease relevant to the patient, should be undertaken. Percutaneous renal biopsy should be performed in all cases in the absence of significant contraindications.[10] Finally, an infection-related exacerbation should be considered in patients with preexisting glomerulonephritis who develop an unexplained flare of their disease.[7]

The likelihood of renal and patient recovery depends on host status, control of infection, and the degree of kidney damage as assessed by both clinical and biopsy parameters. Drug and alcohol withdrawal, malnutrition, immunosuppression, and concurrent infection (both preexisting and hospital acquired) are major contributors to the high rates of morbidity (50%) and mortality (11%) seen in patients with infection-associated glomerulonephritis.[3] Additionally, screening tests for concurrent disease, such as HIV and viral hepatitis, should be undertaken to avoid diagnostic confusion and to optimize management. Cases in which severe crescentic disease has been present on a renal biopsy sample or in which renal dysfunction has persisted or evolved despite clinical eradication of infection have prompted the use of immunosuppressive therapy: 35 cases of infection-associated glomerulonephritis (including 11 cases of classic PSGN) treated with immunosuppressants have been reported[3,11–19] (Table 13-1). Endocarditis was the most frequently associated infection. One controlled trial of prednisolone, cyclophosphamide, dipyridamole, and azathioprine in children with crescentic PSGN showed no benefit over placebo.[18] All other reports involved uncontrolled therapeutic trials of corticosteroids (100%), cyclophosphamide (44%), azathioprine (4%), heparin (4%), dipyridamole (8%), and plasmapheresis (20%), used either singly or in various combinations and always in conjunction with antibiotics. Indices of renal function improved in 52% of cases. No specific reports of therapy-related morbidity or mortality were made; however, 12% of patients progressed to terminal renal failure and 8% of patients died of multiple complications including renal failure. Thus, based on these uncontrolled data, the role of immunosuppressive therapy for infection-associated glomerulonephritis is difficult to determine. Bearing in mind the potential for positive publication bias, these results clearly highlight the need to mount a prospective, controlled clinical trial to examine the safety and efficacy of immunosuppression in this setting. Until then, this form of treatment cannot be broadly recommended, except for consideration in cases of severe renal failure unresponsive to documented clearance of infection.

Table 13-1 Immunosuppressive Treatment of Glomerulonephritis Associated with Bacterial Infection: Published Reports and Trials

Ref.	Infection	No. of Patients	Histology	Treatment	Outcome
Montseny et al[3]	Various, unspecified	17	Crescents (12), Endo (5)	Prednisone (17), cyclophosphamide (8)	5 resolved, 8 CRF, 2 ESRD, 2 deceased
Vanwalleghem et al[11]	*Staphylococcus aureus* prosthesis	1	Crescents, 27%	Prednisone	Improved
Yamashita et al[12]	*S. aureus* pneumonia	1	?	Plasmapheresis, prednisone	Improved late ESRD
Rovzar et al[13]	*Streptococcus viridans* endocarditis	1	Crescents, >50%	Plasmapheresis, prednisone, azathioprine	Improved
McKenzie et al[14]	Endocarditis	1	Crescents, 60%	Plasmapheresis, prednisone	Improved
Ayres et al[15]	Streptococcal endocarditis	1	Crescents, 80%	Prednison, cyclophosphamide, heparin, dipyridamole	Improved
McKinsey et al[16]	*S. aureus* septicemia	1	Some crescents	Prednisone	Improved
Kupari and Teerenhovi[17]	Dental abscess	1	Crescents, 80%	Plasmapheresis, prednisone, cyclophosphamide	Resolved
Roy et al[18]	PSGN	5 treated, 5 controls	Crescents, 70%; crescents, 65%	Prednisone, azathioprine, cyclophosphamide, dipyridamole	Resolved*
Fairley et al[19]	PSGN	1	Crescents, 83%	Plasmapheresis, prednisone, cyclophosphamide, dipyridamole	Resolved

*All patients showed resolution of clinical indicators of renal damage; however, two patients died of causes thought to be unrelated to therapy.[18]

CRF, chronic renal failure; Endo, endoproliferative glomerulonephritis; ESRD, end-stage renal disease; PSGN, poststreptococcal glomerulonephritis.

The prognosis for recovery from infection-associated glomerulonephritis remains linked to the interaction between host factors, the infecting organism, and the amount of kidney damage that is incurred. Recent therapeutic developments have made little impact, with the exceptions of antibiotic prophylaxis for at-risk populations during epidemics of nephritogenic streptococcal infection[2] and the use of antiviral agents for the treatment of glomerulonephritis associated with hepatitis C and B viruses (see Chapters 14 and 24). Thus, the prognosis has changed in line with the epidemiology. In areas where infection-associated glomerulonephritis remains primarily streptococcal, the prognosis remains generally favorable, at least in the short to medium term.[1,20] However, in communities where the majority of cases of infection-associated glomerulonephritis are due to staphylococcal infection occurring in alcoholics or intravenous drug abusers, the prognosis is relatively poor for both patient and renal survival.[3,21]

Is resolution of the clinical episode of acute infection-associated glomerulonephritis all that matters? Long-term follow-up studies of survivors of PSGN have revealed evidence of chronic kidney disease on clinical grounds and on kidney biopsy in a significant proportion and renal failure in a minority.[20,22] Whether these findings are applicable to all forms of infection-associated glomerulonephritis is

unknown. Also unknown is whether such asymptomatic abnormalities indicate a significant increase in the lifetime risk of renal failure, cardiovascular disease, or overall mortality for these patients.[7] This information is required in order to provide accurate prognostic information for both the patient and caring physician and to facilitate the development and use of renoprotective strategies during the acute and recovery phases of infection-associated glomerulonephritis (see Chapter 62).

BACTERIAL INFECTIONS

Streptococcus

Poststreptococcal Glomerulonephritis

The management of classic PSGN involves three phases: (1) the prompt treatment of streptococcal infections in the community, (2) the management of the patient with nephritis, and (3) the prevention or detection of streptococcal disease and PSGN among the patient's contacts.

Animal data have demonstrated that penicillin given within 3 days of the onset of streptococcal infection is able to prevent the development of nephritis, and although there is no conclusive evidence that antibiotic treatment of pharyngitis or impetigo in humans is effective in preventing the development of PSGN, such treatment seems logical to reduce the streptococcal antigenic load. Additionally, antibiotics may prevent the development of suppurative complications in the individual and hopefully reduce the prevalence of pathogenic streptococci in the community. Thus, as the cost and adverse-effect profile of penicillin is favorable, it should be given to patients with clinically probable and/or culture-positive streptococcal pharyngitis or impetigo. The appropriate dose for adults is 1.2 million units of benzathine benzylpenicillin as a single intramuscular injection or 250 mg phenoxymethyl penicillin every 6 hours PO for 10 days. Children should receive half doses, and erythromycin should be given to individuals who are allergic to penicillin.

The diagnosis of PSGN is made in a patient who has historical and/or laboratory evidence of antecedent streptococcal infection, which was followed by a latent period before the development of nephritis. The laboratory finding of decreased C3 is a sensitive, but not specific, supporting feature. Renal biopsy is often required for the diagnosis in endemic cases, although less so in the epidemic situation, to differentiate PSGN from other causes of the nephritic syndrome.

Once the diagnosis is made, patient management involves three phases. First, penicillin is given in an attempt to eliminate streptococcal antigenemia. Second, features of the nephritic syndrome are treated supportively. If hypertension or signs of volume overload are present, sodium intake should be minimized and fluid intake restricted to 1000 mL/day in mild cases and 500 mL/day in moderate to severe cases. Loop diuretics should be used to manage edema. Therapy should be guided by the maintenance of strict fluid balance records including daily weights. In cases of severe volume overload with imminent or actual hypertensive encephalopathy or pulmonary edema, morphine, oxygen, sedation, ventilation, intravenous nitrates, and hydralazine may be required. In this setting, urgent hemodialysis including ultrafiltration is often the most effective and physiologic therapeutic maneuver. With good supportive care, attention to nutrition, and the treatment of intercurrent infection, an acute mortality of less than 1% can be expected.[20] Resolution is spontaneous and generally complete within several months. Patients with adult-onset, nephrotic-range, or persistent proteinuria; extensive crescent formation; and heavy capillary IgG/C3 deposition on biopsy are an exception to this rule and commonly exhibit an incomplete renal recovery. A minority will progress to end-stage renal failure.[20,22]

Combined immunosuppressive and anticoagulant therapy has been tried in severe PSGN in children and was not found to be of benefit.[18] Persisting hypertension should be treated, preferably with an angiotensin-converting enzyme inhibitor. Acute PSGN recurs only rarely, due to the development of type-specific, long-lasting, and protective immunity to streptococcal M protein.

Management of the patient in the long term is less clearly defined. Studies of patients up to 20 years after an episode of acute PSGN reveal conflicting results but clear trends in terms of renal outcome. The vast majority of patients recover acutely, but 5% to 60% will show features of subclinical renal dysfunction (proteinuria or decreased creatinine clearance, fibrosis, and glomerulosclerosis on biopsy) or hypertension during the next 10 to 20 years,[20,22] and almost all patients with resolved PSGN can be shown to have a decreased renal functional reserve. Asymptomatic abnormalities are more common sequelae of PSGN in adults than in children. Whether such abnormalities indicate a significant increase in the lifetime risk of the development of progressive renal failure remains to be determined. It would seem prudent to monitor all patients who recover from PSGN with annual assessment of blood pressure, urinary protein excretion, and creatinine clearance. Hypertension should be treated aggressively, and the development of proteinuria or decreased creatinine clearance should prompt the adoption of general measures for the preservation of renal function (see Chapter 62).

Epidemics of PSGN continue to occur in communities that have relatively poor hygiene and overcrowding. The administration of penicillin (2.4 million units IM for adults, half dose for children) to all community members during such outbreaks appears to be of benefit.[2]

Other Streptococcal Infections

Streptococcus viridans has classically been implicated as the major cause of subacute bacterial endocarditis, whereas *Streptococcus faecalis* (enterococcus) is an increasingly recognized cause of acute endocarditis. These and other groups of streptococci have been documented as causes of proliferative glomerulonephritis, both focal and diffuse, in the setting of infectious endocarditis and other visceral infections. Principles of diagnosis and management are similar to those detailed here for staphylococcal endocarditis. Antibiotic resistance is becoming problematic. The emergence of penicillin-resistant streptococci requires the use of penicillin plus an aminoglycoside until bacterial sensitivities are defined. Enterococci are generally penicillin insensitive and require combination therapy with ampicillin and low-dose gentamycin, which act synergistically. Vancomycin is indicated if enterococci with high-level penicillin resistance are prevalent or are isolated; however, the development of vancomycin-resistant enterococci is a major concern and requires consultation with an antimicrobial expert.[23] Vigilant monitoring of aminoglycoside and vancomycin levels are required to avoid toxicity.

Staphylococcus

Staphylococcal Endocarditis

Staphylococcal endocarditis may occur on normal, damaged, or prosthetic valves on either the left or the right side of the heart. Infection of a previously normal tricuspid valve is particularly commonly seen in intravenous drug abusers. The presentation may be acute, particularly in the case of *Staphylococcus aureus* infection, or chronic, as is typically seen with coagulase-negative staphylococcal endocarditis.

Glomerulonephritis occurs in 20% to 80% of cases of infective endocarditis and may be recognized at any stage of the illness.[4] In cases of infective endocarditis complicated by glomerulonephritis, circulating immune complexes (90% of cases), rheumatoid factors (10%–70%), and cryoglobulins (84%–95%) are present, whereas C3 is frequently reduced in serum. No serologic marker has consistently been shown to have predictive value in identifying the presence or absence of glomerulonephritis in patients with endocarditis. Serology may be more useful for monitoring therapy, as the persistence of circulating immune complexes and C3 depletion, despite antibiotic treatment, has been shown to indicate the failure of therapy and a high probability of persistent infection and glomerulonephritis.[4] Microbiologic identification, including the determination of antibiotic sensitivities, is crucial in establishing a therapeutic plan. Renal biopsy is also crucial to both confirm the diagnosis and provide prognostic information. Biopsy specimens may reveal either focal or diffuse proliferative changes, often accompanied by an exudate of neutrophils. Crescents are less commonly seen. Immunostaining reveals granular C3 deposition, which is often but not always accompanied by IgG or IgM. Staphylococcal antigens have frequently been reported within damaged glomeruli in the absence of immunoglobulin and rarely in the absence of C3, suggesting that staphylococci may induce either direct or complement-mediated renal injury, independent of immunoglobulin.[24]

Treatment involves the intravenous administration of bactericidal antibiotics at dosages appropriate for renal function (see Chapter 91). The role of surgery is to restore valve function and remove foci of infection where necessary. This requires an ongoing evaluation of the patient in consultation with the involved infectious disease and cardiac teams. The persistence of glomerulonephritis, despite the apparent resolution of infection, is an additional indication to reassess the affected heart valve with a view to surgery because the surgical removal of a sterile vegetation has been associated with improvement in renal function.[17] Supportive measures for renal and cardiac function and the optimization of host nutrition and immune status are important components of therapy. As summarized in Table 13-1, the use of immunosuppression after apparent eradication of infection has been reported; however, this approach incurs significant risk of infective relapse and further cardiac decompensation.[3,11,13–15]

Staphylococcal Septicemia

Proliferative glomerulonephritis was documented in 35% of cases of fatal staphylococcal septicemia at autopsy.[25] Treatment is similar to that for infectious endocarditis, in addition to a rigorous search for primary (e.g., skin, bone, joint) and secondary (e.g., heart, lung) sites of infection.

Visceral Abscess

Abscesses within abdominal viscera, bone, joint, lung, and other tissues have been associated with infection-associated glomerulonephritis. *S. aureus*, and, less commonly, other organisms, have been cultured from the abscess fluid. Although blood cultures have frequently been negative in reported cases, bacterial antigens have been identified within glomerular deposits accompanied by immunoglobulin and complement components. Thus, an immune-mediated, infection-associated glomerulonephritis occurs that produces a proliferative renal lesion associated with a nephritic clinical presentation frequently accompanied by severe acute renal failure.[26] Successful eradication of the antigen via surgical evacuation and appropriate antibiotic therapy has resulted in clinical resolution of nephritis in the majority of reported cases.

Shunt Nephritis

Ventriculoatrial shunts, inserted for the treatment of hydrocephalus, may rarely become colonized by coagulase-negative staphylococci or other organisms of low virulence such as *Propionibacterium acnes*.[27] Such colonization is associated with the development of membranoproliferative glomerulonephritis, manifest by heavy proteinuria, hematuria, and renal impairment. The diagnosis may be confirmed by positive culture of blood, cerebrospinal fluid, or the shunt itself. Removal of the shunt, combined with appropriate antibiotic therapy, leads to an improvement in renal function in the majority of cases and is recommended; however, treatment of the infection with antibiotics alone with clearance of infection and restoration of renal function has been reported.[28]

Pneumococcus

Pneumococcal pneumonia, endocarditis, and other infections have been associated with glomerulonephritis. Immune-mediated renal disease is induced via mechanisms similar to those described for staphylococcal infection, although pneumococcal capsular antigen has additionally been detected within a cryoprecipitate obtained from one patient with infection-associated glomerulonephritis. Treatment involves the same principles as discussed for staphylococcal infections. Penicillin is the antibiotic of choice, except in areas of drug-resistant pneumococci, for which initial treatment with vancomycin plus penicillin is advisable pending antibiotic sensitivity determination.[29]

Gram-Negative Bacteria

Salmonella

Although uncommon in typhoid fever, a diffuse proliferative infection-associated glomerulonephritis may occur and is generally associated with a relatively mild nephritic clinical presentation. Glomerulonephritis must be differentiated from cystitis, pyelonephritis, and acute tubular necrosis, all of which may occur in the context of this illness. In contrast, acute infection with various species of *Salmonella* has been associated with the onset of the nephrotic syndrome in patients with coexistent hepatosplenic schistosomiasis. Nephrosis has been found to resolve on the eradication of *Salmonella* carriage by treatment with cotrimoxazole or ampicillin.[30]

Other Bacterial Infections

Glomerulonephritis has been reported following enteritis caused by *Yersinia entercolitica*. Pneumonia or lung abscess due to *Klebsiella pneumoniae*, *Haemophilus influenzae*, *Mycoplasma pneumoniae*, *Pseudomonas aeruginosa*, *Chlamydia psittaci*, and *Legionella pneumophila* have rarely been reported to cause glomerulonephritis. Diarrhea-associated hemolytic-uremic syndrome from *Escherichia coli* O157:H7 is discussed in Chapter 26. *E. coli*, meningococci, and other gram-negative, gram-positive, and anaerobic bacteria causing septicemia, peritonitis, subphrenic abscess, osteomyelitis, meningitis, and septic abortion have also been linked to infection-associated glomerulonephritis. As a generalization, this rare complication of infection has been found to resolve after the eradication of infection with antibiotic treatment and/or surgery.

Mycobacteria

Leprosy

Approximately 10 million people worldwide have leprosy; of these, 6% to 8% can be expected to have glomerulonephritis.[31] Most commonly, a mesangioproliferative lesion has been found on biopsy, with evidence of IgG and C3 deposition on immunofluorescence microscopy; mycobacterial antigens within glomeruli have been documented. Nephritis is generally clinically mild, with low-grade proteinuria and minimal impairment of renal function. Cases of rapidly progressive glomerulonephritis have been reported, generally in the context of an episode of erythema nodosum leprae, in which spontaneous or treatment-associated systemic immune complex disease occurs, superimposed on the course of previously indolent lepromatous leprosy. Standard treatment for erythema nodosum leprae, consisting of 1 mg/kg/day prednisone PO, was reported to produce a rapid resolution.[31] In general, glomerulonephritis due to leprosy responds clinically to bacteriologic cure, although drug treatment may be complicated by the development of erythema nodosum leprae or drug adverse effects.[32] Interstitial nephritis and renal amyloidosis are also documented in patients with leprosy. As opposed to glomerulonephritis, amyloid produces more severe proteinuria and renal impairment and consequently carries a poor prognosis. A recent study with eprosiate, a sulfonated, low molecular weight compound similar to heparan sulfate, has shown promise in slowing the progression of AA (secondary) amyloidosis of the kidney.

Tuberculosis

Tuberculosis may produce direct renal infection and cavitation or glomerular involvement through the development of amyloidosis, but has only rarely been reported as a cause of glomerulonephritis. Treatment involves antituberculous chemotherapy and possibly eprosiate[33] (see Chapter 37).

SPIROCHETES

Syphilis

The prevalence of syphilis is increasing worldwide. As congenital, secondary, and tertiary syphilis have been associated with various forms of glomerulonephritis, renal gumma formation, and amyloidosis, the incidence of renal presentations of syphilis may also be anticipated to increase. Congenital syphilis may result in membranous nephropathy. Acquired secondary and tertiary syphilis in adults may also produce a nephrotic presentation in association with minimal change or membranous features on biopsy. A nephritic presentation may also occur, with typical proliferative glomerular changes of infection-associated glomerulonephritis seen on biopsy. Granular deposition of IgG and C3 is generally demonstrable by immunofluorescence, suggesting an immune complex basis. Treatment of syphilis with penicillin, 2.4 million units by weekly IM injection for 3 weeks, has led to the resolution of proteinuria in the majority of cases.[34]

Leptospirosis

Leptospirosis has been associated with a mesangioproliferative glomerulonephritis, but far more commonly induces acute interstitial nephritis or acute tubular necrosis in the setting of Weil's syndrome. Regardless of the renal lesion produced, treatment involves intensive supportive care and antibiotic treatment, which is of proven benefit if started within the first 5 days of infection. Doxycycline 200 mg/day PO is effective in mild cases. Penicillin, 1.5 million units every 6 hours for 7 days, is preferred for severe disease. Exchange transfusion may have a role in reducing hyperbilirubinemia, which may contribute to the renal toxicity in Weil's syndrome. The renal lesion is entirely reversible on resolution of the infection.[35]

VIRAL INFECTIONS

Viruses in General

Viral infection is almost ubiquitous in humans. However, clinically relevant infection-associated glomerulonephritis due to viral infection is rare. Circulating immune complexes may be found in the serum of patients at some stage in the course of nearly all acute viral infections. Indeed, glomerulonephritis in the setting of viral infection is associated with the glomerular deposition of immune complexes. This is accompanied by endothelial and/or mesangial cell proliferation and rarely by extracapillary crescent formation. Why only a minority of people develop glomerulonephritis on infection with virus is unknown. The probable explanation is that multiple virus-dependent factors (nephritogenicity, virulence, capacity for immunomodulation and chronicity) and host-dependent factors (immune competence, profile of cytokine response, intrarenal kidney cell response) interact to determine the glomerular consequences of infection.[7,36] The management of acute virus-associated glomerulonephritis is directed at clearance of the viral infection, which generally occurs spontaneously, and the provision of supportive care when required. The management of chronic virus-associated glomerulonephritis additionally involves the use of specific antiviral or immunomodulatory therapies, as discussed in Chapter 14 for hepatitis C virus and in Chapter 24 for hepatitis B virus and HIV.

Viral Hepatitis

Hepatitis A has been reported to cause immune complex mesangioproliferative glomerulonephritis. The management of this uncommon complication of hepatitis A virus infection is supportive, and nephritis resolves with recovery from the infection.

Hantaan Virus

Hantaan and related viruses induce an illness known as nephropathia epidemica or hemorrhagic fever with renal syndrome, which is endemic in areas of Southeast Asia and southern Europe and appears in epidemics worldwide.[37] Spread by the inhalation of aerosolized virus-containing particles formed from the excreta of infected mice, these viruses induce a spectrum of disease that ranges from a mild febrile illness to a life-threatening disorder. Severe disease is characterized by several phases. Initially high fever and myalgias dominate, while facial and truncal flushing and petechiae develop in association with thrombocytopenia. Fever suddenly subsides after several days, but profound hypotension develops, associated with oliguric acute renal failure. Systemic hypotension, derangements of intrarenal vasomotor tone, coagulation, and associated interstitial nephritis contribute to renal injury. Membranoproliferative glomerulonephritis has been reported; however, glomerular involvement is generally minor.

The diagnosis is confirmed by an increase in titer of specific antibody to Hantaan virus between serum samples taken 1 week apart. Leptospirosis and scrub typhus should be excluded, also on serologic grounds, because these agents may produce a similar illness but are amenable to treatment with tetracyclines. Treatment of hemorrhagic fever with renal syndrome is supportive only.[37] A specific vaccine is currently under trial in Korea.

Herpes-Type Viruses

Generally mild and spontaneously resolving acute nephritis has been reported as a rare complication of various infections, including infectious mononucleosis, pneumonitis, encephalitis, and congenital infection with Epstein-Barr virus, cytomegalovirus, varicella, and herpes simplex virus. Specific antiviral therapy is indicated for critical organ infection rather than for glomerulonephritis, which tends to resolve after control of the infection.

Other Viruses

Smith and colleagues[38] reported a 3.8% incidence of glomerulonephritis after nonstreptococcal upper respiratory tract infection in American army recruits. Presumably, the majority of these infections were viral in etiology. Recovery was spontaneous and clinically complete (except in one patient with a history of PSGN) but took up to 12 months in some cases. In nephrologic practice, virus-associated glomerulonephritis is a far less frequently encountered cause of glomerulonephritis than these figures would indicate.[36] This is probably due to underdetection. Given the apparently benign clinical course of infection-associated glomerulonephritis after viral upper respiratory tract infection, biopsy does not appear to be indicated except in cases of diagnostic uncertainty. However, the degree of renal functional impairment, as documented above, does indicate a need for follow-up for evidence of chronic kidney disease in such patients. Whether the long-term prognosis of patients with virus-associated glomerulonephritis is similar to that for patients with PSGN is unknown.

Human parvovirus B19 has recently been identified as a possible cause of non–HIV-associated collapsing glomerulopathy. This virus is common and typically causes a mild nonspecific illness, but has been associated with red cell aplasia in a minority of patients. Parvovirus B19 DNA was identified within glomeruli in the majority of cases of supposedly idiopathic collapsing glomerulopathy in one study.[39] The clinical presentation is similar to HIV-associated collapsing glomerulopathy, and progression to renal failure is frequent.

Cases of glomerulonephritis have been reported in association with mumps, measles, and enteroviral infections (Coxsackie B5 virus and echovirus). Generally, these have produced only a mild nephritic illness that resolved spontaneously.

RICKETTSIAL INFECTIONS

Rocky Mountain Spotted Fever

Rocky Mountain spotted fever, in severe cases, results in a multiorgan vasculitis involving the central nervous system, myocardium, and kidney. Renal involvement is predominantly tubulointerstitial because prerenal factors (vasculitis and myocardial depression) combine with a perivascular interstitial nephritis to produce acute renal failure. Glomerular involvement has been described but is overshadowed by the interstitial lesions. Glomerulonephritis has been reported in which a nephritic illness, associated with typical postinfectious changes on biopsy samples, occurred 2 weeks after an acute episode of Rocky Mountain spotted fever. Spontaneous resolution occurred.[40]

Q Fever

Immune complex mesangioproliferative glomerulonephritis has been reported in cases of both endocarditis and sepsis due to *Coxiella burnetii*. Antiphospholipid and anti-DNA autoantibodies have been detected in the sera of these patients, suggesting that the development of antibodies to *Coxiella* antigens cross-reactive to host antigens may have a role in the pathogenesis of Q fever. The diagnosis is based on clinical features and confirmed by serology. Treatment is with doxycycline 100 mg/day PO for 1 week for sepsis, or longer for endocarditis, in which surgical removal of the vegetation, with or without valve replacement, is often required. Renal manifestations have been reported to resolve with cure of the infection.[41]

Scrub Typhus

Rickettsia tsutsugamushi, like other rickettsias, has a predilection for the endothelium. Glomerulonephritis has been reported as a rare sequela of scrub typhus. The clinical illness produced is similar to that seen in infections with leptospirosis and Hantaan virus and should be distinguished on epidemiologic and serologic grounds. Treatment with doxycycline 100 mg/day PO for 1 week is beneficial at any stage of the illness.

FUNGAL INFECTIONS

Mucocutaneous candidiasis has been reported as a cause of immune complex–mediated membranoproliferative glomerulonephritis. Proteinuria and renal function improved on clearance of the infection.[42]

Clinical renal involvement may occur in disseminated histoplasmosis. Proliferative glomerulonephritis, associated with the presence of circulating immune complexes, has been reported in a case of acute primary disseminated histoplasmosis. Renal manifestations resolved following spontaneous recovery from the infection.[43] However, disseminated infection in immunocompromised or nonresolving patients does require therapy with antifungal agents.

PARASITIC INFECTIONS

Malaria

Falciparum Malaria

Transient glomerulonephritis may be a common sequela of infection with *Plasmodium falciparum*, but it is generally mild and undetected. Glomerulonephritis has been demonstrated in 18% of patients with fatal falciparum malaria.[44]

Renal failure is a significant contributor to the mortality of severe falciparum infection; however, acute renal failure in this setting is usually due to acute tubular necrosis, which results from shock, renal vasoconstriction, intravascular coagulation, direct tubular toxicity, and hyperbilirubinemia.[8] Treatment with intravenous quinine and supportive care including hemodialysis is beneficial. Exchange transfusion, designed to reduce parasite load and hyperbilirubinemia, has been reported to be beneficial in selected situations. Elimination of the parasite is accompanied by the resolution of renal abnormalities in surviving patients.[44]

Quartan Malaria

The incidence of childhood nephrotic syndrome is 20 to 60 times more frequent in areas where infection with *Plasmodium malariae* is endemic in comparison with nonendemic areas. A small percentage of patients, mainly children, with quartan malaria develop an immune complex glomerulonephritis. Histologically, this is characterized initially by glomerular capillary wall thickening due to subendothelial immune complex deposition, which evolves to produce capillary collapse and diffuse mesangial sclerosis. The characteristic clinical presentation is with the nephrotic syndrome. Disease progression is the rule, with the development of hypertension and progressive renal failure leading to death in 3 to 5 years. Neither antimalarial treatment nor immunosuppressive therapies have been shown to improve the renal outcome in this condition. Thus, the main therapeutic hope for the future is prevention, either through the development of a vaccine for *P. malariae* or by decreasing the prevalence of the organism.[5]

Schistosomiasis

Chronic schistosomiasis caused by infestation with *Schistosoma haematobium* (endemic in Africa and the Middle East) or *Schistosoma mansoni* (Africa, South America, and the Middle East) has been associated with immune complex glomerulonephritis.[45]

Schistosomiasis due to *S. haematobium* has been associated with membranoproliferative glomerulonephritis and minimal change disease, which responded clinically to antischistosomal treatment. However, the vast majority of cases of renal disease seen in association with *S. haematobium* are due to coinfection with *Salmonella* species, as indicated by the presence of fever and isolation of the organism from blood cultures. In this setting, proteinuria and renal impairment have been shown to respond to treatment of the salmonellosis, with or without antischistosomal treatment.[30] Antischistosomal treatment is indicated because persistence of the schistosomiasis renders these patients susceptible to recurrences of renal disease on reexposure to *Salmonella*.

Glomerular involvement in *S. mansoni* infestation is relatively common. Although rarely reported during the earlier hepatointestinal phase, glomerulopathy is seen in 12% to 15% of patients who develop hepatosplenic disease. Glomerulonephritis is due to immune complex disease. A mesangioproliferative or membranoproliferative lesion may be seen on biopsy and may evolve to focal glomerulosclerosis. Patients are frequently nephrotic. Hypertension and progressive renal failure may develop. Treatment with prednisone, with or without cyclophosphamide, has induced occasional remissions, whereas treatment with antischistosomal drugs has been unsuccessful in altering the course of the renal disease. Amyloidosis may also occur as a complication of chronic schistosomiasis.[45]

Other Parasites

Toxoplasmosis has rarely been associated with glomerulonephritis. Whether nephritis will be increasingly recognized in the setting of toxoplasmosis associated with acquired immunodeficiency syndrome and other immunocompromised states remains to be seen.

Visceral leishmaniasis has been associated with a mild nephritic illness due to mesangioproliferative glomerulonephritis; however, this occurrence is rare and a direct causal link has not been firmly established.

Filariasis due to *Wuchereria bancrofti* has been shown to produce glomerulonephritis with antigen and specific antibody demonstrable within glomeruli. Filariasis caused by *Onchocerca volvulus* and *Loa loa* has also been linked to various types of glomerulonephritis, largely by way of immune complex deposition. Additionally, microfilariae have been demonstrated within glomerular capillaries in association with eosinophilic tubulointerstitial nephritis. The presentation of acute filarial nephropathy is generally nephritic and is responsive to treatment with diethylcarbamazine. Chronic filarial nephropathy more commonly produces a nephrotic presentation and responds poorly to antifilarial drugs.[5]

SUMMARY AND FUTURE DIRECTIONS

Infection with various microbes can cause glomerulonephritis in humans. The percentage of infectious illnesses that result in a clinically apparent episode of infection-associated glomerulonephritis is, however, very small. While the underdiagnosis of infection-associated glomerulonephritis[10] may account for a fraction of this discrepancy, it is clear that a complex interaction of host- and microbe-related factors are involved in determining whether an individual develops glomerulonephritis as a consequence of infection with a particular organism. Such factors remain to be elucidated.

Fortunately, the vast majority of cases of infection-associated glomerulonephritis resolve after either spontaneous or treatment-induced clearance of the underlying infection. A few patients incur progressive renal disease. In some cases, this is caused by a failure of, or a delay in, the clearance of infection. In others, progression may occur despite microbiologic cure. The mechanisms behind progressive disease also remain unclear. As a consequence, therapeutic approaches have been limited to the provision of supportive care and the use of uncontrolled empirical trials of therapy based on regimens that have been successful in the treatment of other forms of glomerulonephritis. Advances in specific therapy for infection-associated glomerulonephritis will require a better understanding of the pathogenetic mechanisms involved. In the interim, if empirical therapies are to be used, then surely it is time for a coordinated effort in mounting a controlled trial of, for example, immunosuppression in infection-associated glomerulonephritis.

Little is known of the long-term consequences of infection-associated glomerulonephritis, with the exception of the follow-up studies of patients after PSGN by Baldwin[22] and Rodriguez-Iturbe[20] and more recently of patients with infection-associated glomerulonephritis of various etiologies by

Montseny and colleagues.[3] The diligent work of these teams has clearly indicated that a significant proportion of patients manifest hypertension, proteinuria, and progressive renal failure as long-term sequelae of infection-associated glomerulonephritis. The risk of developing chronic kidney disease for patients with mild or subclinical infection-associated glomerulonephritis is unknown. What is clear is that patients with infection-associated glomerulonephritis should be followed long term in order to screen for the development of late sequelae amenable to management by conventional renoprotective measures (see Chapter 62). Whether treatment after the acute episode of infection-associated glomerulonephritis with, for example, angiotensin-converting enzyme inhibitors would retard the development of late sequelae is unknown.

In conclusion, several general principles are applicable to the treatment of infection-associated glomerulonephritis, and these are depicted as a treatment algorithm in Figure 13-1. First, prevention should be attempted. This can be accomplished by decreasing the prevalence of infection with nephritogenic organisms in the community, as has been partially achieved in the case of PSGN in developed countries. Prevention remains a difficult issue for many other infections such as neonatal hepatitis B and malaria. Attention to host-dependent risk factors for the development of infection-associated glomerulonephritis, such as alcoholism and intravenous drug abuse, are difficult but potentially modifiable problems of public health. Second, the treatment of cases of infection-associated glomerulonephritis

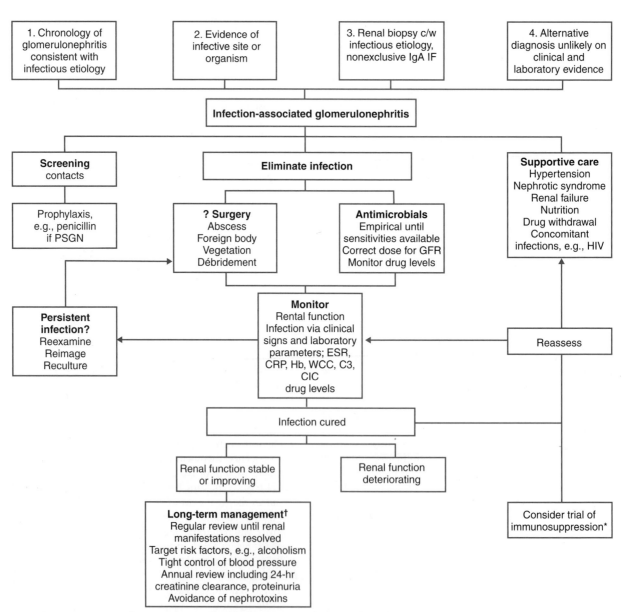

Figure 13-1 Diagnosis and management of infection-associated glomerulonephritis. CIC, circulating immune complex; CRP, C-reactive protein; c/w, combined with; ESR, erythrocyte sedimentation rate; GFR, glomerular filtration rate; Hb, hemoglobin; HIV, human immunodeficiency virus; PSGN, poststreptococcal glomerulonephritis; WCC, white cell count. *Anecdotal evidence only, see text. †See Chapter 62.

should involve the identification and elimination of the infecting organism, combined with supportive care of the patient. Contacts who may be at risk of infection with the same organism should be identified, screened, and given prophylactic treatment if indicated. Long-term follow-up of the patient is indicated. Finally, coordinated investigation into the pathogenesis, natural history, and therapy of this heterogeneous group of disorders is to be supported.

References

1. Tapaneya-Olarn W, Osatakul S, Chatasingh S, Tapaneya-Olarn C: Acute glomerulonephritis in children: A prospective study. J Med Assoc Thai 1989;72(Suppl 1):35–38.
2. Streeton CL, Hanna JN, Messer RD, Merianos A: An epidemic of acute post-streptococcal glomerulonephritis among aboriginal children. J Paediatr Child Health 1995;31:245–248.
3. Montseny J, Meyrier A, Kleinknecht D, Callard P: The current spectrum of infectious glomerulonephritis. Experience with 76 patients and review of the literature. Medicine (Baltimore) 1995;74:63–73.
4. Neugarten J, Baldwin DS: Glomerulonephritis in bacterial endocarditis. Am J Med 1984;77:297–304.
5. Chugh KS, Sakhuja V: Glomerular diseases in the tropics. Am J Nephrol 1990;10:437–450.
6. Keller CK, Andrassy K, Waldherr R, Ritz E: Postinfectious glomerulonephritis: Is there a link to alcoholism? Q J Med 1994;87:97–102.
7. Chadban SJ, Atkins RC: Glomerulonephritis. Lancet 2005;365:1797–1806.
8. Eiam-Ong S, Sitprija V: Falciparum malaria and the kidney: A model of inflammation. Am J Kidney Dis 1998;32:361–375.
9. Rees AJ, Lockwood CM, Peters DK: Enhanced allergic tissue injury in Goodpasture's syndrome by intercurrent bacterial infection. Br Med J 1977;2:723–726.
10. Jones JM, Davison AM: Persistent infection as a cause of renal disease in patients submitted to renal biopsy: A report from the Glomerulonephritis Registry of the United Kingdom MRC. Q J Med 1986;58:123–132.
11. Vanwalleghem J, Maes B, Van Damme B, et al: Steroids for deep-infection-associated glomerulonephritis: A two-edged sword. Nephrol Dial Transplant 1998;13:773–775.
12. Yamashita Y, Tanase T, Terada Y, et al: Glomerulonephritis after methicillin-resistant Staphylococcus aureus infection resulting in end-stage renal failure. Intern Med 2001;40:424–427.
13. Rovzar MA, Logan JL, Ogden DA, Graham AR: Immunosuppressive therapy and plasmapheresis in rapidly progressive glomerulonephritis associated with bacterial endocarditis. Am J Kidney Dis 1986;7:428–433.
14. McKenzie PE, Taylor AE, Woodroffe AJ, et al: Plasmapheresis in glomerulonephritis. Clin Nephrol 1979;12:97–108.
15. Ayres BF, Bastian PD, Haines D, et al: Renal and cardiac complications of drug abuse. Med J Aust 1976;2:489–494.
16. McKinsey DS, McMurray TI, Flynn JM: Immune complex glomerulonephritis associated with Staphylococcus aureus bacteremia: Response to corticosteroid therapy. Rev Infect Dis 1990;12:125–127.
17. Kupari M, Teerenhovi L: Plasma exchanges in the treatment of rapidly progressive glomerulonephritis associated with chronic dental infection. Acta Med Scand 1981;210:511–514.
18. Roy S III, Murphy WM, Arant BS Jr: Poststreptococcal crescenteric glomerulonephritis in children: Comparison of quintuple therapy versus supportive care. J Pediatr 1981;98:403–410.
19. Fairley C, Mathews DC, Becker GJ: Rapid development of diffuse crescents in post-streptococcal glomerulonephritis. Clin Nephrol 1987;28:256–260.
20. Rodriguez-Iturbe B: Epidemic poststreptococcal glomerulonephritis. Kidney Int 1984;25:129–136.
21. Zent R, Van Zyl Smit R, Duffield M, et al: Crescentic nephritis at Groote Schuur Hospital, Cape Town, South Africa—not a benign disease. Clin Nephrol 1994;42:22–29.
22. Baldwin DS: Post-streptococcal glomerulonephritis. A progressive disease? Am J Med 1977;62:1–11.
23. Frieden TR, Munsiff SS, Low DE, et al: Emergence of vancomycin-resistant enterococci in New York City. Lancet 1993;342:76–79.
24. Angangco R, Thiru S, Oliveira DB: Pauci-immune glomerulonephritis associated with bacterial infection. Nephrol Dial Transplant 1993;8:754–756.
25. Powell DE: Non-suppurative lesions in staphylococcal septicaemia. J Pathol Bacteriol 1961;82:141–149.
26. Beaufils M, Morel-Maroger L, Sraer JD, et al: Acute renal failure of glomerular origin during visceral abscesses. N Engl J Med 1976;295:185–189.
27. Beeler BA, Crowder JG, Smith JW, White A: Propionibacterium acnes: Pathogen in central nervous system shunt infection. Report of three cases including immune complex glomerulonephritis. Am J Med 1976;61:935–938.
28. Saíz García F, Zubimendi Herranz A, Silva González C: Nephritis caused by a shunt. Cure of the nephropathy without the need of a surgical replacement of the ventriculo-atrial valve. Rev Clin Esp 1982;164:123–126.
29. Tomasz A: The pneumococcus at the gates. N Engl J Med 1995;333:514–515.
30. Abdul-Fattah MM, Yossef SM, Ebraheem ME, et al: Schistosomal glomerulopathy: A putative role for commonly associated Salmonella infection. J Egypt Soc Parasitol 1995;25:165–173.
31. Ahsan N, Wheeler D, Palmer BF: Leprosy-associated renal disease: Case report and review of the literature. J Am Soc Nephrol 1995;5:1546–1552.
32. Jakeman P: Risk of relapse in multibacillary leprosy. Lancet 1995;345:4–5.
33. Dember LM, Hawkins PN, Hazenberg BP, et al: Eprodisate for the treatment of renal disease in AA amyloidosis. N Engl J Med 2007;356:2349–2360.
34. Hunte W, Al-Ghraoui F, Cohen R: Secondary syphilis and the nephrotic syndrome. J Am Soc Nephrol 1993;3:1351–1355.
35. Kim MJ: Recent advances in leptospirosis research based on molecular biology. Infection 1994;26:109.
36. Glassock RJ: Immune complex-induced glomerular injury in viral diseases: An overview. Kidney Int 1991;40(Suppl 35):S5–S7.
37. Bruno P, Hassell LH, Brown J, et al: The protean manifestations of haemorrhagic fever with renal syndrome. A retrospective view of 26 cases from Korea. Ann Intern Med 1990;113:385–391.
38. Smith MC, Cooke JH, Zimmerman DM, et al: Asymptomatic glomerulonephritis after non-streptococcal upper respiratory infections. Ann Intern Med 1979;91:697–702.
39. Moudgil A, Nast CC, Bagga A, et al: Association of parvovirus B19 infection with idiopathic collapsing glomerulopathy. Kidney Int 2001;59:2126–2133.
40. Quigg RJ, Gaines R, Wakely PE Jr, Schoolwerth AC: Acute glomerulonephritis in a patient with Rocky Mountain spotted fever. Am J Kidney Dis 1991;17:339–342.
41. Tolosa-Vilella C, Rodriguez-Jornet A, Font-Rocabanyera A, Andreu-Navarro X: Mesangioproliferative glomerulonephritis and antibodies to phospholipids in a patient with acute Q fever: A case report. Clin Infect Dis 1995;21:196–198.
42. Chesney RW, O'Regan S, Guyda HJ, Drummond KN: Candida endocrinopathy syndrome with membranoproliferative glomerulonephritis: Demonstration of glomerular Candida antigen. Clin Nephrol 1976;5:232–238.
43. Bullock WE, Artz RP, Bhathena D, Tung KS: Histoplasmosis. Association with circulating immune complexes, eosinophilia, and mesangiopathic glomerulonephritis. Arch Intern Med 1979;139:700–702.

44. Sitprija V: Nephropathy in falciparum malaria. Kidney Int 1988;34:867–877.
45. Barsoum R: Schistosomal glomerulopathies. Kidney Int 1993;44:1–12.

Further Reading

Chadban SJ, Atkins RC: Glomerulonephritis. Lancet 2005;365: 1797–1806.
Chugh KS, Sakhuja V: Glomerular diseases in the tropics. Am J Nephrol 1990;10:437–450.

Montseny J, Meyrier A, Kleinknecht D, Callard P: The current spectrum of infectious glomerulonephritis. Experience with 76 patients and review of the literature. Medicine (Baltimore) 1995;74:63–73.
Neugarten J, Baldwin DS: Glomerulonephritis in bacterial endocarditis. Am J Med 1984;77:297–304.

Chapter 14

Cryoglobulinemia and Hepatitis C–Associated Membranoproliferative Glomerulonephritis

Giuseppe D'Amico and Alessandro Fornasieri

CLINICAL FEATURES, PATHOLOGY, AND PATHOPHYSIOLOGY

Hepatitis C virus (HCV) infection may be associated with the systemic syndrome of mixed cryoglobulinemia or with renal-limited immune complex disease characterized by type 1 membranoproliferative glomerulonephritis (MPGN).

Cryoglobulinemia is a pathologic condition in which the blood contains immunoglobulins that precipitate reversibly in the cold. Two types of mixed cryoglobulinemia (MC), which are composed of at least two immunoglobulins, have been described. In both types, a polyclonal IgG is bound to another immunoglobulin that is an antiglobulin (i.e., it acts as an anti-IgG rheumatoid factor). The important difference between these two types of MC is that in type II MC, the antiglobulin component, which is usually of the IgM class, is monoclonal, whereas in type III MC, it is polyclonal.

It was demonstrated relatively recently that HCV infection can be associated with the clinical syndrome, first described by Meltzer and colleagues[1] in 1966, characterized by purpura, weakness, arthralgia, and, in some cases, glomerular lesions. This had previously been defined as essential mixed cryoglobulinemia because an underlying or associated disease had not been found. HCV induces dysregulation of B lymphocytes toward the production of polyclonal (type III MC) or monoclonal (type II MC) rheumatoid factors with cryoprecipitable properties. This leads to a form of membranoproliferative glomerulonephritis called cryoglobulinemic glomerulonephritis that occurs only when type II MC with an IgMκ monoclonal rheumatoid factor is induced by HCV infection. This lesion is characterized by intense monocyte infiltration and subendothelial and/or intraluminal deposition of the cryoglobulins.[2,3]

Consistent data on the pathogenesis of HCV-related MC suggest that lymphotrophic HCV bound via CD81 receptor can induce cryoprecipitable IgMκ rheumatoid factor production.[4,5] In fact, B cells, protected from apoptosis by HCV-dependent gene translocation, develop oligoclonal monotypic lymphoproliferation.[6] As a consequence, cells expressing oligo- or monoclonal rheumatoid factor infiltrate the portal tracts, spleen, bone marrow,[7] and renal interstitium (personal observation).

Several studies have pointed out the pivotal role of HCV and IgMκ in the formation, transport, deposition, and removal from circulation of cryoprecipitable immune complexes. Immune complexes are formed by HCV–anti-HCV polyclonal IgG (and/or unbound IgG) and IgMκ rheumatoid factor.[8] IgMκ is critical for cryoprecipitation and for glomerular deposition. In fact, cryoprecipitable IgMκ has been shown to have high affinity, in vivo and in vitro, for cellular fibronectin, a normal constituent of the glomerular mesangium.[9,10] In addition, due to the IgMκ component, these immune complexes also escape the normal immune complex erythrocyte transport system[11] and have a direct impact on hepatic and splenic macrophages, which are unable to process them due to abnormalities in the biogenesis of lysosomal enzymes.[12] Although it has been less well studied, it is likely that HCV-associated MPGN arises from similar mechanisms.

Isolated proteinuria with microscopic hematuria is the most frequent presenting renal syndrome in both MC and MPGN and is sometimes associated with signs of moderate chronic renal insufficiency or, less frequently, proteinuria in the nephrotic range. An acute nephritic syndrome, often with macroscopic hematuria, severe proteinuria, hypertension, and a sudden increase in blood urea nitrogen, is present at the onset of the renal disease in approximately 25% of patients, sometimes complicated by acute oliguric renal failure. Arterial hypertension is frequently found at the time of the apparent onset of renal disease, even in patients without nephritic syndrome. Renal and extrarenal vasculitis are frequently present in MC. The corresponding histologic picture is of a membranoproliferative glomerulonephritis with less conspicuous intraluminal deposits and monocyte infiltration, sometimes with a lobular pattern, whereas immunofluorescence shows capillary wall deposits of IgM, IgG, and C3 that are sometimes segmental.[3,13] Electron microscopy shows subendothelial electron dense deposits. Sometimes intraluminal deposits with an organized substructure can be found. A minority of patients present with isolated urinary abnormalities and may have a rather nonspecific picture of mild segmental mesangial proliferation, without significant monocyte infiltration and capillary wall alterations.

In nearly one third of patients, even in those who present with an acute nephritic syndrome or severe nephrotic syndrome, spontaneous remission of renal symptoms may occur. In one third of patients, the renal disease has a rather indolent course and, despite the persistence of urinary abnormalities, does not progress to renal failure for several years. In as many as 20% of patients, recurrent reversible clinical exacerbations such as nephritic syndrome and nephrotic syndrome occur during the course of the disease and are sometimes associated with flare-ups of systemic signs of the disease.

If a moderate degree of renal insufficiency is not already present at clinical onset, it is frequently found during later stages of the disease. However, progression to end-stage renal failure is less common than was believed in the past, even after multiple relapses. Chronic uremia developed in only 10% of patients reported in the literature, usually several years after the onset of renal symptoms. The most frequent causes of death in patients with essential MC are cardiovascular and cerebrovascular accidents, hepatic failure, infection, and systemic vasculitis.[13,14]

TREATMENT

Antiviral Therapy of Hepatitis C Virus Infection in Patients with Mixed Cryoglobulinemia and Moderate Renal Involvement

The currently recommended therapy of HCV infection in patients without MC or renal involvement is a combination of formulations of interferon (IFN)-alfa and ribavirin.[15–18] IFN-alfa is a cytokine that has an important function in the innate antiviral immune response. It should be administered three times per week subcutaneously, usually at the dose of 3 million units (mU). Ribavirin is an oral nucleoside analogue with broad activity against viral pathogens. It is administered orally twice daily at the total dose of 800 to 1200 mg. The overall rate of sustained virologic response, defined as the absence of HCV RNA in serum at least 6 months after the discontinuation of therapy, is low (<20%) with the separate use of the two drugs, but their combination has led to a marked improvement in this rate (as much as 40%–45%).

A further improvement in the rate of sustained virologic response was obtained recently with the development of a long-acting IFN, pegylated IFN, produced by the covalent attachment of polyethylene glycol to the IFN molecule. With its increased half-life, this drug can be given as a weekly dose. Two pegylated IFN formulations are currently approved for the treatment of hepatitis C: alfa-2a, whose recommended weekly dose is 180 µg SC, and alfa-2b, whose recommended dose is 1.5 µg/kg body weight/week SC.

The currently recommended regimen for the treatment of chronic HCV is the combination of weekly subcutaneous injections of pegylated IFN or three times per week subcutaneous injections of IFN-alfa, and twice-daily oral doses of ribavirin. The optimal duration of therapy and dose of ribavirin vary according to the HCV genotype. Although patients with genotype 2 or 3 infection can receive 24 weeks of combination therapy with a dose of 800 mg/day ribavirin, patients with other genotypes, especially genotype 1, should receive ribavirin for 48 weeks at a daily dose of 1000 mg (if their body weight is ≤75 kg) or 1200 mg (if their weight is >75 kg). The weekly dose of IFN-alfa or pegylated IFN does not change according to the genotype.

With the use of these regimens, overall sustained virologic response rates are 75% to 80% among patients with HCV genotype 2 or 3 infection and 40% to 50% among those with genotype 1. The response rate is lower in black patients.

Both IFN-alfa and ribavirin have adverse effects. The most common side effects of IFN-alfa and pegylated IFN are muscle aches and fatigue, but there are sometimes also psychological side effects such as depression, anxiety, irritability, sleep disturbances, and difficulty concentrating. The most common serious side effect of ribavirin is hemolytic anemia, especially if renal insufficiency is present, and is the major reason for dose reduction. Ribavirin is also teratogenic, and strict adherence to an effective means of birth control is mandatory for both women and men who receive this drug.

The available literature suggests that the antiviral therapy may be effective even when cryoglobulinemia and moderate renal involvement complicate the viral infection. As early as 1993 to 1994, three controlled trials[19–21] were published on the effect of IFN-alfa, administered alone, in HCV infection complicated by MC, sometimes associated with moderate signs of renal involvement. The trial of Ferri and colleagues[20] was a crossover, controlled trial in 26 patients with documented HCV infection and clinically active MC (purpura, liver, and/or neurological involvement) but without evident signs of renal involvement. The trial alternated 6 months with IFN-alfa therapy (2 mU daily for a month, then every other day for 5 months) and 6 months without IFN-alfa therapy. The majority of patients were on low-dose steroid treatment before the trial, and this medication was continued during the trial. A significant improvement of purpura, together with a reduction of cryoglobulins and transaminases, was reported during treatment compared with periods without treatment; however, rebound was commonly observed during these drug-free intervals. In three patients, signs of renal involvement appeared during the treatment period. In the randomized, controlled trial of Misiani and colleagues,[21] 53 patients with HCV-associated type II MC, three fourths of whom had some mild renal involvement, were assigned to receive either symptomatic therapy or IFN-alfa for 6 months (1.5 mU/day for 1 week, then 3 mU three times weekly for the next 23 weeks). Many patients in both subgroups were also receiving low-dose steroid treatment before the start of the trial and continued to take it. IFN-alfa eradicated the viremia in 60% of patients, improved the systemic signs of the disease, and reduced the cryocrit, although no beneficial effects on liver damage were documented. With regard to the renal disease, only a small but constant decrease in serum creatinine was reported, without significant change in proteinuria. Despite these beneficial effects in 60% of treated patients, none became completely free of the abnormalities that characterize MC, and all patients relapsed after IFN-alfa was discontinued. In the randomized, controlled trial by Dammacco and colleagues,[19] 65 patients with type II MC due to HCV infection were assigned to four groups: group A, 3 mU of natural IFN-alfa three times per week for 1 year; group B, IFN-alfa as in group A plus 16 mg oral 6-methylprednisolone (MP) on non-IFN-alfa days; group C, 16 mg/day of MP only; group D, no treatment. A good response, arbitrarily defined as decrease in the cryocrit to less than 50% associated with improvement of systemic signs, was obtained in approximately half the patients given IFN-alfa alone or IFN-alfa plus MP, but in only 17% of those given the steroid alone. As in the previous trials, the favorable effect was limited to patients in whom HCV RNA became negative (42% and 50%, respectively, in group A and group B). In patients treated with MP only, despite the demonstration of clinical and biochemical remission in a minority of patients, a significant increase of HCV RNA levels was demonstrated at the end of the treatment in 5 of 13 patients. Recurrence of signs of MP was a frequent phenomenon after discontinuation of the trials, but clinical relapse was delayed in patients receiving the combined treatment (IFN-alfa plus MP) compared with those treated with IFN-alfa alone.

Many subsequent studies[8,22–26] have confirmed the efficacy of antiviral therapy (IFN-alfa with or without ribavirin) in controlling the extrarenal clinical manifestations of cryoglobulinemia, suggesting that improvement in cryoglobulinemia-related symptoms can be achieved even without complete biochemical or virologic responses and that the presence of cryoglobulins does not affect the response to antiviral treatment in patients with HCV infection.

More recently, some uncontrolled studies in patients with cryoglobulinemia and moderate renal involvement have been performed in small numbers of patients, confirming the efficacy of antiviral therapy, especially if IFN-alfa has been combined with ribavirin.

Sabry and colleagues,[27] in a prospective, uncontrolled study, treated 20 patients with HCV-related glomerulonephritis (17 MPGN) with IFN-alfa with or without ribavirin. All patients received IFN 9 mU/week. In the case of persistent HCV RNA at 3 months, ribavirin (15 mg/kg/day) was added to the treatment. Four of 20 patients became HCV RNA negative within 3 months and did not receive ribavirin. Only one of the remaining 16 patients who received ribavirin became HCV RNA negative. A reduction of the ribavirin dose was necessary in seven patients because of an adverse event, especially hemolytic anemia. Proteinuria and HCV RNA levels decreased, while serum complement and albumin levels increased significantly. Renal function remained stable. No data are provided regarding the long-term outcome of the renal disease. Bruchfeld and colleagues[28] treated seven patients with glomerulonephritis and vasculitis and chronic renal insufficiency (glomerular filtration rate between 10 and 65 mL/min) with a combination of IFN-alfa (pegylated IFN in two cases) and ribavirin. Plasma levels of ribavirin were monitored because of the renal insufficiency to avoid overdosing. Six of seven patients became HCV RNA (polymerase chain reaction) negative and four of seven were in virologic and renal remission at the time of publication. One of seven maintained virologic and partial renal remission. One patient who did not tolerate IFN had a renal remission, but relapsed virologically and had a minor vasculitis flare-up after 9 months. Only one patient with vasculitis had low-dose immunosuppression therapy in addition to antiviral therapy. The average daily ribavirin dose was 200 to 800 mg. Alric and colleagues[29] treated 18 patients with HCV-related cryoglobulinemic MPGN with combined therapy of standard or pegylated IFN and ribavirin. After treatment of the acute phase with steroids and/or plasma exchange, antiviral therapy was started in 18 of 25 patients; 7 of these patients did not receive anti-HCV therapy, 14 patients received standard IFN-alfa (3 mU three times per week) plus ribavirin 600 to 1000 mg/day, and 4 received pegylated IFN-alfa 2 (1.5 µg/kg/week) plus ribavirin

Table 14-1 Antiviral Therapy in Hepatitis C Virus–Associated Cryoglobulinemic Glomerulonephritis or Membranoproliferative Glomerulonephritis with Moderate Renal Involvement

Drug	Dose	Duration
Interferon-α	3 million units 3 times weekly SC	
or		
Peginterferon-2α	180 µg once weekly SC	48 wk*
or		
Peginterferon-2β	1.5 µg/kg body weight once weekly SC	
plus		
Ribavirin	800–1200 mg/day in 2 oral doses	

*Treatment can be discontinued after 24 weeks if virus genotype is 2 or 3 or if hepatitis C virus (HCV) RNA is still detectable, and after 12 to 16 weeks if HCV RNA is already undetectable by week 4.

600 to 1000 mg/day. The mean duration of antiviral therapy was 18 months (range, 6–24 months). The patients were followed after antiviral therapy for a mean of 16.7 months (range, 6–30 months). Sustained virologic response was observed in 67% of cases (pegylated IFN had virologic response in three of four patients). After treatment, cryoglobulin levels and proteinuria decreased, while serum albumin level increased in responders compared with nonresponders and to the seven patients who did not receive antiviral treatment. Renal function remained stable in all three groups. Cryoglobulins persisted for a long period after HCV RNA clearance. The authors recommend treating patients for at least 48 weeks and to continue the antiviral therapy even in the absence of a decrease in HCV RNA concentration of 2 log at week 12. To avoid adverse effects, especially hemolysis, ribavirin dose should be adapted to creatinine clearance.

In conclusion, the available experience suggests that in patients with HCV infection and MPGN or glomerulonephritis associated with MC, if there is not an acute flare-up of the disease and even if some impairment of the renal function exists, antiviral treatment with a combination of IFN-alfa and ribavirin is the most valid treatment. When it induces a sustained virologic response, it probably reduces the infection of B cells by the HCV and consequently the production of cryoglobulins and their glomerular and vascular deposition. We propose the schema shown in Table 14-1.

Therapy of Acute Exacerbations of Cryoglobulinemic Glomerulonephritis and Renal Vasculitis

Acute flare-ups of the renal disease, characterized by an acute nephritic syndrome or a nephritic syndrome with less rapid functional deterioration, usually associated with recurrence of the systemic signs of MC (purpura, arthralgia, visceral vasculitis), may occur despite the widespread use of antiviral drugs. In our opinion, they deserve the same aggressive therapy that was used before the viral etiology of the disease became evident. Although these acute manifestations of cryoglobulinemic glomerulonephritis and vasculitis are in some cases spontaneously reversible, in past years, nephrologists who did not aggressively treat this clinical condition observed that irreversible complete loss of renal function can occur. Before the viral origin of essential MC was shown, such misfortunes prompted investigators to use the same anti-inflammatory and cytotoxic drugs that successfully treated other types of rapidly progressive glomerulonephritis as well as antineutrophil cytoplasmic antibody-positive renal vasculitis. Although data from uncontrolled trials using oral steroids and/or cyclophosphamide were initially discouraging, subsequent experience with a regimen based on high-dose intravenous methylprednisolone pulses at the beginning of the steroid treatment,[30] eventually administered with cyclophosphamide, led nephrologists to consider this regimen probably more efficacious because it frequently induced a rapid improvement in the systemic signs of the disease, a progressive regression of the impaired renal function (often with normalization of glomerular filtration rate or serum creatinine), and a decrease in proteinuria.[3]

Plasma exchange or cryofiltration apheresis has been added in more severe cases. Indeed, although a precise relationship between the level of circulating cryoglobulins and severity of renal damage induced by their intraglomerular deposition has not been confirmed by many investigators, the rationale for sharply reducing their level in the blood with such methods appears convincing. Significant amounts of cryoproteins can be removed with this technique, which may prevent local cryoprecipitation in small renal vessels, restore reticuloendothelial system functions that have been saturated by the chronic overload of circulating cryoglobulins, and remove from the blood potentially toxic mediators of inflammation. Many uncontrolled studies have reported rapid improvement in serum creatinine, proteinuria, and cryocrit after plasmapheresis or cryofiltration.[31–34] However, in most trials, this treatment was combined with corticosteroids and cyclophosphamide (to avoid rebound production of cryoglobulins by B cells), so that it is difficult to assess whether the beneficial effects were attributable to the plasmapheresis per se, to the concomitant immunosuppression, to the combination of the two treatments, or to spontaneous recovery.

Over the past 20 years in two renal units in Milan, we have routinely used a therapeutic regimen that includes steroids (short courses of intravenous methylprednisolone pulses, followed by oral prednisone), cyclophosphamide (especially when signs of renal and/or systemic vasculitis were present), and, in the most acute cases, plasmapheresis.[3] No evident signs of worsening of liver involvement, as indicated by the level of hepatic enzymes, were found in more than 50 patients treated as described, nor was there an increased incidence of serious infectious complications, although increasing viral load has been demonstrated after the use of cyclophosphamide.

Obviously a controlled trial is now mandatory to investigate the effect of IFN-alfa or other antiviral drugs given alone compared with the same antiviral drugs combined with anti-inflammatory and cytotoxic drugs plus plasmapheresis. Such a trial must establish, by scientifically rigorous procedures, the superiority of the combination treatment, but at the same time must seek to identify the possible adverse effects on the course of the viral disease and its organ complications (especially liver and nervous system), monitoring also the serum level of viremia by measurement of HCV RNA.

Very recently, rituximab, a human-mouse chimeric monoclonal antibody that binds to B-cell surface antigen CD20, has been used in noncontrolled studies on small numbers of patients in substitution of cyclophosphamide to eliminate the infected B cells that induce oligoclonal monotypic lymphoproliferation and production of type II cryoglobulins. This drug, which is effective and well tolerated in patients with B-cell non-Hodgkin's lymphoma, is expected to interfere with monoclonal IgM production, cryoglobulin synthesis, and their renal deposition. Single cases of such treatment have been described,[35,36] and Roccatello and colleagues[37] described a case series of six patients with HCV-related cryoglobulinemic glomerulonephritis treated with rituximab. One patient received the standard four weekly doses, whereas the other five received two additional doses after 1 and 2 months. Patients invariably showed a decrease in proteinuria, together with a decrease in rheumatoid factor, IgM levels (with unaffected levels of IgG and IgA), and cryocrit. A significant increase in C4 levels was observed while modifications of renal function were not significant. Normalization of bone marrow was also observed in three cases examined. The clinical symptoms purpura, arthralgia, weakness, and paresthesia improved in all cases. No substantial changes in liver enzymes or viral load were observed. Although controlled, randomized studies are required to define the exact indication and dose of rituximab and the

Table 14-2 Treatment of Hepatitis C Virus–Associated Cryoglobulinemic Glomerulonephritis and Vasculitis in the Presence of Severe Acute Signs of Renal Involvement

Drug	Dose	Duration
Interferon-α plus ribavirin plus	Schedule as in Table 14-1	6–12 mo
Steroids plus	0.75–1 g/day methylprednisolone IV for 3 consecutive days, followed by oral prednisolone (0.5 mg/kg body weight/day, tapered over a few weeks until small maintenance doses are achieved)	6 mo
Cyclophosphamide plus	2 mg/kg body weight	3–6 mo
Plasmapheresis	Exchange of 3 L of plasma 3 times weekly	2–3 wk

The anti-inflammatory and immunosuppressive therapy indicated may be substituted in most severe cases of type II cryoglobulinemia and nephritis with rituximab (375 mg/m² IV on days 1, 8, 15, and 22 and eventually two more doses 1 and 2 months later).

long-term effect on liver function, anti-CD20 therapy seems a promising tool in the treatment of acute exacerbation of HCV-related cryoglobulinemic glomerulonephritis and should be preferred to cyclophosphamide. Patients are currently being enrolled in such a study at the National Institute of Allergy and Infectious Diseases.

In conclusion, in the presence of acute signs of renal involvement, intensive anti-inflammatory and cytotoxic treatment must be combined with the antiviral therapy described. The suggested protocol is summarized in Table 14-2.

References

1. Meltzer J, Clauvel JP, Danon F, et al: Biological and clinical significance of cryoglobulins. A report of 86 cases. Am J Med 1974;57:775–778.
2. D'Amico G, Fornasieri A: Cryoglobulinemic glomerulonephritis: A membranoproliferative glomerulonephritis induced by hepatitis C virus. Am J Kidney Dis 1995;25:361–369.
3. D'Amico G: Renal involvement in hepatitis C infection cryoglobulinemic glomerulonephritis. Kidney Int 1998;54:650–671.
4. Fornasieri A, Bernasconi P, Ribero ML, et al: Hepatitis C virus (HCV) in lymphocytes subsets and in B lymphocytes expressing rheumatoid factor cross-reacting idiotype in type II mixed cryoglobulinaemia. Clin Exp Immunol 2000;122:400–403.
5. Pileri P, Uematsu Y, Campagnoli S, et al: Binding of hepatitis C virus to CD81. Science 1998;282:938–941.
6. Zignego AL, Giannelli F, Marrocchi ME, et al: T[14:18] translocation in chronic hepatitis C virus infection. Hepatology 2000;31:474–479.
7. Ramos-Casals M, Trejo O, Garcia-Carrasco M, et al: Mixed cryoglobulinemia: New concepts. Lupus 2000;9:83–91.
8. Zuckerman E, Keren D, Slobodin G, et al: Treatment of refractory, symptomatic, hepatitis C virus related mixed cryoglobulinemia with ribavirin and interferon-alpha. J Rheumatol 2000;27:2172–2178.
9. Fornasieri A, Li M, Armelloni S, et al: Glomerulonephritis induced by human IgMK-IgG cryoglobulins in mice. Lab Invest 1993;69:531–540.
10. Fornasieri A, Armelloni S, Bernasconi O, et al: High binding of immunoglobulin Mk rheumatoid from type II cryoglobulins to cellular fibronectin: A mechanism for induction of in situ immune complex glomerulonephritis? Am J Kidney Dis 1996;27:476–483.
11. Roccatello D, Morsica G, Picciotto G, et al: Impaired hepatosplenic elimination of circulating cryoglobulins in patients with essential mixed cryoglobulinemia and hepatitis C virus (HCV) infection. Clin Exp Immunol 1977;100:9–14.
12. Roccatello D, Isidoro C, Mazzucco G, et al: Role of monocytes in cryoglobulinemia-associated nephritis. Kidney Int 1993;43:1150–1155.
13. Roccatello D, Fornasieri A, Giachino O, et al: Multicenter Study on hepatitis C virus-related cryoglobulinemic glomerulonephritis. Am J Kidney Dis 2007;49:69–82.
14. Tarantino G, Campise M, Banfi G, et al: Long term predictors of survival in essential mixed cryoglobulinemic glomerulonephritis. Kidney Int 1995;47:618–623.
15. Hoofnagle JH, Seeff LB: Peginterferon and ribavirin for chronic hepatitis C. N Engl J Med 2006;355:2444–2451.
16. Hoofnagle JH, Di Bisceglie AM: The treatment of chronic viral hepatitis. Drug Ther 1997;336:347–356.
17. Kamar N, Rostaing L, Alric L: Treatment of hepatitis C-virus-related glomerulonephritis. Kidney Int 2006;69:436–439.
18. Kiyomoto H, Hitomi H, Hosotani Y, et al: The effect of combination therapy with interferon and cryofiltration on mesangial proliferative glomerulonephritis originating from mixed cryoglobulinemia in chronic hepatitis C virus infection. Ther Apher 1999;3:329–333.
19. Dammacco F, Sansonno D, Han JH, et al: Natural interferon-alpha versus its combination with 6-methyl-prednisolone in the therapy of type II mixed cryoglobulinemia: A long-term, randomized, controlled study. Blood 1994;84:3336–3343.
20. Ferri C, Marzo E, Longobardo G, et al: Interferon-alpha in mixed cryoglobulinemia patients: A randomized, crossover-controlled trial. Blood 1993;81:1132–1136.
21. Misiani R, Bellavita P, Fenili D, et al: Interferon alfa-2a therapy in cryoglobulinemia associated with hepatitis C virus. N Engl J Med 1994;330:751–756.
22. Agnello V: Therapy for cryoglobulinemia secondary to hepatitis C virus: The need for tailored protocols and multiclinic studies. J Rheumatol 2000;27:2065–2067.
23. Calleja JL, Albillos A, Moreno-Otero R, et al: Sustained response to interferon-alpha plus ribavirin in hepatitis C virus-associated symptomatic mixed cryoglobulinaemia. Aliment Pharmacol Ther 1999;13:1179–1186.
24. Jefferson JA, Johnson RJ: Treatment of hepatitis C-associated glomerular disease. Semin Nephrol 2000;20:286–292.
25. Lunel F, Cacoub P: Treatment of autoimmune and extra-hepatic manifestation of HCV infection. Ann Med Interne (Paris) 2000;151:58–64.
26. Pellicano R, Marietti G, Leone N, et al: Mixed cryoglobulinaemia associated with hepatitis C virus infection: A predictor factor for treatment with interferon? J Gastroenterol Hepatol 1999;14:1108–1111.
27. Sabry AA, Sobh MA, Sheaashaa HA, et al: Effect of combination therapy (ribavirin and interferon) in HCV-related glomerulopathy. Nephrol Dial Transplant 2002;17:1924–1930.
28. Bruchfeld A, Lindahl K, Ståhle L, et al: Interferon and ribavirin treatment in patients with hepatitis C-associated renal disease and renal insufficiency. Nephrol Dial Transplant 2003;18:1573–1580.
29. Alric L, Plasier E, Thébault S, et al: Influence of antiviral in hepatitis C virus-associated cryoglobulinemic MPGN. Am J Kidney Dis 2004;43:617–623.
30. De Vecchi A, Montagnino G, Pozzi C, et al: Intravenous methylprednisolone pulse therapy in essential mixed cryoglobulinemia nephropathy. Clin Nephrol 1983;19:221–227.
31. Berkaman EM, Orlin JB: Use of plasmapheresis and partial plasma exchange in the management of patients with cryoglobulinemia. Transfusion 1980;20:171–178.
32. Kiyomoto H, Hitomi H, Hosotani Y, et al: The effect of combination therapy with interferon and cryofiltration on mesangial proliferative glomerulonephritis originating from mixed cryoglobulinemia in chronic hepatitis C virus infection. Ther Apher 1999;3:329–333.
33. Siani GA, Siani FS, Ferguson P, et al: Cryofiltration apheresis for treatment of cryoglobulinemia associated with hepatitis C. ASAIO Trans 1995;41:315–318.
34. Sinico RA, Fornasieri A, Fiorini G, et al: Plasma exchange in the treatment of essential mixed cryoglobulinemia nephropathy. Long-term follow up. Int J Artif Organs 1985;2:15–18.
35. Zaja F, Russo D, Fugo O, et al: Rituximab for the treatment of type II mixed cryoglobulinemia. Hematology 1999;84:1157–1158.
36. Lamprecht P, Lerin-Lozano C, Merz H, et al: Rituximab induces remission in refractory HCV associated cryoglobulinaemic vasculitis. Ann Rheum Dis 2003;62:1230–1233.
37. Roccatello D, Baldovino S, Rossi D, et al: Long-term effects of anti-CD20 monoclonal antibody treatment of cryoglobulinemic glomerulonephritis. Nephrol Dial Transplant 2004;19:3054–3061.

Further Reading

Bridoux F, Provot F, Ayache RA, et al: Atteinte rénale au cours des cryoglobulinémies de type II. Presse Med 2003;32:563–569.

D'Amico G: Mixed cryoglobulinemia. In Schrier RW (ed): Diseases of the Kidney and Urinary Tract, 8th ed. Philadelphia: Lippincott Williams & Wilkins, 2007, pp 1776–1786.

Hoofnagle JH, Seeff LB: Peginterferon and ribavirin for chronic hepatitis C. N Engl J Med 2006;355:2444–2451.

Kamar N, Rostaing L, Alric L: Treatment of hepatitis C-virus-related glomerulonephritis. Kidney Int 2006;69:436–439.

Meyers CM, Seeff LB, Stehman-Breen CO, et al: Hepatitis C and renal disease: An update. Am J Kidney Dis 2003;42:631–657.

Roccatello D, Fornasieri A, Giachino O, et al: Multicenter study on hepatitis C virus-related cryoglobulinemic glomerulonephritis. Am J Kidney Dis 2007;49:69-82.

Chapter 15

Lupus Nephritis

James E. Balow, Meryl Waldman, and Howard A. Austin III

BACKGROUND

Systemic lupus erythematosus (SLE) is a complex systemic disease that develops from a massive overproduction of polyclonal antibodies and impaired clearance of immune complexes. Many of the antibodies are autoreactive, either from loss of self-tolerance or from antigenic cross-reactivity, and are used as criteria for the diagnosis of SLE.[1] Renal disease results from deposition of pathogenic immune complexes and infiltration of lymphoid cells within glomeruli, interstitium, and extraglomerular vessels. These humoral and cellular components, along with a host of soluble mediators, evoke a cascade of inflammation, cell death or proliferation, vasculopathy, and fibrogenesis.[2,3] Cumulative evidence indicates that complex interactions between environmental factors and disease susceptibility genes contribute to the pathogenesis of SLE and lupus nephritis.

It is well recognized that renal involvement adversely affects the prognosis of SLE. Indeed, patients often consider kidney disease to be one of the most dreaded complications of SLE. The empathic physician can help the patient realize that the prognosis of lupus nephritis is not uniformly grave and that effective therapies are available for many forms of the disease.[4-9] Patients should know that prognosis varies greatly among the many clinical and pathologic forms of lupus renal disease.[7-9]

Delineation of the specific type of renal involvement is critical to effective clinical management.[10] This process depends on diligent surveillance of patients for hypertension and other clinical and serologic evidence of lupus activity as well as periodic screening by appropriate renal function tests. Urinalysis is clearly one of the most cost-effective methods to detect renal involvement, but special efforts on the part of the clinician are usually needed to verify routine clinical laboratory assessment of urine sediment.[11] Proteinuria is conveniently assessed by measures of protein-to-creatinine ratios on random urine specimens. Renal biopsies are indicated to help delineate the exact type and severity of pathologic lesions early in the course of lupus nephritis.[12,13] A particularly noteworthy study has shown that deferral of renal biopsy is commonly associated with a delay in implementation of cytotoxic drug therapy.[14] Thus, information from early renal biopsy has a substantive impact on the development of a comprehensive treatment plan for patients with lupus nephritis. Management of hypertension and the secondary complications of lupus nephritis are addressed elsewhere in this volume.

The present chapter focuses on immunosuppressive drug treatment of the various pathologically defined forms of lupus nephritis in adults, with an emphasis on class III and IV. The classification system to describe the pathology of lupus nephritis was recently revised.[15,16] One of the goals for the new International Society of Nephrology/Renal Pathology Society classification was to provide a more standardized approach to renal biopsy interpretation that would facilitate the comparison of data across centers. Some of the changes from the earlier World Health Organization classification schemes[17] include the elimination of the normal biopsy category and the subgroups Va–Vd of class V membranous; use of (A) and (C) for designation of active and chronic lesions; and the addition of subcategories within diffuse lupus nephritis (class IV) for predominantly segmental (IV-S) and predominantly global (IV-G) lesions. It is important to keep these differences in mind and to use caution when trying to compare the results of more recent outcome studies based on the newer International Society of Nephrology/Renal Pathology Society classification with older studies using the older World Health Organization classification schemes. A review of the strengths and weaknesses of the new classification system (as well as some of the controversies that have emerged) has recently been published.[18]

REVIEW OF CLINICAL TRIALS

Animal Studies

Important insights into the pathogenesis and treatment of lupus nephritis have emerged from studies of murine models of SLE (e.g., NZB/W, SWR/NZB, MRL/lpr, BXSB). The natural history of SLE is known most precisely from studies of murine models in which death from progressive lupus nephritis occurs predictably unless interdicted by effective immunosuppressive treatments. Comparable knowledge about the natural history of human SLE and lupus nephritis is deficient because of the effects of the host of disease-modifying interventions used in this condition. The different strains of lupus-prone mice appear to have distinct immunologic defects that may have counterparts in the diverse mechanisms underlying human SLE.[19,20] Several strains of lupus mice succumb within a relatively narrow window of time from complications of lupus nephritis; the strain-specific predictable natural history has made them apt subjects for testing new therapies.[21]

Box 15-1 presents a highly simplified overview of experimental therapies that have been tested in the murine models of lupus nephritis. The therapies have been ranked according to their impact on survival (mostly representing amelioration of lupus nephritis). As noted, many therapeutic interventions have a favorable effect on the course of these models. Cyclophosphamide has one of the highest therapeutic indices. Particularly intriguing is a recent study showing that combination of cyclophosphamide and the costimulation inhibitor CTLA4-Ig had a dramatic effect on the advanced stages of murine lupus nephritis.[22,23] Gene therapy is a more complex process that perhaps will offer future prospects for definitive treatment and perhaps a cure for SLE and lupus nephritis.

Human Studies

Although there is general consensus that the outlook for patients with lupus nephritis has improved greatly over the past half century, there remains substantial controversy about which factors are principally responsible for this improvement in prognosis.[24-26] A particularly confounding issue is the tremendous diversity in prognosis among patients in different geographic centers. Descriptions of natural history of lupus nephritis range from dismal odds of renal survival despite aggressive immunosuppressive treatment in some populations[27-30] to excellent long-term survivals with only modest immunosuppressive therapy in other populations.[7,8,25,31] Thus, studies must be of sufficient duration in order to understand important differences in the biology of SLE and the impact of various interventions on the natural history of lupus nephritis among different demographic populations.[32,33] Indeed, studies of therapies for lupus nephritis have been plagued by historical evidence that several immunosuppressive drug regimens, including corticosteroids alone, achieve comparable short- and intermediate-term renal survival outcomes. Thus, reliable attributions of treatment efficacy must be based on the results of prospective, randomized, controlled, long-term clinical trials in lupus nephritis.[34]

Box 15-2 presents a synopsis of the controlled therapeutic trials since 1975 that constitute the foundation for our current recommendations for treatment of proliferative lupus nephritis. The reader may be surprised to learn that fewer than 1200 patients have been enrolled in these various clinical trials to date. Results of the common treatment regimens (drug, route of administration, duration) are grouped together in this box. The criteria for renal disease, the specific treatment regimens, and the conclusions suggested by these major therapeutic trials are presented for each study.

Corticosteroids

The merit of high-dose corticosteroids in patients with various forms of lupus nephritis has never been rigorously proven by modern clinical trial methodology. There have been no controlled clinical trials proving the benefit of corticosteroids over supportive therapy in lupus nephritis, nor have there been any studies directly comparing conventional prednisone

---

Box 15-1   Overview of Experimental Treatments and Survival in Murine Lupus Nephritis

Major Benefit
Cyclophosphamide
T-B cell costimulation inhibitors (anti-CD154 [CD40L], CTLA4-Ig, and other B7 inhibitors)
Total lymphoid irradiation
Bone marrow transplantation
Gene therapy

Moderate Benefit
Sex hormones (in females): Castration, androgens, estrogen antagonists, bromocriptine
Chemical immunosuppression: Glucocorticoids, azathioprine, mycophenolate mofetil, methotrexate, cyclosporin A, tacrolimus, sirolimus, deoxyspergualin, ornithine decarboxylase inhibitors, dimethylthiourea, 5-azacytidine
Inflammation modulators: Prostaglandin E analogues, free radical scavengers, platelet-activating factor receptor antagonists, thromboxane synthase and receptor antagonists, nitric oxide synthase inhibitors, endothelin A receptor antagonists, phosphodiesterase inhibitors, 3-hydroxy-3-methylglutaryl coenzyme A reductase inhibitors
Cytokine and chemokine antagonists against: Interferon gamma, soluble interferon gamma receptors, interleukin-2 receptors, interleukin-6, interleukin-6 receptors, interleukin-10, tumor necrosis factor, B-cell activating factor, transforming growth factor β, soluble interleukin-4 receptors, macrophage chemoattractant protein, fractalkine
Monoclonal antibodies against: Nephritogenic idiotypes, T and B cells, complement
Cell therapy with transfer of T regulatory cells
Anticoagulants: Heparin, heparinoids
Fibrinolytic agents: Ancrod
DNA-related agents: Recombinant murine DNase, bacterial DNA immunization, synthetic oligonucleotide conjugate (LJ-394 DNA toleragen), anti-DNA antibody-based peptide (to manipulate regulatory and suppressor T-cell populations)
Dietary manipulation: Protein, calorie, and fat restriction; vitamin D_3, fish oil, and flaxseed supplements

Box 15-2 Synopsis of Controlled Immunosuppressive Drug and Plasma Exchange Trials in Lupus Nephritis since 1975

Azathioprine: Extended Oral Therapy
Austin and Colleagues (1986)[38] and Steinberg and Steinberg (1991)[44]
Renal disease: Active urinary sediment with lupus nephritis (mostly proliferative) on biopsy. *Treatment:* Prednisone versus prednisone plus azathioprine until major drug toxicity, renal failure, or sustained remission of nephritis. *Conclusions:* Azathioprine did not decrease risk of ESRD compared with prednisone alone during 10 or more years of observation.

Azathioprine plus Cyclophosphamide Combination: Extended Oral Therapy
Austin and Colleagues (1986)[38] and Steinberg and Steinberg (1991)[44]
Renal disease: Active urinary sediment with lupus nephritis (mostly proliferative) on biopsy. *Treatment:* prednisone versus prednisone plus azathioprine and cyclophosphamide combination until major drug toxicity, renal failure, or sustained remission of nephritis. *Conclusions:* After 5 years of observation, azathioprine plus cyclophosphamide significantly decreased the risk of ESRD compared with prednisone alone.

Cyclophosphamide: 6 Months of Oral Therapy
Donadio and Colleagues (1978)[36] and Donadio and Colleagues (1982)[37]
Renal disease: Severe proliferative lupus nephritis on biopsy with clinical evidence of progression. *Treatment:* Prednisone versus prednisone plus oral cyclophosphamide for 6 months. *Conclusions:* The short course of cyclophosphamide significantly improved the probability of a stable renal course over the first 4 years of observation, but there was no difference in late risk of renal failure.

Cyclophosphamide: Oral Therapy Extended Until Complete Remission
Austin and Colleagues (1986)[38] and Steinberg and Steinberg (1991)[44]
Renal disease: Active urinary sediment with lupus nephritis (mostly proliferative) on biopsy. *Treatment:* Prednisone versus prednisone plus cyclophosphamide until major drug toxicity, renal failure, or sustained remission of nephritis. *Conclusions:* After 5 years of observation, cyclophosphamide significantly decreased the risk of ESRD compared with prednisone alone.

Cyclophosphamide: Extended Quarterly Intravenous Pulse Therapy
Austin and Colleagues (1986)[38] and Steinberg and Steinberg (1991)[44]
Renal disease: Active urinary sediment with lupus nephritis (mostly proliferative) on biopsy. *Treatment:* Prednisone versus prednisone plus pulse cyclophosphamide until major drug toxicity, renal failure, or sustained remission of nephritis. *Conclusions:* After 5 years of observation, cyclophosphamide significantly decreased the risk of ESRD compared with prednisone alone and was less toxic than regimens containing daily cyclophosphamide.

Cyclophosphamide: Monthly and Quarterly Pulse Therapies
Boumpas and Colleagues (1992)[45]
Renal disease: Active urinary sediment, reduced renal function, or severely active lupus nephritis on biopsy. *Treatment:* Monthly pulse methylprednisolone for 6 months versus monthly pulse cyclophosphamide for 6 months versus monthly pulse cyclophosphamide for 6 months followed by quarterly pulse cyclophosphamide for 2 years. *Conclusions:* Treatment with the extended course of pulse cyclophosphamide significantly decreased the probability of doubling serum creatinine compared with pulse methylprednisolone; relapse after initial improvement of nephritis was increased after the short course compared with the extended course of pulse cyclophosphamide.

Sesso and Colleagues (1994)[46]
Renal disease: Severe lupus nephritis. *Treatment:* Pulse methylprednisolone versus pulse cyclophosphamide each given monthly for 4 months followed by two quarterly pulse treatments. *Conclusions:* At 18 months, no difference in probability of doubling creatinine or developing ESRD.

Combination Pulse Methylprednisolone and Cyclophosphamide
Gourley and Colleagues (1996)[47] and Illei and Colleagues (2001)[48]
Renal disease: Active urinary sediment, proteinuria, proliferative lupus nephritis on biopsy. *Treatment:* Pulse methylprednisolone monthly for at least 1 year versus pulse cyclophosphamide monthly for 6 months and then quarterly versus combination pulse methylprednisolone and cyclophosphamide therapy. *Conclusions:* Renal remission was least likely with pulse methylprednisolone therapy; remissions tended to be established more rapidly with combination pulse methylprednisolone and cyclophosphamide therapy.

Cyclophosphamide: Low- versus High-Dose Pulse Therapy with Azathioprine Maintenance
Houssiau and Colleagues (2002)[107] and Houssiau and Colleagues (2004)[108]
Renal disease: Proliferative lupus nephritis. *Treatment:* High doses (≤ 1.5 g) pulse cyclophosphamide monthly for 6 months followed by two quarterly doses versus low doses (0.5 g fixed dose) of pulse cyclophosphamide every 2 weeks for six doses. *Conclusions:* After median follow-up of 6 years, there were no substantive differences in the proportions of favorable and unfavorable renal outcomes.

Continued

Box 15-2   Synopsis of Controlled Immunosuppressive Drug and Plasma Exchange Trials in Lupus Nephritis since 1975—cont'd

Cyclophosphamide versus Azathioprine Induction

Grootscholten and Colleagues (2006)[49] and Grootscholten and Colleagues (2007)[109]

Renal disease: Proliferative lupus nephritis (mostly class IV). *Treatment:* Pulse cyclophosphamide (750 mg/m^2) monthly for 6 months and then quarterly for seven doses versus azathioprine with pulse methylprednisolone (1 g for 3 days repeated at 2 and 6 weeks); all received oral corticosteroids; after 2 years, all received azathioprine and low-dose prednisone for 3 years. *Conclusions:* After 2 years, there were no differences in cumulative incidence of complete or partial renal remissions; however, after median follow-up of 5.7 years, there were more relapses, a trend toward a higher incidence of doubling of serum creatinine, and more progression of chronic renal histopathologic lesions in the azathioprine arm.

Mycophenolate Mofetil versus Cyclophosphamide Induction

Chan and Colleagues (2000)[56] and Chan and Colleagues (2005)[55]

Renal disease: Proliferative lupus nephritis with more than 1 g/day proteinuria. *Treatment:* Mycophenolate with a switch to azathioprine at 12 to 24 months versus daily oral cyclophosphamide with a switch to azathioprine at 6 months. *Conclusions:* At 12 months, there were no differences in favorable or unfavorable renal outcomes between the two treatment arms; after an additional year of follow-up into the azathioprine maintenance phase of treatment, patients who initially received mycophenolate had significantly more relapses than did patients receiving cyclophosphamide induction therapy; however, after an extended median follow-up of 63 months, there were no differences in favorable and unfavorable renal outcomes between treatment arms.

Ginzler and Colleagues (2005)[58]

Renal disease: Focal proliferative, diffuse proliferative, and/or membranous with relatively mild renal insufficiency. *Treatment:* Mycophenolate (target dose 3 g/day) for 6 months versus monthly pulse cyclophosphamide (0.5–1 g/m^2) for six doses; all received oral corticosteroids. *Conclusions:* At 24 weeks, there were more complete and overall (complete plus partial) remissions in the mycophenolate treatment arm; at 3-year follow-up, there was a nonsignificant trend toward more renal failure and death in the cyclophosphamide treatment arm.

Ong and Colleagues (2005)[57]

Renal disease: Proliferative lupus nephritis. *Treatment:* Mycophenolate for 6 months versus monthly pulse cyclophosphamide for six doses; all received oral corticosteroids. *Conclusions:* After 6 months, there were no substantive differences in the proportions of favorable and unfavorable renal outcomes or renal histology on repeat biopsy between treatment arms.

Maintenance: Cyclophosphamide Versus Mycophenolate versus Azathioprine

Contreras and Colleagues (2004)[50]

Renal disease: Focal or diffuse proliferative lupus nephritis. *Treatment:* All received induction with monthly pulse cyclophosphamide (four to seven doses) and corticosteroids and then maintenance with mycophenolate (0.5–2 g/day) versus azathioprine (1–3 mg/kg/day) versus IV cyclophosphamide (quarterly) for 25 to 30 months. *Conclusions:* Maintenance with azathioprine or mycophenolate was superior to cyclophosphamide in preventing renal failure and death; relapse-free survival was highest in the mycophenolate arm.

Maintenance: Azathioprine versus Cyclosporine

Moroni and Colleagues (2006)[110]

Renal disease: Proliferative or membranous lupus nephritis. *Treatment:* All received induction with oral cyclophosphamide and corticosteroids for 3 months and then maintenance with cyclosporine versus azathioprine for 2 to 4 years. *Conclusions:* There was no difference in number of lupus flares, decrease in proteinuria, or change in renal function between treatment arms.

Plasma Exchange: With Short-Course Oral Cyclophosphamide

Lewis (1992)[111]

Renal disease: Proliferative or mixed membranous and proliferative lupus nephritis on biopsy. *Treatment:* Prednisone and daily oral cyclophosphamide (8 weeks) only versus prednisone and cyclophosphamide combined with three times weekly plasmapheresis for 4 weeks. *Conclusions:* Plasmapheresis does not improve the clinical outcome in severe lupus nephritis compared with that achieved with prednisone and cyclophosphamide alone.

Plasma Exchange: With Synchronized Intravenous Pulse Cyclophosphamide

Wallace and Colleagues (1998)[112]

Renal disease: Active proliferative lupus nephritis. *Treatment:* Prednisone and six cycles of monthly high-dose pulse cyclophosphamide versus prednisone and six monthly cycles of synchronized plasma exchanges (3 consecutive days) followed by high-dose pulse cyclophosphamide. *Conclusions:* Changes in SLE activity and renal outcomes were comparable in both treatment groups; addition of plasma exchange to a regimen of corticosteroids and pulse cyclophosphamide is not indicated in severe SLE.

with methylprednisolone pulse therapy. Indeed, it is unlikely that prospective clinical trials comparing placebo and low-dose and high-dose corticosteroids for lupus nephritis will ever be performed, because of the potentially confounding effects of the standard clinical practice of using high-dose corticosteroids as first-line treatment for the myriad of extra-renal manifestations and complications of SLE. The best advice for the practitioner is not to withhold corticosteroids for fear of complications, but rather to test regularly the feasibility of reducing doses (preferably to alternate day) and to be willing to substitute alternative immunosuppressive drug strategies if clinical response is delayed. Physicians treating patients with SLE and lupus nephritis should always be inclined to reduce doses of corticosteroids to the lowest necessary for disease control in order to minimize risk of their insidious complications.

The issue whether to use corticosteroids as sole immunosuppressive therapy for the first bout of lupus nephritis has never been resolved. Practices differ considerably, with some arguing that due to the low probability of satisfactory complete remission occurring with corticosteroids alone, one should proceed straight to combination therapy including corticosteroids and a cytotoxic drug as initial therapy, particularly in proliferative lupus nephritis. Others would argue that because corticosteroids occasionally (~10% of cases) may lead to complete remission, one may consider a limited course of high-dose corticosteroids to be rational for previously untreated patients (and those lacking more ominous features such as crescents or fibrinoid necrosis on renal biopsy). The common temptation is to prolong the use of corticosteroids when there is improvement but objectively only partial remission. In our opinion, it is prudent to move to alternative therapy and avoid reliance on corticosteroids unless there is clear-cut complete remission within a time frame before substantive corticosteroid toxicities supervene.

Cyclophosphamide

Daily oral cyclophosphamide has been used as part of several regimens for the treatment of lupus nephritis. Conclusions about efficacy and toxicity have differed dramatically, depending mostly on the duration of cyclophosphamide administration and on the measure of renal outcome. Short-term cyclophosphamide therapy (2–6 months) has been shown to be more efficacious than prednisone alone in decreasing activity and stabilizing lupus nephritis.[35,36] However, the short course of cyclophosphamide did not eliminate the subsequent risk of renal failure.[37] On the other hand, continuation of cyclophosphamide until the patients achieved sustained remission was shown to decrease the risk of late renal failure.[38]

The cumulative toxicity of extended courses of daily cyclophosphamide provides a substantial argument against the use of protracted daily cyclophosphamide therapy for lupus nephritis[39]—a conclusion that emerges from studies of systemic vasculitis.[40] Intermittent pulse therapy has become the preferred method for administering cyclophosphamide, including treatment of children with lupus nephritis.[41,42] This approach is based mostly on experience in oncology where it has long been practice to use high, intermittent dosing as a method of maximizing the therapeutic index of cyclophosphamide as well as other chemotherapeutic drugs. Pulse

cyclophosphamide was tested extensively in murine and human lupus nephritis during the 1970s. The prolongation of survival in lupus mice was dramatic.[1] Demonstration of comparable benefit of cyclophosphamide in a human cohort with moderately severe lupus nephritis required a protracted period of observation and analysis of multiple endpoints, including urinary findings, stabilization of renal pathology,[43] and ultimately decreased risk of renal failure as measures of favorable outcome.[38,44]

After demonstration of the efficacy of prolonged courses of quarterly pulse cyclophosphamide, a subsequent trial was designed to evaluate shorter (6 months), more intense regimens of monthly pulse cyclophosphamide and monthly pulse methylprednisolone for patients with severe proliferative lupus nephritis (presence of renal insufficiency, necrosis, and/or cellular crescents). Neither of these regimens was as effective in preserving renal function or in preventing lupus relapses over a 5-year period as was monthly pulse cyclophosphamide followed by 2 years of quarterly maintenance pulse therapy.[45] Neither this study nor the study by Sesso[46] showed any short-term (i.e., 18 months) differences in renal function outcomes among patients treated with 4 to 6 months of pulse methylprednisolone versus pulse cyclophosphamide.

The most recent National Institutes of Health clinical trial comparing extended courses of pulse methylprednisolone alone, pulse cyclophosphamide alone, and the combination of pulse therapies showed that renal remission was achieved somewhat more rapidly with combination pulse therapy and was least likely with pulse methylprednisolone alone.[47,48] In short, neither pulse methylprednisolone (in either short or extended courses) nor short courses of pulse cyclophosphamide are as efficacious as extended courses of pulse cyclophosphamide in reducing risk of renal progression or in achieving sustained remission of lupus nephritis.

Nonetheless, pulse cyclophosphamide is not universally effective in controlling lupus nephritis. Furthermore, administration of cyclophosphamide is moderately burdensome for the patient, and cumulative doses of cyclophosphamide pose substantial risk of permanent gonadal toxicity. All these concerns have prompted a continued search for more effective, simple, and safe induction and maintenance immunosuppressive drug regimens for lupus nephritis. Two agents that have been tested most extensively in this regard are azathioprine and mycophenolate mofetil.

Azathioprine

The majority of studies indicate that azathioprine adds marginally to the efficacy of prednisone alone. Several studies have shown that azathioprine was not as efficacious as cyclophosphamide, measured by improvement of urine sediment, proteinuria, lupus activity, and serologies. A recently completed controlled trial in the Netherlands also concluded that an induction regimen of azathioprine (with pulse methylprednisolone) is inferior to pulse cyclophosphamide in preserving renal function and preventing renal relapses.[49] However, azathioprine appears to be efficacious as maintenance therapy and continues to be used in many centers around the world for this purpose, often after patients have had substantial improvement or achieved remission of lupus nephritis with cyclophosphamide (or other) therapy. A controlled clinical trial in the United States suggests that azathioprine is as effective as quarterly pulse cyclophosphamide for maintenance therapy.[50]

Mycophenolate Mofetil

Mycophenolic acid was initially tested and shortly abandoned for treatment of several autoimmune diseases in the 1960s. Following its reformulation as mycophenolate mofetil, it was brought to the field of solid organ transplantation as a potential advance over traditional azathioprine. Based principally on studies showing greater efficacy of mycophenolate over azathioprine in reducing transplant rejection, several investigators began exploring the use of mycophenolate in lupus nephritis (particularly for patients averse or refractory to cyclophosphamide).[51–54] Among the most attractive attributes of mycophenolate is its lack of gonadal and urinary bladder toxicity (compared with cyclophosphamide). Several randomized, controlled trials have compared mycophenolate with cyclophosphamide for induction therapy of active lupus nephritis.[55–58] The combined results of these trials have shown that mycophenolate has at least equal efficacy as and less toxicity than cyclophosphamide (oral and IV pulses) for induction therapy. Based on these encouraging findings, many clinicians have already adapted the routine use of mycophenolate for induction. However, potentially important limitations need to be highlighted and addressed before this therapy can be widely accepted for the treatment of severe lupus nephritis. The efficacy of mycophenolate in patients with rapidly progressive crescentic glomerulonephritis, significantly impaired renal function at presentation (creatinine clearance < 30 mL/min) and poor prognostic indicators on biopsy is still unproven, as these patients were excluded from the studies. Follow-up was relatively short; longer term observational data are needed to determine the relapse rate and long-term renal survival in patients treated with mycophenolate compared with cyclophosphamide for which long-term data have been demonstrated. Optimal doses for induction are also not known; many patients may not be able to tolerate the higher doses used in some trials due to gastrointestinal side effects, which might adversely affect outcomes. Pharmacokinetic studies may help to find the ideal doses. Finally, fewer than 200 patients have been treated with mycophenolate for induction therapy (and directly compared with cyclophosphamide) in randomized, controlled trials. Data from a greater number of patients are eagerly awaited.

Mycophenolate appears to be a reasonable option for maintenance therapy. Recent data support the efficacy and safety of mycophenolate after induction with pulse cyclophosphamide[50] or higher doses of mycophenolate.[55] The optimal doses and duration of mycophenolate for maintenance therapy are not known. It is also unclear whether mycophenolate is superior to azathioprine for maintenance. At least based on one study, they perform equally well.[50] The cost of mycophenolate may be a practical limitation, particularly if long-term maintenance is necessary, and may make the less expensive azathioprine more attractive if similar efficacy is confirmed in subsequent trials.

Many of these issues will perhaps be addressed by two trials that are currently in progress. One multicenter international trial will compare mycophenolate with standard pulse cyclophosphamide for induction therapy in patients with severe lupus nephritis. Patients with a satisfactory response after 6 months of induction will be randomized to maintenance with either mycophenolate or azathioprine. Another trial will be comparing efficacy of mycophenolate mofetil and azathioprine as remission-maintaining treatment for proliferative lupus nephritis.

Plasma Exchange

Plasma exchange and immunosuppressive drug therapy have had theoretical appeal as a method to rapidly eliminate pathogenic immune complexes and to inhibit production of autoantibodies.[59,60] Early uncontrolled studies claimed remarkable effectiveness of this dual approach, but this has not been confirmed by controlled therapeutic trials. Neither plasma exchange combined with conventional prednisone and cyclophosphamide[61] nor plasma exchange synchronized with high-dose pulse cyclophosphamide has been found to be superior to immunosuppressive drug therapy alone.

SPECIFIC RECOMMENDATIONS

Assessment of Prognosis and Selection of Patients for Treatment

Lupus nephritis is extremely heterogeneous, both clinically and pathologically. Many variables affect renal prognosis, and a composite of risk factors can be used in justifying treatment strategies. Box 15-3 contains a selected list of factors associated with adverse prognosis and high risk of renal progression in lupus nephritis.[62–66] Some of these factors may be evident at presentation and remain static; others change substantially during the course of lupus nephritis. Although the impact of each factor is different and not easily compared, in general, the greater the number of factors present at any one time, the more unfavorable is the renal prognosis and the stronger are the indications for aggressive immunosuppressive therapy.

Some comments regarding the impact of race on prognosis seem timely. Black race and Hispanic ethnicity have been shown to be associated with poor prognosis of lupus nephritis.[28–30,62,65,67,68] Some studies suggest that black patients with proliferative lupus nephritis respond much less favorably than other racial groups to pulse cyclophosphamide[30] and other interventions.[69] Although this issue clearly warrants continued study, the reader should be mindful that diverse racial mixes may contribute to reported differences in course, prognosis, and treatment responses among studies from different centers around the world.

Treatment Options

Treatment of severe lupus nephritis is generally divided into an initial phase of induction, which is critical to minimize the active immune mediated inflammatory processes, followed by a prolonged maintenance phase aimed at reducing the risk of relapse. The various treatment options and practical recommendations for management of lupus nephritis are presented in condensed format in Boxes 15-4 to 15-7. Nearly all the commonly available immunosuppressive drugs have been used in management of lupus nephritis, and, as described previously, only some have been subjected to scientifically rigorous comparisons. Cyclophosphamide still has the most solid evidence of efficacy for induction of severe lupus nephritis, but mycophenolate is certainly an option for those strongly opposed to

*There is controversy regarding the level of impact of these prognostic factors.
†These prognostic factors per se are not indications for treatment.

cyclophosphamide or with less severe forms of nephritis. At present, it appears that one can justifiably choose among several options of maintenance therapy including quarterly pulse cyclophosphamide, azathioprine, and mycophenolate.

Box 15-4 contains general comments on various choices of immunosuppressive agents, adjunctive therapies for secondary complications of lupus nephritis, and a selective overview of experimental therapies for proliferative and membranous lupus nephropathies.

Box 15-5 provides practical advice for administration of pulse cyclophosphamide therapy. Pulse cyclophosphamide was initially administered during an overnight hospital stay with the intent of ensuring bladder protection through brisk diuresis and control of nausea and vomiting. The newer serotonin receptor antagonists (e.g., ondansetron, granisetron) have revolutionized nausea control and have allowed the safe administration of pulse cyclophosphamide in the outpatient setting. Some risk of complications of pulse cyclophosphamide remains even with careful dose adjustment and meticulous monitoring. Herpes zoster in this patient population is aggravating but rarely life threatening. The risk of gonadal toxicity is dependent on age and total dose.[70–72] Encouraging data from several pilot studies suggest that premature ovarian failure may be reduced by suppressing ovarian function by an analogue of gonadotropin-releasing hormone.[72–74] One such regimen involves monthly intramuscular injections of depot leuprolide acetate at least 10 days before pulse cyclophosphamide infusion. Unfortunately, no consensus has been reached on the optimal approaches to gonadal protection during cytotoxic drug therapy. While fertility status is normally a supercharged issue, the high-risk patient should be thoughtfully counseled not to risk compromise of both future health and fertility (due to renal failure) by rejecting effective therapy for lupus nephritis. Nevertheless, the lowest effective dose and duration of cyclophosphamide should be considered, and alternative agents can be used during maintenance. Malignancy in SLE has been overblown in the past; indeed, cancer diathesis is quite low for both SLE and its treatment with immunosuppressive drugs.[75–78]

Box 15-6 provides a set of practical guidelines for treatment of proliferative lupus nephritis. The recommendations are organized by severity of disease, induction therapies, and maintenance regimens as well as alternative approaches to treatment. Box 15-7 contains guidelines and recommendations for treatment of lupus membranous nephropathy.[79,80]

Relapses of Lupus Nephritis

One of the most perplexing and frustrating aspects of the natural history of SLE is its remitting and relapsing course. Although we now have more treatment options from which to choose, modern treatment neither cures lupus nor completely prevents exacerbations. Furthermore, each major exacerbation is expected to leave residual and cumulative irreversible (often subclinical) damage. Approximately one third to one half of patients have a relapse of nephritis after achieving partial or complete remission of proliferative lupus nephritis.[45,81–89] Nephritic exacerbations clearly have adverse effects on renal prognosis, while proteinuric exacerbations have much less prognostic importance.[82] These observations argue in support of strategies to minimize probabilities of flares of nephritis. One controlled trial has suggested that increases in anti-DNA activity predict impending flares, which could be averted by pre-emptive boosts in corticosteroid therapy. While many agree with the general value of monitoring anti-DNA (or other serologic) activity, most clinicians would use this information as motivation to intensify clinical screening for supportive signs of lupus activity before boosting therapy. This would include assessment of renal function, quantification of proteinuria, dipstick analysis, and microscopy of urine. Nevertheless, it still may be difficult to distinguish between inactive, chronic "fixed" injury and active renal inflammation that necessitates treatment. Renal biopsy is an important tool in reassessing disease activity. In fact, some advocate protocol biopsies to assess disease immunologic activity that may be subclinical. However, the procedure is not without risk, and repeated biopsies may not be practical in the clinical setting. Several recent preliminary studies have identified candidate urinary biomarkers that are associated with lupus disease activity.[90,91] Although these observations need confirmation, such findings raise the possibility that noninvasive monitoring using proteomic profiling assays may help to predict impending relapse and allow more timely intervention.[90,92,93]

Systemic Lupus Erythematosus and End-Stage Renal Failure

None of the current regimens for treatment of lupus nephritis are fully effective in preventing renal failure. However, severe glomerulonephritis with uremia is not synonymous with

Box 15-4   Therapeutic Options for the Management of Lupus Nephritis

Immunosuppressive Drug Therapy

Prednisone: Initiate at 1.0 mg/kg/day, continue for no more than 8 weeks (except when extreme clinical conditions mandate), taper to alternate-day therapy in doses of 0.25 mg/kg every other day, use alternative immunosuppressive drugs rather than continued daily prednisone therapy whenever possible, maintain assiduous surveillance and protection against steroid-induced osteoporosis (i.e., exercise, calcium, bisphosphonates).

Methylprednisolone pulse therapy: Initiate at 1.0 g/m^2 for 3 days for severe activity (rapidly progressive renal failure, crescentic glomerulonephritis) with option to repeat pulse doses at monthly intervals; pulse methylprednisolone is usually used in conjunction with pulse cyclophosphamide.

Cyclophosphamide: Intermittent pulse therapy has the highest therapeutic index, conventional daily cyclophosphamide therapy (2 mg/kg/day) mostly avoided or used for less than 3 months (see Box 15-5 for details on administration of pulse cyclophosphamide).

Azathioprine: Alternative agent in SLE; mostly used for extrarenal disease, in mild lupus nephritis, as maintenance after period of improvement induced by cyclophosphamide or mycophenolate, or as a steroid-sparing agent in patients who require sustained high doses of prednisone or in those unwilling to accept/tolerate cyclophosphamide treatment.

Mycophenolate mofetil: Results are encouraging for use of this drug as an alternative to cyclophosphamide, for both induction and maintenance therapy for proliferative lupus nephritis; expense may be rate limiting; few data are available regarding the value of mycophenolate in membranous lupus nephropathy.

Cyclosporine: Alternative immunosuppressive drug with limited, if any, role in proliferative lupus nephritis; more favorable evidence of use in lupus membranous nephropathy; generally used in low doses (e.g., <5 mg/kg/day); tends to aggravate hypertension and dyslipidemia and worsen renal function; cosmetic side effects (gum hypertrophy, hypertrichosis) are other concerns for its use in young patients with SLE.

Tacrolimus: Another calcineurin inhibitor that shares similar immunosuppressive actions with cyclosporine. Associated with fewer cosmetic side effects than cyclosporine; limited data regarding role in proliferative lupus nephritis; may have benefit in lupus membranous nephropathy; membranous dose titration may be problematic in patients with impaired renal function.

Intravenous immunoglobulins: Expensive, short-term therapy; mostly used in lupus for immune-mediated thrombocytopenia or refractory central nervous system disease; immunosuppressive properties (e.g., suppression of pathogenic anti-DNA idiotypes) under study.

Plasma exchange: Controlled trials have not demonstrated benefit of plasmapheresis in lupus nephritis; mostly used for microangiopathic complications of lupus such as vasculopathy of superimposed thrombotic thrombocytopenic purpura.

Methotrexate: Mostly used as adjunct or alternative anti-inflammatory therapy for extrarenal manifestations of SLE; use in lupus nephritis very limited and mostly anecdotal.

Hydroxychloroquine: Mostly used as adjunct for preventing and alleviating extrarenal manifestations of SLE; it also appears to protect against major disease flares in SLE (including flares of nephritis) and has been shown to be effective in reducing the risk of damage accrual in SLE patients. Inexpensive and widely available even in developing countries. Although serious side effects are rare, retinopathy is an important ophthalmologic complication of therapy—a baseline eye examination and periodic screening are necessary to recognize ocular toxicity and to act accordingly to avoid permanent vision loss; a task force of the American Academy of Ophthalmology has recently published recommendations[113] regarding the intervals for screening, which vary depending on age of the individual, daily and cumulative doses, duration of treatment, coexisting renal or liver disease, and concomitant retinal disease.

Rituximab: Favorable results for proliferative lupus nephritis have been reported in small observational studies, case series, and several pilot studies. Improvement in renal function, proteinuria, serologic activity, and histology has been described even in lupus patients refractory to other conventional immunosuppressives. The data are still limited for both proliferative and membranous lupus nephritis; controlled trials (in progress) are needed to confirm these preliminary results. Development of neutralizing human antichimeric antibodies may influence the efficacy of B-cell depletion. In general, rituximab has an attractive safety profile but in December 2006, the U.S. Food and Drug Administration issued an alert based on two spontaneous reports of fatal progressive multifocal leukoencephalopathy in patients with SLE who had received rituximab therapy. Although extremely rare, candidates for rituximab should be counseled on the possible occurrence of progressive multifocal leukoencephalopathy, and there should be enhanced surveillance for the development of neurological symptoms.

Adjunctive Therapies for Secondary Complications of Renal Disease

Angiotensin antagonists (converting-enzyme inhibitors and receptor antagonists): Glomerular proteinuria persisting after control of active nephritis may be decreased by these agents (this must be balanced against their potential adverse effects on glomerular filtration rate and serum potassium).

Antihypertensives: Treatment of hypertension and drug choices follows standard guidelines; use blood pressure goals appropriate for age of patient (see chapter on hypertension).

Lipid-lowering drugs: These are used for control of hyperlipidemia of nephrotic syndrome. In addition, SLE and lupus nephritis confer a higher risk of accelerated atherosclerosis independent of traditional risk factors. Usually start

Box 15-4 Therapeutic Options for the Management of Lupus Nephritis—cont'd

3-hydroxy-3-methylglutaryl coenzyme A reductase inhibitors and/or fibric acid derivatives if nephrotic syndrome persists for more than 2 to 3 months; 3-hydroxy-3-methylglutaryl coenzyme A reductase inhibitors may also have immunomodulatory properties that are independent of their serum lipid–lowering properties and may help decrease proteinuria (see Chapter 25, "Management of Complications of Nephrotic Syndrome").

Bone protection: Patients with SLE often have low bone mineral density compared with healthy patients. In addition to traditional risk factors, other contributors are long duration of glucocorticoid use, cyclophosphamide, possibly use of gonadotropin-releasing-hormone agonists, and systemic inflammation. Usually start calcium and vitamin D if patients are taking steroids or bisphosphonates if osteopenia or osteoporosis is present on dual-energy x-ray absorptiometry scan.

Thrombotic diathesis: Aspirin should be used if high-titer antiphospholipid antibodies are present; warfarin (Coumadin) anticoagulation should be used if there are thrombotic events related to antiphospholipid syndrome or severe nephrotic syndrome.

Box 15-5 Recommendations for Administration and Monitoring of Pulse Cyclophosphamide Therapy

- Estimate glomerular filtration rate (GFR) by standard methods.
- Calculate body surface area (m^2) by standard methods.
- Cyclophosphamide (CY) dosing and administration:
  Initial dose CY is 0.75 g/m^2 (*important note:* start with 0.5 g/m^2 of CY if glomerular filtration rate is less than one third of expected normal).
  Administer CY in 150 mL normal saline IV over 30 to 60 minutes (*alternative:* equivalent dose of pulse CY may be taken orally in highly motivated and compliant patients).
- Obtain white blood cell count at days 10 and 14 after each CY treatment (*note:* advise patient to delay prednisone until after blood is drawn to avoid transient acute steroid-induced leukocytosis).
- Adjust subsequent doses of CY to keep nadir white blood cell count above 1500/µL (increase CY to maximum dose of 1.0 g/m^2 unless white blood cell count nadir falls below 1500/µL).
- Repeat CY doses monthly (every 3 weeks in patients with extremely aggressive disease) for 6 months and then quarterly for 1 year *after* remission is achieved (defined by inactive urine sediment, proteinuria < 1 g/day, normalization of complement [and ideally anti-DNA], and a state of minimal or no activity of extrarenal lupus).
- Protect bladder against CY-induced hemorrhagic cystitis:
  Induce diuresis with 5% dextrose and 0.45% saline (e.g., 2 L at 250 mL/hr) and encourage frequent voiding; continue high-dose oral fluids through 24 hours; counsel patients to return to clinic if they cannot sustain ingestion of enteral fluids.
  Give mesna (Mesnex) (each dose 20% of total CY dose) intravenously or orally at 0, 2, 4, and 6 hours after CY dosing (*note:* use of mesna strongly urged whenever sustained diuresis may be difficult to achieve or if pulse CY is given in an outpatient setting).
  If patients are anticipated to have difficulty with sustaining diuresis (e.g., severe nephrotic syndrome) or with voiding, insert a three-way Foley catheter with continuous bladder flushing with standard antibiotic irrigating solution (e.g., 3 L) for 24 hours to minimize risk of hemorrhagic cystitis.
- Antiemetics (usually administered orally):
  Dexamethasone (Decadron), 10-mg single dose, plus:
  Serotonin receptor antagonists: e.g., granisetron (Kytril) 1 to 2 mg with CY dose (usually repeat dose in 12 hours); alternatives in this class include ondansetron, dolasetron, palonosetron, and tropisetron
- Monitor fluid balance during diuresis. If patient develops progressive fluid accumulation, use diuretics to re-establish fluid balance.
- Complications of pulse CY
  Expected: Nausea and vomiting (central effect of CY), mostly controlled by serotonin receptor antagonists; transient hair thinning (rarely severe at CY doses < 1 g/m^2).
  Common: Significant infection diathesis only if leukopenia not carefully controlled; modest increase in herpes zoster (very low risk dissemination); infertility (male and female); amenorrhea proportional to age of the patient during treatment and to the cumulative dose of CY.
  Rare: Syndrome of inappropriate antidiuretic hormone (SIADH) (occasionally produces severe hyponatremia during the 24 hours following CY administration in the context of positive fluid balance); transient hepatocellular injury with severe elevations in bilirubin and transaminases (very rare).

Box 15-6 Treatment of Diffuse (and Severe Focal) Proliferative Lupus Nephritis

I. Recommended Initial Treatments
   A. *Moderate disease:* defined by limited number and severity of risk factors (see Box 15-3)
      1. Prednisone (1.0 mg/kg/day): limited trial (up to 8 weeks)
         a. If *complete* response occurs, including clearing of cellular casts and proteinuria, normalization of complement, and minimal lupus activity, simply taper prednisone to alternate day (~0.25 mg/kg) and monitor for flares of nephritis.
         b. If there is no or an incomplete response to prednisone or nephritis worsens, start monthly pulse cyclophosphamide or mycophenolate as outlined in section II. *(Do not delay this therapeutic decision beyond 8 weeks because of a partial response to prednisone.)*
   or
      2. Moderate dose prednisone (0.5 mg/kg/day tapered) plus mycophenolate (target dose 2–3 g/day) for 6 or more months followed by a maintenance regimen (section IV)
   B. *Severe disease:* defined by presence of a constellation of high-risk factors (Box 15-3)
      1. Prednisone (1.0 mg/kg/day tapered) plus:
         a. Monthly pulse cyclophosphamide (0.75 g/m^2; 0.5 g/m^2 if GFR is less than one third normal) for 6 months; increase dose of cyclophosphamide by up to 0.25 g/m^2 increments, to maximum of 1.0 g/m^2 unless total leukocytes fall below 1,500/µL at the 10–14 day nadir point; synchronize with monthly pulse methylprednisolone (1 g/m^2)
   or
         b. Although unproven as an effective alternative in the context of high risk severe disease, mycophenolate has been increasingly used as an alternative induction therapy; target dose 2.0–3.0 g/day for 6 or more months followed by a maintenance regimen (section IV).

II. Alternative Induction Treatment Regimens
   A. *Induction therapy:* prednisone (1.0 mg/kg/day tapered) plus:
      1. Pulse methylprednisolone 1.0 g/m^2/day for three doses; may repeat pulses at 4-week intervals and continue without additional adjunctive therapy for 6 to 12 months if there is steady progress toward remission.
      2. Daily oral cyclophosphamide, 2 mg/kg/day for 2 to 6 months (risk of gonadal and urinary bladder toxicities greater than pulse cyclophosphamide therapy).
      3. Oral pulse cyclophosphamide, ranging from 0.5 g weekly to 1.0 g/m^2 monthly (used only in highly motivated, fastidiously compliant patients).

II. Recommended Transition to Maintenance Immunosuppressive Drug Therapy or Early Discontinuance of Pulse Cyclophosphamide Therapy (at 6 Months)
   A. In selected patients, cyclophosphamide may be stopped and treatment continued with alternate-day prednisone (0.25 mg/kg) alone. Such patients have exquisitely responsive nephritis (defined by complete clearing of cellular casts and proteinuria, normal complement, and minimal lupus activity within the first 6 months). Limited duration of cyclophosphamide therapy is also important for patients giving high priority to maintaining fertility while accepting the risk of low-grade activity of lupus nephritis.
   B. The majority of patients with proliferative lupus nephritis will not be in full remission at 6 months. Convert this group to maintenance therapy using one of the regimens outlined in section IV.
Note: Microscopic hematuria often does not clear for several months, even when most other clinical parameters have remitted; by itself, microscopic hematuria is usually not a sufficient reason to abandon a particular therapeutic program.

IV. Options for Maintenance Therapy
   A. Alternate day prednisone (~0.25 mg/kg) plus:
      1. Azathioprine, 2 mg/kg/day or
      2. Mycophenolate mofetil, 1.0–2.0 g/day or
      3. Pulse cyclophosphamide every 3 months (doses adjusted by same guidelines used during the induction therapy phase).

V. Duration of Therapy
   A. *Cyclophosphamide:* Continue quarterly maintenance cyclophosphamide treatments for 1 year *after* remission of lupus nephritis is achieved (defined by inactive urine sediment, proteinuria < 1 g/day, normalization of complement [and ideally anti-DNA], and a state of minimal or no activity of extrarenal lupus). Patients with isolated fixed proteinuria or persistently elevated anti-DNA (i.e., without other supportive signs of active lupus nephritis) may be considered in remission. If uncertainty persists, findings from a repeat renal biopsy may be extremely useful in defining status of renal disease and indications for ongoing therapy.
   B. *Alternate-day prednisone:* Tapered in very small increments to discontinuance if the patient has been in sustained complete remission for more than 3 years.
   C. *Azathioprine and mycophenolate:* Maintenance for at least 18 to 24 months with subsequent tapering. Would consider criteria described in section V, A, when evaluating duration of maintenance therapy with azathioprine or mycophenolate.

Box 15-7   Treatment of Lupus Membranous Nephropathy*

I. *Mixed membranous and proliferative nephropathies:* Treat as proliferative lupus nephritis (see Box 15-6)
II. *Membranous nephropathy with nephrotic range proteinuria*
   A. First-line treatment is usually high-dose, alternate-day prednisone (e.g., 1–2 mg/kg) for 2 months; taper to approximately 0.25 mg/kg alternate days within 3 to 4 months
   B. Optional adjuncts to prednisone therapy
     1. Cyclosporine, <5 mg/kg/day
     2. Pulse cyclophosphamide, <1 g/m^2 every 1 to 3 months
     3. Pulse methylprednisolone alternating with cyclophosphamide: pulse methylprednisolone, 1.0 g/day for 3 days followed by 27 days of prednisone (0.5 mg/kg/day) alternating with 30 days of cyclophosphamide 2 mg/kg/day; three cycles of each therapy over a 6-month period
     4. Oral cyclophosphamide, 2 mg/kg/day
III. *Membranous nephropathy with nonnephrotic proteinuria:* Treat according to extrarenal disease activity; consider angiotensin antagonists to minimize proteinuria and statins for hyperlipidemia; monitor patients carefully for evidence of progression to nephrotic syndrome or to mixed membranous and proliferative nephropathy.

*Also see Chapter 21, "Idiopathic Membranous Nephropathy."

irreversible end-stage renal failure in lupus nephritis. The rate of evolution of renal failure has very important implications for treatment. Rapidly progressive renal failure, usually due to necrotizing and crescentic glomerulonephritis, is often reversible with effective treatment. Patients with evidence of active nephritis (specifically, nephritic urine sediment), even if oliguric and in advanced renal failure, warrant treatment with pulse methylprednisolone, prednisone, and pulse cyclophosphamide for approximately 3 months into maintenance dialysis therapy.

This disease profile can be contrasted with that of patients who progress slowly and insidiously to irreversible end-stage renal failure. In the latter case, one should avoid the desperate and injudicious use of aggressive immunosuppressive drug therapy in the setting of "burned out" lupus (e.g., renal failure in context of contracted kidneys and urine sediment showing predominantly broad, waxy casts). Conversely, a substantial proportion of patients on maintenance hemodialysis continue to manifest or experience flares of lupus activity, which are clearly indications for continued treatment.[25,94,95] A cautious, incremental prescription of prednisone and immunosuppressive drug therapy in such patients is warranted in order not to increase susceptibility to major infections in the uremic host.

Kidney transplantation is a viable alternative for patients with end-stage renal disease (ESRD) caused by lupus ne-

phritis. Clinically active lupus is uncommon, but evidence of recurrence of lupus nephritis in the allograft is increasingly recognized, although it is a rare cause of allograft loss.[96–99] Indeed, a recent analysis of data from a large-scale transplant registry demonstrated that patients with end-stage renal disease due to lupus nephritis have similar graft, patient, and functional graft survival rates compared with the general transplant recipient population.[100] Nevertheless, it is advisable to avoid transplantation during an acute lupus flare.

FUTURE DIRECTIONS

Experimental Therapies

There are tremendous interest and excitement for use of novel therapies in lupus that allow for more selective targeting of the immune cell subsets, cellular signaling, and molecular pathways believed to be important in disease pathogenesis. Based on encouraging results in lupus mice (see Box 15-1), many biologically based therapies have rapidly evolved from the laboratory to clinical practice. Open-label studies have confirmed the efficacy of some of these therapies for human SLE and lupus nephritis and have led to controlled trials of these agents alone or in combination with conventional immunosuppression agents. Box 15-8 lists some of the therapies that are currently being tested for lupus nephritis in randomized, controlled trials.

There are a number of novel therapies that are candidates for further testing in lupus mice (see Box 15-1) and eventual application to human SLE and lupus nephritis. Translational work has begun employing different methods aimed at overhauling the disordered immune system of patients with severe and conventional treatment-refractory SLE. Recent availability of therapeutic granulocyte colony–stimulating factor has allowed immunoablative regimens involving extreme doses of cyclophosphamide (e.g., 200 mg/kg) with or without adjunctive fludarabine, total body irradiation, antithymocyte globulin, and stem-cell rescue therapy to be tested.[101–106] The original hope of stem-cell transplantation was "going for the cure" in patients with severe lupus. Initial results were encouraging in SLE patients with refractory life-threatening multiorgan disease, but these immunoablative and reconstituting regimens are associated with substantial morbidity, high costs, and not insignificant risk of failure, relapse, and death. Whether this approach represents a definitive advance over more conventional immunosuppressive therapies will need to be answered in ongoing randomized, controlled trials. With the availability of an increasing number of newer immunosuppressive agents and biologic products, stem-cell transplantation is not the first consideration, and judicious selection of appropriate patients is important.

Unanswered Questions

Several issues remain to be addressed in future clinical trials. These include, among others: (1) studies of the comparative benefits of recycling short-term, intense immunosuppressive drug treatment for relapses versus long-term, low-intensity

Box 15-8 Agents (or Approaches) Currently Being Tested Alone or in Combination in Randomized Trials for Lupus Nephritis

Mycophenolate mofetil
Azathioprine
Tacrolimus
Sirolimus
Abatacept (CTLA4-Ig: blockade of T cell costimulation)
Rituximab (anti-CD20)
LJP 394/abetimus (to reduce circulating autoantibodies)
Infliximab (inhibition of tumor necrosis factor α)
Autologous and allogeneic stem-cell transplantation

maintenance therapies to avert relapses and minimize cumulative renal damage in lupus nephritis; (2) identification of maintenance therapy with the best therapeutic index; (3) appropriate use of biologically based therapies; (4) treatment of severe relapses while on maintenance immunosuppression; (5) treatment of refractory lupus; (6) assessment of risks and benefits of early treatment of mesangial disease; and (7) studies to define the optimal treatment of lupus membranous nephropathy.

References

1. Hahn BH: Antibodies to DNA. N Engl J Med 1998;338:1359–1368.
2. Oates JC, Gilkeson GS: Mediators of injury in lupus nephritis. Curr Opin Rheumatol 2002;14:498–503.
3. Kewalramani R, Singh AK: Immunopathogenesis of lupus and lupus nephritis: Recent insights. Curr Opin Nephrol Hypertens 2002;11:273–277.
4. Balow JE, Austin HA 3rd: Progress in the treatment of proliferative lupus nephritis. Curr Opin Nephrol Hypertens 2000;9: 107–115.
5. Esdaile JM: How to manage patients with lupus nephritis. Best Pract Res Clin Rheumatol 2002;16:195–210.
6. Ponticelli C: Treatment of lupus nephritis—the advantages of a flexible approach. Nephrol Dial Transplant 1997;12:2057–2059.
7. Cameron JS: Lupus nephritis. J Am Soc Nephrol 1999;10:413–424.
8. Donadio JV Jr, Hart GM, Bergstralh EJ, et al: Prognostic determinants in lupus nephritis: A long-term clinicopathologic study. Lupus 1995;4:109–115.
9. Huong DL, Papo T, Beaufils H, et al: Renal involvement in systemic lupus erythematosus. A study of 180 patients from a single center. Medicine (Baltimore) 1999;78:148–166.
10. Balow JE: Clinical presentation and monitoring of lupus nephritis. Lupus 2005;14:25–30.
11. Rasoulpour M, Banco L, Laut JM, et al: Inability of community-based laboratories to identify pathological casts in urine samples. Arch Pediatr Adolesc Med 1996;150:1201–1204.
12. Grande JP, Balow JE: Renal biopsy in lupus nephritis. Lupus 1998;7:611–617.
13. Esdaile JM: Current role of renal biopsy in patients with SLE. Baillieres Clin Rheumatol 1998;12:433–448.
14. Esdaile JM, Joseph L, MacKenzie T, et al: The benefit of early treatment with immunosuppressive agents in lupus nephritis. J Rheumatol 1994;21:2046–2051.
15. Weening JJ, D'Agati VD, Schwartz MM, et al: The classification of glomerulonephritis in systemic lupus erythematosus revisited. J Am Soc Nephrol 2004;15:241–250.
16. Weening JJ, D'Agati VD, Schwartz MM, et al: The classification of glomerulonephritis in systemic lupus erythematosus revisited. Kidney Int 2004;65:521–530.
17. Churg J, Bernstein J, Glassock RJ: Lupus nephritis. In Renal Disease: Classification and Atlas of Glomerular Diseases, 2nd ed. New York: Igaku-Shoin, 1995, p 151.
18. Markowitz GS, D'Agati VD: The ISN/RPS 2003 classification of lupus nephritis: An assessment at 3 years. Kidney Int 2007;71: 491–495.
19. Alperovich G, Rama I, Lloberas N, et al: New immunosuppressor strategies in the treatment of murine lupus nephritis. Lupus 2007;16:18–24.
20. Hahn BH: Lessons in lupus: The mighty mouse. Lupus 2001; 10:589–593.
21. Davidson A, Aranow C: Pathogenesis and treatment of systemic lupus erythematosus nephritis. Curr Opin Rheumatol 2006;18: 468–475.
22. Cunnane G, Chan OT, Cassafer G, et al: Prevention of renal damage in murine lupus nephritis by CTLA-4Ig and cyclophosphamide. Arthritis Rheum 2004;50:1539–1548.
23. Daikh DI, Wofsy D: Cutting edge: Reversal of murine lupus nephritis with CTLA4Ig and cyclophosphamide. J Immunol 2001;166:2913–2916.
24. Lewis EJ: The treatment of lupus nephritis: Revisiting Galen. Ann Intern Med 2001;135:296–298.
25. Berden JH: Lupus nephritis. Kidney Int 1997;52:538–558.
26. Donadio JV Jr, Glassock RJ: Immunosuppressive drug therapy in lupus nephritis. Am J Kidney Dis 1993;21:239–250.
27. Bakir AA, Levy PS, Dunea G: The prognosis of lupus nephritis in African-Americans: A retrospective analysis. Am J Kidney Dis 1994;24:159–171.
28. Baqi N, Moazami S, Singh A, et al: Lupus nephritis in children: A longitudinal study of prognostic factors and therapy. J Am Soc Nephrol 1996;7:924–929.
29. Conlon PJ, Fischer CA, Levesque MC, et al: Clinical, biochemical and pathological predictors of poor response to intravenous cyclophosphamide in patients with proliferative lupus nephritis. Clin Nephrol 1996;46:170–175.
30. Dooley MA, Hogan S, Jennette C, et al: Cyclophosphamide therapy for lupus nephritis: Poor renal survival in black Americans. Glomerular Disease Collaborative Network. Kidney Int 1997; 51:1188–1195.
31. Gruppo Italiano per lo Studio della Nefrite Lupica (GISNEL): Lupus nephritis: Prognostic factors and probability of maintaining life-supporting renal function 10 years after the diagnosis. Am J Kidney Dis 1992;19:473–479.
32. Bastian HM, Roseman JM, McGwin G Jr, et al: Systemic lupus erythematosus in three ethnic groups. XII. Risk factors for lupus nephritis after diagnosis. Lupus 2002;11:152–160.
33. Seligman VA, Lum RF, Olson JL, et al: Demographic differences in the development of lupus nephritis: A retrospective analysis. Am J Med 2002;112:726–729.
34. Balow JE: Choosing treatment for proliferative lupus nephritis. Arthritis Rheum 2002;46:1981–1983.
35. Steinberg AD, Decker JL: A double-blind controlled trial comparing cyclophosphamide, azathioprine and placebo in the treatment of lupus glomerulonephritis. Arthritis Rheum 1974;17:923–937.
36. Donadio JV Jr, Holley KE, Ferguson RH, et al: Treatment of diffuse proliferative lupus nephritis with prednisone and combined prednisone and cyclophosphamide. N Engl J Med 1978; 299:1151–1155.
37. Donadio JV Jr, Holley KE, Ilstrup DM: Cytotoxic drug treatment of lupus nephritis. Am J Kidney Dis 1982;2:178–181.
38. Austin HA 3rd, Klippel JH, Balow JE, et al: Therapy of lupus nephritis. Controlled trial of prednisone and cytotoxic drugs. N Engl J Med 1986;314:614–619.
39. Mok CC, Ho CT, Siu YP, et al: Treatment of diffuse proliferative lupus glomerulonephritis: A comparison of two

cyclophosphamide-containing regimens. Am J Kidney Dis 2001;38:256–264.

40. Haubitz M, Schellong S, Gobel U, et al: Intravenous pulse administration of cyclophosphamide versus daily oral treatment in patients with antineutrophil cytoplasmic antibody-associated vasculitis and renal involvement: A prospective, randomized study. Arthritis Rheum 1998;41:1835–1844.

41. Lehman TJ, Onel K: Intermittent intravenous cyclophosphamide arrests progression of the renal chronicity index in childhood systemic lupus erythematosus. J Pediatr 2000;136:243–247.

42. Barbano G, Gusmano R, Damasio B, et al: Childhood-onset lupus nephritis: A single-center experience of pulse intravenous cyclophosphamide therapy. J Nephrol 2002;15:123–129.

43. Balow JE, Austin HA 3rd, Muenz LR, et al: Effect of treatment on the evolution of renal abnormalities in lupus nephritis. N Engl J Med 1984;311:491–495.

44. Steinberg AD, Steinberg SC: Long-term preservation of renal function in patients with lupus nephritis receiving treatment that includes cyclophosphamide versus those treated with prednisone only. Arthritis Rheum 1991;34:945–950.

45. Boumpas DT, Austin HA 3rd, Vaughn EM, et al: Controlled trial of pulse methylprednisolone versus two regimens of pulse cyclophosphamide in severe lupus nephritis. Lancet 1992; 340:741–745.

46. Sesso R, Monteiro M, Sato E, et al: A controlled trial of pulse cyclophosphamide versus pulse methylprednisolone in severe lupus nephritis. Lupus 1994;3:107–112.

47. Gourley MF, Austin HA 3rd, Scott D, et al: Methylprednisolone and cyclophosphamide, alone or in combination, in patients with lupus nephritis. A randomized, controlled trial. Ann Intern Med 1996;125:549–557.

48. Illei GG, Austin HA, Crane M, et al: Combination therapy with pulse cyclophosphamide plus pulse methylprednisolone improves long-term renal outcome without adding toxicity in patients with lupus nephritis. Ann Intern Med 2001;135:248–257.

49. Grootscholten C, Ligtenberg G, Hagen EC, et al: Azathioprine/methylprednisolone versus cyclophosphamide in proliferative lupus nephritis. A randomized controlled trial. Kidney Int 2006;70:732–742.

50. Contreras G, Pardo V, Leclercq B, et al: Sequential therapies for proliferative lupus nephritis. N Engl J Med 2004;350:971–980.

51. Choi MJ, Eustace JA, Gimenez LF, et al: Mycophenolate mofetil treatment for primary glomerular diseases. Kidney Int 2002; 61:1098–1114.

52. Dooley MA, Cosio FG, Nachman PH, et al: Mycophenolate mofetil therapy in lupus nephritis: Clinical observations. J Am Soc Nephrol 1999;10:833–839.

53. Karim MY, Alba P, Cuadrado MJ, et al: Mycophenolate mofetil for systemic lupus erythematosus refractory to other immunosuppressive agents. Rheumatology (Oxford) 2002;41:876–882.

54. Mok CC, Lai KN: Mycophenolate mofetil in lupus glomerulonephritis. Am J Kidney Dis 2002;40:447–457.

55. Chan TM, Tse KC, Tang CS, et al: Long-term study of mycophenolate mofetil as continuous induction and maintenance treatment for diffuse proliferative lupus nephritis. J Am Soc Nephrol 2005;16:1076–1084.

56. Chan TM, Li FK, Tang CS, et al: Efficacy of mycophenolate mofetil in patients with diffuse proliferative lupus nephritis. Hong Kong-Guangzhou Nephrology Study Group. N Engl J Med 2000;343:1156–1162.

57. Ong LM, Hooi LS, Lim TO, et al: Randomized controlled trial of pulse intravenous cyclophosphamide versus mycophenolate mofetil in the induction therapy of proliferative lupus nephritis. Nephrology (Carlton) 2005;10:504–510.

58. Ginzler EM, Dooley MA, Aranow C, et al: Mycophenolate mofetil or intravenous cyclophosphamide for lupus nephritis. N Engl J Med 2005;353:2219–2228.

59. Madore F, Lazarus JM, Brady HR: Therapeutic plasma exchange in renal diseases. J Am Soc Nephrol 1996;7:367–386.

60. Wallace DJ: Apheresis for lupus erythematosus. Lupus 1999;8:174–180.

61. Lewis EJ, Hunsicker LG, Lan SP, et al: A controlled trial of plasmapheresis therapy in severe lupus nephritis. The Lupus Nephritis Collaborative Study Group. N Engl J Med 1992; 326:1373–1379.

62. Korbet SM, Schwartz MM, Evans J, et al: Severe lupus nephritis: Racial differences in presentation and outcome. J Am Soc Nephrol 2007;18:244–254.

63. Austin HA 3rd, Boumpas DT, Vaughan EM, et al: Predicting renal outcomes in severe lupus nephritis: Contributions of clinical and histologic data. Kidney Int 1994;45:544–550.

64. Mok CC: Prognostic factors in lupus nephritis. Lupus 2005; 14:39–44.

65. Barr RG, Seliger S, Appel GB, et al: Prognosis in proliferative lupus nephritis: The role of socio-economic status and race/ethnicity. Nephrol Dial Transplant 2003;18:2039–2046.

66. Contreras G, Pardo V, Cely C, et al: Factors associated with poor outcomes in patients with lupus nephritis. Lupus 2005;14:890–895.

67. Contreras G, Lenz O, Pardo V, et al: Outcomes in African Americans and Hispanics with lupus nephritis. Kidney Int 2006;69:1846–1851.

68. Austin HA 3rd, Boumpas DT, Vaughan EM, et al: High-risk features of lupus nephritis: Importance of race and clinical and histological factors in 166 patients. Nephrol Dial Transplant 1995;10:1620–1628.

69. Lea JP: Lupus nephritis in African Americans. Am J Med Sci 2002;323:85–89.

70. Boumpas DT, Austin HA 3rd, Vaughan EM, et al: Risk for sustained amenorrhea in patients with systemic lupus erythematosus receiving intermittent pulse cyclophosphamide therapy. Ann Intern Med 1993;119:366–369.

71. McDermott EM, Powell RJ: Incidence of ovarian failure in systemic lupus erythematosus after treatment with pulse cyclophosphamide. Ann Rheum Dis 1996;55:224–229.

72. Blumenfeld Z, Shapiro D, Shteinberg M, et al: Preservation of fertility and ovarian function and minimizing gonadotoxicity in young women with systemic lupus erythematosus treated by chemotherapy. Lupus 2000;9:401–405.

73. Manger K, Wildt L, Kalden JR, et al: Prevention of gonadal toxicity and preservation of gonadal function and fertility in young women with systemic lupus erythematosus treated by cyclophosphamide: The PREGO-Study. Autoimmun Rev 2006;5:269–272.

74. Somers EC, Marder W, Christman GM, et al: Use of a gonadotropin-releasing hormone analog for protection against premature ovarian failure during cyclophosphamide therapy in women with severe lupus. Arthritis Rheum 2005;52:2761–2767.

75. Abu-Shakra M, Ehrenfeld M, Shoenfeld Y: Systemic lupus erythematosus and cancer: Associated or not? Lupus 2002;11:137–144.

76. Cibere J, Sibley J, Haga M: Systemic lupus erythematosus and the risk of malignancy. Lupus 2001;10:394–400.

77. Bernatsky S, Boivin JF, Joseph L, et al: The relationship between cancer and medication exposures in systemic lupus erythematosus: A case-cohort study. Ann Rheum Dis 2007;67:74–79.

78. Bernatsky S, Ramsey-Goldman R, Isenberg D, et al: Hodgkin's lymphoma in systemic lupus erythematosus. Rheumatology (Oxford) 2007;46:830–832.

79. Sloan RP, Schwartz MM, Korbet SM, et al: Long-term outcome in systemic lupus erythematosus membranous glomerulonephritis. Lupus Nephritis Collaborative Study Group. J Am Soc Nephrol 1996;7:299–305.

80. Moroni G, Maccario M, Banfi G, et al: Treatment of membranous lupus nephritis. Am J Kidney Dis 1998;31:681–686.

81. Ciruelo E, de la Cruz J, Lopez I, et al: Cumulative rate of relapse of lupus nephritis after successful treatment with cyclophosphamide. Arthritis Rheum 1996;39:2028–2034.

82. Moroni G, Quaglini S, Maccario M, et al: "Nephritic flares" are predictors of bad long-term renal outcome in lupus nephritis. Kidney Int 1996;50:2047–2053.

83. Ponticelli C, Moroni G: Flares in lupus nephritis: Incidence, impact on renal survival and management. Lupus 1998;7:635–638.

84. Swaak AJ, van den Brink HG, Smeenk RJ, et al: Systemic lupus erythematosus. Disease outcome in patients with a disease duration of at least 10 years: Second evaluation. Lupus 2001;10:51–58.

85. Bootsma H, Spronk P, Derksen R, et al: Prevention of relapses in systemic lupus erythematosus. Lancet 1995;345:1595–1599.

86. Hill GS, Delahousse M, Nochy D, et al: Outcome of relapse in lupus nephritis: Roles of reversal of renal fibrosis and response of inflammation to therapy. Kidney Int 2002;61:2176–2186.

87. Illei GG, Takada K, Parkin D, et al: Renal flares are common in patients with severe proliferative lupus nephritis treated with pulse immunosuppressive therapy: Long-term followup of a cohort of 145 patients participating in randomized controlled studies. Arthritis Rheum 2002;46:995–1002.

88. Donadio JV Jr, Holley KE, Wagoner RD, et al: Treatment of lupus nephritis with prednisone and combined prednisone and azathioprine. Ann Intern Med 1972;77:829–835.

89. Mok CC, Ying KY, Tang S, et al: Predictors and outcome of renal flares after successful cyclophosphamide treatment for diffuse proliferative lupus glomerulonephritis. Arthritis Rheum 2004;50:2559–2568.

90. Avihingsanon Y, Phumesin P, Benjachat T, et al: Measurement of urinary chemokine and growth factor messenger RNAs: A noninvasive monitoring in lupus nephritis. Kidney Int 2006;69:747–753.

91. Li Y, Tucci M, Narain S, et al: Urinary biomarkers in lupus nephritis. Autoimmun Rev 2006;5:383–388.

92. Mosley K, Tam FW, Edwards RJ, et al: Urinary proteomic profiles distinguish between active and inactive lupus nephritis. Rheumatology (Oxford) 2006;45:1497–1504.

93. Rovin BH, Song H, Hebert LA, et al: Plasma, urine, and renal expression of adiponectin in human systemic lupus erythematosus. Kidney Int 2005;68:1825–1833.

94. Krane NK, Burjak K, Archie M, et al: Persistent lupus activity in end-stage renal disease. Am J Kidney Dis 1999;33:872–879.

95. Ward MM: Cardiovascular and cerebrovascular morbidity and mortality among women with end-stage renal disease attributable to lupus nephritis. Am J Kidney Dis 2000;36:516–525.

96. Ward MM: Outcomes of renal transplantation among patients with end-stage renal disease caused by lupus nephritis. Kidney Int 2000;57:2136–2143.

97. Lochhead KM, Pirsch JD, D'Alessandro AM, et al: Risk factors for renal allograft loss in patients with systemic lupus erythematosus. Kidney Int 1996;49:512–517.

98. Stone JH, Millward CL, Olson JL, et al: Frequency of recurrent lupus nephritis among ninety-seven renal transplant patients during the cyclosporine era. Arthritis Rheum 1998;41:678–686.

99. Moroni G, Tantardini F, Gallelli B, et al: The long-term prognosis of renal transplantation in patients with lupus nephritis. Am J Kidney Dis 2005;45:903–911.

100. Bunnapradist S, Chung P, Peng A, et al: Outcomes of renal transplantation for recipients with lupus nephritis: Analysis of the Organ Procurement and Transplantation Network database. Transplantation 2006;82:612–618.

101. Traynor A, Burt RK: Haematopoietic stem cell transplantation for active systemic lupus erythematosus. Rheumatology (Oxford) 1999;38:767–772.

102. Pavletic SZ, Illei GG: The role of immune ablation and stem cell transplantation in severe SLE. Best Pract Res Clin Rheumatol 2005;19:839–858.

103. Jayne D, Passweg J, Marmont A, et al: Autologous stem cell transplantation for systemic lupus erythematosus. Lupus 2004;13:168–176.

104. Burt RK, Traynor A, Statkute L, et al: Nonmyeloablative hematopoietic stem cell transplantation for systemic lupus erythematosus. JAMA 2006;295:527–535.

105. Lisukov IA, Sizikova SA, Kulagin AD, et al: High-dose immunosuppression with autologous stem cell transplantation in severe refractory systemic lupus erythematosus. Lupus 2004;13:89–94.

106. Petri M, Brodsky R: High-dose cyclophosphamide and stem cell transplantation for refractory systemic lupus erythematosus. JAMA 2006;295:559–560.

107. Houssiau FA, Vasconcelos C, D'Cruz D, et al: Immunosuppressive therapy in lupus nephritis: The Euro-Lupus Nephritis Trial, a randomized trial of low-dose versus high-dose intravenous cyclophosphamide. Arthritis Rheum 2002;46:2121–2131.

108. Houssiau FA, Vasconcelos C, D'Cruz D, et al: Early response to immunosuppressive therapy predicts good renal outcome in lupus nephritis: Lessons from long-term followup of patients in the Euro-Lupus Nephritis Trial. Arthritis Rheum 2004;50:3934–3940.

109. Grootscholten C, Bajema IM, Florquin S, et al: Treatment with cyclophosphamide delays the progression of chronic lesions more effectively than does treatment with azathioprine plus methylprednisolone in patients with proliferative lupus nephritis. Arthritis Rheum 2007;56:924–937.

110. Moroni G, Doria A, Mosca M, et al: A randomized pilot trial comparing cyclosporine and azathioprine for maintenance therapy in diffuse lupus nephritis over four years. Clin J Am Soc Nephrol 2006;1:925–932.

111. Lewis EJ: Plasmapheresis therapy is ineffective in SLE. Lupus Nephritis Collaborative Study Group. J Clin Apher 1992;7:153.

112. Wallace DJ, Goldfinger D, Pepkowitz SH, et al: Randomized controlled trial of pulse/synchronization cyclophosphamide/apheresis for proliferative lupus nephritis. J Clin Apher 1998;13:163–166.

113. Marmor MF, Carr RE, Easterbrook M, et al: Recommendations on screening for chloroquine and hydroxychloroquine retinopathy: A report by the American Academy of Ophthalmology. Ophthalmology 2002;109:1377–1382.

Further Reading

Balow JE: Clinical presentation and monitoring of lupus nephritis. Lupus 2005;14:5–30.

Bertsias GK, Ioannidis JP, Boletis J, et al: EULAR recommendations for the management of systemic lupus erythematosus (SLE). Report of a task force of the EULAR Standing Committee for International Clinical Studies Including Therapeutics. Ann Rheum Dis 2008;67:195–205.

Chan TM, Li FK, Tang CS, et al: Efficacy of mycophenolate mofetil in patients with diffuse proliferative lupus nephritis. Hong Kong-Guangzhou Nephrology Study Group. New Engl J Med 2000;343:156–162.

Contreras G, Pardo V, Leclercq B, et al: Sequential therapies for proliferative lupus nephritis. N Engl J Med 2004;350:71–80.

Davidson A, Aranow C: Pathogenesis and treatment of systemic lupus erythematosus nephritis. Curr Opin Rheumatol 2006;18:468–475.

Dooley MA, Falk RJ: Human clinical trials in lupus nephritis. Semin Nephrol 2007;27:115–127.

Ginzler EM, Dooley MA, Aranow C, et al: Mycophenolate mofetil or intravenous cyclophosphamide for lupus nephritis. New Engl J Med 2005;353:2219–2128.

Ponticelli C: New therapies for lupus nephritis. Clin J Am Soc Nephrol 2006;1:863–868.

Weening JJ, D'Agati VD, Schwartz MM, et al: The classification of glomerulonephritis in systemic lupus erythematosus revisited. Kidney Int 2004;65:21–30.

Chapter 16

IgA Nephropathy and Henoch-Schönlein Purpura

Jonathan Barratt and John Feehally

BACKGROUND

IgA Nephropathy

IgA nephropathy (IgAN) is a common pattern of glomerulonephritis defined by mesangial IgA deposition.[1] Recurrent macroscopic hematuria is the most frequent clinical presentation and typically occurs in the second and third decades of life. Other patients present with microscopic hematuria, proteinuria, and slowly progressive renal failure. Clinical features at the time of diagnosis indicating a poor prognosis include proteinuria greater than 1 g/24 hr and arterial hypertension.[2] Adverse histopathologic features include glomerular sclerosis, tubular atrophy, and interstitial fibrosis.[2] Rapidly progressive renal failure is unusual; it may result from acute tubular necrosis as a consequence of macroscopic hematuria or superimposed crescentic nephritis. Recurrent IgA deposition after transplantation is common and may be associated with slowly progressive graft failure.[3]

Henoch-Schönlein Nephritis

Henoch-Schönlein purpura (HSP) is a systemic vasculitis with characteristic rash, abdominal pain, and arthralgia; it is particularly common in childhood but may occur at any age. Tissue IgA deposition is a hallmark of HSP. The nephritis that accompanies HSP (HS nephritis) may be histologically indistinguishable from IgAN,[4] although a nephritic/nephrotic presentation with relatively rapid progression to renal failure is more common than in IgAN. It is probable that IgAN is a monosymptomatic form of HSP.[1,4]

Disease Mechanisms in IgA Nephropathy and Henoch-Schönlein Nephritis

IgAN and HSP share many abnormalities of the IgA immune system.[4] Exaggerated polymeric IgA1 responses are typical, although increases in circulating IgA1 are modest. Most evidence suggests that the increased polymeric IgA1 originates from the bone marrow rather than the mucosa.[5] The mechanism of mesangial IgA deposition is not understood, although IgAN and HS nephritis are often regarded as immune complex diseases. Altered O-glycosylation of IgA1 may promote mesangial IgA deposition.[6,7] Mechanisms of ongoing inflammation and scarring are probably common to other forms of chronic glomerulonephritis without IgA deposition. There is increasing evidence of genetic susceptibility to IgAN and HSP, for example, the high prevalence of urinary abnormalities in first- and second-degree relatives of those with IgAN and the substantial number of multiplex families, in some of which both HSP and IgAN occur.[8–10]

TREATMENT APPROACHES

Therapeutic Strategies

With this background, the following approaches to treatment of IgAN could be considered:

- Decrease production of nephrogenic IgA.
- Prevent glomerular IgA deposition or promote its removal.
- Alter early immune and inflammatory events that follow IgA deposition.
- Alter later nonspecific events that promote progressive renal failure.
- Prevent recurrent disease after transplantation.

Therapeutic Endpoints

It is also important to consider how the success of any therapeutic intervention might be judged.

Hematuria

Reduction of episodes of macroscopic hematuria is a clear-cut goal but should not be taken to represent the loss of all disease activity. Properly controlled studies are needed since the natural history of IgAN is that macroscopic hematuria becomes less common with time without intervention.

Proteinuria

Reduction in proteinuria is an attractive short- and long-term goal. If patients are nephrotic, the clinical benefits of reducing proteinuria and correcting serum albumin are unequivocal. However, treatment trial strategy often selects patients using nonnephrotic proteinuria as a marker of poor prognosis. The benefit of modest decreases in proteinuria, even if statistically significant, is uncertain unless accompanied by preservation of renal function.

Prevention of Renal Failure

Prevention of end-stage renal disease (ESRD) is the ultimate goal. However, IgAN is usually so slowly progressive that surrogate markers are required to provide data within an acceptable time frame. Doubling of serum creatinine or decrease in glomerular filtration rate (GFR) can be complemented by histologic data from serial renal biopsies.

Problems of Study Design

Study Group Heterogeneity

It cannot be certain that patients with mesangial IgA deposition always share a common disease process, but, at present, it remains the defining criterion for these studies. Renal histology

can be useful in study recruitment to minimize heterogeneity, but this will be less useful if the interval between biopsy and recruitment is prolonged. Furthermore, the choice of histologic criteria remains controversial. An international consensus on a pathologic classification for IgAN would be of great value in selection for therapeutic trials; the International IgA Nephropathy Network with the Renal Pathology Society, under the auspices of the International Society of Nephrology, are currently developing such a consensus, which it is expected will be announced in 2008.[11] Another factor to be considered in any trial design is the frequency of subclinical IgA nephropathy in supposedly "healthy" control populations. This may be as high as 16% in certain Asian populations.[12] Patients with HSP have been excluded from most available studies; it is therefore still uncertain whether any strategies developed for IgAN are indeed applicable to HS nephritis.

Risk versus Benefit

In slowly progressive disease, the balance of risk versus benefit if prolonged treatment is considered is often unfavorable. Acute immune interventions are also not easy to plan. If there is crescentic nephritis with renal failure, intensive treatment is justifiable; more often, visible hematuria is clinically striking but transient and produces no functional renal impairment, weakening the justification for therapy. In any case, clinically apparent hematuria is likely to represent the tip of an iceberg of ongoing injury, so that shaping and timing the intensity of therapy, even if rational treatments were available, are difficult.

The good prognosis for many patients, particularly those with isolated hematuria, argues against their involvement in prolonged studies of therapies with potential adverse effects. Conversely, the selection of patients by proteinuria can introduce heterogeneity because proteinuria may reflect both active immune injury and fixed chronic damage. Any study using proteinuria as an entry criterion will provide therapeutic guidance for only a minority of patients with IgAN.

Randomized, Controlled Trials

The need for randomized, controlled trials (RCTs) of adequate power to answer questions about the prevention of chronic renal failure in IgAN is pressing. The use of historic controls is of limited value because earlier cohorts of patients may not be comparable, for example, because of changing attitudes over recent years in accepted blood pressure (BP) targets and in the use of medications that interrupt the renin-angiotensin system. It is disappointing, despite the prevalence of IgAN and consensus about its definition and natural history, that there are so few published RCTs. Available studies are clearly defined in this chapter as RCTs and are shown in the tables. Those available in 2006 have been critically reviewed.[13,14] There have been no RCTs in HS nephritis.

Age of Subjects

There is no specific evidence that IgAN is a distinctive disease process when onset is in childhood rather than in adulthood; nevertheless, the application to adult practice of trial findings in children remains uncertain.[15]

Defining Early and Late Disease

The distinction between early inflammatory processes in IgAN and later nonspecific processes leading to renal failure is not easily made and is somewhat artificial. In a disease as indolent as IgAN, such processes will inevitably be concurrent. Diagnosis, defined by the time of renal biopsy, may be many years after the onset of the disease. RCTs of corticosteroids and immunosuppressive regimens have mostly recruited patients with proteinuria and preserved renal function, whereas studies of fish oil have in general recruited those with proteinuria and impaired excretory function.

TREATMENT OF IgA NEPHROPATHY

Decreasing IgA Production

Decreasing Mucosal Antigen Challenge

Attempts have been made in uncontrolled studies to modify food antigen intake or alter mucosal permeability pharmacologically. These have been of little benefit.[16] There is no role for prophylactic antibiotics.

Tonsillectomy

Tonsillectomy may help to prevent episodic macroscopic hematuria in the short term, and proponents of tonsillectomy argue that it also gives long-term renal protection. This view is supported by two large retrospective studies from Japan, although benefit was not apparent until 10 years after tonsillectomy.[17,18] The concomitant use of other treatment modalities and changing therapeutic goals during the follow-up period make these data difficult to interpret; a retrospective study from Germany suggests no benefit of tonsillectomy.[19] Preliminary data from a prospective Japanese RCT of tonsillectomy combined with steroids versus steroids alone has reported improvement in hematuria and proteinuria in the tonsillectomy group, but no difference in doubling of serum creatinine at 24 months.[20]

Phenytoin

Phenytoin reduces serum IgA levels and was given in an RCT for 2 years, but it produced no benefit for renal function or proteinuria nor in renal histology in repeat biopsies after treatment.[21]

Other Approaches to Decreasing IgA Production

There are no other known strategies for reducing relevant IgA production. There is no evidence that any immunosuppressive treatment used in IgAN alters circulating IgA levels, although the possibility cannot be excluded that a number of immune manipulations may reduce a specific subset of nephritogenic polymeric IgA1 molecules. However, no intervention is known to modify the abnormal IgA1 O-glycosylation found in IgAN.

Prevention and Removal of IgA Deposits

The ideal treatment for IgAN would remove IgA from the glomerulus and prevent further IgA deposition. This remains a remote prospect while IgA deposition is so poorly understood. Such a treatment would also need to be extremely safe because it would require application to large numbers of patients with benign disease unless reliable early markers of progression risk were available. The high prevalence of recurrent IgA deposition after transplantation suggests that conventional immunosuppression does not prevent IgA deposition even if it may alter subsequent inflammatory events.

Alteration of Immune and Inflammatory Events That Follow IgA Deposition

Rapidly Progressive Renal Failure Associated with Crescentic IgA Nephritis

In this uncommon situation, the risk-benefit balance is most strongly in favor of intensive immunosuppressive therapy because if crescentic IgA nephritis is not treated, there will almost inevitably be rapid progression to ESRD. Unfortunately, there are no available RCTs.

A number of case series have been reported, and these have been reviewed by Tumlin and Hennigar.[22] The largest single-center experiences in adults are nine cases reported by McIntyre and colleagues,[23] 12 reported by Roccatello and colleagues,[24] 12 reported by Tumlin and colleagues,[25] and 16 reported by Harper and colleagues.[26] Reports in 19 children have been reviewed.[15] Treatment in the majority of cases has included prednisolone and cyclophosphamide, often combined with plasma exchange. It is not possible to make firm conclusions from these data. The decision to treat is usually made based on histologic evidence of aggressive glomerular injury, and most reports include some patients with preserved renal function at the time that treatment is initiated as well as those with rapidly progressive renal failure. Early clinical response is favorable as in other crescentic nephritis, but medium-term results may be disappointing: 60% of treated patients reached ESRD by 12 months in one series[27] and 25% reached ESRD over longer follow-up in another.[26] However, a subset of patients has been reported with circulating IgG antineutrophil cytoplasm antibody who have a more favorable response to immunosuppressive therapy, similar to that seen in other types of antineutrophil cytoplasm antibody–positive crescentic nephritis.[28]

An RCT of immunosuppressive treatments in crescentic IgAN would be particularly valuable, but this is an uncommon condition and such a trial may never be achieved. Based on the available evidence, the use of corticosteroids and cyclophosphamide is justified, but there is insufficient information to recommend the addition of plasma exchange.

Early Treatment with Immunosuppressive/Anti-inflammatory Regimens

Interventions have been made in IgAN soon after diagnosis in those with active disease, even when renal function is still preserved. Treatments have included corticosteroids, cyclophosphamide, azathioprine, mycophenolate mofetil, and pooled human immunoglobulin. In some studies, they have been combined with antiplatelet agents and warfarin. The great majority of such studies are restricted to those with proteinuria greater than 1 g/24 hr, an arbitrary threshold known to be associated with significant risk of progression. The minority with nephrotic syndrome have been excluded from most studies.

Corticosteroids

There has been interest in the potential role of corticosteroids for many years, supported mostly by evidence from uncontrolled trials. In adults with heavy proteinuria,[29] corticosteroids appeared to preserve renal function if initial creatinine clearance was more than 70 mL/min, and the same group reported 10-year follow-up in moderate proteinuria that suggests decreased risk of ESRD with corticosteroids.[30]

However, there have been few RCTs of corticosteroids (Table 16-1). Three months of treatment in children with low-grade proteinuria showed no benefit.[31] Four months of treatment in nephrotic adults showed no overall benefit,[32] although there was a minority with very minor histologic changes who responded rapidly to treatment (see "Nephrotic Syndrome and IgA Nephropathy").

An RCT evaluated 12 months of corticosteroids with antiplatelet agents in nonnephrotic proteinuria with preserved renal function[33]; the control group also received antiplatelet agents. There was a decrease in proteinuria and improvement in histology, but the design and power of the study prevented investigation of any possible protection of renal function.

A larger RCT of 6 months of treatment with corticosteroids showed not only a decrease in proteinuria but also a significant decrease in the risk of a twofold increase in serum creatinine or of ESRD.[34] Further analysis showed that the benefit was sustained for as long as 10 years of follow-up.[35] Angiotensin-converting enzyme (ACE) inhibitors were not used in all patients in this study but were used in equal proportions in both corticosteroid-treated patients and control subjects, although achieved BP was not in line with current recommendations. Remarkably, the authors also report a lack of steroid adverse effects despite the substantial dose over 6 months.

This study remains the only evidence from an RCT that corticosteroids prevent renal failure in IgAN with proteinuria of more than 1 g/24 hr. However, the benefit must be viewed in context; analysis shows that the protection was no greater than that afforded by female gender,[36] emphasizing the need to understand better the many factors that contribute to the highly variable natural history of IgAN. A more recent RCT in which BP was well controlled without renin-angiotensin system blockade showed only a modest decrease in proteinuria with low-dose corticosteroids and no protection of the GFR.[37] It is unclear whether this lack of renoprotection was due to the lower dose of corticosteroid or a genuine lack of effect in patients managed to current BP targets.

The recent review of immunosuppressive treatments for IgAN by the Cochrane Renal Group suggests that corticosteroid therapy may be effective in decreasing proteinuria and the risk of ESRD, although lack of available data meant that the meta-analysis was unable to evaluate the influence of renin-angiotensin system blockade or achieved BP in the analysis.[38]

An interim analysis of a study to assess the additional benefit of azathioprine with corticosteroids has recently reported no improvement in renal outcome at 36 months when azathioprine (1.5 mg/kg/day) is added to prednisone.[39] Unfortunately, this study did not have a control group not receiving corticosteroids.[40] A second study is under way to investigate the additional benefits of 6 months of treatment with corticosteroids in patients with IgAN with proteinuria greater than 1 g/24 hr receiving long-term ACE inhibitor therapy.[41]

Cyclophosphamide

Cyclophosphamide (Table 16-2) has been used in combination with warfarin and dipyridamole in two RCTs that are not consistent. Two studies of very similar design both showed modest decrease in proteinuria,[42,43] but the preservation of renal function in one study[43] could not be confirmed in the other.[42] The use of cyclophosphamide in patients at very high risk of progression (ESRD predicted in all cases

within 5 years) is supported by a single study. Patients received cyclophosphamide followed by azathioprine in conjunction with high-dose prednisolone and were followed for at least 2 years.[44] Notably, BP control and use of renin-angiotensin system blockade in this trial fell well outside current recommendations. Previous RCTs of cyclophosphamide in less severe, slowly progressive IgAN have shown no consistent benefit (reviewed by Feehally[45]), and this is supported by the Cochrane Renal Group meta-analysis that failed to show any significant renal survival benefit from those RCTs incorporating cyclophosphamide, cyclosporine, or other cytotoxic agents, although there was a significant decrease in daily proteinuria.[38]

Cyclophosphamide has not been used alone in IgAN. In any case, many physicians, including us, regard the risk of cyclophosphamide as unacceptable in young adults with IgAN. Further studies have therefore assessed the combination of warfarin and dipyridamole without cyclophosphamide ("Antiplatelet Agents").

Azathioprine

In an open study of children with aggressive disease, azathioprine (see Table 16-2) with prednisolone appeared to preserve renal function.[46] In a long-term, retrospective study, azathioprine with prednisolone preserved renal function, but unfortunately the control group is not comparable.[47] A nonrandomized trial of azathioprine or chlorambucil in adults showed no benefit with either agent.[48] An RCT in children with 2 years of treatment with prednisolone and azathioprine (combined with antiplatelet agents) showed a decrease in proteinuria and lessening of active glomerular injury on repeat renal biopsy.[49] However, all subjects had preserved renal function at recruitment, and the rather short duration of follow-up precluded any investigation of an effect on preservation of renal function.

Cyclosporine

Cyclosporine (see Table 16-2) was used in one RCT.[50] There was a reversible decrease in proteinuria, but this occurred in parallel with a decrease in creatinine clearance, suggesting that the changes were a hemodynamic effect of cyclosporine rather than an immune-modulating effect.

Leflunomide

Leflunomide (see Table 16-2) was used in one RCT.[51] In this short trial, there was a significant decrease in proteinuria with leflunomide, but the trial lasted only 28 weeks, and the study was not designed to evaluate an effect on preservation of renal function.

Mycophenolate Mofetil

Two RCTs report no benefit from mycophenolate mofetil (Table 16-3) in patients either at risk of progression (hypertensive and/or proteinuria > 1 g/24 hr and/or decreased GFR within 5 years of diagnosis)[52] or with more advanced disease (mean serum creatinine at entry 2.6 mg/dL).[53] Both of these studies achieved rigorous BP control with use of an ACE inhibitor. In two separate RCTs, mycophenolate mofetil did decrease proteinuria over an 18-month follow-up period; however, neither study demonstrated a change in the rate of renal decline.[54,55] Again both studies achieved tight BP control with ACE inhibition.

Table 16-1 Randomized, Controlled Trials of Corticosteroid Treatment in IgA Nephropathy

Ref.	Entry Criteria	No. on Active Treatment	Treatment Period (mo)	Follow-up (mo)	Proteinuria before Treatment (mean, g/24 hr)	Proteinuria after Treatment (mean, g/24 hr)	Other Outcomes	Comments
Lai et al[32]	Nephrotic syndrome Cr < 3 mg/dL	17 (adults)	4	12–106	6.5	2.3	Remission of nephrotic syndrome in 6/7 with minor histologic change	40% had steroid-related side effects
Welch et al[31]	Cr < 1.6 mg/dL	20 (children)	3	6	0.7	0.6	None	
Pozzi et al[34,35]	UP 1–3.5 g/24 hr Cr < 1.5 mg/dL	43 (adults)	6	60–120	2.0	0.67	Risk of ESRD reduced	No major adverse effects reported
Shoji et al[33]	UP < 1.5 g/24 hr Cr < 1.5 mg/dL	11 (adults)	12	13	0.8	0.3	Histologic improvement	All received dipyridamole, none received ACEI
Katafuchi et al[37]	Cr < 1.5 mg/dL	43 (adults)	24	65 ± 25	2.3	1.3	Increase in serum albumin and decrease in total cholesterol	No effect on rate of decrease in GFR

ACEI, angiotensin-converting enzyme inhibitor; Cr, serum creatinine; ESRD, endstage renal disease; GFR, glomerular filtration rate; UP, urine protein excretion.

Table 16-2 Randomized, Controlled Trials of Immunosuppressive Treatment in IgA Nephropathy*

Ref.	Entry Criteria	Agent	No. on Active Treatment	Treatment Period (mo)	Follow-up (mo)	Proteinuria before Treatment (mean, g/24 hr)	Proteinuria after Treatment (mean, g/24 hr)	Other Outcomes	Comments
Woo et al[43]	UP < 5 g/24 hr Cr < 1.5 mg/dL	Cyclophosphamide and dipyridamole/warfarin	27	6	60	2.4	0.8	Glomerulosclerosis prevented	Cyclophosphamide for 6 mo, warfarin/dipyridamole for 24 mo
Walker et al[42]	UP >1 g/24 hr Cr 1.1–1.8 mg/dL	Cyclophosphamide and dipyridamole/warfarin	25	6	24	1.7	1.2	Renal function unchanged	Cyclophosphamide for 6 mo, warfarin/dipyridamole for 36 mo
Ballardie and Roberts[44]	Cr > 1.4 mg/dL and increasing by >15% in previous year	Cyclophosphamide, then azathioprine maintenance and prednisone	19	24–60	24–60	3.9	0.7	Decreased rate of decline in GFR at 2 yr, maintained for 5 yr	Cyclophosphamide for 3 mo; target BP < 160/90; limited use of ACEI and ATRA
Yoshikawa et al[49]	Not nephrotic; active biopsy; CrCl normal	Azathioprine + prednisone + dipyridamole + low-dose warfarin	39 (children)	24	24	1.3	0.2	Glomerulosclerosis prevented; intensity of IgA deposits decreased	Control group received dipyridamole/warfarin; renal function normal and unchanged in both groups
Lai et al[50]	UP > 1.5 g/24 hr	Cyclosporine	9	3	6	4.2	1.3	Decrease in proteinuria transient only	Parallel decrease in renal function reversed when cyclosporine withdrawn
Lou et al[51]	UP 1–3 g/24 hr Cr < 4 mg/dL	Leflunomide	30	6	6	1.66	0.6	No difference compared with fosinopril in rate of decline of renal function	Short-term study only but does suggest benefit when used with ACEI and ATRA

*There are no randomized, controlled trials of immunosuppressive agents in crescentic/vasculitic IgA nephropathy; available data are discussed in the text.
ACEI, angiotensin converting enzyme inhibitor; ATRA, angiotensin receptor antagonist; Cr, serum creatinine; CrCl, creatinine clearance; GFR, glomerular filtration rate; UP, urine protein excretion.

Table 16-3 Randomized, Controlled Trials of Mycophenolate Mofetil Treatment in IgA Nephropathy

Ref.	Entry Criteria	No. on Active Treatment	Treatment Period (mo)	Outcomes	Comments
Maes et al[52]	UP > 1 g/24 hr and/or IC 20–70 mL/min and/or BP ≥ 140/90	21	36	No effect on proteinuria, no effect on decrease in GFR	Target BP 125/75; 100% use ACEI
Chen et al[54]	UP > 2 g/24 hr Lee grade IV/V	62	18	Proteinuria reduced (mean, 3.2–0.6 g/24 hr); no effect on decrease in GFR	Target BP 130/80; 100% use ACEI/ATRA
Tang et al[55]	UP > 1 g/24 hr	20	6	Proteinuria reduced (mean, 1.8–1.1 g/24 hr); no effect on decrease in GFR	Target BP 125/85; 100% use ACEI/ATRA
Frisch et al[53]	UP 1–3 g/24 hr with 2 of: male, BP > 150/90, Cr < 4 mg/dL, GScl/TI fibrosis	17	12	No effect on proteinuria or on decrease in GFR	Target BP 130/80; 100% use ACEI/ATRA

ACEI, angiotensin-converting enzyme inhibitor; ATRA, angiotensin receptor antagonist; Cr, serum creatinine; GFR, glomerular filtration rate; GScl, glomerulosclerosis; IC, inulin clearance; TI, tubulointerstitial; UP, urine protein excretion.

The relatively small size and short duration of the studies so far available justify further evaluation, and other studies are in progress.[56]

Mizoribine

A recent retrospective study in Japan showed that mizoribine, which blocks purine synthesis in a manner similar to that of mycophenolate mofetil, resulted in a significant decrease in proteinuria when given to 20 pediatric patients in combination with prednisone, warfarin, and dipyridamole.[57] This was significantly better than the decrease in proteinuria seen in 21 historic control patients who were given only prednisolone, warfarin, and dipyridamole or in 20 historic control patients who also received IV pulses of methylprednisolone. Follow-up renal biopsies in the mizoribine-treated patients showed no progression of chronic lesions, whereas the other two sets of patients had a significant increase in the chronicity index.

Pooled Human Immunoglobulin

The immunomodulatory and anti-inflammatory effects of pooled human immunoglobulin are poorly defined but have some benefit in uncontrolled studies in systemic vasculitis and lupus. Open studies of immunoglobulin have been reported in both severe IgAN (heavy proteinuria with decreasing GFR)[58] and moderate IgAN (persistent proteinuria with GFR > 70 mL/min).[59] Proteinuria decreased, deterioration in GFR slowed in the severe group, and histologic activity scores decreased when repeat renal biopsies were available. There have been no confirmatory studies or prospective, controlled trials of this treatment since 1995. Pooled human immunoglobulin administration is associated with acute kidney injury; however, those studies reporting its use in IgAN have not reported an excessive occurrence of osmotic nephropathy.[60]

Nephrotic Syndrome in IgA Nephropathy

Nephrotic syndrome occurs in only 10% of IgAN. In many of these patients, the heavy proteinuria is a manifestation of significant structural glomerular damage and progressive renal dysfunction. However, a small minority, both adults and children, have nephrosis with minimal glomerular change on renal biopsy, although there are IgA deposits with hematuria; proteinuria remits promptly in response to corticosteroids.[32] In these patients, two common glomerular diseases may coincide: minimal change nephrotic syndrome and IgAN.[61,62] This observation justifies a trial of high-dose corticosteroids, using a regimen appropriate for minimal change disease, in IgAN with nephrotic syndrome and preserved renal function when light microscopy shows minimal glomerular injury. However, there is no evidence to support prolonged exposure to corticosteroids if there is not a prompt response, or their use in nephrotic syndrome in the presence of significant glomerular inflammation. Unfortunately, all recent RCTs of corticosteroids in IgAN have excluded those with nephrotic-range proteinuria, so there is little evidence to inform treatment choices for nephrotic IgAN with significant histologic glomerular injury.

Treatment of Slowly Progressive IgA Nephropathy

There is little to suggest that the events of progressive glomerular injury are unique to IgAN. The growing experimental evidence on mesangial injury and its resolution under the influence of growth factors and cytokines seem to be applicable to mesangial glomerulonephritis, whether or not there are IgA deposits. The adverse influence of hypertension and the likely role of proteinuria in progression likewise are common to all glomerular diseases.

Treatments available are nonspecific. They are reported as treatments for IgAN, but it is more precise to regard them as treatments for chronic glomerular disease, of which IgAN is the most common and most easily defined. (The immunosuppressive stratagems reviewed previously may be equally nonspecific in their efficacy.) The main approaches include treatment of hypertension and the use of antiplatelet agents, anticoagulants, fish oil, and 3-hydroxy-3-methylglutaryl coenzyme A reductase inhibitors.

Predicting Risk of Progression

At diagnosis, conventional clinical and histologic criteria predict cohorts of patients with a poor prognosis.[2] Further refinement of such analyses to improve prediction of outcome early in follow-up for the individual patients would be valuable to identify those who will do badly even if they show none of the known adverse features at diagnosis. This would help to identify those who require more intensive therapy.[63] Genetic markers for risk of progression have been studied, in particular I/D polymorphisms of the ACE gene.[10] However, the association between the ACE DD genotype or any other currently available genetic marker and risk of progression is not reliable enough to influence treatment strategies for the individual patient or to inform stratification in design of treatment trials.

Antiplatelet Agents

The main studies are summarized in Table 16-4. Two studies of dipyridamole/warfarin in combination with cyclophosphamide produced conflicting results (see Table 16-2). In the study in children given azathioprine and corticosteroids, all subjects received dipyridamole/warfarin, so no effect of these agents can be inferred.[49] Two RCTs of dipyridamole/warfarin alone are inconsistent: There was no benefit in one,[64] but some decrease in proteinuria and protection from renal impairment in the other.[65]

Hypertension and the Role of Inhibitors of the Renin Angiotensin System

There is compelling evidence of the benefit of lowering BP in the treatment of chronic progressive glomerular disease.[66] In IgAN, evidence is accumulating that casual clinic BP measurements may underestimate the early impact of hypertension as judged by ambulatory BP monitoring and echocardiographic evidence of increased left ventricular mass.[67] The impact of the early active management of BP on the long-term cardiovascular morbidity and mortality of these patients will be considerable, independent of any effect on the preservation of renal function. There is also powerful evidence of the primary role of ACE inhibitors in chronic proteinuric renal disease in view of their additional benefits in decreasing proteinuria and preserving renal function.[68] However, specific evidence of the role of ACE inhibitors in IgAN is scant (Table 16-5). Short-term randomized studies in normotensive proteinuric IgAN confirm that an ACE inhibitor decreases proteinuria to the same degree as an angiotensin receptor antagonist (ATRA), an effect potentiated by indomethacin.[69,70] A recently completed placebo-controlled RCT of ACE inhibitors in IgAN with proteinuria greater than 1 g/24 hr and creatinine clearance greater than 50 mL/min/1.73 m^2 reported a significant decrease in proteinuria and preservation of renal function independent of systolic or diastolic BP.[71] Likewise a recent RCT of 109 patients reported benefit with an ATRA (valsartan) both in decreasing proteinuria and slowing the rate

of renal deterioration, although the investigators were unable to demonstrate a significant improvement in their primary endpoints of doubling of serum creatinine or ESRD at 2 years.[72] The combination of an ACE inhibitor and ATRA produces a significant additional decrease in proteinuria.[73] Indirect evidence of the benefit from such a combination in IgAN is provided by the COOPERATE study in which an ATRA was given in combination with an ACE inhibitor for nondiabetic proteinuric renal disease. An additional decrease in proteinuria was achieved with no further lowering of BP; 131 of the patients in this large study had IgAN.[74]

The only two RCTs of ACE inhibitors in hypertensive IgAN showed no benefit, although this may be attributable to the relatively short follow-up in one study[75] and the inclusion of patients with advanced disease in the other.[76] However, two retrospective studies in IgAN demonstrated the benefit of using ACE inhibitors for hypertension compared with β-blockers[77] and a wide range of other agents.[78]

ACE inhibitors in combination with ATRA are recommended as the preferred treatment for hypertensive IgAN and should also be considered for normotensive IgAN with significant proteinuria (>1 g/24 hr).

Fish Oil

The available studies are summarized in Table 16-6. The favorable effects of supplementing the diet with ω-3 fatty acids in the form of fish oil include decreases in eicosanoid and cytokine production, changes in membrane fluidity and rheology, and decreased platelet aggregability. These features should significantly decrease the adverse influence of many mechanisms thought to affect progression of chronic glomerular disease. Fish oil treatment does not have the drawbacks associated with immunosuppressive treatment. It is safe apart from a decrease in blood coagulability, which is not usually a practical problem, and an unpleasant taste with flatulence, which may make compliance difficult.

The study of Donadio and colleagues[79] provides convincing evidence of protection with 6 months of treatment with fish oil (12 g/day). However, an unexpected finding was that fish oil did not significantly decrease proteinuria, which is a major risk factor for progression and which has been decreased in all other studies of agents that are renoprotective in IgAN. The benefit was sustained in a longer follow-up of the same cohort, although treatment allocations were not always sustained after the original trial period was completed.[80] A further study showed no difference in outcome between a high (24 g/day) and low (12 g/day) dose of fish oil; once again, proteinuria did not decrease during follow-up.[81] However, these studies conflict with the smaller study of Bennett and colleagues,[82] which showed no benefit from fish oil. Pettersson and colleagues[83] may have failed to show benefit because of the short follow-up period of 6 months. A meta-analysis of these studies suggests that the available evidence does not yet give unequivocal support for the use of fish oil.[84] A recent RCT shows no benefit after 2 years of treatment with fish oil compared with placebo, although a subsequent post hoc analysis of the data in the study revealed a dose-dependent decrease in proteinuria in the fish oil group.[85]

A further confirmatory study of fish oil would be of great value.

Table 16-4   Randomized, Controlled Trials of Antiplatelet/Anticoagulant Treatment in IgA Nephropathy

Ref.	Entry Criteria	Agent	No. on Active Treatment	Treatment Period (mo)	Follow-up (mo)	Outcomes	Comments
Woo et al[43]	UP < 5 g/24 hr Cr < 1.5 mg/dL	Dipyridamole/warfarin (and cyclophosphamide)	27	24	60	Proteinuria decreased (mean, 2.4–0.8 g/24 hr); glomerulosclerosis prevented	Cyclophosphamide for 6 mo
Walker et al[42]	UP > 1 g/24 hr Cr 1.1–1.8 mg/dL	Dipyridamole/warfarin (and cyclophosphamide)	25	36	24	Proteinuria decreased (mean, 1.7–1.2 g/24 hr); renal function unchanged	Cyclophosphamide for 6 mo
Chan et al[64]	UP < 2 g/24 hr Cr < 1.5 mg/dL	Dipyridamole/warfarin	19	33	33	None	
Lee et al[65]	Cr 1.6–3.0 mg/dL	Dipyridamole/warfarin	11	36	60	Proteinuria decreased (mean, 1.4–0.6 g/24 hr); renal function maintained	

Cr, serum creatinine; UP, urine protein excretion.

Table 16-5 Randomized, Controlled Trials of Angiotensin-Converting Enzyme and Angiotensin Receptor Antagonist Inhibitor Treatment in Immunoglobulin A Nephropathy

Ref.	Type of Study	Entry Criteria	No. on Active Treatment	Follow-up (mo)	Outcome	Comments
Maschio et al[69]	Placebo-controlled, crossover	UP 1-2.5 g/24 hr, normotensive	8	8	Proteinuria decreased (mean, 1.8-1.4 g/24 hr)	Short-term study: ? functional importance of minor reduction in proteinuria
Perico et al[70]	RCT: enalapril vs. irbesartan ± indomethacin	UP 0.5-4.0 g/24 hr, Cr < 2.5 mg/dL	10	1	Proteinuria decreased by 55%-61%; effect of enalapril-irbesartan; potentiated by irbesartan	Short-term study
Bannister et al[75]	RCT: enalapril vs. nifedipine	GFR 30-90 mL/min, hypertensive	12	12	Proteinuria decreased (mean, 2.0-1.2 g/24 hr); renal function not different	
Cheng et al[76]	RCT: captopril vs. nadolol/ticlodipine	UP > 1 g/24 hr, Cr 1.3-4.4 mg/dL, hypertensive sclerosis on biopsy	31	>36	No difference in proteinuria, blood pressure, or renal impairment between ACEI and nadolol	Advanced disease at time of study
Coppo et al[71]	RCT: benazepril vs. placebo	UP > 1-3.5 g/24 hr, CrCl > 50 mL/min	32	38	Proteinuria decreased; (55% achieved <0.5 g/24 hr); renal function maintained	Study in children and young adults
Li et al[72]	RCT: valsartan vs. placebo	UP > 1 g/24 hr, Cr 1.4-2.8 mg/dL	54	48	Proteinuria decreased (mean, 1.8-1.2 g/24 hr); reduction in rate of decline of GFR	Target BP 140/90 No difference in primary endpoint (doubling Cr or ESRD)

ACEI, angiotensin-converting enzyme inhibitor; Cr, serum creatinine; CrCl, creatinine clearance; ESRD, end-stage renal disease; GFR, glomerular filtration rate; RCT, randomized controlled trial; UP, urine protein excretion.

Table 16-6   Fish Oil Treatment in IgA Nephropathy

Ref.	Entry Criteria	No. on Active Treatment	Treatment Period (mo)	Outcomes	Comments
Hamazaki et al[94]	No details	10	12	Renal function stabilized	Randomization not described
Bennett et al[82]	Proteinuria	17	24	No benefit	
Cheng et al[95]	Cr 2–6 mg/dL	11	10 (8–12)	No benefit	Advanced renal impairment at recruitment
Petterson et al[83]	UP > 0.5 g/24 hr Cr < 2.8 mg/dL	15	6	No benefit	
Donadio et al[79,80]	UP > 1 g/24 hr Cr < 3 mg/dL	55	24	Fish oils lessened deterioration in renal function	Proteinuria unchanged; poor prognosis in control group
Donadio et al[81]	UP 1.7–3.6 g/24 hr Cr 1.5–4.9 mg/dL	73 (high vs. low dose)	24	No difference between high-dose and low-dose fish oils	No control group not receiving fish oils; protein-uria unchanged
Hogg et al[85]	UP/C > 0.5 eGFR > 50 mL/min	32 (fish oil) 33 (steroids)	24	No difference between fish oil, prednisone, or placebo in rate of de-crease in GFR	Significantly higher UP/C in fish oil group at start of trial

Cr, serum creatinine; eGFR, estimated glomerular filtration rate; UP, urine protein excretion; UP/C, urine protein-to-creatinine ratio.

3-Hydroxy-3-Methylglutaryl Coenzyme A Reductase Inhibitors

One small RCT showed that 6 months of treatment with the 3-hydroxy-3-methylglutaryl coenzyme A reductase inhibitor fluvastatin resulted in a 41% decrease in proteinuria with no effect on the GFR.[86] Further prolonged studies are needed to confirm this effect.

Posttransplantation Recurrence

Mesangial IgA deposition after transplantation is common, occurring in as many as 50% of patients whose primary renal disease was IgAN.[3] Graft survival is no worse in regis-try data than for other primary renal diseases; however, re-cent data indicate that IgA deposition is accompanied by the slow onset of glomerular injury, indistinguishable histo-logically from disease in native kidneys and often at the same tempo. There is no substantial evidence that any par-ticular immunosuppressive regimen decreases the risk of recurrent IgA deposits or prevents any subsequent glomeru-lar injury.[87] One study in Chinese patients suggests that the risk of recurrence may be higher in a transplant from a liv-ing related donor than in a transplant from a live unrelated donor or a cadaver, but numerous other studies do not sup-port this.[88] Based on current evidence, there is no need to recommend any restriction in the use of living as opposed to cadaveric donors.

TREATMENT OF HENOCH-SCHÖNLEIN NEPHRITIS

There are no prospective RCTs to guide the treatment of HS nephritis. Most available data are for children. Most thera-peutic studies of IgAN exclude those with HSP so it is uncer-tain whether a number of potential treatments have a role in HS nephritis. Available studies usually include children whose renal abnormalities have been severe or persistent enough to warrant referral to a nephrologist.

Many patients have transient nephritis during the early phase of HSP that spontaneously remits and requires no treat-ment. It has been proposed that early use of corticosteroids in HSP may prevent nephritis,[89] but this has not been confirmed in other nonrandomized studies.[15]

Rapidly Progressive Renal Failure due to Crescentic Nephritis

Crescentic nephritis is more common in HSP than in IgAN, particularly early in the course. There is little information on treatment in adults; five studies report experience in 81 chil-dren.[15] Regimens are variable and include corticosteroids and cyclophosphamide, with the addition of pulse methylpred-nisolone in some cases; two studies used plasma exchange alone. Precise entry criteria varied in the extent of proteinuria, renal impairment, and histologic injury. Short-term outcomes are encouraging; for example, Oner and colleagues[90] report that 11 of 12 children had a normal GFR at 3 months despite a GFR less than 40 mL/min and more than 60% crescents at presentation. However, in the middle term, 20% of reported cases had an adverse outcome including ESRD.[15]

Active Henoch-Schönlein Nephritis without Renal Failure

In less aggressive HS nephritis, there is little information. Corticosteroids alone have never been shown to be beneficial.[15] Apparently promising findings with combination therapy of corticosteroids, cyclophosphamide, and antiplatelet agents have been reported only in small nonrandomized studies.[15] A recent nonrandomized study reported that the combination of prednisolone and azathioprine preserved renal function and improved histologic appearance, but this relied on comparison with historic controls.[91] There are only five patients with HS nephritis included in the promising studies of pooled immunoglobulin.[58,59]

Slowly Progressive Renal Failure

Although the renal histology and clinical course of slowly progressive HS nephritis and IgAN may be indistinguishable, patients with HS nephritis have not been included in the RCTs of corticosteroids, fish oil, or antiplatelet agents.

Transplant Recurrence

Graft recurrence of HS nephritis is common. There is some evidence that it is more common and more likely to cause graft loss in children receiving kidneys from living related donors than in those receiving cadaver kidneys,[92] although this is not confirmed in adults.[93] No treatment is known to decrease risk of recurrence.

TREATMENT RECOMMENDATIONS

Based on the evidence reviewed here, specific treatment recommendations are described in Figure 16-1 for the different clinical patterns of IgAN and HS purpura.

The most controversial issue remains the treatment of IgAN with proteinuria greater than 1 g/24 hr. Physicians are increasingly using corticosteroids when there is preserved renal function (serum creatinine < 1.5 mg/dL) and fish oils when there is more renal impairment (serum creatinine > 1.5 mg/dL). However, in our opinion, the case is not yet made for either of these therapies. Tight control of BP and decreased proteinuria with ACE inhibitors in combination with ATRAs should be the first line of treatment. If physicians wish to consider additional therapy with fish oil or corticosteroids, this should be contemplated only if proteinuria persists at more than 1 g/24 hr on maximal renin angiotensin system blockade with BP less than 125/75 mm Hg.

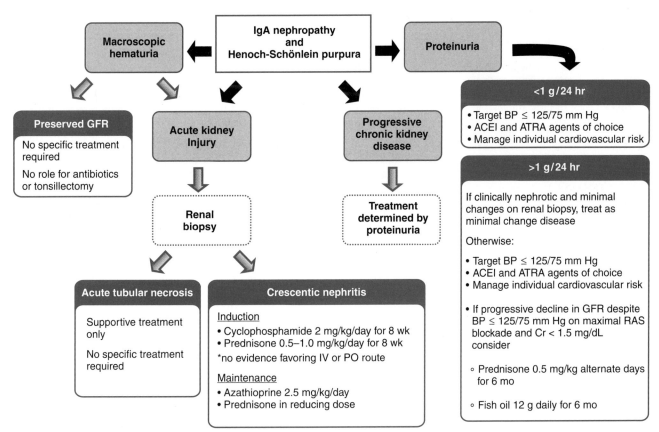

Figure 16-1   Treatment algorithm for the management of IgA nephropathy and Henoch-Schönlein purpura. ACEI, angiotensin-converting enzyme inhibitor; ATRA, angiotensin receptor antagonist; BP, blood pressure; Cr, creatinine; GFR, glomerular filtration rate; RAS, renin-angiotensin system.

FUTURE DIRECTIONS

Specific treatment to prevent mesangial IgA deposition is the ideal goal but remains a remote prospect until the fundamentals of the disease mechanism are understood. It seems unlikely that controlled trials of crescentic IgAN or crescentic HS nephritis will ever be mounted. Prevention of slowly progressive renal failure remains the most promising field, particularly as this may inform the management of chronic glomerular disease other than that associated with IgA deposition. Further studies confirming the value of fish oil and corticosteroids are required. The value of combining ACE inhibitors and ATRAs requires formal confirmation in prospective studies, as does the potential role for 3-hydroxy-3-methylglutaryl coenzyme A reductase inhibitors. Other low-risk strategies need to be developed from an understanding of the mechanisms of progressive renal scarring.

References

1. Barratt J, Feehally J: IgA nephropathy. J Am Soc Nephrol 2005;16:2088–2097.
2. D'Amico G: Natural history of idiopathic IgA nephropathy and factors predictive of disease outcome. Semin Nephrol 2004;24:179–196.
3. Floege J: Recurrent IgA nephropathy after renal transplantation. Semin Nephrol 2004;24:287–291.
4. Davin JC, Ten Berge IJ, Weening JJ: What is the difference between IgA nephropathy and Henoch-Schönlein purpura nephritis? Kidney Int 2001;59:823–834.
5. Barratt J, Feehally J, Smith AC: Pathogenesis of IgA nephropathy. Semin Nephrol 2004;24:197–217.
6. Allen AC, Bailey EM, Brenchley PE, et al: Mesangial IgA1 in IgA nephropathy exhibits aberrant O-glycosylation: Observations in three patients. Kidney Int 2001;60:969–973.
7. Hiki Y, Odani H, Takahashi M, et al: Mass spectrometry proves under-O-glycosylation of glomerular IgA1 in IgA nephropathy. Kidney Int 2001;59:1077–1085.
8. Bisceglia L, Cerullo G, Forabosco P, et al: Genetic heterogeneity in Italian families with IgA nephropathy: Suggestive linkage for two novel IgA nephropathy loci. Am J Hum Genet 2006;79:1130–1134.
9. Gharavi AG, Yan Y, Scolari F, et al: IgA nephropathy, the most common cause of glomerulonephritis, is linked to 6q22-23. Nat Genet 2000;26:354–357.
10. Hsu SI, Ramirez SB, Winn MP, et al: Evidence for genetic factors in the development and progression of IgA nephropathy. Kidney Int 2000;57:1818–1835.
11. Feehally J, Barratt J, Coppo R, et al: International IgA nephropathy network clinico-pathological classification of IgA nephropathy. Contrib Nephrol 2007;157:13–18.
12. Suzuki K, Honda K, Tanabe K, et al: Incidence of latent mesangial IgA deposition in renal allograft donors in Japan. Kidney Int 2003;63:2286–2294.
13. Appel GB, Waldman M: The IgA nephropathy treatment dilemma. Kidney Int 2006;69:1939–1944.
14. Barratt J, Feehally J: Treatment of IgA nephropathy. Kidney Int 2006;69:1934–1938.
15. Wyatt RJ, Hogg RJ: Evidence-based assessment of treatment options for children with IgA nephropathies. Pediatr Nephrol 2001;16:156–167.
16. Feehally J: Immunoglobulin A nephropathy: Fish oils and beyond. Curr Opin Nephrol Hypertens 1996;5:442–446.
17. Hotta O, Miyazaki M, Furuta T, et al: Tonsillectomy and steroid pulse therapy significantly impact on clinical remission in patients with IgA nephropathy. Am J Kidney Dis 2001;38:736–743.
18. Xie Y, Nishi S, Ueno M, et al: The efficacy of tonsillectomy on long-term renal survival in patients with IgA nephropathy. Kidney Int 2003;63:1861–1867.
19. Rasche FM, Schwarz A, Keller F: Tonsillectomy does not prevent a progressive course in IgA nephropathy. Clin Nephrol 1999;51:147–152.
20. Miyazaki M, Hotta O, Komatsuda A, et al: A multicenter prospective cohort study of tonsillectomy and steroid therapy in Japanese patients with IgA nephropathy: A 5-year report. Contrib Nephrol 2007;157:94–98.
21. Clarkson AR, Seymour AE, Woodroffe AJ, et al: Controlled trial of phenytoin therapy in IgA nephropathy. Clin Nephrol 1980;13:215–218.
22. Tumlin JA, Hennigar RA: Clinical presentation, natural history, and treatment of crescentic proliferative IgA nephropathy. Semin Nephrol 2004;24:256–268.
23. McIntyre CW, Fluck RJ, Lambie SH: Steroid and cyclophosphamide therapy for IgA nephropathy associated with crescenteric change: An effective treatment. Clin Nephrol 2001;56:193–198.
24. Roccatello D, Ferro M, Cesano G, et al: Steroid and cyclophosphamide in IgA nephropathy. Nephrol Dial Transplant 2000;15:833–835.
25. Tumlin JA, Lohavichan V, Hennigar R: Crescentic, proliferative IgA nephropathy: Clinical and histological response to methylprednisolone and intravenous cyclophosphamide. Nephrol Dial Transplant 2003;18:1321–1329.
26. Harper L, Ferreira MA, Howie AJ, et al: Treatment of vasculitic IgA nephropathy. J Nephrol 2000;13:360–366.
27. Roccatello D, Ferro M, Coppo R, et al: Report on intensive treatment of extracapillary glomerulonephritis with focus on crescentic IgA nephropathy. Nephrol Dial Transplant 1995;10:2054–2059.
28. Haas M, Jafri J, Bartosh SM, et al: ANCA-associated crescentic glomerulonephritis with mesangial IgA deposits. Am J Kidney Dis 2000;36:709–718.
29. Kobayashi Y, Fujii K, Hiki Y, et al: Steroid therapy in IgA nephropathy: A retrospective study in heavy proteinuric cases. Nephron 1988;48:12–17.
30. Kobayashi Y, Hiki Y, Kokubo T, et al: Steroid therapy during the early stage of progressive IgA nephropathy. A 10-year follow-up study. Nephron 1996;72:237–242.
31. Welch TR, Fryer C, Shely E, et al: Double-blind, controlled trial of short-term prednisone therapy in immunoglobulin A glomerulonephritis. J Pediatr 1992;121:474–477.
32. Lai KN, Lai FM, Ho CP, Chan KW: Corticosteroid therapy in IgA nephropathy with nephrotic syndrome: A long-term controlled trial. Clin Nephrol 1986;26:174–180.
33. Shoji T, Nakanishi I, Suzuki A, et al: Early treatment with corticosteroids ameliorates proteinuria, proliferative lesions, and mesangial phenotypic modulation in adult diffuse proliferative IgA nephropathy. Am J Kidney Dis 2000;35:194–201.
34. Pozzi C, Bolasco PG, Fogazzi GB, et al: Corticosteroids in IgA nephropathy: A randomised controlled trial. Lancet 1999;353:883–887.
35. Pozzi C, Andrulli S, Del Vecchio L, et al: Corticosteroid effectiveness in IgA nephropathy: Long-term results of a randomized, controlled trial. J Am Soc Nephrol 2004;15:157–163.
36. Locatelli F, Pozzi C, Del Vecchio L, et al: Role of proteinuria reduction in the progression of IgA nephropathy. Ren Fail 2001;23:495–505.
37. Katafuchi R, Ikeda K, Mizumasa T, et al: Controlled, prospective trial of steroid treatment in IgA nephropathy: A limitation of low-dose prednisolone therapy. Am J Kidney Dis 2003;41:972–983.

38. Samuels JA, Strippoli GF, Craig JC, et al: Immunosuppressive treatments for immunoglobulin A nephropathy: A meta-analysis of randomized controlled trials. Nephrology (Carlton) 2004;9:177–185.

39. Pozzi C, Del Vecchio L, Andrulli S, et al: Steroids and azathioprine versus steroids alone in IgA nephropathy. Nephrol Dial Transplant 2007;22:FO020,

40. Locatelli F, Pozzi C, Del Vecchio L, et al: Combined treatment with steroids and azathioprine in IgA nephropathy: Design of a prospective randomised multicentre trial. J Nephrol 1999;12: 308–311.

41. Manno C, Gesualdo L, D'Altri C, et al: Prospective randomized controlled multicenter trial on steroids plus ramipril in proteinuric IgA nephropathy. J Nephrol 2001;14:248–252.

42. Walker RG, Yu SH, Owen JE, Kincaid-Smith P: The treatment of mesangial IgA nephropathy with cyclophosphamide, dipyridamole and warfarin: A two-year prospective trial. Clin Nephrol 1990;34:103–107.

43. Woo KT, Lee GS, Lau YK, et al: Effects of triple therapy in IgA nephritis: A follow-up study 5 years later. Clin Nephrol 1991; 36:60–66.

44. Ballardie FW, Roberts IS: Controlled prospective trial of prednisolone and cytotoxics in progressive IgA nephropathy. J Am Soc Nephrol 2002;13:142–148.

45. Feehally J: IgA nephropathy and Henoch-Schönlein purpura. In Brady HR, Wilcox CS (eds): Therapy in Nephrology and Hypertension, 2nd ed. Philadelphia: WB Saunders, 2002.

46. Andreoli SP, Bergstein JM: Treatment of severe IgA nephropathy in children. Pediatr Nephrol 1989;3:248–253.

47. Goumenos D, Ahuja M, Shortland JR, Brown CB: Can immunosuppressive drugs slow the progression of IgA nephropathy? Nephrol Dial Transplant 1995;10:1173–1181.

48. Lagrue G, Bernard D, Bariety J: Traitement par la chlorambucil et azathioprine dans les glomerulonephrites primitives Resultats d'une etude "controlee." J Urol Nephrol 1975;9: 655–672.

49. Yoshikawa N, Ito H, Sakai T, Takekoshi Y, et al: A controlled trial of combined therapy for newly diagnosed severe childhood IgA nephropathy. The Japanese Pediatric IgA Nephropathy Treatment Study Group. J Am Soc Nephrol 1999;10: 101–109.

50. Lai KN, Lai FM, Li PK, Vallance-Owen J: Cyclosporin treatment of IgA nephropathy: A short term controlled trial. Br Med J 1987;295:1165–1168.

51. Lou T, Wang C, Chen Z, et al: Randomised controlled trial of leflunomide in the treatment of immunoglobulin A nephropathy. Nephrology (Carlton) 2006;11:113–116.

52. Maes BD, Oyen R, Claes Ket al: Mycophenolate mofetil in IgA nephropathy: Results of a 3-year prospective placebo-controlled randomized study. Kidney Int 2004;65:1842–1849.

53. Frisch G, Lin J, Rosenstock J, et al: Mycophenolate mofetil (MMF) vs placebo in patients with moderately advanced IgA nephropathy: A double-blind randomized controlled trial. Nephrol Dial Transplant 2005;20:2139–2145.

54. Chen X, Chen P, Cai G, et al: [A randomized control trial of mycophenolate mofetil treatment in severe IgA nephropathy]. Zhonghua Yi Xue Za Zhi 2002;82:796–801.

55. Tang S, Leung JC, Chan LY, et al: Mycophenolate mofetil alleviates persistent proteinuria in IgA nephropathy. Kidney Int 2005;68: 802–812.

56. Hogg RJ, Wyatt RJ: A randomized controlled trial of mycophenolate mofetil in patients with IgA nephropathy [ISRCTN6257616]. BMC Nephrol 2004;5:3.

57. Kawasaki Y, Hosoya M, Suzuki J, et al: Efficacy of multidrug therapy combined with mizoribine in children with diffuse IgA nephropathy in comparison with multidrug therapy without mizoribine and with methylprednisolone pulse therapy. Am J Nephrol 2004;24:576–581.

58. Rostoker G, Desvaux-Belghiti D, Pilatte Y, et al.: High-dose immunoglobulin therapy for severe IgA nephropathy and Henoch-Schönlein purpura. Ann Intern Med 1994;120:476–484.

59. Rostoker G, Desvaux-Belghiti D, Pilatte Y, et al.: Immunomodulation with low-dose immunoglobulins for moderate IgA nephropathy and Henoch-Schönlein purpura. Preliminary results of a prospective uncontrolled trial [see comments]. Nephron 1995;69:327–334.

60. Orbach H, Tishler M, Shoenfeld Y: Intravenous immunoglobulin and the kidney—a two-edged sword. Semin Arthritis Rheum 2004;34:593–601.

61. Clive DM, Galvanek EG, Silva FG: Mesangial immunoglobulin A deposits in minimal change nephrotic syndrome: A report of an older patient and review of the literature. Am J Nephrol 1990;10:31–36.

62. Furuse A, Hiramatsu M, Adachi N, et al: Dramatic response to corticosteroid therapy of nephrotic syndrome associated with IgA nephropathy. Int J Pediatr Nephrol 1985;6:205–208.

63. Feehally J: Predicting prognosis in IgA nephropathy. Am J Kidney Dis 2001;38:881–883.

64. Chan MK, Kwan SY, Chan KW, Yeung CK: Controlled trial of antiplatelet agents in mesangial IgA glomerulonephritis. Am J Kidney Dis 1987;9:417–421.

65. Lee GSL, Choong HI, Chiang GSC, Woo KT: Three-year randomized controlled trial of dipyridamole and low-dose warfarin in patients with IgA nephropathy and renal impairment. Nephrology 1997;3:117–121.

66. Jafar TH, Stark PC, Schmid CH, et al: Progression of chronic kidney disease: The role of blood pressure control, proteinuria, and angiotensin-converting enzyme inhibition: A patient-level meta-analysis. Ann Intern Med 2003;139:244–252.

67. Stefanski A, Schmidt KG, Waldherr R, Ritz E: Early increase in blood pressure and diastolic left ventricular malfunction in patients with glomerulonephritis. Kidney Int 1996;50:1321–1326.

68. Randomised placebo-controlled trial of effect of ramipril on decline in glomerular filtration rate and risk of terminal renal failure in proteinuric, non-diabetic nephropathy. The GISEN Group (Gruppo Italiano di Studi Epidemiologici in Nefrologia). Lancet 1997;349:1857–1863.

69. Maschio G, Cagnoli L, Claroni F, et al: ACE inhibition reduces proteinuria in normotensive patients with IgA nephropathy: A multicentre, randomized, placebo-controlled study. Nephrol Dial Transplant 1994;9:265–269.

70. Perico N, Remuzzi A, Sangalli F, et al: The antiproteinuric effect of angiotensin antagonism in human IgA nephropathy is potentiated by indomethacin. J Am Soc Nephrol 1998;9:2308–2317.

71. Coppo R, Peruzzi L, Amore A, et al: IgACE: A placebo-controlled, randomized trial of angiotensin-converting enzyme inhibitors in children and young people with IgA nephropathy and moderate proteinuria. J Am Soc Nephrol 2007;18:1880–1888.

72. Li PK, Leung CB, Chow KM, et al: Hong Kong study using valsartan in IgA nephropathy (HKVIN): A double-blind, randomized, placebo-controlled study. Am J Kidney Dis 2006;47:751–760.

73. Russo D, Pisani A, Balletta MM, et al: Additive antiproteinuric effect of converting enzyme inhibitor and losartan in normotensive patients with IgA nephropathy. Am J Kidney Dis 1999;33:851–856.

74. Nakao N, Yoshimura A, Morita H, et al: Combination treatment of angiotensin-II receptor blocker and angiotensin-converting-enzyme inhibitor in non-diabetic renal disease (COOPERATE): A randomised controlled trial. Lancet 2003;361:117–124.

75. Bannister KM, Weaver A, Clarkson AR, Woodroffe AJ: Effect of angiotensin-converting enzyme and calcium channel inhibition on progression of IgA nephropathy. Contrib Nephrol 1995;111: 184–192.

76. Cheng IK, Fang GX, Wong MC, et al: A randomized prospective comparison of nadolol, captopril with or without ticlopidine on disease progression in IgA nephropathy. Nephrology (Carlton) 1998;4:19–26.

77. Rekola S, Bergstrand A, Bucht H: Deterioration rate in hypertensive IgA nephropathy: Comparison of a converting enzyme inhibitor and beta-blocking agents. Nephron 1991;59:57–60.

78. Cattran DC, Greenwood C, Ritchie S: Long-term benefits of angiotensin-converting enzyme inhibitor therapy in patients with severe immunoglobulin A nephropathy: A comparison to patients receiving treatment with other antihypertensive agents and to patients receiving no therapy. Am J Kidney Dis 1994; 23:247–254.

79. Donadio JV Jr, Bergstralh EJ, Offord KP, et al: A controlled trial of fish oil in IgA nephropathy. Mayo Nephrology Collaborative Group. N Engl J Med 1994;331:1194–1199.

80. Donadio JV Jr, Grande JP, Bergstralh EJ, et al: The long-term outcome of patients with IgA nephropathy treated with fish oil in a controlled trial. Mayo Nephrology Collaborative Group. J Am Soc Nephrol 1999;10:1772–1777.

81. Donadio JV Jr, Larson TS, Bergstralh EJ, Grande JP: A randomized trial of high-dose compared with low-dose omega-3 fatty acids in severe IgA nephropathy. J Am Soc Nephrol 2001;12: 791–799.

82. Bennett WM, Walker RG, Kincaid-Smith P: Treatment of IgA nephropathy with eicosapentanoic acid (EPA): A two-year prospective trial. Clin Nephrol 1989;31:128–131.

83. Pettersson EE, Rekola S, Berglund L, et al: Treatment of IgA nephropathy with omega-3-polyunsaturated fatty acids: A prospective, double-blind, randomized study. Clin Nephrol 1994;41:183–190.

84. Strippoli GF, Manno C, Schena FP: An "evidence-based" survey of therapeutic options for IgA nephropathy: Assessment and criticism. Am J Kidney Dis 2003;41:1129–1139.

85. Hogg RJ, Lee J, Nardelli N, et al: Clinical trial to evaluate Omega-3 fatty acids and alternate day prednisone in patients with IgA nephropathy: Report from the Southwest Pediatric Nephrology Study Group. Clin J Am Soc Nephrol 2006;1:467–474.

86. Buemi M, Allegra A, Corica F, et al: Effect of fluvastatin on proteinuria in patients with immunoglobulin A nephropathy. Clin Pharmacol Ther 2000;67:427–431.

87. Chandrakantan A, Ratanapanichkich P, Said M, et al: Recurrent IgA nephropathy after renal transplantation despite immunosuppressive regimens with mycophenolate mofetil. Nephrol Dial Transplant 2005;20:1214–1221.

88. Wang AY, Lai FM, Yu AW, et al: Recurrent IgA nephropathy in renal transplant allografts. Am J Kidney Dis 2001;38:588–596.

89. Mollica F, Li Volti S, Garozzo R, Russo G: Effectiveness of early prednisone treatment in preventing the development of nephropathy in anaphylactoid purpura. Eur J Pediatr 1992;151:140–144.

90. Oner A, Tinaztepe K, Erdogan O: The effect of triple therapy on rapidly progressive type of Henoch-Schönlein nephritis. Pediatr Nephrol 1995;9:6–10.

91. Foster BJ, Bernard C, Drummond KN, Sharma AK: Effective therapy for severe Henoch-Schönlein purpura nephritis with prednisone and azathioprine: A clinical and histopathologic study. J Pediatr 2000;136:370–375.

92. Hasegawa A, Kawamura T, Ito H, et al: Fate of renal grafts with recurrent Henoch-Schönlein purpura nephritis in children. Transplant Proc 1989;21:2130–2133.

93. Meulders Q, Pirson Y, Cosyns JP, et al: Course of Henoch-Schönlein nephritis after renal transplantation: Report on ten patients and review of the literature. Transplantation 1994; 58:1179–1186.

94. Hamazaki T, Tateno S, Shishido H: Eicosapentaenoic acid and IgA nephropathy. Lancet 1984;1:1017–1018.

95. Cheng IK, Chan PC, Chan MK: The effect of fish-oil dietary supplement on the progression of mesangial IgA glomerulonephritis. Nephrol Dial Transplant 1990;5:241–246.

Further Reading

Appel GB, Waldman M: The IgA nephropathy treatment dilemma. Kidney Int 2006;69:1939–1944.

Barratt J, Feehally J: Treatment of IgA nephropathy. Kidney Int 2006;69:1934–1938.

Floege J: Is mycophenolate mofetil an effective treatment for persistent proteinuria in patients with IgA nephropathy? Nat Clin Pract Nephrol 2006;2:16–17.

Miyazaki M, Hotta O, Komatsuda A, et al: A multicenter prospective cohort study of tonsillectomy and steroid therapy in Japanese patients with IgA nephropathy: A 5-year report. Contrib Nephrol 2007;157:94–98.

Pozzi C, Andrulli S, Del Vecchio L, et al: Corticosteroid effectiveness in IgA nephropathy: Long-term results of a randomized, controlled trial. J Am Soc Nephrol 2004;15:157–163.

Samuels JA, Strippoli GF, Craig JC, et al: Immunosuppressive treatments for immunoglobulin A nephropathy: A meta-analysis of randomized controlled trials. Nephrology (Carlton) 2004;9:177–185.

Strippoli GF, Manno C, Schena FP: An "evidence-based" survey of therapeutic options for IgA nephropathy: Assessment and criticism. Am J Kidney Dis 2003;41:1129–1139.

Tumlin JA, Hennigar RA: Clinical presentation, natural history, and treatment of crescentic proliferative IgA nephropathy. Semin Nephrol 2004;24:256–268.

Wyatt RJ, Hogg RJ: Evidence-based assessment of treatment options for children with IgA nephropathies. Pediatr Nephrol 2001;16: 156–167.

Chapter 17

Systemic Vasculitis and Pauci-Immune Glomerulonephritis

Jeremy B. Levy and Charles D. Pusey

BACKGROUND

Systemic vasculitis comprises a spectrum of diseases affecting small- and medium-sized blood vessels and can cause severe acute renal failure through glomerular, interstitial, and vascular damage. The diseases can be classified by the size of the blood vessel affected and the organs involved and include microscopic polyangiitis (MP), Wegener's granulomatosis (WG), renal limited vasculitis, and Churg-Strauss syndrome. Pauci-immune glomerulonephritis is the classic histologic diagnosis accompanying all these conditions and allows them to be distinguished clearly from systemic lupus erythematosus, Goodpasture's syndrome, and primary glomerulonephritides with crescentic pathology and rapidly progressive course, because in all these latter conditions, immune deposits are a major feature of the renal histology. Other diseases can also have vasculitic features such as Henoch-Schönlein purpura, essential cryoglobulinemia, rheumatoid arthritis, and Behçet's syndrome, but are not considered further here. It is vital that all patients with rapidly progressive glomerulonephritis (RPGN) have a formal diagnosis confirmed because the potential treatments and outcomes are very different in all these diseases. Most of the vasculitic diseases, especially those affecting the kidneys, are associated with the presence of circulating antineutrophil cytoplasm antibodies (ANCAs), and the generic term ANCA-associated vasculitis is often used. This can be helpful because there is a huge overlap between, for example, WG and MP, and the treatments may be similar, particularly in severe disease with renal involvement. This is less true for localized disease, although induction treatments remain very similar. In general, most patients with pauci-immune crescentic glomerulonephritis behave as if they have vasculitis, have serum ANCA, and are thus treated as a renal-limited vasculitis. In all vasculitides, renal damage is irreversible without treatment and historically has led to significant mortality and the need for renal replacement therapy. Immunosuppression has had a major impact and allows most patients to survive and recover renal function. Until recently, however, treatment recommendations were based on case series with all their inherent problems because of a paucity of controlled clinical trials. Fortunately, over the past 5 years, a series of high-quality randomized, controlled trials have been completed on which treatment decisions can now be based.

DIAGNOSIS

An accurate diagnosis in patients with RPGN is critically important because both the nature of the therapy and the response to treatment will be very different depending on the precise diagnosis. All patients presenting clinically with RPGN or evidence of vasculitis should have a renal biopsy and appropriate serologic investigations performed as a matter of urgency.[1] Assays for anti–glomerular basement membrane (GBM) antibodies, ANCAs, lupus serology, and complement are particularly important, as well as measures of an acute-phase response. ANCAs should be assessed by indirect immunofluorescence on ethanol-fixed neutrophils with confirmation of the antigen specificity by enzyme-linked immunosorbent assay against purified proteinase 3 and myeloperoxidase. The renal biopsy sample should be carefully analyzed for the presence of segmental necrosis and for any immune deposits. Patients with pauci-immune glomerulonephritis usually do have some deposition of complement C3 and immunoglobulin within the mesangium and along the capillary loops, and it is important to try to localize and quantitate the immune deposits to distinguish those patients with truly pauci-immune disease from those who may have underlying primary glomerulonephritis.[2] There is now good evidence that in patients with vasculitis, the presence and proportion of normal glomeruli are an important predictor of renal outcome, in addition to both acute and chronic tubulointerstitial damage.[3] Increasing numbers of patients with crescentic nephritis are being recognized as having both

ANCAs and anti-GBM antibodies, so-called double-positive patients.[4] The outcome in these patients is unclear, but in our experience may be poor and more like that seen with anti-GBM disease. Thus, all anti-GBM antibody-positive patients or those with linear immunoglobulin deposited along the GBM on renal biopsy should have ANCA assays performed because this might influence subsequent management.

CLINICAL TRIALS

The heterogeneity of crescentic glomerulonephritis confounded many early trials of therapy because studies included patients with diseases as diverse as postinfectious nephritis, SLE, WG, and renal-limited vasculitis, and very few studies clearly separated patients into appropriate diagnostic groups. More recently, trials in vasculitis have been very specific about recruiting patients with clearly defined disease, usually based on ANCA serology. Trials in renal disease have generally included patients with ANCA-associated vasculitis regardless of the precise clinical diagnosis, whereas extrarenal studies have been careful to select patients usually with WG. Patients in such studies have been separated according to the extent of disease (localized or generalized) and severity (organ threatening, life threatening) and based on therapy as initial (induction) or maintenance treatment. This has been extremely useful in allowing a better definition of the precise place for various therapies.

Historically, the outcome of patients with vasculitis was dramatically improved with the introduction of oral immunosuppression as induction therapy, particularly the addition of cyclophosphamide to corticosteroids, as described by Fauci and colleagues[5,6] and others,[7,8] at the National Institutes of Health for patients with WG. A similar regimen was subsequently applied to patients with MP[7,9] and has become standard induction therapy for patients presenting with RPGN from renal vasculitis. Introduction of cytotoxic therapy allowed 75% of patients to achieve remission, and more than 85% to survive the acute illness, however at the cost of significant longer term morbidity including infections, bone marrow suppression, and cancer. Treatments used for therapy in vasculitis have evolved from oral and intravenous steroids, oral and intravenous cyclophosphamide, plasma exchange (PE), azathioprine, and methotrexate to mycophenolate mofetil (MMF), infliximab, etanercept, rituximab, and deoxyspergualin, among others.[10]

We concentrate here on treatments supported by good evidence and briefly discuss newer treatments as yet lacking controlled trials. A key feature of all recent trials has been to recognize the difference between induction of remission in patients presenting acutely, maintenance of remission after initial control of disease, and management of relapses, and between disease threatening vital organs and more localized disease, because the relative balance of risks and benefits and the need for intensive acute intervention are clearly different in the two circumstances. Most nephrologists see patients with more severe vasculitis with acute renal failure and RPGN, whereas rheumatologists often see patients with more localized and non–organ-threatening disease.

Induction Treatments

Plasma Exchange

The rationale for the use of PE in MP, WG, and pauci-immune glomerulonephritis was initially based on the similarity of the renal pathology to Goodpasture's syndrome, namely severe focal necrotizing crescentic nephritis and the presumed immune complex etiology. The identification of ANCAs in these conditions strengthens the rationale for the use of PE, although the precise role of the autoantibodies in the pathogenesis of these diseases is not yet clearly defined. Six controlled trials of the value of PE in non–anti-GBM RPGN have been performed.[11–16] Glockner and colleagues[11] could not demonstrate any additional benefit of twice-weekly PE in 14 patients with crescentic RPGN compared with 12 controls treated with oral prednisolone, cyclophosphamide, and azathioprine. However, the patients included in this study were a heterogeneous group, including those with WG, polyarteritis nodosa, systemic lupus erythematosus, scleroderma, and idiopathic RPGN. Furthermore, patients with oliguria were excluded, and three patients in the control group were subsequently successfully treated with PE.

The Hammersmith Hospital controlled trial of PE only treated patients with WG, MP, or idiopathic RPGN, and randomized 48 patients to conventional treatment with oral steroids, cyclophosphamide, and azathioprine, either with or without intensive PE (at least five exchanges in the first 7 days).[12] In this study, PE was of no additional benefit in patients with moderate or severe renal disease who were not dialysis dependent at presentation. However, 10 of 11 dialysis-dependent patients receiving PE discontinued dialysis compared with only three of eight receiving oral immunosuppression alone. Although ANCAs were not routinely measured at that time, these patients fell into diagnostic categories now associated with ANCAs. Rifle and Dechelette[13] also showed a benefit of PE in dialysis-dependent patients: 6 of 8 patients receiving PE recovered renal function but none of six treated with drugs alone.

The Canadian Apheresis Study Group[14] added PE to induction therapy of intravenous methylprednisolone followed by oral prednisolone and azathioprine. This study excluded patients with systemic disease and included one patient with postinfectious RPGN in the PE group. There was no demonstrable benefit of PE in the non–dialysis-dependent patients. However, in dialysis-dependent patients, a nonsignificant trend in benefit was evident: three of four patients receiving PE discontinued dialysis compared with two of seven in the control group. Zauner and colleagues[15] prospectively randomized 39 patients with non–anti-GBM crescentic nephritis to receive PE in addition to standard immunosuppression (pulsed methylprednisolone, oral steroids, and oral cyclophosphamide): 6 of 11 dialysis-dependent patients recovered renal function overall but with no difference in outcome between the two groups. Combining the results from these early controlled trials clearly demonstrates a significant benefit of PE only in dialysis-dependent patients. In total, 25 of 31 dialysis-dependent patients (81%) treated with PE had independent renal function at follow-up compared with 8 of 25 (32%) treated with immunosuppressive drugs alone. A number of single-center cohort studies have shown very similar results for renal recovery with PE.

The small size of these early trials and the combined outcomes suggesting a benefit from PE in patients with severe disease[16] led the European vasculitis study group (EUVAS) to embark on the prospective, randomized, controlled MEPEX trial comparing the use of intravenous methylprednisolone (3 g over 3 days) with PE (seven exchanges in 2 weeks) in 137 patients with serum creatinine greater than 5.8 mg/dL and a new diagnosis of ANCA-associated systemic vasculitis.[17] All patients received oral prednisolone and oral cyclophosphamide. At 3 months, 49% of patients treated with methylprednisolone compared with 69% of those treated with PE were alive and independent of dialysis. PE was also associated with a significantly decreased risk of progression to end-stage renal disease at 12 months (19% versus 43%). Complications and overall survival were identical.

The evidence now seems very strong that patients with ANCA-associated vasculitis and RPGN and a serum creatinine greater than 5.8 mg/dL have a significantly better outcome if treated with PE in addition to cyclophosphamide and oral steroids rather than the widely used alternative of intravenous steroids. This is not necessarily true of all the vasculitides, for example, Churg-Strauss syndrome,[18] or for patients with less severe ANCA-associated renal vasculitis (creatinine < 5.8 mg/dL). Patients with vasculitis and pulmonary hemorrhage have very high mortality rate and also seem to benefit from PE regardless of the serum creatinine level, although there are no randomized trials in this setting.

Alternatives to PE have been investigated in some centers. Stegmayr and colleagues[19] conducted a randomized, controlled trial of PE versus protein A immunoadsorption in 44 patients with RPGN and more than 50% crescents: 7 of 10 dialysis-dependent patients discontinued dialysis, with no difference between the two antibody removal strategies.

Intravenous Methylprednisolone

Intravenous methylprednisolone has also been advocated for the initial therapy of crescentic glomerulonephritis. There has now been one controlled study in patients with severe renal failure (the MEPEX study) comparing intravenous methylprednisolone with PE as induction therapy.[17] As noted above, steroids were significantly less effective than PE, although half the patients treated with intravenous methylprednisolone were able to discontinue dialysis by 3 months. There have been no controlled trials of oral versus intravenous steroids. Bolton and Sturgill[20] reported good results in dialysis-dependent patients with pauci-immune RPGN or vasculitis (excluding WG), with 14 of 19 dialysis-dependent patients treated with intravenous methylprednisolone coming off dialysis. However, this study used very large doses of methylprednisolone (30 mg/kg/day for 3 days, maximum 3 g/day). Andrassy and colleagues[21] also used intravenous methylprednisolone successfully at much lower doses (250 mg/day for 3 days), enabling 11 of 12 dialysis-dependent patients with WG to recover renal function. In contrast, Garrett and colleagues[22] reported improved renal function in only 7 of 17 (41%) patients with ANCA-associated RPGN treated with high-dose intravenous steroids.

Other Treatments for Induction of Remission

Patients with generalized disease but with serum creatinine less than 5.8 mg/dL are often labeled as having generalized organ-threatening disease. These patients historically were treated with oral cyclophosphamide and oral or intravenous steroids, with remission rates between 7% and 100%. However, it became clear that treatment-related morbidity was a significant issue, and over the past decade, trials have focused on identifying less toxic regimens.

Intravenous cyclophosphamide has been tested in several trials in place of oral cyclophosphamide, in view of the successful use of this treatment modality in patients with severe systemic lupus erythematosus.[23–25] There are now 10 non-randomized cohort studies and three randomized trials suggesting equal efficacy of the intravenous route but a lower cumulative dose and thus less likelihood of toxicity, especially infections.[10] A meta-analysis in 2001[26] confirmed a lower infection rate but also suggested an increased risk of relapse in patients treated intravenously, probably also because of the lower cumulative dose. The EUVAS group therefore conducted a prospective, randomized, controlled trial in 160 patients with ANCA-associated vasculitis and serum creatinine less than 5.8 mg/dL comparing oral cyclophosphamide 2 mg/kg/day with intravenous pulses 15 mg/kg every 2 weeks for 6 weeks, and then every 3 weeks for a further seven pulses (CYCLOPS study). Preliminary results suggest both treatments were equally efficacious, and as yet no differences in outcomes have emerged.

Intravenous cyclophosphamide may be less efficacious in successfully limiting severe renal inflammation.[25,27] Guillevin and colleagues[25] and Haubitz and colleagues[27] both reported an inferior rate of recovery from dialysis dependence in patients treated with intravenous cyclophosphamide compared with the response to oral therapy, and Aaserod and colleagues[28] demonstrated an increased relapse rate in more than 108 patients treated with intravenous compared with oral cyclophosphamide.

Cotrimoxazole alone may be able to induce remission in patients with WG localized to the upper airways. Two small nonrandomized studies have shown significant benefits,[29,30] with the majority of patients attaining remission. Cotrimoxazole is well tolerated with few adverse effects. Nephrologists will see very few patients with such limited disease.

Methotrexate has been used in place of cyclophosphamide in a number of patients with WG but without severe crescentic nephritis because methotrexate should be avoided in renal failure.[31,32] Three small uncontrolled studies achieved remission rates of as high as 75%, but with high relapse rates (as high as 57%) and significant toxicity.[10] Most recently, a EUVAS randomized, prospective, controlled trial included 95 patients with generalized non–organ-threatening disease and minimal renal involvement treated with weekly oral methotrexate (≥25 mg/wk) compared with cyclophosphamide, in addition to oral steroids.[33] Complete remissions were achieved in 90% and 94% of patients with methotrexate and cyclophosphamide, respectively (not significant), although patients were slower to achieve remission when treated with methotrexate. Toxicity was no different between the two groups. Relapses were very common, probably because all treatments were stopped at 12 months, and occurred in 69% of those treated with methotrexate and 42% of those receiving cyclophosphamide. Methotrexate, therefore, is certainly an alternative to cyclophosphamide in this setting, especially if patients do not have rapidly progressing disease. It is likely to have less long-term toxicity, but needs to be continued for more than 1 year.

Most recently, patients have been treated with tumor necrosis factor–blocking agents. A pilot study of infliximab in patients with acute disease (including those with renal involvement, but serum creatinine < 5.8 mg/dL) showed significant benefit in inducing remission (88% of patients), although there was concern over the risk of infections.[34] These results were not replicated in a larger trial of the alternative tumor necrosis factor blocker etanercept, which was studied in a prospective, randomized, controlled trial of 181 patients with WG without major renal involvement.[35] Patients were randomized to receive etanercept in addition to either cyclophosphamide or methotrexate and steroids. Seventy percent of patients achieved remission, with no benefit from etanercept, and relapse rates were very high (>50%) regardless of the use of etanercept. Patients in this study had their baseline immunosuppression (steroids) decreased rapidly, and most came off immunosuppressive drugs completely over the first year, despite being at high risk of relapse. There was also a concern over the possibility of an increased risk of cancer in patients receiving etanercept in this study.

A handful of cases of severe crescentic nephritis responding to cyclosporine have also been reported.[36,37] The use of intravenous immunoglobulin (IVIG) appears to be more successful. Jayne and Lockwood[38] treated 26 patients with WG, MP, and rheumatoid vasculitis in whom disease was refractory to conventional steroid and cytotoxic therapy. IVIG was given as Sandoglobulin at a total dose of 2 g/kg over 5 days. By 2 months, 50% of the patients had achieved a full remission, and the remainder had a partial remission of their disease. After 1 year of follow-up, 19 of 26 patients were still in remission and one patient had died of overwhelming sepsis. However, most of these patients were still on oral cyclophosphamide or azathioprine and oral prednisolone. A subsequent randomized, controlled trial of IVIG (2 g/kg total dose) in 34 patients with ANCA-associated vasculitis demonstrated modest treatment responses (14 of 17 patients improved compared with 6 of 17 placebo treated).[39] Benefit was not maintained in the long term, and a reversible increase in serum creatinine was a common complication. Richter and colleagues[40] reported much less promising results in nine patients with ANCA-associated vasculitis who had responded incompletely to conventional therapy. No patient achieved a complete remission with IVIG. The major concern regarding the use of IVIG has been the frequent (usually reversible) deterioration in renal function in patients with an initial creatinine greater than 200 μmol/L.[41] Such nephrotoxicity and questionable efficacy make it difficult to justify the use of IVIG as preferred treatment in patients with severe crescentic nephritis. This contrasts with the successful use of IVIG in another vasculitis, Kawasaki disease.

Mycophenolate has been used to treat patients with a variety of immune-mediated nephritides, usually for chronic disease. Stassen and colleagues[42] used MMF for induction of remission in 32 patients with active WG who could not be treated with cyclophosphamide for various reasons. Mycophenolate was used at 1000 mg twice daily together with oral steroids at 1 mg/kg/day. Seventy-eight percent of patients achieved complete remission, 19% a partial remission, and only one patient did not respond; however, more than 60% had a subsequent relapse. Relapses occurred in patients with complete and partial remissions 6 to 14 months after starting treatment. Adverse effects included leukopenia, anemia, abdominal pain, and diarrhea and were usually dose related.

Rituximab (an anti-CD20 antibody that eliminates B lymphocytes) has been investigated in a very small number of patients with vasculitis and appears promising.[43] Retreatment may be needed as B cells reconstitute after 6 to 9 months, and a randomized trial comparing rituximab with cyclophosphamide for induction (RAVE) is in progress. Deoxyspergualin has also been reported to be beneficial in small numbers of patients, but has to be given as a daily subcutaneous injection and causes predictable transient leukopenia.[44]

Maintenance Therapy

Long-term maintenance therapy is usually required for crescentic nephritis associated with ANCAs. As many as 50% of patients will have a relapse with systemic or local disease.[9] In the Hammersmith series, use of long-term maintenance therapy and tailoring treatment according to ANCA status have decreased the relapse rate at 5 years from 53% to 22%.[9] The majority of patients in this series were still taking a cytotoxic agent in the third year, usually azathioprine. Some recent trials have stopped all immunosuppression by 12 months, for example, the Wegener's Granulomatosis Etanercept Trial of etanercept in WG[35] and the EUVAS trial of methotrexate and cyclophosphamide in nonrenal WG,[33] and relapses occurred in more than 50% of patients within the next year, mostly in the first 6 months after cessation of immunosuppression. Relapses are not trivial, can be life and organ threatening, and expose patients to significantly more immunosuppression with increased treatment-related toxicity. Long-term immunosuppression is therefore crucial, but the precise duration of treatment remains uncertain, and although we have some evidence now about best drugs for maintenance therapy, the place for newer immunosuppressive agents is unclear (Table 17-1).

Cyclophosphamide and Azathioprine

The long-term use of cyclophosphamide has been associated with significant adverse effects,[45] whereas azathioprine is usually well tolerated with a reduced risk of hematologic or urothelial malignancy. The CYCAZAREM randomized, controlled trial in 144 patients with ANCA-associated vasculitis and renal disease (serum creatinine < 5.8 mg/dL) clearly demonstrated that 3 months of cyclophosphamide followed by a switch to oral azathioprine was as effective as cyclophosphamide continued for 9 months after induction of remission.[46] Relapse rates (15.5% and 13.7%, respectively), mortality rates, and end-stage renal disease were identical in both arms of the study, and there was a trend toward less severe complications in patients receiving azathioprine as long-term maintenance therapy. There should therefore no longer be a place for the routine use of long-term cyclophosphamide as maintenance therapy in ANCA-associated RPGN, with the exception of rare patients who are truly cyclophosphamide dependent and have a relapse after switching to all other agents.

Other Agents

In patients taking azathioprine who have a relapse or who are intolerant of it, the use of methotrexate or MMF as maintenance therapy may be considered. Mycophenolate is a more potent immunosuppressive agent than azathioprine and may therefore be more effective than azathioprine in the mainte-

Table 17-1   Drugs Commonly Used in Systemic Vasculitis

Drug	Doses Used	Duration of Use	Adverse Effects
Methylprednisolone and oral prednisolone	15 mg/kg IV, maximum dose 1 g/day 1 mg/kg/day PO, maximum 60 mg	Intravenous given for 3 days; oral continued for at least 1 yr, usually longer, but with decrease in dose; 20 mg by 6 wk, and 10 mg by 6 mo	Infections, hyperglycemia, edema, osteonecrosis, peptic ulcer, psychosis, depression, hypertension, osteoporosis, myopathy, weight gain, bruising
Cyclophosphamide (Cytoxan) (IV)	15 mg/kg every 2 wk ×3, then every 3 wk. Alternatively, 0.5 g/m², maximum 1 g/m²; decrease dose in elderly and if GFR < 50 mL/min	12–25 wk	Infections, leukopenia, thrombocytopenia, bone marrow suppression, hemorrhagic cystitis, carcinoma of the bladder lymphoma, sterility, amenorrhea
Cyclophosphamide (PO)	2 mg/kg/day, reduced to 1.5 mg/kg/day in elderly and decreased GFR	3–6 mo	Infections, leukopenia, thrombocytopenia, bone marrow suppression, carcinoma of the bladder, lymphoma, sterility, amenorrhea
Azathioprine (Imuran)	2 mg/kg/day	At least 9 mo after induction, but often up to 5 yr	Hypersensitivity, leukopenia, bone marrow suppression, myelodysplasia, malignancies, hepatic dysfunction, pancreatitis; levels of thiopurine methyltransferase should ideally be checked before use
Methotrexate	10–25 mg once weekly	At least 12 mo, possibly longer	Leukopenia, bone marrow suppression, hepatic dysfunction, rashes, lung toxicity
Mycophenolate mofetil	500 mg bid–1.5 g bid	At least 12 mo	Leukopenia, anemia, gastrointestinal disturabance especially diarhhea, infections, malignancies (in combination with other immunosuppressants)

GFR, glomerular filtration rate.

nance of remission in systemic vasculitis. Data are, however, currently conflicting. In a pilot study of 11 patients with WG or MP,[47] MMF after standard induction therapy was effective in maintenance of remission in almost all patients. In contrast, in a second study of 14 patients with WG who had been treated with daily cyclophosphamide and steroids to induce remission,[48] MMF was well tolerated but relapses occurred in 43% of cases. An ongoing EUVAS trial is randomizing patients to either azathioprine or MMF after remission induction. Methotrexate may also be used effectively to maintain remission in patients with nonrenal disease initially treated by corticosteroids and cyclophosphamide. This immunosuppressive protocol is attractive because it combines the efficacy of cyclophosphamide in inducing remission together with methotrexate as a drug with a more favorable long-term toxicity profile. Langford and colleagues[49] reported on 31 patients treated in this way who achieved a relapse rate of only 16% at 2 years.

Cyclosporine and deoxyspergualin are also agents that could, in theory, provide useful maintenance immunosuppression; however, data are limited to small uncontrolled case series.

Refractory disease has also been treated with anti–T-lymphocyte antibodies. Lockwood and colleagues[50] used a combination of two humanized monoclonal antibodies, Campath 1H directed against CDw52 and an anti-CD4 antibody, in four patients and achieved a sustained remission in three. Antithymocyte globulin has also achieved a favorable response in a few patients with refractory WG, but, again, relapses were common. In view of the probable importance of ANCAs in the pathogenesis of vasculitis, semi-specific removal of these antibodies has been attempted using L-tryptophan immunoadsorption[51] and, more specifically, with myeloperoxidase-bound immunosorbent columns to remove antimyeloperoxidase ANCAs.[52] Therapy against tumor necrosis factor using infliximab showed promise in the treatment of chronic disease in a small prospective pilot study of 16 patients, with most patients achieving remission despite chronic active disease.[34] Leflunomide has been studied in both pilot studies and a randomized trial compared with methotrexate. Unfortunately, this trial was stopped early as a result of high relapse rates in the methotrexate arm. Leflunomide seemed effective at controlling vasculitis, but toxicity was a significant problem (neuropathy, leukopenia, hypertension). Finally, at least two patients with severe disease have received immunoablation with autologous bone marrow stem-cell transplantation, both of whom were apparently well 6 months after the procedure. Cotrimoxazole has also been used in maintenance therapy and shown to reduce the risk of relapse significantly, especially in WG and especially in patients with extrarenal disease.

In view of the potential toxicity of immunosuppressive therapy and uncertainty over duration of treatment needed, there would clearly be benefit in identifying patients at higher risk of relapse because this might allow targeting of long-term therapy. There is some evidence that patients with persistent ANCA titers and those with anti–proteinase 3 as opposed to myeloperoxidase antibodies have an increased risk of relapse, and patients with a substantial increase in ANCA titers may also be more likely to have a relapse over the coming weeks.[53] Interrogation of immunologic tests can therefore provide some help in guiding maintenance therapy.

Outcome

Crescentic ANCA-positive vasculitis causing RPGN should be controlled with conventional prednisone and cyclophosphamide therapy in more than 70% of patients.[9] Levy and Winearls[54] reported patient survival rates at 1 and 3 years of 86.3% in 31 patients with crescentic glomerulonephritis (of various etiologies) and an overall renal survival rate of 78%. Of these 31 patients, 20 were dialysis dependent at presentation. In the Hammersmith series of 73 patients with WG or MP and an initial creatinine value greater than 500 μmol/L ($>$5.8 mg/dL) who were treated with oral steroids, cyclophosphamide, and PE, 73% were alive with improved renal function 2 months after presentation.[9] Stegmayr and colleagues[19] treated patients with severe renal failure and RPGN in a similar fashion (with PE or immunoadsorption) and were able to show that 70% came off dialysis. Gordon and colleagues[55] reported 82% survival at 3 months in 150 patients with small-vessel vasculitis treated with steroids and oral or intravenous cyclophosphamide, whereas Aaserod and colleagues[28] showed 74% and 75% patient and renal survival at 5 years, respectively, with 55% patients coming off dialysis. In the MEPEX trial of severe ANCA-associated renal disease,[17] 70% of patients treated with PE were alive and off dialysis at 3 months. Renal recovery usually occurs within 1 month but can be delayed substantially after the initiation of therapy (as long as 6 months). In the CYCAZAREM trial, most patients were in remission by 3 months,[46] but a further 16% achieved remission between 3 and 6 months after starting treatment with cyclophosphamide. In this study, the relapse rate was approximately 15% at 18 months; 85% of patients therefore were free of disease activity at this point. In contrast, the randomized trial of methotrexate and cyclophosphamide in nonrenal vasculitis withdrew all therapy by 12 months, and relapses occurred in more than 50% of patients.

Patients with extensive interstitial damage found on their initial renal biopsy sample, marked glomerulosclerosis, or a long history of untreated disease may respond to initial induction therapy but subsequently have declining renal function and ultimately require renal replacement therapy.[3,15,56,57] Increasing age and lack of normal glomeruli on renal biopsy have also been associated with a worse outcome.[3] Patients who achieve a serum creatinine of less than 200 μmol/L (2.3 mg/dL) are subsequently much less likely to require renal support. Patients who suffer relapses of disease with further renal damage are at risk of long-term renal failure, hence, the need to prevent relapses and maintain prolonged remission.

SPECIFIC RECOMMENDATIONS FOR TREATMENT

It is critically important that a specific diagnosis is made in all patients with clinical presentation with RPGN and a renal biopsy sample showing light microscopic changes of crescentic glomerulonephritis. It also helpful to establish ANCA specificity and the spectrum of organ and vascular bed involvement. For example, the recommended treatment regimen will vary considerably between a patient with anti-GBM disease presenting on dialysis (see Chapter 18) and a patient with MP presenting similarly, and long-term therapy may differ between a patient with WG and anti–proteinase 3 ANCA and one with MP and a myeloperoxidase ANCA that has become undetectable. However, it is also important to recognize that as many as 10% of patients with pauci-immune crescentic glomerulonephritis will have a negative test for ANCAs and should be treated in the same way as those with ANCA-positive systemic vasculitis because they have the same renal prognosis.

We recommend that ANCA-positive patients presenting with a creatinine value less than 5.8 mg/dL should be treated with oral prednisolone (1 mg/kg/day, 60 mg maximum dose) and intravenous cyclophosphamide (15 mg/kg, 1.2 g maximum dose) every 2 weeks for the first three infusions and subsequently every 3 weeks for seven further pulses, with a dose decrease in those older than 60 years old and those with a GFR less than 50 mL/min. White blood cell counts should be measured 10 to 14 days after each cyclophosphamide dose, and the dose should be decreased if the white blood cell count has decreased to less than 3×10^9/L. Oral cyclophosphamide is a reasonable alternative and is given at 2 mg/kg/day (150 mg maximum) for 3 months, unless disease is not controlled (6 months maximum), but may be associated with a higher risk of infections. We do not routinely use intravenous methylprednisolone but many centers do, and no trials have addressed this. Oral steroids should be decreased slowly so that patients are on 20 mg/day by approximately 3 months. All patients should receive prophylactic cotrimoxazole 960 mg three times per week, oral antifungals while on cyclophosphamide or high-dose steroids, omeprazole (or alternative) and alendronate, calcium supplements, and vitamin D as bone prophylaxis during steroid therapy.

Patients who present with a creatinine value greater than 5.8 mg/dL or who are dialysis dependent should receive urgent PE using human albumin solution (see Chapter 12) in addition to prednisone and cyclophosphamide. Fresh frozen plasma should be added to the replacement fluids within 3 days of renal biopsy or in the presence of bleeding. PE should be repeated frequently and regularly to provide at least seven 4-L exchanges within the first 2 weeks. If PE is unavailable or delayed in such cases, treatment should begin with intravenous methylprednisolone (15 mg/kg/day, 1 g/day maximum), which should be given for three consecutive days; however, this is not an optimal substitute for PE. All patients with pulmonary hemorrhage should receive PE as well as prednisolone and cyclophosphamide as described previously. Some physicians prefer oral cyclophosphamide in this context based on the MEPEX trial.

Patients with minimal renal involvement can be treated with methotrexate either from induction of therapy or after initial treatment with cyclophosphamide, but response is slower, and treatment certainly needs to be continued for more than 18 months.

Beginning 1 week after initiation of therapy, oral prednisolone should be slowly decreased so that patients are receiving 20 mg by 6 weeks and 10 mg by 5 to 6 months after the initial diagnosis. Cyclophosphamide should only be used for 3 months in most patients and subsequently changed to oral azathioprine (2 mg/kg/day) (as shown by the Cycazarem trial[47]). Renal function, urine sediment, and white blood cell count should be closely monitored, as should inflammatory markers and ANCAs. In our view, treatment should be continued for at least 2 years, and longer if there has been any evidence of disease relapse, high titer serum ANCA, or persistent proteinase 3 ANCA. Early cessation of treatment leads to higher relapse rates. In patients with myeloperoxidase ANCA and well-controlled disease, some physicians would attempt earlier withdrawal of therapy.

Patients with resistant disease can be treated with MMF, IVIG, rituximab, infliximab, leflunomide, or deoxyspergualin in centers with experience with these agents. Relapses can be treated in the same way as induction therapy; however, many centers try to avoid large cumulative cyclophosphamide doses and may use alternative agents. However, severe renal relapses usually do require aggressive induction therapy to prevent irreversible damage. Harder to treat is low-grade chronic grumbling disease, and in this setting, MMF, infliximab, rituximab, and methotrexate may all be useful.

RECURRENCE AFTER TRANSPLANTATION

Despite optimal therapy, approximately 20% of patients with renal vasculitis will develop end-stage kidney failure.[58]

In such cases, kidney transplantation has been shown to be an effective treatment option using standard antirejection protocols (reviewed in Schmitt and van der Woude[58]); however, approximately 17% of patients will experience a relapse of renal or extrarenal vasculitis.[59] Such relapses are generally responsive to treatment with cyclophosphamide, and recent studies have reported excellent 5-year patient and graft survival.[60] Importantly, ANCA titers at the time of transplantation do not appear to predict the likelihood of relapse.[58–60] Thus, in patients with advanced renal failure and extensive scarring found on the renal biopsy sample with little or no clinical or histologic activity, reduction or withdrawal of cytotoxic therapy should be considered in preparation for transplantation. Immunosuppression should not be stopped if there is any evidence of extrarenal disease activity (Boxes 17-1 and 17-2).

FUTURE DIRECTIONS

Over the past 5 years the treatment of vasculitis has been dramatically improved by the completion of multicenter, prospective, randomized, controlled trials that have been adequately powered to answer important questions. Such trials will continue and will test the use of rituximab, MMF, monoclonal antibodies directed against T-cell and endothelial antigens, proinflammatory cytokines, etc., many of which have been shown to be effective in animal models. As the molecular mechanisms involved in crescentic glomerulonephritis are dissected, it will be possible to design more specific forms of immunotherapy, such as analogue peptides involved in the major histocompatibility complex–T-cell receptor trimolecular complex. Minimizing toxicity while retaining treatment potency is a major aim of new therapies as well as reducing relapse rates. Whether this will be achievable remains to be seen.

Box 17-1   Treatment Algorithm for Acute Vasculitis with Renal Involvement (Creatinine < 5.8 mg/dL)

Induction
Cyclophosphamide, 15 mg/kg IV (every 2 wk for 3 doses, then every 3 wk). Alternatively, 2 mg/kg/day PO.
Prednisolone 1 mg/kg/day PO (maximum 60 mg); decrease to 45 mg after 1 wk, then 30 mg, then more slowly (at 2-wk intervals)
Methylprednisolone 500 mg–1 g IV for 3 days is used in some units
Prophylactic cotrimoxazole 960 mg PO 3 times per week; omeprazole, oral nystatin, weekly alendronate, calcium, and vitamin D

Maintenance
Azathioprine 2 mg/kg/day PO; after 3 mo, oral cyclophosphamide if in full remission. If disease activity not fully controlled or PR3 ANCA remains positive, may need 6 mo of oral cyclophosphamide before switching. Continue for at least 18 mo and usually much longer. If using IV cyclophosphamide, switch to oral azathioprine after 10 pulses.
Patients intolerant of azathioprine can use mycophenolate mofetil 1–3 g/day or methotrexate (titrated up to 25 mg once weekly) if renal function good (creatinine, 1.7 g/dL).
Oral prednisolone continued; 20 mg by 3 mo and 10 mg by 6 mo; continue 5–10 mg for at least 1 yr.
Prophylactic oral cotrimoxazole continued in Wegener's granulomatosis only; omeprazole, calcium, and vitamin D

PR3 ANCA, anti–proteinase 3 antineutrophil cytoplasm antibody.

Box 17-2 Treatment Algorithm for Severe Acute Vasculitis (Creatinine > 5.8 mg/dL) or Patients with Pulmonary Hemorrhage and Vasculitis

Induction

Plasma exchange 4 L for human albumin solution 5%, at least 7 exchanges in 2 weeks. Use fresh plasma if ongoing pulmonary hemorrhage, recent surgery, or within 3 days of renal biopsy

If plasma exchange not available, methylprednisolone 500 mg–1 g for 3 days

Cyclophosphamide 2 mg/kg/day PO or 15 mg/kg IV (every 2 weeks for 3 doses, then every 3 weeks)

Prednisolone 1 mg/kg/day; decrease to 45 mg after 1 week, then 30 mg, then more slowly (at 2-week intervals)

Prophylactic cotrimoxazole 960 mg PO 3 times weekly, omeprazole, oral nystatin, weekly alendronate, calcium, and vitamin D

Maintenance

Azathioprine 2 mg/kg/day PO; after 3 months, oral cyclophosphamide if in full remission. If disease activity not fully controlled or PR3 ANCA remains positive, may need 6 months of oral cyclophosphamide before switching. Continue for at least 18 months and usually much longer. If using IV cyclophosphamide, switch to oral azathioprine after 10 pulses.

Patients intolerant of azathioprine can use mycophenolate mofetil 1–3 g/day

Oral prednisolone continued; 20 mg by 3 mo and 10 mg by 6 mo; continue 5–10 mg for at least 1 yr.

Oral prednisolone continued; should be on 20 mg by 3 months and 10 mg by 6 months; continue 5–10 mg for at least 1 year

Prophylactic oral cotrimoxazole continued in Wegener's granulomatosis only; omeprazole, calcium, and vitamin D

PR3 ANCA, anti–proteinase 3 antineutrophil cytoplasm antibody.

References

1. Ferrario F, Rastaldi MP, D'Amico G: The crucial role of renal biopsy in the management of ANCA-associated renal vasculitis. Nephrol Dial Transplant 1996;11:726–728.
2. Jennette JC, Falk RJ: Clinical and pathological classification of ANCA-associated vasculitis: What are the controversies? Clin Exp Immunol 1995;101(Suppl 1):18–22.
3. De Lind van Wijngaarden RA, Hauer HA, Wolterbeek R, et al: Clinical and histologic determinants of renal outcome in ANCA-associated vasculitis: A prospective analysis of 100 patients with severe renal involvement. J Am Soc Nephrol 2006;17:2264–2274.
4. Levy JB, Hammad T, Coulthart A, et al: Clinical features and outcome of patients with both ANCA and anti-GBM antibodies. Kidney Int 2004;66:1535–1540.
5. Fauci AS, Wolff SM: Wegener's granulomatosis: Studies in eighteen patients and a review of the literature. Medicine (Baltimore) 1973;52:535–561.
6. Fauci AS, Haynes BF, Katz P, Wolff SM: Wegener's granulomatosis: Prospective clinical and therapeutic experience with 85 patients for 21 years. Ann Intern Med 1983;98:76–85.
7. Hind CRK, Paraskevakou H, Lockwood CM, et al: Prognosis after immunosuppression of patients with crescentic nephritis requiring dialysis. Lancet 1983;1:263–265.
8. Fuiano G, Cameron JS, Raftery M, et al: Improved prognosis of renal microscopic polyarteritis in recent years. Nephrol Dial Transplant 1988;3:383–391.
9. Gaskin G, Pusey CD: Systemic vasculitis. In Davison A, Cameron JS, Grunfeld JP, et al (eds): Oxford Textbook of Clinical Nephrology, 3rd ed. Oxford: Oxford University Press, 2006.
10. Bosch X, Guilabert A, Espinosa G, Mirapeix E: Treatment of antineutrophil cytoplasmic antibody associated vasculitis: A systematic review. JAMA 2007;298:655–669.
11. Glockner WM, Sieberth HG, Wichmann HE, et al: Plasma exchange and immunosuppression in rapidly progressive glomerulonephritis: A controlled multi-center study. Clin Nephrol 1988;29:1–8.
12. Pusey CD, Rees AJ, Evans DJ, et al: Plasma exchange in focal necrotizing glomerulonephritis without anti-GBM antibodies. Kidney Int 1991;40:757–763.
13. Rifle G, Dechelette E: Treatment of rapidly progressive glomerulonephritis by plasma exchange and methylprednisolone pulses. A prospective randomised trial of cyclophosphamide. Interim analysis. Prog Clin Biol Res 1990;337:263–267.
14. Cole E, Cattran D, Magil A, et al: A prospective randomised trial of plasma exchange as additive therapy in idiopathic crescentic glomerulonephritis. Am J Kidney Dis 1992;20:261–269.
15. Zauner I, Bach D, Kramer BK, et al: Predictive value of initial histology and effect of plasmapheresis on long term prognosis of rapidly progressive glomerulonephritis. Am J Kidney Dis 2002;39:28–35.
16. Levy JB, Pusey CD: Still a role for plasma exchange in rapidly progressive glomerulonephritis? J Nephrol 1997;10:7–13.
17. Jayne DR, Gaskin G, Rasmussen N, et al: Randomized trial of plasma exchange or high dosage methylprednisolone as adjunctive therapy for severe renal vasculitis. J Am Soc Nephrol 2007;18:2180–2188.
18. Guillevin L, Lhote F, Cohen P, et al: Lack of superiority of corticosteroids plus pulse cyclophosphamide and plasma exchanges to corticosteroids plus pulse cyclophosphamide alone in the treatment of polyarteritis nodosa and Churg Strauss syndrome patients with poor prognostic factors. A prospective randomised trial in 62 patients. Arthritis Rheum 1995;38:1638–1645.
19. Stegmayr BG, Almroth G, Berlin G, et al: Plasma exchange or immunoadsorption in patients with rapidly progressive crescentic glomerulonephritis. A Swedish multi-center study. Int J Artif Organs 1999;22:81–87.
20. Bolton WK, Sturgill BC: Methylprednisolone therapy for acute crescentic rapidly progressive glomerulonephritis. Am J Nephrol 1989;9:368–375.
21. Andrassy K, Erb A, Koderisch J, et al: Wegener's granulomatosis with renal involvement: Patient survival and correlations between initial renal function, renal histology, therapy and renal outcome. Clin Nephrol 1991;35:139–147.
22. Garrett PJ, Dewhurst AG, Morgan LS, et al: Renal disease associated with circulating antineutrophil cytoplasmic activity. Q J Med 1992;85:731–749.

23. Austin HA, Klippel JH, Balow JE, et al: Therapy of lupus nephritis. Controlled trial of prednisone and cytotoxic drugs. N Engl J Med 1986;314:614–619.
24. Reinhold-Keller E, Kekow J, Schnabel A, et al: Influence of disease manifestations and antineutrophil cytoplasmic antibody titer on the response to pulse cyclophosphamide therapy in patients with Wegener's granulomatosis. Arthritis Rheum 1994;39:919–924.
25. Guillevin L, Lhote F, Jarrousse B, et al: Treatment of severe Wegener's granulomatosis: A prospective trial comparing prednisone, pulse cyclophosphamide versus prednisone and oral cyclophosphamide [abstract]. Clin Exp Immunol 1995;101 (Suppl 1):43.
26. de Groot K, Adu D, Savage COS: The value of pulse cyclophosphamide in ANCA associated vasculitis: Meta-analysis and critical review. Nephrol Dial Transplant 2001;16:2018–2027.
27. Haubitz M, Schellong S, Gobel U, et al: Intravenous pulse administration of cyclophosphamide versus daily oral treatment in patients with antineutrophil cytoplasmic antibody-associated vasculitis and renal involvement: A prospective, randomized study. Arthritis Rheum 1998;41:1835–1844.
28. Aaserod K, Iversen B, Hammerstrom J, et al: Wegener's granulomatosis: Clinical course in 108 patients with renal involvement. Nephrol Dial Transplant 2000;15:611–618.
29. DeRemee RA, McDonald TJ, Weiland LH: Wegener's granulomatosis: Observations on treatment with antimicrobial agents. Mayo Clin Proc 1985;60:27–32.
30. DeRemee RA: The treatment of Wegener's granulomatosis with trimethoprim/sulfamethoxazole. Arthritis Rheum 1988;31:1068–1074.
31. Hoffman GS, Leavitt RY, Kerr GS, et al: The treatment of Wegener's granulomatosis with glucocorticoids and methotrexate. Arthritis Rheum 1992;35:1322–1329.
32. Sneller MC, Hoffman GS, Talar-Williams C, et al: An analysis of 42 Wegener's granulomatosis patients treated with methotrexate and prednisone. Arthritis Rheum 1995;18:608–613.
33. De Groot K, Rasmussen N, Bacon PA, et al: Randomized trial of cyclophosphamide versus methotrexate for induction of remission in early systemic ANCA associated vasculitis. Arthritis Rheum 2006;65:841–844.
34. Booth A, Harper L, Hammad T, et al: Prospective study of TNF alpha blockade with infliximab in ANCA associated vasculitis. J Am Soc Nephrol 2004;15:717–721.
35. Wegener's Granulomatosis Etanercept Trial (WGET) Research Group: Etanercept plus standard therapy for Wegener's granulomatosis. N Engl J Med 2005;352:351–361.
36. Borleffs JCC, Derksen RHWM, Hene RJ: Treatment of Wegener's granulomatosis with cyclosporin. Ann Rheum Dis 1987;46:175.
37. Gremmel F, Druml W, Schmidt P, Graninger W: Cyclosporin in Wegener's granulomatosis. Ann Intern Med 1988;108:491–492.
38. Jayne DRW, Lockwood CM: Pooled intravenous immunoglobulin in the management of systemic vasculitis. Adv Exp Med Biol 1993;336:469–472.
39. Jayne DRW, Chapel H, Adu D, et al: Intravenous immunoglobulin for ANCA associated systemic vasculitis with persistent disease activity. Q J Med 2000;93:433–439.
40. Richter C, Schnabel A, Csernok E, et al: Treatment of antineutrophil cytoplasmic antibody (ANCA)-associated systemic vasculitis with high-dose intravenous immunoglobulin. Clin Exp Immunol 1995;101:2–7.
41. Levy JB, Pusey CD: Renal failure and intravenous immunoglobulin. Q J Med 2000;93:751–755.
42. Stassen PM, Cohen Tervaert JW, Stegeman CA: Induction of remission in active ANCA associated vasculitis with mycophenolate mofetil in patients who cannot be treated with cyclophosphamide. Ann Rheum Dis 2007;66:798–802.
43. Keogh KA, Ytterberg SR, Fervenza FC, et al: Rituximab for refractory Wegener's granulomatosis. Am J Respir Crit Care Med 2006;173:180–187.
44. Birck R, Warnatz K, Lorenz HM, et al: 15-Deoxyspergulin in patients with refractory ANCA associated systemic vasculitis. J Am Soc Nephrol 2003;14:440–447.
45. Hoffman GS, Leavitt RY, Fleisher TA, et al: Treatment of Wegener's granulomatosis with intermittent high dose intravenous cyclophosphamide. Am J Med 1990;89:403–410.
46. Jayne D, Rasmussen N, Andrassy K, et al: A randomized trial of maintenance therapy for vasculitis associated with antineutrophil cytoplasmic antibodies. N Engl J Med 2003;349:36–44.
47. Nowack R, Gobel U, Klooker P, et al: Mycophenolate mofetil for maintenance therapy of Wegener's granulomatosis and microscopic polyangiitis. J Am Soc Nephrol 1999;10:1965–1971.
48. Langford CA, Talar-Williams C, Sneller MC: Mycophenolate mofetil for remission maintenance in the treatment of Wegener's granulomatosis. Arthritis Rheum 2004;51:278–283.
49. Langford CA, Talar-Williams C, Barron KS, Sneller MC: Use of cyclophosphamide-induction methotrexate maintenance regimen for the treatment of Wegener's granulomatosis. Am J Med 2003;114:463–469.
50. Lockwood CM, Thiru S, Isaacs JD, et al: Long term remission of intractable systemic vasculitis with monoclonal antibody therapy. Lancet 1993;341:1620–1622.
51. Elliott JD, Lockwood CM, Hale G, Waldmann H: Semi-specific immuno-absorption and monoclonal antibody therapy in ANCA positive vasculitis: Experience in four cases. Autoimmunity 1998;28:163–171.
52. Alexandre S, Moguilevsky N, Paindavoine P, et al: Specific MPO immunoabsorption for the treatment of vasculitis. Clin Exp Immunol 2000;120(Suppl 1):43.
53. Buhaescu I, Covic A, Levy JB: Systemic vasculitis: Still a challenging disease. Am J Kidney Dis 2005;43:173–185.
54. Levy JB, Winearls CG: Rapidly progressive glomerulonephritis: What should be first-line therapy? Nephron 1994;67:402–407.
55. Gordon M, Luqmani RA, Adu D, et al: Relapses in patients with systemic vasculitis. Q J Med 1993;86:779–789.
56. Aaserod K, Bostad L, Hammerstrom J, et al: Renal histopathology and clinical course in 94 patients with Wegener's granulomatosis. Nephrol Dial Transplant 2001;16:953–960.
57. Cohen BA, Clark WF: Pauci-immune renal vasculitis: Natural history, prognostic factors and impact of therapy. Am J Kidney Dis 2000;36:914–924.
58. Schmitt WH, van der Woude FJ: Organ transplantation in the vasculitides. Curr Opin Rheumatol 2003;15:22–28.
59. Nachman PH, Segelmark M, Westman K, et al: Recurrent ANCA-associated small vessel vasculitis after transplantation: A pooled analysis. Kidney Int 1999;56:1544–1550.
60. Gera M, Griffin MD, Specks U, et al: Recurrence of ANCA-associated vasculitis following renal transplantation in the modern era of immunosuppression. Kidney Int 2007;71:1296–1301.

Further Reading

Booth AD, Almond MK, Burns A, et al: Outcome of ANCA-associated renal vasculitis: A 5-year retrospective study. Am J Kidney Dis 2003;41:776–784.
Bosch X, Guilabert A, Espinosa G, Mirapeix E: Treatment of antineutrophil cytoplasmic antibody associated vasculitis: A systematic review. JAMA 2007;298:655–669.

Buhaescu I, Covic A, Levy JB: Systemic vasculitis: Still a challenging disease. Am J Kidney Dis 2005;43:173–185.

Hogan SL, Falk RJ, Chin H, et al: Predictors of relapse and treatment resistance in antineutrophil cytoplasmic antibody-associated small-vessel vasculitis. Ann Intern Med 2005;143: 621–631.

Jayne D, Rasmussen N, Andrassy K, et al: A randomized trial of maintenance therapy for vasculitis associated with antineutrophil cytoplasmic antibodies. N Engl J Med 2003;349:36–44.

Jayne DR, Gaskin G, Rasmussen N, et al: Randomized trial of plasma exchange or high dosage methylprednisolone as adjunctive therapy for severe renal vasculitis. J Am Soc Nephrol 2007;18:2180–2188.

Pusey CD: The continuing challenge of anti-neutrophil cytoplasm antibody-associated systemic vasculitis and glomerulonephritis. J Am Soc Nephrol 2006;17:221–223.

Chapter 18

Antiglomerular Basement Membrane Antibody Disease

A. Neil Turner and Andrew J. Rees

BACKGROUND

Goodpasture's syndrome, or antiglomerular basement membrane (anti-GBM) disease, is an uncommon but usually severe disease caused by autoimmunity to a component of certain basement membranes, now identified as NC1 domain of the $\alpha 3$ chain of type IV collagen ($\alpha 3$[IV]NC1). Autoantibodies with specificity for $\alpha 3$(IV)NC1 (usually simply referred to as *anti-GBM antibodies*) have generally been used to define the disorder, although conventional assays for them are negative in rare patients.[1] Anti-GBM antibodies had been used for nearly 100 years to induce experimental nephritis before the human disease was identified, and Goodpasture's syndrome remains one of the few types of human nephritis in which there is considerable understanding of the mechanisms leading to renal injury. It was also the first type of inflammatory glomerulonephritis for which rational rather than empirically based treatment was developed and shown to be effective. This was a landmark because similar therapy was then applied to other types of rapidly progressive glomerulonephritis (RPGN) in which it was often even more effective. Goodpasture's syndrome and its pathogenesis have been reviewed in detail by Turner and Rees.[2]

Clinical and Pathologic Features

Ernest Goodpasture reported a single patient with lung hemorrhage and RPGN in 1919. In retrospect, his patient, like most with this syndrome, probably had systemic vasculitis. Surveys carried out since the introduction of assays for antineutrophil cytoplasm antibodies (ANCAs) have shown that the various types of systemic vasculitis account for about two thirds of cases of lung hemorrhage with RPGN, whereas Goodpasture's syndrome with anti-GBM antibodies accounts for most of the remaining third.

Typical patients present with fulminant disease of short duration, although minor symptoms, particularly of lung disease, may have been present for weeks or occasionally much longer. The phenomenon of a sudden crescendo in disease intensity is common, and it is often only when this occurs that the disease is diagnosed. In such patients, the time window in which treatment can salvage renal function, or even life, is short, and rapid diagnosis and treatment are essential if this is to be achieved.

As well as the classic presentation of Goodpasture's syndrome, patients may present with renal disease alone or with pulmonary disease alone. As the symptoms of minor renal disease are nonspecific, it is common for presentation with isolated renal disease to be late. Lung hemorrhage, conversely, may cause hemoptysis at a relatively early stage, and patients will often seek medical attention at a time when signs of renal involvement may be minimal, although at least microscopic hematuria is usually present. This is important because anti-GBM assays are more likely to be negative in patients with isolated pulmonary disease.[3] Hemoptysis is a poor guide to the severity of pulmonary hemorrhage, and patients may become hypoxic and anemic (typically an iron deficiency anemia if hemorrhage has been occurring for some time) in the absence of gross hemoptysis. Occasionally patients present with subacute renal disease, leading to nephrotic syndrome with hematuria and variable renal impairment. Very mild or rapidly progressive renal disease is much more common. This clinical description was originally based on studies of patients of European Caucasoid descent, but recent large series from China confirm that patients from there have similar clinical features.[4]

Pathologically, the renal disease is of varying severity, but characteristically the glomerular crescents appear to be of a similar age. Even when the diagnosis appears to be obvious, renal biopsy is important for prognostic reasons and thus for guiding therapy. In the lung, the appearance is one of alveolar hemorrhage without specific features.

Diagnosis

Diagnosis rests on the demonstration of anti-GBM antibodies, either fixed to basement membranes of affected organs or in the circulation. Because systemic vasculitis may have a similar clinical picture and even overlap with Goodpasture's syndrome, measurement of ANCAs is essential whenever the diagnosis is contemplated. The most sensitive technique for detection of antibodies is direct immunohistologic examination of a renal biopsy sample. Although linear fixation of immunoglobulin is described in a number of other circumstances, the concurrence of linear antibody fixation and crescentic nephritis occurs only in Goodpasture's syndrome or in systemic vasculitis associated with Goodpasture autoantibodies.[2] However, there are two circumstances in which renal biopsy samples from patients with Goodpasture's syndrome may fail to show linear deposition of immunoglobulin: first, on rare occasions when the intensity of glomerular injury is so severe that the GBM is completely destroyed, and second, in reports of exceptional patients whose initial renal biopsy specimen shows crescentic glomerulonephritis without linear staining who subsequently develop typical Goodpasture's syndrome with circulating anti-GBM antibody linear deposition of IgG.[1,3] Direct immunohistology of lung biopsy samples is less reliable because antibody binding may be patchy.

Immunoassays for circulating anti-GBM antibodies are valuable, but their reliability varies.[5] High titers of antibodies are usually found in patients with fulminant or rapidly progressive disease, and false-negative results should, in these circumstances, be very uncommon. False positives are occasionally found, according to the quality of the antigen used as the ligand. False-negative results are most likely in patients with relatively low antibody titers. These are typically those with isolated lung disease or minor or slowly progressive renal disease. False-negative results may also be encountered in the post-transplantation anti-GBM disease that occurs in some patients with Alport's syndrome, even in the presence of florid disease. This is because anti-GBM antibodies in this setting are alloantibodies directed against the NC1 domain of the $\alpha 5$ collagen chain that is mutated in Alport's syndrome rather than because the $\alpha 3$(IV)NC1 that is targeted by the autoantibodies is Goodpasture's syndrome[6,7] (described later).

As many as one third of patients who present with anti-GBM antibodies also have positive assays for ANCAs, usually but not always perinuclear ANCA with specificity for myeloperoxidase.[4,8] Some of these have clear evidence of small-vessel vasculitis or pulmonary hemorrhage, whereas many do not. The implications for clinical management of double positivity are discussed later.

Basis of Lung Hemorrhage

Lung hemorrhage occurs in approximately 50% of patients at some stage, but, unlike renal injury, its severity and incidence correlate poorly with antibody titers. There is clear evidence from epidemiologic and anecdotal observations and from animal models that local injury to the lung has a powerful influence on whether pulmonary hemorrhage occurs, and this is likely to account for these observations. Several surveys have confirmed a close association of lung hemorrhage with cigarette smoking. Anecdotally, other inhaled substances, notably gasoline and other volatile organic compounds, also appear to precipitate pulmonary hemorrhage. Pulmonary or other infection and volume overload have also been associated with lung hemorrhage.

Circulating anti-GBM antibodies have direct access to the GBM through the fenestrae in the endothelium of glomerular capillaries. Alveolar capillaries are not fenestrated, and in experimental animals, anti-GBM antibodies that are normally excluded from the alveolar basement membrane gain access to it after lung injury induced by gasoline, oxygen toxicity, or the cytokines interferon alfa and interleukin-2.[2]

Measurement of the transfer factor corrected for the patient's lung volume and hemoglobin (kCO) can be useful for detecting the occurrence of subclinical pulmonary hemorrhage and is most useful if related to an initial value.

Alport Post-transplantation Antiglomerular Basement Membrane Disease

Renal transplantation in Alport's syndrome is generally successful, and the overall graft survival rate is at least as good as for other patients. However, as many as 5% may develop crescentic nephritis in the allograft with linear binding of immunoglobulin to the GBM.[9] In the majority of cases, the graft is lost, and retransplantation has been unsuccessful. Typically, the disease develops some months after a first or second allograft and is recognized late, at a stage when the glomeruli have already been destroyed. In subsequent allografts, the disease develops within weeks or even days, and progresses much more rapidly. A few patients have shown less aggressive disease and retained their allografts in these circumstances.[10] Disease is limited to the donor organ.

Most patients with Alport's syndrome lack the network of tissue-specific type IV collagen chains ($\alpha 3/\alpha 4/\alpha 5$) that make up the collagen framework of normal GBM. They are replaced by $\alpha 1/\alpha 2$ chain type IV collagen, the isoforms that form the collagen component of most basement membranes in the body. This seems to be inadequate for long-term structural stability in the GBM, or the cochlea, although Alport lungs do not seem to suffer from the absence of $\alpha 3/\alpha 4/\alpha 5$ from the alveolar basement membrane. Antibodies in Alport anti-GBM disease are therefore directed toward components of the donor GBM that are missing from their own basement membranes, and are therefore allo- rather than autoantibodies. Most cases of Alport's syndrome can be attributed to mutations of the gene encoding the $\alpha 5$ chain of type IV collagen, located on the X chromosome, and our work shows that the usual target of alloantibodies in Alport anti-GBM disease is the NC1 domain of $\alpha 5$ chain type IV collagen.[6] This is distinct from the Goodpasture antigen, which is carried on the 70% homologous NC1 domain of the $\alpha 3$ chain of type IV collagen, and explains why immunoassays optimized to detect the autoantibodies of spontaneous Goodpasture's syndrome may fail to detect the alloantibodies of Alport anti-GBM disease.[7]

RATIONALE AND RESULTS OF THERAPY

Development of Current Regimens

Before the 1970s, a variety of treatments had been suggested for Goodpasture's syndrome, ranging from the use of corticosteroids and azathioprine to bilateral nephrectomy, the latter as a last resort for intractable pulmonary hemorrhage.[2] None had been consistently successful. The observation of Wilson and Dixon[11] that 12.5% of patients survived 1 year or more with functioning kidneys after an episode of Goodpasture's syndrome affecting lungs and kidneys was in keeping with other series of the era.[2] At that time, based on the demonstration that circulating autoantibodies in the disease were directly pathogenic, a potentially highly toxic combination treatment was devised and tested in several patients.[12,13] The combination had three elements: Intensive plasma exchange was undertaken to remove autoantibodies. Cytotoxic therapy, based on cyclophosphamide, was administered to prevent their resynthesis. Corticosteroids were given as an adjunctive anti-inflammatory agent. The initial results were spectacularly good in a group of patients who had previously had an extremely poor prognosis. Lung hemorrhage was arrested, usually within days, and recovery or preservation of renal function was reported. The initial studies were extended, and similar regimens applied elsewhere met with equally impressive results,[14–17] and this has become the standard treatment for Goodpasture's syndrome. None of these studies was controlled, but the improvement in renal function was dramatically different from previous experience and temporally related to the start of treatment.

Effectiveness and Outcome

In subsequent years, the limits of the effectiveness of this therapy and its potential hazards have been delineated. The major cause of morbidity has been infection, often related to neutropenia. The cytotoxic therapy employed in the first series comprised both cyclophosphamide and azathioprine. This usually led to leukopenia, and in recent years most have used cyclophosphamide alone without any obvious loss of effectiveness. Some have used significantly less intensive regimens, with less cyclophosphamide and/or less plasma exchange. It has been our impression, supported to some extent by published results, that this has been less effective, although fair comparison of series from different centers and countries is extremely difficult (Table 18-1).[13,14,16–19]

The mortality of Goodpasture's syndrome is now much improved, but renal survival remains poor. The reason for this is the late stage at which treatment is instituted in most patients. Early treatment is of course difficult in a disease that evolves rapidly and is normally only diagnosed when that evolution occurs, but there is a very clear relationship between the severity of renal disease at presentation and the outcome (see Table 18-1 and Fig. 18-1).

The renal prognosis was originally reported to be better in patients presenting simultaneously with ANCAs as well as anti-GBM antibodies,[20–22] but more extensive experience has shown that this is not always the case. Some double-positive patients have low titers of anti-GBM antibodies that are relatively transient, whereas others have anti-GBM titers similar to those typically found in single-positive patients, and it is this that seems to be the critical determinant of prognosis.[8,23,24] Some double-positive patients have clear evidence of vasculitis outside the kidneys and lungs, and most have anti–myeloperoxidase autoantibodies, and in the latter group, the anti-GBM response is a

Table 18-1   Results of Treatment in Series Using Immunosuppression and Plasma Exchange

Authors	No. of Patients in Study	% WITH INDEPENDENT RENAL FUNCTION AT ONE YEAR ACCORDING TO INITIAL CREATININE LEVEL		Notes on Treatment Given
		<600 μmol/L	≥600 μmol/L	
Briggs et al, 1979	15	36 (4/11)	0 (0/4)	Only 4 of 15 received plasma exchange
Simpson et al, 1982	12	70 (7/10)	0 (0/2)	8 of 12 received plasma exchange
Johnson et al, 1985	17	69 (7/13)	0 (0/4)	Less cyclophosphamide than in Table 18-2; half received plasma exchange, but only every third day and using frozen plasma
Walker et al, 1985	22	82 (9/11)	18 (2/11)	Slightly less cyclophosphamide and plasma exchange than in Table 18-2
Herody et al, 1993	22	93 (13/14)	0 (0/15)	Variable amounts of plasma exchange and different immunosuppressive regimens were used
Hammersmith, 1975–1999	71	95 (18/19)	15 (8/52)	As in Table 18-2, except early patients also received azathioprine 1 mg/kg/day
Cui et al, 1997–2002	69	61 (14/23)	2 (1/46)	Beijing; follow-up at least 6 mo; treatment included pulsed methylprednisolone; only 31 received plasma exchange

Untreated patients have been excluded. Treated patients are divided into two groups according to their creatinine level at the time treatment started or at presentation if this is not available (number in each group in parentheses); 600 μmol/L–6.8 mg/dL. The percentage of patients who were alive and not requiring dialysis at 1 year is shown.
Reproduced with permission from Turner AN, Rees AJ: Antiglomerular basement membrane antibody disease. In Cameron JS, Davison AM, Grunfeld J-P, et al (eds): Oxford Textbook of Clinical Nephrology, 3rd ed. Oxford, UK: Oxford University Press, 2003, pp 647–666.

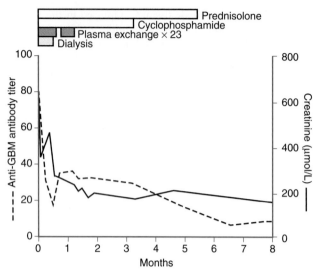

Figure 18-1   Response to treatment of a dialysis-requiring patient with Goodpasture's syndrome (renal disease only, no lung hemorrhage). This patient had 85% crescents but very acute disease. Such a response is unusually good, but many instances have been reported (see text). GBM, glomerular basement membrane.

secondary phenomenon in most, occurring in response to GBM damage caused by small-vessel vasculitis. Other patients, however, clearly develop ANCA-associated disease after presenting with anti-GBM disease and even after its successful treatment.[25] This emphasizes the need for prolonged immunologic monitoring in patients with anti-GBM disease.

Autoantibody levels are usually rapidly suppressed by these treatments and usually remain so after only a short period of therapy. Recurrences are then uncommon. Interestingly, they seem to be particularly likely to occur in patients with lung disease but only minor renal disease.[13] In untreated patients (those with end-stage renal disease but no lung disease), antibodies may persist for 1 or 2 years or even longer. The immune response is therefore usually ultimately self-limiting, but treatment speeds the turn-off of autoantibody synthesis.[26]

Role of Individual Treatment Components

Historical evidence suggests that corticosteroids alone, or azathioprine alone or in combination with corticosteroids, are not effective.[2] Anecdotal accounts of plasma exchange given alone describe rapid resynthesis of autoantibodies.[26] The only randomized, controlled trial in Goodpasture's syndrome addressed the role of plasma exchange.[18] Although the results showed a better outcome in those receiving plasma exchange, the plasma exchange group had less severe renal disease than the drugs-only group, and the authors were justifiably cautious about making firm conclusions. Both the plasma exchange and cyclophosphamide regimens used in that report were less intensive than recommended here, and this may be reflected in the slightly disappointing results (only 69% of patients with creatinine < 6.8 mg/dL recovered renal function; see Table 18-1). Nevertheless, the study did usefully show that patients with mild renal disease could do well with oral cyclophosphamide and prednisolone alone.

Pulses of intravenous methylprednisolone have been widely used in RPGN of other types, and in Goodpasture's syndrome they have sometimes been used in place of plasma exchange after an initial encouraging report.[27] The nonrandomized study of Bolton and Sturgill[28] of the use of pulses of methylprednisolone in crescentic nephritis of various types included 17 patients with Goodpasture's syndrome, but most of these had advanced disease requiring dialysis. The report only discusses effects on renal function. Of the four nonoliguric patients who were treated, only two retained renal function, although methylprednisolone was given without other immunosuppression. Williams and colleagues[29] reported failures of pulse corticosteroid therapy in arresting pulmonary hemorrhage; Johnson and colleagues thought that it may stop pulmonary hemorrhage but that it had no impact on renal disease.[18] Of major concern in the use of very high doses of corticosteroids is the increased risk of secondary infections, sometimes opportunistic, but usually common bacterial infections. There is clear evidence in Goodpasture's syndrome and in animal models that infections may precipitate or exacerbate lung hemorrhage and aggravate renal injury. We do not believe that the safety and efficiency of high-dose steroids have been established as an alternative to plasma exchange in this disease, in which there is a clear basis for removing autoantibodies.

Other Effects of Current Regimens

Although the original rationale for current treatment regimens was to control autoantibody levels, it is clear that therapy does substantially more than this. Plasma exchange depletes clotting factors, complement components, and other known and unknown mediators of renal damage, as well as circulating antibodies. Although immunoadsorption against protein A removes immunoglobulins much more specifically and appears to be equally effective clinically, it has been undertaken in only a few patients, and no real comparison has been made. Similarly, cyclophosphamide suppresses antibody resynthesis but also has profound effects on cell-mediated immunity. It is effective in other autoimmune diseases where there is no evidence of a role for autoantibodies. It is not possible to disentangle these effects of the treatments from the originally intended ones.

Other Agents for Goodpasture's Syndrome

Although cyclosporine, deoxyspergualin, and anti–T-lymphocyte antibodies have been effective in animal models of Goodpasture's syndrome, there is little to suggest that they will be more effective than conventional therapy in the clinic. Cyclosporine has not been uniformly successful in the few patients reported and cannot be recommended. Anti–B-cell therapy with rituximab has obvious rational appeal, and there is at least one report of its use in Goodpasture's syndrome with apparent success,[30] but clearly more data are needed.

Post-transplantation Antiglomerular Basement Membrane Disease

Renal transplantation undertaken in the presence of anti-GBM antibodies has been associated with recurrence of the disease in the allograft, although this has not occurred in all instances.

With the wide availability of immunoassays for anti-GBM antibodies, recurrence now seems to be rare. More frequent is the development of post-transplantation anti-GBM disease in patients in whom the original renal diagnosis was Alport's syndrome.[9] In a proportion of patients, this diagnosis may not have been made beforehand because of a lack of knowledge of family background, new mutations, or autosomal recessive disease. Typical patients are deaf and have developed end-stage renal failure at a relatively young age. They are more likely to have a large gene deletion as the causative mutation. Once the disease has developed, the graft is usually lost despite treatment, although often the disease is recognized late and initial treatments have often been those used for immunosuppression. Thus, many failures of high-dose corticosteroids are recorded, as are some for antilymphocyte antibodies. In those very few reported instances in which the graft has been retained, the treatments used were not particularly unusual.

Children, Pregnancy, and the Elderly

Goodpasture's syndrome is very rare in childhood, but has been reported in those as young as 2 years of age. Lung hemorrhage is rare. The reported numbers are very small, but there is evidence that response to treatment can be at least as good as that of adults.

Three case reports suggest that the fetus may not be directly harmed by maternal anti-GBM disease, although placental transfer of the autoantibodies is to be expected. The fetus will clearly be harmed by maternal pulmonary hemorrhage and renal failure, however, and the prevention of these will usually be the main concern. Anti-GBM disease in the elderly is less likely to be accompanied by lung hemorrhage, but anti-GBM antibodies are more likely to be associated with ANCAs in this age group. The prognosis for renal survival in these circumstances is better, although elderly patients are more susceptible to leukopenia and infection, as well as to other complications of therapy. Doses of cyclophosphamide should be decreased in older patients. The risks of starting or continuing aggressive treatment need to be balanced with these risks.

SPECIFIC RECOMMENDATIONS

Drug Treatment and Antibody Removal

None of the components of currently accepted therapy for Goodpasture's syndrome has been subjected to analysis by rigorous controlled trials, nor are they now likely to be. The recommendations made here are therefore based on theoretical considerations, including the observation that the autoantibodies are directly pathogenic and that this is therefore at least in part an antibody-mediated disease, and on observations of the effects of this and similar treatments. Our regimen for acute severe disease is shown in Table 18-2. The protocol is more intensive than that used by some, but an intensive regimen is required to suppress autoantibody levels as rapidly as possible. Some patients may not require such aggressive therapy, perhaps those with slight lung hemorrhage and no or minimal, nonprogressive renal disease. It is our practice to use full treatment for all patients with severe lung hemorrhage or with significant but potentially recoverable renal disease. The risk of very rapid acceleration of disease is real and can be devastating.

A separate question is whether some patients with severe renal damage but no lung hemorrhage should not be given immunosuppressive treatment or plasma exchange. Given that most dialysis-dependent patients or even those with creatinine greater than 600 μmol/L (6.8 mg/dL) do not recover renal function, there is a strong case for nontreatment in these circumstances.[31] There are several important caveats to following this policy. First, lung hemorrhage may occur as a late development in response to infection, toxic exposure, or other stimuli and should be guarded against and looked for. Second, some patients with ANCAs as well as anti-GBM antibodies have a better renal prognosis with treatment, unless the renal biopsy sample shows advanced scarring, and may be at risk of extrarenal vasculitis. Third, there is strong evidence that treatment shortens the duration of anti-GBM antibody synthesis and consequently not treating lengthens the interval before renal transplantation is possible, sometimes to

Table 18-2   Treatment Recommendations for Acute Goodpasture's Syndrome

Prednisolone	1 mg/kg/24 hr PO. Decrease at weekly intervals to achieve one sixth of this dose by 8 wk (for a starting daily dose of 60 mg, weekly decreases to 45, 30, 25, 20, 15, 12.5, 10 mg). Maintain this dose to 3 months, stop by 4 months.
Cyclophosphamide	2 mg/kg/24 hr PO, rounded down to the nearest 50 mg. Administer by daily IV injection if unable to take orally.
Plasma exchange	Daily exchange of 4 L of plasma for 5% human albumin for 14 days or until the circulating antibody is suppressed. In the presence of pulmonary hemorrhage or within 48 hours of an invasive procedure, 300–400 mL of fresh frozen plasma is given at the end of each treatment. If white blood cell count less than 3.5, stop cyclophosphamide until it recovers. Resume at lower dose if cessation has been necessary.
Monitoring	Daily blood count during plasma exchange and while antibody titer still elevated. At least twice weekly during first month and weekly thereafter. Baseline kCO, with further measurements as indicated. Daily coagulation tests during plasma exchange to monitor for significant depletion of clotting factors. Initially, daily checks of renal and hepatic function and glucose.
Prophylaxis against complications of treatment	Oral nystatin or similar for 1 month. H₂ antagonist during corticosteroid therapy. Prophylaxis against pneumocystis infection during cyclophosphamide therapy. Avoid other antibiotics unless indicated. Close monitoring for signs of infection with full investigation of any fever.

kCO, transfer factor corrected for the patient's lung volume and hemoglobin.

years, because antibody levels subside slowly. Whether treatment with cyclophosphamide and prednisolone (but not plasma exchange) accelerates the disappearance of anti-GBM antibodies in comparison with no treatment has not been clearly shown. Fourth, some patients in these circumstances have recoverable disease, as shown by patients in several series and case reports and as illustrated in Figure 18-1. Some have been shown on renal biopsy to have acute tubular necrosis, so that the nephritis was not as severe as perceived clinically. Others had a very acute and recent onset of severe disease, and the biopsy sample appearance was notable for the very cellular (and uniform) crescents affecting most or all glomeruli. Renal biopsy is therefore an essential part of the assessment of such patients, and if there is any doubt, it is safer to commence treatment until further information is available. There is little hazard from a few days of treatment, but much to lose by delaying.

The specific contribution of plasma exchange to disease that is not immediately life threatening or rapidly progressive is uncertain, as discussed previously. However, it allows more rapid control of anti-GBM antibody levels and thus decreases the risk of an acceleration of disease activity. Immunoadsorption against protein A may permit even more rapid control of autoantibody levels,[32] but it is even more labor intensive and there are no data to suggest it may be more effective.

As discussed earlier, the risks consequent to the use of pulses of methylprednisolone may outweigh potential benefits, and there are no data to suggest they are an adequate substitute for intensive plasma exchange in severe disease. The use of other therapeutic agents must be regarded as experimental in the absence of adequate reported data.

Supportive Treatment

As in other severe illnesses, it is likely that attention to details other than the primary therapy may be critical in determining outcome. These include details of respiratory, renal, and other supportive care.

Lung hemorrhage is precipitated or exacerbated by fluid overload, pulmonary or remote infections, and pulmonary irritants and toxins. Experimentally, this includes oxygen toxicity, so in the intensive care setting, inspired oxygen tension should be kept as low as possible compatible with adequate tissue oxygenation. Patients should be persuaded to stop cigarette smoking.

Infections are the major cause of morbidity and mortality after the first few days. These can be minimized by avoidance of nonessential intravascular lines and obsessive adherence to protocols for the care of those that are in place. Neutrophil counts should be monitored carefully and cyclophosphamide dose adjusted accordingly. Prophylactic agents should be given as indicated (see Table 18-2). Granulocyte-macrophage colony–stimulating factor can be useful for severe neutropenia.

Post-transplantation Antiglomerular Basement Membrane Disease

Recurrences of spontaneous Goodpasture's syndrome are exceptionally uncommon and should respond to treatments similar to those used for the disorder in native kidneys.

As described earlier, anti-GBM disease that occurs after transplantation in patients with Alport's disease is different in that the response is to an alloantigen, not an autoantigen, and there are very few examples of effective therapy on which to base recommendations.[9,10] It is important to appreciate the low sensitivity of standard assays for anti-GBM antibodies in these circumstances as it seems very likely that here, as in spontaneous Goodpasture's syndrome, early recognition and aggressive treatment aimed at suppressing the antibody response must be critical to success. Renal biopsy, including immunofluorescence examination to identify GBM-fixed immunoglobulin, is usually the quickest way to make the diagnosis, and antibody titers can be followed subsequently by using an assay based on crude antigen or by sending samples to a center with access to recombinant or highly purified antigens. Intensive plasma exchange appears to be a critical part of management, and anti–T-cell therapies do not appear to be powerfully effective when used alone. There are obvious problems in using antilymphocyte antibodies in combination with plasma exchange. By analogy with spontaneous anti-GBM disease, cyclophosphamide is likely to be substantially better at suppressing disease than azathioprine. We are aware of one notable success using mycophenolate mofetil after cyclophosphamide had to be stopped because of bone marrow toxicity. Rituximab would be an obvious therapeutic option, but its use in this setting has not yet been reported.

FUTURE DIRECTIONS

Familiarity with treatment regimens and improvements in intensive care have improved death rates in anti-GBM disease, but there has been little further improvement in renal outcome since combination therapy was first described. Indeed, physicians' familiarity with immunosuppressive regimens and the much wider availability of plasma exchange has reduced the rate of referral of patients with this and similar diseases to centers where there is more accumulated experience. This may not be in patients' best interests.

At present, improved outcomes are heavily dependent on rapid recognition and diagnosis and early institution of currently available therapies. It is interesting to speculate why treatment at apparently similar stages of disease is less effective in Goodpasture's syndrome than in other types of RPGN. It may be that although they appear histologically similar, the underlying structural damage is more severe in Goodpasture's syndrome, or there may be other factors to be understood, which could be controlled by additional therapies. Specific immunoadsorption may become a way to remove anti-GBM antibodies without rendering the patient hypogammaglobulinemic,[33] although there is no reason to think that it should be any more effective or technically simpler than immunoadsorption against protein A, which removes most IgG. Therapies directed against B cells, such as rituximab, could be more effective, though.

Work in models of anti-GBM disease has suggested ways in which the inflammatory response may be down-regulated by agents that interfere with the localization of leukocytes to the inflamed glomerulus or by decreasing their activation state once there. Examples in models of anti-GBM disease include interference with leukocyte adhesion, infusions of interleukin-1 receptor antagonist, and infusions of cytokines such as interleukin-4 and interleukin-6, which alter the balance of endogenous synthesis of proinflammatory cytokines and their inhibitors.[34] Several of these approaches could be applicable to human disease. Because of the rarity of Goodpasture's syndrome it is unlikely that randomized clinical trials in that disease alone can be viable, even between multiple centers. However, it remains a disease where information about the immune and inflammatory responses is so much greater than in other types of nephritis, from work in human and in model systems, that further therapies are likely to spring from it.

References

1. Salama AD, Dougan T, Levy JB, et al: Goodpasture's disease in the absence of circulating anti-glomerular basement membrane antibodies as detected by standard techniques. Am J Kidney Dis 2002;39:1162–1167.
2. Turner AN, Rees AJ: Antiglomerular basement membrane disease. In Davidson AM (ed): Oxford Textbook of Clinical Nephrology, 3rd ed. Oxford: Oxford University Press, 2003, pp 647–666.
3. Serisier DJ, Wong RC, Armstrong JG: Alveolar haemorrhage in anti-glomerular basement membrane disease without detectable antibodies by conventional assays. Thorax 2006;61: 636–639.
4. Cui Z, Zhao MH, Xin G, Wang HY: Characteristics and prognosis of Chinese patients with anti-glomerular basement membrane disease. Nephron Clin Pract 2005;99:c49–c55.
5. Sinico RA, Radice A, Corace C, et al: Anti-glomerular basement membrane antibodies in the diagnosis of Goodpasture syndrome: A comparison of different assays. Nephrol Dial Transplant 2006;21:397–401.
6. Brainwood D, Kashtan C, Gubler MC, Turner AN: Targets of alloantibodies in Alport anti-glomerular basement membrane disease after renal transplantation. Kidney Int 1998;53: 762–766.
7. Kang JS, Kashtan CE, Turner AN, et al: The alloantigenic sites of alpha3alpha4alpha5(IV) collagen: Pathogenic X-linked alport alloantibodies target two accessible conformational epitopes in the alpha5NC1 domain. J Biol Chem 2007;282: 10670–10677.
8. Levy JB, Hammad T, Coulthart A, et al: Clinical features and outcome of patients with both ANCA and anti-GBM antibodies. Kidney Int 2004;66:1535–1540.
9. Kashtan CE: Renal transplantation in patients with Alport syndrome. Pediatr Transplant 2006;10:651–657.
10. Browne G, Brown PA, Tomson CR, et al: Retransplantation in Alport post-transplant anti-GBM disease. Kidney Int 2004;65: 675–681.
11. Wilson CB, Dixon FJ: Anti-glomerular basement membrane antibody-induced glomerulonephritis. Kidney Int 1973;3:74–89.
12. Lockwood CM, Rees AJ, Pearson TA, et al: Immunosuppression and plasma-exchange in the treatment of Goodpasture's syndrome. Lancet 1976;1:711–715.
13. Levy JB, Turner AN, Rees AJ, Pusey CD: Long-term outcome of anti-glomerular basement membrane antibody disease treated with plasma exchange and immunosuppression. Ann Intern Med 2001;134:1033–1042.
14. Briggs WA, Johnson JP, Teichman S, et al: Antiglomerular basement membrane antibody-mediated glomerulonephritis and Goodpasture's syndrome. Medicine (Baltimore) 1979;58: 348–361.
15. Johnson JP, Whitman W, Briggs WA, Wilson CB: Plasmapheresis and immunosuppressive agents in antibasement membrane antibody-induced Goodpasture's syndrome. Am J Med 1978;64:354–359.
16. Simpson IJ, Doak PB, Williams LC, et al: Plasma exchange in Goodpasture's syndrome. Am J Nephrol 1982;2:301–311.
17. Walker RG, Scheinkestel C, Becker GJ, et al: Clinical and morphological aspects of the management of crescentic anti-glomerular basement membrane antibody (anti-GBM) nephritis/Goodpasture's syndrome. Q J Med 1985;54:75–89.
18. Johnson JP, Moore J Jr, Austin HA 3rd, et al: Therapy of anti-glomerular basement membrane antibody disease: Analysis of prognostic significance of clinical, pathologic and treatment factors. Medicine (Baltimore) 1985;64:219–227.
19. Herody M, Bobrie G, Gouarin C, et al: Anti-GBM disease: Predictive value of clinical, histological and serological data. Clin Nephrol 1993;40:249–255.
20. Jayne DR, Marshall PD, Jones SJ, Lockwood CM: Autoantibodies to GBM and neutrophil cytoplasm in rapidly progressive glomerulonephritis. Kidney Int 1990;37:965–970.
21. Bosch X, Mirapeix E, Font J, et al: Prognostic implication of anti-neutrophil cytoplasmic autoantibodies with myeloperoxidase specificity in anti-glomerular basement membrane disease. Clin Nephrol 1991;36:107–113.
22. Saxena R, Bygren P, Arvastson B, Wieslander J: Circulating autoantibodies as serological markers in the differential diagnosis of pulmonary renal syndrome. J Intern Med 1995;238: 143–152.
23. Segelmark M, Hellmark T, Wieslander J: The prognostic significance in Goodpasture's disease of specificity, titer and affinity of anti-glomerular-basement-membrane antibodies. Nephron Clin Pract 2003;94:c59–c68.
24. Yang G, Tang Z, Chen Y, et al: Antineutrophil cytoplasmic antibodies (ANCA) in Chinese patients with anti-GBM crescentic glomerulonephritis. Clin Nephrol 2005;63:423–428.
25. Verburgh CA, Bruijn JA, Daha MR, van Es LA: Sequential development of anti-GBM nephritis and ANCA-associated pauci-immune glomerulonephritis. Am J Kidney Dis 1999;34: 344–348.
26. Lockwood CM, Pusey CD, Rees AJ, Peters DK: Plasma exchange in the treatment of immune complex disease. Clin Immunol Allergy 1981;1:433–455.
27. de Torrente A, Popovtzer MM, Guggenheim SJ, Schrier RW: Serious pulmonary hemorrhage, glomerulonephritis, and massive steroid therapy. Ann Intern Med 1975;83:218–219.
28. Bolton WK, Sturgill BC: Methylprednisolone therapy for acute crescentic rapidly progressive glomerulonephritis. Am J Nephrol 1989;9:368–375.
29. Williams PS, Davenport A, McDicken I, et al: Increased incidence of anti-glomerular basement membrane antibody (anti-GBM) nephritis in the Mersey Region, September 1984–October 1985. Q J Med 1988;68:727–733.
30. Arzoo K, Sadeghi S, Liebman HA: Treatment of refractory antibody mediated autoimmune disorders with an anti-CD20 monoclonal antibody (rituximab). Ann Rheum Dis 2002;61: 922–924.
31. Hind CR, Paraskevakou H, Lockwood CM, et al: Prognosis after immunosuppression of patients with crescentic nephritis requiring dialysis. Lancet 1983;1:263–265.
32. Bygren P, Freiburghaus C, Lindholm T, et al: Goodpasture's syndrome treated with staphylococcal protein A immunoadsorption. Lancet 1985;2:1295–1296.
33. Boutaud AA, Kalluri R, Kahsai TZ, et al: Goodpasture syndrome: Selective removal of anti-alpha 3 (IV) collagen autoantibodies. A potential therapeutic alternative to plasmapheresis. Exp Nephrol 1996;4:405–412.
34. Kluth DC, Erwig LP, Rees AJ: Multiple facets of macrophages in renal injury. Kidney Int 2004;66:542–557.

Further Reading

Kashtan CE: Renal transplantation in patients with Alport syndrome. Pediatr Transplant 2006;10:651–657.

Levy JB, Turner AN, Rees AJ, Pusey CD: Long-term outcome of anti-glomerular basement membrane antibody disease treated with plasma exchange and immunosuppression. Ann Intern Med 2001;134:1033–1042.

Levy JB, Hammad T, Coulthart A, et al: Clinical features and outcome of patients with both ANCA and anti-GBM antibodies. Kidney Int 2004;66:1535–1540.

Lockwood CM, Rees AJ, Pearson TA, et al: Immunosuppression and plasma-exchange in the treatment of Goodpasture's syndrome. Lancet 1976;1:711–715.

Turner AN, Rees AJ: Antiglomerular basement membrane disease. In Davidson AM (ed): Oxford Textbook of Clinical Nephrology, 3rd ed. Oxford: Oxford University Press, 2003, pp 647–666.

Chapter 19

Minimal Change Disease

Laura M. Dember and David J. Salant

BACKGROUND

Minimal change disease (MCD) is an idiopathic glomerular disease that accounts for 70% to 90% of cases of idiopathic nephrotic syndrome in children and 10% to 15% of cases in adults.[1] The name MCD has largely superseded the older terms lipoid nephrosis, nil disease, and idiopathic nephrotic syndrome. The disorder is characterized by the rapid onset of severe, symptomatic nephrotic syndrome with well-preserved renal function, almost normal glomerular histology except for generalized podocyte effacement, and a remarkable sensitivity to treatment with glucocorticoids. Because relapse is common and repeated courses of glucocorticoids are associated with significant toxicities, MCD remains one of the major therapeutic challenges in clinical nephrology.

Clinical Features

The clinical presentation of MCD is that of a pure nephrotic syndrome with heavy proteinuria, hypoalbuminemia, hyperlipidemia, and edema formation. Albumin is the predominant urine protein, although moderately selective or nonselective proteinuria has been observed in a significant proportion of adults with MCD.[2] Urinalysis reveals lipiduria, and mild microscopic hematuria may occur, especially in adults. Macroscopic hematuria is rare, and red blood cell casts are not present. Renal tubular cells and granular casts may be seen in the acute renal failure that occurs occasionally in association with MCD. Moderate hypertension is present in 13% to 30% of cases and is more frequent in adults.[1,2] Serum creatinine may be slightly increased at the time of presentation.[2,3] The increase in blood pressure and creatinine typically resolves with remission of the nephrotic syndrome. Adults are more likely to develop acute renal failure than are children.[3–5] The renal failure is usually reversible and often preceded by severe edema formation. Histologic evidence of ischemic tubular injury has been observed in

many cases, but the mechanism of the acute renal failure is not known.[1]

The course of MCD is characterized by multiple remissions and relapses of the nephrotic syndrome and a marked sensitivity to glucocorticoid therapy. In children, the frequency of relapses tends to decrease with age, and in most cases, the episodes cease after several years. The long-term renal outcome of MCD is good, and less than 5% of patients develop end-stage renal disease.[6] In general, the course of the disease is similar in children and adults. Age-related differences in the response to treatment and the frequency of relapses are discussed in detail in subsequent sections of this chapter.

Pathology

Because the diagnosis of MCD is in many respects a diagnosis of exclusion, a challenge lies in avoiding misclassifying lesions of focal and segmental glomerular sclerosis (FSGS) as MCD. Such misclassification has obvious implications for interpreting clinical studies. Those histologic features that should raise suspicion for FSGS are noted in the discussion that follows.

By light microscopy, the glomeruli in MCD usually appear normal. There may be a slight increase in mesangial cellularity, and the visceral epithelial cells may be swollen. The capillaries are patent, and the walls are not thickened. Dilatation of the glomerular capillaries is common and may be due to loss of compliance of the capillary wall resulting from epithelial cell alterations. Glomerular size is usually normal. Enlarged but otherwise normal-appearing glomeruli may be predictive of steroid-unresponsiveness or subsequent development of FSGS.[7] Doubly refractile lipid droplets and periodic acid–Schiff-positive protein droplets may be seen in the cells of the proximal tubule. Focal tubular atrophy and mild segmental interstitial fibrosis are accepted by some authorities as features of MCD; however, if tubulointerstitial changes are diffuse or severe, it is likely that FSGS is present. In adults, particularly elderly patients, vascular changes may be present but are thought to be due to associated conditions such as hypertension rather than MCD.

The results of immunofluorescence studies are negative for immunoglobulin or complement deposition in most cases of MCD. Mesangial IgM, IgG, or C3 deposits have been reported in as many as 20% of cases of MCD in some series and are thought by most investigators to be the result of nonspecific trapping of circulating immunoglobulins.[1] It has been suggested that heavy mesangial IgM deposition, especially in conjunction with some degree of mesangial hypercellularity, may be a marker of glucocorticoid unresponsiveness and/or subsequent development of FSGS. However, this idea remains controversial.

Electron microscopy reveals the major morphologic features of MCD: effacement of the glomerular visceral epithelial cell (podocyte) foot processes and obliteration of the slit-pore complex. These abnormalities are not specific for MCD and occur in other conditions associated with heavy proteinuria. The extent of the foot process effacement and obliteration of the slit-pore complex does not correlate with the amount of proteinuria, but has been shown to correlate with the decrease in glomerular filtration rate.[8] Other electron microscopic features of the podocytes include hypertrophy, increased numbers of pinocytic vesicles and intracytoplasmic lipid and protein droplets, and microvillous transformation of their free surfaces.[1] The endothelial cells lining the capillary loop show normal fenestration, and the glomerular basement membrane is usually of normal thickness.

Pathogenesis

The cause of MCD is unknown. Experimental animal models developed to analyze the mechanisms underlying proteinuria and clearance studies in humans suggest that there is a loss of both charge selectivity and size selectivity of the glomerular filter.[9] Changes in the anionic composition of the glomerular capillary wall are thought to underlie the impairment in charge selectivity and may, in fact, produce defects in size selectivity as well.[10] Whether the primary abnormality occurs in the glomerular basement membrane or in the visceral epithelial cells is not clear. Epithelial cell injury, which is the predominant histologic feature of MCD, may be either the cause or the result of loss of the anionic constituents of the glomerular capillary wall. An immunologic basis of MCD and, more specifically, a disorder of T-lymphocyte function, is suggested by the response to immunosuppressive agents, by the association of minimal change lesions with Hodgkin's disease, and by multiple alterations in the in vitro function of T cells of MCD patients.[1] The observation that supernatants of cultured lymphocytes from patients with MCD can increase capillary wall permeability and induce loss of glomerular polyanions has led to a search for vascular permeability factors secreted by the T cells of these patients.[11,12]

An unresolved question is whether MCD and FSGS represent two distinct clinicopathologic entities or whether they are variants of a single disease process. The differences in responsiveness to glucocorticoids and in long-term renal outcome support the former view. The demonstration of FSGS lesions in subsequent biopsy specimens from patients with an initial histologic diagnosis of MCD has been offered as evidence that MCD can progress to FSGS. However, the possibility of

histologic misclassification due to sampling error limits the conclusions that can be drawn from such observations.

TREATMENT

The impetus for treating MCD arises mainly from the consequences of the nephrotic state, which include malaise from anasarca as well as a predisposition to infection, thrombosis, malnutrition, and possibly atherogenesis. Prior to the availability of antibiotics and glucocorticoids, the mortality of nephrotic syndrome was greater than 50%, with the majority of the deaths during this period resulting from infection.[13] It has been argued that proteinuria itself may be nephrotoxic and contribute to progressive renal injury. Indeed, in MCD, as in other glomerulopathies, the attainment of remission of nephrotic syndrome is associated with good long-term renal outcome.[6,14] Although it is not known whether remission of nephrotic syndrome serves as a favorable prognostic indicator or whether it actually affects the outcome, the latter possibility has been offered as an additional reason to treat MCD.[15]

Because persistent nephrotic syndrome is considered especially harmful in children, most pediatric nephrologists promptly treat the first episode and relapses.[16] The decision to begin treatment in adults is somewhat more complicated because the consequences of the nephrotic syndrome may be less significant, and the therapy is generally less well tolerated.

Terminology

The course of MCD is often described in terms of the response to glucocorticoid treatment. The classification scheme outlined in Box 19-1 evolved from experience with children with idiopathic nephrotic syndrome but is used in the adult literature as well. However, as will become clear later in this

---

Box 19-1 Classification of Minimal Change Disease Based on Response to Glucocorticoid Treatment

Steroid Responsive
Complete remission of proteinuria within 8 weeks of initiating glucocorticoid treatment

Frequently Relapsing
Initially steroid responsive but relapses at rate of two per 6 months or six per 18 months

Steroid Dependent
Initially steroid responsive but relapse during tapering of glucocorticoids or within 2 weeks of discontinuing glucocorticoids

Steroid Resistant
No remission within 8 weeks of initiating glucocorticoid treatment

Complete Remission
Reduction in urinary protein excretion to < 4 mg/hr/m^2 or 0 trace by urine dipstick for 3 consecutive days

Relapse
Reappearance of proteinuria ≥ 4 mg/hr/m^2 for 3 consecutive days

chapter, the definition of steroid-resistant disease should probably differ for children and adults. The criteria for complete remission and relapse shown in Box 19-1 were established by the International Study of Kidney Disease in Children (ISKDC).[17] Although the definitions of these outcomes are relatively uniform in subsequent studies, some variation does exist. Consequently, the ability to generalize from the findings is somewhat limited. Interpretation of the literature is also complicated by the inclusion of patients with primary glomerulopathies other than MCD.

Natural History of Untreated Minimal Change Disease

A clear understanding of the natural history of a disease facilitates both the interpretation of uncontrolled treatment trials and clinical decisions regarding the use of therapies with potential toxicities. Unfortunately, the natural history of untreated MCD has been difficult to establish because the use of glucocorticoids is extremely widespread and data from the preglucocorticoid era is limited by infrequent histologic classification. Spontaneous remissions do occur in MCD and have been reported in 10% to 75% of patients who received only supportive therapy.[18–22] The accuracy of these estimates is limited by the small numbers of untreated patients and, in many cases, the lack of randomization. Although the occurrence of spontaneous remissions has led some investigators to recommend a period of observation before starting treatment, this is impractical because such a remission may not happen until months or years after the onset of disease.

Treatment with Glucocorticoids

Results in Children

Table 19-1 summarizes selected studies that evaluate glucocorticoid therapy for childhood MCD.[17,23–27] Although there are no controlled trials directly comparing glucocorticoid therapy with supportive therapy as initial treatment of childhood MCD, the overwhelming consensus is that both the likelihood and the rapidity of remission are increased with glucocorticoids. In the ISKDC, a multicenter, prospective, uncontrolled trial, 93% of children achieved complete remission with an 8-week course of prednisone.[17] The dose of prednisone used in this study was arbitrarily set at 60 mg/m^2/day (up to 80 mg/day) for 4 weeks followed by 4 weeks of intermittent prednisone at 40 mg/m^2 for three consecutive days out of seven. Subsequently, the Arbeitsgemeinschaft für Pädiatrische Nephrologie (APN), a large multicenter study from Germany, and a single-center study in Japan both showed that a prolonged course of alternate-day prednis(ol)one, given after an initial course of daily prednis(ol)one, resulted in fewer relapses than a short alternate-day course[25] or the intermittent regimen used in the ISKDC trial.[26] The prolonged regimens were not associated with an increase in the cumulative dose or toxicity of glucocorticoids. Bagga and colleagues[27] found a trend toward a longer duration of first remission with an initial 16-week course of prednisolone daily for 8 weeks and alternate days for 8 weeks compared with an initial 8-week course. However, the total number of relapses during a 2-year follow-up period did not differ between the two groups, and

the cumulative glucocorticoid dose was greater in the prolonged therapy group than in the standard therapy group.

Even with more intensive initial treatment protocols, as many as 60% of children will have a relapse within 12 months,[27] and approximately 40% will have a frequently relapsing course[28] (see Box 19-1). Thus, the major challenge in MCD is managing frequently relapsing disease. Using individual frequently relapsing children as their own controls, the APN compared alternate-day prednisolone with intermittent prednisolone (in both cases after 4 weeks of daily therapy) in frequent relapsers and found a lower relapse rate with alternate-day therapy.[23] However, neither treatment was completely satisfactory. Forty-three percent of the alternate-day group suffered at least one relapse during the 6-month treatment period (compared with 72% in the intermittent group), and almost all patients had a relapse during the subsequent 6 months. The use of intravenous methylprednisolone pulse therapy followed by low-dose oral prednisone produced a similar remission rate and relapse rate as the 60 mg/m^2/day standard therapy but was associated with fewer glucocorticoid-associated adverse effects.[24] This study included both children and adults. Although the efficacy data were analyzed separately for adults and children, the adverse events were analyzed together. Given age-related differences in glucocorticoid toxicities, the conclusions that can be drawn from such an analysis are somewhat limited. Induction therapy with alternate-day glucocorticoids has not been studied in children.

Results in Adults

Table 19-2 summarizes results of studies evaluating glucocorticoid treatment of MCD in adults.[2,5,21,29–31] All except one of these studies are retrospective analyses. It should be noted that there was marked variation in the treatment regimens used, particularly with regard to duration and tapering schemes. Remission of nephrotic syndrome was achieved in 70% to 97% of adults treated with glucocorticoids in these studies, a remission rate similar to that of children. However, the time to remission after starting treatment was longer in the adults. In the study by Nolasco and colleagues,[2] 60% of adults were in remission within 8 weeks of starting treatment, and 73% were in remission within 16 weeks. Similar results were reported by Korbet and colleagues.[3] The experience of Fujimoto and colleagues[4] differed somewhat in that a higher percentage (76%) were in remission within 8 weeks, and by 16 weeks, 90% of adults achieved remission. The more rapid response to glucocorticoid treatment in the study by Fujimoto and colleagues may have been due to the younger age of the patients (mean age, 27.7 years in the study by Fujimoto and colleagues versus 40.7 and 42 years in the research by Korbet and colleagues and by Nolasco and colleagues, respectively). The analysis by Korbet and colleagues does, in fact, suggest that the time to remission after initiation of glucocorticoids is shorter in younger adults than in older adults. It is also possible that genetic and environmental factors may influence the outcome. Meyrier and Simon[18] pooled all the published cases of adults treated with glucocorticoids between 1961 and 1987 and found that of 302 patients, 74.8% had complete remission, 7% had partial remission, and 18.2% had no response. The lower rate of complete remission in the pooled data may be due to shorter duration of treatment and the inclusion of patients treated for relapses as well as initial disease.

Table 19-1 Studies of Glucocorticoid Treatment of Minimal Change Disease in Children

Ref.	Design	Clinical Setting*	Mean Follow-up	Treatment	Control	COMPLETE REMISSION (%) Rx	COMPLETE REMISSION (%) Cntrl	RELAPSE (%) Rx	RELAPSE (%) Cntrl	Comments
ISKDC[17] (N = 363)	Prospective, uncontrolled	Initial episode	8 wk	Prednisone daily, then intermittent‡		93		NA		
APN[23] (N = 48)	Prospective, controlled, randomized	Frequently relapsing	12 mo	Prednisone daily then alternate day#	Prednisone daily, then intermittent§	NA	NA	43 $P < .05$	72	Relapse rates refer to those during treatment period; no significant difference during subsequent 6 mo
Imbasciati et al[24] (N = 67)	Prospective, controlled, randomized	Initial episode or relapse	18 mo	IV pulse then low-dose prednisone¶	Prednisone high dose‖	94	97	68	64	Time to response was shorter in the IV methylprednisolone group
APN[25] (N = 61)	Prospective, controlled, randomized	Initial episode	8 mo	Prednisone, short duration**	Prednisone, standard duration††			81 $P = .001$	59	
Ueda et al[26] (N = 46)	Prospective, controlled, randomized	Initial episode	3.8 yr	Prednisolone daily, then long taper‡‡	Prednisolone daily then short intermittent##	100	100	29	62	Relapse rate was significantly lower in the long-duration group within first 6 mo after treatment
Bagga et al[27] (N = 51)	Prospective, controlled, randomized	Initial episode	28 mo	Prednisolone prolonged daily, then alternate day§§	Prednisolone standard daily, then alternate day¶¶	100	100	73	91	Only patients with remission by 4 wk were included; cumulative steroid dose was significantly greater in the prolonged daily group

*See Box 19-1 for general definition of frequently relapsing disease. Criteria in studies may vary somewhat from those in Box 19-1.

†P value is shown if difference is significant ($P < .05$).

‡Prednisone 60 mg/m²/day in divided doses for 4 weeks, then 40 mg/m²/day in divided doses 3 consecutive days out of 7 for 4 weeks.

#Prednisone 60 mg/m²/day in divided doses until remission, then prednisone 35 mg/m² on alternate days for 6 months.

§Prednisone 60 mg/m²/day in divided doses until remission, then 40 mg/m²/day in divided doses 3 consecutive days out of 7 for 6 months.

¶Methylprednisolone 20 mg/kg/day IV for 3 days, prednisone 20 mg/m²/day for 4 weeks, then 20 mg/m² on alternate days, and taper off over 4 months.

‖Prednisone 60 mg/m²/day for 4 weeks, then 40 mg/m² on alternate days, and taper off over 4 months.

**Prednisone 60 mg/m²/day until remission, then prednisone 40 mg/m²/day on alternate days until serum albumin is ≥3.5 g/dL. Relapse treated with same regimen.

††Prednisone 60 mg/m²/day for 4 weeks, then prednisone 40 mg/m²/day on alternate days for 4 weeks. For relapse, 60 mg/m²/day until remission, then 40 mg/m² alternate days for 4 weeks.

‡‡Prednisolone 60 mg/m²/day for 4 weeks, then prednisolone 40 mg/m²/day on alternate days for 4 weeks, then taper off over 5 months.

##Prednisolone 60 mg/m²/day for 4 weeks, then prednisolone 40 mg/m²/day for 3 consecutive days out of 7 for 4 weeks.

§§Prednisolone 2 mg/kg/day for 4 weeks, then 1.5 mg/kg/day for 4 weeks, then 1.5 mg/kg on alternate days for 4 weeks.

¶¶Prednisolone 2 mg/kg/day for 4 weeks, then 1.5 mg/kg/day for 4 weeks, then 1.5 mg/kg on alternate days for 4 weeks.

APN, Arbeitsgemeinschaft für Pädiatrische Nephrologie; Cntrl, control group; ISKDC, International Study of Kidney Diseases in Children; NA, not available; Rx, treatment.

Table 19-2 Studies of Glucocorticoid Treatment of Minimal Change Disease in Adults

Ref.*	Design	Clinical Setting	Mean Follow-up (yr)	Treatment	Complete Remission (%)	RESULTS COMPLETE REMISSION (%) Week			Relapse (%)	Comments
						8	16	28		
Black et al[21] (N = 31)†	Prospective, controlled	Initial episode	>2	Prednisone daily‡	80		NA		NA	Low doses of prednisone used; complete remission rate estimated (refers to treated patients only)
Wang et al[5] (N = 109)	Retrospective, uncontrolled	Initial episode or relapse	2.0	Prednisolone alternate day#	83		NA		NA	Young age at onset (82% had onset of disease before age 30)
Nolasco et al[2] (N = 75)§	Retrospective, uncontrolled	Initial episode	7.5	Prednisone daily¶	77	60	73	77	76	Significantly higher relapse rate in younger patients (age < 45)
Nair et al[29] (N = 58)	Retrospective, uncontrolled	Initial episode	3.0	Prednisolone alternate day||	93	82	93	NA	31	Mean age of patients low (27.7 yr)
Korbet et al[3] (N = 34)	Retrospective, uncontrolled	Initial episode	5.3	Prednisone daily**	91	51	77	85	65	Significantly longer time to achieve remission in older patients (age > 40)
Fujimoto et al[4] (N = 33)	Retrospective, uncontrolled	Initial episode	3.9	Prednisolone daily††	97	76	97	NA	34	Young age at onset (27.7 yr)
Nakayama et al[30] (N = 62)‡‡	Retrospective, uncontrolled	Initial episode	NA	Prednisolone daily##	93	67	77	84	62	Five of 62 patients had spontaneous remission; response rates refer to treated patients only
Waldman et al[31] (N = 95)	Retrospective, uncontrolled	Initial episode	2.5	Prednisone daily or alternate day§§	70	50¶¶	80	88	73.1||||	No detectable differences in outcome between daily and alternate-day groups

*Only patients treated with glucocorticoids alone are included.
†Study compared prednisone with supportive treatment in variety of glomerular diseases. Only patients with minimal change disease included in follow-up. Unable to determine spontaneous remission rate from data because some control group patients received prednisone during follow-up.
‡Prednisone dose varied (mean initial dose, 26 mg/day); treatment duration 6 to 48 months.
#Prednisolone 60 mg/day for 1 week, then 120 mg on alternate days until remission, and tapered off over 10 to 16 months.
§Extension of Cameron et al[33]
¶Prednisone 60 mg/day for 1 week, then 45 mg/day for 4 weeks and taper off over 3 to 15 weeks; mean duration of treatment 13 weeks.
||Prednisolone 2 mg/kg (maximum, 120 mg) on alternate days for 6 to 12 weeks, then tapered off over 12 weeks.
**Prednisone ≥ 60 mg/day for 1 to 3 months and tapered off over 1 to 40 months; mean duration of treatment 8.1 months.
††Prednisolone 1 mg/kg/day for 4 to 8 weeks, then tapered off over approximately 9 months.
‡‡Five patients had spontaneous remission and are not included in the table.
##Prednisolone 60 mg/day in most of the patients, tapered after remission to a maintenance dose of 5 mg/day; mean duration of treatment 3.5 years.
§§Daily dose was approximately 1 mg/kg; alternate-day dose was approximately 2 mg/kg.
¶¶Percentages are estimated from survival curves and refer to complete or partial remission.
||||Includes patients with initial complete or partial remission.
NA, not available.

The results of these studies suggest that similar proportions (70%–80%) of adults and children have at least one relapse. However, adults appear to be less likely than children to have frequently relapsing or steroid-dependent disease (21% in Nolasco and colleagues[2] compared with 40% in the ISKDC[32]).

Initial treatment of MCD with alternate-day glucocorticoids has been evaluated in adults.[5,22,29,31] Nair and colleagues[29] retrospectively analyzed the outcomes of 58 adults treated with prednisolone 2 mg/kg (with maximum of 120 mg) as a single dose every 48 hours. Tapering began once remission was achieved. In contrast to the experience described previously with daily prednisone, 82% of patients in this study were in remission within 6 weeks, 93% were in remission within 12 weeks, and only 31% of patients had a relapse during the follow-up period. The low relapse rate has been attributed to the more gradual tapering regimen used for many of the patients in this study. The experience of Wang and colleagues[5] using alternate-day prednisolone in Malaysian adults with MCD was less impressive. Remission occurred in 78% of 109 patients, but in many cases, it was not achieved until 6 or more months of treatment. Waldman and colleagues[31] found no difference in remission rate, relapse rate, or time to relapse in a retrospective comparison of adults treated with daily versus alternate-day glucocorticoids. The rationale for alternate-day treatment is to decrease the adverse effects of the glucocorticoids. Although Nair and colleagues[29] and Wang and colleagues[4] commented in the reports of their studies that the adverse effects were low using an alternate-day regimen, this claim has not been substantiated by a prospective comparison with daily dosing.

Treatment with Alkylating Agents

Results in Children

The use of therapies other than glucocorticoids has generally been reserved for those patients with frequently relapsing, steroid-dependent, or steroid-resistant MCD. Table 19-3 summarizes selected studies evaluating the efficacy of cyclophosphamide and chlorambucil in such patients.[2,28,33–40] In a prospective, controlled study, the ISKDC compared cyclophosphamide with intermittent prednisone in children with frequently relapsing nephrotic syndrome and found a lower relapse rate in the cyclophosphamide group than in the prednisone group (48% versus 88%).[28] Although this result is consistent with the findings of earlier studies[41,42] and supports the use of alkylating agents in frequently relapsing disease, separate analyses were not performed for the patients with MCD and FSGS, thus preventing firm conclusions regarding MCD per se. Furthermore, the intermittent prednisone regimen used in this study has been shown to be less effective than alternate-day therapy in preventing a relapse.[23]

Alkylating agents appear to be less effective in steroid-dependent disease than in frequently relapsing disease. In one of the APN studies, children with frequently relapsing and steroid-dependent disease were treated with either cyclophosphamide and prednisone or chlorambucil and prednisone.[37] Such treatment produced a remission rate of 72% in those with frequently relapsing disease, but only 28% in the patients with steroid-dependent disease. There is controversy as to whether an increase in the duration of the alkylating agent treatment improves the response in steroid-dependent disease. In a separate study of steroid-dependent children with MCD, the APN found that a 12-week course of cyclophosphamide was associated with a higher 2-year relapse-free rate (67%) than was an 8-week course (22%).[38] However, Ueda and colleagues[39] found no difference in the 5-year relapse-free rates in patients with steroid-dependent MCD treated for 8 or 12 weeks (24% and 25%, respectively).

There are fewer studies of alkylating agents for steroid-resistant MCD. This probably reflects the relative rarity of steroid resistance in true MCD. Uncontrolled studies suggest that steroid-resistant patients with MCD may respond to cyclophosphamide[43,44]; however, in the ISKDC, the early nonresponsive patients (i.e., those whose disease had not remitted after 8 weeks of prednisone) treated with cyclophosphamide plus prednisone did not show a greater remission rate than those treated with prednisone alone.[28] It should be noted, however, that among those who did respond, the remission occurred earlier in the cyclophosphamide group than in the prednisone group (mean interval between beginning of treatment and remission was 38.4 and 95.5 days, respectively). In the one study in which they were directly compared, chlorambucil and cyclophosphamide appeared to be equally effective in frequently relapsing MCD and equally ineffective in steroid-dependent disease.[37]

Results in Adults

In comparison with children, fewer data are available for adults with regard to the response of MCD to alkylating agents. The retrospective analysis by Nolasco and colleagues[2] showed that 69% of adults treated with cyclophosphamide achieved remission. Moreover, 58% of those who had a remission did so within 8 weeks of the initiation of therapy. The duration of remission was longer after treatment with cyclophosphamide than with prednisone in this series. Two thirds of those who responded to cyclophosphamide were still in remission 4 years after treatment. In a small prospective, controlled study, Al-Khader and colleagues[35] treated eight adult patients with MCD with cyclophosphamide and compared the outcome with that in eight patients treated with supportive therapy (diuretics). Seven of those treated with cyclophosphamide attained remission, whereas two of the control patients had a spontaneous remission. None of the patients in either group who achieved remission had a relapse during a mean follow-up period of 6 years. Although this appears to be an impressive outcome, six patients required treatment for longer than 1 month to achieve remission, and it is possible that an equally good result would have been obtained with glucocorticoids.

Toxicity of Alkylating Agents

The bulk of the data in children and adults suggests that cyclophosphamide or chlorambucil therapy, in conjunction with glucocorticoids, will induce remissions of longer duration than those resulting from glucocorticoids alone in patients with frequent relapses, and that these drugs may thus decrease glucocorticoid requirements in steroid-dependent patients. The major toxicities of these agents include reversible alopecia, susceptibility to viral and fungal infections, gonadal failure, and late development of malignancy. Cyclophosphamide can cause hemorrhagic cystitis, and chlorambucil has been associated with the development of seizures. The risk of irreversible gonadal failure increases with patient age (particularly for

Table 19-3 Studies of Alkylating Agents in Minimal Change Disease

Ref.	Design	Clinical Setting*	Mean Follow-up (yr)	Treatment	Control	RESULTS† COMPLETE REMISSION (%) Rx	Cntrl	RELAPSE (%) Rx	Cntrl	Comments
Cameron et al[33] (N = 58)	Retrospective, uncontrolled	Children, FR, MCD	5.8	Cyclophosphamide		98		66		Relapse-free half-life 2.8 yr; duration of treatment variable (2–30 wk)
ISKDC[28] (N = 96)	Prospective, controlled, randomized	Children, FR, SR, NS	NA	Cyclophosphamide ± prednisone, intermittent	Prednisone, intermittent	SR: 56	40	FR: 48 $P < .001$	88	Treatment for FR patients: cyclophosphamide alone; for SR patients: cyclophosphamide + intermittent prednisone
Grupe et al[34] (N = 21)	Prospective, controlled, randomized	Children, FR, SD, NS	1.7	Chlorambucil + prednisone	Prednisone			0 $P < .005$	100	Mean dose of chlorambucil (16.9 mg/kg) above gonadal toxicity limit
Al-Khader et al[35] (N = 14)	Prospective, controlled, randomized	Adults, MCD	6	Cyclophosphamide	Supportive therapy	87	25	0	0	Statistical significance of difference in remission rates not provided in publication
Williams et al[36] (N = 59)	Retrospective, uncontrolled	Children, FR, SD, SR, NS	5	Clorambucil + prednisone				15		Duration of remission same with high (>0.3 mg/kg/day) or low (<0.3 mg/kg/day) dose

Continued

Table 19-3 Studies of Alkylating Agents in Minimal Change Disease—cont'd

Ref.	Design	Clinical Setting*	Mean Follow-up (yr)	Treatment	Control	RESULTS† COMPLETE REMISSION (%) Rx	Cntrl	RELAPSE (%) Rx	Cntrl	Comments
APN[37] (N = 50)	Prospective, controlled, randomized	Children, FR, SD, MCD	2.5	Cyclophosphamide + prednisone taper	Chlorambucil + prednisone taper			FR: 37 SD: 72	12 69	Significantly higher relapse rate in SD patients than in FR patients (cyclophosphamide and chlorambucil patients combined)
Nolasco et al[2] (N = 36)	Retrospective, uncontrolled	Adults, IE, FR, SD, SR, MCD	>4	Cyclophosphamide ± prednisone		69		41		
APN[38] (N = 36)	Prospective, historically controlled	Children, SD, MCD	2	Cyclophosphamide + prednisone taper 12 wk	Cyclophosphamide + prednisone taper 8 wk			33 P = .018	78	Control group comprised the treatment group from APN, 1982[31]
Ueda et al[39] (N = 73)	Prospective, controlled, randomized	Children, SD, MCD	5.3	Cyclophosphamide + prednisolone 12 wk	Cyclophosphamide + prednisolone 8 wk			76	75	As with relapse rate, there was no significant difference in time to relapse between groups
Kyrieleis et al[40] (N = 93)	Retrospective, uncontrolled	Children, SD, FR, MCD	Median (range), 8 (1–39)	Cyclophosphamide 8 wk				65		29% had relapse > 15 yr after initial course of cyclophosphamide

*See Box 19-1 for general definitions of frequently relapsing, steroid dependent, steroid resistant. Criteria in studies may vary somewhat from those in Box 19-1. NS indicates that patient group includes those with idiopathic nephrotic syndrome, not necessarily only patients with minimal change disease.
†P values are shown if <.05.
APN, Arbeitsgemeinschaft für Pädiatrische Nephrologie; Cntrl, control group; CyA, cyclosporine A; FR, frequently relapsing; IE, initial episode; ISKDC, International Study of Kidney Diseases in Children; MCD, minimal change disease; NA, not available; NS, idiopathic nephrotic syndrome; Rx, treatment group; SD, steroid dependent; SR, steroid resistant.

women) and cumulative dose. Gonadal failure is usually reversible if the total cumulative dose of cyclophosphamide or chlorambucil is less than 200 mg/kg or 10 mg/kg, respectively. Most cases of late malignancies after treatment with these agents have occurred in patients treated for at least 1 year. The risk of malignancy with short-term therapy with chlorambucil or cyclophosphamide is not known. The steroid-sparing effect of alkylating agents has been considered a justification for their use in cases of frequently relapsing and steroid-dependent disease. Although patients who enter prolonged remission after such therapy will be spared further steroid toxicity, there is a risk of additive toxicity in those who have a relapse or fail to respond. Therefore, alkylating agents should be limited to those patients with severe steroid toxicity or uncontrolled disease.

Treatment with Calcineurin Inhibitors

Multiple small uncontrolled studies suggesting beneficial effects of cyclosporin A (CyA) in patients with frequently relapsing or steroid-dependent MCD provided the rationale for the larger trials summarized in Table 19-4.[45–51] All but one of these studies included patients with FSGS as well as MCD, and in most cases, separate analyses of the patients with MCD were not performed. Two multicenter, randomized, controlled studies by Ponticelli and colleagues[45,46] showed that CyA at doses of 5 mg/kg/day in adults and 6 mg/kg/day in children is highly effective in maintaining remission in steroid-dependent or frequently relapsing nephrotic syndrome (88% with CyA compared with 68% with cyclophosphamide) and is capable of producing at least a partial remission in 60% of steroid-resistant cases. In the steroid-responsive patients, the relapse rate and glucocorticoid requirement were decreased during treatment with CyA. However, in both of these studies, as well as in a more recent study by El-Husseini and colleagues,[50] relapse occurred in approximately 70% of patients after CyA was discontinued. A limited experience with tacrolimus for MCD does not suggest an advantage of this agent over CyA.[52,53]

The need for prolonged courses of treatment with CyA, owing to the high relapse rate after its discontinuation, has raised concern about chronic cyclosporine nephrotoxicity. Somewhat to the surprise of those involved in the early trials of CyA treatment of MCD, the drug appeared to be well tolerated in the short term, with no discernible alteration in serum creatinine or glomerular filtration rate measurements.[54] It must be recognized, however, that histologic changes have been documented in the absence of changes in the serum creatinine level. Habib and Niaudet[55] reviewed serial renal biopsy specimens from 42 children with nephrotic syndrome (35 with MCD and 7 with FSGS) treated with CyA for 4 to 63 months. Tubulointerstitial lesions developed in 24 patients, and none of the 9 patients with extensive lesions had a decrease in the glomerular filtration rate.

Although the high relapse rate and potential nephrotoxicity of CyA have relegated it to third-line therapy after glucocorticoids and alkylating agents for steroid-dependent or steroid-resistant disease, the results of a long-term study by Meyrier and colleagues[48] in adults with MCD and FSGS give cause to reconsider this position. The essential findings in this study are that adults with MCD (confirmed on repeat biopsy) can be treated with CyA for an extended period (as long as

78 months) without loss of renal function and with scant histologic evidence of CyA nephrotoxicity as long as the dose does not exceed 5.5 mg/kg/day. Not only did this treatment produce complete remission during CyA therapy in 19 of 22 (86%) of these steroid-dependent or steroid-resistant patients, remission was sustained (for 5 months to 6 years) in 10 patients in whom CyA was discontinued after 1 to 5 years. In this study, the factors that were most predictive of histologic CyA nephrotoxicity included dose greater than 5.5 mg/kg/day, the presence of renal insufficiency before treatment, and the percentage of glomeruli with lesions of FSGS on pretreatment biopsy specimen. A similar paucity of CyA nephrotoxicity in adult MCD was reported by Ittel and colleagues.[49] Although these authors did not observe permanent remission in their patients, they were able to maintain partial or complete remission in 15 patients with steroid-dependent or steroid-resistant MCD for 7 to 91 months. Only one patient showed mild interstitial fibrosis suggestive of CyA toxicity. CyA trough whole blood levels were kept at 50 to 150 ng/mL at a mean dose of approximately 4.5 mg/kg/day.

Evaluations of the nephrotoxicity of long-term CyA treatment in children with MCD have included small numbers of patients and have had varied results. Inoue and colleagues[56] found histologic evidence of CyA toxicity in 7 of 13 children after a 2-year course of treatment for steroid-dependent MCD. The changes were considered moderate or severe in five of the patients. Much lower rates of CyA toxicity have been reported by others. Gregory and colleagues[57] performed biopsies on 12 of 22 children with steroid-dependent or steroid-resistant nephrotic syndrome after 12 to 41 months of CyA treatment. Two patients, both with IgM nephropathy, had progression of interstitial fibrosis and tubular atrophy present on pre-CyA biopsy specimens. None of the other patients had histologic evidence of nephrotoxicity. Hino and colleagues[58] found mild tubular atrophy with striped interstitial fibrosis in 2 of 13 children on whom a biopsy was performed after 12 to 43 months of CyA treatment, and Kano and colleagues[59] found such changes in only 1 of 14 children treated with low-dose CyA (1.6–3.1 mg/kg/day) for 2 years. In both of these studies, there was no apparent correlation between either the CyA dose or mean trough level and the development of histologic changes, and the serum creatinine did not increase after CyA treatment in those patients with biopsy evidence of nephrotoxicity. The stability of the serum creatinine was particularly noteworthy in the study by Hino and colleagues[58] because creatinine values were available at 2 to 10.5 years after completion of the CyA treatment.

Thus, although it has yet to be determined whether prolonged treatment with CyA is curative or simply sustains remission until the disease "burns out," it is reasonable to consider maintenance CyA as an alternative to cyclophosphamide in adults with severe steroid-dependent, steroid-resistant, or even frequently relapsing disease, especially those in their reproductive years. Indeed, some authorities argue that short-term, low-dose CyA might even be preferable to glucocorticoids as first-line therapy.

Treatment with Mycophenolate Mofetil

Although there are as yet no controlled studies to support the use of mycophenolate mofetil (MMF) in MCD, several small case series in children and adults[60–64] and personal experience

Table 19-4   Studies of Cyclosporine A in Minimal Change Disease

Ref.	Design	Clinical Setting*	Mean Follow-up (yr)	Treatment	Control	COMPLETE REMISSION (%) Rx	COMPLETE REMISSION (%) Cntrl	RELAPSE (%) Rx	RELAPSE (%) Cntrl	Comments
Ponticelli et al[45] (N = 41)	Prospective, controlled, randomized	Children, adults, SR, MCD, FSGS	1.5 (median)	CyA 6 mo, then taper	Supportive therapy	32 P <.05	0	69‡	NA	Complete or partial remission in 60% of CyA group vs. 16% of Cntrl
Ponticelli et al[46] (N = 66)	Prospective, controlled, randomized	Children, adults, FR, SD, MCD, FSGS	1.7	CyA 9 mo	Cyclophosphamide 8 wk			75	37	P value for % of relapse not provided in publication
Hulton et al[47] (N = 40)	Prospective, uncontrolled	Children, SD, MCD	2	CyA 12–63 mo				72		All patients had relapse after CyA withdrawal
Meyrier et al[48] (N = 36)	Prospective, uncontrolled	Adults, SD, SR, MCD, FSGS	1.6	CyA 6–78 mo (mean, 19.6 mo)		86#				Serial biopsy study, sustained remission in 10 MCD patients after CyA withdrawal
Ittel et al[49] (N = 40)	Prospective, uncontrolled	Adults, FR, SD, SR, MCD, FSGS	2.7 (median)	CyA 6–91 mo (median, 32 mo)		60§				Serial biopsy study, all patients had relapse after CyA withdrawal
El-Husseini et al[50] (N = 117)	Retrospective, uncontrolled	Children, SD, SR, MCD, FSGS	6.1	CyA + prednisolone; all >2 yr (median, 34 mo)		82				Of 29 patients in whom CyA was discontinued, 22 had relapse; of 48 patients with biopsy after treatment, mild CyA nephropathy was present in 2 (4%)
Hoyer et al[51] (N = 152)	Prospective, controlled, randomized	Children, initial episode of nephrotic syndrome		Prednisone plus CyA¶	Prednisone‖	Median sustained remission 22.8 mo	12.5 mo			Only 104 of the 152 randomized patients were included in the primary analysis

*See Box 19-1 for definitions of frequently relapsing, steroid dependent, and steroid resistant. Criteria in studies may vary somewhat from those in Box 19-1.

†P value is shown if difference is significant (i.e., if P <.05).

‡Relapse rate for patients who had complete or partial remission.

#Refers to minimal change disease patients only (N = 22).

§Refers to minimal change disease patients only (N = 15).

¶CyA administered at dose of 150 mg/m²/day for 8 weeks starting when urine was protein free for 3 days. Prednisone was administered at 60 mg/m²/48 hr for 6 weeks.

‖Prednisone was administered at 60 mg/m²/day for 6 weeks followed by 40 mg/m²/48 hr for 6 weeks.

Cntrl, control group; CyA, cyclosporine A; FR, frequently relapsing; FSGS, focal segmental glomerulosclerosis; MCD, minimal change disease; NA, not available; Rx, treatment group; SD, steroid dependent; SR, steroid resistant.

in adults have shown that remission can be maintained in a high proportion of patients with steroid-dependent or frequently relapsing MCD, including patients who have had a relapse after discontinuation of CyA treatment. In the series of MMF-treated adults with proteinuric glomerular diseases reported by Choi and colleagues,[60] five of six patients with steroid-dependent MCD were able to discontinue steroid use. Likewise, durable remission, decrease in relapse rate, and steroid sparing have been reported in children with steroid- and CyA-dependent or frequently relapsing MCD.[61,64] Unfortunately, MMF does not appear to be any better than CyA in effecting a cure, as a high proportion of patients had a relapse after MMF treatment was discontinued.[61,64] Given that MMF is generally better tolerated and is less toxic than CyA and cyclophosphamide, it would be the preferred choice in patients who require long-term maintenance therapy to prevent relapse if future studies confirm the current experience. Unfortunately, MMF has not proved to be effective in inducing remission in steroid-resistant MCD in more than a few anecdotal cases.[61,64]

Treatment with Azathioprine, Levamasole, and Rituximab

Most of the data on the use of azathioprine in MCD comes from anecdotal reports, and the general view is that this drug has limited value in the treatment of this disease. In the only controlled study examining its use in MCD, Abramowicz and colleagues[65] found that azathioprine was ineffective in 31 children with steroid-resistant nephrotic syndrome (only 5 of the patients had MCD). More promising results were reported by Cade and colleagues[66] who treated 13 adults (8 with MCD) with prolonged courses (4 years) of azathioprine and found that all the patients had a progressive decrease in proteinuria and ultimately achieved complete remission. The results of this study and the decreased toxicity profile of azathioprine compared with the alkylating agents led some investigators to argue for further evaluation of its efficacy in MCD.[18] However, interest in azathioprine has lessened in recent years as experience with MMF has accrued for a variety of glomerular diseases.

Levamisole, an immunopotentiating drug, has been used as a steroid-sparing agent in children with frequently relapsing MCD. The British Society of Pediatric Nephrology performed a controlled study of 61 children treated with levamisole or placebo after a steroid-induced remission.[67] Fourteen of 31 patients treated with levamisole were in remission at the end of a 3- to 4-month treatment period compared with three of 30 patients treated with a placebo. However, discontinuation of the drug was associated with a rapid relapse, and only four of the responders were still in remission at the end of the study. A second controlled trial of levamisole found that treatment with this drug resulted in a statistically nonsignificant increase in the proportion of patients with a sustained glucocorticoid-induced remission.[68] Multiple uncontrolled studies suggest a potential role for this drug as a steroid-sparing agent, but adequately powered randomized trials are needed to evaluate its long-term efficacy and safety.[69]

Rituximab is a monoclonal antibody directed against CD20, a cell-surface molecule on B lymphocytes. A case report of attainment of a long-lasting remission with rituximab of frequently relapsing MCD in a 23-year-old woman who had previously been treated with glucocorticoids, CyA, cyclophosphamide, MMF, and basiliximab (an anti-CD25 antibody directed against T lymphocytes) suggests a possible role for B cells in MCD, a disease that has generally been viewed as resulting from disordered T-lymphocyte function.[70]

SPECIFIC RECOMMENDATIONS

Although maintaining MCD patients free of urine protein could probably be accomplished in more than 90% of cases using prednisone, cyclophosphamide, or CyA, such regimens are associated with significant toxicity. Thus, the therapeutic challenge of this disease is to identify the treatment with the highest probability of producing a sustained remission with the lowest risk of toxicity. The literature reviewed earlier is helpful in this regard but is not conclusive. Individual patient variation remains a major factor in choosing among treatment options. Therefore, the recommendations that follow (summarized in Figs. 19-1 and 19-2) should be viewed as flexible guidelines rather than definitive treatment protocols.

Regardless of the specific therapy used, symptomatic management of nephrotic patients should include dietary sodium and fluid restriction to prevent further edema formation. Diuretics may be necessary before specific therapy takes effect, and high doses are often required because of the marked sodium avidity that accompanies nephrotic syndrome. Angiotensin-converting enzyme inhibitors may decrease proteinuria in nephrotic patients and thus may have a role during initial management or in steroid-resistant patients; however, one should be alert to the possibility of an acute reduction in the glomerular filtration rate from alterations in intrarenal hemodynamics. To prevent glucocorticoid-induced osteoporosis, we recommend a daily intake (either through diet or supplements) of 1500 mg of calcium and 400 to 800 IU of vitamin D (with age-appropriate decreases in children) for all patients during glucocorticoid therapy. Additionally, for adult patients receiving long-term glucocorticoid treatment, it is appropriate to obtain a baseline bone mineral density measurement and to consider further prophylactic treatment with bisphosphonates.[71] Although the risk of accelerated atherogenesis in patients with MCD is debated, the use of lipid-lowering agents, preferably 3-hydroxy-3-methylglutaryl coenzyme A reductase inhibitors, should be considered in hyperlipidemic patients with sustained proteinuria. Nephrotic patients are also at risk for thromboembolic disease; however, routine anticoagulation is not recommended for patients with MCD.

Almost all children with idiopathic nephrotic syndrome should be treated empirically with glucocorticoids because of the high probability that they have MCD. A typical regimen for a first attack is as follows: prednisone 60 mg/m^2/day with a maximum of 80 mg/day, given as a single daily dose for 4 weeks. The dose is reduced to 35 to 40 mg/m^2 every other day for the subsequent 4 weeks and then tapered off over an additional 4 weeks. A more gradual tapering scheme consisting of alternate-day dosing at 60 mg/m^2 for 8 weeks after the initial 4 weeks of daily therapy, with tapering over an additional 4 to 6 weeks, such that the total duration of therapy is approximately 4 to 5 months, is preferred by some. A decrease in proteinuria will occur in most children after 2 weeks of treatment. If proteinuria persists in a child after 4 weeks of treatment, a renal biopsy should be performed.

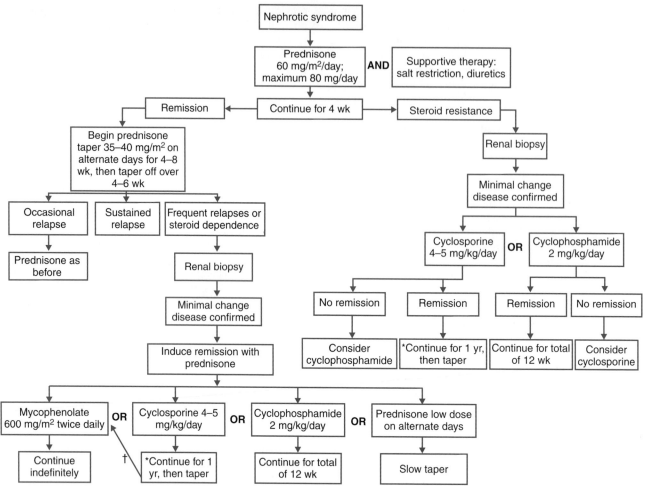

Figure 19-1 Treatment algorithm for children with minimal change disease. *Renal biopsy should be performed to evaluate for cyclosporine toxicity before continuing cyclosporine treatment beyond 1 year. †Patients who relapse after withdrawal of cyclosporine may be maintained on mycophenolate mofetil.

Since MCD accounts for only 10% to 15% of cases of nephrotic syndrome in adults, a renal biopsy should be performed before initiating therapy. If secondary causes of MCD have been eliminated, we recommend treatment with prednisone at 1 mg/kg as a single daily dose. Because the response to glucocorticoids occurs less rapidly in adults than in children, the prednisone therapy should be continued for 12 weeks before the disease is considered to be steroid resistant. A progressive shift to alternate-day dosing beginning at 1 mg/kg should be started 1 week after proteinuria remits and tapered off over 2 to 3 months. Initial treatment with alternate-day prednisone at 2 mg/kg, with a maximum dose of 120 mg every other day, may also be effective and have fewer side effects, but there is less published experience with such a regimen.

Treatment of MCD relapses must take into account their frequency and the severity of glucocorticoid-related toxicities. A first relapse in either a child or adult can usually be treated with a second course of prednisone with tapering beginning as soon as remission occurs. We recommend gradual, rather than rapid, tapering of the second course of prednisone therapy because available data suggest that this results in a lower probability of a subsequent relapse. How-

ever, this approach may not necessarily result in a lower cumulative glucocorticoid dose.

If a relapse occurs during prednisone tapering, the prednisone dose should be increased immediately to the level at which remission occurred. In most cases, remission will result, and a relatively rapid taper can begin. As the dose at which the relapse occurred is approached, the rate of tapering should be made more gradual in order to decrease the likelihood of a second relapse. We recommend that the patient or parent monitor the urine for protein by using a dipstick during the taper to facilitate early detection of relapse.

In some cases of frequently relapsing or steroid-dependent MCD, remission can be sustained with long-term, low-dose, alternate-day prednisone therapy. However, the doses required to maintain remission may be intolerably high, in which case alkylating agents should be considered. Indeed, elderly patients may tolerate cyclophosphamide better than glucocorticoids. Although cyclophosphamide and chlorambucil appear to have similar efficacy, we prefer cyclophosphamide 2 mg/kg/day for 8 to 12 weeks for frequently relapsing disease and 12 weeks for steroid-dependent disease. Prednisone is usually administered with cyclophosphamide, although this may not necessarily improve efficacy. Patients are often already taking glucocorticoids

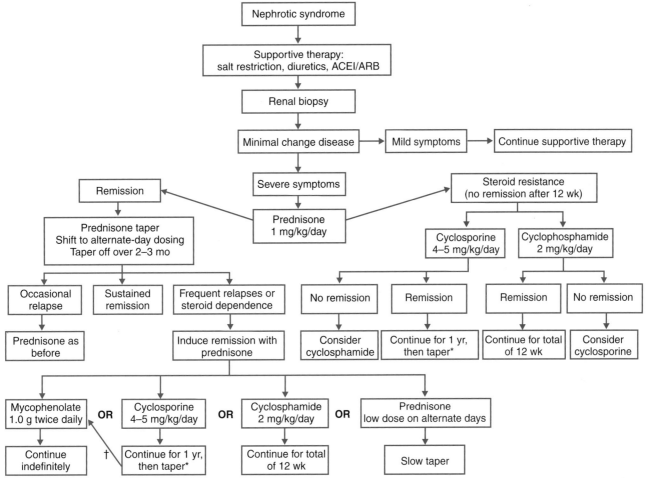

Figure 19-2 Treatment algorithm for adults with minimal change disease. *Renal biopsy should be performed to evaluate for cyclosporine toxicity before continuing cyclosporine treatment beyond 1 year. †Patients who relapse after withdrawal of cyclosporine may be maintained on mycophenolate mofetil. ACEI, angiotensin-converting enzyme inhibitor; ARB, angiotensin receptor blocker.

when the decision is made to start therapy with an alkylating agent. A potential benefit of inducing a remission with glucocorticoids before starting cyclophosphamide therapy is that it may allow the high fluid intake required for protection against cystitis. The usual dose of chlorambucil is 0.1 to 0.2 mg/kg/day. The cumulative doses of cyclophosphamide and chlorambucil should be kept to less than 200 mg/kg and 10 mg/kg, respectively, to avoid gonadal toxicity. The leukocyte count should be monitored during treatment with alkylating agents with dose adjustments as needed to maintain the count between 2000 and 5000 cells/mm³.

CyA is a reasonable option for patients who have a relapse after one or two courses of cyclophosphamide therapy, and we believe that it is a good alternative to an alkylating agent in young adults. The dose of CyA should be initiated at 4 to 5 mg/kg/day in adults and 4 to 6 mg/kg/day in children and adjusted to maintain a whole blood trough level by monoclonal antibody assay of 100 to 150 ng/mL. Treatment should be continued for 1 year and then tapered. If a relapse occurs, CyA should be restarted at the dose that maintained remission but in adults should not exceed 5.5 mg/kg/day. If a response to CyA has not occurred within 3 to 4 months, the drug should be discontinued. It is important to note that the optimal dose

for long-term CyA therapy in children has not been established. In the studies describing outcomes with CyA treatment for longer than 1 year, many of the children had mean trough levels that were less than 100 ng/mL. Steroid-dependent patients may require low doses of prednisone together with CyA to maintain remission and are more likely than those with frequent relapses to have a relapse after discontinuation of CyA therapy. Serum creatinine and creatinine clearance should be monitored periodically during administration of CyA; however, early CyA nephrotoxicity may not be accompanied by changes in these measurements. Therefore, repeat renal biopsy to look for nephrotoxicity is advisable in patients requiring treatment with CyA for more than 1 year.

At present, MMF has a role as maintenance therapy in patients who experience a relapse whenever CyA or cyclophosphamide are discontinued, but if results of several case series are confirmed, it may become the treatment of choice in patients with frequent relapses or steroid-dependent patients.

Steroid-resistant MCD is rare. Children who have nephrotic syndrome that does not remit with prednisone should undergo renal biopsy, as it is likely that they actually have FSGS. Adults who have presumed MCD based on a biopsy performed before treatment may actually have had FSGS that was not apparent on the initial biopsy specimen. Steroid-resistant MCD can be treated with alkylating agents or with CyA using the regimens described for frequently relapsing or steroid-dependent disease, but such patients are less likely to respond.

In conclusion, despite many years of accumulated experience with immunosuppressive agents, the treatment of frequently relapsing MCD remains a challenge. The approach that we have outlined favors a shift from repeated courses of high-dose glucocorticoids or alkylating agents to a maintenance type of treatment with longer courses of low-dose, alternate-day glucocorticoids, CyA, or MMF. In the final analysis, however, treatment must be customized for each patient based on clinical characteristics, disease course, and treatment-associated toxicities.

References

1. Falk RJ, Jennette JC, Nachman PH: Primary glomerular diseases. In Brenner BM (ed): Brenner & Rector's The Kidney, 7th ed. Philadelphia: WB Saunders, 2004, pp 1293–1380.
2. Nolasco F, Cameron JS, Heywood EF, et al: Adult-onset minimal change nephrotic syndrome: A long-term follow-up. Kidney Int 1986;29:1215–1223.
3. Korbet SM, Schwartz MM, Lewis EJ: Minimal-change glomerulopathy of adulthood. Am J Nephrol 1988;8:291–297.
4. Fujimoto S, Yamamoto Y, Hisanaga S, et al: Minimal change nephrotic syndrome in adults: Response to corticosteroid therapy and frequency of relapse. Am J Kidney Dis 1991;17:687–692.
5. Wang F, Looi LM, Chua CT: Minimal change glomerular disease in Malaysian adults and use of alternate day steroid therapy. Q J Med 1982;51:312–328.
6. Tarshish P, Tobin JN, Bernstein J, Edelmann CM Jr: Prognostic significance of the early course of minimal change nephrotic syndrome: Report of the International Study of Kidney Disease in Children. J Am Soc Nephrol 1997;8:769–776.
7. Fogo A, Hawkins EP, Berry PL, et al: Glomerular hypertrophy in minimal change disease predicts subsequent progression to focal glomerular sclerosis. Kidney Int 1990;38:115–123.
8. Guasch A, Myers BD: Determinants of glomerular hypofiltration in nephrotic patients with minimal change nephropathy. J Am Soc Nephrol 1994;4:1571–1581.
9. Guasch A, Deen WM, Myers BD: Charge selectivity of the glomerular filtration barrier in healthy and nephrotic humans. J Clin Invest 1993;92:2274–2282.
10. Bertolatus JA, Hunsicker LG: Glomerular sieving of anionic and neutral bovine albumins in proteinuric rats. Kidney Int 1985;28:467–476.
11. Koyama A, Fujisaki M, Kobayashi M, et al: A glomerular permeability factor produced by human T cell hybridomas. Kidney Int 1991;40:453–460.
12. Maruyama K, Tomizawa S, Seki Y, et al: Inhibition of vascular permeability factor production by cyclosporin in minimal change nephrotic syndrome. Nephron 1992;62:27–30.
13. Parikh C, Gibney E, Thurman JM: The long-term outcome of glomerular diseases. In Schrier RW (ed): Diseases of the Kidney and Urinary Tract, 8th ed. Philadelphia: Lippincott Williams & Wilkins, 2007, pp 1811–1859.
14. Idelson BA, Smithline N, Smith GW, Harrington JT: Prognosis in steroid-treated idiopathic nephrotic syndrome in adults: Analysis of major predictive factors after ten-year follow-up. Arch Intern Med 1977;137:891–896.
15. Glassock RJ: Therapy of idiopathic nephrotic syndrome in adults: A conservative or aggressive therapeutic approach? Am J Nephrol 1993;13:422–428.
16. Brodehl J: Conventional therapy for idiopathic nephrotic syndrome in children. Clin Nephrol 1991;35(Suppl 1):S8–S15.
17. Report of the International Study of Kidney Disease in Children: The primary nephrotic syndrome in children. Identification of patients with minimal change nephrotic syndrome from initial response to prednisone. J Pediatr 1981;98:561–564.
18. Meyrier A, Simon P: Treatment of corticoresistant idiopathic nephrotic syndrome in the adult: Minimal change disease and focal segmental glomerulosclerosis. Adv Nephrol Necker Hosp 1988;17:127–150.
19. Wingen AM, Muller-Wiefel DE, Scharer K: Spontaneous remissions in frequently relapsing and steroid dependent idiopathic nephrotic syndrome. Clin Nephrol 1985;23:35–40.
20. Schena FP, Cameron JS: Treatment of proteinuric idiopathic glomerulonephritides in adults: A retrospective survey. Am J Med 1988;85:315–326.
21. Black D, Rose G, Brewer D: Controlled trial of prednisone in adult patients with the nephrotic syndrome. Br Med J 1970;3:421.
22. Coggins C: Minimal change nephrosis in adults. In Zurukzoglu W (ed): Proceedings of the 8th International Congress of Nephrology. Basel: Karger, 1981, p 336.
23. Arbeitsgemeinschaft fur Padiatrische Nephrologie: Alternate-day prednisone is more effective than intermittent prednisone in frequently relapsing nephrotic syndrome. Eur J Pediatr 1981;135:229–237.
24. Imbasciati E, Gusmano R, Edefonti A, et al: Controlled trial of methylprednisolone pulses and low dose oral prednisone for the minimal change nephrotic syndrome. Br Med J 1985;291:1305–1308.
25. Arbeitsgemeinschaft fur Padiatrische Nephrologie: Short versus standard prednisone therapy for initial treatment of idiopathic nephrotic syndrome in children. Lancet 1988;1:380–383.
26. Ueda N, Chihara M, Kawaguchi S, et al: Intermittent versus long-term tapering prednisolone for initial therapy in children with idiopathic nephrotic syndrome. J Pediatr 1988;112:122–126.
27. Bagga A, Hari P, Srivastava RN: Prolonged versus standard prednisolone therapy for initial episode of nephrotic syndrome. Pediatr Nephrol 1999;13:824–827.
28. Report of the International Study of Kidney Disease in Children: Prospective, controlled trial of cyclophosphamide therapy in children with nephrotic syndrome. Lancet 1974;2:423–427.
29. Nair RB, Date A, Kirubakaran MG, Shastry JC: Minimal-change nephrotic syndrome in adults treated with alternate-day steroids. Nephron 1987;47:209–210.
30. Nakayama M, Katafuchi R, Yanase T, et al: Steroid responsiveness and frequency of relapse in adult-onset minimal change nephrotic syndrome. Am J Kidney Dis 2002;39:503–512.
31. Waldman MCR, Valeri A, Busch J, et al: Adult minimal-change disease: Clinical characteristics, treatment, and outcomes. Clin J Am Soc Nephrol 2007;2:445–453.
32. Report of the International Study of Kidney Disease in Children: Nephrotic syndrome in children: A randomized trial comparing two prednisone regimens in steroid-responsive patients who relapse early. J Pediatr 1979;95:239–243.
33. Cameron JS, Chantler C, Ogg CS, White RH: Long-term stability of remission in nephrotic syndrome after treatment with cyclophosphamide. Br Med J 1974;4:7–11.
34. Grupe WE, Makker SP, Ingelfinger JR: Chlorambucil treatment of frequently relapsing nephrotic syndrome. N Engl J Med 1976;295:746–749.
35. Al-Khader AA, Lien JW, Aber GM: Cyclophosphamide alone in the treatment of adult patients with minimal change glomerulonephritis. Clin Nephrol 1979;11:26–30.
36. Williams SA, Makker SP, Ingelfinger JR, Grupe WE: Long-term evaluation of chlorambucil plus prednisone in the idiopathic nephrotic syndrome of childhood. N Engl J Med 1980;302:929–933.

37. Effect of cytotoxic drugs in frequently relapsing nephrotic syndrome with and without steroid dependence. N Engl J Med 1982;306:451–454.

38. Arbeitsgemeinschaft fur Padiatrische Nephrologie: Cyclophosphamide treatment of steroid dependent nephrotic syndrome: Comparison of eight week with 12 week course. Arch Dis Child 1987;62:1102–1106.

39. Ueda N, Kuno K, Ito S: Eight and 12 week courses of cyclophosphamide in nephrotic syndrome. Arch Dis Child 1990;65:1147–1150.

40. Kyrieleis HA, Levtchenko EN, Wetzels JF: Long-term outcome after cyclophosphamide treatment in children with steroid-dependent and frequently relapsing minimal change nephrotic syndrome. Am J Kidney Dis 2007;49:592–597.

41. Barratt TM, Soothill JF: Controlled trial of cyclophosphamide in steroid-sensitive relapsing nephrotic syndrome of childhood. Lancet 1970;2:479–482.

42. Chiu J, McLaine PN, Drummond KN: A controlled prospective study of cyclophosphamide in relapsing, corticosteroid-responsive, minimal-lesion nephrotic syndrome in childhood. J Pediatr 1973;82:607–613.

43. Bergstrand A, Bollgren I, Samuelsson A, et al: Idiopathic nephrotic syndrome of childhood: Cyclophosphamide induced conversion from steroid refractory to highly steroid sensitive disease. Clin Nephrol 1973;1:302–306.

44. Ponticelli C, Passerini P: Treatment of the nephrotic syndrome associated with primary glomerulonephritis. Kidney Int 1994;46:595–604.

45. Ponticelli C, Rizzoni G, Edefonti A, et al: A randomized trial of cyclosporine in steroid-resistant idiopathic nephrotic syndrome. Kidney Int 1993;43:1377–1384.

46. Ponticelli C, Edefonti A, Ghio L, et al: Cyclosporin versus cyclophosphamide for patients with steroid-dependent and frequently relapsing idiopathic nephrotic syndrome: A multicentre randomized controlled trial. Nephrol Dial Transplant 1993;8:1326–1332.

47. Hulton SA, Neuhaus TJ, Dillon MJ, Barratt TM: Long-term cyclosporin A treatment of minimal-change nephrotic syndrome of childhood. Pediatr Nephrol 1994;8:401–403.

48. Meyrier A, Noel LH, Auriche P, Callard P: Long-term renal tolerance of cyclosporin A treatment in adult idiopathic nephrotic syndrome. Collaborative Group of the Societé de Nephrologie. Kidney Int 1994;45:1446–1456.

49. Ittel TH, Clasen W, Fuhs M, et al: Long-term ciclosporine A treatment in adults with minimal change nephrotic syndrome or focal segmental glomerulosclerosis. Clin Nephrol 1995;44:156–162.

50. El-Husseini A, El-Basuony F, Mahmoud I, et al: Long-term effects of cyclosporine in children with idiopathic nephrotic syndrome: A single-centre experience. Nephrol Dial Transplant 2005;20:2433–2438.

51. Hoyer PF, Brodeh J: Initial treatment of idiopathic nephrotic syndrome in children: Prednisone versus prednisone plus cyclosporine A: A prospective, randomized trial. J Am Soc Nephrol 2006;17:1151–1157.

52. Westhoff TH, Schmidt S, Zidek W, et al: Tacrolimus in steroid-resistant and steroid-dependent nephrotic syndrome. Clin Nephrol 2006;65:393–400.

53. Sinha MD, MacLeod R, Rigby E, Clark AG: Treatment of severe steroid-dependent nephrotic syndrome (SDNS) in children with tacrolimus. Nephrol Dial Transplant 2006;21:1848–1854.

54. Collaborative Study Group of Sandimmune in Nephrotic Syndrome: Safety and tolerability of cyclosporin A (Sandimmune) in idiopathic nephrotic syndrome. Clin Nephrol 1991;35:S48.

55. Habib R, Niaudet P: Comparison between pre- and posttreatment renal biopsies in children receiving cclosporine for idiopathic nephrosis. Clin Nephrol 1994;42:141–146.

56. Inoue Y, Iijima K, Nakamura H, Yoshikawa N: Two-year cyclosporin treatment in children with steroid-dependent nephrotic syndrome. Pediatr Nephrol 1999;13:33–38.

57. Gregory MJ, Smoyer WE, Sedman A, et al: Long-term cyclosporine therapy for pediatric nephrotic syndrome: A clinical and histologic analysis. J Am Soc Nephrol 1996;7:543–549.

58. Hino S, Takemura T, Okada M, et al: Follow-up study of children with nephrotic syndrome treated with a long-term moderate dose of cyclosporine. Am J Kidney Dis 1998;31:932–939.

59. Kano K, Kyo K, Yamada Y, et al: Comparison between pre- and posttreatment clinical and renal biopsies in children receiving low dose cyclosporine-A for 2 years for steroid-dependent nephrotic syndrome. Clin Nephrol 1999;52:19–24.

60. Choi MJ, Eustace JA, Gimenez LF, et al: Mycophenolate mofetil treatment for primary glomerular diseases. Kidney Int 2002;61:1098–114.

61. Bagga A, Hari P, Moudgil A, Jordan SC: Mycophenolate mofetil and prednisolone therapy in children with steroid-dependent nephrotic syndrome. Am J Kidney Dis 2003;42:1114–1120.

62. Barletta GM, Smoyer WE, Bunchman TE, et al: Use of mycophenolate mofetil in steroid-dependent and -resistant nephrotic syndrome. Pediatr Nephrol 2003;18:833–837.

63. Pesavento TE, Bay WH, Agarwal G, et al: Mycophenolate therapy in frequently relapsing minimal change disease that has failed cyclophosphamide therapy. Am J Kidney Dis 2004;43:e3–e6.

64. Mendizabal S, Zamora I, Berbel O, et al: Mycophenolate mofetil in steroid/cyclosporine-dependent/resistant nephrotic syndrome. Pediatr Nephrol 2005;20:914–919.

65. Abramowicz M, Barnett HL, Edelmann CM Jr, et al: Controlled trial of azathioprine in children with nephrotic syndrome. A report for the International Study of Kidney Disease in Children. Lancet 1970;1:959–961.

66. Cade R, Mars D, Privette M, et al: Effect of long-term azathioprine administration in adults with minimal-change glomerulonephritis and nephrotic syndrome resistant to corticosteroids. Arch Intern Med 1986;146:737–741.

67. British Association for Paediatric Nephrology: Levamisole for corticosteroid-dependent nephrotic syndrome in childhood. Lancet 1991;337:1555–1557.

68. Dayal U, Dayal AK, Shastry JC, Raghupathy P: Use of levamisole in maintaining remission in steroid-sensitive nephrotic syndrome in children. Nephron 1994;66:408–412.

69. Davin JC, Merkus MP: Levamisole in steroid-sensitive nephrotic syndrome of childhood: The lost paradise? Pediatr Nephrol 2005;20:10–14.

70. Francois H, Daugas E, Bensman A, Ronco P: Unexpected efficacy of rituximab in multirelapsing minimal change nephrotic syndrome in the adult: First case report and pathophysiological considerations. Am J Kidney Dis 2006;49:158–161.

71. American College of Rheumatology Ad Hoc Committee on Glucocorticoid-Induced Osteoporosis: Recommendations for the prevention and treatment of glucocorticoid-induced osteoporosis: 2001 update. Arthritis Rheum 2001;44:1496–1503.

Further Reading

Eddy AA, Symons JM: Nephrotic syndrome in childhood. Lancet 2003;362:629–639.

Hodson EM, Habashy D, Craig JC: Interventions for idiopathic steroid-resistant nephrotic syndrome in children. Cochrane Database Syst Rev 2006;2:CD003594.

Hodson EM, Craig JC, Willis NS: Evidence-based management of steroid-sensitive nephrotic syndrome. Pediatr Nephrol 2005;20:1523–1530.

Meyrier A: Treatment of idiopathic nephrosis by immunophillin modulation. Nephrol Dial Transplant 2003;18(Suppl 6):79–86.

Chapter 20

Focal Segmental Glomerulosclerosis and Collapsing Glomerulopathy

Monique E. Cho and Jeffrey B. Kopp

Focal segmental glomerulosclerosis (FSGS) is a clinicopathologic entity defined by proteinuria and segmental glomerular scars involving some but not all glomeruli. It is a leading cause of nephrotic syndrome in adults and is the predominant cause of end-stage renal disease (ESRD) among children.[1] The incidence of FSGS has been increasing over the past two decades, with idiopathic FSGS responsible for 3.3% of incident ESRD cases in the United States. FSGS accounts for 7% to 35% of glomerular lesions in children and adults undergoing renal biopsy for nephrotic syndrome.[2–7] Additionally, the prevalence of FSGS in nephrotic black patients is two to four times that in white patients (50%–60% vs. 20%–25%).[6,7]

Few clinical features distinguish patients with new-onset idiopathic nephrotic syndrome due to minimal change nephropathy (MCN) versus FSGS. FSGS is distinguished from MCN by a higher frequency of hematuria and a poorer response to immunosuppressive drug therapies. Although patients with FSGS are more likely to have subnephrotic proteinuria than those with MCN, FSGS patients have a higher frequency of persistent nephrotic syndrome and a greater risk of progression to ESRD. It often progresses over several years to renal insufficiency and hypertension. Approximately 50% of patients with idiopathic FSGS progress to ESRD within 10 years of diagnosis. The progressive nature of this lesion and the high recurrence rate in transplanted kidneys have made the treatment of primary FSGS a serious concern to nephrologists.

FSGS, defined by the characteristic pathologic findings, is a complex syndrome associated with multiple etiologies and variable clinical severity (Table 20-1).[8] FSGS can be classified into idiopathic, genetic, and reactive forms (the last including postadaptive and medication-associated FSGS). Idiopathic FSGS accounts for 10% of all children presenting with nephrotic syndrome.[9] Although FSGS generally carries a poor prognosis, considerable heterogeneity exists in clinical features, renal histology, and outcome. The existing data guiding the treatment of FSGS are mostly drawn from patients with the idiopathic form, and significant uncertainty exists regarding the optimal therapy approach for postadaptive and genetic forms of FSGS.

ETIOLOGY

FSGS is a disease of podocytes with diverse causes. Until recently, the understanding of glomerular injury in FSGS has been limited to more broad concepts and little has been known about biochemical components essential for the glomerular filtration barrier. At the core of pathogenesis of MCN and FSGS, podocyte dysfunction has now been demonstrated as having a particular importance in mediating glomerular permselectivity. The recent series of discoveries has identified specific proteins that are critical to podocyte function, including cellular signaling and maintenance of cytoskeletal structure.

Table 20-1   Taxonomy of the Podocytopathies

	Idiopathic Forms	Genetic Forms	Reactive Forms

Minimal change nephropathy	Idiopathic
	  Steroid sensitive
	  Steroid resistant
		Nonsyndromic
		  NPHS2
		Syndromic
		  DYSF (limb-girdle muscular
		    dystrophy 2B)
			Reactive
			  Hodgkin's disease
			  Immunogenic stimuli
			  Medication associated
			  Nonsteroidal anti-inflammatory agents,
			    gold, penicillamine, lithium, interferon
			    alfa and beta, pamidronate

Focal segmental glomerulosclerosis	Idiopathic	Nonsyndromic
		  NPHS1 + NPHS2
		  NPHS2
		  ACTN4
		  CD2AP
		  TRPC6
		  WT1
		  mtDNA tRNA^{Leu}
		  PLCE1
		Syndromic
		  WT1 (Frasier)
		  mtDNA tRNA^{Leu} (MELAS)
		  PAX2 (renal-coloboma
		    syndrome with
		    oligomeganephronia)
		  LMX1B (nail-patella)
		  COQ2
		  ITGB4
		  COL4A3, A4, A5 (Alport's)
		  GLA (Fabry's)
			Postadaptive
			  Reduced nephron mass
			  Renal dysplasia, surgical renal mass re-
			    duction, reflux nephropathy, chronic
			    interstitial nephritis
			  Initially normal nephron mass
			  Obesity, increased muscle mass, sickle
			    cell anemia, cyanotic congenital
			    heart disease, hypertension*
			Medication associated
			  Cyclosporine, tacrolimus, interferon
			    alfa, lithium, pamidronate

Diffuse mesangial sclerosis	Idiopathic	Nonsyndromic
		  NPHS1 (Congenital nephrotic
		    syndrome, Finnish type)
		  WT1
		  NPHS2
		  PLCE1
		Syndromic
		  LAMB2 (Pierson)
		  WT1 (Denys-Drash)	

Collapsing glomerulopathy	Idiopathic	Nonsyndromic
		  COQ2
		Syndromic
		  ZMPSTEZ4
		  Action myoclonus renal
		    failure
			Infection
			  Viruses (HIV-1, parvovirus B19,*
			    CMV*)
			  Others (Loa loa filiariasis,* visceral
			    leishmaniasis,* *Mycobacterium
			    tuberculosis*)
			Disease associations
			  Adult Still's disease,* thrombotic
			    microangiopathy, multiple myeloma*
			Medication
			  Interferon alfa, pamidronate

*Disease associations for which causation has not been clearly established. The primary podocytopathies are organized into four morphologic patterns and three etiologic categories. Named syndromes are shown. The genes, encoded proteins, and syndrome abbreviations are as follows: *ACTN4*, α-actinin-4; *CD2AP*, CD2-associated protein; *CMV*, cytomegalovirus; *COL4*, type IV collagen; *COQ2*, coenzyme Q synthetase 2; *DYSF*, dysferlin; *GLA*, α-galactosidase A; *HIV-1*, human immunodeficiency virus type 1; *ITGB4*, B$_4$-integrin; *LAMB2*, laminin B$_2$ chain; *LMX1B*, Lim homeobox transcription factor 1B; *MELAS*, mitochondrial myopathy, encephalopathy, lactic acidosis, and strokelike episodes; mtDNA, mitochondrial DNA; *NPHS1*, nephrin; *NPHS2*, podocin; *PAX2*, paired homeobox protein 2; *PLCE1*, phospholipase Cε; *TRPC6*, transient receptor potential cation channel, member 6; *WT1*, Wilms' tumor-1.
Reprinted with permission from Barisoni L, Schnaper HW, Kopp JB: A proposed taxonomy for the podocytopathies: A reassessment of the primary nephrotic diseases. Clin J Am Soc Nephrol 2007;2:529–542.

This exciting and rapidly expanding field of podocyte biology should provide new avenues to gain better understanding of molecular mechanisms underlying foot process effacement, proteinuria, and progressive glomerulosclerosis.

Experimental and clinical studies have shown that podocyte injury can occur from the mutations in podocyte proteins, toxins, viral infections, immunologic factors, and injury from preexisting or ongoing insults (such as obesity and possibly hypertension). Thus, although some forms of FSGS reflect innate abnormalities, others result from the adaptive process of various injuries, including previous glomerular injury.

Idiopathic Focal Segmental Glomerulosclerosis

Like MCN, some cases of idiopathic FSGS may have an immunogenic component in the setting of genetic susceptibility. In some cases of idiopathic FSGS, circulating permeability factor may lead to proteinuria, as suggested by a case of a nephrotic mother who transmitted the factor to her child in utero.[10] In addition, rapid recurrence of proteinuria after transplantation in some cases supports the hypothesis that circulating factor increases the permeability of the glomerular filtration barrier. Permeability factor studies over the past decade, however, have produced conflicting data with limited clinical applicability.

Postadaptive Focal Segmental Glomerulosclerosis

Postadaptive FSGS, or secondary FSGS, arises as a consequence of structural adaptation (glomerular hypertrophy) and/or functional adaptation (glomerular hyperperfusion and hyperfiltration) to either reduced nephron mass or particular disease states (obesity, sickle cell anemia, cyanotic congenital heart disease, and others). The term *postadaptive FSGS* was selected to emphasize that there is believed to be a phase of adaptation that includes glomerular hyperfiltration and glomerulomegaly and that the adaptive phase is followed by the focal and segmental scarring and absolute decrease in podocyte numbers that characterize FSGS. The diagnosis of postadaptive FSGS remains a challenge, given that there are no pathologic hallmarks unique to this form. As the postadaptive form may have different responses to therapy, however, the distinction from the other forms of FSGS becomes important.

Currently available methods to identify postadaptive FSGS include measuring glomerular size, evaluating the degree of foot process effacement on electron microscopy, and determining the fraction of glomeruli with perihilar sclerosis (Table 20-2). Glomerulomegaly may be one of the few distinguishing features of postadaptive FSGS, particularly in obese patients. Obesity is associated with increased renal blood flow, glomerular filtration rate (GFR), and microalbuminuria, features that

Table 20-2 Clinical and Pathological Recognition of Postadaptive Focal Segmental Glomerulosclerosis

Feature	Utility	Limitations
High risk clinical setting		
1. Reduced nephron mass: renal dysplasia, ureteral reflux 2. Initially normal renal mass: sickle cell anemia, cyanotic congenital heart disease	++	The life-time incidence of postadaptive FSGS in these uncommon or rare conditions is probably relatively high, although precise incidence figures are not available
Moderate- or low-risk clinical setting: obesity, hypertension	+	These are common clinical conditions, for which the lifetime incidence of postadaptive FSGS is probably low; idiopathic FSGS may also occur in these individuals.
Nephrotic proteinuria without edema or hypoalbuminemia	+	This pattern is more common is postadaptive FSGS but also occurs in idiopathic FSGS[130]
Perihilar FSGS variant: at least one glomerular showing perihilar hyalinosis and perihilar hyalinosis and/or sclerosis involving > 50% glomeruli	++	Sensitivity and specificity remain to be determined
Glomerulomegaly (average glomerular diameter > 185 μm)	+++	Requires a sufficient number of glomeruli (probably 5–10), multiple levels (possibly 4), and measurement of glomeruli cut at or near hilus.[131]
Podocyte foot process effacement	+	There are significant group differences between idiopathic FSGS and postadaptive FSGS, but there is considerable overlap between the groups, so this has limited utility in a particular cases

When confronted with a renal biopsy specimen that shows FSGS, no history suggesting a genetic cause of FSGS (onset in childhood, family history of FSGS, extrarenal manifestations), and no use of FSGS-associated medication, the pathologist and clinician must weigh the likelihood of idiopathic FSGS versus postadaptive FSGS. Multiple features must be considered in making this distinction.
FSGS, focal segmental glomerulosclerosis.
Reprinted with permission from Schnaper HW, Robson AM, Kopp JB: Nephrotic syndrome: Minimal change nephropathy, focal segmental glomerulosclerosis, and collapsing glomerulopathy. In Schrier RW (ed): Diseases of the Kidney and Urinary Tract: Clinicopathologic Foundations of Medicine, 8th ed. Philadelphia: Lippincott Williams & Wilkins, 2006, pp 1585–1672.

it shares with diabetes mellitus. The mechanisms for these renal abnormalities are not well understood, but the relationship between metabolic syndrome and the risk of renal disease has been well established in recent years. Contributing factors likely include increased renal venous pressure, hyperlipidemia, and increased production of vasoactive and fibrogenic substances by adipocytes, including angiotensin II, insulin, leptin, and transforming growth factor β_1.

It remains unclear whether glomerulomegaly is a necessary precursor lesion to postadaptive FSGS and whether there is a specific genetic susceptibility to developing postadaptive FSGS, as most obese people do not develop glomerulopathy. Whether an individual threshold body mass index for the appearance of glomerulomegaly and FSGS exists is unknown. More research is required to understand the molecular pathways by which increased fat/muscle mass or body mass index lead to glomerular hyperfiltration.

Another differentiating pathologic feature of postadaptive FSGS from idiopathic FSGS is the extent of foot process effacement. Kambham and colleagues[11] found that obesity associated–glomerulopathy in the setting of a body mass index greater than 30 kg/m^2 has a mean foot process effacement of 40% (range, 10%–100%), whereas idiopathic FSGS patients have a mean foot process effacement of 75% (range, 30%–100%). Although there were significant differences in the group means for the extent of podocyte foot process effacement in idiopathic FSGS versus postadaptive FSGS, there was much overlap, so the utility of particular diagnostic criteria (such as podocyte foot process effacement > 50% in the former and < 50% in the latter) is limited.[12]

Another difference in renal histology is that the initial lesion in postadaptive FSGS is preferentially localized to the hilum. Rat models of FSGS that are characterized by increased transcapillary hydraulic pressure, for example, possibly emphasizing the susceptibility of podocytes to injury under increased vascular wall tension.[13,14] Although intriguing, the application of such knowledge is limited in clinical practice, given the difficulty of correctly identifying the location of the sclerosis in limited number of glomeruli. It remains to be determined whether the perihilar variant of idiopathic FSGS also arises as a consequence of glomerular overload from an unrecognized risk factor or biologic process.

Postadaptive FSGS may have a milder clinical course; in comparing obesity-related FSGS and idiopathic FSGS, Khambam and colleagues[11] reported that the patients with obesity-associated glomerulopathy had lower levels of proteinuria and a more indolent course (progression to ESRD 4% vs. 42%). By contrast, Praga and colleagues[15] found that the outcome in obesity-related disease was almost as poor as that of idiopathic FSGS. In this study, 80% of patients had nephrotic range proteinuria at presentation or on follow-up. The level of proteinuria correlated with the body mass index. Despite high proteinuria, hypoalbuminemia and edema were absent, unlike in patients with idiopathic FSGS. The final diagnosis of postadaptive FSGS will depend on carefully integrated data that reflect on medical history, comorbidities, family history, medication history, and the renal pathology.

Genetic Focal Segmental Glomerulosclerosis

One of the areas of intense research has focused on the podocytopathy that underlies FSGS. Investigations illustrating the gene mutations altering protein structure or function crucial to podocytes represented major progress (Table 20-3). The first of the recent discoveries began with the cloning of *NPHS1*, the gene that encodes nephrin and is mutated in congenital nephrotic syndrome.[16] Nephrin localizes to the slit diaphragm and plays a critical role in glomerular permselectivity. Mutations in *ACTN4*, the gene encoding α-actinin 4, an actinfilament cross-linking protein important for cytoskeletal function and highly expressed in the glomerular podocyte, cause an autosomal dominant form of FSGS.[17] Mutations in *NPHS2*, the gene encoding podocin that is an integral podocyte protein, causes autosomal recessive FSGS with early onset (age typically younger than 20 years) and rapid progression to ESRD.[18] Another example leading to defective slit diaphragm is deletion of CD2-associated protein; it leads to nephrotic proteinuria in mice and possibly humans.[19] Some mutations may lead to altered trafficking or intracellular retention of the abnormal proteins, suggesting that potential targets for future therapy include chaperones to ameliorate processing defects.[20] Recent studies suggest that approximately 20% of children with idiopathic FSGS have inherited defects in podocyte proteins that underlie their diseases.[21]

PATHOLOGY

The characteristic renal pathology of FSGS includes segmental areas of podocyte damage and detachment and solidification of glomerular capillaries associated with a marked local increase in collagen accumulation. In many cases, the scar contains areas of hyalinosis. Adhesions or synechiae to Bowman's capsule are common. The uninvolved portions of the glomeruli with segmental sclerosis and the remaining glomeruli in the biopsy are essentially normal.

Immunofluorescence typically shows deposits of IgM and C3 within the segmental scars and concentrated in the hyalinosis lesions. The major ultrastructural finding in nonsclerotic glomerular capillaries is foot process effacement, which varies from mild to severe. In general, the degree of fusion correlates with the severity of proteinuria.

D'Agati and colleagues[22] have proposed a working classification (the Columbia classification) for idiopathic FSGS that comprises five categories: collapsing variant, tip lesion, cellular lesion, perihilar variant, plus a final category for those cases that do not have the diagnostic criteria for the other categories, not otherwise specified, corresponding to classic FSGS. These distinctive pathologic subtypes of FSGS may represent differences in pathogenesis. Collapsing FSGS is a form of FSGS that has been associated with viral infections, notably human immunodeficiency virus, and follows a particularly aggressive course. Patients with the collapsing variant of idiopathic FSGS have a strikingly poor renal survival, with 70% probability of ESRD at 2 years.[23] Because the collapsing variant significantly differs histologically and clinically from other variants, some investigators argue that collapsing glomerulopathy (CG) should be a separate entity from FSGS altogether.[8]

CLINICAL PRESENTATION AND COURSE

The presenting feature in all patients with FSGS is proteinuria, frequently resulting in the nephrotic syndrome, although many patients, particularly adults, may present with nonnephrotic

Table 20-3 Genetic Causes of Human Podocyte Diseases

Gene	Gene Product	Inheritance Chromosome	Function	Renal Syndrome	Prevalence	Extrarenal Findings
NPHS1	Nephrin	AR 19q13.1	Slit-diaphragm complex	Congenital nephrotic syndrome, infantile onset FSGS	Insufficient data	None
NPHS2	Podocin	AR 1q25-31	Slit-diaphragm complex	FSGS onset < 20 yr	Up to 20% of familial or sporadic pediatric FSGS	None
CD2AP	CD2-associated protein	AD 6	Slit-diaphragm complex	FSGS onset > 20 yr	2 reported cases, 1 with family history	None
ACTN4	α-actinin-4	AD 19q13	Cytoskeleton	FSGS onset > 20 yr	3 reported families	None
TRPC6	Transient receptor, cationic, 6	AD 11q21-q22	Channel	FSGS onset > 20 yr	1 reported family	None
PLCE1	Phospholipase Cε	10q23	Signaling protein	DMS or FSGS, onset age ≤4 yr	7 reported families	None
WT1	Wilms' tumor-1	AD 11p13	Transcription factor	DMS or less commonly FSGS (Denys-Drash syndrome), FSGS (Frasier syndrome)	Uncommon	Wilms' tumor, gonadal abnormalities
ITGB4	β1 integrin	AR 17q11-qter	Matrix protein receptor	Congenital FSGS	Uncommon	Epidermolysis bullosa, pyloric atresia
LAMB2	Laminin beta 2	AR 3p21	Basement membrane component	Congenital mesangial sclerosis	5 reported cases	Ophthalmic defects (Pierson syndrome)
PAX2	Pax2 homeobox protein	AR 10q24.3-25.1	Transcription factor	Renal dysplasia, oligomeganephronia		Ophthalmic defects (coloboma)
mtDNA	Mitochondrial tRNA^{leu}	Maternal	Protein synthesis	FSGS	>40 reported cases	MELAS syndrome, diabetes mellitus, cardiomyopathy
Galloway-Mowat syndrome	Unknown	AR	Unknown	DMS or FSGS, congenital, infancy, or early childhood		Microcephaly, hypotonia
Action myoclonus–renal failure syndrome	Unknown	AR	Unknown	Collapsing glomerulopathy, onset 9-30 yr	9 families	Myoclonus, seizures

AD, autosomal dominant; AR, autosomal recessive; DMS, diffuse mesangial sclerosis; FSGS, focal segmental glomerulosclerosis; MELAS syndrome, myocardial myopathy, encephalopathy, lactic acidosis, and strokelike episodes.
Reprinted with permission from Schnaper HW, Robson AM, Kopp JB: Nephrotic syndrome: Minimal change nephropathy, focal segmental glomerulosclerosis, and collapsing glomerulopathy. In Schrier RW (ed): Diseases of the Kidney and Urinary Tract: Clinicopathologic Foundations of Medicine, 8th ed. Philadelphia: Lippincott Williams & Wilkins, 2006, pp 1585–1672.

range proteinuria (<3.5 g/day). In addition, microscopic hematuria, hypertension, and renal insufficiency are common presenting features.

The clinical course and prognosis of FSGS patients are influenced by their presenting features, the histologic characteristics, and response to the therapy. The presence of nephrotic range proteinuria (>3.5 g/day) has been consistently associated with poor outcome, with 50% of patients reaching ESRD within 6 to 8 years (Table 20-4).[24] Massive proteinuria (>10 g/day) is predictive of even worse outcome, with the possibility of reaching ESRD within 3 years of the diagnosis.[25,26] In contrast, nonnephrotic patients tend to have more favorable prognosis, with renal survival of greater than 80% after 10 years. Additional clinical features of prognostic significance include serum creatinine at presentation and race. Patients presenting with serum creatinine greater than 1.3 mg/dL have significantly higher risk of renal demise, irrespective of the degree of proteinuria.[24,27] Some investigators have also noted that black race portends a poorer prognosis with more rapid decline toward ESRD.[6] Others argue that there is no racial difference in renal survival when the analysis is restricted only to nephrotic patients.[28]

Another important predictor of renal outcome is the response to therapy. A retrospective study evaluating a long-term outcome in both children and adults suggested that the achievement of complete remission is the most significant factor determining the clinical course; in both age groups, those with complete remission had a renal survival rate of 100% at 10 years.[29] Those without a complete remission generally progressed with a 10-year renal survival rate of 62% in adults and 58% in children. Achievement of partial remission and its maintenance are also important, with implications for both slowing the progression rate and improving renal survival.[30]

The prognostic importance of histology in FSGS has also been extensively studied.[23,31-33] The degree of interstitial fibrosis (≥20%) has been demonstrated consistently to predict poor renal outcome. In addition, the presence of diffuse mesangial hypercellularity has been associated with more rapid decline of renal function, but this relationship has not been uniformly confirmed in larger studies. The distinct pathologic variants of FSGS, as described by D'Agati,[12] have also been studied to explain the variable clinical course. Among the five pathologic variants of idiopathic FSGS (collapsing, cellular, glomerular tip lesion, perihilar, and not otherwise specified), collapsing FSGS has the highest rate of renal insufficiency at presentation with chronic tubulointerstitial disease, fewest remissions, and highest rate of ESRD.[23,33] In contrast, patients with tip lesion FSGS tend to be older and have the highest remission rate and lowest rate of ESRD. Retrospective analysis has revealed that cellular FSGS also portends poorer prognosis.[31] Patients with the cellular lesion are more often black and severely proteinuric and appear to have higher risk of progressing to ESRD, with poor response to treatment.

Table 20-4 Long-Term Outcome in Focal Segmental Glomerulosclerosis

Location, Year	Population	Average Observation (yr)	Complete Remission (%)	Persistent Renal Abnormalities (%)	CKD (%)	ESRD (%)	Nonrenal Death (%)	Lost to Follow-up (%)	Ref.
London, 1978	12 children, 28 adults	9.5	10	18	20	50	2	0	132
Quebec, 1981	32 children	8	24	40	4	20	12	0	133
Southwest United States, 1985	75 children	4.8	11	37	23	21	0	8	134
Hong Kong, 1991	2 children, 30 adults	6.8	9			16			135
Ontario, Canada, 1998	38 children, 55 adults	11	42	13	11	34	0	0	136
			22	24	13	42	(4)		
Christchurch, New Zealand, 2000	165 adults	6.9	29	8	16	44			46

All reports that included at least 30 patients provided group outcomes after an average duration of more than 4 years. Most patients appear to have had idiopathic focal segmental glomerulosclerosis (FSGS), but some reports included a limited number of postadaptive FSGS or focal global glomerulosclerosis. Children are defined as individuals younger than 15 to 18 years at the time of initial presentation, depending on reference. When data are presented for children and adults separately, the data for children are presented first. Chronic kidney disease (CKD) is defined as an impaired glomerular filtration rate. The proportion of patients experiencing nonrenal deaths is shown in parentheses when these patients are also included in another category. Empty cells indicate that no data were provided from the report.
Reprinted with permission from Schnaper HW, Robson AM, Kopp JB: Nephrotic syndrome: Minimal change nephropathy, focal segmental glomerulosclerosis, and collapsing glomerulopathy. In Schrier RW (ed): Diseases of the Kidney and Urinary Tract: Clinicopathologic Foundations of Medicine, 8th ed. Philadelphia: Lippincott Williams & Wilkins, 2006, pp 1585–1672.

The ability to accurately delineate the prognostic significance of these pathologic variants of idiopathic FSGS will require careful analysis of long-term data of large numbers of patients. The multivariate analyses of all the clinical and histologic features of FSGS suggest that only the achievement of a remission in proteinuria is the independently significant predictor of ESRD. Improving our understanding of the pathophysiology and developing more effective therapy, therefore, is critical to reduce the profound morbidity associated with FSGS.

TREATMENT OF FOCAL SEGMENTAL GLOMERULOSCLEROSIS: BACKGROUND

The goal of treatment of all podocyte diseases is to reduce proteinuria to normal or to the lowest level possible. Regardless of the choice of immunosuppressive therapy, angiotensin-converting enzyme (ACE) inhibitors and angiotensin receptor blockers, given their antiproteinuric and antifibrotic effects, are important components of the treatment of FSGS. Hyperlipidemia and hypertension should also be aggressively treated in nephrotic patients. The following section focuses on the efficacy of immunosuppressive agents.

Initial Therapy of Idiopathic Focal Segmental Glomerulosclerosis

Glucocorticoids

Glucocorticoids remain the main therapeutic agent in nephrotic FSGS, as for MCN. Because children undergo renal biopsy only if they have not responded to glucocorticoids, they may be considered steroid resistant by the time they are diagnosed as having FSGS. Compared with the response rates in MCN, the initial response to conventional doses of glucocorticoid therapy for idiopathic FSGS is poor. The initial treatment for primary FSGS in children has followed the regimen outlined for the treatment of primary nephrotic syndrome by the International Study of Kidney Disease in Children. This consists of prednisone 60 mg/m^2/day (up to 80 mg/day) for 4 to 6 weeks, followed by 40 mg/m^2/day (up to 60 mg/day) every other day for an additional 4 to 6 weeks, and then discontinued.[2] Although this regimen has been found to be satisfactory for the treatment of children with the highly steroid-sensitive lesion of minimal change glomerulopathy, the data suggest that it may be inadequate for those with primary FSGS.

Although pediatric studies of MCN have suggested that longer durations and higher doses of glucocorticoids result in significant decrease in the relapse rate,[34–40] the optimal duration of steroid therapy is not known. Retrospective studies of FSGS have suggested that treatment beyond 6 months does not appear to be beneficial.[29,41] The best predictor of long-term prognosis remains complete remission because the 15-year renal survival rate in both children and adults with complete remission was 100% compared with 51% in those who remain unresponsive.[29] Half of the unresponsive patients had doubled their serum creatinine by 4 years. Based on these data, experts recommend that nephrotic children with idiopathic FSGS be treated with glucocorticoids for up to 6 months. The overall duration of the initial prednisone dose and rapidity of the steroid taper depend on whether and how quickly a complete or partial remission is attained.

Korbet and colleagues,[41–44] who have analyzed the efficacy of steroid therapy in adults with FSGS, have noted that the highest complete remission rates (>30%) were observed in cases treated for longer than 5 months and the lowest rates (≤20%) in patients treated for 2 months or less. Table 20-5 summarizes the results of uncontrolled clinical trials evaluating the efficacy of glucocorticoid therapy in FSGS.[28,29,45–51] These trials include different durations of glucocorticoid therapy, and the overall response rate is typically less than 50%. Importantly, relapse rates are high, from 38% to 67%, although some of these patients may be brought to a second remission by additional glucocorticoid therapy or other therapies.

Because of the possibility of a delayed response, corticosteroid treatment must be sufficiently long. Among nephrotic adult patients with FSGS, approximately 30% may enter complete remission after a course of daily prednisone given at a dose of 1 mg/kg/day for at least 4 months.[44] Given the comorbidities associated with long-term high-dose prednisone therapy, many providers start a slow taper of prednisone after 8 to 12 weeks. Patients who are refractory to steroid therapy tend to have a significant risk of progression to ESRD. Many FSGS patients thus require cytotoxic agents or calcineurin inhibitors to either decrease steroid use or achieve remission.

Mechanisms of Glucocorticoid Efficacy

Glucocorticoids exert potent anti-inflammatory effects on leukocytes and inhibit expression of cytokines and adhesion molecules. Their effectiveness in a noninflammatory disease such as MCN or FSGS is thus difficult to understand. Given the recently discovered significance of the podocyte biology in the pathogenesis of nephrotic syndrome, multiple studies have investigated whether the therapeutic mechanism of glucocorticoids may be through a direct protective effect on podocytes. Using immortalized human podocytes, Xing and colleagues[52] demonstrated that dexamethasone enhanced and accelerated podocyte maturation, with an especially striking effect on up-regulating expression of nephrin. Nephrin, a podocyte protein that plays a key role in regulating signaling pathways, is a critical component of the slit diaphragm regulating glomerular permselectivity. Dexamethasone also down-regulates cyclin kinase inhibitors, augmenting podocyte survival. In addition, dexamethasone treatment led to the down-regulation of vascular endothelial growth factor, which is normally produced by podocytes but is up-regulated in patients with MCN. Other studies have also suggested similar protective effects of glucocorticoids on podocytes to enhance recovery. Dexamethasone has been shown to increase intracellular levels of adenosine 5′ triphosphate through up-regulation of mitochondrial genes, thereby allowing proper glycosylation of nephrin.[53] Other possible therapeutic mechanisms of glucocorticoids include enhancing recovery of podocytes via actin filament stabilization and preventing podocyte apoptosis.[54,55] Therefore, the therapeutic effects of corticosteroids may stem from their direct action on podocytes to promote repair and survival rather than on their immunosuppressive effect. It is possible that the benefit seen with other immunosuppressive agents may also be explained by their direct action on podocyte physiology.

Treatment of Steroid-Refractory or Steroid-Resistant Patients

Cytotoxic Agents

The rationale for using alkylating agents, as with the use of other immunosuppressive agents, is based on the hypothesis that FSGS is a T cell–driven immunologic disease and on empirical data on response. The most common indication for cytotoxic agents such as cyclophosphamide or chlorambucil is steroid dependence. Steroid resistance, in contrast, is highly predictive of resistance to alkylating agents, particularly in adults. Although alkylating agents may yield complete remission in 51% of steroid-sensitive children, they may be effective in only approximately 17% of children who are steroid resistant.[44]

In a randomized, controlled trial involving 60 steroid-resistant FSGS children, the efficacy of prednisone, dosed at 40 mg/m^2 on alternate days for a period of 12 months, and the same prednisone regimen plus a 90-day course of daily cyclophosphamide dosed at 2.5 mg/kg were compared.[56] In both groups, 25% of the children had complete resolution of proteinuria, but those who were treated with cyclophosphamide were 1.6 times more likely to experience a decrease in renal function, suggesting that cyclophosphamide therapy for children with steroid-resistant FSGS may be potentially harmful.

In contrast, there are multiple uncontrolled studies reporting variably beneficial effects of cyclophosphamide in steroid-resistant pediatric patients, with the rate of complete remission ranging from 22% to 66%.[57-59] A recent retrospective study with a follow-up period of more than 10 years suggested that cyclophosphamide leads to complete remission in 43% of steroid-resistant children.[60] The mean duration to enter complete remission was 46 days (range, 8–78 days). More than 60% of the patients who achieved complete remission, however, suffered relapses requiring further immunosuppressive therapy with chlorambucil, vincristine, cyclosporine, or a second course of cyclophosphamide.

Considering the paucity of data from controlled trials and the long-term toxicity, cytotoxic agents are considered mostly inefficient and possibly hazardous in FSGS patients with steroid resistance. The efficacy of alkylating agents, however, may partly depend on certain host factors. In a recent South African retrospective analysis of 223 children, the authors noted that a majority of steroid-resistant Indian children treated with prednisone and cyclophosphamide achieved complete remission, whereas only a minority of steroid-resistant black children responded to the same combination.[61] It is unclear whether the difference in the response truly reflects inherent host differences such as race or uncontrolled biases in a retrospective study design. The data regarding efficacy of alkylating agents stem mostly from uncontrolled studies or retrospective analysis, making it difficult to draw firm conclusions. Nonetheless, cytotoxic agents may be an option for some steroid-resistant nephrotic patients who have otherwise exhausted other options or have contraindications to other medications.

Calcineurin Inhibitors

The generally accepted therapy for patients with steroid-resistant FSGS at the present time is cyclosporine in both children and adults. In a randomized, double-blind, placebo-controlled trial in steroid-resistant children, cyclosporine therapy for 6 months led to 76% decrease in proteinuria compared with no change in the placebo group.[62] Another pediatric prospective, randomized study also suggested that cyclosporine is more effective in decreasing proteinuria compared with chlorambucil, with nearly all patients achieving a decrease in proteinuria with complete remission in 23% of the cohort.[63] In one retrospective study, cyclosporine led to remissions in 40% of steroid-resistant patients.[60]

A randomized, controlled trial demonstrated that cyclosporine is also efficacious in inducing remission in steroid-resistant adult FSGS patients. Cattran and colleagues[64] compared cyclosporine treatment plus low-dose prednisone with placebo plus prednisone and monitored the patients for a mean of 4.2 years. By 26 weeks, 69% (12% complete and 57% partial) of the treatment group versus 4% of the placebo group achieved remission of their proteinuria. Relapses were common, however, occurring in 40% of those who had achieved remission by 1 year and 60% by 18 months. Despite this high relapse rate, renal function was better preserved in the cyclosporine group; the patients treated with cyclosporine were half as likely to experience 50% decrease in their creatinine clearance from baseline. These results suggest that cyclosporine is an effective therapeutic agent in the treatment of steroid-resistant cases of FSGS. In the pediatric literature, limited data also suggest that a combination of steroids and cyclosporine improves the chance of complete remission from 14% with cyclosporine monotherapy to 24% with the combination.[65]

There is more limited experience with tacrolimus in steroid-resistant FSGS patients. In an uncontrolled, prospective trial involving steroid-dependent and steroid-resistant FSGS patients, tacrolimus therapy led to an overall response rate of 90%, with 50% of the patients achieving complete remission and 40% of the patients achieving partial remission.[66] Tacrolimus therapy was, however, associated with small increases in blood glucose, systolic blood pressure, and serum creatinine. Furthermore, as seen with cyclosporine, there was a relapse of nephrotic syndrome in 80% of patients.

Despite recent reports of encouraging short-term success in induction of remission in steroid-resistant FSGS, long-term use of calcineurin inhibitors is associated with nephrotoxicity, progressive interstitial fibrosis, and glomerulosclerosis even in patients who remain in partial remission.[67] Given their additional adverse effects on metabolic profile and blood pressure, it is difficult to assess whether calcineurin inhibitors improve long-term renal survival. Attempts have been made to introduce newer therapies to treat steroid-resistant FSGS, including mycophenolate mofetil (MMF) and sirolimus.

Mycophenolate Mofetil

After the successful use of MMF in the treatment of lupus nephritis, there has been a growing interest in using this agent to treat other proteinuric glomerular disorders. Several small and uncontrolled trials suggest that MMF may be beneficial in patients with FSGS. Choi and colleagues[68] reported that MMF can facilitate steroid withdrawal in otherwise steroid-dependent MCN patients and significantly decrease proteinuria in FSGS patients. A recent prospective study evaluated the efficacy of MMF to induce remission in nephrotic patients who are both steroid and cyclosporine dependent or resistant.[69] After 6 months of MMF therapy, steroid sparing was achieved in 71% of steroid-dependent patients and 42% remained in remission. In steroid-resistant patients, 20% achieved complete

Table 20-5 Clinical Trials of Glucocorticoid Therapy for Adults with Focal Segmental Glomerulosclerosis: Regimen, Remission, Relapse, and Long-Term Outcome

First Author, Location, Year	Design	No. of Patients	Black Subjects (%)	Duration of Therapy
Agarwal, India, 1993	Prospective	65 children, adults (23 lost)	0	High-dose 8-12 wk, taper to 6 mo
Rydel, Illinois, 1995	Retrospective	30 adults	63	High-dose 4-8 wk, total therapy mean, 5 mo
Cattran, Ontario, 1998	Retrospective	18 adults	0	Median, 5 mo; range, 2–50
Ponticelli, Italy, 1999	Retrospective	53 adults	0	A) mean, 24 wk; B) mean, 19 wk
Chitalia, New Zealand, 1999	Retrospective	28	28	High-dose 6–8 wk to 12 wk
Stiles, Washington, DC, 2001	Retrospective	12	83	Mean, 4 mo
Pokhariyal, Lucknow, India, 2003	Retrospective	83 (12 lost)	0	Mean, 3 mo
Franceschini, North Carolina, 2003	Retrospective	36 adults	31	Daily or alternate days for mean of 9 mo
Smith, Bethesda, MD, 2003	Prospective	14 adults	50	Pulse oral dexamethasone for 8 mo

The results of nine uncontrolled studies are summarized. The number of patients treated with glucocorticoids in each study in shown (No). The study of Agarwal et al.[45] included children and adults; the other studies only included adults or, alternatively, only the data from adults are included here. All studies except the study of Cattran et al.[29] stated that one or more forms of postadaptive focal segmental glomerulosclerosis and human immunodefiency virus-type 1–associated nephropathy were excluded. The duration of high-dose glucocorticoid therapy (generally prednisolone or prednisone 1 mg/kg/day) is shown. In the study of Ponticelli et al,[49] patients received either regimen A, prednisone 1 mg/kg/day for 8 weeks, followed by a taper to a mean of 24 weeks, or regimen B, three doses of intravenous methylprednisolone, followed by prednisolone 0.5 mg/kg/day for 8 weeks, and then a taper to a mean of 19 weeks. The definitions of complete remission and

remission. Withdrawal of MMF, however, resulted in immediate relapse in 47%.

MMF may also be used as an adjunctive therapy in those who are resistant to steroids or cyclosporine or to maintain longer remission in those who relapse frequently.[70] In another prospective pediatric study including steroid-dependent MCN and FSGS, MMF therapy led to 70% reduction in relapse rate (from 6.6 to two episodes per year) after 1 year.[71] After discontinuation of MMF treatment, however, 68% of patients had an increased frequency of relapses and recurrence of steroid dependence, requiring treatment with other medications. Long-term therapy with MMF, therefore, may result in significant steroid sparing and a decrease in relapse rates in patients with steroid dependence or in those who are unresponsive to other immunosuppressive therapies, with a response similar to that to cyclosporine. The data, however, are based on small, uncontrolled trials, and further systematic studies are necessary to better understand the indications and efficacy of MMF in the treatment of FSGS. Furthermore, the available current data do not allow direct comparisons of short- and long-term efficacy and safety between MMF and other treatment options.

Sirolimus

Sirolimus, approved for use in organ transplantation by the U.S. Food and Drug Administration in 1999, has antiproliferative and immunosuppressive effects that may be beneficial in FSGS. Sirolimus blocks mesangial, endothelial, and vascular smooth muscle cell proliferation.[72–74] Sirolimus also reduces expression of fibrosis-associated genes in the renal ischemia reperfusion injury model[75] and exerts antifibrotic effects in an experimental model of hepatic fibrosis.[76] Furthermore, preclinical studies and early transplantation literature suggested that sirolimus may lack nephrotoxicity, unlike calcineurin inhibitors.

To determine the efficacy of sirolimus in decreasing proteinuria, Tumlin and colleagues[77] conducted a prospective, open-label trial of 21 patients with idiopathic, steroid-resistant FSGS. After 6 months of therapy, sirolimus induced complete remission in 19% and partial remission in 38%. The GFR was maintained only among the responders, whereas the nonresponders had a mean decrease in the GFR of 3 mL/min/1.73 m^2 during the 6 months.

This favorable effect of sirolimus, however, was not confirmed in two other clinical studies, neither of which was controlled. Fervenza and colleagues[78] evaluated the safety

COMPLETE REMISSION		PARTIAL REMISSION		Complete + Partial Remission (%)	Relapse	Follow-up Status	Ref.
Definition	%	Definition	%				
<0.3 g/day	18	2 g/day	15	33	ND	ESRD: 5% (34 mo)	45
<0.25 g/day	33	<2.5 g/day	17	50	From CR or PR: 67%	CR: 30%, PR: 16%, ESRD: 20% (79 mo)	28
<0.2 g/day	44	ND	ND	ND	From CR: 38%	CR: 44%, CKD/ES RD: 50% (155 mo)	29
<0.2 g/day	40	<2 g/day	19	59	From CR or PR: 55%	ND	49
<0.3 g/day	21	ND	ND	ND	ND	ND	46
<0.2 g/day	0	<3 g/day	42	42	ND	ND	51
<0.3 g/day	25	<2 g/day or 50% decrease if subnephrotic	25	50	ND	ND	48
<0.6 g/day	ND	ND	ND	ND	ND	CR: 11% ESRD: 18% (18 mo)	47
<0.3 g/day	7	<2 g/day	29	36	From CR or PR: 60%	CR: 7%, PR: 14% (20 mo)	50

partial remission are shown. The percentage of subjects in CR is derived from each study; for the study of Agarwal et al.,[45] 23 patients were lost, without endpoint determination, and the calculation of outcome was made here on an intent-to-treat basis (rather than as follow-up). The mean duration of follow-up is shown and the percentage of patients in remission are shown. CKD, chronic kidney disease; ESRD, end-stage renal disease; ND, no data provided.
Reprinted with permission from Schnaper HW, Robson AM, Kopp JB: Nephrotic syndrome: Minimal change nephropathy, focal segmental glomerulosclerosis, and collapsing glomerulopathy. In Schrier RW (ed): Disease of the Kidney and Urinary Tract: Clinicopathologic Foundations of Medicine, 8th ed. Philadelphia: Lippincott Williams & Wilkins, 2006, pp 1585–1672.

and efficacy of sirolimus in treating patients with primary glomerular diseases, including FSGS. Of the 11 patients, 6 developed acute renal failure within 6 weeks of starting sirolimus, with improvement after stopping sirolimus. One patient recovered renal function after discontinuation of the drug but again deteriorated with rechallenge, further strengthening the causal relationship between sirolimus and acute renal failure. In a prospective, open-label study by Cho and colleagues,[79] sirolimus therapy was associated with precipitous fall in GFR in five of six steroid-resistant FSGS patients. In three patients, a decrease in the GFR was also associated with more than a twofold increase in proteinuria, raising concerns that sirolimus may be harmful in some patients with long-standing FSGS.

The discrepancies among the studies may partly reflect differences in study populations. The mechanism underlying sirolimus nephrotoxicity is not clear but appears to involve direct tubular injury. In pathologic conditions characterized by ischemic or chronic tubular injury such as delayed graft function or long-term calcineurin-inhibitor therapy, hindrance of tubular regeneration by sirolimus may severely impair renal recovery. Future studies may help

define the role of sirolimus in glomerular disease and provide better understanding of the risk factors for sirolimus nephrotoxicity.

Other Treatment Considerations

Aggressive control of blood pressure (mean arterial pressure of ≤ 92 mm Hg or ≤ 130/80 mm Hg) and the use of ACE inhibitors have been shown to decrease proteinuria and the rate of decrease in the GFR by as much as 50% in patients with primary glomerulopathies, including FSGS.[80–82] In addition, combining ACE inhibitors with angiotensin receptor blockers may safely slow the progression of nondiabetic renal disease compared with monotherapy.[83]

While blood pressure control and angiotensin antagonists are beneficial in decreasing proteinuria and progression of renal disease, they rarely lead to remission of nephrotic syndrome.[81] Therefore, there is an urgent need for development of more effective therapy options for treating patients with FSGS. The potential future options for treatment of fibrotic renal diseases are listed in Table 20-6. Agents that block fibrotic pathways or mitigate profibrotic

Table 20-6   Potential Novel Therapies for Progressive Glomerulosclerosis

Class	Agent	Molecular Target or Pathway	Animal Model	Ref.	Proteinuria	Matrix	Human Use
Small molecules	Bosentan	ET_A, ET_B receptor antagonist	Ren-2 transgenic rats	137	Reduced	Reduced	Approved
	Darusentan	ET_A receptor antagonist	Puromycin (rate)	138	Reduced	Reduced	IND
	Thiazolidine-diones	PPAR-γ agonist	Remnant nephron (rat)	139	Reduced	ND	Approved
	Eplerenone	Mineralocorticoid-receptor	Uninephrectomy plus NaCl (rat)	140	Reduced	Reduced	Approved
	Isotretinoin	Retinoid acid receptor	Thy-1 nephritis (rat)	141	Reduced	Reduced	Approved
	Gefitinib	EGF-receptor tyrosine kinase inhibitor	L-NAME–induced hypertension (rat)	142	Reduced	Reduced	Approved
	Pirfenidone	TGF-β expression? TNF signaling?	Remnant nephron, KIST mouse	143	Reduced	Reduced	IND
	Tranilast	TGF-β antagonist	Remnant nephron	144	Reduced	Reduced	IND
	AVE 7688	ACE and NEP inhibitor	Remnant nephron	145	Reduced	Reduced	Preclinical
	CDK inhibitors	Cell cycle	HIV-transgenic mouse	146	Reduced	Reduced	Preclinical
	Fasudil	Rho-kinase inhibitor	Dahl rat	147	Reduced	Reduced	Preclinical
	Prolyl hydroxylase inhibitors	Collagen cross-linking	Chronic allograft nephropathy (mouse)	148	ND	Reduced	Preclinical
Peptides	BX471	CCR1 antagonist	Adriamycin	149	No effect	Reduced	Preclinical
	IFN-γ	Fibroblasts	Remnant nephron	150	Reduced	Reduced	Approved
	Bone morphogenetic protein 7	Possible TGF-β antagonist	COL4A3 null mutation mouse	151	Reduced	Reduced	IND
	Hepatocyte growth factor	Possible TGF-β antagonist	ICGN mouse	152	Reduced	Reduced	Preclinical
	Relaxin	Not defined	Remnant nephron (rat)	153	ND	Reduced	Preclinical
	Decorin (proteoglycan)	Binds TGF-β	Thy-1 nephritis	154			
Monoclonal antibodies and others	Etanercept, infliximab	Binds TNF-α	No data	ND			Approved
	Anti-TGF-β	Binds TGF-β	Puromycin	155	ND	Reduced	IND
	Sulodexide (GAG)	Unknown	No data	ND			IND

"Approved" denotes approved by the U.S. Food and Drug Administration (FDA) for a nonrenal indication. "IND" denotes under study for any indication under the Investigational New Drug process of the FDA.

ACE, angiotensin-converting enzyme; CCR1, chemokine receptor; CDK, cyclin-dependent kinase; EGF, endothelial growth factor; ET, endothelin; GAG, glycoscaminoglycan; IFN-γ, interferon gamma; L-NAME, NG-nitro-L-arginine methylester; ND, not determined; PPAR, peroxisome proliferator-activated receptor; TGF, transforming growth factor; TNF, tumor necrosis factor.

effects of various cytokines may serve an important role. Pirfendione, for example, is a potent inhibitor of transforming growth factor β, and a small pilot study has suggested that it may slow the decrease in the GFR in FSGS patients.[84] The safety and efficacy of various antifibrotic agents will need to be defined through controlled clinical trials in the future. Currently, a prospective, randomized, open-label trial sponsored by the National Institutes of Health is ongoing to compare two treatment regimens in children and adults with steroid-resistant FSGS: cyclosporine versus the combination of MMF and dexamethasone over 52 weeks. The treatment regimens in both arms also include ACE inhibitor therapy and alternate-day low-dose prednisone. The results are expected within the next year.

Treatment of Postadaptive Focal Segmental Glomerulosclerosis

ACE inhibitors and angiotensin receptor blockers are important in treating postadaptive FSGS. Praga and colleagues[81] showed that captopril therapy over 12 months decreased proteinuria to a greater extent in postadaptive FSGS (associated with decreased nephron mass and reflux nephropathy) compared with idiopathic FSGS. In addition, Praga and colleagues[85] studied 17 patients with obesity-associated proteinuria with more than 1 g/day. Captopril therapy in eight patients decreased proteinuria by 79% (mean, 3.4 g/day decreasing to 0.7 g/day); interestingly, weight loss in nine patients (mean body mass index decreasing from 37 kg/m^2 to 33 kg/m^2) was associated with a similar decrease in proteinuria by 86%. It is, however, unclear whether the decrease in proteinuria with angiotensin antagonist therapy can be maintained.[15] Early treatment with ACE inhibitors appears to preserve renal function in obesity-associated FSGS, although appropriate controls are lacking. When the diagnosis of postadaptive FSGS is not clear and/or patients are significantly symptomatic from nephrotic proteinuria, the therapeutic approach for idiopathic FSGS is generally applied.

CURRENT THERAPEUTIC RECOMMENDATIONS

Idiopathic Focal Segmental Glomerulosclerosis

The available data suggest that the initial therapy for idiopathic FSGS, unless there are significant contraindications, should be glucocorticoids at 1 mg/kg/day (maximum 80 mg/day) or 2 mg/kg every other day (maximum 120 mg/kg every other day) (Fig. 20-1). Glucocorticoids should be administered long enough to avoid a premature diagnosis of steroid resistance. Many experts recommend a decrease in dose after 2 to 4 months, particularly for those who have not shown a significant decrease in urine protein. Those who do not respond to 16 weeks of glucocorticoid therapy are then diagnosed with steroid resistance and progress to other therapies. Ultimately, the duration of the initial prednisone dose and rapidity of the steroid taper will depend on whether and how rapidly a complete or partial remission is attained.

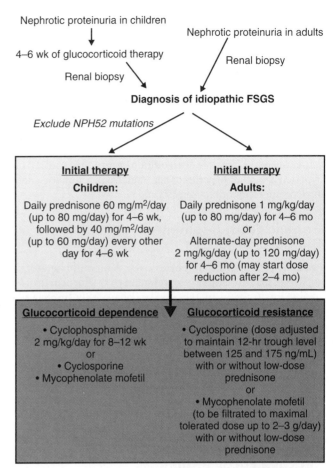

Figure 20-1 Therapy of idiopathic focal segmental glomerulosclerosis (FSGS) in children and adults. The selection of initial therapy and subsequent therapies is shown. The diagnosis of genetic FSGS, postadaptive FSGS, and adaptive FSGS should be considered, in which case therapeutic recommendations will differ (see text). Patients with persistent proteinuria are typically started on angiotensin-converting enzyme inhibitors or angiotensin receptor blockers before, during, or after the first course of glucocorticoids. The dose and duration of glucocorticoid therapy must be modified based on patient factors including age, obesity, diabetes, osteoporosis, and other conditions.

For those who are steroid responsive but become steroid dependent or steroid resistant, cyclosporine should be tried, either as a monotherapy or in addition to a low-dose prednisone (0.15 mg/kg, maximum 15 mg/day). The typical starting dose of cyclosporine is 3 to 4 mg/kg/day given in two divided doses and is generally continued for at least 6 months after attaining complete remission. Some patients require long-term therapy with a low dose (2–3 mg/kg) of cyclosporine to maintain the remission. The utility of calcineurin inhibitors in patients with a GFR less than 40 mL/min/1.73 m^2, significant renal vasculopathy, or significant tubulointerstitial fibrosis is unclear, given the concern for the nephrotoxicity of these agents. While there are fewer data to suggest efficacy of other immunosuppressive agents, these may be considered, particularly in patients who have contraindications to prednisone or cyclosporine. Patients with frequently relapsing or steroid-dependent FSGS may also receive some benefit from cyclophosphamide. Until more data are available, it is difficult to recommend the use of sirolimus for the treatment of FSGS at this time.

Postadaptive Focal Segmental Glomerulosclerosis

Immunosuppressive therapy is generally contraindicated. The therapeutic approach is focused on treating the underlying cause whenever possible. In addition, aggressive control of hypertension and hyperlipidemia, and ACE inhibitors and angiotensin receptor blockers, should be used.

Genetic Focal Segmental Glomerulosclerosis

Pediatric patients with homozygous or compound heterozygous *NPHS2* mutations are refractory to glucocorticoids (defined as 6 weeks of therapy) and have only limited responsiveness to cyclosporine.[86] By contrast, *NPHS2* homozygous and compound heterozygous mutations were absent in 124 children with steroid-sensitive nephrotic syndrome. Immunosuppressive treatment is thus of limited benefit in children with *NPHS2* homozygous and compound heterozygous mutations. It would also likely be prudent to withhold aggressive immunosuppression, particularly glucocorticoids, in patients with *ACTN4*, *CD2AP*, *TRPC6*, and mitochondrial DNA mutations.

Reactive Focal Segmental Glomerulosclerosis

FSGS associated with medication is probably best managed by withdrawing the implicated medication and instituting conservative therapy.

Limitations

Currently, there are no clinical characteristics that can reliably predict the response to a given therapy. Furthermore, there are no published data to determine the balance between the risks and benefits of immunosuppressive therapy in many patient subgroups. Examples include patients with subnephrotic proteinuria at presentation, especially those with proteinuria less than 2 g/day, patients with postadaptive FSGS, and those with idiopathic FSGS who are at significantly increased risk of toxicity associated with glucocorticoid therapy, including those with obesity, diabetes mellitus, severe osteoporosis, or advanced age.

RECURRENT FOCAL SEGMENTAL GLOMERULOSCLEROSIS

In 1972, Hoyer and colleagues[87] published the first report of a rapid recurrence of idiopathic nephrotic syndrome in three patients after renal transplantation. It is now well established that 15% to 50% of patients with FSGS undergoing renal transplantation have a recurrence of the disease, with the average rate of 25% to 30%. The clinical course and outcome have been well documented in both pediatric and adult patients.[88,89]

In a retrospective study analyzing recipients of 78 allografts over a 10-year period, FSGS recurred in approximately 30% of allografts within a mean of 7.5 months (range, 0.5–44 months) after transplantation.[88] Once the diagnosis was made, ESRD eventually developed in 56% of the allografts within an average of 23.7 months (range, 1–65 months). For those who lost their first allograft to recurrent FSGS, the study suggested an even higher risk of a second recurrence of 80%. Risk factors associated with the recurrence of FSGS include young age at initial diagnosis (younger than 15 years), rapid progression of the initial disease (<3 years from diagnosis to ESRD), white race, mesangial hyperplasia, and recurrence in previous allograft within 1 year of transplantation. Patients younger than 5 years of age have a 50% likelihood of a recurrence versus only 10% to 15% in patients older than 30 years.[90] None of these factors, however, is highly predictive in an individual patient.

Although those with genetic causes of FSGS would not be expected to have a recurrence of FSGS after transplantation, multiple reports have described a recurrence in approximately 10% of patients with homozygous or compound heterozygous *NPHS2* mutations.[86,91–93] The mechanism underlying this recurrence is unclear. Recurrence has not been reported in patients with FSGS associated with mutations in *ACTN4* or *TRPC6*, although it is premature to draw any conclusions at the present time.[94,95]

Pathogenesis

The pathogenesis of recurrent FSGS remains unknown. Because prompt institution of plasma exchange after early diagnosis of recurrence can be associated with reversal of epithelial foot process effacement and remission of proteinuria, a circulating permeability factor has long been suspected to initiate injury in recurrent FSGS. Consistent with this hypothesis, rats infused with the serum of a patient with recurrent FSGS develop proteinuria, suggesting that the permeability factor is present in the circulation of FSGS patients and that it can reproduce the glomerular injury when transferred into a normal host.[96] After more than 20 years of research, however, the identity of the permeability factor remains obscure.

Further complicating the attempt to identify the permeability factor is the possibility that the glomerular injury in FSGS patients may stem from the loss of an inhibitor that normally blocks the permeability effect in normal individuals. To determine whether normal serum improves the glomerular albumin permeability in FSGS, Sharma and colleagues[97] incubated isolated rat glomeruli in a mixture of medium containing FSGS serum and normal human serum. Normal human serum prevented the increase in glomerular albumin permeability, and this protective effect diminished as the concentration of normal serum was decreased, suggesting the presence of an inhibitor in the normal serum. Further support for the role of inhibitor loss leading to increased glomerular permeability was provided by Coward and colleagues.[98] The investigators found that the addition of nephrotic FSGS plasma to isolated human podocytes led to an altered distribution of the slit-diaphragm proteins, including selective down-regulation of nephrin and synaptopodin and disruption of intracellular calcium signaling. The altered distribution of nephrin induced by nephrotic plasma could be reversed by co-incubation with nonnephrotic plasma. This work demonstrates that nephrotic plasma seems to be deficient in factors critical for maintaining the physiologic function of the podocyte slit-diaphragm complex.

Given the recurrence of proteinuria after transplantation in genetic forms of FSGS, it is also intriguing to question whether there is an interaction between the molecular defects of the slit diaphragm and permeability factor or whether certain genetic defects actually reflect the loss of certain plasma factors that regulate permselectivity. Due to the surge of interest in podocyte biology stemming from the discovery of disease-associated podocyte genes, the subject of recurrent FSGS provides opportunities to further understand the pathogenesis and thus develop better alternative therapy options.

Treatment

There are no systematic controlled trials to guide the treatment of recurrent FSGS. Clinical practice is based on relatively small series. Immunoabsorption and plasma exchange with or without cyclophosphamide, cyclosporine, glucocorticoids, and intravenous immunoglobulin have been used with limited success.

Plasma Exchange

Although several reports have suggested that plasma exchange can markedly decrease proteinuria in some cases of recurrent FSGS, long-term remission has been difficult to achieve.[88,99–101] A single course of plasma exchange or immunoabsorption may be associated with variable degrees of decrease in proteinuria in approximately half of the cases.[102–104] Although there are no systematic studies to suggest the optimal dosing and frequency of plasma exchange, analysis of 44 cases suggests that the median number of treatments to response is nine.[105] Based on this review, the standard clinical practice is to start early treatment after diagnosis with a regimen of three daily plasmapheresis treatments followed by six treatments on an every-other-day basis. Unfortunately, most patients experience a relapse, and their renal disease progresses. Children, in particular, often require a maintenance schedule of plasma exchange to sustain remission.

The limited efficacy of plasma exchange has led investigators to a trial of cyclophosphamide in children, either with or without plasma exchange. The available data suggest that addition of cyclophosphamide to plasma exchange may lead to sustained remission in 50% to 80% of cases (Table 20-7).[106–111] These studies do not allow firm conclusions, however, given their small size, lack of controls, and often retrospective design.

High-dose cyclosporine has also been used in pediatric patients with recurrent FSGS. Salomon and colleagues[112] adjusted intravenous cyclosporine dose to achieve trough levels of 250 to 350 ng/mL in 17 cases of recurrence. In 14 cases (82%), proteinuria completely disappeared after a mean of 3 weeks. The long-term graft survival at 1 and 5 years was 92% and 70%, respectively. Similar results have been published using oral cyclosporine in children.[113] The safety data in the long term, however, have not been systematically studied, and it is unknown whether any benefit that may be drawn from the prolonged survival of renal graft outweighs the potential complications from the more intensified immunosuppression. Furthermore, there are no published data regarding the efficacy of cyclophosphamide or cyclosporine in adults. Prophylaxis against recurrent FSGS remains a major challenge, and currently there are no methods to reliably decrease the risk of recurrence.

Table 20-7 Use of Increased Immunosuppression for Recurrent Focal Segmental Glomerulosclerosis

Authors	Design	Population	Treatment	No.	Complete Response	Partial Response	No Response	Long-Term Response, Mean No. of Years (Range)
Cochat et al[107]	Prospective	Children	PE + CTX 3 mo	3	3	0	0	3 CR (1 retreatment)
Kershaw et al[109]	Prospective?	Children	CTX 2–3 mo	3	3	0	0	2 CR (1 relapse)
Dall' Amico et al[108]	Retrospective	Children	PE + CTX 2 mo	11	9	0	2	7 CR
Cheong et al[106]	Retrospective	Children	PE + CTX 3 mo	6	3	3	0	2 CR
Saleem et al[111]	Prospective case series	Children	PE + CTX 2 mo (IVIG in 2 of 3 children)	3	0	2	1 (death after 4 mo)	2 PR, 3.25 (3.0–3.5)
Nathanson et al[110]	Retrospective	Children	Variable (PE, IV, CyA, CTX)	14	6	5	3	7 CR, 8.1 (1–14)

CR, complete remission (generally defined as proteinuria < 500 mg/day); CTX, cyclophosphamide; CyA, cyclosporin A; IVIG, intravenous immunoglobulin; PE, plasma exchange; PR, partial remission (generally defined as proteinuria < 2 g/day).

COLLAPSING GLOMERULOPATHY

In 1984, human immunodeficiency virus–associated nephropathy was first recognized as a clinical syndrome and its characteristic histologic features, including podocyte swelling and proliferation, were first characterized.[114] The term CG, however, was not introduced until 1986. The discovery of idiopathic CG soon followed in 1986 by Weiss and colleagues,[115] with subsequent reports from elsewhere within the United States and Europe.[116–120] Since its first recognition, CG has quickly become increasingly common.[117] Although such an epidemiologic pattern strongly suggests a new environmental agent, possibly a virus or toxin, the cause remains unknown.

Idiopathic CG typically presents with a sudden onset of heavy proteinuria, although some patients have subnephrotic proteinuria. Patients have a strikingly poor renal survival, with a 70% probability of ESRD at 2 years, although this is not invariably the case.[23] Some patients report a virus-like prodrome occurring before presentation, with symptoms that may include fever, cough, and diarrhea. Parvovirus B19 infection has been linked with CG, although controversy remains about the strength and specificity of the association.[121–123] CG has also been associated with certain medications, including pamidronate[124] and interferon alfa.[125] The mechanism is unknown.

The pathophysiology of CG remains unclear, although the underlying pathogenic event appears to be injury to podocytes. Podocytes are postmitotic cells in the normal human kidney, and it has been proposed that depletion of podocytes may be critical in the development of FSGS. Unlike the depletion of podocytes as seen in FSGS, however, both human immunodeficiency virus–associated and idiopathic CG are characterized by podocyte dysregulation and proliferation.[126] In contrast to MCN and other glomerulopathies, podocytes undergo characteristic, irreversible ultrastructural changes in CG, including the loss of maturity markers such as synaptopodin. This phenotypic dysregulation of podocytes is associated with cell proliferation, a feature not seen in other glomerular diseases, including idiopathic FSGS. Because CG significantly differs histologically and clinically from other variants, some investigators argue that CG should be a separate entity from FSGS altogether.[8]

There are no published prospective, controlled studies that have examined efficacy of therapy in CG. Unfortunately, the response rate in CG is even lower than that for FSGS, with only 9.6% of patients achieving long-term remission and 15.2% of patients achieving partial remission.[127] As there is no evidence-based treatment of CG, the current therapeutic strategies derive from the empirical approach used for FSGS. According to the available data, response to steroids, cyclosporine, and cyclophosphamide is very poor.[116,117,119] Limited data suggest that early, aggressive treatment may achieve higher remission rates, particularly in patients with better preserved renal function (serum creatinine concentrations < 2.0 mg/dL and < 20% interstitial fibrosis on renal biopsy).[119,128,129]

CONCLUSIONS

MCN, FSGS, and CG represent a complex syndrome with multifactorial causes that culminate in podocyte injury. Although both disorders are considered to have immunologic basis, recent discoveries of the genetic defects associated with podocytopathy have increased the complexity underlying the pathogenesis. Although the diagnosis of MCN and FSGS require careful pathologic examination, considerable variability exists in renal histology, and this heterogeneity may reflect the diverse causes and clinical outcomes of the diseases. The therapeutic responses and prognosis of MCN and FSGS are equally as heterogeneous, reflecting the fact that these disorders do not represent a single clinical or pathologic entity. Most of the patients with MCN and some of those with FSGS are steroid sensitive. The remaining patients with MCN and a larger proportion of those with FSGS and CG are steroid resistant. Steroid resistance is generally associated with poor long-term response with other available therapies, denoting more refractory cases. Much work is needed to better understand the pathophysiology, which may allow identification and development of more specific therapy options in the future. Some of the possible future therapy options are summarized in Table 20-6. Particular areas of interest include molecular pathways involved in initiating podocyte injury and recurrence of nephrotic syndrome after renal transplantation, the molecular determinants of steroid sensitivity, and the relationship between the various histologic variants and clinical outcome.

References

1. Kitiyakara C, Eggers P, Kopp JB: Twenty-one-year trend in ESRD due to focal segmental glomerulosclerosis in the United States. Am J Kidney Dis 2004;44:815–825.
2. The primary nephrotic syndrome in children. Identification of patients with minimal change nephrotic syndrome from initial response to prednisone. A report of the International Study of Kidney Disease in Children. J Pediatr 1981;98:561–564.
3. Bonilla-Felix M, Parra C, Dajani T, et al: Changing patterns in the histopathology of idiopathic nephrotic syndrome in children. Kidney Int 1999;55:1885–1890.
4. Braden GL, Mulhern JG, O'Shea MH, et al: Changing incidence of glomerular diseases in adults. Am J Kidney Dis 2000;35:878–883.
5. Haas M, Spargo BH, Coventry S: Increasing incidence of focal-segmental glomerulosclerosis among adult nephropathies: A 20-year renal biopsy study. Am J Kidney Dis 1995;26:740–750.
6. Ingulli E, Tejani A: Racial differences in the incidence and renal outcome of idiopathic focal segmental glomerulosclerosis in children. Pediatr Nephrol 1991;5:393–397.
7. Korbet SM, Genchi RM, Borok RZ, et al: The racial prevalence of glomerular lesions in nephrotic adults. Am J Kidney Dis 1996;27:647–651.
8. Barisoni L, Schnaper HW, Kopp JB: A proposed taxonomy for the podocytopathies: A reassessment of the primary nephrotic diseases. Clin J Am Soc Nephrol 2007;2:529–542.
9. White RH, Glasgow EF, Mills RJ: Clinicopathological study of nephrotic syndrome in childhood. Lancet 1970;1:1353–1359.
10. Kemper MJ, Wolf G, Muller-Wiefel DE: Transmission of glomerular permeability factor from a mother to her child. N Engl J Med 2001;344:386–387.
11. Kambham N, Markowitz GS, Valeri AM, et al: Obesity-related glomerulopathy: An emerging epidemic. Kidney Int 2001;59:1498–1509.
12. D'Agati V: Pathologic classification of focal segmental glomerulosclerosis. Semin Nephrol 2003;23:117–134.
13. Kriz W, Hosser H, Hahnel B, et al: Development of vascular pole-associated glomerulosclerosis in the Fawn-hooded rat. J Am Soc Nephrol 1998;9:381–396.

14. Kriz W, Lemley KV: The role of the podocyte in glomerulosclerosis. Curr Opin Nephrol Hypertens 1999;8:489–497.
15. Praga M, Hernandez E, Morales E, et al: Clinical features and long-term outcome of obesity-associated focal segmental glomerulosclerosis. Nephrol Dial Transplant 2001;16:1790–1798.
16. Kestila M, Lenkkeri U, Mannikko M, et al: Positionally cloned gene for a novel glomerular protein—nephrin—is mutated in congenital nephrotic syndrome. Mol Cell 1998;1:575–582.
17. Kaplan JM, Kim SH, North KN, et al: Mutations in ACTN4, encoding alpha-actinin-4, cause familial focal segmental glomerulosclerosis. Nat Genet 2000;24:251–256.
18. Boute N, Gribouval O, Roselli S, et al: NPHS2, encoding the glomerular protein podocin, is mutated in autosomal recessive steroid-resistant nephrotic syndrome [erratum appears in Nat Genet 2000;25:125]. Nat Genet 2000;24:349–354.
19. Kim JM, Wu H, Green G, et al: CD2-associated protein haploinsufficiency is linked to glomerular disease susceptibility. Science 2003;300:1298–1300.
20. Liu XL, Done SC, Yan K, et al: Defective trafficking of nephrin missense mutants rescued by a chemical chaperone. J Am Soc Nephrol 2004;15:1731–1738.
21. Ghiggeri GM, Carraro M, Vincenti F: Recurrent focal glomerulosclerosis in the era of genetics of podocyte proteins: Theory and therapy. Nephrol Dial Transplant 2004;19:1036–1040.
22. D'Agati VD, Fogo AB, Bruijn JA, et al: Pathologic classification of focal segmental glomerulosclerosis: A working proposal. Am J Kidney Dis 2004;43:368–382.
23. Thomas DB, Franceschini N, Hogan SL, et al: Clinical and pathologic characteristics of focal segmental glomerulosclerosis pathologic variants. Kidney Int 2006;69:920–926.
24. Korbet SM: Clinical picture and outcome of primary focal segmental glomerulosclerosis. Nephrol Dial Transplant 1999;14(Suppl 3):68–73.
25. Brown CB, Cameron JS, Turner DR, et al: Focal segmental glomerulosclerosis with rapid decline in renal function ("malignant FSGS"). Clin Nephrol 1978;10:51–61.
26. Velosa JA, Holley KE, Torres VE, et al: Significance of proteinuria on the outcome of renal function in patients with focal segmental glomerulosclerosis. Mayo Clin Proc 1983;58:568–577.
27. Wehrmann M, Bohle A, Held H, et al: Long-term prognosis of focal sclerosing glomerulonephritis. An analysis of 250 cases with particular regard to tubulointerstitial changes. Clin Nephrol 1990;33:115–122.
28. Rydel JJ, Korbet SM, Borok RZ, et al: Focal segmental glomerular sclerosis in adults: Presentation, course, and response to treatment. Am J Kidney Dis 1995;25:534–542.
29. Cattran DC, Rao P: Long-term outcome in children and adults with classic focal segmental glomerulosclerosis. Am J Kidney Dis 1998;32:72–79.
30. Troyanov S, Wall CA, Miller JA, et al: Focal and segmental glomerulosclerosis: Definition and relevance of a partial remission. J Am Soc Nephrol 2005;16:1061–1068.
31. Schwartz MM, Evans J, Bain R, et al: Focal segmental glomerulosclerosis: Prognostic implications of the cellular lesion. J Am Soc Nephrol 1999;10:1900–1907.
32. Schwartz MM, Korbet SM, Rydell J, et al: Primary focal segmental glomerular sclerosis in adults: Prognostic value of histologic variants. Am J Kidney Dis 1995;25:845–852.
33. Stokes MB, Valeri AM, Markowitz GS, et al: Cellular focal segmental glomerulosclerosis: Clinical and pathologic features. Kidney Int 2006;70:1783–1792.
34. Bagga A, Hari P, Srivastava RN: Prolonged versus standard prednisolone therapy for initial episode of nephrotic syndrome. Pediatr Nephrol 1999;13:824–827.
35. Ehrich JH, Brodehl J: Long versus standard prednisone therapy for initial treatment of idiopathic nephrotic syndrome in children. Arbeitsgemeinschaft fur Pädiatrische Nephrologie. Eur J Pediatr 1993;152:357–361.
36. Hiraoka M, Tsukahara H, Haruki S, et al: Older boys benefit from higher initial prednisolone therapy for nephrotic syndrome. The West Japan Cooperative Study of Kidney Disease in Children. Kidney Int 2000;58:1247–1252.
37. Jayantha UK: Comparison of ISKDC regime with a six month steroid regime in the treatment of steroid sensitive nephrotic syndrome. Singapore: 7th Asian Congress of Pediatric Nephrology, 2000, November.
38. Ksiazek J, Wyszynska T: Short versus long initial prednisone treatment in steroid-sensitive nephrotic syndrome in children. Acta Paediatr 1995;84:889–893.
39. Norero C, Delucchi A, Lagos E, et al: [Initial therapy of primary nephrotic syndrome in children: Evaluation in a period of 18 months of two prednisone treatment schedules. Chilean Co-operative Group of Study of Nephrotic Syndrome in Children]. Rev Med Chil 1996;124:567–572.
40. Ueda N, Chihara M, Kawaguchi S, et al: Intermittent versus long-term tapering prednisolone for initial therapy in children with idiopathic nephrotic syndrome. J Pediatr 1988;112:122–126.
41. Pei Y, Cattran D, Delmore T, et al: Evidence suggesting undertreatment in adults with idiopathic focal segmental glomerulosclerosis. Regional Glomerulonephritis Registry Study. Am J Med 1987;82:938–944.
42. Korbet SM: Management of idiopathic nephrosis in adults, including steroid-resistant nephrosis. Curr Opin Nephrol Hypertens 1995;4:169–176.
43. Korbet SM: Treatment of primary focal segmental glomerulosclerosis. Kidney Int 2002;62:2301–2310.
44. Korbet SM, Schwartz MM, Lewis EJ: Primary focal segmental glomerulosclerosis: Clinical course and response to therapy. Am J Kidney Dis 1994;23:773–783.
45. Agarwal SK, Dash SC, Tiwari SC, Bhuyan UN: Idiopathic adult focal segmental glomerulosclerosis: A clinicopathological study and response to steroid. Nephron 1993;63:168–171.
46. Chitalia VC, Wells JE, Robson RA, et al: Predicting renal survival in primary focal glomerulosclerosis from the time of presentation. Kidney Int 1999;56:2236–2242.
47. Franceschini N, Hogan SL, Falk RJ: Primum non nocere: Should adults with idiopathic FSGS receive steroids? Semin Nephrol 2003;23:229–233.
48. Pokhariyal S, Gulati S, Prasad N, et al: Duration of optimal therapy for idiopathic focal segmental glomerulosclerosis. J Nephrol 2003;16:691–696.
49. Ponticelli C, Villa M, Banfi G, et al: Can prolonged treatment improve the prognosis in adults with focal segmental glomerulosclerosis? Am J Kidney Dis 1999;34:618–625.
50. Smith D, Branton M, Fervenza F, et al: Pulse dexamethasone for focal segmental glomerulosclerosis. J Am Soc Nephrol 2003;14.
51. Stiles KP, Abbott KC, Welch PG, et al: Effects of angiotensin-converting enzyme inhibitor and steroid therapy on proteinuria in FSGS: A retrospective study in a single clinic. Clin Nephrol 2001;56:89–95.
52. Xing CY, Saleem MA, Coward RJ, et al: Direct effects of dexamethasone on human podocytes. Kidney Int 2006;70:1038–1045.
53. Fujii Y, Khoshnoodi J, Takenaka H, et al: The effect of dexamethasone on defective nephrin transport caused by ER stress: A potential mechanism for the therapeutic action of glucocorticoids in the acquired glomerular diseases. Kidney Int 2006;69:1350–1359.
54. Ransom RF, Lam NG, Hallett MA, et al: Glucocorticoids protect and enhance recovery of cultured murine podocytes via actin filament stabilization. Kidney Int 2005;68:2473–2483.
55. Wada T, Pippin JW, Marshall CB, et al: Dexamethasone prevents podocyte apoptosis induced by puromycin aminonucleoside: role of p53 and Bcl-2-related family proteins. J Am Soc Nephrol 2005;16:2615–2625.

56. Tarshish P, Tobin JN, Bernstein J, et al: Cyclophosphamide does not benefit patients with focal segmental glomerulosclerosis. A report of the International Study of Kidney Disease in Children. Pediatr Nephrol 1996;10:590–593.

57. Martinelli R, Okumura AS, Pereira LJ, et al: Primary focal segmental glomerulosclerosis in children: Prognostic factors. Pediatr Nephrol 2001;16:658–661.

58. Tune BM, Kirpekar R, Sibley RK, et al: Intravenous methylprednisolone and oral alkylating agent therapy of prednisone-resistant pediatric focal segmental glomerulosclerosis: A long-term follow-up. Clin Nephrol 1995;43:84–88.

59. Tune BM, Lieberman E, Mendoza SA: Steroid-resistant nephrotic focal segmental glomerulosclerosis: A treatable disease. Pediatr Nephrol 1996;10:772–778.

60. Abeyagunawardena AS, Sebire NJ, Risdon RA, et al: Predictors of long-term outcome of children with idiopathic focal segmental glomerulosclerosis. Pediatr Nephrol 2007;22: 215–221.

61. Bhimma R, Adhikari M, Asharam K: Steroid-resistant nephrotic syndrome: The influence of race on cyclophosphamide sensitivity. Pediatr Nephrol 2006;21:1847–1853.

62. Lieberman KV, Tejani A: A randomized double-blind placebo-controlled trial of cyclosporine in steroid-resistant idiopathic focal segmental glomerulosclerosis in children. J Am Soc Nephrol 1996;7:56–63.

63. Heering P, Braun N, Mullejans R, et al: Cyclosporine A and chlorambucil in the treatment of idiopathic focal segmental glomerulosclerosis. Am J Kidney Dis 2004;43:10–18.

64. Cattran DC, Appel GB, Hebert LA, et al: A randomized trial of cyclosporine in patients with steroid-resistant focal segmental glomerulosclerosis. North America Nephrotic Syndrome Study Group. Kidney Int 1999;56:2220–2226.

65. Niaudet P: Treatment of childhood steroid-resistant idiopathic nephrosis with a combination of cyclosporine and prednisone. French Society of Pediatric Nephrology. J Pediatr 1994;125: 981–986.

66. Westhoff TH, Schmidt S, Zidek W, et al: Tacrolimus in steroid-resistant and steroid-dependent nephrotic syndrome. Clin Nephrol 2006;65:393–400.

67. Meyrier A, Noel LH, Auriche P, et al: Long-term renal tolerance of cyclosporin A treatment in adult idiopathic nephrotic syndrome. Collaborative Group of the Société de Néphrologie. Kidney Int 1994;45:1446–1456.

68. Choi MJ, Eustace JA, Gimenez LF, et al: Mycophenolate mofetil treatment for primary glomerular diseases. Kidney Int 2002; 61:1098–1114.

69. Mendizabal S, Zamora I, Berbel O, et al: Mycophenolate mofetil in steroid/cyclosporine-dependent/resistant nephrotic syndrome. Pediatr Nephrol 2005;20:914–919.

70. Gellermann J, Querfeld U: Frequently relapsing nephrotic syndrome: Treatment with mycophenolate mofetil. Pediatr Nephrol 2004;19:101–104.

71. Bagga A, Hari P, Moudgil A, et al: Mycophenolate mofetil and prednisolone therapy in children with steroid-dependent nephrotic syndrome. Am J Kidney Dis 2003;42:1114–1120.

72. Wang W, Chan YH, Lee W, et al: Effect of rapamycin and FK506 on mesangial cell proliferation. Transplant Proc 2001; 33:1036–1037.

73. Iwasaki H, Eguchi S, Ueno H, et al: Endothelin-mediated vascular growth requires p42/p44 mitogen-activated protein kinase and p70 S6 kinase cascades via transactivation of epidermal growth factor receptor. Endocrinology 1999;140: 4659–4668.

74. Marx SO, Jayaraman T, Go LO, Marks AR: Rapamycin-FKBP inhibits cell cycle regulators of proliferation in vascular smooth muscle cells. Circ Res 1995;76:412–417.

75. Jain S, Bicknell GR, Whiting PH, et al: Rapamycin reduces expression of fibrosis-associated genes in an experimental model of renal ischaemia reperfusion injury. Transplant Proc 2001;33:556–558.

76. Zhu J, Wu J, Frizell E, et al: Rapamycin inhibits hepatic stellate cell proliferation in vitro and limits fibrogenesis in an in vivo model of liver fibrosis. Gastroenterology 1999;117: 1198–1204.

77. Tumlin JA, Miller D, Near M, et al: A prospective, open-label trial of sirolimus in the treatment of focal segmental glomerulosclerosis. Clin J Am Soc Nephrol 2006;1:109–116.

78. Fervenza FC, Fitzpatrick PM, Mertz J, et al: Acute rapamycin nephrotoxicity in native kidneys of patients with chronic glomerulopathies. Nephrol Dial Transplant 2004;19:1288–1292.

79. Cho ME, Hurley JK, Kopp JB: Sirolimus therapy of focal segmental glomerulosclerosis is associated with nephrotoxicity. Am J Kidney Dis 2007;49:310–317.

80. Maschio G, Alberti D, Janin G, et al: Effect of the angiotensin-converting-enzyme inhibitor benazepril on the progression of chronic renal insufficiency. The Angiotensin-Converting-Enzyme Inhibition in Progressive Renal Insufficiency Study Group. N Engl J Med 1996;334:939–945.

81. Praga M, Hernandez E, Montoyo C, et al: Long-term beneficial effects of angiotensin-converting enzyme inhibition in patients with nephrotic proteinuria. Am J Kidney Dis 1992;20:240–248.

82. Ruggenenti P, Perna A, Zoccali C, et al: Chronic proteinuric nephropathies. II. Outcomes and response to treatment in a prospective cohort of 352 patients: Differences between women and men in relation to the ACE gene polymorphism. Gruppo Italiano di Studi Epidemiologici in Nefrologia (Gisen). J Am Soc Nephrol 2000;11:88–96.

83. Nakao N, Yoshimura A, Morita H, et al: Combination treatment of angiotensin-II receptor blocker and angiotensin-converting-enzyme inhibitor in non-diabetic renal disease (COOPERATE): A randomised controlled trial. Lancet 2003;361:117–124.

84. Cho ME, Smith DC, Branton MH, et al: Pirfenidone slows renal function decline in patients with focal segmental glomerulosclerosis. Clin J Am Soc Nephrol 2007;2:906–913.

85. Praga M, Hernandez E, Andres A, et al: Effects of body-weight loss and captopril treatment on proteinuria associated with obesity. Nephron 1995;70:35–41.

86. Ruf RG, Lichtenberger A, Karle SM, et al: Patients with mutations in NPHS2 (podocin) do not respond to standard steroid treatment of nephrotic syndrome. J Am Soc Nephrol 2004;15:722–732.

87. Hoyer JR, Vernier RL, Najarian JS, et al: Recurrence of idiopathic nephrotic syndrome after renal transplantation. Lancet 1972;2:343–348.

88. Artero M, Biava C, Amend W, et al: Recurrent focal glomerulosclerosis: Natural history and response to therapy. Am J Med 1992;92:375–383.

89. Baum MA: Outcomes after renal transplantation for FSGS in children. Pediatr Transplant 2004;8:329–333.

90. Le Berre L, Godfrin Y, Gunther E, et al: Extrarenal effects on the pathogenesis and relapse of idiopathic nephrotic syndrome in Buffalo/Mna rats. J Clin Invest 2002;109:491–498.

91. Bertelli R, Ginevri F, Caridi G, et al: Recurrence of focal segmental glomerulosclerosis after renal transplantation in patients with mutations of podocin. Am J Kidney Dis 2003;41: 1314–1321.

92. Carraro M, Caridi G, Bruschi M, et al: Serum glomerular permeability activity in patients with podocin mutations (NPHS2) and steroid-resistant nephrotic syndrome. J Am Soc Nephrol 2002;13:1946–1952.

93. Weber S, Gribouval O, Esquivel EL, et al: NPHS2 mutation analysis shows genetic heterogeneity of steroid-resistant nephrotic syndrome and low post-transplant recurrence. Kidney Int 2004;66:571–579.

94. Conlon PJ, Lynn K, Winn MP, et al: Spectrum of disease in familial focal and segmental glomerulosclerosis. Kidney Int 1999;56:1863–1871.

95. Winn MP, Conlon PJ, Lynn KL, et al: A mutation in the TRPC6 cation channel causes familial focal segmental glomerulosclerosis. Science 2005;308:1801–1804.

96. Zimmerman SW: Increased urinary protein excretion in the rat produced by serum from a patient with recurrent focal glomerular sclerosis after renal transplantation. Clin Nephrol 1984;22:32–38.

97. Sharma R, Sharma M, McCarthy ET, et al: Components of normal serum block the focal segmental glomerulosclerosis factor activity in vitro. Kidney Int 2000;58:1973–1979.

98. Coward RJ, Foster RR, Patton D, et al: Nephrotic plasma alters slit diaphragm-dependent signaling and translocates nephrin, podocin, and CD2 associated protein in cultured human podocytes. J Am Soc Nephrol 2005;16:629–637.

99. Artero ML, Sharma R, Savin VJ, et al: Plasmapheresis reduces proteinuria and serum capacity to injure glomeruli in patients with recurrent focal glomerulosclerosis. Am J Kidney Dis 1994;23:574–581.

100. Dantal J, Bigot E, Bogers W, et al: Effect of plasma protein adsorption on protein excretion in kidney-transplant recipients with recurrent nephrotic syndrome. N Engl J Med 1994;330:7–14.

101. Savin VJ, Sharma R, Sharma M, et al: Circulating factor associated with increased glomerular permeability to albumin in recurrent focal segmental glomerulosclerosis. N Engl J Med 1996;334:878–883.

102. Andresdottir MB, Ajubi N, Croockewit S, et al: Recurrent focal glomerulosclerosis: Natural course and treatment with plasma exchange. Nephrol Dial Transplant 1999;14:2650–2656.

103. Dantal J, Baatard R, Hourmant M, et al: Recurrent nephrotic syndrome following renal transplantation in patients with focal glomerulosclerosis. A one-center study of plasma exchange effects. Transplantation 1991;52:827–831.

104. Greenstein SM, Delrio M, Ong E, et al: Plasmapheresis treatment for recurrent focal sclerosis in pediatric renal allografts. Pediatr Nephrol 2000;14:1061–1065.

105. Davenport RD: Apheresis treatment of recurrent focal segmental glomerulosclerosis after kidney transplantation: Re-analysis of published case-reports and case-series. J Clin Apher 2001;16:175–178.

106. Cheong HI, Han HW, Park HW, et al: Early recurrent nephrotic syndrome after renal transplantation in children with focal segmental glomerulosclerosis. Nephrol Dial Transplant 2000;15:78–81.

107. Cochat P, Kassir A, Colon S, et al: Recurrent nephrotic syndrome after transplantation: Early treatment with plasmapheresis and cyclophosphamide. Pediatr Nephrol 1993;7:50–54.

108. Dall'Amico R, Ghiggeri G, Carraro M, et al: Prediction and treatment of recurrent focal segmental glomerulosclerosis after renal transplantation in children. Am J Kidney Dis 1999;34:1048–1055.

109. Kershaw DB, Sedman AB, Kelsch RC, et al: Recurrent focal segmental glomerulosclerosis in pediatric renal transplant recipients: Successful treatment with oral cyclophosphamide. Clin Transplant 1994;8:546–549.

110. Nathanson S, Cochat P, Andre JL, et al: Recurrence of nephrotic syndrome after renal transplantation: Influence of increased immunosuppression. Pediatr Nephrol 2005;20:1801–1804.

111. Saleem MA, Ramanan AV, Rees L: Recurrent focal segmental glomerulosclerosis in grafts treated with plasma exchange and increased immunosuppression. Pediatr Nephrol 2000;14:361–364.

112. Salomon R, Gagnadoux MF, Niaudet P: Intravenous cyclosporine therapy in recurrent nephrotic syndrome after renal transplantation in children. Transplantation 2003;75:810–814.

113. Raafat RH, Kalia A, Travis LB, et al: High-dose oral cyclosporin therapy for recurrent focal segmental glomerulosclerosis in children. Am J Kidney Dis 2004;44:50–56.

114. Pardo V, Aldana M, Colton RM, et al: Glomerular lesions in the acquired immunodeficiency syndrome. Ann Intern Med 1984;101:429–434.

115. Weiss MA, Daquioag E, Margolin EG, et al: Nephrotic syndrome, progressive irreversible renal failure, and glomerular "collapse": A new clinicopathologic entity? Am J Kidney Dis 1986;7:20–28.

116. Detwiler RK, Falk RJ, Hogan SL, et al: Collapsing glomerulopathy: A clinically and pathologically distinct variant of focal segmental glomerulosclerosis. Kidney Int 1994;45:1416–1424.

117. Valeri A, Barisoni L, Appel GB, et al: Idiopathic collapsing focal segmental glomerulosclerosis: A clinicopathologic study. Kidney Int 1996;50:1734–1746.

118. Grcevska L, Polenakovik M: Collapsing glomerulopathy: Clinical characteristics and follow-up. Am J Kidney Dis 1999;33:652–657.

119. Laurinavicius A, Hurwitz S, Rennke HG: Collapsing glomerulopathy in HIV and non-HIV patients: A clinicopathological and follow-up study. Kidney Int 1999;56:2203–2213.

120. Singh HK, Baldree LA, McKenney DW, et al: Idiopathic collapsing glomerulopathy in children. Pediatr Nephrol 2000;14:132–137.

121. Moudgil A, Nast CC, Bagga A, et al: Association of parvovirus B19 infection with idiopathic collapsing glomerulopathy. Kidney Int 2001;59:2126–2133.

122. Tanawattanacharoen S, Falk RJ, Jennette JC, et al: Parvovirus B19 DNA in kidney tissue of patients with focal segmental glomerulosclerosis. Am J Kidney Dis 2000;35:1166–1174.

123. Waldman M, Kopp JB: Parvovirus B19 and the kidney. Clin J Am Soc Nephrol 2007;2:S47–S56.

124. Markowitz GS, Appel GB, Fine PL, et al: Collapsing focal segmental glomerulosclerosis following treatment with high-dose pamidronate. J Am Soc Nephrol 2001;12:1164–1172.

125. Stein DF, Ahmed A, Sunkhara V, et al: Collapsing focal segmental glomerulosclerosis with recovery of renal function: An uncommon complication of interferon therapy for hepatitis C. Dig Dis Sci 2001;46:530–535.

126. Barisoni L, Kriz W, Mundel P, et al: The dysregulated podocyte phenotype: A novel concept in the pathogenesis of collapsing idiopathic focal segmental glomerulosclerosis and HIV-associated nephropathy. J Am Soc Nephrol 1999;10:51–61.

127. Albaqumi M, Soos TJ, Barisoni L, et al: Collapsing glomerulopathy. J Am Soc Nephrol 2006;17:2854–2863.

128. Chun MJ, Korbet SM, Schwartz MM, et al: Focal segmental glomerulosclerosis in nephrotic adults: Presentation, prognosis, and response to therapy of the histologic variants. J Am Soc Nephrol 2004;15:2169–2177.

129. Schwimmer JA, Markowitz GS, Valeri A, et al: Collapsing glomerulopathy. Semin Nephrol 2003;23:209–218.

130. Praga M, Morales E, Herrero JC, et al: Absence of hypoalbuminemia despite massive proteinuria in focal segmental glomerulosclerosis secondary to hyperfiltration. Am J Kidney Dis 1999;33:52–58.

131. Schnaper HW, Robson AM, Kopp JB: Nephrotic syndrome: Minimal change nephropathy, focal segmental glomerulosclerosis, and collapsing glomerulopathy. In Schrier RW (ed): Diseases of the Kidney and Urinary Tract: Clinicopathologic Foundations of Medicine, 8th ed. Philadelphia: Lippincott Williams & Wilkins, 2006, pp 1585–1672.

132. Cameron JS, Turner DR, Ogg CS, et al: The long-term prognosis of patients with focal segmental glomerulosclerosis. Clin Nephrol 1978;10:213–218.

133. Mongeau JG, Corneille L, Robitaille P, et al: Primary nephrosis in childhood associated with focal glomerular sclerosis: Is long-term prognosis that severe? Kidney Int 1981;20:743–746.

134. Group SPNS: Focal segmental glomerulosclerosis in children with idiopathic nephrotic syndrome. A report of the Southwest Pediatric Nephrology Study Group. Kidney Int 1985;27:442–449.

135. Chan PC, Chan KW, Cheng IK, et al: Focal sclerosing glomerulopathy. Risk factors of progression and optimal mode of treatment. Int Urol Nephrol 1991;23:619–629.

136. Cattran DC, Rao P: Long-term outcome in children and adults with classic focal segmental glomerulosclerosis. Am J Kidney Dis 1998;32:72–79.

137. Dvorak P, Kramer HJ, Backer A, et al: Blockade of endothelin receptors attenuates end-organ damage in homozygous hypertensive ren-2 transgenic rats. Kidney Blood Press Res 2004;27:248–258.

138. Ortmann J, Amann K, Brandes RP, et al: Role of podocytes for reversal of glomerulosclerosis and proteinuria in the aging kidney after endothelin inhibition. Hypertension 2004;44:974–981.

139. Ma LJ, Marcantoni C, Linton MF, et al: Peroxisome proliferator-activated receptor-gamma agonist troglitazone protects against nondiabetic glomerulosclerosis in rats. Kidney Int 2001;59:1899–1910.

140. Blasi ER, Rocha R, Rudolph AE, et al: Aldosterone/salt induces renal inflammation and fibrosis in hypertensive rats. Kidney Int 2003;63:1791–1800.

141. Schaier M, Lehrke I, Schade K, et al: Isotretinoin alleviates renal damage in rat chronic glomerulonephritis. Kidney Int 2001;60:2222–2234.

142. Francois H, Placier S, Flamant M, et al: Prevention of renal vascular and glomerular fibrosis by epidermal growth factor receptor inhibition. FASEB J 2004;18:926–928.

143. Park HS, Bao L, Kim YJ, et al: Pirfenidone suppressed the development of glomerulosclerosis in the FGS/Kist mouse. J Korean Med Sci 2003;18:527–533.

144. Kelly DJ, Zhang Y, Gow R, et al: Tranilast attenuates structural and functional aspects of renal injury in the remnant kidney model. J Am Soc Nephrol 2004;15:2619–2629.

145. Benigni A, Zoja C, Zatelli C, et al: Vasopeptidase inhibitor restores the balance of vasoactive hormones in progressive nephropathy. Kidney Int 2004;66:1959–1965.

146. Gherardi D, D'Agati V, Chu TH, et al: Reversal of collapsing glomerulopathy in mice with the cyclin-dependent kinase inhibitor CYC202. J Am Soc Nephrol 2004;15:1212–1222.

147. Nishikimi T, Akimoto K, Wang X, et al: Fasudil, a Rho-kinase inhibitor, attenuates glomerulosclerosis in Dahl salt-sensitive rats. J Hypertens 2004;22:1787–1796.

148. Franceschini N, Cheng O, Zhang X, et al: Inhibition of prolyl-4-hydroxylase ameliorates chronic rejection of mouse kidney allografts. Am J Transplant 2003;3:396–402.

149. Vielhauer V, Berning E, Eis V, et al: CCR1 blockade reduces interstitial inflammation and fibrosis in mice with glomerulosclerosis and nephrotic syndrome. Kidney Int 2004;66:2264–2278.

150. Oldroyd SD, Thomas GL, Gabbiani G, et al: Interferon-gamma inhibits experimental renal fibrosis. Kidney Int 1999;56:2116–2127.

151. Zeisberg M, Bottiglio C, Kumar N, et al: Bone morphogenic protein-7 inhibits progression of chronic renal fibrosis associated with two genetic mouse models. Am J Physiol Renal Physiol 2003;285:F1060–F1067.

152. Mizuno S, Kurosawa T, Matsumoto K, et al: Hepatocyte growth factor prevents renal fibrosis and dysfunction in a mouse model of chronic renal disease. J Clin Invest 1998;101:1827–1834.

153. Garber SL, Mirochnik Y, Brecklin CS, et al: Relaxin decreases renal interstitial fibrosis and slows progression of renal disease. Kidney Int 2001;59:876–882.

154. Border WA, Noble NA, Yamamoto T, et al: Natural inhibitor of transforming growth factor-beta protects against scarring in experimental kidney disease. Nature 1992;360:361–364.

155. Ma LJ, Jha S, Ling H, et al: Divergent effects of low versus high dose anti-TGF-beta antibody in puromycin aminonucleoside nephropathy in rats. Kidney Int 2004;65:106–115.

Further Reading

Barisoni L, Schnaper HW, Kopp JB: A proposed taxonomy for the podocytopathies: A reassessment of the primary nephrotic diseases. Clin J Am Soc Nephrol 2007;2:529–542.

Barisoni L, Kriz W, Mundel P, et al: The dysregulated podocyte phenotype: A novel concept in the pathogenesis of collapsing idiopathic focal segmental glomerulosclerosis and HIV-associated nephropathy. J Am Soc Nephrol 1999;10:51–61.

Cattran DC, Appel GB, Hebert LA, et al: A randomized trial of cyclosporine in patients with steroid-resistant focal segmental glomerulosclerosis. North America Nephrotic Syndrome Study Group. Kidney Int 1999;56:2220–2226.

Kriz W, Lemley KV: The role of the podocyte in glomerulosclerosis. Curr Opin Nephrol Hypertens 1999;8:489–497.

Troyanov S, Wall CA, Miller JA, et al: Focal and segmental glomerulosclerosis: Definition and relevance of a partial remission. J Am Soc Nephrol 2005;16:1061–1068.

Chapter 21

Idiopathic Membranous Nephropathy

Howard A. Austin III

Membranous nephropathy is a common cause of adult-onset nephrotic syndrome, accounting for as many as 33% of cases in which a biopsy was performed to determine the cause of the nephrotic syndrome.[1,2] Characteristic changes in a renal biopsy specimen include diffuse glomerular capillary wall thickening and subepithelial and/or intramembranous electron-dense deposits (described further by Falk and colleagues[3]). Various medications and toxins as well as certain rheumatologic, neoplastic, and infectious diseases account for approximately 20% of membranous nephropathy from developed countries.[4] The underlying cause (e.g., neoplasia or systemic lupus erythematosus) may not be evident at presentation in some patients, requiring an ongoing evaluation to ferret out a specific and, it is hoped, treatable disorder.[4] Treatment of secondary membranous nephropathy is beyond the scope of this chapter.

NATURAL HISTORY

Despite evidence that immunologic mechanisms induce glomerular injury in membranous nephropathy, immunosuppressive drug treatments are not justified for all patients with this disorder. The clinical course of idiopathic membranous nephropathy is highly variable. Although patients with nonnephrotic proteinuria have a favorable prognosis, du Buf-Vereijken and colleagues[5] analyzed 10 studies published during the past 25 years and estimated that nearly 50% of patients with the nephrotic syndrome experienced a decline in renal function. Cattran and colleagues[6] observed that on average approximately 20% of patients in 12 studies progressed to end-stage renal disease within 10 years. Conversely, spontaneous remissions of nephrotic proteinuria occur in approximately one third of cases within 5 years.[7,8]

Patients with persistent proteinuria and hyperlipidemia are at increased risk of cardiovascular and thromboembolic complications of the nephrotic syndrome. Ordonez and colleagues[9] found that patients with the nephrotic syndrome had a fivefold increased risk of myocardial infarction (after statistical adjustment for hypertension and cigarette smoking) compared with age- and sex-matched control subjects who participated in the same health plan. Thus, the nephrotic syndrome is an independent risk factor for accelerated coronary artery disease. The nephrotic syndrome due to membranous nephropathy is also associated with an increased risk of thromboembolic complications.[10,11]

Survival data compiled by Hogan and colleagues[12] illustrate the potential morbidity and mortality attributed to idiopathic membranous nephropathy. A pooled analysis was conducted to estimate renal survival, defined as the probability of not progressing to end-stage renal failure and not succumbing to death due to kidney disease or cardiovascular events associated with persistent nephrotic syndrome. Employing this approach, the probability of renal survival was 86% at 5 years, 65% at 10 years, and 59% at 15 years.

PROGNOSTIC INDICATORS

Generalizations about the prognosis of patients with idiopathic membranous nephropathy are of limited value because the natural history of this disorder is highly variable. To refine estimates of prognosis and to derive relatively objective criteria for instituting therapeutic interventions, investigators have sought to identify high-risk subgroups of patients. Several potentially important prognostic factors have been examined including age, gender, renal function, kidney pathology, and the quantity and types of urinary proteins.[13] Neugarten and colleagues[14] reported a meta-analysis of 21 studies that showed that men with membranous nephropathy experience significantly more rapid deterioration of renal function than women. Zent and colleagues[15] compared renal outcomes in 74 elderly patients (60 years of age and older) with membranous nephropathy with outcomes observed in 249 younger patients. Although the elderly patients were significantly more likely to develop chronic renal insufficiency than the younger patients, there was no difference in the rate of change in renal function or the probability of complete remission in the two groups. Thus, elderly patients with membranous nephropathy are more likely to develop chronic renal insufficiency because of an age-related decrease in renal function reserve at baseline rather than more severe membranous nephropathy. These observations were extended by Troyanov and colleagues[16] who reported that patients with interstitial fibrosis, tubular atrophy, vascular sclerosis, and focal segmental glomerulosclerosis lesions had a lower creatinine clearance at presentation and were more likely to progress to renal failure. Conversely, these chronic histologic features were not correlated with the rate of decline in renal function, nor did they predict the probability of remission in patients treated with immunosuppressive agents. Furthermore, they observed that the stage and pattern (i.e., synchronicity) of electron-dense deposits did not predict the rate of renal function deterioration or renal function survival. The extent of C3 deposition did correlate with the rate of renal function decline but not with renal survival, remissions of proteinuria, or response to immunosuppressive drug therapy.

Clinical observations acquired during a period of time are likely to be stronger predictors of long-term renal function outcome than those obtained at a single time point. Thus, increased serum creatinine at presentation is associated with an increased risk of renal failure, but may reflect age-related changes in renal reserve or readily reversible functional alterations rather than indicate the severity of the membranous nephropathy. Patients observed to have declining renal function due to membranous nephropathy are at particularly high risk of progressive deterioration in renal function.[17] Furthermore, persistent high-grade proteinuria is more predictive than a comparable degree of proteinuria at a single point in time. Pei and colleagues[18] observed that persistent severe proteinuria ($\geq$8 g/day for $\geq$ 6 months) was associated with a 66% probability of progression to chronic renal insufficiency. Less severe proteinuria for longer periods was also associated with an increased risk of developing chronic renal insufficiency. In patients with a moderate level of persistent proteinuria ($\geq$4 g/day for $\geq$18 months), the predictive value of persistent proteinuria was enhanced substantially by considering additional prognostic factors, namely, creatinine clearance at the start of persistent proteinuria and the rate of change in creatinine clearance during the period of persistent proteinuria.

Concern that prolonged observation might delay therapy excessively in some patients has prompted Cattran and colleagues[19] to reassess the predictive models by employing a 6-month period of observation for all levels of persistent proteinuria. A mathematical model was derived and validated by employing data from two additional distinct populations of patients. The algorithm uses the highest level of proteinuria that persisted for a 6-month interval as well as the initial value and the rate of change in creatinine clearance during the period of persistent proteinuria. The equation and examples of how to calculate the probability of progression to chronic renal insufficiency are described by Cattran and colleagues.[19] Based on this equation, Cattran[8] identified low-, medium-, and high-risk groups of patients. Patients with normal renal function and proteinuria 4 g/day or less for 6 months are at low risk (<5%) of renal function decline during the next 5 years. Patients with normal renal function and persistent proteinuria between 4 and 8 g/day for 6 months (despite optimal doses of angiotensin-converting enzyme [ACE] inhibitors and/or angiotensin receptor blockers [ARBs]) are included in the medium-risk group. High-risk patients are identified by declining renal function and/or by persistent severe proteinuria (8 g/day) or more despite optimal conservative management.

Observation of patients for the evolution of time-dependent prognostic factors is recommended for some, but not all, cases of idiopathic membranous nephropathy. Patients who present with combinations of ominous time-independent features (including impaired renal function and/or very severe proteinuria [>10 g/day]) should be considered for treatment without prolonged observation in an effort to reduce the risks of irreversible renal parenchymal injury as well as cardiovascular and thromboembolic complications of the nephrotic syndrome. Quantification of specific urinary proteins at presentation may enhance predictions of clinical outcomes and obviate the need for extended observation before recommending immunosuppressive therapy. Bazzi and colleagues[20] showed that levels of urinary IgG and α_1-microglobulin were significantly associated with the probabilities of remission and progression and could identify those most likely to benefit from immunosuppressive therapy. Branten and colleagues[21] have confirmed and extended these observations. They have also shown that previously established cutoff values for urinary β_2-microglobulin and IgG excretion are useful predictors of renal insufficiency in patients with membranous nephropathy. It will be important to continue to study the predictive value of these and other urinary markers in diverse populations of patients with membranous nephropathy.

CLINICAL TRIALS AND SPECIFIC RECOMMENDATIONS

General Strategy

Patients with membranous nephropathy should be treated with doses of ACE inhibitors and/or ARBs that have been titrated to reduce proteinuria as much as possible and to achieve optimal blood pressure control without excessive increases in serum creatinine and/or potassium.[22] Whereas the response to ACE inhibitors is not consistent in this population, modulation of intrarenal hemodynamic parameters may decrease proteinuria by as much as 50%[23–25] and may decrease the risk of progressive glomerulosclerosis as well. A meta-analysis of 11 randomized, controlled trials showed that ACE inhibitors reduced the risk of progressive renal function deterioration in patients with nondiabetic kidney disease after statistical adjustment for levels of systolic blood pressure and proteinuria.[26] The analysis also showed that the risk of kidney disease progression was lowest in patients whose systolic blood pressure was controlled in the range of 110 to 129 mm Hg and whose protein excretion rate was less than 2 g/day at follow-up visits. If these goals cannot be achieved with an ACE inhibitor, the combination of an ACE inhibitor and an ARB may be beneficial.[27] In a randomized, controlled trial that included 336 patients with nondiabetic renal disease, Nakao and colleagues[28] showed that the combination of an ACE inhibitor and an ARB decreased proteinuria and protected renal function more effectively than either drug alone. The risk of hyperkalemia was not increased by combination therapy compared with ACE inhibitor monotherapy. The ACE inhibitor and ARB monotherapy arms appeared to be equally effective. The incidence of hyperkalemia and nonproductive cough was lowest in the ARB monotherapy group, so ARBs appear to be a reasonable alternative for patients with membranous nephropathy who cannot tolerate ACE inhibitors. Studies in other populations of nephrotic patients suggest that a low-protein diet may augment the hemodynamic effect of blocking the renin-angiotensin system.[29]

It is important to address coronary risk factors in patients with the nephrotic syndrome.[30] Whereas ACE inhibitors may decrease proteinuria and partially correct hyperlipidemia,[31] specific lipid-lowering agents are often indicated as well. 3-Hydroxy-3-methylglutaryl coenzyme A reductase inhibitors are widely used for this purpose and typically lead to 30% to 45% decreases in low-density lipoprotein cholesterol.[32–34]

Concern for the morbidity and mortality associated with pulmonary embolism has led to interest in the possible role of prophylactic anticoagulation for patients with severe nephrotic syndrome due to membranous nephropathy (serum albumin < 2.0–2.5 g/dL).[11] By decision analysis, the risks of life-threatening complications of pulmonary embolism appear to outweigh those associated with prophylactic anticoagulation.[10] However, data from prospective, randomized clinical trials are not available to support this approach.

Patients with membranous nephropathy should be carefully evaluated and started on an individualized regimen of conservative therapies directed at the symptoms and risks of the nephrotic syndrome. Unless there are pressing indications to start immunosuppression sooner, patients should be followed for at least a month on a stable regimen of ACE inhibitors and/or ARBs to assess the response to this intervention. Cattran[8] recommends observation for 6 months on conservative therapies to clarify whether the patient needs immunosuppressive treatment; immunosuppression should start sooner in high-risk patients who manifest declining renal function or other serious complications. It is generally agreed that patients who have low-grade proteinuria (<3.5 or 4 g/day) and normal renal function after the initial assessment and conservative interventions have a low risk of renal function deterioration and should be followed without immunosuppression. At the opposite end of the clinical spectrum, there is consensus that patients with the nephrotic syndrome and declining renal function due to membranous nephropathy should receive immunosuppressive agents.[5,8,13]

Treatment for patients with normal renal function and nephrotic proteinuria has prompted an interesting debate. Some investigators have recommended that immunosuppressive treatments should only be used in patients who develop renal insufficiency or severe intolerable nephrotic syndrome (persistent proteinuria ≥ 8 g/day).[5,35,36] Others have recommended that patients with nephrotic proteinuria (>3.5 or 4 g/day) despite conservative measures should receive immunosuppressive agents.[8,13] Torres and colleagues[35] identified 19 patients with nephrotic proteinuria plus the recent onset of renal insufficiency (serum creatinine ≥ 1.5 mg/dL) and treated them with oral prednisone for 6 months accompanied by chlorambucil (0.15 mg/kg/day) for the first 14 weeks. At the end of follow-up (average 52 months), only 36% were in a complete or partial remission. The probability of renal survival was 90% at 7 years compared with 20% for a group of historical controls who had been managed conservatively. du Buf-Vereijken and colleagues[37] treated 65 patients with renal insufficiency (serum creatinine > 1.5 mg/dL or > 50% increase in serum creatinine) with cyclophosphamide (1.5–2.0 mg/kg/day) for 1 year and concurrent corticosteroids (1 g/day IV methylprednisolone for

3 days at the beginning of the first, third, and fifth months plus prednisone 0.5 mg/kg every other day for the first 6 months). At the end of follow-up (average 51 months), 72% were in a complete or partial remission. Renal survival was 74% at 7 years. Treatment-related complications were reported in 66% of patients, mainly due to bone marrow depression and infection. These studies illustrate the concern that delaying immunosuppressive therapy until renal dysfunction has evolved may decrease the probability of remission and increase the risk of treatment-related complications. In a recent review, du Buf-Vereijken and colleagues[5] indicate that the threshold serum creatinine value of 1.5 mg/dL typically indicates significant renal function impairment, especially in elderly patients. They now seek to start immunosuppression earlier (at lower serum creatinine values) in high-risk patients by estimating the glomerular filtration rate based on the Modification of Diet in Renal Disease study equations and by assessing other prognostic factors such urinary β_2-microglobulin and IgG. Considering that an increased serum creatinine and chronic histologic changes indicate a poor prognosis, moderate- to high-risk patients should be identified as efficiently as possible before the patient experiences an irreversible loss of renal function reserve or serious complications of the nephrotic syndrome.

Nephrotic Syndrome without Renal Insufficiency

The value of alternate-day oral glucocorticoid monotherapy has been studied in three randomized controlled trials.[38–40] Corticosteroids alone failed to increase the rate of long-term remissions of proteinuria in each of these controlled trials. Furthermore, corticosteroids appeared to prevent deterioration in renal function only in the U.S. collaborative trial; the apparent efficacy of corticosteroid therapy in this study may reflect the unusually high incidence of adverse outcomes in the control group. The aggregate impression is that corticosteroid monotherapy offers only marginal benefits, if any. Consequently, investigators have sought to identify alternative immunosuppressive drug regimens that might be more beneficial. Several studies support the value of cytotoxic drug regimens that combine corticosteroids with either chlorambucil or cyclophosphamide for the treatment of patients with idiopathic membranous nephropathy, nephrotic syndrome, and well-preserved renal function (Table 21-1).

Chlorambucil

The most convincing evidence has emerged from the multicenter, prospective, randomized clinical trials of Ponticelli and colleagues.[41–44] They have shown that a 6-month regimen of alternate-month corticosteroids and chlorambucil decreases the risk of deterioration in renal function as well as the duration of the nephrotic syndrome. Ten-year renal survival was 92% in the treatment group compared with 60% among the controls.[44] The recommendation to employ chlorambucil and methylprednisolone for this subset of patients is supported by well-controlled clinical observations. However, a substantial number of patients are unable to tolerate the regimen. Ponticelli and colleagues[44] reported that 4 of 42 patients in one study had to discontinue this therapy because of adverse effects (two because of peptic ulcers that developed while on methylprednisolone, one because of pneumonia, and one

Table 21-1 Selected Randomized, Controlled Trials of Cytotoxic Drug Therapies and Calcineurin Inhibitors

Ref.	Baseline	Treatment	Outcome
Alternate-Month Corticosteroid and Cytotoxic Drug Therapy			
Ponticelli et al[41,42,44]	Plasma creatinine < 150 μmol/L; proteinuria > 3.5 g/day	Methylprednisolone alternating monthly with chlorambucil (N = 42) vs. control (N = 39) for 6 mo	Treatment favored remission of nephrotic syndrome and preservation of renal function
Ponticelli et al[43]	Plasma creatinine < 150 μmol/L; proteinuria > 3.5 g/day	Methylprednisolone alternating monthly with chlorambucil (N = 45) vs. methylprednisolone alone (N = 47) for 6 mo	Combination drug regimen associated with earlier remission of the nephrotic syndrome
Ponticelli et al[45]	Plasma creatinine < 150 μmol/L; proteinuria > 3.5 g/day	Methylprednisolone alternating monthly with either chlorambucil (N = 50) or cyclophosphamide (N = 45) for 6 mo	Regimens were equally effective in inducing remission of the nephrotic syndrome and preserving renal function
Reichert et al[62]	Nephrotic syndrome and deteriorating renal function	Methylprednisolone alternating monthly with chlorambucil (N = 9) vs. monthly pulse cyclophosphamide and pulse methylprednisolone every 2 mo (N = 9) for 6 mo	Renal function improved on chlorambucil regimen but not on pulse cyclophosphamide
Jha et al[46]	Nephrotic syndrome ≥ 6 mo; average MDRD GFR > 80 mL/min	Methylprednisolone alternating monthly with cyclophosphamide (N = 47) vs. control (N = 46) for 6 mo	Treatment favored remission of nephrotic syndrome and preservation of renal function
Calcineurin Inhibitors			
Cattran et al[75]	Declining renal function; persistent proteinuria ≥ 3.5 g/day	Cyclosporine (N = 9) vs. placebo (N = 8)	Average proteinuria and rate of renal function deterioration were decreased in the cyclosporine group, but not the placebo group
Cattran et al[48]	Creatinine clearance ≥ 42 mL/min/1.73 m²; nephrotic-range proteinuria despite at least 8 wk of prednisone ≥ 1 mg/kg/day	Cyclosporine + low-dose prednisone (N = 28) vs. placebo (N = 23) + low-dose prednisone	Complete or partial remissions of proteinuria in 75% of the cyclosporine group and 22% of the placebo group; relapse occurred after 50% of remissions
Praga et al[52]	Nephrotic syndrome ≥ 9 mo; Cockroft-Gault eGFR ≥ 50 mL/min/1.73 m²	Tacrolimus monotherapy (N = 25) vs. control (N = 23) for 18 mo	Treatment favored remission of nephrotic syndrome and preservation of renal function

Cockroft-Gault eGFR, estimated glomerular filtration rate by the Cockroft-Gault formula; MDRD GFR, glomerular filtration rate calculated by the Modification of Diet in Renal Disease study formula.

because of gastric intolerance to chlorambucil). The potential advantage of this approach must be balanced against the risks of malignancy, gonadal toxicity, reversible myelosuppression, infection, gastrointestinal intolerance, and hepatotoxicity associated with chlorambucil. Furthermore, patients should be informed that the long-term toxicities of this and other cytotoxic drug regimens for membranous nephropathy have not been fully defined.

Cyclophosphamide

Because most nephrologists are more familiar with cyclophosphamide than chlorambucil, Ponticelli and colleagues[45] conducted a multicenter controlled clinical trial to compare the efficacy and toxicity of these two alkylating agents when alternated with corticosteroids for the treatment of idiopathic membranous nephropathy. The two regimens appeared to be equally effective, and both are recommended for the treatment of this subset of patients (Box 21-1). The authors observed a complete or partial remission of nephrotic syndrome in 82% of patients in the chlorambucil group and 93% of patients in the cyclophosphamide group. Approximately 30% of patients in each group experienced a relapse between 6 and 30 months after stopping treatment. Renal function tended to improve and then stabilize in both treatment groups. Notably, fewer patients stopped therapy prematurely because of adverse events in the cyclophosphamide group (4.5%) than in the chlorambucil group (12%).

More recently, Jha and colleagues[46] reported a randomized, controlled trial comparing a 6-month regimen of alternate-month prednisolone and cyclophosphamide to supportive treatment in adults with the nephrotic syndrome for at least 6 months. Remissions occurred significantly more frequently in the treatment group (72%) compared with the controls (35%). The 10-year dialysis-free survival rate was 89% in treated patients compared with 65% in controls ($P = .016$). Thus, cytotoxic drug therapy in this study appears to be associated with a renal survival advantage that is comparable with that observed by Ponticelli and colleagues.[44] Although these prospective, controlled trials provide evidence that cytotoxic drug therapy is more effective than supportive treatments or corticosteroids alone, Ponticelli and colleagues[47] report that patients randomized to a potentially less toxic regimen of synthetic corticotropin therapy experienced outcomes comparable with those seen in the patients randomized to cytotoxic drugs. This observation underscores the need for additional randomized, controlled trials to compare the efficacy and toxicity of cytotoxic drugs with those of other regimens described in this chapter.

Calcineurin Inhibitors

A randomized clinical trial reported by Cattran and colleagues[48] compared a 6-month course of cyclosporine with placebo in 51 patients with steroid-resistant idiopathic membranous nephropathy, nephrotic-range proteinuria, and a creatinine clearance of at least 42 mL/min/1.73 m². Adverse effects of cyclosporine included reversible decline in renal function, an increased occurrence and severity of hypertension, and nausea. Two patients in each group progressed to renal insufficiency, defined as a doubling of serum creatinine. A complete or partial remission of proteinuria evolved by week 26 in 75% of the cyclosporine group and 22% of the control group ($P < .001$). By week 72, relapse occurred in approximately 40% of patients in each group. The authors questioned whether the high relapse rate observed in this study was related to the dose (3.5 mg/kg/day) or the duration of treatment (6 months rather than 1 year).

Fritsche and colleagues[49] analyzed data from the German Cyclosporine in Nephrotic Syndrome Study Group in an effort to estimate the optimal duration of cyclosporine therapy for idiopathic membranous nephropathy. They observed that complete remissions occurred up to 20 months after starting cyclosporine; the median treatment period before a complete remission was 225 days in this study. At present, there is insufficient information to determine the optimal duration of cyclosporine therapy for idiopathic membranous nephropathy. The high-risk characteristics of these patients justify a 6- to 12-month course of cyclosporine if the patient can be followed very closely (initially weekly, then biweekly). The risk of chronic cyclosporine nephrotoxicity can be decreased by initiating treatment at 3 mg/kg/day or less[50] and by frequent dose adjustments to avoid clinical and laboratory signs of toxicity. Once a complete or partial remission of proteinuria has been achieved, it is reasonable to taper the dose to approximately 1 to 1.5 mg/kg/day in an effort to maintain remission with a lower risk of nephrotoxicity. Alexopoulos and colleagues[51] observed that relapses occurred significantly more often among patients on low-dose cyclosporine monotherapy compared with those on combination low-dose cyclosporine and prednisolone. Cyclosporine trough levels less than 100 ng/mL appeared to increase the risk of relapse. Most relapses responded to a temporary increase in cyclosporine and/or prednisolone dose.

Recently, Praga and colleagues[52] reported a randomized, controlled trial evaluating tacrolimus monotherapy in patients with Cockroft-Gault estimated glomerular filtration rate of 50 mL/min/1.73 m² or more and the nephrotic syndrome for

---

Box 21-1 Proposed Immunosuppressive Treatments for Idiopathic Membranous Nephropathy: Nephrotic Syndrome without Renal Insufficiency

Recommended Approaches

Alternate-month corticosteroids and cyclophosphamide for 6 months
  Months 1, 3, and 5: methylprednisolone 1 g/day IV for 3 days followed by 0.4 to 0.5 mg/kg/day orally for 27 days
  Months 2, 4, and 6: cyclophosphamide 2.0 to 2.5 mg/kg/day (initial dose) orally for 30 days
Alternate-month corticosteroids and chlorambucil for 6 months
  Months 1, 3, and 5: methylprednisolone (as above)
  Months 2, 4, and 6: chlorambucil 0.2 mg/kg/day (initial dose) orally for 30 days

Alternative Approaches

Cyclosporine 3.5 mg/kg/day in two divided doses (initial dose) and low-dose prednisone for 6 to 12 months
Tacrolimus monotherapy 0.05 mg/kg/day in two divided doses (initial dose), initial target trough 3 to 5 ng/mL, increase target trough to 5 to 8 ng/mL if remission not achieved within 2 months
Mycophenolate mofetil 1 to 2 g/day in two to three divided doses for 6 to 24 months; attempt to taper off corticosteroids
Synthetic corticotropin 1 mg IM every other week (initial dose), gradually increase to 1 mg IM twice weekly for 1 year (see Ponticelli and colleagues[47] and Berg and colleagues[79])
Rituximab four weekly intravenous infusions of 375 mg/m²

at least 9 months despite treatment with maximally tolerated doses of ACE inhibitors or ARBs. The tacrolimus target trough was initially 3 to 5 ng/mL and was increased to 5 to 8 ng/mL after 2 months if the patient was persistently nephrotic. After treatment for 12 months, tacrolimus was tapered off over 6 months. The patients treated with tacrolimus were significantly more likely than controls to achieve a remission by 18 months (94% vs. 35%) and to have stable renal function. No patient in the tacrolimus group had a nephrotic relapse during drug tapering, but 47% had a relapse on average 4 months after tacrolimus was withdrawn.

Mycophenolate Mofetil

Several case series have described mycophenolate mofetil (MMF) treatment for patients who had previously failed to achieve a satisfactory response on corticosteroids, cytotoxic drugs, and/or cyclosporine. Miller and colleagues[53] treated 16 nephrotic patients and observed a 50% decrease in proteinuria in six patients and a sustained partial remission in two patients. MMF was discontinued due to adverse events in two patients (one had persistent diarrhea and the other had varicella-zoster infection). Choi and colleagues[54] treated 17 patients and reported that 2 achieved a complete remission and 8 had a partial remission. Corticosteroids and cyclosporine were successfully withdrawn in 14 of 15 patients who had been steroid or cyclosporine dependent. MMF was discontinued in three patients because of adverse events (severe erosive gastritis, pneumonia, and squamous cell cancer). Additional study is needed to determine the role of MMF in this condition.

Rituximab

Remuzzi and colleagues[55] and Ruggenenti and colleagues[56,57] have described an innovative approach using rituximab (375 mg/m^2 infusions weekly for 4 weeks) to treat patients with the nephrotic syndrome for at least 6 months despite ACE inhibitor therapy. The average protein excretion rate decreased significantly from 9.1 g/day to 4.6 g/day in eight patients with mild or no chronic tubulointerstitial lesions but did not improve significantly in six patients with more severe chronic histologic changes. The authors recommend a prospective trial to compare the efficacy and toxicity of rituximab with other less specific immunosuppressive treatments in patients with mild or no chronic tubulointerstitial changes.

Nephrotic Syndrome with Renal Insufficiency

Several immunosuppressive drug regimens have been proposed for the treatment of nephrotic patients with impaired and declining renal function (Box 21-2); none is clearly superior. Pulse methylprednisolone regimens have yielded favorable short-term outcomes in some patients, but long-term outcomes have been less satisfactory.[58] Combining corticosteroids and azathioprine has led to inconsistent results in this population of patients.[59–61]

Chlorambucil

Although there is considerable experience using alternate-month corticosteroids and chlorambucil for patients with well-preserved renal function, efforts to apply this regimen to patients with a decreased glomerular filtration rate have met with discordant results and a relatively high incidence of adverse events. To address this issue, modified dose schedules have been studied for azotemic patients[62–65] and for elderly patients who are likely to have impaired renal functional reserve.[66,67] A decreased dose of chlorambucil (~0.12 mg/kg/day) appears to ameliorate toxicity in patients with impaired renal function.[68] Concerns regarding the toxicity of corticosteroids in these patients has led several investigators to omit pulse methylprednisolone or to use alternate-day rather than daily oral prednisolone. Because the aggregate experience suggests that intravenous pulse methylprednisolone may contribute to favorable short-term outcomes in patients with declining renal function,[58,64,65] 0.5- to 1-g doses of pulse methylprednisolone are recommended rather than omitting this component of the therapy (see Box 21-2).

Cyclophosphamide

Several regimens that combine corticosteroids and cyclophosphamide may be considered for the treatment of nephrotic patients with impaired renal function (see Box 21-2). There is evidence that cyclophosphamide can be substituted

---

Box 21-2 Proposed Immunosuppressive Treatments for Idiopathic Membranous Nephropathy: Nephrotic Syndrome with Renal Insufficiency

Recommended Approaches

Cyclosporine 3.5 mg/kg/day in two divided doses (initial dose) for 12 months

Alternate-month corticosteroids and cyclophosphamide for 6 months

> Months 1, 3, and 5: methylprednisolone 0.5 to 1.0 g/day IV for 3 days followed by 0.4 mg/kg/day (or 1 mg/kg every other day) orally for 27 days

> Months 2, 4, and 6: cyclophosphamide 1.5 to 2.0 mg/kg/day (initial dose) orally for 30 days

Alternate-month corticosteroids and chlorambucil for 6 months

> Months 1, 3, and 5: methylprednisolone (as above)

> > Months 2, 4, and 6: chlorambucil 0.12 mg/kg/day (initial dose) orally for 30 days

Alternative Approaches

Cyclophosphamide 1.5 to 2 mg/kg/day (initial dose) for 1 year plus prednisone 0.5 mg/kg every other day for 2 to 6 months, then taper to 0.25 mg/kg every other day for the duration of therapy; consider methylprednisolone 1 g/day IV for 3 days at the beginning of months 1, 3, and 5

Mycophenolate mofetil 0.5 to 2 g/day in two to three divided doses plus low-dose prednisone for 6 to 12 months

for chlorambucil in the regimen of Ponticelli and colleagues for patients with well-preserved renal function, but this approach has not been rigorously evaluated in patients with impaired and declining renal function. Intuitively, this appears to be a reasonable (but unproven) approach given the extensive experience employing cyclophosphamide for the treatment of severe glomerular diseases and the relatively brief (3 months) exposure to a cytotoxic drug in the regimen of Ponticelli and colleagues.

Alternatively, several groups[37,69–72] have studied daily oral cyclophosphamide and corticosteroids for a year or more in patients with declining renal function. Renal function stabilized or improved and at least partial remissions of nephrotic proteinuria were observed in most patients treated by investigators in the Netherlands,[37] Toronto,[69,70] and Pittsburgh.[71] These results were superior to those observed among concurrent (nonrandomized) control subjects,[69,70] but serious complications of treatment were observed including leukopenia, infections, amenorrhea, and cancer. Extended oral cyclophosphamide regimens for the treatment of Wegener's granulomatosis have been associated with an 11-fold increase in the incidence of lymphomas and a 33-fold increase in bladder cancers.[73]

In an effort to reduce the toxicity of cytotoxic drug regimens, several investigators have evaluated intermittent pulse regimens of cyclophosphamide and methylprednisolone for high-risk patients with progressive disease. Falk and colleagues[74] observed that an intensive regimen of monthly pulse cyclophosphamide (for 6 months), pulse methylprednisolone (for 3 days), and alternate-day prednisone (starting at 1 mg/kg) was not superior to alternate-day prednisone alone (starting at 2 mg/kg) for patients with deteriorating renal function or persistent proteinuria associated with morbid complications.

A few prospective studies have compared cytotoxic drug regimens for the treatment of patients with nephrotic syndrome and declining renal function. Reichert and colleagues[62] showed that a 6-month regimen of alternate-month methylprednisolone and chlorambucil was more effective than a 6-month regimen of monthly pulse cyclophosphamide and alternate-month pulse methylprednisolone. Branten and colleagues[72] reported that daily oral cyclophosphamide and corticosteroids for 1 year was more effective than alternate-month methylprednisolone and chlorambucil for 6 months. Stable renal function and remissions of proteinuria were observed more frequently after cyclophosphamide treatment for 1 year. Treatment was modified, interrupted, or terminated prematurely because of adverse effects significantly more frequently in the chlorambucil group than in the cyclophosphamide group. Although 60% of the patients were randomly assigned to their treatment groups, this was a complex study in which some patients were not randomized concurrently and others not randomized at all. Additional studies are needed to compare the risks and benefits of various cytotoxic drug regimens for nephrotic patients with declining renal function.

Cyclosporine

Future studies should include comparisons of the long-term efficacy and toxicity of cyclosporine and cytotoxic drug regimens. There has been interest in cyclosporine for patients with idiopathic membranous nephropathy, persistent nephrotic-range proteinuria, and declining renal function since Cattran and colleagues[75] reported the results of a controlled clinical trial in which 17 patients with these characteristics were randomized to receive either cyclosporine (initially 3.5 mg/kg/day in two divided doses) or placebo for 12 months. Proteinuria and the rate of decline in creatinine clearance decreased significantly in the cyclosporine group (but not in the placebo group). Improvement in renal function and proteinuria was sustained in 75% of patients for a mean follow-up period of 21 months after cyclosporine was discontinued. Six of the nine cyclosporine-treated patients experienced elevations in serum creatinine ($\geq$30%) that reversed in five after a decrease in dose. Cyclosporine-treated patients also tended to require additional antihypertensive medication to maintain adequate blood pressure control. Geddes and Cattran[76] have recommended cyclosporine as preferred immunosuppressive therapy for patients with high-grade proteinuria and renal insufficiency. Conversely, Ponticelli and Villa[77] have underscored the nephrotoxic potential of cyclosporine and have suggested that patients with impaired renal function (creatinine clearance < 60 mL/min), severe hypertension, or severe interstitial fibrosis and tubular atrophy should not receive cyclosporine.

SUMMARY

Clearly, the optimal immunosuppressive therapy for patients with persistent high-grade proteinuria and renal insufficiency has not been determined. Meta-analyses published to date do not resolve this issue.[12,78] New studies[46,52] have been reported since those meta-analyses were performed, so this discussion focuses on data from individual studies, especially randomized, controlled trials. Box 21-2 depicts several recommended treatments. Although the recommendation to offer cyclosporine to patients with impaired renal function has been debated,[76,77] evidence supporting this approach includes a small, randomized, controlled clinical trial.[75] Toxicities are largely reversible if the cyclosporine dose is adjusted in response to early signs of toxicity detected by very close follow-up of these patients. Studies supporting the use of alternate-month corticosteroid and cytotoxic drug therapy in patients with renal dysfunction include a small, randomized, controlled clinical trial[62] and several uncontrolled case series.[63–65,68] Renal function has tended to improve or stabilize at least transiently, and toxicity has been modulated by dose reduction. Alternative cytotoxic drug regimens have been studied as well. Intermittent pulse cyclophosphamide has not proven to be effective.[62,74] Daily oral cyclophosphamide and corticosteroids for 1 year or more have been employed as salvage therapy for patients with progressive renal failure. Evidence supporting this approach includes a nonrandomized trial with concurrent controls,[69,70] a clinical study that included randomized and nonrandomized patients,[72] and uncontrolled case series.[37,71] Although Branten and colleagues[72] noted fewer short-term adverse effects among patients receiving daily oral cyclophosphamide and corticosteroids for 1 year than among those treated with alternate-month chlorambucil and corticosteroids for 6 months, it is the long-term toxicities of extended courses of daily oral cytotoxic drug therapy that prompt the greatest concern. Thus, an extended course of daily oral cyclophosphamide and corticosteroids should be reserved for patients manifesting progressive renal insufficiency who understand and accept the potential long-term toxicities of this approach.

At present, the choice of cyclosporine, cytotoxic drug therapy, or no immunosuppression should reflect the priorities of the individual patient as well as comorbid conditions that might affect the risk profile of each approach. Furthermore, attention should be focused on the comprehensive management of cardiovascular risk factors that are frequently observed in this population of patients. Modulation of non-immunologic factors that influence the rate of progression of chronic renal disease are likely to contribute to quality of life and to extend survival by delaying the need for dialysis. Thus, dietary modifications, diuretics, ACE inhibitors, angiotensin II receptor antagonists, and lipid-lowering agents are important therapeutic interventions that should be considered in all patients with membranous nephropathy to decrease the morbidity and mortality associated with the nephrotic syndrome.

References

1. Haas M, Meehan SM, Karrison TG, Spargo BH: Changing etiologies of unexplained adult nephrotic syndrome: A comparison of renal biopsy findings from 1976–1979 and 1995–1997. Am J Kidney Dis 1997;30:621–631.
2. Schena FP: Survey of the Italian Registry of Renal Biopsies. Frequency of the renal diseases for 7 consecutive years. The Italian Group of Renal Immunopathology. Nephrol Dial Transplant 1997;12:418–426.
3. Falk RJ, Jennette JC, Nachman PH: Primary glomerular diseases. In Brenner BM (ed): The Kidney, 7th ed. Philadelphia: WB Saunders, 2004, pp 1293–1380.
4. Glassock RJ: Secondary membranous glomerulonephritis. Nephrol Dial Transplant 1992;7(Suppl 1):64–71.
5. du Buf-Vereijken PWG, Branten AJW, Wetzels JFM: Idiopathic membranous nephropathy: Outline and rationale of a treatment strategy. Am J Kidney Dis 2005;46:1012–1029.
6. Cattran DC, Pei Y, Greenwood C: Predicting progression in membranous glomerulonephritis. Nephrol Dial Transplant 1992;7(Suppl 1):48–52.
7. Glassock RJ: Diagnosis and natural course of membranous nephropathy. Semin Nephrol 2003;23:324–332.
8. Cattran D: Management of membranous nephropathy: When and what for treatment. J Am Soc Nephrol 2005;16:1188–1194.
9. Ordonez JD, Hiatt RA, Killebrew EJ, et al: The increased risk of coronary heart disease associated with nephrotic syndrome. Kidney Int 1993;44:638–642.
10. Sarasin FP, Schifferli JA: Prophylactic oral anticoagulation in nephrotic patients with idiopathic membranous nephropathy. Kidney Int 1994;45:578–585.
11. Glassock RJ: Prophylactic anticoagulation in nephrotic syndrome: A clinical conundrum. J Am Soc Nephrol 2007;18:2221–2225.
12. Hogan SL, Muller KE, Jennette JC, et al: A review of therapeutic studies of idiopathic membranous glomerulopathy. Am J Kidney Dis 1995;25:862–875.
13. Ponticelli C: Membranous nephropathy. J Nephrol 2007;20:268–287.
14. Neugarten J, Acharya A, Silbiger SR: Effect of gender on the progression of nondiabetic renal disease: A meta-analysis. J Am Soc Nephrol 2000;11:319–329.
15. Zent R, Nagai R, Cattran DC: Idiopathic membranous nephropathy in the elderly: A comparative study. Am J Kidney Dis 1997;29:200–206.
16. Troyanov S, Roasio L, Pandes M, et al: Renal pathology in idiopathic membranous nephropathy: A new perspective. Kidney Int 2006;69:1641–1648.
17. Davison AM, Cameron JS, Kerr DNS, et al: The natural history of renal function in untreated idiopathic membranous glomerulonephritis in adults. Clin Nephrol 1984;22:61–67.
18. Pei Y, Cattran D, Greenwood C: Predicting chronic renal insufficiency in idiopathic membranous glomerulonephritis. Kidney Int 1992;42:960–966.
19. Cattran DC, Pei Y, Greenwood CMT, et al: Validation of a predictive model of idiopathic membranous nephropathy: Its clinical and research implications. Kidney Int 1997;51:901–907.
20. Bazzi C, Petrini C, Rizza V, et al: Urinary excretion of IgG and α1—microglobulin predicts clinical course better than extent of proteinuria in membranous nephropathy. Am J Kidney Dis 2001;38:240–248.
21. Branten AJW, du Buf-Vereijken PW, Klasen IS, et al: Urinary excretion of β2-microglobulin and IgG predict prognosis in idiopathic membranous nephropathy: A validation study. J Am Soc Nephrol 2005;16:169–174.
22. Schieppati A, Ruggenenti P, Perna A, Remuzzi G: Nonimmunosuppressive therapy of membranous nephropathy. Semin Nephrol 2003;23:333–339.
23. Thomas DM, Hillis AN, Coles GA, et al: Enalapril can treat the proteinuria of membranous glomerulonephritis without detriment to systemic or renal hemodynamics. Am J Kidney Dis 1991;18:38–43.
24. Gansevoort RT, Heeg JE, Vriesendorp R, et al: Antiproteinuric drugs in patients with idiopathic membranous glomerulopathy. Nephrol Dial Transplant 1992;7(Suppl 1):91–96.
25. Ruggenenti P, Mosconi L, Vendramin G, et al: ACE inhibition improves glomerular size selectivity in patients with idiopathic membranous nephropathy and persistent nephrotic syndrome. Am J Kidney Dis 2000;35:381–391.
26. Jafar TH, Stark PC, Schmid CH, et al: Progression of chronic kidney disease: The role of blood pressure control, proteinuria, and angiotensin-converting enzyme inhibition. A patient-level meta-analysis. Ann Intern Med 2003;139:244–252.
27. Wolf G, Ritz E: Combination therapy with ACE inhibitors and angiotensin II receptor blockers to halt progression of chronic renal disease: Pathophysiology and indications. Kidney Int 2005;67:799–812.
28. Nakao N, Yoshimura A, Morita H, et al: Combination treatment of angiotensin-II receptor blocker and angiotensin-converting-enzyme inhibitor in non-diabetic renal disease (COOPERATE): A randomized controlled trial. Lancet 2003;361:117–124.
29. Ruilope LM, Casal MC, Praga M, et al: Additive antiproteinuric effect of converting enzyme inhibition and a low dose protein intake. J Am Soc Nephrol 1992;3:1307–1311.
30. Radhakrishnan J, Appel AS, Valeri A, et al: The nephrotic syndrome, lipids, and risk factors for cardiovascular disease. Am J Kidney Dis 1993;22:135–142.
31. Ruggenenti P, Mise N, Pisoni R, et al: Diverse effects of increasing lisinopril doses on lipid abnormalities in chronic nephropathies. Circulation 2003;107:586–592.
32. Golper TA, Illingworth DR, Morris CD, et al: Lovastatin in the treatment of multifactorial hyperlipidemia associated with proteinuria. Am J Kidney Dis 1989;13:312–320.
33. Spitalewitz S, Porush JG, Cattran D, et al: Treatment of hyperlipidemia in the nephrotic syndrome: The effects of pravastatin therapy. Am J Kidney Dis 1993;22:143–150.
34. Thomas ME, Harris KPG, Ramaswamy C, et al: Simvastatin therapy for hypercholesterolemic patients with nephrotic syndrome or significant proteinuria. Kidney Int 1993;44:1124–1129.
35. Torres A, Domínguez-Gil B, Carreno A, et al: Conservative versus immunosuppressive treatment of patients with idiopathic membranous nephropathy. Kidney Int 2002;61:219–227.
36. du Buf-Vereijken PWG, Feith GW, Hollander D, et al, Membranous Nephropathy Study Group: Restrictive use of immunosuppressive treatment in patients with idiopathic membranous

nephropathy: High renal survival in a large patient cohort. Q J Med 2004;97:353–360.

37. du Buf-Vereijken PWG, Branten AJW, Wetzels JFM: Cytotoxic therapy for membranous nephropathy and renal insufficiency; improved renal survival but high relapse rate. Nephrol Dial Transplant 2004;19:1142–1148.

38. Collaborative Study of the Adult Idiopathic Nephrotic Syndrome: A controlled study of short-term prednisone treatment in adults with membranous nephropathy. N Engl J Med 1979;301:1301–1306.

39. Cattran DC, Delmore T, Roscoe J, et al: A randomized controlled trial of prednisone in patients with idiopathic membranous nephropathy. N Engl J Med 1989;320:210–215.

40. Cameron JS, Healy MJR, Adu D: The Medical Research Council Trial of short-term high-dose alternate day prednisolone in idiopathic membranous nephropathy with nephrotic syndrome in adults. Q J Med 1990;74:133–156.

41. Ponticelli C, Zucchelli P, Passerini P, et al: A randomized trial of methylprednisolone and chlorambucil in idiopathic membranous nephropathy. N Engl J Med 1989;320:8–13.

42. Ponticelli C, Zucchelli P, Imbasciati E, et al: Controlled trial of methylprednisolone and chlorambucil in idiopathic membranous nephropathy. N Engl J Med 1984;310:946–950.

43. Ponticelli C, Zucchelli P, Passerini P, et al: Methylprednisolone plus chlorambucil as compared with methylprednisolone alone for the treatment of idiopathic membranous nephropathy. N Engl J Med 1992;327:599–603.

44. Ponticelli C, Zucchelli P, Passerini P, et al: A 10-year follow-up of a randomized study with methylprednisolone and chlorambucil in membranous nephropathy. Kidney Int 1995;48:1600–1604.

45. Ponticelli C, Altieri P, Scolar F, et al: A randomized study comparing methylprednisolone plus chlorambucil versus methylprednisolone plus cyclophosphamide in idiopathic membranous nephropathy. J Am Soc Nephrol 1998;9:444–450.

46. Jha V, Ganguli A, Saha TK, et al: A randomized, controlled trial of steroids and cyclophosphamide in adults with nephrotic syndrome caused by idiopathic membranous nephropathy. J Am Soc Nephrol 2007;18:1899–1904.

47. Ponticelli C, Passerini P, Salvadori M, et al: A randomized pilot trial comparing methylprednisolone plus a cytotoxic agent versus synthetic adrenocorticotropic hormone in idiopathic membranous nephropathy. Am J Kidney Dis 2006;47:233–240.

48. Cattran DC, Appel GB, Hebert LA, et al: Cyclosporine in patients with steroid-resistant membranous nephropathy: A randomized trial. Kidney Int 2001;59:1484–1490.

49. Fritsche L, Budde K, Farber L, et al: Treatment of membranous glomerulopathy with cyclosporin A: How much patience is required? Nephrol Dial Transplant 1999;14:1036–1038.

50. Bagnis CI, Du Montcel ST, Beaufils H, et al: Long-term renal effects of low-dose cyclosporine in uveitis-treated patients: Follow-up study. J Am Soc Nephrol 2002;13:2962–2968.

51. Alexopoulos E, Papagianni A, Tsamelashvili M, et al: Induction and long-term treatment with cyclosporine in membranous nephropathy with the nephrotic syndrome. Nephrol Dial Transplant 2006;21:3127–3132.

52. Praga M, Barrio V, Juárez GF, Luno J: Tacrolimus monotherapy in membranous nephropathy: A randomized controlled trial. Kidney Int 2007;71:924–930.

53. Miller G, Zimmerman R, Radhakrishnan J, et al: Use of mycophenolate mofetil in resistant membranous nephropathy. Am J Kidney Dis 2000;36:250–256.

54. Choi MJ, Eustace JA, Gimenez LF, et al: Mycophenolate mofetil treatment for primary glomerular diseases. Kidney Int 2002;61:1098–1114.

55. Remuzzi G, Chiurchiu C, Abbate M, et al: Rituximab for idiopathic membranous nephropathy. Lancet 2002;360:923–924.

56. Ruggenenti P, Chiurchiu C, Brusegan V, et al: Rituximab in idiopathic membranous nephropathy: A one-year prospective study. J Am Soc Nephrol 2003;14:1851–1857.

57. Ruggenenti P, Chiurchiu C, Abbate M, et al: Rituximab for idiopathic membranous nephropathy: Who can benefit? Clin J Am Soc Nephrol 2006;1:738–748.

58. Short CD, Solomon LR, Gokal R, et al: Methylprednisolone in patients with membranous nephropathy and declining renal function. Q J Med 1987;65:929–940.

59. Bone JM, Rostom R, Williams PS: "Progressive" versus "indolent" idiopathic membranous glomerulonephritis. Q J Med 1997;90:699–706.

60. Ahuja M, Goumenos D, Shortland JR, et al: Does immunosuppression with prednisolone and azathioprine alter the progression of idiopathic membranous nephropathy? Am J Kidney Dis 1999;34:521–529.

61. Brown JH, Douglas AF, Murphy BG, et al: Treatment of renal failure in idiopathic membranous nephropathy with azathioprine and prednisolone. Nephrol Dial Transplant 1998;13:443–448.

62. Reichert LJM, Huysmans FTM, Assmann K, et al: Preserving renal function in patients with membranous nephropathy: Daily oral chlorambucil compared with intermittent monthly pulses of cyclophosphamide. Ann Intern Med 1994;121:328–333.

63. Mathieson PW, Turner AN, Maidment CGH, et al: Prednisolone and chlorambucil treatment in idiopathic membranous nephropathy with deteriorating renal function. Lancet 1988;2:869–872.

64. Warwick GL, Geddes CC, Jones Boulton JM: Prednisolone and chlorambucil therapy for idiopathic membranous nephropathy with progressive renal failure. Q J Med 1994;87:223–229.

65. Brunkhorst R, Wrenger E, Koch KM: Low-dose prednisolone/chlorambucil therapy in patients with severe membranous glomerulonephritis. Clin Invest 1994;72:277–282.

66. Ponticelli C, Passerini P, Cresseri D: Primary glomerular diseases in the elderly. Glomerulonephritis in the elderly. Geriatr Nephrol Urol 1996;6:105–112.

67. Cameron JS: Nephrotic syndrome in the elderly. Semin Nephrol 1996;16:319–329.

68. Mathieson P: Treating progressive and indolent MGN. Q J Med 1998;91:167.

69. West ML, Jindal KK, Bear RA, et al: A controlled trial of cyclophosphamide in patients with membranous glomerulonephritis. Kidney Int 1987;32:579–584.

70. Jindal K, West M, Bear R, et al: Long-term benefits of therapy with cyclophosphamide and prednisone in patients with membranous glomerulonephritis and impaired renal function. Am J Kidney Dis 1992;19:61–67.

71. Bruns FJ, Adler S, Fraley DS, et al: Sustained remission of membranous glomerulonephritis after cyclophosphamide and prednisone. Ann Intern Med 1991;114:725–730.

72. Branten AJW, Reichert LJM, Koene RAP, et al: Oral cyclophosphamide versus chlorambucil in the treatment of patients with membranous nephropathy and renal insufficiency. Q J Med 1998;91:359–366.

73. Hoffman GS, Kerr GS, Leavitt RY, et al: Wegener granulomatosis: An analysis of 158 patients. Ann Intern Med 1992;116:488–498.

74. Falk RJ, Hogan SL, Muller KE, et al: Treatment of progressive membranous glomerulopathy. A randomized trial comparing cyclophosphamide and corticosteroids with corticosteroids alone. Ann Intern Med 1992;116:438–445.

75. Cattran DC, Greenwood C, Ritchie S, et al: A controlled trial of cyclosporine in patients with progressive membranous nephropathy. Kidney Int 1995;47:1130–1135.

76. Geddes CC, Cattran DC: The treatment of idiopathic membranous nephropathy. Semin Nephrol 2000;20:299–308.

77. Ponticelli C, Villa M: Does cyclosporin have a role in the treatment of membranous nephropathy? Nephrol Dial Transplant 1999;14:23–25.

78. Perna A, Schieppati A, Zamora J, et al: Immunosuppressive treatment for idiopathic membranous nephropathy: A systemic review. Am J Kidney Dis 2004;44:385–401.

79. Berg A-L, Nilsson-Ehle P, Arnadottir M: Beneficial effects of ACTH on the serum lipoprotein profile and glomerular function in patients with membranous nephropathy. Kidney Int 1999;56:1534–1543.

Further Reading

Cattran D: Management of Membranous Nephropathy: When and what for treatment. J Am Soc Nephrol 2005;16:1188–1194.

du Buf-Vereijken PWG, Branten AJW, Wetzels JFM: Idiopathic membranous nephropathy: Outline and rationale of a treatment strategy. Am J Kidney Dis 2005;46:1012–1029.

Glassock RJ: Diagnosis and natural course of membranous nephropathy. Semin Nephrol 2003;23:324–332.

Ponticelli C: Membranous nephropathy. J Nephrol 2007;20:268–287.

Schieppati A, Ruggenenti P, Perna A, Remuzzi G: Nonimmunosuppressive Therapy of Membranous Nephropathy. Semin Nephrol 2003;23:333–339.

Chapter 22

Idiopathic Membranoproliferative Glomerulonephritis

Peter Hewins, Richard J.H. Smith, and Caroline O.S. Savage

CHAPTER CONTENTS

NEW INSIGHTS INTO PATHOGENESIS AND RATIONAL BASIS FOR TREATMENT

Membranoproliferative glomerulonephritis (MPGN) is an uncommon disease, although its prevalence varies and is reportedly much higher in less prosperous countries.[1–5] It most often affects older children or young adults who present with acute nephritis, nephrosis, or abnormal urine analysis. Based on differences resolved by electron microscopy, three types of MPGN are recognized, a simple classification belying considerable etiologic heterogeneity. MPGN type 1 and some cases of MPGN type 3 are immune complex diseases and may be associated with infection, systemic lupus erythematosus, or malignancy, although in other instances, MPGN type 3 appears to be unrelated to immune complex deposition.[6–9] Serum complement profiles reflect classic pathway activation in at least some cases of MPGN types 1 and 3.[10,11] Interestingly, the incidence of MPGN type 1, the most common variant of the three, is decreasing in a number of countries for reasons that are unclear but may reflect changing patterns of infectious disease.[1,3,12] MPGN type 1 can be triggered by hepatitis C virus infection, an observation made primarily in Japan and the United States; this association is less frequent in some parts of Europe.[13,14] (See Chapter 14 for detailed discussion and treatment of hepatitis C virus–associated renal disease). Unrecognized pathogens may be causally linked to many cases of idiopathic MPGN types 1 and 3. MPGN type 2 (more appropriately known as dense deposit disease [DDD]) is characterized by intramembranous glomerular basement membrane (GBM) deposits of unknown composition, but C3 deposition without immunoglobulin is another consistent glomerular abnormality.[15]

A series of observations in animals deficient in the complement regulator factor H (CFH) and a few families segregating mutations in the same gene have definitively established dysregulation of the alternative pathway (AP) of complement as a pathogenetic mechanism for DDD.[15–18] These studies validate earlier hypotheses based on the frequency of C3 hypocomplementemia and C3 nephritic factors ([CeNeFs] autoantibodies that stabilize the C3 convertase) in a significant proportion of MPGN patients together with rare examples of DDD in individuals with acquired AP dysfunction (Fig. 22-1).[19,20] Patient data, however, indicate that familial AP dysregulation may be associated with all types of MPGN.[21–24] The complexity of CFH-associated renal disease is revealed by its association with atypical hemolytic uremic syndrome (aHUS)[25] (see Chapter 26 for detailed discussion and treatment of aHUS): homozygous CFH mutations associated with decreased CFH serum levels are observed in some patients with DDD, whereas heterozygous mutations, especially of the C-terminus of CFH, are found in patients with aHUS.[26] Interestingly, some aHUS patients have decreased CFH serum levels, and there are reports of not only sequential development of MPGN type 1 and aHUS in a single individual but also of MPGN patients with mutations or polymorphisms in regions of the CFH gene usually associated with aHUS.[27–29]

The functional importance of the polymorphisms in CFH (and CFH-related protein 5) that have been linked to DDD can be inferred from their overrepresentation in individuals with age-related macular degeneration, another condition strongly associated with the complement cascade and indeed identical retinal abnormalities arise prematurely in some patients with DDD.[27,30] Mutations in other *CFHR* genes, such as *CFRH1* and *CFRH3*, have been described in aHUS but remain to be examined in MPGN.[31] The potential influence of AP dysregulation on the classic complement pathway may also be relevant because experimental models of immune complex glomerulonephritis emphasize the impact of AP amplification on complement activation triggered through the classic pathway.[32–34] It is feasible that mutations or polymorphisms in genes encoding AP-regulatory proteins

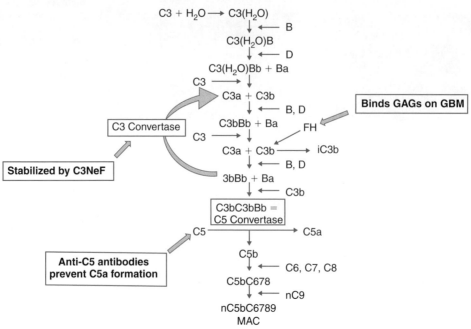

Figure 22-1 Membranoproliferative glomerulonephritis (MPGN) is caused by dysregulation of the alternative pathway (AP) of complement activation in some individuals, particularly those with dense-deposit disease (DDD). Normally, the AP is constitutively active at low levels through the hydrolysis of the thioester in C3 to $C3(H_2O)$. Hydrolyzed C3 combines with factor B, and in the presence of factor D, $C3(H_2O)Bb$ is formed. This intermediate convertase leads to the production of C3a and C3b from C3, and C3b enters the C3bBb amplification loop, which is indicated by the curved arrow. Amplification by fluid phase C3bBb occurs with low efficiency because free C3b is rapidly inactivated by factors H and I. However, C3b can also bind covalently to surfaces or to IgG as a covalent dimer. C3bC3bIgG is partially protected from inactivation by factors H and I by steric hindrance and is 7 to 10 times more efficient in generating a C3 convertase than surface-bound monomeric C3b. On surfaces or on IgG in the fluid phase, C3 convertase can become a C5 convertase by acquiring an additional C3b in its vicinity, which increases affinity for C5. Since factor H is required to control levels of C3b in the fluid phase, the *Cfh−/−* mouse mutant develops DDD. Factor B is also critical to the formation of C3bBb, and consequently the *Cfh−/−.Cfb−/−* mouse mutant does not develop DDD. In the *Cfh−/−.C5−/−* mouse mutant and the *Cfh−/−* mouse mutant treated with anti-C5 antibodies, the degree of kidney disease is decreased compared with the degree of kidney disease seen in the *Cfh−/−* mutant. This decrease is due to the prevention of C5a formation. The complement-regulating properties of factor H are as a decay-accelerating factor (destabilizing C3bBb) and as a cofactor for factor I. In addition to regulating the AP in the fluid phase, factor H binds polyanionic surfaces and regulates attached C3bBb. The glomerular basement membrane (GBM) lacks constitutive membrane-bound complement regulators and is particularly dependent on factor H for protection from the AP. GAGs, glycosaminoglycans.

contribute to the development of MPGN types 1 and 3 in individuals exposed to stimuli that incite IC deposition.

Genetic predisposition to MPGN may arise through mutations in other components of the complement system including membrane cofactor protein (MCP, CD46), and various factors in the classic and terminal pathways.[29,35] The mechanisms underlying these associations remain to be determined but may include susceptibility to infection and impaired IC processing and clearance, which are likely to be important in MPGN types 1 and 3. Finally, MPGN has been linked to genes seemingly unrelated to complement regulation (X-linked MPGN and *LMNA* associated with partial lipodystrophy and DDD in the absence of C3NeF or hypocomplementemia).[36,37]

The prognosis for patients with MPGN is guarded, with 40% to 50% requiring permanent renal replacement therapy in many series with extended follow-up (≥10 years). The impact of treatment has been at best limited (no significant effect on renal survival in most trials), and recurrence with graft loss is frequent in transplant recipients.[14,38–41] A review of published data in 1999 advocated corticosteroid and antiplatelet therapy for selected children and adults with MPGN,

respectively, but the evidence for these recommendations is not compelling.[42] There have been no subsequent sizable or prospective, randomized trials of treatment of MPGN, and, given the decreasing incidence of at least MPGN type 1, there are obstacles to future studies. Nevertheless, the remarkable developments in understanding the molecular basis for MPGN hold the promise of novel, targeted therapies that can be rapidly translated into patient care. As we learn more about the pathophysiology of MPGN, there may also be rationale for replacing current histologic classifications with pathogenetic descriptions to recognize homogeneous conditions with logical targets for treatment.[43] On that basis, we believe that there is good reason to collect DNA from all individuals with "idiopathic" MPGN and to perform CFH genotyping in at least all individuals with DDD, irrespective of serum complement levels because these are not invariably depressed in the context of abnormal complement regulation. Every opportunity should be taken to understand the basis of these increasingly uncommon conditions if we are to avoid relying solely on the results of historical trials in patient treatment. Herein we briefly review evidence relating to classical treatments of MPGN and highlight experimental data that point toward future directions in therapy.

WHEN IS TREATMENT OF MEMBRANOPROLIFERATIVE GLOMERULONEPHRITIS NECESSARY?

The aggressive natural history and low (<5%) spontaneous remission rate of MPGN suggest that treatment is desirable. Indeed, data from Japan, where early detection of MPGN has been possible through school urinary screening programs, suggest that treatment can be highly effective.[44] In most countries, however, there is a delay in diagnosis, and, coupled with the uncertain efficacy, long duration, and potential toxicity of immunosuppressant protocols, treatment decisions can be difficult. Identifying patients with perceived adverse prognostic features is desirable, but the evidence base on which these decisions can be made remains limited. For example, heavy proteinuria and/or the presence of the nephrotic syndrome have been highlighted as markers of poor outcome in many but not all studies.[14,38,39,41,45,46] Similarly, the impact of impaired renal function, hypertension, hypocomplementemia, C3NeF, and histologic features of DDD have also been contested.[38,40,41,47–49] A recent retrospective series of 70 children and adults from Ireland used a multivariate analysis to show that nephrosis-range proteinuria, interstitial fibrosis, cellular crescents, and mesangial proliferation are independently associated with end-stage renal disease, which ranged from 12% for those with the most favorable composite histologic features to 92% for those with nephrosis-range proteinuria and cellular crescents at 10-year follow-up. DDD was associated with a comparatively worse outcome, but this was not independent of histologic parameters, an observation that is consistent with early reports.[45] In a retrospective series of 53 U.K. children, nephrotic syndrome and 20% chronic damage or more on biopsy at presentation predicted a worse outcome as did renal function at 1 year but not initial renal function.[46] MPGN type also did not predict outcome in this series.

Given our current understanding of the role of angiotensin II and proteinuria in progressive kidney disease, meticulous blood pressure control and generic strategies to decrease albuminuria based on angiotensin-converting enzyme (ACE) inhibitors or angiotensin II antagonists seem prudent in all patients with MPGN.[50] Smoking cessation, dietary salt restriction, and statin therapy where appropriate should not be overlooked. In practice, a high proportion of patients with MPGN, particularly children, continue to receive immunosuppressive therapy, which is most often corticosteroid based.[46,51]

CORTICOSTEROID THERAPY

During the past 35 years, there have been a number of trials of prolonged steroid therapy for MPGN, primarily conducted in children. Methylprednisolone and alternate-day prednisolone have been the most often used treatments, but the results are not persuasive. In the largest randomized trial of extended alternate-day prednisolone in proteinuric children with MPGN ($N = 80$), improved renal survival in the treatment group at 130 months was marginal (62% vs. 12%, $P = .07$) and even less clear at earlier time points.[52] Among 71 children treated predominantly with extended alternate-day prednisolone in uncontrolled studies by West and colleagues,[53] 10- and 20-year renal survival rates were 82% and 56%, respectively, from disease onset. Notably subcapsular cataracts and growth failure occurred in 11 and 17% respectively. The same authors have suggested that MPGN type 3 is less responsive to alternate-day prednisolone than MPGN type 1, but the mean GFR of the two groups at entry was significantly different, which may have influenced outcome.[54] Patients with DDD in general do not respond to corticosteroid therapy,[9] although children with juvenile acute nonproliferative glomerulonephritis, which may be a distinct entity or a rare crescentic variant of DDD, have been suggested to benefit.[55,56] Data on the treatment of adult MPGN with steroids are extremely limited.

ANTIPLATELET AGENTS AND ANTICOAGULANTS

Antiplatelet and anticoagulant therapies have been advocated in MPGN based on platelet activation and reduced half-life. In a crossover trial ($N = 18$), unpaired analysis of warfarin plus dipyridamole versus placebo showed stabilization of serum creatinine and decreased proteinuria in the treatment group compared with the placebo group. However, analysis of patients completing crossover did not support an overall benefit of treatment, and there were significant risks, with a 37% hemorrhagic complication rate and one death from intracranial hemorrhage.[57] Encouraging results at 1 and 4 years from a randomized trial ($N = 40$) of aspirin plus dipyridamole versus placebo were not maintained in longer term follow-up (10-year renal survival rate was 49 ± 11.5% with treatment versus 41 ± 11% with placebo, not significant).[58,59] A subsequent study comparing aspirin plus dipyridamole to placebo for nephrotic adults with MPGN ($N = 18$) reported a significant decrease in proteinuria with treatment and no excess bleeding.[60] Sizable but comparable decreases in blood pressure were achieved in the two groups, and more patients in the placebo arm received ACE inhibitors. Serum creatinine was unchanged at 36 months in both arms of the study.

CYTOTOXIC THERAPIES

A number of largely uncontrolled trials have combined cyclophosphamide with anticoagulant or antiplatelet treatments since the 1970s.[61,62] Although none of these studies demonstrates a convincing advantage and serious adverse effects were not uncommon, cytotoxic agents are probably still in use because in two cohort studies that commenced in the 1980s, 11% and 17% of children received cyclophosphamide.[46,51] Published data on the use of newer agents such as mycophenolate mofetil are extremely limited and are insufficiently well controlled to permit any definitive conclusions to be reached.[63]

PLASMA EXCHANGE

Interest in the use of plasma exchange and infusion has been renewed by increased understanding of the role of dysregulated complement activation in MPGN. There are no sizable or controlled trials of these therapies, but case reports in both

MPGN and aHUS signal its potential efficacy where deficiencies or mutations in circulating complement regulators such as CFH are implicated.[64–66] The half-life of factor H is approximately 6 days, and thus plasma infusions of 10 to 20 mL/kg every 14 days have been described.

KIDNEY TRANSPLANTATION

Concern persists over comparatively high rates of recurrence and consequent graft loss in patients undergoing transplantation for MPGN. MPGN type 1 and DDD recur in at least approximately 30% and approximately 50% of allograft recipients, respectively.[67–69] United States Renal Data System data on graft loss with MPGN type 1 ($N = 1574$) demonstrate that the 5-year incidence of graft failure due to recurrent disease has increased from 3.5% in 1988 to 1994 to 7.2% in 1995 to 2003 ($P = .02$), whereas graft loss from other causes has decreased.[70] Five-year graft survival in North American children with DDD has been reported to be less favorable than that of pediatric allograft recipients as a whole ($50.0 \pm 7.5\%$ vs. $74.3 \pm 0.6\%$, $P < .001$) with 14.7% of grafts lost to recurrent disease.[51] Glomerular crescents on transplant biopsy samples were associated with graft loss in that study. Little and colleagues[14] reported that crescents on native renal biopsy were negatively correlated with allograft survival in a multivariate analysis and that this adverse histologic parameter accounted for a trend toward worse outcome of patients with DDD.

POTENTIAL THERAPEUTIC TARGETS IN THE COMPLEMENT CASCADE

Animal models of DDD and available human data provide clear rationale for attempting to correct uncontrolled activation of the alternative complement pathway in patients. The replacement of deficient or defective CFH by plasma infusion or exchange has been discussed and is likely to be most appropriate when CFH levels are decreased or genotyping identifies mutations known to impair CFH protein function. In the future, administration of purified or recombinant CFH may become feasible. Plasma exchange will also deplete circulating nephritic factors, although at present, there is limited evidence to suggest that removal of C3NeF is beneficial. Nephritic factors capable of stabilizing the AP convertase were first recognized more than 30 years ago, but their importance has remained in doubt because neither hypocomplementemia nor the presence/persistence of C3NeF appear to have prognostic value in most series, and there is no evidence to suggest that nephritic factors form part of the immune deposits in patients with MPGN.[47,49] Nevertheless, because it is now clear that abnormal stabilization of the AP convertase (through CFH deficiency or defect) is sufficient to incite disease, interest in nephritic factors has been revived.

Considerable heterogeneity exists in the function of C3NeFs, which may well be relevant to the selection of patients most likely to benefit from therapeutic intervention targeting these autoantibodies.[71–73] Meyers, West, and colleagues[74,75] have argued that an autoantibody (terminal pathway NeF), which stabilizes the C3/5 convertase is largely restricted to patients with MPGN type 3 and is likely to have pathogenetic significance, although others have disputed that it is invariably present. The serum complement profile and composition of glomerular immune deposits in patients with terminal pathway NeF and MPGN type 3 typically resemble those seen with factor H deficiency (in both humans and animals) with marked activation of the terminal pathway.[7,11,16,17,22,76] In contrast, the C3NeF found in more than 80% patients with DDD (C3 amplifying NeF) stabilizes the C3 convertase but not the C3/C5 convertase. West and colleagues[77] have demonstrated that glomerular immune deposits in at least some patients with DDD are derived from circulating C3 convertase that is not accompanied by C5 deposition and consequently their pathologic significance is unknown. Mice deficient in both CFH and C5 still develop proteinuria implying that C3 deposition alone is sufficient to damage the GBM, although the severity of renal disease is greater in mice with intact C5 expression.[78] Nephritic factors are least frequently observed in patients with MPGN type 1 but may still occur and can stabilize both AP and classic pathway convertases.[8,79–81] Once the pathogenetic significance of these various nephritic factors is better comprehended, there will be a clearer rationale for plasma exchange and B cell–targeted therapies (e.g., rituximab) in selected patients.[82]

As we have indicated (see Fig. 22-1), AP dysregulation of various origins impinges on the terminal complement pathway, which leads to assembly of the membrane attack complex and production of the anaphylatoxin C5a, and this identifies another potential therapeutic target. Preventing C5 activation has a protective effect in CFH-deficient mice and a humanized monoclonal anti-C5 antibody, eculizumab, has been shown to be clinically efficacious in another disease defined by defective complement regulation, paroxysmal nocturnal hemoglobinuria.[78,83] There is a clear rationale for considering eculizumab in patients with MPGN and documented abnormal AP activation (in particular, those with DDD, CFH dysfunction associated with any clinicopathologic variant of MPGN, or MPGN type 3 with terminal pathway C3NeF). There is also reason to consider eculizumab in patients with MPGN types 1 and 3 associated with IC deposition and/or classic pathway activation because again recruitment of the terminal pathway may well incite glomerular injury. Notably, there has been interest in the use of eculizumab to treat both lupus nephritis and membranous nephropathy in which similar mechanisms are operational, although experience in membranous nephropathy suggests that adequate dosing may be critical to achieve benefit.[84,85] Careful exclusion of occult infection is essential before considering modulation of this arm of the innate immune system.

Correction of complement dysregulation is theoretically possible through liver transplantation, and combined kidney/liver transplantation have been reported in patients with recurrent aHUS.[86] Perioperative plasma exchange is probably advisable given the apparent increased potential for graft thrombosis in the setting of CFH deficiency.[87] It seems likely that such strategies will be attempted in MPGN.

Finally, the GBM may be another potential therapeutic target in MPGN even when the precipitants of complement activation cannot be readily identified. Complement activation is

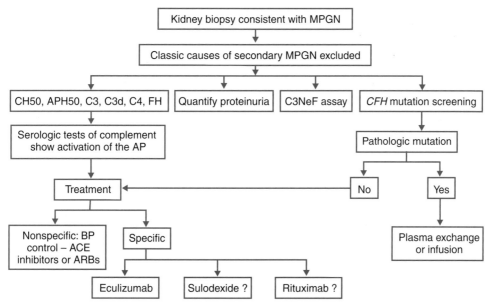

Figure 22-2 Flow diagram for the diagnostic evaluation and possible treatment of idiopathic membranoproliferative glomerulonephritis (MPGN) in which there is evidence of dysregulation of alternate pathway (AP) activity (e.g., dense-deposit disease). Diagnosis requires a renal biopsy, which must show pathognomic electron-dense deposits. Serologic tests should include C3 (expected to be low), C3d (a breakdown product of C3, expected to be increased), C4 (may be low), and CH50 and APH50, two general tests of activity of the classic and APs, respectively. Screening should also include assaying C3NeF and determining levels and the nucleotide sequence of factor H. The rationale for the treatment options presented is discussed in the text. Serologic markers of AP activity and serologic and urinary markers of kidney function should be monitored regularly. Suggested drug regimens are eculizumab 600 mg IV once weekly for 4 weeks followed by maintenance dosing with 900 mg IV every 2 weeks (based on its use in paroxysmal nocturnal hemoglobinuria[57]); sulodexide 200 mg/day PO; rituximab 375 mg/m² IV weekly for 4 weeks (based on its use in hepatitis C virus–associated cryoglobulinemia and idiopathic membranous nephropathy; monthly maintenance doses may also be considered). ACE, angiotensin-converting enzyme; ARBs, angiotensin receptor blockers; BP, blood pressure.

known to cause loss of heparin sulfate from cells and extracellular matrices and could mediate GBM injury during ischemia reperfusion.[88] Furthermore, polymorphisms in the CFH gene that may affect its interaction with heparin and other glycosaminoglycans have been described in patients with DDD, and up-regulation of GBM-associated heparanase occurs in the context of DDD.[27,89] Therefore, the efficacy of sulodexide, a highly purified glycosaminoglycan now being tested in diabetic nephropathy where the glycosaminoglycan composition of GBM is also altered may be relevant to MPGN.[90] Potential indications for these new therapeutic options are shown in Figure 22-2.

SUMMARY

The treatment of MPGN remains a clinical challenge because the available evidence base is limited in scope and offers only qualified endorsement for conventional treatments. At least some forms of MPGN are becoming less common and the current classification system may benefit from restructuring. The importance of the alternative complement pathway in DDD is clear and is potentially amenable to novel therapeutic manipulations. Furthermore, these same observations may well be pertinent to many cases of MPGN types 1 and 3: patients with terminal pathway C3NeF exhibit overt

AP dysregulation, activation of the terminal complement pathway through either classic pathways or APs probably mediates glomerular damage, and polymorphisms in AP-regulator genes could influence amplification of classic pathway activation. At present, the comparative benefits of treatments such as plasma infusion/exchange, eculizumab, and rituximab have not been examined, and although plasma infusion/exchange seems most logical for patients with identified CFH deficiency or functional mutation, definitive protocols cannot be offered. However, we believe that these options are therapeutically attractive and should be considered in the context of the limited efficacy of conventional therapies. A key question that remains to be addressed is the appropriate timing for the use of newer complement-modulating therapies. Reserving treatment for patients who have not responded to generic treatments may decrease cost and risk of treatment-related adverse events in patients with disease that has a favorable natural history, but at the same time irreversible glomerular scarring and recruitment of nonimmunologic mechanisms of injury may occur, thus limiting the effectiveness of new treatments in those with more aggressive disease. Clearly there is a need for further investigation of pathogenetic mechanisms, and this may well be the most successful strategy for improving outcomes in uncommon diseases for which the organization of large, controlled therapeutic trials is problematic.

USEFUL LINKS

www.fh-hus.org. The interactive factor H atypical hemolytic uremic syndrome mutation database and website that includes information on MPGN associated mutations for both professionals and patients.

genome.uiowa.edu/ddd. The newly established Dense Deposit Disease Outcome Database intended to provide physicians with real-time data on treatment outcomes of patients with DDD.

References

1. Simon P, Ramee MP, Boulahrouz R, et al: Epidemiologic data of primary glomerular diseases in western France. Kidney Int 2004;66:3:905–908.
2. Rivera F, Lopez-Gomez JM, Perez-Garcia R: Clinicopathologic correlations of renal pathology in Spain. Kidney Int 2004;66: 898–904.
3. Covic A, Schiller A, Volovat C, et al: Epidemiology of renal disease in Romania: A 10 year review of two regional renal biopsy databases. Nephrol Dial Transplant 2006;21:419–424.
4. Gesualdo L, Di Palma AM, Morrone LF, et al: The Italian experience of the national registry of renal biopsies. Kidney Int 2004;66:890–894.
5. Razukeviciene L, Bumblyte IA, Kuzminskis V, et al: Membranoproliferative glomerulonephritis is still the most frequent glomerulonephritis in Lithuania. Clin Nephrol 2006;65:87–90.
6. Rennke HG: Secondary membranoproliferative glomerulonephritis. Kidney Int 1995;47:643–656.
7. West CD, McAdams AJ. Membranoproliferative glomerulonephritis type III: Association of glomerular deposits with circulating nephritic factor-stabilized convertase. Am J Kidney Dis 1998;32:56–63.
8. Jackson EC, McAdams AJ, Strife CF, et al: Differences between membranoproliferative glomerulonephritis types I and III in clinical presentation, glomerular morphology, and complement perturbation. Am J Kidney Dis 1987;9:115–120.
9. Meyers KE, Finn L, Kaplan BS: Membranoproliferative glomerulonephritis type III. Pediatr Nephrol 1998;12:512–522.
10. Ooi YM, Vallota EH, West CD: Classical complement pathway activation in membranoproliferative glomerulonephritis. Kidney Int 1976;9:46–53.
11. Varade WS, Forristal J, West CD: Patterns of complement activation in idiopathic membranoproliferative glomerulonephritis, types I, II, and III. Am J Kidney Dis 1990;16:196–206.
12. Iitaka K, Saka T, Yagisawa K, et al: Decreasing hypocomplementemia and membranoproliferative glomerulonephritis in Japan. Pediatr Nephrol 2000;14:794–796.
13. Giannico G, Manno C, Schena FP: Treatment of glomerulonephritides associated with hepatitis C virus infection. Nephrol Dial Transplant 2000;15(Suppl 8):34–38.
14. Little MA, Dupont P, Campbell E, et al: Severity of primary MPGN, rather than MPGN type, determines renal survival and post-transplantation recurrence risk. Kidney Int 2006;69:504–511.
15. Appel GB, Cook HT, Hageman G, et al: Membranoproliferative glomerulonephritis type II (dense deposit disease): An update. J Am Soc Nephrol 2005;16:1392–1403.
16. Hegasy GA, Manuelian T, Hogasen K, et al: The molecular basis for hereditary porcine membranoproliferative glomerulonephritis type II: Point mutations in the factor H coding sequence block protein secretion. Am J Pathol 2002;161:2027–2034.
17. Pickering MC, Cook HT, Warren J, et al: Uncontrolled C3 activation causes membranoproliferative glomerulonephritis in mice deficient in complement factor H. Nat Genet 2002;31:424–428.
18. Licht C, Schlotzer-Schrehardt U, Kirschfink M, et al: MPGN II—genetically determined by defective complement regulation? Pediatr Nephrol 2007;22:2–9.
19. Meri S, Koistinen V, Miettinen A, et al: Activation of the alternative pathway of complement by monoclonal lambda light chains in membranoproliferative glomerulonephritis. J Exp Med 1992;175:939–950.
20. West CD: Nephritic factors predispose to chronic glomerulonephritis. Am J Kidney Dis 1994;24:956–963.
21. Marder HK, Coleman TH, Forristal J, et al: An inherited defect in the C3 convertase, C3b,Bb, associated with glomerulonephritis. Kidney Int 1983;23:749–758.
22. Levy M, Halbwachs-Mecarelli L, Gubler MC, et al: H deficiency in two brothers with atypical dense intramembranous deposit disease. Kidney Int 1986;30:949–956.
23. Neary JJ, Conlon PJ, Croke D, et al: Linkage of a gene causing familial membranoproliferative glomerulonephritis type III to chromosome 1. J Am Soc Nephrol 2002;13:2052–2057.
24. Dragon-Durey MA, Fremeaux-Bacchi V, Loirat C, et al: Heterozygous and homozygous factor H deficiencies associated with hemolytic uremic syndrome or membranoproliferative glomerulonephritis: Report and genetic analysis of 16 cases. J Am Soc Nephrol 2004;15:787–795.
25. Atkinson JP, Goodship TH: Complement factor H and the hemolytic uremic syndrome. J Exp Med 2007; 204:1245–1248.
26. Saunders RE, Abarrategui-Garrido C, Fremeaux-Bacchi V, et al: The interactive factor H-atypical hemolytic uremic syndrome mutation database and website: Update and integration of membrane cofactor protein and factor I mutations with structural models. Hum Mutat 2007;28:222–234.
27. Abrera-Abeleda MA, Nishimura C, Smith JL, et al: Variations in the complement regulatory genes factor H (CFH) and factor H related 5 (CFHR5) are associated with membranoproliferative glomerulonephritis type II (dense deposit disease). J Med Genet 2006;43:582–589.
28. Vaziri-Sani F, Holmberg L, Sjoholm AG, et al: Phenotypic expression of factor H mutations in patients with atypical hemolytic uremic syndrome. Kidney Int 2006;69:981–988.
29. Servais A, Fremeaux-Bacchi V, Lequintrec M, et al: Primary glomerulonephritis with isolated C3 deposits: A new entity which shares common genetic risk factors with haemolytic uraemic syndrome. J Med Genet 2007;44:193–199.
30. Hageman GS, Anderson DH, Johnson LV, et al: A common haplotype in the complement regulatory gene factor H (HF1/CFH) predisposes individuals to age-related macular degeneration. Proc Natl Acad Sci U S A 2005;102:7227–7232.
31. Zipfel PF, Edey M, Heinen S, et al: Deletion of complement factor H-related genes CFHR1 and CFHR3 is associated with atypical hemolytic uremic syndrome. PLoS Genet 2007;3:e41.
32. Watanabe H, Garnier G, Circolo A, et al: Modulation of renal disease in MRL/lpr mice genetically deficient in the alternative complement pathway factor. Br J Immunol 2000;164:786–794.
33. Alexander JJ, Aneziokoro OG, Chang A, et al: Distinct and separable roles of the complement system in factor H-deficient bone marrow chimeric mice with immune complex disease. J Am Soc Nephrol 2006. 17:1354–1361.
34. Alexander JJ, Pickering MC, Haas M, et al: Complement factor H limits immune complex deposition and prevents inflammation and scarring in glomeruli of mice with chronic serum sickness. J Am Soc Nephrol 2005;16:52–57.
35. Coleman TH, Forristal J, Kosaka T, et al: Inherited complement component deficiencies in membranoproliferative glomerulonephritis. Kidney Int 1983;24:681–690.
36. Stutchfield PR, White RH, Cameron AH, et al: X-linked mesangiocapillary glomerulonephritis. Clin Nephrol 1986;26:150–156.
37. Owen KR, Donohoe M, Ellard S, et al: Mesangiocapillary glomerulonephritis type 2 associated with familial partial lipodystrophy (Dunnigan-Kobberling syndrome). Nephron Clin Pract 2004;96:c35–c38.

38. Swainson CP, Robson JS, Thomson D, et al: Mesangiocapillary glomerulonephritis: A long-term study of 40 cases. J Pathol 1983;141:449–468.

39. D'Amico G, Ferrario F: Mesangiocapillary glomerulonephritis. J Am Soc Nephrol 1992;2(10 Suppl):S159–S166.

40. Schwertz R, de Jong R, Gretz N, et al: Outcome of idiopathic membranoproliferative glomerulonephritis in children. Arbeitsgemeinschaft Padiatrische Nephrologie. Acta Paediatr 1996;85:308–312.

41. Schmitt H, Bohle A, Reineke T, et al: Long-term prognosis of membranoproliferative glomerulonephritis type I. Significance of clinical and morphological parameters: An investigation of 220 cases. Nephron 1990;55:242–250.

42. Levin A: Management of membranoproliferative glomerulonephritis: Evidence-based recommendations. Kidney Int Suppl 1999;70:S41–S46.

43. Walker PD, Ferrario F, Joh K, et al: Dense deposit disease is not a membranoproliferative glomerulonephritis. Mod Pathol 2007;20:605–616.

44. Yanagihara T, Hayakawa M, Yoshida J, et al: Long-term follow-up of diffuse membranoproliferative glomerulonephritis type I. Pediatr Nephrol 2005;20:585–590.

45. Habib R, Kleinknecht C, Gubler MC, et al: Idiopathic membranoproliferative glomerulonephritis in children. Report of 105 cases. Clin Nephrol 1973;1:194–214.

46. Cansick JC, Lennon T, Cummins CL, et al: Prognosis, treatment and outcome of childhood mesangiocapillary (membranoproliferative) glomerulonephritis. Nephrol Dial Transplant 2004;19:2769–2777.

47. Bennett WM, Fassett RG, Walker RG, et al: Mesangiocapillary glomerulonephritis type II (dense-deposit disease): Clinical features of progressive disease. Am J Kidney Dis 1989;13: 469–476.

48. Pedersen RS: Long-term prognosis in idiopathic membranoproliferative glomerulonephritis. Scand J Urol Nephrol 1995; 29:265–272.

49. Schwertz R, Rother U, Anders D, et al: Complement analysis in children with idiopathic membranoproliferative glomerulonephritis: A long-term follow-up. Pediatr Allergy Immunol 2001;12:166–172.

50. Kent DM, Jafar TH, Hayward RA, et al: Progression risk, urinary protein excretion, and treatment effects of angiotensin-converting enzyme inhibitors in nondiabetic kidney disease. J Am Soc Nephrol 2007;18:1959–1965.

51. Braun MC, Stablein DM, Hamiwka LA, et al: Recurrence of membranoproliferative glomerulonephritis type II in renal allografts: The North American Pediatric Renal Transplant Cooperative Study experience. J Am Soc Nephrol 2005;16: 2225–2233.

52. Tarshish P, Bernstein J, Tobin JN, et al: Treatment of mesangiocapillary glomerulonephritis with alternate-day prednisone—a report of the International Study of Kidney Disease in Children. Pediatr Nephrol 1992;6:123–130.

53. West CD, McAdams AJ, Witte DP, Acute non-proliferative glomerulitis: A cause of renal failure unique to children. Pediatr Nephrol 2000;14:786–793.

54. Braun MC, West CD, Strife CF: Differences between membranoproliferative glomerulonephritis types I and III in long-term response to an alternate-day prednisone regimen. Am J Kidney Dis 1999;34:1022–1032.

55. McEnery PT: Membranoproliferative glomerulonephritis: The Cincinnati experience—cumulative renal survival from 1957 to 1989. J Pediatr 1990;116:S109–S114.

56. Hoschek JC, Dreyer P, Dahal S, et al: Rapidly progressive renal failure in childhood. Am J Kidney Dis 2002;40:1342–1347.

57. Zimmerman SW, Moorthy AV, Dreher WH, et al: Prospective trial of warfarin and dipyridamole in patients with membranoproliferative glomerulonephritis. Am J Med 1983;75:920–927.

58. Donadio JV Jr, Anderson CF, Mitchell JC 3rd, et al: Membranoproliferative glomerulonephritis. A prospective clinical trial of platelet-inhibitor therapy. N Engl J Med 1984;310:1421–1426.

59. Donadio JV Jr, Offord KP: Reassessment of treatment results in membranoproliferative glomerulonephritis, with emphasis on life-table analysis. Am J Kidney Dis 1989;14:445–451.

60. Zauner I, Bohler J, Braun N, et al: Effect of aspirin and dipyridamole on proteinuria in idiopathic membranoproliferative glomerulonephritis: A multicentre prospective clinical trial. Collaborative Glomerulonephritis Therapy Study Group (CGTS). Nephrol Dial Transplant 1994;9:619–622.

61. Cameron JS, Turner DR, Heaton J, et al: Idiopathic mesangiocapillary glomerulonephritis. Comparison of types I and II in children and adults and long-term prognosis. Am J Med 1983;74:175–192.

62. Cattran DC, Cardella CJ, Roscoe JM, et al: Results of a controlled drug trial in membranoproliferative glomerulonephritis. Kidney Int 1985;27:436–441.

63. Jones G, Juszczak M, Kingdon E, et al: Treatment of idiopathic membranoproliferative glomerulonephritis with mycophenolate mofetil and steroids. Nephrol Dial Transplant 2004;19:3160–3164.

64. McGinley E, Watkins R, McLay A, et al: Plasma exchange in the treatment of mesangiocapillary glomerulonephritis. Nephron 1985;40:385–390.

65. Kurtz KA, Schlueter AJ: Management of membranoproliferative glomerulonephritis type II with plasmapheresis. J Clin Apher 2002;17:135–137.

66. Licht C, Heinen S, Jozsi M, et al: Deletion of Lys224 in regulatory domain 4 of factor H reveals a novel pathomechanism for dense deposit disease (MPGN II). Kidney Int 2006;70: 42–50.

67. Shimizu T, Tanabe K, Oshima T, et al: Recurrence of membranoproliferative glomerulonephritis in renal allografts. Transplant Proc 1998;30:3910–3913.

68. Andresdottir MB, Assmann KJ, Hoitsma AJ, et al: Renal transplantation in patients with dense deposit disease: Morphological characteristics of recurrent disease and clinical outcome. Nephrol Dial Transplant 1999;14:1723–1731.

69. Andresdottir MB, Assmann KJ, Hoitsma AJ, et al: Recurrence of type I membranoproliferative glomerulonephritis after renal transplantation: Analysis of the incidence, risk factors, and impact on graft survival. Transplantation 1997;63:1628–1633.

70. Kasiske BL, Snyder J, Peng Y, et al: Changes in outcomes for kidney transplant patients with type 1 membranoproliferative glomerulonephritis [abstract 1765]. Am J Transplant 2006;6 (Suppl 2):654.

71. Mollnes TE, Ng YC, Peters DK, et al: Effect of nephritic factor on C3 and on the terminal pathway of complement in vivo and in vitro. Clin Exp Immunol 1986;65:73–79.

72. Clardy CW, Forristal J, Strife CF, et al: A properdin dependent nephritic factor slowly activating C3, C5, and C9 in membranoproliferative glomerulonephritis, types I and III. Clin Immunol Immunopathol 1989;50:333–347.

73. Tanuma Y, Ohi H, Hatano M: Two types of C3 nephritic factor: Properdin-dependent C3NeF and properdin-independent C3NeF. Clin Immunol Immunopathol 1990;56:226–238.

74. Meyers KE, Strife CF, Witzleben C, et al: Discordant renal histopathologic findings and complement profiles in membranoproliferative glomerulonephritis type III. Am J Kidney Dis 1996;28:804–810.

75. West CD, McAdams AJ: The alternative pathway C3 convertase and glomerular deposits. Pediatr Nephrol 1999;13:448–453.

76. Strife CF, Jackson EC, McAdams AJ: Type III membranoproliferative glomerulonephritis: Long-term clinical and morphologic evaluation. Clin Nephrol 1984;21:323–334.

77. West CD, Witte DP, McAdams AJ: Composition of nephritic factor-generated glomerular deposits in membranoproliferative glomerulonephritis type 2. Am J Kidney Dis 2001;37:1120–1130.

78. Pickering MC, Warren J, Rose KL, et al: Prevention of C5 activation ameliorates spontaneous and experimental glomerulonephritis in factor H-deficient mice. Proc Natl Acad Sci U S A 2006;103:9649–9654.

79. Ohi H, Yasugi T: Occurrence of C3 nephritic factor and C4 nephritic factor in membranoproliferative glomerulonephritis (MPGN). Clin Exp Immunol 1994;95:316–321.

80. Tanuma Y, Ohi H, Watanabe S, et al: C3 nephritic factor and C4 nephritic factor in the serum of two patients with hypocomplementaemic membranoproliferative glomerulonephritis. Clin Exp Immunol 1989;76:82–85.

81. Strife CF, Prada AL, Clardy CW, et al: Autoantibody to complement neoantigens in membranoproliferative glomerulonephritis. J Pediatr 1990;116:S98–S102.

82. Salama AD, Pusey CD: Drug insight: Rituximab in renal disease and transplantation. Nat Clin Pract Nephrol 2006;2:221–230.

83. Hillmen P, Young NS, Schubert J, et al: The complement inhibitor eculizumab in paroxysmal nocturnal hemoglobinuria. N Engl J Med 2006;355:1233–1243.

84. Bao L, Quigg RJ: Complement in lupus nephritis: The good, the bad, and the unknown. Semin Nephrol 2007;27:69–80.

85. Cattran D: Management of membranous nephropathy: When and what for treatment. J Am Soc Nephrol 2005;16:1188–1194.

86. Saland JM, Emre SH, Shneider BL, et al: Favorable long-term outcome after liver-kidney transplant for recurrent hemolytic uremic syndrome associated with a factor H mutation. Am J Transplant 2006. 6:1948–1952.

87. Remuzzi G, Ruggenenti P, Colledan M, et al: Hemolytic uremic syndrome: A fatal outcome after kidney and liver transplantation performed to correct factor H gene mutation. Am J Transplant 2005;5:1146–1150.

88. Stefanidis I, Heintz B, Stocker G, et al: Association between heparan sulfate proteoglycan excretion and proteinuria after renal transplantation. J Am Soc Nephrol 1996;7:2670–2676.

89. Smith RJ, Alexander J, Barlow PN, et al: New approaches to the treatment of dense deposit disease. J Am Soc Nephrol 2007;18:2447–2456.

90. Lauver DA, Lucchesi BR: Sulodexide: A renewed interest in this glycosaminoglycan. Cardiovasc Drug Rev 2006;24:214–226.

Further Reading

Appel GB, Cook HT, Hageman G, et al: Membranoproliferative glomerulonephritis type II (dense deposit disease): An update. J Am Soc Nephrol 2005;16:1392–1403.

Licht C, Schlötzer-Schrehardt U, Kirschfink M, et al: MPGN II—genetically determined by defective complement regulation? Pediatr Nephrol 2007;22:2–9.

Saunders RE, Abarrategui-Garrido C, Frémeaux-Bacchi V, et al: The interactive Factor H-atypical hemolytic uremic syndrome mutation database and website: Update and integration of membrane cofactor protein and Factor I mutations with structural models. Hum Mutat 2007;28:222–234.

Smith RJ, Alexander J, Barlow PN, et al: New approaches to the treatment of dense deposit disease. J Am Soc Nephrol 2007;18:2447–2456.

Zipfel PF, Heinen S, Jzsi M, Skerka C: Complement and diseases: Defective alternative pathway control results in kidney and eye diseases. Mol Immunol 2006;43:97–106.

Chapter 23

Amyloidosis and Other Fibrillary and Monoclonal Immunoglobulin-Associated Kidney Diseases

Joline L.T. Chen and Laura M. Dember

CHAPTER CONTENTS

Several disorders fall into the broad category of fibrillary and monoclonal immunoglobulin-associated kidney diseases (Table 23-1). Fibrillary kidney diseases include all types of amyloidosis that affect the kidney, fibrillary glomerulonephritis (GN), and immunotactoid glomerulopathy. Monoclonal immunoglobulin–associated kidney disorders include AL amyloidosis, light-chain or heavy-chain deposition disease (LCDD and HCDD, respectively), and myeloma cast nephropathy. There is probably a monoclonal immunoglobulin component in at least some cases of immunotactoid glomerulopathy, and thus, like AL amyloidosis, this disorder should be considered both fibrillary and monoclonal immunoglobulin–associated. Type I and II cryoglobulinemias are monoclonal immunoglobulin–associated diseases that are covered in Chapter 14.

AMYLOIDOSIS

Classification, Clinical Features, and Kidney Histology

Amyloidosis is a group of diseases in which proteins that are normally soluble form insoluble fibrils in tissues. The fibrils have a specific structure that renders them morphologically indistinguishable regardless of the protein from which they form. Amyloid fibrils are composed of four to six protofilaments with a high β-pleated sheet content that interact in a highly ordered manner. The ultrastructure of amyloid fibrils is responsible for the binding by Congo red dye and the amyloid-defining birefringence when Congo red–stained fibrils are viewed under polarized light.[1]

The amyloidoses are classified based on the precursor protein that forms the fibrils and by the distribution of amyloid deposition as either systemic or localized. Localized amyloidosis refers to disease in which the amyloid is deposited only at the site of synthesis of the amyloidogenic protein. Localized disease does not affect the kidney and is not covered in this chapter. The major types of systemic amyloidosis are immunoglobulin light chain (AL), amyloid A (AA), the familial or hereditary amyloidoses, senile systemic amyloidosis, and β_2-microglobulin amyloidosis (Table 23-2). Immunoglobulin heavy chain (AH) amyloidosis is extremely rare and is not discussed separately from the much more common AL amyloidosis. Senile systemic and β_2-microglobulin amyloidosis do not affect the kidney and also are not discussed further in this chapter.

The clinical manifestations of amyloidosis depend on the organs involved.[2] Organ involvement can be widespread, as is frequent in AL amyloidosis, or restricted to one or two

Table 23-1 Fibrillary and Monoclonal Immunoglobulin Diseases of the Kidney

Disease	Fibril Diameter and Orientation	Congo Red Staining	Detectable Monoclonal Immunoglobulin Protein*	Urinary Findings	Kidney Pathology	Extrarenal Manifestations
Amyloidosis	8–10 nm, randomly arrayed	Yes	AL or AH: yes†; light-chain isotype more often λ than κ; other amyloidoses: no	Albumin, usually nephrotic range	Mesangial expansion and/or nodules, weakly PAS positive; reactivity by IF to single light-chain isotype; fibrils by EM	Yes
Fibrillary glomerulonephritis	15–20 nm, randomly arrayed	No	Usually not	Albumin, nephrotic or subnephrotic range; microscopic hematuria	Mesangial expansion by PAS-positive material, capillary wall thickening, double contours; reactivity by IF to Ig, light chains, complement, usually without restriction to single heavy-chain subclass or light-chain isotype; fibrils by EM	Rare
Immunotactoid glomerulopathy	30–60 nm microtubules, organized parallel distribution	No	Sometimes‡	Albumin, nephrotic, or subnephrotic range; microscopic hematuria	Mesangial expansion with PAS-positive material, mild mesangial hypercellularity, thickening of glomerular capillary walls; reactivity by IF to complement and Ig; can be restricted to single heavy-chain subclass and light-chain isotype; electron-dense deposits with substructure and fibrils by EM	Rare
Light or heavy chain deposition disease	No fibrils	No	Usually§; light-chain isotype more often κ than λ	Albumin, often nephrotic range, unless isolated tubular involvement; microscopic hematuria in some patients	Strongly PAS-positive nodular glomerulosclerosis; reactivity by IF along glomerular and tubular basement membranes to single light-chain isotype (LCDD) or immunoglobulin class (HCDD); large, granular electron-dense deposits along basement membranes and in mesangium	Yes
Myeloma cast nephropathy	No fibrils	No	Yes; high plasma cell burden; light-chain isotype more often κ than λ	Light-chain proteinuria	Intratubular highly refractile and often fractured casts, interstitial inflammatory cells and fibrosis	Yes

*Methods for detection of monoclonal immunoglobulin protein include serum immunofixation electrophoresis and urine immunofixation electrophoresis, quantitative serum-free light-chain assay, and bone marrow biopsy.
†Plasma cell burden is usually low, unless occurring in conjunction with multiple myeloma.
‡Lymphoproliferative disorder is evident in some patients.
§Plasma cell burden is usually low, unless occurring in conjunction with multiple myeloma. Serum immunofixation electrophoresis or urine immunofixation electrophoresis usually reveals monoclonal protein but in some cases the only evidence of monoclonality is single light chain isotype or heavy chain class in tissue biopsy.
EM, electron microscopy; HCDD, heavy-chain deposition disease; IF, immunofluorescence; LCDD, light-chain deposition disease; PAS, periodic acid-Schiff.

Table 23-2 Types of Systemic Amyloidosis

Disease	Amyloidogenic Protein	Organ Involvement
AL amyloidosis	Monoclonal immunoglobulin light chain or fragment	Kidney, heart, liver, gastrointestinal tract, spleen, nervous system, soft tissue, thyroid, adrenal gland
AH amyloidosis	Monoclonal immunoglobulin heavy chain or fragment	Rare; kidney involvement predominates in the small number of reported cases
AA amyloidosis	Serum amyloid A fragment	Kidney, liver, gastrointestinal tract, spleen, autonomic nervous system, thyroid
Hereditary amyloidoses		
Transthyretin amyloidosis	Transthyretin	Peripheral nervous system, heart, vitreous opacities; kidney involvement is not typical
Fibrinogen Aα amyloidosis	Fibrinogen Aα chain	Kidney, liver, spleen; hypertension is common; kidney involvement is predominantly glomerular
Apolipoprotein A1 amyloidosis	Apolipoprotein A1	Kidney, liver, heart, skin, larynx; kidney involvement is predominantly medullary
Apolipoprotein A2 amyloidosis	Apolipoprotein A2	Kidney
Lysozyme amyloidosis	Lysozyme	Kidney, liver, gastrointestinal tract, spleen, lymph nodes, lung, thyroid, salivary glands
Gelsolin amyloidosis	Gelsolin	Cranial nerves, cornea
Senile systemic amyloidosis	Transthyretin (wild type)	Heart, soft tissue
Dialysis-related amyloidosis	β_2-microglobulin	Osteoarticular tissue; less commonly involves gastrointestinal tract, blood vessels, heart

organs or tissue types (see Table 23-2). The kidney is the most common site of amyloid deposition for AL, AA, apoA1, and apoA2 amyloidosis and also is often involved in fibrinogen Aα disease. Nephrotic syndrome with progressive loss of glomerular filtration rate and eventual development of end-stage renal disease (ESRD) is the typical clinical course for amyloid nephropathy, although nonproteinuric disease does occur when amyloid deposition is confined to the tubulointerstitium or vasculature. Nephrotic syndrome from amyloidosis can be severe with urinary protein excretion in the range of 10 to 20 g/day, marked hypoalbuminemia, and diuretic-resistant anasarca. Amyloid deposition in the heart produces a restrictive cardiomyopathy with thickening of the ventricular walls. Because the wall thickening is caused by an infiltrative rather than a hypertrophic process, the electrocardiographic signal typically is of low voltage. The finding of low voltage on the electrocardiogram can help distinguish amyloid heart disease from hypertensive heart disease. Autonomic nervous system involvement typically causes orthostatic hypotension, impaired motility of the gastrointestinal tract manifested as early satiety, diarrhea or constipation, and erectile dysfunction. Hepatic involvement is characterized by an enlarged liver and elevated alkaline phosphatase blood concentration, but preserved liver function in most cases. Sensory neuropathy, soft-tissue amyloid deposition, and ecchymoses from capillary fragility are other common disease manifestations in some, but not all, types of amyloidosis.

Amyloid can deposit anywhere in the kidney. Glomerular involvement tends to predominate but is not always present, particularly in certain types of hereditary amyloidosis. By light microscopy, glomerular amyloid appears as amorphous material in the mesangium and capillary loops. Mesangial deposits can produce nodules that resemble lesions of diabetic nephrop-

athy or LCDD. However, in contrast to diabetic nephropathy or LCDD, nodules in amyloid-associated nephropathy stain weakly with periodic acid–Schiff because they are composed of amyloid protein rather than extracellular matrix. Amyloid deposition in the tubulointerstitium produces tubular atrophy and interstitial fibrosis. By electron microscopy, amyloid fibrils appear to be randomly arrayed without an ordered orientation; they are nonbranching and have diameters of 8 to 10 nm.

Light or electron microscopic examination of a kidney biopsy specimen does not enable determination of the type of amyloidosis. Immunofluorescence examination can, but does not necessarily, reveal deposition of a single light-chain isotype in AL amyloidosis and should be negative for reactivity against intact immunoglobulins or complement. AA protein can be detected by immunofluorescence or immunohistochemistry with commercially available antibodies.[3]

Treatment of Amyloidosis

AL Amyloidosis

AL amyloidosis is the most common of the systemic amyloidoses. The disease course varies substantially among patients; however, in general, AL disease tends to progress more rapidly than other types of amyloidosis and, if not effectively treated, is usually fatal. There have been tremendous advances in the treatment of AL amyloidosis during the past decade, and it is now possible to produce remission of the hematologic disease, or at least a reduction in the production of the amyloidogenic light chain, in a significant proportion of patients.

Current treatments for AL amyloidosis are summarized in Table 23-3.[4–17] The treatments are all directed at the clonal

Table 23-3   Treatments for AL Amyloidosis

Regimen	Study	Description	Result	Utility
		REPRESENTATIVE STUDIES (REF.)		
Cyclic oral melphalan with prednisone	Skinner et al,[4] N = 100 (2 treatment groups)	Randomized, controlled trial of melphalan/prednisone/colchicine vs. colchicine	Extended survival from 7 to 12 mo	Reserve for patients unable to tolerate more effective treatments
	Kye et al,[5] N = 220 (3 treatment groups)	Randomized, controlled trial of melphalan/prednisone/colchicine vs. melphalan/prednisone vs. colchicine	Extended survival from 8 to 18 mo	
IV high-dose melphalan and autologous stem cell transplantation (HDM/SCT)	Comenzo et al,[6] N = 25	Single-center observational study	Established feasibility of the approach	Reasonable to consider as first-line treatment for selected patients Treatment at centers specializing in amyloidosis is recommended because of treatment-associated toxicity
	Dispenzieri et al,[7] N = 126	Single-center case-control study of HDM/SCT vs. oral melphalan/prednisone	4-yr survival 71% vs. 41% in HDM/SCT and melphalan/prednisone groups, respectively	
	Skinner et al,[8] N = 312	Single-center observational study	Complete hematologic response: 40%; median survival: 4.6 yr; TRM: 13%	
	Goodman et al,[9] N = 92	Multicenter observational study	Median survival: 5.3 yr; TRM: 23%	
	Sanchorawala et al,[10] N = 53	Single-center observational study of tandem transplantation	5 of 17 patients (31%) who had 2nd HDM/SCT converted from partial to complete hematologic response	
	Jaccard et al,[11] N = 100	Multicenter randomized, open-label trial of HDM/SCT vs. oral melphalan plus dexamethasone	Median survival: 22.2 and 56.9 mo in HDM/SCT and melphalan/dexamethasone groups, respectively; TRM with HDM/SCT was 24% (higher than that seen in most single-center studies)	
Oral melphalan with high-dose dexamethasone	Palladini et al,[12] N = 46	Single-center observational study of patients not eligible for HDM/SCT	33% had complete hematologic response; median time to response; 4.5 mo	First-line treatment for patients too ill to tolerate HDM/SCT or for patients receiving treatment at center that does not specialize in amyloidosis
	Jaccard et al,[11] N = 100	Multicenter, randomized, open-label trial of HDM/SCT vs. oral melphalan plus dexamethasone	Median survival: 22.2 and 56.9 mo in HDM/SCT and melphalan/dexamethasone groups, respectively, TRM with HDM/SCT was 24% (higher than that seen in most single-center studies)	Duration of hematological response and tolerability of repeated courses of dexamethasone not established

Continued

	Study	Design	Results	Comments
Thalidomide/dexamethasone	Seldin et al,[13] N = 16	Single-center observational study of thalidomide as single agent	None of the patients had complete hematologic response; 50% of patients discontinued treatment because of drug-related toxicity (e.g., pulmonary edema, peripheral neuropathy, renal impairment, sedation)	Thalidomide is poorly tolerated in AL amyloidosis; lenalidomide, a thalidomide analogue, appears to be as effective and better tolerated (see below)
	Dispenzieri et al,[14] N = 12	Single-center observational study of thalidomide as single agent	All patients withdrew from the study because of treatment-related toxicity	
	Palladini et al,[15] N = 31	Single-center observational study of thalidomide with intermediate-dose dexamethasone	31% of patients had complete hematologic response; 65% of patients had treatment-related toxicity	
Lenalidomide/dexamethasone	Sanchorawala et al,[16] N = 34	Single-center observational study	29% of assessable patients had complete hematologic response; toxicities included fatigue, myelosuppression, and thromboembolic events	Based on small published experience, appears to be good option for patients unable to tolerate or unresponsive to HDM/SCT or melphalan with high-dose dexamethasone
	Dispenzieri et al,[17] N = 23	Single-center observational study	40% of patients had hematologic response (partial or complete); toxicities were fatigue, myelosuppression, and rash	

TRM, treatment-associated mortality.

plasma cells producing the amyloidogenic light chain. Treatment efficacy is usually evaluated based on the hematologic response and patient survival. A complete hematologic response is defined as the absence of detectable monoclonal light chain by serum and urine immunofixation electrophoresis, normal serum concentrations or ratios of κ and λ light chains by a quantitative nephelometric assay, and a bone marrow biopsy specimen without increased plasma cells or evidence of plasma cell clonality. Because the toxicities of the treatments differ in both quality and severity, selection of treatment requires careful consideration of the distribution of organ involvement and the level of organ dysfunction in an individual patient.

For many years, the standard treatment of AL amyloidosis consisted of repeated cycles of oral melphalan with prednisone.[4,5] Although such treatment has been shown in randomized, controlled trials to extend survival, its benefit is modest, increasing median survival by only approximately 5 to 10 months (see Table 23-3). Multiple cycles of treatment are required before there is benefit; during this period, progression of organ dysfunction is likely. Importantly, attainment of a complete hematologic response is exceedingly rare with this approach. Although the use of cyclic oral melphalan and prednisone is appropriate for patients who cannot tolerate more aggressive alternatives, the regimen has been replaced, to a large extent, by more effective treatments.

High-dose melphalan and autologous stem-cell transplantation (HDM/SCT) is currently viewed by many as the treatment most likely to produce a complete hematologic remission.[7,8,18] This treatment approach consists of mobilization of peripheral stem cells using growth factor, typically granulocyte colony–stimulating factor, collection of stem cells with leukopheresis, intravenous administration of myeloablative doses of melphalan, and infusion of the stem cells to support bone marrow recovery. In single-center series, complete hematologic remission rates with this approach range from to 25% to 67%, and median survival, in those studies that reported it, is approximately 5 years.[8,19–24] The eligibility criteria for treatment with HDM/SCT vary among these series, and it is important to recognize that in most of the studies, the treatment was conducted at referral centers with particular expertise in treating patients with amyloidosis. Treatment-associated mortality appears to be higher in multicenter studies than in single-center studies, probably because in the former, many of the patients received care at centers that do not have extensive experience treating amyloidosis.[9,25]

The toxicities of HDM/SCT include those associated with the chemotherapy (e.g., mucositis, cytopenia, infection, bleeding), as well as toxicities related to stem-cell mobilization and collection. The administration of growth factor for stem-cell mobilization can cause substantial fluid retention that is poorly tolerated in patients with heart involvement or severe nephrotic syndrome. Collection of stem cells can trigger arrhythmias or hemodynamic alterations, particularly in individuals with heart involvement. Treatment-related mortality is substantially higher when HDM/SCT is used for AL amyloidosis (approximately 14% in amyloidosis referral centers) than when used for multiple myeloma (<5%), undoubtedly because of the underlying organ dysfunction in patients with amyloidosis.[26] Advanced cardiac disease, reduced renal function, hypotension from autonomic nervous system dysfunction, involvement of more than two organs, and poor performance status by oncologic assessment scales are predictors of treatment-associated morbidity and mortality with HDM/SCT.

For patients who have a partial, but not complete, hematologic response to HDM/SCT, tandem cycles of high-dose melphalan can be performed if adequate stem cells for two courses of chemotherapy are collected initially. A single-center study evaluating this approach in 53 patients was recently published.[10] Twenty-seven (55%) of the enrolled patients attained a complete hematologic response after the first cycle of high-dose melphalan and thus did not undergo tandem transplantation. Of the 22 patients who did not achieve a full response after initial treatment, 17 received a second treatment with HDM/SCT. One of these patients died during the peritransplantation period, and five (31%) achieved a complete hematologic response. These findings suggest that for some individuals, a second stem-cell transplantation can convert a partial hematologic response to a full response.

An alternative to myeloablative doses of melphalan with stem-cell transplantation that is gaining increasing attention is cyclic oral melphalan with high-dose dexamethasone (40 mg/day), typically administered for 4 consecutive days every 4 weeks. Experience with this approach was initially reported by Palladini and colleagues[12] in a study of 46 patients who were not eligible for HDM/SCT. Fifteen patients (33%) had a complete hematologic response and 31 (67%) had a partial hematologic response after a median of four cycles. The treatment was well tolerated in this series, although fluid retention, particularly in patients with amyloid cardiomyopathy or nephrotic syndrome, and myopathy are potential problems associated with repeated courses of high-dose dexamethasone. A multicenter, randomized trial comparing HDM/SCT to cyclic oral melphalan with dexamethasone was recently published.[11] The trial randomized 50 patients to each treatment arm. Median survival, the primary endpoint of the trial, was 22.2 months in the HDM/SCT group compared with 56.9 months in the cyclic oral melphalan with high-dose dexamethasone group, a statistically significant and clinically important difference. Importantly, 47% of the 38 patients in the melphalan plus dexamethasone group who received at least three cycles of melphalan with high-dose dexamethasone had a complete hematologic response, suggesting that the treatment approach can, at least temporarily, eradicate the clonal plasma cells. This study is the first multicenter, randomized trial comparing two different treatments for AL amyloidosis, and that alone makes it important. Although the findings of the trial suggest that the efficacy of oral melphalan with high-dose dexamethasone is as good as or better than that of HDM/SCT, it is important to note that (1) the treatment-related mortality with HDM/SCT was higher in this trial than that observed in single-center studies carried out at referral centers, (2) the median survival with HDM/SCT was substantially lower in this trial than in several previously reported single-center experiences, and (3) the durability of hematologic response after discontinuation of melphalan/dexamethasone was not reported. Clarification of the respective roles of HDM/SCT and oral melphalan with dexamethasone should emerge over the next few years with additional experience and additional studies.

Thalidomide is an immunomodulatory agent with activity against plasma cells that has been used either alone or in combination with dexamethasone for patients with AL amyloidosis who either are too ill to undergo HDM/SCT or have not responded to the treatment. Although the drug appears to have some efficacy, it has been found to be poorly tolerated in patients with AL amyloidosis.[13,14] Lenalidomide is a thalidomide analogue that patients with amyloidosis seem to tolerate better as it is less sedating and less likely than thalidomide to cause peripheral neuropathy. Small studies suggest that lenalidomide has efficacy in AL amyloidosis.[16,17] Bortezomib, a proteosome inhibitor approved for the treatment of multiple myeloma, is starting to be studied as a treatment for AL amyloidosis, but its efficacy has not been established.

An important finding from the HDM/SCT experience is that improvements in function of affected organs can occur in AL amyloidosis and that the improvements are much more likely for patients who achieve a complete hematologic response than for those with persistent hematologic disease. With regard to kidney disease, substantial reductions in proteinuria and other features of nephrotic syndrome occur in the majority of patients if production of the amyloidogenic light chain is halted.[27,28] Because of the variability among patients in the rate of decline in GFR, as well as high mortality rates among patients who do not respond to treatment, it has been more difficult to evaluate the impact of hematologic response on progression of renal impairment; such studies are under way.

AA Amyloidosis

AA amyloidosis occurs in the setting of long-standing inflammation when a proteolytic fragment of the acute phase reactant serum amyloid A forms amyloid. The most common inflammatory conditions underlying AA amyloidosis are rheumatoid arthritis, familial Mediterranean fever, inflammatory bowel disease, and chronic infections such as osteomyelitis. The current treatment approach for AA amyloidosis is to treat the underlying inflammatory disease and thereby reduce production of serum amyloid A. In familial Mediterranean fever, a disease associated with a high rate of development of AA amyloidosis, lifelong treatment with colchicine to inhibit familial Mediterranean fever–associated inflammation prevents amyloidosis in many patients.[29] Marked reductions in proteinuria have been reported in individuals with AA amyloidosis–associated kidney disease from a variety of underlying inflammatory conditions after treatment with cytotoxic agents or tumor necrosis factor receptor blockers.[30–32] These functional improvements are presumed to be due to suppression of serum amyloid A production and resultant decrease in AA amyloid formation. However, it is possible that these agents also have additional antiamyloid effects through suppression of cytokine production or by altering the expression of specific mediators of amyloid fibril–induced cellular toxicity.

For many individuals with AA amyloidosis, adequate suppression of serum amyloid A production is not possible. Fibrillogenesis inhibition using small molecules that have structural similarity to glycosaminoglycan moieties is a treatment approach that is currently under investigation. Because of the role of glycosaminoglycans in promoting amyloid fibril formation and tissue deposition, interfering with interactions between glycosaminoglycans and amyloidogenic proteins or fibrils should decrease new amyloid formation and might promote degradation of existing amyloid deposits. A multicenter, randomized placebo-controlled trial of 183 individuals with AA amyloidosis–associated kidney disease found that eprodisate treatment reduced the risk of a composite endpoint of renal decline or death.[33] The results of this trial are promising; however, the drug is not yet approved for use by either the U.S. Food and Drug Administration or the European Agency for the Evaluation of Medicinal Products.

Hereditary Amyloidoses

Because transthyretin (TTR) is synthesized by the liver, production of amyloidogenic variants of TTR can be eliminated by orthotopic liver transplantation. The abnormal amyloidogenic TTR variant disappears from the circulation after the liver is removed and replaced with a liver expressing only wild-type TTR. Orthotopic liver transplantation has been performed in more than 660 individuals with TTR amyloidosis and is considered the definitive treatment for the disease.[34] Unfortunately, amyloid deposition sometimes persists because wild-type TTR can deposit as amyloid at sites of preexisting amyloid deposits. Nonetheless, disease progression usually is slowed, and in many patients, clinical manifestations improve after liver transplantation. There is substantially less experience using liver transplantation for fibrinogen Aα amyloidosis, a disease that is more likely than TTR amyloidosis to involve the kidney. Case reports describe individuals with fibrinogen Aα disease who have undergone combined liver and kidney transplantation.[35–37] In all these patients, liver and kidney failure from amyloid disease was present, as fibrinogen amyloidosis, in contrast with TTR disease, often involves the liver. Outcomes were considered satisfactory without evidence of amyloid in the transplanted organs at 2 to 6 years. Liver transplantation is not appropriate for lysozyme amyloidosis because lysozyme is synthesized by polymorphonuclear cells and macrophages. Similarly, for apolipoprotein AI amyloidosis, because apolipoprotein AI is synthesized by the intestine in addition to the liver, amyloid formation would be anticipated to continue after liver transplantation, although perhaps at a slower rate.

The renal response to orthotopic liver transplantation has been evaluated in a small series of patients with TTR amyloidosis and kidney involvement.[38] Proteinuria did not change significantly in these patients, but serum creatinine levels remained relatively stable over several years. Although these patients had histologically evident renal amyloid, the clinical manifestations were mild before liver transplantation, limiting extrapolation of the findings to patients with more pronounced kidney manifestations.

Amyloidosis-Associated End-Stage Renal Disease

For any of the types of amyloidosis, dialysis dependence should not preclude aggressive treatment aimed at reducing ongoing amyloid production. Although amyloidosis-associated ESRD is not reversible, treatment can prevent progression of extrarenal disease. Concern has been expressed about the appropriateness of offering HDM/SCT to dialysis-dependent patients with AL amyloidosis because of treatment-associated toxicities. However, experience with treating selected patients with HDM/SCT suggests that both the hematologic response rate and treatment-associated mortality are similar in dialysis-dependent patients compared with the overall population of patients undergoing this treatment.[39] Furthermore, attainment of a complete hematologic response has enabled subsequent kidney transplantation in some of these patients.

Because of the likelihood of recurrence of amyloid nephropathy in renal allografts, under most circumstances, kidney transplantation should be restricted to patients with inactive disease, that is, those in whom ongoing amyloid production has been eliminated with treatment. However, proceeding with kidney transplantation might be reasonable if disease is limited to the kidney and if the progression to ESRD occurred over many years rather than rapidly.

Summary of Treatment Recommendations for Amyloidosis

The treatments that are currently available for amyloidosis all target the source of the amyloidogenic protein. For AL amyloidosis, treatments are directed against the clonal plasma cells, the source of the amyloidogenic immunoglobulin light chains. It is now clear that cyclic oral melphalan and prednisone, the main treatment for this disease for many years, is less effective than newer, more aggressive approaches such as HDM/SCT, oral melphalan with high-dose dexamethasone, and possibly lenalidamide-based regimens. Because of the variability of organ involvement and severity of organ dysfunction, as well as the toxicities associated with different treatment regimens, decisions about which approach to use must be individualized. Because of the unique toxicities associated with HDM/SCT in patients with AL amyloidosis, it is our opinion that, for most patients, HDM/SCT should be performed only at centers with experience caring for patients with amyloidosis. The relative benefits of HDM/SCT and oral melphalan with high-dose dexamethasone are not clear at present but should emerge as additional experience accumulates. For AA amyloidosis, the goal of treatment should be to suppress the underlying inflammatory disease. If regulatory approval for eprodisate is obtained, this drug will provide an additional treatment option for patients with AA amyloidosis. For hereditary TTR amyloidosis, a disease that sometimes involves the kidney, orthotopic liver transplantation is an effective treatment. The much more limited experience with liver transplantation for fibrinogen Aα disease suggests that it is reasonable to consider the approach, possibly in conjunction with kidney transplantation.

LIGHT-CHAIN DEPOSITION DISEASE

Nomenclature, Clinical Features, and Histology

LCDD is a plasma cell disorder in which monoclonal light chains deposit in glomerular and tubular basement membranes. The light chains do not form fibrils. Related but much rarer disorders are HCDD and light and heavy chain deposition disease (LHCDD). In HCDD, monoclonal heavy chains form deposits similar to those seen in LCDD, and in LHCDD both monoclonal heavy and monoclonal light chains form deposits. The pathogenesis of these disorders is probably

similar, and as a group, they are often referred to as monoclonal immunoglobulin deposition diseases (MIDD). The discussion that follows is restricted for the most part to LCDD but probably is applicable to all forms of MIDD.

LCDD can occur in association with multiple myeloma or in the absence of an overt plasmacytosis. In some patients, the plasma cell burden is sufficiently low that restricted expression by plasma cells of light chains of one isotype is not evident. Additionally, in some patients, the combination of a low plasma cell burden and a high avidity of the monoclonal light chain for tissue can result in the absence of detectable monoclonal light chain in the serum or urine even with sensitive immunofixation studies or quantitative free light-chain assays. In such cases, the evidence of a plasma cell dyscrasia may be limited to the kidney biopsy findings. However, usually a monoclonal light chain is detected by serum or urine immunofixation electrophoresis. The light chain is more often κ than λ.

Most patients with LCDD have proteinuria, which is often in the nephrotic range. The urinary protein is composed mostly of albumin; thus, patients often have other manifestations of nephrotic syndrome. Light chain deposition can be restricted to the tubular basement membranes, in which case proteinuria will be minimal. Microscopic hematuria is present in some patients. Many patients have renal impairment at the time of diagnosis, and progression to ESRD is frequent. The rate of decline in GFR varies. Most patients progress to ESRD over many months to years; however, rapid progression can occur. Importantly, small series suggest that recurrence in renal allografts is nearly universal.[40] Extrarenal disease is present in a substantial proportion of patients but is often not appreciated. The liver and heart are probably the most common sites of extrarenal disease, but clinical or histologic evidence of light-chain deposition in many other tissues has been reported.[41–44]

The kidney biopsy findings in LCDD usually involve both the glomeruli and tubules. Mild mesangial expansion with thickened glomerular capillary walls or full-blown nodular glomerulosclerosis can be seen by light microscopy. In contrast to amyloidosis, the nodules are strongly periodic acid–Schiff positive because they are composed of extracellular matrix rather than the light chains. Thickened tubular basement membranes and interstitial fibrosis are often evident. By immunofluorescence, deposition of light chain of a single isotype is present along the capillary walls, mesangium, and tubular basement membranes. The staining often has a linear, ribbon-like appearance. Electron microscopy reveals granular, and often large, deposits along glomerular and tubular basement membranes and, to a lesser extent, in the mesangium. The glomerular capillary deposits are predominantly subendothelial.[44,45]

Treatment of Light-Chain Deposition Disease

Until recently, LCDD occurring in the absence of multiple myeloma was viewed by many as a renal-limited disorder rather than a systemic disease. An appreciation for the poor renal prognosis, the frequency of extrarenal involvement, and the disease pathogenesis has altered this perception at least to some extent. Aggressive treatment directed at the clonal plasma cells, although not in widespread use, is beginning to be recognized as a justified approach to the management of this disease.[46]

The published experience with HDM/SCT for LCDD is limited to a few case reports and two small case series. Royer and colleagues[47] reported the outcomes of 11 patients with LCDD or HCDD treated with HDM/SCT. Ten of the patients had multiple myeloma, seven patients had extrarenal manifestations, and four patients were dialysis dependent. Six patients had a complete hematologic response after HDM/SCT, and a decrease in proteinuria or improvement in renal function occurred in four patients. Extrarenal manifestations improved in the six patients who had heart or liver involvement. A description of the outcomes after HDM/SCT of nine patients with LCDD without multiple myeloma was included in a recent publication.[46] Seven of the patients had a complete hematologic remission. One of the patients was dialysis dependent at the time of treatment and underwent kidney transplantation after attaining a hematologic remission. All the patients were alive at a median follow-up of 17 months. Several reports have documented regression of histologic lesions in the kidney, heart, and liver after treatment, suggesting that end-organ damage from LCDD is potentially reversible.[48,49]

Summary of Treatment Recommendations for Light-Chain Deposition Disease

The results from the admittedly limited experience treating LCDD with high-dose chemotherapy, together with the poor prognosis associated with untreated disease, provides a compelling argument for aggressive treatment of this disorder. Additional experience with HDM/SCT as well as the use of alternative treatments that have been found to be effective for AL amyloidosis or multiple myeloma should enable refinement of treatment approaches, a decrease in treatment-related toxicities, and improved outcomes for this disease.

MYELOMA CAST NEPHROPATHY

Multiple Myeloma and the Kidney

Multiple myeloma is a hematologic malignancy that results from clonal expansion of plasma cells in the bone marrow. The clinical manifestations of multiple myeloma result from both the high burden of proliferating plasma cells as well as from the immunoglobulin molecules secreted by the clonal plasma cells. Kidney disease in the setting of multiple myeloma can be caused by the plasma cells themselves (e.g., hypercalcemia-induced acute renal failure) or the secreted monoclonal immunoglobulin molecules. Most myeloma-associated immunoglobulin-mediated kidney disease is caused by light chains or light-chain fragments. However, intact monoclonal immunoglobulin molecules can cause type I cryoglobulinemia or noncryoglobulinemic proliferative GN, and monoclonal heavy chains can cause HCDD or AH amyloidosis. Two of the light-chain–associated disorders, AL amyloidosis and LCDD, are discussed in separate sections of this chapter; this section of the chapter addresses myeloma cast nephropathy, the most common myeloma-associated light-chain disorder. Fanconi syndrome resulting from damage to proximal tubular cells by filtered light chains is an additional light-chain–mediated kidney process that can occur in multiple myeloma.

Diagnosis, Clinical Features, and Kidney Histology

The diagnosis of multiple myeloma requires the combination of a bone marrow biopsy with a cellular composition of at least 10% plasma cells, demonstration of a monoclonal immunoglobulin protein in the blood or urine, and myeloma-related end-organ damage such as renal insufficiency, hypercalcemia, anemia, and lytic bone lesions. Diagnostic criteria and staging systems have been published by the International Myeloma Working Group.[50,51] Although a definitive diagnosis of cast nephropathy requires a kidney biopsy, the diagnosis is often made based on clinical suspicion.

Cast nephropathy typically occurs in individuals with a high plasma cell burden and a high concentration of monoclonal light chains in the serum and urine. Thus, unlike AL amyloidosis or LCDD, cast nephropathy usually occurs in the presence of overt multiple myeloma. Patients with cast nephropathy present with an increased serum creatinine concentration that can be either acute or chronic. Proteinuria is present but, because the urinary protein is composed of light chains and not albumin, the urine dipstick will be negative for protein, and nephrotic syndrome will not be present. The presence of nonalbumin urinary protein in a patient with multiple myeloma and renal impairment makes cast nephropathy a more likely diagnosis than myeloma-associated AL amyloidosis or LCDD, both of which usually, but not always, cause high-grade albuminuria (see Table 23-1). Many factors have been implicated as triggers of cast nephropathy; these include volume depletion, hypercalciuria, low urine pH, diuretics, and intravenous administration of radiographic contrast media.

The major histologic findings of cast nephropathy are casts within distal tubules, tubular dilatation, and tubular atrophy. By light microscopy, the casts are eosinophilic and refractile and often appear fractured. Macrophages and, in some cases, giant cells are often present in the interstitium surrounding the occluded tubules. The interstitial inflammation and fibrosis contribute to the renal failure in patients with cast nephropathy and may be more important in terms of long-term renal prognosis than the intratubular obstruction. By immunofluorescence, the casts show reactivity to immunoglobulin light chain of the same isotype as that of the circulating monoclonal protein.

Treatment of Cast Nephropathy

The main objectives in treating cast nephropathy are to minimize the propensity of filtered light chains to form intratubular casts, to decrease production of the light chains by the clonal plasma cells, and to enhance removal of the light chains from the circulation. Aggressive hydration to increase urinary flow will decrease the concentration of the light chains in the tubular fluid. Alkalinization of the urine by administration of sodium bicarbonate in an effort to decrease cast formation is often recommended; however, it should be recognized that the benefit of raising urine pH depends on the characteristics of the specific light chain. Decreasing production of light chains is accomplished with chemotherapy. Although a detailed discussion of chemotherapeutic regimens for multiple myeloma is beyond the scope of this chapter, issues that have particular relevance to cast nephropathy or to the treatment of patients with renal failure are addressed. Removal of light chains with plasma exchange or hemodialysis has received recent attention and is the major focus of this section of the chapter.

Plasma Exchange for Cast Nephropathy

The objective of plasma exchange is to rapidly remove circulating light chains and prevent ongoing renal injury before chemotherapy effectively eliminates or decreases monoclonal light-chain production. Case reports from as far back as 30 years ago have documented the use of plasma exchange to treat acute renal failure due to cast nephropathy.[52–58] Over the subsequent years, case series and small controlled trials have suggested a benefit of plasma exchange in this setting. Key features of these studies are summarized in Table 23-4.[59–65]

With the exception of the study by Movilli and colleagues,[65] all the small retrospective studies that compared renal outcomes in patients who received plasma exchange in addition to chemotherapy with those for patients who received chemotherapy alone reported a benefit of plasmapheresis. The limitations of all these studies include their retrospective nature, the lack of randomization to treatment approach, and small sample size. In addition, for several of the studies, follow-up was too short to allow assessment of long-term outcomes.

One of the first randomized, controlled trials of plasma exchange evaluated 29 patients with multiple myeloma and acute renal failure. Fifteen patients were randomized to plasma-exchange treatment in addition to cyclophosphamide therapy and glucocorticoids, whereas the control group received only cytotoxic therapy and glucocorticoids. Among dialysis-dependent patients, 11 of 13 in the plasma exchange group compared with 2 of 11 in the group receiving chemotherapy alone were

Table 23-4   Representative Studies of Plasma Exchange for Myeloma Cast Nephropathy

Study (Ref.)	Design	Treatment	Findings
Pozzi et al,[59] N = 50	Retrospective review	Chemotherapy/plasma exchange vs. chemotherapy	Recovery of renal function occurred in 61% of patients who received plasma exchange compared with 27% of patients who received chemotherapy alone
Misiani et al,[60] N = 23	Retrospective review	Chemotherapy/plasma exchange	8 of 10 patients with acute renal failure had recovery of renal function; 11 of 13 patients with chronic renal failure had improvement in renal function
Zucchelli et al,[61] N = 29	Randomized trial	Plasma exchange/chemotherapy vs. chemotherapy	11 of 15 patients in the plasma exchange group compared with 2 of 14 patients in the control group had improved renal function; 1-year survival rates were 66% and 28% in the plasma exchange and control groups, respectively
Johnson et al,[62] N = 21	Randomized trial	Plasma exchange/hydration/chemotherapy vs. hydration/chemotherapy	10 of 11 patients in plasma exchange group compared with 5 of 10 patients in control group had improved renal function
Moist et al,[63] N = 26	Retrospective review	Hydration/plasma exchange/chemotherapy	15 of the 26 patients had improved renal function by 3 mo
Clark et al,[64] N = 97 (104 patients randomized; 97 patients included in analyses)	Randomized, controlled, multicenter trial	Plasma exchange/conventional therapy vs. conventional therapy	No statistically significant difference between groups in the composite outcome of death, estimated glomerular filtration rate < 30 mL/min/1.73m^2 or dialysis dependence; 42% of dialysis-dependent patients in the plasma exchange group compared with 37% of dialysis-dependent patients in the control group became dialysis independent (difference not statistically significant)
Movilli et al,[65] N = 55	Retrospective review	Plasma exchange vs. no plasma exchange	No difference between groups in renal or patient survival

able to discontinue dialysis. Patient survival at 1 year was also higher in the plasma exchange group. The authors concluded that plasma exchange provides both renal and overall survival benefit. Interestingly, the dialysis-dependent patients in the plasma exchange group were treated with hemodialysis, whereas the patients in the control group received peritoneal dialysis. This source of bias might be expected to favor the plasma exchange group if hemodialysis is more effective than peritoneal dialysis at removing light chains.

A second trial randomized 11 patients to plasmapheresis and 10 patients to control therapy.[62] A greater number of patients in the plasmapheresis group than in the control group had a favorable renal response. There was no survival difference at 1 year. Drawbacks of this study are its small sample size, heterogeneity of plasma exchange regimens, and exclusion from the trial of patients with melphalan-resistant disease.

The Canadian Apheresis Group performed a multicenter trial that evaluated 104 patients with newly diagnosed multiple myeloma and acute renal failure.[64] Patients were randomly assigned to conventional therapy plus four to seven plasma exchange treatments or conventional therapy alone. Approximately 30% of patients in both groups were dialysis dependent at study entry. During follow-up, 66% and 50% of dialysis-dependent patients in the plasma exchange group and control group, respectively, were able to discontinue dialysis, and approximately 20% of patients in both groups initiated dialysis. There was no difference between treatment groups in the composite endpoint of death, dialysis dependence, or severe renal impairment at 6 months, and the investigators interpreted the trial as showing no benefit of plasma exchange. This trial had several strengths including its multicenter nature and the sample size that was substantially larger than that of earlier randomized trials. However, the study has been criticized because approximately 20% of patients did not have detectable monoclonal light chain in the urine, and biopsy documentation of cast nephropathy was not required. If cast nephropathy was not the cause of renal failure in many of the patients, the ability to detect a benefit of plasma exchange would be reduced.

In summary, there is not strong evidence supporting a role for plasma exchange in cast nephropathy. Although earlier retrospective case series and small randomized trials suggested a benefit, a more recent, larger multicenter, randomized trial found similar outcomes among patients treated with or without plasma exchange. It is possible that because of a more rapid decrease in production of the pathogenic light chains, current chemotherapeutic approaches have lessened the impact of plasma exchange. It is also possible that plasma exchange, at least as currently performed, is not sufficiently effective at removing light chains.[66] The recent availability of a quantitative assay for measuring serum light-chain concentrations should enable better assessment of efficacy of interventions aimed at light-chain removal.

Hemodialysis for Cast Nephropathy

The molecular weight of light chains (approximately 25 kD for κ and λ light-chain monomers and 50 kD for λ dimers) precludes their passage through the pores of conventional or high-flux hemodialyzer membranes. However, adsorption of light chains by dialyzer membranes has been demonstrated, so it is possible that some light-chain removal does occur with standard hemodialysis treatments. Indeed, one of the limita-

tions of the studies of plasma exchange is that they did not standardize the dialyzer membranes or dialysis regimens for those patients who were dialysis dependent. A recently proposed approach to the treatment of cast nephropathy is the use of "superflux" or "protein-leaking" dialyzer membranes.[67] These membranes have pore sizes that are substantially larger than high-flux membranes. In the only published study evaluating large-pore dialyzers for cast nephropathy, the mean in vitro decreases in κ and λ light-chain concentrations by a superflux dialyzer were 96% and 94%, respectively, after 4 hours. Use of the dialyzers in a small number of patients with acute renal failure from cast nephropathy suggested that extended daily dialysis in combination with chemotherapy might be more effective at light-chain removal than is plasma exchange. The findings from this pilot study are intriguing, but as the authors acknowledge, further study is required to establish a role of such dialyzers in the treatment of cast nephropathy.

Chemotherapy for Multiple Myeloma: Kidney-Specific Issues

The general approach to treating patients with newly diagnosed multiple myeloma is to start with an induction regimen such as thalidomide and dexamethasone to decrease the plasma cell burden, followed by high-dose chemotherapy (usually melphalan) with SCT. Although SCT extends survival and results in a hematologic remission in a substantial proportion of patients, most patients eventually experience a relapse and require additional treatment. Tandem SCT, thalidomide, lenalidomide, dexamethasone, and bortezomib, all of which are discussed in the AL amyloidosis section, are currently being used as salvage treatment for patients with resistant or relapsed disease or as initial treatment in individuals who are not eligible for SCT.[68]

A general observation is that multiple myeloma patients with renal impairment have greater treatment-associated toxicity and decreased overall survival than those with preserved renal function.[69-71] There are several potential contributors to the relatively poor outcomes. Renal impairment may be a marker of high tumor burden or aggressive disease. Additionally, renal failure increases susceptibility to infection, bleeding, and other complications of chemotherapy. Finally, renal failure often excludes patients from aggressive treatments or leads to administration of lower and therefore less effective doses of drugs.

For many of the agents used to treat multiple myeloma, optimal dosing in patients with renal impairment has not been determined. For example, although melphalan elimination is the result of degradation and very little is excreted by the kidney, studies evaluating pharmacokinetics of melphalan in individuals with renal impairment have yielded conflicting results.[72] Some studies suggest that melphalan clearance is decreased in the setting of renal failure and others have not. Moreover, information about clearance of many of these drugs by hemodialysis or peritoneal dialysis is limited or nonexistent. Most centers decrease the dose of melphalan when it is administered as part of a myeloablative regimen from 200 mg/m^2 to 140 or 100 mg/m^2 in individuals with significant renal impairment. Thalidomide clearance is not dependent on renal function. Lenalidomide dosing is adjusted based on renal function, but there is little information to guide dosing in patients undergoing dialysis.[73] Clearance of bortezomib is dependent on both the liver and the kidney, and decreased dosing may be required if the creatinine clearance is less than

30 mL/min. Bisphosphonates, which are typically administered long term to patients with multiple myeloma, are contraindicated when the glomerular filtration rate is decreased, and among patients with multiple myeloma and normal renal function, rare complications of bisphosphonate treatment include focal and segmental glomerulosclerosis, collapsing glomerulopathy, and acute tubular necrosis.[74–76]

Kidney Transplantation in Multiple Myeloma

Malignancy is generally a contraindication for kidney transplantation; however, for multiple myeloma, combined kidney and allogeneic stem-cell transplantation from the same donor has been performed in a small number of individuals. Three case reports describe a total of seven patients with multiple myeloma and ESRD who underwent dual kidney and stem-cell transplantation from HLA-identical siblings.[77–79] These patients all received nonmyeloablative preparative therapy with intravenous cyclophosphamide, antithymocyte globulin, and thymic irradiation with the goal of attaining donor-specific allotolerance and temporary chimerism. Long-term patient and renal survival in six of these patients has been maintained, even in the presence of donor marrow rejection.[79]

Summary of Treatment for Cast Nephropathy

Multiple myeloma is a common malignancy with frequent kidney involvement. The goal of treatment is to eliminate the malignant clone of plasma cells using cytotoxic agents, immunomodulatory agents, and proteosome inhibitors. A benefit of plasma exchange in conjunction with anti–plasma cell treatment for cast nephropathy has not been demonstrated, although one could argue that it might be helpful to some individuals and that its utility has not been adequately assessed. The use of superflux hemodialysis to remove light chains may have benefit, but experience with this approach is limited to a single pilot study.

FIBRILLARY GLOMERULONEPHRITIS AND IMMUNOTACTOID GLOMERULOPATHY

Classification, Clinical Features, and Kidney Histology

Fibrillary GN and immunotactoid glomerulopathy are relatively rare disorders in which immunoglobulin-containing fibrillary deposits are present in the mesangium and glomerular capillary walls. The fibrils do not stain with Congo red dye, thereby distinguishing them from amyloid. The major discriminating features between fibrillary GN and immunotactoid glomerulopathy are the size and distribution patterns of the fibrils. In fibrillary GN, the fibrils are 15 to 20 nm in diameter and deposit in what appears to be a random array. In immunotactoid glomerulopathy, the fibrils are actually microtubules with hollow centers and diameters of 30 to 60 nm. The microtubules deposit in organized, parallel arrays providing a substructure to the deposits evident by electron microscopy.[80] Although there is controversy about whether the two disorders differ pathogenetically,[81] it does appear that immunotactoid glomerulopathy is more likely than fibrillary GN to occur in association with a lymphoproliferative disorder. Additionally, the microtubules of immunotactoid glomerulopathy are often composed of what appears to be monoclonal immunoglobulin molecules, whereas the immunoglobulin components of the fibrils of fibrillary GN more often appear to be polyclonal, albeit with some restriction of the heavy-chain subtype.

The clinical manifestations of fibrillary GN and immunotactoid glomerulopathy are similar. Proteinuria is always present and is often in the nephrotic range, microscopic hematuria is common, and patients are often hypertensive. Creatinine is often elevated at presentation. The rate of decline of renal function is variable; in several series, approximately 50% of patients with fibrillary GN or immunotactoid glomerulopathy had progressed to ESRD within 2 to 4 years.[80,82–84] Extrarenal manifestations of these disorders are rare, but patients with associated lung, heart, or liver involvement have been reported.[85,86]

Renal histologic findings vary but are predominantly glomerular. In both fibrillary GN and immunotactoid glomerulopathy, light microscopy usually reveals mesangial expansion with periodic acid–Schiff-positive material and focal or diffuse glomerular capillary wall thickening with double contours or spikes. Proliferative GN, sometimes with cellular or fibrocellular crescents, can occur. Immunofluorescence reveals complement and immunoglobulin heavy and light chains in the mesangium and along capillary walls. In fibrillary GN, the immunoglobulin appears to be polyclonal, although subtyping suggests some restriction to IgG subtypes 1 and 4. In a substantial proportion of biopsy specimens from patients with immunotactoid glomerulopathy, the immunoglobulin deposits appear to be monoclonal intact immunoglobulin (usually IgG κ). By electron microscopy, the deposits are present in the mesangium, within the glomerular capillary walls, and rarely in the tubular basement membranes or interstitium. Ultrastructural examination reveals fibrils or microtubules in the same location as the electron-dense deposits. The glomerular capillary fibrils are usually within the basement membrane but can also have a subepithelial or subendothelial distribution.

Both fibrillary GN and immunotactoid glomerulopathy have been found in association with systemic diseases such as diabetes mellitus, solid tumors, human immunodeficiency virus, and hepatitis C, but pathophysiologic links between the systemic illnesses and the glomerulopathy are not established. Lymphoproliferative disorders with or without a circulating paraprotein are present in some patients with immunotactoid glomerulopathy.[80,87–91]

Treatment of Fibrillary Glomerulonephritis and Immunotactoid Glomerulopathy

There are no established treatments for fibrillary GN or immunotactoid glomerulopathy. The published experience regarding treatment of these disorders is restricted to case reports and small series. Because of the apparent involvement of immunoglobulin, various immunosuppressive therapies have been tried. Case reports and anecdotal evidence suggest that glucocorticoids alone or in combination with cyclophosphamide, cyclosporine, or plasma exchange may occasionally be effective.[80,83,84,89,92–97] However, the response rate is probably less than 10%,[84] and among those who do respond with remission of nephrotic syndrome, many relapse after treatment is discontinued.[89] Some authors have suggested that steroid treatment may be particularly helpful for patients with preserved renal function[94] and that more aggressive treatment with cyclophosphamide therapy should be attempted if there are cellular crescents and/or diffuse proliferation on kidney biopsy.[95] It is our opinion that evaluation for an underlying lymphoproliferative disorder with bone marrow biopsy and immunofixation electrophoretic studies of the serum and urine should be performed in all individuals with a histologic diagnosis of fibrillary GN or immunotactoid glomerulopathy. If there is evidence of an associated lymphoproliferative disorder, treating the underlying malignancy may have a beneficial effect on the kidney process.[80]

Kidney Transplantation

Individuals with fibrillary GN or immunotactoid glomerulopathy have undergone kidney transplantation. Recurrence of disease in the allograft has been reported in approximately 50% of patients in small case series.[82,98–100] However, it appears that despite recurrent disease, deterioration of allograft function is slow, perhaps because of the administration of immunosuppressive therapies.[82,99]

Summary of Treatment Recommendations for Fibrillary Glomerulonephritis and Immunotactoid Glomerulopathy

There is no specific treatment for fibrillary GN or immunotactoid glomerulopathy. All patients with these disorders should undergo evaluation for a lymphoproliferative disorder with bone marrow biopsy, immunofixation electrophoresis of the serum and urine, and quantitative serum-free light-chain assay. If a disorder is identified, appropriate chemotherapy should be administered. In the absence of an underlying hematologic disease, we recommend supportive care but do not believe that evidence justifies the use of immunosuppressive or cytotoxic agents. Kidney transplantation should be considered if there is progression to ESRD because adequate renal function may be sustained even in the setting of recurrent disease.

References

1. Merlini G, Bellotti V: Molecular mechanisms of amyloidosis. N Engl J Med 2003;349:583–596.
2. Falk RH, Comenzo RL, Skinner M: The systemic amyloidoses. N Engl J Med 1997;337:898–909.
3. Dember LM: Amyloidosis-associated kidney disease. J Am Soc Nephrol 2006;17:3458–3471.
4. Skinner M, Anderson J, Simms R, et al: Treatment of 100 patients with primary amyloidosis: A randomized trial of melphalan, prednisone, and colchicine versus colchicine only. Am J Med 1996;100:290–298.
5. Kyle RA, Gertz MA, Greipp PR, et al: A trial of three regimens for primary amyloidosis: Colchicine alone, melphalan and prednisone, and melphalan, prednisone, and colchicine. N Engl J Med 1997;336:1202–1207.
6. Comenzo RL, Vosburgh E, Falk RH, et al: Dose-intensive melphalan with blood stem-cell support for the treatment of AL (amyloid light-chain) amyloidosis: Survival and responses in 25 patients. Blood 1998;91:3662–3670.
7. Dispenzieri A, Kyle RA, Lacy MQ, et al: Superior survival in primary systemic amyloidosis patients undergoing peripheral blood stem cell transplantation: A case-control study. Blood 2004;103:3960–3963.
8. Skinner M, Sanchorawala V, Seldin DC, et al: High-dose melphalan and autologous stem-cell transplantation in patients with AL amyloidosis: An 8-year study. Ann Intern Med 2004;140:85–93.
9. Goodman HJ, Gillmore JD, Lachmann HJ, et al: Outcome of autologous stem cell transplantation for AL amyloidosis in the UK. Br J Haematol 2006;134:417–425.
10. Sanchorawala V, Wright DG, Quillen K, et al: Tandem cycles of high-dose melphalan and autologous stem cell transplantation increases the response rate in AL amyloidosis. Bone Marrow Transplant 2007;40:557–562.
11. Jaccard A, Moreau P, Leblond V, et al: High-dose melphalan versus melphalan plus dexamethasone for AL amyloidosis. N Engl J Med 2007;357:1083–1093.
12. Palladini G, Perfetti V, Obici L, et al: Association of melphalan and high-dose dexamethasone is effective and well tolerated in patients with AL (primary) amyloidosis who are ineligible for stem cell transplantation. Blood 2004;103:2936–2938.
13. Seldin DC, Choufani EB, Dember LM, et al: Tolerability and efficacy of thalidomide for the treatment of patients with light chain-associated (AL) amyloidosis. Clin Lymphoma 2003;3:241–246.
14. Dispenzieri A, Lacy MQ, Rajkumar SV, et al: Poor tolerance to high doses of thalidomide in patients with primary systemic amyloidosis. Amyloid 2003;10:257–261.
15. Palladini G, Perfetti V, Perlini S, et al: The combination of thalidomide and intermediate-dose dexamethasone is an effective but toxic treatment for patients with primary amyloidosis (AL). Blood 2005;105:2949–2951.
16. Sanchorawala V, Wright DG, Rosenzweig M, et al: Lenalidomide and dexamethasone in the treatment of AL amyloidosis: Results of a phase 2 trial. Blood 2007;109:492–496.
17. Dispenzieri A, Lacy MQ, Zeldenrust SR, et al: The activity of lenalidomide with or without dexamethasone in patients with primary systemic amyloidosis. Blood 2007;109:465–470.
18. Sanchorawala V: Light-chain (AL) amyloidosis: diagnosis and treatment. Clin J Am Soc Nephrol 2006;1:1331–1341.
19. van Gameren II, Hazenberg BP, Jager PL, et al: AL amyloidosis treated with induction chemotherapy with VAD followed by high dose melphalan and autologous stem cell transplantation. Amyloid 2002;9:165–174.
20. Blum W, Khoury H, Lin HS, et al: Primary amyloidosis patients with significant organ dysfunction tolerate autologous transplantation after conditioning with single-dose total body irradiation alone: A feasibility study. Biol Blood Marrow Transplant 2003;9:397–404.
21. Gertz MA, Lacy MQ, Dispenzieri A, et al: Risk-adjusted manipulation of melphalan dose before stem cell transplantation in patients with amyloidosis is associated with a lower response rate. Bone Marrow Transplant 2004;34:1025–1031.
22. Mollee PN, Wechalekar AD, Pereira DL, et al: Autologous stem cell transplantation in primary systemic amyloidosis: The impact of selection criteria on outcome. Bone Marrow Transplant 2004;33:271–277.
23. Perz JB, Schonland SO, Hundemer M, et al: High-dose melphalan with autologous stem cell transplantation after VAD induction chemotherapy for treatment of amyloid light chain amyloidosis: A single centre prospective phase II study. Br J Haematol 2004;127:543–551.
24. Chow LQ, Bahlis N, Russell J, et al: Autologous transplantation for primary systemic AL amyloidosis is feasible outside a major amyloidosis referral centre: The Calgary BMT Program experience. Bone Marrow Transplant 2005;36:591–596.
25. Moreau P, Leblond V, Bourquelot P, et al: Prognostic factors for survival and response after high-dose therapy and autologous stem cell transplantation in systemic AL amyloidosis: A report on 21 patients. Br J Haematol 1998;101:766–769.

26. Dember LM: Emerging treatment approaches for the systemic amyloidoses. Kidney Int 2005;68:1377–1390.

27. Dember LM, Sanchorawala V, Seldin DC, et al: Effect of dose-intensive intravenous melphalan and autologous blood stem-cell transplantation on al amyloidosis-associated renal disease. Ann Intern Med 2001;134:746–753.

28. Leung N, Dispenzieri A, Fervenza FC, et al: Renal response after high-dose melphalan and stem cell transplantation is a favorable marker in patients with primary systemic amyloidosis. Am J Kidney Dis 2005;46:270–277.

29. Ozen S: Renal amyloidosis in familial Mediterranean fever. Kidney Int 2004;65:1118–1127.

30. Elkayam O, Hawkins PN, Lachmann H, et al: Rapid and complete resolution of proteinuria due to renal amyloidosis in a patient with rheumatoid arthritis treated with infliximab. Arthritis Rheum 2002;46:2571–2573.

31. Mpofu S, Teh LS, Smith PJ, et al: Cytostatic therapy for AA amyloidosis complicating psoriatic spondyloarthropathy. Rheumatology (Oxford) 2003;42:362–366.

32. Gottenberg JE, Merle-Vincent F, Bentaberry F, et al: Anti-tumor necrosis factor alpha therapy in fifteen patients with AA amyloidosis secondary to inflammatory arthritides: A followup report of tolerability and efficacy. Arthritis Rheum 2003;48: 2019–2024.

33. Dember LM, Hawkins PN, Hazenberg BP, et al: Eprodisate for the treatment of renal disease in AA amyloidosis. N Engl J Med, 356:2349-60, 2007.

34. Ericzon BG, Larsson M, Herlenius G, Wilczek HE: Report from the Familial Amyloidotic Polyneuropathy World Transplant Registry (FAPWTR) and the Domino Liver Transplant Registry (DLTR). Amyloid 2003;10(Suppl 1):67–76.

35. Gillmore JD, Booth DR, Rela M, et al: Curative hepatorenal transplantation in systemic amyloidosis caused by the Glu-526Val fibrinogen alpha-chain variant in an English family. Q J Med 2000;93:269–275.

36. Zeldenrust S, Gertz M, Uemichi T, et al: Orthotopic liver transplantation for hereditary fibrinogen amyloidosis. Transplantation 2003;75:560–561.

37. Mousson C, Heyd B, Justrabo E, et al: Successful hepatorenal transplantation in hereditary amyloidosis caused by a frameshift mutation in fibrinogen Aalpha-chain gene. Am J Transplant 2006;6:632–635.

38. Snanoudj R, Durrbach A, Gauthier E, et al: Changes in renal function in patients with familial amyloid polyneuropathy treated with orthotopic liver transplantation. Nephrol Dial Transplant 2004;19:1779–1785.

39. Casserly LF, Fadia A, Sanchorawala V, et al: High-dose intravenous melphalan with autologous stem cell transplantation in AL amyloidosis-associated end-stage renal disease. Kidney Int 2003;63:1051–1057.

40. Leung N, Lager DJ, Gertz MA, et al: Long-term outcome of renal transplantation in light-chain deposition disease. Am J Kidney Dis 2004;43:147–153.

41. Pozzi C, Locatelli F: Kidney and liver involvement in monoclonal light chain disorders. Semin Nephrol 2002;22:319–330.

42. Croitoru AG, Hytiroglou P, Schwartz ME, Saxena R: Liver transplantation for liver rupture due to light chain deposition disease: A case report. Semin Liver Dis 2006;26:298–303.

43. Peng SK, French WJ, Cohen AH, Fausel RE: Light chain cardiomyopathy associated with small-vessel disease. Arch Pathol Lab Med 1988;112:844–846.

44. Ronco P, Plaisier E, Mougenot B, Aucouturier P: Immunoglobulin light (heavy)-chain deposition disease: From molecular medicine to pathophysiology-driven therapy. Clin J Am Soc Nephrol 2006;1:1342–1350.

45. Lin J, Markowitz GS, Valeri AM, et al: Renal monoclonal immunoglobulin deposition disease: The disease spectrum. J Am Soc Nephrol 2001;12:1482–1492.

46. Salant DJ, Sanchorawala V, D'Agati VD: A case of atypical light chain deposition disease—diagnosis and treatment. Clin J Am Soc Nephrol 2007;2:858–867.

47. Royer B, Arnulf B, Martinez F, et al: High dose chemotherapy in light chain or light and heavy chain deposition disease. Kidney Int 2004;65:642–648.

48. Mariette X, Clauvel JP, Brouet JC: Intensive therapy in AL amyloidosis and light-chain deposition disease. Ann Intern Med 1995;123:553.

49. Komatsuda A, Wakui H, Ohtani H, et al: Disappearance of nodular mesangial lesions in a patient with light chain nephropathy after long-term chemotherapy. Am J Kidney Dis 2000;35:E9.

50. Criteria for the classification of monoclonal gammopathies, multiple myeloma and related disorders: A report of the International Myeloma Working Group. Br J Haematol 2003;121:749–757.

51. Greipp PR, San Miguel J, Durie BG, et al: International staging system for multiple myeloma. J Clin Oncol 2005;23:3412–3420.

52. Feest TG, Burge PS, Cohen SL: Successful treatment of myeloma kidney by diuresis and plasmapheresis. Br Med J 1976;1:503–1504.

53. Fortuny IE, McCullough J: Plasma exchange by continuous flow centrifugation. Minn Med 1977;60:25–26.

54. Isbister JP, Biggs JC, Penny R: Experience with large volume plasmapheresis in malignant paraproteinaemia and immune disorders. Aust N Z J Med 1978;8:154–164.

55. Misiani R, Remuzzi G, Bertani T, et al: Plasmapheresis in the treatment of acute renal failure in multiple myeloma. Am J Med 1979;66:684–688.

56. Locatelli F, Pozzi C, Pedrini L, et al: Steroid pulses and plasmapheresis in the treatment of acute renal failure in multiple myeloma. Proc Eur Dial Transplant Assoc 1980;17:690–694.

57. Morse EE, Pisciotto PT: Therapeutic plasmapheresis in patients with renal disease. Ann Clin Lab Sci 1981;11:361–366.

58. Zucchelli P, Pasquali S, Cagnoli L, Rovinetti C: Plasma exchange therapy in acute renal failure due to light chain myeloma. Trans Am Soc Artif Intern Organs 1984;30:36–39.

59. Pozzi C, Pasquali S, Donini U, et al: Prognostic factors and effectiveness of treatment in acute renal failure due to multiple myeloma: A review of 50 cases. Report of the Italian Renal Immunopathology Group. Clin Nephrol 1987;28:1–9.

60. Misiani R, Tiraboschi G, Mingardi G, Mecca G: Management of myeloma kidney: An anti-light-chain approach. Am J Kidney Dis 1987;10:28–33.

61. Zucchelli P, Pasquali S, Cagnoli L, Ferrari G: Controlled plasma exchange trial in acute renal failure due to multiple myeloma. Kidney Int 1988;33:1175–1180.

62. Johnson WJ, Kyle RA, Pineda AA, et al: Treatment of renal failure associated with multiple myeloma. Plasmapheresis, hemodialysis, and chemotherapy. Arch Intern Med 1990;150: 863–869.

63. Moist L, Nesrallah G, Kortas C, et al: Plasma exchange in rapidly progressive renal failure due to multiple myeloma. A retrospective case series. Am J Nephrol 1999;19:45–50.

64. Clark WF, Stewart AK, Rock GA, et al: Plasma exchange when myeloma presents as acute renal failure: A randomized, controlled trial. Ann Intern Med 2005;143:777–784.

65. Movilli E, Guido J, Silvia T, et al: Plasma exchange in the treatment of acute renal failure of myeloma. Nephrol Dial Transplant 2007;22:1270–1271.

66. Cserti C, Haspel R, Stowell C, Dzik W: Light chain removal by plasmapheresis in myeloma-associated renal failure. Transfusion 2007;47:511–514.

67. Hutchison CA, Cockwell P, Reid S, et al: Efficient removal of immunoglobulin free light chains by hemodialysis for multiple myeloma: In vitro and in vivo studies. J Am Soc Nephrol 2007;18:886–895.

68. Singhal S, Mehta J: Multiple myeloma. Clin J Am Soc Nephrol 2006;1:1322–1330.
69. San Miguel J, Lahuerta JJ, Garcia-Sanz R, et al: Are myeloma patients with renal failure candidates for autologous stem cell transplantation? Haematol J 2000;1:28–36.
70. Badros A, Barlogie B, Siegel E, et al: Results of autologous stem cell transplant in multiple myeloma patients with renal failure. Br J Haematol 2001;114:822–829.
71. Knudsen LM, Nielsen B, Gimsing P, Geisler C: Autologous stem cell transplantation in multiple myeloma: Outcome in patients with renal failure. Eur J Haematol 2005;75:27–33.
72. Tricot G, Alberts DS, Johnson C, et al: Safety of autotransplants with high-dose melphalan in renal failure: A pharmacokinetic and toxicity study. Clin Cancer Res 1996;2:947–952.
73. Niesvizky R, Naib T, Christos PJ, et al: Lenalidomide-induced myelosuppression is associated with renal dysfunction: Adverse events evaluation of treatment-naive patients undergoing front-line lenalidomide and dexamethasone therapy. Br J Haematol 2007;138:640–643.
74. Desikan R, Veksler Y, Raza S, et al: Nephrotic proteinuria associated with high-dose pamidronate in multiple myeloma. Br J Haematol 2002;119:496–469.
75. Barri YM, Munshi NC, Sukumalchantra S, et al: Podocyte injury associated glomerulopathies induced by pamidronate. Kidney Int 2004;65:634–641.
76. Markowitz GS, Fine PL, Stack JI, et al: Toxic acute tubular necrosis following treatment with zoledronate (Zometa). Kidney Int 2003;64:281–289.
77. Spitzer TR, Delmonico F, Tolkoff-Rubin N, et al: Combined histocompatibility leukocyte antigen-matched donor bone marrow and renal transplantation for multiple myeloma with end stage renal disease: The induction of allograft tolerance through mixed lymphohematopoietic chimerism. Transplantation 1999;68:480–484.
78. Buhler LH, Spitzer TR, Sykes M, et al: Induction of kidney allograft tolerance after transient lymphohematopoietic chimerism in patients with multiple myeloma and end-stage renal disease. Transplantation 2002;74:1405–1409.
79. Fudaba Y, Spitzer TR, Shaffer J, et al: Myeloma responses and tolerance following combined kidney and nonmyeloablative marrow transplantation: in vivo and in vitro analyses. Am J Transplant 2006;6:2121–2133.
80. Rosenstock JL, Markowitz GS, Valeri AM, et al: Fibrillary and immunotactoid glomerulonephritis: Distinct entities with different clinical and pathologic features. Kidney Int 2003;63: 1450–1461.
81. Ivanyi B, Degrell P: Fibrillary glomerulonephritis and immunotactoid glomerulopathy. Nephrol Dial Transplant 2004;19:2166–2170.
82. Pronovost PH, Brady HR, Gunning ME, et al: Clinical features, predictors of disease progression and results of renal transplantation in fibrillary/immunotactoid glomerulopathy. Nephrol Dial Transplant 1996;11:837–842.
83. Brady HR: Fibrillary glomerulopathy. Kidney Int 1998;53: 1421–1429.
84. Schwartz MM, Korbet SM, Lewis EJ: Immunotactoid glomerulopathy. J Am Soc Nephrol 2002;13:1390–1397.
85. Masson RG, Rennke HG, Gottlieb MN: Pulmonary hemorrhage in a patient with fibrillary glomerulonephritis. N Engl J Med 1992;326:36–39.
86. Rovin BH, Bou-Khalil P, Sedmak D: Pulmonary-renal syndrome in a patient with fibrillary glomerulonephritis. Am J Kidney Dis 1993;22:713–716.
87. Amir-Ansari B, O'Donnell P, Nelson SR, Cairns HS: Fibrillary glomerulonephritis in a patient with adenocarcinoma of stomach. Nephrol Dial Transplant 1997;12:210–2101.
88. Haas M, Rajaraman S, Ahuja T, et al: Fibrillary/immunotactoid glomerulonephritis in HIV-positive patients: A report of three cases. Nephrol Dial Transplant 2000;15:1679–1683.
89. Bridoux F, Hugue V, Coldefy O, et al: Fibrillary glomerulonephritis and immunotactoid (microtubular) glomerulopathy are associated with distinct immunologic features. Kidney Int 2002;62:1764–1775.
90. Guerra G, Narayan G, Rennke HG, Jaber BL: Crescentic fibrillary glomerulonephritis associated with hepatitis C viral infection. Clin Nephrol 2003;60:364–368.
91. Gielen GA, Wetzel JF, Steenbergen EJ, Mudde AH: Fibrillary glomerulonephritis in a patient with type 2 diabetes mellitus. Neth J Med 2006;64:119–123.
92. Kurihara I, Saito T, Sato H, et al: Successful treatment with steroid pulse therapy in a case of immunotactoid glomerulopathy with hypocomplementemia. Am J Kidney Dis 1998;32:E4.
93. Kurosu M, Ando Y, Takeda S, et al: Immunotactoid glomerulopathy characterized by steroid-responsive massive subendothelial deposition. Am J Kidney Dis 2001;37:E21.
94. Dickenmann M, Schaub S, Nickeleit V, et al: Fibrillary glomerulonephritis: Early diagnosis associated with steroid responsiveness. Am J Kidney Dis 2002;40:E9.
95. Blume C, Ivens K, May P, et al: Fibrillary glomerulonephritis associated with crescents as a therapeutic challenge. Am J Kidney Dis 2002;40:420–425.
96. Rihova Z, Honsova E, Spicka I, et al: Immunotactoid glomerulonephritis as a cause of acute renal failure. Nephrol Dial Transplant 2004;19:1016–1017.
97. Mahajan S, Kalra V, Dinda AK, et al: Fibrillary glomerulonephritis presenting as rapidly progressive renal failure in a young female: A case report. Int Urol Nephrol 2005;37:561–564.
98. Korbet SM, Rosenberg BF, Schwartz MM, Lewis EJ: Course of renal transplantation in immunotactoid glomerulopathy. Am J Med 1990;89:91–95.
99. Carles X, Rostaing L, Modesto A, et al: Successful treatment of recurrence of immunotactoid glomerulopathy in a kidney allograft recipient. Nephrol Dial Transplant 2000;15:897–900.
100. Samaniego M, Nadasdy GM, Laszik Z, Nadasdy T: Outcome of renal transplantation in fibrillary glomerulonephritis. Clin Nephrol 2001;55:159–166.

Further Reading

Dember LM: Amyloidosis-associated kidney disease. J Am Soc Nephrol 2006;17:3458–3471.
Korbet SM, Schwartz MM: Multiple myeloma. J Am Soc Nephrol 2006;17:2533–2545.
Ronco P, Plaisier E, Mougenot B, Aucouturier P: Immunoglobulin light (heavy)-chain deposition disease: from molecular medicine to pathophysiology-driven therapy. Clin J Am Soc Nephrol 2006;1:1342–1350.
Rosenstock JL, Markowitz GS, Valeri AM, et al: Fibrillary and immunotactoid glomerulonephritis: Distinct entities with different clinical and pathologic features. Kidney Int 2003;63:1450–1461.
Singhal S, Mehta J: Multiple myeloma. Clin J Am Soc Nephrol 2006;1:1322–1330.

Chapter 24

Hepatitis B– and HIV-Related Renal Diseases

Brian D. Radbill, Christina M. Wyatt, Joseph A. Vassalotti, Mary E. Klotman, and Paul E. Klotman

CHAPTER CONTENTS

HEPATITIS B VIRUS AND RENAL DISEASE

Background

Hepatitis B virus (HBV), a partially double-stranded circular DNA hepadnavirus first discovered in 1966,[1] is a major cause of acute and chronic hepatitis, cirrhosis, and hepatocellular carcinoma. An estimated 350 million people are chronically infected with HBV worldwide.[2] Although HBV remains endemic in Southeast Asia and sub-Saharan Africa with reported prevalence rates of 3% to 26%,[3] the United States has significantly lower levels of infection with a prevalence rate of less than 0.5% or approximately 1.25 million chronic carriers.[4] Since the implementation of a national vaccination strategy in 1991, the incidence of HBV infection in the United States has decreased by an estimated 80%.[5] Continued universal vaccination of the general populations in the United States and Western Europe should ultimately eliminate incident HBV infection in those areas.

Hepatitis B Virus–Associated Renal Disease

An association between HBV and renal disease was first recognized in 1971 when hepatitis B surface antigen (HBsAg) was demonstrated in immune complexes deposited in the glomeruli of a 53-year-old man with membranous nephropathy.[6] Since then, HBV has been associated with a variety of renal diseases, including membranous nephropathy (MN), membranoproliferative glomerulonephritis (MPGN), mesangial proliferative glomerulonephritis, IgA nephropathy, and polyarteritis nodosa (PAN) (Table 24-1). The frequency of HBV-associated renal disease correlates with the prevalence of HBV in the general population and is higher in countries where HBV is endemic. Although there are few data documenting the actual prevalence of HBV-associated renal disease, it is thought to affect only a small percentage of the large number of chronic carriers worldwide.[7]

Pathogenesis

The pathogenesis of HBV-associated renal disease is classically believed to be mediated by the formation of circulating immune complexes composed of viral antigens and host antibodies that are passively trapped within the glomerular basement membrane.[8] Alternatively, studies demonstrating the presence of HBV DNA and RNA in the glomeruli and renal tubular epithelial cells of patients with HBV-associated glomerulonephritis suggest HBV-associated renal disease could be the result of local expression of viral antigens with subsequent in situ immune complex formation.[9,10] Although HBsAg, hepatitis B core antigen, and hepatitis B early antigen (HBeAg) have all been identified in the glomerular deposits of patients with HBV-associated renal disease, HBeAg is considered the most highly correlated with HBV-associated nephropathy, particularly HBV-associated MN (HBV MN).[10–12] The pathogenic role of HBeAg in HBV-associated renal disease is supported by the

Table 24-1 Estimated Frequency of Glomerular Diseases Associated with Viral Hepatitis and Human Immunodeficiency Virus

	HBV	HCV	HIV
Minimal change disease	+/−	+/−	+
IgA nephropathy	+/−	+/−	++
Membranous nephropathy	+++	+	+
MPGN	++	++	+
MPGN plus cryoglobulinemia	+/−	+++	+/−
MesPGN	++	++	+/−
Focal and segmental glomerulosclerosis	+/−	+/−	+++
Polyarteritis nodosa	+++	+	+
Thrombotic microangiopathy	−	+/−	++

+/−, case reports without clear association; +, isolated case reports; ++, occasional reports; +++, common association. HBV, hepatitis B virus; HCV, hepatitis C virus; HIV, human immunodeficiency virus; MesPGN, mesangial proliferative glomerulonephritis. MPGN, membranoproliferative glomerulonephritis.

remission of proteinuria that typically occurs with clearance of the HBeAg and seroconversion to anti-HBe.[13,14]

Indications for Renal Biopsy

All patients with suspected HBV-associated renal disease should undergo a kidney biopsy to confirm the diagnosis and rule out other virally mediated renal diseases (e.g., cryoglobulinemic glomerulonephritis secondary to hepatitis C virus) that may be present in co-infected individuals. Magnetic resonance angiography may be preferred over a percutaneous renal biopsy or conventional angiography in diagnosing renal disease in HBV-associated PAN because it avoids both the potential to puncture a renal arterial aneurysm and the risk of radiocontrast-induced nephrotoxicity; however, care should be taken in using gadolinium-containing contrast agents in patients with severe renal insufficiency due to their reported association with nephrogenic systemic fibrosis.[15]

Membranous Nephropathy

HBV MN is most often observed in children, predominantly males, living in HBV endemic areas.[16,17] Patients typically present with proteinuria, commonly in the nephrotic range and often complicated by the nephrotic syndrome. Serologic studies in the majority of patients reveal hepatitis B surface and hepatitis B early antigenemia. The natural course of HBV MN in children has been associated with a 30% to 60% rate of spontaneous remission,[11] and the overall prognosis is considered favorable with one retrospective study reporting a cumulative probability of remission in 84% of children after 10 years.[13] In contrast, adult-onset HBV MN has a poorer prognosis and spontaneous remission is rare. In one study of 21 patients, 29% developed progressive renal failure and 10% required long-term renal replacement therapy after a mean follow-up of 60 months.[18]

Membranoproliferative Glomerulonephritis

HBV MPGN is the most common HBV-associated renal disease in adults.[16] Both type I and III MPGN have been described in the setting of HBV but not type II (dense deposit disease).[10] HBV MPGN usually occurs in the absence of cryoglobulins, and most reported cases of HBV associated with cryoglobulinemia involves patients co-infected with the hepatitis C virus or patients who presented before hepatitis C virus testing was available.[19] Spontaneous improvement is rare, and prognosis with this lesion is poorer than with HBV MN.

Polyarteritis Nodosa

Patients with HBV-associated PAN typically present with fever, rash, abdominal pain, new-onset or severe hypertension, mononeuritis multiplex, hematuria, and renal failure. The clinical manifestations of HBV-associated PAN are essentially the same as PAN in HBV-negative patients except that malignant hypertension, renal infarction, and orchiepididymitis may be more common in the setting of HBV.[20] The characteristic renal lesions of PAN are aneurysms of the medium-sized arteries of the kidney.[21,22] Serologic studies typically reveal high levels of HBV DNA and the absence of antineutrophil cytoplasmic antibody. Wild-type HBV, characterized by HBeAg, accounts for most but not all cases.[23] Proteinuria, elevated serum creatinine, and gastrointestinal involvement confer the highest mortality, with death usually following gastrointestinal hemorrhage, infarction, or perforation.[24]

Treatment

Antiviral Therapy

Antiviral therapy is the cornerstone of treatment for HBV-related kidney disease. Although our experience is limited to earlier antiviral agents, such as interferon alfa (IFN-α) and lamivudine (Table 24-2), newer nucleoside/nucleotide analogues are available and more are in development. Optimal treatment of HBV-related renal disease may require several antiviral agents, either alone or in combination, and we recommend consulting a hepatologist or an infectious disease specialist before initiating therapy.

Nucleoside/Nucleotide Analogues

Nucleoside/nucleotide analogues act on the HBV polymerase to inhibit viral DNA replication.[25] There are currently three nucleoside/nucleotide analogues approved for the treatment of chronic hepatitis in patients with HBV: lamivudine (3TC), adefovir, and entecavir[25] (Table 24-3). Lamivudine (3TC), a cytosine analogue reverse transcriptase inhibitor developed in 1989, was the first nucleoside analogue approved for the treatment of HBV in 1998 and has been demonstrated to lower HBV DNA levels, induce seroconversion, and yield an hepatic histologic response.[26] Several anecdotal case reports have demonstrated the efficacy of lamivudine in HBV-associated renal disease.[27–30] A recent Chinese cohort study compared 10 patients with biopsy-proven HBV MN treated with oral lamivudine (100 mg/day) versus 12 historic controls from the pre–lamivudine era.[31] The baseline demographics and clinical characteristics of both groups were similar, and all patients received either an angiotensin-converting enzyme inhibitor or an angiotensin II receptor blocker.[31] After 12 months of

Table 24-2   Summary of Intervention Trials for Hepatitis B Virus– and Human Immunodeficiency Virus–Related Renal Disease

Design	Treated (N)	Control (N)	Therapy	Outcome	Comment	Ref.: Disease
Retrospective	15	None	IFN-α	Decreased proteinuria and HBeAg clearance in 53%	Better response with MN than MPGN	32: HBV MN and MPGN
Prospective, randomized	20	20	IFN-α	100% proteinuria resolution, 80% HBeAg cleared	All subjects were children with steroid-resistant disease	33: HBV MN
Retrospective	6	None	IFN-α	100% PAN recovery, 66% HBeAg cleared	Concomitant steroids and PE	34: HBV PAN
Retrospective	10	12	Lamivudine 100 mg/day	60% in remission by 1 yr, 100% renal survival at 3 yr	All patients on ACEI or ARB	41: HBV MN
Retrospective	10	None	Lamivudine 100 mg/day	70% HBeAg cleared	Concomitant steroids and PE	23: HBV PAN
Retrospective	8	11	Protease inhibitor	Slower decline in CrCl	Only 6 biopsy-proven cases, ACEI and prednisone in some	84: HIVAN
Retrospective	26	10	HAART	Renal survival improved	Higher baseline Scr in controls	85: HIVAN
Prospective, nonrandomized	12	8	Fosinopril 10 mg/day	SCr and proteinuria improved	Controls refused ACEI	88: HIVAN
Retrospective	9	9	Captopril 6.25–25 mg tid	Renal survival improved	One suicide in ACEI group	89: HIVAN
Retrospective	20	None	Prednisone	SCr improved in 17/20 60 mg/day	Infectious complications common	90: HIVAN
Retrospective	15	87	Prednisone 1 mg/kg/day	Renal survival improved	No significant improvement in proteinuria	91: HIVAN
Retrospective	13	8	Prednisone 60 mg/day	Renal survival improved	No mortality benefit, increased hospital days	92: HIVAN

ACEI, angiotensin-converting enzyme inhibitor; ARB, angiotensin II receptor blocker; CrCl, creatinine clearance; HAART, highly active antiretroviral therapy; HBeAg, hepatitis B early antigen; HBV, hepatitis B virus; HIVAN, HIV-associated nephropathy; IFN-α, interferon alfa; MN, membranous nephropathy; MPGN, membranoproliferative glomerulonephritis; PAN, polyarteritis nodosa; PE, plasma exchange; SCr, serum creatinine.

therapy, 60% of lamivudine-treated patients were in complete remission (defined as having <300 mg of proteinuria/day) as compared with 25% of patients in the control group.[31] Furthermore, the cumulative 3-year renal survival rate was 100% in the lamivudine-treated group compared with 58% in the control group.[31] There are few data involving the use of nucleoside analogues for the treatment of HBV PAN; however, in one as yet unpublished report, of 10 patients treated with oral lamivudine (100 mg/day) as part of an HBV PAN regimen (which includes initiation corticosteroid therapy for 1–2 weeks), nine recovered and seven achieved HBeAg/Hbe antibody seroconversion.[23] Although there are no data concerning the use of the newer antivirals in the treatment of HBV-associated renal disease, given the direct role of the virus in the pathogenesis of the renal lesions and the increased incidence of resistance with prolonged lamivudine use (15%–20% per year

with an estimated 70% at 5 years), it is reasonable to assume that adefovir and entecavir, in combination with lamivudine or as monotherapy, should play key roles in the treatment of HBV-associated nephropathy.[25] Of note, in higher doses (30–120 mg), adefovir is associated with renal tubular toxicity; however, this complication has not been reported in the lower doses (10 mg) proposed for long-term HBV therapy.[32]

Interferon

A meta-analysis of 16 randomized, controlled trials in which subcutaneous IFN-α was used to treat patients with chronic HBV (without known renal disease) showed benefit with high-dose (more than 15 million units/m^2 per week) IFN-α therapy for 3 to 6 months.[33] A retrospective National Institutes of Health study of 15 patients with chronic HBV and

Table 24-3 Dosing Recommendations for Anti–Hepatitis B Virus–Approved Agents in Renal Impairment

Antiviral Agents (HBV)	Creatinine Clearance (mL/min)	Recommended Dose
Lamivudine	≥50	300 mg once daily
	30–49	150 mg once daily
	15–29	150 mg first dose, then 100 mg once daily
	5–14	150 mg first dose, then 50 mg once daily
	<5	50 mg first dose, then 25 mg once daily
Adefovir	≥50	10 mg once daily
	20–49	10 mg q 48 hr
	10–19	10 mg q 72 hr
	Hemodialysis	10 mg once weekly (after hemodialysis)
Entecavir	≥50	Treatment naive: 0.5 mg once daily
		Lamivudine refractory: 1 mg once daily
	30–49	Treatment naive: 0.25 mg once daily
		Lamivudine refractory: 0.5 mg once daily
	10–29	Treatment naive: 0.15 mg once daily
		Lamivudine refractory: 0.3 mg once daily
	<10	Treatment naive: 0.05 mg once daily
		Lamivudine refractory: 0.1 mg once daily
	Hemodialysis	Dose for creatinine clearance <10 (after hemodialysis)

glomerulonephritis (10 patients with HBV MN, 4 patients with HBV MPGN, 1 with unknown biopsy result) treated with 16 weeks of daily or alternate-day subcutaneous IFN-α2b (5 million units) demonstrated resolution of HBeAg and reduction in proteinuria in eight patients (53%).[34] Of note, all eight responders had HBV MN, whereas four of the seven nonresponders were the patients with known HBV MPGN.[34] An open trial of 40 Chinese children with heavy proteinuria and biopsy-proven steroid-resistant HBV MN also showed benefit with IFN-α therapy.[35] Patients were randomized to three times weekly subcutaneous IFN-α2b (5 or 8 million units, based on weight) versus supportive treatment alone.[35] After 12 months of therapy, proteinuria resolved in 100% of patients in the IFN-α–treated group compared with only 10% of patients in the control group.[35] Furthermore, although 80% of the IFN-α–treated patients became HBeAg negative, none of the patients in the control group achieved seroconversion.[35] In a review of 41 patients with HBV PAN, approximately 30% of whom had either renal failure or the nephrotic syndrome, six patients received treatment with IFN-α2b in addition to a short course of steroids and plasma exchange therapy.[36] All the IFN-α–treated patients recovered from PAN and 66% demonstrated HBeAg seroconversion.[36]

Adjunctive Therapy

Corticosteroids
Use of corticosteroids in vitro and in vivo promotes HBV replication and transcription, and up-regulates viral antigen expression, including HBsAg and HBeAg.[37-39] Although there are few published data regarding corticosteroid use in HBV MPGN, HBV MN responds poorly to corticosteroid therapy, and even a short course of corticosteroids may exacerbate hepatocellular injury in an HBV-infected patient.[11,13,40] Corticosteroid therapy should therefore be avoided in HBV MN and HBV MPGN. However, a short course (2 weeks) of corticosteroids (oral prednisone 1 mg/kg), with or without pulse methylprednisolone (15 mg/kg for 1–3 days), rapidly tapered after 1 week and withdrawn completely by the end of 2 weeks and followed by plasma exchange and antiviral therapy, is recommended to control the life-threatening manifestations of HBV PAN.[41,42]

Plasma Exchange
Alternate-day plasma exchange is used to clear immune complexes in HBV PAN and is part of the protocol described previously.[36,41,42] The duration of plasma exchange therapy should be tailored to the severity of the PAN manifestations.

Hepatitis B Virus and Renal Replacement Therapy

Management of Hepatitis B Virus in End-Stage Renal Disease

The incidence and prevalence of HBs antigenemia in U.S. hemodialysis patients has decreased dramatically since the 1970s[43,44] as a result of improved adherence to infection control practices, strict segregation of HBsAg-positive patients and their hemodialysis equipment from HBV-susceptible (HBsAb-negative) patients, and routine vaccination of HBV-susceptible patients and staff. Routine serologic testing for HBV (monthly HBsAg) in all HBV-susceptible hemodialysis patients is recommended to rapidly detect and isolate newly infected patients.[43] Due to what is likely an impaired cellular immune response, seroconversion after conventional HBV vaccination is suboptimal in dialysis patients compared with the general population (50%–73% versus > 90%), and it is therefore recommended that end-stage renal disease (ESRD) patients receive a four-dose (40 μg/dose) vaccination schedule as opposed to the conventional three-dose (20 μg/dose) schedule.[45] Diagnosing active liver disease in an HBV-positive ESRD patient is complicated by the fact that dialysis patients tend to have lower transaminase levels as compared with non-uremic patients and a liver biopsy is often the only way to correctly grade the degree of hepatic damage.[45] Although the impact of HBV infection on ESRD mortality may often be overshadowed by cardiovascular disease and other comorbidities, cirrhosis imparts a 35% increased risk of death in ESRD patients,[45,46] and antiviral treatment should be considered in all HBV-infected ESRD patients.

Management of Hepatitis B Virus in Renal Transplantation

Although immunosuppressive therapy is known to increase viral replication and worsen underlying liver disease,[47] there are conflicting data regarding the effect of chronic HBV infection on patient and graft survival after renal transplantation. Earlier studies comparing HBsAg-positive and HBsAg-negative kidney transplant recipients reported no difference in patient survival and demonstrated no difference or an increase in graft survival.[47–50] More recently, a large French case-control study comparing long-term outcomes in HBV-infected versus noninfected kidney transplant recipients demonstrated that, in addition to age and biopsy-proven cirrhosis, HBsAg positivity was independently associated with decreased 10-year patient and graft survival rates.[51] A recent meta-analysis of six retrospective cohort studies also concluded that HBsAg-positive renal transplant recipients have decreased patient and graft survival rates.[52] Therefore, although HBsAg is not a contraindication to renal transplantation, most centers perform a liver biopsy before transplantation, and antiviral therapy should be initiated if there is histologic evidence of active disease. Furthermore, a post-transplantation immunosuppressive regimen that avoids the use of antilymphocyte globulin is recommended because it may trigger fulminant hepatic failure in HBV-infected renal transplant recipients.[53] Nucleoside/nucleotide analogues are currently the agents of choice in the treatment of both pre- and post-transplantation HBV, as IFN-α is poorly tolerated in patients on dialysis and may precipitate graft rejection in the post-transplantation setting.[54] Lamivudine therapy before renal transplantation (prophylactic), at the time of renal transplantation (preemptive), and after renal transplantation in response to recurrent hepatic dysfunction (reactive)[53,55,56] have all proven successful, as measured by the elimination of serum HBV DNA, but data suggest that prophylactic or preemptive lamivudine use may be superior. One nonrandomized study reported a recurrence of viremia in 10% of patients treated with lamivudine before or at the time of renal transplantation compared with 42% of patients in the group not treated with lamivudine.[55] Another small retrospective study reported that 100% of patients prophylactically or preemptively treated with lamivudine remained negative for HBV DNA compared with 50% of untreated patients.[57] However, due to the risk of developing antiviral resistance with prolonged use and the risk of potentially inducing a hepatitis flare with antiviral withdrawal, the optimal timing and duration of pretransplantation lamivudine therapy require further study.

HUMAN IMMUNODEFICIENCY VIRUS AND RENAL DISEASE

Background

The human retrovirus human immunodeficiency virus (HIV) type 1 (HIV) was discovered in 1983,[58] 2 years after the first published reports of acquired immunodeficiency syndrome (AIDS).[59] In 2006, an estimated 40 million people were living with HIV infection worldwide, with nearly 25 million affected individuals living in sub-Saharan Africa.[60]

HIV-Associated Renal Disease

The spectrum of kidney disease associated with HIV infection includes acute renal failure, electrolyte abnormalities, medication nephrotoxicity, and glomerular disease. This section focuses on the glomerular diseases associated with HIV infection, primarily HIV-associated nephropathy (HIVAN) and HIV-associated immune complex disease (see Table 24-1).

Pathogenesis

The pathogenesis of HIVAN involves HIV infection of the kidney. HIV mRNA and DNA can be detected in tubular and glomerular epithelial cells in biopsy tissue from patients with HIVAN,[61,62] and mouse models expressing HIV transgenes develop kidney disease that closely resembles human HIVAN.[63–65] Two specific retroviral genes, HIV *nef* and *vpr,* contribute to the pathogenesis of HIVAN.[66,67] The strong association with black race also suggests a role for host genetic factors, and studies in the mouse model have identified a potential genetic susceptibility locus on chromosome 3.[68]

Indications for Renal Biopsy

Kidney biopsy is required for the definitive diagnosis of HIV-infected patients with significant proteinuria or renal failure of unknown etiology because a significant proportion of patients with suspected HIVAN will have an alternative diagnosis.[69] This is particularly true in the aging antiretroviral-treated HIV population in the United States and Western Europe, in whom comorbid kidney disease due to diabetes, hypertension, or viral hepatitis is increasingly common.

HIV-Associated Nephropathy

Classically, HIVAN presents with heavy proteinuria and progressive renal failure, with the rapid onset of ESRD in the absence of treatment. Hypertension and edema may be less common than in other rapidly progressive glomerular diseases, and ultrasonography often reveals normal or increased kidney size. Although presentation can occur at any time, HIVAN is most often a complication of advanced HIV infection.[70] The epidemiology of HIVAN is most remarkable for the striking predominance of black race, with nearly 90% of the ESRD attributed to HIV occurring in blacks.[60] Classic renal pathology includes focal and segmental glomerulosclerosis with capillary collapse, tubular microcystic dilatation, and interstitial infiltration.[69] Endothelial tubuloreticular inclusions, a characteristic finding in untreated cases of HIVAN, are uncommon in highly active antiretroviral therapy (HAART)–treated patients. The glomerular lesion of HIVAN is distinguished by podocyte proliferation rather than podocyte loss.[71] When these characteristics are found in aggregate, the diagnosis of HIVAN is highly likely; however, similar pathology has been reported in HIV-negative patients and has been associated with the bisphosphonate pamidronate.[72] HIV testing should be offered to all patients with suggestive biopsy findings.

HIV-Associated Immune Complex Disease

A variety of glomerular diseases are described in HIV-infected patients, including minimal change disease, IgA nephropathy or other mesangial proliferative glomerulonephritis, MN, MPGN, and crescentic glomerulonephritis. In contrast to HIVAN, patients with HIV-associated immune complex disease are more likely to have hematuria, hypocomplementemia, mild to moderate proteinuria, and a more indolent course. Unlike HIVAN, immune complex glomerular disease is not strongly associated with black race.[73,74] Although evidence supporting a pathogenic role for HIV has been demonstrated in rare cases,[75] the relationship between HIV infection and immune complex disease is not well established. Because of the association with hepatitis B and C viruses, immune complex disease should prompt serologic testing for hepatitis virus co-infection.

HIV and Thrombotic Microangiopathy

The classic pentad of microangiopathic hemolytic anemia, thrombocytopenia, renal dysfunction, neurological signs, and noninfectious fever is found in a minority of HIV-infected patients with thrombotic microangopathy.[76] Microangiopathic hemolytic anemia, thrombocytopenia, and increased serum lactate dehydrogenase are required to establish the diagnosis.[76] Before the introduction of HAART, the 1-year mortality rate after the development of HIV-related thrombotic microangiopathy approached 100%.[76–78] This complication is increasingly rare in populations with access to HAART.[79]

Treatment

Antiretroviral Therapy

Treatment of the underlying cause is a primary principle in the management of secondary glomerular disease. Improvement in HIVAN has been demonstrated in patients receiving HAART, and the annual incidence of ESRD attributed to HIV decreased substantially after the widespread introduction of HAART.[60] Pre- and post-HAART kidney biopsies in two severe HIVAN cases demonstrated dramatic improvement in renal pathology, with associated improvement in kidney function.[61,80] Although HAART-related improvements have also been reported in HIV-related pediatric nephrotic syndrome and MN,[81,82] the benefit of HAART in

non-HIVAN kidney disease is less clear.[83] The role of HAART in the treatment of HIV-related kidney disease is primarily supported by epidemiologic data and cohort studies,[84,85] with no data from rigorous clinical trials. Randomized, placebo-controlled clinical trials are no longer ethical given the established benefits of HAART for HIV infection, and expert guidelines recommend consideration of HAART in all patients with HIV and chronic kidney disease based on existing data.[86]

Nephrologists involved in the care of HIV patients should be familiar with HAART agents with potential nephrotoxic effects, as well as those agents that require dose adjustment in patients with reduced kidney function. For example, the protease inhibitors indinavir and atazanavir have been associated with nephrolithiasis and obstructive nephropathy, and the nucleotide reverse transcriptase inhibitor tenofovir has been associated with Fanconi syndrome and acute renal failure.[87] In general, the nucleoside and nucleotide reverse-transcriptase inhibitors require dose adjustment in patients with a decreased glomerular filtration rate, whereas protease inhibitors and most nonnucleoside reverse-transcriptase inhibitors do not require dose adjustment.[87] Interested readers are encouraged to consult recent review articles and package inserts because of the rapid pace of antiretroviral drug development.

Adjunctive Therapy: Angiotensin System Blockade and Corticosteroids

Nonrandomized studies of adult HIVAN patients have shown improvements in proteinuria and delayed progression using angiotensin-converting enzyme inhibitors (see Table 24-2).[88,89] Because of the known benefits of angiotensin system blockade in other proteinuric kidney diseases, many nephrologists consider these agents the standard of care for the treatment of HIVAN. As such, randomized clinical trials are unlikely to be performed, and current guidelines recommend these agents for first-line therapy of hypertension or proteinuria in patients with HIV and chronic kidney disease.[86]

Case reports and retrospective series have shown improvement in kidney function and modest improvement in proteinuria with corticosteroids in adults with HIVAN.[90–92] The presumed role of corticosteroids is improvement in interstitial inflammation.[93,94] The potential risks of therapy and unknown long-term effects make these third-line agents in selected cases (see Table 24-2).

HIV and Renal Replacement Therapy

Management of HIV in End-Stage Renal Disease

HIVAN is an important cause of ESRD in young African Americans, who represent 90% of the incident ESRD cases attributed to HIV in the United States.[60] The prevalence of HIV infection in the dialysis population varies with center location and the demographics of the local ESRD population. Voluntary HIV testing should be offered to all new dialysis patients because HAART may be associated with improved survival and potential improvement in kidney function. Survival of HIV-positive dialysis patients has dramatically improved in the HAART era,[95] with similar outcomes with peritoneal dialysis and hemodialysis.[96]

Effects of HIV in Renal Transplantation

With improved long-term survival in the HAART era, kidney transplantation is now a reasonable alternative in selected patients with preserved immune function and undetectable viral load on HAART.[97,98] Ongoing studies are investigating whether the long-term survival advantage conferred by kidney transplantation in the general ESRD population is also realized in patients with HIV. Communication between transplantation nephrologists and HIV providers is essential to avoid significant interactions between antiretroviral and immunosuppressive agents. Potential transplant recipients should be referred to a transplantation center with experience in the evaluation and management of HIV-positive recipients.

References

1. Purcell RH: The discovery of the hepatitis viruses. Gastroenterology 1993;104:955–963.
2. Lee WM: Hepatitis B virus infection. N Engl J Med 1997;337:1733–1745.
3. Ayodele OE, Salako BL, Kadiri S, et al: Hepatitis B virus infection: Implications in chronic kidney disease, dialysis and transplantation. Afr J Med Med Sci 2006;35:111–119.
4. McQuillan GM, Coleman PJ, Kruszon-Moran D, et al: Prevalence of hepatitis B virus infection in the United States: The National Health and Nutrition Examination Surveys, 1976 through 1994. Am J Public Health 1999;89:14–18.
5. Wasley A, Miller JT, Finelli L, Centers for Disease Control and Prevention (CDC): Surveillance for acute viral hepatitis—United States, 2005. MMWR Surveill Summ 2007;56:1–24.
6. Combes B, Shorey J, Barrera A, et al: Glomerulonephritis with deposition of Australia antigen-antibody complexes in glomerular basement membrane. Lancet 1971;2:234–237.
7. Levy M, Chen N: Worldwide perspective of hepatitis B-associated glomerulonephritis in the 80s. Kidney Int Suppl 1991;35:S24–S33.
8. Takekoshi Y, Tochimaru H, Nagata Y, Itami N: Immunopathogenetic mechanisms of hepatitis B virus-related glomerulopathy. Kidney Int Suppl 1991;35:S34–S39.
9. Lai KN, Ho RT, Tam JS, Lai FM: Detection of hepatitis B virus DNA and RNA in kidneys of HBV related glomerulonephritis. Kidney Int 1996;50:1965–1977.
10. Bhimma R, Coovadia HM: Hepatitis B virus-associated nephropathy. Am J Nephrol 2004;24:198–211.
11. Lin CY: Clinical features and natural course of HBV-related glomerulopathy in children. Kidney Int Suppl 1991;35:S46–S53.
12. Lin CY: Hepatitis B virus-associated membranous nephropathy: Clinical features, immunological profiles and outcome. Nephron 1990;55:37–44.
13. Gilbert RD, Wiggelinkhuizen J: The clinical course of hepatitis B virus-associated nephropathy. Pediatr Nephrol 1994;8:11–14.
14. Lai KN, Lai FM: Clinical features and the natural course of hepatitis B virus-related glomerulopathy in adults. Kidney Int Suppl 1991;35:S40–S45.
15. Grobner T, Prischl FC: Gadolinium and nephrogenic systemic fibrosis. Kidney Int 2007;72:260–264.
16. Lee HS, Choi Y, Yu SH, et al: A renal biopsy study of hepatitis B virus-associated nephropathy in Korea. Kidney Int 1988;34:537–543.
17. Lai KN, Lai FM, Chan KW, et al: The clinico-pathologic features of hepatitis B virus-associated glomerulonephritis. Q J Med 1987;63:323–333.
18. Lai KN, Li PK, Lui SF, et al: Membranous nephropathy related to hepatitis B virus in adults. N Engl J Med 1991;324:1457–1463.
19. Gower RG, Sausker WF, Kohler PF, et al: Small vessel vasculitis caused by hepatitis B virus immune complexes. Small vessel vasculitis and HBsAG. J Allergy Clin Immunol 1978;62:222–228.
20. Lhote F, Cohen P, Guillevin L: Polyarteritis nodosa, microscopic polyangiitis and Churg-Strauss syndrome. Lupus 1998;7:238–258.
21. Bron KM, Strott CA, Shapiro AP: The diagnostic value of angiographic observations in polyarteritis nodosa. A case of multiple aneurysms in the visceral organs. Arch Intern Med 1965;116:450–454.
22. Hekali P, Kajander H, Pajari R, et al: Diagnostic significance of angiographically observed visceral aneurysms with regard to polyarteritis nodosa. Acta Radiol 1991;32:143–148.
23. Trepo C, Guillevin L: Polyarteritis nodosa and extrahepatic manifestations of HBV infection: The case against autoimmune intervention in pathogenesis. J Autoimmun 2001;16:269–274.
24. Guillevin L, Lhote F, Gayraud M, et al: Prognostic factors in polyarteritis nodosa and Churg-Strauss syndrome. A prospective study in 342 patients. Medicine (Baltimore) 1996;75:17–28.
25. Dusheiko G, Antonakopoulos N: Treatment of hepatitis B. Gut 2007;57:105–124.
26. Olsen SK, Brown RS Jr: Hepatitis B treatment: Lessons for the nephrologist. Kidney Int 2006;70:1897–1904.
27. Okuse C, Yotsuyanagi H, Yamada N, et al: Successful treatment of hepatitis B virus-associated membranous nephropathy with lamivudine. Clin Nephrol 2006;65:53–56.
28. Kanaan N, Horsmans Y, Goffin E: Lamivudine for nephrotic syndrome related to hepatitis B virus (HBV) infection. Clin Nephrol 2006;65:208–210.
29. Wen YK, Chen ML: Remission of hepatitis B virus-associated membranoproliferative glomerulonephritis in a cirrhotic patient after lamivudine therapy. Clin Nephrol 2006;65:211–215.
30. Izzedine H, Massard J, Poynard T, Deray G: Lamivudine and HBV-associated nephropathy. Nephrol Dial Transplant 2006;21:828–829.
31. Tang S, Lai FM, Lui YH, et al: Lamivudine in hepatitis B-associated membranous nephropathy. Kidney Int 2005;68:1750–1758.
32. Fung SK, Lok AS: Drug insight: Nucleoside and nucleotide analog inhibitors for hepatitis B. Nat Clin Pract Gastroenterol Hepatol 2004;1:90–97.
33. Wong DK, Cheung AM, O'Rourke K, et al: Effect of alpha-interferon treatment in patients with hepatitis B e antigen-positive chronic hepatitis B. A meta-analysis. Ann Intern Med 1993;119:312–323.
34. Conjeevaram HS, Hoofnagle JH, Austin HA, et al: Long-term outcome of hepatitis B virus-related glomerulonephritis after therapy with interferon alfa. Gastroenterology 1995;109:540–546.
35. Lin CY: Treatment of hepatitis B virus-associated membranous nephropathy with recombinant alpha-interferon. Kidney Int 1995;47:225–230.
36. Guillevin L, Lhote F, Cohen P, et al: Polyarteritis nodosa related to hepatitis B virus. A prospective study with long-term observation of 41 patients. Medicine (Baltimore) 1995;74:238–253.
37. Tur-Kaspa R, Laub O: Corticosteroids stimulate hepatitis B virus DNA, mRNA and protein production in a stable expression system. J Hepatol 1990;11:34–36.
38. Lai FM, Tam JS, Li PK, Lai KN: Replication of hepatitis B virus with corticosteroid therapy in hepatitis B virus related membranous nephropathy. Virchows Arch A Pathol Anat Histopathol 1989;414:279–284.
39. Lai KN, Tam JS, Lin HJ, Lai FM: The therapeutic dilemma of the usage of corticosteroid in patients with membranous nephropathy and persistent hepatitis B virus surface antigenaemia. Nephron 1990;54:12–17.
40. Hoofnagle JH, Davis GL, Pappas SC, et al: A short course of prednisolone in chronic type B hepatitis. Report of a randomized, double-blind, placebo-controlled trial. Ann Intern Med 1986;104:12–17.

41. Guillevin L, Mahr A, Cohen P, et al: Short-term corticosteroids then lamivudine and plasma exchanges to treat hepatitis B virus-related polyarteritis nodosa. Arthritis Rheum 2004;51:482–487.

42. Guillevin L, Mahr A, Callard P, et al: Hepatitis B virus-associated polyarteritis nodosa: Clinical characteristics, outcome, and impact of treatment in 115 patients. Medicine (Baltimore) 2005;84: 313–322.

43. Recommendations for preventing transmission of infections among chronic hemodialysis patients. MMWR Recomm Rep 2001;50(RR-5):1–43.

44. Finelli L, Miller JT, Tokars JI, et al: National surveillance of dialysis-associated diseases in the United States, 2002. Semin Dial 2005;18:52–61.

45. Wong PN, Fung TT, Mak SK, et al: Hepatitis B virus infection in dialysis patients. J Gastroenterol Hepatol 2005;20:1641–1651.

46. Marcelli D, Stannard D, Conte F, et al: ESRD patient mortality with adjustment for comorbid conditions in Lombardy (Italy) versus the United States. Kidney Int 1996;50:1013–1018.

47. Fornairon S, Pol S, Legendre C, et al: The long-term virologic and pathologic impact of renal transplantation on chronic hepatitis B virus infection. Transplantation 1996;62:297–299.

48. Flagg GL, Silberman H, Takamoto SK, Berne TV: The influence of hepatitis B infection on the outcome of renal allotransplantation. Transplant Proc 1987;19:2155–2158.

49. Friedlaender MM, Kaspa RT, Rubinger D, et al: Renal transplantation is not contraindicated in asymptomatic carriers of hepatitis B surface antigen. Am J Kidney Dis 1989;14:204–210.

50. Nelson SR, Snowden SA, Sutherland S, et al: Outcome of renal transplantation in hepatitis BsAg-positive patients. Nephrol Dial Transplant 1994;9:1320–1323.

51. Mathurin P, Mouquet C, Poynard T, et al: Impact of hepatitis B and C virus on kidney transplantation outcome. Hepatology 1999;29:257–263.

52. Fabrizi F, Martin P, Dixit V, et al: HBsAg seropositive status and survival after renal transplantation: Meta-analysis of observational studies. Am J Transplant 2005;5:2913–2921.

53. Lee WC, Wu MJ, Cheng CH, et al: Lamivudine is effective for the treatment of reactivation of hepatitis B virus and fulminant hepatic failure in renal transplant recipients. Am J Kidney Dis 2001;38:1074–1081.

54. Gane E, Pilmore H: Management of chronic viral hepatitis before and after renal transplantation. Transplantation 2002;74:427–437.

55. Han DJ, Kim TH, Park SK, et al: Results on preemptive or prophylactic treatment of lamivudine in HBsAg+ renal allograft recipients: Comparison with salvage treatment after hepatic dysfunction with HBV recurrence. Transplantation 2001;71:387–394.

56. Kletzmayr J, Watschinger B, Muller C, et al: Twelve months of lamivudine treatment for chronic hepatitis B virus infection in renal transplant recipients. Transplantation 2000;70:1404–1407.

57. Filik L, Karakayali H, Moray G, et al: Lamivudine therapy in kidney allograft recipients who are seropositive for hepatitis B surface antigen. Transplant Proc 2006;38:496–498.

58. Barre-Sinoussi F, Chermann JC, Rey F, et al: Isolation of a T-lymphotropic retrovirus from a patient at risk for acquired immune deficiency syndrome (AIDS). Science 1983;220:868–871.

59. Siegal FP, Lopez C, Hammer GS, et al: Severe acquired immunodeficiency in male homosexuals, manifested by chronic perianal ulcerative herpes simplex lesions. N Engl J Med 1981;305:1439–1444.

60. UNAIDS. 2006 AIDS Epidemic Update. Available online: www.unaids.org/en/KnowledgeCentre/HIVData/GlobalReport/. Accessed April 10, 2008.

61. Winston JA, Bruggeman LA, Ross MD, et al: Nephropathy and establishment of a renal reservoir of HIV type 1 during primary infection. N Engl J Med 2001;344:1979–1984.

62. Bruggeman LA, Ross MD, Tanji N, et al: Renal epithelium is a previously unrecognized site of HIV-1 infection. J Am Soc Nephrol 2000;11:2079–2087.

63. Dickie P, Felser J, Eckhaus M, et al: HIV-associated nephropathy in transgenic mice expressing HIV-1 genes. Virology 1991;185:109–119.

64. Bruggeman LA, Dikman S, Meng C, et al: Nephropathy in human immunodeficiency virus-1 transgenic mice is due to renal transgene expression. J Clin Invest 1997;100:84–92.

65. Zhong J, Zuo Y, Ma J, et al: Expression of HIV-1 genes in podocytes alone can lead to the full spectrum of HIV-1-associated nephropathy. Kidney Int 2005;68:1048–1060.

66. Husain M, Gusella GL, Klotman ME, et al: HIV-1 nef induces proliferation and anchorage-independent growth in podocytes. J Am Soc Nephrol 2002;13:1806–1815.

67. Zuo Y, Matsusaka T, Zhong J, et al: HIV-1 genes *vpr* and *nef* synergistically damage podocytes, leading to glomerulosclerosis. J Am Soc Nephrol 2006;17:2832–2843.

68. Gharavi AG, Ahmad T, Wong RD, et al: Mapping a locus for susceptibility to HIV-1-associated nephropathy to mouse chromosome 3. Proc Natl Acad Sci U S A 2004;101:2488–2493.

69. D'Agati V, Appel GB: Renal pathology of human immunodeficiency virus infection. Semin Nephrol 1998;18:406–421.

70. Winston JA, Klotman ME, Klotman PE: HIV-associated nephropathy is a late, not early, manifestation of HIV-1 infection. Kidney Int 1999;55:1036–1040.

71. Barisoni L, Kriz W, Mundel P, D'Agati V: The dysregulated podocyte phenotype: A novel concept in the pathogenesis of collapsing idiopathic focal segmental glomerulosclerosis and HIV-associated nephropathy. J Am Soc Nephrol 1999;10:51–61.

72. Markowitz GS, Appel GB, Fine PL, et al: Collapsing focal segmental glomerulosclerosis following treatment with high-dose pamidronate. J Am Soc Nephrol 2001;12:1164–1172.

73. Casanova S, Mazzucco G, Barbiano di Belgiojoso G, et al: Pattern of glomerular involvement in human immunodeficiency virus-infected patients: An Italian study. Am J Kidney Dis 1995;26:446–453.

74. Nochy D, Glotz D, Dosquet P, et al: Renal disease associated with HIV infection: A multicentric study of 60 patients from Paris hospitals. Nephrol Dial Transplant 1993;8:11–19.

75. Kimmel PL, Phillips TM, Ferreira-Centeno A, et al: Brief report: Idiotypic IgA nephropathy in patients with human immunodeficiency virus infection. N Engl J Med 1992;327:702–706.

76. Thompson CE, Damon LE, Ries CA, Linker CA: Thrombotic microangiopathies in the 1980s: Clinical features, response to treatment, and the impact of the human immunodeficiency virus epidemic. Blood 1992;80:1890–1895.

77. Ucar A, Fernandez HF, Byrnes JJ, et al: Thrombotic microangiopathy and retroviral infections: A 13-year experience. Am J Hematol 1994;45:304–309.

78. Gadallah MF, el-Shahawy MA, Campese VM, et al: Disparate prognosis of thrombotic microangiopathy in HIV-infected patients with and without AIDS. Am J Nephrol 1996;16: 446–450.

79. Becker S, Fusco G, Fusco J, et al: HIV-associated thrombotic microangiopathy in the era of highly active antiretroviral therapy: An observational study. Clin Infect Dis 2004;39(Suppl 5): S267–S275.

80. Wali RK, Drachenberg CI, Papadimitriou JC, et al: HIV-1-associated nephropathy and response to highly-active antiretroviral therapy. Lancet 1998;352:783–784.

81. Viani RM, Dankner WM, Muelenaer PA, Spector SA: Resolution of HIV-associated nephrotic syndrome with highly active antiretroviral therapy delivered by gastrostomy tube. Pediatrics 1999;104:1394–1396.

82. Dellow E, Unwin R, Miller R, et al: Protease inhibitor therapy for HIV infection: The effect on HIV-associated nephrotic syndrome. Nephrol Dial Transplant 1999;14:744–747.

83. Szczech LA, Gupta SK, Habash R, et al: The clinical epidemiology and course of the spectrum of renal diseases associated with HIV infection. Kidney Int 2004;66:1145–1152.

84. Szczech LA, Edwards LJ, Sanders LL, et al: Protease inhibitors are associated with a slowed progression of HIV-related renal diseases. Clin Nephrol 2002;57:336–341.

85. Atta MG, Gallant JE, Rahman MH, et al: Antiretroviral therapy in the treatment of HIV-associated nephropathy. Nephrol Dial Transplant 2006;21:2809–2813.

86. Gupta SK, Eustace JA, Winston JA, et al: Guidelines for the management of chronic kidney disease in HIV-infected patients: Recommendations of the HIV Medicine Association of the Infectious Diseases Society of America. Clin Infect Dis 2005;40:1559–1585.

87. Wyatt CM, Klotman PE: Antiretroviral therapy and the kidney: Balancing benefit and risk in patients with HIV infection. Expert Opin Drug Saf 2006;5:275–287.

88. Burns GC, Paul SK, Toth IR, Sivak SL: Effect of angiotensin-converting enzyme inhibition in HIV-associated nephropathy. J Am Soc Nephrol 1997;8:1140–1146.

89. Kimmel PL, Mishkin GJ, Umana WO: Captopril and renal survival in patients with human immunodeficiency virus nephropathy. Am J Kidney Dis 1996;28:202–208.

90. Smith MC, Austen JL, Carey JT, et al: Prednisone improves renal function and proteinuria in human immunodeficiency virus-associated nephropathy. Am J Med 1996;101:41–48.

91. Laradi A, Mallet A, Beaufils H, et al: HIV-associated nephropathy: Outcome and prognosis factors. Groupe d'Etudes nephrologiques d'Ile de France. J Am Soc Nephrol 1998;9:2327–2335.

92. Eustace JA, Nuermberger E, Choi M, et al: Cohort study of the treatment of severe HIV-associated nephropathy with corticosteroids. Kidney Int 2000;58:1253–1260.

93. Briggs WA, Tanawattanacharoen S, Choi MJ, et al: Clinicopathologic correlates of prednisone treatment of human immunodeficiency virus-associated nephropathy. Am J Kidney Dis 1996;28:618–621.

94. Ross MJ, Fan C, Ross MD, et al: HIV-1 infection initiates an inflammatory cascade in human renal tubular epithelial cells. J Acquir Immune Defic Syndr 2006;42:1–11.

95. Abbott KC, Hypolite I, Welch PG, Agodoa LY: Human immunodeficiency virus/acquired immunodeficiency syndrome-associated nephropathy at end-stage renal disease in the United States: Patient characteristics and survival in the pre highly active antiretroviral therapy era. J Nephrol 2001;14:377–383.

96. Ahuja TS, Collinge N, Grady J, Khan S: Is dialysis modality a factor in survival of patients with ESRD and HIV-associated nephropathy? Am J Kidney Dis 2003;41:1060–1064.

97. Stock PG, Roland ME, Carlson L, et al: Kidney and liver transplantation in human immunodeficiency virus-infected patients: A pilot safety and efficacy study. Transplantation 2003;76:370–375.

98. Kumar MS, Sierka DR, Damask AM, et al: Safety and success of kidney transplantation and concomitant immunosuppression in HIV-positive patients. Kidney Int 2005;67:1622–1629.

Further Reading

Dusheiko G, Antonakopoulos N: Treatment of hepatitis B. Gut 2007;57:105–124.

Fabrizi F, Bunnapradist S, Martin P: HBV infection in patients with end-stage renal disease. Semin Liver Dis 2004;24(Suppl 1):63–70.

Guillevin L, Mahr A, Callard P, et al: Hepatitis B virus-associated polyarteritis nodosa: Clinical characteristics, outcome, and impact of treatment in 115 patients. Medicine 2005;84:5313–5322.

Han SH: Extrahepatic manifestations of chronic hepatitis B. Clin Liver Dis 2004;8:2403–2418.

Izzedine H, Launay-Vacher V, Deray G: Antiviral drug-induced nephrotoxicity. Am J Kidney Dis 2005;45:804–817.

Pelletier SJ, Norman SP, Christensen LL, et al: Review of transplantation in HIV patients during the HAART era. Clin Transpl 2004:63–82.

Tang S, Lai FM, Lui YH, et al: Lamivudine in hepatitis B-associated membranous nephropathy. Kidney Int 2005;68:41750–41758.

Wyatt CM Klotman PE: Antiretroviral therapy and the kidney: balancing benefit and risk in patients with human immunodeficiency virus infection. Expert Opin Drug Saf 2006;5:275–287.

Wyatt CM, Klotman PE: HIV-associated nephropathy in the era of antiretroviral therapy. Am J Med 2007;120:488–492.

Chapter 25

Management of Complications of Nephrotic Syndrome

Yvonne M. O'Meara and Jerrold S. Levine

BACKGROUND

Nephrotic syndrome (NS) is a clinical complex characterized by proteinuria of more than 3.5 g/1.73 m^2/24 hr (in practice > 3.0–3.5 g/24 hr), hypoalbuminemia, edema, hyperlipidemia, and lipiduria.[1–4] The key component is proteinuria, which results from altered permeability of the glomerular filtration barrier, namely the glomerular basement membrane and podocytes with their slit diaphragms. Proteinuria sets in motion a series of homeostatic and compensatory mechanisms that result in the clinical features of NS.[1,2] These features can occur with lesser degrees of proteinuria or may be absent even in patients with massive proteinuria. Although the diseases and pathogenic mechanisms underlying NS are diverse, the result is alteration in the charge- and/or size-selective properties of the glomerular capillary wall such that permeability to albumin and other intermediate-sized macromolecules is enhanced.[3,4]

Management of NS focuses on (1) treatment of the causative disease where possible, generally with a combination of immunosuppressive drugs such as corticosteroids, cytotoxic agents, and calcineurin inhibitors, and (2) treatment of the complications that are responsible for much of the morbidity associated with this condition. In this chapter, we discuss management of the complications of NS. Specifically, we address the treatment of hypoalbuminemia, edema, hyperlipidemia, abnormalities of calcium homeostasis, thromboembolic phenomena, and increased susceptibility to infection. It must be stressed that in many areas, there is a dearth of prospective, controlled clinical trials, so that recommendations on treatment remain somewhat empirical. Where there is controversy or inadequate data regarding the management of a particular problem, the authors' view is presented.

HYPOALBUMINEMIA/PROTEINURIA

It is becoming increasingly clear that proteinuria per se may be deleterious to the kidney and play a role in the progression of renal disease.[5] The rate of progression is increased in patients with heavy proteinuria, and interventions that reduce urinary protein excretion have been demonstrated to slow the rate of decline of glomerular filtration rate (GFR) in both diabetic and nondiabetic renal disease.[6,7] The sequelae of hypoalbuminemia include an increased risk of acute renal failure (from renal hypoperfusion and filtration failure), systemic and renal drug toxicity (because of alterations in free and protein-bound drug levels), enhanced platelet aggregability, hyperlipidemia, and edema formation.[1] Protein malnutrition is an important complication, particularly in children in whom normal growth and development may become stunted. Although outside the scope of this chapter, drug dosing needs to be approached with care in patients with NS, especially those with hypoalbuminemia and impaired renal function.[8] Not only will hepatic and renal clearances be affected, but the range of therapeutic levels will need to be lowered for drugs having a high degree of protein binding because therapeutic ranges are typically based on total drug concentration rather than the bioactive free portion.

In general, the greater the magnitude of the proteinuria, the lower the serum albumin concentration. However, this relationship is not constant, and many patients do not develop hypoalbuminemia even in the presence of persistent heavy proteinuria. Other factors that may contribute to decreased serum albumin levels in patients with nephrotic-range proteinuria include an inappropriately low rate of hepatic albumin synthesis and, although controversial, an increased rate of renal albumin catabolism.[1]

Management

Therapeutic strategies employed to decrease proteinuria and increase serum albumin levels include manipulations of dietary protein intake and treatment with a combination of angiotensin-converting enzyme inhibitors (ACEIs), angiotensin receptor blockers (ARBs), nonsteroidal anti-inflammatory drugs (NSAIDs), and aldosterone antagonists. The antiproteinuric mechanisms are thought to involve both hemodynamic and local factors affecting glomerular permselectivity characteristics. These measures may confer substantial benefit in patients with severe NS, for whom much of the morbidity derives from persistent heavy proteinuria. Furthermore, a decrease in proteinuria may be associated with slowing of the rate of progression of the underlying renal disease (see later).

Manipulation of Dietary Protein Intake

Although early reports advocated the use of high-protein diets to treat hypoalbuminemia, more recent work has called into question the rationale and efficacy of such an approach. In general, it appears that a high-protein diet results in increases in the rates of both hepatic albumin synthesis and urinary protein loss such that the plasma albumin level fails to increase and may actually decrease.[1,9,10] Furthermore, a high protein intake, by increasing glomerular capillary pressures, has been implicated in the progression of a variety of renal diseases.[11]

Early studies suggested that ingestion of a low-protein diet may reduce urinary protein loss, although this effect was offset by a concomitant decline in hepatic albumin synthesis, so that serum albumin concentrations were not consistently increased.[9,12,13] Recent studies have failed to show a consistent effect of dietary protein restriction on proteinuria. In a randomized, crossover trial, Remuzzi and colleagues[14] found that protein restriction (0.6 mg/kg/day) had no effect on renal hemodynamics or proteinuria in nephrotic patients with membranous nephropathy. D'Amico and colleagues[15] reported similarly disappointing results with a protein-restricted diet that was supplemented with essential amino acids and contained a high ratio of polyunsaturated to saturated fats. At variance with these results, Giordano and colleagues[16] reported a significant decrease in proteinuria (38%) and a small but significant increase in serum albumin in seven patients with NS ingesting a low-protein diet for 4 weeks (0.55 g/kg/day plus 1 g of dietary protein per gram of daily protein excretion). Walser and colleagues[17] studied 16 nephrotic patients fed a very low protein diet (0.33 g/kg/day) supplemented with 10 to 20 g/day of essential amino acids for an average of 10 months. All patients had a decrease in proteinuria and an increase in serum albumin. Indeed, for the five patients with an initial GFR higher than 30 mL/min, the response was especially dramatic, with the serum albumin increasing from 2.5 to 3.8 g/dL and proteinuria declining from 9.1 to 1.9 g/day.

Debate also continues about the potential risk of increasing protein malnutrition by restriction of dietary protein intake in patients who are already severely hypoalbuminemic.[13,18,19] A lack of patient tolerability and the need for close nutritional monitoring are additional factors that may dissuade prescription of such regimens.

Until the benefits and potential risks of dietary protein manipulation are further clarified, it would appear reasonable to advise a moderate dietary protein intake of 0.8 to 1.0 g/kg/day in adults. In children, a greater intake, of approximately 1.2 g/kg/day, may be preferable to avoid the hazards of growth retardation. Several studies suggest a lack of risk with such moderate restriction. Lim and colleagues[20] showed that nephrotic patients ingesting 0.84 g/kg/day protein maintained a positive nitrogen balance of 0.5 g/day. Similarly, Maroni and colleagues[21] demonstrated positive nitrogen balance in a group of patients consuming 0.8 g/kg/day protein plus 1 g protein per gram of urine protein. Giordano and colleagues[22] showed that the rate of synthesis of IgG was unchanged in seven nephrotic patients whose protein intake was decreased from 1.2 to 0.66 g/kg/day. Finally, to achieve optimal nutrition, an adequate energy intake ($\geq$35 kcal/kg/day) must also be ensured.

Angiotensin Antagonists

ACEIs can decrease proteinuria by as much as 50% in a variety of proteinuric states without decreasing GFR or effective renal plasma flow.[23,24] The mechanism of this effect is still debated, but appears to entail both hemodynamic and structural factors. Structural factors may predominate because the maximal antiproteinuric effect takes 4 to 8 weeks to develop. This would also explain why short-term infusion of angiotensin reversed the renal and systemic hemodynamic effects of ACEIs without affecting the decrease in proteinuria.[25] Moreover, ACEIs have been shown to decrease selectively the fractional clearance of large molecular weight dextrans, suggesting a direct improvement in the size-selective properties of the filtration barrier.[26,27] Whether this effect is mediated via inhibition of angiotensin or other angiotensin-independent effects of ACEIs is not yet clear.

The antiproteinuric effect of ACEIs is dose dependent and apparently independent of changes in systemic blood pressure. Other antihypertensive agents that lower blood pressure to a comparable degree do not similarly decrease proteinuria. The degree of decrease in proteinuria varies considerably among patients, and some may not respond at all. Importantly, the antiproteinuric effect of ACEIs appears to depend on sodium restriction. Heeg and colleagues[23] showed that a high sodium intake (200 mmol/day) abrogated the decrease in proteinuria mediated by lisinopril during a period of low salt intake (50 mmol/day). Buter and colleagues[28] demonstrated that addition of a thiazide diuretic to patients ingesting a high-sodium diet can reverse the blunting effect of a high sodium intake on the decrease in proteinuria. Finally, the effects of ACEIs tend to be greater in patients with higher baseline proteinuria, probably because of the greater room for a measurable reduction.[29]

It is now well established that ACEIs slow the progression of both diabetic and nondiabetic renal disease.[6,7,30–37] In the REIN trial of ACEIs in proteinuric renal disease, the renoprotective effect of ramipril correlated with the observed decrease in proteinuria.[6] Four recent meta-analyses involving the same pool of 1860 nondiabetic patients from 11 randomized, controlled trials analyzed closely the beneficial effect of ACEIs in slowing the progression of renal disease, an effect that again was more pronounced in patients with higher levels of baseline proteinuria.[34–37] These meta-analyses suggest that proteinuria may be a specific marker identifying patients with renal disease for whom ACEIs possess an added benefit over other antihypertensive agents that lower blood pressure to a comparable degree.[34–36] Indeed, the specific benefit of ACEIs appeared to be limited to patients with significant proteinuria

($\geq$500 mg/day).[37] Among patients at high risk of progression of renal disease, but lacking significant proteinuria (<500 mg/day), ACEIs showed no advantage over other antihypertensive regimens.[37]

Although debate continues as to the superiority of ACEIs versus ARBs,[38,39] it appears that, at optimal doses, the antiproteinuric and renoprotective effects of these two classes of drugs are fairly equivalent.[40,41] In the COOPERATE study of 263 patients with nondiabetic renal disease and proteinuria exceeding 300 mg/day, an ACEI (trandolapril 3 mg/day) and an ARB (losartan 300 mg/day) were equally effective in preventing a doubling of creatinine and/or end-stage renal disease.[40] ACEIs and ARBs not only lowered proteinuria equivalently (~45% decrease of median maximum), but their effects occurred with similar kinetics and were sustained for the 3 years of the study.[40] The recent ROAD study compared an ACEI (benazepril) and an ARB (losartan), each dosed according to one of two regimens: conventional (benazepril 10 mg/day vs. losartan 50 mg/day) or optimal (benazepril up to 200 mg/day [median, 100 mg/day] vs. losartan up to 40 mg/day [median, 20 mg/day]).[41] The study population of 339 nondiabetic patients with chronic renal insufficiency and proteinuria (>1 g/day) were followed for a median of 3.7 years. The ACEI and ARB performed equivalently for all endpoints. Optimal doses of each agent were more effective than conventional doses in decreasing proteinuria (50%–55% vs. 35%–40%).[41] Compared with conventional doses, optimal doses also decreased by approximately 50% the number of patients reaching the combined primary endpoint of death, end-stage renal disease, and/or doubling of creatinine.[41] Importantly, the number of adverse events, such as hyperkalemia and acute decreases in the GFR, did not differ between patients given an ACEI and ARB or between conventional and optimal dosing.[41] The ROAD study suggests that ACEIs and ARBs may currently be used at doses that incompletely inhibit the renin-angiotensin-aldosterone axis.

Given that ACEIs and ARBs antagonize the effects of angiotensin through different mechanisms and have distinct effects beyond the renin-angiotensin-aldosterone axis,[39] a clear rationale exists for using these drugs in combination. Most studies examining this issue (including several meta-analyses and systematic reviews) have indicated a superiority of a combination of an ACEI and ARB over either agent alone.[39,40,42–73] The major endpoint in these studies, most of which were of short duration (<6 months), was proteinuria reduction, although blood pressure lowering and renoprotection were also examined in several.[39,40,72,73] Overall, the data are most convincing for patients with nondiabetic proteinuric renal disease, largely based on the COOPERATE study[39,40,72] because of its superior design (parallel group vs. crossover), longer duration (3 years vs. <1 year), larger sample size (263 patients), and clearly defined endpoints. Among patients receiving combination therapy with ACEI and ARB (trandolapril plus losartan), 11% reached the combined primary endpoint (end-stage renal disease and/or doubling of creatinine) compared with 23% of patients who received either agent alone. A similar advantage was observed for lowering of proteinuria (~76% reduction in median maximum change for combination therapy versus ~45% reduction for either agent alone). Although it seems likely that a similar result will apply to diabetic patients with proteinuric renal disease, available studies involving diabetic patients preclude a definitive conclusion because of their short duration (<12 weeks).[73]

These studies unfortunately leave unresolved the basis for the superiority of combination therapy. Two major possibilities, not mutually exclusive, exist: an additive benefit may be attributable to nonoverlapping pharmacologic effects of ACEIs and ARBs[39] or to suboptimal dosing as individual agents.[41] The latter important possibility has been inadequately addressed. As discussed earlier, titrating the dose of an ACEI or ARB upward led to significant further renoprotection and decreases in proteinuria.[41] On average, this added benefit was obtained by a doubling of the daily dose of either agent. Until the basis for the superiority of combined therapy is determined, we recommend that an ACEI and an ARB be used together at conventional doses, especially in patients with nondiabetic proteinuric renal disease. ACEIs and ARBs have a number of important adverse effects in patients with renal disease, including a decrease in the GFR and hyperkalemia. Although the prevalence of these adverse effects does not appear to be increased by combination therapy, patients should be monitored carefully after the introduction of an ACEI and an ARB, either alone or in combination.

Nonsteroidal Anti-inflammatory Drugs

NSAIDs decrease proteinuria to a comparable degree as ACEIs.[74,75] The mechanism of action is not clear, although the decrease in proteinuria likely depends on inhibition of renal prostaglandin synthesis. In a small study of seven nephrotic patients, a significant correlation was observed between the decrease in proteinuria and decreased renal prostaglandin E_2 excretion.[76] Indomethacin improved the profile of fractional dextran clearance and decreased flux through the shunt pathway, a major source of abnormal proteinuria in NS.[77]

The beneficial effect of NSAIDs occurs more rapidly than that of ACEIs (1–3 days). In some studies, decreased proteinuria is associated with decreases in both the GFR and effective renal plasma flow.[75] Sodium depletion enhanced both the antiproteinuric effect and the decrease in the GFR.[74] Although lisinopril and indomethacin had an additive effect in decreasing proteinuria, the combination produced a pronounced decrease in the GFR and significant hyperkalemia.[75] In another study, indomethacin had an additive antiproteinuric effect in combination with either the ACEI enalapril or the ARB irbesartan.[78] No adverse effect on renal hemodynamics was seen with short-term administration.[78] NSAIDs have a number of adverse renal effects, including hyperkalemia, acute renal failure, and salt and water retention. In general, we recommend that ACEIs and ARBs be used as preferred antiproteinuric agents and that NSAIDs be reserved for patients who are refractory to other measures.

Aldosterone Antagonists

Addition of the aldosterone antagonist spironolactone at 25 mg/day to the regimen of nondiabetic patients with chronic renal disease and proteinuria (>1 g per gram of creatinine per day) led to a decrease in both proteinuria (~50%) and the rate of decrease in the estimated GFR (~30%) after 1 year compared with a control group not given spironolactone.[79] Before the start of the study, patients had been stably treated with conventional doses of an ACEI and an ARB, either alone or in combination. Baseline aldosterone levels correlated with the level of proteinuria and predicted the degree of proteinuria decrease, in support of the authors' contention that ACEIs and/or ARBs incompletely inhibit aldosterone synthesis.[79] Similar results were observed in a smaller study of diabetic patients.[80]

Although these results are encouraging, it remains unclear whether circulating aldosterone in the presence of an ACEI and/or an ARB represents true escape or merely incomplete inhibition of the renin-angiotensin-aldosterone axis from suboptimal doses of an ACEI and/or an ARB. Also, the addition of spironolactone is not without risk, especially of hyperkalemia. Although the addition of spironolactone to an ACEI and/or an ARB increased serum potassium from a mean of 4.2 mEq/L at baseline to 5.0 mEq/L after 12 months of treatment, this necessitated discontinuation of the drug in only a few patients.[79] Conversely, serious hyperkalemia from the combination of spironolactone and an ACEI has been previously reported.[81]

Measures to Ablate Renal Function in Refractory Nephrotic Syndrome

Therapeutic ablation of renal function may be considered in occasional patients with refractory complications of NS, particularly when renal function is already depressed. A variety of measures have been used, including medical nephrectomy with high doses of NSAIDs, percutaneous transfemoral embolization using artificial agents or autologous blood clot, balloon occlusion of the renal arteries, and surgical nephrectomy.[82–85] Bilateral renal arterial embolization with autologous blood clot is probably the safest of the methods but should be considered only as a last resort in intractable cases.[85]

EDEMA

Edema is one of the most common symptoms of NS and often the reason patients come to medical attention. Fluid accumulates predominantly in areas of dependency or low tissue pressure. Hence, periorbital edema is common in the morning and leg edema at the end of the day. Pleural effusions and ascites occur frequently. Pulmonary edema does not occur in the presence of normal cardiac function, although in patients with very low plasma oncotic pressure (<8 mm Hg), minor elevations in left atrial filling pressure may lead to pulmonary congestion, despite the normally protective low-pressure features of the pulmonary circuit.[3]

The classic theory of edema formation in NS postulates that hypoalbuminemia leads to decreased intravascular oncotic pressure, with leakage of extracellular fluid from the blood into the interstitium and a decrease in blood volume. Hypovolemia then leads to activation of both the renin-angiotensin-aldosterone axis and the sympathetic nervous system, as well as release of antidiuretic hormone and suppression of atrial natriuretic peptide, thereby signaling the kidney to retain salt and water.[86] However, it is now clear that this classic theory applies to a minority of patients because the majority of patients with established NS have normal or even elevated blood volumes and stimulation of the renin-angiotensin-aldosterone axis is not consistently present.[87,88] Hence, primary renal sodium retention must also contribute to edema formation, although the factors responsible for this sodium avidity and the role of hypoalbuminemia in its genesis remain unclear.[88,89] Given the heterogeneity of NS in terms of patient age, the underlying pathophysiologic process, and the level of renal function, it is likely that different mechanisms of sodium retention exist in different patients.[88,90]

Management

Treatment of edema involves restriction of dietary sodium and the judicious use of diuretics (see Chapter 33). Considerable improvement should be possible for nearly all patients. For many patients, however, complete resolution of edema is not only unattainable but also undesirable because of the risk of volume contraction. In cases of mild edema, dietary sodium restriction to 100 to 150 mEq/day may be sufficient by itself. Restriction to less than 100 mEq/day is indicated in patients with more severe edema. Compliance with sodium restriction can be ascertained by measuring 24-hour urinary excretion of sodium. Institution of diuretic therapy is indicated in patients with symptomatic edema unresponsive to sodium restriction.

Furosemide pharmacokinetics and pharmacodynamics are often abnormal in patients with NS, many of whom show a degree of diuretic resistance. Although the following discussion focuses on the loop diuretic furosemide, similar principles apply to nearly all other diuretics in common clinical use, including the loop diuretic bumetanide, the thiazide diuretics, and the potassium-sparing diuretics amiloride and triamterene. The diuretic effect of furosemide depends on binding to, and inhibition of, a specific transporter located in the luminal membrane of the loop of Henle. Because furosemide is highly protein bound ($>90\%$), it cannot enter the urine by glomerular filtration. Entry into the urine occurs instead via secretion by the proximal tubule. Binding of furosemide to albumin aids secretion in two ways: (1) because of its tight association with albumin, furosemide is restricted to the vascular space and therefore has a higher rate of delivery to the kidney and (2) optimal secretion of furosemide may depend on the presence of albumin.

Thus, several mechanisms probably account for the diuretic resistance observed in patients with NS and hypoalbuminemia.[91,92]

1. Oral bioavailability may be decreased because of bowel wall edema and impaired absorption.
2. In the presence of hypoalbuminemia, furosemide will be incompletely bound to albumin and therefore diffuse out of the vascular space, thereby decreasing delivery of furosemide to the kidney.[93]
3. Even that fraction of furosemide that makes it into the urinary space may be limited in efficacy because tubular furosemide may bind to filtered albumin, thereby limiting the availability of free drug to interact with its receptor on the luminal brush border.[94]
4. Short-term hemodynamic and long-term renal structural changes may further diminish the diuretic response to furosemide. Structural changes include hypertrophy of distal tubular cells, leading to enhanced sodium reabsorption at sites distal to the loop, as well as intrinsic changes in the activity of the target of furosemide, the $Na^+/K^+/2Cl^-$ cotransporter.[95] In some instances, resistance may reflect the coexistence of renal impairment, with resulting impaired secretion of furosemide into the proximal tubular lumen.[96]
5. A continued high dietary sodium intake and the ingestion of NSAIDs may also cause an inadequate diuretic response.

A recent study casts doubt on the contribution of urinary protein binding of loop diuretics to diuretic resistance in NS.[97] In this study, coadministration of sulfisoxazole with furosemide was used to displace furosemide from binding to urinary albumin, but failed to enhance the natriuretic effect. Moreover, despite an observed increase in the volume of distribution of furosemide, there was no decrease in the rate of diuretic excretion, thereby questioning the pharmacodynamic role of hypoalbuminemia per se. These results suggest that normal renal compensatory mechanisms to diuretic use and/or a primary increase of sodium avidity may play a predominant role in the diuretic resistance of NS.

Dosing recommendations for diuretics in NS are empirically derived and will vary according to the degree of diuretic resistance.[92,98] Short-term diuretic resistance may be overcome by increasing the diuretic dose and frequency of administration, or by switching to a continuous intravenous infusion. Long-term resistance may require sequential nephron blockade through the combined use of loop and distal diuretics. In many cases, a lack of appreciation of the pharmacokinetic properties of diuretics can lead to improper dosing and seeming resistance in an otherwise responsive patient.[99] We have reviewed extensively the pharmacology and principles of diuretic use as well as strategies to overcome resistance extensively elsewhere.[99]

Some authors advocate intravenous coadministration of furosemide and albumin for patients with severe refractory edema. The use of such a regimen presumes that pharmacokinetic factors contribute importantly to diuretic resistance. In the most successful study, an equimolar infusion of salt-poor albumin (40 mg furosemide premixed with 6 g of salt-poor albumin) increased recovery of furosemide from the urine and led to an enhanced diuretic response.[93] More recent studies have provided less encouraging results.[100] Fliser and colleagues[101] infused 60 mg furosemide plus 200 mL of 20% human albumin to a group of nephrotic patients. The rate of urinary furosemide excretion was unchanged, suggesting that the observed modest increase in sodium excretion and urine volume was secondary to alterations in renal hemodynamics. Other workers failed to find any potentiation of furosemide by intravenous albumin.[102–104] Some of this lack of effect may be due to the fact that the albumin and furosemide were not admixed before infusion or that furosemide was administered at submaximal doses. In addition, in some studies, the natriuretic response to furosemide alone was substantial, suggesting that the patients studied may not have been truly diuretic resistant. Taken together, these studies are consistent with a critical role for primary sodium retention in the pathophysiology of the edema of NS. Based on current evidence, we recommend that the combination of furosemide and albumin should be reserved for patients with refractory edema. When used in combination, the drugs should probably be admixed before intravenous administration.

If the response to furosemide alone is inadequate, a thiazide diuretic can be added. The combination of two drugs acting at different sites may yield a synergistic response with enhanced natriuresis.[105] Thiazide diuretics are generally ineffective in the presence of renal impairment (GFR < 20–30 mL/min). Some patients may show an exaggerated response to the combination of a thiazide and loop diuretic, and severe volume contraction and dangerous hypokalemia can result. Careful monitoring for the first few days is therefore essential. Metolazone may also be useful in the treatment of nephrotic edema, either alone or combined with a loop diuretic.[106]

As discussed previously, activity of the renin-angiotensin-aldosterone system is highly variable in patients with NS, so that the response to aldosterone antagonists is highly inconsistent.[86] Aldosterone antagonists may be most useful in conjunction with loop diuretics to prevent hypokalemia. Conversely, hyperkalemia is always a risk with this class of diuretics, particularly in patients with diminished renal function.

Intravenous infusion of salt-poor albumin is also sometimes employed for the treatment of intractable nephrotic edema and in some patients appears to restore diuretic responsiveness (300 mL of 15% albumin infused over 45 minutes, followed by a furosemide bolus to establish a diuresis, given on alternate days).[107] This treatment is expensive, and any benefit is short-lived because the injected albumin is rapidly excreted in the urine or redistributes to extravascular tissue spaces. Despite these considerations, some authors recommend that a therapeutic trial of 50 to 75 g of albumin be undertaken over 2 to 3 days in patients in whom diuretics have effected no improvement in their edema or in whom complications of diuretic therapy preclude further increases in drug dose.[2] As the infusion of hyperoncotic albumin can precipitate pulmonary edema in patients with severe hypoproteinemia and any degree of cardiac impairment, patients should be monitored closely during therapy. The use of ultrafiltration for the treatment of edema resistant to standard therapy has also been described.[108]

All patients must be monitored carefully for adverse effects of diuretic therapy. Particular attention should be paid to intravascular volume and renal perfusion because of the risk of precipitating prerenal failure. Changes in orthostatic blood pressure, neck vein distention, and the ratio of blood urea nitrogen to serum creatinine may be helpful in assessing renal perfusion. In patients who have evidence of volume depletion and in whom diuretics exacerbate a prerenal state, bed rest and the use of support stockings may help mobilize edema.

HYPERLIPIDEMIA

A host of abnormalities of lipid metabolism exist in patients with NS.[109–112] These include elevations in all the following: total plasma cholesterol, very low density lipoprotein, intermediate-density lipoprotein, low-density lipoprotein (LDL), and lipoprotein (a). Triglyceride levels may also be elevated, particularly in patients with very heavy proteinuria. Although levels of high-density lipoprotein (HDL) are variable, the distribution among subclasses is altered such that HDL2 is decreased and HDL3 is increased. Elevated levels of apoproteins B, C, and E have also been shown, whereas the levels of apoproteins AI and AII, the major apoproteins in HDL, have been reported as normal. Qualitative abnormalities in lipoprotein composition are also described.[109]

The mechanisms of hyperlipoproteinemia in NS have not been fully elucidated. Increased hepatic synthesis of apoprotein B–containing lipoproteins, stimulated by decreased plasma oncotic pressure, may be an important factor.[109] In general, however, decreased lipid catabolism is thought to play a more important role than hepatic overproduction of lipoproteins.[113–115] Depletion of endothelium-bound lipoprotein lipase and alterations in the binding capacity of very low density lipoprotein are thought to contribute importantly to decreased catabolism.[115] Lowered plasma viscosity, decreased oncotic pressure, decreased plasma tonicity, urinary loss of liporegulatory substances, and decreased lipoprotein lipase activity may all play a role in the genesis of hyperlipidemia.[2]

Although the same lipid abnormalities in nonnephrotic populations have been associated with an increased incidence of cardiovascular disease, there is controversy as to whether these findings can be extrapolated to NS. Most reports on cardiovascular disease in NS are small, retrospective, and lacking in appropriate control groups, perhaps accounting for their conflicting results.[116,117] A more recent retrospective study of 142 patients with NS documented a 5.5-fold increased risk of myocardial infarction after controlling for other risk factors such as hypertension and smoking.[118] Hyperlipidemia has also been implicated in accelerating glomerular injury.[109,119] Indeed, similar pathophysiologic mechanisms are thought to contribute to progression of both glomerulosclerosis and atherosclerosis.[120] Such considerations provide an additional rationale for the treatment of nephrotic hyperlipidemia. Until the results of prospective, controlled trials dictate otherwise, it seems prudent to treat severe and/or prolonged hyperlipidemia, particularly in patients with other cardiovascular risk factors.[113,121]

Management

The approach to management of nephrotic hyperlipidemia is similar to that for nonnephrotic patients and consists of dietary measures, oral lipid-lowering agents, and modification of associated risk factors such as smoking and hypertension.[110,121,122] Available studies are small, mostly uncontrolled, and of short duration. Most studies were designed to test short-term efficacy and safety of specific therapeutic interventions rather than long-term benefits in cardiac or progressive renal disease. Thus, recommendations regarding treatment are based on limited data, much of which awaits confirmation in long-term, prospective, controlled studies.

Dietary Manipulations

Given the magnitude of hyperlipidemia seen in association with NS, dietary measures alone, unless highly restrictive, are usually ineffective as sole therapy.[15,122–124] Institution of a moderately restricted diet, low in cholesterol (<300 mg) and fat, with a high ratio of polyunsaturated to saturated fats, during the run-in phase of small trials of lipid-lowering agents failed to effect any significant improvement in lipid parameters.[125–127] More impressive results have been reported with more restricted diets. After 6 months on a diet low in cholesterol (<200 mg), low in fat (<30% total calories), and rich in polyunsaturated fatty acids, total and LDL cholesterol decreased by 24% and 27%, respectively.[15] A vegetarian soy-based diet low in fat and protein and essentially cholesterol free decreased total cholesterol by 28% and LDL by 33% in 20 nephrotic patients over an 8-week period.[128] It is doubtful that such strict diets would be tolerated by most patients with NS. Moreover, the long-term safety of such diets has not been assessed. Uncontrolled human studies have suggested that a diet high in long-chain ω-3 polyunsaturated fatty acids (e.g., enriched in fish oil) may decrease total plasma triglycerides and cholesterol as well as decrease proteinuria.[129,130] As other studies have failed to confirm this effect,[123] further evaluation

is needed before the routine use of fish oil supplementation can be recommended.

Pharmacologic Therapy

A variety of agents have been used in the treatment of nephrotic hyperlipidemia, including bile acid sequestrants, fibric acid derivatives, probucol, and 3-hydroxy-3-methylglutaryl coenzyme A reductase inhibitors. The bile acid sequestrants cholestyramine and colestipol lowered LDL cholesterol by 19% to 32% and total cholesterol by 8% to 20%.[131,132] However, these drugs are not ideal first-line agents because of a high incidence of gastrointestinal adverse effects and a tendency to increase triglyceride levels. The fibric acid derivative gemfibrozil decreased triglycerides by 51%, total cholesterol by 15%, and LDL by 12.5%, while increasing HDL by 18%, in a 6-week randomized, double-blind, placebo-controlled trial in 11 patients.[133] Addition of the resin colestipol led to further improvements in lipid parameters, but the combination was poorly tolerated. Gemfibrozil alone was well tolerated, although one patient developed a markedly elevated creatine phosphokinase after vigorous exercise. Clofibrate, an older fibric acid derivative, has been associated with severe adverse effects in patients with renal impairment and should be avoided.[134] The use of probucol effected a moderate decrease in total and LDL cholesterol in two studies, but decreases also occurred in HDL cholesterol.[133,135]

3-Hydroxy-3-methylglutaryl coenzyme A (HMG-CoA) reductase inhibitors decrease hepatic cholesterol production by inhibiting the rate-limiting enzyme involved in cholesterol synthesis. These agents decrease total cholesterol, LDL cholesterol, and very low density lipoprotein triglycerides, and in some studies also increase HDL cholesterol.[124–127,131,136–148] Lipoprotein (a) levels were decreased in one study in patients with high baseline levels,[145] but they were unchanged in two other studies.[127,144] In general, HMG-CoA reductase inhibitors are well tolerated and appear to be safe in studies up to 2 years in duration. Occasional patients have developed mild asymptomatic increases in aspartate aminotransferase[125,137] or creatine phosphokinase,[124,126,140,141,144,147] but in most instances, these did not necessitate withdrawal of the drug. In a recent meta-analysis of studies on the treatment of nephrotic hyperlipidemia, HMG-CoA reductase inhibitors were found to be the most effective therapy.[149]

Data from experimental studies in vitro and in animal models suggest that the pleiotropic effects of statins may have additional benefits by decreasing proteinuria and delaying the progression of renal disease.[150,151] However, conclusive data to support these findings in humans are lacking. In a meta-analysis of 12 trials in which lipid-lowering agents were administered to patients with proteinuric renal diseases, a significant reduction in the rate of decrease of the GFR was observed that correlated with study duration.[152] A nonsignificant trend toward a decrease in proteinuria was also found. A number of other small studies of up to 2 years' duration also demonstrated a decrease in proteinuria with statin treatment.[124,146] However, this is not a consistent finding.[138,140] More recently, a prospective, controlled study by Bianchi and colleagues[153] looked at the effects of treatment with atorvastatin for 1 year in a group of 56 patients with proteinuria and chronic kidney disease. A significant decrease in proteinuria and slowing of the rate of decrease in the GFR were observed that were additive to the effects of an ACEI or an ARB.

No large randomized trials have specifically looked at progression of renal disease as a primary outcome, but a slowing of the decrease in the GFR has been suggested in post hoc analyses of subgroups of patients in large cardiovascular trials. A recent meta-analysis of 15 placebo-controlled, randomized trials found a significant decrease in proteinuria with statins, the effect being more pronounced in subjects with higher baseline protein excretion.[154] A secondary analysis of data from the Cholesterol and Recurrent Events trial found that pravastatin significantly slowed the rate of decline in renal function in subjects with a GFR less than 40 mL/min and in those with a GFR less than 50 mL/min who also had proteinuria.[155] In contrast, an analysis of data from the PREVEND cohort study and the PREVEND-IT trial failed to demonstrate an effect of statin therapy on either proteinuria or GFR.[156] In a recent meta-analysis of 27 trials in 39,704 participants, a modest effect of statins in decreasing proteinuria and slowing the rate of loss of renal function was observed.[157] There was considerable heterogeneity among trials, and the observed decrease in the rate of loss of renal function was confined to patients with cardiovascular disease. No effect was seen in patients with other causes of chronic kidney disease, such as hypertension, diabetes mellitus, or glomerulonephritis.[157] The true role of statins as renoprotective agents awaits confirmation in long-term trials specifically designed to look at prespecified renal endpoints.

Finally, there is some evidence to suggest that antiproteinuric treatment with ACEIs may be accompanied by an improvement in lipid parameters. Keilani and colleagues[158] reported 13% and 15% decreases in total and LDL cholesterol, respectively, in a group of patients with moderate proteinuria without NS. A reduction in lipoprotein (a) also occurred, but only three patients had frankly elevated levels at the start of the trial. The combination of an ACEI and an NSAID effected decreases in total cholesterol, LDL cholesterol, and lipoprotein (a) in nine patients with nephrosis-range proteinuria.[159] These alterations in lipid parameters correlated with decreases in proteinuria.

A reasonable approach to the management of nephrotic hyperlipidemia is to institute therapy with an HMG-CoA reductase inhibitor in conjunction with a low-cholesterol diet. Modification of other risk factors, such as smoking and obesity, is also important. If this regimen is inadequate, a bile acid sequestrant may be added as long as triglyceride levels are not excessive. If triglycerides are very high and/or HDL levels are low, a fibric acid analogue such as gemfibrozil could be added. Although these strategies will undoubtedly lower lipid levels, whether they will translate into a decrease in cardiovascular morbidity or a slowing of progression of renal disease awaits confirmation in long-term controlled trials.

ABNORMALITIES OF CALCIUM HOMEOSTASIS

Hypocalcemia (both total and ionized) and secondary hyperparathyroidism have been variably described in NS. Potential mechanisms include decreased intestinal absorption of calcium and a blunted calcemic response to parathyroid hormone.[1] Moreover, levels of 25-hydroxycholecalciferol (25-OH-D), the precursor of the active vitamin, are decreased in most patients with NS, probably because of loss of this metabolite in the urine bound to its vitamin D

carrier protein.[160,161] Levels of the physiologically active 1,25-dihydroxycholecalciferol (1,25-[OH]$_2$-D) are more variable, being normal in some studies and low in others.[1]

Despite these alterations in calcium and vitamin D metabolism, studies have yielded conflicting data regarding the incidence of bone disease in patients with NS.[161,162] In one study, bone structure was largely normal among patients with normal renal function. Severe demineralization and bone resorption occurred only in association with deterioration of renal function.[163] Nevertheless, bone abnormalities were more pronounced in patients with NS than in a control group with comparable azotemia but lacking proteinuria. Others have reported evidence of osteomalacia and secondary hyperparathyroidism even in patients with normal renal function.[164] A more recent study of 30 adults with NS and normal renal function documented normal bone histology in one third of patients and osteomalacia in 57% of the group.[161] The presence of osteomalacia correlated with the degree of proteinuria and the duration of NS.[161] It seems clear that the potential for osteomalacia exists in these patients and may increase as renal failure supervenes. The known deleterious effects of glucocorticoids on bone mineral density may be of relevance in patients who receive prolonged or frequent courses of steroids for treatment of NS. It is of interest in this regard that a recent study of bone density in a group of 60 children and adolescents with steroid-sensitive NS, who had received an average of 23,000 mg prednisone, failed to show evidence of osteoporosis.[165] Bone mineral content of the lumbar spine and of the whole body were not different from a group of 195 control subjects.[165]

Management

Treatment with oral vitamin D therapy should be prescribed for patients with evidence of osteomalacia or secondary hyperparathyroidism, patients with persistently low serum ionized calcium levels, patients in whom progressive renal insufficiency is anticipated, and patients who have unremitting or frequently relapsing NS.[166] Unfortunately, there is little information available on the optimal formulation or dose for vitamin D replacement in NS. In one study, vitamin D$_3$ (25 mg) was administered daily for a period of 4 to 52 weeks to nine nephrotic patients with documented low levels of 25-OH-D and 1,25-(OH)$_2$-D.[167] Normalization of 25-OH-D levels occurred in eight of nine patients, and normalization of 1,25-(OH)$_2$-D levels in five patients in whom the baseline serum creatinine was normal. Serum calcium levels should be monitored closely in patients on vitamin D replacement therapy. Measurement of bone mineral density should be considered in patients with persistent NS, particularly if they have received high doses of corticosteroids or have additional risk factors for osteoporosis.

HYPERCOAGULABILITY AND THROMBOEMBOLISM

Numerous defects in coagulation factors, clotting inhibitors, the fibrinolytic system, and platelet function have been invoked to explain the hypercoagulable state that exists in patients with NS.[168–171] There is a distinct lack of uniformity among the various studies. In general, levels of fibrinogen, factor V, factor VII, and α_2-antiplasmin are increased, whereas those of factor IX, factor XI, factor XII, antithrombin III, plasminogen, and α_1-antitrypsin are decreased. Disturbances in platelet physiology that could promote clotting include increased aggregability, increased levels of β-thromboglobulin (a protein released at the time of platelet aggregation), and increased levels of von Willebrand's factor. The cause of enhanced platelet aggregability is most likely multifactorial, with hypoalbuminemia, hyperlipidemia, and hyperfibrinogenemia all playing a role.[172] Despite these multiple abnormalities, a direct relationship has yet to be established between any specific defect and the occurrence of thromboembolic complications.[173]

Approximately 20% (range, 8%–44%) of adult NS patients develop thromboembolic complications other than renal vein thrombosis (RVT). As many as 50% of these episodes are clinically silent.[168] Arterial thromboses occur much less frequently than venous thromboses and have been described in the pulmonary, femoral, mesenteric, and coronary arteries. The incidence of RVT varies in different series from 2% to 60%, with an average of 35%. RVT is most common in membranous nephropathy.[174] Chronic RVT is usually asymptomatic and can only be diagnosed with certainty by renal venography, although computed tomography is also useful diagnostically and is less invasive.[171] Long-term follow-up of established cases indicates that chronic RVT is generally benign, with a low incidence of thromboembolic episodes in patients who are anticoagulated.[174,175] Moreover, there appear to be no adverse effects on renal function or the degree of proteinuria.[2] Acute RVT is less frequent. Patients usually present with flank pain and tenderness, macroscopic hematuria, and deterioration in renal function. Routine venography is not recommended in NS patients. Venography should be reserved for patients with features suggestive of acute RVT, an unexplained rapid deterioration in renal function, or symptoms suggestive of an acute thromboembolic event such as pulmonary embolus.

Management

Management of the thrombotic tendency in NS involves preventive measures such as avoiding immobilization or volume depletion, both of which increase the risk of clotting. Patients with a history of thromboembolism before the onset of NS should receive prophylactic anticoagulation if they are immobilized or have other major risk factors for clotting. In patients who experience an episode of thrombus or embolus, anticoagulants should be continued for as long as the nephrotic state persists.[169] Intravenous heparin followed by warfarin is the standard treatment for acute RVT.[169,174,175] The international normalized ratio must be carefully monitored in nephrotic patients as warfarin kinetics are affected by NS, and dose adjustment may be necessary with changes in serum albumin level.[176] Recent case reports describe successful treatment of RVT with low molecular weight heparin continued in the outpatient setting.[177,178] Fibrinolytic therapy, both systemic and local, has been successfully used in isolated patients,[179–182] but does not appear to be superior to standard anticoagulant therapy. A more recent report described successful treatment of RVT with percutaneous catheter-directed thrombectomy in seven cases of acute RVT followed by thrombolysis in five cases.[183] Such direct percutaneous approaches are probably best reserved for patients with acute symptomatic RVT.[171]

The issue of prophylactic anticoagulation in NS is controversial. Prophylaxis with the low molecular weight heparin enoxaparin was recently studied in 55 adult patients for periods of 2 to 48 months.[184] No thrombotic episodes occurred during therapy, as evidenced by renal vein Doppler ultrasonography, lower leg Doppler ultrasonography, and lung ventilation-perfusion scintigraphy. There were no documented adverse effects, and patients found self-administration of the once-daily dose to be tolerable. Some authors advocate the use of prophylaxis in patients with membranous nephropathy because these are the patients at highest risk of thrombotic complications.[4,185,186] A recent study using a decision analysis model concluded that the benefits of prophylactic anticoagulation begun at the time of diagnosis of NS due to membranous nephropathy outweighed the risks of bleeding.[185] Despite the arguments in favor of prophylactic anticoagulation, its routine use in all nephrotic patients cannot be recommended. Further prospective, controlled studies are indicated to determine both the necessity and optimal prophylactic anticoagulant regimens for patients with NS.

INCREASED SUSCEPTIBILITY TO INFECTION

A number of immunologic abnormalities have been documented in patients with NS. These include depressed immunoglobulin levels due to urinary loss, impaired antibody generation, defective opsonization due to depressed levels of complement factor B, and abnormalities of cell-mediated immunity.[1] In many patients, nonspecific depression of immune responses may occur because of malnutrition, vitamin D deficiency, or immunosuppressive therapy. These abnormalities may result in an increased susceptibility to infection, with the peritoneum and lungs being the sites most frequently involved.

Before the introduction of antibiotics, pulmonary, meningeal, or peritoneal infection with encapsulated organisms, such as *Streptococcus*, *Haemophilus*, and *Klebsiella* species, was a common cause of death, particularly in children. In recent years, the incidence of infection with these agents has decreased, although adult patients continue to display an increased incidence of infection with gram-negative bacteria.[187]

Management

Aggressive antibiotic therapy should be instituted at the first suspicion of infection. Prophylactic use of antibiotics, pneumococcal vaccine, or intravenous administration of hyperimmunoglobulin should be considered in high-risk cases. Vaccination should be given whenever possible during periods of remission because NS may impair the antibody response to vaccination.[188] Despite an adequate initial response to vaccination, many vaccinated patients do not maintain adequate antibody titers over time.[189,190] Nonetheless, pneumococcal vaccination is still recommended for children older than 2 years of age and for adults with severely depressed immunoglobulins, particularly if NS is likely to be persistent or if renal failure supervenes.[1,2] Although intravenous immunoglobulin has been used in NS,[187] insufficient data preclude specific recommendations.

References

1. Bernard DB: Extra-renal manifestations of nephrotic syndrome. Kidney Int 1988;33:1184–1202.
2. Harris RC, Ismail N: Extrarenal complications of the nephrotic syndrome. Am J Kidney Dis 1994;23:447–497.
3. Falk RJ, Jennette JC, Nachman PH: Primary glomerular disease. In Brenner BM (ed): The Kidney, 6 ed. Philadelphia: WB Saunders, 2000, pp 1263–1349.
4. Orth SR, Ritz E: The nephrotic syndrome. N Engl J Med 1998;338:1202–1211.
5. Ruggenenti P, Remuzzi G: The role of protein traffic in the progression of renal diseases. Annu Rev Med 2000;51:315–327.
6. The GISEN Group (Gruppo Italiano di Studi Epidemiologici in Nefrologia): Randomised placebo-controlled trial of effect of ramipril on decline in glomerular filtration rate and risk of terminal renal failure in proteinuric, non-diabetic nephropathy. Lancet 1997;349:1857–1863.
7. Lewis EJ, Hunsicker LG, Bain RP, et al: The effect of angiotensin-converting enzyme inhibition in diabetic nephropathy. N Engl J Med 1993;329:1456–1462.
8. Gugler R, Shoeman DW, Huffman DH, et al: Pharmacokinetics of drugs in patients with the nephrotic syndrome. J Clin Invest 1975;55:1182–1189.
9. Kaysen GA, Kirkpatrick WG, Couser WG: Albumin homeostasis in the nephrotic rat: Nutritional considerations. Am J Physiol 1984;247:F192–F202.
10. Kaysen GA, Gambertoglio J, Jiminez I, et al: Effect of dietary protein intake on albumin homeostasis in nephrotic patients. Kidney Int 1986;29:572–577.
11. Brenner BM, Meyer TW, Hostetter TH: Dietary protein intake and the progressive nature of kidney disease: The role of hemodynamically mediated glomerular injury in the pathogenesis of progressive glomerulosclerosis in aging, renal ablation, and intrinsic renal disease. N Engl J Med 1982;307:652–659.
12. Aparicio M, Bouchet JL, Gin H, et al: Effect of a low-protein diet on urinary albumin excretion in uremic patients. Nephron 1988;50:288–291.
13. Don BR, Kaysen GA, Hutchinson FN, et al: The effect of angiotensin-converting enzyme inhibition and dietary protein restriction in the treatment of proteinuria. Am J Kidney Dis 1991;17:10–17.
14. Remuzzi A, Perticucci E, Battaglia C, et al: Low-protein diet and glomerular size-selective function in membranous glomerulopathy. Am J Kidney Dis 1991;17:317–322.
15. D'Amico G, Remuzzi G, Maschio G, et al: Effect of dietary proteins and lipids in patients with membranous nephropathy and nephrotic syndrome. Clin Nephrol 1991;35:237–242.
16. Giordano M, de Feo P, Lucidi P, et al: Effects of dietary protein restriction on fibrinogen and albumin metabolism in nephrotic patients. Kidney Int 2001;60:235–242.
17. Walser M, Hill S, Tomalis EA: Treatment of nephrotic adults with a supplemented, very low-protein diet. Am J Kidney Dis 1996;28:354–364.
18. Feehally J, Baker F, Walls J: Dietary protein manipulation in experimental nephrotic syndrome. Nephron 1988;50:247–252.
19. Aparicio M, Chauveau P, Combe C: Are supplemented low-protein diets nutritionally safe? Am J Kidney Dis 2001;37 (Suppl 2):S71–S76.
20. Lim VS, Wolfson M, Yarasheski KE, et al: Leucine turnover in patients with nephrotic syndrome: Evidence suggesting body protein conservation. J Am Soc Nephrol 1998;9:1067–1073.
21. Maroni BJ, Staffeld C, Young VR, et al: Mechanisms permitting nephrotic patients to achieve nitrogen equilibrium with a protein-restricted diet. J Clin Invest 1997;99:2479–2487.
22. Giordano M, Lucidi P, De Feo P, et al: Dietary protein intake does not affect IgG synthesis in patients with nephrotic syndrome. Nephrol Dial Transplant 2004;19:2494–2498.
23. Heeg JE, De Jong PE, van der Hem GK, et al: Efficacy and variability of the antiproteinuric effect of ACE inhibition by lisinopril. Kidney Int 1989;36:272–279.
24. Brunner HR: ACE inhibitors in renal disease. Kidney Int 1992;42:463–479.
25. Heeg JE, de Jong PE, van der Hem GK, et al: Angiotensin II does not acutely reverse the reduction of proteinuria by long-term ACE inhibition. Kidney Int 1991;40:734–741.
26. Meyer TW, Morelli E, Loon N, et al: Converting enzyme inhibition and glomerular size selectivity in diabetic nephropathy. J Am Soc Nephrol 1990;1:S64–S68.
27. Thomas DM, Hillis AN, Coles GA, et al: Enalapril can treat the proteinuria of membranous glomerulonephritis without detriment to systemic or renal hemodynamics. Am J Kidney Dis 1991;18:38–43.
28. Buter H, Hemmelder MH, Navis G, et al: The blunting of the antiproteinuric effect of ACE inhibition by high sodium intake can be restored by hydrochlorothiazide. Nephrol Dial Transplant 1998;13:1682–1685.
29. Jafar TH, Stark PC, Schmid CH, et al: Proteinuria as a modifiable risk factor for the progression of non-diabetic renal disease. Kidney Int 2001;60:1131–1140.
30. Maschio G, Alberti D, Janin G, et al: Effect of the angiotensin-converting-enzyme inhibitor benazepril on the progression of chronic renal insufficiency. N Engl J Med 1996;334:939–945.
31. Ruggenenti P, Perna A, Gherardi G, et al: Renal function and requirement for dialysis in chronic nephropathy patients on long-term ramipril: REIN follow-up trial. Lancet 1998;352: 1252–1256.
32. Ruggenenti P, Perna A, Gherardi G, et al: Renoprotective properties of ACE-inhibition in non-diabetic nephropathies with non-nephrotic proteinuria. Lancet 1999;354:359–364.
33. Ruggenenti P, Perna A, Gherardi G, et al: Chronic proteinuric nephropathies: Outcomes and response to treatment in a prospective cohort of 352 patients with different patterns of renal injury. Am J Kidney Dis 2000;35:1155–1165.
34. Jafar TH, Schmid CH, Landa M, et al: Angiotensin-converting enzyme inhibitors and progression of nondiabetic renal disease. A meta-analysis of patient-level data. Ann Intern Med 2001;135:73–87.
35. Jafar JT, Stark PC, Schmid CH, et al., AIPRD Study Group: Angiotensin-converting enzyme inhibition and progression of renal disease: Proteinuria as a modifiable risk factor for the progression of non-diabetic renal disease. Kidney Int 2001;60:1131–1140.
36. Jafar JT, Stark PC, Schmid CH, et al., AIPRD Study Group: Progression of chronic kidney disease: The role of blood pressure control, proteinuria, and angiotensin-converting enzyme inhibition—a patient level meta-analysis. Ann Intern Med 2003;139:244–252.
37. Kent DM, Jafar TH, Hayward RA, et al., AIPRD Study Group: Progression risk, urinary protein excretion, and treatment effects of angiotensin-converting enzyme inhibitors in nondiabetic kidney disease. J Am Soc Nephrol 2007;18:1959–1965.
38. Wilmer WA, Rovin BH, Herbert CJ, et al: Management of glomerular proteinuria: A commentary. J Am Soc Nephrol 2003;14:3217–3232.
39. Wolf G, Ritz E: Combination therapy with ACE inhibitors and angiotensin II receptor blockers to halt progression of chronic renal disease: pathophysiology and indications. Kidney Int 2005;67:799–812.
40. Nakao N, Yoshimura A, Morita H, et al: Combination treatment of angiotensin-II receptor blocker and angiotensin-converting enzyme inhibitor in non-diabetic renal disease (COOPERATE): A randomised controlled trial. Lancet 2003;361:117–124 [published erratum in Lancet 2003;361:1230].
41. Hou FF, Xie D, Zhang X, et al: Renoprotection of optimal antiproteinuric doses (ROAD) study: A randomized controlled

study of benazepril and losartan in chronic renal insufficiency. J Am Soc Nephrol 2007;18:1889–1898.

42. Zoccali C, Valvo E, Russo D, et al: Antiproteinuric effect of losartan in patients with chronic renal diseases. Nephrol Dial Transplant 1997;12:234–235.

43. Russo D, Pisani A, Balletta MM, et al: Additive antiproteinuric effect of converting enzyme inhibitor and losartan in normotensive patients with IgA nephropathy. Am J Kidney Dis 1999;33:851–856.

44. Hebert LA, Falkenhain M, Nohman N, et al: Combination ACE inhibitor and angiotensin II receptor antagonist in diabetic nephropathy. Am J Nephrol 1999;19:1–6.

45. Mogensen CE, Neldam S, Tikkanen I, et al: Randomized controlled trial of dual blockade of renin-angiotensin system in patients with hypertension, microalbuminuria, and non-insulin dependent diabetes: The Candesartan and Lisinopril Microalbuminuria (CALM) study. Br Med J 2000;321:1440–1444.

46. Tutuncu NB, Gurlek A, Gedik O: Efficacy of ACE inhibitors and ATII receptor blockers in patients with microalbuminuria: A prospective study. Acta Diabetol 2001;38:157–161.

47. Russo D, Minutolo R, Pisani A, et al: Coadministration of losartan and enalapril exerts additive antiproteinuric effects in IgA nephropathy. Am J Kidney Dis 2001;38:18–25.

48. Agarwal R: Add-on angiotensin receptor blockade with maximized ACE inhibition. Kidney Int 2001;59:2282–2289.

49. Agarwal R, Siva S, Dunn SR, et al: Add-on angiotensin II receptor blockade lowers urinary transforming growth factor-levels. Am J Kidney Dis 2002;39:486–492.

50. Luño J, Barrio V, Goicoechea MA, et al: Effects of dual blockade of the renin-angiotensin system in primary proteinuric nephropathies. Kidney Int 2002;62(Suppl 82):S47–S52.

51. Rossing K, Christensen PK, Jensen BR, et al: Dual blockade of the renin-angiotensin system in diabetic nephropathy: A randomized double-blind crossover trial. Diabetes Care 2002;25:95–100.

52. Berger ED, Bader BD, Ebert C, et al: Reduction of proteinuria; combined effects of receptor blockade and low dose angiotensin-converting enzyme inhibition. J Hypertens 2002;20:739–743.

53. Laverman GD, Navis G, Henning RH, et al: Dual renin-angiotensin system blockade at a optimal doses for proteinuria. Kidney Int 2002;62:1020–1025.

54. Jacobsen P, Andersen S, Rossing K, et al: Dual blockade of the renin-angiotensin system in type 1 patients with diabetic nephropathy. Nephrol Dial Transplant 2002;17:1019–1024.

55. Kincaid-Smith P, Fairley K, Packham D: Randomized controlled crossover study of the effect on proteinuria and blood pressure of adding an angiotensin II receptor antagonist to an angiotensin converting enzyme inhibitor in normotensive patients with chronic renal disease and proteinuria. Nephrol Dial Transplant 2002;17:597–601.

56. Ferrari P, Marti HP, Pfister M, et al: Additive antiproteinuric effect of combined ACE inhibition and angiotensin II receptor blockade. J Hypertens 2002;20:125–130.

57. Kuriyama S, Tomonari H, Tokudome G, et al: Anti-proteinuric effects of combined anti-hypertensive therapies in patients with overt type 2 diabetic nephropathy. Hypertens Res 2002;25:849–855.

58. Tylicki L, Rutkowski P, Renke M, et al: Renoprotective effect of small doses of losartan and enalapril in patients with primary glomerulonephritis. Short-term observation. Am J Nephrol 2002;22:356–362.

59. Jacobsen P, Andersen S, Jensen BR, et al: Additive effect of ACE inhibition and angiotensin II receptor blockade in type I diabetic patients with diabetic nephropathy. J Am Soc Nephrol 2003;14: 992–999.

60. Campbell R, Sangalli F, Perticucci E, et al: Effects of combined ACE inhibitor and angiotensin II antagonist treatment in human chronic nephropathies. Kidney Int 2003;63:1094–1103.

61. Iodice C, Balletta MM, Minutolo R, et al: Maximal suppression of renin-angiotensin system in nonproliferative glomerulonephritis. Kidney Int 2003;63:2214–2221.

62. Jacobsen P, Anderson S, Rossing K, et al: Dual blockade of the renin-angiotensin system versus maximal recommended dose of ACE inhibition in diabetic nephropathy. Kidney Int 2003;63:1874–1880.

63. Rossing K, Jacobsen P, Pietraszek L, et al: Renoprotective effects of adding angiotensin II receptor blocker to maximal recommended doses of ACE inhibitor in diabetic nephropathy: A randomized double-blind crossover trial. Diabetes Care 2003;26:2268–2274.

64. Kim MJ, Song JH, Suh JH, et al: Additive anti-proteinuric effect of combination therapy with ACE inhibitor and angiotensin receptor antagonist: Differential short-term response between IgA nephropathy and diabetic nephropathy. Yonsei Med J 2003;44:463–472.

65. Song JH, Lee SW, Suh JH, et al: The effects of dual blockade of the renin-angiotensin system on urinary protein and transforming growth factor-beta excretion in 2 groups of patients with IgA and diabetic nephropathy. Clin Nephrol 2003;60:318–326.

66. Segura J, Praga M, Campo C, et al: Combination is better than monotherapy with ACE inhibitor or angiotensin receptor antagonist at recommended doses. J Renin Angiotensin Aldosterone Syst 2003;4:43–47.

67. Cetinkaya R, Odabas AR, Selcuk Y: Anti-proteinuric effects of combination therapy with enalapril and losartan in patients with nephropathy due to type II diabetes. Int J Clin Pract 2004;58:432–435.

68. Rutkowski P, Tylicki L, Renke M, et al: Low-dose dual blockade of the renin-angiotensin system in patients with primary glomerulonephritis. Am J Kidney Dis 2004;43:260–268.

69. Horita Y, Tadokoro M, Taura K, et al: Low-dose combination therapy with temocapril and losartan reduces proteinuria in normotensive patients with immunoglobulin a nephropathy. Hypertens Res 2004;27:963–970.

70. Matos JP, de Lourdes Rodrigues M, Ismerim VL, et al: Effects of dual blockade of the renin angiotensin system in hypertensive type 2 diabetic patients with nephropathy. Clin Nephrol 2005;64:180–189.

71. Song JH, Cha SH, Lee HJ, et al: Effect of low-dose dual blockade of renin-angiotensin system on urinary TGF-(beta) in type 2 diabetic patients with advanced kidney disease. Nephrol Dial Transplant 2006;21:683–689.

72. MacKinnon M, Shurraw S, Akbari A, et al: Combination therapy with an angiotensin receptor blocker and an ACE inhibitor in proteinuric renal disease: A systematic review of the efficacy and safety data. Am J Kidney Dis 2006;48:8–20.

73. Jennings DL, Kalus JS, Coleman CI, et al: Combination therapy with an ACE inhibitor and an angiotensin receptor blocker for diabetic nephropathy: A meta-analysis. Diabet Med 2007;24:486–493.

74. Donker AJM, Brentjens JRH, van der Hem GK, et al: Treatment of the nephrotic syndrome with indomethacin. Nephron 1978;22:374–381.

75. Heeg JE, de Jong PE, Vriesendorp R, et al: Additive antiproteinuric effect of the NSAID indomethacin and the ACE inhibitor lisinopril. Am J Nephrol 1990;10(Suppl 1):94–97.

76. Vriesendorp R, de Zeeuw D, de Jong PE, et al: Reduction of urinary protein and prostaglandin E2 excretion in the nephrotic syndrome by non-steroidal anti-inflammatory drugs. Clin Nephrol 1986;25:105–110.

77. Golbetz H, Black V, Shemesh O, et al: Mechanism of the antiproteinuric effect of indomethacin in nephrotic humans. Am J Physiol 1989;256:F44–F51.

78. Perico N, Remuzzi A, Sangalli F, et al: The antiproteinuric effect of angiotensin antagonism in human IgA nephropathy is potentiated by indomethacin. J Am Soc Nephrol 1998;9:2308–2317.

79. Bianchi S, Rigazzi R, Campese VM: Long-term effects of spironolactone on proteinuria and kidney function in patients with chronic kidney disease. Kidney Int 2006;70:2116–2123.

80. van den Meiracker AH, Baggen RGA, Pauli S, et al: Spironolactone in type 2 diabetic nephropathy: Effects on proteinuria, blood pressure and renal function. J Hypertension 2006;24:2285–2292.

81. Schepkens H, Vanholder R, Billiouw JM, et al: Life-threatening hyperkalemia during combined therapy with angiotensin-converting enzyme inhibitors and spironolactone. Am J Med 2001;110:438–441.

82. Avram MM, Lepner HI, Gan AC: Medical nephrectomy. The use of metallic salts for the control of massive proteinuria in the nephrotic syndrome. Proc Am Soc Artif Intern Organs 1976;22:431–438.

83. McCarron DA, Rubin RJ, Barnes BA, et al: Therapeutic bilateral renal infarction in end-stage renal disease. N Engl J Med 1976;294:652.

84. Baumelou A, Legrain M: Medical nephrectomy with anti-inflammatory non-steroidal drugs. Br Med J 1982;284:234.

85. Olivero JL, Pedro Frommer J, Gonzalez JM: Medical nephrectomy: The last resort for intractable complications of the nephrotic syndrome. Am J Kidney Dis 1993;21:260–263.

86. Abraham WT, Schrier RW: Edematous disorders: Pathophysiology of renal sodium and water retention and treatment with diuretics. Curr Opin Nephrol Hypertens 1993;2:798–805.

87. Palmer BF, Alpern RJ: Pathogenesis of edema formation in the nephrotic syndrome. Kidney Int 1997;51(Suppl 59):S21–S27.

88. Hamm LL, Batuman V: Edema in the nephrotic syndrome: New aspect of an old enigma. J Am Soc Nephrol 2003;14:3288–3289.

89. Dorhout Mees EJ, Koomans HA: Understanding the nephrotic syndrome: What's new in a decade? Nephron 1995;70:1–10.

90. Vande Walle JGJ, Donckerwolcke RA, Koomans HA: Pathophysiology of edema formation in children with nephrotic syndrome not due to minimal change disease. J Am Soc Nephrol 1999;10:323–331.

91. Wilcox CS: Diuretics. In Brenner BM (ed): The Kidney, 5th ed. Philadelphia: WB Saunders, 2000, pp 2219–2252.

92. Brater DC: Diuretic therapy. N Engl J Med 1998;339:387–395.

93. Inoue M, Okajima K, Itoh K, et al: Mechanism of furosemide resistance in analbuminemic rats and hypoalbuminemic patients. Kidney Int 1987;32:198–203.

94. Kirchner KA, Voelker JR, Brater DC: Binding inhibitors restore furosemide potency in tubule fluid containing albumin. Kidney Int 1991;40:418–424.

95. Sjostrom PA, Odlind BG, Beermann BA, et al: Pharmacokinetics and effects of furosemide in patients with the nephrotic syndrome. Eur J Clin Pharmacol 1989;37:173–180.

96. Danielsen H, Pedersen EB, Madsen M, et al: Abnormal renal sodium excretion in the nephrotic syndrome after furosemide: Relation to glomerular filtration rate. Acta Med Scand 1985;217:513–518.

97. Agarwal R, Gorski JC, Sundblad K, et al: Urinary protein binding does not affect response to furosemide in patients with nephrotic syndrome. J Am Soc Nephrol 2000;11:1100–1105.

98. Rose BD: Diuretics. Kidney Int 1991;39:336–352.

99. Levine JS, Iglesias J: Diuretic use and fluid management. In Murray PT, Hall JB, Brady HR (eds): Intensive Care in Nephrology. London: Taylor & Francis, 2006, pp 315–337.

100. Elwell RJ, Spenser AP, Eisele G: Combined furosemide and human albumin treatment for diuretic-resistant edema. Ann Pharmacother 2003;37:695–700.

101. Fliser D, Zurbruggen I, Mutschler E, et al: Coadministration of albumin and furosemide in patients with the nephrotic syndrome. Kidney Int 1999;55:629–634.

102. Akcicek F, Yalniz T, Basci A, et al: Diuretic effect of frusemide in patients with nephrotic syndrome: Is it potentiated by intravenous albumin? Br Med J 1995;310:162–163.

103. Sjostrom PA, Odlind BG: Effect of albumin on diuretic treatment in the nephrotic syndrome. Br Med J 1995;310:1537.

104. Chalasani N, Gorski JC, Horlander JC, et al: Effects of albumin/furosemide mixtures on responses to furosemide in hypoalbuminemic patients. J Am Soc Nephrol 2001;12:1010–1016.

105. Nakahama H, Orita Y, Yamazaki M, et al: Pharmacokinetic and pharmacodynamic interactions between furosemide and hydrochlorothiazide in nephrotic patients. Nephron 1988;49:223–227.

106. Dargie HJ, Allison MEM, Kennedy AC, et al: Efficacy of metolazone in patients with renal edema. Clin Nephrol 1974;2:157–160.

107. Davison AM, Lambie AT, Verth AH, et al: Salt-poor human albumin in management of nephrotic syndrome. Br Med J 1974;1:481–484.

108. Fauchald P, Noddeland H, Norseth J: An evaluation of ultrafiltration as treatment of diuretic-resistant oedema in nephrotic syndrome. Acta Med Scand 1985;217:127–131.

109. Wheeler DC, Bernard DB: Lipid abnormalities in the nephrotic syndrome: Causes, consequences and treatment. Am J Kidney Dis 1994;23:331–346.

110. Warwick GL, Packard CJ: Pathogenesis of lipid abnormalities in patients with nephrotic syndrome/proteinuria: Clinical implications. Miner Electrolyte Metab 1993;19:115–126.

111. Kronenberg F, Lingenhel A, Lhotta K, et al: Lipoprotein(a)- and low-density lipoprotein-derived cholesterol in nephrotic syndrome: Impact on lipid-lowering therapy? Kidney Int 2004;66:348–354.

112. Vaziri ND: Molecular mechanisms of lipid disorders in nephrotic syndrome. Kidney Int 2003;63:1964–1976.

113. Keane WF, St Peter JV, Kasiske BL: Is the aggressive management of hyperlipidemia in nephrotic syndrome mandatory? Kidney Int 1992;42(Suppl 38):134–141.

114. Kaysen GA, de Sain-van der Velden MGM: New insights into lipid metabolism in the nephrotic syndrome. Kidney Int 1999;55(Suppl 71):S18–S21.

115. Shearer GC, Stevenson FT, Atkinson DN, et al: Hypoalbuminemia and proteinuria contribute separately to reduced lipoprotein catabolism in the nephrotic syndrome. Kidney Int 2001;59:179–189.

116. Wass V, Cameron JS: Cardiovascular disease and the nephrotic syndrome: The other side of the coin. Nephron 1981;27:58–61.

117. Mallick NP, Short CD: The nephrotic syndrome and ischaemic heart disease. Nephron 1981;27:54–57.

118. Ordonez JD, Hiatt RA, Killebrew EJ, et al: The increased risk of coronary heart disease associated with nephrotic syndrome. Kidney Int 1993;44:638–642.

119. Keane WF, Kasiske BL, O'Donnell MP, et al: The role of altered lipid metabolism in the progression of renal disease: Experimental evidence. Am J Kidney Dis 1991;17(Suppl 1):38–42.

120. Diamond JR, Karnovsky MJ: Focal and segmental glomerulosclerosis: Analogies to atherosclerosis. Kidney Int 1988;33:917–924.

121. Olbricht CJ, Koch KM: Treatment of hyperlipidemia in nephrotic syndrome: Time for a change? Nephron 1992;62:125–129.

122. Grundy SM: Management of hyperlipidemia of kidney disease. Kidney Int 1990;37:847–853.

123. D'Amico G, Gentile MG: Influence of diet on lipid abnormalities in human renal disease. Am J Kidney Dis 1993;22:151–157.

124. Rayner BL, Byrne MJ, van Zyl Smit R: A prospective clinical trial comparing the treatment of idiopathic membranous nephropathy and nephrotic syndrome with simvastatin and diet, versus diet alone. Clin Nephrol 1996;46:219–224.

125. Kasiske BL, Velosa JA, Halstenson CE, et al: The effects of lovastatin in hyperlipidemic patients with nephrotic syndrome. Am J Kidney Dis 1990;15:8–15.

126. Biesenbach G, Zazgornik J: Lovastatin in the treatment of hypercholesterolemia in nephrotic syndrome due to diabetic nephropathy stage IV–V. Clin Nephrol 1992;37:274–279.

127. Spitalewitz S, Porush JG, Cattran D, et al: Treatment of hyper-lipidemia in the nephrotic syndrome: The effects of pravastatin therapy. Am J Kidney Dis 1993;22:143–150.

128. D'Amico G, Gentile MG, Manna G, et al: Effect of vegetarian soy diet on hyperlipidemia in nephrotic syndrome. Lancet 1992;339:1131–1134.

129. Hall AV, Parbtani A, Clark WF, et al: Omega-3 fatty acid sup-plementation in primary nephrotic syndrome: Effects on plasma lipids and coagulopathy. J Am Soc Nephrol 1992;2:1321–1329.

130. De Caterina R, Caprioli R, Giannessi D, et al: n-3 Fatty acids reduce proteinuria in patients with chronic glomerular disease. Kidney Int 1993;44:843–850.

131. Rabelink AJ, Hene RJ, Erkelens DW, et al: Effects of simvastatin and cholestyramine on lipoprotein profile in hyperlipidemia of nephrotic syndrome. Lancet 1988;ii:1335–1338.

132. Valeri A, Gelfand J, Blum C, et al: Treatment of the hyperlipid-emia of the nephrotic syndrome: A controlled trial. Am J Kidney Dis 1986;8:388–396.

133. Groggel GC, Cheung AK, Ellis-Benigni K, et al: Treatment of nephrotic hyperlipoproteinemia with gemfibrozil. Kidney Int 1989;36:266–271.

134. Bridgman JF, Rosen SM, Thorp JM: Complications during clofibrate treatment of nephrotic-syndrome hyperlipoprotein-emia. Lancet 1972;2:506–509.

135. Iida H, Izumino K, Asaka M, et al: Effect of probucol on hy-perlipidemia in patients with nephrotic syndrome. Nephron 1987;47:280–283.

136. Vega GL, Grundy SM: Lovastatin therapy in nephrotic hyper-lipidemia: Effects on lipoprotein metabolism. Kidney Int 1988;33:1160–1168.

137. Golper TA, Illingworth RD, Morris CD, et al: Lovastatin in the treatment of multifactorial hyperlipidemia associated with proteinuria. Am J Kidney Dis 1989;13:312–320.

138. Elisaf M, Dardamanis M, Pappas M, et al: Treatment of nephrotic hyperlipidemia with lovastatin. Clin Nephrol 1991;36:50–51.

139. Bazzato G, Landini S, Fracasso A, et al: Treatment of nephrotic syndrome hyperlipidemia with simvastatin. Curr Ther Res 1991;50:744–752.

140. Chan PC, Robinson JD, Yeung WC, et al: Lovastatin in glomer-ulonephritis patients with hyperlipidaemia and heavy protein-uria. Nephrol Dial Transplant 1992;7:93–99.

141. Warwick GL, Packard CJ, Murray L, et al: Effect of simvastatin on plasma lipid and lipoprotein concentrations and low-density lipoprotein metabolism in the nephrotic syndrome. Clin Sci 1992;82:701–708.

142. Thomas ME, Harris KPG, Ramaswamy C, et al: Simvastatin therapy for hypercholesterolemic patients with nephrotic syn-drome or significant proteinuria. Kidney Int 1993;44:1124–1129.

143. Martins Prata M, Nogueira AC, Reimao Pinto J, et al: Long-term effect of lovastatin on lipoprotein profile in patients with primary nephrotic syndrome. Clin Nephrol 1994;41:277–283.

144. Wanner C, Bohler J, Eckardt HG: Effects of simvastatin on lipoprotein (a) and lipoprotein composition in patients with nephrotic syndrome. Clin Nephrol 1994;41:138–143.

145. Brown CD, Azrolan N, Thomas L, et al: Reduction of lipopro-tein (a) following treatment with lovastatin in patients with unremitting nephrotic syndrome. Am J Kidney Dis 1995;26:170–177.

146. Rabelink AJ, Hene RJ, Erkelens DW, et al: Partial remission of nephrotic syndrome in patients on long-term simvastatin. Lancet 1990;335:1045–1046.

147. Olbricht CJ, Wanner C, Thiery J, et al: Simvastatin in nephrotic syndrome. Kidney Int 1999;56:(Suppl 71):S113–S116.

148. Matzkies FK, Bahner U, Teschner M, et al: Efficiency of 1-year treatment with fluvastatin in hyperlipidemic patients with nephrotic syndrome. Am J Nephrol 1999;19:492–494.

149. Massy ZA, Ma JZ, Louis TA, et al: Lipid-lowering therapy in patients with renal disease. Kidney Int 1995;48:188–198.

150. D'Amico G: Statins and renal diseases: From primary preven-tion to renal replacement therapy. J Am Soc Nephrol 2006;17:S148–S152.

151. Trevisan R, Dodesini AR, Lepore G: Lipids and renal disease. J Am Soc Nephrol 2006;17:S145–S147.

152. Fried LF, Orchard TJ, Kasiske BL, et al: Effect of lipid reduction on the progression of renal disease: A meta-analysis. Kidney Int 2001;59:260–269.

153. Bianchi S, Bigazzi R, Caiazza A, et al: A controlled, prospective study of the effects of atorvastatin on proteinuria and progres-sion of kidney disease. Am J Kidney Dis 2003;41:565–570.

154. Douglas K, O'Malley PG, Jackson JL: Meta-analysis: The effect of statins on albuminuria. Ann Int Med 2006;145:117–124.

155. Tonelli M, Moye L, Sacks FM, et al: Effect of pravastatin on loss of renal function in people with moderate chronic renal insufficiency and cardiovascular disease. J Am Soc Nephrol 2003;14:1605–1613.

156. Atthobari J, Brantsma AH, Gansevoort RT, et al: The effect of statins on urinary albumin excretion and glomerular filtration rate: Results from both a randomized clinical trial and an ob-servational cohort study. Nephrol Dial Transplant 2006;21:3106–3114.

157. Sandhu S, Wiebe N, Fried LF, et al: Statins for improving renal outcomes: A meta-analysis. J Am Soc Nephrol 2006;17:2006–2016

158. Keilani T, Schlueter WA, Levin ML, et al: Improvement of lipid abnormalities associated with proteinuria using fosinopril, an angiotensin-converting enzyme inhibitor. Ann Intern Med 1993;118:246–254.

159. Gansevoort RT, Heeg JE, Dikkeschei FD, et al: Symptomatic anti-proteinuric treatment decreases serum lipoprotein (a) concentration in patients with glomerular proteinuria. Nephrol Dial Transplant 1994;9:244–250.

160. Sato KA, Gary RW, Lemann J: Urinary excretion of 25-hydroxyvitamin D in health and nephrotic syndrome. J Lab Clin Med 1980;69:325–330.

161. Mittal SK, Dash SC, Tiwari SC, et al: Bone histology in patients with nephrotic syndrome and normal renal function. Kidney Int 1999;55:1912–1919.

162. Korkor A, Schwartz J, Bergfeld M, et al: Absence of metabolic bone disease in adult patients with the nephrotic syndrome and normal renal function. J Clin Endocrinol Metab 1983;56:496–500.

163. Tessitore N, Bonucci E, D'Angelo A, et al: Bone histology and calcium metabolism in patients with nephrotic syndrome and normal or reduced renal function. Nephron 1984;37:153–159.

164. Malluche HH, Goldstein DA, Massry SG: Osteomalacia and hyperparathyroid bone disease in patients with nephrotic syndrome. J Clin Invest 1979;63:494–500.

165. Leonard MB, Feldman HI, Shults J, et al: Long-term, high-dose glucocorticoids and bone mineral content in childhood glucocorticoid-sensitive nephrotic syndrome. N Engl J Med 2004;351:868–875.

166. Alon U, Chan JCM: Calcium and vitamin D homeostasis in the nephrotic syndrome: Current status. Nephron 1984;36:1–4.

167. Haldimann B, Trechsel U: Vitamin D replacement therapy in patients with nephrotic syndrome. Miner Electrolyte Metab 1983;9:154–156.

168. Llach F: Hypercoagulability, renal vein thrombosis and other thrombotic complications of nephrotic syndrome. Kidney Int 1985;28:429–439.

169. Cameron JS: Coagulation and thromboembolic complications in the nephrotic syndrome. Adv Nephrol 1984;13:75–114.

170. Rabelink TJ, Zwaginga JJ, Koomans HA, et al: Thrombosis and hemostasis in renal disease. Kidney Int 1994;46:287–296.

171. Singhal R, Brimble KS: Thromboembolic complications in the nephrotic syndrome: pathophysiology and clinical management. Thromb Res 2006;118:397–407.

172. Machleidt C, Mettang T, Starz E, et al: Multifactorial genesis of enhanced platelet aggregability in patients with nephrotic syndrome. Kidney Int 1989;36:1119–1124.

173. Robert A, Olmer M, Sampol J, et al: Clinical correlation between hypercoagulability and thromboembolic phenomena. Kidney Int 1987;31:830–835.

174. Llach F, Papper S, Massry SG: The clinical spectrum of renal vein thrombosis: acute and chronic. Am J Med 1980;69:819–827.

175. Wagoner RD, Stanson AW, Holley KE, et al: Renal vein thrombosis in idiopathic membranous glomerulopathy and nephrotic syndrome: Incidence and significance. Kidney Int 1983;23:368–374.

176. Ganeval D, Fischer AM, Barre J, et al: Pharmacokinetics of warfarin in the nephrotic syndrome and effect on vitamin K-dependent clotting factors. Clin Nephrol 1986;25:75–80.

177. Yang S-H, Lee C-H, Ko S-F, et al: The successful treatment of renal-vein thrombosis by low-molecular-weight heparin in a steroid-sensitive nephrotic patient. Nephrol Dial Transplant 2002. 17:2017–2019.

178. Wu C-H, Ko S-F, Lee C-H, et al: Successful outpatient treatment of renal vein thrombosis by low-molecular weight heparins in 3 patients with nephrotic syndrome. Clin Nephrol 2006;65:443–440.

179. Burrow CR, Walker G, Bell WR, et al: Streptokinase salvage of renal function after renal vein thrombosis. Ann Intern Med 1984;100:237–238.

180. Crowley JP, Matarese RA, Quevedo SF, et al: Fibrinolytic therapy for bilateral renal vein thrombosis. Arch Intern Med 1984;144:159–160.

181. Morrisey EC, McDonald BR, Rabetoy GM: Resolution of proteinuria secondary to bilateral renal vein thrombosis after treatment with systemic thrombolytic therapy. Am J Kidney Dis 1997;29:615–619.

182. Lam K-K, Lui C-C: Successful treatment of acute inferior vena cava and unilateral renal vein thrombosis by local infusion of recombinant tissue plasminogen activator. Am J Kidney Dis 1998;32:1075–1079.

183. Kim HS, Fine DM, Atta MG: Catheter-directed thrombectomy and thrombolysis for acute renal vein thrombosis. J Vasc Interv Radiol 2006;17:815–822.

184. Rostoker G, Durand-Zaleski I, Petit-Phar M, et al: Prevention of thrombotic complications of the nephrotic syndrome by the low-molecular-weight heparin enoxaparin. Nephron 1995;69:20–28.

185. Sarasin FP, Schifferli JA: Prophylactic oral anticoagulation in nephrotic patients with idiopathic membranous nephropathy. Kidney Int 1994;45:578–585.

186. Bellomo R, Atkins RC: Membranous nephropathy and thromboembolism: Is prophylactic anticoagulation warranted? Nephron 1993;63:249–254.

187. Ogi M, Yokoyama H, Tomosugi N, et al: Risk factors for infection and immunoglobulin replacement therapy in adult nephrotic syndrome. Am J Kidney Dis 1994;24:427–436.

188. Garin EH, Sausville PJ, Richard GA: Impaired primary antibody response in experimental nephrotic syndrome. Clin Exp Immunol 1983;52:595–598.

189. Spika JS, Halsey NA, Le CT, et al: Decline of vaccine-induced antipneumococcal antibody in children with nephrotic syndrome. Am J Kidney Dis 1986;7:466–470.

190. Guven AG, Akman S, Bahat E, et al: Rapid decline of antipneumococcal antibody levels in nephrotic children. Pediatr Nephrol 2004;19:61–65.

Further Reading

Crew RJ, Radhakrishnan J, Appel G: Complications of the nephrotic syndrome and their treatment. Clin Nephrol 2004;62:245–259.

D'Amico G: Statins and renal diseases: From primary prevention to renal replacement therapy. J Am Soc Nephrol 2006;17:S148–S152.

Jennings DL, Kalus JS, Coleman CI, : Combination therapy with ACE inhibitor and an angiotensin receptor blocker for diabetic nephropathy: A meta-analysis. Diabetic Med 2007;24:486–493.

Singhal R, Brimble KS: Thromboembolic complications in the nephrotic syndrome: pathophysiology and clinical management. Thrombosis Res 2006;118:397–407.

Vaziri ND: Molecular mechanisms of lipid disorders in nephrotic syndrome. Kidney Int 2003;63:1964–1976.

Wilmer WA, Rovin BH, Hebert CJ,: Management of glomerular proteinuria: A commentary. J Am Soc Nephrol 2003;14:3217–3232.

Wolf G, Ritz E: Combination therapy with ACE inhibitors and angiotensin II receptor blockers to halt progression of chronic renal disease: Pathophysiology and indications. Kidney Int 2005;67: 799–812.

Chapter 26

Thrombotic Microangiopathies

Piero Ruggenenti, Marina Noris, and Giuseppe Remuzzi

BACKGROUND

The term thrombotic microangiopathy (TMA) defines a lesion of vessel-wall thickening (mainly arterioles and capillaries), intraluminal platelet thrombosis, and partial or complete obstruction of the vessel lumina. Depending on whether renal or brain lesions prevail, two pathologically indistinguishable, but somehow clinically different, entities have been described: hemolytic uremic syndrome (HUS) and thrombotic thrombocytopenic purpura (TTP). Injury to the endothelial cell is the central and likely inciting factor in the sequence of events leading to TMA. Loss of physiologic thromboresistance, leukocyte adhesion to damaged endothelium, complement consumption, abnormal von Willebrand factor (vWF) release and fragmentation, and

increased vascular shear stress may then sustain and amplify the microangiopathic process. Intrinsic abnormalities of the complement system and of the vWF factor pathway may account for a genetic predisposition to the disease that may play a paramount role in particular in familial and recurrent forms. Due to their poor outcome and response to treatment, these congenital (genetic) forms are considered separately from acquired forms, whose outcome is strongly dependent on the possibility to treat or remove the underlying cause. The pathogenesis of acquired forms is only briefly reviewed to provide the background to different specific treatments. Mechanisms of genetic forms are discussed in more detail because they have been clarified only recently and will certainly have major relevance in identifying specific treatment modalities in the next few years. Forms

Table 26-1   Classification of Thrombotic Microangiopathies

Forms	Clinical Features
Acquired	
Shigatoxin associated	HUS
Neuraminidase associated	HUS
Immune-mediated ADAMTS-13 defective activity associated	TTP (often recurrent)
Immune-mediated CFH defective activity associated	HUS (recurrent)
Pregnancy associated	HUS, TTP, HELLP syndrome
Systemic disease associated	HUS, TTP
Drug associated	HUS, TTP
Bone marrow and solid organ transplantation associated	HUS (de novo or recurrent)
Genetic	
CFH, CFI, MCP abnormalities associated	HUS (often recurrent and familial)
ADAMTS-13 deficiency associated	HUS, TTP (often recurrent and familial)
Abnormal cobalamin metabolism associated	HUS
Others	HUS, TTP (often recurrent and familial)
Idiopathic	HUS, TTP

CFH, complement factor H; CFI, complement factor I; HELLP, hemolysis, elevated liver enzymes, and low platelet count; HUS, hemolytic uremic syndrome; MCP, membrane cofactor protein; TTP, thrombotic thrombocytopenic purpura.

without a recognized genetic predisposition or precipitating agent are referred to as idiopathic forms and discussed separately from acquired and genetic forms (Table 26-1).

ACQUIRED

These are by far the most common forms of TMA. Toxins, autoantibodies, pregnancy, systemic diseases, and drugs have been associated with TMAs that may present with the clinical features of both HUS and TTP. In most of these cases, early recognition and removal or treatment of the underlying condition is therefore of paramount importance to achieve remission.

Shiga Toxin–Associated Thrombotic Microangiopathy

Shiga toxin (Stx)–associated HUS (Stx-HUS), the most frequent form of TMA, may follow infection by certain strains of *Escherichia coli* or *Shigella dysenteriae*, which produce a powerful exotoxin (Stx).[1] The term *Shiga toxin* was initially used to describe the exotoxin produced by *S. dysenteriae* type 1. Then, some strains of *E. coli* (mostly the serotype O157:H7) isolated from human cases with diarrhea were found to produce a toxin similar to the one of *S. dysenteriae*. This toxin was subsequently given different names such as Shiga-like toxin for its similarities with Stx or verotoxin for its cytopathic effect on Vero cells (i.e., African green monkey kidney cells). The terms Shiga-like toxin and verotoxin should now be abandoned and only the term Stx should be used to encompass the exotoxins produced both by *S. dysenteriae* and *E. coli*. After food contaminated by Stx-producing *E. coli* or

S. dysenteriae is ingested, the toxin is released in the gut and may cause watery or most often bloody diarrhea because of a direct effect on the intestinal mucosae. When Stx, via the intestinal mucosae, reaches the systemic circulation, full-blown HUS may develop. Stx-HUS is usually considered a disease with a good outcome, with complete recovery in approximately 90% of cases. However, a recent meta-analysis of 49 studies including 3476 patients showed that 12% of patients die during the acute phase of the disease or remain dialysis dependent, 16% have residual kidney insufficiency with glomerular filtration rate values ranging from 5 to 80 mL/min/1.73 m^2, 15% are proteinuric, and 10% are hypertensive.[2] Age younger than 2 years, severe gastrointestinal prodromes, elevated white blood cell count, and anuria early in the course of the disease are predictors of the severity of HUS. Anuria for more than 10 days or the need for dialysis in the acute phase, as well as proteinuria at 12-month follow-up have been associated with an increased risk of chronic renal failure in the long term. Patched cortical necrosis or involvement of more than 50% glomeruli are further predictors of poor outcome.

Diagnosis rests on detection of *E. coli* O157:H7 in stool cultures. Serologic tests for antibodies to Stx and O157 lipopolysaccharide can be done in research laboratories, and tests are being developed for rapid detection of *E. coli* O157:H7 and Stx in stools.

Undercooked ground beef is the most common source of infection, but ham, turkey, cheese, unpasteurized milk, juice, water, and fresh vegetables irrigated with contaminated water have also been implicated. Secondary person-to-person contact is an important way to spread infection in institutions, particularly day-care centers and nursing homes. Infected patients should be excluded from day-care centers until two consecutive stool cultures are negative for *E. coli* O157:H7 to prevent further transmission. However, the most important preventive measure in child-care centers is supervised hand washing.

Supportive Therapy

In children, the mortality rate from typical Stx-HUS has significantly decreased over the past 40 years, probably as the result of better supportive management of anemia, renal failure, hypertension, and electrolyte and water imbalance. Intravenous isotonic volume expansion as soon as an *E. coli* O157:H7 infection is suspected, that is, within the first 4 days of illness, even before culture results are available, may limit the severity of kidney dysfunction and the need for renal replacement therapy.[3] Bowel rest is important for the hemorrhagic colitis associated with Stx-HUS. Antimotility agents should be avoided because they may prolong the persistence of *E. coli* in the intestinal lumen and therefore increase patient exposure to Stx. The use of antibiotics should be restricted to the very limited number of patients presenting with bacteremia[4] because in children with *E. coli* enteritis, they may increase the risk of HUS by 17-fold.[5] A possible explanation is that antibiotic-induced injury to the bacterial membrane might favor the acute release of large amounts of preformed toxin. Alternatively, antibiotic therapy might give *E. coli* O157:H7 a selective advantage if these organisms are not as readily eliminated from the bowel as are the normal intestinal flora. Moreover, several antimicrobial drugs, particularly the quinolones, trimethoprim, and furazolidone, are potent inducers of the expression of the Stx 2 gene and may increase the level of toxin in the intestine. Although the possibility of a cause-and-effect relationship between antibiotic therapy and increased risk of HUS has been challenged by a recent meta-analysis of 26 reports,[6] there is no reason to prescribe antibiotics because they do not improve the outcome of colitis, and bacteremia is rare in Stx-HUS. However, these considerations do not necessarily apply to many cases of bloody diarrhea, in particular in South America and India, that are precipitated by *E. coli* strains different from O157:H7 or by other bacteria, such as *Shigella* dysentery type 1. For instance, when hemorrhagic colitis is caused by *Shigella* dysentery type 1, early and empirical antibiotic treatment shortens the duration of diarrhea and decreases the incidence of complications and the risk of transmission by shortening the duration of bacterial shedding. Thus, in developing countries where *Shigella* is the most frequent cause of hemorrhagic colitis, antibiotic therapy should be started early and even before the involved pathogen is identified.

Careful blood pressure control and renin-angiotensin system blockade may be particularly beneficial long-term treatment for those patients who suffer chronic renal disease after an episode of Stx-HUS. A study in 45 children with renal sequelae of HUS followed for 9 to 11 years documented that early restriction of proteins and use of angiotensin-converting enzyme inhibitors may have a beneficial effect on long-term renal outcome, as documented by a positive slope of 1/Cr values over time in treated patients.[7] In another study, treatment with angiotensin-converting enzyme inhibitors for 8 to 15 years after severe Stx-HUS normalized blood pressure, reduced proteinuria, and improved the glomerular filtration rate.[8]

Shiga Toxin Binding

An oral Stx binding agent composed of repeated synthetic carbohydrate determinants that mimic the Stx receptor linked to colloidal silica (Synsorb Pk) has been developed with the rationale of inhibiting intestinal absorption of the toxin. However, after preliminary studies showing that the drug is well tolerated and effectively binds the toxin, a prospective, randomized, double-blind, placebo-controlled clinical trial of 145 children with diarrhea-associated HUS failed to demonstrate any beneficial effect of treatment on disease outcome.[9] This may have been because the drug is only effective in the gut and in most cases, Synsorb was administered only after the onset of HUS and target organs had been already exposed to Stx. Alternatively, impaired gastrointestinal motility may have limited delivery of the drug to the distal intestine were *E. coli* localize, or the affinity of Synsorb may be too low to compete with endogenous receptors. Whatever the explanation, this study suggests that strategies aimed at interfering with gastrointestinal absorption of Stx may have limited ability to prevent or limit HUS in children with gastrointestinal O157:H7 infection unless given before the onset of HUS to all those affected by an outbreak of diarrhea.

Plasma Manipulation and Other Specific Treatments

No specific therapy aimed at preventing or limiting the microangiopathic process has been proved to affect the course of Stx-HUS in children. Two prospective, controlled trials found that plasma therapy may limit short-term renal lesions, but does not affect long-term renal outcome and patient survival[10,11] (Table 26-2). Heparin and antithrombotic agents may increase the risk of bleeding and should be avoided. Whether tissue type plasminogen activator, discriminating between fibrin and fibrin-bound plasminogen, gives a better risk-benefit profile in the treatment of HUS is worth investigating.

The efficacy of specific treatments in adult patients is difficult to evaluate because most information is derived from uncontrolled series that may also include non–Stx-HUS cases (see Table 26-2). In particular, no prospective, randomized trials are available to definitely establish whether plasma infusion or exchange may offer some specific benefit compared with supportive treatment alone. However, comparative analyses of two large series of patients treated[12] or not treated[13] with plasma suggest that plasma therapy may dramatically decrease overall mortality of Stx *E. coli* O157:H7–associated HUS. These findings lead us and others to consider plasma infusion or exchange suitable for adult patients, in particular, in those with severe renal insufficiency and central nervous system involvement.

Rescue Treatments

Bilateral Nephrectomy

In occasional patients, increased shear stress and platelet activation in the damaged renal microvasculature may sustain the microangiopathic process even after the precipitating factor has been exhausted.[1] In these rare cases, persistent thrombocytopenia associated with severe refractory hypertension and signs of hypertensive encephalopathy may put the patient in imminent danger of death. In such dramatic cases, bilateral nephrectomy was followed within 2 weeks by complete hematologic and clinical remission.[14]

The rationale of the procedure rests on evidence that removing the kidneys eliminates a major site of vWF fragmentation, which would limit platelet activation and protect patients from the further spreading of microvascular lesions.[14] However, bilateral nephrectomy is irreversible and should be

Table 26-2 Controlled Studies of Specific Treatments of Different Forms of Thrombotic Microangiopathy

Ref.	Design	Clinical Features	No. of Patients	TREATMENT		Outcome
				Case	Controls	
Child Series						
Loirat et al[78]	Prospective, randomized, multicenter	HUS	33	Heparin, urokinase	Supportive	Comparable survival, clinical outcomes, and histologic changes in cases and controls
Van Damme-Lombaerts et al[79]	Prospective, randomized, monocenter	HUS	58	Heparin, dipyridamole	Supportive	Comparable survival, clinical outcomes, and histologic changes in cases and controls
Loirat et al[80]	Prospective, randomized, monocenter	HUS	79	FFP (10 mL/kg/day)	Supportive	Lower serum creatinine at 6 mo (63 ± 21 vs. 48 ± 13 μmol/L, $P < .005$) and fewer cases of cortical necrosis (0 vs. 7, $P < .02$) in cases than in controls
Rizzoni et al[10]	Prospective, randomized, multicenter	HUS	32	FFP (10–30 mL/kg/day)	Supportive	Comparable survival, clinical outcomes, and histologic changes in cases and controls
Gianviti et al[81]	Retrospective, multicenter	HUS (with ARF)	33	PE (3–10 exch.)	Supportive	Less residual renal insufficiency (glomerular filtration rate < 80 mL/min) in cases than in controls (18% vs. 43%)
Adult Series						
Italian group[82]	Retrospective, multicenter	TTP	29	PE (3–15 exch.)	Steroids, antiplatelets	Less mortality (18% vs. 43%) and more remissions (86% vs. 57%) in cases than in controls
French group[83]	Retrospective, multicenter	HUS	53	PE (2–21 exch.)	Supportive	Less mortality (0% vs. 23%) and less end-stage renal disease (26% vs. 64%) in cases than in controls
Henon[84]	Prospective, randomized, multicenter	TTP (with ARF)	40	PE (3–35 exch.)	FFP, ASA, dipyridamole	Less mortality (15% vs. 43%) and more remissions (80% vs. 52%) in cases than in controls
Rock et al[29]	Prospective, randomized, multicenter	TTP	102	PE (3–36)	FFP, ASA, dipyridamole	Less mortality (22% vs. 37%) and more remissions (78% vs. 49%) in cases than in controls

ARF, acute renal failure; ASA, acetylsalicylic acid; exch., replacement of one plasma volume; FFP, fresh frozen plasma; HUS, hemolytic uremic syndrome; PE, plasma exchange; TTP, thrombotic thrombocytopenic purpura.

considered only for patients in whom all other approaches have failed. Potential candidates are patients who are plasma resistant (defined as > 20 procedures with no improvement of clinical and laboratory findings) or plasma dependent (patients who have to be continuously infused with plasma to remain in remission and in whom the platelet count invariably drops, with signs of hemolysis, within a few days after plasma is discontinued).

Nephrectomy should not be considered unless a renal biopsy specimen, obtained as soon as the platelet count increases, even transiently, with plasma to a level where the procedure is safe, shows chronic diffuse lesions associated with signs of the disease, meaning arteriolar thrombosis and myointimal proliferation. Finally, nephrectomy should be considered only in the presence of life-threatening signs such as major neurological dysfunction or coma or uncontrolled bleeding as a consequence of refractory thrombocytopenia.

Kidney Transplantation

Kidney transplantation should be considered as an effective and safe treatment for those children who progress to end-stage renal disease (ESRD). Indeed, the outcome of renal transplantation is good in children with Stx-HUS, recurrence rates range from 0% to 10%,[15,16] and graft survival at 10 years is even better than in control children with other diseases.[17]

Neuraminidase-Associated Thrombotic Microangiopathy

This is a rare but potentially fatal disease that may complicate pneumonia or, less frequently, meningitis caused by *Streptococcus pneumoniae*. Neuraminidase produced by *S. pneumoniae*, by removing sialic acid from the cell membranes, exposes Thomsen-Friedenreich antigen to preformed circulating IgM antibodies.[18] Then, binding of circulating preformed IgM antibodies to this cryptic antigen exposed on platelet and endothelial cell surface would cause platelet aggregation and endothelial damage. Binding of IgM antibodies to the antigen expressed on circulating erythrocytes may also explain why Coombs-positive hemolytic anemia is so frequently reported in patients with neuraminidase-induced HUS. The clinical picture is usually severe, with respiratory distress, neurological involvement, and coma.

Therapy

The outcome is greatly dependent on the effectiveness of antibiotic therapy. In theory, plasma, either infused or exchanged, is contraindicated because adult plasma contains antibodies against the Thomsen-Friedenreich antigen that may accelerate polyagglutination and hemolysis.[18] Thus, patients should be treated only with antibiotics and washed red cells. In some cases, however, plasma therapy, occasionally in combination with steroids, has been associated with recovery.

Thrombotic Microangiopathy Associated with Immune-Mediated Defective Activity of Complement Regulatory Proteins

Recurrent, atypical HUS has been recently reported[19] in three children with circulating IgG autoantibodies against complement factor H (CFH), a circulating glycoprotein that modu-

lates the activity of the alternative complement pathway (see "Thrombotic Microangiopathy Associated with Congenital Defects" and Chapter 30) (Fig. 26-1). Anti-CFH antibodies were captured by enzyme-linked immunosorbent assay using purified human factor H–coated plates. Subsequent studies in five unrelated patients found that the binding epitopes for CFH autoantibodies localize in the cell-binding C terminus of CFH.[20]

Of interest, the children showed an increased titer of circulating antinuclear antibodies, a finding that supports the possibility of an autoimmune pathogenesis of the disease. One child had two recurrences with pancreas and liver involvement, progressed to ESRD, and eventually required a bilateral nephrectomy to control refractory hypertension. The other two children recovered from the first episode with plasma exchange, then had four and three relapses, respectively, and recovered again with plasma exchange. These two children were maintained on long-term therapy with a steroid and azathioprine, respectively.

Treatment

Available information is insufficient to provide clear guidelines for treatment of this rare form of HUS. Conceivably, however, when anti-CFH autoantibodies are detected, plasma exchange and steroids or other immunosuppressive agents should be considered with the rationale of removing the pathogenic antibody from the circulation as soon as possible and inhibiting its synthesis.

Thrombotic Microangiopathy Associated with Immune-Mediated Deficiency of von Willebrand's Factor–Cleaving Protease (ADAMTS-13) Activity

This is an immune-mediated, nonfamilial form of TMA that most likely accounts for the majority of cases so far reported as acute idiopathic or sporadic TTP. The disease is characterized by a severe deficiency of a plasma metalloprotease, ADAMTS-13, that in normal individuals cleaves ultralarge vWF multimers as soon as they are secreted[21] and in TTP patients is inhibited by a specific autoantibody that develops transiently and tends to disappear during remission.[22–25] These inhibitory anti-ADAMTS-13 antibodies, characterized either as IgG or IgM and IgA, have been detected in 50% to 90% of patients with acquired TTP.[25,26] Recent studies found inhibitory antiprotease antibodies reacting against the cysteine-rich and spacer domains of recombinant ADAMTS-13 in all considered patients with acquired TTP.[25] In some cases, the antibodies were directed only against these epitopes, but in the majority of plasma samples from TTP patients, different combinations of antibodies against the propeptide, the Tsp-1, and the CUB domains[25] were found, suggesting a polyclonal autoantibody response.

Further evidence of the pathogenetic role of these autoantibodies is derived from finding that they usually disappear from the circulation when remission is achieved with effective treatment, and this occurs in parallel with the normalization of ADAMTS-13 activity. Although TTP associated with ADAMTS-13 inhibitors is usually sporadic, recurrent episodes have also been reported due to the reappearance of the inhibitor in the circulation several weeks or even months after the resolution of the presenting episode. Of note, autoantibodies

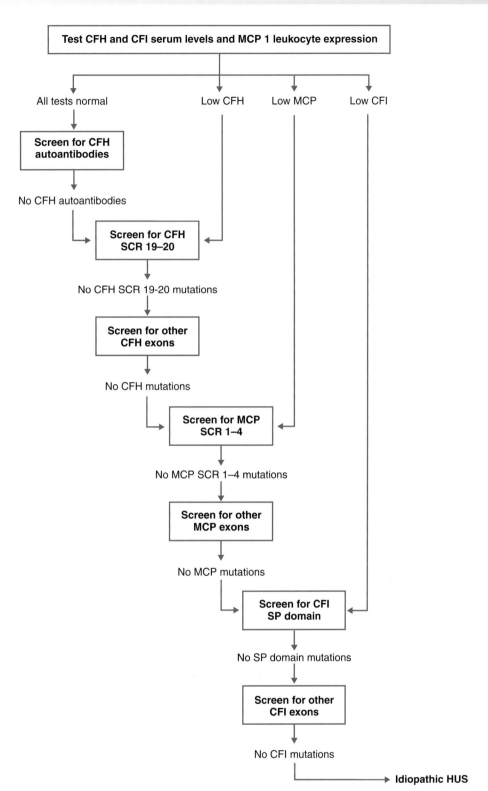

Figure 26-1   Flow diagram of the steps suggested to optimize the cost-effectiveness of screening for genetic defects in patients with hemolytic uremic syndrome not associated with Shiga toxin and suspected, genetically determined abnormalities in complement regulatory proteins. A preliminary screen for serum complement factor H (CFH) and complement factor I (CFI) levels by either enzyme-linked immunosorbent assay or RID, and for membrane cofactor protein (MCP) expression in peripheral blood leukocytes by fluorescence-activated cell sorter is recommended to identify which is the candidate gene to evaluate. If no abnormalities are detected, we suggest screening for anti-CFH autoantibodies and then if no autoantibodies are detected, looking for mutations of candidate genes, starting to evaluate the *CFH* gene, which is more frequently affected by pathogenic mutations, followed by *MCP* and *CFI* genes, respectively. Within each gene, the exons where the mutations tend to localize more frequently should be studied first. HUS, hemolytic uremic syndrome; RID, radial immunodiffusion; SCR, short consensus repeat; SP, serine protease.

against the ADAMTS-13 have also been observed in patients developing TTP during treatment with antiplatelet drugs such as ticlopidine (see "Drug-Associated Thrombotic Microangiopathy").

The clinical picture is usually severe, with an abrupt onset of neurological signs, purpura, and fever.[27] Neurological symptoms usually dominate the clinical picture and may be fleeting and fluctuating, probably because of continuous thrombus formation and dispersion in the brain microcirculation. Coma and seizures complicate more severe forms.

Supportive Therapy, Plasma Manipulation, and Other Specific Treatments

In the early 1960s, TTP was almost invariably fatal, but now, thanks to earlier diagnosis, improved intensive care facilities, and new techniques such as plasma therapy, survival may reach 90%.[28,29]

Plasma manipulation is a cornerstone of the therapy of the acute episode. Plasma may serve to induce remission of the disease by replacing defective protease activity. In theory, compared with infusion, exchange may offer the advantage of also rapidly removing anti–ADAMTS-13 antibodies. This, however, needs to be proved in controlled trials. In addition, corticosteroids might inhibit the synthesis of antiprotease autoantibodies. In a series of 33 patients with anti–ADAMTS-13 antibodies and undetectable ADAMTS-13 activity, combined treatment with plasma exchange and steroids was associated with disease remission in approximately 90% of cases.[26] The rationale of combined treatment is that plasma exchange will have only a temporary effect on the presumed autoimmune basis of the disease and additional immunosuppressive treatment may cause a more lasting response. Thirty of 108 patients with either TTP or HUS were reported to have recovered after treatment with corticosteroids alone. All of them, however, had mild forms, and none of them were tested for ADAMTS-13 activity.

Rescue Treatments

Plasma Cryosupernatant

Cryosupernatant fraction (i.e., plasma from which a cryoprecipitate containing the largest plasma vWF multimers, fibrinogen, and fibronectin has been removed) instead of fresh frozen plasma has been successful in treating a small number of patients who did not respond to repeated exchanges or infusions with fresh frozen plasma.[30] The rationale for this approach is that plasma cryosupernatant may provide the same beneficial factor(s) found in whole plasma (for instance, in this specific case, the defective/inhibited ADAMTS-13 activity), but does not contain those factors (including large vWF multimers) that may actually sustain the microangiopathic process until remission is achieved. Based on this, the use of plasma cryosupernatant has been suggested as first-line therapy. Results of preliminary uncontrolled studies seem encouraging.[31]

Rituximab

Recently, the infusion of rituximab, an antibody directed against B cells, has been proven to be effective in inducing remission in TTP patients with ADAMTS-13 antibodies refractory to any other treatment[25] and in maintaining patients in remission when used as prophylactic therapy. Longitudinal evaluation of ADAMTS-13 activity and autoantibody levels may help monitor patient response to treatment.

Splenectomy

Before the discovery of the efficacy of plasma exchange for the treatment of TTP, splenectomy was quite frequently performed, but most patients still died. More recent studies in patients refractory to plasma therapy cast further doubt on the efficacy of splenectomy because of high morbidity and mortality.[28,32] However, the patients in these studies were unselected, and splenectomy might be expected to achieve persistent remission by removing a major site of antibody synthesis in those with autoantibodies against ADAMTS-13 that persist in the circulation despite plasma and immunosuppressive therapy. This appears to have been the case in two reports in which patients with autoimmune TTP who had failed to respond to plasma exchange and immunosuppression or had repeated relapses entered a stable remission with disappearance of the ADAMTS-13 protease inhibitor.[22,33] These reports, however, are far from conclusive, and further studies with a larger number of patients are needed to assess the therapeutic value of this invasive procedure.

Platelet Transfusions

The severe thrombocytopenia in TTP has led many physicians to administer platelet transfusions with the aim of preventing severe bleeding complications. However, reports of sudden death, decreased survival, and delayed recovery after platelet transfusion dramatically document the danger of giving platelets to patients with active TTP. Thus, platelet transfusions are contraindicated in acute TTP, except in cases of life-threatening bleeding.

Pregnancy-Associated Thrombotic Microangiopathies

TMA associated with pregnancy includes TTP (usually in the early phases of pregnancy), HELLP syndrome (hemolysis, elevated liver enzymes, and low platelet count) (usually near term), and HUS (usually postpartum).[34] The disease is considered a specific complication of pregnancy, but reports of women with familial recurrence or defective ADAMTS-13 activity without a demonstrable inhibitor provide convincing evidence that, at least in a proportion of cases, an underlying genetic predisposition plays a central role in the pathogenesis of TMA and pregnancy may just represent a precipitating event.[35] Changes observed during normal pregnancy, such as progressively decreasing fibrinolytic activity, loss of endothelial thrombomodulin, increasing levels of procoagulant factors, and decreasing ADAMTS-13 activity, may contribute to precipitate the disease in those at risk.

Thrombotic Thrombocytopenic Purpura

TTP develops during the antepartum period in 89% of cases, usually within 24 weeks. Later in the course of pregnancy, clinical features of TTP and preeclampsia may overlap. Despite limited experience, available series show that the maternal mortality rate has decreased from 68% to almost zero with the institution of plasma therapy.[34] Delivery is recommended only for those patients who do not respond to plasma therapy.

Measurement of plasma antithrombin III activity has been suggested as a useful tool to differentiate TTP and preeclampsia. Before gestational week 28 and when antithrombin III plasma activity is normal, TTP is most likely. Plasma therapy could be tried, and, if effective, it should be continued until term and/or complete remission of the disease. Delivery can be considered as rescue after failure of plasma therapy. The role of other treatments often employed in idiopathic TTP remains elusive.

After week 34 of gestation, preeclampsia is most likely and is usually associated with decreased plasma antithrombin III activity. Delivery is the treatment of choice and is usually followed by complete recovery within 24 to 48 hours. Persistent disease may be an indication to attempt a course of plasma therapy. Between 28 and 34 weeks, the optimal treatment is controversial. It is some times held that delivery should always be considered as first-line therapy, whereas others believe that if there is no evidence of fetal distress and plasma antithrombin III activity is normal, a course of plasma therapy can be reasonably attempted before inducing delivery.[36]

HELLP Syndrome

HELLP syndrome is simply a form of severe preeclampsia in which, in addition to hypertension and renal dysfunction, there is evidence of microangiopathic hemolysis and liver involvement. The syndrome is most common in white multiparous women with a history of poor pregnancy outcome. It arises in the antepartum period in 70% of cases. Symptoms usually arise within 24 to 48 hours postpartum, occasionally after an uncomplicated pregnancy.[34]

Diagnosis is based on (1) hemolysis (defined as fragmented erythrocytes in the circulation and lactic dehydrogenase of at least 600 U/L), (2) elevated liver enzymes (serum glutamic oxaloacetic transaminase > 70 U/L), and (3) low platelet count (<100 × 10³/mm³).[33] Overt disseminated intravascular coagulation is reported in 25% of cases. Intrahepatic hemorrhage, subcapsular liver hematoma, and liver rupture are rare life-threatening complications. The maternal and perinatal mortality rates range from 0% to 24% and from 7.7% to 60%, respectively. Most of the perinatal deaths are related to abruptio placentae, intrauterine asphyxia, and extreme prematurity. As many as 44% of the infants are growth retarded.

Termination of pregnancy is the only definitive therapy. Hydralazine or dihydralazine is the first-choice drug to control pregnancy-induced hypertension, and magnesium sulfate prevents and treats convulsions. Both peritoneal dialysis and hemodialysis have been used to treat acute renal failure. Platelet transfusions are needed for clinical bleeding or severe thrombocytopenia (platelet count < 20,000/μL).

In approximately 5% of patients with HELLP syndrome, symptoms and laboratory abnormalities do not improve after delivery. These are cases with central nervous system abnormalities associated with renal and cardiopulmonary dysfunction and activation of coagulation. Uncontrolled studies suggest that plasma exchange may help recovery in patients with persistent evidence of disease 72 hours or more after delivery. However, plasma therapy is ineffective during pregnancy and may increase fetal and maternal risk when used to delay delivery. Preliminary evidence suggests that, postpartum, corticosteroids may speed up disease recovery and, antepartum, may postpone delivery of previable fetuses and reduce the mother's need for blood products.

Postpartum Hemolytic Uremic Syndrome

By definition, postpartum HUS follows a normal delivery by no more than 6 months.[1] The clinical course is usually fulminant. Supportive care including dialysis, transfusions,

and careful fluid management remains the most important form of treatment. Whether plasma therapy improves survival or limits renal sequelae has not been established so far. Antiplatelet agents, heparin, and antithrombotic therapy may enhance the risk of bleeding and have no proven efficacy.

Systemic Disease–Associated Thrombotic Microangiopathy

Prevention and treatment of TMA associated with systemic diseases largely rest on specific treatment of the underlying conditions.

Antiphospholipid Syndrome, Systemic Lupus Erythematosus, Scleroderma, and Malignant Hypertension

Plasma therapy should always be attempted in TMA associated with systemic diseases even if its efficacy in this setting is poorly defined. Regarding antiphospholipid syndrome, until the relationships between the various antiphospholipid antibodies identified so far and clinical manifestations of the disease are clarified, oral anticoagulation remains the only treatment of proven efficacy, even if concomitant thrombocytopenia may increase the risk of hemorrhagic complications, to prevent and treat micro- and macrovascular thromboses. Blood pressure control is the keystone of treatment of TMA associated with scleroderma crisis and malignant hypertension.

Human Immunodeficiency Virus

Both HUS and TTP are among the complications of acquired immunodeficiency syndrome (AIDS), which may account for as many as 30% of hospitalized HUS/TTP patients. Plasma manipulation appears to be the only feasible approach. Uncontrolled series provide evidence that the survival rate in patients with human immunodeficiency virus without AIDS is comparable with that of those with idiopathic TTP. By contrast, patients with AIDS associated with TTP almost invariably have a poor outcome and do not appear to benefit from plasma therapy.[36]

Cancer

TMA complicates almost 6% of cases of metastatic carcinoma. The prognosis is extremely poor and most patients die within a few weeks. Therapy is minimally effective. Administration of blood products to correct symptomatic anemia often results in exacerbation of the syndrome, with rapid worsening of hemolysis, deterioration of renal function, and pulmonary edema.

Drug-Associated Thrombotic Microangiopathy

Mitomycin and Anticancer Drugs

A form of TMA resembling HUS has been described in cancer patients treated with mitomycin C. Disease manifestation is dose related, and renal dysfunction is reported in less than 2% of patients given a cumulative dose lower than 50 mg/m² and in more than 28% of those given more than 50 mg/m² or receiving more than one course of therapy.

Platinum- and bleomycin-containing combinations have also been reported to induce HUS. The fatality rate is close to 79%, and the median time to death is approximately 4 weeks. Patients surviving the acute phase often remain on long-term dialysis or die later of a recurrence of the tumor or metastases. The possibility of preventing the syndrome by giving steroids during mitomycin treatment has been suggested and needs to be confirmed in prospective, controlled trials. Plasma exchange is usually attempted, but its effectiveness is unproven. Regimens that contain platinum and bleomycin have also been reported to induce HUS.

Antiplatelet Drugs

TMA has been reported in 1 of every 1600 to 5000 patients treated with ticlopidine. Neurological abnormalities occur within 1 month of treatment in 80% of cases. The overall survival rate is 67% and is improved by early treatment withdrawal and plasma therapy. Generation of an autoantibody against ADAMTS-13 protease may be involved in the pathogenesis of ticlopidine-associated TTP. In seven patients who developed TTP 2 to 7 weeks after initiation of ticlopidine therapy, severely decreased levels of ADAMTS-13 activity were reported along with the appearance of IgG molecules in their blood, which inhibited ADAMTS-13 activity.[37] The deficiency resolved after ticlopidine therapy was discontinued and plasmapheresis was instituted. Eleven cases have been reported during treatment with clopidogrel, a new antiaggregating agent that has achieved widespread clinical use for its safety profile. All patients had neurological involvement and were treated with plasma exchange: eight fully recovered, two had relapses that rapidly recovered after retreatment with plasma exchange, and one died. Half the patients were concomitantly treated with cholesterol-lowering drugs. Conceivably, these drugs should be avoided in clopidogrel-treated patients.

Quinine

Quinine is one of the drugs more frequently associated with TMA. The disease typically occurs in patients presensitized by previous exposure to quinine and rapidly follows reingestion of the drug. Quinine is generally used to treat muscle cramps, but it is also contained in beverages (tonic water and bitter lemon drinks). Quinine-dependent antiplatelet, antierythrocyte, and antigranulocyte antibodies have been involved in the pathogenesis of the disease. Presenting symptoms are often severe, and death or irreversible kidney failure are common outcomes unless quinine is immediately withdrawn and plasma exchange is promptly provided. Avoidance of successive quinine use is necessary to prevent recurrences.

Interferon Alfa

Renal impairment is the predominant feature of TMA associated with interferon alfa. Recovery of the TMA has been reported to follow early discontinuation of the drug and prompt supportive therapy[38]; however, the prognosis for renal recovery is poor, resulting in ESRD in approximately half of the cases. Because of the few cases reported, it is not possible to evaluate the effectiveness of specific therapies such as plasma exchange or infusion.

Bone Marrow and Solid Organ Transplantation–Associated Thrombotic Microangiopathy

Among acquired forms of HUS, post-transplantation HUS is being reported with continuously increasing frequency and appears to affect a progressively increasing number of patients worldwide. Albeit poorly defined, the incidence of the disease is remarkably higher in the transplant recipient than in the general population, most likely because of the clustering of several risk factors in this particular setting of patients. In renal transplants, HUS may ensue for the first time in patients who never had the disease (de novo post-transplantation HUS) or may affect patients whose primary cause of ESRD was HUS (recurrent post-transplantation HUS). Treatment of post-transplantation HUS rests on removal of the inciting factor(s), relief of symptoms, and plasma infusion or exchange. No other approach has proven effective.

De Novo Posttransplantation Hemolytic Uremic Syndrome

This form occurs in renal and extrarenal transplant recipients and is usually triggered by immunosuppressive drugs such as calcineurin inhibitors,[29] less frequently by virus infections, and, specifically in renal transplant recipients by acute vascular rejection. A peculiar form of de novo post-transplantation HUS may affect the recipients of a bone marrow transplant, usually in the setting of a graft–versus-host disease or of intensive graft-versus-host disease prophylaxis, including total body irradiation.

Therapy

Drug withdrawal or dose reduction is the first-line therapy for de novo cyclosporin A– or tacrolimus-associated forms, but is effective in less than 50% of cases.[39] A remarkably higher success rate (84%) has been reported with adjunctive plasma infusion or exchange. A similar response rate, but in much smaller series, has been reported with intravenous IgG infusion given with the rationale to neutralize hypothetical circulating cytotoxic or platelet agglutinating factors. Once remission is achieved, patient rechallenge with decreased doses of cyclosporin A or tacrolimus, with switching from one drug to the other one, or, finally, with replacement of both drugs with mycophenolate mofetil has been anecdotally reported to maintain adequate immunosuppression without further disease recurrences. Very recently, compassionate treatment with rapamycin has been associated with a remarkably good outcome in 15 patients with cyclosporin A– or tacrolimus-associated posttransplantation HUS, with no patient requiring rapamycin withdrawal because of disease recurrence.[40] Monoclonal anti–interleukin-2 receptor antagonists may also be a valid option to maintain adequate immunosuppression, avoiding the toxic effects of calcineurin inhibitors. The outcome of de novo forms occurring in the setting of viral infection parallels the response to treatment of the underlying disease. Despite intensive plasma therapy or rescue treatment with plasma cryosupernatant or protein A immune adsorption, the outcome of de novo forms complicating BMT is still dramatically poor, with a mortality rate closed to 90%. In addition to the severity of the microangiopathic process, quantified by serum lactate dehydrogenase levels and the percentage of circulating fragmented erythrocytes, infection, progressive graft-versus-host disease or relapse of the underlying disease may account for such discouraging figures.

Recurrent Posttransplantation Hemolytic Uremic Syndrome

This form is most frequently reported in patients who progressed to ESRD because of non–Stx-HUS, in particular, in those with genetic forms. Whether the precipitating factors associated with the novo HUS may contribute also to disease recurrence on the kidney graft is still a debated question. This is consistent with, albeit not proved by, evidence that a precipitating factor is often observed or suspected in patients with recurrent disease.

Therapy

Recurrent forms usually do not respond to any type of therapy and are associated with a graft loss rate close to 100%. Based on these data, kidney transplantation should be considered as an effective and safe treatment of ESRD only for patients with Stx-HUS, but should be considered with extreme caution in those with non–Stx-HUS, in particular, in genetic forms. In particular, until new strategies to effectively limit or prevent recurrence become available, kidney transplantation is contraindicated in familial/relapsing forms and in all cases with a well-characterized genetic abnormality predisposing to the disease (see later).

GENETIC (THROMBOTIC MICROANGIOPATHY ASSOCIATED WITH CONGENITAL DEFECTS)

These forms are rare, often occur in families, occur mainly but not exclusively in children, and frequently relapse even after complete recovery of the presenting episode. Depending on the involved defect and the age at disease onset, these forms may present with the clinical features of HUS or TTP or both in different members of the same family or in different episodes in the same patient. ESRD, permanent neurological sequelae, or death is the outcome in the majority of cases.[1] Therapy seldom achieves persistent remission of the disease. Genetic counseling is therefore of paramount importance. In cases with recognized genetic mutations, antenatal diagnosis by amniocentesis or chorionic villus biopsy is possible and the carrier state can be identified.

Thrombotic Microangiopathy Associated with Genetic Abnormalities in Complement Regulatory Proteins

In 1998, Warwicker and colleagues[41] studied three families with non–Stx-HUS and established linkage in the affected individuals to the regulator of complement activation gene cluster on human chromosome 1q32, which encodes for several complement regulatory proteins. The first examined candidate gene in this region was factor H (*CFH*), due to the fact that an association between familial HUS and CFH abnormalities had been reported previously.

Since the first report by Warwicker and colleagues, more than 100 different *CFH* mutations in patients with non–Stx-HUS[42] have been described. In sporadic forms, the mutation was either inherited from a clinically unaffected parent or, more rarely—only four cases reported—arose de novo in the proband.[43] The mutation frequency is approximately 30%.[44,45]

CFH is a plasma glycoprotein that plays an important role in the regulation of the alternative pathway of complement. It serves as a cofactor for the C3b-cleaving enzyme complement factor I (CFI) in the degradation of newly formed C3b molecules and controls decay, formation, and stability of the C3b convertase C3bBb. CFH consists of 20 homologous short consensus repeats (SCRs). The complement regulatory domains needed to prevent fluid-phase alternative pathway amplification have been localized within the N-terminal SCR1-4.[46] The inactivation of surface-bound C3b is dependent on the binding of the C-terminal domain of CFH to polyanionic molecules, which increases CFH affinity for C3b and exposes its complement regulatory N-terminal domain.[47]

The vast majority of CFH mutations in HUS patients are heterozygous and cause either single amino acid changes or premature translation interruptions, mainly clustering in the C-terminal domains, and are commonly associated with normal CFH plasma levels. Expression and functional studies demonstrated that CFH proteins carrying HUS-associated mutations have a severely reduced capability to interact with polyanions and with surface-bound C3b[47], which results in a lower density of mutant CFH molecules bound to endothelial cell surfaces and a diminished complement regulatory activity on their cell membranes.[47] In contrast, these mutants have a normal capacity to control activation of the complement in plasma, as indicated by data showing that they retain a normal cofactor activity in the proteolysis of fluid-phase C3b.

In a recent study,[48] a heterozygous hybrid gene derived from a crossing over between intron 21 of CFH and intron 4 of CFHR1 (CFH-related 1) was found in five patients. The hybrid gene consists of the first 21 exons of CFH (encoding SCRs 1–18 of CFH) and the last two exons of CFHR1 (encoding SCRs 4 and 5 of CFHR1). The protein product of the hybrid gene is identical to the CFH mutant S1191L/V1197A, which arises by gene conversion and lacks surface complement regulatory activity. The frequency of this abnormality in non–Stx-HUS patients is estimated to be approximately 6%.

Abnormalities in two additional genes encoding for complement regulatory proteins have been recently involved in predisposition to non–Stx-HUS. Two reports from independent groups described mutations in MCP (encoding membrane cofactor protein) in affected individuals of four families.[49,50] MCP is a widely expressed transmembrane glycoprotein that serves as a cofactor for CFI to cleave C3b and C4b deposited on the host cell surface.[51] To date, approximately 40 MCP mutations in non–Stx-HUS have been reported, with a mutation frequency of 10% to 15%.[45] Evaluation of mutant protein expression and function showed either severely decreased protein expression on the cell surface, decreased C3b binding capability, and/or capacity to prevent complement activation.[45]

Twenty-four mutations in CFI, encoding a plasma serine protease that cleaves and inactivates C3b and C4b, have been reported in patients with non–Stx-HUS, with a frequency of 5% to 12% in different studies.[45,52,53] All of them are heterozygous mutations, 80% cluster in the serine-protease domain and either cause greatly decreased protein secretion or result in mutant proteins with decreased cofactor activity.

The list of published and unpublished mutations in CFH, MCP, and CFI is continuously updated in the Factor H–HUS database (www.fh-hus.org). The database includes also CFH, MCP, and CFI single nucleotide polymorphisms.

More recently, two gain-of-function mutations in the gene encoding complement factor B (CFB), a zymogen that carries the catalytic site of the complement alternative pathway convertase, have been found in two families from a Spanish HUS cohort.[54]

Although genotype-phenotype correlations are often inexact, analysis of published reports[44,45,55,56] indicates that the course and outcome of non–Stx-HUS are influenced by the gene involved. Non–Stx-HUS associated with CFH mutations most often presents early in childhood, although adult onset is reported in approximately 30% of cases. The clinical course is characterized by a high rate of relapses and 60% to 80% of patients die or develop ESRD after the presenting episode or progress to ESRD as a consequence of relapses. Non–Stx-HUS associated with MCP mutations presents mostly in childhood; the acute episode is in general milder than in CFH mutation carriers, and 80% of patients undergo complete remission. Recurrences are very frequent, but their effect on long-term outcome is rather mild, with approximately 60% to 70% of patients remaining dialysis free even after several recurrences. However, there are some exceptions; a subgroup of patients lost renal function either during the first episode or later in life. The clinical course of patients with CFI mutations is more variable. The onset is in childhood in half of the patients. Fifty-eight percent of patients eventually develop ESRD.

Therapy

Genetic characterization of patients could potentially help in tailoring treatment. Plasma infusion or exchange has been used in patients with HUS due to CFH mutations, with the rationale to provide the patients with normal CFH to correct the genetic deficiency. In published studies, some patients with CFH mutations did not respond at all to plasma infusion and died or developed ESRD. Others required plasma infusion at weekly intervals to raise CFH plasma levels sufficiently to maintain remission.[57,58] Stratton and Warwicker[59] were able to induce sustained remission in a patient with a CFH mutation with 3 months of weekly plasma exchange in conjunction with intravenous immunoglobulins. At 1 year after stopping plasma therapy, the patient remained disease free and dialysis independent. In our series,[45] approximately 50% of patients with CFH mutations treated with plasma underwent either complete or partial hematologic remission. However, half of the patients did not respond at all to plasma infusion and 20% died during an acute episode.

Because CFI and CFB are plasma proteins, plasma infusion and plasma exchange would be expected to be of value in patients with defects in the corresponding genes. Published data in small numbers of patients document that approximately half the patients with either CFI[45] or CFB mutations[54] underwent remission after plasma infusion, exactly as observed in patients with CFH mutations.

There is less rationale for using plasma in patients with MCP mutations because MCP is a transmembrane cell–associated protein and theoretically plasma infusion or exchange would

not correct the MCP defect. Published data[45,50] indicate that the majority (70%–80%) of patients experienced remission after plasma infusion or exchange; however, complete recovery from the acute episode was also observed in 70% to 80% of patients not treated with plasma.

Transplantation

The role of kidney transplantation in patients with non–Stx-HUS who have progressed to ESRD is still a matter of debate. Actually, approximately 50% of the patients who underwent a renal transplantation had a recurrence of the disease in the grafted organ.[56] There is no effective treatment for recurrences, and graft failure occurs in more than 90% of patients. Genotyping for CFH, MCP, and CFI mutations should be performed in all patients with ESRD secondary to non–Stx-HUS being considered for transplantation to help determine graft prognosis. In patients with CFH mutations, the graft outcome is poor; the recurrence rate ranges from 30% to 100% according to different surveys and is significantly higher than in patients without CFH mutations.[44,56,60] As CFH is mainly produced by the liver, kidney transplantation alone will not correct the CFH genetic defect. Simultaneous kidney and liver transplantation has been performed in two young children with non–Stx-HUS and CFH mutations, with the objective of correcting the genetic defect to prevent disease recurrences.[56] However, both cases treated with this procedure were complicated by premature irreversible liver failure. The patient in the first case recovered after a second uneventful liver transplantation. The child, who had experienced monthly recurrences before transplantation, has had no symptoms of HUS at more than 2 years of follow-up. The second patient died of fatal primary nonfunction of the liver graft followed by multiorgan failure. Increased susceptibility of the transplanted liver to ischemic or immune injury related to uncontrolled complement activation may have been responsible for the liver failure. Two more cases of combined kidney and liver transplantation in patients with CFH mutations have been subsequently reported.[61] In both cases, the post-transplantation outcome was favorable with good renal and liver function recorded at 2-year follow-up. In those two cases, extensive plasma exchange was given before surgery to provide patients with enough normal CFH to prevent liver graft damage. Thus, in this setting, combined liver and kidney transplantation may be an effective way to gain independence from long-term dialysis and may be lifesaving in those infants who, on dialysis, have a poor life expectancy.

As CFI and CFB are plasma proteins, one could speculate that HUS recurrence may take place in the transplanted kidney, and patients may experience graft failure. The few data available are in line with this hypothesis, as graft failures for recurrence occurred in 7 of 8 patients with CFI mutations and in one patient with CFB mutation.[45,62] Conversely, kidney graft outcome is favorable in patients with MCP mutations, as found in four patients who successfully underwent transplantation with no disease recurrence.[56] There is a strong theoretical rationale for this: MCP is a transmembrane protein highly expressed in the kidney. Transplantation of a kidney expressing normal MCP not surprisingly corrects the defects in these patients.

Thrombotic Microangiopathy Associated with Congenital Deficiency of ADAMTS-13

This rare form of TMA is associated with a congenital defect of ADAMTS-13, a plasma metalloprotease that cleaves ultra-large vWF multimers into smaller multimers. The defect was originally described in TTP[21,22]; however, emerging data indicate that patients with HUS[24] may also have a complete lack of ADAMTS-13 activity, albeit less frequently. Thus, on clinical grounds, a possible congenital defect of ADAMTS-13 cannot be excluded only on the basis of predominant renal localization of disease manifestation. TMA associated with congenital ADAMTS-13 deficiency presents either in families or in patients with no familial history of the disease.[21,22,24,63] In both cases, the disease is inherited as an autosomal recessive trait, as documented by ADAMTS-13 levels in healthy relatives of patients who fell into bimodal distribution with a group with half normal values, consistent with carriers, and the other half with normal values.[63]

Recurrences are very frequent and may occur even after symptom-free periods of months or years. Although they are more frequent in adults, relapsing forms of TMA have also been reported in children with congenital ADAMTS-13 deficiency in whom renal symptoms are predominant.[64]

To date, more than 50 ADAMTS-13 mutations have been identified in patients with familial TTP.[63,65] Affected individuals within families were either homozygous for the same mutation or compound heterozygous for two different mutations, confirming that the disease was inherited as a recessive trait.

The mutations have been found along the entire ADAMTS-13 gene and no clustering is evident, although more than 70% of them are located from the metalloprotease through the Tsp-1-2 domains.[25] Studies on secretion and activity of the mutated forms of the protease showed that most of these mutations impair secretion from the cells.[66] In those cases in which the mutated proteins are secreted, their proteolytic activity is greatly decreased.[66]

Therapy

At present, therapy of ADAMTS-13–associated TMA involves plasma infusion or exchange to replenish the active protease. Actually, providing just 5% of normal enzymatic activity may be sufficient to degrade large vWF multimers, which may be relevant to induce remission of the microangiopathic process, and this effect is sustained over time due to the relatively long half-life (2–4 days) of the protease. In two brothers with complete deficiency of the protease and relapsing TTP, disease remission was achieved by plasmapheresis and was concurrent with an almost full recovery of ADAMTS-13 activity. Both patients achieved a long-lasting remission, although protease activity decreased to less than 20% over 20 days after plasma therapy withdrawal.[67] One patient of ours with relapsing TTP due to congenital ADAMTS-13 deficiency[64] who had more than 100 relapses over 7 years was given different forms of treatment on different occasions: exchange, plasma infusion alone or plasma removed and replaced with albumin and saline. Clinical remission and normalization of platelet count within a few days were invariably obtained by plasma exchange or infusion, but plasma removal never increased the platelet count. Thus, plasma infusion is likely an established first-line treatment for HUS or TTP forms associated with congenital ADAMTS-13 protease deficiency. Although individual attacks usually respond to treatment, long-term prognosis is invariably poor if therapy fails to achieve a lasting remission.

Thrombotic Microangiopathy Associated with Inborn Abnormal Cobalamin Metabolism

This is a rare autosomal recessive form of HUS associated with an inborn abnormality of cobalamin metabolism.[68] The disease manifests in the first days or months of life. Children fail to thrive, have poor feeding and vomiting, and may present neurological symptoms of fatigue, delirium, psychosis, and seizures. In cases with early onset, the disease has a fulminant evolution and occasionally involves the pulmonary vasculature, but when it occurs later in childhood, it may follow a more chronic course. The hallmarks of defective cobalamin metabolism are hyperhomocysteinemia and methylmalonic aciduria, and the extremely high homocysteine levels have been suggested to have a role in the pathogenesis of the vascular lesions. Without treatment, the disease is fatal, and it is likely that some children die undiagnosed.

Therapy

Treatment is directed at correcting the metabolic disorder as effectively as possible.[69] Daily intramuscular administration of hydroxycobalamin may reduce both homocysteine levels and methylmalonic aciduria, whereas oral hydroxycobalamin and cyanocobalamin are ineffective. Oral betaine further reduces serum homocysteine levels by activating betaine-homocysteine methyltransferase. Supplementation of folic acid to avoid folate deficiency induced by 5-methyltetrahydrofolate trapping and of L-carnitine to increase propionyl carnitine excretion has been recommended, but it is unclear whether they improve disease outcome. Despite treatment, the majority of children with early-onset disease die or have severe neurological sequelae. Intensified treatment in older children with less acute disease may achieve remission of the microangiopathic process and amelioration of the other clinical manifestations of the metabolic disorder. It is not known whether plasma therapy would improve disease outcome.

Other Genetic Forms

Conceivably, the mutations described account for approximately 50% of genetic forms of TMA. Patients with decreased C3 but no evidence of CFH, MCP, CFI, or CFB abnormalities have been described. In these rare cases, uncontrolled activation of the alternative complement pathway may be due to genetic defects in other complement regulatory proteins, including DAF, CR1, CR2, and C4 binding protein. Other cases may be associated with still unrecognized genetic defects. Among these are familial forms transmitted with a dominant or recessive pattern of inheritance that may manifest with the features of HUS or TTP in different members of the same family or in different recurrences in the same patient.

Therapy

Plasma infusion or exchange is the only therapy that may have some effect. Regardless of treatment, however, disease outcome is usually poor.

IDIOPATHIC

These are forms of unknown etiology with progressive renal function deterioration and neurological involvement that may resemble TTP. They may follow a progressive course to end-stage renal failure or death and very likely constitutes a disease closer to TTP that requires more specific therapies to stop the progression of the microangiopathic process. These cases recur more often after kidney transplantation.[70]

Therapy

Plasma infusion and exchange have been retrospectively found to limit residual renal insufficiency or the risk of end-stage renal failure in children. Uncontrolled studies suggest that plasma infusion or exchange may markedly lower the mortality rate and risk of end-stage renal failure in adults.[1,71] Intravenous immunoglobulins have been suggested to limit neurological involvement, but their effectiveness too is still unproven. Bilat-

eral nephrectomy (see "Shiga-Toxin–Associated Thrombotic Microangiopathy") may be attempted as rescue therapy in patients with severe renal involvement, refractory hypertension/thrombocytopenia, and hypertensive encephalopathy.

SPECIFIC RECOMMENDATIONS

In addition to symptomatic treatment, various specific therapies have been suggested for the different forms of TMA (Tables 26-2, 26-3 and 26-4), but, until recently, no clear-cut guidelines were available to identify which patients should be treated, which therapies should be chosen, and how these should be administered. Over the past decade, however, the identification of at least two broad categories of patients, those with genetically determined and those with acquired immune-mediated disease, has allowed, at least in some circumstances, targeting the therapeutic intervention to specific pathogenic mechanisms and therefore to optimize the

Table 26-3 Specific Therapies Most Commonly Used in Thrombotic Microangiopathy, Doses, and Routes of Administration

Therapy	Dose	Route of Administration
Antiplatelet Agents		
Aspirin	325–1300 mg/day	Oral
Dipyridamole	400–600 mg/day	Oral
Dextran 70	500 mg bid	IV injection
Prostaglandin I_2	10–20 ng/kg/min	Continuous IV infusion
Antithrombotic Agents		
Heparin	5000 U	IV bolus injection
	750–1000 U/hr	Continuous IV infusion
Streptokinase	250,000 U	IV bolus injection
	100,000 U/hr	Continuous IV infusion
Antioxidant Agents		
Vitamin E	1000 mg/m²/day	Oral
Immunosuppressive Agents		
Prednisone	200 mg tapered to 60 mg/day, then 5 mg decrease per week	Oral during active disease, oral after remission
Prednisolone	200 mg tapered to 60 mg/day, then 5 mg decrease per week	IV during active disease, IV after remission
Immunoglobulins	400 mg/kg/day	IV infusion
Vincristine	1.4 mg/m² on day 1	IV injection
	1 mg every 4 days	IV injection up to 4 doses
Fresh Frozen Plasma		
Infusion	20–30 mL/kg on day 1	IV infusion
	10–20 mL/kg/day	IV infusion until remission
Exchange	1–2 plasma volumes/day	IV until remission
Cryosupernatant	See plasma infusion/exchange	See plasma infusion/exchange
Sodium detergent treated	See plasma infusion/exchange	See plasma infusion/exchange

Table 26-4 Indications for Specific Therapy in the Different Forms of Thrombotic Microangiopathy

Disease	Comment
Acquired	
Shiga-toxin associated	
Childhood forms	No indication (possibly with the exception of plasma infusion/exchange for severe forms with anuria and neurological signs)
Adult forms	Plasma infusion/exchange (to minimize the risk of sequelae)
Neuraminidase associated	Possible indication for plasma infusion/exchange (combined with steroids to minimize adverse reactions)
Immune-mediated defective CFH activity	Plasma infusion/exchange combined with steroid or immunosuppressive therapy
Immune-mediated defective ADAMTS-13 activity	Plasma infusion/exchange combined with steroid or immunosuppressive therapy (life saving)
Pregnancy associated	
TTP	Plasma infusion/exchange (life saving)
HELLP syndrome	Plasma infusion/exchange (in selected cases and after delivery)
Postpartum HUS	Plasma infusion/exchange (often ineffective)
Systemic disease associated	Plasma infusion/exchange (combined with treatment of underlying disease)
Drug associated	Plasma infusion/exchange (combined with drug withdrawal)
Transplant associated	Plasma infusion/exchange (often ineffective)
Genetic	
CFH, CFI, CFB abnormalities	Plasma infusion/exchange (often ineffective)
MCP abnormalities	Probably no indication for plasma infusion/exchange (relatively good outcome also with conservative therapy alone)
ADAMTS-13 deficiency	Plasma infusion/exchange (life saving)
Abnormal cobalamin metabolism	Correction of the metabolic abnormalities; possible indication for plasma infusion/exchange
Others	Plasma infusion/exchange (often ineffective)
Idiopathic	Plasma infusion/exchange (often ineffective)

CFB, complement factor B; CFH, complement factor H; CFI, complement factor I; HELLP, hemolysis, elevated liver enzymes, and low platelet count; HUS, hemolytic uremic syndrome; MCP, membrane cofactor protein; TTP, thrombotic thrombocytopenic purpura.

risk-benefit profile of intervention. Thus, plasma exchange is especially beneficial for patients with immune-mediated deficiency of ADAMTS-13 or factor H because it provides an excess of the plasma components that may saturate and neutralize the autoantibody activity and partially restore their circulating levels while removing the autoantibody from the circulation. Similar considerations apply to steroids, vincristine, immunoglobulins, immunosuppressants, and splenectomy. In particular, steroids have been extensively used in the past to treat patients with so-called idiopathic TTP or with atypical forms of HUS, with inconsistent results. Although these treatments may have a role in immune forms of TMA by inhibiting the production of the autoantibody and, in combination with plasma exchange, effecting clearance of the autoantibody from the circulation, they definitely have no role in the treatment of genetic forms. Trials that included both the immune and genetic forms of TMA invariably diluted the potential benefits of steroids or immunosuppressive therapy in subjects with immune-mediated disease. This may explain the inconclusive results of previous studies in HUS and TTP. Fut-ure studies should likely focus on the role of steroids as first-line therapy for immune-mediated forms and on vincristine, high-dose immunoglobulins, or other immunosuppressants as second-line therapy, with splenectomy being considered only rarely as rescue therapy for those patients with refractory disease and life-threatening thrombocytopenia or neurological involvement. Conversely, patients with genetically determined ADAMTS-13 deficiency may benefit from both plasma infusion or exchange because both procedures may re-place the defective activity, with the exchange procedure offering the possibility of supplying larger amounts of plasma without the risk of fluid overload. This applies also to patients with forms of HUS associated with genetic abnormalities of circulating complement regulators such as factors H and I.

Conversely, there is less rationale or evidence for plasma therapy, either as infusion or exchange, in forms associated with abnormalities of membrane-bound regulatory proteins such as MCP.

Finally, when a given intervention is being considered in an individual patient, the risks and benefits of add-on therapy with a specific treatment should always be evaluated compared with conservative therapy alone. Thus, the use of invasive and potentially toxic treatments such as plasma exchange or immunosuppressive agents aimed at stopping the microangiopathic process should be restricted to cases that, without intervention, are expected to have a poor outcome. The risk of sensitization, which may limit the possibility of a successful transplantation in those progressing to ESRD, should also be taken into account at the time the option of plasma therapy is being considered. Along this line, conservative therapy alone is the intervention of choice in most cases of childhood STx-HUS, which usually recover spontaneously. Similarly, waiting before considering plasma therapy is the best strategy in cases associated with MCP mutations because these forms appear to have a high rate of spontaneous remission that does not appear to be appreciably increased by plasma therapy.

Whenever indicated, specific therapy should be started as soon as diagnosis is established to speed up disease recovery and minimize morbidity and mortality. Treatment should be continued until complete disease remission is achieved.

Platelet count and serum lactate dehydrogenase are the most sensitive markers for monitoring the response to therapy. In conditions associated with decreased platelet production (cancer- or AIDS-associated TMA), serum lactate dehydrogenase concentration is a more reliable indicator of disease activity than platelet count. In pregnancy-associated TMA, monitoring serum transaminases may be helpful.

Screening and Diagnosis

Understanding of the genetic basis of non–Stx-HUS has its implications for patient management, in particular, in the perspective of kidney transplantation for those who progress to ESRD; thus the demand for genetic screening has been progressively increasing. However, a full analysis for mutations in the four complement proteins so far recognized to be involved in the disease is extremely expensive and time-consuming. To optimize cost-effectiveness of genetic studies and guarantee timely delivery of the results, an initial screen based on protein levels (either serum levels or surface expression) appears a rational approach to rapidly identify the gene likely involved (see Fig. 26-1). Even when complement regulator levels are normal, both the titer of anti-CFH antibodies and possibly involved genes should be studied according to the expected frequency of mutations. Thus, the CFH gene should be considered first because it may be mutated in approximately 30% of cases, followed by MCP and CFI genes, which may be mutated in approximately 10% and 2% to 5% of cases, respectively. Then, to minimize cost and detection time, the exons where the mutations are more frequently identified within a given gene should be studied first: thus, the analysis of CFH gene should start with the study of the SCRs 19 and 20, where the majority of CFH mutations tend to cluster; the same applies to SCRs 1 to 4 of MCP, where 90% of

mutations are identified, and to the serine protease domain, which accounts for 60% of CFI mutations.

Plasma Manipulation

The infusion is intended to deliver the equivalent of one plasma volume ($\approx$30 mL/kg of body weight) over the first 24 hours and approximately 20 mL/kg of body weight daily thereafter. To avoid fluid overload, diuretics or ultrafiltration may be employed. The exchange procedure is usually intended to replace one to two plasma volumes every day.

Two procedures are available for plasma separation in the setting of plasma exchange: filtration and centrifugation. The total extracorporeal volume of the plasma circuit affects the choice of the procedure. It is estimated that the total extracorporeal volume should not exceed 8% to 10% of total blood volume of the patient (taken as 100 mL/kg in infants < 10 kg and 80 mL/kg in children > 10 kg). Thus, the filtration system, which has an extracorporeal volume less than 100 mL, is preferred for small children and in patients with cardiovascular instability. Plasma centrifugation is the standard procedure for all other cases.

Other Specific Treatments

In a large series of TTP patients,[29] 200 mg/day of oral prednisone (or 200 mg/day of intravenous prednisolone in patients with evidence of hepatic dysfunction) were given until complete normalization of the markers of hemolysis, when corticosteroids were rapidly tapered to 60 mg/day and then more slowly by 5 mg/week. In HELLP syndrome, dexamethasone was given, 10 mg intravenously every 12 hours until delivery and for 36 hours thereafter.

The recommended initial dose of vincristine is 1.4 mg/m^2 (not to exceed 2 mg) by intravenous injection, followed by 1 mg intravenously every 4 days until complete remission is achieved. Because of its severe neurotoxicity, the drug should be used with caution.

Antiplatelet agents have been given by a variety of schedules. Dipyridamole (400 mg/day) and aspirin (325 mg/day) are usually given for at least 2 weeks and until disease remission.[28]

Prostaglandin I$_2$ (epoprostenol), infused at the recommended doses of 10 to 20 ng/kg/min, may cause hypotension, headache, facial flushing, and diarrhea. Stable analogues have recently been developed, but their effectiveness remains to be investigated in controlled trials.

The suggested doses of antithrombotic agents used in HUS are given in Table 26-3. Oral vitamin E is usually given, 1000 mg/m^2/day until complete remission of the disease. Other antioxidants available for trial include allopurinol, desferoxamine, and superoxide dismutase.

Rescue Treatments

When cryosupernatant fraction (i.e., plasma from which the cryoprecipitate containing the largest plasma vWF multimers, fibrinogen, and fibronectin has been removed) is used, during the infusion or exchange procedure, patients should be given the same volumes as stated previously for whole plasma (see Table 26-2).

Bilateral nephrectomy and splenectomy are irreversible procedures and should be considered only for patients at imminent risk of death or with disabling disease. In patients at increased risk of bleeding because of severe refractory thrombocytopenia, platelet transfusion may be indicated before surgery.

FUTURE DIRECTIONS

Acquired Forms

Research efforts are aimed at identifying more specific approaches that may interfere with the causes of endothelial injury and the sequence of events triggered by endothelial damage. Along this line, several agents aimed at interrupting the pathogenic cascade starting with the ingestion of Stx-producing *E. coli* strains and eventually culminating in full-blown HUS are currently under investigation.[1] Molecular decoys such as orally administered nonpathogenic recombinant *E. coli*, genetically engineered to display a Stx receptor on the surface,[72–74] have been successfully used to bind and inactivate the toxin in the intestines of mice. In another study, a plant-based oral vaccination with nicotiana tabacum cells transfected with the gene encoding inactivated Stx2 fully protected mice from challenge with a lethal dose of the toxin.[75] Yet another approach is to use Stx inhibitors; among them is STARFISH, an oligobivalent, water-soluble carbohydrate ligand that can simultaneously engage all five B subunits of Stx, which might help to prevent toxin that already has entered the circulation from binding to specific receptors.[76] Others have ameliorated disease in pigs by injection of toxin-neutralizing antibodies.[77] Although natural infection with *E. coli* O157 does not confer immunity and no human vaccine is currently available, Shiga toxoid vaccines have been shown effective in preventing related diseases in animals.

At present, however, prevention remains the most efficient strategy to decrease the morbidity and mortality associated with Stx–*E. coli* infection. A multifaceted approach is required including novel ways of decreasing Stx–*E. coli* carrier rate in livestock and implementing a zero-tolerance policy for contaminated foods and beverages. Generalized pasteurization of ground beef through irradiation will probably help to limit/prevent *E. coli* O157 and other food-borne pathogen infections.

Agents to prevent shear-induced, vWF-mediated platelet aggregation in vitro may hold promise in the therapy of TMA, in which high shear stress forces in damaged microvessels may sustain vWF-mediated intravascular platelet thrombosis. These agents include aurin tricarboxylic acid, a potent inhibitor of large vWF multimers binding to the platelet surface glycoprotein Ib receptor that is now under investigation as an arterial antithrombotic agent; recombinant fragments of the vWF monomer competitively block the binding of vWF multimers to GP1b, as do monoclonal antibodies to the arginine-glycine-aspartate-binding region for glycoprotein IIb/IIIa on monomeric subunits of vWF multimers.

An alternative approach is aimed at identifying the plasma component(s) that might induce remission of HUS and TTP (examples of these might be ADAMTS-13 and CFH, found to be defective in some forms of TMA). A plasma fraction that substantially retains the beneficial activity of whole plasma would reduce the total amount of plasma proteins infused, limiting the risk of allergic reactions and fluid overload. The active plasma fraction in lyophilized form could be made available to centers that lack facilities for plasma exchange: It would allow better and more prompt treatment of the disease at considerably lower cost and would limit the risk of viral infection. Novel techniques such as the solvent-detergent virus inactivation method by which viruses are inactivated by a lipid solvent and detergent that disrupt the lipid envelope are under evaluation to assess the possibility of limiting viral contamination of plasma without lowering its effectiveness.

Clinical trials to assess the effectiveness of these treatments are, however, difficult to design properly. In view of the good outcome of childhood diarrhea-associated HUS, trials invariably require several hundreds of patients to ensure that they have the power to demonstrate an additional beneficial effect of the treatment under evaluation compared with supportive therapy alone. Conversely, adult HUS and TTP patients are often so ill that treatments are usually attempted in combination, thus confounding data interpretation. This may explain why, so far, the majority of information on the treatment of TMA comes from retrospective and often uncontrolled trials rather than from prospective, randomized trials.

Genetic Forms

New information derived from recent genetic studies will perhaps open the perspective on new specific treatments for patients with genetic forms of HUS and TTP. Specific replacement therapies with recombinant factor H and ADAMTS-13 could become a viable alternative to plasma treatment. This is reasonably feasible for patients with ADAMTS-13 gene mutations because even low (5% of normal) vWF-cleaving protease activity may be sufficient to degrade large vWF multimers. Finally, the full definition of factor H and ADAMTS-13 gene sequence will soon render gene therapy a realistic option for patients with inherited HUS or TTP.

References

1. Ruggenenti P, Noris M, Remuzzi G: Thrombotic microangiopathy, hemolytic uremic syndrome, and thrombotic thrombocytopenic purpura. Kidney Int 2001;60:831–846.
2. Garg AX, Suri RS, Barrowman N, et al: Long-term renal prognosis of diarrhea-associated hemolytic uremic syndrome: A systematic review, meta-analysis, and meta-regression. JAMA 2003;290:1360–1370.
3. Ake JA, Jelacic S, Ciol MA, et al: Relative nephroprotection during *Escherichia coli* O157:H7 infections: Association with intravenous volume expansion. Pediatrics 2005;115:e673–e680.
4. Chiurchiu C, Firrincieli A, Santostefano M, et al: Adult nondiarrhea hemolytic uremic syndrome associated with Shiga toxin *Escherichia coli* O157:H7 bacteremia and urinary tract infection. Am J Kidney Dis 2003;41:E4.
5. Wong CS, Jelacic S, Habeeb RL, et al: The risk of the hemolytic-uremic syndrome after antibiotic treatment of *Escherichia coli* O157:H7 infections. N Engl J Med 2000;342:1930–1936.
6. Safdar N, Said A, Gangnon RE, Maki DG: Risk of hemolytic uremic syndrome after antibiotic treatment of *Escherichia coli* O157:H7 enteritis: A meta-analysis. JAMA 2002;288:996–1001.
7. Caletti MG, Lejarraga H, Kelmansky D, Missoni M: Two different therapeutic regimes in patients with sequelae of hemolytic-uremic syndrome. Pediatr Nephrol 2004;19:1148–1152.
8. Van Dyck M, Proesmans W: Renoprotection by ACE inhibitors after severe hemolytic uremic syndrome. Pediatr Nephrol 2004;19:688–690.

9. Trachtman H, Cnaan A, Christen E, et al: Effect of an oral Shiga toxin-binding agent on diarrhea-associated hemolytic uremic syndrome in children: A randomized controlled trial. JAMA 2003;290:1337–1344.

10. Rizzoni G, Claris-Appiani A, Edefonti A, et al: Plasma infusion for hemolytic-uremic syndrome in children: Results of a multicenter controlled trial. J Pediatr 1988;112:284–290.

11. Loirat C, Veyradier A, Foulard M, et al: von Willebrand factor (vWF)-cleaving protease activity in pediatric hemolytic uremic syndrome (HUS) [abstract]. Pediatr Nephrol 2001;16:617A.

12. Dundas S, Murphy J, Soutar RL, et al: Effectiveness of therapeutic plasma exchange in the 1996 Lanarkshire Escherichia coli O157:H7 outbreak. Lancet 1999;354:1327–1330.

13. Carter AO, Borczyk AA, Carlson JA, et al: A severe outbreak of Escherichia coli O157:H7–associated hemorrhagic colitis in a nursing home. N Engl J Med 1987;317:1496–1500.

14. Remuzzi G, Galbusera M, Salvadori M, et al: Bilateral nephrectomy stopped disease progression in plasma-resistant hemolytic uremic syndrome with neurological signs and coma. Kidney Int 1996;49:282–286.

15. Artz MA, Steenbergen EJ, Hoitsma AJ, et al: Renal transplantation in patients with hemolytic uremic syndrome: High rate of recurrence and increased incidence of acute rejections. Transplantation 2003;76:821–826.

16. Loirat C, Niaudet P: The risk of recurrence of hemolytic uremic syndrome after renal transplantation in children. Pediatr Nephrol 2003;18:1095–1101.

17. Ferraris JR, Ramirez JA, Ruiz S, et al: Shiga toxin-associated hemolytic uremic syndrome: Absence of recurrence after renal transplantation. Pediatr Nephrol 2002;17:809–814.

18. McGraw ME, Lendon M, Stevens RF, et al: Haemolytic uraemic syndrome and the Thomsen Friedenreich antigen. Pediatr Nephrol 1989;3:135–139.

19. Dragon-Durey MA, Loirat C, Cloarec S, et al: Anti-factor H autoantibodies associated with atypical hemolytic uremic syndrome. J Am Soc Nephrol 2005;16:555–563.

20. Jozsi M, Strobel S, Dahse HM, et al: Anti-factor H autoantibodies block C-terminal recognition function of factor H in hemolytic uremic syndrome. Blood 2007;110:1516–1518.

21. Furlan M, Robles R, Lamie B: Partial purification and characterization of a protease from human plasma cleaving von Willebrand factor to fragments produced by in vivo proteolysis. Blood 1996;87:4223–4234.

22. Furlan M, Robles R, Galbusera M, et al: von Willebrand factor-cleaving protease in thrombotic thrombocytopenic purpura and the hemolytic-uremic syndrome. N Engl J Med 1998;339:1578–1584.

23. Tsai HM, Lian EC: Antibodies to von Willebrand factor-cleaving protease in acute thrombotic thrombocytopenic purpura. N Engl J Med 1998;339:1585–1594.

24. Veyradier A, Obert B, Houllier A, et al: Specific von Willebrand factor-cleaving protease in thrombotic microangiopathies: A study of 111 cases. Blood 2001;98:1765–1772.

25. Galbusera M, Noris M, Remuzzi G: Thrombotic thrombocytopenic purpura—then and now. Semin Thromb Hemost 2006;32:81–89.

26. Ferrari S, Scheiflinger F, Rieger M, et al: Prognostic value of anti-ADAMTS 13 antibody features (Ig isotype, titer, and inhibitory effect) in a cohort of 35 adult French patients undergoing a first episode of thrombotic microangiopathy with undetectable ADAMTS 13 activity. Blood 2007;109:2815–2822.

27. Caletti MG, Gallo G, Gianantonio CA: Development of focal segmental sclerosis and hyalinosis in hemolytic uremic syndrome. Pediatr Nephrol 1996;10:687–692.

28. Bell WR, Braine HG, Ness PM, Kickler TS: Improved survival in thrombotic thrombocytopenic purpura-hemolytic uremic syndrome. Clinical experience in 108 patients. N Engl J Med 1991;325:398–403.

29. Rock GA, Shumak KH, Buskard NA, et al: Comparison of plasma exchange with plasma infusion in the treatment of thrombotic thrombocytopenic purpura. Canadian Apheresis Study Group. N Engl J Med 1991;325:393–397.

30. Byrnes JJ, Moake JL, Klug P, Periman P: Effectiveness of the cryo-supernatant fraction of plasma in the treatment of refractory thrombotic thrombocytopenic purpura. Am J Hematol 1990;34:169–174.

31. Rock G, Shumak KH, Sutton DM, et al: Cryosupernatant as replacement fluid for plasma exchange in thrombotic thrombocytopenic purpura. Members of the Canadian Apheresis Group. Br J Haematol 1996;94:383–386.

32. Hayward CP, Sutton DM, Carter WH Jr, et al: Treatment outcomes in patients with adult thrombotic thrombocytopenic purpura-hemolytic uremic syndrome. Arch Intern Med 1994;154:982–987.

33. Furlan M, Robles R, Solenthaler M, Lammle B: Acquired deficiency of von Willebrand factor-cleaving protease in a patient with thrombotic thrombocytopenic purpura. Blood 1998;91:2839–2846.

34. Weiner CP: Thrombotic microangiopathy in pregnancy and the postpartum period. Semin Hematol 1987;24:119–129.

35. George JN: The association of pregnancy with thrombotic thrombocytopenic purpura-hemolytic uremic syndrome. Curr Opin Hematol 2003;10:339–344.

36. Ruggenenti P, Remuzzi G: The pathophysiology and management of thrombotic thrombocytopenic purpura. Eur J Haematol 1996;56:191–207.

37. Tsai HM, Rice L, Sarode R, et al: Antibody inhibitors to von Willebrand factor metalloproteinase and increased binding of von Willebrand factor to platelets in ticlopidine-associated thrombotic thrombocytopenic purpura. Ann Intern Med 2000;132:794–799.

38. Ohashi N, Yonemura K, Sugiura T, et al: Withdrawal of interferon-alpha results in prompt resolution of thrombocytopenia and hemolysis but not renal failure in hemolytic uremic syndrome caused by interferon-alpha. Am J Kidney Dis 2003;41:E10.

39. Taylor CM: Complement factor H and the haemolytic uraemic syndrome. Lancet 2001;358:1200–1202.

40. Ruggenenti P, Galli M, Remuzzi G: Hemolytic uremic syndrome, thrombotic thrombocytopenic purpura, and antiphospholipid antibody syndromes. In Neilson EG, Couser WG (eds): Immunologic Renal Diseases. Philadelphia: Lippincott Williams & Wilkins, 2001, pp 1179–1208.

41. Warwicker P, Goodship TH, Donne RL, et al: Genetic studies into inherited and sporadic hemolytic uremic syndrome. Kidney Int 1998;53:836–844.

42. Saunders RE, Abarrategui-Garrido C, Fremeaux-Bacchi V, et al: The interactive Factor H-atypical hemolytic uremic syndrome mutation database and website: Update and integration of membrane cofactor protein and factor I mutations with structural models. Hum Mutat 2007;28:222–234.

43. Perez-Caballero D, Gonzalez-Rubio C, et al: Clustering of missense mutations in the C-terminal region of factor H in atypical hemolytic uremic syndrome. Am J Hum Genet 2001;68:478–484.

44. Neumann HP, Salzmann M, Bohnert-Iwan B, et al: Haemolytic uraemic syndrome and mutations of the factor H gene: A registry-based study of German speaking countries. J Med Genet 2003;40:676–681.

45. Caprioli J, Noris M, Brioschi S, et al: Genetics of HUS: The impact of MCP, CFH, and IF mutations on clinical presentation, response to treatment, and outcome. Blood 2006;108:1267–1279.

46. Rodriguez de Cordoba S, Esparza-Gordillo J, Goicoechea de Jorge E, et al: The human complement factor H: Functional roles, genetic variations and disease associations. Mol Immunol 2004;41:355–367.

47. Jozsi M, Manuelian T, Heinen S, et al: Attachment of the soluble complement regulator factor H to cell and tissue surfaces: Relevance for pathology. Histol Histopathol 2004;19:251–258.

48. Venables JP, Strain L, Routledge D, et al: Atypical haemolytic uraemic syndrome associated with a hybrid complement gene. PLoS Med 2006;3:e431.

49. Noris M, Brioschi S, Caprioli J, et al: Familial haemolytic uraemic syndrome and an MCP mutation. Lancet 2003;362:1542–1547.

50. Richards A, Kemp EJ, Liszewski MK, et al: Mutations in human complement regulator, membrane cofactor protein (CD46), predispose to development of familial hemolytic uremic syndrome. Proc Natl Acad Sci U S A 2003;100:12966–12971.

51. Goodship TH, Liszewski MK, Kemp EJ, et al: Mutations in CD46, a complement regulatory protein, predispose to atypical HUS. Trends Mol Med 2004;10:226–231.

52. Fremeaux-Bacchi V, Dragon-Durey MA, Blouin J, et al: Complement factor I: A susceptibility gene for atypical haemolytic uraemic syndrome. J Med Genet 2004;41:e84.

53. Kavanagh D, Kemp EJ, Mayland E, et al: Mutations in complement factor I predispose to development of atypical hemolytic uremic syndrome. J Am Soc Nephrol 2005;16:2150–2155.

54. Goicoechea de Jorge E, Harris CL, Esparza-Gordillo J, et al: Gain-of-function mutations in complement factor B are associated with atypical hemolytic uremic syndrome. Proc Natl Acad Sci U S A 2007;104:240–245.

55. Caprioli J, Castelletti F, Bucchioni S, et al: Complement factor H mutations and gene polymorphisms in haemolytic uraemic syndrome: The C-257T, the A2089G and the G2881T polymorphisms are strongly associated with the disease. Hum Mol Genet 2003;12:3385–3395.

56. Noris M, Bucchioni S, Galbusera M, et al: Complement factor H mutation in familial thrombotic thrombocytopenic purpura with ADAMTS13 deficiency and renal involvement. J Am Soc Nephrol 2005;16:1177–1183.

57. Landau D, Shalev H, Levy-Finer G, et al: Familial hemolytic uremic syndrome associated with complement factor H deficiency. J Pediatr 2001;138:412–417.

58. Cho HY, Lee BS, Moon KC, et al: Complete factor H deficiency-associated atypical hemolytic uremic syndrome in a neonate. Pediatr Nephrol 2007;22:874–880.

59. Stratton JD, Warwicker P: Successful treatment of factor H-related haemolytic uraemic syndrome. Nephrol Dial Transplant 2002;17:684–685.

60. Bresin E, Daina E, Noris M, et al., International Registry of Recurrent and Familial HUS/TTP: Outcome of renal transplantation in patients with non-Shiga toxin-associated haemolytic uremic syndrome: Prognostic significance of genetic background. Clin J Am Soc Nephrol 2006;1:88–99.

61. Saland JM, Emre SH, Shneider BL, et al: Favorable long-term outcome after liver-kidney transplant for recurrent hemolytic uremic syndrome associated with a factor H mutation. Am J Transplant 2006;6:1948–1952.

62. Geelen J, van den Dries K, Roos A, et al: A missense mutation in factor I (IF) predisposes to atypical haemolytic uraemic syndrome. Pediatr Nephrol 2007;22:371–375.

63. Levy GG, Nichols WC, Lian EC, et al: Mutations in a member of the ADAMTS gene family cause thrombotic thrombocytopenic purpura. Nature 2001;413:488–494.

64. Ruggenenti P, Galbusera M, Cornejo RP, et al: Thrombotic thrombocytopenic purpura: Evidence that infusion rather than removal of plasma induces remission of the disease. Am J Kidney Dis 1993;21:314–318.

65. Fujikawa K, Suzuki H, McMullen B, Chung D: Purification of human von Willebrand factor-cleaving protease and its identification as a new member of the metalloproteinase family. Blood 2001;98:1662–1666.

66. Donadelli R, Banterla F, Galbusera M, et al: In-vitro and in-vivo consequences of mutations in the von Willebrand factor cleaving protease ADAMTS13 in thrombotic thrombocytopenic purpura. Thromb Haemost 2006;96:454–464.

67. Furlan M, Robles R, Morselli B, et al: Recovery and half-life of von Willebrand factor-cleaving protease after plasma therapy in patients with thrombotic thrombocytopenic purpura. Thromb Haemost 1999;81:8–13.

68. Baumgartner ER, Wick H, Maurer R, et al: Congenital defect in intracellular cobalamin metabolism resulting in homocysteinuria and methylmalonic aciduria. I. Case report and histopathology. Helv Paediatr Acta 1979;34:465–482.

69. Van Hove JL, Van Damme-Lombaerts R, Grunewald S, et al: Cobalamin disorder Cbl-C presenting with late-onset thrombotic microangiopathy. Am J Med Genet 2002;111:195–201.

70. Remuzzi G, Ruggenenti P, Codazzi D, et al: Combined kidney and liver transplantation for familial haemolytic uraemic syndrome. Lancet 2002;359:1671–1672.

71. George JN: How I treat patients with thrombotic thrombocytopenic purpura-hemolytic uremic syndrome. Blood 2000;96:1223–1229.

72. Paton AW, Morona R, Paton JC: A new biological agent for treatment of Shiga toxigenic Escherichia coli infections and dysentery in humans. Nat Med 2000;6:265–270.

73. Pinyon RA, Paton JC, Paton AW, et al: Refinement of a therapeutic Shiga toxin-binding probiotic for human trials. J Infect Dis 2004;189:1547–1555.

74. Takahashi M, Taguchi H, Yamaguchi H, et al: The effect of probiotic treatment with Clostridium butyricum on enterohemorrhagic Escherichia coli O157:H7 infection in mice. FEMS Immunol Med Microbiol 2004;41:219–226.

75. Wen SX, Teel LD, Judge NA, O'Brien AD: A plant-based oral vaccine to protect against systemic intoxication by Shiga toxin type 2. Proc Natl Acad Sci U S A 2006;103:7082–7087.

76. Mulvey GL, Marcato P, Kitov PI, et al: Assessment in mice of the therapeutic potential of tailored, multivalent Shiga toxin carbohydrate ligands. J Infect Dis 2003;187:640–649.

77. Matise I, Cornick NA, Booher SL, et al: Intervention with Shiga toxin (Stx) antibody after infection by Stx-producing Escherichia coli. J Infect Dis 2001;183:347–350.

78. Loirat C, Beaufils F, Sonsino E, et al: [Treatment of childhood hemolytic-uremic syndrome with urokinase. Cooperative controlled trial]. Arch Fr Pediatr 1984;41:15–19.

79. Van Damme-Lombaerts R, Proesmans W, Van Damme B, et al: Heparin plus dipyridamole in childhood hemolytic-uremic syndrome: A prospective, randomized study. J Pediatr 1998;113:913–918.

80. Loirat C, Sonsino E, Hinglais N, et al: Treatment of the childhood haemolytic uremic syndrome with plasma. A multicentre randomized controlled trial. The French Society of Paediatric Nephrology. Pediatr Nephrol 1988;2:279–285.

81. Gianviti A, Perna A, Caringella A, et al: Plasma exchange in children with hemolytic-uremic syndrome at risk of poor outcome. Am J Kidney Dis 1993;22:264–266.

82. Italian Cooperative Group for the Study of Thrombotic Thrombocytopenic Purpura: Thrombotic thrombocytopenic purpura (TTP) treatment: Italian cooperative retrospective study on 29 cases. Haematologica 1986;71:39–43.

83. Adult hemolytic uremic syndrome with renal microangiopathy. Outcome according to therapeutic protocol in 53 cases. French Cooperative Study Group for Adult HUS. Ann Med Interne (Paris) 1992;143(Suppl 1):27–32.

84. Henon P: [Treatment of thrombotic thrombopenic purpura. Results of a multicenter randomized clinical study]. Presse Med 1991;20:1761–1767.

Further Reading

Besbas N, Karpman D, Landau D, et al., European Paediatric Research Group for HUS: A classification of hemolytic uremic syndrome and thrombotic thrombocytopenic purpura and related disorders. Kidney Int 2006;70:423–431.

Espinosa G, Bucciarelli S, Cervera R, et al: Thrombotic microangio-pathic haemolytic anaemia and antiphospholipid antibodies. Ann Rheum Dis 2004;63:730–736.

George JN: Clinical practice. Thrombotic thrombocytopenic purpura. N Engl J Med 2006;354:1927–1935.

MacConnachie AA, Todd WTA: Potential therapeutic agents for the prevention and treatment of haemolytic uraemic syndrome in Shiga toxin producing *Escherichia coli infection.* Curr Opin Infect Dis 2004;17:479–482.

O'Brian JM, Barton JR: Controversies with the diagnosis and man-agement of HELLP syndrome. Clin Obstet Gynecol 2005;48: 460–477.

Richards A, Liszewski KM, Kavanagh D, et al: Implications of the initial mutations in membrane cofactor protein (MCP; CD46) leading to atypical hemolytic uremic syndrome. Mol Immunol 2007;44:111–122.

Siegler R, Oakes R: Hemolytic uremic syndrome; pathogenesis, treatment, and outcome. Curr Opin Pediatr 2005;17:200–2004.

Tsai HM: The molecular biology of thrombotic microangiopathy. Kidney Int 2006;70:16–23.

Zakarija A, Bennet C: Drug-induced thrombotic microangiopathy. Semin Thromb Hemost 2005;31:681–690.

Zipfel PF, Skerka C: Complement dysfunction in hemolytic uremic syndrome. Curr Opin Rheumatol 2006;18:548–555.

Chapter 27

Treatment of Acute Interstitial Nephritis

James P. Smith and Eric G. Neilson

Acute interstitial nephritis (AIN) leads to renal failure following persistent autoimmunity in the tubulointerstitium. Since the classic description of AIN by W.T. Councilman in 1898,[1] the epidemiology of the disorder has changed significantly and so have the therapeutic implications. In the preantibiotic era, AIN was a complicating feature of scarlet fever, diphtheria, tuberculosis, or other infections, whereas today it is far more likely to result from an immunologic response to drug therapy, except perhaps in children or renal transplant recipients in whom infectious AIN is still seen. The role of the immune system in the pathophysiology of AIN was established more than 30 years ago through experiments in animal models, and the rationale for current therapy largely rests on these classic studies. Unfortunately, randomized, controlled trials of various therapies are notably absent from the medical literature. Therefore, one must consider therapeutic options based on knowledge of the pathophysiology of this disease.

Retrospective series suggest that among patients with acute renal failure, AIN accounts for the primary process in 1% to 4% of all cases or 10% to 15% of those in which a biopsy was performed.[2,3] It is likely that this is an underestimate due to underreporting and the avoidance of renal biopsy in presumed cases of AIN, a practice that we discourage. Some estimate that almost 25% of patients with end-stage renal disease suffer from primary tubulointerstitial injury.[4] Furthermore, a recent case series of adult AIN at a tertiary referral center suggests that the burden of AIN may be increasing, as the annual incidence increased from 1% to 4% over the 12 years analyzed.[2] This increase probably reflects a growth in the polypharmacy of patient care.[5]

Although a complete discussion of the histology and pathophysiology of AIN is beyond the scope of this chapter, many aspects of this disease resemble characteristics of other forms of autoimmune tissue injury. A nephritogenic immune response is initiated when the host reacts to a foreign antigen (e.g., a hapten-protein conjugate[6]), loses tolerance to a self-antigen (e.g., the glycoprotein 3M-1 in the case of antitubular basement membrane [TBM] disease[7]), responds to a neoantigen produced by a toxic insult, or identifies a self-antigen as foreign due to molecular mimicry with an infectious agent.[8] Mononuclear cells, primarily CD4[+] helper T cells and macrophages, infiltrate the interstitium and effect the immune response by inducing a delayed-type hypersensitivity response with the release of inflammatory mediators and by stimulating CD8[+] T cell–mediated cytotoxicity.[4] Although not absolute, parenchymal eosinophils suggest the presence of drug-induced AIN. If neutrophils predominate, one should search for an infectious cause. Tubulitis, characterized by disruption of the TBM and lymphocytic invasion, is more common. The parenchymal inflammation is accompanied by interstitial edema and distortion of the normal architecture. With continued injury, tubular epithelial cells undergo epithelial-mesenchymal transition and join the pool of fibroblasts that produce extracellular matrix and subsequent renal fibrosis.[9] Immune deposits are rarely observed by immunofluorescence or electron microscopy, except in the rare cases of anti-TBM disease in which the TBMs demonstrate linear staining with IgG antibodies.

For the purposes of therapy, AIN may be classified into three major categories: (1) drug-induced AIN, accounting for approximately 70% of cases in recent series; (2) infectious causes, accounting for approximately 8%; and (3) systemic immune disorders among the remainder.[10] A large number of drugs have been associated with AIN, and many have reasonable foundation based on pathophysiology. For example, it was demonstrated in 1975 that methicillin forms a hapten conjugate with proteins along the TBM, leading to a drug-induced form of anti-TBM disease and AIN.[6] The contribution of a detrimental immune response in drug-induced AIN is also suggested by the observations that a reaction to a given drug only occurs in a small percentage of the population, is not dose dependent, is occasionally associated with extrarenal signs and symptoms of hypersensitivity, and usually recurs with rechallenge.[11] Exciting recent data support a direct link between drugs and the immune response; peripheral T cells isolated from patients with AIN activate and proliferate ex vivo when incubated with a specific drug from their regimen.[12] A comprehensive listing of offenders may be found elsewhere, but commonly implicated drugs include β-lactam antibiotics, sulfonamides, nonsteroidal anti-inflammatory drugs, proton pump inhibitors, anticonvulsants, rifampin, allopurinol, cimetidine, and thiazides.[11,13,14]

Infection-related AIN may result from multiple pathogens, but viruses (including BK virus in transplant recipients), leptospirosis, legionella, diphtheria, and tuberculosis are among some of the most frequently seen. AIN may also be observed in conjunction with Sjögren's syndrome, systemic lupus erythematosus, and sarcoidosis. When found in association with uveitis, although not always temporally concordant, it is classified as tubulointerstitial nephritis-uveitis syndrome. Although these causes may seem disparate, the common denominator is the putative role of the immune response in renal inflammation and subsequent destruction. Therefore, attempts at therapeutic intervention have focused on immunomodulators.

CLINICAL APPROACH

Renal fibrosis may develop within 2 weeks of the onset of AIN, and the extent of tubulointerstitial fibrosis correlates with renal survival. This provides the rationale for early definitive diagnosis and treatment.[4] The diagnosis of AIN is suggested by the classic presentation of a patient who has defervesced in response to antibiotic therapy for an infectious illness and then develops a recrudescence of fever associated with a skin rash and a decline in renal function. Although methicillin tended to produce this monomorphic clinical picture, the classic triad of fever, rash, and eosinophilia is found in less than 5% of patients in the current era.[2] Urinary eosinophils detected with Hansel stain and gallium scintigraphy have been proposed to aid in the diagnosis of AIN, but neither is sensitive nor specific enough for routine clinical use. The difficulty in making a clinical diagnosis of AIN is highlighted in a retrospective study by Buysen and colleagues.[15] In a biopsy series of 25 clinically suspected cases of AIN, the diagnosis was confirmed in 11 (44%). They also reviewed the clinical charts of 18 biopsy-proven AIN cases and discovered that the diagnosis had been clinically suspected in only 11 (61%). This bedside error rate demonstrates the potential value of a renal biopsy in establishing the diagnosis, as long as the patient can undergo the procedure without excessive risk and would be a suitable candidate for immunosuppressive therapy. Histological examination of renal tissue with specific attention to the degree of inflammation and tubulointerstitial fibrosis may provide prognostic information and influence the choice or timing of therapy.

THERAPY

The use of immunosuppressive drugs in the treatment of AIN remains controversial because there are no prospective, randomized, controlled trials that evaluate this therapeutic option. Given the varied causes of AIN, the relative scarcity of clinical cases, and the ethical dilemma of withholding potentially beneficial drug therapy from a patient who does not improve after withdrawal of the putative offending agent, it seems unlikely that any such trials will be conducted in the future. Current recommendations for therapy, therefore, are based on numerous case reports and several small, retrospective case series that demonstrate the occasional benefit of immunosuppression. The collective experience is greatest with corticosteroids, and few human data have been published for other immunomodulating drugs such as mycophenolate mofetil (MMF), cyclosporine, and cyclophosphamide.

Withdrawal of the Offending Agent

The initial treatment of AIN is not controversial. Every effort must be made to remove the suspected offending agent immediately after making a diagnosis. In the case of infection-associated AIN, treatment of the underlying infection is analogous to the discontinuation of a medication in drug-induced AIN. The duration of renal injury has been shown to affect the renal outcome; one study reported that AIN patients who suffered acute renal failure for 2 weeks or less had a significantly better renal outcome than those who had ARF for 3 weeks or more (serum creatinine ~1 mg/dL vs. ~3 mg/dL at the end of follow-up).[16] Similarly, continued exposure to a drug responsible for AIN can result in significant irreversible damage, including the need for long-term dialysis.[17–19]

Even though the prompt withdrawal of the offending agent often leads to clinical improvement, it is not known whether this acute improvement suggests the cessation of indolent injury. It is certainly plausible that the destructive immune response is perpetuated by a proinflammatory cytokine milieu that lingers for varying periods of time after the antigen has been removed. Furthermore, the nature and course of the immune response may vary depending on the target moiety. For example, in the era of methicillin-induced AIN, complete recovery of renal function was the rule with the serum creatinine returning to baseline in approximately 90% of reported patients even though the mean duration of renal failure was 1.5 months.[11] In the recent summary by Baker and Pusey[10] of three modern series totaling 128 patients, however, only 64% made a full recovery (serum creatinine < 1.5 mg/dL), 23% made a partial recovery, and 13% remained on renal replacement therapy at the end of follow-up. Whether this difference in prognosis is inherent to the antigen is speculative, but the modern experience supports our belief that AIN can no longer be considered a benign disease.

Corticosteroids

Corticosteroids have been used as immunosuppressive agents for several decades. They effectively attenuate the inflammatory response by suppressing both the innate (macrophage and dendritic cell–mediated) and adaptive (T and B cell–mediated) immune response. Upon binding to glucocorticoid receptors, the receptor-corticosteroid complex translocates to the nucleus, binds to specific DNA sequences (glucocorticoid response elements) that reside in the promoter regions of glucocorticoid-regulated gene products, and recruits coactivator or corepressor proteins, all of which modulate the transcription of inflammatory mediators. By this mechanism, transcription of IκB is up-regulated, leading to the inhibition of the proinflammatory transcription factor nuclear factor-κB. Interestingly, the receptor-corticosteroid complex also directly interacts with nuclear factor-κB, preventing the transcription of cytokines such as interleukin-1, -2, and -6 and tumor necrosis factor α. Corticosteroids also attenuate the production of inflammatory prostaglandins by inhibiting nuclear factor-κB–mediated transcription of cyclooxygenase-2 and through the up-regulation of annexin I (lipocortin-1) and mitogen-activated protein kinase phosphatase 1, two proteins that inhibit cytosolic phospholipase A_{2a}. Last, corticosteroids exert posttranslational effects such as reducing the mRNA stability of inflammatory cytokines and chemokines.[20] These mechanisms provide the scientific rationale for using these drugs to treat AIN.

Perhaps the most often quoted study that demonstrates a beneficial effect of corticosteroids in AIN is a retrospective review by Galpin and colleagues[21] of 14 patients with methicillin-induced AIN (8 biopsy proven). In addition to the withdrawal of methicillin, eight patients received prednisone (mean oral dose, 60 mg/day) for a mean duration of 9.6 days. Compared with the six patients who did not receive prednisone, those in the treated group were more likely to return to their previous normal serum creatinine level (six of eight treated vs. two of six not treated) and achieved their new baseline with greater rapidity (9.3 days vs. 54 days).

Following this report, Linton and colleagues[22] published their experience with nine cases of drug-induced AIN. Withdrawal of the inciting drug led to improvement in only two cases. The seven nonresponders were treated with prednisone 60 mg/day for periods of 6 to 12 days, and all exhibited a prompt diuresis and improvement in renal function within 2 days of initiating steroid therapy. Within 10 days, all treated patients returned to their previous baseline level of renal function. Several other reports describe a similar brisk response to the initiation of steroids in AIN. Pusey and colleagues[23] treated seven episodes of biopsy-proven AIN with high-dose intravenous methylprednisolone (500–1000 mg/day) in a regimen similar to that used for the treatment of acute renal allograft rejection. All patients responded with a remarkable diuresis and/or improvement in renal function within 72 hours of treatment without major side effects. In two additional episodes not treated with steroids, one patient was left with advanced, chronic renal failure and the other achieved normal renal function more slowly than those in the steroid-treated group.

A larger case series evaluated 27 patients with biopsy-proven AIN (15 drug induced, 9 associated with infection, and 3 idiopathic). Seventeen of these patients improved with drug discontinuation or treatment of the associated infection. Ten demonstrated continued renal decline after 5 to 20 days (mean, 10 days) and were then treated with three daily doses of intravenous methylprednisolone or a 3- to 4-week course of oral prednisone (40–60 mg/day). Six (60%) of these patients achieved a normal serum creatinine at a mean of 1 month, and the remaining had a partial improvement in renal function. A plot of renal function over time demonstrates a dramatic correlation between the initiation of steroids and the improvement in serum creatinine in every patient treated.[15]

Enriquez and colleagues[24] observed a similar temporal association of steroid administration and improved renal function. A woman with acute renal failure due to biopsy-proven idiopathic AIN demonstrated rapid improvement in renal function after treatment with three boluses of intravenous methylprednisolone (1000 mg daily) followed by 1 mg/kg/day of oral prednisone. Renal function worsened when steroids were discontinued (serum creatinine: 1.7–5.0 mg/dL), but improved again following their reintroduction. This pattern repeated during the second steroid taper, and the patient again responded favorably to steroids. Eventually, steroids were successfully discontinued and renal function remained stable for an additional year of follow-up with a serum creatinine of 0.9 mg/dL. In a separate dramatic case report, a patient who had been hemodialysis dependent for more than 3 months due to AIN was treated with high-dose methylpred-

nisolone; surprisingly, renal function improved and dialysis was discontinued.[25]

Not all reports describe a beneficial effect of corticosteroids on the prognosis of AIN.[2,19,26,27] The largest published series to date that specifically addresses the role of corticosteroid therapy in the management of AIN is a retrospective analysis by Clarkson and colleagues.[2] Reviewing 2598 adult native renal biopsy specimens at a tertiary referral center over a 12-year period, the authors identified 42 patients with AIN. Patients were excluded if they had findings consistent with acute pyelonephritis, a connective tissue disorder, or sarcoidosis or were found to have a coexisting glomerular disease (except minimal change disease, which is associated with nonsteroidal anti-inflammatory–induced AIN). As expected in a retrospective study of this duration, steroid regimens varied but were initiated within 4 days of renal biopsy and typically comprised intravenous methylprednisolone (500 mg for 2–4 days) followed by oral prednisone (0.75 mg/kg/day tapered over 3–6 weeks). Twenty-six of 42 (60%) patients received corticosteroid therapy, and the remainder received supportive care. Although not a randomized study, the reported baseline characteristics between the conservatively managed and corticosteroid-treated groups were similar. No difference in median serum creatinine was observed between the two groups at 1, 6, and 12 months after diagnosis.[2]

It is important to recognize that although corticosteroid therapy may be associated with side effects such as hypertension, hyperglycemia, psychiatric disturbance, weight gain, and increased risk of infection, none of the studies described herein reported major adverse events due to corticosteroid use. Therefore, we believe that the risk-benefit ratio favors a corticosteroid trial for most patients with biopsy-proven AIN who fail to show an improvement in renal function within days of discontinuing the offending agent. Clinical judgment is required in cases in which this risk-benefit ratio may be higher, such as those already showing marked interstitial fibrosis and/or minimal active inflammation at the time of biopsy. If renal biopsy is absolutely contraindicated, an empirical trial of corticosteroids may be reasonable if the history and evaluation are strongly suggestive of AIN and removal of the inciting agent does not produce a satisfactory clinical response.

Mycophenolate Mofetil

It is somewhat surprising that the largest reported human experience with immunomodulatory agents other than corticosteroids for AIN is a retrospective, single-center study of MMF use in eight patients.[28] MMF is widely used in solid-organ transplantation and has been shown to reduce the incidence of acute rejection in renal allograft recipients.[29] It is a prodrug of mycophenolic acid (MPA), an inhibitor of the rate-limiting enzyme inosine monophosphate dehydrogenase in the de novo pathway of purine synthesis. Since T and B cells are more dependent on this pathway than most other cells, they are especially prone to the antiproliferative effects of MPA. Moreover, MPA is an especially potent inhibitor of type II inosine monophosphate dehydrogenase, which is expressed in activated lymphocytes. It also induces apoptosis of activated T cells and suppresses the expression of cell adhesion molecules, thereby decreasing mononuclear cell recruitment to sites of inflammation.[30]

Preddie and colleagues[28] published the first case series of MMF use in steroid-dependent biopsy-proven AIN. These eight patients received at least 6 months of steroids (in one or two courses) and experienced a worsening of the serum creatinine when steroids were tapered or discontinued. Acute interstitial nephritis was attributed to drugs in two patients, mixed connective tissue disease in one, and an idiopathic cause in three; granulomatous interstitial nephritis was observed in the remaining two patients, associated with sarcoid in one and with perinuclear antineutrophil cytoplasmic antibody seropositivity in the other. MMF was initiated at 500 to 1000 mg twice daily and titrated to 1000 mg twice daily as tolerated by the leukocyte count and gastrointestinal side effects. Renal function improved in six of the eight patients, defined as a decrease in serum creatinine of at least 0.3 mg/dL, and the remaining two experienced no significant change in function. At the most recent follow-up before the authors published their experience (mean, 28 months; range, 14–40), all had discontinued corticosteroids and five patients had discontinued MMF as well. In another isolated case report, a pediatric patient with renal-limited sarcoidosis was maintained successfully on MMF after induction therapy with corticosteroids.[31] Although we do not recommend MMF for initial treatment of AIN, it may find future use in select cases characterized by a relapsing steroid-responsive pattern.

Cyclophosphamide and Cyclosporine

Not all patients with AIN experience improved renal function after removal of the offending agent and a trial of corticosteroids. In these unfortunate circumstances, there are no published human trials or case series to guide further therapy with alternative immunomodulatory agents. Convincing experimental evidence in animal models and anecdotal human reports, however, suggest that cyclophosphamide and cyclosporine may have a role in the treatment algorithm for select cases of steroid-resistant AIN.

Cyclophosphamide is an alkylating agent that gained popularity in the 1970s for the treatment of lupus and vasculitis. It forms covalent bonds and cross-links a variety of macromolecules, with DNA likely being the most important. Cross-linking DNA impairs replication and transcription and ultimately leads to cell death or dysfunction. This makes cyclophosphamide one of the most potent immunosuppressant drugs available, but also one that carries a substantial risk of toxicity.

The level of evidence available for cyclophosphamide use in AIN comes primarily from experimental animals. Brown Norway rats immunized with rabbit renal TBMs provide an experimental model of severe tubulointerstitial nephritis. The appearance of anti-TBM antibodies is followed by an intense mononuclear cell infiltrate (mainly T cells and macrophages) within several weeks. Agus and colleagues[32] demonstrated that treatment with daily oral cyclophosphamide beginning at the time of immunization prevented the development of anti-TBM antibodies and histologic lesions. More important, when therapy was initiated after established interstitial disease, progression of histologic lesions halted. With administration early in the course of established disease, there was even a trend toward regression of histological severity and decreased serum creatinine. To extrapolate this rat model of anti-TBM disease to human AIN is not easy, but the study does provide

a rationale for a therapeutic trial in select cases. The published use of cyclophosphamide in human AIN consists of anecdotal experience mainly in the setting of sarcoidosis and a single case report of presumed drug-induced granulomatous AIN in the setting of concomitant chronic lymphocytic leukemia.[33] In the latter case, the authors assumed their regimen of corticosteroids and a single dose of intravenous cyclophosphamide treated the patient's AIN and chronic lymphocytic leukemia, respectively. The patient, who was dialysis dependent due to acute renal failure, recovered her renal function after 6 weeks of hemodialysis and achieved a baseline serum creatinine of 2.8 mg/dL 9 months after diagnosis.[33] It is unknown what effect the cyclophosphamide had, if any, on the course of AIN in this case.

A full discussion of the use of cyclophosphamide is beyond the scope of this chapter, and the reader is referred to Chapter 10 ("Immunosuppressive Agents for the Therapy of Glomerular and Tubulointerstitial Disease") for additional information. The patient should be made aware of the risks of cyclophosphamide therapy, including teratogenicity, hematologic toxicity, infection, malignancy (bladder cancer being the most common tumor associated with daily oral therapy), hemorrhagic cystitis, alopecia, and gonadal toxicity (in both men and women, with the incidence among women increasing with age).[34] Some physicians will bank sperm or eggs if the patient is of child-bearing age. These risks increase with cumulative dose and length of treatment and must be reflected in the risk-benefit ratio for an individual patient.

The risk of malignancy secondary to cyclophosphamide therapy is difficult to quantify, as retrospective analyses are plagued by confounding variables such as concomitant carcinogenic drug exposure, other therapies (e.g., external radiation), and the oncogenic potential of the underlying disease process. Noting these limitations, a case-control study of breast cancer patients suggests that even after adjustment for radiation exposure, a cumulative dose of cyclophosphamide greater than 20 g may be associated with an increased risk of hematological malignancy.[35] Most reports of malignancy, however, report greater cumulative doses and durations of therapy than we would suggest for treating AIN. For example, in a retrospective study of 119 patients with rheumatoid arthritis, the mean total dose and duration of cyclophosphamide was 74.9 g over 43.8 months in those who developed a subsequent malignancy compared with 45.8 g over 28.1 months in control patients.[36] In a National Institutes of Health cohort of 145 patients with Wegener's granulomatosis treated with oral cyclophosphamide, eight patients (6%) developed transitional-cell carcinoma of the bladder. The duration from initiation of therapy to diagnosis of bladder cancer ranged from 7 months to 17 years, and seven of the eight patients had received a total of more than 100 g of cyclophosphamide.[37] Regarding the treatment of AIN, if a comparatively short course of cyclophosphamide successfully improves renal function in a patient with severe renal dysfunction after other therapies have failed, the benefit of avoiding the morbidity and mortality of end-stage renal disease may outweigh the potential therapeutic risks. Generally, we attempt oral cyclophosphamide 2 mg/kg/day and stop therapy if the serum creatinine does not decrease by 6 to 8 weeks. If the patient responds, a reasonable approach would be to continue therapy for 4 months, at which time an alternative agent (such as MMF) could be substituted to minimize cyclophosphamide exposure.

Cyclosporin A has been used in transplantation and immune-mediated diseases since the 1980s. This fungus-derived endecapeptide binds to cyclophilin, and the resulting complex subsequently inhibits the serine/threonine phosphatase calcineurin. The loss of calcineurin's phosphatase activity prevents the translocation of cytosolic nuclear factor of activated T cells to the nucleus for transcription of interleukin-2, thereby inhibiting T-cell activation.[34] The effectiveness of cyclosporine to treat established AIN was tested in the Brown Norway rat model of anti-TBM disease described previously.[38] Similar to cyclophosphamide, multiple investigators have demonstrated that cyclosporine halts disease progression, even when initiated after disease is established, by inhibiting the cell-mediated immune response.[38–40]

Cyclosporine has been used in a few cases of the tubulointerstitial nephritis-uveitis syndrome, but these reports do not provide adequate data to assess renal response; in fact, with the exception of one case, most attribute renal improvement to preceding courses of corticosteroids.[41–43] One case report of a severe vancomycin-associated hypersensitivity reaction with skin rash and visceral involvement (hepatitis and acute renal failure with pyuria, eosinophiluria, and low-grade proteinuria) attributed a dramatic clinical improvement to a 5-day course of cyclosporine (100 mg twice daily) after 3 weeks of steroid administration had failed. The skin rash resolved within a week and was accompanied by a slow, but stable, improvement in renal function. The patient, who had been dialysis dependent for 6 weeks at the time of cyclosporine initiation, was able to discontinue renal replacement therapy 5 weeks later and had a serum creatinine of 1.0 mg/dL 20 months after initial presentation.[44] Although the rapid resolution of skin lesions was temporally related to cyclosporine treatment, it is speculative as to whether the drug also led to the improvement in renal function. In addition, when contemplating the use of cyclosporine, the drug's nephrotoxic potential must be considered as well as its proclivity to stimulate the renal fibrogenesis that one is attempting to suppress.[45]

SPECIFIC RECOMMENDATIONS

It is important to establish a definitive diagnosis of AIN early in its course. There are no clinical, laboratory, or imaging features with adequate sensitivity or specificity to rule out the diagnosis. With a good clinical story, we favor the use of early renal biopsy if the procedure and the use of immunosuppressive therapy are not contraindicated by the patient's general medical condition. In addition to providing the diagnosis, histologic analysis may guide therapy. For example, the presence of a diffuse cellular infiltrate or granulomatous inflammation may encourage the use of immunosuppressive agents, whereas the presence of significant fibrosis may favor withholding potentially toxic therapy.

As outlined in Figure 27-1, the putative agent(s) responsible for the inflammatory response must be discontinued or treated as soon as the diagnosis is suspected.

In patients who do not demonstrate substantial improvement within several days of removing the inciting agent, we recommend a trial of corticosteroids (Table 27-1). Prednisone 1 mg/kg/day (maximum 80 mg/day) should be initiated, preceded in severe cases by pulse high-dose intravenous methylprednisolone (250–1000 mg/day for 1–3 days) at the clinician's

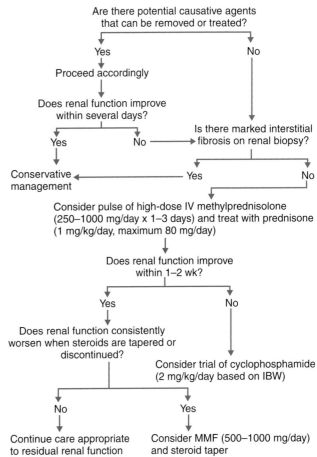

Figure 27-1 Suggested treatment algorithm for acute interstitial nephritis. IBW, ideal body weight. See text for details.

discretion. If renal function improves within 7 to 10 days, the drug should be continued for approximately 2 months and then tapered over the next several weeks.

If renal function improves with steroid use but repeatedly worsens during the taper or with discontinuation, MMF may be administered as a steroid-sparing alternative. We recommend an initial dose of 500 mg twice daily, titrated to 1000 mg twice daily if gastrointestinal symptoms and the leukocyte count permit.

In cases of severe AIN that do not respond to corticosteroid therapy within 1 to 2 weeks, cyclophosphamide may be considered if histologic examination of the renal parenchyma suggests potential salvage. In these difficult cases, we suggest the addition of oral cyclophosphamide (2 mg/kg/day based on ideal body weight) with steroids. In nonresponders, the drug should be discontinued after 6 to 8 weeks to minimize toxicity. In responders, there are no data to guide duration of therapy, but it would not be unreasonable to continue cyclophosphamide for 4 months, at which time a switch to another immunosuppressant agent, such as MMF, could be considered, akin to induction and maintenance therapy for lupus nephritis. In our opinion, corticosteroids may be maintained at lower doses (20–40 mg/day) while initially treating with cyclophosphamide. Vigilance for leukopenia, infections, and microscopic hematuria is exceedingly important.

Supportive therapy for patients with acute renal failure includes dialysis as necessary. For patients who recover partial

Table 27-1 Immunosuppressive Drugs and Level of Evidence for Use in Acute Interstitial Nephritis

Drug	Initial Dose / Route / Duration*	Level of Evidence
Methylprednisolone	250 to 1000 mg/day for 1–3 days (IV), followed by oral prednisone	Retrospective case series
Prednisone	1 mg/kg/day (max. 80 mg daily; oral) for 7–10 days, frequently assessing for response	Retrospective case series
Mycophenolate mofetil	500 mg twice daily, titrating to 1000 mg twice daily, as steroids are tapered	Retrospective case series (relapsing steroid-responsive cases only)
Cyclophosphamide	2 mg/kg/day (based on IBW; oral) for 6–8 weeks, frequently assessing for response and toxicity	Experimental animal data; anecdotal human reports
Cyclosporine	3 mg/kg/day in divided doses twice daily (based on IBW; oral) for 4–6 weeks, frequently assessing for response and toxicity	Experimental animal data; anecdotal human reports

*Initial doses and therapeutic trial durations are provided; see text for details. Given the lack of adequate evidence regarding the use of immunosuppressant drugs in AIN, the treating physician must rely on clinical judgment, involve the patient in the decision making, and individualize therapy.
IBW, ideal body weight.

renal function, appropriate attention should be given to chronic kidney disease care, including the use of renin-angiotensin system blockade, in an attempt to obviate renal progression.

FUTURE DIRECTIONS

We have witnessed an impressive growth of knowledge in the field of immunology over the past several years, and many new immunomodulatory agents have entered routine clinical use, testing, or active development. Given that not one randomized, controlled trial has been performed for AIN therapy to date, however, we are not optimistic that these new agents will take positions outside of the occasional case report or small series. Because tubulointerstitial fibrosis is the final common pathway to all chronic kidney diseases, it is likely that the development of drugs targeting fibrogenesis will have more of an impact on the prognosis of these patients. For example, we are encouraged by recent elegant work that suggests that bone morphogenic protein-7 administration reverses transforming growth factor β_1–mediated epithelial-mesenchymal transition and renal pathology in an animal model of chronic kidney disease.[46] Other mediators of transforming growth factor β signaling may also hold promise, such as a transforming growth factor β type I receptor kinase (ALK5) inhibitor that ameliorated fibrosis in an animal model of obstructive nephropathy.[47] These approaches are far from routine clinical application but hold considerable promise for the future.

References

1. Councilman WT: Acute interstitial nephritis. J Exp Med 1898;3: 393–420.
2. Clarkson MR, Giblin L, O'Connell FP, et al: Acute interstitial nephritis: Clinical features and response to corticosteroid therapy. Nephrol Dial Transplant 2004;19:2778–2783.
3. Wilson DM, Turner DR, Cameron JS, et al: Value of renal biopsy in acute intrinsic renal failure. Br Med J 1976;2:459–461.
4. Neilson EG: Pathogenesis and therapy of interstitial nephritis. Kidney Int 1989;35:1257–1270.
5. Neilson EG: The downside of a drug-crazed world. J Am Soc Nephrol 2006;17:2650–2651.
6. Border WA, Lehman DH, Egan JD, et al: Antitubular basement-membrane antibodies in methicillin-associated interstitial nephritis. N Engl J Med 1974;291:381–384.
7. Clayman MD, Martinez-Hernandez A, Michaud L, et al: Isolation and characterization of the nephritogenic antigen producing anti-tubular basement membrane disease. J Exp Med 1985;161:290–305.
8. Sherlock JE: Interstitial nephritis in rats produced by E. coli in adjuvant: immunological findings. Clin Exp Immunol 1977;30:154–159.
9. Kalluri R, Neilson EG: Epithelial-mesenchymal transition and its implications for fibrosis. J Clin Invest 2003;112: 1776–1284.
10. Baker RJ, Pusey CD: The changing profile of acute tubulointerstitial nephritis. Nephrol Dial Transplant 2004;19:8–11.
11. Rossert J: Drug-induced acute interstitial nephritis. Kidney Int 2001;60:804–817.
12. Spanou Z, Keller M, Britschgi M, et al: Involvement of drug-specific T cells in acute drug-induced interstitial nephritis. J Am Soc Nephrol 2006;17:2919–2927.
13. Geevasinga N, Coleman PL, Webster AC, Roger SD: Proton pump inhibitors and acute interstitial nephritis. Clin Gastroenterol Hepatol 2006;4:597–604.
14. Murray KM, Keane WR: Review of drug-induced acute interstitial nephritis. Pharmacotherapy 1992;12:462–467.
15. Buysen JG, Houthoff HJ, Krediet RT, Arisz L: Acute interstitial nephritis: A clinical and morphological study in 27 patients. Nephrol Dial Transplant 1990;5:94–99.
16. Laberke HG, Bohle A: Acute interstitial nephritis: Correlations between clinical and morphological findings. Clin Nephrol 1980;14:263–273.
17. Baldwin DS, Levine BB, McCluskey RT, Gallo GR: Renal failure and interstitial nephritis due to penicillin and methicillin. N Engl J Med 1968;279:1245–1252.
18. Jensen HA, Halveg AB, Saunamaki KI: Permanent impairment of renal function after methicillin nephropathy. Br Med J 1971;4:406.
19. Schwarz A, Krause PH, Kunzendorf U, et al: The outcome of acute interstitial nephritis: Risk factors for the transition from acute to chronic interstitial nephritis. Clin Nephrol 2000;54:179–190.

20. Rhen T, Cidlowski JA: Antiinflammatory action of glucocorticoids—new mechanisms for old drugs. N Engl J Med 2005;353:1711–1723.
21. Galpin JE, Shinaberger JH, Stanley TM, et al: Acute interstitial nephritis due to methicillin. Am J Med 1978;65:756–765.
22. Linton AL, Clark WF, Driedger AA, et al: Acute interstitial nephritis due to drugs: Review of the literature with a report of nine cases. Ann Intern Med 1980;93:735–741.
23. Pusey CD, Saltissi D, Bloodworth L, et al: Drug associated acute interstitial nephritis: Clinical and pathological features and the response to high dose steroid therapy. Q J Med 1983;52:194–211.
24. Enriquez R, Gonzalez C, Cabezuelo JB, et al: Relapsing steroid-responsive idiopathic acute interstitial nephritis. Nephron 1993;63:462–465.
25. Frommer P, Uldall R, Fay WP, Deveber GA: A case of acute interstitial nephritis successfully treated after delayed diagnosis. CMAJ 1979;121:585–586, 591.
26. Bhaumik SK, Kher V, Arora P, et al: Evaluation of clinical and histological prognostic markers in drug-induced acute interstitial nephritis. Ren Fail 1996;18:97–104.
27. Koselj M, Kveder R, Bren AF, Rott T: Acute renal failure in patients with drug-induced acute interstitial nephritis. Ren Fail 1993;15:69–72.
28. Preddie DC, Markowitz GS, Radhakrishnan J, et al: Mycophenolate mofetil for the treatment of interstitial nephritis. Clin J Am Soc Nephrol 2006;1:718–722.
29. The Tricontinental Mycophenolate Mofetil Renal Transplantation Study Group: A blinded, randomized clinical trial of mycophenolate mofetil for the prevention of acute rejection in cadaveric renal transplantation. Transplantation 1996;61:1029–1037.
30. Allison AC, Eugui EM: Mycophenolate mofetil and its mechanisms of action. Immunopharmacology 2000;47:85–118.
31. Moudgil A, Przygodzki RM, Kher KK: Successful steroid-sparing treatment of renal limited sarcoidosis with mycophenolate mofetil. Pediatr Nephrol 2006;21:281–285.
32. Agus D, Mann R, Clayman M, et al: The effects of daily cyclophosphamide administration on the development and extent of primary experimental interstitial nephritis in rats. Kidney Int 1986;29:635–640.
33. Pena de la Vega L, Fervenza FC, Lager D, et al: Acute granulomatous interstitial nephritis secondary to bisphosphonate alendronate sodium. Ren Fail 2005;27:485–489.
34. Stein CM: Immunoregulatory drugs. In Harris ED, Ruddy S, Kelley WN (eds): Kelley's Textbook of Rheumatology, 7th ed. Philadelphia: Elsevier/Saunders, 2005, pp 922–924.
35. Curtis RE, Boice JD Jr, Stovall M, et al: Risk of leukemia after chemotherapy and radiation treatment for breast cancer. N Engl J Med 1992;326:1745–1751.
36. Baker GL, Kahl LE, Zee BC, et al: Malignancy following treatment of rheumatoid arthritis with cyclophosphamide. Long-term case-control follow-up study. Am J Med 1987;83:1–9.
37. Talar-Williams C, Hijazi YM, Walther MM, et al: Cyclophosphamide-induced cystitis and bladder cancer in patients with Wegener granulomatosis. Ann Intern Med 1996;124:477–484.
38. Shih W, Hines WH, Neilson EG: Effects of cyclosporin A on the development of immune-mediated interstitial nephritis. Kidney Int 1988;33:1113–1118.
39. Gimenez A, Leyva-Cobian F, Fierro C, et al: Effect of cyclosporin A on autoimmune tubulointerstitial nephritis in the brown Norway rat. Clin Exp Immunol 1987;69:550–556.
40. Thoenes GH, Umscheid T, Sitter T, Langer KH: Cyclosporin A inhibits autoimmune experimental tubulointerstitial nephritis. Immunol Lett 1987;15:301–306.
41. Gion N, Stavrou P, Foster CS: Immunomodulatory therapy for chronic tubulointerstitial nephritis-associated uveitis. Am J Ophthalmol 2000;129:764–768.
42. Guerriero S, Vischi A, Giancipoli G, et al: Tubulointerstitial nephritis and uveitis syndrome. J Pediatr Ophthalmol Strabismus 2006;43:241–243.
43. Sanchez-Burson J, Garcia-Porrua C, Montero-Granados R, et al: Tubulointerstitial nephritis and uveitis syndrome in southern Spain. Semin Arthritis Rheum 2002;32:125–129.
44. Zuliani E, Zwahlen H, Gilliet F, Marone C: Vancomycin-induced hypersensitivity reaction with acute renal failure: Resolution following cyclosporine treatment. Clin Nephrol 2005;64:155–158.
45. Burdmann EA, Andoh TF, Yu L, Bennett WM: Cyclosporine nephrotoxicity. Semin Nephrol 2003;23:465–476.
46. Zeisberg M, Hanai J, Sugimoto H, et al: BMP-7 counteracts TGF-beta1-induced epithelial-to-mesenchymal transition and reverses chronic renal injury. Nat Med 2003;9:964–968.
47. Moon JA, Kim HT, Cho IS, et al: IN-1130, a novel transforming growth factor-beta type I receptor kinase (ALK5) inhibitor, suppresses renal fibrosis in obstructive nephropathy. Kidney Int 2006;70:1234–1243.

Further Reading

Baker RJ, Pusey CD: The changing profile of acute tubulointerstitial nephritis. Nephrol Dial Transplant 2004;19:8–11.
Clarkson MR, Giblin L, O'Connell FP, et al: Acute interstitial nephritis: Clinical features and response to corticosteroid therapy. Nephrol Dial Transplant 2004;19:2778–2783.
Michel DM, Kelly CJ: Acute interstitial nephritis. J Am Soc Nephrol 1998;9:506–515.
Neilson EG: Pathogenesis and therapy of interstitial nephritis. Kidney Int 1989;35:1257–1270.
Rossert J: Drug-induced acute interstitial nephritis. Kidney Int 2001;60:804–817.

PART III

Diabetic Nephropathy

CONTENTS

Chapter 28

Therapy for Diabetic Nephropathy

William L. Whittier, Julia B. Lewis, and Edmund J. Lewis

Diabetic nephropathy (DN) is the single most common cause of end-stage renal disease (ESRD) in the United States and Europe. According to the World Health Organization, more than 171 million people worldwide have diabetes mellitus (DM) (www.who.int/diabetes/facts/world_figures/en, accessed June 2007) and approximately 30% to 40% will develop DN.[1] Many of these patients will reach ESRD, although in the United States, the number of patients entering the Medicare ESRD program with DM appears to have plateaued.[2] Many patients with early DN die of cardiovascular events before reaching ESRD. DM and chronic kidney disease (CKD) are independent risk factors for increased cardiovascular (CV) morbidity and mortality. Patients with DM and CKD have even higher mortality rates than patients without DM and CKD.[3] The CV risk associated with CKD is present with an estimated glomerular filtration rate (GFR) as high as 60 mL/min, and the risk increases with declining renal function.[4] This chapter reviews strategies to care for the patient with DN and impede the devastating progression of DN.

PREVENTION

The clinical course of DN has been best defined in patients with type 1 DM, as the time of onset of the disease in these patients is so readily apparent. Studies of type 2 DM and nephropathy are less readily defined; however, the reported experience in the type 2 diabetics seen in Native Americans, specifically the Pima Indians of Arizona, would indicate that the clinical course in these patients who develop type 2 DM at an early age mirrors that of the type 1 population.[5–7] The natural history of DN is summarized in Figure 28-1. After a period of glomerular hyperfiltration, the earliest clinically detectable stage of DN is microalbuminuria. Generally, patients have the onset of abnormal urine albumin excretion from 5 to 10 years after the onset of DM. Microalbuminuria is defined as the excretion of small amounts of albumin, below the level that can be detected by a traditional urinary dipstick evaluation. This level is quantified (Table 28-1) and arbitrarily determined to be clinically relevant if within the range of 20 to 200 mg albumin per gram of creatinine in a spot urine specimen or 30 to 300 mg of albumin in a 24-hour urine collection. When microalbuminuria is the result of DM, it progresses to overt nephropathy, defined by urinary albumin excretion rates of 300 mg or more in 24 hours, in up to 50% of patients in 5 to 10 years.[8–12] Clinical predictors of the development of microalbuminuria and progression to overt nephropathy include increased age, male gender, African American or Hispanic race, smoking, increased body mass index, elevated glycosylated hemoglobin, presence of proliferative diabetic retinopathy, duration of DM, dyslipidemias, and systolic hypertension.[13–17] Once albuminuria is established, if untreated, a decrease in GFR of up to 50% will occur within 2 years.[18]

With the advent of medications that slow progression of DN, the primary cause of death has shifted from renal failure to CV disease. Patients with DM who have never had a CV event are at greater risk of having one than a patient without DM but with a known history of a CV event.[19] The risk of a CV event is higher in a diabetic patient with nephropathy and progressively increases as GFR decreases.[20–22] Treatment that prevents the progression of renal disease becomes the cornerstone of therapy for delaying ESRD with all of its attendant CV risks.

Glycemic Control for the Prevention of Diabetic Nephropathy

Poorly controlled glucose carries an inherent risk of complications in patients with DM. Impaired fasting glucose is an established risk factor for developing CV complications.[19,23] Furthermore, data from observational studies have demonstrated a consistent association of poorly controlled blood sugars and the development and progression of DN.[24–27]

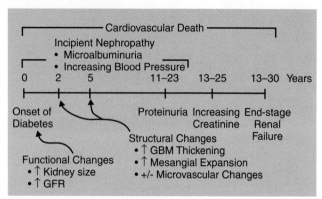

Figure 28-1 Typical natural history of diabetic nephropathy for a patient with type 2 diabetes mellitus. Glomerular filtration rate (GFR) is elevated at the onset of diabetes mellitus. Structural changes follow. With the development of microalbuminuria, there is typically an increase in blood pressure, and advancing structural damage appears in the kidney and vasculature elsewhere. With progression to overt proteinuria, the GFR starts to decrease usually in a linear fashion and, without intervention, the patient reaches end-stage renal failure. The risk of cardiovascular death is present early in the course of diabetic nephropathy and progresses as the renal disease advances. GBM, glomerular basement membrane. (Modified from Lewis JB: Diabetic nephropathy in patients with type II diabetes. Geriatr Nephrol Urol 1999;9:168.)

Treating poorly controlled glucose is therefore essential, and several studies have evaluated the impact of intensive glycemic control on preventing the complications of DM.

Two clinical trials have examined the hypothesis that intensive blood glucose control could slow or prevent the development of complications of DM including nephropathy.[28,29] The Diabetes Control and Complications Trial[28] was a prospective trial randomizing 1441 patients with type 1 DM to conventional versus intensive blood glucose control. The patients were followed for an average of 6.5 years and achieved mean hemoglobin A1C values of 7.2% and 9.1% for the intensive and conventional arms, respectively. Patients in the intensive group had a significantly lower incidence of developing microalbuminuria and overt albuminuria compared with the conventional group. Interestingly, the beneficial effect persisted even after the trial ended, when, on long-term follow-up, the group of patients in the intensive arm during the study period had a sustained beneficial effect on preventing the development of microalbuminuria, overt albuminuria, and

hypertension despite a lack of persistent difference in achieved hemoglobin A1C values on follow-up.[30,31] The Diabetes Control and Complications Trial was a landmark study demonstrating conclusively that intensive blood glucose control in patients with type 1 DM will slow or prevent the development of DN as well as other complications of DM.

This same hypothesis was tested in the United Kingdom Prospective Diabetes Study (UKPDS) in patients with type 2 DM.[29] The investigators randomized 3867 patients with newly diagnosed type 2 DM to receive intensive therapy with oral hypoglycemic agents or insulin versus conventional therapy with diet alone. The average hemoglobin A1C values achieved were 7.0% in the intensive arm versus 7.9% in the conventional arm. Patients randomized to the intensive therapy group had a significant decrease in any diabetes-related endpoint, but no statistically significant decrease in the development of microalbuminuria, albuminuria, or twofold increase in the serum creatinine. However, renal function was tested infrequently. These data did not demonstrate a positive effect of aggressive glycemic control in the prevention of DN in type 2 DM in the UKPDS population. In another study of intense glucose control in 110 Japanese patients with type 2 DM, intensive insulin therapy reduced the development of microalbuminuria and overt albuminuria compared with less intensive insulin therapy.[32] This effect persisted at follow-up of 8 years.[32,33]

Although the optimal level of glycemic control is unknown, the current American Diabetes Association guidelines recommend that the hemoglobin A1C level be kept at less than 7% in patients with type 1 and 2 DM.[34]

Control of Blood Pressure for the Prevention of Diabetic Nephropathy

Profound evidence exists of the importance of blood pressure control and choice of antihypertensive therapy in patients with existing DN (see "Therapy of Diabetic Nephropathy"). The answer to the question of whether patients with established type 1 or 2 DM are less likely to develop progressive nephropathy if their blood pressure is well controlled is not as clear. Observational studies have linked the presence of hypertension and uncontrolled blood pressure to the development of microalbuminuria or proteinuria in patients with DM.[8,9,16,17,24,27] Randomized, controlled trials have had conflicting results. Embedded within the UKPDS study was a trial comparing two levels of blood pressure control with regard to the development of macrovascular and microvascular complications in 1148 hypertensive patients with type 2 DM and a normal GFR.[35] During the

Table 28-1 Categories of Urinary Protein Excretion

	Dipstick Protein	24-Hour Protein	24-Hour Albumin	Spot Collection	Timed Collection
Normal	Negative	<150 mg	<30 mg	<30 μg albumin/mg creatinine	<20 μg/min
Microalbuminuria	Negative	150–500 mg	30–300 mg	30–300 μg albumin/mg creatinine	20–200 μg/min
Overt nephropathy	1(+) to 4(+)	≥500 mg	≥300 mg	≥300 μg albumin/mg creatinine	≥200 μg/min

mean follow-up of 8.4 years, the mean blood pressure in those patients with more active blood pressure control (mean achieved blood pressure, 144/82 mm Hg) was lower than the group with less tight control (mean achieved blood pressure, 154/87 mm Hg). The risk of any complication or death from diabetes, myocardial infarction, and the composite of microvascular complications was less with lower systolic blood pressure.[36] This study was unable to demonstrate a statistically significant benefit of lower blood pressure on the renal endpoints of proteinuria or twofold increase in the serum creatinine. However, it is important to emphasize that the UKPDS was not designed as a trial to examine renal endpoints.

The Appropriate Blood Pressure in Diabetes study[37] was carried out to determine the importance of blood pressure control in an attempt to prevent the onset of progressive renal dysfunction. The investigators randomized 480 normotensive patients with type 2 DM to intensive blood pressure or moderate blood pressure control and observed these patients over 5 years. There was a significant decrease in the development of albuminuria in the group randomized to the intensive therapy. However, the primary endpoint of the study was a change in creatinine clearance, and no difference was noted between the groups.

As noted below, intensive blood pressure control is an important therapeutic goal in the diabetic population, particularly with respect to the prevention of CV events and treatment of the course of established renal disease. However, the value of blood pressure control as a preventive measure with respect to the onset of nephropathy remains an open question.

Blockade of the Renin-Angiotensin System to Prevent Diabetic Nephropathy

Before the onset of microalbuminuria, the initial mechanism in the development of DN is renal hypertrophy, hyperfunction, and glomerular hyperfiltration. Evidence derived from the measurement of glomerular hemodynamic parameters in experimental diabetes in the rat reveals increased intraglomerular pressures from the direct transmission of pressure along a dilated afferent arteriole as well as vasoconstriction due to the effects of increased angiotensin II on the efferent arteriole. Blockade of the angiotensin II effect on the efferent arteriole with angiotensin-converting enzyme (ACE) inhibitors leads to an improvement in the elevated intraglomerular pressure, which may well account for the preservation of glomerular structure and function in DM.[38-41]

In view of the apparent central role of angiotensin II antagonism in the interruption of a pathogenic pathway in DM, which can result in glomerular damage, the question has arisen whether blockade of the renin-angiotensin system (RAS) prevents the development of clinically detectable DN. The Bergamo Nephrologic Diabetes Complications Trial[42,43] was a multicenter, controlled trial designed to investigate whether blood pressure control and choice of blood pressure agent could prevent the onset of microalbuminuria in patients with hypertension and type 2 DM. A total of 1204 patients were randomized to receive the ACE inhibitor trandolapril, the calcium channel blocker verapamil, a combination of trandolapril and verapamil, or placebo and followed for a median of 3.6 years. The primary outcome of developing microalbuminuria was the defined endpoint of the development of DN, and this was less in the groups receiving trandolapril. The verapamil arm was equivalent to placebo. A post hoc analysis

revealed that treatment with the ACE inhibitor trandolapril prevented microalbuminuria independent of blood pressure control.[43] This study supports the recommendation that treatment of patients with type 2 DM without clinically detectable DN with an ACE inhibitor is effective in reducing the development of early nephropathy.

Cardiovascular Risk Reduction

Patients with DM, and even more so for patients with DN, are prone to CV complications and death. Targeting a global decrease in CV risk, especially early in the course of the disease, is instrumental in promoting the long-term health of these patients. Unfortunately, although there is much evidence demonstrating the benefit of a variety of interventions to reduce CV events in patients with DM, patients with DN are typically excluded from these trials. However, the Steno-2 trial evaluated such an approach for patients with type 2 DM and microalbuminuria.[44] One hundred sixty patients were randomly assigned to either an intensified treatment plan of lifestyle modification, smoking cessation, pharmacologic therapy for hyperglycemia, hypertension, dyslipidemia, microalbuminuria, and aspirin or conventional therapy and followed for an average of 7.8 years. Patients who received intensive therapy had a significant decrease in CV death and events, peripheral vascular disease, urinary albumin excretion, as well as retinopathy and neuropathy. Although this study was not designed to detect which therapy was responsible for the greatest effect, clearly an organized global approach to decrease in CV risk was beneficial.

More specific therapy of blocking the RAS for decreasing CV events has also been tested. The Heart Outcomes Prevention Evaluation trial was a randomized, controlled study of patients with vascular disease or DM performed in an attempt to ascertain a CV effect of the ACE inhibitor ramipril versus placebo. Compared with placebo, treatment with ramipril significantly reduced the primary outcome of a composite of myocardial infarction, stroke, or death from CV causes over a 5-year period.[45] The trial enrolled 9297 patients, 3577 (38%) of whom had DM. The MICRO-Heart Outcomes Prevention Evaluation substudy of the Heart Outcomes Prevention Evaluation trial examined these 3577 patients for the same primary outcome with the addition of the development of overt nephropathy. The study was halted early because of the consistent benefit of ramipril for all CV outcomes as well as nephropathy.[46] Additional evidence was supplied by the Reduction in End-Points in Non-Insulin Dependent Diabetes Mellitus with the Angiotensin II Antagonist Losartan trial investigators.[47] In this study, over a follow-up period of 3.4 years, 1513 patients with overt DN from type 2 DM were randomized to receive angiotensin antagonism with losartan 100 mg/day or placebo. The primary outcome of the composite of doubling of the serum creatinine, ESRD, or death was significantly lower in the group assigned to losartan. A secondary analysis of this study[48,49] demonstrated that albuminuria was the strongest predictor of CV outcome. There was an 18% decrease in CV risk for every 50% decrease in albuminuria, and a 27% decrease in heart failure risk for every 50% decrease in albuminuria. This lends additional support for the cardioprotective role of blockade of the RAS and decrease in albuminuria in the patient with DN.

Patients with DM have the same risk of cardiac mortality as patients with known coronary artery disease.[19] As patients with CKD and ESRD from DN have an even greater risk,[3,50] it remains essential to reduce this risk with lifestyle modification, smoking cessation, aspirin, and pharmacologic therapy for hyperglycemia, hypertension, dyslipidemia, and albuminuria.

THERAPY OF DIABETIC NEPHROPATHY

The natural history of DN has been altered by therapeutic interventions that reduce the malignant course and delay the progression to ESRD. Blockade of the RAS, blood pressure control, and blood glucose control all have a role in maintaining preservation of renal function. As the nephropathy progresses, treating the sequelae of CKD and adjusting medications for the decrease in GFR become important aspects of patient care. With these therapies, there has been a remarkable decrease in new onset ESRD from DN since 1995.[2,51]

Blood Pressure Control

Initial studies of blood pressure reduction in patients with DN were performed with small numbers of patients but demonstrated an overall benefit of blood pressure control. In 1982, Mogensen[52] evaluated the effects of blood pressure control on progression of DN. He reported that lowering blood pressure from a mean of 162/103 mm Hg to 144/95 mm Hg in six patients reduced the rate of loss of GFR from 1.23 mL/min/month to 0.49 mL/min/month. Others confirmed these findings.[53–55] In 1987, Parving and colleagues[54] reported that treating blood pressure from a mean of 143/96 mm Hg to 129/84 mm Hg in 11 patients with type 1 DM and DN decreased the rate of GFR decline from 0.89 mL/min/month to 0.22 mL/min/month.

These promising results suggested further study would be necessary to determine the optimal blood pressure range to prevent the pathologic progression of DN. The UKPDS randomized patients to two different blood pressure goals and found an impressive risk reduction in CV and diabetes-related events with the lower achieved blood pressure (144/82 mm Hg), but was unable to detect a renoprotective effect of being randomized to the lower blood pressure.[35,54] However, this may have reflected the limitation of study design in the UKPDS. A further trial,[37] the Appropriate Blood Pressure in Diabetes study, not only demonstrated a decrease in the development of albuminuria, but also a decrease in the progression to overt nephropathy in the group that achieved a mean blood pressure of $128 \pm 0.8/75 \pm 0.3$ mm Hg. Finally, a smaller study[56] investigated the effects of lowering blood pressure in patients with type 1 DM and advanced DN by randomizing them to a mean arterial pressure of 92 mm Hg or less versus 100 to 107 mm Hg. Patients were followed for 2 years, and those randomized to the lower mean arterial pressure goal experienced an improvement in proteinuria from an average of 1043 mg/day to 535 mg/day compared with the group with the higher mean arterial pressure goal that developed an average increase in urinary protein excretion from 1140 mg/day to 1723 mg/day. Based on this randomized study, renal remission was achieved, defined as a 24-hour urine protein excretion of less than 500 mg/day coupled with a loss of GFR of less than 2 mL/min per year. Blood pressure control was achieved using

ramipril, which was titrated up to a dose of 20 mg/day before the addition of other antihypertensive agents. Therefore, those patients with the best outcome had better blood pressure control and were on average treated with the higher dose of the ACE inhibitor.

The Irbesartan Diabetic Nephropathy Trial (IDNT) revealed that the application of angiotensin receptor blockade in patients with overt nephropathy significantly slowed the rate of progression to loss of renal function in type 2 DM (see later).[57] When the impact of the patients' blood pressure at the time of entry into the study was examined, it was clear that patients who entered the study with more poorly controlled blood pressure were more likely to develop renal failure. Despite this relationship between the lack of historical blood pressure control and an adverse renal outcome, it was demonstrated in the IDNT that the achieved blood pressure had a more profound effect on outcome than did the baseline blood pressure.[58] Hence, despite a history of undertreatment of the blood pressure, achieving blood pressure control was an important and effective therapeutic goal.

Intensive blood pressure control therefore has substantial benefits for treatment of nephropathy in patients with DM; however, how far should the clinician attempt to lower it? Is there CV harm in lowering blood pressure too much? In 1988, the concept of the J curve was introduced.[59] This was based on the fact that lowering blood pressure diminished CV disease and death, but there was a definable plateau where blood pressure control lacked a benefit for CV mortality. In fact, decreasing the diastolic blood pressure below this plateau was associated with an increase in mortality. This relationship between blood pressure control and clinical outcome therefore was depicted graphically as a U- or J-shaped curve and was compatible with the observation that during diastole, lower blood pressures could limit coronary perfusion.[59,60] This concept is essential to apply to patients with DM and DN who have a well-established CV risk. Attempting to control the systolic pressure in this population can lead to the potential danger of decreasing diastolic pressure too far. The post hoc analysis of the IDNT confirmed the J-curve relationship in the patient with DN, as a plateau was reached in the development of renal outcomes at a systolic blood pressure of less than 130 mm Hg, and, more importantly, all-cause mortality increased below a systolic blood pressure of 120 mm Hg.[58] In this same population of overt DN, CV deaths and congestive heart failure events increased at an achieved systolic blood pressure of less than 120 mm Hg, and the relative risk of a myocardial infarction was higher in those patients who achieved a lower diastolic blood pressure.[61] An additional trial, not a post hoc analysis, was performed by Osher and colleagues.[62] The investigators attempted to treat patients with DM and hypertension to the blood pressure goal of less than 130/85 mm Hg as recommended by the most recent Joint National Commission on the Prevention, Detection, Evaluation, and Treatment of High Blood Pressure.[63] The diastolic blood pressure goal was achieved in 90% of the patients and the systolic goal in 33%. The achievement of a diastolic blood pressure of less than 70 mm Hg was more likely in patients who were older, had a higher systolic blood pressure, or a history of coronary artery disease.

Treatment of blood pressure in the patient with DN should therefore be targeted between the range of 120 to

130/80 to 90 mm Hg, with care to not excessively lower the diastolic pressure.

Blockade of the Renin-Angiotensin System

Angiotensin receptor blockers (ARB) and ACE inhibitors block the deleterious renal effects of angiotensin II while simultaneously lowering blood pressure, and, as lowering blood pressure has been shown to improve renal outcomes, debate could exist as to which effect is renoprotective. The first large human clinical trial to examine this hypothetical effect of renoprotection with RAS blockade in DN was in 409 patients with type 1 DM and overt DN.[64] Overt DN was defined as the excretion of 500 mg proteinuria/day or more and serum creatinine of 2.5 mg/dL or less. The patients were randomized to receive captopril 25 mg three times daily or placebo, and blood pressures were similar in the two groups. The results were a dramatic 43% decrease in the doubling of serum creatinine (Fig. 28-2) as well as a statistically significant decrease in time to death, dialysis, or transplantation with captopril compared with placebo. Thus, in patients with type 1 DM and DN, ACE inhibitors provide renoprotection superior to that with blood pressure treatment alone.

The data in DN associated with type 2 DM is also compelling. The Effect of Irbesartan in the Development of Diabetic Nephropathy in Patients with Type 2 Diabetes investigators[65] randomized 590 patients with type 2 DM and microalbuminuria to receive either placebo, irbesartan 150 mg, or irbesartan 300 mg for 2 years. The primary endpoint of albuminuria more than 200 mg/day was statistically lower ($P < .001$) in the irbesartan 150-mg group and 300-mg group compared with the placebo group, with the greatest decrease at the highest

dose (Fig. 28-3). This study demonstrated not only the importance of blockade of the RAS for the renal outcome, but also the importance of dose on efficacy, with the higher dose being more efficacious.

More advanced DN from type 2 DM was studied by the IDNT group,[57] who randomized 1715 hypertensive patients with overt DN (median baseline serum creatinine, 1.67 mg/dL; median baseline urinary protein excretion, 2.9 g/24 hr) to receive one of three treatment regimens: (1) irbesartan 300 mg/day, (2) amlodipine 10 mg/day, or (3) placebo. Patients were followed for an average of 2.6 years. Antihypertensive agents with the exception of ACE inhibitors, ARBs, and calcium channel blockers were used as needed in each group to target a blood pressure of less than 135/85 mm Hg. The primary composite endpoint of doubling of the serum creatinine, development of end-stage renal disease, or death was significantly lower in the irbesartan arm compared with the amlodipine or placebo arm. Blood pressure control was similar in all three arms and equivalent in the amlodipine and irbesartan groups.

Similar results were demonstrated in the Reduction in End-Points in Non-Insulin Dependent Diabetes Mellitus with the Angiotensin II Antagonist Losartan trial,[47] in which randomization to angiotensin antagonism with losartan produced a decrease in the primary outcome of the composite of doubling of the serum creatinine, ESRD, or death. The benefit was greater than that attributed to blood pressure decrease alone. These two independent trials gave extraordinarily similar results, providing remarkable attestation for the use of ARBs for renoprotection in overt DN from type 2 DM.

These data established the blood pressure–independent effects of renoprotection with blockade of the RAS for DN in patients with type 1 and 2 DM. Figure 28-4 represents renal

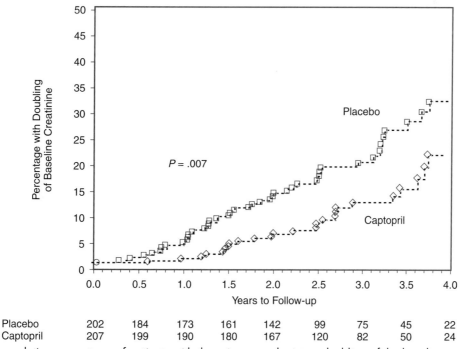

Placebo	202	184	173	161	142	99	75	45	22
Captopril	207	199	190	180	167	120	82	50	24

Figure 28-2 The cumulative percentage of patients with the primary endpoint: a doubling of the baseline serum creatinine concentration to at least 2.0 mg/dL. (From Lewis EJ, Hunsicker LG, Bain RP, Rohde RD: The effect of angiotensin-converting-enzyme inhibition on diabetic nephropathy. The Collaborative Study Group. N Engl J Med 1993;329:1456–1462.)

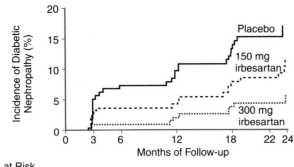

Figure 28-3   Incidence of progression to diabetic nephropathy during treatment with 150 mg/day irbesartan, 300 mg/day irbesartan, or placebo in hypertensive patients with type 2 diabetes and persistent microalbuminuria. The difference between the placebo group and the 150-mg group was not significant (P = .08 by the log-rank test), but the difference between the placebo group and the 300-mg group was significant (P < .001 by the log-rank test). (From Parving HH, Lehnert H, Brochner-Mortensen J, et al: The effect of irbesartan on the development of diabetic nephropathy in patients with type 2 diabetes. N Engl J Med 2001;345:870.)

outcomes from the IDNT, stratified by treatment assignment and systolic blood pressure quartiles.[58] It is apparent that, in addition to randomization to the irbesartan group, the lower quartiles of achieved systolic blood pressure were associated with improved renal outcomes. Thus, blood pressure control

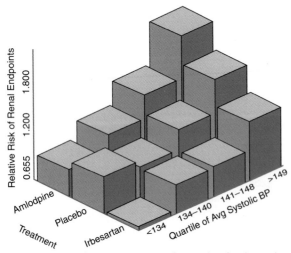

Figure 28-4   Simultaneous impact of quartile of achieved systolic blood pressure (BP) and treatment modality on the relative risk for reaching a renal endpoint (doubling of baseline serum creatinine or end-stage renal disease, defined as serum creatinine ≤ 6.0 mg/dL or renal replacement therapy). Avg, average. (From Pohl MA, Blumenthal S, Cordonnier DJ, et al: Independent and additive impact of blood pressure control and angiotensin II receptor blockade on renal outcomes in the irbesartan diabetic nephropathy trial: Clinical implications and limitations. J Am Soc Nephrol 2005;16:3031.)

and inhibition of the RAS offer independent and additive effects to prevent progression of DN.

In addition to blood pressure, proteinuria is reduced in patients with DN treated with RAS blockade. In the IDNT, baseline proteinuria was a strong and linear determinant of developing a renal endpoint (Fig. 28-5A). More importantly, improved renal outcomes were associated with a decrease in proteinuria (see Fig. 28-5B).[66] Data from the Reduction in End-Points in Non-Insulin Dependent Diabetes Mellitus with the Angiotensin II Antagonist Losartan trial also demonstrated a significant decrease in proteinuria in those patients assigned to losartan.[47] The baseline proteinuria was predictive of a renal endpoint and ESRD, and decrease in the protein excretion was associated with fewer renal outcomes and ESRD.[49] This emphasizes that proteinuria may be another potential target for therapy in DN, as more evidence is emerging for the association of proteinuria as an independent modifiable risk factor for progression of advanced DN.[48,49]

Blockade of the RAS with ACE inhibitors or ARBs has been well established in slowing the progression of DN, and therapies that antagonize this system further by other maneuvers have been evaluated. Most of these trials are small in sample size and/or contain confounding variables. Higher doses of ARBs than those approved by the U.S. Food and Drug Administration have been shown to decrease microalbuminuria to a greater degree than the accepted doses.[67] Studies of combining ACE inhibitors and ARBs have shown a decrease in proteinuria below what was established with either agent alone.[68–75] Blockade of aldosterone receptors with spironolactone[76] and eplerenone[77] has been shown in small trials to reduce proteinuria in patients with DN independent of their effects on blood pressure. The renin inhibitor aliskiren, currently approved by the U.S. Food and Drug Administration for control of blood pressure, has preliminarily shown reduction in proteinuria additive to the effects of RAS blockade by losartan.[78] At present, however, no study of these alternative and novel maneuvers to block the RAS has been shown to be associated with a decrease in the rate of decline of renal function. Proteinuria reduction alone has been associated with improved renoprotection, and therefore long-term studies with further blockade of other agents that interfere with the RAS to document significant delay in the progression to ESRD are eagerly anticipated.

Care must be taken to monitor and treat the potential development of hyperkalemia when using any agent to block the RAS. Given the fact that many of these patients have a decreased GFR or even hyporeninemic hypoaldosteronism, maximally blocking the RAS at multiple sites may lead to an increased incidence of hyperkalemia. The rigorous nature of follow-up in a clinical trial typically would follow this closely; however, widespread application of clinical trial data to patients in the general public who may not meet criteria for the study and/or may not follow up as closely can be dangerous,[79] especially with the known consequence of sudden death seen with hyperkalemia. It is prudent to check the serum potassium 7 to 14 days after establishing therapy with these agents.

Overwhelming evidence from statistically valid clinical trials supports blockade of the RAS with ACE inhibitors or ARBs to decrease the rate of progression of DN. They are considered the first-line therapy for the patient with microalbuminuria or overt DN. Evidence exists proving a beneficial effect of ACE inhibition in patients with overt nephropathy from type 1 DM

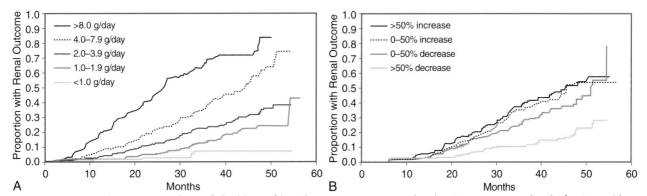

Figure 28-5 **A,** Kaplan-Meier analysis of doubling of baseline serum creatinine level, serum creatinine level of 6.0 mg/dL, or the development of end-stage renal disease by baseline proteinuria values. **B,** Kaplan-Meier analysis of doubling of baseline serum creatinine level, serum creatinine level of 6.0 mg/dL, or the development of end-stage renal disease by level of proteinuria change in the first 12 months. (**B,** From Atkins RC, Briganti EM, Lewis JB, et al: Proteinuria reduction and progression to renal failure in patients with type 2 diabetes mellitus and overt nephropathy. Am J Kidney Dis 2005;45:283, 285.)

and reduction in albuminuria in DN from type 2 DM. Evidence of angiotensin II blockade with ARBs proves the beneficial effect in patients with microalbuminuria and overt nephropathy from type 2 DM. Further evidence and safety data must exist before recommending the use of additional novel maneuvers to block the RAS in patients with DN.

Diet

The modern diabetic diet of low fat, low sodium, moderately low protein, and high fiber has been shown to decrease blood pressure in patients with type 2 DM and hypertension.[80] This has not been formally evaluated for patients with DN. Studies on dietary protein restriction have had mixed results.[81–85] Due to the dietary restrictions of fat and simple carbohydrates in diabetic patients, restricting protein may increase the risk of protein malnutrition. A reasonable recommendation is to follow a low sodium (<2 g/day) diet with moderate protein intake (0.8 g/kg/day).

Treating Chronic Kidney Disease and Avoiding Acute Kidney Injury

In addition to focusing on slowing or reversing the progression of DN, care must be taken to treat the sequelae of CKD. This therapy is beyond the scope of this chapter and can be reviewed in Part XII: Chronic Renal Failure and Its Systemic Manifestations. However, certain precautions are unique to evaluating the diabetic patient. As the GFR decreases, dosing for insulin and other oral hypoglycemic agents with renal excretion needs adjustment. Metformin should be held when the creatinine clearance decreases to less than 60 mL/min as the risk of type B lactic acidosis develops.[86] Diabetic patients, and especially those with DN, are at increased risk of developing acute kidney injury.[87] These acute insults can often lead to an irrecoverable loss of renal function and have a direct correlation with a higher mortality.[88] It is sensible to avoid, if possible, situations that may cause acute kidney injury, such as iodinated contrast exposure, atheroemboli, and nonsteroidal anti-inflammatory agents, as these may accelerate the progression of CKD. As the diabetic patient has a

high risk of vascular disease and congestive heart failure, control of coronary risk factors and volume status is prudent. Finally, dialysis education, preparation for transplantation, or palliative care should begin early in the course of CKD in patients with diabetes to allow for an informative and effective evaluation.[89]

Future Strategies

Despite the established therapies for reducing progressive nephropathy, the patient with diabetes is still at risk of eventual renal failure and CV complications. New medications to reduce and perhaps reverse this risk may be developed in the future. One such drug is sulodexide, a glycosaminoglycan that has shown promise in pilot studies to reduce albuminuria in patients with DN.[90] Endothelin antagonism is another novel target for treatment of DN; however, trials with these agents were recently halted due to side effects associated with the use of the study drug. Inhibitors of transforming growth factor β, such as pirfenidone, may have promise in inhibiting fibrosis in the kidney as DN progresses.[91,92] Ruboxistaurin, a protein kinase C inhibitor, has also been shown to decrease proteinuria in patients with DN in preliminary pilot studies.[93] Agents that reduce or inhibit glycosylation end products also show promise.[94–97] In light of limitations of maximally blocking the RAS system, such as hyperkalemia, these future therapies for DN are attractive. There must be further study with rigorous clinical trials and safety data must exist before recommendation of these novel therapies in addition to RAS blockade.

TREATMENT OF THE DIABETIC PATIENT WITH END-STAGE RENAL DISEASE

Hemodialysis, peritoneal dialysis, renal transplantation, and palliative care are all options for the diabetic patient with ESRD. These are discussed in detail in Parts XIII and XIV. The choice of renal replacement therapy is individualized for each patient, but the treating physician and the patient should be aware of the specific risks that a diabetic patient carries.

The diabetic patient with ESRD has a higher morbidity, mostly from cardiac and vascular disease, compared to a nondiabetic patient with ESRD.[51] Furthermore, mortality is nearly double for a diabetic with ESRD compared with a nondiabetic with ESRD.[3,51] Although kidney transplantation is associated with an improved mortality, no proven difference in overall mortality exists between those patients on hemodialysis versus peritoneal dialysis.[51] The studies evaluating a difference in dialysis modality for the mortality of diabetic patients have demonstrated conflicting results,[98–103] which can be explained by the nature of their observational and/or retrospective study designs. To date, there has not been an appropriately powered randomized trial to define a difference in mortality with respect to modality of dialysis for patients with DM and ESRD.

Other practical factors are involved when choosing the dialysis modality for the patient with DN. Blindness from proliferative diabetic retinopathy may limit a patient's ability to perform peritoneal dialysis.[104] Rates of recurrent peritonitis are also higher in patients with DM.[104] Patients with DM have an accelerated course to peritoneal membrane failure.[105] Systemic glucose absorption from the dialysate may lead to worsening hyperglycemia and increasing insulin requirements in patients undergoing peritoneal dialysis. In patients undergoing hemodialysis, the preponderance of vascular disease in those with diabetes limits the maturity and increases the rate of complications of vascular access.[106] The increased rate of cardiac disease, left ventricular hypertrophy, and autonomic insufficiency observed in patients with diabetes can contribute to intradialytic hypotension, arrhythmias, or even sudden death on hemodialysis.[104] Therefore, the choice of dialysis modality in diabetic patients with ESRD should remain individualized.

Transplantation in patients with DM remains an attractive alternative to dialysis. In patients with type 1 DM, pancreas transplantation is a viable option to restore euglycemia. Survival for patients with diabetes with a renal transplant is markedly higher than survival on dialysis. The survival for diabetic patients undergoing renal transplantation is approximately 80% at 5 years,[2] and the unadjusted 5-year patient survival rate is 83.4% for diabetics undergoing living donor transplantation in the United States (the scientific registry of transplant recipients, www.ustransplant.org, accessed June 2007). This is a lower percentage compared with those reported for living donation or renal failure from other etiologies, such as polycystic kidney disease (94.5%) or glomerular disease (94.1%) at 5 years. These less favorable results are chiefly due to the increased CV disease in diabetic patients. However, according to the U.S. Renal Data Systems report, the survival rate of patients with DM on dialysis is approximately 25% at 5 years,[2] an astounding difference compared with transplantation. This cannot be entirely explained by selection bias, as those patients who are eligible for transplantation but remain on the transplantation waiting list have a lower survival compared with transplant recipients, but a higher survival than those on dialysis who are not on the waiting list.[107]

CONCLUSION

The management of the patient with diabetes is complex and suited to a multidisciplinary approach. Glycemic and blood pressure control is necessary to assist in the prevention of DN.

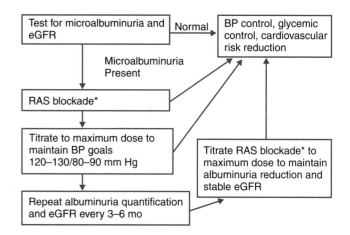

*Provided no contraindication: persistent hyperkalemia, angioedema, prerenal azotemia, pregnancy

Figure 28-6 Treatment algorithm for diabetic nephropathy. BP, blood pressure; eGFR, estimated glomerular filtration rate; RAS, renin-angiotensin system blockade.

Once nephropathy has developed, substantial evidence exists for blockade of the RAS to delay the onset of ESRD as first-line therapy. Blood pressure control clearly remains important as the disease progresses. Exciting novel therapies beyond blockade of the RAS are eagerly anticipated and must be tested through rigorous clinical study for safety and efficacy. Treating the sequelae of CKD and preparing the patient for ESRD become more relevant as the GFR decreases. Throughout the entire course of DM and DN, CV risk reduction for this high-risk population remains vital. The therapies discovered in the past 30 years have helped improve the devastating progression of DN (Fig. 28-6).

References

1. Krolewski M, Eggers PW, Warram JH: Magnitude of end-stage renal disease in IDDM: A 35 year follow-up study. Kidney Int 1996;50:2041–2046.
2. Collins AJ, Kasiske B, Herzog C, et al: Excerpts from the United States Renal Data System 2006 Annual Data Report. Am J Kidney Dis 2007;49:A6–A7, S1–S296.
3. Ritz E, Rychlik I, Locatelli F, Halimi S: End-stage renal failure in type 2 diabetes: A medical catastrophe of worldwide dimensions. Am J Kidney Dis 1999;34:795–808.
4. Go AS, Chertow GM, Fan D, et al: Chronic kidney disease and the risks of death, cardiovascular events, and hospitalization. N Engl J Med 2004;351:1296–1305.
5. Nelson RG, Morgenstern H, Bennett PH: An epidemic of proteinuria in Pima Indians with type 2 diabetes mellitus. Kidney Int 1998;54:2081–2088.
6. Pavkov ME, Bennett PH, Sievers ML, et al: Predominant effect of kidney disease on mortality in Pima Indians with or without type 2 diabetes. Kidney Int 2005;68:1267–1274.
7. Pavkov ME, Knowler WC, Bennett PH, et al: Increasing incidence of proteinuria and declining incidence of end-stage renal disease in diabetic Pima Indians. Kidney Int 2006;70:1840–1846.
8. Cooper ME, Frauman A, O'Brien RC, et al: Progression of proteinuria in type 1 and type 2 diabetes. Diabet Med 1988;5:361–368.

9. Haneda M, Kikkawa R, Togawa M, et al: High blood pressure is a risk factor for the development of microalbuminuria in Japanese subjects with non-insulin-dependent diabetes mellitus. J Diabetes Complications 1992;6:181–185.

10. John L, Rao PS, Kanagasabapathy AS: Rate of progression of albuminuria in type II diabetes. Five-year prospective study from south India. Diabetes Care 1994;17:888–890.

11. Mogensen CE: Microalbuminuria predicts clinical proteinuria and early mortality in maturity-onset diabetes. N Engl J Med 1984;310:356–360.

12. Ravid M, Savin H, Jutrin I, et al: Long-term stabilizing effect of angiotensin-converting enzyme inhibition on plasma creatinine and on proteinuria in normotensive type II diabetic patients. Ann Intern Med 1993;118:577–581.

13. Grundy SM, Benjamin IJ, Burke GL, et al: Diabetes and cardiovascular disease: A statement for healthcare professionals from the American Heart Association. Circulation 1999;100:1134–1146.

14. Grundy SM, Howard B, Smith S Jr, et al: Prevention Conference VI: Diabetes and Cardiovascular Disease: Executive summary: Conference proceeding for healthcare professionals from a special writing group of the American Heart Association. Circulation 2002;105:2231–2239.

15. Olivarius NF, Beck-Nielsen H, Andreasen AH, et al: Randomised controlled trial of structured personal care of type 2 diabetes mellitus. Br Med J 2001;323:970–975.

16. Parving HH, Lewis JB, Ravid M, et al: Prevalence and risk factors for microalbuminuria in a referred cohort of type II diabetic patients: A global perspective. Kidney Int 2006;69:2057–2063.

17. Savage S, Nagel NJ, Estacio RO, et al: Clinical factors associated with urinary albumin excretion in type II diabetes. Am J Kidney Dis 1995;25:836–844.

18. Kussman MJ, Goldstein H, Gleason RE: The clinical course of diabetic nephropathy. JAMA 1976;236:1861–1863.

19. Haffner SM, Lehto S, Ronnemaa T, et al: Mortality from coronary heart disease in subjects with type 2 diabetes and in nondiabetic subjects with and without prior myocardial infarction. N Engl J Med 1998;339:229–234.

20. Borch-Johnsen K, Feldt-Rasmussen B, Strandgaard S, et al: Urinary albumin excretion. An independent predictor of ischemic heart disease. Arterioscler Thromb Vasc Biol 1999;19:1992–1997.

21. Dinneen SF, Gerstein HC: The association of microalbuminuria and mortality in non-insulin-dependent diabetes mellitus. A systematic overview of the literature. Arch Intern Med 1997;157:1413–1418.

22. Gerstein HC, Mann JF, Yi Q, et al: Albuminuria and risk of cardiovascular events, death, and heart failure in diabetic and nondiabetic individuals. JAMA 2001;286:421–426.

23. Laakso M, Lehto S: Epidemiology of risk factors for cardiovascular disease in diabetes and impaired glucose tolerance. Atherosclerosis 1998;137(Suppl):S65–S73.

24. Barzilay J, Warram JH, Bak M, et al: Predisposition to hypertension: Risk factor for nephropathy and hypertension in IDDM. Kidney Int 1992;41:723–730.

25. Gilbert RE, Tsalamandris C, Bach LA, et al: Long-term glycemic control and the rate of progression of early diabetic kidney disease. Kidney Int 1993;44:855–859.

26. Dahl-Jorgensen K, Bjoro T, Kierulf P, et al: Long-term glycemic control and kidney function in insulin-dependent diabetes mellitus. Kidney Int 1992;41:920–923.

27. Krolewski AS, Canessa M, Warram JH, et al: Predisposition to hypertension and susceptibility to renal disease in insulin-dependent diabetes mellitus. N Engl J Med 1988;318:140–145.

28. The effect of intensive treatment of diabetes on the development and progression of long-term complications in insulin-dependent diabetes mellitus. The Diabetes Control and Complications Trial Research Group. N Engl J Med 1993;329:977–986.

29. Intensive blood-glucose control with sulphonyl ureas or insulin compared with conventional treatment and risk of complications in patients with type 2 diabetes (UKPDS 33). UK Prospective Diabetes Study (UKPDS) Group. Lancet 1998;352:837–853.

30. Retinopathy and nephropathy in patients with type 1 diabetes four years after a trial of intensive therapy. The Diabetes Control and Complications Trial/Epidemiology of Diabetes Interventions and Complications Research Group. N Engl J Med 2000;342:381–389.

31. Writing Team for the Diabetes Control and Complications Trial/Epidemiology of Diabetes Interventions and Complications Research Group: Sustained effect of intensive treatment of type 1 diabetes mellitus on development and progression of diabetic nephropathy: The Epidemiology of Diabetes Interventions and Complications (EDIC) study. JAMA 2003;290:2159–2167.

32. Ohkubo Y, Kishikawa H, Araki E, et al: Intensive insulin therapy prevents the progression of diabetic microvascular complications in Japanese patients with non-insulin-dependent diabetes mellitus: A randomized prospective 6-year study. Diabetes Res Clin Pract 1995;28:103–117.

33. Shichiri M, Kishikawa H, Ohkubo Y, Wake N: Long-term results of the Kumamoto Study on optimal diabetes control in type 2 diabetic patients. Diabetes Care 2000;23(Suppl 2):B21–B29.

34. American Diabetes Association: Standards of medical care in diabetes—2007. Diabetes Care 2007;30(Suppl 1):S4–S41.

35. Tight blood pressure control and risk of macrovascular and microvascular complications in type 2 diabetes: UKPDS 38. UK Prospective Diabetes Study Group. Br Med J 1998;317:703–713.

36. Adler AI, Stratton IM, Neil HA et al: Association of systolic blood pressure with macrovascular and microvascular complications of type 2 diabetes (UKPDS 36): Prospective observational study. Br Med J 2000;321:412–419.

37. Schrier RW, Estacio RO, Esler A, Mehler P: Effects of aggressive blood pressure control in normotensive type 2 diabetic patients on albuminuria, retinopathy and strokes. Kidney Int 2002;61:1086–1097.

38. Dunn BR, Zatz R, Rennke HG, et al: Prevention of glomerular capillary hypertension in experimental diabetes mellitus obviates functional and structural glomerular injury. J Hypertens Suppl 1986;4:S251–S254.

39. Hommel E, Parving HH, Mathiesen E, et al: Effect of captopril on kidney function in insulin-dependent diabetic patients with nephropathy. Br Med J 1986;293:467–470.

40. Parving HH, Hommel E, Damkjaer NM, Giese J: Effect of captopril on blood pressure and kidney function in normotensive insulin dependent diabetics with nephropathy. Br Med J 1989;299:533–536.

41. Zatz R, Dunn BR, Meyer TW, et al: Prevention of diabetic glomerulopathy by pharmacological amelioration of glomerular capillary hypertension. J Clin Invest 1986;77:1925–1930.

42. Ruggenenti P, Fassi A, Ilieva AP, et al: Preventing microalbuminuria in type 2 diabetes. N Engl J Med 2004;351:1941–1951.

43. Ruggenenti P, Perna A, Ganeva M, et al: Impact of blood pressure control and angiotensin-converting enzyme inhibitor therapy on new-onset microalbuminuria in type 2 diabetes: A post hoc analysis of the BENEDICT trial. J Am Soc Nephrol 2006;17:3472–3481.

44. Gaede P, Vedel P, Larsen N, et al: Multifactorial intervention and cardiovascular disease in patients with type 2 diabetes. N Engl J Med 2003;348:383–393.

45. Yusuf S, Sleight P, Pogue J, et al: Effects of an angiotensin-converting-enzyme inhibitor, ramipril, on cardiovascular events in high-risk patients. The Heart Outcomes Prevention Evaluation Study Investigators. N Engl J Med 2000;342:145–153.

46. Effects of ramipril on cardiovascular and microvascular outcomes in people with diabetes mellitus: Results of the HOPE study and MICRO-HOPE substudy. Heart Outcomes Prevention Evaluation Study Investigators. Lancet 2000;355:253–259.

47. Brenner BM, Cooper ME, de ZD et al: Effects of losartan on renal and cardiovascular outcomes in patients with type 2 diabetes and nephropathy. N Engl J Med 2001;345:861–869.

48. de Zeeuw D, Remuzzi G, Parving HH, et al: Albuminuria, a therapeutic target for cardiovascular protection in type 2 diabetic patients with nephropathy. Circulation 2004;110:921–927.

49. de Zeeuw D, Remuzzi G, Parving HH, et al: Proteinuria, a target for renoprotection in patients with type 2 diabetic nephropathy: Lessons from RENAAL. Kidney Int 2004;65:2309–2320.

50. Rodriguez JA, Cleries M, Vela E: Diabetic patients on renal replacement therapy: Analysis of Catalan Registry data. Renal Registry Committee. Nephrol Dial Transplant 1997;12:2501–2509.

51. Friedman EA, Friedman AL, Eggers P: End-stage renal disease in diabetic persons: Is the pandemic subsiding? Kidney Int Suppl 2006;S51–S54.

52. Mogensen CE: Long-term antihypertensive treatment inhibiting progression of diabetic nephropathy. Br Med J 1982;285:685–688.

53. Nyberg G, Blohme G, Norden G: Constant glomerular filtration rate in diabetic nephropathy. Correlation to blood pressure and blood glucose control. Acta Med Scand 1986;219:67–72.

54. Parving HH, Andersen AR, Smidt UM, et al: Effect of antihypertensive treatment on kidney function in diabetic nephropathy. Br Med J 1987;294:1443–1447.

55. Parving HH, Andersen AR, Smidt UM, Svendsen PA: Early aggressive antihypertensive treatment reduces rate of decline in kidney function in diabetic nephropathy. Lancet 1983;1: 1175–1179.

56. Lewis JB, Berl T, Bain RP, et al: Effect of intensive blood pressure control on the course of type 1 diabetic nephropathy. Collaborative Study Group. Am J Kidney Dis 1999;34:809–817.

57. Lewis EJ, Hunsicker LG, Clarke WR, et al: Renoprotective effect of the angiotensin-receptor antagonist irbesartan in patients with nephropathy due to type 2 diabetes. N Engl J Med 2001;345: 851–860.

58. Pohl MA, Blumenthal S, Cordonnier DJ, et al: Independent and additive impact of blood pressure control and angiotensin II receptor blockade on renal outcomes in the irbesartan diabetic nephropathy trial: Clinical implications and limitations. J Am Soc Nephrol 2005;16:3027–3037.

59. Cruickshank JM: Coronary flow reserve and the J curve relation between diastolic blood pressure and myocardial infarction. Br Med J 1988;297:1227–1230.

60. Cruickshank JM, Thorp JM, Zacharias FJ: Benefits and potential harm of lowering high blood pressure. Lancet 1987;1:581–584.

61. Berl T, Hunsicker LG, Lewis JB, et al: Impact of achieved blood pressure on cardiovascular outcomes in the Irbesartan Diabetic Nephropathy Trial. J Am Soc Nephrol 2005;16:2170–2179.

62. Osher E, Greenman Y, Tordjman K, et al: Attempted forced titration of blood pressure to <130/85 mm Hg in type 2 diabetic hypertensive patients in clinical practice: The diastolic cost. J Clin Hypertens (Greenwich) 2006;8:29–34.

63. Chobanian AV, Bakris GL, Black HR, et al: Seventh report of the Joint National Committee on Prevention, Detection, Evaluation, and Treatment of High Blood Pressure. Hypertension 2003;42:1206–1252.

64. Lewis EJ, Hunsicker LG, Bain RP, Rohde RD: The effect of angiotensin-converting-enzyme inhibition on diabetic nephropathy. The Collaborative Study Group. N Engl J Med 1993;329:1456–1462.

65. Parving HH, Lehnert H, Brochner-Mortensen J, et al: The effect of irbesartan on the development of diabetic nephropathy in patients with type 2 diabetes. N Engl J Med 2001;345:870–878.

66. Atkins RC, Briganti EM, Lewis JB, et al: Proteinuria reduction and progression to renal failure in patients with type 2 diabetes mellitus and overt nephropathy. Am J Kidney Dis 2005;45:281–287.

67. Rossing K, Schjoedt KJ, Jensen BR, et al: Enhanced renoprotective effects of ultrahigh doses of irbesartan in patients with type 2 diabetes and microalbuminuria. Kidney Int 2005;68:1190–1198.

68. Andersen NH, Poulsen PL, Knudsen ST, et al: Long-term dual blockade with candesartan and lisinopril in hypertensive patients with diabetes: The CALM II study. Diabetes Care 2005;28:273–277.

69. Jacobsen P, Andersen S, Jensen BR, Parving HH: Additive effect of ACE inhibition and angiotensin II receptor blockade in type I diabetic patients with diabetic nephropathy. J Am Soc Nephrol 2003;14:992–999.

70. Jacobsen P, Andersen S, Rossing K, et al: Dual blockade of the renin-angiotensin system in type 1 patients with diabetic nephropathy. Nephrol Dial Transplant 2002;17:1019–1024.

71. Jacobsen P, Andersen S, Rossing K, et al: Dual blockade of the renin-angiotensin system versus maximal recommended dose of ACE inhibition in diabetic nephropathy. Kidney Int 2003;63:1874–1880.

72. Mogensen CE, Neldam S, Tikkanen I, et al: Randomised controlled trial of dual blockade of renin-angiotensin system in patients with hypertension, microalbuminuria, and non-insulin dependent diabetes: The candesartan and lisinopril microalbuminuria (CALM) study. Br Med J 2000;321:1440–1444.

73. Rossing K, Christensen PK, Jensen BR, Parving HH: Dual blockade of the renin-angiotensin system in diabetic nephropathy: A randomized double-blind crossover study. Diabetes Care 2003;25:95–100.

74. Rossing K, Jacobsen P, Pietraszek L, Parving HH: Renoprotective effects of adding angiotensin II receptor blocker to maximal recommended doses of ACE inhibitor in diabetic nephropathy: A randomized double-blind crossover trial. Diabetes Care 2003;26:2268–2274.

75. Song JH, Cha SH, Lee HJ, et al: Effect of low-dose dual blockade of renin-angiotensin system on urinary TGF-beta in type 2 diabetic patients with advanced kidney disease. Nephrol Dial Transplant 2006;21:683–689.

76. Schjoedt KJ, Rossing K, Juhl TR, et al: Beneficial impact of spironolactone on nephrotic range albuminuria in diabetic nephropathy. Kidney Int 2006;70:536–542.

77. Epstein M: Aldosterone receptor blockade and the role of eplerenone: evolving perspectives. Nephrol Dial Transplant 2003;18:1984–1992.

78. Parving H-H, Lewis JB, Lewis EJ, Hollenberg NK: Aliskiren in Evaluation of Proteinuria in Diabetes (AVOID). N Engl J Med 2008, in press.

79. Juurlink DN, Mamdani MM, Lee DS, et al: Rates of hyperkalemia after publication of the Randomized Aldactone Evaluation Study. N Engl J Med 2004;351:543–551.

80. Dodson PM, Pacy PJ, Bal P, et al: A controlled trial of a high fibre, low fat and low sodium diet for mild hypertension in type 2 (non-insulin-dependent) diabetic patients. Diabetologia 1984;27:522–526.

81. Hansen HP, Tauber-Lassen E, Jensen BR, Parving HH: Effect of dietary protein restriction on prognosis in patients with diabetic nephropathy. Kidney Int 2002;62:220–228.

82. Pomerleau J, Verdy M, Garrel DR, Nadeau MH: Effect of protein intake on glycaemic control and renal function in type 2 (non-insulin-dependent) diabetes mellitus. Diabetologia 1993;36:829–834.

83. Shichiri M, Nishio Y, Ogura M, Marumo F: Effect of low-protein, very-low-phosphorus diet on diabetic renal insufficiency with proteinuria. Am J Kidney Dis 1991;18:26–32.

84. Walker JD, Bending JJ, Dodds RA, et al: Restriction of dietary protein and progression of renal failure in diabetic nephropathy. Lancet 1989;2:1411–1415.

85. Zeller K, Whittaker E, Sullivan L, et al: Effect of restricting dietary protein on the progression of renal failure in patients with insulin-dependent diabetes mellitus. N Engl J Med 1991;324:78–84.

86. DeFronzo RA: Pathogenesis of type 2 diabetes: Implications for metformin. Drugs 1999;58(Suppl 1):29–30.

87. Parfrey PS, Griffiths SM, Barrett BJ, et al: Contrast material-induced renal failure in patients with diabetes mellitus, renal insufficiency, or both. A prospective controlled study. N Engl J Med 1989;320:143–149.

88. Rihal CS, Textor SC, Grill DE, et al: Incidence and prognostic importance of acute renal failure after percutaneous coronary intervention. Circulation 2002;105:2259–2264.

89. Gaston RS, Basadonna G, Cosio FG, et al: Transplantation in the diabetic patient with advanced chronic kidney disease: A task force report. Am J Kidney Dis 2004;44:529–542.

90. Gambaro G, Kinalska I, Oksa A, et al: Oral sulodexide reduces albuminuria in microalbuminuric and macroalbuminuric type 1 and type 2 diabetic patients: The Di.N.A.S. randomized trial. J Am Soc Nephrol 2002;13:1615–1625.

91. McGowan TA, Zhu Y, Sharma K: Transforming growth factor-beta: A clinical target for the treatment of diabetic nephropathy. Curr Diab Rep 2004;4:447–454.

92. Zhu Y, Usui HK, Sharma K: Regulation of transforming growth factor beta in diabetic nephropathy: Implications for treatment. Semin Nephrol 2007;27:153–160.

93. Tuttle KR, Bakris GL, Toto RD, et al: The effect of ruboxistaurin on nephropathy in type 2 diabetes. Diabetes Care 2005;28:2686–2690.

94. Coughlan MT, Cooper ME, Forbes JM: Can advanced glycation end product inhibitors modulate more than one pathway to enhance renoprotection in diabetes? Ann N Y Acad Sci 2005;1043:750–758.

95. Coughlan MT, Thallas-Bonke V, Pete J, et al: Combination therapy with the advanced glycation end product cross-link breaker, alagebrium, and angiotensin converting enzyme inhibitors in diabetes: Synergy or redundancy? Endocrinology 2007;148:886–895.

96. Jandeleit-Dahm KA, Lassila M, Allen TJ: Advanced glycation end products in diabetes-associated atherosclerosis and renal disease: Interventional studies. Ann N Y Acad Sci 2005;1043:759–766.

97. Voziyan PA, Hudson BG: Pyridoxamine as a multifunctional pharmaceutical: Targeting pathogenic glycation and oxidative damage. Cell Mol Life Sci 2005;62:1671–1681.

98. Bloembergen WE, Port FK, Mauger EA, Wolfe RA: A comparison of mortality between patients treated with hemodialysis and peritoneal dialysis. J Am Soc Nephrol 1995;6:177–183.

99. Fenton SS, Schaubel DE, Desmeules M, et al: Hemodialysis versus peritoneal dialysis: A comparison of adjusted mortality rates. Am J Kidney Dis 1997;30:334–342.

100. Heaf JG, Lokkegaard H, Madsen M: Initial survival advantage of peritoneal dialysis relative to haemodialysis. Nephrol Dial Transplant 2002;17:112–117.

101. Held PJ, Port FK, Turenne MN, et al: Continuous ambulatory peritoneal dialysis and hemodialysis: Comparison of patient mortality with adjustment for comorbid conditions. Kidney Int 1994;45:1163–1169.

102. Jaar BG, Coresh J, Plantinga LC, et al: Comparing the risk for death with peritoneal dialysis and hemodialysis in a national cohort of patients with chronic kidney disease. Ann Intern Med 2005;143:174–183.

103. Vonesh EF, Snyder JJ, Foley RN, Collins AJ: The differential impact of risk factors on mortality in hemodialysis and peritoneal dialysis. Kidney Int 2004;66:2389–2401.

104. Passadakis P, Oreopoulos D: Peritoneal dialysis in diabetic patients. Adv Ren Replace Ther 2001;8:22–41.

105. Locatelli F, Pozzoni P, Del VL: Renal replacement therapy in patients with diabetes and end-stage renal disease. J Am Soc Nephrol 2004;15(Suppl 1):S25–S29.

106. Prischl FC, Kirchgatterer A, Brandstatter E, et al: Parameters of prognostic relevance to the patency of vascular access in hemodialysis patients. J Am Soc Nephrol 1995;6:1613–1618.

107. Wolfe RA, Ashby VB, Milford EL, et al: Comparison of mortality in all patients on dialysis, patients on dialysis awaiting transplantation, and recipients of a first cadaveric transplant. N Engl J Med 1999;341:1725–1730.

Further Reading

de Zeeuw D: Albuminuria: A target for treatment of type 2 diabetic nephropathy. Semin Nephrol 2007;27:172–181.

Grundy SM, Howard B, Smith S Jr, et al: Prevention Conference VI: Diabetes and Cardiovascular Disease: executive summary: Conference proceeding for healthcare professionals from a special writing group of the American Heart Association. Circulation 2002;105:2231–2239.

Lewis EJ: Treating hypertension in the patient with overt diabetic nephropathy. Semin Nephrol 2007;2:182–194.

Locatelli F, Pozzoni P, Del VL: Renal replacement therapy in patients with diabetes and end-stage renal disease. J Am Soc Nephrol 2004;15(Suppl 1):S25–S29.

Parving HH: Diabetic nephropathy: Prevention and treatment. Kidney Int 2001;60:2041–2055.

PART IV

Disorders of Fluid, Electrolyte, and Acid-Base Homeostasis

CONTENTS

Chapter 29

Therapy of Dysnatremic Disorders

Joshua M. Thurman and Tomas Berl

Abnormalities of the serum sodium concentration (S_{Na}) are the most common electrolyte disorders encountered in clinical medicine.[1] Collectively referred to as the dysnatremias, they represent disturbances in the control of the body's relative amount of water to sodium. In some settings, treatment must be prompt and judicious, because symptoms may be life-threatening and inappropriate therapy can be deleterious. Skilled management of these disorders requires an understanding of the normal control of the serum sodium, the pathologic settings in which dysnatremias occur, and the ability to quantify the disturbances in order to prescribe safe and effective treatment.

PLASMA SODIUM CONCENTRATION

The plasma sodium value only reflects the relative amount of sodium to water.[2] It cannot therefore be used to assess total body sodium (TB_{Na}). The S_{Na} is determined by TB_{Na}, total body potassium (TB_K), and total body water (TBW):

$$S_{Na} = \frac{(TB_{Na} + TB_K)}{TBW} \qquad \text{(Eq. 29-1)}$$

Careful analysis by Nguyen and Kurtz[3] has led to more sophisticated formulas describing how the S_{Na} is established, but this simple equation is still very useful in clinical evaluation of the patient. From Equation 29-1, it can be seen that

hyponatremia can occur as a consequence of a decrease in the body's content of monovalent cations, an increase in TBW, or a combination of these. Overall, the dysnatremias should be viewed primarily as disturbances in water balance, with a variable component of negative solute balance.

The sodium concentration is a primary determinant of plasma osmolality (P_{osm}):

$$P_{osm} = 2[Na] + glucose/18 + BUN/2.8 \qquad \text{(Eq. 29-2)}$$

where BUN represents blood urea nitrogen. Normally, the osmolality of body fluids can be estimated as twice the S_{Na} plus approximately 10 mOsm to account for other solutes. The addition of solutes to the extracellular fluid will increase its measured osmolality. However, the permeability of a solute across cell membranes determines whether it will cause water to be redistributed between the intracellular and extracellular compartments. Solutes that are permeable across cell membranes, such as urea, ethanol, methanol, and ethylene glycol, do not induce water movement and thus cause hyperosmolality without cellular dehydration. In contrast, the addition of impermeable solutes such as glucose (in an insulinopenic state) or mannitol establishes an effective gradient for water to leave the cell. This process lowers the S_{Na}, producing a translocational hyponatremia in the setting of either an isotonic or even hypertonic state, and leads to cellular dehydration. Conversely, when hyponatremia occurs as a consequence of an increase in TBW (hypotonic hyponatremia), water flows into cells causing increased cell volume and decreased intracellular osmolality.

THERAPEUTIC APPROACH TO THE HYPONATREMIC PATIENT

Although most hyponatremic patients are asymptomatic, severe hyponatremia is a medical emergency that may lead to cerebral edema, tentorial herniation, and death.[4–6] Surveys of severe symptomatic hyponatremia suggest high mortality rates in the absence of aggressive intervention.[7] In some patients, however, the treatment itself may result in central nervous system demyelination, producing permanent neurological sequelae or even death. Safe treatment therefore requires an understanding of cerebral adaptation to hypotonicity and knowledge of the patient groups at greatest risk of poor outcomes.

Cerebral Adaptation to Hypotonicity

Due to the unyielding confines of the skull, the brain is the primary site of symptoms in acute hyponatremia. Decreases in extracellular osmolality cause water to flow into the intracellular space, and the resultant cellular edema within the fixed volume of the cranium produces an increase in intracranial pressure. Fortunately, the brain possesses adaptive mechanisms that defend against such increases in intracranial pressure, making overt neurological manifestations infrequent.[8] The first protective mechanism, occurring early in hyponatremia (1–3 hours), involves a decrease in cerebral extracellular fluid volume. As cellular volume expands, the resultant increase in interstitial pressure stimulates flow of extracellular fluid into the cerebrospinal fluid, which is shunted into the systemic circulation, effectively relieving some of the elevation of intracranial pressure. This mechanism protects against mild acute changes in hyponatremia. A second protective mechanism involves a reduction in intracellular solutes. This starts approximately 3 hours after the onset of hypotonicity with the loss of cellular potassium. This is followed over the next 72 hours by the loss of organic solutes, including glutamate, taurine, myo-inositol, and glutamine.[9] Although some of the osmolyte losses occur within 24 hours, the loss of such solutes becomes more marked in subsequent days and accounts for almost complete restoration of cerebral water.

The benefits afforded by cerebral adaptation are also the source of the problems encountered in the treatment of hyponatremia. The increase in plasma tonicity that accompanies correction of chronic hyponatremia requires a reversal of the adaptive process to prevent cellular dehydration. The rate at which the brain reverses this process and restores lost solutes is of great pathophysiologic importance. Although brain sodium and chloride levels recover rapidly, the reaccumulation of osmolytes is considerably delayed. The process of increasing or restoring cellular electrolytes and accumulating organic osmolytes in the face of increasing extracellular sodium concentration is less efficient in brains previously adapted to hypotonic conditions compared with those in normonatremic states. This is reflected by the greater cerebral water loss sustained by adapted brains.[10]

Correction of chronic hyponatremia with resultant cerebral dehydration correlates with the delayed appearance of severe neurological deficits and the pathologic finding of foci of demyelination. This finding, called the osmotic demyelination syndrome (ODS), was initially observed in the central basis pontis but also occurs elsewhere throughout the central nervous system. The typical clinical presentation is for patients to show an initial improvement in mental status after the start of correction, with subsequent deterioration and development of (1) motor abnormalities, sometimes progressing to flaccid quadriplegia and even respiratory paralysis; (2) pseudobulbar palsy; and (3) mental status or behavioral changes, including progressive loss of consciousness. The diagnosis of this ODS is made through confirmation of foci of demyelination on head computed tomography or magnetic resonance imaging, although the radiographic findings may lag behind clinical findings by several weeks. Although survival without residual deficits is becoming more common, ODS frequently has a fatal course within 3 to 5 weeks, making this a dreaded complication of therapy. It must be noted that the diagnosis of ODS is made primarily based on clinical findings because the radiographic features can be absent.

RISK FACTORS FOR NEUROLOGICAL COMPLICATIONS OF HYPONATREMIA AND ITS CORRECTION

Mortality estimates of inpatient hyponatremia range from 10% to 50%, although the contribution of the hypotonicity to poor outcome is difficult to separate from other underlying causes. Oh and colleagues[11] suggest that most patients dying of complications related to acute hyponatremia may already be brain dead at the time of diagnosis, further supporting need for careful monitoring and a high index of suspicion in making the diagnosis.

Symptoms of hyponatremia, such as gastrointestinal complaints, lethargy, apathy, agitation, and cramps, occur most commonly with rapid decreases in S_{Na} to less than 125 mEq/L. Seizures and coma usually result from rapid decreases to levels below 110 mEq/L. Conversely, hyponatremia usually needs to be present for at least 72 hours to set the stage for complications related to treatment. Despite these generalizations, there is tremendous variation in the physiologic responses to water intoxication and the likelihood of suffering complications during correction. Clinical surveys and experimental data suggest that there are subgroups of patients at greatest risk of either acute cerebral edema or osmotic demyelination (Box 29-1).

Risk Factors for Acute Cerebral Edema

Hypoxia

The combination of hyponatremia and hypoxia may be particularly dangerous.[12,13] In experimental animals, hypoxia abrogates the volume adaptive response to hyponatremia, therefore resulting in increased brain edema.[14] Patients with symptomatic hyponatremia and hypoxia who are corrected at

Box 29-1 Patient Groups at Increased Risk of Neurological Complications of Hyponatremia

Acute Cerebral Edema	Osmotic Demyelination
Hypoxic patients	Alcoholics
Postoperative premenopausal women	Malnourished patients
	Hypokalemic patients
Elderly women on thiazide diuretics	Burn patients
	Patients with previous hypoxic episodes
Polydipsic patients	Elderly women on thiazide diuretics
Children	
Marathon runners	Serum Na < 105 mEq/L

rates slower than 0.55 mEq/L/hr may have greater mortality than those corrected faster,[13] even though this rate of correction is similar to what is commonly recommended for patients with chronic hyponatremia.

Hospital-Acquired Hyponatremia in Premenopausal Women

In the hospital setting, hyponatremic premenopausal women are more symptomatic at higher sodium levels than other groups and appear to be at increased risk of neurological complications related to acute hyponatremia. Although hyponatremia appears to develop with almost equal frequency in men and women, Ayus and colleagues[15] reported that of 307 men with postoperative hyponatremia, only one had an outcome of permanent cerebral dysfunction or death; in contrast, 33 of 367 women with hyponatremia had such outcomes. Experimental data support gender differences in arginine vasopressin (AVP) release and its cerebral action, including the process of cerebral adaptation. In female rats, AVP decreases high-energy phosphates and pH in the brain and increases mortality relative to male rats. Some of these effects may be related to female sex hormones, which can stimulate release of AVP, compared with male sex hormones, whose action may be inhibitory.[16] Studies in rabbits suggest that cellular adaptation may be less efficient in females than in males, perhaps due to decreased potassium extrusion. Synaptosomes obtained from females demonstrated lower levels of sodium transport and Na^+/K^+-ATPase activity than those obtained from males.[17]

Patients on Thiazide Diuretics

Thiazide diuretics are a common cause of hyponatremia. These agents reduce electrolyte-free water clearance by inhibiting sodium reabsorption in the early distal tubule and also induce sodium, potassium, and magnesium losses. They may also directly stimulate thirst. Occasionally, thiazides can cause severe hyponatremia, with levels below 115 mEq/L. The majority of affected patients reach these levels within 2 weeks of starting the diuretic, although approximately one third require fewer than 5 days.[18] These patients seem to have a predisposition to thiazide-induced hyponatremia, as rechallenge with the drug can rapidly reinduce the hypotonic state.

Sonnenblick and colleagues[18] reported 12 deaths in a group of 129 patients with diuretic-induced severe hyponatremia. These deaths were directly related to the hyponatremia and were associated with a lower mean sodium level on presentation (103 mEq/L) compared with those patients who recovered (108 mEq/L). In most studies, the patients at greatest risk are elderly women with low body mass. This may be related to decreased body water at the start of therapy, but possibilities also include altered hypothalamic responses and intrarenal water excretion defects in this group. Of note, some elderly women may have a habitually increased water intake and low solute intake as described by the "tea and toast" diet. Low solute excretion impairs the ability to excrete the ingested water load, resulting in hyponatremia.

Polydipsia

Polydipsia, particularly in psychiatric patients, is a common cause of hyponatremia. Approximately 6% to 17% of all chronically ill psychiatric patients exhibit features of polydipsia, consuming 4 to 25 L of water per day. Most of these patients have schizophrenia, although associations with affective disorders, mental retardation, and alcoholism are also observed. Only a subgroup of polydipsic patients becomes hyponatremic; estimates range from 25% to 50%.[19] Hyponatremic patients who compulsively drink water frequently have increased circulating levels of AVP and defects in intrarenal water handling. These abnormalities may be related to antipsychotic medications, but some evidence suggests the presence of defects in water homeostasis even in the absence of pharmacotherapeutic agents.[20] Excessive water intake also increases the risk of hyponatremia in marathon runners.[21]

Children

Children are at risk of becoming hyponatremic because of either excessive dietary intake of hypotonic fluids (such as plain water or diluted formula) or the inappropriate use of hypotonic fluids during hospital admission.[22] Use of hypotonic fluids in children may overestimate their requirements and also may not take into account nonosmotic release of vasopressin due to stimuli such as pain and nausea.[23] In the United States, hyponatremia is the primary cause of nonfebrile seizures and may also cause respiratory failure. Keating and colleagues[24] reviewed 34 cases of water intoxication in infants and found that an inability to pay for formula was the most common reason given by caretakers for diluting the formula or substituting water.

Risk Factors for Osmotic Demyelination

Several factors appear to increase the treated individual's susceptibility to ODS (see Table 29-1). First, ODS is rarely observed in patients with S_{Na} of more than 120 mEq/L and occurs only if hyponatremia has been present for at least 24 hours and probably for 48 hours. Serum sodium less than 105 mEq/L also increases the risk of this complication. In addition, severely hyponatremic patients with alcoholism, malnutrition, or hypokalemia as well as elderly women taking thiazide diuretics appear to be at increased risk of osmotic demyelination.[25] Hypoxia or anoxia may also contribute.[14]

TREATMENT STRATEGIES IN HYPONATREMIA

The optimal treatment of hyponatremia involves attention to four factors: (1) the presence of symptoms, (2) the duration of the hypo-osmolality, (3) the volume status, and (4) the degree of hyponatremia.

Urine electrolytes and calculation of electrolyte-free water clearance can help predict how the kidney will handle the salt and water administered during therapy and the changes in serum sodium that ensue. If the urine sodium concentration (U_{Na}) is less than 10 mEq/L, the kidney is sodium avid and the patient will likely retain any sodium that is administered. Conversely, if U_{Na} is more than 50 mEq/L, the kidney will likely excrete any sodium that is administered, and the concentration at which it excretes this sodium will determine the change in the patient's S_{Na}.

For patients who are euvolemic and who will likely excrete the administered sodium, the electrolyte-free water clearance can be calculated to predict the resultant change in the relative amount of TBW to sodium. Urine flow (V) can be divided into two components. The first component is the urine volume needed to excrete electrolytes at the concentration of electrolytes in plasma (i.e., isotonic). The second component is any remaining urine volume, which represents electrolyte-free water (cH$_2$Oe). Because sodium and potassium contribute to the osmolality of urine and sodium is the primary determinant of osmolality in serum, the fraction of urine volume that is isotonic can be calculated as:

$$\frac{(U_{Na}+U_K)}{S_{Na}} \tag{Eq. 29-3}$$

The electrolyte-free water can therefore be calculated as:

$$cH_2Oe = V\left[1-\frac{(U_{Na}+U_K)}{S_{Na}}\right] \tag{Eq. 29-4}$$

The cH$_2$Oe is negative when $U_{Na} + U_K > S_{Na}$, indicating that the kidney is producing urine with an electrolyte concentration greater than that of plasma. Formation of urine with this composition will tend to decrease the S_{Na}. Conversely, if $U_{Na} + U_K < S_{Na}$, cH$_2$Oe is positive and S_{Na} will increase.

Treatment of Acute Symptomatic Hyponatremia

In view of the potentially life-threatening complications of acute hyponatremia as described previously, there is a wide consensus that rapid correction of hyponatremia is indicated in patients in whom hyponatremia has developed in less than 48 hours (Fig. 29-1). Generally, the presence of symptoms indicates that hyponatremia has developed too quickly for the adaptive mechanisms to compensate, and symptomatic patients have probably developed hyponatremia over a short period. Because patients who have acutely developed hyponatremia have not had time to adapt to the change in tonicity, they also arc at less risk of developing complications from correction of the hyponatremia (ODS).

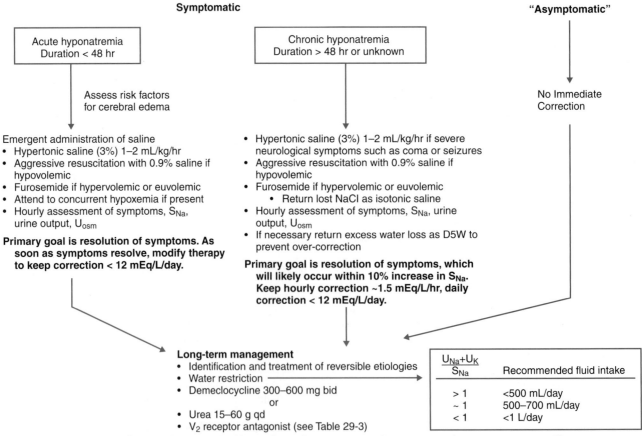

Figure 29-1   Treatment of severe (<125 mEq/L) euvolemic hyponatremia. S_{Na}, serum sodium concentration; U_K, urine potassium concentration; U_{Na}, urine sodium concentration.

Therapy should be initiated immediately in symptomatic patients, particularly in those at increased risk of complications, such as those with hypoxia. For patients with hyponatremia of less than 48 hours' duration and/or risk factors for the development of cerebral edema, treatment is aimed at achieving the following (Box 29-2):

1. Initial sodium administration should increase the serum sodium by approximately 2 mEq/L/hr. A rapid increase in the S_{Na} can be achieved by administering hypertonic saline (3% saline contains 513 mEq/L of Na). Hypertonic saline is often started at 1 to 2 mL/kg/hr. The primary goal for the administration of 3% saline is not the restoration of a sodium deficit but the rapid reversal of potentially life-threatening cerebral edema.
2. For patients in whom the duration is known to be less than 48 hours, full correction is probably safe, but probably should be continued only until symptoms resolve. After that, correction can be slowed to keep the total daily correction at less than 12 mEq/L.
3. Address and correct concurrent hypoxemia.

A clinical case is described to illustrate the approach to such a patient and to highlight the following principles:

1. In the setting of antidiuresis, $U_{Na} + U_K$ can exceed 150 mEq/L, and the electrolyte-free water clearance is negative. Thus, if isotonic saline is infused, the body may excrete the infused sodium in a more concentrated form, possibly even worsening the hyponatremia.
2. The administration of hypertonic saline with furosemide ensures electrolyte-free water excretion while preventing volume expansion.

Case History

A 31-year-old, 60-kg woman with normal preoperative laboratory values underwent an elective hysterectomy with minimal intraoperative blood loss. During a 4-hour period encompassing the surgery and recovery room care, she received 2 L of 0.9% normal saline. Thereafter, 125 mL/hr of 0.45% normal saline was administered. Her total urine output for the 12 hours after surgery was 1500 mL. The patient suffered progressively worsening abdominal pain and intermittent vomiting, for which she received meperidine (Demerol) and prochlorpera-

zine (Compazine). At 30 hours postoperatively, mental status changes developed and S_{Na} was 114 mEq/L. Her intravenous orders were changed to 200 mL/hr of 0.9% normal saline for 5 hours, during which time the patient's urine output was 750 mL, U_{Na} was 140 mEq/L, and U_K was 60 mEq/L. The patient then had a seizure and respiratory arrest. The repeat S_{Na} was 112 mEq/L.

Case Analysis

Because preoperative S_{Na} was 140 mEq/L and preoperative TBW was 30 L (50% of body weight), rearranging Equation 29-1 gives

$$TB_{Na} + TB_K = S_{Na} \times TBW$$
$$= 140 \times 30$$
$$= 4200 \text{ mEq}$$

Postoperatively, when S_{Na} was 114 mEq/L (assuming solute balance), the patient's new TBW would have been:

$$TBW = \frac{(U_{Na} + U_K)}{S_{Na}}$$
$$= \frac{4200 \text{ mEq}}{114 \text{ mEq/L}}$$
$$= 36.8 \text{ L}$$

Therefore, a rough estimate of positive water balance would have been $36.8 - 30 = 6.8$ L.

Even after the patient's hyponatremia was recognized and the hypotonic fluids were replaced by isotonic saline, the patient's S_{Na} continued to decrease. The following table is an analysis of water and solute balance during the 5 hours of isotonic saline infusion.

	Water (L)	Solute (Na + K) (mEq)
Intake (0.9% saline at 200 mL/hr)	1.00	150 Na
Output	0.75	105 Na + 45 K
Balance (intake − output)	+0.25	0

Box 29-2 General Guidelines for the Treatment of Symptomatic Hyponatremia

Acute Hyponatremia (duration < 48 hr)	**Chronic Hyponatremia (duration > 48 hr)**
Increase S_{Na} rapidly by ~2 mEq/L/hr until resolution of symptoms	Initial rapid increase in S_{Na} by 10% or 10 mEq/L
Full correction probably safe but not necessary	Perform frequent neurological evaluations; correction rate may be reduced with improvement in symptoms
Limit correction to 12 mEq/24 hr	At no time after initial increment should correction exceed rate of 1.5 mEq/L/hr or total increment of 12 mEq/L/day
Treat coexistent hypoxia	Hypotonic fluids, and even DDAVP, should be administered to prevent correction in excess of desired daily goal

The sum of urinary cations ($U_{Na} + U_K$) should be less than the concentration of infused sodium to ensure excretion of electrolyte-free water.
DDAVP, 1-desamine-8-D-arginine vasopressin; U_{Na}, urine sodium concentration; U_K, urine potassium concentration.

The resultant TBW is now 36.8 + 0.25 = 37.05 L. The S_{Na}, assuming essentially unchanged solute balance, would be

$$S_{Na} = \frac{(TB_{Na} + TB_K)}{TBW}$$
$$= \frac{4200\,mEq}{37.05\,L}$$
$$= 113\,mEq/L$$

This example illustrates that, in a patient with high AVP levels, the infusion of isotonic saline not only fails to correct hyponatremia but can further aggravate it. The correction of hyponatremia requires the excretion of electrolyte-free water, that is, the sum of urinary sodium and potassium must be less than the sodium of the infusing fluid.

The administration of furosemide promotes such electrolyte-free water excretion. When combined with the infusion of hypertonic saline, S_{Na} can be promptly increased. The following table illustrates what would have happened if the patient had received 100 mL/hr of 3% saline for 2 hours and 40 mg furosemide, with urine output of 1000 mL, U_{Na} 70 mEq/L, and U_K 30 mEq/L.

	Water (mL)	Solute (Na + K) (mEq)
Intake (3% saline at 100 mL/hr)	200	100 Na
Output	1000	70 Na + 30 K
Balance (intake − output)	−800	0

Therefore, TBW is 36.8 − 0.8 = 36 L. Because solute balance is unchanged:

$$S_{Na} = \frac{(TB_{Na} + TB_K)}{TBW}$$
$$= \frac{4200\,mEq}{36\,L}$$
$$= 117\,mEq/L$$

Thus, rather than decreasing, the patient's S_{Na} has increased and has done so at an acceptable rate (~2 mEq/L/hr).

Treatment of Chronic Symptomatic Hyponatremia

Symptomatic hyponatremia that has persisted for longer than 48 hours or is of unknown duration must be treated with great caution. Neurological symptoms, such as depressed sensorium or seizures, reflect cerebral dysfunction and the need for some correction, yet overly rapid correction puts the patient at risk of osmotic demyelination (see Fig. 29-1). Various studies have attempted to resolve whether it is the rate or magnitude of correction that determines the risk of complications (Table 29-1). However, these two variables are not readily dissociated because a rapid correction rate is usually accompanied by a greater absolute magnitude of correction over a given time period.

Several animal studies indicate that the daily absolute change may be the primary determinant of the risk of osmotic demyelination and that correction by less than 25 mEq/L in the first 24 hours correlates best with survival. Soupart and colleagues[26] showed that in rats corrected over 48 hours, 95% of the hyponatremic animals developed brain lesions when the daily absolute change in S_{Na} reached 20 mEq/L/day. Below this limit, the incidence and severity of brain lesions were very low, even in the group corrected rapidly with bolus injections. In another study, hyponatremic rats treated with rapid correction (2.7 mEq/L/hr) but an absolute change in S_{Na} of less than 25 mEq/L/day had a lower mortality rate (95% survival) compared with rats treated with rapid correction and an absolute change in S_{Na} of more than 25 mEq/L/day (15% survival).[27] Verbalis and Martinez[28] have shown that in rats with hyponatremia of 19 days' duration, demyelination might be a function of both the rate and magnitude of correction. Demyelination was not observed in any rats in which the maximal correction rate was less than 2.5 mEq/L/hr and the magnitude of increase in S_{Na} was less than 25 mEq/L/day. If either of these limits was exceeded, the demyelination rate was 60%.

What is known about this subject in humans? Obviously, the potentially severe consequences make controlled clinical trials in humans impossible. Most retrospective studies indicate that demyelinating lesions are rare in patients who are corrected at a rate less than 0.5 mEq/L/hr and a magnitude less than 12 mEq/L/day (see Table 29-1). Sterns and colleagues[29] reported eight hyponatremic patients who developed the ODS after being corrected by more than 12 mEq/L in 24 hours. In a subsequent study, Sterns[25] reviewed 54 patients with chronic hyponatremia who underwent treatment. Seven of these patients developed neurological complications after treatment. Those who developed neurological complications had experienced a wide range of corrections (<0.7 mEq/L/hr in three patients), but all had been corrected by more than 12 mEq/L in 24 hours (mean correction, 17 mEq/L in 24 hours). In another retrospective study of 56 patients, 14 developed neurological complications, although there were no neurological complications in patients corrected by less than 0.55 mEq/L/hr and less than 12 mEq/L/day.[30] In a retrospective analysis of the literature, Ayus and colleagues[31] initially found that patients treated slowly (<0.7 mEq/L/hr) had a greater mortality than those corrected at a rate of 2 mEq/L/hr. However, this was based on case reports that may have included patients with acute hyponatremia, and the deaths were typically due to brain edema and herniation as one would expect with acute hyponatremia corrected too slowly.[4] In a combined prospective and retrospective analysis of patients with demyelinating lesions, Ayus and colleagues[32] later showed that an increase in S_{Na} of more than 25 mEq/L in the initial 48 hours was the primary risk factor for the development of cerebral lesions.

A more recent study by Ayus and Arieff[33] also highlights the risks of delaying therapy in symptomatic patients. The outcomes of 53 postmenopausal women with chronic symptomatic hyponatremia were compared based on whether they were treated promptly with saline, treated with saline only after the onset of respiratory insufficiency, or treated with fluid restriction only. The group treated promptly had no long-term neurological sequelae, whereas those whose treatment was delayed until after the onset of respiratory insufficiency had significant morbidity and mortality, particularly in the group treated by fluid restriction alone. Thus, although the rate and magnitude of correction must be controlled, treatment should be initiated promptly.

Table 29-1 Studies of Patients with Chronic Hyponatremia

Ref.	Type of Study	No. of Patients	Initial S_Na (mEq/L)	Rate of Correction (mmol/L/hr)	Magnitude of Correction (mmol/L/day)	No. of Patients with Neurological Complications
Sterns et al[29]	Retrospective	8 (duration of hyponatremia uncertain)	107		Average 21.5, all corrected > 12	8
	Literature review	51				22/38 of those corrected >12 mmol/L/day; 0/13 corrected <12 mmol/L/day
Sterns[25]	Retrospective	54 chronic cases	107	0.59	17 in those with neurological complications	7 (2 had demyelination)
		10 acute cases (defined as 2-4 days)	105	1.57		None
Ayus et al[32]	Prospective	33 (30 of whom had hyponatremia for >24 hr)	108 ± 1	1.3 ± 0.2 (in 5 patients, correction was 1.6-4.7)	20 ± 1 (2 acute patients were corrected to 27 and 38 mmol/L, raising the average)	None
	Retrospective	12 (four with hepatic encephalopathy and only mild hyponatremia)	107 ± 4	1 ± 0.2	37 ± 3 (over 41 ± 3 hr)	8
	Literature review	17	107 ± 2	0.7 ± 0.1	27 ± 2 (over 39 ± 4 hr)	17 (11 with evidence of demyelination)
Sterns et al[30]	Retrospective	56	<105	No complications if <0.55	No complications if <12 mmol/L/day	14
Ayus and Arieff[33]	Prospective	17	111	0.7	14	None
		22	103	0.8	22	14 died or had permanent neurological sequelae
		14	109	0.1	3	11 died, three had permanent neurological sequelae

The question of whether the process that leads to brain demyelination is reversible has significant clinical importance. This issue has been studied by Soupart and colleagues.[34] Hyponatremic rats were submitted to an excessive correction (>25 mEq/L) with hypertonic saline during a single intraperitoneal infusion. This osmotic stress was maintained for 12 hours. Next, hypotonic fluid was administered to maintain the total magnitude of correction at less than 20 mEq/L/day. Mild brain lesions were noted in 20% of the treated group and in 100% of the control rats that did not receive hypotonic fluids. This experiment implies that, at least in animals, subsequent brain damage can be prevented in asymptomatic rats by early lowering of S_{Na}, provided that the final correction is maintained at less than 20 mEq/L/day. Soupart and colleagues[35] have also published a case report of a patient with chronic symptomatic hyponatremia who received hypotonic fluid and 1-desamine-8-D-arginine vasopressin (DDAVP) to lower the serum sodium after she had initially been overcorrected. The patient was reported to have had neurological deterioration after the overcorrection, but after the sodium was relowered and allowed to correct slowly, she recovered without neurological deficits. Other similar reports have also been published.[36,37]

The rate at which S_{Na} will increase depends on the rate of administration and electrolyte content of infused fluids as well as on the rate of production and electrolyte content of urine. The initial increment may be achieved with cautious infusion of hypertonic or normal saline and furosemide, with frequent determinations of S_{Na} and urinary electrolytes. Hypertonic saline is rarely needed in this clinical setting and should be reserved for patients who have seizures. A number of formulas have been put forth to predict the change in serum sodium that would ensue with various saline infusion rates.[3,38,39] These formulas may be helpful as a guide to initial therapy, but because they fail to account for ongoing renal and extrarenal losses, their use is limited.[40] Recent attempts to determine the validity of the Adrogue-Madias formula[38] revealed that it accurately predicts changes in S_{Na} under most clinical settings with a tendency to underestimate the achieved S_{Na} concentration, sometimes by significant amounts.[41] If correction occurs at an inappropriately rapid rate, free water should be administered. After the desired increment is attained, therapy can continue in the form of water restriction.

These data lead us to propose the following guidelines for treating chronic hyponatremia (see Fig. 29-1 and Box 29-2).

1. Correction of S_{Na} should be undertaken without delay in symptomatic patients, particularly those experiencing seizures. Because cerebral water is only increased by approximately 10% in severe chronic hyponatremia, S_{Na} should be increased by 10% or approximately 10 mEq/L over approximately 8 to 12 hours, followed by water restriction. Rapid correction of S_{Na} should only continue until symptoms resolve or until this 10% change is achieved.
2. After the initial correction, the rate should not exceed 1 to 1.5 mEq/L/hr and probably should be less than 0.5 mEq/L/hr.
3. S_{Na} should not be increased by more than 12 mEq/L/day.
4. If the patient has reached the desired rate or magnitude of correction yet is excreting hypotonic urine, hypotonic fluids and even DDAVP can be administered to prevent correction in excess of the desired daily goal. Calculation of the electrolyte-free water and attention to urine volume can be used to predict the patient's free water requirement.

Example

A 50-kg man with altered mental status is found to have an S_{Na} of 110 mEq/L. The initial goal of therapy is to increase the patient's S_{Na} by 10% or to approximately 120 mEq/L. If the patient is thought to be euvolemic, correction can be achieved via electrolyte-free water excretion without a significant change in total body osmoles.

For men, TBW $\cong$ 0.6 × weight (kg). Because the osmoles remain constant, Equation 29.1 can be rearranged to yield:

$$\frac{\text{Desired } S_{Na}}{S_{Na}} = \frac{\text{TBW}}{\text{Desired TBW}}$$

Because TBW = 0.6 × 50 = 30 L,

$$\text{Desired TBW} = \frac{S_{Na} \times \text{TBW}}{\text{Desired } S_{Na}}$$

$$= \frac{110 \times 30}{120}$$

$$= 27.5 \text{ L}$$

Therefore, 2.5 L of electrolyte-free water must be excreted. If the water is to be excreted over 10 hours, the urine should contain 250 mL/hr of electrolyte-free water. This can be achieved by administering furosemide and replacing any sodium, potassium, and excess free water lost in the urine. The balance during the first 2 hours is shown in the following table.

	Water (mL)	Solute (Na + K) (mEq)
Intake (500 mL normal saline + 100 mL D5W with 20 mEq KCl)	600	75/20
Output	1000	75/20
Balance	−400	0

D5W, 5% dextrose in water.

Continuing to replace urine electrolyte or excess electrolyte-free water losses, the balance during the subsequent 2 hours is shown in the following table.

	Water (mL)	Solute (Na + K) (mEq)
Intake (400 mL normal saline + 100 mL D5W with 20 mEq KCl)	500	60/20
Output	800	60/25
Balance	−300	−5

D5W, 5% dextrose in water.

The patient's TBW has decreased by approximately 700 mL, total body osmoles are essentially unchanged, and one can estimate S_{Na} as approximately 113 mEq/L.

Asymptomatic Euvolemic Hyponatremia

Even those hyponatremic patients who appear asymptomatic may have subtle neurological findings. For example, one study of such patients found that rigorous examination often detected unsteady gait or attention deficits, and they had a significantly increased risk of falls.[42] Nevertheless, patients without obvious deficits should be corrected very cautiously as cerebral adaptation has likely occurred (see Fig. 29-1). Nonedematous asymptomatic hyponatremia should invoke a search for reversible causes. If indicated, thyroid or glucocorticoid replacement should be initiated. If the syndrome of inappropriate secretion of antidiuretic hormone (SIADH) is present, identification of reversible causes should be undertaken with subsequent removal of offending agents. If the aforementioned strategies are not attainable, then fluid restriction should be prescribed. An initial restriction of 1 L/day is often prescribed. In most patients, this will be adequate to allow net free water excretion. In some patients, however, such an intake still exceeds insensible and urinary losses and does not result in improvement. Furst and colleagues[43] described a patient whose S_{Na} decreased from 121 to 117 mEq/L over 24 hours even though his fluid intake was limited to 1 L/day. This patient had a U_{Na} of 100 mEq/L and a U_K of 66 mEq/L and produced 900 mL of urine over the 24 hours. Using Equation 29-4, net electrolyte-free water can be calculated as follows:

$$cH_2Oe = V\left[1 - \frac{(U_{Na} + U_K)}{S_{Na}}\right]$$
$$= 0.9\left[1 - \frac{(100+66)}{121}\right]$$
$$= -0.33\,L$$

Unless his intake is less than insensible losses plus electrolyte-free water excretion (which is negative in this case), his S_{Na} will decrease even more. The authors therefore propose guidelines for therapy based on urine and serum electrolytes (incorporated in Fig. 29-1).

Restricting fluid intake to 1 L/day or less is difficult to attain in the outpatient setting, and pharmacologic therapy may be necessary. SIADH impairs the renal capacity for urine dilution, but pharmacologic agents that impair urinary concentration increase free water excretion.

Lithium carbonate and demeclocycline hydrochloride have been used in the treatment of chronic hyponatremia. The nephrotoxicity and unwanted central nervous system effects of lithium have limited its usefulness. Demeclocycline, however, is safer and effective for the treatment of SIADH.[44] Administered in doses of 300 to 600 mg twice daily, demeclocycline interferes with the renal action of AVP and promotes maximal water diuresis after 1 to 2 weeks of therapy. To ensure adequate gastrointestinal absorption, the drug should be given at least 1 to 2 hours after eating, and antacids that contain aluminum, calcium, or magnesium should be avoided. Once diuresis begins, the dose may be tapered to 150 to 300 mg twice daily to minimize toxicity. Additionally, water intake should be allowed to increase, thus preventing diabetes insipidus–induced dehydration. Nephrotoxicity may be observed in patients with liver disease. Azotemia independent of renal function may result from mild antianabolic effects. It may be associated with severe photosensitivity and should not be used in pregnant patients or children due to abnormalities in bone or enamel formation.

Urea has also been used in the treatment of SIADH.[45] Assume that a patient has an S_{Na} of 134 mEq/L, a fixed urine concentration of 800 mOsm/day, an obligatory solute load of 500 mOsm/day, a dietary sodium intake of 100 mmol/day, and a potassium intake of 40 mmol/day. Calculation of the volume required to excrete the daily solute load at baseline reveals:

$$V = \frac{\text{solute excretion}}{U_{Osm}}$$
$$= \frac{500\,\text{mOsm/day}}{800\,\text{mOsm/kg H}_2O}$$
$$= 0.625\,\text{L/day}$$

Urinary sodium and potassium concentrations can be determined as follows:

$$U_{Na} = 100\,\text{mmol}/0.625\,L = 160\,\text{mmol/L}$$
$$U_K = 40\,\text{mmol}/0.625\,L = 64\,\text{mmol/L}$$

These values may then be inserted into Equation 29-4 to compute the electrolyte-free water clearance:

$$cH_2Oe = V\left[1 - \frac{(U_{Na} + U_K)}{S_{Na}}\right]$$
$$= 0.625\left[1 - \frac{(160+64)}{134}\right]$$
$$= -0.418\,\text{/day}$$

The negative value for excretion of electrolyte-free water clearance implies net free water absorption, which could worsen hyponatremia.

Under the same conditions, administration of urea (30 g/day) adds approximately 500 mOsm/day to the obligatory solute load that must be excreted. This has a profound effect on electrolyte-free water clearance:

Volume required for excretion of solute load

$$= \frac{1000\,\text{mOsm/day}}{800\,\text{mOsm/kg H}_2O}$$
$$= 1.25\,\text{L/day}$$

As a result of the increased volume for solute clearance, urinary electrolyte concentrations decrease:

$$U_{Na} = \frac{100\,\text{mmol}}{1.25\,L} = 80\,\text{mmol/L}$$

$$U_K = \frac{40\,\text{mmol}}{1.25\,L} = 32\,\text{mmol/L}$$

Note the resultant changes in electrolyte-free water clearance:

$$cH_2Oe = V\left[1 - \frac{(U_{Na} + U_K)}{S_{Na}}\right]$$

$$= 1.25\left[1 - \frac{(80 + 32)}{134}\right]$$

$$= -1.25(1 - 0.83) = 0.21 \text{ L/day}$$

Thus, the administration of urea has altered this patient's water handling from net reabsorption to excretion of electrolyte-free water. Without altering urinary concentration, the increase in urine flow allows for more liberal water intake without the danger of worsening hyponatremia. Urea administration at doses more than 60 g is limited by gastrointestinal adverse effects such as gastric distress and diarrhea. A similar effect can be obtained by increasing salt intake (200 mEq/day) in combination with furosemide. Because this combination is likely to result in high potassium losses, serum potassium needs to be monitored and potassium replacement should be provided.

More recently, several small nonpeptide vasopressin antagonists have been developed that block the function of AVP at the V_2 receptor (Table 29-2). Several studies have demonstrated that they can induce a water diuresis and effectively increase the S_{Na} in patients with SIADH.[46,47] In the recently published Study of Ascending Levels of Tolvaptan in Hyponatremia I and II (SALT I/II) trials, 91 patients with SIADH were treated with tolvaptan for 30 days, and the S_{Na} in these patients increased by a greater degree than those who received placebo.[48] In another study,[49] patients received the oral vasopressin antagonist satavaptan for 1 year without any major side effects. Conivaptan is the only drug in this class to have U.S. Food and Drug Administration approval for the treatment of euvolemic hyponatremia.[50,51] It can only be administered intravenously, and it also blocks the V_1 receptor. As there is not yet much experience with these agents, they should be initiated at the lowest available dose. The urine osmolality can be monitored, and the dose can gradually be increased. These drugs should permit easing of the free water restriction and may increase the achievable S_{Na}. At this time, they appear to be safe, and ODS has not been reported. However, with further experience, possible adverse affects may emerge as the use of the drug increases.

Hypovolemic and Hypervolemic Hyponatremia

Hypovolemic hyponatremia results from the loss of both water and solute, with a greater relative loss of solute. The nonosmotic release of AVP in response to reduced effective circulating volume perpetuates the hyponatremia by producing antidiuresis. Patients with this type of hyponatremia are usually asymptomatic, probably because the losses of sodium and water limit the development of cerebral edema. The cornerstone of therapy is the administration of isotonic saline while also treating the underlying disturbance (Box 29-3). Resolution of the volume disturbance removes the stimulus for AVP and restores normal S_{Na}.

Hypervolemic hyponatremia is observed when both water and solute are increased, but water is increased to a greater extent. This condition is very difficult to treat because it often reflects severe irreversible dysfunction of the liver, heart, or kidney. In heart failure, cirrhosis, and nephrotic syndrome, decreased effective arterial volume results in the nonosmotic stimulation of AVP and an increase in thirst. Therefore, compliance with water restriction is difficult. Diuretics are the primary therapeutic agents for edema, but caution must be used in selecting the appropriate regimen. Whereas thiazide diuretics impair urinary dilution and may exacerbate hyponatremia, loop diuretics increase free water excretion and can improve S_{Na}. Correction of the underlying disturbances is usually not attainable.

The vasopressin antagonists can be employed to induce a water diuresis in patients with nonosmotic release of AVP. These agents can reduce the total body water and reduce the need for free water restriction. Because it blocks both the V_1 and V_2 receptors (see Table 29-2), Conivaptan has vasodilatory and aquaretic effects, both of which may be beneficial in congestive heart failure (CHF), although its vasodilatory effects are probably inappropriate for patients with cirrhosis.[52] It has been shown to decrease the pulmonary capillary wedge pressure in patients with CHF,[53] and currently it is approved by the U.S. Food and Drug Administration for the treatment of hypervolemic hyponatremia. The oral V_2 receptor antagonists lixivaptan[54] and tolvaptan[48,55] have also successfully been used to induce a water diuresis in patients with CHF. In the recently published Efficacy of Vasopressin Antagonism in Heart Failure Outcome Study with Tolvaptan (EVEREST) trial, patients with CHF and hyponatremia who received tolvaptan had significant increases in their S_{Na}.[56] However, the drug did not alter long-term all-cause

Table 29-2 Nonpeptide Arginine Vasopressin Receptor Antagonists

	Tolvaptan	Lixivaptan	Stavaptan	Conivaptan
Receptor	V_2	V_2	V_2	V_{1a}/V_2
Route of administration	Oral	Oral	Oral	IV
Urine volume	↑	↑	↑	↑
Urine osmolality	↓	↓	↓	↓
Na excretion	↔	↔ low dose, ↑ high dose	↔	↔
Manufacturer	Otsuka	CardioKine	Sanofi-Aventis	Astellas

Adapted with permission from Lee CR, Watkins ML, Patterson JH, et al: Vasopressin: A new target for the treatment of heart failure. Am Heart J 2003;146:9–18.

Box 29-3 Treatment of Noneuvolemic Hyponatremia

Hypovolemic Hyponatremia	**Hypervolemic Hyponatremia**
Volume restoration with isotonic saline	Water restriction
Identify and correct cause of water and sodium losses	Sodium restriction
	Substitute loop diuretics in place of thiazide diuretics
sodium and water retention	Treatment of stimulus for
V_2 receptor antagonists	

mortality, cardiovascular mortality, or CHF hospitalizations in the full study cohort, most of whom were not hyponatremic. Vasopressin antagonists have also been successfully used to increase the serum sodium concentration in patients with cirrhosis and dilutional hyponatremia.[57]

Patients with cirrhosis and CHF typically have only mild hyponatremia, and the optimal S_{Na} is not known. The increased TBW associated with hyponatremia in these conditions contributes to vascular congestion,[58] however, and may also limit the use of diuretics. Furthermore, there is evidence that correction of hyponatremia can improve symptoms and mortality, even beyond the benefits attributable to improvements in the volume status.[59] Thus, there is reason to expect that the use of vasopressin antagonists may improve outcomes in these patients, but conclusive clinical trials have not yet been performed and the target S_{Na} has not been determined.

THE HYPERNATREMIC PATIENT

Hypernatremia is defined as S_{Na} greater than 146 mEq/L. The presence of hypernatremia implies both extracellular hyperosmolality and, more importantly, hypertonicity, which produces central nervous system injury through cell shrinkage. The reported incidence of hypernatremia ranges from 0.65% to 2.23% of all hospitalized patients. Morbidity and mortality estimates in hypernatremic adults range from 42% to more than 70%, with approximately 10% mortality in chronic hypernatremia compared with 75% mortality in severe acute elevations of S_{Na} (>160 mEq/L). Unfortunately, even in survivors, neurological sequelae are common, especially in children in whom two thirds may show long-term deficits. As with hyponatremia, correcting hypernatremia too rapidly may be as dangerous as allowing the condition to persist.

TREATMENT OF THE HYPERNATREMIC PATIENT

Cerebral Response to Hypernatremia

Cellular dehydration is the primary basis of brain injury, as fluid shifts from the cellular compartment into the extracellular fluid. Neurological symptoms ensue, with initial changes in sensorium potentially culminating in seizures, coma, or death. Although alterations of cellular fluid and solute balance likely contribute to these signs and symptoms, pathologic evidence demonstrates

a variety of underlying anatomic derangements. Loss of brain cell volume places mechanical stress on cerebral vessels and supporting tissues, potentially leading to damage of vascular structures. This is supported by autopsy evidence of hypernatremia-related capillary and venous congestion, subcortical and subarachnoid bleeding, and venous sinus thrombosis.[60]

Cellular adaptation to extracellular hypertonicity results in an increase in intracellular osmolality. This is achieved through events that mirror those described previously for adaptation to hyponatremia. Within seconds, the brain is protected from severe water loss by an increase in cellular sodium, potassium, and chloride content.[60] Thereafter, cerebral dehydration is further attenuated by the accumulation of osmolytes such as glutamine, glycerolphosphorylcholine, and myo-inositol.[61] As cellular adaptation requires a period of days to reach full effect, the rate and severity of developing hypernatremia alter the degree of cell shrinkage and injury. Because it also takes several days for cells to reverse the accumulation of these organic osmolytes, treatment of chronic hypernatremia requires a gradual reduction of extracellular fluid tonicity to avoid treatment-induced cerebral edema.

Prevention

Hypernatremia occurs in predictable clinical settings (Box 29-4). Elderly persons, hospitalized patients receiving hypertonic infusions, those suffering increased insensible losses or undergoing osmotic losses, those with diabetes, and patients with previous symptoms of polydipsia and polyuria should invoke a high index of suspicion when displaying neurological alterations, especially in periods of stress.

Geriatric patients have impaired thirst responses, decreased urinary concentrating ability, and lower baseline levels of TBW. As a result, elderly patients are the group most likely to develop severe hypernatremia in the outpatient setting, and hypernatremia in the elderly accounts for 1% to 2% of all hospital admissions.[62] The most common scenario is that of a debilitated patient with a febrile illness. Increased insensible losses are not compensated because of impaired access to free water. Recognition of mental status changes in settings of increased insensible losses should prompt close attention to S_{Na} and increased administration of free water.

Hospitalized patients are also susceptible to the development of hypernatremia. Individuals developing hypernatremia during hospital admission are more likely to be younger and to have an iatrogenic cause.[63] In a careful survey of hyponatremia in the intensive care unit, Polderman and colleagues[64] noted

Box 29-4 Patient Groups at Increased Risk of Development of Severe Hypernatremia

Elderly patients
Hospitalized patients
   Hypertonic infusions
   Tube feedings
   Osmotic diuretics
   Lactulose
   Mechanical ventilation
   Patients with decreased baseline levels of consciousness
Patients with uncontrolled diabetes
Patients with underlying polyuric disorders

that those who acquired the electrolyte disorder in the hospital had longer stays in the intensive care unit and higher mortality. Inpatients with high insensible losses (e.g., patients on mechanical ventilators) develop hypernatremia due to restricted access to water and inadequate fluid prescriptions. Hypertonic fluid administration (e.g., sodium bicarbonate) and osmotic diuretics including mannitol and urea may also result in hypertonicity. Hyperosmolar tube feedings may induce diarrhea and gastrointestinal water losses, and the large daily osmolar load may lead to increased electrolyte-free water losses. Palevsky and colleagues[63] noted that despite frequent S_{Na} measurements, treatment of hypernatremia was often delayed. Of patients with S_{Na} values more than 150 mEq/L, 50% did not receive hypotonic fluid within 24 hours of becoming hypernatremic and only 36% were corrected within 72 hours.

Patients with both type 1 and 2 diabetes frequently develop hypernatremia in the setting of diabetic ketoacidosis or hyperosmotic nonketotic coma. In both disorders, a relative deficiency in insulin with respect to increased basal requirements produces hyperglycemia and glucosuria. The ensuing osmotic diuresis and decreased fluid intake produce a state of hypovolemic hypernatremia. The S_{Na} must be interpreted with caution because it may not reflect the actual degree of hyperosmolality. Hyperglycemia leads to the translocation of cellular water into the extracellular fluid and may cause a dilutional hyponatremia. New-onset hyperglycemia associated with decreases in mental status should invoke prompt evaluation and therapy of both volume and free water deficits. However, the simultaneous administration of both insulin and free water can lead to a rapid decrease in extracellular osmolality and can result in cerebral edema.[65] To prevent an excessively rapid decrease in serum osmolality, isotonic fluids can be used until the serum glucose is only mildly elevated, at which point hypotonic saline can be administered to start correcting the free water deficit.[66]

Polyuric patients should undergo evaluation for defects in urinary concentration because previous knowledge of such disorders can avert serious hypernatremia. In diabetes insipidus, patients compensate for water losses by consuming large amounts of water, thus maintaining relatively normal osmolality. If an illness increases water losses or restricts access to water, hypernatremia will result. Patients at risk of diabetes insipidus include those with central nervous system disease or trauma and those receiving lithium or amphotericin B.

TREATMENT STRATEGIES IN HYPERNATREMIA

The keys to detection and treatment of hypernatremia are (1) recognition of symptoms, when present; (2) correct identification of the underlying defects of water metabolism; (3) correction of volume disturbances; and (4) correction of hypertonicity (Fig. 29-2). Treatment should be initiated promptly to avoid worsening of hypernatremia and increased risk of poor outcome. Once the condition has been stabilized, steps may be taken for long-term prevention.

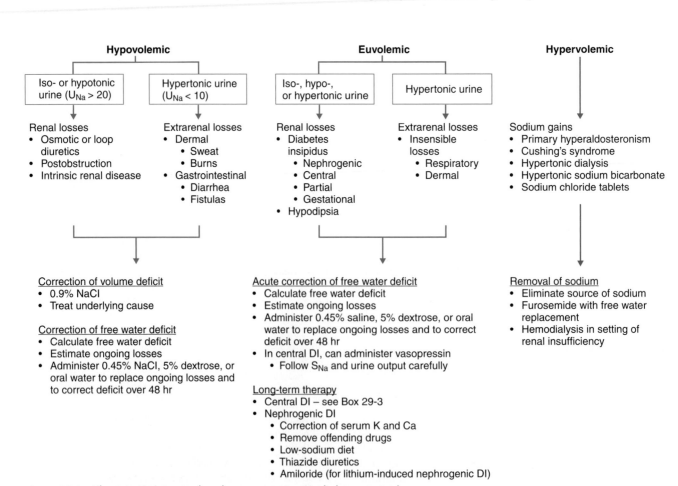

Figure 29-2   Therapeutic approach to hypernatremia. DI, diabetes insipidus.

Box 29-5   General Guidelines for the Treatment of Symptomatic
Hypernatremia

> Correct at rate of 2 mEq/L/hr
> Replace half calculated water deficit over first 12–24 hr
> Replace remaining deficit over the next 24 hr
> Perform serial neurological examinations; prescribed rate
>   of correction can be decreased with improvement in
>   symptoms
> Perform measurements of serum and urine electrolytes
>   every 1–2 hr

Early signs and symptoms of hypernatremia are nonspecific and primarily manifest as changes in mental status. These include restlessness, irritability, lethargy, confusion, and somnolence. Progression of neurological injury may produce muscular twitching, hyperreflexia, seizures, coma, or even death. If corresponding mechanisms are intact, patients may complain of intense thirst. As previously asserted, mental status changes related to hypernatremia may be difficult to differentiate from neurological manifestations of other underlying illnesses. Therefore, a high index of suspicion is required for consistent diagnosis.

The rate of correction of hypernatremia depends on its rate of development and on the presence or absence of symptoms. As a general rule, the rate of correction should parallel the rate of development. Cerebral adaptation to chronic hypernatremia results in the generation of organic intracellular solutes.[61] If extracellular tonicity is rapidly decreased, water moves into brain cells producing cerebral edema. A slower rate of correction likely prevents these events by allowing time for dissipation of these solutes. Two studies in children suggest that correction of hypernatremia should occur at 0.5 mEq/L/hr or less.[67,68] No seizures occurred in those corrected at this rate, whereas seizures occurred in nearly 20% of the patients in the group corrected more rapidly. If symptoms are present and the time course of hypernatremia is acute, then rapid correction with resolution of hypernatremia over several hours is appropriate. It is generally recommended that half of the deficit be replaced in 12 to 24 hours as the neurological status is carefully monitored (Box 29-5). Thereafter, the remaining deficit can be corrected during the ensuing 48 hours. The maximum correction rate should not exceed 2 mEq/L/hr. Because ongoing fluid losses are difficult to estimate, frequent determinations of S_{Na} should be made during the course of treatment.

Therapy, like diagnosis, is categorized by extracellular volume status. The chief goals are initial correction of underlying volume disturbances and subsequent correction of hypertonicity.

Euvolemic Hypernatremia

The guiding principles in the treatment of euvolemic hypernatremia are (1) restoration of the water deficit and (2) decrease in ongoing losses of hypotonic fluids.

The presence of such losses is not always obvious. The measurement of urinary osmolality can suggest the excretion of isotonic or even hypertonic urine despite continued electrolyte-free water losses.

For example, a patient has the following laboratory values: S_{Na} = 146 mEq/L, U_{osm} = 320 mOsm/kg H_2O, S_{osm} = 310 mOsm/kg, U_{Na} = 40 mEq/L, U_K = 30 mEq/L, and urine volume = 2 L. U_{osm} greater than S_{osm} might suggest that no free water is being excreted. However, using Equation 29-4, calculation of electrolyte-free water clearance reveals the following:

$$cH_2Oe = V\left[1 - \frac{(U_{Na} + U_K)}{S_{Na}}\right]$$

$$cH_2Oe = V\left[\frac{70}{146}\right]$$

$$= 2\,L \times 0.52 = 1.04\,L$$

Therefore, this individual is excreting more than 1 L of electrolyte-free water during the period of this urine collection. If this water is not replaced, S_{Na} will increase further. Replacement can be with oral cold water or infusion of 5% dextrose in water.

The water deficit can be calculated based on the S_{Na} and the assumption that 60% of body weight is water.

$$\text{Water deficit} = 0.6 \times \text{Body weight} \times \left[\frac{S_{Na}}{140} - 1\right]$$

For example, the water deficit of a 70-kg male with an S_{Na} of 156 mEq/L would be

$$0.6 \times 70 \times \left[\frac{156}{140} - 1\right] = 4.8\,L$$

This is the net positive water balance that needs to be achieved over approximately 48 hours, not including ongoing losses that must also be replaced, as estimated by the electrolyte-free water clearance. The water deficit can be replaced orally or parenterally, using solutions such as 0.45% sodium chloride or 5% dextrose in water (see Box 29-4 and Fig. 29-2). Central diabetes insipidus may be treated by hormone replacement or pharmacologic agents (Table 29-3). In acute settings where renal water losses are extensive, aqueous vasopressin is preferable. Its short duration of action allows for more careful monitoring and decreases the likelihood of complications such as water intoxication. An initial dose of 5 μg may be given subcutaneously, with quantification of its effect on S_{Na} and urine output used to guide additional dosing. Vasopressin activates vascular V_1 receptors and may produce coronary spasm, uterine contraction, gastrointestinal cramping, and pallor. Caution must therefore be used in patients with known coronary artery disease or peripheral vascular disease. In chronic settings, DDAVP is the agent of choice because of its long half-life, diminished V_1 receptor stimulation, and its availability in an oral formulation. It is conveniently administered intranasally in doses of 10 to 20 μg every 12 to 24 hours, and a single dose may induce antidiuresis for 8 to 12 hours. It is also available in 0.1- or 0.2-mg tablets, which can be started at 0.05 mg every 12 to 24 hours and titrated depending on the response. DDAVP may also be given intravenously or subcutaneously, especially during periods of upper respiratory disease or surgery. For patients who are converted from the intranasal to the

Table 29-3 Therapeutic Regimens for the Treatment of Diabetes Insipidus

	Drug	Dose
Complete central diabetes insipidus	DDAVP	10–20 μg intranasally every 12–24 hr 0.1–0.8 mg orally in divided doses; start with 0.05 mg orally every 12 hr and adjust as needed
Partial central diabetes insipidus	DDAVP	10–20 μg intranasally every 12–24 hr
	Aqueous vasopressin	5–10 U SC every 4–6 hr
	Chlorpropamide	250–500 mg/day
	Clofibrate	500 mg tid to qid
	Carbamazepine	400–600 mg/day
Nephrogenic diabetes insipidus	Thiazide diuretics	25–50 mg/day
	NSAIDs	Indomethacin 1–2 mg/kg/day
	Amiloride (for lithium-related disease)	5 mg/day
Gestational diabetes insipidus	DDAVP	As above

DDAVP, 1-desamine-8-D-arginine vasopressin; NSAIDs, nonsteroidal anti-inflammatory drugs.
Adapted from Lanese D, Teitelbaum I: Hypernatremia. In Jacobson HR, Striker GE, Klahr S (eds): The Principles and Practice of Nephrology. Philadelphia: CV Mosby, 1998, pp 884–887.

injectable form, the dose should be reduced to 10% of the intranasal administration. Dosing regimens need to be tailored individually, with a bias toward undertreatment. The lowest dose that decreases polyuria to acceptable levels should be used, and the return of polyuria should be noted before repeat dosing to prevent hyponatremia. The drug appears to be safe for use in pregnancy and is resistant to degradation by increased circulating vasopressinases. DDAVP is usually tolerated extremely well, but in very large doses may cause hypertension, headache, and abdominal cramping. Unfortunately, the agent is very expensive, and adjunctive measures may be used to decrease the required dose.

When the quantity of DDAVP available for treatment is limited and in cases of partial central diabetes insipidus, circulating AVP may be increased by pharmacologic agents that potentiate its release. These drugs include chlorpropamide, clofibrate, and carbamazepine. When used alone, these agents are not usually adequate to control polyuria, but when combined with hormonal therapy, decreased solute intake, or diuretic administration, they prove very useful in the treatment of diabetes insipidus. It is interesting that chlorpropamide has been used to normalize S_{Na} by increasing water intake and has also been used to treat primary polydipsia. Although other agents such as thioridazine and benzodiazepines appear to increase water intake, they are not of practical use.

Nephrogenic diabetes insipidus does not respond to increased circulating levels of AVP. Initial therapeutic maneuvers should be focused on identifying reversible etiologies of impaired water conservation and, if possible, correcting them. This includes treatment of hypokalemia, hypercalcemia, or the withdrawal of drugs such as lithium, demeclocycline, glyburide, or colchicine. Because of its therapeutic benefits, lithium may be difficult to discontinue in some bipolar patients. In such cases, amiloride may attenuate water losses by blocking entry of lithium into the collecting tubule cell.[69] Thiazide diuretics may

decrease polyuria related to nephrogenic diabetes insipidus by reducing the delivery of dilute urine to the distal collecting tubule. This seems to occur by inducing mild extracellular fluid volume contraction with a decreased glomerular filtration rate and increased proximal tubular reabsorption, and by diminishing sodium reabsorption in the diluting segment of the distal nephron. Another method of reducing renal water losses is by reducing oral solute intake in the form of a low-sodium diet. The polyuria of congenital nephrogenic diabetes insipidus may be attenuated by nonsteroidal anti-inflammatory drug–mediated inhibition of cyclooxygenase. Potential future therapies may include agents that modulate the insertion of aquaporin-2 into the tubular epithelial cells.[70]

A rare form of diabetes insipidus may occur during pregnancy. This is related to the production of a vasopressinase by the placenta.[71] These patients respond to treatment with DDAVP, which is not subject to degradation by the enzyme.

Hypovolemic Hypernatremia

When hypernatremia coexists with low TB_{Na} and physical evidence of hypovolemia, the primary goal is fluid resuscitation because the extracellular fluid volume contraction may be more life threatening than the hypertonicity. Such patients should receive initial therapy with normal saline or other plasma expanders until signs of hypovolemia are no longer present. In states of hypernatremia, isotonic saline is actually hypotonic compared with the existing extracellular fluid and can lower plasma osmolality, although not significantly. Serial examinations of volume status should demonstrate the return of normal neck veins and improvement of orthostatic hypotension or tachycardia. Once intravascular volume depletion has been corrected, administration of 0.45% saline or 5% dextrose may be used for further correction of hypertonicity.

Hypervolemic Hypernatremia

When the patient is hypervolemic and hypernatremic, the therapeutic goal is to remove the excess sodium. Natriuresis is likely to be present if renal function is normal but can be further enhanced by diuretics such as furosemide with 5% dextrose. Care must be taken not to reduce S_{Na} too rapidly with concomitant diuretic and hypotonic fluid administration. The rate of urine flow and calculation of electrolyte-free water clearance can help estimate free water requirements. If renal function is impaired, volume overload and hypertonicity may require treatment by dialysis.

References

1. Anderson RJ, Chung HM, Kluge R, Schrier RW: Hyponatremia: A prospective analysis of its epidemiology and the pathogenetic role of vasopressin. Ann Intern Med 1985;102:164–168.
2. Berl T, Verbalis JG: Pathophysiology of water metabolism. In Brenner B (ed): The Kidney, 7th ed. Philadelphia: WB Saunders; 2004, pp 857–920.
3. Nguyen MK, Kurtz I: New insights into the pathophysiology of the dysnatremias: A quantitative analysis. Am J Physiol Renal Physiol 2004;287:F172–F180.
4. Arieff AI: Hyponatremia, convulsions, respiratory arrest, and permanent brain damage after elective surgery in healthy women. N Engl J Med 1986;314:1529–1535.
5. Arieff AI, Ayus JC, Fraser CL: Hyponatraemia and death or permanent brain damage in healthy children. Br Med J 1992;304:1218–1222.
6. Arieff AI, Guisado R: Effects on the central nervous system of hypernatremic and hyponatremic states. Kidney Int 1976;10:104–116.
7. Ayus J, Krothapalli R, Arieff A: Treatment of hyponatremia: The case for rapid correction. In Narins R (ed): Controversies in Nephrology and Hypertension. New York: Churchill Livingstone, 1984, pp 393–407.
8. Verbalis JG: Hyponatremia: Epidemiology, pathophysiology, and therapy. Curr Opin Nephrol Hypertens 1993;2:636–652.
9. Sterns RH, Baer J, Ebersol S, et al: Organic osmolytes in acute hyponatremia. Am J Physiol 1993;264:F833–F836.
10. Berl T: Treating hyponatremia: Damned if we do and damned if we don't. Kidney Int 1990;37:1006–1018.
11. Oh MS, Kim HJ, Carroll HJ: Recommendations for treatment of symptomatic hyponatremia. Nephron 1995;70:143–150.
12. Ayus JC, Armstrong D, Arieff AI: Hyponatremia with hypoxia: Effects on brain adaptation, perfusion, and histology in rodents. Kidney Int 2006;69:1319–1325.
13. Kokko JP: Symptomatic hyponatremia with hypoxia is a medical emergency. Kidney Int 2006;69:1291–1293.
14. Vexler ZS, Ayus JC, Roberts TP, et al: Hypoxic and ischemic hypoxia exacerbate brain injury associated with metabolic encephalopathy in laboratory animals. J Clin Invest 1994;93:256–264.
15. Ayus JC, Wheeler JM, Arieff AI: Postoperative hyponatremic encephalopathy in menstruant women. Ann Intern Med 1992;117:891–897.
16. Stone JD, Crofton JT, Share L: Sex differences in central adrenergic control of vasopressin release. Am J Physiol 1989;257:R1040–R1045.
17. Fraser CL, Kucharczyk J, Arieff AI, et al: Sex differences result in increased morbidity from hyponatremia in female rats. Am J Physiol 1989;256:R880–R885.
18. Sonnenblick M, Friedlander Y, Rosin AJ: Diuretic-induced severe hyponatremia. Review and analysis of 129 reported patients. Chest 1993;103:601–606.
19. Illowsky BP, Kirch DG: Polydipsia and hyponatremia in psychiatric patients. Am J Psychiatry 1988;145:675–683.
20. Goldman MB, Luchins DJ, Robertson GL: Mechanisms of altered water metabolism in psychotic patients with polydipsia and hyponatremia. N Engl J Med 1988;318:397–403.
21. Almond CS, Shin AY, Fortescue EB, et al: Hyponatremia among runners in the Boston Marathon. N Engl J Med 2005;352:1550–1556.
22. Bhalla P, Eaton FE, Coulter JB, et al: Lesson of the week: Hyponatraemic seizures and excessive intake of hypotonic fluids in young children. Br Med J 1999;319:1554–1557.
23. Durward A, Tibby SM, Murdoch IA: Hyponatraemia can be caused by standard fluid regimens. Br Med J 2000;320:943.
24. Keating JP, Schears GJ, Dodge PR: Oral water intoxication in infants. An American epidemic. Am J Dis Child 1991;145:985–990.
25. Sterns RH: Severe symptomatic hyponatremia: Treatment and outcome. A study of 64 cases. Ann Intern Med 1987;107:656–664.
26. Soupart A, Penninckx R, Stenuit A, et al: Treatment of chronic hyponatremia in rats by intravenous saline: Comparison of rate versus magnitude of correction. Kidney Int 1992;41:1662–1667.
27. Ayus JC, Krothapalli RK, Armstrong DL: Rapid correction of severe hyponatremia in the rat: Histopathological changes in the brain. Am J Physiol 1985;248:F711–F719.
28. Verbalis JG, Martinez AJ: Neurological and neuropathological sequelae of correction of chronic hyponatremia. Kidney Int 1991;39:1274–1282.
29. Sterns RH, Riggs JE, Schochet SS Jr: Osmotic demyelination syndrome following correction of hyponatremia. N Engl J Med 1986;314:1535–1542.
30. Sterns RH, Cappuccio JD, Silver SM, Cohen EP: Neurologic sequelae after treatment of severe hyponatremia: A multicenter perspective. J Am Soc Nephrol 1994;4:1522–1530.
31. Ayus JC, Krothapalli RK, Arieff AI: Changing concepts in treatment of severe symptomatic hyponatremia. Rapid correction and possible relation to central pontine myelinolysis. Am J Med 1985;78:897–902.
32. Ayus JC, Krothapalli RK, Arieff AI: Treatment of symptomatic hyponatremia and its relation to brain damage. A prospective study. N Engl J Med 1987;317:1190–1195.
33. Ayus JC, Arieff AI: Chronic hyponatremic encephalopathy in postmenopausal women: Association of therapies with morbidity and mortality. JAMA 1999;281:2299–2304.
34. Soupart A, Penninckx R, Crenier L, et al: Prevention of brain demyelination in rats after excessive correction of chronic hyponatremia by serum sodium lowering. Kidney Int 1994;45:193–200.
35. Soupart A, Ngassa M, Decaux G: Therapeutic relowering of the serum sodium in a patient after excessive correction of hyponatremia. Clin Nephrol 1999;51:383–386.
36. Goldszmidt MA, Iliescu EA: DDAVP to prevent rapid correction in hyponatremia. Clin Nephrol 2000;53:226–229.
37. Oya S, Tsutsumi K, Ueki K, Kirino T: Reinduction of hyponatremia to treat central pontine myelinolysis. Neurology 2001;57:1931–1932.
38. Adrogue HJ, Madias NE: Hyponatremia. N Engl J Med 2000;342:1581–1589.
39. Janicic N, Verbalis JG: Evaluation and management of hypo-osmolality in hospitalized patients. Endocrinol Metab Clin North Am 2003;32:459–481.
40. Barsoum NR, Levine BS: Current prescriptions for the correction of hyponatraemia and hypernatraemia: Are they too simple? Nephrol Dial Transplant 2002;17:1176–1180.
41. Liamis G, Kalogirou M, Saugos V, Elisaf M: Therapeutic approach in patients with dysnatraemias. Nephrol Dial Transplant 2006;21:1564–1569.

42. Renneboog B, Musch W, Vandemergel X, et al: Mild chronic hyponatremia is associated with falls, unsteadiness, and attention deficits. Am J Med 2006;119:71 e1–e8.

43. Furst H, Hallows KR, Post J, et al: The urine/plasma electrolyte ratio: A predictive guide to water restriction. Am J Med Sci 2000;319:240–244.

44. Forrest JN Jr, Cox M, Hong C, et al: Superiority of demeclocycline over lithium in the treatment of chronic syndrome of inappropriate secretion of antidiuretic hormone. N Engl J Med 1978;298:173–177.

45. Decaux G, Brimioulle S, Genette F, Mockel J: Treatment of the syndrome of inappropriate secretion of antidiuretic hormone by urea. Am J Med 1980;69:99–106.

46. Decaux G: Long-term treatment of patients with inappropriate secretion of antidiuretic hormone by the vasopressin receptor antagonist conivaptan, urea, or furosemide. Am J Med 2001;110:582–584.

47. Saito T, Ishikawa S, Abe K, et al: Acute aquaresis by the nonpeptide arginine vasopressin (AVP) antagonist OPC-31260 improves hyponatremia in patients with syndrome of inappropriate secretion of antidiuretic hormone (SIADH). J Clin Endocrinol Metab 1997;82:1054–1057.

48. Schrier RW, Gross P, Gheorghiade M, et al: Tolvaptan, a selective oral vasopressin V2-receptor antagonist, for hyponatremia. N Engl J Med 2006;355:2099–2112.

49. Soupart A, Gross P, Legros J, et al: Successful long-term treatment of hyponatremia in syndrome of inappropriate antidiuretic hormone secretion with satavaptan (SR121463B), an orally active nonpeptide vasopressin V2-receptor antagonist. Clin J Am Soc Nephrol 2006;1:1154–1560.

50. Ellison DH, Berl T: Clinical practice. The syndrome of inappropriate antidiuresis. N Engl J Med 2007;356:2064–2072.

51. Greenberg A, Verbalis JG: Vasopressin receptor antagonists. Kidney Int 2006;69:2124–2130.

52. Sica DA: Hyponatremia and heart failure—treatment considerations. Congest Heart Fail 2006;12:55–60.

53. Udelson JE, Smith WB, Hendrix GH, et al: Acute hemodynamic effects of conivaptan, a dual V(1A) and V(2) vasopressin receptor antagonist, in patients with advanced heart failure. Circulation 2001;104:2417–2423.

54. Abraham WT, Shamshirsaz AA, McFann K, et al: Aquaretic effect of lixivaptan, an oral, non-peptide, selective V2 receptor vasopressin antagonist, in New York Heart Association functional class II and III chronic heart failure patients. J Am Coll Cardiol 2006;47:1615–1621.

55. Gheorghiade M, Niazi I, Ouyang J, et al: Vasopressin V2-receptor blockade with tolvaptan in patients with chronic heart failure: Results from a double-blind, randomized trial. Circulation 2003;107:2690–2696.

56. Konstam MA, Gheorghiade M, Burnett JC Jr, et al: Effects of oral tolvaptan in patients hospitalized for worsening heart failure: The EVEREST Outcome Trial. JAMA 2007;297:1319–1331.

57. Gerbes AL, Gulberg V, Gines P, et al: Therapy of hyponatremia in cirrhosis with a vasopressin receptor antagonist: A randomized double-blind multicenter trial. Gastroenterology 2003;124:933–939.

58. Schrier RW: Role of diminished renal function in cardiovascular mortality: Marker or pathogenetic factor? J Am Coll Cardiol 2006;47:1–8.

59. Licata G, Di Pasquale P, Parrinello G, et al: Effects of high-dose furosemide and small-volume hypertonic saline solution infusion in comparison with a high dose of furosemide as bolus in refractory congestive heart failure: Long-term effects. Am Heart J 2003;145:459–466.

60. McManus ML, Churchwell KB, Strange K: Regulation of cell volume in health and disease. N Engl J Med 1995;333:1260–1266.

61. Lien YH, Shapiro JI, Chan L: Effects of hypernatremia on organic brain osmoles. J Clin Invest 1990;85:1427–1435.

62. Snyder NA, Feigal DW, Arieff AI: Hypernatremia in elderly patients. A heterogeneous, morbid, and iatrogenic entity. Ann Intern Med 1987;107:309–319.

63. Palevsky PM, Bhagrath R, Greenberg A: Hypernatremia in hospitalized patients. Ann Intern Med 1996;124:197–203.

64. Polderman KH, Schreuder WO, Strack van Schijndel RJ, Thijs LG: Hypernatremia in the intensive care unit: An indicator of quality of care? Crit Care Med 1999;27:1105–1108.

65. Silver SM, Clark EC, Schroeder BM, Sterns RH: Pathogenesis of cerebral edema after treatment of diabetic ketoacidosis. Kidney Int 1997;51:1237–1244.

66. Harris GD, Fiordalisi I, Harris WL, et al: Minimizing the risk of brain herniation during treatment of diabetic ketoacidemia: A retrospective and prospective study. J Pediatr 1990;117:22–31.

67. Blum D, Brasseur D, Kahn A, Brachet E: Safe oral rehydration of hypertonic dehydration. J Pediatr Gastroenterol Nutr 1986;5:232–235.

68. Kahn A, Brachet E, Blum D: Controlled fall in natremia and risk of seizures in hypertonic dehydration. Intensive Care Med 1979;5:27–31.

69. Wells BG: Amiloride in lithium-induced polyuria. Ann Pharmacother 1994;28:888–889.

70. Fujiwara TM, Bichet DG: Molecular biology of hereditary diabetes insipidus. J Am Soc Nephrol 2005;16:2836–2846.

71. Durr JA, Hoggard JG, Hunt JM, Schrier RW: Diabetes insipidus in pregnancy associated with abnormally high circulating vasopressinase activity. N Engl J Med 1987;316:1070–1074.

Further Reading

Berl T: Treatment of the syndrome of inappropriate antidiuretic hormone secretion and the emergence of vasopressin antagonists for hyponatremic disorders. May 2007, volume 5, issue 5, www.nephrologyrounds.org.

Kurtz I, Nguyen MK: Evolving concepts in the quantitative analysis of the determinants of the plasma water sodium concentration and the pathophysiology and treatment of the dysnatremias. Kidney Int 2005;68:1982–1993.

Schrier RW: Water and sodium retention in edematous disorders: Role of vasopressin and aldosterone. Am J Med 2006;119(7 Suppl 1):S47–S53.

Verbalis JG, Berl T: Disorders of water balance. In Brenner BM (ed): Brenner and Rector's The Kidney, vol I, 8th ed. Philadelphia: WB Saunders, 2007, pp 859–904.

Verbalis JG: The syndrome of inappropriate antidiuretic hormone secretion and other hypoosmolar disorders. In Schrier RW (ed): Diseases of the Kidney and Urinary Tract, 8th ed. Philadelphia: Lippincott Williams & Wilkins, 2007, pp 2214–2248.

Chapter 30

Treatment of Hypokalemia and Hyperkalemia

Kamel S. Kamel, Man S. Oh, Shih-Hua Lin, and Mitchell L. Halperin

BRIEF OVERVIEW OF K$^+$ PHYSIOLOGY

It is important to recognize at the outset that hyperkalemia or hypokalemia are common laboratory findings in a heterogeneous group of disorders. Therefore, it is not appropriate to have a "one-size-fits-all" recommendation for therapy that will apply to all patients with these electrolyte disorders. Accordingly, our objective is to provide an approach to therapy that is based on the pathophysiology of the disorder in an individual patient.[1,2] There are three areas of emphasis: First, one must define and deal with emergencies that are present when the patient seeks medical attention (with regard to the dyskalemias, the dangers usually are due to cardiac arrhythmia or respiratory muscle weakness). Second, one needs to anticipate and prevent risks that may be caused by the initial therapy. Third, in the long term, measures need to be taken to return the potassium (K$^+$) level in body compartments to normal and reverse the abnormal physiologic processes. Overviews of two aspects of K$^+$ physiology are outlined briefly to provide the background needed for the design of therapy: first, the events at the interface between the extracel-lular fluid (ECF) and the intracellular fluid (ICF) compartments (control of the transcellular distribution of K$^+$) and second, the concepts concerning the regulation of renal K$^+$ excretion.

Interface between Extracellular Fluid and Intracellular Fluid

K$^+$ ions are retained inside cells by a negative voltage. When this voltage becomes more negative, K$^+$ will shift into cells; the converse is also true. The electrogenic cation pump, the Na$^+$/K$^+$-ATPase (Na/K-ATPase) generates this negative voltage by pumping out three Na$^+$ ions while importing only two K$^+$ ions; hence, there is an export of one third of a positive charge per Na$^+$ that exits from the cell via this pump.[3] It follows that an abnormal shift of K$^+$ across cell membranes can be anticipated when the activity of the Na/K-ATPase deviates from its expected physiology; this is usually due to altered hormone levels. The main hormones that cause a shift of K$^+$ into cells are β_2-adrenergic agonists, insulin, and thyroid hormone; aldosterone may also cause a shift of K$^+$ into cells when given to patients who lack this hormone. The Na/K-ATPase is activated directly by β_2-adrenergics, which phosphorylate the Na/K-ATPase, whereas thyroid hormone increases the number of the Na/K-ATPase units in the cell membrane. Flux through the Na/K-ATPase will increase substantially when more Na$^+$ enters cells. For this to result in an increase in the negative voltage inside cells, the entry of Na$^+$ must be electroneutral; this occurs when Na$^+$ enters the cell via the Na$^+$/H$^+$ ion exchanger (NHE) (Fig. 30-1).[4]

It appears that the NHE is normally inactive in cells; this can be deduced from the fact that the concentrations of its substrates (Na$^+$ in the ECF compartment and H$^+$ in the ICF compartment) are considerably higher than those of its products (Na$^+$ in the ICF compartment and H$^+$ in the ECF compartment) at steady state (see Fig. 30-1). There are two major activators of the NHE: insulin and a higher concentration of H$^+$ in the ICF compartment.

Renal Regulation

Control of the rate of K$^+$ excretion occurs primarily in the late cortical distal nephron, including the cortical collecting duct (CCD).[5] The excretion of a large quantity of K$^+$ requires a high flow rate in the CCD. A lumen-negative transepithelial voltage must be generated and open K$^+$ channels must be present in the apical membranes of the principal cells in this nephron segment to secrete K$^+$. To generate this voltage, the reabsorption of Na$^+$ must occur at a faster rate than the accompanying anion (chloride [Cl$^-$]).[2] The pathway for Na$^+$ reabsorption is via an epithelial Na$^+$ channel (ENaC) in the apical membrane of principal cells.[6] Stimulation of the reabsorption of Na$^+$ and/or the secretion of K$^+$ is influenced to a major extent by the hormone aldosterone,[7]

CLINICAL ASSESSMENT OF THE CONCENTRATION OF K$^+$ IN THE CORTICAL COLLECTING DUCT

The two parameters affecting the net secretion of K$^+$ in the CCD can be assessed in a semiquantitative fashion as illustrated in Figure 30-2 (Equation 30-1).[8] To estimate the concentration of K$^+$ in fluid traversing the terminal CCD ([K$^+$]$_{CCD}$), one needs to adjust the measured concentration of K$^+$ in the urine (U$_K$) for the reabsorption of water in the medullary collecting duct. This can done by dividing U$_K$ by the ratio of the urine osmolality to osmolality in fluid exiting the terminal CCD (equal to the plasma osmolality when vasopressin acts) (Equation 30-1). A

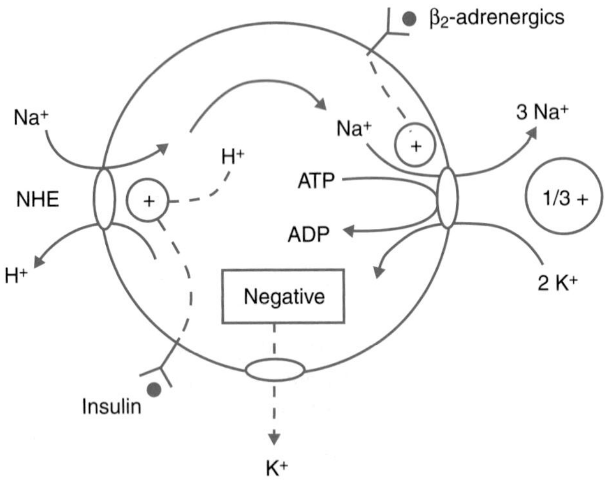

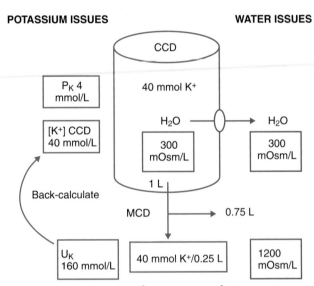

Figure 30-2 Assessment of components of K$^+$ excretion in the cortical collecting duct (CCD). The barrel-shaped structures represent the CCD and the *arrow* below it is the medullary collecting duct (MCD). In this example, the luminal K$^+$ concentration in the CCD is 40 mmol/L or 10-fold greater than the peritubular K$^+$ concentration of 4.0 mmol/L (equal to the plasma potassium concentration [P$_K$]). When 1 L of fluid traverses the MCD and 75% of the water is reabsorbed, if no K$^+$ is reabsorbed or secreted in the MCD, the potassium concentration in the urine (U$_K$) and the urine osmolality are both fourfold higher (U$_K$ increases from 40 to 160 mmol/L; urine osmolality increases from 300 mOsm/kg H$_2$O (equal to the plasma osmolality when vasopressin acts) to 1200 mOsm/kg H$_2$O. This should be taken into account in assessing the [K$^+$]$_{CCD}$. Similarly, an estimate of the minimum flow rate in the terminal CCD can be obtained by dividing the osmole excretion rate by the plasma osmolality. (From Halperin ML: The ACID Truth and Basic Facts: With a Sweet Touch, an enLYTEnment, 5th ed. Toronto, Ontario: RossMark Medical Publishers, 2004, with permission.)

Figure 30-1 Na/K-ATPase activity and the creation of an intracellular negative voltage. The Na/K-ATPase generates the electrical driving force for K$^+$ entry into cells providing that the source of the Na$^+$ pumped out was either Na$^+$ that existed in cells or Na$^+$ that entered cells in an electroneutral fashion via the NHE (Na$^+$/H$^+$ ion exchanger). Two hormones that cause more Na$^+$ pumping by the Na/K-ATPase are shown; the first is insulin, which activates the NHE, and the second is catecholamines (β_2-adrenergic actions), which activate the Na/K-ATPase by phosphorylation. The increase in negative voltage in cells will diminish the exit of K$^+$ from cells via K$^+$ channels. ADP, adenosine diphosphate; ATP, adenosine triphosphate. (From Halperin ML: The ACID Truth and Basic Facts: With a Sweet Touch, an enLYTEnment, 5th ed. Toronto, Ontario: RossMark Medical Publishers, 2004, with permission.)

similar calculation is done to estimate the flow rate in the terminal CCD (Equation 30-2). One premise in these calculations is the absence of a large reabsorption of osmoles in the medullary collecting duct. While this is true for electrolyte, it may be not the case for urea, as recent findings suggest that the amount of urea that is delivered to the distal convoluted tubule is about threefold larger that that excreted in the urine. Although there are no normal values for the excretion of K^+ in steady state because normal subjects excrete all the K^+ that they ingest, there are expected responses in the presence of hypokalemia or hyperkalemia; the expected value in a patient with hypokalemia is less than 15 mmol/day ($U_K/U_{creatinine} < 1.5$ in mmol/mmol terms), and in a patient with hyperkalemia is more than 200 mmol/day ($U_K/U_{creatinine} > 20$ in mmol/mmol terms)

$$[K^+]_{CCD} = U_K/(U/P)_{osm} \qquad \text{(Eq. 30-1)}$$
$$\text{Flow rate}_{CCD} = \text{osmole excretion rate}/P_{osm} \qquad \text{(Eq. 30-2)}$$

Hypokalemia with a High $[K^+]_{CCD}$

The usual value for the $[K^+]_{CCD}$ is less than 6 and that for the transtubular potassium gradient is less than 2 if hypokalemia is of nonrenal origin. A $[K^+]_{CCD}$ that is inappropriately high for the presence of hypokalemia indicates a higher luminal negative voltage in CCD due to a higher rate of electrogenic Na^+ reabsorption (and/or an altered K^+ conductance). We divide these patients into two subgroups based on their renal handling of Na^+.[1] The first one is a primary lesion affecting Na^+ where the reabsorption of Na^+ is accelerated. In this setting, the effective arterial blood volume is expanded, renin activity in plasma is low (with exception of conditions such as renal artery stenosis and renin-secreting tumors), and there is an ability to have low concentrations of Na^+ and Cl^- in the urine, but only when the ECF volume is contracted. In the second subgroup, there is slower reabsorption of Cl^-. It is characterized by a contracted effective arterial blood volume and high renin activity in plasma.

Faster Reabsorption of Na^+

When there is an increase in the number of open ENaC units in the luminal membrane of the cortical distal nephron, the lumen could become more electronegative. Causes of an overabundance of active ENaCs in the luminal membrane of principal cells include an inborn error (e.g., Liddle syndrome), the presence of too much aldosterone (e.g., primary hyper-reninemic hyperaldosteronism, primary hyperaldosteronism, glucocorticoid-remediable aldosteronism, and drugs or hormones that have mineralocorticoid actions). Cortisol may act as a mineralocorticoid when there is insufficient activity of the enzyme 11β-hydroxysteroid dehydrogenase in principal cells, which converts intracellular cortisol to its inactive metabolite cortisone.[9] This occurs when there is massive overproduction (or administration of large doses) of cortisol, when inhibitors of this enzyme are present (e.g., by glycyrrhizic acid from licorice[10] or carbenoxolone) or if there are inborn errors that diminish the activity of 11β-hydroxysteroid dehydrogenase (apparent mineralocorticoid excess).

Slower Reabsorption of Cl^-

A slower Cl^- type of lesion may be due to a low distal delivery of Cl^- to the CCD or the presence of luminal HCO_3^- and/or an alkaline luminal fluid, which seems to decrease the reabsorption of Cl^- in the CCD.[11] A slower Cl^- type of lesion may also be due to a large increase in the delivery of Na^+ and Cl^- to the CCD along with a retained stimulus for the reabsorption of Na^+ via ENaCs due to the continuing presence of aldosterone (a low effective arterial blood volume); hence, the rate of reabsorption of Na^+ by ENaCs exceeds that for Cl^- (see Fig. 30-2). Examples include the use of diuretics or diseases such as Bartter and Gitelman's syndromes in which there is inhibition of NaCl reabsorption at a site upstream of a CCD.

Hyperkalemia with a Low $[K^+]_{CCD}$

The usual value for the $[K^+]_{CCD}$ is greater than 30 and that of the transtubular potassium is greater than 7 gradient if hyperkalemia is of nonrenal origin. The $[K^+]_{CCD}$ that is inappropriately low for the presence of hyperkalemia usually indicates that there is a smaller negative luminal voltage in CCD, which is almost always due to a decreased electrogenic reabsorption of Na^+; rarely, the major problem can be lower K^+ conductance in these nephron segments. We divide patients into two subgroups based on their renal handling of Na^+. In the first subgroup, the Na^+ reabsorption is slower in the CCD in which the effective arterial blood volume is contracted, the renin activity in plasma is high, and there is an inability to have low concentrations of Na^+ and Cl^- in the urine when the effective arterial blood volume is contracted. In the second subgroup, there is faster reabsorption of Cl^-. It is characterized by an expanded effective arterial blood volume, low renin activity in plasma, and an ability to have low concentrations of Na^+ and Cl^- in the urine when the effective arterial blood volume is contracted.

Slower Reabsorption of Na^+

This disorder can be seen in a number of settings. Examples include when there is an inborn error that decreases the availability of ENaCs (e.g., pseudohypoaldosteronism type I), low production of aldosterone (e.g., Addison's disease), drugs that interfere with the synthesis of aldosterone (e.g., nonsteroidal anti-inflammatory drugs, angiotensin-converting enzyme inhibitors, angiotensin II receptor blockers, heparin, and ketoconazole), blockers of the aldosterone receptor in principal cells of the cortical distal nephron (e.g., spironolactone), ENaCs inhibited by luminal acting K^+-sparing diuretics (e.g., amiloride, triamterene), and when certain drugs block ENaCs (e.g., trimethoprim and pentamidine).

Faster Reabsorption of Cl^-

There are two possible reasons for having the reabsorption of Na^+ fail to exceed that of Cl^- in the *late* cortical distal nephron. First, there could be an increased permeability for Cl^- in the late cortical distal nephron (i.e., a Cl shunt disorder).[12] Examples may include the hyperkalemia in some patients with type 2 diabetes mellitus and patients on cyclosporine or tacrolimus. Second, there could be an enhanced reabsorption of Na^+ and Cl^- in the distal convoluted tubule, which diminishes the delivery of Na^+ and Cl^- to the late cortical distal nephron (called Gordon's syndrome). The molecular basis for this latter disorder has been attributed to deletions in the genes encoding for WNK kinase-1 and WNK kinase-4 (WNK stands for "with no lysine" [K is the abbreviation for lysine]).[13]

HYPOKALEMIA

General Considerations for the Treatment of Hypokalemia

Causes of hypokalemia are listed in Box 30-1. The steps to take in the treatment of patients with an emergency related to hypokalemia are illustrated in Figure 30-3.

Medical Emergencies

There are two potentially life-threatening circumstances that require aggressive therapy: The most common is a cardiac arrhythmia and the other is extreme weakness involving the respiratory muscles, especially when respiratory acidosis or metabolic acidosis (e.g., distal renal tubular acidosis due to a low rate of secretion of H^+ or an accelerated secretion of HCO_3^- in the distal neph-

---

Box 30-1   Causes of Hypokalemia

Decreased Intake of K^+
Rarely a primary cause unless K^+ intake is very low and duration is prolonged
Can augment the degree of hypokalemia if there is ongoing K^+ loss

Shift of K^+ into Cells
Hormones (insulin and β-adrenergics are the most important ones)
Metabolic alkalosis
Anabolic state (e.g., recovery from diabetic ketoacidosis)
Other (anesthesia, hereditary hypokalemic periodic paralysis)

Increased Urine K^+ Loss
High $[K^+]_{CCD}$
Faster reabsorption of Na^+ in the CCD
Constitutively active epithelial Na^+ channel (ENaC) (e.g., Liddle syndrome), artificial ENaC (e.g., amphotericin B)

High aldosterone levels
Cortisol acts as a mineralocorticoid
Low 11β-hydroxysteroid dehydrogenase activity (apparent mineralocorticoid excess), inhibitors of 11β-hydroxysteroid dehydrogenase (e.g., licorice), very high cortisol level (e.g., corticotropin-producing tumor)
Relatively slower reabsorption of Cl^- in the CCD
Delivery of Na^+ without Cl^- to the CCD and a contracted effective arterial blood volume
Inhibition of Cl^- reabsorption in the CCD (e.g., bicarbonaturia)
High delivery of Na^+ and Cl^- to the CCD and a maximum rate of Na^+ reabsorption that exceeds that for Cl^- (e.g., states with inhibition of NaCl reabsorption of an upstream nephron segment plus effective arterial blood volume contraction, e.g., use of diuretics, Bartter or Gitelman's syndrome)

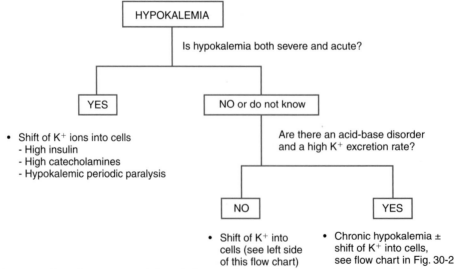

Figure 30-3 Initial approach to the patient with hypokalemia. The initial aim is to determine whether there is a major component of shift of K^+ into cells. This is suggested from the time course and a clinical history of the presence of factors associated with a shift of K^+ into cells. Laboratory assessment of the rate of excretion of K^+ and the presence of an acid-base disorder help to confirm this diagnosis. (From Halperin ML: The ACID Truth and Basic Facts: With a Sweet Touch, an enLYTEnment, 5th ed. Toronto, Ontario: RossMark Medical Publishers, 2004, with permission.)

ron or severe diarrhea) is present. Having decided that hypokalemia requires urgent therapy, enough K^+ must be given to increase the plasma K^+ concentration (P_K) quickly and to a high enough level (~3.0 mM) to avert these dangers; the total K^+ deficit should be replaced *much* more slowly. Because large doses and a high concentration of K^+ may need to be infused at the outset, K^+ must be administered via a large central vein and the patient should be connected to a cardiac monitor. Unless otherwise indicated, the infusion should not contain glucose or HCO_3^- because this may lead to a shift of K^+ into cells, which may aggravate an already severe degree of hypokalemia.

Illustrative Example

A patient fell from a great height and sustained a serious head injury.[14] While in the intensive care unit, his P_K decreased to 1.3 mmol/L over 30 minutes, and this led to a ventricular tachycardia. This sudden and marked shift of K^+ into cells was likely due to the extreme adrenergic response from the head injury and the administration of adrenergic agents to support his hemodynamic state. In this setting, we would try to increase his P_K by 1 mmol/L in 1 minute, recognizing the fact that the increase would be much smaller in the interstitial fluid bathing cardiac myocytes. Therefore, we would infuse 3 mmol K^+/min for the first 5 minutes (blood volume: 5 L; cardiac output: 5 L/min; 60% of blood volume is plasma, i.e., 3 L). At this time, we would decrease the rate of infusion of K^+ to 1 mmol/min and measure the P_K (stopping the infusion for 60 seconds to avoid a spuriously high P_K). If the electrocardiographic changes did not improve and there was little increase in the P_K, we would repeat this procedure.

No Medical Emergency

The initial emphasis in our approach to patients with hypokalemia is to determine whether there is an important shift of K^+ into cells; the steps to take are shown in Figure 30-3. Conversely, if the problem is due to an excessive excretion of K^+, the diagnostic approach differs and the steps are illustrated in Figure 30-4. In both of these categories, there is no generic therapy for hypokalemia because this is a finding rather than a specific disease. There is a different emphasis in the therapy of patients who have hypokalemia due to a shift of K^+ into cells (Fig. 30-5). Because these patients do not have a large deficit of K^+, we begin by discussing our management of these patients. This is followed by general comments about replacing a large deficit of K^+ and concluded with a discussion of specific therapy for some of the common disorders that are associated with hypokalemia.

Hypokalemic Periodic Paralysis

Typically, these patients have very low rates of K^+ excretion and they do not have an acid-base disorder.[15] In the Western world, most cases of hypokalemic periodic paralysis are sporadic or familial and therapy is simply to infuse enough KCl to increase the P_K to more than 3.0 mmol/L. A high-carbohydrate meal or an adrenergic surge may precipitate the attack. In contrast, Asian patients are most frequently young males who have hyperthyroidism. Other causes of an attack of hypokalemic periodic paralysis include a high and prolonged adrenergic surge, the use of amphetamines, or a very large intake of beverages containing caffeine.[16] The most important issue for therapy is to decide whether an adrenergic

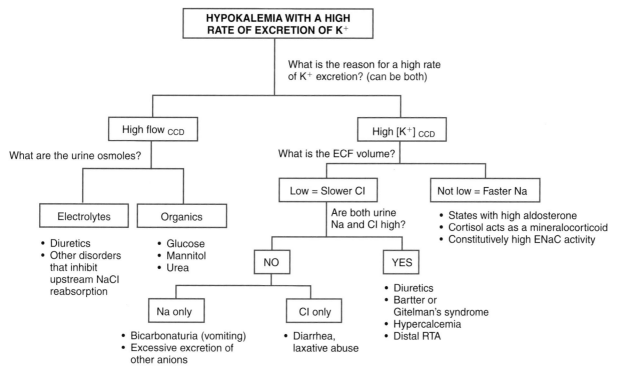

Figure 30-4 Renal causes of hypokalemia and a low rate of excretion of K^+. Assessment of the components of K^+ excretion in the cortical collecting duct (CCD) is obtained by back-calculating the flow rate and the concentration of K^+ in the urine to values in fluid traversing the terminal CCD, as shown in Figure 30-2. A list of likely causes of a high rate of excretion of K^+ is provided below the diagnostic categories. ECF, extracellular fluid; ENaC, epithelial Na channel; RTA, renal tubular acidosis. (From Halperin ML: The ACID Truth and Basic Facts: With a Sweet Touch, an enLYTEnment, 5th ed. Toronto, Ontario: RossMark Medical Publishers, 2004, with permission.)

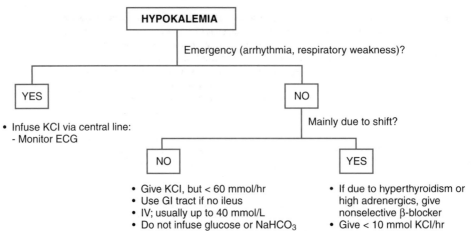

Figure 30-5   Treatment of the patient with hypokalemia. If an emergency is present (usually cardiac), intravenous KCl must be given promptly, and this usually means via a central vein. The electrocardiogram (ECG) must be monitored to guide therapy. Longer term strategies are to determine whether there is an important shift of K^+ into cells, especially if its cause is too much adrenaline or hyperthyroidism as the treatment now is with a nonselective β-blocker and much lower doses of KCl. In other settings, the goal is to administer sufficient KCl, and the oral route is preferred. If given in a peripheral vein, the K^+ should not exceed 40 mmol/L. In either case, and the amount given should not usually exceed 60 mmol/L/hr. Substances that cause K^+ to shift into cells such as glucose, via the release of insulin and $NaHCO_3$, should not be given at this stage of therapy. GI, gastrointestinal. (From Halperin ML: The ACID Truth and Basic Facts: With a Sweet Touch, an enLYTEnment, 5th ed. Toronto, Ontario: RossMark Medical Publishers, 2004, with permission.)

surge may be the cause of the hypokalemia. This is suggested by findings such as tachycardia and a wide pulse pressure on physical examination. Plasma phosphate levels are usually low. If that were the case, we would administer a nonselective β-blocker (propranolol 3 mg/kg) as their first-line treatment, especially if the patient had thyrotoxic hypokalemic periodic paralysis because it can cause a prompt increase in P_K (within 2 hours).[17] If effective, much smaller doses of KCl may be needed for therapy. In retrospective, case-controlled studies, rebound hyperkalemia (>5.0 mmol/L) was observed in 30% to 70% of patients with thyrotoxic hypokalemic periodic paralysis if more than 90 mmol of KCl were given within 24 hours or at a rate of more than 10 mmol/hr.[18] Hence we prefer to give less than this amount unless the P_K fails to increase to a safe level of approximately 3 mmol/L. Acetazolamide may be useful to prevent attacks of hypokalemic periodic paralysis patients with the sporadic or familial types of this disorder; nevertheless, its mechanism of action is not clear.

Specific Issues in K^+ Replacement Therapy

Magnitude of the K^+ Deficit

It is common practice to infer that there is a deficit of 100 to 400 mmol K^+ if the P_K has decreased from 4.0 to 3.0 mmol/L and that a P_K of 2 mmol/L suggests that there is a much greater deficit of K^+ (as high as 800 mmol in a 70-kg adult). However, this is not supported with solid data because a component of the hypokalemia is due to a shift of K^+ into cells in many patients. In our view, there is no useful quantitative relationship between P_K and the total body K^+ deficit in an individual patient. Hence, careful monitoring of P_K during replacement of the K^+ deficit is mandatory.

Route of K^1 Administration

The oral route is the preferred one to administer K^+. Certain factors may necessitate using the intravenous route, including the urgency of therapy, the level of consciousness, and the presence of gastrointestinal problems. As a rule, the concentration of K^+ should not be more than 40 mmol/L if infused peripherally because higher K^+ concentrations may irritate veins with a lower rate of blood flow; the rate of administration of K^+ should not exceed 60 mmol/hr in most settings.

K^+ Preparations

Most preparations that are in tablet form release K^+ slowly (Table 30-1). Although usually well tolerated, they occasionally cause ulcerative or stenotic lesions in the gastrointestinal tract due to a high local K^+ concentration. Oral KCl can also be given in a crystalline form (e.g., salt substitutes such as Co-salt (equal amounts of NaCl and KCl), which provide 14 mmol K^+/g); this is generally well tolerated and is an inexpensive form of K^+ supplementation.

For electroneutrality, a deficit of K^+ must be accompanied by the loss of Cl^- or HCO_3^- or a gain of Na^+. With a KCl deficit (e.g., due to chronic vomiting or diuretic use), KCl is needed; in contrast, with a $KHCO_3$ deficit (e.g., due to diarrhea), K^+ with HCO_3 (or a HCO_3^- equivalent, e.g., citrate) is needed. A note of caution is necessary: The administration of HCO_3^- may cause a shift of K^+ into cells in certain settings. Therefore, in a patient who is markedly hypokalemic and acidemic, KCl should be given initially; alkali in the form of $NaHCO_3$ may then be administered after the P_K approaches a safer level (>3 mmol/L). In conditions in which K^+ loss is matched by Na^+ retention (e.g., in a patient with primary hyperaldosteronism), K^+ is usually given as KCl while measures are taken to ensure that NaCl

Table 30-1 Commonly Used Potassium Supplements

	K$^+$ Salt	Unit
Oral Preparations		
Apo-K	KCl	8 mEq/tablet
Slow-K	KCl	8 mEq/tablet
Micro-K	KCl	8 mEq/capsule
K-Dur	KCl	20 mEq/tablet
K-Lyte/Cl	KCl	25 mEq/effervescent tablet
K-Lyte	K citrate	25 mEq/effervescent tablet
K-Lor	KCl	20 mEq/packet
Polycitra K	K citrate	2 mEq/mL
K-10	KCl	1.33 mEq/mL
Roychlor	KCl	1.33 mEq/mL
Intravenous Preparations		
K chloride	KCl	2 mEq/mL
K acetate	K acetate	4 mEq/mL
K phosphate	K phosphate	4.4 mEq/10mL

will be excreted. The need for K$^+$ as its phosphate salt is most evident when there is rapid anabolism; examples include patients on nutritional support or those in the acute recovery phase of a catabolic disorder such as diabetic ketoacidosis. If given, phosphate should not be administered too rapidly (<50 mmol in 8 hours) because a large phosphate load has the risk of inducing metastatic calcification and hypocalcemia. We give K$^+$ as KCl in the treatment of patients who have diabetic ketoacidosis and rely on the patient's diet to supply the phosphate needed for the anabolic phase of the illness, which occurs later.

Although it may seem reasonable on superficial analysis to increase the intake of K$^+$-rich foods (e.g., bananas, fruit juice), this is not an effective way to replace a K$^+$ deficit. A few centimeters of banana provides only about 1 mmol of K$^+$, so it will take a true banana lover to consume enough bananas to provide 50 mmol K$^+$ each day. The calories in this quantity of bananas could add 22.5 to 45 kg to the patient's body weight in a year. Conversely, a large amount of K$^+$ can be obtained through dietary means by ingesting vegetables, which have a high ratio of potassium to calories.

Adjuncts to Therapy

Administering K$^+$-sparing diuretics to patients with hypokalemia can decrease renal loss of K$^+$. However, this is only useful on a long-term therapy basis and not during the treatment of acute hypokalemia, when the rate of K$^+$ excretion is usually less than 10 mmol/hr. Amiloride and triamterene are better tolerated than spironolactone because they lack the gastrointestinal and hormonal complications of spironolactone (amenorrhea, gynecomastia, decreased libido). Eplerenone is a highly selective mineralocorticoid receptor antagonist that is associated with a lower incidence of endocrine side effects, but is also significantly more expensive than spironolactone.[19] When using the ENaC blockers amiloride and triamterene, the patient should have a low intake

of NaCl because this leads to a lower delivery of osmoles to the CCD and thereby a lower flow rate.[20] With a lower flow rate, the concentration of the drug near the ENaC will be higher. There is an important note of caution; hyperkalemia can develop when K$^+$ is given along with K$^+$-sparing diuretics, especially if other conditions that may compromise K$^+$ excretion are present; it should also be recognized that these drugs have a long half-life.

Risks of Therapy

With prolonged hypokalemia, the CCD may become hyporesponsive to the kaliuretic effect of aldosterone (probably due to fewer luminal K$^+$ ion channels for the secretion of K$^+$); this would allow aldosterone to continue to be a NaCl-retaining hormone while diminishing its kaliuretic effect.[21] Hence, it is important to monitor the P$_K$ frequently during the treatment of hypokalemia.

Hyperkalemia has been observed in approximately 4% of patients taking K$^+$ supplements. The risk is highest in patients with renal failure and diabetes mellitus. The simultaneous use of angiotensin-converting enzyme inhibitors, β-blockers, or nonsteroidal anti-inflammatory drugs may also predispose to the development of hyperkalemia.

Specific Causes of Hypokalemia

A summary of the causes of hypokalemia is provided in Box 30-1. We only comment briefly on those that are common or because new strides have been made in understanding their pathophysiology, which have implications for therapy. A summary of the specific issues in therapy of these disorders is provided in Table 30-2.

Diuretic-Induced Hypokalemia

When hypokalemia develops in this setting, it is usually modest in degree.[22] A decrease in P$_K$ to less than 3 mmol/L occurs in less than 10% of patients on the usual doses of thiazide-type diuretics and usually occurs in the first 2 weeks of therapy. Although there is some controversy, it is our view that patients with chronic diuretic-induced hypokalemia, even if it is mild in degree, should be treated.

There are several ways to minimize the degree of diuretic-induced hypokalemia. First, give the lowest effective dose of diuretic because the risk of hypokalemia is dose dependent. In most patients with essential hypertension, 12.5 to 25 mg of hydrochlorothiazide produces as great a decrease in blood pressure as higher doses. Second, the intake of K$^+$ should not be low. Salt substitutes such as Co-salt (14 mmol K$^+$/g) are an inexpensive way to provide K$^+$ while decreasing the intake of Na$^+$. Third, lowering the rate of K$^+$ excretion can minimize the degree of hypokalemia. This may be achieved in part by limiting the intake and thereby the excretion of NaCl to approximately 100 mmol/day. The renal loss of K$^+$ can be reduced with the use of K$^+$-sparing diuretics. Nevertheless, their dose may need to be adjusted independently because a higher distal flow rate lowers the luminal concentration of this class of drugs and hence they become less effective blockers of ENaCs. Therefore, we do not favor the use of tablets of combination of thiazide or a loop diuretic plus a K$^+$-sparing diuretic.

Primary Hyperaldosteronism

This should be suspected when there is both hypertension and hypokalemia with renal K$^+$ wasting in patients who have low

Table 30-2 Specific Issues in Therapy of Some Disorders of Hypokalemia

Disorder	Specific Issues in Therapy
Diuretic-induced hypokalemia	Use lowest effective dose of diuretics
	K supplements (e.g., Co-salt)
	Restrict NaCl intake to <100 mmol/day
	Add K^+-sparing diuretics
Primary hyperaldosteronism	Unilateral adrenal adenoma: laparoscopic adrenalectomy
	Bilateral adrenal hyperplasia: mineralocorticoid receptor antagonists (preferred), ENaC blockers
Bartter and Gitelman's syndromes	K^+ supplements, in frequent divided doses
	K^+-sparing diuretics: may aggravate salt wasting, high doses of amiloride needed
	Mg supplements if hypomagnesemia
	ACE inhibitors, ARBs: limited by hypotension
	Prostaglandin inhibitors: risk of chronic renal dysfunction with prolonged use
Glucocorticoid-remediable aldosteronism	Glucocorticoids
Liddle syndrome	ENaC blockers, high doses required
Apparent mineralocorticoid excess	Mineralocorticoid receptor antagonists
	ENaC blockers; must have low intake of NaCl

For details, see the text.
ACE, angiotensin-converting enzyme; ARBs, angiotensin receptor blockers; ENaC, epithelial Na^+ channel

plasma renin activity. A poorly explained fact is that a significant number of patients with primary hyperaldosteronism do not have hypokalemia. Laparoscopic unilateral adrenalectomy is generally the preferred treatment in a patient with an adrenal adenoma.[23] If successful, it should induce a marked reduction in aldosterone secretion, a decrease in blood pressure, and correction of the hypokalemia. Notwithstanding, hypertension persists in as many as 40% to 65% of patients after unilateral adrenalectomy, especially those with a family history of hypertension and those who were taking two or more antihypertensive medications prior to surgery.[24] In patients with bilateral adrenal hyperplasia or those with an adrenal adenoma but who are not candidates for surgery, medical therapy is the preferred treatment.[25] The goals of therapy, however, are not only to control blood pressure and correct the hypokalemia, but also to reverse the unwanted effects of hyperaldosteronism on the heart. The administration of a mineralocorticoid receptor antagonist (spironolactone or eplerenone) is the preferred therapy. Amiloride is an alternative in those who are intolerant of these drugs. The issue about the need for a low intake of NaCl to decrease the flow rate in CCD applies in this setting.

Bartter Syndrome and Gitelman's Syndrome

The current therapy for both Bartter and Gitelman's syndromes includes KCl supplements, K^+-sparing agents, and the use of angiotensin-converting enzyme inhibitors or angiotensin II receptor blockers. Correction of hypokalemia in these patients is rather difficult, even with large K^+ supplements.[20] One might be able to maintain a somewhat higher P_K in these patients by giving the same daily amount of K^+ supplements but using a more frequent dosing schedule. This is perhaps because a large dose of K^+ may induce a sufficient increase in the P_K to cause the insertion of K^+ channels into the luminal membrane in CCD cells and hence an

increase in K^+ secretion.[26,27] Hypomagnesemia may be a contributing factor in the enhanced kaliuresis in some patients with Gitelman's syndrome.[28] Again, correction of hypomagnesemia with oral magnesium is usually difficult and also limited by gastrointestinal side effects. K^+-sparing diuretics (amiloride, spironolactone) may help conserve K^+. A common clinical observation is that even high doses of amiloride fail to curtail the excessive kaliuresis in patients with Bartter and Gitelman's syndromes. Part of the explanation of this diminished effect could be related to the higher flow in the CCD due to inhibition of NaCl reabsorption in upstream nephron segments. This higher volume delivery to the CCD lowers the concentration of ENaC blockers, thus diminishing their effectiveness.[20] A potential concern using these agents in patients with Bartter or Gitelman's syndromes is that they may aggravate their salt wasting. This may become evident if, for example, dietary salt intake is decreased or there is a nonrenal cause of the loss of NaCl. Angiotensin-converting enzyme inhibitors have been used to decrease levels of angiotensin II and aldosterone with variable success; if effective, hypotension becomes an important concern. In prenatal Bartter syndrome, prostaglandin E_2 synthesis can be reduced with cyclooxygenase inhibitors such as indomethacin.[29] Inhibition of prostaglandin E_2 synthesis attenuates salt wasting with hypokalemia and minimizes the systemic symptoms of prostaglandin excess. Caution is advised using these agents in the neonatal period as acute renal failure and patent ductus arteriosus are documented complications. Because of the potential for causing chronic renal dysfunction, the lowest possible effective dose of these drugs should be used.

Glucorticoid-Remediable Aldosteronism

Glucocorticoid-remediable aldosteronism is an autosomal dominant form of hypertension caused by a chimeric gene, which results in aldosterone synthesis being under the control of corticotropin rather than its normal regulator, angiotensin II.[30] In this disorder, exogenous glucocorticoids may suppress the release of corticotropin and thereby the secretion of aldosterone.

Liddle Syndrome

Liddle syndrome is an autosomal dominant disorder that is caused by mutations in either the β or the γ subunit of the ENaC that leads to its defective degradation and thereby an increased number of active ENaC units in the luminal membrane of principal cells in the CCD.[31] The channel is amiloride and triamterene sensitive providing that their concentrations are high enough in luminal fluid, explaining the efficacy of these K$^+$-sparing diuretics in the treatment of this syndrome. Conversely, aldosterone receptor antagonists are not effective in these patients.

Apparent Mineralocorticoid Excess

Apparent mineralocorticoid excess is the result of a mutation in the gene encoding for 11β-hydroxysteroid dehydrogenase type 2,[32] the enzyme responsible for converting cortisol to its inactive metabolite, cortisone, in principal cells of the CCD. This enzyme is inhibited by glycyrrhetinic acid in licorice. These patients can be treated with ENaC blockers (e.g., amiloride, triamterene), with the same caveat for the need for salt restriction noted previously. In contrast to patients with Liddle syndrome, patients with apparent mineralocorticoid excess usually have a good response to spironolactone.

HYPERKALEMIA

The steps to identify the major diagnostic categories for patients with hyperkalemia are summarized in Figure 30-6. It is necessary to make the specific diagnosis because the mode

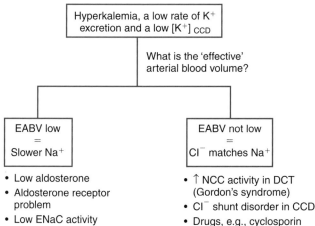

Figure 30-6 Renal causes for hyperkalemia and a low rate of excretion of K$^+$. For details, see legend to Figure 30-4. A list of likely causes of a low rate of excretion of K$^+$ is provided below the diagnostic categories. CCD, cortical collecting duct; DCT, distal convoluted tubule; EABV, effective arterial blood volume; ENaC, epithelial Na$^+$ channel; Na$^+$-Cl$^-$ cotransporter. (From Halperin ML: The ACID Truth and Basic Facts: With a Sweet Touch, an enLYTenment, 5th ed. Toronto, Ontario: RossMark Medical Publishers, 2004, with permission.)

and emphasis of therapy are strongly influenced by the diagnostic category.

General Considerations for Treatment of Hyperkalemia

Medical Emergencies

The major danger for the patient with hyperkalemia is a cardiac arrhythmia. Because minor electrocardiographic changes may progress rapidly to a dangerous arrhythmia, any patient with an electrocardiographic abnormality related to hyperkalemia should be treated as a medical emergency. We would also treat patients with a severe degree of hyperkalemia (e.g., $P_K > 7.0$ mmol/L) aggressively, even in the absence of electrocardiographic changes. A note of caution, however, is needed: a severe degree of hyperkalemia is well tolerated in certain settings such as extremes of exercise (the supermarathon) and in infants.

The steps to take in the treatment of patients with an emergency related to hyperkalemia are discussed below and are illustrated in Figure 30-7.

Antagonize the Cardiac Effects of Hyperkalemia

Calcium is the best agent and its effects should be evident within minutes. It is usually given as 20 to 30 mL of a 10% calcium gluconate solution (two to three ampoules) or 10 mL of 10% calcium chloride (one ampoule). Both solutions are equally effective, but the former is safer than the latter in case of infiltration of the needle during an intravenous infusion because at high concentrations calcium gluconate is mostly undissociated, whereas calcium chloride is nearly completely dissociated. Once calcium gluconate enters the circulation and gets diluted greatly, it also becomes mostly dissociated. This dose can be repeated in 5 minutes if electrocardiographic changes persist. The effect may last 30 to 60 minutes. Extreme caution should be exerted using Ca^{2+} in patients on digitalis because hypercalcemia may precipitate digitalis toxicity.

Induce a Shift of K$^+$ into the Intracellular Fluid

Use of Insulin

Many studies support the use of insulin in the treatment of acute hyperkalemia in patients with end-stage renal disease (ESRD).[33–36] For example, Blumberg and colleagues[33] studied 10 patients with ESRD on hemodialysis after an overnight fast before their regularly scheduled hemodialysis. The patients were treated on different occasions with approximately 20 units of intravenous regular insulin plus glucose, NaHCO$_3$ at 4 mmol/min, epinephrine 0.05 μg/kg/min, or hemodialysis. The P_K was followed for 60 minutes. Hemodialysis was the most effective modality that lowered the P_K, decreasing it from 5.6 to 4.3 mmol/L. Insulin with glucose also caused the P_K to decrease rapidly from 5.6 to 4.7 mmol/L. Of note, epinephrine caused only a minor decrease in the P_K. Intravenous NaHCO$_3$ failed to lower the P_K. Large doses of insulin are needed for maximal K$^+$ shift into cells. In the study by Blumberg and colleagues,[33] 20 units of regular insulin were given to increase the plasma insulin level to 300 to 400 mU/L. One cannot overemphasize the need to give enough glucose to prevent the development of hypoglycemia and to monitor blood glucose levels for a sufficient period of time.

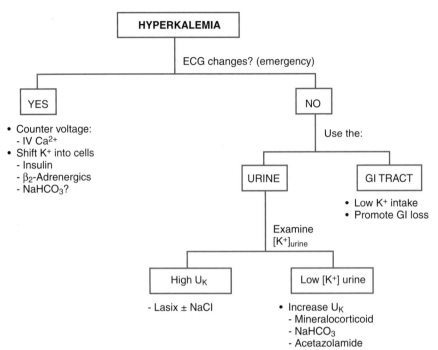

Figure 30-7 Treatment of the patient with hyperkalemia. If an emergency is present (usually cardiac), intravenous Ca^{2+} must be given. This treatment should act promptly. Efforts are now made to shift K^+ into cells with insulin and glucose. Longer term strategies are to limit the intake of K^+, increase its excretion in the gastrointestinal (GI) tract, and promote its excretion in the urine. In this latter context, examine the potassium concentration in the urine (U_K) and flow rate to decide leverage for therapy (see Fig. 30-2 for details). ECG, electrocardiogram; ICF, intracellular fluid. (From Halperin ML: The ACID Truth and Basic Facts: With a Sweet Touch, an enLYTEnment, 5th ed. Toronto, Ontario: RossMark Medical Publishers, 2004, with permission.)

We recommend insulin with glucose as initial therapy to induce a shift of K^+ into cells in the emergency treatment of hyperkalemia. Although some suggest treating nondiabetic, hyperkalemic patients with a bolus of glucose without exogenous insulin, we believe that this strategy is unwise because the high levels of insulin required to induce an adequate shift of K^+ into cells might not be achieved without giving insulin. In addition, hypertonic glucose may cause K^+ to shift out of cells in patients with inadequate insulin reserves, leading to a paradoxical increase in the P_K.[37]

β2-Adrenergic Agonists

β2-Agonists stimulate the Na/K-ATPase via a cyclic adenosine monophosphate–dependent pathway (see Fig. 30-1). The ability of β2-adrenergic stimulation to lower the P_K in patients with renal failure has been demonstrated in a number of studies.[34–36,38,39] Montoliu and colleagues[38] gave 20 patients on maintenance hemodialysis 0.5 mg albuterol intravenously over 15 minutes, which caused the mean P_K to decrease from 5.6 to 4.5 mmol/L within 30 minutes. Of note, eight of these patients developed tremors and six had minor ill-defined discomfort. In a second part of the study, consecutive patients with acute or chronic renal failure were given intravenous albuterol (0.5 mg over 15 minutes). Their mean P_K decreased from 7.0 to 5.6 mmol/L within 30 minutes, and the effect was sustained for 3 hours. Reversal of the electrocardiographic manifestations of hyperkalemia was documented in most of the patients, and only minor adverse effects were noted. It was recognized, however, that there was considerable individual variation in the response of the P_K to albuterol, although the data for individual patients were not shown.

A number of studies have examined nebulized β2-agonists as therapy for hyperkalemia. In a study by Allon and colleagues,[40] 10 hyperkalemic ESRD patients on hemodialysis were treated with 10 mg of nebulized albuterol, 20 mg of nebulized albuterol, or placebo on three separate occasions. After the administration of albuterol, the P_K decreased within 30 minutes and this decrease was sustained for at least 2 hours. The maximum decreases in P_K were 0.6 mmol/L with the 10-mg dose and 1.0 mmol/L with the 20-mg dose. However, two of the 10 patients were resistant to the hypokalemic effects of albuterol. There was a minimal increase in heart rate and a notable absence of cardiovascular adverse effects.

Although these studies suggest that β2-agonists are effective in rapidly lowering the P_K, we do not recommend their use as preferred therapy in the emergency treatment of hyperkalemia for two reasons. First, they are not effective in a significant proportion of patients; 20% to 40% of patients studied had a decrease in P_K of less than 0.5 mmol/L. It is unclear why some patients do not exhibit a decrease in P_K after the administration of β2-agonists, and it is not possible to predict which patients will respond. Second, we are concerned about the safety of these drugs in the doses used for the treatment of hyperkalemia, which are four to eight times those prescribed for the treatment of acute asthma. Although no severe adverse events were reported in the studies noted here, most were performed in stable patients with a mild degree of hyperkalemia before their regular hemodialysis session. A number of these studies excluded patients on β-blockers and selected those with no significant coronary heart disease or unstable heart rhythms. Therefore, the safety of these agents was determined in a group of patients who may not resemble the general ESRD population, which has a high prevalence of cardiac disease.

Whether the effect of nebulized β_2-agonists in lowering P_K is additive to that of insulin has been examined by Allon and Copkney.[34] In a crossover design, 12 patients on maintenance hemodialysis who had predialysis P_K values that were greater than 5 mmol/L received 10 units of regular insulin plus glucose as an intravenous bolus or 20 mg of nebulized albuterol over 10 minutes, or both. Insulin decreased P_K in 15 minutes and albuterol decreased P_K within 30 minutes. There was a similar decrease in P_K with insulin (0.65 mmol/L) or albuterol (0.66 mmol/L). However, four of 10 patients treated with albuterol had a mean decrease in P_K of less than 0.5 mmol/L. There was a substantially greater decrease in P_K with the combined regimen (1.2 mmol/L) compared with either agent alone. One should note, however, that only 10 units of intravenous regular insulin were given in this study, the plasma insulin level was only 40 mU/L at 60 minutes, and the magnitude of the decrease in P_K was lower than that observed in other studies when higher doses of insulin were used. Blumberg and colleagues[33] administered 20 units of intravenous insulin and achieved a similar decrease in P_K ($\sim$1 mmol/L) as Allon and Copkney[34] with their combined therapy of 10 units of intravenous insulin and albuterol. Thus, it remains uncertain whether β_2-agonists would have a P_K-lowering effect additive to that of insulin if insulin were given at the higher doses.

NaHCO$_3$

The first step in the action of NaHCO$_3$ is to decrease the concentration of H^+ in the ECF compartment and thereby promote the exit of H^+ and entry of Na^+ into cells via the NHE (see Fig. 30-1). However, because the NHE is normally inactive in most cell membranes, this will not cause a decrease in the P_K. Thus, only if the NHE were active would the administration of NaHCO$_3$ have the potential to lower the P_K. One major activator of the NHE is intracellular acidosis because H^+ ions are not only a substrate for the NHE, but they also bind to a modifier site that activates it.

The potential value of NaHCO$_3$ for therapy of patients with a severe degree of hyperkalemia is not clear. NaHCO$_3$ therapy did not lower the P_K acutely in a number of studies.[33,41,42] In more detail, Blumberg and colleagues[33] administered 100 to 215 mmol of intravenous NaHCO$_3$ as either an isotonic or a hypertonic solution to 10 patients with ESRD on hemodialysis who had mild hyperkalemia (mean P_K close to 5.5 mmol/L). Although the mean plasma HCO$_3^-$ concentration increased from 21 to 34 mmol/L, there was no change in P_K after 60 minutes, a time frame during which this intervention must have a significant effect if it were to be used in a potentially life-threatening situation. In a subsequent study, Blumberg and colleagues[41] infused 390 mmol of NaHCO$_3$ over 6 hours in 12 patients with ESRD on hemodialysis. There was a moderate decrease in P_K from 6.0 to 5.4 mmol/L, but only after 4 hours of starting the NaHCO$_3$ infusion. It is noteworthy that the studies that found a lack of effect of NaHCO$_3$ were performed in stable hemodialysis patients without significant acidosis. In other words, these studies examined the effect of NaHCO$_3$ when the NHE was presumably in an inactive mode. The question remains as to whether NaHCO$_3$ would be effective in patients with a more significant degree of acidosis, when the NHE is likely to become activated. There are limited data in the literature to answer this question. A report by Schwarz and colleagues[43] described four uremic patients with P_K values ranging from 5.9 to 8.5 mmol/L associated with electrocardiographic changes attributable to hyperkalemia and a profound degree of acidosis (plasma HCO$_3^-$ 1.3–7.3 mmol/L). In all four patients, an infusion of 150 to 400 mmol NaHCO$_3$ caused a significant decrease in the P_K and improvement of their electrocardiogram. Although it is difficult to draw definite conclusions, this study identifies a potential value for NaHCO$_3$ in certain settings. Accordingly, we would administer NaHCO$_3$ to treat dangerous hyperkalemia in patients with significant acidosis, but we would not use it as the only emergency therapy to shift K^+ into cells. However, the excessive administration of NaHCO$_3$ should be avoided due to the risk of inducing hypernatremia, ECF volume expansion, carbon dioxide retention, and a decrease in ionized serum calcium, which may aggravate the effect of hyperkalemia.

Studies that examined the combined use of NaHCO$_3$ with insulin have also produced conflicting results. Allon and Shanklin[35] found that the addition of NaHCO$_3$ did not enhance the P_K-lowering effects of insulin in their study of eight patients on hemodialysis. In this study, the mean P_K before therapy was 4.5 mmol/L and the mean plasma HCO$_3^-$ was 22 mmol/L. In contrast, Kim[44] compared insulin, NaHCO$_3$, or both in eight patients with a predialysis P_K of more than 6 mmol/L. There was no change in the P_K with NaHCO$_3$ as the sole therapy after 60 minutes, and insulin caused the P_K to decrease from 6.3 to 5.7 mmol/L. The combination of insulin and NaHCO$_3$ led to the greatest decline in P_K (from 6.2 to 5.2 mmol/L). It is unclear why Kim[44] found a synergistic effect of NaHCO$_3$ with insulin, yet Allon and Shanklin[35] did not; it should be noted, however, that the patients studied by these authors were not hyperkalemic.

No Medical Emergency: Removal of K$^+$ from the Body

It is important to appreciate that to lower the P_K from 7.0 to 6.0 mmol/L requires very much less K^+ loss than that needed to lower the P_K from 6.0 to 5.0 mmol/L. Hence, it is important to cause even a small K^+ loss when there is a severe degree of hyperkalemia.

Diuretics and/or Mineralocorticoids

There are two aspects to consider in this context. If the excretion of K^+ is low because of a low urine volume with a high concentration of K^+, a loop diuretic may be able to induce a kaliuresis by increasing the flow rate in the CCD. One can avoid unwanted ECF volume contraction by replacing the NaCl lost in the urine. Conversely, if the urine K^+ concentration is unduly low, giving a mineralocorticoid (100 μg of fludrocortisone acetate) and inducing bicarbonaturia with the carbonic anhydrase inhibitor acetazolamide may cause substantial kaliuresis (the HCO$_3^-$ lost in the urine might need to be replaced).

Cation-Exchange Resins

A cation-exchange resin is a cross-linked polymer with negatively charged structural units. The resin can exchange bound Na$^+$ (Kayexalate) or Ca^{2+} (calcium resonium) for cations including K^+. The purpose of using resins is to enhance the elimination of K^+ from the gastrointestinal tract. The cation-exchange resin Kayexalate contains 4 mEq of Na^+/g. This Na^+ is theoretically exchangeable for 4 mEq of K^+. Thus, 30 g Kayexalate could theoretically remove 120 mEq of K^+. However, this degree of exchange does not occur at the Na^+ and K^+ concentrations found in the gastrointestinal tract. In more detail, Emmet and colleagues[45] examined the in vitro binding characteristics of Kayexalate and found that the Na^+ and K^+ concentrations at which 50% of Na^+ is exchanged for K^+ were 65 and 40 mmol/L, respectively. With a higher concentration of Na^+ and/or a lower concentration of K^+, less exchange would be expected to take place. If one considers the concentrations of Na^+ and K^+ in the duodenum (110 and 15 mmol/L, respectively), jejunum (140 and 5 mmol/L. respectively), ileum (130 and 20 mmol/L, respectively), and rectum (10 and 80 mmol/L, respectively),[46] it seems that the only favorable location for the exchange of Na^+ for K^+ is in the lumen of the rectum. Because there is little absorption of K^+ in the rectum, there is no significant advantage to having the K^+ in its luminal fluid excreted in an ionic form or bound to a resin. Furthermore, normal fecal K^+ excretion is approximately 9 mmol/day; subjects with ESRD excrete only slightly more K^+ (an extra 2–3 mmol/day) in their feces than do normal subjects.

In humans, active secretion of K^+ in the gastrointestinal tract occurs in the rectosigmoid portion of the colon. One possible theoretical benefit for the use of cation-exchange resins is if they were to lower the K^+ concentration in luminal water, thereby enhancing the net secretion of K^+ in this portion of the colon. However, a number of factors limit the magnitude of this process. Other cations are available to exchange for resin-bound Na^+ apart from K^+, including NH_4^+, Ca^{2+}, and Mg^{2+}. The concentration of NH_4^+ in stool water may be high in patients with ESRD as a result of their high blood urea levels and because of bacterial urease activity in the lumen of the gastrointestinal tract. Cations such as Ca^{2+} and Mg^{2+} have an even greater affinity for the resin than K^+ because of their divalent positive charge. In addition, resins are usually given with cathartics because of their tendency to cause constipation, which can increase the concentration of Na^+ in stool water, leading to conditions even more unfavorable for the exchange of Na^+ for K^+. Colonic secretion of K^+ in normal subjects is approximately 4 mmol/day. It has been suggested that patients with ESRD have enhanced colonic secretion of K^+ that is perhaps mediated by aldosterone.[47,48] Balance data are conflicting, and the evidence of increased removal of K^+ by the gastrointestinal tract in patients with ESRD is not convincing.[49] Even if there were an adaptive increase in colonic K^+ secretion, stool volume will be limiting for the total removal of K^+. If one assumes a transepithelial voltage as high as 90 mV (measured values are significantly lower, close to 40 mV), and a P_K of 5 mmol/L, the concentration of K^+ in stool water would be close to 100 mmol/L. With a usual stool weight of 125 g/day, of which 75% is water, only 10 mmol of K^+ will be excreted. In experiments in which dialysis bags were placed into the rectum of patients with chronic renal failure,[48] the rate of net K^+ secretion was 1.5 $\mu mol/hr/cm^2$ of rectal surface area. Thus, with an average rectal surface area of 100 cm^2, the net K^+ secretion would be only 4 mmol/day. If, however, this high rate of K^+ secretion could be present unabated throughout the entire colon, fecal K^+ excretion could be as high as 70 mmol/day if stool volume were not limiting. Thus, from a theoretical point of view, resins would

seem of little use in inducing a loss of K^+ from the gastrointestinal tract unless lowering of the stool K^+ concentration plays an important role in this process and, more importantly, the patient has diarrhea.

Two reports are commonly cited to support the use of resins for treatment of hyperkalemia.[50,51] Although the authors of both studies concluded that resins were useful for treating hyperkalemia, it is difficult to determine their exact role. It should be noted that several doses were given, sometimes for a number of days, and that the effect on P_K was noted after 1 to 5 days. Furthermore, it is not clear whether the effect was due to the resin or merely to the induction of diarrhea with hypertonic glucose or other cathartics.

Two studies have reexamined the effect of cathartics and/or resins on fecal K^+ excretion. First, Emmett and colleagues[45] gave nine normal human subjects 60 or 120 g sorbitol, 100 mmol sodium sulfate, or eight phenolphthalein/docusate tablets; each with and without 30 g Kayexalate. Stool water and Na^+ and K^+ concentrations were followed over the next 12 hours. Phenolphthalein resulted in the highest stool K^+ excretion rate (37 mmol in 12 hours) compared with the other laxatives. The addition of 30 g Kayexalate to phenolphthalein increased stool K^+ excretion only modestly to 49 mmol in 12 hours. The addition of the resin to sorbitol or sodium sulfate did not significantly increase stool K^+ excretion compared with either laxative alone. The results of this study suggest that the majority of K^+ excretion with cathartics and resins is due to the induction of diarrhea. Second, Gruy-Kapral and colleagues[52] studied the effect of a single dose of cathartic and/or resin on fecal K^+ excretion and the P_K in patients with renal failure. The results of the study support the argument that resins do not contribute to fecal K^+ excretion above the induction of diarrhea alone and that single-dose resin/cathartic therapy is of no value in the management of acute hyperkalemia.

In summary, we do not recommend the use of resins for acute hyperkalemia. In the setting of chronic hyperkalemia, the addition of resins to cathartics adds little to the induction of diarrhea alone. One other point merits emphasis: there is convincing evidence that the hypertonic sorbitol may cause colonic necrosis.[53]

Dialysis

Hemodialysis is more effective than peritoneal dialysis for removing K^+. Removal rates of K^+ can approximate 35 mmol/hr with a dialysate bath K^+ concentration of 1 to 2 mmol/L. A glucose-free dialysate is preferable to avoid the glucose-induced release of insulin and the subsequent shift of K^+ into cells, lessening the removal of K^+.

Specific Causes of Hyperkalemia

As mentioned earlier, hyperkalemia is a laboratory finding and not a specific disorder. Hence, the settings where hyperkalemia is present are heterogeneous in pathophysiology, and thus the treatment for each group is different. Accordingly, they are discussed under separate headings.

Syndrome of Hyporeninemic Hypoaldosteronism

Patients in this diagnostic category are heterogeneous with regard to the pathophysiology of their disorder and therefore require different approaches to the treatment of their hyperkalemia.[54]

Group with a Low Capacity to Produce Renin

The basis of this group of disorders may be destruction of or a biosynthetic defect in the juxtaglomerular apparatus. The net result is hyporeninemia and thereby a low plasma aldosterone level. Accordingly, there is a relatively slower reabsorption of Na^+ in the CCD. Hyperkalemia will develop if there is a sufficiently large intake of K^+ such that an increase in the P_K must be present to permit the kidneys to excrete the daily K^+ load because of the chronic low aldosterone levels. The effective arterial blood volume will tend to be low. With respect to treatment, patients with this group of disorders are expected to have a significant decrease in their P_K due to an increase in their $[K^+]_{CCD}$ after the administration of exogenous mineralocorticoids for several days (e.g., fluodrocortisone 100 μg/day). The administration of diuretics to these patients will aggravate the degree of contraction of their effective arterial blood volume.

Group with Low Stimulus to Produce Renin

There are two subtypes in this group of patients.

Enhanced Reabsorption of Na^+ and Cl^- in the Distal Convoluted Tubule

This is due to an abnormal regulation of the signal system that affects the distribution of the Na^+, Cl^- cotransporter in this nephron segment with more active units ending up in the luminal membrane. This seems to be the underlying pathophysiology in patients with pseudohypoaldosteronism type II (Gordon's syndrome).[55] When there is an enhanced upstream reabsorption of Na^+ and Cl^-, this results in a low delivery of Na^+ and Cl^- to the CCD, which compromises the ability of this nephron segment to reabsorb Na^+ faster than Cl^- and thereby leads to a diminished excretory capacity for K^+. ECF volume expansion is a hallmark of the pathophysiology and results in hyporeninemia and thus a lower than expected plasma aldosterone level given the hyperkalemia. These patients do not have an appreciable increase in their K^+ excretion with exogenous mineralocorticoids, but their K^+ excretion should increase when thiazide diuretics are given (higher Na^+ and Cl^- delivery to the CCD) if ENaCs are open. Of note, mineralocorticoids may aggravate the hypertension in patients who have excessive reabsorption of Na^+ and Cl^- in the distal convoluted tubule.

Cl Shunt Disorder

This subtype is most commonly seen in patients with diabetic nephropathy. Although the basis of the disorder remains to be established, it is possible that the reabsorption of Na^+ and Cl^- may be augmented in the distal convoluted tubule or these patients may have a Cl shunt disorder in the CCD.[56] With the former pathophysiology, the ideal treatment would be with a thiazide diuretic as described above. Conversely, patients with a Cl shunt have a significant increase in their K^+ excretion with the induction of bicarbonaturia (perhaps secondary to the inhibition of the reabsorption of Cl^- in the CCD).[11] Hence, inducing bicarbonaturia with acetazolamide may increase K^+ excretion; HCO_3^- loss may have to be replaced to avoid the development of metabolic acidosis.

Cyclosporine-Induced Hyperkalemia

Hyperkalemia develops in some patients receiving cyclosporine after organ transplantation. Even though cyclosporine can lead to inhibition of Na/K-ATPase in vitro, we favor the hypothesis that the pathophysiology of hyperkalemia in these patients resembles a Cl shunt disorder in the CCD.[57] A kaliuresis could be enhanced in these patients with the administration of a loop diuretic to increase the flow rate in the CCD or the administration of acetazolamide to induce bicarbonaturia.

Trimethoprim-Induced Hyperkalemia

Trimethoprim and pentamidine cause hyperkalemia by blocking ENaCs in the CCD.[58] Although frequently reported in patients who have acquired immunodeficiency syndrome and have received high doses of trimethoprim for the treatment of *Pneumocystis carinii* pneumonia, trimethoprim causes an increase in P_K even when used in conventional doses. Patients with acquired immunodeficiency syndrome might also have other causes that make them prone to the development of a more severe degree of hyperkalemia (shift of K^+ from cells, decreased K^+ excretion because of low flow in the CCD due to a low rate of delivery of osmoles (NaCl and urea) to the CCD[2]).

Use of a loop diuretic may help by increasing the volume delivered to the CCD, which will lower the concentration of trimethoprim in its lumen; enough NaCl administration will be required to defend ECF volume. Because trimethoprim only blocks ENaCs when the drug is in its charged (protonated) form, increasing luminal fluid pH in the CCD should decrease the cationic form of trimethoprim and minimize the antikaliuretic effect of this drug.[59] Inducing bicarbonaturia with acetazolamide and the use of a loop diuretic are rational therapeutic options in a patient with hyperkalemia in whom continuation of trimethoprim is necessary. However, sufficient NaCl and $NaHCO_3$ would need to be given to avoid a contracted ECF volume and metabolic acidosis, respectively.

Addison's Disease

Adrenal crisis is an emergency that requires immediate restoration of the intravascular volume (intravenous saline) and correction of the cortisol deficiency (administer dexamethasone or hydrocortisone). Beware of increasing the plasma sodium concentration too rapidly if hyponatremia is present because of the risk of osmotic demyelination in a catabolic patient. Both expansion of the effective arterial blood volume and the administration of cortisol can lead to a decrease in the circulating level of vasopressin. Therefore, we prefer to give 1-desamine-8-D-arginine vasopressin at the outset to avoid a large water diuresis. Water intake must be restricted while DDAVP acts.

Patients with chronic adrenal insufficiency should receive replacement therapy with both a glucocorticoid and a mineralocorticoid.[60] For the former, hydrocortisone 25 mg (15 mg in the morning and 10 in the afternoon) is usually given. For mineralocorticoid replacement, fludrocortisone in a single dose of 50 to 200 μg is usually used. Dose adjustments are made based on patients' symptoms, ECF volume status, blood pressure measurements, and P_K.

It is interesting to note that a lack of hyperkalemia is not uncommon because almost one third of patients with Addison's disease did not have high P_K values. Hence, this should not be an absolute diagnostic criterion.[61]

CONCLUDING REMARKS

Hyperkalemia and hypokalemia are common electrolyte disorders that may cause life-threatening cardiac arrhythmias. Therefore, our approach to therapy emphasizes first measures to deal with an emergency related to hypokalemia or hyperkalemia. In the long term, the design of appropriate therapy requires an understanding of the pathophysiology of the disorder in the individual patient because hypokalemia and hyperkalemia are not specific diagnoses, but rather findings in a heterogeneous group of disorders.

References

1. Kamel KS, Davids MR, Lin S-H, Halperin ML: Interpretation of electrolytes and acid-base parameters in blood and urine. In Brenner BM (ed): Brenner and Rector's The Kidney, vol 1, 8th ed. Philadelphia: WB Saunders, 2007, pp 749–774.
2. Halperin ML, Kamel KS: Potassium. Lancet 1998;352:135–142.
3. Clausen T, Everts ME: Regulation of the Na,K-pump in skeletal muscle. Kidney Int 1989;35:1–13.
4. Counillon LL, Pouyssegur RJ: The members of the Na+/H+ exchanger gene family: Their structure, function, expression, and regulation. In Seldin DW, Giebisch G (eds): The Kidney: Physiology & Pathophysiology, vol 1. Philadelphia: Lippincott Williams & Wilkins, 2000, pp 223–234.
5. Giebisch G, Malnic G, Berliner R: Control of renal potassium excretion. In Brenner BM (ed): Brenner and Rector's The Kidney, vol 1, 5th ed, Philadelphia: WB Saunders, 1996, pp 371–407.
6. Rossier BC: Cum grano salis: The epithelial sodium channel and the control of blood pressure. J Am Soc Nephrol 1997;8:980–992.
7. Halperin ML, Kamel KS: Dynamic interactions between integrative physiology and molecular medicine: The key to understand the mechanism of action of aldosterone in the kidney. Can J Physiol Pharmacol 2000;78:587–594.
8. Kamel KS, Quaggin S, Scheich A, Halperin ML: Disorders of potassium homeostasis: An approach based on pathophysiology. Am J Kidney Dis 1994;24:597–613.
9. Funder JW: 11β-Hydroxysteroid dehydrogenase and the meaning of life. Mol Cell Endocrinol 1990;68:C3–C5.
10. Edwards CRW: Lessons from licorice. N Engl J Med 1991;24: 1242–1243.
11. Carlisle EJF, Donnelly SM, Ethier J, et al: Modulation of the secretion of potassium by accompanying anions in humans. Kidney Int 1991;39:1206–1212.
12. Schambelan M, Sebastian A, Rector FC Jr: Mineralocorticoid-resistant renal hyperkalemia without salt wasting (type II pseudohypoaldosteronism): Role of increased renal chloride reabsorption. Kidney Int 1981;19:716–727.
13. Kahle KT, Wilson FH, Lalioti M, et al: WNK kinases: Molecular regulators of integrated epithelial ion transport. Curr Opin Nephrol Hypertens 2004;557–562.
14. Schaefer M, Link J, Hannemann L, Rudolph KH: Excessive hypokalemia and hyperkalemia following head injury. Intensive Care Med 1995;21:235–237.
15. Lin SH, Lin YF, Halperin ML: Hypokalemia and paralysis. Q J Med 2001;94:133–139.
16. Al-Alazami M, Lin S, Chih-Jen C, et al: Unusual causes of hypokalaemia and paralysis. Q J Med 2006;99:181–192.
17. Lin SH, Lin YF: Propranolol rapidly reverses paralysis, hypokalemia and hypophosphatemia in thyrotoxic periodic paralysis. Am J Kidney Dis 2001;37:620–624.
18. Lin S-H, Halperin ML: Hypokalemia: A practical approach to diagnosis and its genetic basis. Clin Med Chem 2007;14:1551–1565.
19. Pitt B, Remme W, Zannad F, et al: Eplerenone Post-Acute Myocardial Infarction Heart Failure Efficacy and Survival Study Investigators. Eplerenone, a selective aldosterone blocker, in patients with left ventricular dysfunction after myocardial infarction. N Engl J Med 2003;348:1309–1321.
20. Kamel KS, Oh MS, Halperin ML: Bartter's, Gitelman's, and Gordon's syndromes: From physiology to molecular biology and back, yet still some unanswered questions. Nephron 2002;92:18–27.
21. Vasuvattakul S, Quaggin SE, Scheich AM, et al: Kaliuretic response to aldosterone: Influence of potassium in the diet. Am J Kidney Dis 1993;21:152–160.
22. Tannen RL: Diuretic-induced hypokalemia. Kidney Int 1985;28: 988–1000.
23. Meria P, Kempf BF, Hermieu JF, et al: Laparoscopic management of primary hyperaldosteronism: Clinical experience with 212 cases. J Urol 2003;169:32–35.
24. Sawka AM, Young WF, Thompson GB, et al: Primary aldosteronism: factors associated with normalization of blood pressure after surgery. Ann Intern Med 2001;135:258–261.
25. Ghose RP, Hall PM, Bravo EL: Medical management of aldosterone-producing adenomas. Ann Intern Med 1999;131:105–108.
26. Wang WH: Regulation of renal K transport by dietary K intake. Annu Rev Physiol 2004;66:547–569.
27. Cheema-Dhadli S, Lin S-H, Chong CK, et al: Requirements for a high rate of potassium excretion in rats consuming a low electrolyte diet. J Physiol Lond 2006;572.2:493–501.
28. Kamel KS, Harvey E, Douek K, Halperin ML: Studies on the pathogenesis of hypokalemia in Gitelman's syndrome: Role of bicarbonaturia and hypomagnesemia. Am J Nephrol 1998;18:42–49.
29. Nusing RM, Seyberth HW: The role of cyclooxygenases and prostanoid receptors in furosemide-like salt losing tubulopathy: The hyperprostaglandin E syndrome. Acta Physiol Scand 2004;181: 523–528.
30. Rich GM, Ulick S, Cook S, et al: Glucocorticoid-remediable aldosteronism in a large kindred: Clinical spectrum and diagnosis using a characteristic biochemical phenotype. Ann Intern Med 1992;116:813–820.
31. Warnock DG: Liddle's syndrome: 30 years later. J Nephrol 1993;6:142–148.
32. Funder JW, Pearce PT, Smith R, Smith AI: Mineralocorticoid action: Target tissue specificity is enzyme, not receptor, mediated. Science 1998;242:583–585.
33. Blumberg A, Weidmann P, Shaw S, Gnadinger M: Effect of various therapeutic approaches on plasma potassium and major regulating factors in terminal renal failure. Am J Med 1988;85: 507–512.
34. Allon M, Copkney C: Albuterol and insulin for treatment of hyperkalemia in hemodialysis patients. Kidney Int 1990;38:869–872.
35. Allon M, Shanklin N: Effect of bicarbonate administration on plasma potassium in dialysis patients: Interactions with insulin and albuterol. Am J Kidney Dis 1996;28:508–514.
36. Lens XM, Montoliu J, Cases A, et al: Treatment of hyperkalemia in renal failure: Salbutamol v. insulin. Nephrol Dial Transplant 1989;4:228–232.
37. Conte G, Dal Canton A, Imperatore P, et al: Acute increase in plasma osmolality as a cause of hyperkalemia in patients with renal failure. Kidney Int 1990;38:301–307.
38. Montoliu J, Lens XM, Revert L: Potassium-lowering effect of albuterol for hyperkalemia in renal failure. Arch Intern Med 1987;147:713–717.
39. Liou HH, Chiang SS, Wu SC, et al: Hypokalemic effects of intravenous infusion or nebulization of salbutamol in patients with chronic renal failure. Am J Kidney Dis 1994;23:266–270.
40. Allon M, Dunlay R, Copkney C: Nebulized albuterol for acute hyperkalemia in patients on hemodialysis. Ann Intern Med 1989;110:426–429.
41. Blumberg A, Weidmann P, Ferrari P: Effect of prolonged bicarbonate administration on plasma potassium in terminal renal failure. Kidney Int 1992;41:369–374.
42. Guttierez R, Schlessinger F, Oster JR, et al: Effect of hypertonic versus isotonic sodium bicarbonate on plasma potassium concentration in patients with end-stage renal disease. Miner Electrolyte Metab 1991;17:297–302.
43. Schwarz KC, Cohen BD, Lubash GD, Rubin AL: Severe acidosis and hyperpotassemia treated with sodium bicarbonate infusion. Circulation 1959;19:215–220.

44. Kim HJ: Combined effect of bicarbonate and insulin with glucose in acute therapy of hyperkalemia in end-stage renal disease patients. Nephron 1996;72:476–482.

45. Emmett M, Hootkins RE, Fine KD: Effect of three laxatives and a cation exchange resin on fecal sodium and potassium excretion. Gastroenterology 1995;108:752–760.

46. Johnson LR: Fluid and electrolyte absorption. In Johnson LR (ed): Gastrointestinal Physiology, 5th ed. Philadelphia: Mosby-Yearbook, 1997, pp 135–145.

47. Sandle GI, Gaiger E, Tapster S, Goodsphip THJ: Evidence for large intestinal control of potassium homeostasis in uremic patients undergoing long term dialysis. Clin Sci 1987;73:247–252.

48. Martin RS, Panease S, Virginillo M, et al: Increased secretion of potassium in the rectum of man with chronic renal failure. Am J Kidney Dis 1986;8:105–110.

49. Agarwal R, Afzalpurkar R, Fordtran J: Pathophysiology of potassium absorption and secretion by the human intestine. Gastroenterology 1994;107:548–571.

50. Flinn RB, Merrill JP, Welzant WR: Treatment of the oliguric patient with a new sodium-exchange resin and sorbitol. N Engl J Med 1961;264:111–115.

51. Scherr L, Ogden DA, Mead AW: Management of hyperkalemia with a cation-exchange resin. N Engl J Med 1961;264:115–119.

52. Gruy-Kapral C, Emmett M, Santa Ana CA: Effect of single dose resin-cathartic therapy on serum potassium concentration in patients with end-stage renal disease. J Am Soc Nephrol 1998;9:1924–1930.

53. Gerstman BB, Kirkman P, Platt R: Intestinal necrosis associated with postoperative orally administered sodium polystyrene sulfonate in sorbitol. Am J Kidney Dis 1992;20:159–161.

54. Kamel KS, Lin S-H, Halperin ML: Clinical disorders of hyperkalemia. In Alpern R, Hebert SC (eds): The Kidney, vol 1. New York: Raven Press, 2008, pp 1387–1405.

55. Wilson FH, Disse-Nocodeme S, Choate KA, et al: Human hypertension caused by mutations in WNK kinases. Science 2001;293:1107–1112.

56. Kaiser UB, Ethier JH, Kamel KS, Halperin ML: Persistent hyperkalemia in a patient with diabetes mellitus: Presumptive evidence for a chloride shunt type of disorder. Clin Invest Med 1992;15:187–193.

57. Kamel K, Ethier JH, Quaggin S, et al: Studies to determine the basis for hyperkalemia in recipients of a renal transplant who are treated with cyclosporin. J Am Soc Nephrol 1992;2:1279–1284.

58. Choi MJ, Fernandez PC, Patnaik A, et al: Trimethoprim induced hyperkalemia in a patient with AIDS. N Engl J Med 1993;328:703–706.

59. Schreiber MS, Chen C-B, Lessan-Pezeshki M, et al: Antikaliuretic action of trimethoprim is minimized by raising urine pH. Kidney Int 1996;49:82–87.

60. Orth DN, Kovacs WJ: The adrenal cortex. In Wilson JD, Foster DW, Kronenberg HM, Larsen PR (eds): Williams Textbook of Endocrinology, 9th ed. Philadelphia: WB Saunders, 1998, p 550.

61. Gagnon RF, Halperin ML: Possible mechanisms to explain the absence of hyperkalemia in a patient with Addison's disease. Nephrol Dial Transplant 2001;16:1280–1284.

Further Reading

Al-Alazami M, Lin S, Chih-Jen C, et al: Unusual causes of hypokalaemia and paralysis. Q J Med 2006;99:181–192.

Kamel KS, Davids MR, Lin S-H, Halperin ML: Interpretation of electrolytes and acid-base parameters in blood and urine. In Brenner BM (ed): Brenner and Rector's The Kidney, Vol. 1, 8th ed. Philadelphia: WB Saunders, 2007, pp 749–774.

Kamel KS, Lin S-H, Halperin ML: Clinical disorders of hyperkalemia. In Alpern R, Herbert SC (eds): The Kidney, vol 1. New York, Raven Press, 2008, pp 1387–1405.

Kamel KS, Wei C: Controversial issues in treatment of hyperkalemia. Nephrol Dial Transplant 2003;18:2215–2218.

Lin SH, Lin YF, Halperin ML: Hypokalemia and paralysis. Q J Med 2001;94:133–139.

Chapter 31

Metabolic and Respiratory Acidosis

Thomas D. DuBose, Jr.

PATHOPHYSIOLOGY OF ACID-BASE DISORDERS

Definition and Fundamental Concepts

Metabolic acidosis occurs when there is increased production of endogenous acid (e.g., lactic acid and ketoacids), loss of bicarbonate (HCO_3^-) in diarrhea, or a sustained inability to generate new bicarbonate by the kidney (renal failure and renal tubular acidosis). Metabolic acidosis is recognized by the co-occurrence of acidemia (pH < 7.35) and a low serum bicarbonate concentration (total CO_2 concentration). Metabolic acidosis may also be recognized by an elevated anion gap (AG), even in the face of normal values for pH and HCO_3^- in plasma. Two broad types of metabolic acidoses are recognized by consideration of the AG: (1) high AG acidoses and (2) normal AG or hyperchloremic acidoses.[1] The AG is defined as:

$$AG = Na^+ - (Cl^- + HCO_3^-) = 10 \text{ mEq/L (range, 8–12 mEq/L)}$$

A flow diagram outlining the diagnostic approach to metabolic acidosis, in which the initial consideration is the AG, is displayed in Figure 31-1.

When there is a primary decrease in plasma $[HCO_3^-]$, an increase in alveolar ventilation and thereby a decrease in $Paco_2$ (respiratory compensation) are expected because the medullary chemoreceptors are stimulated by acidemia to invoke an increase in ventilation. The ratio of $[HCO_3^-]$ to $Paco_2$ and the subsequent pH will be returned toward, but not to, normal. This hypocapnic response to acidemia is predictable in simple acid-base disturbances and blunts the magnitude of the decline in blood pH that would occur otherwise.[1]

Respiratory and metabolic compensation can be predicted for metabolic and respiratory acid-base disturbances from the formulas in Table 31-1. The degree of respiratory compensation expected in uncomplicated or "simple" metabolic acidosis was derived empirically and can be predicted from the relationship:

$$Paco_2 = (1.5 \times HCO_3^-) + 8 \pm 2 \text{ mm Hg.}$$

The diagnostic approach to the patient with a low HCO_3^- is outlined in Figure 31-1. Thus, in a patient with metabolic acidosis and a plasma $[HCO_3^-]$ of 12 mEq/L, a $Paco_2$ between 24 and 28 mm Hg would be anticipated. Values for $Paco_2$ less than 24 or more than 28 mm Hg denote a mixed disturbance (metabolic acidosis and respiratory alkalosis, or metabolic acidosis and respiratory acidosis, respectively). Although this relationship is reliable, the $Paco_2$ can be estimated more conveniently by adding 15 to the patient's serum $[HCO_3^-]$.

Renal Response to Acidosis

The kidneys regulate plasma $[HCO_3^-]$ through three processes: (1) reabsorption of the filtered HCO_3^-; (2) excretion of titratable acidity; and (3) biochemical synthesis and excretion of NH_4^+. The sum of the last two processes represents net acid excretion (net acid excretion = titratable acidity + $NH_K^+ - HCO_3^-$). Approximately 80% to 90% of the filtered HCO_3^- is reabsorbed in the proximal tubule. Under normal conditions, the distal nephron reabsorbs the remainder of the filtered HCO_3^- (5%–10%). The quantity of acidic amino acids produced on a daily basis from metabolism and digestion of dietary protein is approximately 40 to 60 mEq. Thus, an equal amount of acid must be secreted by the collecting duct to prevent the development of chronic positive hydrogen ion balance and metabolic acidosis. NH_4^+ excretion, a major component of net acid excretion, is regulated by both NH_4^+ production and NH_4^+ transport within the kidney.[1,2]

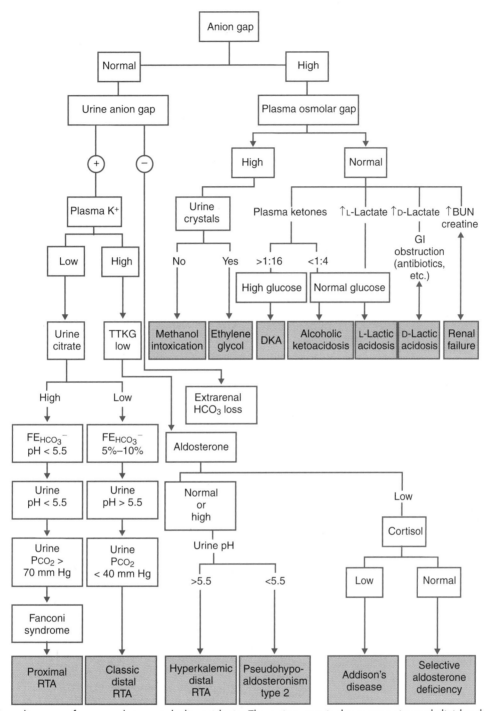

Figure 31-1 Flow diagram of approach to metabolic acidosis. The anion gap is the entry point and divides the types of metabolic acidoses into high anion gap and normal anion gap categories. Final diagnoses are displayed in shaded boxes. BUN, blood urea nitrogen; DKA, diabetic ketoacidosis; $FE_{HCO_3^-}$, fractional excretion of bicarbonate; GI, gastrointestinal; RTA, renal tubular acidosis; TTKG, transtubular potassium.

Because the filtered load of phosphate is relatively constant, the 20 to 30 mEq excreted as titratable acid daily (primarily phosphate) is fixed and not subject to the robust regulatory mechanisms governing ammoniagenesis and ammonium excretion. Therefore, for practical purposes, NH_4^+ excretion is the most sensitive index of the kidney's response to systemic acidosis.

When renal function is normal, the kidney responds to chronic metabolic acidosis by increasing NH_4^+ production and excretion; therefore, NH_4^+ production and excretion are much less than normal in the face of chronic renal failure, hyperkalemia, and renal tubular acidosis (RTA). Therefore, a normal renal response to metabolic acidosis must be distinguished from a subnormal response to determine whether the kidney is

Table 31-1 Respiratory and Metabolic Compensation

Disorder	Prediction of Compensation
Metabolic acidosis	$Paco_2 = (1.5 \times HCO_3^-) + 8$ or $Paco_2$ will ↓ 1.25 mm Hg per mmol/L ↓ in $[HCO_3^-]$ or $Paco_2 = [HCO_3^-] + 15$
Metabolic alkalosis	$Paco_2$ will ↑ 0.75 mm Hg per mmol/L ↑ in $[HCO_3^-]$ or $Paco_2$ will ↑ 6 mm Hg per 10 mmol/L ↑ in $[HCO_3^-]$ or $Paco_2 = [HCO_3^-] + 15$
Respiratory alkalosis	
Acute	$[HCO_3^-]$ will ↓ 2 mmol/L per 10 mm Hg ↓ in $Paco_2$
Chronic	$[HCO_3^-]$ will ↓ 4 mmol/L per 10 mm Hg ↓ in $Paco_2$
Respiratory acidosis	
Acute	$[HCO_3^-]$ will ↑ 1 mmol/L per 10 mm Hg ↑ in $Paco_2$
Chronic	$[HCO_3^-$ will ↑ 4 mmol/L per 10 mm Hg ↑ in $Paco_2$

responding appropriately or is responsible for the acidosis. NH_4^+ excretion can be estimated from a spot urine sample by consideration of the urine anion gap (UAG) and/or the urinary osmolal gap. The UAG, a commonly applied surrogate for the measurement of $[NH_4^+]_u$, is defined as the difference between the concentrations of chloride (Cl^-) and the sum of the urinary cations Na^+ and K^+, that is, $UAG = [Na^+ + K^+]_u - [Cl^-]_u$. In chronic metabolic acidosis of nonrenal origin (such as diarrhea), the expected response by the kidney is to increase NH_4^+ production and excretion. The increase in $[NH_4^+]$ in the urine in this condition is detected, clinically manifested as an increase in the UAG (i.e., the urinary Cl^- exceeds the sum of urinary $Na^+ + K^+$). In contrast, in hyperchloremic metabolic acidosis of renal origin (i.e., RTA), the UAG is expected to be zero or positive, denoting no increase in, or minimal, NH_4^+ in the urine, signifying an inappropriate renal response to the metabolic acidosis or a tubular defect in H^+ secretion.[2] Caution is warranted with this test because ketonuria or the presence of drug anions or toxins (such as toluene metabolites) in the urine invalidates this method.

The urinary NH_4^+ may be estimated more precisely from the measured urine osmolality (U_{osm}), urine $[Na^+ + K^+]$, and urine urea and glucose:

$$Urinary\ NH_4^+ = 0.5(U_{osm} - 2\ [Na^+ + K^+] + [blood\ urea\ nitrogen/2.8] + [glucose/18])$$

If the difference in measured and calculated osmolality were 150 mOsm/kg H_2O, the ammonium concentration would be 150×0.5 or 75 mEq/L. Values less than 20 mEq/L suggest impaired ammonium excretion.

CLINICAL EXAMPLES OF METABOLIC ACIDOSIS

Clinical Settings for Mixed Acid-Base Disorders

Mixed acid-base disorders are commonly observed in patients in critical care units and may lead to dangerous extremes of pH or, conversely, a normal pH in the face of grossly abnormal values for $Paco_2$ and HCO_3^-. Mixed acid-base disorders can be distinguished from simple (single) disturbances by prediction of the respiratory compensatory response (as explained previously), by comparison of the decrease in AG with the increase in serum HCO_3^-, or by the use of clinical nomograms.

High Anion Gap Acidosis (Anion Gap > 12 mEq/L)

There are five major causes of a high AG acidosis: (1) ketoacidoses, (2) L-lactic acidosis, (3) acute and chronic renal failure, (4) ingested drugs and toxins, and, rarely (5) gastrointestinal overproduction of organic acids (D-lactic acidosis) (Box 31-1 and Fig. 31-2).[3] Identification of the underlying cause of a high AG acidosis is facilitated by consideration of the clinical setting and associated laboratory values. Initial screening to differentiate the high AG acidoses should include the following:

1. A careful history or other evidence of drug or toxin ingestion;
2. Arterial blood gas measurement to detect coexisting respiratory alkalosis;
3. Oxalate crystals in the urine plus an osmolal gap in the patient with a high AG acidosis suggest ethylene glycol ingestion;
4. Historical evidence of diabetes mellitus (diabetic ketoacidosis);
5. Evidence of alcoholism or increased levels of β-hydroxybutyrate (alcoholic ketoacidosis);
6. Observation for clinical signs of uremia and determination of blood urea nitrogen and creatinine (uremic acidosis);

Box 31-1 Clinical Causes of High Anion Gap

Ketoacidosis
Diabetic ketoacidosis (acetoacetate)
Alcoholic ketoacidosis (β-hydroxybutyrate)
Starvation ketoacidosis

Lactic Acidosis
L-Lactic acid acidosis (types A and B)
D-Lactic acid acidosis

Toxins
Ethylene glycol
Methyl alcohol
Salicylate
Propylene glycol
Pyroglutamic acidosis

Renal Failure
Acute
Chronic

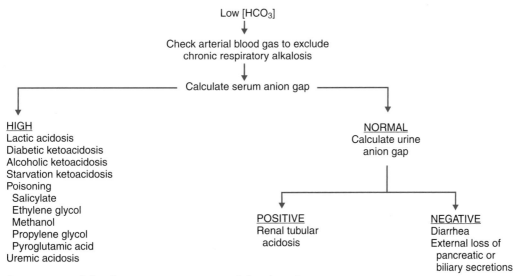

Figure 31-2 Diagnostic path for the patient presenting with low bicarbonate.

7. Recognition of the numerous settings in which L-lactate levels may be increased (hypotension, cardiac failure, drugs, leukemia, cancer);
8. Appreciation of the possibility of accumulation of D-lactate in the presence of low gastrointestinal motility, gastrointestinal obstruction, gastrointestinal pouches, antibiotic therapy, and bacterial overgrowth;

The distinguishing features of high AG acidoses are outlined in Figure 31-2.

Diabetic Ketoacidosis

Pathophysiology
Diabetic ketoacidosis is due to increased fatty acid metabolism and accumulation of acetoacetate and β-hydroxybutyrate, the consequences of insulin deficiency and relative excess of glucagon. An absence of insulin stimulates lipolysis and fatty acid release, whereas glucagon stimulates the hepatic metabolism of fatty acids to ketoacids.

Key Diagnostic Points
Diabetic ketoacidosis (most often in insulin-dependent diabetes mellitus) is seen in association with an intercurrent illness, particularly infections, which increase insulin requirements temporarily and acutely. The diagnosis is confirmed by the concurrence of a metabolic acidosis, strongly positive plasma ketones in undiluted serum, hyperglycemia, extracellular fluid (ECF) volume depletion, and Kussmaul's respiration. Although hyperchloremic acidosis may occur in patients who remain euvolemic, the majority of patients will have an AG acidosis, a consequence of buffering by bicarbonate of the H^+ from ketoacids released into the plasma.

Therapeutic Options
Therapy consists of insulin to inhibit ketoacid production and intravenous fluids for ECF volume restoration and correction of electrolyte deficits. Low-dose intravenous insulin therapy (0.1 U/kg/hr) reduces plasma glucose, smoothly corrects the ketonemia, lowers the elevated AG, and repairs the acidosis. Although regular insulin may also be administered intramus-

cularly (0.2 mg/kg initially, then 6 units every hour), it should be noted that intramuscular insulin may not be effective in volume-depleted and/or hypotensive patients, as is often the case in ketoacidosis. Most, if not all, patients with diabetic ketoacidosis require correction of the ECF volume depletion that predictably accompanies the osmotic diuresis and ketoacidosis. Initiate therapy with IV isotonic saline at a rate of 1000 mL/hr. The usual ECF deficit in adults is in the range of 3 L of isotonic saline. When the pulse and blood pressure have stabilized and the corrected serum $[Na^+]$ is 130 to 135 mEq/L, switch to 0.45% NaCl. Ringer's lactate should be avoided. If the blood sugar decreases to less than 250 to 300 mg/dL, 0.45% NaCl with 5% dextrose should be administered.[4]

Total body potassium depletion is usually present. Nevertheless, the serum potassium is usually elevated at admission, indicating that potassium replacement therapy must be individualized. Normal or decreased $[K^+]$ on admission, which is found in certain patients (e.g., where vomiting was a prominent prodromal symptom), indicates severe potassium depletion. Potassium depletion occurs as a result of osmotic diuresis, decreased dietary intake, and vomiting, which accompanies diabetic ketoacidosis. Administration of saline, insulin, and alkali will cause the potassium level to decrease further by enhancing renal K^+ excretion. Frequent monitoring (hourly) of the serum potassium is mandatory and a precise recipe is difficult to provide. Caution should be exercised in the presence of hyperkalemia, especially in the patient with renal insufficiency; withhold potassium as long as the serum level is more than 5.0 mEq/L. Nevertheless, when urine output has been established, 20 mEq KCl may be administered in each liter of intravenous fluid as long as the plasma $[K^+]$ is less than 3.8 mEq/L. Monitor and record plasma concentrations of K^+, glucose, HCO_3^-, Na^+, and Cl^- hourly.

Controversial Points
The routine administration of phosphate (usually as potassium phosphate) is not advised because of the potential for hyperphosphatemia and hypocalcemia. A significant number of patients with diabetic ketoacidosis will display hyperphosphatemia before initiation of therapy. In virtually all patients, the increased phosphate concentration on admission is followed by

a decrease in plasma phosphate levels within 2 to 6 hours after initiation of therapy. In this circumstance, phosphate should be replaced as neutral potassium phosphate (10–20 mmol per liter of intravenous fluids) unless hyperkalemia coexists, in which case neutral sodium phosphate should be used. Bicarbonate therapy is usually not necessary unless the acidosis is very severe (pH < 7.0 and Paco$_2$ is low). In general, the increase in AG above normal represents potential bicarbonate or that bicarbonate that will be realized when circulating ketones are metabolically converted to bicarbonate following primary therapy (insulin). Nevertheless, during therapy it is difficult to predict to what extent ketones will be converted back to bicarbonate before being lost in the urine when glomerular filtration rate is normalized. If exogenous bicarbonate is administered, that amount of bicarbonate will be added to that produced endogenously so that an "overshoot alkalosis" may develop. Therefore, a prudent goal is to administer small amounts of bicarbonate (50–100 mEq IV in 250 mL of 0.25% NaCl) until the pH reaches approximately 7.2 or [HCO$_3^-$] is 10 to 12 mEq/L. Because bicarbonate therapy has been associated with cerebral edema in children with diabetic ketoacidosis, it should be avoided in young children except for extreme acidemia (pH < 7.0) and then in very small amounts. Bicarbonate has never been demonstrated to improve the outcome in diabetic ketoacidosis. With exogenous bicarbonate therapy, additional potassium will be needed.[4]

Alcoholic Ketoacidosis

Pathophysiology and Diagnostic Points

This relatively common but underappreciated disorder occurs in alcoholics, particularly binge drinkers. Ketoacidosis develops when alcohol consumption is abruptly curtailed, usually as a result of vomiting or abdominal pain. In association with starvation and metabolism of ethanol (which inhibits gluconeogenesis), the glucose concentration is frequently low or normal. When ECF volume depletion is pronounced, the acidosis may be severe. The AG value is increased because of increased ketones, predominantly β-hydroxybutyrate. Mild lactic acidosis may coexist because of alteration in the redox state caused by ethanol or severe hypoxia. The nitroprusside ketone reaction (Acetest) can detect acetoacetic acid but not β-hydroxybutyrate, so the initial degree of ketosis and ketonuria may not be appreciated. Typically, insulin levels are low and levels of triglyceride, cortisol, glucagon, and growth hormone are increased, leading to ketoacidosis.

Therapeutic Options

The mainstay of therapy is intravenous normal saline to expand the ECF. Glucose is necessary if hypoglycemia is present. Insulin is obviously contraindicated, illustrating why the diagnosis of alcoholic ketoacidosis must not be mistaken for diabetic ketoacidosis. Intravenous replacement of potassium, phosphate, and magnesium deficits, as well as vitamin supplementation (thiamine 100 mg IV), are usually necessary and should be given as needed later in the course, particularly in the face of chronic alcoholism and malnutrition. Hypophosphatemia usually emerges several hours after admission, so the need for therapy can be overlooked, especially if the serum phosphate concentration on admission is normal. Profound hypophosphatemia may provoke aspiration, rhabdomyolysis, and coagulopathy. Phosphate should be replaced as either neutral sodium or potassium phosphate 10 to 20 mmol per liter of intravenous fluids, as dictated

by plasma [K$^+$]. Upper gastrointestinal hemorrhage, pancreatitis, and pneumonia may accompany alcoholic ketoacidosis.[4]

L-Lactic Acidosis

Pathophysiology

L-Lactic acidosis occurs in a diverse group of disorders that are recognized by an increase in plasma L-lactate concentration (normal venous levels < 1.8 mmol/L or 16 mg/dL). Brain, muscle, gastrointestinal tract, skin, and red cells produce lactate, whereas the liver is the major organ that participates in lactate disposal. Lactate synthesis is altered by changes in systemic pH, which control the rate of glycolysis by acting on the rate-limiting enzyme, phosphofructokinase. Acidosis decreases while alkalosis increases lactate production. The major determinants of plasma L-lactate levels include the concentration of pyruvate, the reduced nicotinamide adenine dinucleotide–to–oxidized nicotinamide adenine dinucleotide ratio, and the pH. Clinically significant L-lactic acidosis (plasma L-lactate > 4.0 mmol/L) is most often the result of tissue hypoxia; other causes include metabolic disorders, drugs, toxins, or hereditary defects. The accumulation of L-lactate may be secondary to an obvious cause of tissue hypoxia, for example, cardiac arrest, cardiogenic shock hemorrhage, sepsis, carbon monoxide poisoning, severe asthma, and severe anemia; this is called type A L-lactic acidosis. Conversely, type B L-lactic acidosis may accompany disorders in which tissue hypoperfusion or hypoxia are absent, such as diabetes mellitus, ethanol poisoning, liver failure, mitochondrial diseases, thiamine deficiency, malignancies, and drug and toxin overdose (e.g., metformin, salicylates, cocaine, fructose, cyanide, nonnucleoside reverse transcriptase inhibitors, nitroprusside). Lactic acidosis in combination with respiratory alkalosis can be observed early in the development of septic shock and may be one of the few harbingers of this entity.[5]

Treatment

The basic principle of therapy is that the underlying condition initiating the disruption in normal L-lactate metabolism must first be corrected. Every attempt should be made to restore tissue perfusion. Vasoconstricting agents should be administered only when absolutely necessary and at the lowest feasible dose because they potentiate the hypoperfused state. Alkali therapy is generally recommended for acute severe acidemia (pH < 7.15) to improve cardiac function and lactate utilization. However, the use of bicarbonate therapy is of only marginal value. Excess bicarbonate may depress cardiac performance and can even exacerbate the acidemia through increased phosphofructokinase activity. Thus, attempts to normalize the pH or [HCO$_3^-$] by exogenous bicarbonate therapy is deleterious.[5] One approach is to provide, by slow infusion over 30- to 40-minute intervals, sufficient bicarbonate to increase the arterial pH to no more than 7.2, that is, correct [HCO$_3^-$] to 8 mEq/L. Despite initial enthusiasm for the use of dichloroacetate, a beneficial effect has not been substantiated. Similarly, no benefit is derived from administration of THAM (tromethamine). Thiamine should also be administered (50–100 mg) in patients with chronic malnutrition or alcoholism.

Fluid overload occurs with excessive bicarbonate therapy because the amount required is often massive when production of lactic acid is relentless. This complication may require slow continuous ultrafiltration, continuous venovenous hemodialysis, or acute intermittent hemodialysis. There is no evidence from controlled studies that would support one form of renal replacement therapy over the others. Theoretically, all three should correct volume overload, remove lactate, and add bicarbonate. It has been the author's experience that continuous renal replacement therapy is more successful in controlling these parameters but offers no documentable improvement in overall mortality. Lactate-containing dialysate should be avoided, which obviates the use of typical peritoneal dialysis solutions. Unabated severe L-lactic acidosis in patients receiving large amounts of bicarbonate carries a very high mortality. If the underlying cause of the L-lactic acidosis can be corrected, the blood lactate will be reconverted to bicarbonate. Bicarbonate derived from lactate conversion in addition to any new bicarbonate generated by renal mechanisms during acidosis and from exogenous alkali therapy are additive and may result in an "overshoot" alkalosis.

D-Lactic Acidosis

Pathophysiology

D-Lactate, which is not an endogenous metabolite in vertebrates, is produced by bacterial overgrowth in the gastrointestinal tract in association with jejunoileal bypass, intestinal obstruction, antibiotic therapy, or decreased gastrointestinal motility. The diagnosis of D-lactic acidosis requires measurement of D-lactate levels specifically because it is not measured as L-lactate. The acid-base disturbance may consist of both an increased AG and hyperchloremia.[6]

Treatment

Because the potential danger in D-lactic acidosis is from accumulation of toxic products and not the acidosis, initial therapy should include (1) cessation of feeding, (2) eradication of bacterial overgrowth by administration of appropriate oral antibiotics (metronidazole or neomycin) or intravenous vancomycin, and (3) enhanced gastrointestinal motility. Longer term therapy may necessitate reversal of intestinal bypass if stasis and bacterial overgrowth persist or are recurrent.

Drug-Induced Acidosis

Salicylates

Aspirin overdose usually gives rise to a complex acid-base disturbance, in which respiratory alkalosis predominates (due to stimulation of respiration by salicylates) and a high AG may occur concomitantly. Only a portion of the increased AG can be attributed to the increased plasma salicylate concentration, for example, a toxic salicylate level of 100 mg/dL can only account for an increase in AG of 7 mEq/L. Lactic acid production is also often increased, partly as a direct effect of the drug and partly as a result of the decrease in P_{CO_2} induced by salicylate.[3,4]

Treatment

The initial step in therapy should include vigorous gastric lavage followed by activated charcoal administration via a nasogastric tube. The mainstay of therapy is an alkaline diuresis to allow the relatively impermeant anionic form of salicylate to be trapped in tubular fluid and excreted in the urine. To facilitate removal of salicylate, intravenous sodium bicarbonate in amounts adequate to alkalinize the urine and maintain urine output is necessary (urine pH $>$ 7.5). An alkaline diuresis may be induced by infusion of half-isotonic saline plus two ampoules of sodium bicarbonate (7.5% = 44.6 mEq or 8.4% = 50 mEq). Although this form of therapy is straightforward in acidotic patients, alkalemia from respiratory alkalosis

may make this approach hazardous. Arterial pH should be monitored and not allowed to increase to more than 7.55. Acetazolamide in small doses (250 mg) is recommended only when an alkaline diuresis cannot be achieved or when the pH exceeds 7.55 because larger doses may result in systemic metabolic acidosis if sodium bicarbonate is not given concomitantly. Moreover, acetazolamide and salicylates compete for binding sites on albumin. Coexisting metabolic acidosis greatly impedes salicylate clearance and enhances salicylate entry into the central nervous system and must be avoided. Hypokalemia may occur as a result of alkaline diuresis from either sodium bicarbonate or acetazolamide and should be treated promptly. If renal failure prevents rapid clearance of salicylate or if salicylate levels remain in the toxic range ($>$40–50 mg/dL), hemodialysis against a bicarbonate dialysate (35 mEq/L) should be performed.

Toxin-Induced Acidosis: Ethylene Glycol and Methyl Alcohol and the Osmolal Gap

Pathophysiology

Plasma osmolality (mOsm/kg H_2O) is calculated according to the following expression:

$$P_{osm} = 2Na^+ + glucose/18 + blood\ urea\ nitrogen/2.8,$$

where blood urea nitrogen and glucose are expressed in milligrams per deciliter. The calculated and determined osmolality should agree to within 10 to 15 mOsm/kg. When the measured osmolality exceeds the calculated osmolality by more than 15 to 20 mOsm/kg, one of two circumstances prevails: (1) the serum sodium may be spuriously low, as occurs with hyperlipidemia or hyperproteinemia (pseudohyponatremia), or (2) osmolytes other than sodium salts, glucose, or urea have accumulated in plasma. Examples include the accumulation of solutes that can increase plasma osmolality, such as the alcohols ethylene glycol and methyl alcohol. Less commonly, mannitol or retained radiocontrast agents increase the osmolal gap. In these examples, the difference between the calculated osmolality and the measured osmolality is proportional to the concentration of the unmeasured solute (osmolal gap). With an appropriate clinical history and index of suspicion, the osmolal gap becomes a very helpful screening tool in poison-associated AG acidosis.[4]

Ethylene Glycol

Diagnostic Points Ingestion of ethylene glycol (commonly used in antifreeze) leads to a metabolic acidosis and severe damage to the central nervous system, heart, lungs, and kidneys. Ethylene glycol (molecular mass 62 d) increases the osmolal gap ($>$10 mOsm/kg H_2O). The increased AG and osmolal gap are attributable to ethylene glycol and its metabolites oxalic acid, glycolic acid, and other organic acids. Lactic acid production increases secondary to inhibition of the tricarboxylic acid cycle and altered intracellular redox state. Diagnosis is facilitated by recognizing oxalate crystals in the urine, the presence of an osmolal gap in serum, and a high AG acidosis. Ethylene glycol ingested as antifreeze may be detected in the urine sample by use of Wood's light. Treatment should not be delayed while awaiting measurement of ethylene glycol levels in this setting. Propylene glycol, used as a vehicle for certain intravenous medications (e.g., lorazepam) has been associated with toxin-induced metabolic acidosis. Pyroglutamic acidosis has also been observed in critically ill patients receiving acetaminophen.[4]

Treatment

The principles of treatment of ethylene glycol intoxication (and propylene glycol intoxication) are to stop production of toxic metabolites by competitive inhibition of alcohol dehydrogenase using intravenous administration of fomepizole or ethanol, coupled with removal of the accumulated toxins. Immediate therapy is necessary to prevent irreversible central nervous system and renal toxicity. Ethanol (20% solution) 0.6 g/kg IV is given over 30 to 45 minutes followed by a maintenance infusion of 5% ethanol 110 mg/kg/hr to produce a serum ethanol level of 100 to 150 mg/dL. A saline or osmotic diuresis should be initiated and the patient given thiamine and pyridoxine supplements, fomepizole or ethanol, and hemodialysis. During dialysis, it is necessary to increase the rate of ethanol infusion. The intravenous administration of the alcohol dehydrogenase inhibitor fomepizole (4-methylpyrazole) (7 mg/kg as a loading dose) or ethanol serves to lessen toxicity because they compete with ethylene glycol for metabolism by alcohol dehydrogenase. Fomepizole, although expensive, offers the advantage of a predictable decrease in ethylene glycol levels without the adverse effects, such as excessive obtundation, associated with ethanol infusion.

Methyl Alcohol

Ingestion of methyl alcohol, as wood alcohol or paint thinners, causes metabolic acidosis and severe optic nerve and central nervous system manifestations when methyl alcohol is metabolized to formaldehyde and formic acid. Lactic acid, ketoacids, and other unidentified organic acids may contribute to the acidosis.[4]

Diagnostic Points Nausea, vomiting, and abdominal pain are usually present. Lactic acids and ketoacids as well as other unidentified organic acids may contribute to the high AG. Because of its high retention and low molecular mass (32 d), an osmolal gap is usually present.

Treatment The treatment of methyl alcohol intoxication is generally similar to that for ethylene glycol intoxication, including ethanol or fomepizole administration, general supportive measures, volume expansion, and hemodialysis. Initiation of a saline diuresis is less of an issue with methyl alcohol than with ethylene glycol intoxication because renal toxicity is not a direct effect of methyl alcohol intoxication and crystals are not present in the urine.[4]

Acute and Chronic Renal Failure

Pathophysiology

Progressive renal insufficiency will eventually convert the hyperchloremic acidosis of moderate renal insufficiency to the typical high AG acidosis of advanced renal failure. Low glomerular filtration, continued reabsorption of organic anions, and low NH_4^+ excretion all contribute to the pathogenesis of this metabolic disturbance. As functional renal mass is compromised in the relentless progression of renal disease, the number of functioning nephrons eventually becomes insufficient to maintain NH_4^+ excretion to the extent necessary to balance net acid production. Thus, $[HCO_3^-]$ declines but rarely decreases to less than 15 mEq/L, and the AG rarely is more than 20 mEq/L. The acid retained in patients with chronic renal disease is buffered in part by alkaline salts derived from bone, resulting in

loss of bone calcium carbonate that contributes to the skeletal demineralization seen with renal acidosis. In addition, chronic acidosis increases urinary calcium excretion to a level proportional to the degree of cumulative acid retention and is corrected with repair of the acidosis.[7]

Treatment

Both uremic acidosis and hyperchloremic acidosis of renal insufficiency require oral alkali replacement to maintain $[HCO_3^-]$ between 20 and 24 mEq/L. This can usually be accomplished with relatively modest amounts of alkali (1–1.5 mEq/kg/day). Sodium citrate (Shohl's Solution or Bicitra) has been shown to enhance the absorption of aluminum from the gastrointestinal tract and should never be administered to patients receiving aluminum-containing antacids because of the risk of aluminum intoxication. If hyperkalemia persists, furosemide (60–80 mg/day) should be added.

Hyperchloremic Metabolic Acidosis (Normal Anion Gap Acidosis)

Pathogenesis and Differential Diagnosis

Alkali may be lost from the gastrointestinal tract (diarrhea) or from the kidneys (RTA). In these disorders (Box 31-2), reciprocal changes in chloride and bicarbonate result in a normal AG. In a pure form of simple hyperchloremic acidosis, therefore, the increase in chloride above the normal value equals approximately the decrease in bicarbonate. The absence of such a relationship suggests a mixed disturbance. Diarrhea results in the loss of large quantities of HCO_3^- and further HCO_3^- depletion occurs by its reaction with organic acids. Instead of an acid urine pH, as often anticipated with diarrhea, a pH of 6.0 is usually observed because metabolic acidosis and hypokalemia increase renal NH_4^+ synthesis and excretion, thus providing more urinary buffer, which increases urine pH. Metabolic acidosis due to gastrointestinal losses with a high urine pH can be differentiated from RTA because urinary NH_4^+ excretion is low in RTA and high in patients with diarrhea. Urinary NH_4^+ levels can be estimated by calculating the UAG or the urine osmolal gap (see previously). With extrarenal bicarbonate loss, $[Cl^-]$ in urine exceeds $[Na^+ + K^+]$ in urine. If urine $[Na^+ + K^+]$ exceeds $[Cl^-]$, urine $[NH_4^+]$ is low, a finding compatible with RTA. The distinguishing features of hyperchloremic acidoses are outlined in Table 31-2.[2]

Hyperchloremic Acidosis of Chronic Renal Failure

Pathophysiology

Loss of functioning renal parenchyma due to progressive renal failure is commonly associated with metabolic acidosis, which is typically hyperchloremic when the glomerular filtration rate is 20 to 50 mL/min but may convert to the classic high AG acidosis of uremia with more advanced renal failure, that is, when the glomerular filtration rate is less than 15 mL/min. The major defect in acidification with advanced renal failure is that ammoniagenesis is reduced in proportion to the loss of functional renal mass. In addition, medullary NH_4^+ accumulation and trapping in the medullary collecting duct are impaired. Because of adaptive increases in K^+ secretion by the collecting duct and colon, the acidosis of chronic renal insufficiency is typically normokalemic.[6]

Box 31-2   Differential Diagnosis of Hyperchloremic Metabolic Acidosis

Gastrointestinal Bicarbonate Loss
Diarrhea
External pancreatic or small bowel drainage
Uterosigmoidostomy, jejunal loop
Drugs
Calcium chloride (acidifying agent)
Magnesium sulfate (diarrhea)
Cholestyramine (bile acid diarrhea)

Renal Acidosis
Hypokalemia
  Proximal RTA (type 2)
  Distal (classic) RTA (type 1)
Hyperkalemia
  Generalized distal nephron dysfunction (type 4 RTA)
  Mineralocorticoid deficiency
  Mineralocorticoid resistance (PHA I autosomal dominant)
  Voltage defects (PHA I autosomal recessive)
  PHA II
    ↓ Na^+ delivery to distal nephron
  Tubulointerstitial disease

Drug-induced hyperkalemia
  Potassium-sparing diuretics (amiloride, triamterene, spirono-lactone)
  Trimethoprim
  Pentamidine
  ACE inhibitors and ARBs
  NSAIDs
  Cyclosporine, tacrolimus
Normokalemia
  Early renal insufficiency

Other
Acid loads (ammonium chloride, hyperalimentation)
Loss of potential bicarbonate: ketosis with ketone excretion
Dilution acidosis (rapid saline administration)
Hippurate
Cation exchange resins

ACE, angiotensin-converting enzyme; ARBs, angiotensin II receptor blockers; NSAIDs, nonsteroidal anti-inflammatory drugs; PHA, pseudohypoaldosteronism; RTA, renal tubular acidosis.

Table 31-2   Distinguishing Features of Hyperchloremic Acidoses

	Proximal RTA (Type 2 RTA)	Classic Distal RTA (Type 1 RTA)	Generalized Distal Defect (Type 4 RTA)	Extrarenal Bicarbonate Loss
Anion gap	Normal	Normal	Normal	Normal
Plasma [K^+]	Low (with therapy)	Low	High	Low
Urine osmolal gap or urine anion gap	Low (positive)	Low (positive)	Very low (positive)	High (negative)
Urine pH	Low	High	Low or high	Low or high
Urine P_{CO_2} (mm Hg)	>70	<40	<40	>70
$FE_{HCO_3}^-$	>15% (with therapy)	5%–10%	10%–15%	<5%
Urine citrate	High	Low	Low	Normal
TTKG	High	High	Low	Low
Treatment	K-Shohls or $KHCO_3$ and thiazide	Shohls or $NaHCO_3$ Tabs	Low K^+ diet; Avoid K^+-retaining drugs; Furosemide; $NaHCO_3$; Treat underlying CKD	$NaHCO_3$

$FE_{HCO_3}^-$, fractional excretion of bicarbonate; RTA, renal tubular acidosis; TTKG, transtubular potassium gradient.

Renal Tubular Acidosis

Proximal Renal Tubular Acidosis
Diagnostic Points   The majority of cases of proximal RTA fit into the category of generalized proximal tubular dysfunction with glycosuria, generalized aminoaciduria, hypercitraturia, and phosphaturia. The generalized failure of proximal tubular function is referred to as Fanconi syndrome. The diagnosis is confirmed by demonstrating an inappropriately high rate of bicarbonate excretion in the face of a slow or normal plasma bicarbonate (>10%–15%). Causes of acquired proximal RTA include the dysproteinemias, heavy metal intoxication, vitamin D deficiency or resistance, cancer chemotherapeutic drugs (such as ifosfamide), and

genetically transmitted systemic diseases (Wilson's disease, hereditary fructose intolerance).[2]

Treatment The treatment of proximal RTA is directed toward amelioration of, or improvement in, the fluid, electrolyte, and acid-base abnormalities. In patients with proximal RTA, large amounts of exogenous bicarbonate are required to correct the $[HCO_3^-]$ to normal. Moreover, because bicarbonate absorption in the proximal tubule is impaired, the increase in distal bicarbonate delivery results in enhanced renal potassium wasting and hypokalemia. Therefore, large alkali loads are not advised; rather, smaller amounts of alkali therapy may be provided as Shohl's Solution (one to two tablespoons three times daily) or sodium bicarbonate tablets (650 mg, one to two tablets three times daily or 5–10 mEq/kg/day). If there is a compelling necessity to correct the plasma bicarbonate (growing children with proximal RTA), hydrochlorothiazide may be added to enhance proximal bicarbonate absorption. Most children and some adults will require potassium supplementation (K-Shohl's Solution or Polycitra, or -Lyte), particularly if larger doses of alkali are provided.

Classic Distal Renal Tubular Acidosis

Pathophysiology and Diagnostic Points The typical findings in classic distal RTA include hypokalemia, hyperchloremic acidosis, an abnormally low excretion of urinary NH_4^+ (positive UAG or low urinary osmolal gap), and, in contradistinction to proximal RTA, an inappropriately high urine pH in the face of systemic metabolic acidosis. Recently, the genetic bases of inherited forms of classic distal RTA have been elucidated. A number of patients in families with autosomal recessive distal RTA have been shown to have point mutations in the gene that encodes the basolateral HCO_3^-/Cl^- exchanger (or band 3 protein) in A-type intercalated cells of the collecting duct. Other families with inherited sensorineural deafness and classic distal RTA have been shown to have defects in the H^+-ATPase (Box 31-3). Finally, an inherited form not associated with hearing impairment has been associated with an abnormality of a unique subunit of the H^+-ATPase. Under a number of different circumstances, including acute acid infusion, patients with classic hypokalemic distal RTA are unable to acidify their urine to a pH less than 5.5. Most patients with acquired distal RTA and many with inherited forms of distal RTA (except those with the HCO_3^-/Cl^- exchanger defect)

Box 31-3 Disorders with Dysfunction of Renal Acidification—Selective Defect in Net Acid Excretion: Classic Distal Renal Tubular Acidosis

Primary
Familial
  1. Autosomal dominant
    a. *AE1* gene
  2. Autosomal recessive
    a. With deafness (rd RTA1 or *ATP6B1* gene)
    b. Without deafness (rd RTA2 or *ATP6N1B*)
Sporadic

Endemic
Northeastern Thailand

Secondary to Systemic Disorders
Autoimmune Diseases
Hyperglobulinemic purpura
Cryoglobulinemia
Sjögren's syndrome
Thyroiditis
Human immunodeficiency virus nephropathy
Fibrosing alveolitis
Chronic active hepatitis
Primary biliary cirrhosis
Polyarteritis nodosa

Hypercalciuria and Nephrocalcinosis
Primary hyperparathyroidism
Hyperthyroidism
Medullary sponge kidney
Fabry's disease
X-linked hypophosphatemia
Vitamin D intoxication
Idiopathic hypercalciuria
Wilson's disease
Hereditary fructose intolerance

Drug- and Toxin-Induced Disease
Amphotericin B
Cyclamate
Hepatic cirrhosis
Ifosfamide
Foscarnet
Toluene
Mercury
Vanadate lithium
Classic analgesic nephropathy

Tubulointerstitial Diseases
Balkan nephropathy
Chronic pyelonephritis
Obstructive uropathy
Vesicoureteral reflux
Kidney transplantation
Leprosy
Jejunoileal bypass with hyperoxaluria

Associated with Genetically Transmitted Diseases
Ehlers-Danlos syndrome
Sickle cell anemia
Medullary cystic disease
Hereditary sensorineural deafness
Osteopetrosis with carbonic anhydrase II deficiency
Hereditary elliptocytosis
Marfan syndrome
Jejunal bypass with hyperoxaluria
Carnitine palmitoyltransferase

uniformly display a lower urinary PCO_2 than normal subjects. These abnormalities suggest that one or both of the transporters in the collecting duct involved in bicarbonate absorption (H^+-ATPase or H^+/K^+-ATPase) are defective. In contrast, patients with the inherited HCO_3^-/Cl^- exchanger abnormality have been reported to have higher than normal urinary PCO_2. This finding suggests that the HCO_3^-/Cl^- exchanger may be mistargeted to the apical membrane in these patients. With the exception of the gradient lesion (insertion of a leak pathway) that accompanies amphotericin B intoxication, most patients with distal RTA studied with dynamic tests of urinary acidification, such as urinary PCO_2, have been shown to have a defect in H^+ secretion or a pump defect rather than the "gradient" or "leak" defect as proposed initially.[2]

Hypokalemia and hypercalciuria often accompany this disorder, but proximal tubule reabsorptive function is preserved. Thus, hypocitraturia is common, and the combination of hypercalciuria and hypocitraturia enhance urinary stone formation and nephrocalcinosis. Nephrocalcinosis is a marker of classic distal RTA because it does not occur with proximal RTA or the generalized dysfunction of the nephron associated with hyperkalemia. Nephrocalcinosis aggravates further the decrease in net acid excretion by impairing the transfer of NH_4^+ from Henle's loop to the collecting duct.

Most patients with distal RTA have distal RTA in association with a systemic illness, which is referred to as secondary distal RTA.

Treatment Correction of chronic metabolic acidosis can usually be achieved in patients with classic distal RTA by administration of alkali in an amount sufficient to neutralize the production of metabolic acids derived from the diet. In adult patients with distal RTA, this is usually equal to no more than 1 mEq/kg/day or 10 to 30 mL with water after meals and at bedtime, as Shohl's Solution or sodium bicarbonate tablets. Preparations include (1) Shohl's Solution (Bictra) (sodium citrate 500 mg and citric acid 334 mg/5 mL) and (2) sodium bicarbonate tablets (325 and 650 mg contain 3.8 and 7.6 mEq, respectively). In patients with distal RTA, correction of acidosis with alkali therapy reduces urinary potassium excretion, and hypokalemia and sodium depletion may resolve without additional therapy. Frank wasting of potassium may occur in a minority of patients in association with secondary hyperaldosteronism despite correction of the acidosis by the alkali therapy. A major benefit of correction of the acidosis is that the renal failure should not progress, especially when nephrocalcinosis accompanies distal RTA. The frequency of nephrolithiasis, when present, is usually markedly reduced by alkali therapy.[2]

Generalized Distal Nephron Dysfunction (Type 4 Renal Tubular Acidosis)

Pathophysiology and Diagnostic Points Although hyperchloremic metabolic acidosis and hyperkalemia occur with regularity in advanced renal insufficiency, patients with type 4 RTA have hyperkalemia that is disproportionate to the decrease in the glomerular filtration rate. In such patients, a generalized dysfunction of potassium and acid secretion by the collecting tubule is present. In this group of disorders, urinary NH_4^+ excretion is depressed and renal function often compromised at the time of diagnosis. Patients with renal insufficiency and hyperkalemia (>5.0 mEq/L) have hyperkalemia that is disproportionate to the decrease in the glomerular filtration rate. The causes of type 4 RTA are listed in Box 31-4.

The transtubular potassium gradient = $(U_K/P_K)/(U/P)_{osm}$, where U represents urine values and P represents plasma values. The transtubular potassium gradient is abnormally low in patients with this disorder, indicating that the collecting tubule is not responding appropriately to the prevailing hyperkalemia. Impaired NH_4^+ production and excretion, in part due to hyperkalemia, leads to impaired net acid excretion and systemic metabolic acidosis. This form of generalized distal tubule dysfunction with hyperkalemia is acquired with diabetic nephropathy, obstructive uropathy, sickle cell nephropathy, tubulointerstitial diseases, and transplant rejection (see Box 31-4).[2]

A number of patients have been reported with hyperkalemia, hyperchloremic metabolic acidosis, hypertension, undetectable plasma renin activity, and low aldosterone levels (type 2 pseudohypoaldosteronism). These patients generally have not exhibited glomerular or tubulointerstitial disease. The acidosis in such patients is mild and can be accounted for by the magnitude of hyperkalemia. Renal potassium secretion is resistant to mineralocorticoid administration. Renin and aldosterone levels both increase if volume expansion is corrected by diuretics or salt restriction. This autosomal dominant disorder is the result of an increase in expression and function of the sodium chloride cotransporter (NCCT) in the distal convoluted tubule. Specifically, the interacting proteins WNK1 and WNK4 normally responsible for regulating apical membrane localization of NCCT are defective. The hyperkalemia that follows depresses, in turn, NH_4^+ production and excretion and may result in hyperchloremic metabolic acidosis, especially in the face of even mild renal insufficiency. The result of this defect is constitutive activation of NCCT causing volume expansion, shunting of voltage, and a decrease in delivery of Na^+ and Cl^- to the cortical collecting tubule, causing decreased $K+$ secretion.

In addition to this specific genetic abnormality, voltage defects may be acquired. For example, impaired operation of the sodium channel can also occur as a result of drugs that interfere with sodium channel function such as amiloride, triamterene, pentamidine, and trimethoprim, as a result of conditions that alter sodium absorption indirectly such as aldosterone resistance, or as a result of cyclosporine or tacrolimus administration. Nonsteroidal anti-inflammatory drugs and the angiotensin-converting enzyme inhibitors may also produce hyperkalemia and metabolic acidosis, particularly in patients with preexisting renal insufficiency or volume depletion or in the elderly. Therefore, drugs should always be considered as a possible cause of hyperkalemia and metabolic acidosis in such patients.[2]

Treatment A decrease in serum potassium enhances renal ammoniagenesis and NH_4^+ excretion, increasing net acid excretion and thus improving or correcting the metabolic acidosis. Treatment of patients with mild chronic hyperkalemia and metabolic acidosis with chronic renal insufficiency is not always necessary, and the decision to treat is often based on the severity of the hyperkalemia and acidosis, when present. Patients with combined glucocorticoid and mineralocorticoid deficiency should receive both adrenal steroids in replacement doses. Patients with hyporeninemic hypoaldosteronism may respond to a cation-exchange resin (sodium polystyrene sulfonate 15 g orally once daily *without sorbitol*), alkali therapy (Shohl's Solution, one to two tablespoons twice daily), or a loop diuretic (furosemide 40–80 mg/day) to induce renal potassium and salt excretion. Mineralocorticoid replacement

Box 31-4   Disorders with Dysfunction of Renal Acidification: Generalized Abnormality of Distal Nephron with Hyperkalemia

Mineralocorticoid Deficiency

Primary Mineralocorticoid Deficiency

Combined deficiency of aldosterone, desoxycorticosterone, and cortisol
  Addison's disease
  Bilateral adrenalectomy
  Bilateral adrenal destruction
  Hemorrhage or carcinoma
Congenital enzymatic defects
  21-Hydroxylase deficiency
  3β-Hydroxydehydrogenase deficiency
  Desmolase deficiency
Isolated (selective) aldosterone deficiency
  Chronic idiopathic hypoaldosteronism
  Heparin (low molecular weight or unfractionated) in critically ill patient
  Familial hypoaldosteronism
  Coricosterone methyloxidase deficiency, types 1 and 2
  Primary zona glomerulosa defect
  Transient hypoaldosteronism of infancy
  Persistent hypotension and/or hypoxemia in critically ill patient
Angiotensin II–converting enzyme inhibition
  Endogenous
  Angiotensin-converting enzyme inhibitors and angiotensin I receptor antagonists

Secondary Mineralocorticoid Deficiency

Hyporeninemic hypoaldosteronism
  Diabetic nephropathy

Tubulointerstitial nephropathies
Nephrosclerosis
Nonsteroidal anti-inflammatory drugs
Acquired immunodeficiency syndrome
IgM monoclonal gammopathy

Mineralocorticoid Resistance

PHA I, autosmal dominant (hMR defect)

Renal Tubular Dysfunction (Voltage Defect)

PHA I, autosomal recessive
PHA II, autosomal dominant
Drugs that interfere with Na^+ channel function in CCTs
  Amiloride
  Triamterene
  Trimethoprim
  Pentamidine
Drugs that interfere with Na^+/K^+-ATPase in CCTs
  Cyclosporine, tacrolimus
Drugs that inhibit aldosterone effect on CCTs
  Spironolactone
Disorders associated with tubulointerstitial nephritis and renal insufficiency
  Lupus nephritis
  Methicillin nephrotoxicity
  Obstructive nephropathy
  Kidney transplant rejection
  Sickle cell disease
  Williams syndrome with uric acid nephrolithiasis

CCTs, cortical collecting tubules; PHA, pseudohypoaldosteronism

---

with 9α-fludrocortisone (0.1–0.3 mg/day) can theoretically improve net acid excretion. However, mineralocorticoid administration is contraindicated in the face of coexisting hypertension or congestive heart failure. Volume depletion should be avoided unless the patient is volume overexpanded or hypertensive. Pseudohypoaldosteronism in children (type I) should be treated with avid dietary sodium chloride intake, whereas pseudohypoaldosteronism in adults (type II) responds to thiazide diuretics and dietary salt restriction. Because bicarbonate is not avidly absorbed in the distal nephron, administration of bicarbonate in sufficient quantity to induce bicarbonaturia may reverse the voltage defect induced by amiloride, pentamidine, or trimethoprim by enhancing K^+ and H^+ secretion by the collecting duct.[2]

RESPIRATORY ACIDOSIS

Diagnostic Points

Respiratory acidosis can be due to severe pulmonary disease, respiratory muscle fatigue, or abnormalities in ventilatory control and is recognized by an increase in $Paco_2$ and a decrease in pH (Box 31-5). In acute respiratory acidosis, there is an immediate compensatory increase (due to cellular buffering mechanisms) in $[HCO_3^-]$, which increases by 1 mmol/L for every

10-mm Hg increase in $Paco_2$. In chronic respiratory acidosis (>24 hours), renal adaptation increases the $[HCO_3^-]$ by 4 mmol/L for every 10-mm Hg increase in $Paco_2$. The serum $[HCO_3^-]$ usually does not increase to more than 38 mmol/L.[4,8]

The clinical features vary according to the severity and duration of the respiratory acidosis, the underlying disease, and whether there is accompanying hypoxemia. A rapid increase in $Paco_2$ may cause anxiety, dyspnea, confusion, psychosis, and hallucinations and may progress to coma. Lesser degrees of dysfunction in chronic hypercapnia include sleep disturbances, loss of memory, daytime somnolence, personality changes, impairment of coordination, and motor disturbances such as tremor, myoclonic jerks, and asterixis. Headaches and other signs that mimic increased intracranial pressure, such as papilledema, abnormal reflexes, and focal muscle weakness, are due to vasoconstriction secondary to loss of the vasodilator effects of CO_2.

Depression of the respiratory center by a variety of drugs, injury, or disease can produce respiratory acidosis. This may occur acutely with general anesthetics, sedatives, and head trauma or chronically with sedatives, alcohol, intracranial tumors, and the syndromes of sleep-disordered breathing (e.g., primary alveolar and obesity hypoventilation syndromes). Abnormalities or disease in the motor neurons, neuromuscular junction, and skeletal muscle can cause hypoventilation via respiratory muscle fatigue. Mechanical ventilation, when not

Box 31-5   Respiratory Acidosis

Central
Drugs (anesthetics, morphine, sedatives)
Stroke
Infection

Airway
Obstruction
Asthma

Parenchyma
Emphysema/chronic obstructive pulmonary disease
Pneumoconiosis
Bronchitis
Adult respiratory distress syndrome
Barotrauma

Mechanical Ventilation
Hypoventilation
Permissive hypercapnia

Neuromuscular
Poliomyelitis
Kyphoscoliosis
Myasthenia
Muscular dystrophies
Multiple sclerosis

Miscellaneous
Obesity
Hypoventilation

properly adjusted or supervised, may result in respiratory acidosis, particularly if CO_2 production suddenly increases (because of fever, agitation, sepsis, or overfeeding) or alveolar ventilation decreases because of worsening pulmonary function. High levels of positive end-expiratory pressure in the presence of reduced cardiac output may cause hypercapnia as a result of large increases in alveolar dead space. Permissive hypercapnia is used to decrease barotrauma compared with conventional mechanical ventilation. It seems prudent to keep the pH in the range of 7.2 to 7.3 by administration of sodium bicarbonate.[4,8]

Acute hypercapnia follows sudden occlusion of the upper airway or generalized bronchospasm as in severe asthma, anaphylaxis, inhalational burn, or toxin injury. Chronic hypercapnia and respiratory acidosis occur in end-stage obstructive lung disease. Restrictive disorders involving both the chest wall and the lungs can cause respiratory acidosis because the high metabolic cost of respiration causes ventilatory muscle fatigue. Advanced stages of intrapulmonary and extrapulmonary restrictive defects present as chronic respiratory acidosis.

The diagnosis of respiratory acidosis requires the measurement of $Paco_2$ and arterial pH. A detailed history and physical examination often indicate the cause.

Treatment

The management of respiratory acidosis depends on its severity and rate of onset. Acute respiratory acidosis can be life threatening, and measures to reverse the underlying cause should be undertaken simultaneously with restoration of adequate alveolar ventilation. This may necessitate tracheal intubation and assisted mechanical ventilation. Oxygen administration should be titrated carefully in patients with severe obstructive pulmonary disease and chronic CO_2 retention who are breathing spontaneously. When oxygen is used injudiciously, these patients may experience progression of the respiratory acidosis. Aggressive and rapid correction of hypercapnia should be avoided because the decreasing $Paco_2$ may provoke the same complications noted with acute respiratory alkalosis (i.e., cardiac arrhythmias, reduced cerebral perfusion, and seizures). The $Paco_2$ should be lowered gradually in chronic respiratory acidosis, aiming to restore the $Paco_2$ to baseline levels and to provide sufficient Cl^- and K^+ to enhance the renal excretion of HCO_3^-.

Chronic respiratory acidosis is frequently difficult to correct, but measures aimed at improving lung function such as cessation of smoking, use of oxygen, bronchodilators, glucocorticoids, diuretics, and physiotherapy can help some patients and forestall further deterioration in most. The use of respiratory stimulants may be useful in selected patients, particularly if hypercapnia is out of proportion to the abnormality in lung function.

References

1. Alpern RJ, Hamm LL: Urinary acidification. In DuBose TD, Hamm LL (eds): Acid-Base and Electrolyte Disorders: A Companion to Brenner and Rector's The Kidney. Philadelphia: WB Saunders, 2002, pp 23–40.
2. Bidani A, Tauzon DM, Heming TA: Regulation of whole body acid-base balance. In DuBose TD, Hamm LL (eds): Acid-Base and Electrolyte Disorders: A Companion to Brenner and Rector's The Kidney. Philadelphia: WB Saunders, 2002, pp 1–21.
3. DuBose TD, McDonald GA: Renal tubular acidosis. In DuBose TD, Hamm LL (eds): Acid-Base and Electrolyte Disorders: A Companion to Brenner and Rector's The Kidney. Philadelphia: WB Saunders, 2002, pp 189–206.
4. Jorens PG, Demey HE, Schepens PJ, et al: Unusual D-lactic acid acidosis from propylene glycol metabolism in overdose. J Toxicol Clin Toxicol 2004;42:163–169.
5. Krapf R, Alpern RJ, Seldin DW: Clinical syndromes of metabolic acidosis. In Seldin DW and Giebisch G (eds): The Kidney, 3rd ed. Philadelphia: Lippincott Williams & Wilkins, 2000, pp 2055–2072.
6. Kraut JA, Kurtz I: Metabolic acidosis of CKD: Diagnosis, clinical characteristics, and treatment. Am J Kidney Dis 2005;45:978–993.
7. Laski ME, Wesson DE: Lactic acidosis. In DuBose TD, Hamm LL (eds): Acid-Base and Electrolyte Disorders: A Companion to Brenner and Rector's The Kidney. Philadelphia: WB Saunders, 2002, pp 68–83.
8. Whitney GM, Szerlip HM: Acid-base disorders in the critical care setting. In: DuBose TD, Hamm LL (eds): Acid-Base and Electrolyte Disorders: A Companion to Brenner and Rector's The Kidney. Philadelphia: WB Saunders, 2002, pp 165–187.

Further Reading

DuBose TD Jr: Acid-base disorders. In Brenner BM (ed): Brenner and Rector's The Kidney, 8th ed. Philadelphia: WB Saunders, 2007, pp 505–546.

DuBose TD Jr: Acidosis and alkalosis. In Kasper DL, Braunwald E, Fauci AS, et al (eds): Harrison's Principles of Internal Medicine, 17th ed. New York: McGraw-Hill, 2007, pp 287–295.

DuBose TD Jr, Alpern RJ: Renal tubular acidosis. In Scriver CR, Beaudet AL, Valle D, et al. (eds): The Metabolic and Molecular Bases of Inherited Diseases, 8th ed. New York: McGraw-Hill, 2000, pp 4983–5021.

Emmett M: Diagnosis of simple and mixed disorders. In DuBose TD, Hamm LL (eds): Acid-Base and Electrolyte Disorders. Philadelphia: WB Saunders, 2002, pp 41–53.

Halperin M, Cherney DZI, Kamel KS: Ketoacidosis. In DuBose TD, Hamm LL (eds): Acid-Base and Electrolyte Disorders. Philadelphia: WB Saunders, 2002, pp 67–82.

Hamm LL, Alpern RJ: Cellular mechanisms of renal tubular acidification. In Seldin DW, Giebisch G (eds): The Kidney: Physiology and Pathophysiology, 3rd ed. New York: Lippincott, Williams & Wilkins, 2000, pp 1935–1979.

Laski ME, Wesson DW: Lactic acidosis. In DuBose TD, Hamm LL (eds): Acid-Base and Electrolyte Disorders. Philadelphia: WB Saunders, 2002, pp 83–108.

Toews GB: Respiratory acidosis. In DuBose TD, Hamm LL (eds): Acid-Base and Electrolyte Disorders. Philadelphia: WB Saunders, 2002, pp 129–146.

Chapter 32

Treatment of Metabolic and Respiratory Alkalosis

Biff F. Palmer

CHAPTER CONTENTS

METABOLIC ALKALOSIS

The pathogenesis of metabolic alkalosis involves both the generation and maintenance of this disorder.[1] The generation of metabolic alkalosis refers to the addition of new HCO_3^- to the blood as a result of either loss of acid or gain of alkali. New HCO_3^- may be generated by either renal or extrarenal mechanisms. Because the kidneys have an enormous capacity to excrete HCO_3^-, even vigorous HCO_3^- generation may not be sufficient to produce sustained metabolic alkalosis. To maintain a metabolic alkalosis, the capacity of the kidney to correct the alkalosis must be impaired, or, equivalently, the capacity to reclaim HCO_3^- must be enhanced. After correcting the underlying cause, the treatment of metabolic alkalosis is directed toward removing those factors responsible for maintaining the alkalosis.

Clinical Consequences of Metabolic Alkalosis

Metabolic alkalosis is generally considered a benign condition by most physicians. However, there is evidence to suggest that under certain circumstances, metabolic alkalosis can contribute significantly to mortality. In fact, a direct relationship has been shown between increasing blood pH and hospital mortality in patients with a pH of greater than 7.48.[2,3] The demonstration that high arterial blood pH correlates with mortality does not establish a cause-and-effect relationship. It is certainly plausible that conditions associated with high mortality cause metabolic and respiratory alkalosis, making alkalosis merely a marker of a poor prognosis. However, there are a number of reasons to believe that high blood pH can contribute to the poor prognosis. This is based on

some of the known pathophysiological effects of a high blood pH (Box 32-1).

First, increases in blood pH (alkalemia) cause respiratory depression. This effect of metabolic pH changes on respiration is mediated via both central and peripheral chemoreceptors. Although the effects of metabolic alkalosis on respiration are well appreciated, the effects of alkalosis to decrease tissue oxygen delivery are less well appreciated. Alkalosis can decrease oxygen delivery by two possible mechanisms. First, by the Bohr effect, alkalosis leads to a shift in the oxygen dissociation curve of hemoglobin, which decreases the ability of hemoglobin to release oxygen in peripheral tissues. Thus, even in the absence of changes in blood flow, alkalosis can lead to marked decreases in oxygen delivery to tissues.

In addition to the Bohr effect, alkalosis is a potent vasoconstrictor. Numerous studies have shown that increases in pH associated with decreases in P_{CO_2} (respiratory alkalosis) lead to vasoconstriction and decreased perfusion of the brain, heart, and peripheral circulation. Respiratory alkalosis is used clinically to decrease cerebral blood flow in patients with cerebral edema. Although it is unclear from studies in humans and whole animals whether pH changes due to metabolic alkalosis have the same effect, in vitro studies show that pH is the critical determinant of vascular smooth muscle tone irrespective of whether pH is altered by changes in P_{CO_2} or HCO_3^- concentration.[4,5]

Alkalosis-induced vasoconstriction together with the Bohr effect may cause clinical tissue hypoxia in certain settings. For example, hyperventilation has been shown to precipitate chest pain, ST segment increase, and spasm on coronary angiography in patients with Prinzmetal's angina.[6] Similarly, hyperventilation has been shown to cause angina in the presence or absence of coronary artery disease.[7] Alkalosis has also been

Box 32-1 Systemic Effects of Metabolic Alkalosis

I. Cardiovascular
  A. Heart: Arrhythmias, especially in patients with emphysema
  B. Vascular: Arteriolar vasoconstriction
II. Pulmonary
  A. Ventilation: Hypoventilation
  B. Oxygen delivery: Decreased in acute alkalosis (Bohr effect)
III. Renal
  A. Antinatriuretic effect
IV. Nervous system
  A. Peripheral: Neuromuscular irritability
  B. Central: Confusion, lethargy, seizures

---

reported to induce cardiac arrhythmias that are unresponsive to antiarrhythmics and respond only to correction of the alkalosis. Unfortunately, this is only substantiated by a number of case reports, and it is difficult to prove an increased incidence.

In summary, evidence suggests that alkalemia can decrease oxygen delivery to tissues, and this may become a key factor in some critically ill patients. Alkalemia constricts vascular smooth muscle in vitro and appears to decrease tissue perfusion in vivo. This, along with inhibition of oxygen release from hemoglobin, leads to decreased tissue oxygen delivery, which is demonstrable clinically with regard to the heart where coronary artery spasm, angina, arrhythmias, and congestive heart failure may be precipitated. Most likely, oxygen delivery to the brain is also compromised in ill patients with alkalosis, but it is frequently clinically difficult to distinguish brain hypoxia from other causes of encephalopathy. Given these considerations, alkalosis should be aggressively corrected in critically ill patients in whom perfusion of the heart and brain is essential.

Treatment

Metabolic alkalosis is best approached according to the mechanism of maintenance because correction of the maintenance mechanism leads to correction of the metabolic alkalosis. Reduced effective arterial blood volume is the mechanism responsible for the maintenance of metabolic alkalosis in the majority of patients. In those settings where effective blood volume can be restored with saline, the metabolic alkalosis is easily corrected.[8]

A number of conditions are poorly responsive to the administration of NaCl. These conditions are generally maintained by a combination of increased mineralocorticoid levels along with high distal Na^+ delivery and hypokalemia. The distinction between these entities relies on assessment of the effective arterial volume. Effective arterial volume is assessed by physical examination (postural changes in blood pressure and pulse), the blood urea nitrogen-to-creatinine ratio, serum uric acid concentration, and urinary electrolytes. Although the urine Na^+ concentration is useful in most patients to assess effective arterial volume, the urinary Cl^- is actually more helpful in this situation.

The advantage of urinary Cl^- is because many patients with metabolic alkalosis may have intermittent bicarbonaturia. HCO_3^- functions as a nonreabsorbable anion and carries a varying combination of Na^+ and K^+ into the urine causing urinary Na^+ to be increased even though the patient may be volume contracted. In this setting, urinary Cl^- remains low and thus is more reflective of the volume contracted state. A urinary Cl^- less than 15 mEq/L is suggestive of metabolic alkalosis maintained by a low effective arterial volume, whereas a urinary Cl^- greater than 20 mEq/L is suggestive of metabolic alkalosis maintained by other mechanisms (Table 32-1).

Approach to the Patient with Decreased Effective Arterial Volume: Saline Responsive

Gastrointestinal Acid Loss

Loss of acid as occurs with vomiting or nasogastric suction is a common cause of metabolic alkalosis maintained by volume contraction. The loss of gastric acid generates a metabolic alkalosis, whereas the loss of NaCl in the gastric fluid leads to volume contraction. During active vomiting, the plasma HCO_3^- concentration tends to be higher than the threshold for reabsorption in the proximal nephron. The resultant bicarbonaturia leads to increased excretion of $NaHCO_3$ and $KHCO_3$, resulting in further total body Na^+ depletion and development of K^+ depletion. During this active phase, urinary electrolytes show a urine Cl^- less than 15 mEq/L, in the presence of a high urine Na^+, a high urine K^+, and a urine pH of 7 to 8. When the patient stops vomiting, an equilibrium is established such that bicarbonaturia disappears but a metabolic alkalosis is maintained by the volume contraction, K^+ depletion, and decreased glomerular filtration rate. Of these factors, the effective arterial volume contraction is clearly the main factor in maintenance of metabolic alkalosis. At this time, urine Na^+ and Cl^- are both low. Administration of NaCl results in bicarbonaturia and the metabolic alkalosis is corrected.

The amount of saline required to correct the alkalotic state should be determined by an ongoing assessment of the volume status of the patient. This assessment should include frequent monitoring for the presence of orthostatic changes in blood pressure and pulse, examination of the neck veins to assess jugular venous pressure, and determination of skin turgor. In addition to a decrease in the serum bicarbonate concentration, laboratory data indicating the effectiveness of therapy include a decrease in the blood urea nitrogen-to-creatinine ratio and evidence of less hemoconcentration as reflected by a decrease in albumin concentration and hematocrit.

K^+ can be given orally or intravenously as KCl salt. The safest way to administer KCl is orally. KCl can be given in doses of 100 to 150 mEq/day. Liquid KCl is bitter tasting and like the tablet can be irritating to the gastric mucosa. The microencapsulated or wax-matrix forms of KCl are better tolerated. Intravenous administration of K may be necessary if the patient cannot take oral medications or if the K deficit is large and is resulting in cardiac arrhythmias, respiratory paralysis, or rhabdomyolysis. Intravenous KCl should be given at a

Table 32-1 Classification of Metabolic Alkalosis According to Mechanism, Cause, and Response to Administration of Saline

Effective Arterial Volume	Low	Low	High
Urine Cl concentration (mEq/L)	<15	>15	>15
Response to saline	Corrects (saline responsive)	No correction (saline resistant)	No correction (saline resistant)
Maintenance	Low effective arterial volume	Low effective arterial volume + high distal Na⁺ delivery and mineralocorticoid effect	High distal Na⁺ delivery and mineralocorticoid effect
	I. Gastrointestinal acid loss	I. Primary increase in distal delivery of Na⁺	Primary increase in mineralocortoid or mineralocorticoid-like effect
	A. Vomiting/nasogastric suction	A. Active diuretic use (loop and thiazide)	
	B. Congenital chloridorrhea	B. Mg²⁺ deficiency	
	C. Villous adenoma	C. Bartter syndrome	
		D. Gitelman's syndrome	
	II. Posthypercapneic alkalosis		
	III. Diuretics		
	IV. Nonreabsorbable anions		

maximum rate of 20 mEq/hr and maximum concentration of 40 mEq/L.

Diuretics

Thiazide and loop diuretics are another common cause of a metabolic alkalosis. These diuretics lead to a metabolic alkalosis that is generated in the distal nephron by the combination of high aldosterone levels and enhanced distal delivery of Na⁺. If diuretics are stopped and the patient is maintained on a low-salt diet, the alkalosis will be maintained despite the fact that distal delivery is no longer increased. In this setting, patients tend to be volume contracted and K⁺ deficient. Once again, it is the contraction of the effective arterial volume that is the major factor leading to the maintenance of metabolic alkalosis. Saline infusion in this setting corrects the metabolic alkalosis.

Posthypercapneic Alkalosis

Another saline-responsive metabolic alkalosis is posthypercapneic alkalosis. When a patient becomes hypercapneic, the kidney retains $NaHCO_3$. The retention of $NaHCO_3$ leads to increased urinary excretion of NaCl in an attempt to maintain extracellular fluid volume unchanged. When the Pco_2 is then returned to normal, the kidney will attempt to correct the metabolic alkalosis by excreting $NaHCO_3$. However, if the patient is on a low-salt diet, as these patients frequently are for prevention of right-sided heart failure, the $NaHCO_3$ diuresis will lead to volume contraction, causing the bicarbonaturia to abate. The patient will be left with a metabolic alkalosis, once again maintained by decreased effective arterial volume. Administration of saline corrects the metabolic alkalosis.

In certain patients, it may be difficult to correct the factors responsible for maintenance of metabolic alkalosis. This most frequently occurs in patients whose metabolic alkalosis is maintained by decreased effective arterial volume, but whose cardiovascular system cannot tolerate administration of NaCl. In these situations, one must ask how important it is to correct the metabolic alkalosis. Based on the previous discussion, patients in whom one would want to aggressively correct metabolic alkalosis would include (1) those with chronic lung disease in whom intubation is imminent or extubation is difficult and metabolic alkalosis needs to be corrected to improve the drive to respiration; (2) those with myocardial ischemia with evolving myocardial infarction, those who are having chest pain post-infarction, or those with unstable angina; and (3) ill patients with cerebral dysfunction in whom cerebral hypoperfusion is a possible contributing factor.

If metabolic alkalosis needs to be treated aggressively and cannot be treated by correcting the cause of the generation or maintenance, a number of options still exist. First, ammonium chloride can be given.[9] This is generally a safe way to administer acid if given orally. However, if given intravenously, especially in patients with liver disease, ammonium chloride administration may cause ammonia toxicity. Arginine hydrochloride has been used in the past to lower the plasma $[HCO_3^-]$ but has been removed from the market because of life-threatening hyperkalemia.

The most commonly used approach to correcting alkalosis in these difficult patients is administration of carbonic anhydrase inhibitors such as acetazolamide. Carbonic anhydrase catalyzes the dehydration of luminal carbonic acid (produced when filtered HCO_3^- reacts with secreted H^+) to water and CO_2 and the hydration of cellular CO_2 to carbonic acid, allowing the formation of H^+ for secretion into the luminal fluid. The uncatalyzed dehydration of carbonic acid occurs very slowly. By inhibiting the activity of this enzyme, carbonic anhydrase inhibitors inhibit renal acidification and thus cause the kidney to at least partially correct the metabolic alkalosis.[10]

The magnitude of the bicarbonaturia induced is directly related to the serum HCO_3^- concentration. As the HCO_3^- concentration decreases, the clinical effectiveness of the drug declines in a parallel fashion. As a result, only rarely does the plasma HCO_3^- concentration return to normal.

Acetazolamide is frequently used in patients with chronic respiratory acidosis who develop a metabolic alkalosis. Normally, in patients with chronic respiratory acidosis, the capacity of the kidney to reabsorb bicarbonate increases, resulting in an increase in plasma HCO_3^- concentration. Use of loop diuretics in such patients, as in the treatment of cor pulmonale, can result in further increases in the serum HCO_3^- concentration. In this setting, the induction of a metabolic alkalosis can depress ventilation, aggravating both the hypoxemia and hypercapnia. Normally the metabolic alkalosis can be treated by discontinuing the diuretic and administering NaCl. In the patient who is significantly edematous, however, this approach may not be practical. In this circumstance, acetazolamide can be used to inhibit HCO_3^- reabsorption and thus lower serum HCO_3^- concentration.

A potential problem that is associated with use of carbonic anhydrase inhibitors in patients with lung disease is a worsening of hypercapnia. Carbonic anhydrase is normally present within red blood cells and is involved in CO_2 movement into red cells in peripheral tissues and movement from red cells into the alveoli in the lungs. Thus, carbonic anhydrase inhibition can prevent red-cell uptake of CO_2 in peripheral tissues and can prevent CO_2 release in the lung. The latter can lead to an increase in the Pco_2 of the arterial blood, whereas the former leads to an even further increase in Pco_2 in peripheral tissues. Generally, patients with normal lungs can respond to this by increasing respiration and preventing the increase in the Pco_2 of the arterial blood. However, patients with lung disease cannot respond adequately and further increases in arterial Pco_2 as well as even larger increases in unmeasured tissue Pco_2 may be dangerous to the patient.

A safe approach to the aggressive treatment of metabolic alkalosis that has gained support is the use of hydrochloric acid (HCl) infusions.[11,12] In general, HCl can be safely administered as a 0.15 to 0.25 normal solution in normal saline or 5% dextrose in water given through a central line. Due to the sclerosing properties of HCl, it is imperative that the position of the central line in the superior vena cava be verified by chest radiograph before initiating infusion. Infusion rates should be no more than 0.2 mmol/kg of body weight per hour. One should use a bicarbonate space of 50% of ideal body weight when calculating the amount of HCl to be given. As an example, to decrease the plasma bicarbonate from 50 to 40 mmol/L in a 70-kg patient, the amount of HCl required is 350 mmol ($10 \times 70 \times 0.5$). If the physician wishes, the HCl can be added to an amino acid solution in total parenteral nutrition and given centrally.[13] In addition, there is also a report in which HCl was given in an amino acid solution with intralipid through a peripheral vein.[14]

Approach to the Patient with Decreased Effective Arterial Volume: Saline Resistant

In some forms of metabolic alkalosis, the alkalosis is maintained by a decreased effective arterial volume, but because other maintenance factors are also present, the alkalosis is not completely saline responsive. In these patients, saline infusions may improve the metabolic alkalosis but will not completely correct it. In general, these patients may have a low effective arterial volume but typically do not have a low urine Cl^-. One cause of this syndrome is continued use of thiazide or loop diuretics. Diuretic-induced volume contraction contributes to maintenance, but an additional factor, the combination of high distal Na^+ delivery without suppressed mineralocorticoid levels, also contributes to maintenance. Other conditions, such as magnesium deficiency, Gitelman's syndrome, and Bartter syndrome, are similar to this in that NaCl absorption in Henle's loop or distal convoluted tubule is inhibited. Once again, volume contraction contributes to maintenance of metabolic alkalosis, but the alkalosis is also maintained by high distal Na^+ delivery with high mineralocorticoid levels. The treatments of these conditions are summarized in Table 32-2.

Approach to the Patient with Increased Effective Arterial Volume: Saline Resistant

The last type of metabolic alkalosis is not maintained by a decreased effective arterial volume, but rather maintained by high

Table 32-2 Treatment of Various Saline-Resistant Causes of Metabolic Alkalosis

↓EABV		↑EABV	
Cause	**Treatment**	**Cause**	**Treatment**
Thiazide and loop diuretics	Discontinue drug, replete EABV	Renin-secreting tumor	Remove tumor
Mg^{2+} deficiency	Replete Mg^{2+} deficit	Primary hyperaldosteronism	Remove tumor, spironolactone for BAH
Gitelman's syndrome	Amiloride, triamterene, or spironolactone, K^+ supplements, Mg^{2+} supplements	Glucocorticoid-suppressible hyperaldosteronism	Dexamethasone
Bartter syndrome	Amiloride, triamterene, or spironolactone, K^+ supplements, Mg^{2+} supplements in some	Liddle syndrome	Amiloride or triamterene

BAH, bilateral adrenal hyperplasia; EABV, effective arterial blood volume.

mineralocorticoid levels (in the presence of maintained distal delivery of Na^+) and K^+ deficiency. The most common cause of this saline-resistant alkalosis is a primary increase in mineralocorticoid levels not related to volume contraction. The mechanism of the generation of the alkalosis described previously, enhanced Na^+ delivery with high mineralocorticoid activity, is also responsible for maintenance of the metabolic alkalosis in this setting. In addition, K^+ deficiency, which also occurs in this setting, exacerbates the tendency to alkalosis.

The preferred treatment of metabolic alkalosis in patients with volume expansion and primary mineralocorticoid excess is to remove the underlying cause of the persistent mineralocorticoid activity (see Table 32-2). When this is not possible, therapy is directed at blocking the actions of the mineralocorticoid at the level of the kidney. The potassium-sparing diuretics are effective agents in blocking the actions of mineralocorticoids in the kidney and are commonly used in the treatment of these disorders. Mineralocorticoid receptor blockers such as spironolactone are effective in these patients, with the exception of Liddle syndrome, in which the defect is distal to the receptor. Spironolactone inhibits Na^+ reabsorption by blocking the binding of aldosterone to its cytoplasmic receptor thereby inhibiting aldosterone-induced Na^+ reabsorption. The decrease in luminal electronegativity impairs distal acidification as a result of the decrease in the electrical driving force for H^+ secretion into the tubular lumen. Spironolactone can further limit distal H^+ secretion because this drug not only inhibits aldosterone-stimulated Na^+ reabsorption but also blocks the direct stimulatory effect of aldosterone on the H^+ secretory pump.

Na^+ channel blockers such as amiloride and triamterene are also effective in these patients. These drugs directly inhibit the luminal membrane Na^+ channel, decreasing the luminal electronegativity of the collecting duct and secondarily impairing renal K^+ and H^+ losses. The net result is inhibition of renal Na^+ retention, K^+ loss, and increases in renal net acid excretion, resulting in prevention of hypertension and hypokalemic alkalosis.

Liddle syndrome is characterized by hypokalemic metabolic alkalosis and volume expansion but is not due to mineralocorticoid excess. Rather, this disorder results from overactivity of the Na^+ channel in the distal nephron. Predictably, use of spironolactone to block the mineralocorticoid receptor is without effect in this disorder. By contrast, the electrolyte abnormalities and hypertension are normalized by use of the sodium channel blockers triamterene and amiloride.

RESPIRATORY ALKALOSIS

Primary respiratory alkalosis results from hypocapnia and is defined by a $Paco_2$ of less than 35 mm Hg in the setting of alkalemia. Primary respiratory alkalosis needs to be differentiated from secondary hypocapnia, which is a compensatory mechanism in the setting of primary metabolic acidosis.

Cause

An increase in alveolar ventilation relative to CO_2 production gives rise to respiratory alkalosis. Because changes in CO_2 production are negligible, almost all cases of hypocapnia result from increased CO_2 elimination, which is the equivalent of increased alveolar hyperventilation.

In the majority of cases, primary hypocapnia reflects pulmonary hyperventilation due to increased ventilatory drive. The latter might result from signals arising from the lung, the peripheral chemoreceptors (carotid and aortic), the brainstem chemoreceptors, or influences originating in other centers of the brain. The response to CO_2 of the brainstem chemoreceptors can be augmented by systemic diseases (e.g., sepsis, liver disease), pharmacological agents, anxiety, volition, and other influences. Hypoxemia is a major stimulus to pulmonary ventilation, but Pao_2 values less than 60 mm Hg are required to elicit this effect consistently.

Primary hypocapnia is probably the most frequent acid-base disturbance encountered. In critically ill patients, its presence might be a grave prognostic sign, especially if Pco_2 levels are less than 20 to 25 mm Hg.[15] Furthermore, respiratory alkalosis is the most common acid-base abnormality in patients hospitalized in intensive care units, occurring either as the simple disorder or as a component of mixed disturbances.

Hepatic failure is a common and important cause of primary hypocapnia.[16] The severity of hypocapnia correlates with the level of blood ammonia and has prognostic significance. Systemic infections arising from gram-positive and gram-negative bacteria are also a major cause of respiratory alkalosis. Direct stimulation of central chemoreceptors by bacterial toxins from gram-negative organisms accounts, at least in part, for the hyperventilation observed in some patients with sepsis. Thus, unexplained respiratory alkalosis in a hospitalized patient calls for evaluation for the presence of gram-negative sepsis. The presence of respiratory alkalosis can be an important clue to the presence of salicylate intoxication. High progesterone levels (pregnancy) can also cause respiratory alkalosis.

Clinical Manifestation of Respiratory Alkalosis

Although there is overlap in the clinical manifestations of metabolic and respiratory alkalosis, this section discusses those features specific to respiratory alkalosis. Mild respiratory alkalosis causes lightheadedness, palpitations, and paresthesias of the extremities and the circumoral area.[17] Acute hypocapnia decreases cerebral blood flow and produces decreased acidity in all body fluids as well as hypocalcemia, hypokalemia, and a pH-induced shift of oxyhemoglobin dissociation curve; all these alterations have been implicated as determinants of the clinical manifestations of this acid-base disorder.[18,19] The acute hypocapnia-induced reduction in cerebral blood flow might reach values less than 50% of normal, resulting in an increased lactate output by the brain due to cerebral hypoxia. A decrease in intracranial pressure, which is generally not harmful, and electroencephalographic changes consisting of generalized slowing and high-voltage waves are also present in acute respiratory alkalosis. The effects of acute hypocapnia on the cerebral circulation have been used in the treatment of brain edema resulting from neurosurgical procedures, head trauma, meningitis, and encephalitis. Unfortunately, the hypocapnia-induced reduction in intracranial pressure is short lasting, and blood flow returns to normal in sustained hypocapnia.

Hypocapnia leads to alkalemia, which causes binding of free calcium to albumin in the blood. Thus, patients with acute respiratory alkalosis might present clinically in a similar way as patients with hypocalcemia. Chvostek's and Trousseau's signs are well-known clinical tests that can be occasionally elicited in patients with acute respiratory alkalosis.

The cardiovascular manifestations of respiratory alkalosis might be also very prominent. A major reduction in cardiac output accompanied by arteriolar vasoconstriction, tissue hypoperfusion, and a large increment in plasma lactate is frequently attributed to severe acute hypocapnia. This syndrome is typically observed in surgical patients under general anesthesia or those having depression of the central nervous system and receiving mechanical respiratory assistance; in all likelihood, it reflects the effects of passive hyperventilation. Normal volunteers with active hyperventilation do not develop clinical manifestations of coronary insufficiency or cardiac arrhythmias. Patients with ischemic heart disease might occasionally develop cardiac arrhythmias, ischemic electrocardiographic changes, and even angina pectoris during acute hypocapnia. None of the previously described hemodynamic effects seems to be present in uncomplicated chronic hypocapnia.

Treatment

Primary respiratory alkalosis is treated by correcting the underlying cause (Box 32-2). A patient with anxiety-hyperventilation syndrome should be treated by providing reassurance. Rebreathing into a paper bag or any other closed system will cause the PCO_2 to increase with each breath taken and lead to a partial correction of hypocapnia and improvement of symptoms. In the rare case in which there is no response to conservative management, sedatives can be used.

In mechanically ventilated patients the PCO_2 can be increased by either increasing the inspired CO_2 tension or by increasing the dead space of the ventilator circuit. Correction of respiratory alkalosis may prove helpful in correcting arrhythmias in patients with underlying coronary disease. By contrast, one needs to be cautious in increasing the PCO_2 in patients with brain injury because cerebral perfusion may increase and cause further worsening of intracranial pressure.

Respiratory alkalosis frequently develops as a complication of hypoxia. Administration of oxygen or return to lower altitudes can reverse the respiratory alkalosis that develops in this setting.

Aspirin (acetylsalicylic acid) has a direct stimulatory effect on the respiratory center. In the overdose setting, increased ventilation decreases the PCO_2 and results in respiratory alkalosis. In addition to conservative management, the initial goal of therapy is to correct systemic acidemia and to alkalinize the urine pH. By increasing systemic pH, the ionized fraction of salicylic acid will increase, and, as a result, there will be less accumulation of the drug in the central nervous system. Similarly, an alkaline urine pH will favor increased urinary excretion because the ionized fraction of the drug is poorly reabsorbed by the tubule. At serum concentrations of more than 80 mg/dL or in the setting of severe clinical toxicity, hemodialysis can be used to accelerate the removal of the drug from the body.

Box 32-2   Treatment of Respiratory Alkalosis

I. Treatment begins with correcting underlying cause
II. Hypoxemia
  A. Supplemental oxygen
  B. Return to lower altitude
III. Mechanical ventilation
  A. Increase dead space in ventilatory circuit
  B. Sedation and/or use of paralytic agent
IV. Psychogenic hyperventilation
  A. Rebreathe into closed system (paper bag)
  B. Antianxiety medications where indicated
V. Salicylate toxicity
  A. Urinary alkalinization
  B. Hemodialysis with severe clinical toxicity or level >80 mg/dL

References

1. Palmer BF, Alpern RJ: Metabolic alkalosis. J Am Soc Nephrol 1997;8:1462–1469.
2. Wilson RF, Gibson D, Percinel AK, et al: Severe alkalosis in critically ill surgical patients. Arch Surg 1972;105:197–203.
3. Anderson LE, Henrich WL: Alkalemia-associated morbidity and mortality in medical and surgical patients. South Med J 1987;80:729–733.
4. Rinaldi GJ, Cattaneo EA, Cingolani HE: Interaction between calcium and hydrogen ions in canine coronary arteries. J Mol Cell Cardiol 1987;19:773–784.
5. Yasue H, Omote S, Takizawa A, et al: Alkalosis-induced coronary vasoconstriction: Effects of calcium, diltiazem, nitroglycerin, and propranolol. Am Heart J 1981;102:206–210.
6. Yasue H, Nagao M, Omote S, et al: Coronary arterial spasm and Prinzmetal's variant form of angina induced by hyperventilation and Tris-buffer infusion. Circulation 1978;58:56–62.
7. Lary D, Goldschlager N: Electrocardiographic changes during hyperventilation resembling myocardial ischemia in patients with normal coronary arteriograms. Am Heart J 1974;87:383–390.
8. Cohen JJ: Correction of metabolic alkalosis by the kidney after isometric expansion of extracellular fluid. Am J Med 1968;47:1181–1192.
9. Zintel HA, Rhoads JE, Ravdin IS: The use of intravenous ammonium chloride in the treatment of alkalosis. Surgery 1943;14:728–731.
10. Preisig PA, Toto RD, Alpern RJ: Carbonic anhydrase inhibitors. Renal Physiol 1987;10:136–159.
11. Worthley L: Intravenous hydrochloric acid in patients with metabolic alkalosis in hypercapnia. Arch Surg 1986;121:1195–1198.
12. Brimioulle S, Vincent J, Dufaye P, et al: Hydrochloric acid infusion for treatment of metabolic alkalosis: Effects on acid-base balance and oxygenation. Crit Care Med 1985;13:738–742.
13. Finkle D, Dean R: Buffered hydrochloric acid: A modern method of treating metabolic alkalosis. Am Surg 1981;47:103–106.
14. Knutsen O: New method for administration of hydrochloric acid in metabolic alkalosis. Lancet 1983;1:953–956.
15. Mazzara J, Ayers S, Grace W: Extreme hypocapnia in the critically ill patient. Am J Med 1974;56:450–456.
16. Ahya S, Jose Soler M, Levitsky J, et al: Acid-base and potassium disorders in liver disease. Semin Nephrol 2006;26:466–470.
17. Laffey J, Kavanagh B: Hypocapnia. N Engl J Med 2002;347:43–53.

18. Nevin M, Colchester A, Adams S, Pepper J: Evidence for involvement of hypocapnia and hypoperfusion in aetiology of neurological deficit after cardiopulmonary bypass. Lancet 1987;2:1493–1495.

19. Ayres S, Grace W: Inappropriate ventilation and hypoxemia as causes of cardiac arrhythmias. The control of arrhythmias without antiarrhythmic drugs. Am J Med 1969;46:495–505.

Further Reading

Ahya SN, Jose Soler M, Levitsky J, et al: Acid-base and potassium disorders in liver disease. Semin Nephrol 2006;26:466–470.

Foster GT, Vaziri ND, Sassoon CS: Respiratory alkalosis. Respir Care 2001;46:384–391.

Khanna A, Kurtzman NA: Metabolic alkalosis. J Nephrol 2006;19(Suppl 9):S86–S96.

Laski ME, Sabatini S: Metabolic alkalosis, bedside and bench. Semin Nephrol 2006;26:404–421.

Leaf DE, Goldfarb DS: Mechanisms of action of acetazolamide in the prophylaxis and treatment of acute mountain sickness. J Appl Physiol 2007;102:1305–1307.

Palmer BF, Alpern RJ: Liddle's syndrome. Am J Med 1998;104: 301–309.

Palmer BF, Alpern RJ: Metabolic alkalosis. J Am Soc Nephrol 1997;8:1462–1469.

Chapter 33

Diuretic Use in Edema and the Problem of Resistance

David H. Ellison and Christopher S. Wilcox

CHAPTER CONTENTS

"Flooding of the heart" was described by the ancient Egyptians, and cures were often heroic.[1] The term diuretic is derived from the Greek *diouretikos* ("promoting urine"), and diuretics have been employed for hundreds of years. Paracelsus recognized the diuretic properties of mercury.[1] The modern era of diuretics began with the synthesis of thiazides and loop diuretics, which were developed empirically. Although few new diuretics have become available during the past 10 years, our understanding of diuretic-sensitive transport pathways has exploded, and progress in rational therapeutic approaches to edematous conditions has continued. This chapter reviews uses of diuretic drugs to treat edematous conditions. Where data from controlled trials support particular approaches or where consensus recommendations on therapy are available, they are emphasized. Otherwise, the authors provide their personal recommendation. The reader is referred elsewhere for a discussion of diuretic treatment of hypertension and nonedematous disorders (Chapters 29, 30, 35, and 51).

SITES, MECHANISMS OF ACTION, AND RECOMMENDED DIURETIC DOSES

The sites and mechanisms of action of the most commonly used diuretics are shown in Figure 33-1. Recommended doses are summarized in Table 33-1. The subject has been reviewed.[2,3]

Most diuretic drugs in clinical use act primarily on the renal tubules to inhibit Na^+ reabsorption and increase fractional Na^+ excretion. Active NaCl reabsorption is driven by the Na^+/K^+-ATPase pump, which is expressed at the basolateral membrane (the blood side) of epithelial cells along the nephron, keeping the intracellular Na^+ concentration low. Each nephron segment possesses unique apical mechanisms that permit Na^+ to move across the luminal membrane; these specific transport pathways at the luminal membrane form the molecular bases of most diuretic action. Together, active Na^+ extrusion from the basolateral membrane and passive Na^+ entry across the luminal membrane permit vectoral Na^+ absorption.[4]

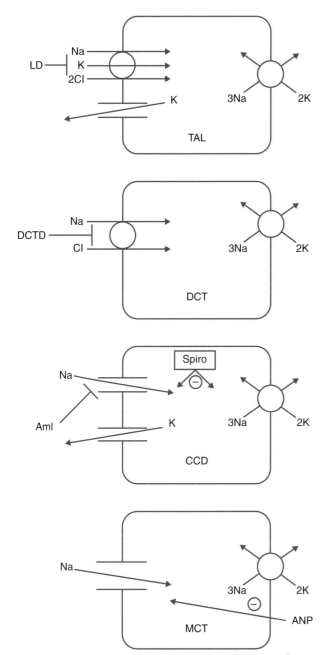

Figure 33-1 Principal cellular sites and mechanisms of action of the most commonly used classes of diuretics. Aml, amiloride; ANP, atrial natriuretic peptide; CCD, cortical collecting duct; DCT, distal convoluted tubule; DCTD, distal convoluted tubule diuretics; LD, loop diuretics; MCT, medullary collecting tubule; Spiro, spironolactone; TAL, thick ascending limb.

Proximal Tubule Diuretics

An important pathway by which Na^+ crosses the luminal membrane of proximal tubule cells involves electroneutral exchange of Na^+ for H^+. Protons then titrate filtered bicarbonate, forming carbonic acid, which dehydrates to CO_2 and H_2O, a reaction catalyzed by carbonic anhydrase.[5,6] Carbonic anhydrase inhibitors interfere with enzyme activity both inside the cell and within the brush border. The net result is impaired Na^+, HCO_3^-, Cl^-, and water reabsorption by the proximal tubule and increased renal Na^+, Cl^-, HCO_3^-, and water excretion (for more details, see Ellison and Wilcox[2]). The use of carbonic anhydrase inhibitors is limited by the development of tolerance and unwanted adverse effects.[2,7–12]

Loop Diuretics

Approximately 25% of the filtered NaCl is reabsorbed along Henle's loop. An electroneutral $Na^+/K^+/2Cl^-$ transport pathway generates net NaCl reabsorption because much of the absorbed K^+ is recycled via a luminal K^+ channel. Loop diuretics such as furosemide, bumetanide, and torsemide inhibit the $Na^+/K^+/2Cl^-$ pathway directly (see Fig. 33-1).[2,13,14] Loop diuretics are potent (high-ceiling) drugs that promote the excretion of Na^+ and Cl^-. Although they inhibit K^+ reabsorption along the thick ascending limb, their effects on K^+ excretion reflect predominantly an increase in K^+ secretion along the distal nephron. Loop diuretics increase Mg^{2+} and Ca^{2+} excretion.[15–17] Loop diuretics also impair the ability of the kidney to concentrate and dilute urine and have important hemodynamic effects, both within the kidney and systemically. They increase secretion of vasodilatory prostaglandins[18] and, when administered intravenously, often decrease cardiac preload owing to venodilation. Loop diuretics block the tubuloglomerular feedback mechanism.[19] In normal subjects, they increase renal blood flow but have little effect on glomerular filtration rate (GFR).[20]

Distal Convoluted Tubule Diuretics

Distal convoluted tubule (DCT) diuretics (thiazides and thiazide-like drugs) bind to the Na^+/Cl^- transporter expressed at the apical membrane of cells along the distal tubule (see Fig. 33-1).[21] DCT diuretics impair urinary diluting capacity, but have no effect on urinary concentrating ability. Most DCT diuretics become less effective when the GFR decreases to less than 30 to 40 mL/min. DCT diuretics increase Mg^{2+} excretion but, in contrast to loop diuretics, decrease Ca^{2+} excretion.[22]

Potassium-Sparing Distal Diuretics

Sodium reabsorption along the aldosterone-sensitive distal nephron (ASDN) (comprising the late DCT, the connecting tubule, and the cortical collecting duct), which amounts to only 3% to 5% of the filtered NaCl load, is primarily electrogenic (current generating), unlike transport along more proximal segments. Two groups of diuretics act predominantly in the ASDN. Sodium channel blockers (see Fig. 33-1), such as triamterene and amiloride,[3,23] act from the lumen to inhibit Na^+ movement through Na^+ channels in cells of the ASDN. Because these drugs impair Na^+ movement along the ASDN, the lumen-negative transepithelial voltage decreases, thereby inhibiting K^+ secretion. This accounts for their potassium-sparing action. The second class is represented by spironolactone and eplerenone, competitive antagonists of mineralocorticosteroid receptors. Aldosterone stimulates Na^+ reabsorption and K^+ secretion along the ASDN and increases the lumen-negative transepithelial voltage. By inhibiting the action of aldosterone, these drugs cause mild natriuresis and K^+ retention. Spironolactone has troubling estrogenic side effects.[24]

Table 33-1   Commonly Prescribed Classes of Diuretic and Recommended Dose Range

Class of Diuretic	Available Dose Sizes	Daily Dose Range (Starting Dose to Maximum Recommended* Dose)
Carbonic Anhydrase Inhibitors		
Acetazolamine	125, 250, 500 mg	125–375 mg
Loop Diuretics		
Furosemide	20, 40, 500 mg; 1 mg/mL (pediatric); 10 mg/mL (injection)	20–500 mg
Bumetanide	1, 5; 1 mg/5 mL (liquid); 0.5 mg/mL (injection)	0.5–10 mg
Torsemide	5, 10, 20, 100 mg; 5 mg/mL (injection)	5–200 mg
Ethacrynic acid	50 mg; 50 mg (powder for injection)	25–400 mg
Distal Convoluted Tubule Diuretics		
Bendrofluazide	2.5, 5 mg	2.5–10 mg
Chlorothiazide	250, 500 mg	250–2000 mg
Cyclopenthiazide	25, 50 mg	25–100 mg
Hydrochlorothiazide	12.5, 25, 50 mg	12.5–200 mg
Hydroflumethiazide	50 mg	25–200 mg
Indapamide	1.25, 2.5 mg	1.25–5 mg
Methychlorthiazide	2.5, 5 mg	2.5–10 mg
Polythiazide	1, 2, 4 mg	0.5–4 mg
Chlorthalidone	15, 25, 50, 100 mg	15–200 mg
Mefruside	25 mg	12.5–100 mg
Metolazone	2.5, 5, 10 mg	2.5–10 mg (up to 150 mg has been used in renal failure)
Distal Potassium-Sparing Diuretics **Na$^+$ Channel Blockers**		
Amiloride	5 mg	5–20 mg
Triamterene	50, 100 mg	50–250 mg
Mineralocorticoid Antagonists		
Spironolactone	25, 50, 100 mg	50–400 mg
Eplerenone	25, 50, 100 mg	50–200 mg
Aquaretics		
Conivaptan (IV)	20-mg load, then 20–40 mg/day	20 mg/4 mL
Natriuretic Peptides		
Nesiritide (IV)	1.5 mg powder	2 μg/kg bolus, then 0.01–0.03 μg/kg/min
Osmotic Diuretics		
Mannitol (IV)	5, 10, 15, 20, 25%	25–200 g

*The maximum safe dose of most diuretics is rarely indicated or advantageous.

Eplerenone is a more selective aldosterone antagonist without these adverse effects.[25]

Natriuretic Peptides

Atrial natriuretic peptide (ANP) and B-type natriuretic peptide act at many sites in the kidney and elsewhere to decrease left atrial pressure and blood pressure and increase renal salt excretion. As shown in Figure 33-1, a major site of ANP action in the kidney is along the medullary collecting tubule. Natriuretic peptides are metabolized by endopeptidases. Drugs that inhibit neutral endopeptidase increase plasma ANP concentrations. In hypertensive patients, this decreases blood pressure, increases the GFR and renal Na^+ excretion, and decreases the plasma renin activity.[26] Nesiritide is a recombinant B-type natriuretic peptide that is approved for use in patients with decompensated heart failure.[27]

Osmotic Diuretics

Osmotic diuretics, such as mannitol, do not interfere directly with specific transport proteins but rather act as osmotic particles in tubule fluid. This inhibits both fluid and NaCl reabsorption (for more details, please see Ellison and Wilcox,[2] Better and colleagues,[28] and Warren and Blantz[29]). Thus, these drugs increase the excretion not only of fluid but also of Na^+, K^+, Cl^-, bicarbonate, and other solutes. The urinary osmolality during osmotic diuresis approaches that of plasma, regardless of the state of hydration. Osmotic diuretics increase renal blood flow and wash out the medullary solute gradient, effects that contribute to the diuretic-induced impairment in urinary concentrating capacity.

Aquaretics

Arginine vasopressin receptor antagonists (aquaretics) are new therapeutic agents to treat euvolemic and hypervolemic hyponatremia. Unlike the other diuretics discussed previously, these drugs enhance the excretion of electrolyte-free water by blocking arginine vasopressin binding to vasopressin receptors. In the kidney, vasopressin type 2 receptors (V_2 receptors) at the basolateral membrane of collecting duct cells transduce an increase in apical water permeability, thereby increasing water reabsorption; conversely, blocking this receptor increases water excretion when vasopressin is present. Conivaptan is the first aquaretic approved for clinical use in the United States. It is a combined V_2 and V_{1a} antagonist that is available only as an intravenous preparation. In a controlled trial of patients with euvolemic and hypervolemic hyponatremia, it caused a dose-dependent increase in serum sodium concentration (S_{Na}),[30] whereas in patients with heart failure, it increased urine volume and decreased the pulmonary capillary wedge pressure.[31] It is currently approved to treat both euvolemic and hypervolemic hyponatremia, but its route of administration means that its use is restricted to hospitalized patients. Although its nonselective properties make hypotension a potential side effect, owing to the blockade of vascular V1 receptors, this has not been prominent in clinical studies to date.

Orally active vasopressin receptor antagonists cause free water diuresis without appreciable natriuresis in water-deprived human subjects.[32] They increase urine volume, free water clearance, and S_{Na} in hyponatremic patients with syndrome of inappropriate secretion of antidiuretic hormone (SIADH).[33] One such agent, lixivaptan, is an oral vasopressin receptor antagonist that is selective for aquaretic (V_2) receptors and increases S_{Na} in patients with syndrome of inappropriate secretion of antidiuretic hormone, congestive heart failure (CHF), or cirrhosis.[34] Tolvaptan is another agent that has been subjected to controlled trials. When given to patients with heart failure, it increases the urine volume, decreases the body weight, and decreases edema at 7 days[35] and maintains the S_{Na} within the normal range for as long as 25 days.[36] In the second study of hospitalized patients with an ejection fraction less than 40%, it decreased the body weight on the first day. Although it did not modify CHF outcomes at 2 months, it corrected hyponatremia and appeared beneficial in subgroups of patients with azotemia or those with clinical signs of congestion at baseline. A recent study in patients with New York Heart Association class II to III CHF has shown that 30 mg tolvaptan produces a diuresis similar to that with 80 mg furosemide, but, unlike furosemide, does not increase renal Na^+ and K^+ excretion and does not decrease renal blood flow.[37] A recent large controlled international trial of tolvaptan in hospitalized patients with worsening heart failure failed to detect a decrease in long-term mortality or heart failure–related mortality over 9 months.[38] A third oral V_2 receptor antagonist, satavaptan, was effective in controlling S_{Na} for as long as 12 months in an open-label study.[39] Thus, arginine vasopressin antagonists appear to be an effective means to treat acute or chronic conditions associated with dilutional hyponatremia.

New Agents

Aminophylline is an adenosine receptor antagonist that inhibits NaCl reabsorption in the proximal tubule and diluting segments and causes a modest increase in GFR.[40] Highly selective adenosine type 1 receptor antagonists are natriuretic[41] and antihypertensive, and potentiate furosemide-induced natriuresis in normal humans[42] and in patients with diuretic-resistant CHF. Adenosine type 1 receptor antagonists disrupt glomerulotubular balance and tubuloglomerular feeedback, thereby decreasing proximal reabsorption and maintaining the GFR.[41]

PHARMACOKINETICS

Most diuretics in clinical use have their predominant site of action on the luminal membrane of the nephron. Therefore, to be effective, they must be absorbed across the gastrointestinal tract, reach the systemic circulation in active form, and be concentrated in tubular fluid; the final process usually requires secretion across the proximal tubule.[43]

Most diuretics are well absorbed. The bioavailability of furosemide is 50% to 69%,[2] whereas the bioavailability of bumetanide and torsemide is approximately 90% (Table 33-2). Loop diuretics circulate bound to albumin (95%–99%). Therefore, loop diuretics do not enter kidney tubules by glomerular filtration and instead undergo secretion along the proximal tubule. Carbonic anhydrase inhibitors, loop diuretics, and thiazides are weak organic anions (OA^-) that are taken up across the basolateral membrane of the proximal tubule by an organic anion transporter (OAT) (Fig. 33-2).[44] Four OAT genes are

Table 33-2 Pharmacokinetics of Diuretic Drugs

Diuretic	Oral Bioavailability (%)	ELIMINATION HALF-LIFE (HR)			
		Normal	CKD	Cirrhosis	Heart Failure
Loop Diuretics					
Furosemide	50	1.5–2	2.8	2.5	2.7
Bumetanide	90	1	1.6	2.3	1.3
Torsemide	90	3–4	4–5	8	6
DCT Diuretics					
Chlorthiazide	40	1.5	ND	ND	ND
Chlorthalidone	64	24–55	ND	ND	ND
Hydrochlorothiazide	70	2.5	↑	ND	ND
Hydroflumethiazide	73	6–25	ND	ND	6–28
Indapamide	93	15–25	ND	ND	ND
Polythiazide	ND	26	ND	ND	ND
Trichlormethiazide	ND	1–4	5–10	ND	ND
Potassium-Sparing Distal Diuretics					
Amiloride	CD	17–26	100	NC	ND
Triamterene	>80	2–5	Prolonged	NC	ND
Spironolactone	CD	1.5	NC	NC	ND
Active metabolites*		>15	ND	ND	ND

*Values for the active metabolite of spironolactone.
CD, conflicting data; CKD, chronic kidney disease; DCT, distal convoluted tubule; NC, no change; ND, not determined.
Data adapted from Brater DC: Diuretic therapy. N Engl J Med 1998;339:387–395.

expressed in the kidney.[44] OAT-1 and OAT-3 have been shown to have high affinity for loop, thiazide, and carbonic anhydrase diuretics[45,46]; genetic disruption of OAT-1 leads to furosemide resistance in mice, indicating that OAT-1 plays an important role in diuretic secretion by the proximal tubule.[44] OA transport across the basolateral cell membrane is a tertiary active system in which OAs are exchanged for intracellular α-ketoglutarate. The intracellular levels of α-ketoglutarate are kept high by a parallel cotransporter of Na^+/α-ketoglutarate. This uses the favorable electrochemical gradient for Na^+ created by the operation of the basolateral Na^+/K^+-ATPase and a negative membrane potential created by a basolateral K^+ conductase.

The luminal brush border secretory pathway for OA^- and diuretics is less well defined. Two mechanisms have been identified. One is a voltage-driven OAT^- that derives energy from the negative membrane potential.[47] This process can transport loop diuretics and thiazides in addition to p-aminohippurate and urate.[47] There is also an OA:urate/hydroxyl anion countertransport mechanism that could provide an exit route for diuretics from the proximal tubule cells.[44]

Several factors alter secretion of loop diuretics, thereby affecting their actions. Other OAs can compete with diuretics for transport by OAT. These include β-lactam and sulfonamide antibiotics, nonsteroidal anti-inflammatory drugs,[48] antiviral agents such as adefovir, p-aminohippurate, methotrexate, uric acid, and a number of endogenous organic anions.[49] In contrast, uptake of loop diuretics into the proximal tubule cells is stimulated by alkalosis[50] and by albumin across the range found in plasma.[51,52] Therefore, chronic kidney disease impairs loop diuretic secretion because of the

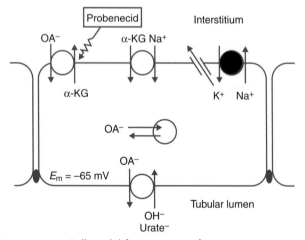

Figure 33-2 Cell model for secretion of organic anions (OA^-) by proximal tubule cells. For description, see text. Carbonic anhydrase, loop, and thiazide diuretics can all be transported by the organic anion transporter (OAT) in exchange for α-ketoglutarate (α-KG). E_m, membrane potential.

accumulation of OAs and urate, the development of acidosis, and often a decrease in serum albumin concentration.[53]

Approximately one half of an intravenous dose of furosemide is eliminated unchanged by the kidney, whereas one half is eliminated as the inactive glucuronide. In contrast, bumetanide and torsemide are not subjected to major glucuronidation, but instead are metabolized by a cytochrome P-450 process in the liver to inactive metabolites.[43,54] Thiazide diuretics are mostly excreted in active form. As noted, proximal tubule cells possess mechanisms to bioinactivate furosemide specifically.[55–57] Studies in experimental animals have shown that, after peritubular uptake into the early segment of the proximal tubule, furosemide is metabolized by uridine diphosphate-glucuronyl transferase to the inactive glucuronide, which is secreted into the proximal lumen.[58] In experimental animals, this uptake process is inhibited by serum albumin,[53] in contrast to the stimulation by albumin of the uptake process that transports active furosemide into the tubular lumen. Therefore, a decrease in serum albumin concentration may decrease the secretion of active furosemide and increase the renal uptake and metabolism to the inactive glucuronide. These studies in animals have yet to be confirmed by clinical investigation.

The relationship between the log of the plasma or urinary loop diuretic concentration and the fractional sodium excretion is normally sigmoidal (Fig. 33-3). This is analogous to a dose-response curve. Inhibition of proximal secretion with probenecid decreases diuretic secretion into the urine and natriuresis, but does not perturb the relationship between natriuresis and diuretic excretion. This is consistent with the effect of probenecid to inhibit diuretic secretion rather than blocking the diuretic action on the nephron.[49] A similar interaction occurs with indomethacin,[48] although the main effect of nonsteroidal anti-inflammatory drugs is to decrease the responsiveness of the tubule to furosemide.[48] This is predominantly the result of decreased generation of prostaglandin E2 because the natriuretic response to furosemide can be restored in indomethacin-treated rats by microperfusion of prostaglandin E2 into the nephron.[59] A reduced dietary salt intake and repeated administration of furosemide during salt restriction cause a shift in the natriuresis-drug concentration curve to the right and thereby diminish the natriuretic responsiveness to a unit delivery of diuretic to the tubule lumen.[60]

There are some pharmacokinetic differences between loop diuretics. Bumetanide is more extensively metabolized than furosemide, which accounts for its shorter half-life.[43] Torsemide is less extensively metabolized and more bioavailable than other loop diuretics and has a rather longer half-life.[54,61–63] The more lipid-soluble drugs (e.g., bendroflumethiazide and polythiazide) are more potent, have a more prolonged action, and are more extensively metabolized.[64] DCT diuretics are handled at the kidney similarly to loop diuretics.[64]

Of the distal potassium-sparing agents, triamterene is well absorbed. It is rapidly hydroxylated to metabolites that retain some diuretic activity.[65,66] The drug and its metabolite are excreted by the kidney, with a half-life of approximately 3 to 5 hours, which is delayed in renal failure.[67] Amiloride is incompletely absorbed. It is secreted in active form into tubular fluid.[68] It has a longer duration of action, approximately 18 hours. Spironolactone is an aldosterone antagonist. It is metabolized to active compounds (canrenones).[69,70] It is readily absorbed and bound to plasma proteins. Although spironolactone itself has a relatively short half-life, the half-life of pharmacologically active metabolites is approximately 20 hours, meaning that effects of spironolactone on serum potassium can persist for several days after discontinuation. Spironolactone takes as long as 48 hours to become fully effective.

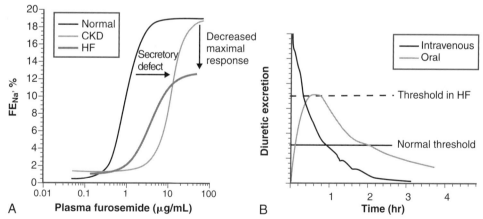

Figure 33-3   Dose-response curve for loop diuretics. **A,** The fractional Na$^+$ excretion (FE$_{Na}$) as a function of plasma loop diuretic concentration. Compared with normal subjects, patients with chronic kidney disease (CKD) show a rightward shift in the curve owing to impaired diuretic secretion. The maximal response is preserved when expressed as FE$_{Na}$ (but not when expressed as absolute Na$^+$ excretion). Patients with congestive heart failure (CHF) demonstrate a rightward and downward shift, even when expressed as FE$_{Na}$, and thus are relatively diuretic resistant. **B,** Comparison of the response to intravenous and oral doses of loop diuretics. In a normal individual (Normal), an oral dose may be as effective as an intravenous dose because the time above the natriuretic threshold (indicated by the Normal threshold line) is approximately equal. If the natriuretic threshold increases (as indicated by the Heart Failure threshold line), then the oral dose may not provide a high enough serum level to elicit natriuresis.

Nesiritide (B-type natriuretic peptide) is approved only for intravenous use. It exhibits biphasic disposition from the plasma. The mean terminal half-life is approximately 18 minutes. The mean initial half-life is approximately 2 minutes.

CLINICAL USE OF DIURETICS

A general approach to diuretic treatment of edema and diuretic resistance is presented in Figure 33-4. Use of diuretics to treat specific disorders is discussed in the following.

Acute Renal Failure

Acute renal failure is frequently associated with a decrease in urine output. Obstruction of kidney tubules by casts and sloughed cells can contribute to renal dysfunction. Patients who develop oliguria in the setting of acute renal failure have mortality rates that are higher than those in whom oliguria does not develop. For all these reasons, diuretic drugs have been used commonly in attempts to prevent or treat acute renal failure[71] (see also Chapter 3). However, a review of 11 randomized trials found no benefit of loop

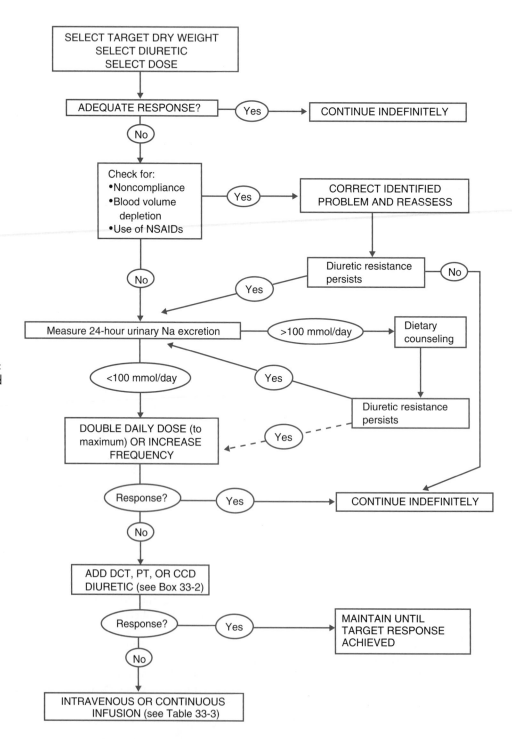

Figure 33-4 Algorithm for treating patients with ascites. TIPS, transjugular intrahepatic portosystemic shunting. Based in part on recommendations of Runyon.[136]

diuretics or mannitol for the prevention or treatment of acute renal failure.[71]

Prevention

Several studies have examined the ability of diuretics, including mannitol, to prevent renal failure in high-risk situations. Mannitol decreases the risk of acute renal failure after renal transplantation.[72] Mannitol is also commonly used as prophylaxis for patients undergoing vascular surgery, although data in support of its efficacy are mixed.[73] Mannitol may also be effective as part of a regimen of forced alkaline diuresis in the setting of crush injuries and rhabdomyolysis,[74] although controlled studies are not available. In a subset of patients with diabetic kidney disease, mannitol was found to decrease the likelihood of acute renal failure after cardiac catheterization, but the number of patients studied was small.[75] Conversely, in several situations, mannitol provides no prophylactic benefit. In a well-controlled study of radiocontrast-induced acute renal failure, both mannitol and furosemide were inferior to 0.45% NaCl as prophylaxis.[76] Furthermore, mannitol itself may induce acute renal failure.[77] In reviewing data concerning mannitol and acute renal failure, Conger[73] concluded that mannitol has an established role only in preventing primary transplant dysfunction. Most clinicians would also use mannitol (initial dose of 12.5 g followed by 50–100 g/24–48 hr) to prevent myoglobinuric acute renal failure.

Furosemide does not appear to have a role in prophylaxis for radiocontrast-induced acute renal failure.[76] Lassnigg and colleagues[78] reported that neither dopamine nor furosemide was superior to saline to prevent renal failure after cardiac surgery. Thus, loop diuretics are not indicated for prophylaxis for acute renal failure.

Treatment

High doses of loop diuretics (2–15 mg/kg) can increase urine output in some patients with oliguric acute renal failure.[79,80] This may be a useful effect because increasing water and electrolyte excretion makes controlling extracellular fluid (ECF) volume easier. Although initial reports showed that patients whose urine output increases after diuretic administration have lower mortality than those whose output does not increase, the effect is not causal. Shilliday and colleagues[81] randomized 92 patients with acute renal failure to either loop diuretics or placebo. All patients received dopamine and mannitol. The results showed that loop diuretics significantly increased urine output, but did not affect the requirement for dialysis or the time until renal recovery. These data suggest that a positive response to diuretics identifies a less severely affected subgroup of patients. A cohort study of patients in intensive care units with acute renal failure showed a positive association between diuretic use and mortality, raising the possibility that these drugs may have adverse effects in this clinical setting.[82] A subsequent randomized, controlled study of dialysis-dependent patients with acute renal failure did not show a significant effect of diuretics on mortality.[83] These conflicting results and the continuing use of diuretics in this clinical setting have led to calls for larger multicenter randomized trials.[84]

High-dose loop diuretic infusion in the setting of acute renal failure is not necessarily benign. In one study, deafness occurred in 3.4% of patients treated with high doses of furosemide (3 g/day in addition to an initial bolus).[85] Renal failure

impairs metabolic clearance of loop diuretics, especially furosemide. Thus, renal failure is a risk factor for loop diuretic–induced ototoxicity.

To summarize, several studies indicate that loop diuretics can increase urine output in the setting of oliguric acute renal failure. Continuous infusion may be especially effective in this regard. Despite increasing urine output, there is no evidence that loop diuretics (or mannitol) improve prognosis, lessen the need for dialysis, or speed recovery from acute renal failure. Some investigators recommend a trial of loop diuretics for patients with oliguric acute renal failure to attempt to increase urine output. If diuresis does not ensue or if excessive doses are required, diuretic treatment should be stopped. One protocol is to give 40 mg furosemide, 1 mg bumetanide, or 25 mg torsemide IV and to double the dose every hour if there is no response to a total daily dose of 1 g furosemide or equivalent.[71] Bumetanide or torsemide are hepatically metabolized and therefore may be preferred to furosemide, which is metabolized by the kidney and accumulates to a greater degree in patients with renal insufficiency.

In experimental animals, ANP speeds recovery from a renal insult.[86] Unfortunately, this effect was not replicated in a trial of acute renal failure in humans,[87] although a subgroup analysis suggested a beneficial effect in oliguric patients. At this time, ANP cannot be recommended to treat patients with acute renal failure.

Chronic Renal Insufficiency

This has been reviewed recently.[88,89] Sodium and water retention occurs very commonly in the setting of chronic kidney disease. Dietary NaCl restriction is important to control hypertension and edema, but diuretic therapy is often necessary. Loop diuretics are preferred because DCT diuretics alone are usually ineffective when the GFR is less than 30 mL/min and distal potassium-sparing diuretics can cause serious hyperkalemia and acidosis in patients with renal insufficiency.

The ability of loop diuretics to increase fractional Na^+ excretion (FE_{Na}) is preserved as the GFR decreases (see Fig. 33-3).[62,90,91] This indicates that the absolute increase in renal Na^+ excretion elicited by a ceiling dose of loop diuretic decreases in proportion to the decrease in the GFR. In addition, the dose of drug required to achieve a given increment in NaCl excretion in chronic kidney disease increases because accumulated organic acids compete with diuretics for proximal tubule secretion, as shown in Figure 33-3. When the GFR is 15 mL/min, only one fifth to one tenth as much loop diuretic is secreted as in a normal individual.[62]

Patients with chronic renal insufficiency, however, usually do remain responsive to loop diuretics, even when the GFR is as low as 10 to 15 mL/min, providing they are prescribed at a higher dose. DCT diuretics, conversely, are relatively ineffective for patients whose GFRs are less than 30 mL/min when they are administered by themselves. However, these drugs remain effective in renal failure when added to a regimen that includes a loop diuretic, as discussed later,[91] but at the cost of a sharp further increase in the serum creatinine and blood urea nitrogen concentrations and a high incidence of hypokalemia and electrolyte disorders.[92] For refractory patients, a loop diuretic infusion (e.g., bumetanide, 1 mg/hr for 12 hours) produces a greater natriuresis and less myalgia than two bolus injections.[93]

Nephrotic Syndrome

Nephrotic syndrome is a combination of proteinuria of 3.5 g/24 hr or more, hypoalbuminemia, and edema. Hypoalbuminemia may contribute to edema by reducing plasma oncotic pressure and permitting a shift of fluid out of the capillaries and into the interstitium. In this case, one would anticipate that the plasma volume would be lower than normal.[94] Although this mechanism may be of central importance for patients with minimal change nephropathy or severe hypoalbuminemia,[95] many nephrotic patients do not show evidence of plasma volume depletion. This has led to an alternative "overflow hypothesis," which posits that primary renal salt retention underlies the edema of nephrotic syndrome.[96,97] Evidence in support of this hypothesis includes observations that the sympathetic nervous system and the renin-angiotensin-aldosterone axis are often not strongly stimulated in nephrotic patients, as would be expected if they had a decreased blood volume,[98,99] that many such patients are hypertensive, and that natriuresis during treatment often begins before plasma oncotic pressure increases. Yet, primary renal salt retention alone causes hypertension but not edema because escape occurs.[100] Thus, it seems likely that fluid shift out of the vascular tree is a necessary component of nephrotic edema.[94] In many patients, and especially in diabetic nephrosis, primary renal salt retention plays an important role.

Regardless of the mechanism, diuretics are important for treating nephrotic edema. As with other causes of edema, dietary salt restriction plays a central role in treatment. Because most nephrotic patients are significantly diuretic resistant,[62] DCT diuretics are generally not used as first-line agents. Loop diuretics, such as furosemide 40 to 60 mg/day, can be administered orally and increased to a maximum of 240 mg/day as single or divided doses.

Intravenous albumin has been used to treat nephrotic edema for more than 50 years. Early work showed that some nephrotic patients achieve natriuresis with albumin alone, presumably because plasma volume increases.[101] After loop diuretics were introduced into clinical practice, albumin was no longer used by itself because diuretic drugs were found to be more effective. Nevertheless, despite concerns about efficacy, safety, and expense, the combination of albumin and loop diuretics is commonly used to treat nephrotic edema, especially in pediatric patients. Controlled studies in adults suggest that albumin may potentiate diuresis or natriuresis when combined with a loop diuretic, but only modestly.[102–104] Studies in children, in whom the diagnosis is often minimal change nephropathy, suggest that combined loop diuretics and albumin infusion effectively reduce ECF volume.[105,106] This effect is transient, unless remission is achieved, and complications are common. Several concepts for rational albumin use can be advanced. First, the therapeutic approach should be based on a careful assessment of the vascular volume. Many adult patients or those with diabetes or focal and segmental glomerulosclerosis have ECF volume expansion. In this setting, albumin use should be discouraged.[102,106,107] In contrast, for patients who appear to be volume depleted, especially patients with minimal change disease and profound hypoalbuminemia, albumin may be indicated. For children, albumin is generally administered as a 25% solution (1 g/kg body weight for 1–4 hours) together with furosemide 1.5 mg/kg. Such treatment has been reported to induce a 0.4-kg weight loss per infusion and can be repeated five or more times.[105,108]

Hypoalbuminemia decreases the binding of furosemide to plasma proteins and thereby increases its volume of distribution.[109] Although one study reported that premixing furosemide with 6 g albumin in the syringe before intravenous injection enhanced the diuresis of patients with the nephrotic syndrome,[110] this has not been confirmed.[102,103,111] Indeed, two studies have shown that patients with a serum albumin of 2 g/100 dL can deliver normal quantities of furosemide into the urine.[109,112] Although diuretic resistance in nephrotic patients can result from impairments in diuretic delivery into tubular fluid, patients with nephrotic syndrome usually demonstrate normal diuretic clearance,[113] suggesting that other mechanisms predominate. Diuretics may bind to albumin in the tubule lumen. Kirchner and colleagues[114] showed that albumin in tubule fluid blunts the ability of loop diuretics to inhibit Na^+ and Cl^- transport. In animal models, inhibiting diuretic binding restores a normal response, but a study in human nephrotic syndrome suggests that this is not a predominant mechanism. Thus, binding inhibitors should not be considered therapeutic options.[113]

Heart Failure

Heart failure affects 5 million people in the United States. General aspects of heart failure diagnosis and treatment are beyond the scope of this chapter (see Consensus Recommendations for the Management of Chronic Heart Failure[115]). The following discussion focuses on the role of diuretics in treating heart failure. Systolic dysfunction (left ventricular ejection fraction ≤40%) is the best understood form of heart failure. When left ventricular function is impaired, cardiac output decreases. This leads to a decrease in mean arterial pressure and activation of neurohumoral systems, including the renin-angiotensin-aldosterone axis, which, together with other factors, lead to salt and fluid retention, with resulting symptoms of dyspnea, exercise intolerance, and edema.[116]

Diuretic drugs have been used to treat CHF for more than 500 years. It is clear that, except in mild cases, most patients with CHF require diuretic treatment to control symptoms of fluid overload. It is not possible to conduct placebo-controlled trials to determine whether diuretics reduce mortality. However, a meta-analysis of trials in CHF concluded that diuretics decreased the odds ratio for death to 0.25 and for hospitalization to 0.31.[117] Results of the recent Antihypertensive and Lipid-Lowering Treatment to Prevent Heart Attack Trial in hypertensive subjects show that randomization to a thiazide diuretic decreases the risk of hospitalization or dying of heart failure compared with an angiotensin-converting enzyme inhibitor (ACEI) or a calcium channel blocker.[118] Early attempts to withdraw diuretics and treat CHF ACEIs alone frequently led to recrudescence of volume overload.[119] However, because diuretics have not been shown to affect mortality except in the Antihypertensive and Lipid-Lowering Treatment to Prevent Heart Attack Trial, they should not be employed as monotherapy for patients with systolic dysfunction. Instead, they should be used for symptomatic control as supplementary but essential agents. They should always be combined with moderate restriction of dietary Na^+ (approximately 2 g Na^+/day).

The goal of diuretic treatment of CHF is to eliminate symptoms and signs of fluid retention.[115,120,121] Azotemia or symptomatic hypotension should prompt a slowing or temporary cessation of diuretic treatment. Once the patient has stabilized, additional attempts to control ECF volume expansion should be made. The dry weight can be estimated as the weight at which symptoms of orthopnea and paroxysmal nocturnal dyspnea disappear, the jugular venous pressure returns to normal, and edema disappears. Once this weight is determined, diuretic therapy is adjusted to achieve this weight. The GFR should be expected to decrease modestly (10%–20%) as the patient achieves dry weight.

Either thiazides[62] or loop diuretics can be used for mild CHF.[122] The efficacy and safety of loop and DCT diuretics appear to be similar.[123–125] A lower incidence of postural hypotension has been reported when treating elderly patients with loop rather than DCT diuretics,[126] but other studies suggest that DCT diuretics are tolerated better.[125]

A dose of 25 to 50 mg/day of hydrochlorothiazide can be used to treat patients with mild heart failure. For patients with more severe disease and normal renal function, a typical regimen is 20 mg furosemide twice daily.[62] Because the dose-response curve for loop diuretics is steep, it is important to ensure that the chosen dose exceeds the diuretic threshold. This is established by doubling the diuretic dose until a clear natriuretic response ensues or a safe maximal dose is obtained. Most ambulatory patients can detect such an effect within 4 hours and can identify the effective dose in this manner. Thereafter, furosemide can be administered two times or more daily to ensure adequate contraction of the ECF volume. There is sufficient postdiuretic salt retention after a short-acting loop diuretic that it is difficult to achieve a negative salt balance if the diuretic is given once daily unless dietary salt is very severely restricted.[60] Therefore, patients unable to restrict dietary salt intake require more frequent dosing. Indeed, during high salt intake, furosemide may fail to contract the ECF volume because postdiuretic NaCl retention overcomes initial natriuresis.[60]

Patients with uncompensated congestive heart failure may develop diuretic resistance owing to impaired diuretic absorption across the gastrointestinal tract (see Fig. 33-3). Brater[127] showed that absorption of furosemide and bumetanide is slowed in CHF, leading to a 50% decrease in peak urinary diuretic concentrations. In contrast, the bioavailability (which is the percentage of total dose absorbed in active form) is unchanged.[128] Inasmuch as loop diuretics must achieve a critical threshold concentration to inhibit salt transport effectively, slowed gastrointestinal absorption may lead to diuretic resistance. This provides some rationale for intravenous diuretic therapy in patients resistant to oral agents. Absorption generally improves with clearance of edema.[129] Bowel wall edema, impaired gastrointestinal motility, and altered bowel wall perfusion may all contribute to delayed diuretic absorption.

Nesiritide is a recombinant human B-type natriuretic peptide that was approved by the U.S. Food and Drug Administration for the treatment of acute decompensated CHF.[130] Studies of natriuretic peptide receptor A–deficient mice implicate this system in the natriuretic response to blood volume expression[131] and provide a rationale for B-type natriuretic peptide in the treatment of decompensated CHF. Nesiritide given short term to patients with decompensated CHF can decrease the pulmonary capillary wedge pressure.[27] However, subsequent studies have shown that nesiritide is not a diuretic in patients with chronic heart failure and, when compared with placebo, may increase the risk of death and worsening renal function.[132–134] Until more data are available, nesiritide cannot be recommended as a primary therapy for decompensated CHF.

Cirrhosis and Ascites

Ascites, which commonly accompanies hepatic cirrhosis, results primarily from three mutually reinforcing processes. First, systemic and splanchnic vasodilation reduce the effective arterial pressure (predominantly determined by the mean arterial pressure), leading to renal salt retention. Second, fluid transudes from the plasma to the interstitium owing to hypoalbuminemia and vasodilation. Third, increased blood volume and portal resistance lead to portal hypertension. Together, these processes lead to ECF volume expansion, with a predominance of fluid in the peritoneal cavity (ascites).[116,135]

Nonhepatic causes of ascites may be responsible in as many as 20% of cases (such as peritoneal carcinomatosis). These do not respond to diuretic treatment. An algorithm for treating cirrhotic ascites is shown in Figure 33-4. The first component is abstinence from alcohol, which decreases portal pressure in some patients.[136] The second factor is to restrict the dietary Na^+ intake to 2 g/day (86 mEq/day). A more severe Na^+ restriction will promote a more rapid decrease in ECF volume, but is considerably less palatable. Restricting water intake is usually not necessary, unless the serum Na^+ level is less than 120 mmol/L. Bed rest is not generally recommended.

For patients with tense ascites, large-volume (4–6 L) paracentesis is usually indicated. This treatment is usually tolerated well, improves well-being, and leads to rapid resolution of ascites,[137] although the prognosis is not affected. The use of colloid during or after paracentesis remains a subject of debate.[138–140] Many investigators suggest that a single paracentesis of 4 to 6 L can be tolerated without administering albumin, if edema is present. If there is no edema and if paracentesis is repeated, then albumin (25–50 g) can be administered.[136] Following paracentesis, diuretics must be continued to decrease reaccumulation of edema.[141]

Although large-volume paracentesis has assumed an important role in treating patients with tense ascites, approximately 90% of patients with ascites can be controlled with diuretics and salt restriction.[142] Thus, practice guidelines approved by the American Association for the Study of Liver Disease emphasize the primary role of diuretics to treat cirrhotic ascites. Spironolactone has traditionally been the drug of choice. Concerns about hyperkalemia, slow onset of action, half-life, and side effects have prompted investigation of other agents for these patients. Amiloride does not induce painful gynecomastia, as does spironolactone, but is less effective.[143] In randomized, controlled trials, spironolactone was also shown to be more effective than furosemide when given alone and had a lower incidence of side effects.[144,145] When ascites is mild, spironolactone may be administered at 25 to 50 mg/day or eplerenone at 50 to 100 mg/day. There is no pharmacokinetic justification for the common practice of administering spironolactone more than once daily.[146] When ascites is more pronounced, spironolactone or eplerenone is usually initiated together with furosemide. A regimen of spironolactone and furosemide, in a ratio of 100 mg to 40 mg, has been found empirically to lead to the highest ratio of efficacy to side effects.[136] The rapid onset of furosemide action initiates diuresis before the peak effect of spironolactone action (at approximately 2 weeks[144]). Spironolactone attenuates furosemide-induced hypokalemia and alkalosis, which can precipitate encephalopathy. Furosemide attenuates spironolactone-induced hyperkalemia. Doses can be increased to a maximum of 400 mg spironolactone/160 mg furosemide. Furosemide can be withheld initially from hypokalemic patients. Conversely, spironolactone must be used carefully for patients with intrinsic renal disease, especially diabetic nephropathy. Eplerenone, a more selective aldosterone antagonist, is more expensive, equally effective, but does not have estrogenic side effects.

Treatment is documented by daily weight loss. For patients who have peripheral edema, there is no ceiling for daily weight loss. For patients without edema, daily weight losses should not exceed 0.5 kg.[147] Severe hyponatremia (<120 mmol/L), prerenal azotemia (creatinine > 2.0 mg/dL), or encephalopathy should prompt cessation of diuretics.

Patients who are refractory to diuretic treatment or who require repeated paracenteses should be considered for transjugular intrahepatic portosystemic shunting.[148] A recent systematic meta-analysis concluded that transjugular intrahepatic portosystemic shunting is more effective at removing ascites compared with paracentesis without a significant difference in mortality, gastrointestinal bleeding, infection, and acute renal failure. However, transjugular intrahepatic portosystemic shunting patients develop hepatic encephalopathy significantly more often than patients treated with paracentesis.[149] Definitive therapy of cirrhotic ascites often involves liver transplantation.

Idiopathic Edema

Idiopathic edema is diagnosed by excluding other systemic and local (venous, lymphatic, and neural) causes.[150] The classic features of idiopathic edema include periodic swelling of the legs, hands, and face and abdominal bloating, occurring almost exclusively in women. Idiopathic edema is frequently associated with eating disorders. When present in obese individuals, it often disappears or improves if weight is lost. Many patients with idiopathic edema are already taking diuretics when first evaluated. Diuretic abuse may be a component of the disorder.[151,152] It is not clear whether diuretics should be used as treatment. A low-salt diet should be prescribed, and adherence to the prescribed regimen can be confirmed by measuring renal sodium excretion. If diuretics are used, they may be given at night, when they may be more effective. Spironolactone is a good choice because its action is prolonged, making rebound edema less of a problem and because it prevents the effects of secondary hyperaldosteronism. Potassium-sparing diuretics such as amiloride will also help to address the hypokalemia that frequently accompanies idiopathic edema. Unfortunately, diuretics usually fail to control the edema.[150]

TOXICITY AND USE IN SPECIAL CIRCUMSTANCES

The main metabolic adverse effects of diuretics are listed in Box 33-1; these and other adverse side effects are discussed elsewhere in more detail.[2] Toxic effects can be divided into metabolic effects, which are often dose related, and idiosyncratic effects, which are dose independent. The latter usually manifest as allergic sulfonamide-like skin reactions that can occasionally develop into severe and life-threatening Stevens-Johnson syndrome.[153–155]

Box 33-1 Adverse and Clinically Useful Metabolic Effects of Diuretics

DCT Diuretics	Loop Diuretics	Potassium-sparing Distal Diuretics
Hypokalemia	Hypokalemia	Hyperkalemia
Hyponatremia	Hyperglycemia	Metabolic acidosis
Hyperglycemia	Hyperlipidemia	Hypomagnesuria
Hyperlipidemia	Metabolic alkalosis	
Metabolic alkalosis	Hypercalciuria	
Hypocalciuria and hypercalcemia	Hypocalciuria	
Hypermagnesuria	Hypermagnesuria	
Hyperuricemia		

DCT, distal convoluted tubule.

Azotemia and Extracellular Fluid Volume Depletion

Diuretics are frequently administered to treat edema, which can result in a decrease in the effective arterial blood volume. Overzealous diuretic use or intercurrent complicating illnesses can lead to excessive contraction of the intravascular volume, orthostatic hypotension, renal dysfunction, and sympathetic overactivity. Although patients with CHF usually require diuretic therapy, the combination of diuretics and ACEIs is especially likely to cause renal dysfunction. High diuretic doses or extreme dietary NaCl restriction may predispose to renal dysfunction during therapy with diuretics and ACEIs for CHF.[156,157] It is important to attempt to continue ACEIs because they are shown to decrease mortality. Functional renal failure in such patients often responds to a decrease in diuretic dose or a liberalization in dietary NaCl intake. Other patients at increased risk for relative contraction of the intravascular volume during loop diuretic therapy include the elderly,[158] patients with preexisting renal insufficiency,[159] patients with right-sided heart failure or pericardial disease, and patients taking nonsteroidal anti-inflammatory drugs.

Hypokalemia

Hypokalemia occurs commonly during therapy with both loop and DCT diuretics. A decline in serum K^+ concentration is common in patients given DCT diuretics, but most patients do not become frankly hypokalemic.[160] The clinical significance of diuretic-induced hypokalemia continues to be debated.[161–167] Hypokalemia may be more common during treatment with long-acting DCT diuretics, such as chlorthalidone, than with shorter acting DCT diuretics, such as hydrochlorothiazide, or with the very short acting loop diuretics.[168] DCT diuretics also increase renal Mg^{2+} excretion and can lead to hypomagnesemia, which contributes to the hypokalemia observed under these conditions.[169,170] Some studies suggest that maintenance magnesium therapy can prevent or attenuate the development of hypokalemia,[171] but this has not been supported universally. Hypokalemia also occurs commonly during therapy with loop diuretics, although the magnitude is smaller than that induced by DCT diuretics (loop diuretics 0.3 mmol/L compared with DCT diuretics 0.5–0.9

mmol/L[168,172]). During prolonged therapy with loop diuretics, the degree of potassium wasting correlates best with volume contraction and serum aldosterone levels.[173]

Hyponatremia

Diuretics have been reported to contribute to more than one half of all hospitalizations for serious hyponatremia. Potentially life-threatening hyponatremia is relatively common during treatment with DCT diuretics.[174] Several factors contribute. DCT diuretics inhibit solute transport in the diluting segment of the kidney, can reduce the GFR, contract the ECF volume, and lead to hypokalemia.[175] Hyponatremia is less common with loop diuretics because these drugs block the concentrating mechanism. In fact, loop diuretics can be used to treat hyponatremia, when combined with hypertonic saline, for the SIADH.[176,177] The combination of loop diuretics and ACEIs can correct hyponatremia in the setting of heart failure.[178]

Glucose Intolerance

Glucose intolerance is a dose-related complication of DCT diuretic use.[179,180] The pathogenesis remains unclear, but several contributory factors have been suggested.[181] First, diuretic-induced hypokalemia may decrease insulin secretion by the pancreas via effects on the membrane voltage of pancreatic beta cells. Prevention of hypokalemia by oral potassium supplementation normalizes the insulin response to hyperglycemia.[182] Hypokalemia interferes with insulin-mediated glucose uptake by muscle, but most patients demonstrate relatively normal insulin sensitivity.[183] Recently, it has been suggested that DCT diuretics directly activate calcium- or adenosine triphosphate–activated potassium channels on pancreatic beta cells that inhibit insulin secretion.[184] In a large randomized study, fasting glucose was not significantly different after 4 years of treatment with chlorthalidone versus amlodipine.[185]

Hyperlipidemia

DCT diuretics increase levels of total cholesterol, total triglyceride, and low-density lipoprotein cholesterol and reduce high-density lipoprotein.[183] Definitive information about the mechanisms by which DCT diuretics alter lipid metabolism is not available, but many of the mechanisms that affect glucose homeostasis have been suggested to contribute. Hyperlipidemia, like hyperglycemia, is a dose-related side effect and one that wanes with time.[186] In some clinical studies, the effect of low-dose DCT diuretic treatment on serum low-density lipoprotein was not significantly different from that of placebo,[187] whereas in others, total cholesterol was higher during diuretic treatment (1.6 mg/dL higher, $P = .009$, in the group treated with chlorthalidone than amlodipine).[185] Hypertension treatment with DCT diuretics has now been shown clearly to reduce the risk of stroke, coronary heart disease, CHF, and cardiovascular mortality.[188]

Metabolic Alkalosis

Diuretics cause metabolic alkalosis via several mechanisms. They increase the excretion of bicarbonate-free acidic urine and stimulate the renin-angiotensin-aldosterone pathway. Al-dosterone stimulates H^+ secretion by the medullary collecting tubule[189] and increases the magnitude of the transepithelial voltage in the ASDN. Hypokalemia contributes to metabolic alkalosis by increasing ammonium production,[190] stimulating bicarbonate reabsorption by proximal tubules,[191,192] and increasing the activity of the H^+/K^+-ATPase in the distal nephron.[193] Finally, contraction of the ECF volume stimulates Na^+/H^+ exchange in the proximal tubule and may decrease the filtered load of bicarbonate. All these factors may contribute to the metabolic alkalosis observed during chronic loop diuretic treatment.

Hyperuricemia and Gout

Thiazide and loop diuretics increase the plasma uric acid concentration because they reduce the ECF volume and increase the proximal tubule fluid reabsorption. They also compete with the urate secretory mechanism. Thus, they can aggravate or precipitate gout.

Ototoxicity

Ototoxicity is the most common toxic effect of loop diuretics unrelated to their effects on the kidney. Deafness, although usually temporary, can be permanent.[194,195] All loop diuretics can cause ototoxicity.[194,195] The mechanism involves inhibition of the secretory isoform of the $Na^+/K^+/2Cl^-$ in the stria vascularis.[196-199] Ototoxicity appears to be related to the peak serum concentration of loop diuretics and therefore tends to occur during rapid drug infusion of high doses. For this reason, this complication is most common in patients with uremia.[200] Furosemide infusion should be limited to 240 mg/hr.[201] The incidence is higher in patients with renal failure and cirrhosis and in those receiving aminoglycosides or cisplatin, as well as in infants.[200]

Impotence

Impotence is a common side effect of thiazide diuretics[202] and responds to sildenafil.[203]

DIURETIC RESISTANCE

General Causes

Resistance to a diuretic implies an inadequate reduction in ECF volume during treatment with moderate to high diuretic doses. The evaluation and management of diuretic resistance are summarized in Table 33-3 and Figure 33-4.

The first step is to ensure that the patient has renal edema. This must be differentiated from lymphatic or venous obstruction, from idiopathic edema, or from a complication of therapy, such as with a calcium entry blocker that redistributes fluid from the plasma to the interstitial compartment.

The second step is to assess compliance. Therapy with a loop diuretic or thiazide is almost invariably accompanied by a decrease in serum K^+ concentration and an increase in plasma bicarbonate and urate concentrations. Therefore, failure to detect these changes from pretreatment values suggests noncompliance. Noncompliance with the diuretic prescription often results from adverse effects, including impotence. However, the most common cause of resistance to diuretics is

Table 33-3   Identification and Management of General Causes of Diuretic Resistance

Cause or Example	Identification	Management
Nonrenal Edema		
Lymphatic or venous obstruction	Diagnose from clinical history and examination	Institute appropriate nondiuretic therapy
Cyclic edema	Ask about periodicity (women)	Institute appropriate therapy
CCB therapy	Obtain drug history	Reduce dose of CCB, substitute another agent, or add an ACEI
Noncompliance		
With diuretic prescription	Check for decrease in S_K, increase in plasma HCO_3 and urate levels with loop or thiazide therapy; urinary diuretic screen	Counsel patient and ask direct questions concerning adverse effects and problems with impotence
With diet	Measure 24-hr Na^+ excretion, corrected for creatinine excretion. Goal (mmol Na^+/24 hr) is: mild hypertension or edema, <100; severe hypertension or edema, <80	Obtain dietary consultation; repeat 24-hr urine to ensure that problem is corrected
Pharmacokinetic Alterations		
Incomplete or delayed absorption	Measure plasma levels	Change to more bioavailable drug, increase does or administer intravenously
Decreased renal function	Quantify GFR	Increase dose in proportion to decrease in GFR
Pharmacodynamic Alterations		
Edematous states	Clinical examination	Increase diuretic dose
Activation of RAA axis	Measure PRA	Consider ACEI, AT_1 antagonist, or spironolactone
Intranephronal adaptation to primary diuretic		Consider concurrent use of second diuretic
Adverse Drug Interactions		
NSAIDs	Obtain drug history	Decrease dose or discontinue NSAIDs

ACEI, angiotensin-converting enzyme inhibitor; AT_1, angiotensin I receptor blocker; CCB, calcium entry blockers; GFR, glomerular filtration rate; NSAIDs, nonsteroidal anti-inflammatory drugs; PRA, plasma renin activity; RAA, renin-angiotensin axis; S_k, serum potassium concentration.

failure to comply with restriction of NaCl intake. For patients with mild edema, a diet with no added salt, using a KCl substitute, and abstinence from salted or canned foods is usually sufficient to reduce Na^+ intake to a target of 100 mmol/24 hr (2.3 g Na^+/24 hr). For patients with diuretic resistance or severe edema, the help of a dietitian is necessary to reduce daily Na^+ intake to levels of 80 mmol or less. Dietary Na^+ compliance can be assessed by a 24-hour urine collection for Na^+ excretion (with concurrent estimation of creatinine to judge the adequacy of the collection), providing the patient is stable and has not just started or stopped diuretic therapy.

The third step is to search for pharmacokinetic or pharmacodynamic limitations of diuretic action. Diuretic absorption in patients with severe edema may be incomplete or delayed because of edema or poor blood flow to the intestines. A decrease in the GFR limits the fraction of diuretic eliminated in active form via the tubular lumen. Doses of loop diuretics should be increased in proportion to the decrease in GFR. Patients with severe edema typically exhibit diuretic resistance because of

salt-retaining mechanisms in nephron segments whose reabsorptive processes are not blocked by the diuretic. There may be pronounced activation of the renin-angiotensin-aldosterone axis that can be assessed by measurement of plasma renin activity and that is caused by the combined actions of the underlying disease state and the diuretic. Intranephronal adaptations occur during diuretic therapy that enhance reabsorption at other sites. This can be addressed rationally by adding a second diuretic, as described in the following. Finally, nonsteroidal anti-inflammatory drugs can limit both the natriuretic and antihypertensive action of diuretics.

Therapeutic Approaches

High-Dose and Intravenous Diuretic Therapy

High doses of loop diuretics are frequently used to treat severe volume overload, especially when treatment is urgent. Ceiling doses of furosemide, bumetanide, and torsemide have been estimated (Table 33-4). When given as a bolus, ceiling doses of furosemide range from 80 mg IV in hepatic cirrhosis to 500 mg IV in severe acute renal failure. The ceiling dose is that which provides maximal inhibition of the $Na^+/K^+/2Cl^-$ co-transporter, thereby reaching the plateau of the loop diuretic dose-response curve. Administering doses above the ceiling may increase 24-hour NaCl excretion because the time during which the urinary diuretic concentration is above the natriuretic threshold is prolonged. However, the effects of higher doses are marginal. It is better to increase the frequency of administration rather than administer extremely large doses.

High doses of loop diuretics given intravenously lead to capacitance vessel vasodilation that may be useful in patients with CHF who experience symptomatic relief before significant volume and NaCl losses have occurred. In one study,[204] patients with ECF volume expansion after an acute myocardial infarction experienced a decrease in left ventricular filling pressure and an improvement in dyspnea within 5 to 15 minutes of receiving 0.5 to 1.0 mg/kg of intravenous furosemide. The early decrease in left ventricular filling pressure resulted from increased venous capacitance rather than diuresis. Pretreatment of animals with indomethacin greatly attenuates furosemide-induced venodilation, suggesting that prostaglandin secretion contributes importantly to the effects of loop diuretics on vascular tone.[205]

Although venodilation and improvements in cardiac hemodynamics frequently result from intravenous loop diuretic therapy in acute left ventricular failure, other reports indicate that the hemodynamic response may be more complex. Loop diuretics stimulate renin secretion both by activating the macula densa mechanism and by reducing ECF volume. In two series, 1.0- to 1.5-mg/kg furosemide boluses, administered to patients with chronic CHF, resulted in transient deterioration in hemodynamics (during the first hour), with a decrease in stroke volume index, an increase in left ventricular filling pressure, and exacerbation of CHF symptoms.[206,207] These changes were attributed to activation of the renin-angiotensin system because ACEIs attenuated the pressor response. Johnston and colleagues[208] reported that low-dose intravenous furosemide increased venous capacitance but that higher doses did not,

perhaps because angiotensin II generation overwhelms the prostaglandin-mediated vasodilatory effects. Nevertheless, intravenous loop diuretics remain the primary therapy for patients in acute pulmonary edema because symptoms usually do improve before natriuresis, suggesting that, even when cardiac output decreases, most patients experience a rapid decrease in left ventricular filling pressure. Further symptomatic improvement occurs later with natriuresis.

The major limitation of high doses of loop diuretics is drug toxicity. Fluid and electrolyte complications result directly from the diuresis and natriuresis. For diuretic-resistant patients, ototoxicity may occur during high-dose therapy,[209] especially when administered as a bolus.[210] Furosemide toxicity is minimized by administering the diuretic less than 10 mg/min.[209,211] Myalgias may occur after high doses of bumetanide. Continuous infusion of diuretics avoids high peak levels and the concomitant toxicity (see "Continuous Diuretic Infusion") in diuretic-resistant patients.

Another complication of high-dose furosemide treatment can be thiamine deficiency.[212] Chronic furosemide administration has been reported to lead to thiamine deficiency in animals and, in some reports, in humans. In one study,[213] patients with CHF who had received 80 mg/day furosemide for at least 3 months were randomized to receive intravenous thiamine or placebo. Intravenous thiamine improved hemodynamics, natriuresis, and indices of thiamine status. This work must be confirmed before thiamine can be recommended routinely for patients using prolonged high-dose loop diuretic treatment, but it raises the possibility that loop diuretics may predispose to nutritional deficiencies.

Combined Diuretic Therapy

Diuretic resistance can often be treated with two classes of diuretic used simultaneously. Controlled trials[214] suggest little or no benefit from giving two agents of the same class (e.g., ethacrynic acid and furosemide). In contrast, adding a proximal tubule diuretic or a DCT diuretic to a loop diuretic is often dramatically effective. DCT diuretics added to loop diuretics are synergistic (the combination is more effective than

Table 33-4 Ceiling Daily Doses of Loop Diuretics

	FUROSEMIDE		BUMETANIDE		TORSEMIDE	
	IV	PO	IV	PO	IV	PO
Chronic kidney disease						
GFR 20–50 mL/min	80–160	160	4–8	4–8	50	50
GFR <20 mL/min	200	240	8–10	8–10	8–10	100
Severe acute renal failure	500	NA	12	NA	200	NA
Nephrotic syndrome	120	240	3	3	20–50	20–50
Cirrhosis	40–80	80–160	1	1–2	10–20	20
Congestive heart failure	40–80	80–160	1–2	1–2	10–20	20

Ceiling dose indicates the dose that produces the maximal increase in fractional Na^+ excretion (FE_{Na}). Larger doses may increase net daily natriuresis by increasing the duration of natriuresis without increasing the maximal rate. All doses are in milligrams.
GFR, glomerular filtration rate; NA, not available.
Based on Brater DC: Diuretic therapy. N Engl J Med 1998;339:387–395.

Box 33-2   Combination Diuretic Therapy

To a ceiling dose of a loop diuretic (Table 33–1) add:
    Distal convoluted tubule diuretics
        Metolazone 2.5–10 mg/day PO*
        Hydrochlorothiazide (or equivalent) 25–100
            mg/day PO
        Chlorothiazide 500–1000 mg IV
    Proximal tubule diuretics
        Acetazolamide 250–375 mg/day or up to 500
            mg IV
    Collecting duct diuretics
        Spironolactone 100–200 mg/day
        Eplerenone 100–200 mg/day
        Amiloride 5–10 mg/day

*Metolazone is generally best given for a limited period of time (3–5 days) or should be reduced in frequency to three times per week once extracellular fluid volume has decreased to the target level. Only in patients who remain volume expanded should full doses be continued indefinitely, based on the target weight.

the sum of the effects of each drug alone) (see Box 33-2 for regimens).[2,91,215–219]

DCT diuretics do not alter the pharmacokinetics or the bioavailability of loop diuretics. The addition of a DCT diuretic to a loop diuretic enhances NaCl excretion via several mechanisms (for a review, see Ellison[4]). The most important mechanism is probably by inhibiting NaCl transport along the distal tubule, where tubular Na^+ and Cl^- uptake is stimulated by the loop diuretic. During prolonged use of loop diuretics for resistant edema, distal nephron cells become hypertrophic and hyperplastic,[220] and there is an increase in the density of Na^+/K^+-ATPase pump sites,[221,222] in the density of Na^+/Cl^- cotransporters,[223] and in the intrinsic capacity to reabsorb Na^+ and Cl^-.[224] Thus, when microperfused with a standard NaCl load, distal tubules from animals treated long term with loop diuretics reabsorb Na^+ and Cl^- as much as three times more rapidly than those of control animals.[225] Because DCT diuretics can inhibit apical Na^+/Cl^- cotransport by the distal tubule even under these stimulated conditions, the effects of these diuretics will be greatly magnified in patients in whom high doses of loop diuretics have led to hypertrophy and hyperplasia. Loon and coworkers[219] showed that the natriuretic effect of chlorothiazide in humans was enhanced after treatment with furosemide for 1 month. These data suggest that daily oral furosemide treatment, even in modest doses, may be sufficient to induce adaptive changes along the distal nephron and that these may be treated with combination drug therapy.

When a second class of diuretic is added, the dose of loop diuretic should not be altered because the shape of the loop diuretic dose-response curve is not affected by addition of other classes of diuretic. Thus, the loop diuretic should be given in an effective or ceiling dose (see Table 33-4). The choice of DCT diuretic is arbitrary. Many clinicians choose metolazone because its half-life is longer than some classic thiazide diuretics and because metolazone has been reported to remain effective even when the GFR is low. Yet, direct comparisons between metolazone and classic thiazides have shown little difference in natriuretic potency when combined

with loop diuretics in patients with nephrotic edema, heart failure, or azotemia.[91,226,227]

DCT diuretics may be added in full doses (see Box 33-2) when a rapid and robust response is needed, but this is likely to lead to complications and an extremely close follow-up is mandatory. We advocate hospitalizing patients when initiating aggressive combination therapy because fluid and electrolyte depletion, sometimes massive, occurs commonly during combination diuretic therapy. Serious side effects are noted in as many as two thirds of published reports describing combination therapy.[228] One reasonable approach is to establish a therapeutic target weight and achieve control of the expanded ECF volume by adding escalating daily doses of a DCT diuretic. When the target weight is attained, the DCT diuretic can be prescribed three times weekly and the dose adjusted based on the patient's weight.

Another approach to combination therapy may be a short fixed course. Comparison was made of adding a thiazide-type diuretic to furosemide for either a fixed 3-day period or adjusting the dose to achieve targeted volume losses during 5 to 7 days. Both regimens were equally effective in decreasing ECF volume and symptoms. Surprisingly, natriuresis and diuresis continued even after the thiazide-type diuretic was discontinued during the fixed regimen.[226] For outpatients requiring combined therapy, one approach is to add a modest dose of a DCT diuretic, such as 2.5 to 5.0 mg/day of metolazone, for 3 days only. Higher doses or longer time periods are effective but probably too dangerous for routine outpatient use. Because DCT diuretics are absorbed more slowly than loop diuretics (peak levels at 1.5–4.0 hours for DCT diuretics compared with 0.5–2.0 hours for loop diuretics), it is rational to administer the DCT diuretic 0.5 to 1 hour before the loop diuretic.

Drugs that act on the ASDN, such as amiloride, spironolactone, and eplerenone, can be added to a regimen of loop diuretics, but their effects are generally less dramatic than those of DCT diuretics.[229] The combination of spironolactone and loop diuretics has not been shown to be synergistic, but can prevent hypokalemia while maintaining renal Na^+ excretion. Potassium-sparing distal diuretics are used commonly to treat patients with cirrhosis of the liver in whom hypokalemia must be avoided because it predisposes to hepatic encephalopathy. A combination of furosemide and spironolactone or eplerenone is now considered the preferred regimen for cirrhotic ascites.[136] Potassium-sparing distal diuretics also reduce Mg^{2+} excretion, making hypomagnesemia less likely than when combined with loop diuretics.

It is now clear that blockade of mineralocorticoid receptors can improve mortality of patients with systolic dysfunction.[230] Although this effect has been attributed to direct cardiac or vascular effects, renal effects also contribute. Barr and colleagues[231] randomized 42 patients with New York Heart Association class II to III CHF to either 50 to 100 mg/day spironolactone or placebo added to a regimen of loop diuretics and ACEIs. Spironolactone increased Na^+ excretion, increased the urinary Na^+-to-K^+ ratio, increased the serum Mg^{2+} concentration, and decreased ventricular arrhythmias. Others have reported similar results.[232,233] Nevertheless, hyperkalemia is a concern when adding spironolactone to ACEI therapy, especially in those patients with renal insufficiency.[234] In one study, potentially life-threatening hyperkalemia during spironolactone treatment was found to be predicted by renal insufficiency, diabetes, older age, dehydration, and concomitant use of other medications that may cause hyperkalemia.[235] Similar effects likely accompany eplerenone therapy.

Combination diuretic therapy is often indicated for hospitalized patients in an intensive care unit who need urgent diuresis because of diuretic resistance in the setting of obligate fluid and solute loads. Two intravenous drugs are available to supplement loop diuretics: chlorothiazide (500–1000 mg once or twice daily) and acetazolamide (250–375 mg as many as four times daily). Chlorothiazide has relatively potent carbonic anhydrase–inhibiting capacity in the proximal tubule and also blocks the thiazide-sensitive Na^+/Cl^- cotransporter in the DCT. It has a longer half-life than some other thiazides. Both chlorothiazide and acetazolamide can act synergistically with loop diuretics. Acetazolamide is especially useful when metabolic alkalosis complicates the treatment of edema because this may make it difficult to correct hypokalemia or to wean a patient from a ventilator.[236] The use of acetazolamide can correct alkalosis without the need to administer saline but often requires replacement of K^+ losses with additional KCl. In other situations, combination diuretic therapy may be targeted at the underlying disease process. Theophylline is a mild diuretic acting at adenosine type 1 receptors in the proximal tubule,[30,31] but acts synergistically with loop diuretics and may be useful when bronchospasm and edema are present together. For patients with left ventricular dysfunction, afterload reduction may enhance diuresis.

Continuous Diuretic Infusion

Continuous diuretic infusion can be considered for hospitalized patients who are resistant to diuretic therapy.[237] There are several potential advantages. First, it prevents the postdiuretic NaCl retention that complicates intermittent administration. Second, constant infusion yields greater acute natriuresis than bolus therapy. In one study of patients with chronic kidney disease, a continuous infusion of bumetanide was 32% more efficient than a bolus of the same dose.[238] In another study of patients with severe CHF, 60 to 80 mg/day furosemide was more effective when given as a continuous infusion after a loading dose (30–40 mg) than when given as bolus doses three times daily. Bumetanide has a short half-life, torsemide has a longer half-life, and furosemide is intermediate. Therefore, the ratio of the efficiency of continuous infusion to bolus is greatest for bumetanide and least for torsemide. Indeed, bolus torsemide is an alternative approach to continuous bumetanide infusion. Third, poorly documented observations suggest that some patients who are resistant to large doses of diuretics given by bolus may respond to continuous infusion.[239,240] These studies have failed to compare equivalent doses or to randomize the treatments, but Van Meyel and colleagues[240] showed natriuresis during constant infusion in patients who had failed to respond to 250 mg furosemide given as a bolus. Fractional Na^+ excretion varied in a linear manner with total daily furosemide dose between 480 and 3840 mg/day. Fourth, the diuretic response can be more easily titrated and is smoother with continuous diuretic infusion. Magovern and Magovern[241] reported successful diuresis of hemodynamically compromised patients after cardiac surgery by continuous furosemide infusion. Infusing loop diuretics continuously may decrease the sympathetic discharge and activation of the renin-angiotensin system and may moderate the abrupt solute and fluid losses that occur after a large intravenous bolus. Finally, drug toxicity from loop diuretics, such as ototoxicity (observed with all loop diuretics) and myopathies (with bumetanide), appears to be less common when the drugs are administered as continuous infusions. Total daily furosemide doses exceeding 2 g have been well tolerated when administered over 24 hours, but these high infusion rates may lead to toxic serum concentrations if continued for prolonged periods in patients with renal failure. Torsemide, which has a relatively greater clearance by hepatic metabolism, may be preferred for prolonged high-dose therapy.

Additional Measures in Specific Circumstances

Endopeptidase Inhibitors and Atrial Peptides

ANP and other biologically active peptides are degraded by neutral endopeptidases. Therefore, drugs that inhibit these enzymes increase plasma ANP levels and cause natriuresis. Indeed, neutral endopeptidase inhibitors given to hypertensive subjects do increase plasma ANP concentrations, lower blood pressure,[242] and, when given to normotensive subjects, increase glomerular filtration and Na^+ excretion and decrease the plasma renin activity.[26] Therefore, such therapy might potentiate diuretic-induced Na^+ and fluid loss. This hypothesis was tested in a dog model of acute CHF. Furosemide alone caused natriuresis, but decreased the GFR and activated the renin-angiotensin axis. During low-dose ANP infusion, the furosemide-induced natriuresis was potentiated, the GFR was stabilized and the renin-angiotensin-aldosterone axis was maintained.[243] Therefore, endopeptidase inhibition or ANP infusion might be effective in treating loop diuretic resistance, but this requires validation in human subjects. As discussed previously, brain natriuretic peptide has recently been approved for use in decompensated CHF.[27] However, follow-up studies have been quite discouraging.[132–135]

Aquaretics

As noted previously, oral vasopressin receptor antagonists have been developed but are not yet available in the United States. An intravenous nonselective vasopressin antagonist, however, is available to treat euvolemic and hypervolemic hyponatremia. These agents may become useful in promoting free-water excretion and normalizing S_{Na} in patients with diuretic-induced hyponatremia. However, they will have to be used with care because in these circumstances, the hyponatremia can represent renal free-water retention, which is a final line of volume defense during forced diuretic-induced natriuresis.

Circulatory Support and Inotropic Agents

Dopamine, dobutamine, and milrinone are used commonly to increase urinary Na and water excretion. Their use to prevent acute renal failure was described earlier in this chapter. Acute dopamine infusion increases renal plasma flow, urinary sodium excretion, the GFR, and the functional status of patients with moderate to severe CHF. Beregovich and coworkers[244] showed that cardiac output and Na^+ excretion increase progressively as dopamine infusion is increased from 1 to 5 and 10 mg/kg/min in patients with classes III and IV CHF. However, stroke volume and urinary flow rate peak at 5 mg/kg/min, and several patients develop sinus tachycardia or striking increases in systemic vascular resistance at doses of 5 mg/kg/min or more. Although acute effects of dopamine infusion on renal sodium excretion and cardiac hemodynamics are often dramatic, natriuretic effects typically wane after 12 to 24 hours.[245]

Dobutamine is a dopamine derivative that is a potent inotrope without significant effects on mesenteric or systemic vascular tone or blood pressure. Both dopamine and dobutamine have been reported to improve cardiac output, renal perfusion, and, in some situations, Na^+ excretion. Hilberman and colleagues[246] compared the effects of dopamine and dobutamine in 12 patients who had undergone open heart surgery and developed depressed left ventricular performance postoperatively. The drugs were administered in random order in doses that increased cardiac output equally (dopamine 5.0 ± 1.8 and dobutamine 3.5 ± 1.8 mg/kg/min). Although they had similar effects on renal plasma flow, renal vascular resistance, and glomerular filtration rate, dopamine increased urinary flow rate by 2.8-fold and Na^+ excretion by 4.6-fold more than dobutamine. Because dopamine can increase Na^+ and water excretion during treatment with dobutamine in patients with CHF, it appears to have unique natriuretic properties. These studies provide a rationale for combining low doses (2–5 mg/kg/min) of dopamine and dobutamine in critically ill patients.

Two other studies limit the enthusiasm for dopamine when added to a loop diuretic to treat CHF. In one study of six patients with chronic stable CHF, neither dopamine nor dobutamine was more effective than placebo in increasing urine volume.[247] In a randomized, crossover study,[248] dopamine (1–3 mg/kg/min) did not increase urinary solute and water excretion when added to a maximally effective dose of furosemide given to patients with stable heart failure, but did lead to potentially serious tachyarrhythmias in several patients. Although this study does not provide evidence supporting the use of low-dose dopamine in patients with CHF, the patients studied were stable and did respond to furosemide alone. Whether dopamine might elicit diuresis in patients who become refractory to furosemide alone was not addressed. According to the most recent guidelines of the Heart Failure Society of America, intravenous inotropes (dobutamine or milrinone) may be considered to relieve symptoms and improve end-organ function in patients with advanced heart failure characterized by left ventricular dilation, reduced left ventricular ejection fraction, and diminished peripheral perfusion or end-organ dysfunction (low output syndrome), particularly if these patients have marginal systolic blood pressure (<90 mm Hg), have symptomatic hypotension despite adequate filling pressure, or are unresponsive to or intolerant of intravenous vasodilators. These agents may be considered in similar patients with evidence of fluid overload if they respond poorly to intravenous diuretics or manifest diminished or worsening renal function. The same group does not make a recommendation with respect to dopamine.

Another situation in which dopamine is often employed is in critically ill patients with mild to moderate renal dysfunction. In two uncontrolled studies of critically ill patients, dopamine (1.5–2.5 mg/kg/min) increased urine output by 42% to 50% in patients with baseline urinary outputs less than 0.5 to 1 mL/kg/hr.[249,250] In a controlled, crossover study of critically ill patients comparing dopamine (200 mg/min) with dobutamine (175 mg/min) or placebo, dopamine increased urine output significantly without affecting creatinine clearance, whereas dobutamine increased creatinine clearance significantly without affecting urine output.[251] Taken together, these data suggest that dopamine may increase renal Na^+ and water excretion in some patients with mild to moderate renal dysfunction.

In summary, dopamine and dobutamine are effective inotropes that increase cardiac output and can improve renal perfusion and Na^+ and water excretion when administered to patients with systolic dysfunction. In contrast, data supporting a role for low (renal)-dose dopamine to protect against acute renal failure, to treat stable CHF, or to treat diuretic resistance are lacking.

Ultrafiltration

Most patients who appear to be resistant to diuretics respond to one of the approaches outlined (see Table 33-4 and Fig. 33-4). Side effects of diuretic therapy such as prerenal azotemia and metabolic alkalosis, rather than diuretic resistance, usually limit the ability to reduce ECF volume further. When pharmacologic therapy fails, plasma ultrafiltration, with or without accompanying hemodialysis, may be used to remove ECF. Agostoni and colleagues[252] randomized patients with CHF to equal volume removal by ultrafiltration or furosemide. The ECF volume remained contracted after ultrafiltration but rebounded to baseline after the intravenous diuretic treatment was discontinued. The ECF volume rebound after loop diuretic use was associated with a brisk increase in plasma renin and angiotensin II levels. ECF volume contraction induced by diuretics or ultrafiltration stimulates renin secretion via effects on vascular fullness, but loop diuretics additionally stimulate renin secretion directly via the macula densa. This loop diuretic–induced counterregulatory hormonal response may contribute to more rapid fluid reaccumulation. Recently, ultrafiltration was compared with intravenous diuretics in a randomized study of patients hospitalized with heart failure. The results showed that net fluid losses were greater in the ultrafiltration group and at 90 days, and fewer ultrafiltration patients had been hospitalized.[253] These results suggest a role for ultrafiltration in selected patients with heart failure.

General Approach to Patients with Diuretic Resistance

A general approach to diuretic resistance is given in Figures 33-4 and 33-5 and Table 33-3. It is important to establish a target response. This can be defined by a set weight, by clearance of peripheral edema, or by improvement in respiratory or other symptoms. Some patients require modest edema to maintain renal perfusion and general well-being, but recent recommendations for treating heart failure recommended keeping patients quite dry.

Noncompliance with dietary prescription can be determined by measuring the sodium excretion rate over 24 hours. If excretion exceeds 100 mmol (43 mmol Na^+ = 1 g Na^+; 100 mmol = 2.3 g), then excessive dietary NaCl intake is likely contributing to the apparent resistance.

If diuretic resistance persists despite effective NaCl restriction, the dose of loop diuretic should be doubled until a response is obtained or until the ceiling dose (see Table 33-5) is attained. A distinct increase in urinary output should be noted within 4 hours of an oral diuretic dose if a clinical response has been attained. If the response is still inadequate, poor gastrointestinal absorption should be considered and a drug with a higher and more consistent bioavailability, such as torsemide, should be selected or the diuretic should be given intravenously.

If the response remains inadequate, combination diuretic therapy should be considered (see Box 33-1). This is best initiated under observation in hospital. The most potent combina-

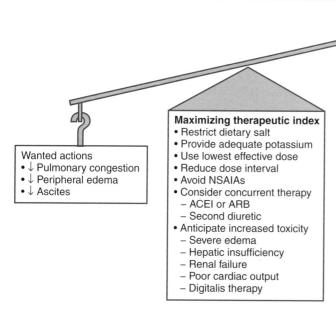

Wanted actions
- ↓ Pulmonary congestion
- ↓ Peripheral edema
- ↓ Ascites

Maximizing therapeutic index
- Restrict dietary salt
- Provide adequate potassium
- Use lowest effective dose
- Reduce dose interval
- Avoid NSAIAs
- Consider concurrent therapy
  - ACEI or ARB
  - Second diuretic
- Anticipate increased toxicity
  - Severe edema
  - Hepatic insufficiency
  - Renal failure
  - Poor cardiac output
  - Digitalis therapy

Unwanted actions
Biochemical
- ↓Serum potassium, ↓ serum magnesium
- ↑ Glucose, ↑ lipids
- ↑ BUN
Symptomatic
- Weakness and lethargy
- Impotence

Figure 33-5 Balancing the desirable and undesirable actions of diuretics. ACEI, angiotensin-converting enzyme inhibitor; ARB, angiotensin receptor blocker; BUN, blood urea nitrogen; NSAIAs, nonsteroidal anti-inflammatory agents.

tion is metolazone or a thiazide added to a loop diuretic, but this approach carries a significant risk of hypokalemia, azotemia, and severe volume depletion. For patients whose serum potassium concentration or blood pressure is low, adding a collecting duct diuretic, such as spironolactone, eplerenone, and amiloride, is preferable. These patients must be followed for the potential development of hyperkalemia, especially those who are on concomitant ACEI therapy.

For those patients who remain unresponsive, more aggressive therapy in the hospital is indicated with intravenous loop diuretic infusions that can be combined, if necessary, with intravenous or oral DCT diuretics or carbonic anhydrase inhibitors. While the role of ultrafiltration remains unclear, it should be considered in selected unresponsive patients with intractable congestive cardiac failure.

References

1. Eknoyan G: A history of diuretics. In Seldin DW, Giebisch G (eds): Diuretic Agents: Clinical Physiology and Pharmacology. San Diego: Academic Press, 1997, pp 3–28.
2. Ellison DH, Wilcox CS: Diuretics. In Brenner BM (ed): Brenner and Rector's The Kidney, 7th ed. Philadelphia: WB Saunders, 2008, pp 1646–1678.
3. Velazquez H, Wright FS: Effects of diuretic drugs on Na, Cl, and K transport by rat renal distal tubule. Am J Physiol 1986;250: F1013–F1023.
4. Ellison DH: Diuretic resistance: Physiology and therapeutics. Semin Nephrol 1999;19:581–597.
5. Kaunisto K, Parkkila S, Rajaniemi H, et al: Carbonic anhydrase XIV: Luminal expression suggests key role in renal acidification. Kidney Int 2002;61:2111–2118.
6. Maren TH: Carbonic anhydrase: General perspective and advances in glaucoma research. Drug Dev Res 1987;10:255.
7. Swenson ER, Robertson HT, Hlastala MP: Effects of carbonic anhydrase inhibition on ventilation-perfusion matching in the dog lung. J Clin Invest 1993;92:702–709.
8. Heller I, Halevy J, Cohen S, Theodor E: Significant metabolic acidosis induced by acetazolamide. Not a rare complication. Arch Intern Med 1985;145:1815–1817.
9. Webster LT, Davidson CS: Production of impending hepatic coma by a carbonic anhydrase inhibitor, diamox. Proc Soc Exp Biol Med 1956;91:27–31.
10. Kass MA, Kolker AE, Gordon M, et al: Acetazolamide and urolithiasis. Ophthalmology 1981;88:261–265.
11. Krivoy N, Ben-Arieh Y, Carter A, Alroy G: Methazolamide-induced hepatitis and pure RBC aplasia. Arch Intern Med 1981;141:1229–1230.
12. Mallette LE: Acetazolamide-accelerated anticonvulsant osteomalacia. Arch Intern Med 1977;137:1013–1017.
13. Hannaert P, Alvarez-Guerra M, Pirot D, et al: Rat NKCC2/ NKCC1 cotransporter selectivity for loop diuretic drugs. Naunyn Schmiedebergs Arch Pharmacol 2002;365:193–199.
14. Isenring P, Forbush B: Ion transport and ligand binding by the Na-K-Cl cotransporter, structure-function studies. Comp Biochem Physiol A Mol Integr Physiol 2001;130:487–497.
15. Quamme GA: Control of magnesium transport in the thick ascending limb. Am J Physiol 1989;256:F197–F210.
16. Suki WN, Rouse D, Ng, RC, Kokko JP: Calcium transport in the thick ascending limb of Henle. Heterogeneity of function in the medullary and cortical segments. J Clin Invest 1980;66:1004–1009.
17. Quamme GA: Effect of furosemide on calcium and magnesium transport in the rat nephron. Am J Physiol 1981; 241:F340–F347.
18. Gerber JG: Role of prostaglandins in the hemodynamic and tubular effects of furosemide. Fed Proc 1983;42:1707–1710.
19. Wright FS, Schnermann J: Interference with feedback control of glomerular filtration rate by furosemide, triflocin, and cyanide. J Clin Invest 1974;53:1695–1708.
20. Epstein M, Hollenberg NK, Guttmann RD, et al: Effect of ethacrynic acid and chlorothiazide on intrarenal hemodynamics in normal man. Am J Physiol 1971;220:482–487.
21. Okusa MD, Ellison DH: Physiology and pathophysiology of diuretic action. In Seldin DW, Giebisch G (eds): The Kidney: Physiology & Pathophysiology. Amsterdam: Academic Press 2000, pp 2877–2922.
22. Dai L-J, Friedman PA, Qumme GA: Cellular mechanism of chlorothiazide and cellular potassium depletion on Mg2+ uptake in mouse distal convoluted tubule cells. Kidney Int 1996;51:1008–1017.
23. Busch AE, Suessbrich H, Kunzelmann K, et al: Blockade of epithelial Na+ channels by triamterenes—underlying mechanisms and molecular basis. Pflugers Arch 1996;432:760–766.
24. Rose LI, Underwood RH, Newmark SR, et al: Pathophysiology of spironolactone-induced gynecomastia. Ann Intern Med 1977;87:398–403.
25. Delyani JA, Rocha R, Cook CS, et al: Eplerenone: A selective aldosterone receptor antagonist (SARA). Cardiovasc Drug Rev 2001;19:185–200.

26. Wilkins MR, Unwin RJ, Kenny AJ: Endopeptidase-24.11 and its inhibitors: Potential therapeutic agents for edematous disorders and hypertension. Kidney Int 1993;43:273–285.

27. Colucci WS, Elkayam U, Horton DP, et al: Intravenous nesiritide, a natriuretic peptide, in the treatment of decompensated congestive heart failure. N Engl J Med 2000;343:246–253.

28. Better OS, Rubinstein I, Winaver JM, Knochel JP: Mannitol therapy revisited (1940–1997). Kidney Int 1997;51:886–894.

29. Warren SE, Blantz RC: Mannitol. Arch Intern Med 1981;141:493–497.

30. Zeltser D, Rosansky S, van Rensburg H, et al: Assessment of the efficacy and safety of intravenous conivaptan in euvolemic and hypervolemic hyponatremia. Am J Nephrol 2007;27:447–457.

31. Udelson JE, Smith WB, Hendrix GH, et al: Acute hemodynamic effects of conivaptan, a dual V(1A) and V(2) vasopressin receptor antagonist, in patients with advanced heart failure. Circulation 2001;104:2417–2423.

32. Shimizu K: Aquaretic effects of the nonpeptide V2 antagonist OPC-31260 in hydropenic humans. Kidney Int 1995;48:220–226.

33. Sato T, Ishikawa S, Abe K, et al: Acute aquaresis by nonpeptide arginine vasopressin (AVP) antagonist OPC-31260 improves hyponatremia in patients with syndrome of inappropriate secretion of antidiuretic hormone (SIADH). J Clin Endocrinol Metab 1997;82:1054–1057.

34. Gerbes AL, Gülberg V, Ginès P, et al.; the VPA Study Group: Therapy of hyponatremia in cirrhosis with vasopressin receptor antagonist: A randomized double-blind multicenter trial. Gastroenterology 2003;124:933–939.

35. Gheorghiade M, Konstam MA, Burnett JC Jr, et al: Efficacy of Vasopressin Antagonism in Heart Failure Outcome Study With Tolvaptan (EVEREST) Investigators: Short-term clinical effects of tolvaptan, an oral vasopressin antagonist, in patients hospitalized for heart failure: The EVEREST Clinical Status Trials. JAMA 2007;297:1332–1343.

36. Gheorghiade M, Niazi I, Ouyang J, et al: Vasopressin V2-receptor blockade with tolvaptan in patients with chronic heart failure: Results from a double-blind, randomized trial. Circulation 2003;107:2690–2696.

37. Costello-Boerrigter LC, Smith WB, Boerrigter G, et al: Vasopressin-2-receptor antagonism augments water excretion without changes in renal hemodynamics or sodium and potassium excretion in human heart failure. Am J Physiol Renal Physiol 2006;290:F273–F278.

38. Konstam MA, Gheorghiade M, Burnett JC Jr, et al: Efficacy of Vasopressin Antagonism in Heart Failure Outcome Study With Tolvaptan (EVEREST) Investigators: Effects of oral tolvaptan in patients hospitalized for worsening heart failure: The EVEREST Outcome Trial. JAMA 2007;297:1319–1331.

39. Soupart A, Gross P, Legros J-J, et al: Successful long-term treatment of hyponatremia in syndrome of inappropriate antidiuretic hormone secretion with satavaptan (SR121463b), an orally active nonpeptide vasopressin V2-receptor antagonist. Clin J Am Soc Nephrol 2006;1:1154–1160.

40. Brater DC, Kaojaren S, Chennavasin P: Pharmacodynamics of the diuretic effects of aminophylline and acetazolamide alone and combined with furosemide in normal subjects. J Pharmacol Exp Ther 1983;227:92–97.

41. Wilcox CS, Welch WJ, Schreiner GF, Belardinelli L: Natriuretic and diuretic actions of a highly selective adenosine A1 receptor antagonist. J Am Soc Nephrol 1999;10:714–720.

42. Welch WJ: Adenosine A1 receptor antagonists in the kidney: Effects in fluid-retaining disorders. Curr Opin Pharmacol 2002;2:165–170.

43. Brater DC: Disposition and response to bumetanide and furosemide. Am J Cardiol 1986;57:20A–25A.

44. Sweet DH, Bush KT, Nigam SK: The organic anion transporter family: From physiology to ontogeny and the clinic. Am J Physiol 2001;281:F197–F205.

45. Cha SH, Sekine T, Fukushima JI, et al: Identification and characterization of human organic anion transporter 3 expressing predominantly in the kidney. Mol Pharmacol 2001;59:1277–1286.

46. Uwai Y, Saito H, Hashimoto Y, Inui KI: Interaction and transport of thiazide diuretics, loop diuretics, and acetazolamide via rat renal organic anion transporter rOAT1. J Pharmacol Exp Ther 2000;295:261–265.

47. Krick W, Wolff NA, Burckhardt G: Voltage-driven p-aminohippurate, chloride, and urate transport in porcine renal brush-border membrane vesicles. Pflugers Arch 2000;441:125–132.

48. Chennavasin P, Seiwell R, Brater DC: Pharmacokinetic-dynamic analysis of the indomethacin-furosemide interaction in man. J Pharmacol Exp Ther 1980;215:77–81.

49. Chennavasin P, Seiwell R, Brater DC, Liang WM: Pharmacodynamic analysis of the furosemide-probenecid interaction in man. Kidney Int 1979;16:187–195.

50. Loon NR, Wilcox CS: Mild metabolic alkalosis impairs the natriuretic response to bumetanide in normal human subjects. Clin Sci 1998;94:287–292.

51. Pichette V, Geadah D, du Souich P: The influence of moderate hypoalbuminaemia on the renal metabolism and dynamics of furosemide in the rabbit. Br J Pharmacol 1996;119:885–890.

52. Besseghir K, Mosig D, Roch-Ramel F: Facilitation by serum albumin of renal tubular secretion of organic ions. Am J Physiol 1989;256:F475–F484.

53. Rose HJ, O'Malley K, Pruitt AW: Depression of renal clearance of furosemide in man by azotemia. Clin Pharmacol Ther 1977;21:141–146.

54. Blose JS, Adams Jr KF, Patterson JH: Torsemide: A pyridine-sulfonylurea loop diuretic. Ann Pharmacother 1995;29:396–402.

55. Sear JW: Drug biotransformation by the kidney: How important is it, and how much do we really know? Br J Anaesth 1991;67:369–372.

56. Sommers DK, Meyer EC, Moncrieff J: The influence of co-administered organic acids on the kinetics and dynamics of furosemide. Br J Clin Pharmacol 1991;32:489–493.

57. Schali C, Roch-Ramel F: Transport and metabolism of [3H]morphine in isolated, nonperfused proximal tubular segments of the rabbit kidney. J Pharmacol Exp Ther 1982;223:811–815.

58. Pichette V, du Souich P: Role of the kidneys in the metabolism of furosemide: Its inhibition by probenecid. J Am Soc Nephrol 1996;7:345–349.

59. Kirchner KA, Martin CJ, Bower JD: Prostaglandin E2 but not I2 restores furosemide response in indomethacin-treated rats. Am J Physiol 1986;250:F980–F985.

60. Wilcox CS, Mitch WE, Kelly RA, et al: Response of the kidney to furosemide: I, Effects of salt intake and renal compensation. J Lab Clin Med 1983;102:450–458.

61. Brater DC: Clinical pharmacology of loop diuretics. Drugs 1991;41:14–22.

62. Brater DC: Diuretic therapy. N Engl J Med 1998;339:387–395.

63. Brunner G, Von Bergmann K, Häcker W, Von Möllendorff E: Comparison of diuretic effects and pharmacokinetics of torasemide and furosemide after a single oral dose in patients with hydropically decompensated cirrhosis of the liver. Arzneim Forsch Drug Res 1998;38:176–179.

64. Welling PG: Pharmacokinetics of the thiazide diuretics. Biopharm Drug Dispos 1986;7:501–535.

65. Mutschler E, Gilfrich HJ, Knauf H, et al: Pharmacokinetics of triamterene. Clin Exp Hypertens 1983;5:249–269.

66. Villeneuve JP, Rocheleau F, Raymond G: Triamterene kinetics and dynamics in cirrhosis. Clin Pharmacol Ther 1984;35:831–837.

67. Knauf H, Mohrke W, Mutschler E: Delayed elimination of triamterene and its active metabolite in chronic renal failure. Eur J Clin Pharmacol 1983;24:453–456.

68. Somogyi AA, Hovens CM, Muirhead MR, Bochner F: Renal tubular secretion of amiloride and its inhibition by cimetidine

in humans and in an animal model. Drug Metab Dispos 1989;17:190–196.

69. Andriulli A, Arrigoni A, Gindro T, et al: Canrenone and androgen receptor-active materials in plasma of cirrhotic patients during long-term K-canrenoate or spironolactone therapy. Digestion 1989;44:155–162.

70. Cook CS, Hauswald C, Oppermann JA, Schoenhard GL: Involvement of cytochrome P-450IIIA in metabolism of potassium canrenoate to an epoxide: Mechanism of inhibition of the epoxide formation by spironolactone and its sulfur-containing metabolite. J Pharmacol Exp Ther 1993;266:1–7.

71. Smirnakis KV, Yu AS: Diuretics in acute renal failure. In Brady HR, Wilcox CS (eds): Therapy in Nephrology and Hypertension, 2nd ed. Philadelphia: WB Saunders, 2003, pp 33–37.

72. Bonventre JV, Weinberg JM: Kidney preservation ex vivo for transplantation. Annu Rev Med 1992;43:523–553.

73. Conger JD: Interventions in clinical acute renal failure: What are the data? Am J Kidney Dis 1995;26:565–576.

74. Better OS, Stein JH: Early management of shock and prophylaxis of acute renal failure in traumatic rhabdomyolysis. N Engl J Med 1990;322:825–829.

75. Weisberg LS, Kurnik PB, Kurnik BRC: Risk of radiocontrast nephropathy in patients with and without diabetes mellitus. Kidney Int 1994;45:259–265.

76. Solomon R, Werner C, Mann D, et al: Effects of saline, mannitol and furosemide on acute decreases in renal function induced by radiocontrast agents. N Engl J Med 1994;331:1416–1420.

77. Dorman HR, Sondheimer JH, Cadnapaphornchai P: Mannitol-induced acute renal failure. Medicine 1990;69:153–159.

78. Lassnigg A, Donner E, Grubhofer G, et al: Lack of renoprotective effects of dopamine and furosemide during cardiac surgery. J Am Soc Nephrol 2000;11:97–104.

79. Anderson RJ, Linas SL, Berns AS, et al: Nonoliguric acute renal failure. N Engl J Med 1977;296:1134–1138.

80. Brown CB, Ogg CS, Cameron JS: High dose frusemide in acute renal failure: A controlled trial. Clin Nephrol 1981;15:90–96.

81. Shilliday IR, Quinn KJ, Allison ME: Loop diuretics in the management of acute renal failure: A prospective, double-blind, placebo-controlled, randomized study. Nephrol Dial Transplant 1997;12:2592–2596.

82. Mehta RL, Pascual MT, Soroko S, Chertow GM; PICARD Study Group. Diuretics, mortality, and nonrecovery of renal function in acute renal failure. JAMA 2002;288:2547–2553.

83. Uchino S, Doig GS, Bellomo R, et al; Beginning and Ending Supportive Therapy for the Kidney (B.E.S.T. Kidney) Investigators: Diuretics and mortality in acute renal failure. Crit Care Med 2004;32:1669–1677.

84. Cantarovich F, Rangoonwala B, Lorenz H, et al; High-Dose Furosemide in Acute Renal Failure Study Group. High-dose furosemide for established ARF: A prospective, randomized, double-blind, placebo-controlled, multicenter trial. Am J Kidney Dis 2004;44:402–409.

85. Conger JD, Falk SA, Hammond WS: Atrial natriuretic peptide and dopamine in established acute renal failure in the rat. Kidney Int 1991;40:21–28.

86. Allgren RL, Marbury TC, Rahman SN, et al: Anaritide in acute tubular necrosis. N Engl J Med 1997;336:828–834.

87. Wilcox CS: New insights into diuretic use in patients with chronic renal disease. J Am Soc Nephrol 2002;13:798–805.

88. Sica DA, Gehr TW: Diuretic use in stage 5 chronic kidney disease and end-stage renal disease. Curr Opin Nephrol Hypertens 2003;12:483–490.

89. Van Olden RW, van Meyel JJM, Gerlag PGG: Sensitivity of residual nephrons to high dose furosemide described by diuretic efficiency. Eur J Clin Pharmacol 1995;47:483–488.

90. Voelker JR, Cartwright Brown D, Anderson S, et al: Comparison of loop diuretics in patients with chronic renal insufficiency. Kidney Int 1987;32:572–578.

91. Fliser D, Schroter M, Neubeck M, Ritz E: Coadministration of thiazides increases the efficacy of loop diuretics even in patients with advanced renal failure. Kidney Int 1994;46:482–488.

92. Wollam GL, Tarazi RC, Bravo EL, Dustan HP: Diuretic potency of combined hydrochlorothiazide and furosemide therapy in patients with azotemia. Am J Med 1982;72:929–938.

93. Copeland JG, Campbell DW, Plachetka JR, et al: Diuresis with continuous infusion of furosemide after cardiac surgery. Am J Surg 1983;146:796–799.

94. Schrier RW, Fassett RG: A critique of the overfill hypothesis of sodium and water retention in the nephrotic syndrome. Kidney Int 1998;53:1111–1117.

95. Oliver WJ, Owings CL: Sodium excretion in the nephrotic syndrome. Relation to serum albumin concentration, glomerular filtration rate, and aldosterone excretion rate. Am J Dis Child 1967;113:352–362.

96. Ichikawa I, Rennke HG, Hoyer JR, et al: Role for intrarenal mechanisms in the impaired salt excretion of experimental nephrotic syndrome. J Clin Invest 1983;71:91–103.

97. Bernard DB, Alexander EA, Couser WG, Levinsky NG: Renal sodium retention during volume expansion in experimental nephrotic syndrome. Kidney Int 1978;14:478–485.

98. Meltzer JI, Keim HJ, Laragh JH, et al: Nephrotic syndrome: Vasoconstriction and hypervolemic types indicated by renin-sodium profiling. Ann Intern Med 1979;91:688–696.

99. Brown EA, Markandu ND, Sagnella GA, et al: Evidence that some mechanism other than the renin system causes sodium retention in nephrotic syndrome. Lancet 1982;2:1237–1240.

100. Reinhardt HW, Boemke W, Palm U, Kaczmarczyk G: What causes escape from sodium retaining hormones? Acta Physiol Scand Suppl 1990;591:12–17.

101. Luetscher JA, Hall AD, Kremer VL: Treatment of nephrosis with concentrated human serum albumin. I. Effects on the proteins of body fluids. J Clin Invest 1949;28:700–712.

102. Akcicek F, Yalniz T, Basci A, et al: Diuretic effect of frusemide in patients with nephrotic syndrome: Is it potentiated by intravenous albumin? Br Med J 1995;310:162–163.

103. Fliser D, Zurbruggen I, Mutschler E, et al: Coadministration of albumin and furosemide in patients with the nephrotic syndrome. Kidney Int 1999;55:629–634.

104. Sjostrom PA, Odlind BG: Effect of albumin on diuretic treatment in the nephrotic syndrome. Br Med J 1995;310:1537.

105. Baum M: Ask the expert. Pediatr Nephrol 2000;14:184–185.

106. Haws RM, Baum M: Efficacy of albumin and diuretic therapy in children with nephrotic syndrome. Pediatrics 1993;91:1142–1146.

107. Mees EJD: Does it make sense to administer albumin to the patient with nephrotic oedema? Nephrol Dial Transplant 1996;11:1224–1226.

108. Weiss RA, Schoeneman M, Greifer I: Treatment of severe nephrotic edema with albumin and furosemide. NY State J Med 1984;84:384–386.

109. Keller E, Hoppe-Seyler G, Schollmeyer P: Disposition and diuretic effect of furosemide in the nephrotic syndrome. Clin Pharmacol Ther 1982;32:442–449.

110. Inoue M, Okajima K, Itoh K, et al: Mechanism of furosemide resistance in analbuminemic rats and hypoalbuminemic patients. Kidney Int 1987;32:198–203.

111. Chalasani N, Gorski JC, Horlander JC Sr, et al: Effects of albumin/furosemide mixtures on responses to furosemide in hypoalbuminemic patients. J Am Soc Nephrol 2001;12:1010–1016.

112. Rane A, Villeneuve JP, Stone WJ, et al: Plasma binding and disposition of furosemide in the nephrotic syndrome and in uremia. Clin Pharmacol Ther 1978;24:199–207.

113. Agarwal R, Gorski JC, Sundblad K, Brater DC: Urinary protein binding does not affect response to furosemide in patients with nephrotic syndrome. J Am Soc Nephrol 2000;11:1100–1105.

114. Kirchner KA, Voelker JR, Brater DC: Binding inhibitors restore furosemide potency in tubule fluid containing albumin. Kidney Int 1991;40:418–424.

115. Consensus Recommendations for the Management of Chronic Heart Failure. On behalf of the membership of the advisory council to improve outcomes nationwide in heart failure. Am J Cardiol 1999;83:1A–38A.

116. Schrier RW, Gurevich AK, Cadnapaphornchai MA: Pathogenesis and management of sodium and water retention in cardiac failure and cirrhosis. Semin Nephrol 2001;21:157–172.

117. Faris R, Flather M, Purcell H, et al: Current evidence supporting the role of diuretics in heart failure: A meta analysis of randomised controlled trials. Int J Cardiol 2002;82:149–158.

118. Davis BR, Piller LB, Cutler JA, et al: Role of diuretics in the prevention of heart failure: The Antihypertensive and Lipid-Lowering Treatment to Prevent Heart Attack Trial. Circulation 2006;113:2201–2210.

119. Richardson A, Scriven AJ, Poole-Wilson PA, et al: Double-blind comparison of captopril alone against frusemide plus amiloride in mild heart failure. Lancet 1987;2:709–711.

120. Rasool A, Palevsky PM: Treatment of edematous disorders with diuretics. Am J Med Sci 2000;319:25–37.

121. Andreoli TE: Edematous states: An overview. Kidney Int 1997;51(Suppl 59):S2–S10.

122. Gomberg-Maitland M, Baran DA, Fuster V: Treatment of congestive heart failure: Guidelines for the primary care physician and the heart failure specialist. Arch Intern Med 2001;161:342–352.

123. Gillies A, Morgan T, Myers J: Comparison of piretanide and chlorothiazide in the treatment of cardiac failure. Med J Aust 1980;1:170–172.

124. Levy B: The efficacy and safety of furosemide and a combination of spironolactone and hydrochlorothiazide in congestive heart failure. J Clin Pharmacol 1977;17:420–430.

125. Viherkoski M, Huikko M, Varjoranta K: The effect of amiloride/hydrochlorothiazide combination vs furosemide plus potassium supplementation in the treatment of oedema of cardiac origin. Ann Clin Res 1981;13:11–15.

126. Heseltine D, Bramble MG: Loop diuretics cause less postural hypotension than thiazide diuretics in the frail elderly. Curr Med Res Opin 1988;11:232–235.

127. Brater DC: Pharmacokinetics of loop diuretics in congestive heart failure. Br Heart J 1994;72:S40–S43.

128. Brater DC, Day B, Burdette A, Anderson S: Bumetanide and furosemide in heart failure. Kidney Int 1984;26:183–189.

129. Vasko MR, Cartwright DB, Knochel JP, et al: Furosemide absorption is altered in decompensated congestive heart failure. Ann Intern Med 1985;102:314–318.

130. Topol EJ: Nesiritide—not verified. N Engl J Med 2005;353:113–116.

131. Shi SJ, Vellaichamy E, Chin SY, et al: Natriuretic peptide receptor A mediates renal sodium excretory responses to blood volume expansion. Am J Physiol Renal Physiol 2003;285:F694–F702.

132. Sackner-Bernstein JD: Short-term risk of death after treatment with nesiritide for decompensated heart failure: A pooled analysis of randomized controlled trials. JAMA 2005;293:1900–1905.

133. Sackner-Bernstein JD, Skopicki HA, Aaronson KD: Risk of worsening renal function with nesiritide in patients with acutely decompensated heart failure. Circulation 2005;111:1487–1491.

134. Teerlink JR, Massie BM: Nesiritide and worsening of renal function: The emperor's new clothes? Circulation 2005;111:1459–1461.

135. Gines P, Cardenas A, Arroyo V, Rodes J: Management of cirrhosis and ascites. N Engl J Med 2004;350:1646–1654.

136. Runyon BA: Management of adult patients with ascites caused by cirrhosis. Hepatology 1998;27:264–272.

137. Gines P, Arroyo V, Quintero E, Planas R, et al: Comparison of paracentesis and diuretics in the treatment of cirrhotics with tense ascites. Results of a randomized study. Gastroenterology 1987;93:234–241.

138. Luca A, Garcia-Pagan JC, Bosch J, et al: Beneficial effects of intravenous albumin infusion on the hemodynamic and humoral changes after total paracentesis. Hepatology 1995;22:753–758.

139. Peltekian KM, Wong F, Liu PP, et al: Cardiovascular, renal, and neurohumoral responses to single large-volume paracentesis in patients with cirrhosis and diuretic-resistant ascites. Am J Gastroenterol 1997;92:394–399.

140. Tito L, Gines P, Arroyo V, et al: Total paracentesis associated with intravenous albumin management of patients with cirrhosis and ascites. Gastroenterology 1990;98:146–151.

141. Fernandez-Esparrach G, Guevara M, Sort P, et al: Diuretic requirements after therapeutic paracentesis in non-azotemic patients with cirrhosis. A randomized double-blind trial of spironolactone versus placebo. J Hepatol 1997;26:614–620.

142. Stanley MM, Ochi S, Lee KK, et al: Peritoneovenous shunting as compared with medical treatment in patients with alcoholic cirrhosis and massive ascites. Veterans Administration Cooperative Study on Treatment of Alcoholic Cirrhosis with Ascites. N Engl J Med 1989;321:1632–1638.

143. Angeli P, Dalla PM, De BE, et al: Randomized clinical study of the efficacy of amiloride and potassium canrenoate in nonazotemic cirrhotic patients with ascites. Hepatology 1994;19:72–79.

144. Fogel MR, Sawhney VK, Neal EA, et al: Diuresis in the ascitic patient: A randomized controlled trial of three regimens. J Clin Gastroenterol 1981;3(Suppl 1):73–80.

145. Perez-Ayuso RM, Arroyo V, Planas R, et al: Randomized comparative study of efficacy of furosemide versus spironolactone in nonazotemic cirrhosis with ascites. Relationship between the diuretic response and the activity of the renin-aldosterone system. Gastroenterology 1983;84:961–968.

146. Sungaila I, Bartle WR, Walker SE, et al: Spironolactone pharmacokinetics and pharmacodynamics in patients with cirrhotic ascites. Gastroenterology 1992;102:1680–1685.

147. Pockros PJ, Reynolds TB: Rapid diuresis in patients with ascites from chronic liver disease: The importance of peripheral edema. Gastroenterology 1986;90:1827–1833.

148. Rossle M, Ochs A, Gulberg V, et al: A comparison of paracentesis and transjugular intrahepatic portosystemic shunting in patients with ascites. N Engl J Med 2000;342:1701–1707.

149. Saab S, Nieto JM, Lewis SK, Runyon BA: TIPS versus paracentesis for cirrhotic patients with refractory ascites. Cochrane Database Syst Rev 2006;(4):CD004889.

150. Kay A, Davis CL: Idiopathic edema. Am J Kidney Dis 1999;34:405–423.

151. MacGregor GA, Markandu ND, Roulston JE, et al: Is "idiopathic" edema idiopathic? Lancet 1979;1:397–400.

152. Young JB, Brownjohn AM, Lee MR: Diuretics and idiopathic oedema. Nephron 1986;43:311–312.

153. Addo HA, Ferguson J, Frain Bell W: Thiazide-induced photosensitivity: A study of 33 subjects. Br J Dermatol 1987;116:749–760.

154. Heydenreich G, Pindborg T, Schmidt H: Bullous dermatosis among patients with chronic renal failure on high dose frusemide. Acta Med Scand 1977;202:61–64.

155. Dominguez-Ortega J, Martinez-Alonso JC, Dominguez-Ortega C, et al: Anaphylaxis to oral furosemide. Allergol Immunopathol (Madr) 2003;31:345–347.

156. Packer M: Identification of risk factors predisposing to the development of functional renal insufficiency during treatment with converting-enzyme inhibitors in chronic heart failure. Cardiology 1989;76:50–55.

157. Packer M, Lee WH, Medina N, et al: Functional renal insufficiency during long-term therapy with catopril and enalapril in severe chronic heart failure. Ann Intern Med 1987;106:346–354.

158. Smith WE, Steele TH: Avoiding diuretic-related complications in older patients. Geriatrics 1983;38:117–119.

159. Kaufman AM, Levitt MF: The effect of diuretics on systemic and renal hemodynamics in patients with renal insufficiency. Am J Kidney Dis 1985;5:A71–A78.

160. Siegel D, Hulley SB, Black DM, et al: Diuretics, serum and intracellular electrolyte levels, and ventricular arrhythmias in hypertensive men. JAMA 1992;267:1083–1089.

161. Flaker G, Villarreal D, Chapman D: Is hypokalemia a cause of ventricular arrhythmias. J Crit Illness 1986;2:66–74.

162. Freis ED: Critique of the clinical importance of diuretic-induced hypokalemia and elevated cholesterol level. Arch Intern Med 1989;149:2640–2648.

163. Harrington JT, Isner JM, Kassinger JP: Our national obsession with potassium. Am J Med 1982;73:155–159.

164. Kaplan NM: Our appropriate concern about hypokalemia. Am J Med 1984;77:1–4.

165. Kaplan NM: How bad are diuretic-induced hypokalemia and hypercholesterolemia? Arch Intern Med 1989;149:2649.

166. Kassirer JP, Harrington JT: Diuretics and potassium metabolism: A reassessment of the need, effectiveness and safety of potassium therapy. Kidney Int 1977;11:505–515.

167. Myers MG: Diuretic therapy and ventricular arrhythmias in persons 65 years of age and older. Am J Cardiol 1990;65:599–603.

168. Ram CVS, Garrett BN, Kaplan NM: Moderate sodium restriction and various diuretics in the treatment of hypertension. Arch Intern Med 1981;141:1015–1019.

169. Dorup I: Magnesium and potassium deficiency. Its diagnosis, occurrence and treatment in diuretic therapy and its consequences for growth, protein synthesis and growth factors. Acta Physiol Scand Suppl 1994;618:1–55.

170. Rude RK: Physiology of magnesium metabolism and the important role of magnesium in potassium deficiency. Am J Cardiol 1989;63:31G–34G.

171. Dorup I, Skajaa K, Thybo NK: Oral magnesium supplementation restores the concentrations of magnesium, potassium and sodium-potassium pumps in skeletal muscle of patients receiving diuretic treatment. J Intern Med 1993;233:117–123.

172. Palmer B: Potassium disturbances associated with the use of diuretics. In Seldin DW, Giebisch G (eds): Diuretic Agents: Clinical Physiology and Pharmacology. San Diego: Academic Press, 1997, pp 571–583.

173. Wilcox CS, Mitch WE, Kelly RA, et al: Factors affecting potassium balance during frusemide administration. Clin Sci 1984;67:195–203.

174. Ashraf N, Locksley R, Arieff AI: Thiazide-induced hyponatremia associated with death or neurologic damage in outpatients. Am J Med 1981;70:1163–1168.

175. Fichman MP, Vorherr H, Kleeman CR, Telfer N: Diuretic-induced hyponatremia. Ann Intern Med 1971;75:853–863.

176. Hantman D, Rossier B, Zohlman R, Schrier R: Rapid correction of hyponatremia in the syndrome of inappropriate secretion of antidiuretic hormone: An alternative treatment to hypertonic saline. Ann Intern Med 1973;78:870–875.

177. Schrier RW: New treatments for hyponatremia. N Engl J Med 1978;298:214–215.

178. Dzau VJ, Hollenberg NK: Renal response to captopril in severe heart failure: Role of furosemide in natriuresis and reversal of hyponatremia. Ann Intern Med 1984;100:777–782.

179. Carlsen JE, Kober L, Torp-Pedersen C, Johansen P: Relation between dose of bendrofluazide, antihypertensive effect, and adverse biochemical effects. Br Med J 1990;300:975–978.

180. Shalev H, Ohali M, Abramson O: Nephrocalcinosis in pseudohypoaldosteronism and the effect of indomethacin therapy. J Pediatr 1994;125:246–248.

181. Zillich AJ, Garg J, Basu S, et al: Thiazide diuretics, potassium, and the development of diabetes: A quantitative review. Hypertension 2006;48:219–224.

182. Helderman JH, Elahi D, Andersen DK, et al: Prevention of the glucose intolerance of thiazide diuretics by maintenance of body potassium. Diabetes 1983;32:106–111.

183. Toto R: Metabolic derangements associated with diuretic use: Insulin resistance, dyslipidemia, hyperuricemia, and anti-adrenergic effects. In Seldin DW, Giebisch G (eds): Diuretic Agents: Clinical Physiology and Pharmacology. San Diego: Academic Press, 1997, pp 621–636.

184. Pickkers P, Schachter M, Hughes AD, et al: Thiazide-induced hyperglycaemia: A role for calcium-activated potassium channels? Diabetologia 1996;39:861–864.

185. ALLHAT Officers and Coordinators for the ALLHAT Collaborative Research Group: The Antihypertensive and Lipid-Lowering Treatment to Prevent Heart Attack Trial. Major outcomes in high-risk hypertensive patients randomized to angiotensin-converting enzyme inhibitor or calcium channel blocker vs diuretic: The Antihypertensive and Lipid-Lowering Treatment to Prevent Heart Attack Trial (ALLHAT). JAMA 2002;288:2981–2997.

186. Ott SM, LaCroix AZ, Ichikawa LE, et al: Effect of low-dose thiazide diuretics on plasma lipids: Results from a double-blind, randomized clinical trial in older men and women. J Am Geriatr Soc 2005;51:1003–1013.

187. Grimm RH Jr, Flack JM, Grandits GA, et al: Long-term effects on plasma lipids of diet and drugs to treat hypertension. Treatment of Mild Hypertension Study (TOMHS) Research Group. JAMA 1996;275:1549–1556.

188. Psaty BM, Smith NL, Siscovick DS, et al: Health outcomes associated with antihypertensive therapies used as first-line agents. JAMA 1997;277:739–745.

189. Stone DK, Seldin DW, Kokko JP, Jacobson HR: Mineralocorticoid modulation of rabbit medullary collecting duct acidification. A sodium-independent effect. J Clin Invest 1983;72:77–83.

190. Tannen RL: The effect of uncomplicated potassium depletion on urine acidification. J Clin Invest 1970;49:813–827.

191. Soleimani M, Aronson PS: Ionic mechanism of $Na+$-$HCO3-$ cotransport in rabbit renal basolateral membrane vesicles. J Biol Chem 1989;264:18302–18308.

192. Soleimani M, Grassi SM, Aronson PS: Stoichiometry of $Na+$-$HCO-3$ cotransport in basolateral membrane vesicles isolated from rabbit renal cortex. J Clin Invest 1987;79:1276–1280.

193. Wingo CS: Active proton secretion and potassium absorption in the rabbit outer medullary collecting duct. Functional evidence for proton-potassium-activated adenosine triphosphatase. J Clin Invest 1989;84:361–365.

194. Maher JF, Schreiner GF: Studies on ethacrynic acid in patients with refractory edema. Ann Intern Med 1965;62:15–29.

195. Nochy D, Callard P, Bellon B, et al: Association of overt glomerulonephritis and liver disease: A study of 34 patients. Clin Nephrol 1976;6:422–427.

196. Bosher SK: The nature of the ototoxic actions of ethacrynic acid upon the mammalian endolymph system. I. Functional aspects. Acta Otolaryngol 1980;89:407–418.

197. Hidaka H, Oshima T, Ikeda K, et al: The Na-K-Cl cotransporters in the rat cochlea: RT-PCR and partial sequence analysis. Biochem Biophys Res Commun 1996;220:425–430.

198. Ikeda K, Oshima T, Hidaka H, Takasaka T: Molecular and clinical implications of loop diuretic ototoxicity. Hear Res 1997;107:1–8.

199. Mizuta K, Adachi M, Iwasa KH: Ultrastructural localization of the Na-K-Cl cotransporter in the lateral wall of the rabbit cochlear duct. Hear Res 1997;106:154–162.

200. Star RA: Ototoxicity. In Seldin DW, Giebisch G (eds): Diuretic Agents: Clinical Physiology and Pharmacology. San Diego: Academic Press, 1997, pp 637–642.

201. Wigand ME, Heidland A: Ototoxic side-effects of high doses of frusemide in patients with uraemia. Postgrad Med J 1971;47:54–56.

202. Chang SW, Fine R, Siegel D, et al: The impact of diuretic therapy on reported sexual function. Arch Intern Med 1991;151:2402–2408.

203. Pickering TG, Shepherd AMM, Puddy I, et al: Sildenafil citrate for erectile dysfunction in men receiving multiple antihypertensive agents: A randomized controlled trial. Am J Hypertens 2004;17:1135–1142.

204. Dikshit K, Vyden JK, Forrester JS, et al: Renal and extrarenal hemodynamic effects of furosemide in congestive heart failure after acute myocardial infarction. N Engl J Med 1973;288:1087–1090.

205. Wilcox CS: Diuretics. In Brenner BM, Rector FC (eds): The Kidney, 5th ed. New York: Raven Press, 1996, pp 2299–2330.

206. Curran KA, Hebert MJ, Cain BD, Wingo CS: Evidence for the presence of a K-dependent acidifying adenosine triphosphatase in the rabbit renal medulla. Kidney Int 1992;42:1093–1098.

207. Francis GS, Siegel RM, Goldsmith SR, et al: Acute vasoconstrictor response to intravenous furosemide in patients with chronic congestive heart failure. Activation of the neurohumoral axis. Ann Intern Med 1985;103:1–6.

208. Johnston GD, Nicholls DP, Leahey WJ: The dose-response characteristics of the acute non-diuretic peripheral vascular effects of frusemide in normal subjects. Br J Clin Pharmacol 1984;18:75–81.

209. Rybak LP: Ototoxicity of loop diuretics. Otolaryngol Clin North Am 1993;26:829-844.

210. Dormans TP, Gerlag PG: Combination of high-dose furosemide and hydrochlorothiazide in the treatment of refractory congestive heart failure. Eur Heart J 1996;17:1867–1874.

211. Nierenberg DW: Furosemide and ethacrynic acid in acute tubular necrosis. West J Med 1980;133:163–170.

212. Lubetsky A, Winaver J, Seligmann H, et al: Urinary thiamin excretion in the rat: Effects of furosemide, other diuretics and volume load. J Lab Clin Med 1999;134:232–237.

213. Shimon I, Almog S, Vered Z, et al: Improved left ventricular function after thiamine supplementation in patients with congestive heart failure receiving long-term furosemide therapy. Am J Med 1995;98:485–490.

214. Chemtob S, Doray J-L, Laudignon N, et al: Alternating sequential dosing with furosemide and ethacrynic acid in drug tolerance in the newborn. Am J Dis Child 1989;143:850–854.

215. Ellison DH: The physiologic basis of diuretic synergism: Its role in treating diuretic resistance. Ann Intern Med 1991;114:886–894.

216. Brater DC, Pressley RH, Anderson SA: Mechanisms of the synergistic combination of metolazone and bumetanide. J Pharmacol Exp Ther 1985;233:70–74.

217. Knauf H, Mutschler E: Diuretic effectiveness of hydrochlorothiazide and furosemide alone and in combination in chronic renal failure. J Cardiovasc Pharmacol 1995;26:394–400.

218. Nakahama H, Orita Y, Yamazaki M, et al: Pharmacokinetic and pharmacodynamic interactions between furosemide and hydrochlorothiazide in nephrotic patients. Nephron 1988;49:223–227.

219. Loon NR, Wilcox CS, Unwin RJ: Mechanism of impaired natriuretic response to furosemide during prolonged therapy. Kidney Int 1989;36:682–689.

220. Kaissling B, Bachmann S, Kriz W: Structural adaptation of the distal convoluted tubule to prolonged furosemide treatment. Am J Physiol 1985;248:F374–F381.

221. Scherzer P, Wald H, Popovtzer MM: Enhanced glomerular filtration and Na+-K+-ATPase with furosemide administration. Am J Physiol 1987;252:F910–F915.

222. Barlet-Bas C, Khadouri C, Marsy S, Doucet A: Enhanced intracellular sodium concentration in kidney cell recruits a latent pool of Na-K-ATPase whose size is modulated by corticosteroids. J Biol Chem 1990;265:7799–7803.

223. Garg LC, Kapturczak M: Renal compensatory response to hydrochlorothiazide changes Na-K-ATPase in distal nephron. In Puschett JB, Greenberg A (eds): Diuretics II: Chemistry, Pharmacology, and Clinical Applications. Amsterdam: Excerpta Medica, 1987, pp 188–194.

224. Stanton BA, Kaissling B: Adaptation of distal tubule and collecting duct to increased Na delivery. II. Na+ and K+ transport. Am J Physiol 1988;255:F1269–F1275.

225. Ellison DH, Velazquez H, Wright FS: Adaptation of the distal convoluted tubule of the rat: Structural and functional effects of dietary salt intake and chronic diuretic infusion. J Clin Invest 1989;83:113–126.

226. Channer KS, McLean KA, Lawson-Matthew P, Richardson M: Combination diuretic treatment in severe heart failure: A randomised controlled trial. Br Heart J 1994;71:146–150.

227. Garin EH: A comparison of combinations of diuretics in nephrotic edema. Am J Dis Child 1987;141:769–771.

228. Oster JR, Epstein M, Smoller S: Combined therapy with thiazide-type and loop diuretic agents for resistant sodium retention. Ann Intern Med 1983;99:405–406.

229. Jeunemaitre X, Charru A, Chatellier G, et al: Long-term metabolic effects of spironolactone and thiazides combined with potassium-sparing agents for treatment of essential hypertension. Am J Cardiol 1988;62:1072–1077.

230. The Randomized Aldactone Evaluation Study [RALES]: Effectiveness of spironolactone added to an angiotensin-converting enzyme inhibitor and a loop diuretic for severe chronic congestive heart failure. Am J Cardiol 1996;78:902–907.

231. Barr CS, Lang CC, Hanson J, et al: Effects of adding spironolactone to an angiotensin-converting enzyme inhibitor in chronic congestive heart failure secondary to coronary artery disease. Am J Cardiol 1995;76:1259–1265.

232. Dahlstrom U, Karlsson E: Captopril and spironolactone therapy for refractory congestive heart failure. Am J Cardiol 1993;71:29A–33A.

233. van Vliet AA, Donker AJ, Nauta JJ, Verheugt FW: Spironolactone in congestive heart failure refractory to high-dose loop diuretic and low-dose angiotensin-converting enzyme inhibitor. Am J Cardiol 1993;71:21A–28A.

234. Zannad F: Angiotensin-converting enzyme inhibitor and spironolactone combination therapy: New objectives in congestive heart failure treatment. Am J Cardiol 1993;71:34A–39A.

235. Schepkens H, Vanholder R, Billiouw JM, Lameire N: Life-threatening hyperkalemia during combined therapy with angiotensin-converting enzyme inhibitors and spironolactone: An analysis of 25 cases. Am J Med 2001;110:438–441.

236. Miller PD, Berns AS: Acute metabolic alkalosis perpetuating hypercarbia. A role for acetazolamide in chronic obstructive pulmonary disease. JAMA 1977;238:2400–2401.

237. Martin SJ, Danziger LH: Continuous infusion of loop diuretics in the critically ill: A review of the literature. Crit Care Med 1994;22:1323–1329.

238. Rudy DW, Voelker JR, Greene PK, et al: Loop diuretics for chronic renal insufficiency: A continuous infusion is more efficacious than bolus therapy. Ann Intern Med 1991;115:360–366.

239. Gerlag PGG, VanMeijel JJM: High-dose furosemide in the treatment of refractory congestive heart failure. Arch Intern Med 1988;148:286–291.

240. van Meyel JJM, Smits P, Dormans T, et al: Continuous infusion of furosemide in the treatment of patients with congestive heart failure and diuretic resistance. J Intern Med 1994;235:329–334.

241. Magovern JA, Magovern, GJ Jr: Diuresis in hemodynamically compromised patients: Continuous furosemide infusion. Ann Thorac Surg 1990;50:482–484.

242. Ogihara T, Rakugi H, Masuo K, et al: Antihypertensive effects of the neutral endopeptidase inhibitor SCH 42495 in essential hypertension. Am J Hypertens 1994;7:943–947.

243. Fett DL, Cavero PG, Burnett JC: Low-dose atrial natriuretic factor and furosemide in experimental acute congestive heart failure. J Am Soc Nephrol 1993;4:162–167.

244. Beregovich J, Bianchi C, Rubler S, et al: Dose-related hemodynamic and renal effects of dopamine in congestive heart failure. Am Heart J 1974;87:550–557.

245. Braun GG, Bahlmann F, Brandl M, Knoll R: Long term administration of dopamine: Is there a development of tolerance? Prog Clin Biol Res 1989;308:1097–1099.

246. Hilberman M, Maseda J, Stinson EB, et al: The diuretic properties of dopamine in patients after open-heart operation. Anesthesiology 1984;61:489–494.

247. Good J, Frost G, Oakley CM, Cleland JG: The renal effects of dopamine and dobutamine in stable chronic heart failure. Postgrad Med J 1992;68 Suppl 2:S7–S11.

248. Vargo DL, Brater C, Rudy DW, Swan SK: Dopamine does not enhance furosemide-induced natriuresis in patients with congestive heart failure. J Am Soc Nephrol 1996;7:1032–1037.

249. Flancbaum L, Choban PS, Dasta JF: Quantitative effects of low-dose dopamine on urine output in oliguric surgical intensive care unit patients. Crit Care Med 1994;22:61–68.

250. Parker S, Carlon GC, Isaacs M, et al: Dopamine administration in oliguria and oliguric renal failure. Crit Care Med 1981;9:630–632.

251. Duke GJ, Briedis JH, Weaver RA: Renal support in critically ill patients: Low-dose dopamine or low-dose dobutamine? Crit Care Med 1994;22:1919–1925.

252. Agostoni P, Marenzi G, Lauri G, et al: Sustained improvement in functional capacity after removal of body fluid with isolated ultrafiltration in chronic cardiac insufficiency: Failure of furosemide to provide the same result. Am J Med 1994;96:191–199.

253. Costanzo MR, Guglin ME, Saltzberg MT, et al; UNLOAD Trial Investigators: Ultrafiltration versus intravenous diuretics for patients hospitalized for acute decompensated heart failure. J Am Coll Cardiol 2007;49:675–683.

Further Reading

Brater DC: Pharmacology of diuretics. Am J Med Sci 2000;319:38–50.

Brater DC: Use of diuretics in cirrhosis and nephrotic syndrome. Semin Nephrol 1999;19:575–580.

Davis BR, Piller LB, Cutler JA, et al: Role of diuretics in the prevention of heart failure: The Antihypertensive and Lipid-Lowering Treatment to Prevent Heart Attack Trial. Circulation 2006;113:2201–2210.

Ellison DH, Wilcox CS: Diuretics. In Brenner BM (ed): Brenner & Rector's The Kidney, 7th ed. Philadelphia: WB Saunders, 2008, pp 1646–1678.

Okusa MD, Ellison DH: Physiology and pathophysiology of diuretic action. In Seldin DW, Giebisch G (eds): The Kidney: Physiology & Pathophysiology. Amsterdam, Academic Press, 2000, pp 2877–2922.

Salvetti A, Ghiadoni L: Thiazide diuretics in the treatment of hypertension: An update. J Am Soc Nephrol 2006;17:S25–S29.

Wilcox CS: New insights into diuretic use in patients with chronic renal disease. J Am Soc Nephrol 2002;13:798–805.

Wilcox CS: Metabolic and adverse effects of diuretics. Semin Nephrol 1999;19:557–568.

Chapter 34

Hypercalcemia, Hypocalcemia, and Other Divalent Cation Disorders

Pouneh Nouri and Francisco Llach

CHAPTER CONTENTS

CALCIUM DISORDERS

Homeostasis

The adult human body contains approximately 1200 g of calcium, of which more than 99% is within bone. The remaining 1% is distributed in three different plasma fractions: approximately 50% is bound to serum albumin, 10% is complexed to various serum anions (phosphate, bicarbonate, citrate, lactate), and 40% is free and ionized. Ionized calcium is the physiologically active form. Its concentration is tightly regulated by the endocrine system. Normal total serum calcium concentration (S_{Ca}) ranges from 8.5 to 10.5 mg/dL (2.1–2.5 mmol/L), whereas ionized S_{Ca} is approximately 5 mg/dL (1.2 mmol/L). A decrease in serum albumin lowers the total S_{Ca}, although the ionized fraction remains normal. A correction for hypoalbuminemia may be made by adding 0.8 mg/dL to the total S_{Ca} for every 1-g/dL drop in serum albumin concentration less than 4 g/dL. Conversely, falsely elevated S_{Ca} may result from hemoconcentration and may be found in rare patients with multiple myeloma who produce calcium-binding paraproteins.[1] In contrast to changes in serum albumin, which affect only total S_{Ca}, changes in pH affect the ionized but not total S_{Ca}. Acidosis increases ionized calcium by decreasing its binding to albumin, whereas alkalosis has the opposite effect. A direct measurement of ionized S_{Ca} is preferred in patients who have combined changes in pH and serum albumin.

The S_{Ca} normally reflects a balance between the entry of calcium into the extracellular fluid (ECF) from the gastrointestinal tract, skeleton, and kidneys and its removal by renal excretion and deposition into the skeleton. The precise regulation of

S_{Ca} is largely controlled by parathyroid hormone (PTH) and the highly-active-vitamin D_3 metabolite 1,25-dihydroxycholecalciferol (1,25[OH]$_2$D$_3$, also called cholecalcitriol). Dietary calcium is absorbed in the proximal intestine via both active and passive processes. Absorption is enhanced by calcitriol, the principal hormonal regulator of intestinal absorption. In the kidneys, 99% of the filtered load of calcium is reabsorbed. Approximately 90% of reabsorption occurs passively in the proximal tubule and Henle's loop; the remaining 10% occurs in the distal tubule under the regulation of PTH. A decrease in free S_{Ca} stimulates the release of PTH, which increases renal calcium reabsorption. PTH also mediates the hydroxylation of calciferol (dihydroxyvitamin D_3) to calcitriol. The effects of S_{Ca} on PTH secretion are mediated via a calcium-sensing receptor. This cell-surface receptor is coupled with guanine-nucleotide regulatory G proteins and is expressed in the parathyroid, kidney, brain, and other organs.[2]

Hypercalcemia

Pathophysiology, Clinical Features, and Cause

Hypercalcemia is usually caused by an increase in ionized S_{Ca}. Hypercalcemia develops when the rate of entry of calcium into the ECF exceeds its excretion into urine or deposition in bone. An increase in influx can result from increased absorption from either intestine or bone, or both. However, multiple sites can be involved. For example, hypervitaminosis D increases both intestinal calcium absorption and bone resorption. Primary hyperparathyroidism (PHP) increases reabsorption from bone and renal tubules and increases renal synthesis of calcitriol. The major causes of hypercalcemia are PHP and malignancy: PHP accounts for more than 90% of cases in ambulatory patients, whereas in hospitalized patients, cancer accounts for approximately 65% of cases.[3]

Clinical presentation of hypercalcemia depends on the magnitude and rapidity of the elevation in S_{Ca}. Mild hypercalcemia (10.6–2 mg/dL) accompanying PHP is generally asymptomatic.[4] More severe hypercalcemia is frequently associated with neurological, gastrointestinal, and renal manifestations. Neurological symptoms may range from subtle changes in concentration to depression, confusion, increased somnolence, and even coma. Gastrointestinal symptoms are often prominent, with constipation, anorexia, nausea, and vomiting. The most important renal manifestations are nephrolithiasis, renal tubular dysfunction (particularly decreased concentrating ability[5]), and acute and chronic renal insufficiency. Nephrolithiasis has been reported in 20% of patients with PHP, whereas 4% to 5% of stone formers have PHP.[6] Increased calcitriol production may contribute to both hypercalciuria and stone formation.

Rarely, familial hypocalciuric hypercalcemia (FHH), also known as familial benign hypercalcemia, is easily confused with milder cases of the more common PHP. FHH is generally asymptomatic and does not require treatment. However, it is important to identify patients with FHH to avoid unnecessary parathyroidectomy for presumable PHP. Because most cases of FHH are associated with loss-of-function mutations in a single gene (*CASR* or calcium-sensing receptor), genetic testing can assist in the diagnosis of FHH.

Diagnosis

PHP and malignancy account for 80% to 90% of cases. Longstanding asymptomatic hypercalcemia suggests FHH. An elevated serum intact PTH concentration (measured by immunoradiometric assay) indicates the presence of PHP or a patient taking lithium.[7] If the plasma PTH level is below normal, a neoplastic disorder should be strongly considered (Fig. 34-1). The diagnosis of humoral hypercalcemia of malignancy can be confirmed by demonstrating an elevated serum PTH–related protein. The serum levels of the vitamin D metabolites calcitriol and 25-hydroxycholecalciferol (calcidiol) should be measured if there is no obvious malignancy and neither PTH nor PTH-related protein levels are elevated. An elevated serum calcidiol is indicative of vitamin D intoxication due to the ingestion of either vitamin D or calcidiol itself. Conversely, increased levels of calcitriol may be induced by direct intake of this metabolite, extrarenal production in granulomatous diseases or lymphoma, or increased renal production by PTH.

Treatment

Overview

The definitive treatment of hypercalcemia depends on the treatment of the underlying disease, for example, parathyroidectomy for PHP and chemotherapy for a malignancy. The initial treatment can be instituted without a specific diagnosis. General measures include rapid mobilization and hydration. Volume depletion, by limiting renal calcium excretion, perpetuates a vicious circle and worsens acute hypercalcemia. Medications that worsen hypercalcemia, such as thiazide diuretics, should be discontinued. Volume expansion with isotonic saline usually decreases S_{Ca} by enhancing renal calcium excretion. Only after volume repletion should loop diuretics be used to enhance sodium and calcium excretion

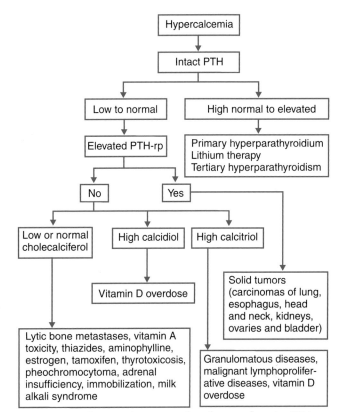

Figure 34-1 Diagnostic approach to hypercalcemia. PTH, parathyroid hormone; PTH-rp, PTH-related protein.

(Fig. 34-2). In patients with renal failure, dialysis effectively removes calcium from the ECF. Careful monitoring of cardiac function and serum electrolytes is necessary with both saline diuresis and dialysis treatment. Hypercalcemia can be divided into mild (S_{Ca} < 12 mg/dL), moderate (S_{Ca} 12–14 mg/dL), and severe (S_{Ca} > 14 mg/dL).[8]

Mild Hypercalcemia

Most cases of mild hypercalcemia are caused by PHP. All patients with PHP and symptomatic hypercalcemia who are surgical candidates should be referred to an experienced parathyroid surgeon for parathyroidectomy. Few would disagree that the best management for the patient with obvious symptoms or associated conditions of the disease or profound hypercalcemia (>12 mg/dL) is parathyroidectomy.[9] Patients with FHH require no therapy.

There is a debate surrounding the issue of the best management of asymptomatic patients or those with mild symptoms and no associated conditions of PHP. To address this issue, in 1990, the National Institutes of Health together with the National Institute of Diabetes and Digestive and Kidney Diseases defined a set of guidelines for operative interventions in these patients. These include markedly elevated serum calcium (>12 mg/dL); history of an episode of life-threatening hypercalcemia; decreased creatinine clearance by 30% compared with age-matched normal subjects; markedly elevated 24-hour urine calcium (>400 mg/day); nephrolithiasis; age older than 50; osteitis fibrosa cystica; bone mass more than 2 SD below controls matched for age, gender, and ethnic

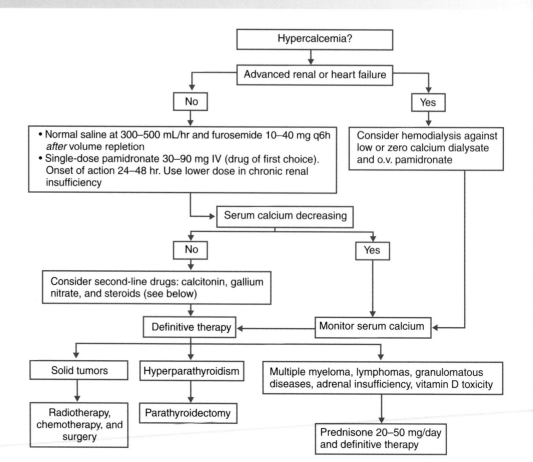

Figure 34-2 Treatment of hypercalcemia. IV, intravenous.

group; and neuromuscular symptoms (i.e., documented proximal weakness, atrophy, hyperreflexia, and gait disturbance).[9] However, management of patients with asymptomatic PHP remains controversial.[10] Immediate intervention is not necessary. Surgery may be beneficial in patients with vertebral osteopenia, in whom parathyroidectomy may lead to a dramatic improvement (as much as 20%) in bone density.[11] Consideration of parathyroidectomy should also be given to patients with PHP who are vitamin D deficient because the loss of inhibition by calcitriol on the PTH gene worsens the PHP.[12] Replacement of vitamin D in face of hypercalcemia and/or hypercalciuria can be risky. Estrogen-progestin therapy is beneficial in postmenopausal women with PHP because it decreases bone resorption and decreases S_{Ca} by 0.5 to 1.0 mg/dL and increases bone density modestly.[13] Estrogen-progestin therapy decreases urinary calcium and hydroxyproline excretion and serum alkaline phosphatase, indicating decreased bone resorption, without changes in PTH.[14]

Diuretics should not be used to treat patients with mild PHP. Loop diuretics increase calcium excretion in the urine but may induce volume depletion. Thiazide diuretics are contraindicated because they decrease urinary calcium excretion and increase S_{Ca}. Oral inorganic phosphates can effectively lower S_{Ca}, but the resultant ectopic calcification is harmful to kidneys, blood vessels, and soft tissues. Thus, inorganic phosphates are reserved for patients who are not candidates for or who have failed alternate therapies and those who are moderately hypophosphatemic. The use of β-adrenergic blockers such as propranolol, H_2 receptor antagonists such as cimetidine, and

progestin has been unsuccessful in decreasing S_{Ca} in patients with PHP.

Bisphosphonates are potent inhibitors of bone but are rarely required for mild hypercalcemia. However, risedronate, a newer bisphosphonate that can be given orally, inhibits bone resorption and decreases fasting S_{Ca} in patients with PHP.[15] It may become the drug of choice for patients with PHP, particularly those with osteoporosis. However, long-term benefit has not been documented (see "Severe Hypercalcemia"). Drugs under development include those that activate the calcium-sensing receptor in the parathyroid gland, thereby inhibiting PTH secretion,[16] calcitriol analogues that inhibit PTH secretion directly but do not stimulate gastrointestinal calcium or phosphate absorption,[17] and drugs that block the PTH receptor.[18]

Moderate Hypercalcemia

Moderate hypercalcemia (S_{Ca} 12–14 mg/dL) should be treated aggressively if there are signs or symptoms. The severity of the symptoms correlates with the rate of increase in S_{Ca}. In patients with few or mild symptoms, treatment of the underlying cause should be instituted while embarking on hydration and mobilization. When neurological symptoms are the sole manifestation of hypercalcemia, other causes of an altered mental status must be excluded.[19]

The rationale for the use of normal saline for initial treatment is that volume depletion impairs glomerular filtration and increases sodium and calcium reabsorption in the proximal tubule. Normal saline should be administered to replenish volume and decrease proximal tubule calcium reabsorption. Occasional patients may become hypernatremic and require hypotonic fluids because of the relative resistance to antidiuretic hormone in hypercalcemia combined with impairment of thirst if they are confused. If congestive heart failure develops or a more rapid decrease in S_{Ca} is desired, small doses of a loop diuretic may be added (e.g., furosemide 10–20 mg every 6 hours). Diuretic-induced ECF depletion should be avoided as this worsens hypercalcemia. Higher doses of loop diuretics may be required in patients with renal insufficiency. The combination of intravenous normal saline and loop diuretics should decrease S_{Ca} rapidly, by approximately 1 to 3 mg/dL, within 1 to 2 days. If the symptoms persist or hypercalcemia worsens, the treatment plan for severe hypercalcemia should be instituted.

Severe Hypercalcemia

When S_{Ca} exceeds 14 mg/dL, therapy should be initiated regardless of whether the patient has signs or symptoms of hypercalcemia, except in terminally ill patients. Therapy involves a combination of volume replenishment, enhanced renal calcium excretion, reduced bone resorption, and management of the underlying disease.

Patients with an elevated PTH should be referred for prompt parathyroidectomy after S_{Ca} has been decreased sufficiently for safe surgery. Excessive preoperative correction of hypercalcemia leads to postoperative hypocalcemia due to a decrease in osteoclastic bone resorption and marked influx of calcium into unmineralized osteoid.

Malignancy is usually responsible for severe hypercalcemia. Specific treatment of tumors with radiation or chemotherapy should not be delayed. Mobilization and oral sodium chloride and water, although still helpful, are unlikely alone to correct hypercalcemia. The first step is replacement of ECF volume with 0.9% saline at 300 to 500 mL/hr, decreased after volume deficit has been partially corrected. At least 3 to 4 L should be given in the first 24 hours to achieve a positive fluid balance of at least 2 L. Caution is required in patients who are elderly and those with compromised cardiac or renal function. Saline infusion increases the delivery of sodium chloride, fluid, and calcium to Henle's loop. Therefore, a loop diuretic is used to block transport at this site. Furosemide (40–160 mg/day in divided doses) is given after the ECF volume has been replenished. Thiazide diuretics are contraindicated because they decrease renal calcium excretion. The patient's hemodynamic and electrolyte status (potassium, phosphate, and magnesium replenishment are usually required) must be monitored closely, often in an intensive care unit.

Concomitant measures to reduce osteoclastic bone resorption should be initiated because there is usually a marked enhancement of osteoclast-mediated bone resorption in patients with hypercalcemia. Bisphosphonates are analogues of pyrophosphate that are resistant to phosphatases. These bone-seeking compounds bind to hydroxyapatite and prevent its dissolution. They have a very long half-life. Because they are poorly absorbed (1%–5% of an oral dose), they should be given with water on an empty stomach at least 30 minutes before food.[20] Approximately 80% of the absorbed bisphosphonate is cleared by the kidney. The remaining 20% is taken up by bone, and this is enhanced by high bone turnover. Although the plasma half-life is only 1 hour, bisphosphonates may persist in bone for the patient's lifetime.[20] Intravenous

administration of bisphosphonate should be given as 500 mL over at least 4 hours to dilute the precipitated calcium bisphosphonate that likely accounts for much of the nephrotoxicity.[21] In patients with renal insufficiency, therapy should be initiated with lower doses diluted in larger volumes of fluid with additional doses given if renal function remains stable.

Etidronate is given intravenously (7.5 mg/kg/day in saline over 4 hours) for at least three consecutive days. Prolonging treatment to 5 days increases the response rate from 60% to 100% of patients. Therapy should be interrupted if S_{Ca} decreases rapidly (2–3 mg/dL in the first 2–3 days) or normalizes to avoid hypocalcemia. Normocalcemia may persist for 1 to 7 weeks. Some patients can be maintained on oral etidronate (20 mg/kg/day). Prolonged administration has been associated with osteomalacia[22] and hyperphosphatemia due to increased tubular reabsorption of phosphate. The dose of etidronate should be decreased by 50% in patients with renal insufficiency because some is excreted in the urine.

As pamidronate is more potent and long-lasting than etidronate, it is the bisphosphonate of choice.[22] A single injection of pamidronate is more effective in ameliorating hypercalcemia than a 3-day regimen of intravenous etidronate.[23] The intravenous dose of pamidronate depends on the degree of hypercalcemia: 30 mg if S_{Ca} is less than 12 mg/dL (3 mmol/L), 60 mg if S_{Ca} is 12 to 13.5 mg/dL (3.0–3.4 mmol/L), and 90 mg if S_{Ca} is higher. It is usually given in isotonic saline as a single intravenous infusion over 4 to 24 hours.[24] The dose should not be repeated in less than 7 days. Pamidronate is well tolerated, although a few patients develop fever. It is excreted by the kidney. Although not approved for use in patients with renal failure, pamidronate seems to be safe and effective for the treatment of patients on dialysis who have severe hypercalcemia induced by the combination of calcium carbonate and calcitriol,[25] provided that the dose does not exceed 30 mg. Pamidronate produces sustained normocalcemia for 15 days. In patients with cancer, the duration of hypocalcemic effect correlates inversely with serum PTH-related protein concentrations, with values more than 12 pmol/L usually indicating a short-lived response.[26]

Clodronate (4–6 mg/kg/day infused over 2–4 hours) is widely used in Europe but is not available in the United States.

Alendronate, although very potent when administered intravenously, is approved only for oral therapy of osteoporosis.

Zolendronic acid (Zometa) has been recently approved by U.S. Food and Drug Administration for the treatment of the hypercalcemia of malignancy. A single 4- to 8-mg dose of zolendronic acid is more effective than 90 mg pamidronate. The duration of normocalcemia is 32 to 43 days. In addition, a 4-mg dose of zolendronic acid offers the convenience of a 15-minute infusion time compared with 2 to 24 hours for pamidronate. Zolendronic acid also decreases the skeleton-related events in patients with metastatic breast cancer, multiple myeloma, Paget's disease, and bone metastasis from prostate and lung cancers.[27]

Risedronate, a potent third-generation oral bisphosphonate, is being evaluated for treatment of hypercalcemia. It decreases S_{Ca} in mild PHP, but its long-term utility remains to be determined.

Ibandronate (Boniva) is approved by U.S. Food and Drug Administration as once per month oral treatment for osteoporosis. Its intravenous administration as a bolus within a few minutes for the treatment of hypercalcemia of malignancy and skeleton-related events of solid tumors has been approved in Europe without an increased risk of nephrotoxicity compared with other intravenous forms of bisphosphonates (i.e., zolendronic acid and pamidronate).[28,29]

Osteochemonecrosis of jaws is a well-described side effect of bisphosphonates. The oral preparations (i.e., alendronate and risedronate) are considered low risk of osteonecrosis. Nephrotoxicity is a rare but important reported side effect of zolendronic acid, which should be avoided in patients with any degree of renal failure. Other bisphosphonates need dose adjustments for creatinine clearance less than 30 mL/min.[30]

Plicamycin (mithramycin) inhibits osteoclastic RNA synthesis and decreases osteoclastic bone resorption. It is given intravenously (15–25 µg/kg) over 3 to 6 hours and repeated in 1 to 2 days if required. S_{Ca} begins to decrease within 12 hours, usually reaching a nadir by 48 hours. The hypocalcemic effect lasts for several days. Repeated doses can be given at 3- to 7-day intervals. Use of mithramycin is limited by its toxicity, particularly in patients with liver, bone marrow, or kidney disease. It is rarely used.

Calcitonin inhibits osteoclastic bone resorption and enhances renal calcium excretion. The most potent form of the drug is salmon calcitonin, which is given intramuscularly or subcutaneously (4–8 U/kg every 6–12 hours). It is safe and nontoxic and acts rapidly within 4 to 6 hours. Unfortunately, calcitonin is effective in only 60% to 70% of patients, most of whom then develop tachyphylaxis rapidly.[22] It is additive with bisphosphonates.

Gallium nitrate inhibits bone resorption by binding to bone, decreasing hydroxyapatite crystal solubility, and decreasing S_{Ca}. Because it also inhibits PTH secretion, it may be particularly effective in the treatment of hyperparathyroidism. It is administered intravenously over 5 days at a dose of 200 mg/m²/day in 1 L of saline over 24 hours. Like bisphosphonates, there is a latent period of 6 to 8 days before a nadir in S_{Ca} is seen, with the effect lasting approximately 1 week. However, adverse effects are more frequent and more severe, with nephrotoxicity being common as well as hypophosphatemia and anemia. The drug should be avoided in patients with renal insufficiency or those receiving concomitant nephrotoxic agents.

Glucocorticoids decrease S_{Ca} by inhibiting cytokine release, by direct cytolytic effects on select tumor cells, by inhibiting intestinal calcium absorption, and by increasing renal calcium excretion. They are effective in hypercalcemia due to myeloma, other hematologic malignancies, sarcoidosis, and vitamin D intoxication. Other tumors rarely respond. The initial oral dose of prednisone is 20 to 50 mg twice daily. The S_{Ca} may take 5 to 10 days to decrease, after which the dose should be gradually decreased. Toxicity limits the usefulness of glucocorticoids for long-term therapy.

Hemodialysis, with little or no calcium in the dialysis fluid, and peritoneal dialysis, albeit slower, are both very effective modes of therapy for hypercalcemia. Dialysis is particularly useful in patients with renal insufficiency or congestive heart failure who cannot safely be given intravenous saline.

Inorganic phosphates, although effective, are not recommended for therapy of hypercalcemia because of the precipitation of calcium phosphate crystals in blood vessels and soft tissues.

Future therapies for cancer-induced hypercalcemia include noncalcemic analogues of calcitriol (e.g., 22-oxacalcitriol)

that reduce the release of PTH-related protein. A calcimimetic agent, such as norcalcin, that binds to the calcium-sensing receptor and suppresses the release of PTH is being evaluated for PHP.

Hypocalcemia

Clinical Features, Pathophysiology, and Cause

The symptoms and signs of acute hypocalcemia include latent tetany, tetany, papilledema, and seizures. By comparison, ectodermal and dental changes, cataracts, basal ganglia calcification, and extrapyramidal disorders are features of chronic hypocalcemia.[31] Hypocalcemia can cause emotional instability, anxiety, depression, confusional states, hallucinations, and frank psychosis. Hypocalcemia characteristically causes prolongation of the QT interval on the electrocardiogram. Because the ST segment rather than the T wave is affected, the interval to the onset of the T wave (QoTc interval) may be a more sensitive indicator of hypocalcemia.[32] Hypocalcemia impairs the response to digitalis. Ventricular arrhythmias and congestive heart failure can occur. Chronic hypocalcemia, particularly when associated with hypophosphatemia and vitamin D deficiency, causes growth plate abnormalities in children (rickets) and defects in the mineralization of new bone. Severe symptomatic hypocalcemia requires immediate intervention.

Falsely low S_{Ca} due to hypoalbuminemia should first be excluded by measuring ionized S_{Ca}. The most common causes of hypocalcemia in hospital include magnesium deficiency, pancreatitis, sepsis, acute and chronic renal failure, hypoparathyroidism, vitamin D deficiency, and complexing of calcium with infused phosphate, citrate, or albumin[33] (Fig. 34-3).

Treatment

Rationale and Overview

Treatment of hypocalcemia varies with its severity, the rapidity with which it develops, and the underlying cause. At one end of the spectrum, an asymptomatic patient with mild hypocalcemia (7.5–8.5 mg/dL, 1.9–2.1 mmol/L) may

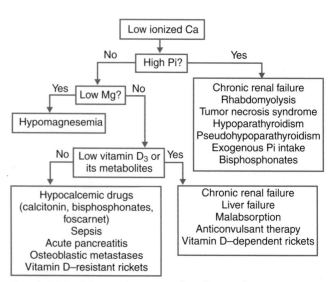

Figure 34-3 Diagnostic approach to hypocalcemia.

warrant cautious observation and require only oral calcium supplements (500–1000 mg elemental calcium every 6 hours ingested between meals). In contrast, a patient with tetany, a sign of severe hypocalcemia, must be treated aggressively with intravenous calcium. Patients with S_{Ca} less than 7.5 mg/dL, or any symptoms, require parenteral therapy (Fig. 34-4). Administration of calcium alone is only effective transiently. PTH is not available for clinical use; therefore, patients with PTH deficiency are treated with calcium and vitamin D.

Investigation into the underlying cause for hypocalcemia should include the serum phosphate (high in renal failure and tumor lysis and low in hypomagnesemia, osteoblastic metastatic disease, and vitamin D–deficient states such as osteomalacia), creatinine, and alkaline phosphatase (high in renal osteodystrophy, osteoblastic metastatic disease, and osteomalacia).

Hypocalcemia is often associated with other electrolyte and acid-base disorders. Hypomagnesemia should be treated as needed (see "Hypomagnesemia"). When metabolic acidosis is present, S_{Ca} must be corrected before acidosis because the treatment of acidosis decreases the ionized S_{Ca}, thereby precipitating problems such as tetany or cardiac arrest. Moreover, sodium bicarbonate and calcium salts must be administered in different intravenous lines to avoid precipitation of calcium carbonate. Because the administration of calcium potentiates digoxin toxicity, such patients should be monitored closely.

Hyperphosphatemia may accompany hypocalcemia in patients with hypoparathyroidism, renal disease, rhabdomyolysis, or tumor lysis. To avoid precipitation of calcium and phosphate, calcium supplementation must be given with phosphorus binders. By decreasing the fraction of calcium bound to phosphate, a decrease in the serum phosphate improves ionized S_{Ca}. When hypocalcemia persists, it is best to delay calcium supplementation until the serum phosphate is less than 6 mg/dL.

Acute Hypocalcemia

Patients with symptomatic hypocalcemia should be treated immediately. Many patients have symptoms when ionized S_{Ca} is less than 2.8 mg/dL or total S_{Ca} is less than 7 mg/dL. In general, the intravenous infusion of 15 mg/kg of elemental calcium over 4 to 6 hours will increase total S_{Ca} by approximately 2 to 3 mg/dL.[30] Thus, a 70-kg patient with S_{Ca} of 6 mg/dL will require approximately 1 g of elemental calcium to increase S_{Ca} to 8 mg/dL. Several forms of calcium can be used for intravenous administration.

Calcium gluconate (10% in 10-mL ampoules containing 94 mg of elemental calcium) is given in emergency situations as one ampoule over 4 minutes followed by a calcium gluconate drip, if necessary. Solutions concentrated to greater than 200 mg (two ampoules) of calcium per 100 mL should be avoided because calcium is irritating to veins. Ten ampoules (100 mL) may be combined with 1000 mL of 5% dextrose and infused at 50 mL/hr (45 mg of elemental calcium per hour), titrating the rate as needed. For a symptomatic 70-kg patient, calcium may be infused more rapidly until symptoms subside, then the infusion is decreased to 50 mL/hr to achieve a low-normal calcium level within 8 to 18 hours. If necessary, all 10 ampoules may be infused over 4 to 6 hours.[34]

Calcium gluceptate (10%) is similar to calcium gluconate but provides 90 mg of elemental calcium in a 5-mL ampoule, which is useful in patients who cannot tolerate large volumes

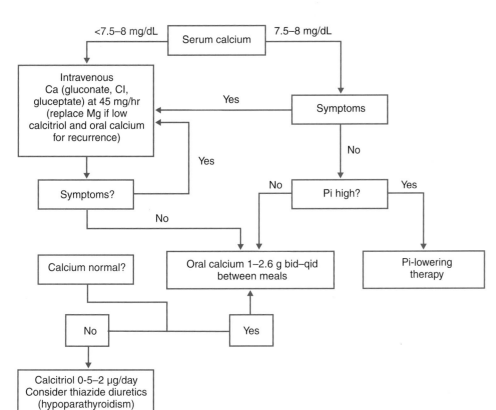

Figure 34-4 Treatment of hypocalcemia. S_{Ca}, serum calcium concentration.

of fluid. Ten ampoules (50 mL) may be added to 450 mL of 5% dextrose as 1.8 mg/mL. A dose of 45 mg of calcium (half an ampoule) can be infused in 25 mL of fluid.

Calcium chloride (10%) provides more calcium per ampoule (272 mg per 10-mL ampoule) and is more bioavailable than either calcium gluconate or calcium gluceptate. Although this results in a more rapid elevation in S_{Ca}, which may be preferable in emergency situations, it is more irritating to veins, thus rendering it less desirable for prolonged infusion.

Calcium glubionate (Neo-Calglucon) is an oral liquid that provides 23 mg of calcium per milliliter or 115 mg per teaspoon (5 mL). It is readily absorbed in the gastrointestinal tract and is well tolerated. It is an excellent supplement for hypocalcemic neonates and infants and for adults who lack intravenous access.

Patients with hypocalcemia following elective parathyroidectomy for renal osteodystrophy may require emergency vitamin D therapy. When the excessive PTH stimulation is withdrawn suddenly, calcium and phosphate accumulate rapidly in healing bone lesions and osteoclastic bone resorption is decreased. These effects cause a dramatic decrease in S_{Ca} (hungry bone syndrome). The failed kidneys cannot increase calcitriol, so that intestinal calcium absorption remains low. Intravenous calcium is often required initially and is replaced with oral calcium supplements and calcitriol. Calcitriol is the vitamin D metabolite with the greatest potency and most rapid onset of action. It is available in oral (Rocaltrol) and intravenous (Calcijex) preparations. Initially, large intravenous doses are generally required ($\sim$1–2 μg/day), decreasing to maintenance oral daily doses or three times weekly intravenous doses at dialysis of 0.2 to 1.0 μg.[33]

Chronic Hypocalcemia

This requires treatment with oral calcium supplementation and, if necessary, vitamin D to enhance intestinal calcium absorption. Calcium is available with carbonate, gluconate, lactate, acetate, citrate, glubionate, and phosphate, although absorption varies with the preparation and timing of ingestion. Treatment is usually started at a dose of 1000 to 2600 mg two to four times daily between meals, adjusted according to S_{Ca}. Calcium carbonate is available in tablets containing 500 to 750 mg of calcium. Calcium citrate is well absorbed but should not be used in patients taking aluminum-containing medications because it enhances aluminum absorption. Calcium glubionate is well absorbed but expensive. Calcium phosphate should be avoided because it exacerbates hyperphosphatemia and metastatic calcification.[35]

Patients with hypoparathyroidism may develop hypercalciuria with treatment because they lack the normal stimulatory effect of PTH on renal tubular calcium reabsorption and therefore excrete excessive calcium. This may cause nephrolithiasis, nephrocalcinosis, or chronic renal insufficiency. Therefore, the dose of calcium should be adjusted to maintain S_{Ca} slightly below normal range and calcium excretion should be measured periodically. A few patients with hypoparathyroidism can be treated with a thiazide diuretic.

In disorders associated with insufficient vitamin D (e.g., hypoparathyroidism, osteomalacia, chronic renal failure), calcitriol acts rapidly because it requires no further metabolism to function. Administration of 0.5 to 1.0 μg/day is usually sufficient, although in extreme cases, such as immediately after parathyroidectomy, more may be required (2–3 μg). Calcitriol is more expensive than the parent vitamin D compounds vitamin D_2 (ergocalciferol) and vitamin D_3 (cholecalciferol), which are adequate for nutritional deficiency at doses of approximately 400 U/day or for malabsorption at higher doses (50,000–100,000 U/day). However, their action may be delayed for several weeks because they require conversion to calcitriol. They are ineffective for diseases in which 25- or 1α-hydroxylation is impaired, such as liver and renal failure, hypoparathyroidism, and vitamin D–dependent rickets type 1. In contrast to the rapid elimination of calcitriol and calcidiol (within days), vitamins D_2 and D_3 may continue to function for several weeks after dosing, potentially resulting in hypervitaminosis D.[35]

PHOSPHATE DISORDERS

Homeostasis

Phosphate is the most abundant intracellular anion: approximately 80% is contained within bone mineral, 19% in cells, and approximately 1% in the ECF. Plasma phosphate concentrations are 2.5 to 4.5 mg/dL (0.81–1.45 mmol/L) in adults and 4.0 to 7.0 mg/dL (1.3–2.3 mmol/L) in children. Thus, changes in serum phosphate concentration (S_{Pi}) may not reflect total body content. The majority ($\sim$70%) of S_{Pi} is organic and present mainly in phospholipids, and the remainder is inorganic. Approximately 15% of inorganic phosphate is bound to protein and is therefore not available for ultrafiltration by the kidneys. The remainder exists mainly in the monohydrogen (HPO_4^{2-}) and dihydrogen ($H_2PO_4^-$) forms in a ratio of 4:1 at a physiologic pH of 7.4. Small amounts are complexed to sodium, magnesium, and calcium.

S_{Pi} is not as tightly regulated as S_{Ca}. It varies with dietary intake, age (higher in infants and children, decreasing with adolescence), time of day (peak at 4 AM and nadir 6–7 hours later), and hormonal status (higher in postmenopausal women). Phosphate is prevalent in meats, dairy products, and grains. Some 65% of ingested phosphate (800–1600 mg/day) is absorbed in the small intestine, both passively and by calcitriol-mediated active transport. Normally, phosphate transport occurs primarily through unregulated paracellular diffusive pathways. However, when luminal phosphate concentrations are low, absorption is by active sodium-dependent transport via a Na^+/P cotransporter that is secondarily active and uses the favorable sodium gradient from the basolateral Na^+/K^+-ATPase.[36] Phosphate egress is passive. Calcitriol enhances phosphate absorption, whereas PTH stimulates intestinal phosphate absorption indirectly by increasing the synthesis of calcitriol. Other factors that increase intestinal phosphate absorption include low phosphate intake, acidosis, bile salts, lactose, prolactin, thyroid hormone, and the acute effect of glucocorticoids. Calcium, magnesium, and aluminum decrease phosphate absorption by binding to phosphate. Hypophosphatemia stimulates production of calcitriol, which subsequently enhances phosphate and calcium absorption. Hyperphosphatemia increases PTH secretion and decreases calcitriol production.

Renal phosphate excretion generally equals phosphate absorption. Some 85% of phosphate reabsorption occurs in the proximal tubule, where the brush-border membrane phosphate transporter is secondarily active via the Na^+/P cotransporter.[37]

Growth hormone, insulin-like growth factor I, insulin, epidermal growth factor, thyroid hormone, and calcitriol stimulate renal phosphate reabsorption. PTH, PTH-related protein, calcitonin, atrial natriuretic factor, transforming growth factors α and β, and glucocorticoids inhibit phosphate absorption.[21] Intravascular volume expansion and high-phosphate diets enhance phosphate excretion.

S_{Pi} can be decreased acutely by stimulating cellular uptake with intravenous glucose or insulin, ingestion of carbohydrate-rich meals, acute respiratory alkalosis, epinephrine, and rapid cell proliferation (e.g., neoplasia).[38] Conversely, S_{Pi} is increased by metabolic acidosis and intravenous infusion of calcium.

Hyperphosphatemia

Clinical Features, Pathophysiology, and Cause

Hyperphosphatemia (S_{Pi} > 4.5 mg/dL in adults, >7 mg/dL in children) is most commonly caused by decreased renal phosphate excretion due to renal failure (i.e., glomerular filtration rate < 20–25 mL/min). Hyperphosphatemia due to defective renal phosphate clearance also occurs with hypoparathyroidism, pseudohypoparathyroidism, increased growth hormone or insulin-like growth factor I, bisphosphonate therapy, and a variety of rare inherited diseases.[19] Acidosis redistributes cellular phosphate to the plasma. Hyperphosphatemia can also occur during increased release of intracellular phosphate in acute tumor lysis or rhabdomyolysis coupled with acute renal failure[39] (Fig. 34-5).

In advanced renal failure, hyperphosphatemia is a universal finding. As the glomerular filtration rate decreases, fractional tubular phosphate excretion increases progressively, under the influence of PTH, to 60% to 90%. This maintains S_{Pi} until the glomerular filtration rate decreases to less than 25 mL/min. The ensuing hyperphosphatemia and loss of functioning kidney mass suppress the production of calcitriol, thus decreasing intestinal absorption of calcium. The ensuing

decrease in S_{Ca} and increase in S_{Pi} decrease calcitriol and increase PTH secretion, which may aggravate hyperphosphatemia by release of calcium and phosphate from bone. The eventual parathyroid hyperplasia and excessive PTH action cause high-turnover bone disease.[39]

The rapid turnover of malignant tumors stimulated by chemotherapy releases intracellular potassium, uric acid, and phosphate. Uric acid precipitation in the renal tubules can cause acute renal failure, which may worsen the hyperphosphatemia and hyperkalemia. Increasing the urine pH with intravenous alkaline sodium bicarbonate solubilizes the uric acid but may enhance calcium phosphate precipitation, which can cause nephrocalcinosis or nephrolithiasis.

Pseudohyperphosphatemia due to hyperglobulinemia, hyperlipidemia, hemolysis, and hyperbilirubinemia can be assessed by serum analysis after deproteinization.

The manifestations of acute severe hyperphosphatemia are related mainly to accompanying hypocalcemia and tetany caused by precipitation of calcium phosphate. In addition, hyperphosphatemia inhibits the activity of 1α-hydroxylase in the kidney. The resulting decrease in calcitriol aggravates hypocalcemia further by impairing intestinal calcium absorption, inducing skeletal resistance to PTH. Profound hypocalcemia and tetany are occasionally observed during the early phase of the tumor lysis syndrome and rhabdomyolysis. When the (calcium ∞ phosphate) product exceeds approximately 65, patients may develop metastatic calcification in the skin, cornea, blood vessels, myocardium, heart valves, and other organs.[39] Patients on maintenance dialysis may also develop premature coronary artery calcification.[40] An extreme case of metastatic calcification, acral calciphylaxis, is rapid occlusion of small-sized arteries with necrosis and gangrene of the digits. Parathyroidectomy is recommended if PTH levels are extremely elevated.[39] Hyperphosphatemia is critical in the development of secondary hyperparathyroidism and renal osteodystrophy in chronic renal failure.

Treatment

Correction of the cause is the primary aim. Acute hyperphosphatemia in patients who do not have renal failure is treated by saline diuresis. Proximally acting diuretics, such as acetazolamide, are the most phosphaturic. Correction of acidosis or treatment of hyperglycemia with insulin promotes cellular phosphate uptake.

In patients with impaired renal function, S_{Pi} may be decreased by dietary phosphate restriction. Because phosphate is ubiquitous, severe dietary restriction is impractical. The average American diet contains 800 to 1600 mg of phosphate; restriction to 1000 to 1250 mg does not cause protein-calorie malnutrition.[39] In patients with end-stage renal disease or severe acute renal failure, S_{Pi} may be decreased by dialysis. Although dialysis membranes are permeant to phosphate, there is only a slow phosphate efflux from the large intracellular phosphate stores. Hemodialysis removes only approximately 2 to 3 g of phosphate per week. Nocturnal hemodialysis improves control of S_{Pi}.[41] Peritoneal dialysis is more effective in eliminating phosphate but is still unable to match the dietary phosphate intake of most patients.

Phosphate binders form insoluble nonabsorbable compounds with phosphate in the intestines that are lost in stool. They must be ingested immediately before, during, or after the meal. Calcium, aluminum, and magnesium all bind phosphate,

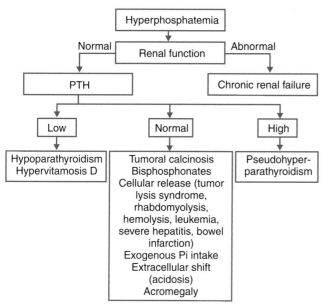

Figure 34-5 Diagnostic approach to hyperphosphatemia. PTH, parathyroid hormone.

although magnesium is relatively weak and is avoided in renal insufficiency. Oral calcium carbonate and the more potent calcium acetate are preferred to calcium citrate because the latter enhances intestinal aluminum absorption. Calcium carbonate is available in 500- and 1000-mg tablets. The initial dose is 1 g with each meal three times daily. If S_{Pi} does not decrease, the dose is gradually increased to 8 to 12 g/day. Persistent hyperphosphatemia may be due to incomplete dissolution of the tablets in the gastrointestinal tract, excessive phosphate intake, or noncompliance. Hypercalcemia is more likely if a vitamin D preparation is also given or if there is decreased bone turnover due to osteomalacia or adynamic bone disease.[42] Absorption of calcium promotes coronary arterial calcification, which is associated with coronary atherosclerosis.[41] If hypercalcemia develops or if the (calcium phosphate) product exceeds 65, the therapy should be replaced by noncalcium-based phosphate binders (Sevelamer or Fosrenol). Decreasing the dialysate calcium to 2.5 mg/L or less is useful when large doses of calcium are required.[36,39] However, extended treatment with a low-calcium dialysate increases the risk of severe hyperparathyroidism. Aluminum hydroxide can cause aluminum intoxication, with vitamin D–resistant osteomalacia, a refractory microcytic anemia, bone and muscle pain, and dementia. It is no longer recommended.

Sevelamer (Renagel) is a nonabsorbable agent that contains neither calcium nor aluminum. It is a cationic polymer that binds phosphate through ion exchange. It is as effective as calcium carbonate or calcium acetate but does not affect S_{Ca}.[43] It lowers total cholesterol concentration by 15%. Gastrointestinal adverse effects may limit its use in some patients. At present, it is reserved for patients with hypercalcemia because of its considerable cost. The usual recommended dose is 800 to 1600 mg with meals three times per day.

Lanthanum carbonate (Fosrenol) is a first-line calcium-free phosphate binder that helps lower serum phosphate levels. The initial recommended dose is 750 to 1500 mg of Fosrenol tablets with each meal. It is in chewable form only, which is good for dialysis patients trying to watch their fluid intake. The active ingredient in Fosrenol is two to three times more potent than sevelamer hydrochloride on a gram-for-gram basis. Lanthanum carbonate showed a safety profile that is similar to the overall profile of the standard therapy with calcium carbonate during 3 years of treatment.[44,45]

Treatment of secondary hyperparathyroidism begins with a decrease in S_{Pi} while maintaining the (calcium ∞ phosphate) product less than 65. Thereafter, pulse oral or intravenous calcitriol two to three times per week can reduce PTH secretion. To prevent adynamic bone disease, most investigators recommend that intact PTH should be maintained in a mildly elevated range (<250 pg/mL).[46] Mild hyperparathyroidism (intact PTH 250–400 pg/mL) should be treated first with better control of S_{Pi}. If PTH continues to increase, calcitriol (intravenous Calcijex or oral Rocaltrol) is initiated at a dose of 1 μg three times weekly. For PTH greater than 600 to 700 pg/mL, an increase in calcitriol dose to 2 μg or more three times weekly is required. Calcitriol may cause hypercalcemia and may exacerbate hyperphosphatemia. Paricalcitol (Zemplar) in an active form of vitamin D for the treatment of secondary hyperparathyroidism in chronic kidney disease. The oral form is approved for stage 3 and 4 chronic kidney disease, and the intravenous form for patients on renal replacement therapy. The starting dose is 0.04 to 0.1 μg/kg. Paricalcitol, a selective new vitamin D analogue that is as effective in decreasing PTH, is equal to calcitriol but

with one tenth of the risk of inducing hypercalcemia, hyperphosphatemia, and elevated CaXP product to more than 65. The selectivity of paricalcitol makes this agent the analogue of choice in patients with chronic kidney disease.

Another recently approved novel agent for the treatment of secondary hyperparathyroidism in dialysis patients is Sensipar (cinacalcet hydrochloride), a calcimimetic agent. The major physiologic action of cinacalcet is that increases the sensitivity of the calcium-sensing receptor to activation by extracellular calcium. The result is a safe direct inhibition of PTH synthesis and secretion. In addition, cinacalcet has a mild effect in patients with chronic kidney disease in decreasing S_{Ca} and S_{Pi}. The starting dose is 30 mg once daily, which should be titrated up not more than every 2 to 4 weeks to 60, 90, 120, and 180 mg to achieve normal serum calcium and target PTH.[47] Cinacalcet should be used in combination with paricalcitol. S_{Ca} may also be decreased by decreasing dialysate calcium concentrations. Patients with refractory secondary hyperparathyroidism or those who develop severe hypercalcemia require parathyroidectomy.[48]

Hypophosphatemia

Clinical Features, Pathophysiology, and Cause

Moderate hypophosphatemia (S_{Pi} 1–2.5 mg/dL, 0.32–0.81 mmol/L) is usually asymptomatic. Severe hypophosphatemia (S_{Pi} < 1 mg/dL or 0.32 mmol/L) indicates total body phosphate depletion and is potentially fatal. Numerous cellular mechanisms require phosphate (e.g. 2,3-diphosphoglycerate and adenosine triphosphate).[36,39] Clinical features include erythrocyte, leukocyte, and platelet dysfunction; myopathy; confusion; ataxia; seizures and coma; respiratory insufficiency; osteomalacia; metabolic acidosis; cardiac arrhythmias; and cardiomyopathy. Hypophosphatemia may result from decreased intestinal phosphate absorption, increased renal phosphate losses, and a shift of phosphate to intracellular compartments (Fig. 34-6).

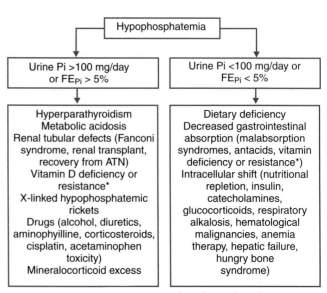

Figure 34-6 Diagnostic approach to hypophosphatemia. *More than one mechanism involved. ATN, acute tubular necrosis; FE$_{Pi}$, fractional excretion of phosphate.

Alcoholism and Alcohol Withdrawal

As many as 10% of chronic alcoholics are hypophosphatemic.[36,39] The causes include insufficient phosphate intake, use of phosphate-binding antacids for gastrointestinal disorders, emesis, hypomagnesemia, diarrhea, and excessive alcohol-induced renal phosphate excretion, as well as intracellular shifts due to hyperventilation or glucose infusion in patients with alcoholic cirrhosis or in acute abstinence.[36]

Nutritional Repletion

This may result in severe hypophosphatemia due to cellular phosphate uptake and utilization in anabolic tissue if sufficient amounts of phosphate are not provided. Phosphate requirements often exceed those provided in either enteral or parenteral feeds.[36,39]

Diabetes Mellitus

Patients with decompensated diabetes associated with ketoacidosis excrete excessive phosphate due to osmotic diuresis. The plasma level is usually maintained because of large shifts of phosphate from cells into plasma. Administration of insulin, fluids, and correction of ketoacidosis causes S_{Pi} to decrease sharply. Patients with very low S_{Pi} usually require phosphate supplementation during correction of hyperglycemia and acidosis.[36]

Acute Respiratory Alkalosis

Acute hyperventilation can reduce S_{Pi} to very low levels as phosphate enters muscle. Such a decrease in S_{Pi} is not observed in acute metabolic alkalosis. Paradoxically, chronic hyperventilation causes hyperphosphatemia.[48]

Treatment

Rationale and Overview

The appropriate management of hypophosphatemia usually requires phosphate supplementation and diagnosis of the cause to prevent recurrence. Phosphate replacement can cause diarrhea (with oral supplements), hyperphosphatemia, and hypocalcemia.[36,39] Therefore, replacement should be used cautiously. Diarrhea is uncommon in patients with severe phosphate deficiency, especially when daily doses of phosphate are less than 1 g and given four times daily. Hypophosphatemia should be seen as a marker of an underlying disorder for which evaluation and therapy may be necessary. Hypophosphatemia should be anticipated in patients receiving enteral or parenteral nutrition, malnourished patients receiving glucose-containing intravenous fluids, and alcoholics.

Oral replacement is preferred in asymptomatic patients, even those with very low phosphate levels (Table 34-1). Correction of any associated hypokalemia and hypomagnesemia decreases phosphaturia (Fig. 34-7). Milk provides 1 g/L (33 mmol/L) of inorganic phosphate. It is usually better tolerated than phosphate tablets.[36,39]

Mild Hypophosphatemia Mild hypophosphatemia ($S_{Pi} > 2$ mg/dL), especially when ascribed to intracellular shifts, usually resolves without pharmacologic intervention.

Moderate Hypophosphatemia Moderate hypophosphatemia ($S_{Pi} > 1$ mg/dL in adults, >2 mg/dL in children) responds to oral supplementation. Patients receiving total parenteral nutrition should receive at least 1000 mg/day (32 mmol) of phosphate. Lactose and lipids are poorly tolerated in malnourished patients with lactose or fat intolerance. Therefore, skim milk is preferable. With each 8-oz serving (containing ~235 mg of phosphate), most people can replenish their stores with four to eight glasses per day for 7 to 10 days.[36,39]

Severe Hypophosphatemia In general, S_{Pi} less than 0.5 mg/dL reflects a phosphate deficit of more than 3 g; in the presence of symptoms, this deficit is more than 10 g.[36] In asymptomatic patients, severe hypophosphatemia is treated with oral supplements of phosphate (6–10 g) over several days. Oral supplements are available as monobasic, dibasic, and acid sodium and potassium salts. Neutral potassium and sodium

Table 34-1   Phosphate Preparations

	Phosphate	Sodium	Potassium
Oral Preparations			
Skim milk	1 g/L	28 mEq/L	38 mEq/L
Neutra-Phos	250 mg/packet	7.1 mEq/packet	7.1 mEq/packet
Phospho-Soda	150 mg/mL	4.8 mEq/mL	0
Neutra-Phos K	250 mg/capsule	0	14.25 mEq/capsule
K-Phos Original	150 mg/capsule	0	3.65 mEq/capsule
K-Phos Neutral	250 mg/tablet	13 mEq/tablet	1.1 mEq/tablet
Intravenous Preparations			
Neutral sodium potassium phosphate	1.1 mmol/mL	0.2 mEq/mL	0.02 mEq/mL
Neutral sodium phosphate	0.09 mmol/mL	0.2 mEq/mL	0
Sodium phosphate	3.0 mmol/mL	4.0 mEq/mL	0
Potassium phosphate	3.0 mmol/mL	0	4.4 mEq/mL

From Subramanian R, Khardori R: Severe hypophosphatemia: Pathophysiologic implications, clinical presentations, and treatment. Medicine 2000;79:1–8.

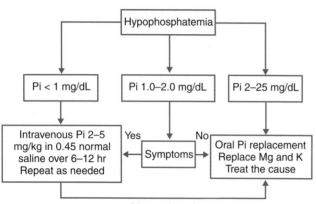

Figure 34-7 Treatment of hypophosphatemia.

preparations (Neutraphos, K-Phos Neutral) provide 250 mg of phosphate per tablet (see Table 34-1) but also contain large amounts of sodium. Phosphate enemas are also available (Fleet Enema) for patients intolerant of oral supplements. Because of the high sodium content, laxative effect, and erratic absorption, enemas are not primary therapy. In symptomatic patients, intravenous supplementation is usually required to increase S_{Pi} to more than 1.0 to 1.5 mg/dL, at which point oral supplements may be given. The usual starting dose is 2 mg/kg IV infused in half-normal saline over 6 hours or 5 mg/kg over 12 hours, checking S_{Pi} frequently and discontinuing the infusion when necessary. In symptomatic, severely hypophosphatemic patients, 1 g of phosphate in 1 L of fluid may be infused over 8 to 12 hours.[36,39] Intravenous phosphate can precipitate with calcium and produce hypocalcemia, renal failure, and serious arrhythmias. Intravenous phosphate supplements are also available in combination with sodium or potassium.

MAGNESIUM DISORDERS

The normal body content of magnesium is approximately 1000 mmol or 22.66 g, of which 50% to 60% is contained in bone; extracellular magnesium accounts for only 1%. The normal serum magnesium concentration is 1.7 to 2.2 mg/dL (0.75–0.95 mmol/L). Approximately 55% is ionized and 15% complexed to bicarbonate, citrate, and phosphate; the remaining 30% is protein bound and thus is not available for ultrafiltration by the kidneys.

Magnesium is essential for the function of important enzymes, including those involved in the transfer of phosphate groups, all reactions that require ATP, and every step in the replication and transcription of DNA and translation of mRNA. Magnesium is also required for cellular energy metabolism and has an important role in membrane stabilization, nerve conduction, ion transport, and calcium channel activity.

Homeostasis

Maintenance of normal magnesium levels depends on gastrointestinal absorption and renal excretion. Daily magnesium intake is 300 to 350 mg. Absorption is by saturable and passive systems. Absorption is reduced by phosphate in the diet and enhanced by calcitriol.

Daily renal excretion of magnesium averages 100 mg. The thick ascending limb of Henle's loop reabsorbs 60% to 70%. Reabsorption in the thick ascending limb and distal tubule (~10%) is closely regulated by the serum magnesium concentration. Reabsorption in the thick ascending limb is regulated by the calcium/magnesium-sensing receptor, located on the basolateral membrane of the thick ascending limb.[49]

Hypermagnesemia

Clinical Features, Pathophysiology, and Cause

Patients with renal insufficiency are susceptible to hypermagnesemia. Most cases are caused by magnesium ingestion. Hypermagnesemia due to cellular release complicates tumor lysis syndrome, rhabdomyolysis, acidosis, and catecholamine excess. Mild hypermagnesemia complicates FHH, Addison's disease, hyperparathyroidism, and lithium therapy.[50] Hypermagnesemia causes mild hypotension, nausea, flushing, and loss of deep tendon reflexes, somnolence, weakness, lethargy, and ultimately apnea due to muscular paralysis. Cardiac manifestations include prolongation of PR, QRS, and QT intervals, bradycardia, complete heart block, and even cardiac arrest.

Treatment

Patients with mild hypermagnesemia and normal renal function require only discontinuation of magnesium supplementation (Fig. 34-8). For those with severe symptoms of hypermagnesemia, intravenous calcium (100–200 mg) is the initial treatment. Glucose and insulin can shift magnesium intracellularly. Patients with a serum magnesium concentration in excess of 8 to 9 mg/dL should have cardiac monitoring and be considered for ventilatory support. Hemodialysis against a low-magnesium dialysate is more effective than peritoneal dialysis in rapidly decreasing the serum magnesium concentration in patients with renal failure.[51]

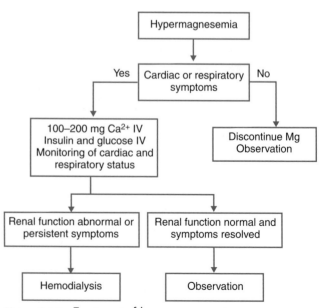

Figure 34-8 Treatment of hypermagnesemia.

Hypomagnesemia

Clinical Features, Pathophysiology, and Cause

Hypomagnesemia occurs in 12% of hospitalized patients.[51] Gastrointestinal depletion occurs during acute or chronic diarrhea or during malabsorption. Thiazide and loop diuretics inhibit tubular magnesium reabsorption, although hypomagnesemia is usually mild because of increased proximal tubular magnesium reabsorption induced by the volume depletion. Diabetes mellitus is the most common cause of hypomagnesemia, probably secondary to glycosuria and osmotic diuresis (Fig. 34-9).

The possibility of cellular magnesium depletion despite a maintained serum magnesium concentration should be considered as a possible cause of refractory hypokalemia or unexplained hypocalcemia. This is detected by demonstrating a low renal magnesium excretion (<24 mg/day) or a low fractional excretion of magnesium (<2%).

Magnesium deficiency causes neuromuscular irritability, with tremor, tetany, asterixis, myoclonus, seizures, muscular weakness, prolongation of PR and QT intervals, ventricular and supraventricular arrhythmias, and diminished response to digoxin. Accompanying hypokalemia or hypocalcemia can be refractory to therapy unless magnesium deficiency is corrected.

Treatment

Mild hypomagnesemia can be treated with oral replacement (Fig. 34-10) using a sustained-release preparation such as Slow Mag, containing magnesium chloride, or Mag-Tab SR, containing magnesium lactate (2.5–3.5 mmol or 60–84 mg of magnesium per tablet). Patients with severe magnesium deficiency require six to eight tablets daily, whereas those with mild asymptomatic disease require only two to four tablets daily. Patients with renal magnesium wasting due to loop diuretics benefit from a magnesium-sparing diuretic such as amiloride (5–10 mg/day). Amiloride is also used for the persistent renal magnesium wasting associated with Bartter or

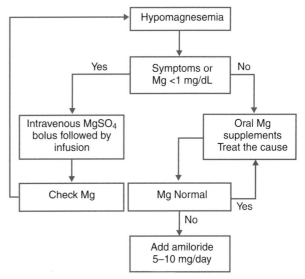

Figure 34-10   Treatment of hypomagnesemia.

Gitelman's syndrome or cisplatin nephrotoxicity. Adults with malabsorption may require daily magnesium supplementation of as much as 50 mmol (~1 g); children with malabsorption may require as much as 30 mmol (720 mg).

Patients with symptomatic or more severe hypomagnesemia require parenteral magnesium. Magnesium sulfate (2.1 mmol/mL) as a 50% solution is effective intramuscularly but should preferably be given intravenously. For life-threatening cardiac arrhythmias or seizures, 4 to 8 mmol (100–200 mg) of magnesium sulfate may be given intravenously over 5 to 10 minutes, followed by an intravenous infusion of 0.5 mmol/kg/day (12 mg/kg) or 4 mmol (~100 mg) intramuscularly every 3 to 4 hours. Approximately half of the administered magnesium will be excreted, and therapy may need to be continued for several days. The dose should be decreased in patients with renal insufficiency who require close monitoring.[51]

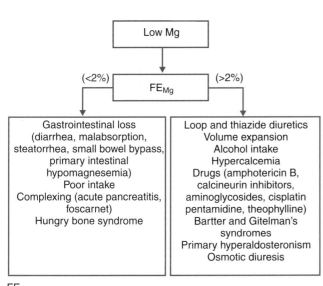

FE_{Mg}
$$\text{(fractional excretion of Mg)} = \frac{\text{Urinary Mg} \times \text{plasma creatinine} \times 100}{(0.7 \times \text{plasma Mg}) \times \text{urinary creatinine}}$$

Figure 34-9   Diagnostic approach to hypomagnesemia.

References

1. Pearce CJ, Hine TJ, Peek K: Hypercalcemia due to Ca^{2+} binding by a polymeric IgA kappa paraprotein. Ann Clin Biochem 1991;28:229–234.
2. Brown EM, Pollak M, Seidman CE, et al: Calcium ion-sensing cell-surface receptors. N Engl J Med 1995;333:234–240.
3. Walls J, Ratcliffe WA, Howell A, et al: Parathyroid hormone and parathyroid hormone-related protein in the investigation of hypercalcemia in two hospital populations. Clin Endocrinol 1994;41:407–413.
4. Bilezikian JP: Management of hypercalcemia. J Clin Endocrinol Metab 1993;77:1445–1449.
5. Earm JH, Christensen BM, Frokiaer J, et al: Decreased aquaporin-2 expression and apical plasma membrane delivery in kidney collecting ducts of polyuric hypercalcemic rats. J Am Soc Nephrol 1998; 9:2181–2193.
6. Parks J, Coe F, Favus M: Hyperparathyroidism in nephrolithiasis. Arch Intern Med 1980;140:1479–1481.
7. Haden ST, Stoll AL, McCormick S, et al: Alterations in parathyroid dynamics in lithium-treated subjects. J Clin Endocrinol Metab 1997;82:2844–2848.
8. Favus MJ (ed): Primer on the Metabolic Bone Diseases and Disorders of Mineral Metabolism. Philadelphia: Lippincott–Raven, 1996, p 179.

9. Eigelberger MS, Cheah WK, Ituarte PH, et al: The NIH criteria for parathyroidectomy in asymptomatic primary hyperparathyroidisim, are they too limited? Ann Surg 2004;239: 528–535.

10. NIH conference. Diagnosis and management of asymptomatic primary hyperparathyroidism: Consensus Development Conference statement. Ann Intern Med 1991;114:593–597.

11. Silverberg SJ, Gartenberg F, Jacobs TP, et al: Increased bone mineral density after parathyroidectomy in primary hyperparathyroidism. J Clin Endocrinol Metab 1995;80:729–734.

12. Silverberg SJ, Shane E, Dempster DW, Bilezikian JP: The effects of vitamin D insufficiency in patients with primary hyperparathyroidism. Am J Med 1999;107:561–567.

13. Marcus R, Madvig P, Crim M, et al: Conjugated estrogens in the treatment of postmenopausal women with hyperparathyroidism. Ann Intern Med 1984;100:633–640.

14. Grey AB, Stapleton JP, Evans MC, et al: Effect of hormone replacement therapy on bone mineral density in postmenopausal women with mild primary hyperparathyroidism. A randomized, controlled trial. Ann Intern Med 1996;125:360–368.

15. Reasner CA, Stone MD, Hosking DJ, et al: Acute changes in calcium homeostasis during treatment of primary hyperparathyroidism with risedronate. J Clin Endocrinol Metab 1993;77:1067–1071.

16. Silverberg SJ, Bone HG 3rd, Marriott TB, et al: Short-term inhibition of parathyroid hormone secretion by a Ca^{2+}-receptor agonist in patients with primary hyperparathyroidism. N Engl J Med 1997;337:1506–1510.

17. Finch JL, Brown AJ, Slatopolsky E: Differential effects of 1,25-dihydroxy-vitamin D3 and 19-nor-1,25-dihydroxy-vitamin D2 on calcium and Pi resorption in bone. J Am Soc Nephrol 1999;10:980–985.

18. Rosen HN, Lim M, Garber J, et al: The effect of PTH antagonist BIM-44002 on S_{Ca} and PTH levels in hypercalcemic hyperparathyroid patients. Calcif Tissue Int 1997;61:455–459.

19. Shane E: Hypercalcemia: Pathogenesis, clinical manifestations, differential diagnosis and management. In Favus MJ (ed): Primer on the Metabolic Bone Diseases and Disorders of Mineral Metabolism. Philadelphia: Lippincott–Raven, 1996, pp 171–181.

20. Agarwal R, Knochell JP: Hypophosphatemia and hyperphosphatemia. In Brenner BM (ed): Brenner and Rector's The Kidney, 6th ed. Philadelphia: WB Saunders, 2000, pp 1071–1114.

21. Tenenhouse H: Cellular and molecular mechanisms of renal phosphate transport. J Bone Miner Res 1997;12:159–164.

22. Bilezikian JP: Management of acute hypercalcemia. N Engl J Med 1992;326:1196–1203.

23. Gucalp R, Ritch P, Wiernik PH, et al: Comparative study of pamidronate disodium and etidronate disodium in the treatment of cancer-related hypercalcemia. J Clin Oncol 1992;10:134–142.

24. Gucalp R, Theriault R, Gill I, et al: Treatment of cancer-associated hypercalcemia. Double-blind comparison of rapid and slow intravenous infusion regimens of pamidronate disodium and saline alone. Arch Intern Med 1994;154:1935–1944.

25. Davenport A, Goel S, Mackenzie JC: Treatment of hypercalcaemia with pamidronate in patients with end stage renal failure. Scand J Urol Nephrol 1993;27:447–451.

26. Gurney H, Grill V, Martin TJ: Parathyroid hormone-related protein and response to pamidronate in tumour-induced hypercalcaemia. Lancet 1993;341:1611–1613.

27. Major P, Lortholary A, Hon J, et al: Zoledronic acid is superior to pamidronate in the treatment of hypercalcemia of malignancy: A pooled analysis of two randomized, controlled clinical trials. J Clin Oncol 2001;19:558–567.

28. Guay DR: Ibandronate, an experimental intravenous bisphosphonate for osteoporosis, bone metastasis, and hypercalcemia of malignancy. Pharmacotherapy 2006;26:655–673.

29. Pecherstorfer M, Steinhauer EU, Rizzoli R, et al: Efficacy and safety of ibandronate in the treatment of hypercalcemia of malignancy: A randomized multicentric comparison to pamidronate. Support Care Cancer 2003;11:539–547.

30. Von Moos R: Bisphosphonate treatment recommendations for oncologists. Oncologist 2005;10(Suppl 1):19–24.

31. Fonseca OA, Calverley JR: Neurological manifestations of hypoparathyroidism. Arch Intern Med 1967;120:202–206.

32. Colletti RB, Pan MW, Smith EW, Genel M: Detection of hypocalcemia in susceptible neonates: The QoTc interval. N Engl J Med 1974;290:931–935.

33. Shane E: Hypocalcemia: Pathogenesis, clinical manifestations, differential diagnosis and management. In Favus MJ (ed): Primer on the Metabolic Bone Diseases and Disorders of Mineral Metabolism. Philadelphia: Lippincott–Raven, 1996, pp 217–219.

34. Pak CYC: Calcium disorders: Hypercalcemia and hypocalcemia. In Kokko JP, Tannen RL (eds): Fluids and Electrolytes. Philadelphia: WB Saunders, 1990, pp 596–630.

35. Hruska KA, Connolly J: Hyperphosphatemia and hypophosphatemia. In Favus MJ (ed): Primer on the Metabolic Bone Diseases and Disorders of Mineral Metabolism. Philadelphia: Lippincott–Raven, 1996, pp 238–245.

36. Cross HS, Debiec H, Peterlik M: Mechanism and regulation of intestinal phosphate reabsorption. Miner Electrolyte Metab 1990;16:115–124.

37. Murer H, Biber J: Molecular mechanisms in renal phosphate reabsorption. Nephrol Dial Transplant 1995;10:1501–1504.

38. Mostellar ME, Tuttle EP: Effects of alkalosis on plasma concentration and urinary excretion of inorganic phosphate in man. J Clin Invest 1964;43:138–149.

39. Llach F, Felsenfeld AJ, Haussler MR: The pathophysiology of altered calcium metabolism in rhabdomyolysis-induced acute renal failure. Interactions of parathyroid hormone, 25-hydroxycholecalciferol, and 1,25-dihydroxycholecalciferol. N Engl J Med 1981;305:117–123.

40. Goodman WG, Goldin J, Kuizon BD, et al: Coronary-artery calcification in young adults with end-stage renal disease who are undergoing dialysis. N Engl J Med 2000;342:1478–1483.

41. Mucsi I, Hercz G, Uldall R, et al: A control of serum phosphate without any phosphate binders in patients treated with nocturnal hemodialysis. Kidney Int 1998;53:1399–1404.

42. Kurz P, Monier-Faugere MC, Bognar B, et al: Evidence for abnormal calcium homeostasis in patients with adynamic bone disease. Kidney Int 1994;46:855–861.

43. Chertow GM, Burke SK, Lazarus JM, et al: Poly[allylamine hydrochloride] (RenaGel): A noncalcemic phosphate binder for the treatment of hyperphosphatemia in chronic renal failure. Am J Kidney Dis 1997;29:66–71.

44. Hutchinson AJ, Maes B, Vanwalleghem J, et al: Long-term efficacy and tolerability of lanthanum carbonate: Results from a three year study. Nephron Clin Pract 2006;102:61–71.

45. Finn WF, Joy MS: A long-term, open-label extension study on the safety of treatment with lanthanum carbonate, a new phosphate binder, in patients receiving hemodialysis. Curr Med Res Opin 2005;21:657–664.

46. Coburn JW, Frazao J: Calcitriol in the management of renal osteodystrophy. Semin Dial 1996;9:316–320.

47. Lindberg JS, Culleton B, Wong G, et al: Cinacalcet HCl, an oral calcimimetic agent for the treatment of secondary hyperparathyroidism in hemodialysis and peritoneal dialysis: A randomized, double-blind, multicenter study. J Am Soc Nephrol 2005;16:800–807.

48. Krapg R, Jaeger P, Hulter HN: Chronic respiratory alkalosis induced renal PTH-resistance, hyperphosphatemia and hypocalcemia in humans. Kidney Int 1992;42:727–734.

49. Quamme GA: Renal magnesium handling: New insights in understanding old problems. Kidney Int 1997;52:1180–1195.

50. Rude RK: Magnesium depletion and hypermagnesemia. In Favus MJ (ed): Primer on the Metabolic Bone Diseases and Disorders of Mineral Metabolism. Philadelphia: Lippincott–Raven, 1996, pp 234–238.

51. Wong ET, Rude RK, Singer FR, Shaw ST Jr: A high prevalence of hypomagnesemia and hypermagnesemia in hospitalized patients. Am J Clin Pathol 1983;79:348–352.

Further Reading

Agus ZS, Berenson JR: Treatment of hypercalcemia of malignancy with bisphosphonates. Semin Oncol 2002;29(6 Suppl 21):12–18.

Nouri P, Nikakhtar B, Llach F: Uremic osteodystrophy. In Nissenson A, Fine R (eds): Handbook of Dialysis Therapy, 4th ed. Philadelphia: Elsevier, 2007.

Schwarz S, Trivedi BK, Kalantar-Zadeh K, Kovesdy CP: Association of disorders in mineral metabolism with progression of kidney disease. Clin J Am Soc Nephrol 2006;1:825–831.

Sitges-Serra A, Bergenfelz A. Clinical update: Sporadic primary hyperparathyroidism. Lancet 2007;370:468–470.

Von Moos R: Bisphosphonate treatment recommendations for oncologists. Oncologist 2005;10(Suppl 1):19–24.

PART V

Nephrolithiasis

CONTENTS

Chapter 35

Evaluation and Management of Kidney Stone Disease

Eric N. Taylor and Gary C. Curhan

CHAPTER CONTENTS

Kidney stones are a major cause of morbidity. The lifetime prevalence of symptomatic nephrolithiasis exceeds 10% in men and 5% in women,[1,2] and more than $2 billion is spent on treatment each year.[3] Appropriate evaluation and intervention are required to prevent recurrent kidney stones.

DIAGNOSIS OF STONE DISEASE

Clinical and Laboratory Manifestations

Symptomatic nephrolithiasis classically presents with unilateral flank pain of sudden onset. The pain is precipitated by the passage of a kidney stone from the renal pelvis to the ureter and is due to ureteral spasm. Because the waxing and waning pain of a symptomatic stone does not completely remit, the term renal colic is technically inaccurate.[4] The pain is often severe and can be accompanied by nausea and vomiting. The location of the pain depends on the location of the kidney stone: A stone in the upper ureter may cause pain to radiate anteriorly to the abdomen, whereas a stone in the lower ureter can cause pain to radiate to the ipsilateral testicle in men or to the ipsilateral labium in women. If the stone is lodged at the ureterovesical junction, the patient may experience urinary frequency and urgency. Less commonly, nephrolithiasis can manifest as gross hematuria without pain.

On physical examination, the patient will be in obvious pain and may constantly adjust position in an unsuccessful attempt to alleviate the discomfort. Ipsilateral costovertebral angle tenderness may be present. Signs and symptoms of sepsis can occur in cases of obstruction with infection.

Serum chemistries are usually normal, but leukocytosis may be present due to stress or infection.[5] Although the urinalysis will often reveal hematuria and pyuria (and occasionally crystalluria),[5] the absence of red cells in the urine does not exclude a stone, particularly in cases in which a stone causes complete ureteral obstruction.[6]

Imaging

Helical computed tomography scan (HCT) is the preferred radiographic test to confirm or exclude the diagnosis of nephrolithiasis.[7] HCT does not require radiocontrast and can visualize uric acid stones (traditionally considered radiolucent).[7] Typically, the HCT will show a ureteral stone or evidence of recent passage (e.g., perinephric stranding or hydronephrosis). HCT can detect small stones that may be missed by intravenous urography.[8,9]

Few studies have compared HCT with ultrasonography (US). However, in patients presenting with presumed renal colic, the sensitivity of HCT was 96% compared with 61% for US; the specificity for each was 100%.[10] Although US has the advantage of avoiding radiation, it can only image the kidney and proximal ureter. Thus, ureteral stones can be missed on US. US may also miss renal stones less than 3 mm in size.[11]

The conventional abdominal x-ray (x-ray examination of the kidney and upper bladder) is inadequate for diagnosis. It can miss a stone in the ureter or kidney (even when radiopaque) and provides no information on obstruction or recent stone passage.

Differential Diagnosis

In general, a kidney stone must pass into the ureter to cause pain. Therefore, the isolated presence of a renal stone on radiography is an inadequate explanation for acute abdominal or flank pain.[5] The differential diagnosis of a patient with suspected renal colic includes musculoskeletal pain, herpes zoster, acute cholecystitis, duodenal ulcer, appendicitis, diverticulitis, pyelonephritis, abdominal aortic aneurysm, gynecologic disease, and ureteral obstruction due to blood clot, sloughed papilla, or ureteral stricture.[4,5]

MANAGEMENT IN THE ACUTE SETTING

Medical Treatment

Because renal colic is excruciating, analgesia is a primary goal in the acute setting. Randomized, controlled trials suggest that parenteral nonsteroidal anti-inflammatory drugs are as effective as narcotics in treating renal colic.[12] Newer medications that may be effective include antispasmodics,[13] trigger point injection with lidocaine,[14] desmopressin,[15] and nonsteroidal anti-inflammatory drugs combined with nitrates.[16] However, data on the utility of these interventions are limited.

Medical therapy has also been directed at treating kidney stones or hastening ureteral stone passage. Alkalinization of the urine may dissolve uric acid stones,[17] and some experts believe that volume expansion will increase the likelihood of stone passage,[18] but this is not proven. α-Blockers and calcium channel blockers also may facilitate the passage of ureteral stones.[19]

Surgical Treatment

See Chapter 36 for details.

Larger and more proximal ureteral stones are less likely to pass spontaneously and are more likely to require urologic intervention. If a stone does not pass rapidly, the patient can be sent home with oral analgesia and instructions to return for fever or uncontrollable pain. Most urologists prefer to wait several days before intervention unless there is evidence of infection, low likelihood of spontaneous passage (e.g., stone > 6 mm), presence of an anatomic abnormality that would prevent passage, or unrelenting pain.[20] Infection in the setting of obstruction is a surgical emergency and mandates emergent drainage.

The initial urologic approach may be directed at the relief of obstruction (generally by cystoscopic placement of a ureteral stent) rather than stone removal. Anatomy of the urologic tract, availability of technology, experience of the urologist, and the size, location, and composition of the stone determine the best option for stone removal. Extracorporeal shock wave lithotripsy is the least invasive option and is most effective for smaller calcium stones (<1 cm) located in the renal pelvis or proximal ureter.[21-23] Cystoscopic stone removal by basket extraction or fragmentation is invasive but effective and can now be used to remove stones in the proximal ureter or kidney.[24] Percutaneous nephrostolithotomy is more invasive but may be necessary for large stone burdens or stones that cannot be removed cystoscopically.[25] It is rare that a patient requires open ureterolithotomy or nephrolithotomy.

CLINICAL AND METABOLIC EVALUATION

The First Stone

Disagreement exists about the benefit of performing a full clinical and metabolic evaluation after the first episode of nephrolithiasis.[26] Assuming that the patient is willing to participate in a diagnostic work-up and to adhere to treatment recommendations, we encourage a full evaluation for most stone formers for the following reasons. First, although recurrence rates are uncertain, the chance of passing a second calcium stone may be as high as 30% to 50% after 5 years.[1,27,28] Second, treatable systemic diseases of clinical importance, such as osteoporosis and primary hyperparathyroidism, may be diagnosed during the metabolic evaluation.[29] Third, allowing a stone former to progress to recurrence may hinder the effectiveness of subsequent prophylaxis.[30] Finally, some analyses suggest that medical prevention may be cost saving.[31]

For individuals with a large stone burden or at very high risk of recurrence, little disagreement exists about the utility of a complete work-up. Specifically, patients with a large first stone (e.g., >10 mm), multiple stones on initial imaging, recurrent stones, or stones requiring invasive intervention should be offered a complete evaluation.

Stone Composition

Because treatment recommendations vary by stone type, every effort should be made to retrieve a passed stone for chemical analysis. Approximately 80% of kidney stones contain calcium, and the majority of calcium stones consist primarily of calcium oxalate.[21] Although most calcium oxalate stones contain some calcium phosphate, only 5% of kidney stones have hydroxyapatite or brushite (calcium monohydrogen phosphate) as their main constituent.[21,32] Approximately 10% of calcium stones contain some uric acid.[21] Other types of stones, such as pure uric acid, struvite, and cystine are less common but merit careful attention because of recurrence risk.

History and Laboratory Testing

Evaluation should be directed toward identifying risk factors for stone formation with the goal of devising appropriate, individualized therapy (Box 35-1 delineates risk factors for calcium oxalate nephrolithiasis). The evaluation should start with a detailed history, which will provide information crucial for treatment recommendations. The following should be covered: medical history to identify potentially predisposing conditions (e.g., gout, diabetes, bowel disease, obesity, primary hyperparathyroidism), dietary intake, vitamin and supplement use (particularly vitamin C), medication use before the stone event, family history of stone disease, total number of stones, evidence of residual stones, number and types of procedures, and types and success of previous preventive treatments. More severe stone disease will lower the threshold for early medical intervention in addition to recommended dietary changes.

The metabolic evaluation should include a determination of serum electrolytes, creatinine, calcium, phosphorus, and uric acid. Although usually normal, a low serum bicarbonate should prompt consideration of type 1 renal tubular acidosis, which is classically associated with calcium phosphate stones. Intact parathyroid hormone should be measured if the serum calcium is elevated or in the high normal range, if the serum phosphorus is low, or if the urinary excretion of calcium is elevated.

A urinalysis should be performed as part of the initial evaluation. A urine pH more than 7 with phosphate crystals

Box 35-1   Risk Factors for Calcium Oxalate Stone Formation

Urinary Risk Factors
High levels
  Calcium
  Oxalate
Low levels
  Citrate
  Total volume

Dietary Risk Factors
High intake
  Sodium
  Animal protein
  Sucrose/fructose
  Vitamin C
  Oxalate
Low intake
  Fluid
  Calcium (dietary)
  Potassium
  Phytate
  Magnesium

Other Risk Factors
Anatomical abnormalities (e.g., medullary sponge kidney)
Family history of calcium stone disease
Obesity

suggests calcium phosphate or struvite stones. The presence of hexagonal cystine crystals is pathognomic for cystinuria. Uric acid or calcium oxalate crystalluria can be seen in individuals without stones and therefore is less informative. Red and white cells are frequently seen in the urine of asymptomatic individuals with residual kidney stones.

The cornerstone of the metabolic evaluation is the 24-hour urine collection. To tailor initial intervention and determine response to treatment, 24-hour urine collections are necessary even if the stone composition is known. The stone-forming patient should wait at least 6 weeks before performing 24-hour urine collection because individuals frequently alter their dietary habits immediately after an episode of nephrolithiasis.[33] In addition, two collections are necessary because of substantial day-to-day variability in urinary parameters: A single 24-hour urine collection is insufficient.[34] The factors that should be measured include total volume, creatinine (to assess the adequacy of collection), calcium, oxalate, citrate, uric acid, sodium, potassium, phosphorus, and pH. Algorithms for the evaluation and management of the patient with calcium stone disease, according to urinary abnormality, are provided in Box 35-2 and Figures 35-1, 35-2, and 35-3.

Estimates of relative supersaturation, based on measurements of the urine factors described, are offered by some laboratories and should be obtained whenever possible. The relative supersaturation can guide selection of and determine response to therapy. Because of controversy over the clinical importance of the classic schemata of Pak and colleagues,[35] most clinicians do not attempt to categorize individuals with

idiopathic hypercalciuria into absorptive, resorptive, or renal subtypes.

The Normal Metabolic Evaluation

Because kidney stones can remain asymptomatic for many years before they pass into the ureter and cause renal colic, the actual time of stone formation is usually unknown. Therefore, the metabolic evaluation may be completely normal. In this case, no intervention is required. However, repeat imaging in 1 year to identify active stone formation, in conjunction with another 24-hour urine, is warranted in recurrent stone formers.

PREVENTION OF STONE RECURRENCE: CALCIUM OXALATE NEPHROLITHIASIS

Fluid Intake

Nephrolithiasis is a disease of concentration. Modifying the concentration of lithogenic factors is the focus of stone prevention. The concentration of calcium, for example, can be lowered by reducing urinary calcium or by increasing urine volume. Thus, fluid intake is a critical component of stone prevention. Observational studies[36–38] and a randomized, controlled trial[39] have demonstrated that higher fluid intake decreases the risk of stone formation. However, patients need to be given specific advice on how much to drink to form at least 2 L of urine per day. In addition to fluid intake, other factors such as insensible loss and water contained in foods influence urine volume. Rather than broadly recommending eight glasses of water per day, the recommendation can be tailored to the individual patient by using the information on total volume from the 24-hour urine collections. For example, if an individual produces 1.5 L of urine per day, consuming an additional two 8-oz (240 mL) glasses of water would increase their output to the target of 2 L.

Patients often want to know what they should and should not drink. Despite previous beliefs to the contrary, alcoholic beverages, coffee, and tea do not increase the risk of stone formation.[40,41] Individuals with stone disease should not drink sugar-sweetened soda. The intake of milk should not be restricted.

Some clinicians believe that a patient should have urine that is very light in color and should wake up at least once per night to void. There are no data to support the use of color as a guide, and the desire to have constantly dilute urine needs to be balanced against the need for sleep.

Dietary Recommendations

Individuals with calcium oxalate stone disease and elevated urinary calcium should restrict their intake of sodium and animal protein.[42] Additional dietary recommendations should be based on the results of the 24-hour urine collection. For example, dietary oxalate restriction or discontinuation of vitamin C supplementation may be of limited utility in a calcium oxalate stone former with lower urinary excretion of oxalate. For low urinary citrate, the patient should increase intake of dietary alkali (fruits and vegetables) and decrease intake of

Box 35-2 Treatment of Idiopathic Hypercalciuria

Dietary Changes	Medications	Comments
Increase total fluid intake to maintain urine volume > 2 L/day Adequate dietary calcium intake Decrease animal protein intake (≤5 servings of animal flesh per week) Decrease sodium intake (<2.4 g/day)	Chlorthalidone or hydrochlorothiazide 25 mg/day; titrate to 50–100 mg/day as needed	Administer hydrochlorothiazide twice daily to maximize hypocalciuric effect Hypokalemia secondary to diuretic therapy can precipitate hypocitraturia High sodium intake may result in failure of thiazide to decrease urinary calcium

acid-producing foods such as animal protein. Of note, there is no evidence that dietary calcium restriction alone is helpful in preventing the formation of calcium stones, and there is substantial evidence that it may be harmful. Observational data showing an inverse relationship between dietary calcium and the risk of incident kidney stones suggest that dietary calcium may bind to oxalate in the gut, thereby limiting intestinal oxalate absorption (and subsequent urinary oxalate excretion). Indeed, the inhibitory effect of calcium ingestion on urinary oxalate excretion has been demonstrated in oxalate-loading studies.[43,44] The role of calcium supplements deserves comment because their use is so common. A patient with calcium nephrolithiasis who wishes to continue calcium supplementation should collect 24-hour urine samples on and off the supplement. If the urinary supersaturation of the calcium salt in question increases during the period of supplement use, the supplement should be discontinued.

Drug Therapy

Medications are indicated for the stone-forming patient with severe disease or whose urinary abnormalities persist despite attempted lifestyle changes. Because the goal of

therapy is to prevent the additional formation and growth of calcium oxalate stones and because an existing calcium stone will not dissolve, the passage of another stone does not necessarily reflect failure of dietary interventions. As with dietary modification, the 24-hour urine collection is essential to select intervention and to gauge the success or failure of treatment.

Thiazide diuretics can lower the urinary excretion of calcium by as much as 150 mg/day, and treatment with a thiazide may reduce the rate of stone recurrence by as much as 90%.[45,46] The diuretic dose is usually started at chlorthalidone or hydrochlorothiazide 25 mg/day (or its equivalent), but many patients will require 50 to 100 mg/day (with twice-daily dosing for hydrochlorothiazide) to achieve satisfactory decreases in urinary calcium excretion. Without dietary sodium restriction, the reduction in urinary calcium excretion obtained with treatment may be inadequate. In addition, serum potassium levels should be closely monitored during therapy because hypokalemia can result in a decrease in urinary citrate excretion. Thiazide diuretics may be beneficial even in patients without overt hypercalciuria.[45,46]

Calcium stone formers with hyperuricosuria may be treated with allopurinol (100–300 mg/day). Allopurinol may reduce

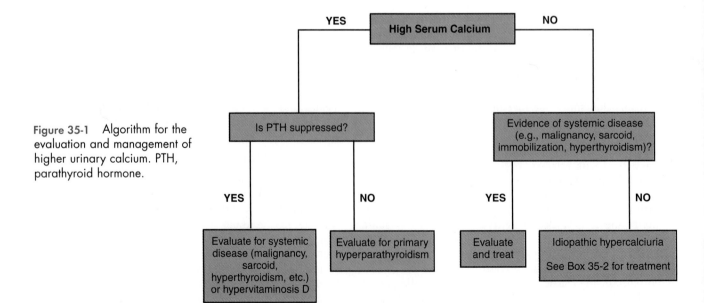

Figure 35-1 Algorithm for the evaluation and management of higher urinary calcium. PTH, parathyroid hormone.

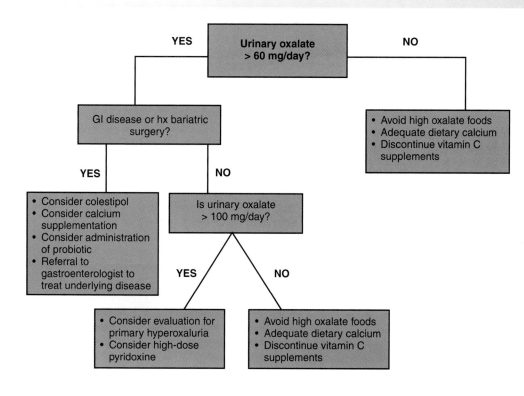

Figure 35-2   Algorithm for the evaluation and management of higher urinary oxalate. GI, gastrointestinal; hx, history.

new stone formation by as much as 80% in individuals with isolated hyperuricosuria.[47]

Urinary citrate excretion can be increased by the administration of an oral alkali load, usually in the form of potassium citrate started at 20 mEq three times daily.[48,49] In one study, stone recurrence in a group of hypocitraturic patients treated with potassium citrate decreased from 1.2 to 0.1 per patient year (versus no change with placebo).[49] Potassium salts should be administered cautiously to patients with chronic kidney disease or those taking drugs that decrease urinary potassium excretion.

To date, no satisfactory drug treatment exists to decrease the urinary excretion of oxalate. For patients with increased intestinal absorption of oxalate secondary to bowel disease, clinicians sometimes administer oxalate binders such as calcium carbonate or colestipol. Experimental therapies include the oral administration of oxalate-consuming bacteria and the administration of high-dose pyridoxine (to decrease the endogenous production of oxalate).[50,51]

PREVENTION OF STONE RECURRENCE: OTHER STONE TYPES

For the less common stone types, few data exist to support the role of specific dietary recommendations, and trial evidence for medical therapies is generally absent. Therefore, the following recommendations are based on the pathophysiology of the different stone types and clinical experience.

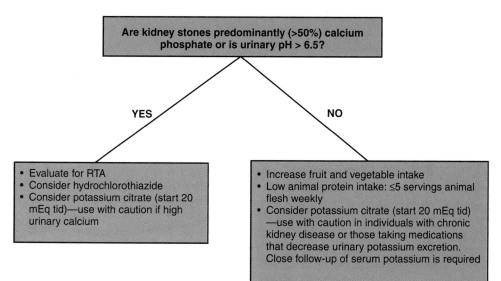

Figure 35-3   Algorithm for the evaluation and management of lower urinary citrate. RTA, renal tubular acidosis.

Uric Acid Stones

The primary risk factor for uric acid nephrolithiasis is low urinary pH, and alkali supplementation is the most effective treatment for pure uric acid stones.[17] If urine pH is maintained at 6.5 or higher (which may require 30–40 mEq of supplemental alkali dosed three times daily), pure uric acid stones will dissolve. A lower pH target can be used to prevent new uric acid stone formation. If the patient has marked hyperuricosuria and is unable to maintain an elevated urine pH, allopurinol should be added to the medical regimen.

Decreasing the consumption of meat, chicken, and seafood will decrease purine intake and uric acid production and will also decrease the amount of endogenous acid production from the metabolism of sulfur-containing amino acids. Higher intake of fruits and vegetables, which are high in potential base (such as citrate), may increase the urine pH and decrease the risk of uric acid crystal formation.

Because of the relationships between insulin resistance, obesity, and low urinary pH,[52–54] as well as data linking both obesity and diabetes to a higher risk of uric acid stones,[55,56] patients with uric acid stone disease may benefit from weight loss. Currently, there is no evidence supporting the role for insulin-sensitizing agents as a modality for the treatment of uric acid nephrolithiasis.

Cystine Stones

Cystine stones result from cystinuria, an autosomal recessive disorder, and usually require medication for prevention. Tiopronin and penicillamine increase the solubility of filtered cystine, but have a high frequency of adverse side effects. Supplemental alkali may provide some benefit by increasing urinary pH,[57] but is rarely sufficient as the sole treatment.

Restricting dietary sodium may reduce the urinary excretion of cystine. Because the solubility of cystine increases as urinary pH increases, fruit and vegetable consumption may be beneficial. There is little evidence to support the dietary restriction of proteins high in cystine. However, reducing animal protein intake may be beneficial by increasing urine pH.

Struvite Stones

Struvite stones form in the setting of upper urinary tract infection with urease-producing bacteria. Struvite stones can be very large ("staghorn calculi") and usually require urologic intervention. In addition to complete removal of all residual fragments, prevention of recurrent urinary tract infection is crucial to prevent recurrence. Acetohydroxamic acid inhibits urease, but has frequent and serious side effects.[58]

Calcium Phosphate Stones

Information on dietary factors related to calcium phosphate stone formation is limited. Patients with type 1 RTA benefit from the administration of alkali supplementation, generally in the form of potassium citrate. However, alkali supplementation should be used with caution because an increase in urinary pH can increase the risk of calcium phosphate crystal formation. Thiazides can be used to decrease the excretion of urinary calcium using an approach similar to that recommended for calcium oxalate stones.

FOLLOW-UP

Close follow-up is essential to determine the efficacy of treatment and gauge the need for additional intervention. We recommend a repeat 24-hour urine collection 6 to 8 weeks after initiation of treatment. If a stone former is symptom free and on a treatment regimen that has adequately reduced urine lithogenicity, we recommend a follow-up 24-hour urine collection annually. Because x-ray examination of the kidney and upper bladder or US can identify new kidney stones or an increase in the size of a previous stone, annual imaging is a reasonable way to detect treatment failure in an asymptomatic patient. We do not recommend routine follow-up with HCT for asymptomatic individuals because of radiation dose and cost.

CONCLUSION

Nephrolithiasis is common, costly, and painful. Advances in imaging and urologic techniques have improved the diagnosis and management of stone disease in the acute setting. Because recurrence is common, a clinical and metabolic evaluation should be offered to patients willing to adhere to specific dietary and/or pharmacologic recommendations. Even if stone composition is known, a thorough evaluation requires at least two 24-hour urine specimens collected at least 6 weeks after resolution of an acute episode. The initial choice of dietary or medical intervention should be tailored to the individual patient based on stone type, if known, and the 24-hour urine results. Subsequent 24-hour urine collections are necessary to gauge the adequacy of treatment. Prevention of stone recurrence is an achievable goal with individualized therapy and regular follow-up.

References

1. Johnson CM, Wilson DM, O'Fallon WM, et al: Renal stone epidemiology: A 25-year study in Rochester, Minnesota. Kidney Int 1979;16:624–631.
2. Hiatt RA, Dales LG, Friedman GD, Hunkeler EM: Frequency of urolithiasis in a prepaid medical care program. Am J Epidemiol 1982;115:255–265.
3. Pearle M, Calhoun E, Curhan GC: Urolithiasis. In Litwin MS, Saigal CS (eds): Urologic Diseases in America. Washington, DC: U.S. Dept of Health and Human Services, 2004, p 34.
4. Gupta M: Acute and chronic renal pain. In Coe FL, Favus MJ, Pak C, et al (eds): Kidney Stones: Medical and Surgical Management. Philadelphia: Lippincott–Raven, 1996, pp 463–500.
5. Asplin J, Chandhoke P: The stone forming patient. In Coe FL, Favus MJ, Pak C, et al (eds): Kidney Stones: Medical and Surgical Management. Philadelphia: Lippincott–Raven, 1996, pp 773–786.
6. Li J, Kennedy D, Levine M, et al: Absent hematuria and expensive computerized tomography: Case characteristics of emergency urolithiasis. J Urol 2001;165:782–784.
7. Vieweg J, Teh C, Freed K, et al: Unenhanced helical computerized tomography for the evaluation of patients with acute flank pain. J Urol 1998;160:679–684.
8. Wong SK, Ng LG, Tan BS, et al: Acute renal colic: Value of unenhanced spiral computed tomography compared with intravenous urography. Ann Acad Med Singapore 2001;30:568–572.
9. Lang EK, Macchia RJ, Thomas R, et al: Improved detection of renal pathologic features on multiphasic helical CT compared

with IVU in patients presenting with microscopic hematuria. Urology 2003;61:528–532.

10. Sheafor DH, Hertzberg BS, Freed KS, et al: Nonenhanced helical CT and US in the emergency evaluation of patients with renal colic: Prospective comparison. Radiology 2000;217:792–797.

11. Fowler KA, Locken JA, Duchesne JH, Williamson MR: US for detecting renal calculi with nonenhanced CT as a reference standard. Radiology 2002;222:109–113.

12. Labrecque M, Dostaler L-P, Rouselle R, et al: Efficacy of nonsteroidal anti-inflammatory drugs in the treatment of acute renal colic: A meta-analysis. Arch Intern Med 1994;154:1381–1387.

13. Romics I, Molnar DL, Timberg G, et al: The effect of drotaverine hydrochloride in acute colicky pain caused by renal and ureteric stones. BJU Int 2003;92:92–96.

14. Iguchi M, Katoh Y, Koike H, et al: Randomized trial of trigger point injection for renal colic. Int J Urol 2002;9:475–479.

15. Lopes T, Dias JS, Marcelino J, et al: An assessment of the clinical efficacy of intranasal desmopressin spray in the treatment of renal colic. BJU Int 2001;87:322–325.

16. Kekec Z, Yilmaz U, Sozuer E: The effectiveness of tenoxicam vs isosorbide dinitrate plus tenoxicam in the treatment of acute renal colic. BJU Int 2000;85:783–785.

17. Rodman J, Sosa R, Lopez M: Diagnosis and treatment of uric acid calculi. In Coe FL, Favus MJ, Pak C, et al. (eds): Kidney Stones: Medical and Surgical Management. Philadelphia: Lippincott–Raven, 1996, pp 973–989.

18. Bihl G, Meyers A: Recurrent renal stone disease—advances in pathogenesis and clinical management. Lancet 2001;358:651–656.

19. Hollingsworth JM, Rogers MA, Kaufman SR, et al: Medical therapy to facilitate urinary stone passage: A meta-analysis. Lancet 2006;368:1171–1179.

20. Curhan G, Fitzpatrick J: Nephrolithiasis: Lithotripsy and surgery. In Brady H, Wilcox C (eds): Therapy in Nephrology and Hypertension, 2nd ed. New York: Elsevier, 2003, pp 405–411.

21. Coe FL, Parks JH, Asplin JR: The pathogenesis and treatment of kidney stones. N Engl J Med 1992;327:1141–1152.

22. Smith LH, Drach G, Hall P, et al: National High Blood Pressure Education Program (NHBPEP) review paper on complications of shock wave lithotripsy for urinary calculi. Am J Med 1991;91:635–641.

23. Ehreth JT, Drach GW, Arnett ML, et al: Extracorporeal shock wave lithotripsy: Multicenter study of kidney and upper ureter versus middle and lower ureter treatments. J Urol 1994;152:1379–1385.

24. Rudnick DM, Bennett PM, Dretler SP: Retrograde renoscopic fragmentation of moderate-size (1.5–3.0-cm) renal cystine stones. J Endourol 1999;13:483–485.

25. Albala DM, Assimos DG, Clayman RV, et al: Lower pole I: A prospective randomized trial of extracorporeal shock wave lithotripsy and percutaneous nephrostolithotomy for lower pole nephrolithiasis—initial results. J Urol 2001;166:2072–2080.

26. Uribarri J, Oh MS, Carroll HJ: The first kidney stone. Ann Intern Med 1989;111:1006–1009.

27. Williams RE: Long-term survey of 538 patients with upper urinary tract stone. Br J Urol 1963;35:416–437.

28. Coe FL, Keck J, Norton ER: The natural history of calcium urolithiasis. JAMA 1977;238:1519–1523.

29. Pak CY, Poindexter JR, Adams-Huet B, Pearle MS: Predictive value of kidney stone composition in the detection of metabolic abnormalities. Am J Med 2003;115:26–32.

30. Parks JH, Coe FL: An increasing number of calcium oxalate stone events worsens treatment outcome. Kidney Int 1994;45:1722–1730.

31. Parks JH, Coe FL: The financial effects of kidney stone prevention. Kidney Int 1996;50:1706–1712.

32. Levy FL, Adams-Huet B, Pak CY: Ambulatory evaluation of nephrolithiasis: An update of a 1980 protocol. Am J Med 1995;98:50–59.

33. Hess B, Hasler-Strub U, Ackermann D, Jaeger P: Metabolic evaluation of patients with recurrent idiopathic calcium nephrolithiasis. Nephrol Dial Transplant 1997;12:1362–1368.

34. Parks JH, Goldfisher E, Asplin JR, Coe FL: A single 24-hour urine collection is inadequate for the medical evaluation of nephrolithiasis. J Urol 2002;167:1607–1612.

35. Pak CY, Kaplan R, Bone H, et al: A simple test for the diagnosis of absorptive, resorptive and renal hypercalciurias. N Engl J Med 1975;292:497–500.

36. Curhan GC, Willett WC, Rimm EB, Stampfer MJ: A prospective study of dietary calcium and other nutrients and the risk of symptomatic kidney stones. N Engl J Med 1993;328:833–838.

37. Curhan G, Willett W, Speizer F, et al: Comparison of dietary calcium with supplemental calcium and other nutrients as factors affecting the risk for kidney stones in women. Ann Intern Med 1997;126:497–504.

38. Curhan GC, Willett WC, Knight EL, Stampfer MJ: Dietary factors and the risk of incident kidney stones in younger women (Nurses' Health Study II). Arch Intern Med 2004;164:885–891.

39. Borghi L, Meschi T, Amato F, et al: Urinary volume, water and recurrences in idiopathic calcium nephrolithiasis: A 5-year randomized prospective study. J Urol 1996;155:839–843.

40. Curhan GC, Willett WC, Rimm EB, et al: Prospective study of beverage use and the risk of kidney stones. Am J Epidemiol 1996;143:240–247.

41. Curhan GC, Willett WC, Speizer FE, Stampfer MJ: Beverage use and risk for kidney stones in women. Ann Intern Med 1998;128:534–540.

42. Borghi L, Schianchi T, Meschi T, et al: Comparison of two diets for the prevention of recurrent stones in idiopathic hypercalciuria. N Engl J Med 2002;346:77–84.

43. Hess B, Jost C, Zipperle L, et al: High-calcium intake abolishes hyperoxaluria and reduces urinary crystallization during a 20-fold normal oxalate load in humans. Nephrol Dial Transplant 1998;13:2241–2247.

44. Liebman M, Chai W: Effect of dietary calcium on urinary oxalate excretion after oxalate loads. Am J Clin Nutr 1997;65:1453–1459.

45. Ettinger B, Citron JT, Livermore B, Dolman LI: Chlorthalidone reduces calcium oxalate calculous recurrence but magnesium hydroxide does not. J Urol 1988;139:679–684.

46. Laerum E, Larsen S: Thiazide prophylaxis of urolithiasis. A double-blind study in general practice. Acta Med Scand 1984;215:383–389.

47. Ettinger B, Tang A, Citro J, et al: Randomized trial of allopurinol in the prevention of calcium oxalate calculi. N Engl J Med 1986;315:1386–1389.

48. Sakhaee K, Alpern R, Jacobson HR, Pak CY: Contrasting effects of various potassium salts on renal citrate excretion. J Clin Endocrinol Metab 1991;72:396–400.

49. Barcelo P, Wuhl O, Servitge E, et al: Randomized double-blind study of potassium citrate in idiopathic hypocitraturic calcium nephrolithiasis. J Urol 1993;150:1761–1764.

50. Lieske JC, Goldfarb DS, De Simone C, Regnier C: Use of a probiotic to decrease enteric hyperoxaluria. Kidney Int 2005;68:1244–1249.

51. Monico CG, Rossetti S, Olson JB, Milliner DS: Pyridoxine effect in type I primary hyperoxaluria is associated with the most common mutant allele. Kidney Int 2005;67:1704–1709.

52. Abate N, Chandalia M, Cabo-Chan AV Jr, et al: The metabolic syndrome and uric acid nephrolithiasis: Novel features of renal manifestation of insulin resistance. Kidney Int 2004;65:386–392.

53. Cameron MA, Maalouf NM, Adams-Huet B, et al: Urine composition in type 2 diabetes: Predisposition to uric acid nephrolithiasis. J Am Soc Nephrol 2006;17:1422–1428.

54. Maalouf NM, Sakhaee K, Parks JH, et al: Association of urinary pH with body weight in nephrolithiasis. Kidney Int 2004;65:1422–1425.

55. Daudon M, Lacour B, Jungers P: Influence of body size on urinary stone composition in men and women. Urol Res 2006;34:193–199.

56. Daudon M, Traxer O, Conort P, et al: Type 2 diabetes increases the risk for uric acid stones. J Am Soc Nephrol 2006;17:2026–2033.

57. Goldfarb DS, Coe FL, Asplin JR: Urinary cystine excretion and capacity in patients with cystinuria. Kidney Int 2006;69:1041–1047.

58. Williams JJ, Rodman JS, Peterson CM: A randomized double-blind study of acetohydroxamic acid in struvite nephrolithiasis. N Engl J Med 1984;311:760–764.

Further Reading

Borghi L, Meschi T, Amato F, et al: Urinary volume, water and recurrences in idiopathic calcium nephrolithiasis: A 5-year randomized prospective study. J Urol 1996;155:839–843.

Borghi L, Schianchi T, Meschi T, et al: Comparison of two diets for the prevention of recurrent stones in idiopathic hypercalciuria. N Engl J Med 2002;346:77–84.

Curhan GC, Taylor EN: 24-h uric acid excretion and the risk of kidney stones. Kidney Int 2008;73:489–496.

Curhan GC, Willett WC, Rimm EB, Stampfer MJ: A prospective study of dietary calcium and other nutrients and the risk of symptomatic kidney stones. N Engl J Med 1993;328:833–838.

Curhan GC, Willett WC, Speizer FE, Stampfer MJ: Beverage use and risk for kidney stones in women. Ann Intern Med 1998;128:534–540.

Ettinger B, Citron JT, Livermore B, Dolman LI: Chlorthalidone reduces calcium oxalate calculous recurrence but magnesium hydroxide does not. J Urol 1988;139:679–684.

Ettinger B, Tang A, Citron JT, et al: Randomized trial of allopurinol in the prevention of calcium oxalate calculi. N Engl J Med 1986;315:1386–1389.

Taylor EN, Curhan GC: Diet and fluid prescription in stone disease. Kidney Int 2006;70:835–839.

Taylor EN, Curhan GC: Oxalate intake and the risk for nephrolithiasis. J Am Soc Nephrol 18:2007:2198–2204.

Chapter 36

Nephrolithiasis: Lithotripsy and Surgery

John M. Fitzpatrick

During the past 15 years, the management of urinary calculi has undergone revolutionary changes as a result of the increasing number and availability of nonsurgical therapeutic approaches. Pyelolithotomy, ureterolithotomy, and retrograde blind endoscopic procedures were previously the only treatment options for removal of symptomatic stones. Fortunately, the development of extracorporeal shock wave lithotripsy (SWL), percutaneous nephrolithotomy (PCNL), and ureteroscopic lithotripsy has provided urologists with less invasive and safer treatment possibilities. The use of SWL and PCNL has led to a dramatic reduction in morbidity and mortality and has hastened recovery and return to usual activities. Remarkable technologic advances in the methods of SWL and endourology have continued with the introduction of smaller and less expensive devices. Although new technology has rendered stone management safer and less invasive, the appropriate role of each modality remains unsettled and merits careful individualized consideration.

This chapter discusses the role of lithotripsy and surgery in the management of nephrolithiasis. All the procedures described require the skill of an experienced urologist. For a more detailed discussion of these techniques, there are several excellent reviews.[1,2]

TYPES OF LITHOTRIPSY

There are two main categories of lithotripsy: extracorporeal and intracorporeal.

Extracorporeal Shock Wave Lithotripsy

Extracorporeal SWL, the most common technique, is performed by the generation of shock waves external to the body that are transmitted through the skin and soft tissues and focused on the stone. The energy delivered causes fragmentation of the stone into smaller pieces that can then be passed spontaneously or removed endoscopically by the urologist. The original lithotriptors required the patient to be immersed in water to transmit the shock wave through the body to the stone; however, newer generation machines require only a small water cushion. Although SWL is often referred to as noninvasive lithotripsy, cystoscopic placement of ureteral stents before treatment may be needed to relieve obstruction or allow passage of a large (>1.5 cm) stone burden.

Intracorporeal Lithotripsy

Intracorporeal lithotripsy is performed through a nephroscope or cystoscope and is therefore more invasive than extracorporeal SWL. The four types of device currently available for intracorporeal lithotripsy (electrohydraulic, ultrasonic, laser, and pneumatic) differ according to the manner in which the energy for fragmentation is generated and delivered to the stone.

Electrohydraulic Lithotripsy

Electrohydraulic lithotripsy, the first method of intracorporeal lithotripsy to be introduced, fragments stones by the transfer of energy from the generated shock wave to the stone at the fluid-stone interface. An electrical spark vaporizes water and creates a shock wave. Ureteral damage may occur from exposure to the spark produced during shock wave generation.

Ultrasonic Lithotripsy

Ultrasonic lithotripsy makes use of mechanical vibration to break stones into smaller fragments that may be aspirated with specialized probes. This method requires direct contact between the probe and the stone and has several drawbacks. For example, it is often necessary to ensnare the stone in a basket before treatment because pressure exerted on the stone during the procedure may cause upward migration of stone fragments. In addition, heat produced within the ureter by the probe may lead to the formation of ureteral strictures. Furthermore, the rigidity and large size of the probes prevent the use of small ureteroscopes.

Laser Lithotripsy

The flexibility and fine caliber of the fibers used to deliver the laser energy have allowed remarkable miniaturization of ureteroscopes. Moreover, laser fragmentation of stones can be performed with greater precision and control than by other methods and without propulsion of fragments or damage to surrounding tissue.

A number of laser types are available for stone fragmentation. The susceptibility to fragmentation by laser energy is dependent on stone composition and physical factors specific to each type of laser, such as pulse duration and wavelength. For example, the energy delivered by the pulsed dye laser has proved to be useful in the disruption of most stones and has the advantage of sparing the ureter from damage. Although this laser type does not fragment cystine stones well, its effectiveness can be enhanced by staining the cystine stone with an absorbing dye. In contrast, the holmium laser effectively disintegrates the surface of any stone with minimal propulsion, gradually cracking or boring a hole through the stone. However, ureteral tissue may absorb the wavelength from the holmium laser and is thus vulnerable to injury.

Pneumatic Lithotripsy

The Swiss Lithoclast, the least expensive intracorporeal device, has been used effectively for stone fragmentation at all levels of the urinary tract. Under direct visualization, a solid rigid probe is applied directly to the stone to cause mechanical disruption by repeated percussion of the probe tip, similar to the mechanical action of a pneumatic jackhammer. Grasping instruments may then be used to remove the stone fragments. However, retrograde displacement of a ureteral stone is a potential drawback of this procedure, and the precise positioning required to prevent tissue damage and the need for a rigid or semirigid endoscope limit its usefulness as well.

EFFICACY OF LITHOTRIPSY

Although there is general agreement that both extracorporeal and intracorporeal lithotripsy are effective, there are no large randomized, controlled trials comparing these two methods. A recent small randomized trial of 64 patients found comparable success rates for SWL compared with ureteroscopy for the treatment of distal ureteral calculi of 1.5 cm or smaller.[3] Results from studies of the individual methods must be compared with caution because the success or effectiveness of treatment is not uniformly defined. Although stone free is the gold standard for a successful procedure, there is great variability in the ascertainment of this outcome with respect to both the time of assessment (e.g., immediately after the procedure, after 7 days, after 3 months) and the imaging modalities employed (e.g., radiograph of the kidneys, ureter, and bladder, intravenous pyelography, ultrasonography, computed tomography). When SWL was first introduced, a treatment session that produced clinically insignificant fragments was deemed a success. However, this definition has fallen out of favor owing to its ambiguity and the reality that the retention of small fragments results in regrowth and recurrence of symptomatic stone disease. The definition of a treatment failure may vary as well, yet is most commonly defined as the need for a repeated treatment or another type of procedure.

Extracorporeal Shock Wave Lithotripsy

The success of SWL depends on the location, size, and composition of the stone. Thus, a comparison of success rates between different studies must consider all three of these factors. Stones in the kidney are treated with slightly greater success than are ureteral stones, and success rates are higher for proximal ureteral stones than for distal stones. Small stones, usually smaller than 2 cm, are more easily treated with SWL than are larger stones. Softer stones (calcium oxalate dihydrate, uric acid, apatite, and struvite) are more easily fragmented with SWL than are harder stones (calcium oxalate monohydrate, brushite, and cystine).

SWL is the treatment of choice for most renal stones, and success rates as high as 90% have been reported.[4] However, further procedures may be necessary in as many as 20% of patients with stones of 1 to 2 cm. In general, SWL is more effective in the treatment of stones in the renal pelvis than in the calyces and, depending on size, composition, calyceal configuration, and infundibular pelvic angle, is least effective in treating lower pole stones.

There is an inverse relationship between stone size and stone-free rates. Stones larger than 2 cm in diameter are rarely successfully treated with SWL alone and may best be removed by PCNL in the upper urinary tract and ureteroscopically in the lower tract.

Stone-free rates of more than 80% for calcium oxalate and uric acid stones (softer stones) have been reported, although no distinction was made based on stone size.[5] A study of retreatment rates in patients with stones of known composition, 1 to 3 cm in diameter, and treated with SWL found that calcium oxalate monohydrate calculi (hard stones) required the greatest number of retreatment procedures (10%), followed by struvite (6%), and calcium oxalate dihydrate (3%).[6]

First-generation lithotriptors caused enough pain to require anesthesia, either general or epidural. Most patients treated with newer generation devices require only moderate intravenous analgesia while undergoing SWL.

The early complications of SWL have been well described and are generally minor, with pain and hematuria most commonly reported. Direct injury to the kidney and surrounding tissues as well as complications due to the passage of stone fragments may also occur. Much less information is available on the long-term effects of SWL because most follow-up efforts have focused only on the short-term results and complications.

The morphologic changes that may occur after SWL and their mechanisms have been studied by a variety of imaging techniques. Imaging by computed tomography or magnetic resonance reveals that more than 75% of treated patients have changes in renal tissue and demonstrate edema in and around the kidney, as well as intraparenchymal, subcapsular, or perirenal hemorrhage. Although damage to nonrenal tissues has been rarely reported, pancreatitis, gastric erosions, ecchymoses of the colonic mucosa, splenic rupture, pulmonary contusions, and cardiac arrhythmias may occur. Although there have been no reported adverse effects of SWL on fertility or the risk of birth defects, the impact of SWL on the reproductive tract, if any, has yet to be established. SWL should not be used on pregnant women.

Functionally, biochemical evidence of kidney damage directly after SWL has been documented. Although the results of these laboratory studies generally return to near-normal levels within days, it is unclear whether these changes represent only transient dysfunction or more consequential chronic damage. A small prospective, randomized study suggested that pretreatment with nifedipine or allopurinol may protect the kidney from shock wave–induced renal damage.[7] Nevertheless, there is no clear evidence to indicate that SWL is associated with any long-term effect on renal function in humans.[8]

Ureteral stone fragments may cause obstruction after incomplete stone fragmentation or fragmentation of a large stone burden resulting in steinstrasse, literally "stone street." Typically, partially obstructing steinstrasse will clear spontaneously within 2 to 4 weeks in asymptomatic patients. Otherwise, percutaneous nephrostomy tube decompression, ureteroscopic manipulation, PCNL, repeated SWL, or even open ureterolithotomy may be necessary to clear the stone fragments. Repeated SWL is often attempted in patients with minimal symptoms and no evidence of infection. In contrast, emergency decompression of the collecting system with a percutaneous nephrostomy tube is necessary for symptomatic patients or asymptomatic patients with significant obstruction. Steinstrasse that persist for longer than 1 or 2 weeks after placement of the percutaneous nephrostomy tube may be relieved with repeated SWL, ureteroscopy, or intracorporeal lithotripsy.

Although it has been suggested that SWL is associated with new-onset hypertension, this connection is not supported by all studies. The most persuasive study demonstrated that the incidence of hypertension is not higher in patients treated with SWL compared with other methods of stone removal. Nevertheless, there was a statistically significant increase in diastolic blood pressure of just less than 1 mm Hg in SWL-treated patients.[9] This increase may be more pronounced in older patients.

To date, the safe upper limit of shock wave energy that can be delivered to one kidney during one session, the total amount of energy that can be delivered cumulatively, and the minimum safe interval between treatment sessions have yet to be defined. The variables to be considered include the number of shock waves and the power at which they are delivered. These vary for each type of machine and have not been standardized. However, despite these variations, there are few reports of renal injury to the hundreds of thousands of patients treated with SWL. Available data suggest that if chronic kidney damage does occur, it is most likely to be incurred by patients with some degree of preexisting renal dysfunction.[10]

SURGICAL MODALITIES

Stone surgery has changed so considerably over the past decade that the term has almost dropped out of use. The percutaneous approach was then introduced, which involved new technology both to approach the kidney and to enter it without damaging vital structures, and then to remove the stone if small or to fragment and aspirate it if larger.

Percutaneous Nephrolithotomy

The fact that stone removal from the kidney required an extensive flank incision long frustrated urologists. Eventually, the task was performed using a combination of radiographic and minimally invasive surgical techniques.[11]

The procedure is usually performed in a single session with general anesthesia. A fine needle is inserted into the renal pelvis under ultrasound or radiographic guidance: the track is not made directly into the pelvis but through the parenchyma of the lower pole of the kidney, so that the track into the lower pole calyx is supported by the renal tissue itself. A nephroscope is passed, and if the stone is visualized, it can be broken up by intracorporeal lithotripsy. The fragments are then evacuated, and a non–self-retaining nephrostomy tube is inserted and sutured to the skin.[12]

Failure to remove the stone fragments completely is uncommon, particularly with increasing experience. The overall success rate of 95% throughout the world shows that this technique is an excellent way to clear, using one single method, all but the most refractory of stones.[13–15]

The complication rate is low: hemorrhage requiring blood transfusion or surgical intervention is seen in 1% to 3% of patients, and residual stones are left behind in 2% to 8%.[15] Sepsis can develop, especially if the preoperative urine culture is positive. In this case, antibiotic prophylaxis is needed.[16]

Open Surgery

The newer techniques for removing and fragmenting stones, alone or in combination, have eliminated the requirement for open surgery except in a small number of cases. The actual percentage of cases that today require open surgery is not known but is unlikely to be greater than 12%. Stones of large bulk and complexity should be managed in stone centers by urologists who have the experience required for this type of surgery.

One of two methods is used to incise the renal cortical tissue and to approach the peripheral stone fragments in the calyces: radical paravascular nephrotomy[17] and anatrophic nephrolithotomy.[18] In the former approach, incisions are made between the branches of the renal artery. The calyx is approached and the fragments are removed. Several of these nephrotomies may have to be made, placed laterally in the kidney on either the anterior or posterior surface. After complete removal of the stone, the nephrotomies are closed with a fine suture, aiming to close only the renal capsule.

In anatrophic nephrolithotomy, the incision follows the avascular line between the segments of the kidney that are supplied by the anterior and posterior segmented branches of the renal artery. After complete removal of the stone, the kidney incision is sutured and closed completely.

EFFECT OF SURGICAL APPROACHES ON RENAL FUNCTION

The overall effect on renal function of PCNL is usually minimal. Although there is a potential risk that increases with the size of the access track, no studies have reported any serious postoperative loss of function.

Two aspects of open surgery may interfere with postoperative renal function: renal ischemia and parenchymal incisions. To prevent excessive hemorrhage when the renal parenchyma is incised, the renal artery is traditionally clamped, exposing the kidney to ischemia. If the ischemic period is longer than 20 minutes, irreversible renal damage may occur. A number of methods have been described to preserve renal function during ischemia of more than 20-minute duration, including renal cooling and vasoactive agents. In a canine model, the function of kidneys subjected to radial paravascular nephrotomy was unchanged compared with that of controls.[19] There was a statistically significant difference in postoperative function when the anatrophic nephrotomy was compared with control kidneys.

RECOMMENDATIONS

Contemporary Indications for Intervention

The generally accepted indications for intervention for the treatment of urinary calculi are summarized in Box 36-1. Absolute indications include persistent or progressive high-grade obstruction by the stone, urinary tract infection, and intractable pain. Infection in the face of obstruction is a medical emergency that requires immediate intervention to relieve the obstruction before SWL. Relative indications for intervention include occupational factors, significant hematuria requiring transfusion, substantial stone growth despite appropriate medical management, stone size judged too large to pass spontaneously, or failure of a ureteral stone to move during a 6-week period.

A finding of hydronephrosis, a sign of ureteral obstruction, at initial presentation is not necessarily an indication for intervention. However, if follow-up studies reveal a lack of improvement during a 1- to 2-week period, intervention is usually required whether or not symptoms are present.

The location, size, and composition of the stone are the most important factors guiding the decision to treat and with which method (Box 36-2). Realistically, the cost of purchasing and maintaining the different types of lithotripsy equipment is substantial, and most hospitals, even large academic centers, have only one extracorporeal and one or two intracorporeal lithotripsy devices available. Thus, treatment with

---

Box 36-1   Indications for Urological Intervention in Nephrolithiasis

Absolute Indications
Persistent obstruction
Urinary tract infection
Intractable pain

Relative Indications
Failure of ureteral stone to progress
Significant hematuria
Stone growth despite optimal medical treatment
Social, economic, or occupational factors
Stone too large to pass spontaneously

Box 36-2   Factors Influencing Choice of Intervention

Stone Characteristics
Size
Location
Composition

Urinary Tract Anatomy
Duplicated collecting system
Horseshoe kidney
Medullary sponge kidney
Solitary kidney
Transplanted kidney
Pediatric patient

Availability of Technology
Experience of urologist

---

extracorporeal or intracorporeal lithotripsy is the first decision to be made, based on the availability of devices. Second, the skill and familiarity of the treating urologist with the different methods are important. Third, the choice of approach depends on both economic factors and individual preferences (e.g., travel, time lost from work, retreatment rates). Fourth, other medical conditions, such as morbid obesity and severe scoliosis or kyphosis, and conditions associated with an increased risk of general anesthesia must be taken into consideration.

Renal Calculi

The majority of patients with renal stones smaller than 2 cm may be successfully managed with outpatient SWL and return to routine activities within 48 hours. In contrast, SWL treatment of stones 2 cm or larger presents a substantial risk of ureteral obstruction from stone fragments; therefore, PCNL is extremely effective and is the procedure of choice. Depending on stone composition and other clinical circumstances, stones 2 to 3 cm in size may occasionally be treated with SWL. A treatment algorithm for the management of renal calculi is presented in Figure 36-1.

Bilateral Stones

In the setting of bilateral stone disease, each kidney is commonly treated individually in separate sessions. However, patients with symptomatic bilateral stones may require bilateral intervention and can be treated with SWL during a single session if the stone burden is not too large and renal function is normal.[10] Patients with abnormal renal function before bilateral SWL treatment may be more likely to develop acute renal failure.[10] Potentially, patients with normal renal function and asymptomatic large bilateral stones may undergo bilateral SWL by an experienced endourologist in a single session for economic, social, or medical reasons (e.g., risk of anesthesia).

Calyceal Diverticula

Stones in calyceal diverticula are generally asymptomatic. Nevertheless, intervention is necessary in the setting of local symptoms such as pain, associated infection, hematuria, or progressive stone growth. Rarely, if there is adequate drainage from the calyceal diverticulum, SWL is the treatment of choice

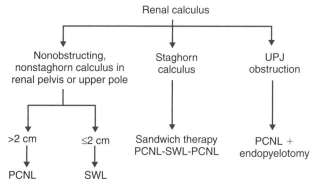

Figure 36-1 Treatment algorithm for the initial management of renal calculi. PCNL, percutaneous nephrolithotomy; SWL, shock wave lithotripsy; UPJ, ureteropelvic junction.

for stones smaller than 1.5 cm. PCNL is recommended for stones 1.5 cm or larger.

The management of asymptomatic calyceal calculi is more of a problem. One study suggested that 30% of patients with asymptomatic calyceal stones will present with a symptomatic episode within 3 years and 50% within 5 years of the initial evaluation.[20] Most urologists recommend a conservative approach and observe patients with asymptomatic calyceal diverticuli with calculi.

Horseshoe Kidney

Approximately 20% of individuals with a horseshoe kidney form a stone at some time. These stones may be composed of struvite, the result of infection due to abnormal urinary drainage, or calcium oxalate. SWL can be attempted if it is anatomically feasible. PCNL may be used as a primary or adjunctive procedure, particularly for larger stones. In general, stones 2 cm or smaller may be treated with either a first-generation lithotriptor or PCNL; PCNL is the treatment of choice for stones larger than 2 cm.[21]

Medullary Sponge Kidney

SWL may be attempted for the treatment of renal calculi in patients with medullary sponge kidney, although the data on its effectiveness are limited.[22] It is noteworthy that residual calcifications will likely be evident on kidney ureter bladder film owing to the presence of parenchymal calcifications. Thus, radiographic assessment of the success of the procedure and preventive medical therapies is difficult.

Staghorn Calculi

Struvite staghorn calculi are particularly concerning because they arise from infected urine and the stones harbor infection. Struvite staghorn calculi that fill the major part of the collecting system should be treated with a combination of percutaneous stone removal and SWL. The assessment of overall and split renal function is important when choosing which treatment to offer. The American Urological Association's treatment guidelines state that for struvite staghorn calculi, PCNL should be performed to debulk the stone mass occupying the renal pelvis, followed by SWL or flexible nephroscopy at a later date to remove fragments remaining in the calyces.[23] In

experienced hands, the stone-free rates with the combined approach should exceed 80%.[21]

Solitary Kidney

A solitary kidney, whether congenital or acquired, presents a unique set of difficulties. Obstruction of a solitary kidney can lead to acute renal failure. SWL with or without cystoscopic assistance is the best approach in this setting because it is preferable to avoid the use of a percutaneous nephrostomy owing to potential damage to the renal parenchymal tissue. Otherwise, the same criteria for treatment selection apply to a solitary kidney.

Transplanted Kidney

Fortunately, renal calculi form in less than 2% of transplanted kidneys. Hyperparathyroidism and nonabsorbable sutures are the most important risk factors. As for the native solitary kidney, it is preferable to avoid a percutaneous approach in a transplanted kidney. The transplanted kidney is typically located in the right or left lower quadrant of the abdomen and therefore is accessible by SWL. Alternatively, cystoscopic treatment with one of the intracorporeal methods may be attempted by an experienced endourologist.[24]

Ureteral Calculi

Renal colic from a ureteral stone is the most frequent reason for a patient to present to a physician for acute treatment of nephrolithiasis. At the time of presentation, a radiographic study will usually be obtained that may consist of an intravenous pyelogram (also known as intravenous urogram) or an ultrasound examination; many centers have replaced these with the preferred spiral computed tomography, which is more rapid and provides greater resolution. For patients with a known history of stones whose renal and ureteral anatomy is known, kidney ureter bladder film may be sufficient to identify a new stone.

The size of the ureteral calculus is an important factor in the determination of the need for intervention. Historically, ureteral stones 4 mm or smaller were observed, in anticipation of their spontaneous passage. However, recent data suggest that both size and location influence the likelihood of spontaneous passage.[25] In a retrospective study of 378 patients with ureteral stones, overall 60% of the stones passed without requiring intervention. Notably, the more proximal the stone is, the lower the passage rate. For example, a 4-mm stone passed spontaneously only 20% of the time if it were located in the proximal ureter, whereas the same size stone in the distal ureter passed spontaneously in 55% of cases.[25] Currently, even with the new technology available, patients with stones 4 mm or smaller rarely undergo intervention because of the excellent chance of spontaneous passage. However, improvements in technology have altered the indications for intervention for those patients with slightly larger stones who in the past would have been observed expectantly.

When intervention is deemed necessary, the location of the stone within the ureter is an important consideration that influences the selection of the method to be used (Fig. 36-2). Approximately 70% to 80% of proximal ureteral stones (above the iliac vessels) can be successfully treated with extracorporeal SWL. Although there are no large prospective, randomized

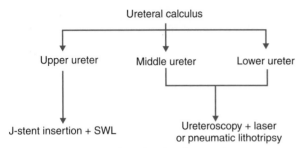

Figure 36-2 Treatment algorithm for the initial management of ureteral calculi. SWL, shock wave lithotripsy.

trials that compare SWL with other methods of removal, SWL is a reasonable choice for the initial management of proximal ureteral stones because of safety, noninvasiveness, and observed high success rates. Complications from SWL for proximal ureteral stones often result from stone manipulation before treatment, and ureteral stent placement does not increase the efficacy of treatment. However, in the setting of ureteral calculi larger than 1.5 cm, urosepsis, or complete ureteral obstruction, the placement of a ureteral stent or nephrostomy tube is often necessary. If SWL alone is unsuccessful, retrograde approaches are indicated. If the stone still cannot be removed, an antegrade (percutaneous) approach may be attempted. PCNL is a highly effective yet much more invasive option for the removal of a proximal ureteral stone.

The optimal treatment of distal ureteral stones is also controversial, primarily because of the lack of any prospective, randomized, controlled studies comparing SWL and ureteroscopy. SWL and endoscopic lithotripsy are both acceptable treatments of distal ureteral stones. SWL requires many more repeated treatments than endoscopic lithotripsy, but the latter is more invasive and occasionally may result in ureteral stricture formation.

SWL treatment of stones located in the distal ureter is technically more difficult than for stones in the renal pelvis or calyces. Thus, some urologists still employ ureteroscopy to manipulate the stone retrogradely into the renal pelvis and then proceed with SWL (referred to as "push-bang"). However, data suggest that this more invasive technique does not yield substantially higher stone-free rates than does SWL alone.[26]

As with renal stones, the comparative efficacy of the different approaches to treatment of ureteral calculi is difficult to assess. Most likely, the choice of treatment will be based on availability and experience with the various methods. Similarly, the choice of ureteroscopic technique often depends on the availability of the equipment and the experience of the urologist. If it is available, the pulsed dye laser may be used for fragmentation of most ureteral calculi. However, ultrasonic lithotripsy may be more effective for the treatment of a calcium oxalate monohydrate stone larger than 1 cm. Small durile stones are best treated by grasping with forceps or a basket followed by extraction. Treatment of cystine stones is more easily performed by electrohydraulic lithotripsy or holmium laser than by coating with dye and fragmentation by the pulsed dye laser.[27]

The treatment of infants, pregnant women, or extremely obese individuals merits special consideration. Minimal invasiveness and radiation exposure are particularly important in pediatric and obstetric patients, and conservative management is prudent. SWL, preferably with ultrasound localization, may be used in infants. Ureteroscopic techniques are another treatment option. Nevertheless, pregnant patients who present with symptomatic ureteral stones may require urgent treatment because of the increased risk to the fetus from systemic maternal infection or premature labor. The potential for serious complications and the technical difficulties involved in the treatment of infants and pregnant women demand care by only the most experienced endourologists. Although endoscopic treatment of distal calculi can be accomplished under local anesthesia in pregnant women, the most prudent approach is to insert an indwelling stent and allow the patient to complete the pregnancy. Extreme obesity, conversely, may impede SWL localization and the ability of the shock wave to reach the calculus; thus, ureteroscopic methods are preferable in this setting.[28]

Antibiotics and Shock Wave Lithotripsy

Historically, routine antimicrobial prophylaxis has been administered even in the absence of infection in the urinary tract. However, a prospective, randomized trial involving 360 patients revealed that the incidence of urinary tract infection after SWL was low in patients with sterile urine before intervention and suggested that prophylactic antibiotics may be unnecessary.[29] If bacteriuria is associated with calculi, prophylactic antibiotics are required whatever the planned surgical procedure.

References

1. Lingeman JE, Preminger GM (eds): New Developments in the Management of Urolithiasis. New York: Igaku-Shoin Medical Publishers, 1996.
2. Coe F, Favus M, Pak C, et al (eds): Kidney Stones: Medical and Surgical Management. Philadelphia: Lippincott-Raven, 1996.
3. Pearle MS, Nadler R, Bercowsky E, et al: Prospective randomized trial comparing shock wave lithotripsy and ureteroscopy for management of distal ureteral calculi. J Urol 2001;166:1255–1260.
4. Dawson C, Whitfield HN: The long-term results of treatment of urinary stones. Br J Urol 1994;74:397–404.
5. Graf J, Deiderichs W, Schulze H: Long-term follow-up in 1003 extracorporeal shock wave lithotripsy patients. J Urol 1988;140: 479–483.
6. Dretler SP: Stone fragility: A new therapeutic distinction. J Urol 1988;139:1124–1127.
7. Li B, Zhou W, Li P: Protective effects of nifedipine and allopurinol on high energy shock wave induced acute changes of renal function. J Urol 1995;153:596–598.
8. Liou LS, Streem SB: Long-term renal functional effects of shock wave lithotripsy, percutaneous nephrolithotomy and combination therapy: A comparative study of patients with solitary kidney. J Urol 2001;166:36–37.
9. Lingeman JE, Woods JR, Toth PD: Blood pressure changes following extracorporeal shock wave lithotripsy and other forms of treatment for nephrolithiasis. JAMA 1990;263: 1789–1794.
10. Lingeman JE, Newmark J: Adverse bioeffects of shock-wave lithotripsy. In Coe F, Favus M, Pak C, et al (eds): Kidney Stones: Medical and Surgical Management. Philadelphia: Lippincott-Raven, 1996, pp 605–614.
11. Fernstrom I, Johansson B: Percutaneous pyelolithotomy. A new extraction technique. Scand J Urol Nephrol 1976;10:257–259.

12. Marberger M: Percutaneous renal surgery: Its role in stone management. In Krane RJ, Siroky MB, Fitzpatrick JM (eds): Clinical Urology. Philadelphia: JB Lippincott, 1994, pp 254–265.

13. Alken P: Teleskopbougierset zur perkutanen Nephrostomie. Akt Urol 1981;12:216.

14. Segura JW, Patterson DE, LeRoy AJ, et al: Percutaneous lithotripsy. J Urol 1983;130:1051-1054.

15. Marberger M, Stackl W, Hruby W, et al: Late sequelae of ultrasonic lithotripsy of renal calculi. J Urol 1985;133:170–173.

16. Marberger M: Disintegration of renal and ureteral calculi with ultrasound. Urol Clin North Am 1983;10:729–742.

17. Wickham JE, Coe N, Ward JP: One hundred cases of nephrolithotomy under hypothermia. J Urol 1974;112:702–705.

18. Boyce WH, Elkins IB: Reconstructive renal surgery following anatrophic nephrolithotomy: Followup of 100 consecutive cases. J Urol 1974;111:307–312.

19. Fitzpatrick JM, Sleight MW, Braack A, et al: Intrarenal access: Effects on renal function and morphology. Br J Urol 1980;52:409–414.

20. Glowacki LS, Beecroft ML, Cook R J, et al: The natural history of asymptomatic urolithiasis. J Urol 1992;147:319–321.

21. Pearle M, Clayman M: Outcomes and selection of surgical therapies of stones in the kidney and ureter. In Coe F, Favus M, Pak C, et al (eds): Kidney Stones: Medical and Surgical Management. Philadelphia: Lippincott-Raven, 1996, pp 705–755.

22. Fuchs G, Patel A, Tognoni P: Management of stones associated with anatomic abnormalities of the urinary tract. In Coe F, Favus M, Pak C, et al (eds): Kidney Stones: Medical and Surgical Management. Philadelphia: Lippincott-Raven, 1996, pp 1037–1057.

23. Segura JW, Preminger GM, Assimos DG, et al: Nephrolithiasis Clinical Guidelines Panel summary report on the management of staghorn calculi. The American Urological Association Nephrolithiasis Clinical Guidelines Panel. J Urol 1994;151:1648–1651.

24. Benoit G, Blanchet P, Eschwege P, et al: Occurrence and treatment of kidney graft lithiasis in a series of 1500 patients. Clin Transplant 1996;10:176–180.

25. Morse RM, Resnick MI: Ureteral calculi: Natural history and treatment in an era of advanced technology. J Urol 1991;145:263–265.

26. Cass AS: Do upper ureteral stones need to be manipulated (push back) into the kidneys before extracorporeal shock wave lithotripsy? J Urol 1992;147:349–351.

27. Dretler SP: Modes of intracorporeal lithotripsy. In Coe F, Favus M, Pak C, et al (eds): Kidney Stones: Medical and Surgical Management. Philadelphia: Lippincott-Raven, 1996, pp 651–663.

28. Aso Y, Minowada S: Management of ureteral calculi. In Coe F, Favus M, Pak C, et al (eds): Kidney Stones: Medical and Surgical Management. Philadelphia: Lippincott-Raven, 1996, pp 665–679.

29. Ilker Y, Turkeri LN, Korten V, et al: Antimicrobial prophylaxis in management of urinary tract stones by extracorporeal shock-wave lithotripsy: Is it necessary? Urology 1995;46:165–167.

Further Reading

Smith D, Badlani GH, Bagley DH, et al (eds): Smith's Textbook of Endourology, 2nd ed. Hamilton, Ontario: BC Decker, 2007, pp 79–368.

Stoller ML, Meng MV (eds): Urinary Stone Disease. Totowa, NJ: Humana Press, 2007, pp 555–660.

Wein AJ, Kavoussi LR, Novick AC, et al (eds): Campbell-Walsh Urology, 9th ed. Philadelphia: Saunders-Elsevier, 2007, pp 1361–1564.

PART VI

Genitourinary Infections, Malignancy, and Obstruction

CONTENTS

Chapter 37

Therapy of Urinary Tract Infection

Nina E. Tolkoff-Rubin and Robert H. Rubin

The term urinary tract infection (UTI) encompasses a group of clinical disorders that are quite diverse and that, together, constitute the most common form of bacterial infection affecting humans throughout their life span. UTI is primarily an infection of females (both adult and pediatric). Males have a significant incidence of UTI only at the two extremes of life because of the higher incidence of urogenital anomalies among male babies and the effects of prostatic disease in the geriatric population.[1] More than 7 million women seek medical attention each year for acute, uncomplicated UTI (cystitis), with more than 100,000 hospital admissions each year for the care of pyelonephritis at a total cost of more than $1 billion per year. The incidence of cystitis in sexually active young women is 0.5% to 0.7% per year. Approximately 50% of women will have at least one UTI in their lifetime.[2,3] UTI may involve deep tissue infection of the kidney and/or the prostate gland, or superficial mucosal infection of the bladder; an estimated 90% of infections in males involve tissue invasion, whereas 70% or more of UTIs in females represent superficial mucosal infection. Clinically, UTIs may be symptomatic or asymptomatic, may cause bloodstream invasion, and may occur in anatomically normal or abnormal urinary tract anatomy or in persons with or without underlying renal disease.[1–5]

Over the years, it has been postulated that UTI, even if asymptomatic, had important effects beyond the inflammatory consequences of microbial invasion: hypertension, progressive renal disease, an increased mortality, and complications of pregnancy being the most notable. UTI does not by itself cause these effects. However, when UTI is combined with other conditions such as vesicoureteral reflux or obstruction, it will accelerate the damage to the kidneys, particularly in children. As far as increased mortality is concerned, which has been studied most in the elderly, it appears that UTI is a marker of ill health and other significant disease, but by itself does not cause increased mortality with or without antimicrobial therapy. In contrast, pregnant women should be screened for bacteriuria and aggressively treated because UTI during pregnancy can be associated with fetal loss, prematurity, and pyelonephritis in the mother. In renal transplant recipients, UTI is associated with allograft rejection. Treatment of asymptomatic bacteriuria is not associated with a decrease in mortality.[1,6–12]

Not surprisingly, different clinical syndromes of UTI require different patient management strategies. The purpose of this chapter is to outline the current concepts of pathogenesis, diagnosis, prevention, and treatment of this most common of human infections.

PATHOGENESIS OF URINARY TRACT INFECTION

Although bacteremia with such virulent organisms as *Staphylococcus aureus*, *Pseudomonas aeruginosa*, and *Salmonella typhi* can infect the kidneys through the hematogenous route, more than 95% of UTIs occur because of ascension of organisms from the distal urethra to the bladder, the ureters, and, finally, the kidneys. Both bacterial virulence factors and certain host factors determine whether sustained infection is to occur. Gender is a major determinant of the incidence of UTI. In males with normal urinary tract anatomy and function, the incidence of UTI is quite low, at least in part due to the physical separation of the distal urethra from the fecal reservoir of bacteria and perhaps to the presence of antibacterial substances in the secretions of the normal prostate. In men, lack of circumcision, homosexual activity that involves anal intercourse, and, uncommonly, heterosexual vaginal intercourse with a woman colonized with a uropathogen have been associated with an increased risk of UTI. However, because sustained colonization of the distal urethra in males is difficult to accomplish, bacteriuria is unusual in the absence of prostatic dysfunction or other urogenital abnormalities.[1]

Virtually all the studies of the pathogenesis of UTI have been carried out in women with *Escherichia coli* infection. However, the data that are clinically available now suggest that similar mechanisms are operative in males with UTI and also in other not uncommon bacterial causes of UTI such as *Proteus* and *Klebsiella* organisms. Therefore, it is not unreasonable to base our discussion of the pathogenesis of UTI primarily on the data generated in females with *E. coli* infection. A few clones of *E. coli*, termed uropathogenic or nephritogenic *E. coli*, possess a variety of virulence properties that appear to be important in mediating the key steps in the pathogenesis of UTI in the normal urinary tract: sustained intestinal carriage, persistence in the vagina, and ascension and invasion of the urinary tract despite normal urine output.[1,3,13]

These virulence properties are closely linked on the bacterial chromosome and are found in only a restricted number of *E. coli* serotypes (O1, O2, O4, O6, O7, O75, and O150 cause the majority of UTIs). The virulence properties of *E. coli* include the following: an intact O (somatic) antigen, a K (capsular) antigen, the production of hemolysin, the presence of the iron-binding protein aerobactin, the ability to resist the bactericidal effect of normal human serum, the production of colicin V, increased adherence to vaginal and uroepithelial cells, the production of both cytotoxic necrotizing factor type 1 and hemolysin, and the ability to induce an inflammatory response. Genes mediating these urovirulence factors are usually linked to large multigene chromosomal segments called pathogenicity islands and are absent in *E. coli* found in normal fecal flora.[14–20] The most important of these bacterial virulence factors are adhesins present on the surfaces of the uropathogenic strains that mediate attachment and adherence via specific receptors on the uroepithelium. Although a variety of bacterial adhesin-host receptor systems have been defined, the best studied (and probably most important) surface adhesins are the p-fimbriae (also known as p-pili, or type II pili), which bind to the globoseries of glycolipid receptors that have a common disaccharide $\alpha Gal(1-4)\beta Gal$. These receptors are identical to the glycosphingolipids of the P blood group system and are found on the epithelial cells of the vagina, urinary tract, kidneys, and large intestine, but not on phagocytic cells.[21–27]

Uropathogenic strains are able to attach to the host mucosal cells (thus effecting sustained carriage in the large intestine and adherence to the vaginal and uroepithelium) while avoiding binding to host polymorphonuclear cells.[21,28–30] Type I fimbriae bind to mannose epitopes, for example, those found on such glycoproteins as secretory IgA and Tamm-Horsfall protein, and are thought to play a role in urovirulence in the presence of other virulence factors. In addition, there are uropathogenic strains that adhere in the absence of fimbriae.[31–34]

Recently, a single clone of uropathogenic *E. coli* has been identified as the cause of a large number of UTIs in individual communities. Isolates of these bacteria were identified initially by being trimethoprim-sulfamethoxazole resistant (generally associated with multidrug resistance). Epidemiologic studies have suggested that the source of this clonal outbreak is contaminated food or water. Prolonged colonization of the intestine is the first step in the pathogenesis of these infections, and it is possible that long-term intestinal carriage provides the opportunity for acquiring plasmids that mediate drug resistance. That this is an important phenomenon is shown by the fact that this single clone accounted for 10% of all UTIs in California, Minnesota, and Michigan and for 38% to 51% of trimethoprim-sulfamethoxazole–resistant strains. Similar clusters of cases have occurred in south London, UK, and St. Louis, MO, and this clone has also been shown to be endemic in Barcelona, Spain. This clone (termed clone A) has played a significant role in the spread of antimicrobial resistance. A hitherto unusual stereotype to be isolated from the urinary tract, O15:K52:H1, is characteristic of this phenomenon. The epidemiologic pattern of this particular clone is very reminis-

cent of that seen when hemorrhagic enterocolitis due to *E. coli* O157:H7 was identified as a community-wide outbreak owing to the ingestion of contaminated food, and it is postulated that a similar epidemiologic pattern is operational here.[35,36]

Host factors are at least as important as bacterial virulence factors in the pathogenesis of UTI. These include the following:

1. Normal vaginal flora, particularly the presence of lactobacilli, plays an important role in preventing the colonization of the vaginal vestibule with uropathogenic strains. Such colonization is a necessary, although not sufficient, first step in the pathogenesis of UTI. It is estimated that approximately 8% of patients with uropathogen colonization of the vagina develop UTI, and when it occurs, it is the same organism that is colonizing. Thus, spermicides, used with condoms or diaphragms for contraception, inhibit the normal flora, and the metabolic changes induced by menopause have a similar effect—the result being an increased propensity to recurrent UTI. Sexual intercourse will regularly introduce distal urethral and vaginal flora into the bladder. If the organisms are so introduced, they will be quickly eliminated by local host defenses, including voiding. If uropathogens are present, they will adhere, and sexual activity will have played an important role in the development of sustained UTI.

2. The normally functioning bladder has a significant capacity for eliminating bacteria that have been introduced. Three factors appear to contribute significantly to this ability: the elimination of bacteria by voiding, the presence of bacteriostatic substances in the urine, and the intrinsic mucosal defense mechanisms (including the ability to mount an inflammatory response starting when the bacteria adhere to the mucosal lining). It is worth emphasizing that these defenses are greatly attenuated when there is a significant postvoiding residual.[37–41]

3. The ability to secrete blood group antigens into body fluids, including the urine and vaginal secretions, is an important host defense against UTI. These blood group antigens appear to block the adherence of bacterial adhesions to uroepithelial receptors and thus protect against the initiation of infection. Women who are nonsecretors have an increased incidence of recurrent UTI, and uropathogens have been shown to adhere to periurethral and vaginal mucosal cells from these women in much greater numbers than do those in women who are secretors.[42–45]

4. A competent ureterovesical junction provides significant protection against the reflux of both sterile and infected urine into the kidney.[1]

Thus, there are a number of conditions that predispose to UTI and do so by overcoming the host defenses delineated. These conditions either promote the occurrence of UTI or amplify its clinical impact. A corollary of these observations is that different antimicrobial programs are necessary for the prevention and treatment of UTI in patients with one or more of the following conditions:

1. Impedance of urine flow due to anatomic obstruction (e.g., a stone or an enlarged prostate gland) or a functional inability to empty the bladder (e.g., a neurogenic bladder due to spinal cord injury or neuropathy due to diabetes or multiple sclerosis) greatly increases the susceptibility to and the impact of UTI.[1]

2. Vesicoureteral reflux predisposes to the spread of infection to the kidney, and the combination of reflux and infection appears to be synergistic in terms of producing chronic renal injury, especially in children, and most particularly in children younger than the age of 5.[1]

3. The presence of foreign bodies such as an indwelling bladder catheter markedly increases the incidence of UTI. Even with modern closed drainage systems, once such a catheter is in place, after the first 3 days of its presence, there is an incidence of bacteriuria at a rate of 1% to 3% per day, with most patients becoming bacteriuric by the end of 1 month.[1]

Notable by their absence from this analysis are immunosuppressed states. Defects in T-cell, B-cell, and polymorphonuclear leukocyte function do not appear to be associated with an increased incidence of UTI, although the impact of any infections that do occur may be increased in the face of such conditions. Similarly, there is little evidence that conditions such as diabetes mellitus are associated with an increased incidence of UTI until diabetic neuropathy affecting bladder function develops.[1]

DIAGNOSIS OF URINARY TRACT INFECTION

The range of possible symptom complexes caused by UTI is very broad, ranging from asymptomatic bacteriuria to symptomatic abacteriuria (the acute urethral syndrome), from symptoms related to the lower urinary tract (dysuria and frequency) to symptoms suggesting kidney invasion and pyelonephritis (e.g., loin pain and costovertebral angle tenderness), to full-blown septic shock. The relationship of symptoms to the presence of bacteriuria and the anatomic site of infection is incomplete. Thus, 30% of women with symptoms of dysuria and frequency will have covert kidney involvement, whereas a similar or higher percentage of men with bacterial prostatitis will also have covert kidney involvement. Because the relationship between symptoms and either the presence of true infection or the anatomic site of infection is incomplete, the laboratory plays an important role in the diagnosis and management of UTI. This is particularly true given the difficulty of acquiring a voided urine specimen that is not contaminated by distal urethral or vaginal flora. The following observations can be used in deciding whether true UTI is present and that treatment is indicated.[1,2]

In patients without bladder or ureteral catheters, more than 95% of infections are caused by a single species at any one time, with the *Enterobacteriaceae*, *P. aeruginosa*, enterococci, and *Staphylococcus saprophyticus* (this last being a particularly important uropathogen in sexually active young women) causing virtually all these infections. In contrast, the organisms that commonly colonize the distal urethra and skin of both men and women and the vagina of women (*Staphylococcus epidermidis*, diphtheroids, lactobacilli, *Gardnerella vaginalis*, and a variety of anaerobes) rarely cause UTI. The rare exception to this rule are patients with such complicating factors as an infarcted kidney or a necrotic tumor mass that has been invaded by these commensal organisms, particularly the anaerobes. Otherwise, the presence of one or more of these organisms in the urine suggests primarily a contaminated culture.[1,15]

In the adult patient who has urinary symptoms, the presence of pyuria correlates closely with UTI. The measurement of leukocyte esterase activity in the urine may be used as a screening technique, but the preferred method is to examine the unspun urine in a counting chamber, with more than 10 leukocytes/mm³ being highly associated with true infection. The traditional method of testing for pyuria, by microscopic examination of spun urine, is fraught with error, carrying a high rate of both false positives and false negatives. A similarly useful low-technology approach to the diagnosis of UTI is to examine under a light microscope a Gram stain of unspun urine. The presence of one or more organisms per oil immersion field correlates with the presence of 10^5 bacteria/mL or more in urine (otherwise known as significant bacteriuria).[1,2,46–48]

The cornerstone of the diagnostic approach to UTI is the quantitative urine culture. More than four decades ago, Kass[48] and Savage and colleagues[49] defined the concept of significant bacteriuria ($>10^5$ colony-forming units [CFU]/mL of a single uropathogenic species) as an epidemiologic tool for diagnosing true infection. However, it is now clear that, in as many as 20% to 30% of true bacterial UTIs in women with symptoms of infection, fewer organisms are present in the urine. These women respond appropriately to antibiotic therapy for the particular bacteria identified, just as those with significant bacteriuria do. The quantitative urine culture remains a useful diagnostic tool, however, but the guidelines have been revised, based on careful studies of patients who are symptomatic and respond to antimicrobial intervention.[2,50,51]

1. *Acute, uncomplicated UTI in women.* A diagnostic criterion of more than 10^5 CFU/mL has a specificity of 99%, but a sensitivity of 51%. Particularly in the symptomatic patient, a more appropriate criterion appears to be 10^3 CFU/mL or more, which has a sensitivity of approximately 80% and a specificity of approximately 90%.

2. *Acute urethral syndrome in women* (also called *symptomatic abacteriuria*). This entity is probably a variant of acute, uncomplicated UTI in that symptoms of dysuria and frequency predominate, with two major causes being noted: bacterial infection with the usual uropathogens but with fewer (10^2–10^4 CFU/mL) being present or *Chlamydia trachomatis* infection. Patients from both these groups have pyuria on urinalysis and respond to appropriate antimicrobial therapy. It has been suggested that those patients with low-count bacteriuria have early UTI, with increasing counts as time passes without therapy. Occasionally, patients with *Neisseria gonorrhoeae* infection or vaginitis will present with symptoms of dysuria and frequency, but cultures and vaginal examinations should permit these individuals to be distinguished from the others. In addition, there is a group of women with similar symptoms but who lack pyuria on urinalysis. These appear not to have a microbial basis to their symptoms, do not respond to antimicrobial therapy, and should be managed symptomatically.

3. *Acute, uncomplicated pyelonephritis in women.* Approximately 80% of patients will have more than 10^5 CFU/mL in their urine; 10% to 15% will have 10^4 to 10^5 CFU/mL in their urine; and the remainder will have fewer than 10^4 CFU/mL in their urine. Thus, 10^4 CFU/mL of a single uropathogen is the usual requirement for the laboratory diagnosis of acute, uncomplicated pyelonephritis.

4. *Urinary tract infection in men.* A diagnostic threshold of 10^4 CFU/mL or more offers sensitivity and specificity of more than 90%.

5. *Particular infections.* Infections due to *S. saprophyticus* and *Candida* species (as well as other fungal pathogens, presumably) usually have organism counts in the 10^2 to 10^4 CFU/mL range.

CLINICAL MANAGEMENT OF URINARY TRACT INFECTION

Acute, Uncomplicated Urinary Tract Infection in Women

Patients with this form of UTI are defined by their presenting symptom complex: symptoms of lower urinary tract inflammation (i.e., dysuria, frequency, urgency, or suprapubic discomfort) in the absence of signs and symptoms of vaginitis (vaginal discharge or odor, pruritus, dyspareunia, external dysuria without frequency, and vulvovaginitis on examination). Therapy for this form of UTI has three objectives: eradication of the lower UTI that is producing symptoms, identification of the minority of patients (~30%) who have silent renal infection and require more intensive therapy, and eradication of uropathogenic clones from the vaginal and gastrointestinal reservoirs that could produce rapid reinfection of the urinary tract.[52,53]

The cornerstone of therapy for this clinical syndrome in otherwise healthy women is a short course of therapy (3 days) with trimethoprim-sulfamethoxazole, trimethoprim, or a fluoroquinolone (e.g., ofloxacin, ciprofloxacin, and undoubtedly other fluoroquinolones that have not as yet been subjected to rigorous study). β-Lactams appear to be far less effective, both in terms of eliminating the bacteriuria and in clearing the uropathogens of interest from the vaginal and colonic reservoirs, thus predisposing to recurrence. The macrocrystals of nitrofurantoin have not been studied as rigorously as the other compounds, but currently available information suggests that 3 days of therapy with this compound is not as effective as the recommended compounds, but that 7 days of therapy may yield results similar to those obtained with 3 days of trimethoprim-sulfamethoxazole. Another option would appear to be single-dose fosfomycin therapy. Although, at present, the standard of care is 3 days of trimethoprim-sulfamethoxazole therapy, the specter of resistance looms. If the incidence of resistance in a particular community is more than 20%, then a fluoroquinolone would become the empiric (before sensitivity data are known) treatment of choice. Because of the importance of the fluoroquinolones in the treatment of prostatitis and other forms of complicated infection, the recently published guidelines for the management of acute, uncomplicated UTI in women has recommended the use of other drugs to delay the emergence of resistance to the fluoroquinolones.[52,53]

Because acute, uncomplicated UTI in healthy women is so common, and the efficacy, cost, and side-effects of short-course therapy so favorable, an efficient approach to such infections that minimizes laboratory studies and visits to the physician can be defined. The first step is to initiate short-course therapy in response to the complaint of dysuria and frequency without symptoms of vaginitis. If a urine specimen is readily available, a leukocyte esterase dipstick test can be carried out (which has a reported sensitivity of 75%–96% in this clinical setting); urine culture and microscopic examination of the urine are reserved for the patient with an atypical presentation. Alternatively, a reliable patient who reports a typical clinical presentation by telephone should have short-course therapy prescribed without initial examination of the urine.[1,52,53]

The important patient-physician interaction comes after completion of the therapy. If the patient is asymptomatic, nothing further needs to be done. If the patient is still symptomatic, both urinalysis and urine culture are necessary. If both of these results are negative and no clear microbial cause of symptoms is present, symptomatic relief is prescribed and attention is directed toward sexual practices, gynecologic conditions, personal hygiene, allergy to clothing dyes, and the like. If the patient is pyuric but not bacteriuric, then the differential diagnosis includes *C. trachomatis* (common in sexually active, reproductive-age individuals), tuberculosis, systemic fungal infection, and intra-abdominal inflammatory processes such as a diverticular abscess abutting the urinary tract. The presence of bacteriuria and pyuria should trigger a 10- to 14-day course of therapy, provided that the isolate was sensitive to the drug previously prescribed. If it has been resistant, then another trial of short-course therapy with a suitable drug would be appropriate.[1,52–58]

Short-course therapy is prescribed for the eradication of superficial mucosal infection of the bladder and is contraindicated in patients with a high probability of tissue-invading infection. The following groups of patients, therefore, should never be considered as candidates for short-course therapy: any man with a UTI (tissue invasion of the prostate, kidney, or both should be assumed, and, as predicted, short-course therapy fails in men more than 80% of the time, even when both groups have identical presenting symptoms), patients with overt pyelonephritis, patients with symptoms of longer than 7 days' duration, patients with underlying structural or functional defects of the urinary tract, immunosuppressed individuals, and patients with indwelling catheters.[1]

Acute, Uncomplicated Pyelonephritis in Women

The clinical syndrome in these patients includes recurrent rigors and fever; back and loin pain (with tenderness on percussion of the costovertebral angle), often with associated colicky abdominal pain; nausea and vomiting; dysuria; and frequency. These individuals, by definition, have invasive tissue infection, have or are at risk of bacteremia, and merit intensive antimicrobial therapy. The three goals of therapy in this group of individuals are control of possible urosepsis (bacteremia and its consequences), eradication of the invading organism, and prevention of recurrences. The therapeutic approach to acute, uncomplicated pyelonephritis can be divided into two parts: immediate control and final eradication of the process.[1,2]

The initial antimicrobial program prescribed should have a more than 99% probability of being effective against the infecting organism. A urine Gram stain should be part of the initial evaluation. If a gram-positive organism is responsible, then ampicillin or amoxicillin/clavulanic acid therapy would be reasonable. More likely would be a gram-negative bacillus, with a variety of regimens then being useful: a fluoroquinolone, a β-lactam/aminoglycoside combination, or an advanced-spectrum β-lactam alone (e.g., imipenem, ceftazidime, piperacillin/tazobactam) can be prescribed to achieve this goal. Although parenteral therapy is usually prescribed to ensure the prompt achievement of therapeutic blood levels, it should be recognized that, in patients with milder disease oral agents such as fluoroquinolones and trimethoprim-sulfamethoxazole with excellent antimicrobial spectrum and oral bioavailability can be employed throughout the course of treatment if the GI tract is functioning adequately. At present, provided adequate blood levels are achieved, there is no evidence that any one of the regimens listed is better than any other in terms of accomplishing the first task: initial control of systemic sepsis.[1,2,52,53]

Following the establishment of control over sepsis, usually signaled by the temperature curve returning to a near-normal level, oral therapy can be instituted. Failure of this to occur within 72 hours of initiating therapy should trigger a search for some complicating problem (e.g., a stone, obstruction from any cause, poor bladder function). Once evidence of improvement has occurred, prescription of trimethoprim-sulfamethoxazole or a fluoroquinolone to complete a 14-day course of therapy appears to be the most effective means of eradicating both tissue infection and residual clones of uropathogen present in the gastrointestinal tract, which could cause early recurrence if left in place.[1,2,52,53]

Urinary Tract Infection in Pregnancy

Pregnant women constitute the one group in whom screening for asymptomatic bacteriuria, and subsequent treatment, if found, is justified to prevent adverse consequences for both mother and fetus: a risk of symptomatic pyelonephritis later in pregnancy that can induce premature onset of labor and delivery. Some experts have attributed increased fetal loss and prematurity to UTI in the mother as well. Treatment of either asymptomatic infection or infection associated with symptoms of bladder inflammation is similar to that for nonpregnant women with acute, uncomplicated UTI, that is, short-course therapy. However, there are two major differences in the overall management when compared with the management of nonpregnant women with UTIs: (1) The drugs that can be used safely are somewhat limited because of toxicity issues and (2) continuing follow-up throughout pregnancy with treatment and prophylaxis instituted for positive cultures is indicated.[59]

There is extensive experience with sulfonamides, nitrofurantoin, ampicillin, and cephalexin in the treatment of UTI during pregnancy, with sulfonamides being avoided near term because of their possible contribution to the development of kernicterus in the newborn. Fluoroquinolones are avoided because of possible adverse effects on fetal cartilage development. In pregnant women with overt pyelonephritis, hospital admission and parenteral therapy with β-lactam drugs and aminoglycosides should be considered the standard of care.[1]

Recurrent Urinary Tract Infection in Women

The majority of recurrent UTIs in women of all ages are due to reinfection. The first steps in preventing such infections do not involve the use of antimicrobial agents. They do include voiding immediately after sexual intercourse and changing contraceptive practice to one in which a spermicide (which eliminates

the normal protective flora in the vagina, increasing the potential for colonization with a uropathogen) is not required (e.g., from a diaphragm to oral contraceptives).[1,37–40] In postmenopausal women, two further measures have been shown to be of value: (1) local or systemic estrogen replacement, which will change the pH of the vagina, promotes the reappearance of the normal flora (particularly the lactobacilli) and protects against colonization with uropathogens[60] and (2) ingestion of moderate amounts of cranberry or blueberry juice, which has been shown to have a marked protective effect against UTI owing to the secretion in the urine and the vagina of organic molecules that block the critical interaction of uropathogen surface adhesions to epithelial receptors, the first step in the invasion of the anatomically normal urinary tract.[61–63] Although the data supporting the use of cranberry juice have come primarily from studies of postmenopausal women, our anecdotal experience with reproductive-age women suggests efficacy in this population as well.

Despite the institution of the previously listed maneuvers, there remains a group of otherwise healthy women who are subject to recurrent symptomatic infection. A small minority of these will have recurrent infection owing to a sequestered focus within the kidney that causes relapsing infection after courses of therapy of 14 days or less. Such relapsing infections deserve at least one attempt at cure with an extended course (4–6 weeks) of therapy, preferably with trimethoprim-sulfamethoxazole or a fluoroquinolone to which the infecting organism is susceptible. If some predisposing factor such as a renal calculus is present, the intensive antimicrobial therapy should be carried out in conjunction with correction of the underlying abnormality. Patients with relapsing symptomatic infection that only derives temporary benefit from extended treatment courses usually can be kept symptom free with long-term suppressive therapy.[1]

The majority of women (at least 85%) with recurrent UTI have repeated reinfection. There are basically three antimicrobial strategies that are effective in this situation:

1. Low-dose, long-term prophylaxis with either trimethoprim-sulfamethoxazole or a fluoroquinolone (e.g., ciprofloxacin 250 mg or ofloxacin 200 mg) at bedtime. The efficacy of these prophylactic regimens is further delineated by their effectiveness in preventing UTI in the more challenging population of kidney transplant recipients.
2. A variant of continuous prophylaxis is for the woman to take a single dose of a fluoroquinolone or trimethoprim-sulfamethoxazole as postcoital prophylaxis.
3. Finally, many of these women prefer not to take antimicrobial drugs so continuously. These women may be given a supply of drug (again, either a fluoroquinolone or trimethoprim-sulfamethoxazole is preferable over other classes of drug in terms of efficacy) for single-dose therapy with the onset of symptoms of UTI.[1,54,64–67]

Urinary Tract Infection in Men

UTI in men should always be assumed to mean tissue invasion of the prostate, kidney, or both. Thus, the standard of care is 10 to 14 days of fluoroquinolone or trimethoprim-sulfamethoxazole unless antimicrobial intolerance or an unusual pathogen requires an alternative approach. In men younger than 50 years, the following conditions are associated with an increased risk of UTI: anal intercourse, intercourse with women colonized with uropathogens, and acquired immunodeficiency syndrome with a CD4 lymphocyte count of less than 200/mm³. Men without one of these risk factors, particularly those with recurrent infection after an appropriate treatment course, merit a urologic evaluation as well as a more intensive treatment course: 4 to 6 weeks at a minimum. Recurrent infection in men usually suggests a sustained focus within the prostate that is difficult to eradicate for one or more of the following reasons: many antimicrobial agents do not diffuse well across the prostatic epithelium into the prostatic fluid where the infection lies, the prostate may harbor calculi that can block drainage of portions of the prostate gland or act as foreign bodies around which persistent infection can be hidden, and an enlarged (and inflamed) prostate gland can cause bladder outlet obstruction, resulting in incomplete emptying and difficulty in eradicating infection.[1,2,13,68,69]

Complicated Urinary Tract Infection

The term complicated UTI is used to describe a heterogeneous group of patients who have a wide variety of underlying structural and functional defects of the urinary tract. As a consequence, the range of organisms causing UTI is much greater than that for the general population, and antimicrobial resistance is common. As a result, the therapeutic principles employed in this patient population are somewhat different from those for other patient groups. In general, asymptomatic bacteriuria should not be treated, the major exception being when the bacteriuric patient is scheduled to undergo urinary tract manipulation; in this circumstance, sterilization of the urine before manipulation and continuation of antimicrobial therapy for 3 to 7 days after manipulation can prevent urosepsis.[1,2]

Acutely septic patients with complicated UTI merit initial broad-spectrum therapy (e.g., ampicillin plus gentamicin, imipenem/cilastin, piperacillin/tazobactam) until bacteriologic data are available and permit a more precise choice of therapy. For more subacutely ill individuals, a fluoroquinolone appears to be optimal initial therapy. In conjunction with antimicrobial therapy, thought should be given to correcting the abnormalities that led to the infection, whenever possible. If this can be accomplished, a prolonged 4- to 6-week curative course of therapy in conjunction with the surgical manipulation is appropriate. If such correction is not possible, shorter courses of therapy (7–14 days), aimed at controlling the symptoms, appear to be more reasonable. Spinal cord injury patients represent a particular challenge. In these patients, intermittent self-catheterization with clean catheters and methenamine prophylaxis has been shown to decrease the morbidity associated with UTI in this population.[1,2,13,70]

Candidal Infection of the Urinary Tract

Candidal UTI has become increasingly common in recent years, particularly in individuals who are diabetic, have bladder catheters in place, or are receiving corticosteroids. Well-validated guidelines for managing candidal UTI are not available, particularly criteria for distinguishing trivial colonization from clinically significant infection. The following represents the approach that we take at present, pending the availability of more data.[1,2,71,72]

1. The first step is the correction of the underlying conditions that led to the infection in the first place: removal of the catheter, correction of the hyperglycemia, cessation of broad-spectrum antibacterial therapy, and marked reduction in corticosteroid dose, if possible. Once these are accomplished, if candiduria is persistent, then further therapy can be considered.
2. If an indwelling bladder catheter is still required, it is reasonable to insert a three-way catheter and administer an amphotericin or a nystatin rinse to the bladder; this has an efficacy rate of approximately 50% to 60%. However, if a catheter is not required, it is far better to treat with systemic antifungal therapy to avoid the risk of other organisms being introduced because of the catheter.
3. Fluconazole, at a dose of 200 to 400 mg/day, is an effective therapy for candidal UTI caused by *Candida albicans*, *Candida tropicalis*, and most of the other candidal species, because of the extremely high concentrations that are delivered into the urine. The two organisms associated with fluconazole failure are *Candida krusei* and *Candida glabrata*.
4. In individuals who do not respond to fluconazole, the combination of low-dose systemic amphotericin (e.g., 10 mg/day) plus flucytosine at full doses (100 mg/kg/day in three or four divided doses) is quite effective when prescribed for a 10- to 14-day course. Flucytosine administered alone results in the rapid emergence of resistance, so the role of the low-dose amphotericin (which penetrates the urine poorly) is primarily to protect the flucytosine, which reaches quite high concentrations in the urine.

SUMMARY

Improved understanding of the pathogenesis and impact of UTI has led to improved therapy. Perhaps the most important lessons of the past few decades are the following:

1. The normal vaginal flora in women is an important host defense against the occurrence of UTI, and strategies to reconstitute it (e.g., elimination of spermicides in premenopausal women and estrogen replacement in postmenopausal women) can be quite effective in preventing recurrent UTI.
2. The critical first step in the pathogenesis of UTI is adherence to the uroepithelium through the specific interaction of bacterial surface adhesions to specific receptors on the epithelial cell, and strategies such as the ingestion of cranberry juice (which delivers organic substances to the site that block such adhesions) can help prevent UTI.
3. Different clinical syndromes associated with UTI require different modes of antimicrobial prescription, although the optimal drugs for the treatment and prevention of UTI are trimethoprim-sulfamethoxazole and the fluoroquinolones.
4. In this regard, tissue-invasive infection (as all UTI in men should be assumed to be) needs more extended therapy than acute, uncomplicated UTI in women, for which the cornerstone of treatment is short-course therapy (3 days).

References

1. Rubin RH, Cotran RS, Tolkoff-Rubin NA: Urinary tract infection, pyelonephritis, and reflux nephropathy. In Brenner BM (ed): Brenner & Rector's The Kidney, 8th ed. Philadelphia: WB Saunders, 2007.

2. Hooten TM, Stamm WE: Diagnosis and treatment of uncomplicated urinary tract infection Infect. Dis Clin North Am 1997;11:551–581.

3. Hooton TM, Scholes D, Hughes JP, et al: A prospective study of risk factors for symptomatic urinary tract infection in young women. N Engl J Med 1996;335:468–474.

4. Zinner SH: Management of urinary tract infections in pregnancy: A review with comments on single dose therapy. Infection 1992;20 (Suppl 4):S280–S285.

5. Banhidy F, Achs N, Puho EH, Czeizel AE: Pregnancy complications and birth outcomes of pregnant women with infections and related drug treatments. Scand J Infect Dis 2007;39:390–397.

6. Hazhir H: Asymptomatic bacteriuria in pregnant women. Urol J 2007;4:24–27.

7. Hooton TM, Scholes D, Stapleton AE, et al: A prospective study of asymptomatic bacteriuria in sexually active young women. N Engl J Med 2000;343:992–997.

8. Nicolle LE, Bradley S, Colgan R, et al: Infectious Diseases Society of America guidelines for the diagnosis and treatment of asymptomatic bacteriuria in adults. Clin Infect Dis 2005;40: 643–654.

9. Garin EH, Olavarria F, Garcia Nieto V, et al: Clinical significance of primary vesicoureteral reflux and urinary prophylaxis after acute pyelonephritis. Pediatrics 2006;117:626–632.

10. Blumenthal I: Vesicoureteric reflux and urinary tract infection in children. Postgrad Med J 2006;82:31–35.

11. Valera B, Gentil MA, Cabello V, et al: Epidemiology of urinary infections in renal transplant recipients. Transplant Proc 2006; 38:2414–2415.

12. Rice JC, Peng T, Kuo YF, et al: Renal allograft injury is associated with urinary tract infection due to Escherichia coli bearing adherence factors. Am J Transplant 2006;6:2375–2383.

13. Roberts JA: Etiology and pathogenesis of pyelonephritis. Am J Kidney Dis 1991;17:1–9.

14. Sabate M, Moreno E, Perezt T, et al: Pathogenicity island markers in commensal and uropathogenic isolates. Clin Microbiol Infect 2006;12;880–886.

15. Fischer H, Yamamoto M, Akira S, et al: Mechanism of pathogen-specific TLRA activation in mucosal recognition receptors and adaptor protein selection. Eur J Immunol 2006;36:267–277.

16. Chassin C, Goucon JM, Darche S, et al: Renal collecting duct epithelial cells react to pyelonephritis-associated E. coli by activating distinct TLR4-dependent and independent pathways. J Immunol 2006;177:4773–4774.

17. Engel D, Dobrindt D, Tittel A, et al: Tumor necrosis factor alpha- and inducible nitric oxide synthase cells are rapidly recruited to the bladder in urinary tract infection dispensable for bacterial clearance. Infect Immun 2006;74:6100–6107.

18. Chowdhury P, Sacks SH, Sheerin NS: Toll-like receptors TLR2 and TLR4 initiate the innate immune response of the tubular epithelium to bacterial products. Clin Exp Immunol 2006;145: 346–356.

19. Davis JM, Carvalho HM, Rasmussen SB, O'Brien AD: Cytotoxic necrotizing factor type 1 delivered by outer membranes of uropathogenic Escherichia coli attenuates polymorphonuclear leukocyte antimicrobial activity and chemotaxis. Infect Immun 2006;74:4401–4408.

20. Schroppel B, He JC: Expression of Toll-like receptors in the kidney. Their potential role in fighting infection. Kidney Int 2006;69: 815–822.

21. Svanborg C, Bergsten G, Fischer H, et al: Uropathogenic Escherichia coli as a model of host-parasite interaction. Curr Opin Microbiol 2006;9:33–39.

22. Svensson M, Platt FM, Svanborg C: Glycolipid receptor depletion as an approach to specific antimicrobial action. FEMS Microbiol Lett 2006;258:1–8.

23. Iwahi T, Abe Y, Nakao M, et al: Role of type 1 fimbriae in the pathogenesis of ascending urinary tract infection induced by Escherichia coli in mice. Infect Immunol 1983;40:265–315.

24. Hagberg L, Hull S, Hull R, et al: Contribution of adhesin to bacterial persistence in the mouse urinary tract. Infect Immun 1983;40:265–272.

25. Svanborg-Eden C, Eriksson B, Hanson LA: Adhesion of Escherichia coli to human uroepithelial cells in vitro. Infect Immun 1977;18:767–774.

26. Kallenius G, Molby R, Svensson SB, et al: Occurrence of P-fimbriated Escherichia coli in urinary tract infections. Lancet 1981;2:1369–1372.

27. Leffler H, Svanborg-Eden C: Glycolipid receptors for uropathogenic Escherichia coli binding to human erythrocytes and uroepithelial cells. Infect Immun 1981;34:920–929.

28. Johnson JR: Virulence factors in Escherichia coli urinary tract infection. Clin Microbiol Rev 1991;4:80–128.

29. Agace W, Hedges S, Andersson U, et al: Selective cytokine production by epithelial cells following exposure to Escherichia coli. Infect Immun 1993;61:602–609.

30. Hedges S, Agace W, Svanborg C: Epithelial cytokine responses and mucosal cytokine networks. Trends Microbiol 1995;3:266–270.

31. Pere A, Nowicki B, Saxen H, et al: Expression of P_1 type-1 and type 1_c fimbriae of Escherichia coli in the urine of patients with acute urinary tract infection. J Infect Dis 1987; 156:567–574.

32. Nowicki B, Labigne A, Moseley S, et al: The Dr hemagglutinin, afimbrial adhesins AFA-1 and AFA-III, and F1845 fimbriae of uropathogenic and diarrhea-associated Escherichia coli belong to a family of hemagglutinins with Dr receptor recognition. Infect Immun 1990;58:279–281.

33. Goluszka P, Popov V, Selvarangan R: Dr Fimbriae operon of uropathogenic Escherichia coli mediate microtubule dependent invasion to the HeLa epithelial cell line. J Infect Dis 1997;176: 158–167.

34. Zafriri D, Gron Y, Eisenstein BI, et al: Growth advantages and enhanced toxicity of Escherichia coli adherent to tissue culture cells due to restricted diffusion of products secreted by the cells. J Clin Invest 1987;79:1210–1216.

35. Manges AR, Johnson JR, Foxman B, et al: Widespread distribution of urinary tract infection caused by a multidrug-resistant Escherichia coli clonal group. N Engl J Med 2001;345: 1007–1013.

36. Stamm WE: An epidemic of urinary tract infections? N Engl J Med 2001;345:1055–1057.

37. Hooton TM, Hillier S, Johnson C, et al: Escherichia coli bacteriuria and contraceptive method. JAMA 1991;265:64–69.

38. Strom BL, Collins M, West SL, et al: Sexual activity, contraceptive use, and other risk factors for systematic and asymptomatic bacteriuria: A case-control study. Ann Intern Med 1987;107: 816–823.

39. Fihn SD, Latham RH, Roberts P, et al: Association between diaphragm use and urinary tract infection. JAMA 1985;254: 240–245.

40. Stamm WE, Hooton TM: Management of urinary tract infections in adults. N Engl J Med 1993;329:1328–1334.

41. Raz R, Stamm WE: A controlled trial of intravaginal estriol in postmenopausal women with recurrent urinary tract infections. N Engl J Med 1993;329:753–756.

42. Sheinfeld J, Schaeffer AJ, Cordon-Cardo C, et al: Association of the Lewis blood group phenotype with recurrent urinary tract infections in women. N Engl J Med 1989;320:773–777.

43. Jantausch BA, Criss VR, O'Donnell R, et al: Association of Lewis blood group phenotypes with urinary tract infection in children. J Pediatr 1994;124:863–868.

44. Navas EL, Venegas MF, Duncan JL, et al: Blood group antigen expression on vaginal cells and mucus in women with and without a history of urinary tract infections. J Urol 1994;152:345–349.

45. Hooton TM, Scholes D, Hughes JP, et al: A prospective of risk factors for symptomatic urinary tract infections in young women. N Engl J Med 1996;335:468–474.

46. Pollack HM: Laboratory techniques for detection of urinary tract infection and assessment of value. Am J Med 1983;75:79–84.

47. Stamm WE: Measurement of pyuria and its relation to bacteriuria. Am J Med 1983;75:53–58.

48. Kass EH: Bacteriuria and the diagnosis of infections of the urinary tract: With observations on the use of methionine as a urinary antiseptic. Arch Intern Med 1957;100:709–714.

49. Savage WE, Hajj SN, Kass EH: Demographic and prognostic characteristics of bacteriuria in pregnancy. Medicine (Baltimore) 1967;46:385–407.

50. Stamm WE, Wagner KF, Amsel R, et al: Causes of the acute urethral syndrome in women. N Engl J Med 1980;303:409–415.

51. Stamm WE, Counts GW, Running KR, et al: Diagnosis of coliform infection in acutely dysuric women. N Engl J Med 1982;307:463–468.

52. Warren JW, Abrutyn E, Hebel JR, et al: Guidelines for antimicrobial treatment of uncomplicated acute bacterial cystitis and acute pyelonephritis in women. Clin Infect Dis 1999;29:745–758.

53. Saint S, Scholes D, Fihn SD, et al: The effectiveness of a clinical practice guideline for the management of pressured uncomplicated urinary tract infection in women. Am J Med 1999;106:636–641.

54. Stamm WE, Hooton TM: Management of urinary tract infections in adults. N Engl J Med 1993;329:1328–1334.

55. Johnson JR, Stamm WE: Urinary tract infections in women: Diagnosis and treatment. Ann Intern Med 1989;111:906–917.

56. Inter-Nordic Urinary Tract Infection Study Group: Double-blind comparison of 3-day versus 7-day treatment with norfloxacin in symptomatic urinary tract infections. Scand J Infect Dis 1988;20:619.

57. Hooton TM, Johnson C, Winter C, et al: Single dose and three day regimens of ofloxacin versus trimethoprim-sulfamethoxazole for acute cystitis in women. Antimicrob Agents Chemother 1991;35:1479–1483.

58. Norrby SR: Short term treatment of uncomplicated lower urinary tract infection in women. Rev Infect Dis 1990;12:458–467.

59. Zinner SH: Management of urinary tract infections in pregnancy: A review with comments on single dose therapy. Infection 1992;20(Suppl 4):S280–S285.

60. Raz R, Stamm WE: A controlled trial of intravaginal estriol in postmenopausal women with recurrent urinary tract infections. N Engl J Med 1993;329:753–756.

61. Avorn J, Monane M, Gurwitz JH, et al: Reduction of bacteriuria and pyuria after ingestion of cranberry juice. JAMA 1994;271:751–754.

62. Zafriri D, Ofek I, Adar R, et al: Inhibitory activity of cranberry juice on adherence of type 1 and P fimbriated *Escherichia coli* to eukaryotic cells. Antimicrob Agents Chemother 1989;33:92–98.

63. Ofek I, Goldhar J, Zafriri D, et al: Anti-*Escherichia* adhesin activity of cranberry and blueberry juices. N Engl J Med 1991;324:1599.

64. Ronald AR, Harding GKM: Urinary infection prophylaxis in women. Ann Intern Med 1981;9:268–270.

65. Harding GKM, Buckwald FJ, Marrie TJ, et al: Prophylaxis of recurrent urinary tract infection in female patients: Efficacy of low dose, thrice weekly therapy with trimethoprim-sulfamethoxazole. JAMA 1979;242:1975–1977.

66. Stapleton A, Latham RH, Johnson C, Stamm WE: Postcoital antimicrobial prophylaxis for recurrent urinary tract infection: A randomized, double-blind, placebo-controlled trial. JAMA 1990;264:703–706.

67. Wong ES, McKevitt M, Running K, et al: Management of recurrent urinary tract infections with patient-administered single dose therapy. Ann Intern Med 1985;102:302–307.

68. Wong ES, Stamm WE: Sexual acquisition of urinary tract infection in a man. JAMA 1983;250:3087–3088.

69. Hoepelman AI, van Buren M, van den Broek J, Borleffs JC: Bacteriuria in men infected with HIV-1 is related to their immune status (CD4+ cell count). AIDS 1992;6:179–184.

70. Abrutyn E, Mossey J, Berlin JA, et al: Does asymptomatic bacteriuria predict mortality and does antimicrobial treatment reduce mortality in elderly ambulatory women? Ann Intern Med 1994;120:827–833.

71. Jacobs LG, Skidmore EA, Cardoso LA, Ziv F: Bladder irrigation with amphotericin B for treatment of fungal urinary tract infections. Clin Infect Dis 1994;18:313–318.

72. Hibberd PH, Rubin RH: Clinical aspects of fungal infection in organ transplant recipients. Clin Infect Dis 1994;19(Suppl 1):S33–S40.

Further Reading

Hooton TM, Samadpour M: Is acute uncomplicated urinary tract infection a foodborne illness and are animals the source? Clin Infect Dis 2005;40:258–259.

Manges AR, Dietrich PS, Riley LW: Multi-drug resistant *Escherichia coli* clonal groups in causing community-acquired pyelonephritis. Clin Infect Dis 2004;38:329–334.

Manges AR, Johnson JR, Foxman B, O'Bryan TT: Widespread distribution of urinary tract infection caused by a multidrug resistant Escherichia coli clonal group. N Engl J Med 2001;345:1007–1013.

Raz R, Chazan B, Dan M: Cranberry juice and urinary tract infection. Clin Infect Dis 2004;38:1413–1419.

Stamm WE: Estrogens and urinary tract infection. J Infect Dis 2007;195:623–624.

Chapter 38

Primary Neoplasms of the Kidney

Marc B. Garnick

Carcinoma of the kidney is perhaps one of the most enigmatic of cancers. The myriad presenting features, which include paraneoplastic phenomena, can challenge the most astute diagnostician.[1–3] The disease is typically diagnosed during the sixth and seventh decades with a male-to-female ratio of 2:1. It is estimated that there will be 39,000 newly diagnosed cases with an estimated 13,000 deaths in 2007.[4,5] Today, many renal cancers can be diagnosed at early, and potentially curable, stages owing to the more widespread use of ultrasonography and computed tomography (CT) of the abdomen, which may pick up early asymptomatic lesions of the kidney. Most malignant cancers of the kidney are adenocarcinomas; other pathologic varieties include transitional carcinomas of the renal pelvis and Wilms' tumor in children.[6]

RISK FACTORS

Risk factors for the development of renal cancer include cigarette smoking, occupational exposure to cadmium, obesity, excessive exposure to analgesics, acquired cystic disease in dialysis patients, adult polycystic kidney disease, and other industrial exposures, such as asbestos, leather tanning, and certain petroleum products. Genetic and familial forms of the disease occur, most notably with von Hippel-Lindau disease, an autosomal dominant disease characterized by the development of multiple tumors of the central nervous system, pheochromocytomas, and bilateral renal carcinomas.[7] Several families have also been reported with a high incidence of renal cancer. Genetic analyses of these patients demonstrate a balanced translocation between the short arm of chromosome 3 and either chromosome 6 or chromosome 8. Tuberous sclerosis may also be associated with a risk of developing renal cell cancer, but this risk is considerably less than that of von Hippel-Lindau disease. Other abnormalities have been reported.[8]

More recent genetic advances have identified the *RASSF1* gene, a Ras association family 1 gene, which may possess tumor-suppressor activity. In one study, abnormalities of this gene were identified in a high percentage of patients with primary clear-cell cancers.[9]

PRESENTATION

Patients with renal cell cancer present with symptoms produced by the local neoplasm, with signs and symptoms of paraneoplastic phenomena, or by other aspects of systemic disease. Likewise, the patient may be totally asymptomatic and, as is quite common today, may be diagnosed by a radiographic abnormality detected on ultrasound or abdominal CT scanning. Less than 10% of patients present with the classic triad of hematuria, abdominal mass, and flank pain. In the patient who presents with signs or symptoms (as opposed to the diagnosis secondary to the asymptomatic finding radiographically), most common features include hematuria (70%), flank pain (50%), palpable mass (20%), fever (15%), and erythrocytosis (infrequent). Other features may include acute onset of lower extremity edema, or, in males, the presence of a left-sided varicocele, indicating an obstruction of the left gonadal vein at its point of entry into the left renal vein by a tumor thrombus. Other paraneoplastic/systemic manifestations include liver function abnormalities, high-output congestive failure, cachexia, fever, amyloidosis, anemia erythrocytosis, thrombocytosis, hypercalcemia, and manifestations of the secretion of substances such as prostaglandins, renin, glucocorticoids, and cytokines such as interleukin-6.

At presentation, a very small percentage of tumors are bilateral, whereas less than one third of patients have demonstrable metastatic disease in almost any organ of the body. The most common sites of metastases include the lung, bone, liver, and brain, but other sites such as the thyroid may be affected.

PATHOLOGY

In the past, renal carcinomas were divided pathologically into a classification that evaluated cell type and growth pattern. The former included clear-cell, spindle, and oncocytic types, whereas the latter included acinar, papillary, or sarcomatoid varieties. This classification has undergone a transformation to more accurately reflect the morphology and the histochemical and molecular bases of different types of adenocarcinomas.[10,11] Based on these studies, five distinct carcinoma types have been identified, including clear-cell (75%–85% of tumors), chromophilic (15%), chromophobic (5%), oncocytic (uncommon), and collecting (Bellini's) duct (very rare) varieties. Each of these carcinoma types has a unique growth pattern, cell of origin, and cytogenetic characteristics. Table 38-1 summarizes this information and more accurately reflects the increased knowledge on molecular and genetic abnormalities of these lesions.

DIAGNOSTIC EVALUATION AND STAGING

Evidence from the history or physical examination that suggests a renal abnormality should be followed by either an abdominal ultrasound or abdominal CT scan. In the past, intravenous pyelography was commonly used, but this procedure has largely been replaced. There are emerging data using abdominal magnetic resonance imaging. Often, however, evidence of a space-occupying lesion in the kidney is found incidentally during radiographic testing for other unrelated conditions for which an ultrasound or abdominal CT scan is performed. Indeed, renal cancer, once dubbed the "internist's tumor" because of its multiple manifestations at presentation, can now be called the "radiologist's tumor" because many lesions are detected during radiographic evaluations.

Renal ultrasonography may help to distinguish simple cysts from more complex abnormalities. A simple cyst is defined sonographically by a lack of internal echoes, the presence of smooth borders, and the transmission of the ultrasound wave. If these three features exist, a benign cyst is most likely to be present. At one time, cyst puncture was used but seems to be unnecessary today in the asymptomatic patient without hematuria. Periodic repeat ultrasound scans are suggested for follow-up. If a change occurs in the lesion, cyst puncture, needle aspiration, or CT should be considered to further evaluate the lesion.

If the criteria for a simple sonographic cyst are not met or the ultrasound scan suggests a solid or complex mass, a CT scan should be performed. If a renal neoplasm is demonstrated by CT scan, renal vein or caval involvement should be assessed by CT or by magnetic resonance imaging. Although used frequently in the past, selective renal arteriography has assumed a more limited use, mainly in further evaluating the renal vasculature in patients who are to undergo partial nephrectomy (nephron-sparing surgery). CT is also very helpful in determining the presence of lymphadenopathy. Figure 38-1 illustrates a modern-day algorithm for the diagnostic evaluation of a renal mass.

The differential diagnosis of a renal mass detected on a CT scan includes primary renal cancers, metastatic lesions to the kidney, and benign lesions. The latter two groups include angiomyolipomas (renal hamartomas), oncocytomas, and other rare unusual growths. If a renal cancer is considered based on the radiographic studies of the kidney, the patient should undergo a preoperative staging evaluation to assess the presence of metastases in the lung, bone, or brain. The operative and diagnostic approaches may be dictated dependent on the preoperative stage of the patient. For example, the patient who presents with stage IV disease by virtue of a positive bone scan may need only a needle biopsy of either the kidney lesion or the bone lesion to establish the tissue diagnosis and thus avoid more extensive surgery on the kidney. In contrast, a patient with an isolated pulmonary lesion may be considered for both a nephrectomy and a pulmonary nodulectomy in one operative intervention.

Table 38-1   Pathologic Classification of Renal Cell Carcinoma

| Carcinoma Type | Growth Pattern | Cell of Origin | CYTOGENETIC CHARACTERISTICS | | Incidence (%) |
			Major	Minor	
Clear cell	Acinar or sarcomatoid	Proximal tubule	3p−	+5, +7, +12, −6q, −8p, −9, −14q, −Y	75–85
Chromophilic*	Papillary or sarcomatoid	Proximal tubule	+7, +17, −Y	+12, +16, +20, −14	12–14
Chromophobic	Solid, tubular, or sarcomatoid	Intercalated cell of cortical collecting duct†	Hypodiploid	—	4–6
Oncocytic	Typified by tumor nests	Intercalated cell of cortical collecting duct	Undetermined	—	2–4
Collecting duct	Papillary or sarcomatoid	Medullary collecting duct	Undetermined	—	1

*These tumors were previously classified as papillary tumors.
†This classification is based on the work of Storkel and associates.[10]
From Motzer RJ, Bander NH, Nanus DM: Renal-cell carcinoma. N Engl J Med 1996;335:865–875. Copyright 1996 Massachusetts Medical Society. All rights reserved.

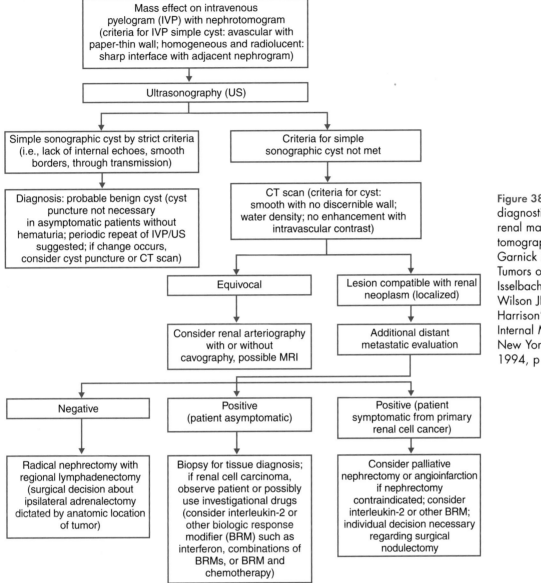

Figure 38-1 Algorithm for the diagnostic evaluation of a renal mass. CT, computed tomography. (Modified from Garnick MB, Brenner BM: Tumors of the urinary tract. In Isselbacher KJ, Braumwald E, Wilson JD, et al [eds]: Harrison's Principles of Internal Medicine, 13th ed. New York: McGraw-Hill, 1994, p 1337.)

Renal cell cancer can be staged using one of two systems that are in common use.[6] The TNM (tumor, nodes, metastasis) system has the advantage of being more specific but has the disadvantage of being cumbersome; a modification of the Robson staging system is more practical and more widely used in the United States. In this latter system, stage I represents cancer that is confined to the kidney capsule, stage II indicates invasion through the renal capsule but not beyond Gerota's fascia, stage III reflects involvement of regional lymph nodes and the ipsilateral renal vein or the vena cava, and stage IV indicates the presence of distant metastases. In the sixth edition of the AJCC Cancer Staging Manual, the American Joint Committee on Cancer subdivides stage T1 into T1a, tumors as 4 cm or less; and T1b, tumors greater than 4 cm but less than 7 cm and all tumor limited to the kidney. Table 38-2 illustrates both systems. Other, newer staging systems used by the Eastern Cooperative Oncology Group have integrated the TNM classification with other variables such as performance status and histologic grade of the tumor. These systems provide prognostic categories and more accurately predict 2- and 5-year survival rates.[12,13]

CLINICAL TRIALS AND SPECIFIC RECOMMENDATIONS

The standard therapy for localized renal cell carcinoma is radical nephrectomy, which includes removal of the kidney, Gerota's fascia, the ipsilateral adrenal gland, and regional hilar lymph nodes. The value of an extended hilar lymphadenectomy seems to be related to its ability to provide prognostic information because there is rarely a therapeutic reason for performing this portion of the operation. In the past, the removal of the ipsilateral adrenal gland was performed routinely; however, most data suggest that it is involved in less than 5% of cases and occurs most frequently with large upper pole lesions.[14] Therefore, ipsilateral adrenalectomy is reserved for patients with glands that appear to be abnormal or enlarged on the CT scan or for those patients with large upper pole renal lesions in whom the probability of direct extension of the tumor to the adrenal gland is more likely.

The surgical technique of performing a partial nephrectomy (nephron-sparing surgery) has become more popular,

Table 38-2 Comparison of Modified Robson and TNM Staging Systems for Renal Adenocarcinoma

Modified Robson Stage		T	N	M
I	Confined by renal capsule	T1 (small) T2 (large)	N0	M0
II	Through renal capsule confined by Gerota's fascia	T3a	N0	M0
IIIa	Renal vein involvement	T3b	N0	M0
IIIb	Lymphatic involvement	T1–3b	N1–4	M0
IV	Contiguous organ involvement or	T1–3b	N0–4	M0
	Metastatic spread	T1–3b	N0–4	M1

TNM, tumor, node, metastasis.
From McDougal WS, Garnick MB: Clinical signs and symptoms of kidney cancer. In Vogelzang NJ, Scardino PT, Shipley WU, et al (eds): Comprehensive Textbook of Genitourinary Oncology. Baltimore: Williams & Wilkins, 1996, p 546.

especially for patients with small tumors, for those at risk of developing bilateral tumors, or for patients in whom the contralateral kidney is at risk of other systemic diseases such as diabetes or hypertension.[15,16] The main concern associated with partial nephrectomy is the likelihood of tumor recurrence in the operated kidney because many renal cancers may be multicentric. Local recurrence rates of 4% to 10% have been reported, and even lower rates have been reported when a partial nephrectomy was performed for smaller lesions (<3 cm with a normal contralateral kidney). Lesions that are centrally located, however, still require a radical nephrectomy. Frequent follow-up, usually with CT or ultrasonography, is necessary for patients who undergo a partial nephrectomy.

Renal cancer involving the inferior vena cava occurs more frequently with right-sided tumors and is associated with metastases in almost 50% of patients. Obstruction of the vena cava may lead to the diagnosis; symptoms include abdominal distention with ascites, hepatic dysfunction, nephrotic syndrome, abdominal wall venous collaterals, varicocele, malabsorption, and pulmonary embolus. The anatomic location of the caval thrombus is important prognostically. Supradiaphragmatic lesions, which may involve the heart, can be resected, but the prognosis is poor; patients with subdiaphragmatic lesions have a better 5-year survival rate, but this usually occurs in less than 50% of cases.[3] When approaching the surgical management of these patients, a team of specialists is required, especially if a cardiac tumor thrombectomy is contemplated.

The role of surgery in the management of metastatic disease, either at the initial presentation or later, remains controversial. Although most data that support nephrectomy plus metastasectomy are anecdotal, many patients with synchronous renal cell cancer and an isolated pulmonary nodule may be considered for surgical resection of both lesions. Likewise, patients who develop an isolated lesion in the liver or lung some time after the removal of the kidney may also be considered for surgical removal of the metastasis. Nevertheless, even when such vigorous surgery is carried out, most patients do poorly. Additional controversy surrounds the practice of performing a nephrectomy on patients with widespread metastatic disease as a means of potentially improving their response to systemic therapy. Many investigative programs require such resection; at this point, the practice should be considered investigational. However, a patient who does experience an excellent response to systemic therapy should be considered for a nephrectomy after the response. Finally, because many renal tumors can become quite large, consideration should be given to palliative nephrectomy (in the setting of metastatic disease), especially if the patient experiences uncontrollable hematuria or pain or is catabolic secondary to the sheer mass of the tumor.

Systemic Management of Advanced Stages of Renal Cell Cancer

The management of patients with either locally advanced renal cancer or with metastatic disease provides a great challenge to physicians and clinical investigators. Although chemotherapy and hormone treatments have been studied extensively in patients with metastatic renal cancer, no single treatment protocol or program has been uniformly effective. Therefore, most physicians treating the disease usually rely on novel modalities of treatment, including biologic response modifiers, investigational anticancer agents, differentiation agents (e.g., retinoic acid), vaccines, and gene therapy.

It has been known for a long time that renal cancer may occasionally incite an immune response in the host, leading to spontaneous remissions of cancer. Although rare, this observation has led many to study agents that can augment the body's immune system. The agents that have been studied most extensively include the interferons, interleukins, cytokines, cell-based therapies, and combinations of the aforementioned.

Cytokine Therapies

Interferon therapy with interferon alfa, beta, or gamma moieties has led to responses in approximately 12% to 20% of treated patients.[17,18] Although their effects are numerous, interferons demonstrate antiproliferative activity against renal cell cancers in vitro, are stimulatory to immune cell function, and can modulate the expression of major histocompatibility complex molecules. Although patients' responses have been seen in many anatomic areas, patients who have had a previous nephrectomy with isolated pulmonary metastases and who are otherwise well may have a higher response rate. The duration of the response is usually less than 2 years, although longer lasting remissions have been noted in a few selected patients. Interferons have been combined with other immune modifiers and with chemotherapy agents, with no real improvement in patient outcome in larger scale trials. However, several smaller trials have combined interferon with interleukin-2 chemotherapy agents (e.g., 5-fluorouracil), and the preliminary results have been encouraging in some cases. Today, most centers will reserve the use of interleukin-2 for those with clear-cell histologies, as its effectiveness is less in other histologies.

The toxicity of interleukin-2 is related to alterations in vascular permeability, leading to a capillary leak-type syndrome. Although the drug is approved for the management of patients with metastatic renal cell cancer by the U.S. Food and Drug Administration, its use should be restricted to patients who can tolerate the side effect profile and to patients with acceptable cardiac, renal, pulmonary, and hepatic function.

Tyrosine Kinase Inhibitors

The most important information surrounding the systemic management of renal cell cancer has been the introduction and approval of two new multikinase inhibitors. These agents inhibit a variety of tyrosine kinases including vascular endothelial growth factor receptors and platelet-derived growth factors. These factors play a critical role in cell signaling that enable cellular proliferation and the development of new blood vessel formation. The two drugs that have gained approval are sunitinib and sorafenib. Response rates in cytokine-refractory, previously treated patients have been in the range of 35% to 40% with sunitinib, with median time to progression of 8 months. The clinical data with sorafenib have demonstrated a longer progression-free survival compared with placebo in cytokine-resistant patients. Fatigue, diarrhea, hand-foot syndrome, skin discoloration, and abnormalities of pancreatic enzymes (rarely with pancreatitis) have been observed with this new class of agents.[19,20]

These agents can be considered for either first- or second-line therapy (after development of cytokine resistance) in patients with metastatic renal cell cancer. Clear-cell histologies respond more favorably. The use of tyrosine kinase inhibitors will continue to be evaluated in a wide spectrum of circumstances, both as monotherapy and in combination with other biologic agents.

Investigational therapies continue to be studied for renal cell cancer.[21] Many such approaches are under investigation and include novel cytokines such as interleukin-12, combinations of biologic agents with or without chemotherapeutic agents, circadian timing of chemotherapy administration, vaccine therapy, various forms of cellular therapy, and gene therapy. Although all these approaches have a solid scientific preclinical rationale, none, unfortunately, can be considered standard treatment. The sobering fact remains that almost 50% of patients diagnosed with renal cell cancer die of their disease within 5 years of diagnosis, and a substantial proportion initially present with advanced stages of cancer spread.

Wilms' Tumor (Nephroblastoma) and Neuroblastoma

Wilms' tumor and neuroblastoma are the two most common pediatric kidney tumors.[2] Wilms' tumor is usually found in children younger than 5 years of age and usually presents with abdominal mass, pain, hematuria, elevations in blood pressure, and systemic manifestations (e.g., fever). Genetic alterations of chromosome 11 have been associated with the disease. The diagnosis is usually established by CT or magnetic resonance imaging, identifying bilaterality in approximately 5% of patients. Less than 20% of patients have metastases at initial presentation; if they are found, metastases are usually in the lung and liver.

Neuroblastoma has many characteristics in common with Wilms' tumor, but is characterized by an elevation of catecholamines, vanillylmandelic acid, and homovanillic acid in most patients. Both diseases are highly curable with a multimodal approach using aggressive surgery, multiagent chemotherapy (with or without bone marrow transplantation), and selective use of radiation therapy.

FUTURE DIRECTIONS

Clearly, the most important prognostic feature for a cure in managing renal cell cancers is the stage and the genetic makeup of the individual tumor. Identification of high-risk patient populations, such as those with a strong family history or genetic predisposition, should be attempted to allow an earlier diagnosis and a potential cure. However, for most patients, additional research is needed to develop strategies for eradication of metastatic deposits. Further testing of biologic modifiers, gene therapy, and chemotherapies directed at eliminating neoplastic cells are the ultimate goal, and patients should be encouraged to enter these types of clinical investigations.

References

1. Garnick MB: Bladder, renal and testicular cancer. Sci Am Med 1995;12:1–5.
2. Shapiro CL, Garnick MB, Kantoff PW: Tumors of the kidney, ureter, and bladder. In Bennett JC (ed): Cecil Textbook of Medicine, 20th ed. Philadelphia: WB Saunders, 1996, p 867.
3. McDougal WS, Garnick MB: Clinical signs and symptoms of kidney cancer. In Vogelzang NJ, Scardino PT, Shipley WU, et al (eds): Comprehensive Textbook of Genitourinary Oncology. Baltimore: Williams & Wilkins, 1996, p 546.
4. Cohen HT, McGovern FJ: Renal cell carcinoma. N Engl J Med 2005:353:2477–2490.
5. Sokoloff MH, deKernion JB, Figlin RA, Belldegrun A: Current management of renal cell carcinoma. CA Cancer J Clin 1996; 46:284–302.
6. Beahrs OH, Henson DE, Hutter RVP, et al: Handbook for the Staging of Cancer, 4th ed. Philadelphia: JB Lippincott, 1993.
7. Latif F, Tory K, Gnarra J, et al: Identification of the von Hippel-Lindau tumor suppressor gene. Science 1993;260:1317–1320.
8. Olsson CA, Sawczuk IS: Urologic cancer. Urol Clin North Am 1993;20.
9. Dreijerink K, Braga E, Kuzmin I, et al: The candidate tumor suppressor gene RASSF1A, from human chromosome 3p21.3 is involved in kidney tumorigenesis. Proc Natl Acad Sci U S A 2001;98:7504–7509.
10. Storkel S, Stearata PV, Drenckhaln D, Thoenes W: The human chromophobe cell renal carcinoma: Its probable relation to intercalated cells of the collecting duct. Virchows Arch B Cell Pathol Incl Mol Pathol 1989;56:237–245.
11. Storkel S, van den Berg E: Morphologic classification of renal cancer. World J Urol 1995;13:153–158.
12. Zisman A, Pantuck A, Dorey F, et al: Improved prognostication of renal cell carcinoma using an integrated staging system. J Clin Oncol 2001;19:1649–1657.
13. Motzer RJ, Mazumdar M, Bacik J, et al: Survival and prognostic stratification of 670 patients with advanced renal cell carcinoma. J Clin Oncol 1999;17:2530–2540.
14. Shalev M, Cipolla B, Guille F, et al: Is ipsilateral adrenalectomy a necessary component of radical nephrectomy? J Urol 1995; 153:1415–1417.
15. Licht MR, Novick AC, Goormastic M: Nephron sparing surgery in incidental versus suspected renal cell carcinoma. J Urol 1994;152:39–42.

16. Thrasher JB, Paulson DF: Prognostic factors in renal cancer. Urol Clin North Am 1993;20:247–262.

17. Nanus DM, Pfeffer LM, Bander NH, et al: Antiproliferative and antitumor effects of alpha-interferon in renal cell carcinomas: Correlation with the expression of a kidney-associated differentiation glycoprotein. Cancer Res 1990;50:4190–4194.

18. Minasian LM, Motzer RJ, Gluck L, et al: Interferon alpha-2a in advanced renal cell carcinoma: Treatment results and survival in 159 patients with long-term follow-up. J Clin Oncol 1993;11:1368–1375.

19. Motzer RJ, Hutson TE, Tomczak P, et al: Sunitinib versus interferon alfa in metastatic renal cell carcinoma. N Engl J Med 2007;356:115–124.

20. Escudier B, Eisen T, Stadler WM, et al: Sorafenib in advanced clear-cell renal-cell carcinoma. N Engl J Med 2007:356:125–134.

21. Wigginton JM, Komschlies KL, Back TC, et al: Administration of interleukin 12 with pulse interleukin 2 and the rapid and complete eradication of murine renal carcinoma. J Natl Cancer Inst 1996;88:38–43.

Further Reading

Vogelzang NJ, Scardino PT, Shipley WU, et al (eds): Comprehensive Textbook of Genitourinary Oncology. Baltimore: Williams & Wilkins, 1996, p 546.

Chapter 39

Myeloma and Secondary Involvement of the Kidney in Dysproteinemias

Paul W. Sanders

This chapter reviews the current potential approaches to management of the three major renal lesions associated with immunoglobulin light-chain deposition: AL-type amyloidosis, monoclonal light-chain deposition disease, and cast nephropathy. A review of Waldenström's macroglobulinemia is also included. Detailed discussions of cryoglobulinemia, fibrillary glomerulonephritis, immunotactoid glomerulonephritis, and amyloidosis related to other causes are discussed in other chapters.

IMMUNOGLOBULIN LIGHT-CHAIN METABOLISM AND ASSOCIATED RENAL LESIONS

Renal failure is a common occurrence in multiple myeloma; in one large series, nearly half of the 1027 patients with newly diagnosed myeloma had associated serum creatinine concentrations that were 1.3 mg/dL or greater.[1] In the necropsy study of kidneys of 57 patients by Iványi,[2] the most common renal lesion was cast nephropathy or myeloma kidney (65%), whereas 21% had AL-type amyloidosis and 11% had monoclonal light-chain deposition disease. Although the traditional view has been to treat patients who have features of overt myeloma, the focus in recent years has shifted from estimating disease burden using techniques that assess the size of the clonal population of plasma cells to recognition that the circulating monoclonal protein product should also be addressed when it produces organ dysfunction. Although most, if not all, patients with documented cast nephropathy have multiple myeloma, only approximately 20% of patients with primary (AL-type) amyloidosis had multiple myeloma,[3] and 26% of patients with monoclonal light-chain deposition disease manifested either myeloma or another lymphoproliferative disease over time.[4] In some patients, renal failure may be the only clinical manifestation of an otherwise silent, but deadly, clone of plasma cells or occult malignancy.[5] Despite the absence of extrarenal manifestations and degree of bone marrow plasmacytosis, as discussed in subsequent sections, the combined data support a therapeutic approach that decreases monoclonal light-chain production in all patients with documented renal failure related to monoclonal light chains.

An understanding of the pathophysiology of the disease processes is important in the therapeutic interventions in this spectrum of diverse conditions. Although immunoglobulins and immunoglobulin heavy chains can be pathogenic, the immunoglobulin light chain is usually at the center of the pathogenesis of these diverse renal lesions. Identification of the nature of the renal injury allows tailoring of subsequent treatment (Table 39-1). The variable effects on the glomeruli, tubulointerstitium, and vasculature that are responsible for an inconstant set of presenting renal manifestations are related to sequence variations in the variable domain of the light chain. These sequence variations, for example, confer the propensity to polymerize to form AL-type amyloid.[6-8] Only very rarely do heavy chains alone form amyloid.[9] Amyloid expands the glomerular mesangium, compressing the capillary loops and subsequently producing the clinical manifestations of progressive kidney failure. Monoclonal light-chain deposition disease, the second most common glomerular lesion associated with monoclonal gammopathies, is characterized by deposition of monoclonal light chain, typically κ isotype, in the mesangium. Occasionally, heavy chains may also be present, prompting some authors to describe this lesion as monoclonal light-chain and light- and heavy-chain deposition disease. Very rarely, heavy chains alone can cause monoclonal heavy-chain deposition disease. Light chains from patients with monoclonal light-chain deposition disease stimulate mesangial cells to produce transforming growth factor β, which then serves as an autacoid to stimulate mesangial cell production of extracellular matrix proteins.[10] Continued expansion of the mesangium compresses the capillary loops, which decreases glomerular filtration and ultimately produces glomerulosclerosis. Hydrophobic amino acid residues in the complementarity-determining region 1 and abnormal glycosylation of the variable domain have been identified in light chains responsible for monoclonal light-chain deposition diseases.[11-14]

With a molecular mass of 22 kd (approximately one third that of albumin), monomeric free light chains are filtered at the

Table 39-1 Potential Therapies for Monoclonal Light Chain–Related Kidney Diseases*

Kidney Lesion	Treatment
AL-type amyloidosis	HDT/SCT
	Chemotherapy
	Dialysis
	Kidney transplantation
Monoclonal light-chain deposition disease	HDT/SCT
	Chemotherapy
	Dialysis
	Kidney transplantation
Cast nephropathy	HDT/SCT
	Chemotherapy ± plasmapheresis
	Maintain normocalcemia
	Hydration
	Avoid exposure to radiocontrast material, nonsteroidal anti-inflammatory agents, and diuretics
	Dialysis
	Kidney transplantation
Waldenström's macroglobulinemia	Chemotherapy
	Plasmapheresis

*See text for details.
HDT/SCT, high-dose chemotherapy with autologous peripheral stem-cell transplantation.

glomerulus. Filtered light chains enter the proximal tubule where low molecular mass proteins are endocytosed and hydrolyzed, and the constituent amino acids are returned to the circulation. Some pathologic light chains undergo a similar reabsorption process but are hydrolyzed poorly and accumulate in lysosomes. Clinical manifestations of this altered process can include renal failure from proximal tubular cell necrosis or, in less severe cases, acquired Fanconi syndrome. Unusual nonpolar amino acid residues in complementarity-determining region 1 and absence of accessible side chains in the complementarity-determining region 3 loop appear to be responsible for the homotypic crystallization of the light chain in the proximal tubule in Fanconi syndrome.[15,16]

Cast nephropathy is the most common kidney disease associated with monoclonal light chains, occurring in approximately one third of patients with myeloma. Light chains secreted by these patients are unique in that they demonstrate specific binding to Tamm-Horsfall glycoprotein in vitro. The complementarity-determining region 3 domain in the variable domain of the light chain determines binding to Tamm-Horsfall glycoprotein.[17] Nephrotoxic light chains that escape proximal tubular reabsorption enter the thick ascending limb of Henle's loop, bind to Tamm-Horsfall glycoprotein, and produce casts that obstruct flow of tubule fluid. This results in proximal tubule

atrophy, interstitial inflammation and fibrosis, and subsequent renal failure.[18–20]

In recent years, a quantitative immunoassay for serum free light chains has been developed and tested.[21,22] This assay provides indication of response to treatment and removal of the offending light chain. Baseline serum free monoclonal light chain levels greater than 75 mg/dL correlated with depressed renal function (serum creatinine concentration ≥2 mg/dL) and more aggressive myeloma.[23] Patients with documented renal involvement from AL-type amyloidosis or monoclonal light-chain deposition disease can present a challenge in the identification of the monoclonal protein in the circulation,[4,5,24–26] although the use of the serum free light chain assay offers promise in the detection of the abnormal protein and the response to treatment.[27,28]

AL-TYPE AMYLOIDOSIS

The management of AL-type amyloidosis is in a state of flux. After the initial randomized trial that suggested improved survival in a subset of patients who did not have rapidly progressive disease and received chemotherapy in the form of melphalan and prednisone,[29] more aggressive anti–plasma cell therapy has been undertaken.[30,31] A longitudinal analysis of six separate trials performed over 8 years suggested that patients with AL-type amyloidosis respond to high-dose chemotherapy with autologous peripheral stem-cell transplantation (HDT/SCT).[31] Subjects with multiple myeloma were excluded from these trials. Although renal dysfunction was not an exclusion criterion, there were several other exclusion criteria that included age 80 years and older, uncompensated congestive heart failure, left ventricular ejection fraction less than 0.40, persistent pleural effusions, systolic blood pressure less than 90 mm Hg, oxygen saturation less than 95% on room air, and significant overall functional impairment. Median survival of the 312 patients who underwent HDT/SCT was 4.6 years with 46% achieving a complete hematologic response, and this 46% demonstrated improved long-term survival. Thus, HDT/SCT appeared to produce greater survival rates and opportunity for a hematologic response compared with historical controls who received other forms of therapy.[29,32] Those patients who had evidence of multiorgan system dysfunction, particularly cardiac disease, and were considered ineligible for HDT/SCT, had a median survival of 4 months with only 16% (35 of the 225) alive at the time of publication.[31] In a follow-up quality-of-life analysis from this group, those patients who underwent HDT/SCT had demonstrably sustained improvement in their quality of life; this outcome was particularly true for those patients who achieved a complete hematologic response.[33]

In another retrospective case-control study, 63 patients with AL-type amyloidosis undergoing standard therapy were matched according to a series of biochemical and functional parameters to 63 consecutive patients with AL-type amyloidosis undergoing HDT/SCT. A good attempt was made to match the characteristics of two groups, including age, gender, degree of organ involvement (primarily cardiac, renal, neural), and time from diagnosis to initiation of therapy. After 4 years of follow-up, those patients who received HDT/SCT demonstrated a significantly greater survival rate compared with the control group.[34] Although these studies support a more aggressive treatment intervention for AL-type amyloidosis in suitable patients, the limitation of these observations is the lack of a randomized, prospective trial.

A consistent finding from therapeutic trials was the observation that survival was adversely affected by functional involvement of two or more organs (cardiac, renal, gastrointestinal, neurological, and soft tissue) by amyloid infiltration at the time of presentation. Cardiac involvement in particular was a major predictor of overall survival.[35] Another important observation was that organ function could improve with successful chemotherapy. At 1 year, 42% of patients treated with HDT/SCT therapy demonstrated improved organ function, including those patients with kidney disease.[35] Other investigators have reported complete resolution of nephrotic syndrome as well as acute kidney injury after HDT/SCT.[36] Despite reports that amyloid deposition may regress with successful treatment and recent demonstration that endogenous cysteine proteases can degrade AL-type amyloid in vitro,[37] functional kidney improvement can occur without regression of glomerular AL-type amyloid deposition.[38]

Although patients with AL-type amyloidosis die of organ dysfunction and not tumor burden, the current approach to treatment is a therapeutic regimen that targets the monoclonal plasma cell population and is available in the community.[39] Increasingly, the approach will consist of HDT/SCT if the patient is younger than 70 years of age and renal functional impairment is not severe (creatinine clearance > 50 mL/min or serum creatinine concentration < 3.0–4.0 mg/dL).[39] A beneficial renal response—decrease in proteinuria and stabilization or improvement in renal function—was associated with prolonged survival.[40] Some centers report that the presence of severe disease requiring renal replacement therapy is not a contraindication, and recovery from kidney failure and nephrotic syndrome can occur, but because procedure-related mortality is increased, HDT/SCT should probably be performed at centers with special expertise.[39,41] Patients who have systolic blood pressures less than 90 mm Hg or who have poor overall functional capability have exceedingly high procedure-related mortality rates with HDT/SCT.[42]

The recent success of thalidomide as an alternative treatment of multiple myeloma[43] has led to more frequent treatment of AL-type amyloidosis with this agent in an uncontrolled fashion. Because thalidomide is not well tolerated in these patients, some authors have recommended initial doses of 50 mg/day.[44] Although dose modifications of thalidomide are not required in renal failure, caution is advised[45]; hyperkalemia, perhaps related to tumor lysis, may occur, especially during the first few weeks of treatment.[46,47] Randomized, controlled trials are needed to guide therapy of AL-type amyloidosis, but the limitations of long-term treatment with alkylating agents make HDT/SCT, thalidomide, and the analogue lenalidomide[48] potentially attractive therapies in AL-type amyloidosis.

Kidney transplantation is an option in patients with end-stage kidney failure due to AL-type amyloidosis, although experience with this approach is limited and evidence of a lasting (12-month) reduction in the offending light chain should be confirmed before proceeding with transplantation. This approach might be particularly beneficial for those patients who manifest renal-limited amyloidosis. In one study of 62 patients, eight of whom had AL-type amyloidosis, 65% survived 5 years after kidney allograft implantation. In this study, amyloid was found to involve the graft in 10% and 3% lost the graft as a result of this involvement at the time of publication.[49] Another small study performed living donor kidney transplantation followed by HDT/SCT in eight patients; this study demonstrated the feasibility of this approach, but the early mortality rate was significant (two of eight) and kidney function worsened in one patient after HDT/SCT.[50]

MONOCLONAL LIGHT-CHAIN DEPOSITION DISEASE

As reviewed by Ronco and colleagues,[51] monoclonal light-chain deposition disease represents a prototypical model of glomerulosclerosis whose pathogenesis is related to production of transforming growth factor β.[10] The dominant clinical manifestation is progressive renal failure, although the disease is systemic and other organs, including heart and liver, may be involved.[51] Randomized, controlled trials for treatment of monoclonal light-chain deposition disease are unavailable, but these patients appear to benefit from the same chemotherapy as that given for multiple myeloma, particularly if the renal failure is mild at presentation.[4] The 5-year patient survival rate approaches 70%,[4] but is decreased by coexistent myeloma. The serum creatinine concentration at presentation is an important predictor of subsequent kidney function: five of eight patients with serum creatinine concentrations less than 354 μmol/L (4.0 mg/dL) did not progress with chemotherapy, whereas 9 of 11 patients with creatinine concentrations greater than 354 μmol/L at presentation progressed to end-stage kidney injury despite therapy.

Encouraged by the early success of melphalan/prednisone,[4] three small nonrandomized trials examined the use of HDT/SCT in monoclonal light-chain deposition disease.[52,53] The first study consisted of a retrospective analysis of 11 patients; 10 were considered to have myeloma and most were stage I. All patients had clinically apparent renal disease, with four manifesting severe kidney failure requiring renal replacement therapy at the start of treatment. Four patients had congestive heart failure. Despite the high frequency of renal and cardiac involvement, procedure-related death from stem-cell harvesting and HDT/SCT did not occur. Three of the four patients on dialysis, however, developed morbid complications from which they eventually recovered. Five patients had a complete hematologic response as well as improvement in organ function. Histologic confirmation of regression of the light-chain deposits in affected organs was also shown. During the median follow-up period of 51 months, three patients required additional treatment because of a relapse of myeloma; one patient died 93 months after HDT/SCT from complications related to myeloma.[52] The second report[53] also described the feasibility and success of HDT/SCT in five patients with monoclonal light-chain deposition disease. In the third report, all patients had concomitant myeloma and advanced renal disease requiring renal replacement therapy, but successful therapy improved renal function in a subset; 5 of 10 patients with biopsy-proven monoclonal light-chain deposition disease became dialysis independent after HDT/SCT.[54]

The high incidence of progressive kidney disease in monoclonal light-chain deposition disease has prompted treatment with kidney transplantation at several institutions, but the disease will recur in the allograft if the underlying plasma-cell dyscrasia is not addressed.[55–57] The largest collection[57] reported the outcome of seven patients who received kidney transplants (four deceased donor and three living related). Recurrence of the disease was observed in five of the seven allografts. The median time to reach end-stage kidney failure after recurrence was 33.3 months, with an overall median graft survival of 37.3 months. Median patient survival was 6.1 years, which is worse than age-matched kidney transplant recipients. However, one patient remained alive with a functioning allograft and no evidence of recurrence 13 years after transplantation. The authors concluded that long-term kidney allograft survival is significantly decreased in monoclonal light-chain deposition disease, emphasizing the need to control monoclonal light-chain production before kidney transplantation.

CAST NEPHROPATHY

A cornerstone of acute management of cast nephropathy is prevention of aggregation of light chains with Tamm-Horsfall glycoprotein. Volume repletion, normalization of electrolytes, and avoidance of complicating factors such as furosemide, radiocontrast material, and nonsteroidal anti-inflammatory agents are mainstays of therapy in the prevention of cast nephropathy. Tubule fluid flow rates should be kept high to avoid obstruction from light chains.[20,58] Daily fluid intake of as much as 3 L in the form of free water should be encouraged as long as defects in osmoregulation do not manifest. Although alkalinization of the urine prevents renal failure due to light chains in rats,[59] in one inadequately controlled trial in humans, alkalinization of the urine was not beneficial.[60] Until better studies are available, because increasing the ambient sodium concentration also facilitates binding in vitro,[20] administration of sodium bicarbonate (or citrate) should probably be avoided.

Hypercalcemia develops in 20% to 30% of patients with multiple myeloma. Hypercalcemia is both directly nephrotoxic and enhances the nephrotoxicity of light chains.[19,20] For these reasons, aggressive intervention to achieve normalization of the serum ionized calcium concentration is necessary. Initial management includes volume expansion with 0.9% NaCl intravenously, provided kidney function is not irreversibly impaired. Loop diuretics facilitate renal calcium excretion, but may facilitate nephrotoxicity from light chains.[20] Consequently, loop diuretics should be administered judiciously and only after the patient is clinically euvolemic. Glucocorticoid treatment, such as intermittent high-dose dexamethasone, is frequently helpful for the management of hypercalcemia. Bisphosphonates, particularly pamidronate and zoledronic acid, are used to treat moderate hypercalcemia (serum calcium > 3.25 mmol/L or 13 mg/dL). Although hypercalcemia of myeloma responds to bisphosphonates, these agents are nephrotoxic and should be administered only to euvolemic patients. Bisphosphonates have also been used to treat myeloma. In one prospective study, patients who received monthly intravenous infusions of pamidronate 90 mg had fewer skeletal events (pathologic fractures, cord compression, bone radiotherapy) and less bone pain with improved quality of life compared with the group who received placebo.[61] Many authorities recommend the use of monthly pamidronate therapy, particularly in those patients with advanced myeloma. Kidney function and proteinuria should be monitored during treatment with these agents and the dose adjusted accordingly should kidney function or proteinuria worsen.

Virtually all patients with cast nephropathy have criteria for the diagnosis of multiple myeloma, and the primary approach to treatment is antitumor therapy. The traditional treatment, which consisted of alkylating agents and steroids, has been replaced, particularly in younger patients, with high-dose chemotherapy with autologous peripheral stem-cell transplantation (HDT/SCT). A randomized trial showed that patients who received HDT/SCT had improved event-free survival and overall survival rates than did patients who received conventional chemotherapy. The mean serum creatinine of patients at the time of entry into this study was 1.3 mg/dL (113 μmol/L).[62] A multicenter, randomized trial determined that, compared with conventional chemotherapy, HDT/SCT was a more effective first-line treatment for myeloma when patients were younger than 65 years of age at diagnosis.[63] Patients with advanced renal disease were accepted into this trial, and, perhaps not surprisingly, survival rates were higher among patients who had serum creatinine levels less than 1.7 mg/dL than among patients with creatinine concentrations 1.7 mg/dL or greater.[63] As experience with the use of HDT/SCT has increased, more institutions are using this approach even in patients with advanced renal disease.[64] HDT/SCT performed on 59 dialysis-dependent patients with myeloma resulted in improvement in kidney function in 24%; the rate of recovery was higher in patients who were on dialysis for less than 6 months.[54] Twenty-eight patients had a kidney biopsy in this study, and 15 had biopsy-proven cast nephropathy; of these 15 patients, six became dialysis independent after HDT/SCT.[54]

At present, most clinicians prefer to treat myeloma with a combination of vincristine, doxorubicin, and dexamethasone (VAD) before HDT/SCT because this combination of agents can produce a rapid decrease in the plasma cell clone.[64–66] Typically, long-term treatment with alkylating agents is avoided before HDT/SCT because these drugs may impede peripheral stem-cell harvest and are associated with myelodysplasia and acute myelogenous leukemia.[67]

Several as yet unproven therapies are on the horizon. Patients with advanced renal failure and refractory myeloma have been treated with bortezomib[68] and thalidomide,[69] with encouraging results. Both agents are now in experimental use in induction chemotherapeutic regimens before HDT/SCT[70,71] and may eventually replace the combination of vincristine, doxorubicin, and dexamethasone. Myeloablative therapy with allogeneic stem-cell transplantation may prove effective in controlling kidney failure in myeloma, but has significant mortality and is currently limited to a small population who are deemed suitable for such treatment and have an HLA-compatible relative. Whether nonmyeloablative allogeneic stem-cell transplantation, so-called mini-allograft therapy, will provide beneficial results in myeloma[72,73] without the attendant complications such as severe graft-versus-host disease remains uncertain. However, a recent nonrandomized study enrolled 162 patients who had newly diagnosed myeloma and were younger than 65 years of age to examine the potential benefit of tandem transplants. After therapy with vincristine, doxorubicin, and dexamethasone and HDC/APSCT, they were divided into two groups, with patients who had HLA-identical siblings receiving nonmyeloablative total-body irradiation and allogeneic stem-cell transplantation and the remaining patients receiving a second HDT/SCT using autologous stem cells. In follow-up, the 80 patients who received the allografts fared significantly better than the 82 patients who received two HDT/SCT. Graft-versus-host disease accounted for most of the treatment-related mortality in the allograft group.[74]

Plasmapheresis in the setting of acute renal failure related to cast nephropathy is controversial. The standard protocol has consisted of five daily plasma exchange sessions, with an additional exchange on days 7 and 10 if necessary. Zucchelli and colleagues[75] randomized 29 patients with myeloma, light-chain proteinuria, and acute renal failure to receive either plasma exchanges with chemotherapy or chemotherapy alone. Plasmapheresis dramatically decreased light-chain proteinuria and increased urine output; 13 of 15 patients recovered renal function. Of the 14 patients who did not receive plasma exchange therapy, only two recovered function. As a result, plasma exchange therapy significantly improved survival at 1 year post-treatment. An uncontrolled, nonrandomized study has also suggested that patients with advanced multiple myeloma (stage IIIB) and coexistent renal failure may benefit from plasma exchange therapy performed every 5 weeks on three consecutive days just before combination chemotherapy; survival in the plasmapheresis group improved compared with a group who received melphalan and prednisone alone (median survival, 17 vs. 2 months).[76] A recent randomized trial suggested no clinical benefit from plasma exchange for patients with acute kidney injury,[77] although there were limitations to this study that should be considered. Kidney biopsy was not a prerequisite for entry into the study, and in perhaps one third of patients with myeloma and acute kidney injury, the cause was not cast nephropathy but related instead to obstruction (nephrolithiasis, papillary necrosis, and amyloid deposition in the ureters), hypercalcemia, and hyperviscosity syndrome, in addition to other causes seen in the general population, such as drug-related allergic interstitial nephritis and contrast nephropathy. Serum free light chains were not determined either before or after the plasma exchange. Despite the significant number of patients, the study may have been underpowered to detect differences between the groups, especially because biopsy-proven cast nephropathy was not a criterion for inclusion in the study. Until additional data are provided, it is prudent not to recommend plasmapheresis for every patient with acute kidney injury, although there may be a subset of patients who do respond to plasmapheresis. If plasma exchange is performed, demonstration of the efficacy of treatment by quantifying changes in serum free light-chain levels should be performed. Finally, hyperviscosity syndrome remains an indication for plasma exchange.

A significant issue related to plasma exchange therapy is the relatively inefficient removal of circulating light chains, and other techniques for rapid decrease in serum light-chain concentrations may become available in the near future. In a recent nonrandomized trial, eight patients who had acute kidney injury from biopsy-proven cast nephropathy received dialysis using a dialyzer with a very large effective pore size (~50 kd). This approach effectively decreased serum free light-chain concentrations, providing the potential to accelerate recovery

from acute kidney injury. In this trial, 5 of 13 patients recovered kidney function by the time of publication of the report.[78]

Renal replacement therapy in the form of hemodialysis or peritoneal dialysis is generally recommended in patients with kidney failure from monoclonal light chain–related renal diseases. Recovery of kidney function sufficient to survive without dialysis occurs in as many as 5% of patients with multiple myeloma, although in some patients, this requires months to achieve, probably because the traditional chemotherapeutic regimens slowly reduce circulating light-chain levels. Despite the susceptibility to infection in multiple myeloma, the peritonitis rate for continuous ambulatory peritoneal dialysis (one episode every 14.4 months) was not unacceptably high.[79] Neither peritoneal dialysis nor hemodialysis appears to provide a superior survival advantage in patients with myeloma.

Kidney transplantation has also been successfully performed in highly selected patients with multiple myeloma. Extrarenal manifestations should be absent and serum light-chain levels controlled for more than 1 year in patients before considering kidney transplantation. Despite rigorous pre-transplantation surveillance, however, myeloma may recur and cast nephropathy can occur in the allograft. These complications notwithstanding, kidney transplantation remains a therapeutic option in highly selected patients who have persistent end-stage kidney disease after treatment.

WALDENSTRÖM'S MACROGLOBULINEMIA

This rare disorder constitutes approximately 5% of monoclonal gammopathies and is a monoclonal B-cell malignancy whose transcription profile resembles that of chronic lymphocytic leukemia.[80] This condition clinically behaves more like lymphoma, although the malignant lymphoplasmacytic cell line also secretes IgM (macroglobulin), which is usually responsible for the renal symptoms at presentation. IgM is a large molecule that is not excreted and accumulates in plasma to produce hyperviscosity syndrome and cryoglobulinemia. Neurological symptoms (headaches, dizziness, deafness, stupor), visual impairment (from hemorrhages and exudates and sluggish flow through the venous system), bleeding diathesis (complexed clotting factors with IgM and platelet dysfunction), kidney failure, and symptoms of hypervolemia are classic manifestations of this disease. Osteolytic lesions are uncommon. Kidney failure is usually mild but occurs in approximately 30% of patients. Although lymphoplasmacytic cell infiltration can produce nephromegaly and renal failure, hyperviscosity syndrome and precipitation of IgM in the glomerular capillaries are the most common causes of renal failure. Approximately 10% to 15% of patients also develop AL-type amyloidosis, but cast nephropathy is rare in these patients.

The typical course of Waldenström's macroglobulinemia is protracted, but occasionally the disease is more aggressive. Prognostic modeling of Waldenström's macroglobulinemia suggested that age older than 65 years, organomegaly, and perhaps elevated β_2-microglobulin levels (>4 mg/L) were adverse prognostic factors that were associated with a reduction in life span. Patients with none of these risk factors had a median survival of 10.6 years, whereas the group who were of advanced age or had organomegaly had a median survival of 4.2 years.[81] In sorting out this process further, molecular analysis may also be of benefit; for example, a 6q gene deletion may discriminate Waldenström's macroglobulinemia from IgM monoclonal gammopathy of undetermined significance.[82] In the typical presentation consisting of an advanced age (sixth to seventh decades) and slowly progressive course, the major therapeutic goal is relief of symptoms. Randomized, controlled therapeutic trials are lacking in this disorder. Plasmapheresis is indicated for hyperviscosity syndrome, followed by alkylating agents alone. All patients with monoclonal IgM levels greater than 3 g/dL should have serum viscosity checked. A relative serum viscosity more than 4 or whole blood viscosity more than 8 centipoise usually correlates with symptoms of hyperviscosity, although significant individual variation exists.[83] Occasionally, clinically apparent hyperviscosity syndrome is associated with only mild increases in serum viscosity, particularly if the IgM forms cryoprecipitate and the serum viscosity is determined at room temperature. Alternatively, some patients with marked increases in serum viscosity manifest no symptoms. Plasmapheresis is indicated in symptomatic patients only and should be continued until symptoms resolve and serum viscosity normalizes. Blood transfusions, which can further increase viscosity, should be avoided in patients with hyperviscosity syndrome. Initial chemotherapy is usually chlorambucil 0.1 mg/kg/day PO, with titration to control serum IgM concentration and organomegaly without inducing cytopenias. More aggressive chemotherapy (cyclophosphamide, vincristine, prednisone), given monthly, has also been used in patients who do not respond to chlorambucil. However, a recognized complication of long-term therapy with alkylating agents is the development of myelodysplasia and acute myelogenous leukemia.[84] Other agents have been tried in small clinical studies, including rituximab, because, unlike plasma cells, the lymphoplasmacytic cells appear to express CD20.[85] Severe renal failure requiring renal replacement therapy is uncommon in this disorder.

SUMMARY

Advances in understanding the pathophysiology of monoclonal light chain–related kidney diseases have produced improvements in management and prolongation of survival in this population. Approaches designed to lower circulating monoclonal light chains and attack the basic mechanisms of kidney damage, along with judicious use of renal replacement therapies, provide the best results. For most monoclonal light chain–related kidney diseases, the most aggressive cytotoxic therapies appear to offer the best long-term kidney prognosis but also produce greater morbidity and mortality, particularly in elderly patients. As is true for most diseases, the treating physician must weigh the risks of a particular treatment versus the potential benefit for the individual patient. Even with the recent advances in treatment, however, overall prognosis remains suboptimal, so the clinician should remain receptive to new therapies for this unique family of potentially reversible kidney lesions.

References

1. Kyle RA, Gertz MA, Witzig TE, et al: Review of 1027 patients with newly diagnosed multiple myeloma. Mayo Clin Proc 2003; 78:21–33.
2. Iványi B: Frequency of light chain deposition nephropathy relative to renal amyloidosis and Bence Jones cast nephropathy in a necropsy study of patients with myeloma. Arch Pathol Lab Med 1990;114:986–987.
3. Kyle RA, Greipp PR: Amyloidosis (AL): Clinical and laboratory features in 229 cases. Mayo Clin Proc 1983;58:665–683.
4. Heilman RL, Velosa JA, Holley KE, et al: Long-term follow-up and response to chemotherapy in patients with light-chain deposition disease. Am J Kidney Dis 1992;20:34–41.
5. Sanders PW, Herrera GA, Kirk KA, et al: Spectrum of glomerular and tubulointerstitial renal lesions associated with monotypical immunoglobulin light chain deposition. Lab Invest 1991;64:527–537.
6. Solomon A, Frangione B, Franklin EC: Bence Jones proteins and light chains of immunoglobulins: Preferential association of the V$_{IVI}$ subgroup of human light chains with amyloidosis AL(l). J Clin Invest 1982;70:453–460.
7. Schormann N, Murrell JR, Liepnieks JJ, Benson MD: Tertiary structure of an amyloid immunoglobulin light chain protein: A proposed model for amyloid fibril formation. Proc Natl Acad Sci U S A 1995;92:9490–9494.
8. Wall JS, Gupta V, Wilkerson M, et al: Structural basis of light chain amyloidogenicity: Comparison of the thermodynamic properties, fibrillogenic potential and tertiary structural features of four V$_l$6 proteins. J Mol Recognit 2004;17:323–331.
9. Eulitz M, Weiss DT, Solomon A: Immunoglobulin heavy-chain-associated amyloidosis. Proc Natl Acad Sci U S A 1990;87: 6542–6546.
10. Zhu L, Herrera GA, Murphy-Ullrich JE, et al: Pathogenesis of glomerulosclerosis in light chain deposition disease: Role for transforming growth factor-β. Am J Pathol 1995;147: 375–385.
11. Rocca A, Khamlichi AA, Aucouturier P, et al: Primary structure of a variable region of the V$_{kI}$ subgroup (ISE) in light chain deposition disease. Clin Exp Immunol 1993;91:506–509.
12. Bellotti V, Stoppini M, Merlini G, et al: Amino acid sequence of k Sci, the Bence Jones protein isolated from a patient with light chain deposition disease. Biochim Biophys Acta 1991;1097: 177–182.
13. Cogné M, Preud'homme J-L, Bauwens M, et al: Structure of a monoclonal kappa chain of the V kappa IV subgroup in the kidney and plasma cells in light chain deposition disease. J Clin Invest 1991;87:2186–2190.
14. Khamlichi AA, Rocca A, Touchard G, et al: Role of light chain variable region in myeloma with light chain deposition disease: Evidence from an experimental model. Blood 1995;86:3655–3659.
15. Deret S, Denoroy L, Lamarine M, et al: Kappa light chain-associated Fanconi's syndrome: Molecular analysis of monoclonal immunoglobulin light chains from patients with and without intracellular crystals. Protein Eng 1999;12:363–369.
16. Decourt C, Bridoux F, Touchard G, Cogné M: A monoclonal V kl light chain responsible for incomplete proximal tubulopathy. Am J Kidney Dis 2003;41:497–504.
17. Ying W-Z, Sanders PW: Mapping the binding domain of immunoglobulin light chains for Tamm-Horsfall protein. Am J Pathol 2001;158:1859–1866.
18. Huang Z-Q, Kirk KA, Connelly KG, Sanders PW: Bence Jones proteins bind to a common peptide segment of Tamm-Horsfall glycoprotein to promote heterotypic aggregation. J Clin Invest 1993;92:2975–2983.
19. Huang Z-Q, Sanders PW: Biochemical interaction of Tamm-Horsfall glycoprotein with Ig light chains. Lab Invest 1995;73: 810–817.

20. Sanders PW, Booker BB, Bishop JB, Cheung HC: Mechanisms of intranephronal proteinaceous cast formation by low molecular weight proteins. J Clin Invest 1990;85:570–576.

21. Bradwell AR, Carr-Smith HD, Mead GP, et al: Highly sensitive, automated immunoassay for immunoglobulin free light chains in serum and urine. Clin Chem 2001;47:673–680.

22. Mead GP, Carr-Smith HD, Drayson MT, et al: Serum free light chains for monitoring multiple myeloma. Br J Haematol 2004;126:348–354.

23. van Rhee F, Bolejack V, Hollmig K, et al: High serum free-light chain levels and their rapid reduction in response to therapy define an aggressive multiple myeloma subtype with poor prognosis. Blood 2007;110:827–832.

24. van Ingen G, van Bronswijk H, Meijer CJLM, Stel HV: Light chain deposition disease without detectable light chains in serum or urine. Report of a case and review of the literature. Neth J Med 1991;39:142–147.

25. Preud'homme J-L, Aucouturier P, Touchard G, et al: Monoclonal immunoglobulin deposition disease (Randall type). Relationship with structural abnormalities of immunoglobulin chains. Kidney Int 1994;46:965–972.

26. Buxbaum JN, Chuba JV, Hellman GC, et al: Monoclonal immunoglobulin deposition disease: Light chain and light and heavy chain deposition diseases and their relation to light chain amyloidosis. Ann Intern Med 1990;112:455–464.

27. Katzmann JA, Clark RJ, Abraham RS, et al: Serum reference intervals and diagnostic ranges for free kappa and free lambda immunoglobulin light chains: Relative sensitivity for detection of monoclonal light chains. Clin Chem 2002;48:1437–1444.

28. Abraham RS, Katzmann JA, Clark RJ, et al: Quantitative analysis of serum free light chains. A new marker for the diagnostic evaluation of primary systemic amyloidosis. Am J Clin Pathol 2003;119:274–278.

29. Skinner M, Anderson JJ, Simms R, et al: Treatment of 100 patients with primary amyloidosis: A randomized trial of melphalan, prednisone, and colchicine versus colchicine only. Am J Med 1996;100:290–298.

30. Comenzo RL, Vosburgh E, Falk RH, et al: Dose-intensive melphalan with blood stem-cell support for the treatment of AL (amyloid light-chain) amyloidosis: Survival and responses in 25 patients. Blood 1998;91:3662–3670.

31. Skinner M, Sanchorawala V, Seldin DC, et al: High-dose melphalan and autologous stem-cell transplantation in patients with AL amyloidosis: An 8-year study. Ann Intern Med 2004;140:85–93.

32. Kyle RA, Gertz MA, Greipp PR, et al: A trial of three regimens for primary amyloidosis: Colchicine alone, melphalan and prednisone, and melphalan, prednisone, and colchicine. N Engl J Med 1997;336:1202–1207.

33. Seldin DC, Anderson JJ, Sanchorawala V, et al: Improvement in quality of life of patients with AL amyloidosis treated with high-dose melphalan and autologous stem cell transplantation. Blood 2004;104:1888–1093.

34. Dispenzieri A, Kyle RA, Lacy MQ, et al: Superior survival in primary systemic amyloidosis patients undergoing peripheral blood stem cell transplantation: A case-control study. Blood 2004;103:3960–3963.

35. Sanchorawala V, Wright DG, Seldin DC, et al: High-dose intravenous melphalan and autologous stem cell transplantation as initial therapy or following two cycles of oral chemotherapy for the treatment of AL amyloidosis: Results of a prospective randomized trial. Bone Marrow Transplant 2004;33:381–388.

36. Snanoudj R, Mamzer-Bruneel MF, Hermine O, et al: Recovery of acute renal failure and nephrotic syndrome following autologous stem cell transplantation for primary (AL) amyloidosis. Nephrol Dial Transplant 2003;18:2175–2177.

37. Bohne S, Sletten K, Menard R, et al: Cleavage of AL amyloid proteins and AL amyloid deposits by cathepsins B, K, and L. J Pathol 2004;203:528–537.

38. Zeier M, Perz J, Linke RP, et al: No regression of renal AL amyloid in monoclonal gammopathy after successful autologous blood stem cell transplantation and significant clinical improvement. Nephrol Dial Transplant 2003;18:2644–2647.

39. Durie BG, Kyle RA, Belch A, et al: Myeloma management guidelines: A consensus report from the Scientific Advisors of the International Myeloma Foundation. Hematol J 2003;4:379–398.

40. Leung N, Dispenzieri A, Fervenza FC, et al: Renal response after high-dose melphalan and stem cell transplantation is a favorable marker in patients with primary systemic amyloidosis. Am J Kidney Dis 2005;46:270–277.

41. Badros A, Barlogie B, Siegel E, et al: Results of autologous stem cell transplant in multiple myeloma patients with renal failure. Br J Haematol 2001;114:822–829.

42. Mollee PN, Wechalekar AD, Pereira DL, et al: Autologous stem cell transplantation in primary systemic amyloidosis: The impact of selection criteria on outcome. Bone Marrow Transplant 2004;33:271–277.

43. Barlogie B, Desikan R, Eddlemon P, et al: Extended survival in advanced and refractory multiple myeloma after single-agent thalidomide: Identification of prognostic factors in a phase 2 study of 169 patients. Blood 2001;98:492–494.

44. Gertz MA, Lacy MQ, Dispenzieri A: Therapy for immunoglobulin light chain amyloidosis: The new and the old. Blood Rev 2004;18:17–37.

45. Izzedine H, Launay-Vacher V, Deray G: Thalidomide for the nephrologist. Nephrol Dial Transplant 2005;20:2011–2012.

46. Fakhouri F, Guerraoui H, Presne C, et al: Thalidomide in patients with multiple myeloma and renal failure. Br J Haematol 2004;125:96–97.

47. Harris E, Behrens J, Samson D, et al: Use of thalidomide in patients with myeloma and renal failure may be associated with unexplained hyperkalaemia. Br J Haematol 2003;122:160–161.

48. Sanchorawala V, Wright DG, Rosenzweig M, et al: Lenalidomide and dexamethasone in the treatment of AL amyloidosis: Results of a phase 2 trial. Blood 2007;109:492–496.

49. Hartmann A, Holdaas H, Fauchald P, et al: Fifteen years' experience with renal transplantation in systemic amyloidosis. Transplant Int 1992;5:15–18.

50. Leung N, Griffin MD, Dispenzieri A, et al: Living donor kidney and autologous stem cell transplantation for primary systemic amyloidosis (AL) with predominant renal involvement. Am J Transplant 2005;5:1660–1670.

51. Ronco PM, Alyanakian MA, Mougenot B, Aucouturier P: Light chain deposition disease: A model of glomerulosclerosis defined at the molecular level. J Am Soc Nephrol 2001;12:1558–1565.

52. Royer B, Arnulf B, Martinez F, et al: High dose chemotherapy in light chain or light and heavy chain deposition disease. Kidney Int 2004;65:642–648.

53. Weichman K, Dember LM, Prokaeva T, et al: Clinical and molecular characteristics of patients with non-amyloid light chain deposition disorders, and outcome following treatment with high-dose melphalan and autologous stem cell transplantation. Bone Marrow Transplant 2006;38:339–343.

54. Lee CK, Zangari M, Barlogie B, et al: Dialysis-dependent renal failure in patients with myeloma can be reversed by high-dose myeloablative therapy and autotransplant. Bone Marrow Transplant 2004;33:823–828.

55. Howard AD, Moore J, Tomaszewski M-M: Occurrence of multiple myeloma three years after successful renal transplantation. Am J Kidney Dis 1987;10:147–150.

56. Alpers CE, Marchioro TL, Johnson RJ: Monoclonal immunoglobulin deposition disease in a renal allograft: Probable recurrent disease in a patient without myeloma. Am J Kidney Dis 1989;13:418–423.

57. Leung N, Lager DJ, Gertz MA, et al: Long-term outcome of renal transplantation in light-chain deposition disease. Am J Kidney Dis 2004;43:147–153.

58. Sanders PW, Booker BB: Pathobiology of cast nephropathy from human Bence Jones proteins. J Clin Invest 1992;89:630–639.

59. Holland MD, Galla JH, Sanders PW, Luke RG: Effect of urinary pH and diatrizoate on Bence Jones protein nephrotoxicity in the rat. Kidney Int 1985;27:46–50.

60. MRC Working Party on Leukemia in Adults: Analysis and management of renal failure in fourth MRC myelomatosis trial. Br Med J 1984;288:1411–1416.

61. Berenson JR, Lichtenstein A, Porter L, et al: Efficacy of pamidronate in reducing skeletal events in patients with advanced multiple myeloma. N Engl J Med 1996;334:488–493.

62. Attal M, Harousseau J-L, Stoppa A-M, et al: A prospective, randomized trial of autologous bone marrow transplantation and chemotherapy in multiple myeloma. N Engl J Med 1996;335:91–97.

63. Child JA, Morgan GJ, Davies FE, et al: High-dose chemotherapy with hematopoietic stem-cell rescue for multiple myeloma. N Engl J Med 2003;348:1875–1883.

64. Barlogie B, Shaughnessy J, Tricot G, et al: Treatment of multiple myeloma. Blood 2004;103:20–32.

65. Barlogie B, Smith L, Alexanian R: Effective treatment of advanced multiple myeloma refractory to alkylating agents. N Engl J Med 1984;310:1353–1356.

66. Kyle RA: Update on the treatment of multiple myeloma. Oncologist 2001;6:119–124.

67. Govindarajan R, Jagannath S, Flick JT, et al: Preceding standard therapy is the likely cause of MDS after autotransplants for multiple myeloma. Br J Haematol 1996;95:349–353.

68. Jagannath S, Barlogie B, Berenson JR, et al: Bortezomib in recurrent and/or refractory multiple myeloma. Initial clinical experience in patients with impaired renal function. Cancer 2005;103:1195–1200.

69. Singhal S, Mehta J, Desikan R, et al: Antitumor activity of thalidomide in refractory multiple myeloma. N Engl J Med 1999;341:1565–1571.

70. Harousseau JL, Attal M, Leleu X, et al: Bortezomib plus dexamethasone as induction treatment prior to autologous stem cell transplantation in patients with newly diagnosed multiple myeloma: Results of an IFM phase II study. Haematologica 2006;91:1498–1505.

71. Breitkreutz I, Lokhorst HM, Raab MS, et al: Thalidomide in newly diagnosed multiple myeloma: Influence of thalidomide treatment on peripheral blood stem cell collection yield. Leukemia 2007;21:1294–1299.

72. Ma SY, Lie AK, Au WY, et al: Non-myeloablative allogeneic peripheral stem cell transplantation for multiple myeloma. Hong Kong Med J 2004;10:77–83.

73. Badros A, Barlogie B, Siegel E, et al: Improved outcome of allogeneic transplantation in high-risk multiple myeloma patients after nonmyeloablative conditioning. J Clin Oncol 2002;20:1295–1303.

74. Bruno B, Rotta M, Patriarca F, et al: A comparison of allografting with autografting for newly diagnosed myeloma. N Engl J Med 2007;356:1110–1120.

75. Zucchelli P, Pasquali S, Cagnoli L, Ferrari G: Controlled plasma exchange trial in acute renal failure due to multiple myeloma. Kidney Int 1988;33:1175–1180.

76. Wahlin A, Löfvenberg E, Holm J: Improved survival in multiple myeloma with renal failure. Acta Med Scand 1987;221:205–209.

77. Clark WF, Stewart AK, Rock GA, et al: Plasma exchange when myeloma presents as acute renal failure: A randomized, controlled trial. Ann Intern Med 2005;143:777–784.

78. Hutchison CA, Cockwell P, Reid S, et al: Efficient removal of immunoglobulin free light chains by hemodialysis for multiple myeloma: In vitro and in vivo studies. J Am Soc Nephrol 2007;18:886–895.

79. Shetty A, Oreopoulos DG: Continuous ambulatory peritoneal dialysis in end-stage renal disease due to multiple myeloma. Perit Dial Int 1995;15:236–240.

80. Chng WJ, Schop RF, Price-Troska T, et al: Gene-expression profiling of Waldenstrom macroglobulinemia reveals a phenotype more similar to chronic lymphocytic leukemia than multiple myeloma. Blood 2006;108:2755–2763.

81. Ghobrial IM, Fonseca R, Gertz MA, et al: Prognostic model for disease-specific and overall mortality in newly diagnosed symptomatic patients with Waldenstrom macroglobulinaemia. Br J Haematol 2006;133:158–164.

82. Schop RF, Van Wier SA, Xu R, et al: 6q deletion discriminates Waldenström macroglobulinemia from IgM monoclonal gammopathy of undetermined significance. Cancer Genet Cytogenet 2006;169:150–153.

83. MacKenzie MR, Lee TK: Blood viscosity in Waldenström macroglobulinemia. Blood 1977;49:507–510.

84. Rodriguez JN, Fernandez-Jurado A, Martino ML, Prados D: Waldenström's macroglobulinemia complicated with acute myeloid leukemia. Report of a case and review of the literature. Haematologica 1998;83:91–92.

85. Byrd JC, White CA, Link B, et al: Rituximab therapy in Waldenström's macroglobulinemia: Preliminary evidence of clinical activity. Ann Oncol 1999;10:1525–1527.

Further Reading

Barlogie B, Shaughnessy J, Tricot G, et al: Treatment of multiple myeloma. Blood 2004;103:20–32.

Child JA, Morgan GJ, Davies FE, et al: High-dose chemotherapy with hematopoietic stem-cell rescue for multiple myeloma. N Engl J Med 2003;348:1875–1883.

Clark WF, Stewart AK, Rock GA, et al: Plasma exchange when myeloma presents as acute kidney injury: A randomized, controlled trial. Ann Intern Med 2005;143:777–784.

Dispenzieri A, Kyle RA, Lacy MQ, et al: Superior survival in primary systemic amyloidosis patients undergoing peripheral blood stem cell transplantation: A case-control study. Blood 2004;103:3960–3963.

Durie BG, Kyle RA, Belch A, et al: Myeloma management guidelines: A consensus report from the Scientific Advisors of the International Myeloma Foundation. Hematol J 2003;4:379–398.

Gertz MA: Waldenström macroglobulinemia: A review of therapy. Am J Hematol 2005;79:147–157.

Mead GP, Carr-Smith HD, Drayson MT, et al: Serum free light chains for monitoring multiple myeloma. Br J Haematol 2004;126:348–354.

Ronco PM, Alyanakian MA, Mougenot B, Aucouturier P: Light chain deposition disease: A model of glomerulosclerosis defined at the molecular level. J Am Soc Nephrol 2001;12:1558–1565.

Skinner M, Sanchorawala V, Seldin DC, et al: High-dose melphalan and autologous stem-cell transplantation in patients with AL amyloidosis: An 8-year study. Ann Intern Med 2004;140:85–93.

van Rhee F, Bolejack V, Hollmig K, et al: High serum free-light chain levels and their rapid reduction in response to therapy define an aggressive multiple myeloma subtype with poor prognosis. Blood 2007;110:827–832.

Chapter 40

Obstructive Uropathy

Christopher J. Cutie and W. Scott McDougal

Obstructive uropathy is defined as any functional impedance to the anterograde flow of urine. This obstruction may occur in the upper tract (renal pelvis, ureters), lower tract (bladder, urethra), or both, and may be the result of an intrinsic defect or extrinsic process. A common cause of renal function compromise, urinary obstruction may be diagnosed and treated with multiple modalities, depending on the nature and location of the obstruction. Timely diagnosis and treatment of acute obstruction, as well as the appropriate management of chronic obstruction, is a multidisciplinary effort requiring contributions by primary care providers, internists, nephrologists, urologists, and radiologists.

OVERVIEW

The degree of urinary obstruction typically correlates with the patient's clinical presentation. Complete bilateral obstruction results in anuria, whereas partial or unilateral obstruction may present with intermittent episodes of oliguria and polyuria. Clinical symptoms of urinary obstruction may include flank, suprapubic, or groin discomfort; recurrent urinary tract infections; dysuria; hematuria; stranguria; and acute or chronic renal failure. Acute bilateral obstruction results in postrenal failure. The serum blood urea nitrogen-to-creatinine ratio approximates 10:1 and the urine-to-plasma urea and urine-to-plasma creatinine ratios are indistinguishable from intrarenal failure. Complete anuria requires a prompt evaluation for an obstructing process.

Management of obstruction relies on adequate drainage of the urinary system. Bladder decompression may be achieved by placement of either a urethral catheter or suprapubic cystotomy tube. Drainage of the renal collecting system is possible both endoscopically in a retrograde fashion with a ureteral stent or percutaneously with a nephrostomy tube. Endoscopic procedures typically require administration of spinal or general anesthesia. In the setting of a critically ill patient with other significant comorbidities, nephrostomy tube placement is often the preferred technique because this can be performed under ultrasound guidance with either minimal intravenous sedation or local anesthesia. In either scenario, definitive intervention is necessary for the ultimate preservation of renal function.

Although acute urinary obstruction must be managed expeditiously, chronic urinary tract obstruction also requires timely diagnosis and management. Chronic obstruction may predispose the afflicted patient to a variety of conditions that are wide-ranging in severity. Urine stasis often leads to bacterial colonization, with sequelae ranging from urinary tract infections and pyelonephritis to fulminant urosepsis and concomitant cardiovascular collapse. Long-standing partial obstruction may also compromise the functional integrity of various structures, particularly the bladder and upper tracts of the renal collecting system, both of which are fairly sensitive to intraluminal pressure changes. This chapter discusses the multiple causes of urinary obstruction as well as the diagnostic considerations and available treatment modalities of each.

CALCULI

Urolithiasis is the most common cause of urinary obstruction, accounting for approximately \$2.1 billion in health care expenditures annually.[1] In the United States, 13% of men and 7% of women will be diagnosed with kidney stones at some point throughout their lifetime.[2] Peak age at diagnosis in men is 30 years, whereas women exhibit a bimodal distribution, with peaks at 35 and 55 years. Although many of these stones are found incidentally and are not associated with symptoms of pain, obstruction, or infection, the risk of hospitalization and surgical intervention is ever present and increasing as the general population grows. Furthermore, 50% of patients with a history of urolithiasis will re-form stones within 5 years.[2]

The majority of calculi are composed of uric acid, calcium oxalate monohydrate, calcium oxalate dihydrate, cystine, or ammonium magnesium phosphate (struvite) or some combination thereof. Stones typically form within the collecting system of the kidney and subsequently travel to distal portions of the urinary tract. However, they may also form at the site of a foreign body (i.e., stent, catheter, suture material, human hair). Depending on their size, composition, and conformation, stones may either pass spontaneously in the urine or impact anywhere along the course of the urinary tract. The three most common sites for stone impaction are the ureteropelvic junction (UPJ), the mid-ureter at the level of the iliac vessels, and the ureterovesicle junction. The ureteric caliber at the UPJ and ureterovesicle junction is generally smaller than that along the course of the ureter. Extrinsic compression by the iliac vessels where the mid-ureter crosses causes a narrowing of the ureteral lumen at this level.

The likelihood of spontaneous passage of calculi is dependent on several criteria. These include stone size and shape, as well as patient anatomy and history of stone passage.[3] However, due to the intrinsic variability of an individual's ureteral caliber, as well as the conformation of calculi, these criteria serve merely as a guide and must be appropriately incorporated into each clinical setting. Reported percentages of spontaneous stone passage vary widely in the literature, ranging from 29% to 98% for stones 0.5 cm or smaller located in the proximal ureter compared with rates of 71% to 98% for those of comparable size located in the distal ureter.[3] Stones ranging from 0.5 to 1.0 cm have a lower likelihood of spontaneous passage, with rates ranging from 10% to 53% for those in the proximal ureter; rates are somewhat better for the distal ureter, ranging from 23% to 53%.[3] Moreover, recent studies have demonstrated the utility of α-adrenergic blockers, calcium channel blockers, and nonsteroidal anti-inflammatory medications in facilitating spontaneous stone passage via ureteral smooth muscle relaxation.[4,5]

Treatment Options

Dissolution therapy is an appropriate first-line treatment modality for uric acid and cystine stones. Uric acid stones, comprising 5% to 10% of all urinary stones, typically form in an acidic urine (pH $\leq$ 5.5).[6] They are relatively soft compared with calcium oxalate and cystine stones and are associated with hyperuricosuria, low urinary volume, and persistently acidic urine. These stones are often radiolucent on radiographic imaging and measure a density of 500 Hounsfield units or less on computed tomography. Dissolution therapy with oral urine alkalinizing medications (potassium citrate) has been shown to be efficacious in as many as 80% of patients.[6] Those patients failing dissolution therapy may then be further treated with a surgical intervention.

Cystine stones, which account for approximately 1% of all urinary calculi, also form in acidic urine. Cystinuria results from a defect in the renal tubular absorption of the amino acids cystine, ornithine, lysine, and arginine. Patients with the inherited autosomal recessive disorder excrete in excess of 600 mg of cystine daily in their urine (normal < 100 mg/day). In addition to increasing urine volume, first-line therapy remains urine alkalization with a goal urine pH of more than 7.0. Should dissolution therapy be ineffective, patients may also be treated with oral chelating agents, such as D-penicillamine (250 mg

every 6 hours) or α-mercaptopropionylglycine (250 mg every 6 hours) to increase urine cystine solubility.[7] Cystine stone formers will often present with staghorn calculi. These stones are extremely dense (> 1200 Hounsfield units) and are therefore not amenable to certain treatment modalities, such as extracorporeal shock wave therapy (ESWL).

Struvite stones, in comparison, form in alkaline urine. Commonly associated with chronic urinary tract infections secondary to urea-splitting pathogens (*Proteus mirabilis, Klebsiella pneumoniae, Pseudomonas aeruginosa*), these stones exist in a urine pH of more than 7.5. Urease splits urea into component ammonia groups, resulting in alkaline urine. Because these stones are closely associated with infection, definitive treatment relies on clearance of all stone burden and maintenance of a sterile urine, typically through antibiotic prophylaxis.

Prevention

Prevention of recurrent urolithiasis is based on maintaining high urine volume, increasing the concentration of stone-inhibiting substances in the urine, and decreasing the concentration of lithogenic substances. Patients are encouraged to consume more than 2.5 L of fluid daily and to supplement their fluid intake with citrate-rich fluids, such as lemonade.[8] Citrate binds calcium in the urine and inhibits calcium oxalate crystal formation. Foods rich in oxalate, such as tea, coffee, leafy green vegetables (spinach), rhubarb, nuts, and beer should be avoided. Meats and other protein-rich foods should also be consumed in moderation, as degradation of these purine-heavy foods results in elevated serum uric acid concentrations. Allopurinol may also be prescribed for those patients with hyperuricemia. Cystine stone formers should be counseled to reduce their intake of methionine-containing foods, such as meats and dairy products.

Surgical Intervention

Recent advances in the endoscopic treatment of calculi and the significant improvement of lithotripsy devices have allowed the majority of surgical treatments to be performed in an outpatient setting. Holmium pulsed-dye lasers have become ever more powerful and are relatively easy to use. Furthermore, ureteroscopes and imaging equipment have dramatically improved, allowing excellent visualization of ureteral and renal pelvic anatomy and calculi. Renal stones measuring as large as 2 cm may now be treated with staged ureteroscopic procedures or ESWL, depending on the location and hardness of the stone. Selection criteria for surgical stone management include stone location, size, composition, collecting system/ureteral anatomy, patient health/performance status, and patient preference.

ESWL involves delivery of shock waves generated by electromagnetic energy sources. These shock waves are propagated through water and delivered to the stone burden under direct, real-time fluoroscopic imaging. To reliably use ESWL, patient selection is vitally important. The stone must be radiopaque and visualized on standard radiographs because fluoroscopy or ultrasonography is used intraoperatively to identify and target the stone. Shock waves are then delivered to the stone until evidence of fragmentation is identified. ESWL may often be performed under conscious sedation, although some patients may require administration of general anesthesia for improved tolerability. Although ESWL is noninvasive, it has been associated with specific risks, including cardiac arrhythmias, renal contusions, hemorrhage, and bruising. Recent studies also suggest that ESWL may be associated with the delayed development of diabetes due to pancreatic fibrosis secondary to shock wave injury.[9]

ESWL is appropriate for stones measuring as much as 1.5 cm located above the bony pelvis. The ischial body may impede shock wave propagation and mute the fragmentation effects on stones located in the distal ureter. Moreover, patients undergoing ESWL treatment must be warned of the risks of steinstrasse, literally translated as "a road of stone." This occurs when a stone is broken into multiple smaller fragments and the lead fragment is unable to spontaneously pass, which causes ureteral obstruction proximal to the stone burden. Classic symptoms of flank pain, dysuria, and hematuria may result, and a secondary procedure (e.g., stent or nephrostomy tube placement, salvage ureteroscopy) is often necessary because the lead fragment will not pass.

Ureteroscopy is defined as any endoscopic manipulation of the ureter and its contents. Since its development in the early 1980s, ureteroscopy has revolutionized the treatment of ureteral and renal stones.[10] Whereas open ureterolithotomy for stone extraction was commonly performed through the 1970s and required an inpatient hospitalization, ureteroscopy allows outpatient treatment of most urinary stones today. Rigid and flexible ureteroscopes are currently available and are used either independently or in tandem depending on stone size and location. Standard ureteroscopes measure approximately 8 French in size and are introduced via the urethra to the level of the stone. Various tools, including holmium lasers and nitinol extraction baskets, are then used to fragment, retrieve, and remove the stone. A ureteral stent is typically placed for temporary renal decompression and to allow residual stone fragments to pass. This stent also mitigates the risk of ureteral obstruction from posttreatment ureteral inflammation and edema.

If dissolution therapy fails or is not feasible, staghorn calculi and large renal stones are best treated with percutaneous nephrolithotomy, which requires nephrostomy access to the kidney via the flank. This procedure allows for high stone-free rates with fewer secondary procedures necessary.[11] Open surgery, including pyelolithotomy and anatrophic nephrolithotomy, is rarely performed and reserved for those patients with highly complicated anatomy (e.g., crossed-fused ectopia, horseshoe kidney) or grossly enlarged stone burden (>5 cm). With the increased popularity of laparoscopic procedures, minimally invasive pyelolithotomy is also frequently offered for large renal pelvic or ureteropelvic junction stones.

URETEROPELVIC JUNCTION OBSTRUCTION

UPJ obstruction accounts for approximately 50% of prenatally diagnosed hydronephrosis. Classically, UPJ obstruction presents as a unilateral process; however, bilateral obstruction may occur. Causes of UPJ obstruction may be both intrinsic and extrinsic in nature. In some instances, there is a crossing anatomic vessel (an accessory renal artery or vein), which kinks the ureter at the level of the UPJ. Surgical correction of the anomaly with pyeloplasty and vessel transposition is the definitive treatment. Intrinsic defects within the ureter, including an aperistaltic segment secondary to malformation of the ureteral musculature as well as ureteral valves (Ostling's valves) are a cause of UPJ obstruction in children.[12] Diagnosis typically is made based on a ^{99m}Tc-mercaptoacetylglycine study or intravenous pyelography. Again, treatment involves a pyeloplasty and excision of this aperistaltic segment. Impacted ureteral stones and previous endoscopic ureteral manipulation, with concomitant ureteral inflammation and fibrosis, may also result in ureteral strictures, leading to UPJ obstruction. Excision of this stenotic segment and primary reanastomosis is the recommended treatment. Endopyelotomy or ureteroscopic incision of ureteral strictures and balloon dilatation have been reported as other initial management options with varying degrees of success.[13]

Before a major surgical repair, the degree of function in the affected kidney should be calculated. This is commonly performed using a dimercaptosuccinic acid scan, a radionuclide study that measures the uptake of tracer material within the renal tubules and is a reliable means of assessing renal function. Because the goal of therapy is to maintain existing renal function, which is not apt to improve after pyeloplasty, a simple nephrectomy as definitive treatment should be considered.

BENIGN PROSTATIC HYPERPLASIA

Benign prostatic hyperplasia (BPH) is a commonly diagnosed condition that is responsible for a significant proportion of lower urinary tract complaints in middle-aged and elderly men. In the United States in 2000, this condition accounted for 117,000 emergency department visits and 105,000 hospitalizations, accounting for $1.1 billion in expenditures.[1] A consequence of persistent testosterone stimulation, BPH occurs as a result of growth of adenomatous prostatic tissue. This is a benign condition and may be managed expectantly, pharmacologically, or surgically. Chronic obstruction, left untreated, results in recurrent bladder overdistention, which may lead to bladder trabeculation and formation of diverticula and cellules. These outpouchings of bladder epithelium can further predispose the patient to urinary tract infections, stone formation, and, most importantly, deterioration of the upper tracts leading to compromised renal function and ultimately renal failure.

Patients with significant lower urinary tract symptoms should be evaluated by a urologist. Although symptoms of urinary frequency, hesitancy, and urgency may be attributed to BPH, evaluation of the lower urinary tract is required. Thorough physical examination should include suprapubic palpation and inspection of the penis for evidence of meatal stenosis or phimosis. A digital rectal examination is required, and patients are encouraged to complete a symptom score questionnaire. This questionnaire rates symptoms of nocturia, urgency, frequency, stranguria, force of urine stream, intermittency, and the need for second voiding and serves as a baseline for subsequent comparison after initiation of medical therapy or surgery. Cystoscopy is recommended for specific indications, such as hematuria, suspected bladder stones, or early bladder cancer. Transition cell carcinoma in situ is often associated with irritative urinary symptoms.[14] A postvoid residual and uroflow are also important studies in the diagnosis of BPH. A postvoid residual greater than 200 mL is significant, as is a uroflow rate of less than 15 mL/sec.[15] Ultimately, because this is a benign condition, informed treatment decisions should be based on patient satisfaction and perceived quality of life.

Treatment Options

Medications

There are two main classes of medications prescribed for treatment of symptoms of BPH: α_1-adrenergic receptor blockers and 5α-reductase inhibitors. α-Blockers (terazosin, doxazosin, tamsulosin, alfuzosin) result in blockade of sympathetic peripheral α_1 receptors, resulting in relaxation of both prostatic and bladder neck smooth muscle. These medications are generally well tolerated but, given their mechanism of action, may cause hypotension, dizziness, or syncope. α-Blockers have been definitively shown to exhibit efficacy in the treatment of men with urinary symptoms attributable to BPH, but do not decrease the incidence of acute urinary retention episodes.[16]

5α-Reductase inhibitors (finasteride, dutasteride) inhibit the enzyme 5α-reductase, thus preventing conversion of testosterone to dihydrotestosterone, which is chemically active within the prostate and stimulates prostatic tissue growth. Such deprivation of dihydrotestosterone results in prostatic epithelial atrophy. Dutasteride (Avodart) inhibits both the type I and II forms of 5α-reductase and may provide an increased benefit to patients.[17] These medications are often used in tandem with α-blockers and have been shown to demonstrate great efficacy in multiple studies.[16,18] 5α-Reductase inhibitors do affect serum prostate-specific antigen (PSA) levels, typically decreasing them by 50%. Therefore, this decrease must be noted before initiation of 5α-reductase therapy because treatment may influence the subsequent care of patients managed with routine PSA screening and monitoring tests. Furthermore, patients applying topical 5α-reductase for hair growth (Propecia) must be informed that their serum PSA level will be reduced, typically by 50% as well.[19] Combination therapy with both α-blockers and 5α-reductase inhibitors appears to have a synergistic effect, as studies have shown an approximately 50% decrease in disease progression compared with monotherapy.[16] Of note, medications are not effective in patients with enlarged prostatic median lobes. The median lobe may serve as a ball valve, intermittently obstructing the bladder neck, resulting in outflow obstruction. These patients are best served by transurethral resection of this tissue.

BPH may result in an elevated PSA, although not typically to the levels seen in aggressive prostate cancer. However, an elevated PSA may not simply be attributed to prostatic hyperplasia, and an appropriate evaluation and work-up is warranted.

Surgery

Several technologic advances have vastly improved the urologist's armamentarium of surgical options for treatment of BPH. In addition to the standard transurethral resection of prostate tissue using the electrosurgical resectoscope, new devices incorporating laser and microwave energy have resulted in safer, faster, and more cost-effective treatment strategies. Various laser vaporization technologies, including holmium

and KTP (potassium titanyl phosphate), allow for significantly smaller intraoperative blood loss as well as fewer risks of postprocedure absorptive hyponatremia.[20] Many patients are catheter free after these procedures and do not require an inpatient hospitalization. These devices use a wavelength of light (523 nm) that is absorbed by both blood and tissue, allowing for more exact tissue destruction and simultaneous hemostasis. Microwave therapy has also exhibited efficacy as an office-based treatment modality, using a special urethral catheter with a thermal coil that delivers highly focused energy to the prostatic bed with resultant tissue necrosis. After administration of mild sedatives and topical urethral lidocaine, this catheter is inserted in the standard fashion by a urologist and left in place for approximately 30 to 60 minutes.

Expanding titanium urethral stents (UroLume) have also been developed for treatment of bladder outlet obstruction. These devices are endoscopically placed within the prostatic urethra and serve to stent open the urethral lumen by inhibiting coaptation of the prostatic lobes. Although success rates vary considerably for this procedure, these stents are associated with significant morbidity and are difficult to remove once urothelium has grown into them.[21] These devices are often reserved for poor surgical candidates who are unable to endure general anesthesia for more invasive procedures, such as transurethral resection.

GENITOURINARY MALIGNANCY

Occasionally, bladder, prostate, and urethral tumors may cause urinary obstruction. Muscle invasive bladder cancer arising from the trigone or base of the bladder can obstruct the ureteral orifices, resulting in hydroureteronephrosis. Transurethral resection of the tumor may alleviate this obstruction, but the cancer may recur if the resection is incomplete. Highly advanced prostate cancer may present with bladder outlet obstruction. Transurethral resection of the obstructing lesion is again the preferred treatment of choice. Both bladder and prostate cancers may often present in this situation with gross hematuria or clot retention. Urethral tumors, albeit rare, may also result in an intrinsic obstruction of urinary flow. Often, a catheter may be placed around the obstructing lesion as a temporary measure, followed by further workup and definitive treatment.

URETHRAL STRICTURE/STENOSIS

A urethral stricture is a narrowing of the urethral lumen, resulting in a slowing or cessation of urine flow.[22] Urethral strictures are significantly more common in males, given the far longer course of the male urethra compared with that of the female. Risk factors for urethral stricture disease include recurrent urinary tract infections or urethritis (i.e., gonococcal), trauma, previous urethral instrumentation or surgery, pelvic irradiation, and advanced age. Diagnosis is typically based on direct vision with cystoscopy as well as retrograde urethrography to delineate the anatomic location and length of the stricture. Treatment modalities include manual dilatation (metal sounds, balloon dilators), transurethral incision/resection, and open primary repair. Because these strictures are typically composed of dense scar tissue, they tend to recur in the absence of definitive open surgery. A biopsy of the tissue at the stricture site should always be performed to rule out a coincident urethral tumor as the obstructing lesion.

Presenting symptoms of urethral strictures often include urinary urgency and hesitancy, decreased force or caliber of the urine stream, persistent suprapubic fullness, recurrent urinary infections, the need for frequent second voids, and urinary retention. In some patients, the stricture is such that urethral catheter placement in the standard blind fashion is not possible, requiring placement of a catheter over a wire under cystoscopic guidance or placement of a suprapubic cystostomy tube for acute bladder decompression.

BLADDER DYSFUNCTION

In the normal state, voiding is a reflex function under voluntary control. Coordinated voiding, characterized by external sphincter relaxation and subsequent detrusor contraction, is controlled by the pontine micturition complex's effect on the sacral cord (S2-S4).[23] The pontine micturition complex, in turn, is under cortical control. Detrusor hyperreflexia with coordinated external sphincter activity results from suprapontine lesions (e.g., stroke, Parkinson's disease). This is in contrast to detrusor hyperreflexia without coordinated external sphincter activity, which is caused by a suprasacral spinal lesion (e.g., myelodysplasia, multiple sclerosis). Detrusor areflexia is caused by damage to the sacral reflex arc (e.g., neuropathy, disk herniation), and also occurs during the acute spinal shock phase after a spinal cord injury. Urodynamics, a real-time study that measures bladder pressure, abdominal pressure, sphincter activity, bladder compliance, and flow rate, is commonly used to delineate these disorders.

Optimal bladder function relies on adequate maintenance of filling and emptying pressures in both the storage and expulsion of urine. During the filling stage, bladder pressures must be low enough to allow for transit of urine from the ureter to the bladder. Should the bladder pressure exceed the ureteral and renal pelvic pressures, urine will reflux in a retrograde fashion, resulting in ureteral dilatation. The ureter can withstand continuous intravesicle pressures as high as approximately 40 cm H_2O. Higher resting pressures lead to ureteral damage and resultant renal compromise.

The voiding stage is dependent on an important interplay between the bladder detrusor smooth muscle and the external skeletal muscle sphincter. At the initiation of a void, the external sphincter is relaxed under voluntary control, followed by contraction of the detrusor muscle. This allows for the coordinated flow of urine in an anterograde fashion. A defect in the detrusor muscle, external sphincter, or signaling neuron pathways therein results in bladder dysfunction. The result is a high-pressure bladder with inadequate voiding. Treatment modalities include anticholinergic medications (e.g., tolterodine, oxybutynin) to inhibit detrusor contraction.

Clean intermittent catheterization is the ideal modality for bladder decompression in the patient with urinary obstruction secondary to neurogenic bladder dysfunction.[24] Long-term indwelling catheters are not recommended because these can result in a host of complications, including recurrent urinary tract infections, urethral meatal erosion,

orchitis, epididymitis, prostatitis, bladder calculi, and squamous metaplasia of the bladder epithelium, a premalignant condition.[25] Clean intermittent catheterization requires diligent attention to patient hygiene, catheter care, and catheterization technique.

Those patients with detrusor-sphincter dyssynergia, characterized by bladder hyperreflexia with coordinated external sphincter relaxation, are plagued by poor bladder compliance and outlet obstruction. Bladder augmentation with subsequent clean intermittent catheterization may be recommended for these patients to ensure adequate urine storage and drainage. However, in those not suitable for augmentation or the necessary maintenance techniques required, urinary diversion is also a viable option. A sphincterotomy may also be performed, but this ultimately results in incontinence.

EXTRINSIC COMPRESSION

A variety of other oncologic and inflammatory conditions may result in obstructive uropathy as a result of extrinsic compression of one or both ureters, the bladder, or the urethra. Gynecologic malignancies arising from pelvic organs, such as the cervix, ovary, and uterus, may result in a mass effect on the ureters or trigone of the bladder, resulting in urinary obstruction. This may also result from masses of the colon and inflammatory processes, such as sigmoid diverticulitis, Crohn's disease, and ulcerative colitis. Such inflammatory reaction may result in a reactive fibrosis around one or both ureters, leading to proximal obstruction of urine. With regards to tumor compression, this typically occurs as a chronic process, with the gradual onset of flank pain. Ultrasonography or computed tomography will often demonstrate unilateral or bilateral hydronephrosis in the setting of an enlarging pelvic mass, potentially in the absence of symptoms (silent hydronephrosis). Decompression of the renal collecting system with either a percutaneous nephrostomy tube or ureteral stent is indicated, as this obstruction may predispose the patient to renal failure in the setting of chemotherapy for the primary tumor. Moreover, as many of these patients are immunosuppressed due to immunotherapy or as a consequence of the disease, an obstructed collecting system may be a setup for urinary tract infections and subsequent urosepsis, which may prove fatal in the debilitated patient.

POSTOBSTRUCTIVE DIURESIS

Urinary obstruction, either unilateral or bilateral, may result in fluid overload, renal insufficiency, and electrolyte abnormalities. However, relief of this obstruction may also result in profound effects on the patient's volume status and electrolyte homeostasis. Acute decompression of the bladder will often result in polyuria and, in some cases, hematuria. This hematuria is due to decompression of previously dilated mucosal cystic vessels, which rupture in the setting of intravesicle pressure changes. It may be fairly significant and require clot evacuation and continuous bladder irrigation.

Postobstructive diuresis may be physiologic, pathologic, or a combination of the two. Physiologic diuresis occurs as a result of fluid overload and elevated urea levels, which are excreted when the obstruction is relieved. Pathologic diuresis occurs as a result of increased tubule permeability and lack of an osmotic gradient in the renal medulla. Postobstructive polyuria is characterized by increased salt and water excretion and may vary widely with respect to volume. As many as 10% of patients will exhibit excessive diuresis, requiring intravenous fluid replacement. To accurately assess clinical improvement and normalization of volume status, daily weight, urine output, and orthostatic blood pressures are recorded. Plasma electrolytes should be monitored carefully (every 6–12 hours in the acute setting), particularly potassium, sodium, and magnesium, because these values demonstrate the degree of nephron recovery post-obstruction. Urine output is replaced with half normal saline, as the sodium content of the diuresis is typically approximately 70 mEq/L. Careful attention must be paid to avoid overhydration of the patient, thereby perpetuating the disease. Many patients with modest diuresis may eat and drink their way back to a normal volume state. Intermittent bladder drainage, once believed to mitigate hematuria, is not recommended as this typically serves only to confuse the accurate recording of urine output.

FETAL AND PEDIATRIC UROPATHIES

Advances in diagnostic and treatment modalities for fetuses, infants, and children have had a tremendous impact on the management of urinary obstruction in this patient population. Congenital malformations, such as posterior urethral valves, a persistent prostatic utricle, or the sequelae of such neurological disorders as spina bifida may all result in obstruction. Posterior urethral valves, present in males, are remnant flaps of mucosal tissue within the urethra, typically at the level of the veru montanum in the prostatic urethra. These patients often present with prenatal oligohydramnios, bladder distention, and bilateral hydronephrosis. Diagnosis is confirmed with a voiding cystourethrogram, and treatment includes endoscopic valve ablation. Temporary decompression of the obstructed bladder in the setting of posterior urethral valves may be accomplished with a cutaneous vesicostomy, which is an incontinent urinary diversion. Long-term sequelae of renal obstruction may include an inability of the kidney to maximally concentrate urine. This predisposes affected children to polydipsia and intolerance to fluid deprivation.

References

1. Litwin MS, Saigal CS, Yano EM, et al: Urologic Diseases in America Project: Analytical methods and principal findings. J Urol 2005;173:933–937.
2. Pearle MS, Calhoun EA, Curhan GC, Urologic Disease in America Project: Urolithiasis. J Urol 2005;173:848–857.
3. Segura JW, Preminger GM, Assimos DG, et al: Ureteral stones clinical guidelines panel summary: Report on the management of ureteral calculi. J Urol 1997;158:1915–1921.
4. Yilmaz E, Batislam E, Basar MM, et al: The comparison and efficacy of 3 alpha1-adrenergic blockers for distal ureteral stones. J Urol 2005;173:2010–2012.
5. Porpiglia F, Ghignone G, Fiori C, et al: Nifedipine versus tamsulosin for the management of lower ureteral stones. J Urol 2004; 172:568–571.
6. Shekarriz B, Stoller ML: Uric acid nephrolithiasis: Current concepts and controversies. J Urol 2002;168:1307–1314.
7. Barbey F, Joly D, Rieu P, et al: Medical treatment of cystinuria: Critical reappraisal of long-term results. J Urol 2000;163: 1419–1423.
8. Seltzer MA, Low RK, McDonald M, et al: Dietary manipulation with lemonade to treat hypocitrauric calcium nephrolithiasis. J Urol 1996;156:907–909.
9. Krambeck AE, Gettman MT, Rohlinger AL, et al: Diabetes mellitus and hypertension associated with shock wave lithotripsy of renal and proximal ureteral stones at 19 years of follow-up. J Urol 2006; 175:1742–1747.
10. Harmon WJ, Sherson PD, Blute ML, et al: Ureteroscopy: Current practice and long-term complications. J Urol 1997;157: 42–43.
11. Preminger GM, Assimos DG, Lingeman JE, et al: Chapter 1: AUA guideline on management of staghorn calculi: Diagnosis and treatment recommendations. J Urol 2005;173: 1991–2000.
12. Park JM, Bloom DA: The pathophysiology of UPJ obstruction. Current concepts. Urol Clin North Am 1998;25: 161–169.
13. Gerber GS, Kim JC: Ureteroscopic endopyelotomy in the treatment of patients with ureteropelvic junction obstruction. Urology 2000;55:198–202.
14. Utz DC, Zincke H: The masquerade of bladder cancer in situ as interstitial cystitis. J Urol 1974. 111:160–161.
15. Kaplan SA, Roehrborn CG, McConnell JD, et al: Baseline symptoms, uroflow and post-void residual urine as predictors of BPH clinical progression in the medically treated arms of the MTOPS trial. J Urol 2003;169(4 Suppl):332–333.
16. McConnell JD, Roehrborn CG, Bautista OM, et al: The long-term effect of doxazosin, finasteride and combination therapy on the clinical progression of benign prostatic hyperplasia. N Engl J Med 2003;349:2387–2398.
17. Hagerty J, Ginsberg P, Harkaway R: A prospective, comparative study of the onset of symptomatic benefit of dutasteride versus finasteride in men with benign prostatic hyperplasia in everyday clinical practice (Abstract 1353). Presented at the Annual Meeting of American Urological Association, San Francisco, CA, 2004.
18. Roehrborn CG, Boyle P, Bergner D, et al: Serum prostate-specific antigen and prostate volume predict long-term changes in symptoms and flow rate: Results of a four-year randomized trial comparing finasteride to placebo. PLESS Study Group. Urology 1999;54:662–669.
19. DiAmico A, Roehrborn C: Effect of 1 mg/day finasteride on concentrations of serum prostate-specific antigen in men with androgenic alopecia: A randomized controlled trial. Lancet Oncol 2007;8:21–25.
20. Malek RS, Kuntzman RS, Barrett DM: High power potassium-titinyl-phosphate laser vaporization prostatectomy. J Urol 2000; 163:1730–1733.
21. Masood S, Djaladat H, Kouriefs C, et al: The 12-year outcome analysis of an endourethral wallstent for treating benign prostatic hyperplasia. BJU Int 2004;94:1271–1274.
22. Santucci RA, Joyce GF, Wise M: Male urethral stricture disease. In Litwin MS, Saigal CS (eds): Urologic Diseases in America. U.S. Department of Health and Human Services, Public Health Service, National Institutes of Health, National Institute of Diabetes and Digestive and Kidney Diseases. Washington, DC: U.S. Government Printing Office, NIH Publication No. 07-5512, pp 533–551.
23. Weiss RM, George NJR, O'Reilly PH: Comprehensive Urology. New York: Mosby International, 2001.
24. Lapides J, Diokno AC, Silber SJ, Lowe BS: Clean, intermittent self-catheterization in the treatment of urinary tract disease. Trans Am Assoc Genitourin Surg 1971;63:92–96.

25. Kaufman JM, Fam B, Jacobs SC, et al: Bladder cancer and squamous metaplasia in spinal cord injury patients. J Urol 1977;118:967–971.

Further Reading

Jones DA, George NJR, O'Reilly PH, Barnard RJ: The biphasic nature of renal functional recovery following relief of chronic obstructive uropathy. Br J Urol 1988;61:192–197.

Klahr S: Obstructive uropathy. In Giebisch GH, Seldin DW (eds): The Kidney: Physiology and Pathophysiology, 3rd ed. Philadelphia: Lippincott–Raven, 2000, pp 2473–2512.

Preminger GM, Harvey JA, Pak CY: Comparative efficacy of 'specific' potassium citrate therapy versus conservative management in nephrolithiasis of mild to moderate severity. J Urol 1985; 135:658–661.

Renal Disease and Pregnancy

CONTENTS

Chapter 41

Hypertension in Pregnancy

Mounira Habli and Baha M. Sibai

Hypertensive disorders are the most common medical complications of pregnancy, affecting 5% to 10% of all pregnancies.[1,2] The incidence of disease depends on many different demographic parameters including maternal age, race, and associated underlying medical conditions. These disorders are responsible for approximately 16% of maternal mortality in developed countries. Classification of hypertensive disorders in pregnancy includes chronic hypertension and the group of hypertensive disorders unique to pregnancy called gestational hypertension and preeclampsia. Approximately 30% of hypertensive disorders in pregnancy are due to chronic hypertension and 70% are due to gestational hypertension.[1] The spectrum of disease ranges from mildly elevated blood pressures with minimal clinical significance to severe hypertension and multiorgan dysfunction. Understanding the disease process and the impact of hypertensive disorders on pregnancy is of the utmost importance because these disorders remain a major cause of maternal and perinatal morbidity and mortality worldwide.

DEFINITIONS AND CLASSIFICATIONS

Making an appropriate diagnosis can be difficult at times in the gravid patient; however, adhering to the following definitions and classification schemes will help to eliminate confusion. Hypertension in pregnancy is defined as a systolic blood pressure of 140 mm Hg or greater or a diastolic blood pressure of 90 mm Hg or greater. These measurements must be present on at least two occasions at least 6 hours apart, but no more than a week apart.

Abnormal proteinuria in pregnancy is defined as the excretion of 300 mg or more of protein in 24 hours. The most accurate measurement of proteinuria is obtained with a 24-hour urine collection. A value of 1+ or greater correlates with 30 mg/dL. Proteinuria by dipstick is defined as 1+ or more on at least two occasions at least 6 hours apart but no more than 1 week apart. The accuracy of semiquantitative dipstick measurements on spot urine samples compared with 24-hour urine collections is highly variable. Therefore, should time allow, a 12- or 24-hour urine collection should be performed as part of the diagnostic criteria to define

proteinuria. Care should be taken when obtaining urine protein measurements to use a clean sample because blood, vaginal secretions, and bacteria can increase the amount of protein in the urine.[1-3]

Edema is a common finding in the gravid patient, occurring in approximately 50% of women. Lower extremity edema is the most typical form. Pathologic edema is seen in nondependent regions such as the face, hands, or lungs. Excessive, rapid weight gain of 5 pounds or more per week may be sign of fluid retention.[1,2]

The classification system of hypertension in pregnancy was proposed originally by the American College of Obstetricians and Gynecologists Committee on Terminology in 1972. Further modifications by the National High Blood Pressure Education Program Working Group in 2000 arrived at the classification scheme used today, which offers simple, concise, and clinically relevant features for each of the four categories. This system recognizes four major categories of hypertension in pregnancy: gestational hypertension, preeclampsia or eclampsia, chronic hypertension, and preeclampsia superimposed on chronic hypertension. Table 41-1 lists these categories and the features of each.[1-3]

Gestational Hypertension

Gestational hypertension is the most frequent cause of hypertension during pregnancy. The rate ranges between 6% and 17% in healthy nulliparous women and between 2% and 4% in multiparous women.[4] Gestational hypertension is considered severe if there is sustained systolic blood pressure to at least 160 mm Hg and/or diastolic blood pressure to at least 110 mm Hg for at least 6 hours without proteinuria.[4] Treatment generally is not warranted because most patients have mild hypertension. However, approximately 46% of patients diagnosed with preterm gestational hypertension will develop proteinuria and progress to preeclampsia. In general, the majority of cases of mild gestational hypertension are diagnosed at or beyond 37 weeks and have a pregnancy outcome similar to term normotensive pregnancies. However, higher rates of induction and cesarean sections are seen in pregnancies complicated by gestational hypertension.[4]

Table 41-1 Classification of Hypertension in Pregnancy with Definitions

Diagnosis	Definition
Gestational hypertension	Hypertension developing after 20 wk of gestation or during the first 24 hr postpartum without proteinuria or other signs of preeclampsia
Transient hypertension	Hypertension resolves by 12 wk postpartum
Chronic hypertension	Hypertension that does not resolve by 12 wk postpartum
Preeclampsia or eclampsia	Hypertension typically developing after 20 wk of gestation with proteinuria; eclampsia is the occurrence of seizure activity without other identifiable causes
Chronic hypertension	Hypertension diagnosed before pregnancy, before 20 wk of gestation, or after 12 wk postpartum
Preeclampsia superimposed	The development of preeclampsia or eclampsia in a woman with preexisting on chronic hypertension

Based on data from references 1, 2, and 3.

Chronic Hypertension

Chronic hypertension is defined by increased blood pressure occurring before pregnancy or increased blood pressure measurements before 20 weeks of gestation.[5] The rate of chronic hypertension is 1% to 5% in pregnancy. This number is affected by factors such as maternal age, obesity, and race.[5] The incidence of chronic hypertension among African Americans is 2.5% compared with 1% among other racial groups. Given the trend in delayed childbearing as women pursue careers and educational goals and the epidemic of obesity, increasing numbers of pregnancies will be complicated by chronic hypertension.

Determination of associated underlying medical conditions and the classification of hypertension are important in the management and counseling of patients with chronic hypertension in pregnancy. The cause of chronic hypertension can be either primary or secondary.[3] Primary hypertension, also referred to as idiopathic hypertension or essential hypertension, occurs in 90% of pregnancies. Secondary hypertension occurs in the remaining 10% of pregnancies and is associated with the following underlying medical conditions: renal disease, endocrine disease, collagen vascular disease, and coarctation of the aorta.[3]

Women with chronic hypertension in pregnancy are at increased risk of the development of superimposed preeclampsia, abruptio placentae, intrauterine growth restriction, and preterm delivery.[6-8] The rate of superimposed preeclampsia in women with chronic hypertension is 15% to 25%.[7,8] If the patient has chronic hypertension of more than 4 years' duration or renal insufficiency or had hypertension in a previous pregnancy, the rate of superimposed preeclampsia increases. Overall, abruptio placentae occurs in 1.5% of pregnancies complicated by chronic hypertension.[6,9] This rate varies from 1% in women with uncomplicated chronic hypertension to 3% in women with superimposed preeclampsia. Proteinuria is an independent risk factor for an adverse perinatal outcome, regardless of the development of superimposed preeclampsia. A maternal serum creatinine level greater than 1.4 mg/dL at conception is another risk factor for increased fetal loss and progressive worsening of maternal renal disease. Fetal loss is increased 10-fold in women with uncontrolled chronic hypertension and impaired renal function at conception compared with normotensive women and women with well-controlled hypertension.[10] Therefore, management of women with chronic hypertension should begin before conception.

Women with chronic hypertension should be counseled regarding the increased risk of adverse maternal and fetal outcomes as discussed previously. The diagnosis of superimposed preeclampsia may be difficult to make in the patient with chronic hypertension, particularly with baseline nephropathy. To make the diagnosis, the patient should have increasing or difficult-to-control blood pressure, thrombocytopenia, significant increase in liver enzymes, new-onset proteinuria, or significant increase in preexisting proteinuria. Any patient with chronic hypertension who develops headache, right upper quadrant pain, or visual disturbances requires further evaluation for superimposed preeclampsia. If superimposed preeclampsia develops in a patient with chronic hypertension, she should be hospitalized for close maternal and fetal evaluation.

Management

The management of pregnancies complicated by chronic hypertension differs for the low-risk group versus the high-risk group. Patients considered in the low-risk group have, by definition, mild hypertension without evidence of organ damage (Fig. 41-1). The high-risk group has either severe hypertension (systolic blood pressure > 160 mm Hg or diastolic blood pressure > 110 mm Hg) or mild hypertension with evidence of organ involvement (Fig. 41-2). Patients with low-risk chronic hypertension who do not develop superimposed preeclampsia have pregnancy outcomes similar to those of the general population. Prenatal care in low-risk patients should include 24-hour urine collection for total protein determination in the first trimester and at least monthly visits in the first and second trimesters. Visits should be every 1 to 2 weeks after 32 weeks, looking carefully for the development of superimposed preeclampsia.

Central to the management of the high-risk chronic hypertensive pregnancy is the use of antihypertensive pharmacotherapy (Table 41-2). The choice of agent depends on the pharmacologic actions and is covered in the next section. Prenatal care of the high-risk patient includes a first-trimester 24-hour urine collection for total protein level. The frequency

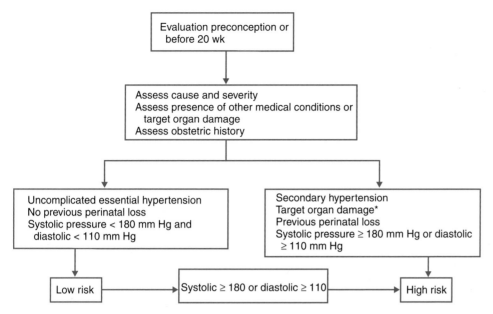

Figure 41-1 Initial evaluation of women with chronic hypertension. (From Sibai BM: Chronic hypertension in pregnancy. Obstet Gynecol 2002;100:369–377.)

*Left ventricular dysfunction, retinopathy, dyslipdemia, maternal age older than 40 years, microvascular disease, stroke.

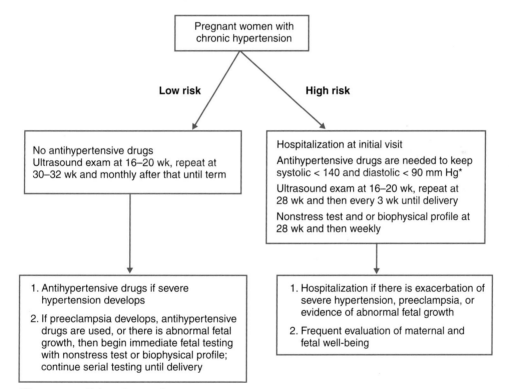

Figure 41-2 Antepartum management of chronic hypertension.

of visits in the first and second trimesters should be every 2 weeks and weekly in the third trimester if clinically indicated. In general, pregnancies in patients with high-risk chronic hypertension should not be continued past 40 weeks. As for fetal surveillance for low- or high-risk patients, there is general agreement to perform them as described in Figure 41-2.

Preeclampsia and Eclampsia

The rate of preeclampsia ranges between 2% and 7% in healthy nulliparous women.[11] The rate is substantially higher in women with twin gestation (14%) and those with previous preeclampsia (18%).[11] Preeclampsia may be subdivided further into mild

Table 41-2   Antihypertensive Medications: Indications/Precautions

Drug	Starting Dose	Maximum Dose	Comments
Acute Treatment of Severe Hypertension			
Hydralazine	5–10 mg IV every 20 mim	30 mg	
Labetalol	20–40 mg IV every 10–15 min	220 mg	Avoid in women with asthma or congestive heart failure
Nifedipine	10–20 mg PO every 30 min	50 mg	
Long-Term Treatment of Hypertension			
Methyldopa	250 mg bid	4/day	Rarely indicated
Labetalol	100 mg bid	2400 mg/day	First choice
Atenolol	50 mg qd	100 mg/day	Associated with IUGR
Propanolol	40 mg bid	640 mg/day	To be used with associated thyroid disease
Hydralazine	10 mg tid	100 mg/day	To be used in cases of left ventricular hypertrophy
Nifedipine/diltiazem	10 mg bid	120 mg/day	To be used in women with diabetes
	120–180 mg qd	540 mg/day	
Thiazide diuretic	12.5 mg bid	50 mg/day	Use in salt-sensitive hypertension and/or CHF; may be added as second agent; not to be used if preeclampsia develops or IUGR present
ACE inhibitors/ARB			Not to be used due to teratogenicity

CHF, congestive heart failure; IUGR, Intrauterine growth restriction.
Based on data from references 1, 2, 4, 10, and 19.

and severe forms. The distinction between the two is made based on the degree of hypertension and proteinuria and the involvement of other organ systems. The criteria for mild preeclampsia and severe preeclampsia are presented in Box 41-1. A particularly severe form of preeclampsia is the HELLP syndrome, which is an acronym for hemolysis, elevated liver enzymes, and low platelet count. This syndrome is manifest by laboratory findings consistent with hemolysis, elevated levels of liver function, and thrombocytopenia. The diagnosis may be deceptive because hypertension and proteinuria might be absent in 10% to 15% of women who develop HELLP and in 20% to 25 % of those who develop eclampsia. A patient diagnosed with HELLP syndrome is automatically classified as having severe preeclampsia.[12] Another severe form of preeclampsia is eclampsia, which is the occurrence of seizures not attributable to other causes.

Several risk factors for preeclampsia have been identified such as advanced maternal age (older than 35 years), especially if conception was secondary to assisted reproductive technology, and primigravid. Obesity is another important factor.[11] The causal agent responsible for the development of preeclampsia remains unknown. The syndrome is characterized by vasospasm, hemoconcentration, and ischemic changes in the placenta, kidney, liver, and brain. These abnormalities usually are seen in women with severe preeclampsia.[13] Theories as to the causative mechanisms include placental origin, immunologic origin, and genetic predisposition, among others.[13]

No good screening test for the prediction of preeclampsia exists. Doppler ultrasonography is a useful method to assess the velocity of uterine blood flow in the second trimester. Abnormal velocity waveform is characterized by a high resis-

Box 41-1   Criteria for the Diagnosis of Preeclampsia

Mild
SBP > 140 mm Hg and/or DBP > 90 mm Hg on two occasions at least 6 hours apart, typically occurring after 20 weeks of gestation (no more than 1 week apart)
Proteinuria of 300 mg in a 24-hour urine collection or >1+ on two random sample urine dispsticks at least 6 hours apart (no more than 1 week apart)

Severe
SBP > 160 mm Hg and/or DBP > 110 mm Hg on two occasions at least 6 hours apart
Proteinuria of ≥5 g in a 24-hour urine specimen or 3+ or greater on two random urine samples collected at least 4 hours apart
Oliguria < 500 mL/24 hours
Thrombocytopenia platelet count < 100,000/mm^3
Elevated liver function test results with persistent epigastric or right upper quadrant pain
Pulmonary edema
Persistent severe cerebral or visual disturbances

DBP, diastolic blood pressure; SBP, systolic blood pressure.
Based on data from references 2 and 11.

tance index or an early diastolic notch (unilateral or bilateral). Data still do not support this test for routine screening. Recently, investigators have begun to examine soluble fms-like tyrosine kinase-1 receptors (sFlt-1) and placental growth factor as early markers for preeclampsia.[14] Future studies done using proteomic and other markers as soluble endoglin and fms-like tyrosine kinase receptors (sFlt) are still ongoing.

Preventive interventions for preeclampsia could affect maternal and perinatal morbidity and mortality worldwide. As a result, during the past decade, several randomized trials reported several methods to reduce the rate and/or severity of preeclampsia. In summary, several trials assessed protein or low-salt diets, diuretics, bed rest, zinc, magnesium, fish oil or vitamin C and E supplementation, and heparin to prevent preeclampsia in women, but results showed minimal to no effect.[11,15]

Maternal and Perinatal Outcome

Maternal and neonatal outcome in patients with preeclampsia relates largely to one or more of the following factors: the gestational age at delivery, severity of disease, quality of management and presence of preexisting disease. Perinatal mortalities are increased in those who develop the disease before 34 weeks of gestation. Risk to the mother can be significant and includes the possible development of disseminated intravascular coagulation, intracranial hemorrhage, renal failure, retinal detachment, pulmonary edema, liver rupture, abruptio placentae, and death.[11] Therefore, experienced clinicians should be caring for women with preeclampsia.

Management of Mild and Severe Preeclampsia

Ideally, a patient having preeclampsia should be hospitalized at the time of the diagnosis. Management of the patient with mild preeclampsia should include baseline laboratory evaluation including 24-hour urine collection for protein, hematocrit, platelet count, serum creatinine value, and aspartate aminotransferase level. At the time of diagnosis, ultrasonography should be performed to evaluate amniotic fluid volume and estimated fetal weight and confirm gestational age. The only definitive cure for preeclampsia is delivery. The main objective of the management of preeclampsia must always be the safety of the mother and a mature newborn who will not require intensive and prolonged neonatal care. The general consensus for management of mild preeclampsia and severe preeclampsia are listed in Figures 41-3 and 41-4.

Intrapartum Management

While in labor, patients with severe preeclampsia will receive intravenous magnesium sulfate for seizure prophylaxis. This is controversial in regard to mild preeclampsia. There are only two double-blind, placebo-controlled trials evaluating the use of magnesium sulfate in patients with mild preeclampsia.[16,17] In both trials, patients with well-defined mild preeclampsia were randomized during labor or postpartum, and there was no difference in the percentage of women who progressed to severe preeclampsia (12.5% vs. 13.8%; relative risk = 0.90; 95% confidence interval: 0.52–1.54). There were no instances of eclampsia among 181 patients assigned to placebo. Thus, we recommend individualizing the use of magnesium sulfate in each case.

Pain management in labor should be individualized as well. Intravenous narcotics and regional anesthesia are both appropriate options. Close monitoring of blood pressure intrapartum is necessary. Antihypertensive medications may be needed to keep blood pressure less 160 mm Hg systolic and less than 110 mm Hg diastolic. The most commonly used intravenous medications for this purpose are labetalol and hydralazine. The recommended doses of medications for the immediate treatment of hypertension are listed in Table 41-2. Care should be taken not to decrease the blood pressure too rapidly because a marked decrease in mean arterial pressure may lead to decreased renal perfusion and decreased placental perfusion. Preeclamptic women receiving magnesium sulfate are also at risk of postpartum hemorrhage due to uterine atony.

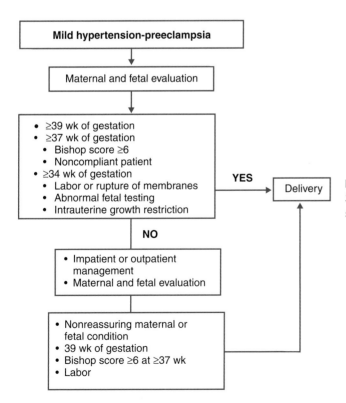

Figure 41-3 Management of mild preeclampsia. (From Sibai BM: Diagnosis and management of gestational hypertension and preeclampsia. Obstet Gynecol 2003;102:181–192.)

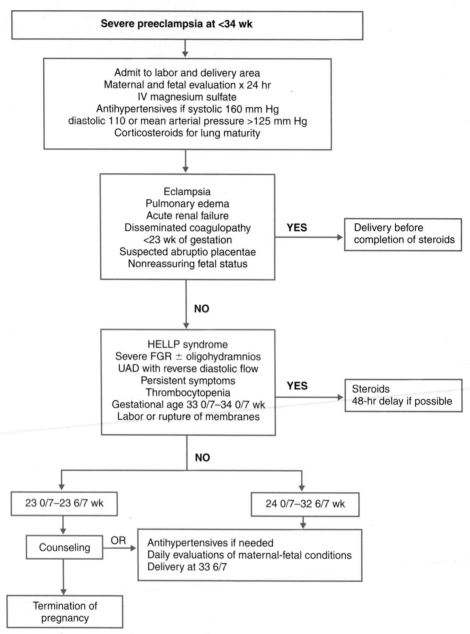

Figure 41-4 Management of severe preeclampsia. FGR, fetal growth restriction; HELLP, hemolysis, elevated liver enzymes, and low platelet count (syndrome). UAD, umbilical artery Doppler. (From Sibai BM, Barton JR: Expectant management of severe preeclampsia remote from term: Patient selection, treatment, and delivery indications. Am J Obstet Gynecol 2007;196:514:e1–e9.)

Patients should be monitored closely for at least 12 to 24 hours postpartum. Postpartum eclampsia occurs in 25% of patients. There is no need for continued seizure prophylaxis beyond 24 hours postpartum.

Counseling

Any patient diagnosed with preeclampsia is at significantly greater risk of having an underlying medical condition than is a normotensive gravida. A study by Dekker and Sibai[18] found 39% of patients with a history of early-onset severe preeclampsia developed chronic hypertension. Another study by Nisell and coworkers[19] found that 37% of patients with a history of pregnancy-induced hypertension and 20% of patients with a history of preeclampsia were noted to have hypertension at

7-year follow-up. It is thus essential that women diagnosed with preeclampsia receive close follow-up. With regard to future pregnancies, patients with preeclampsia are at increased risk of developing preeclampsia during subsequent gestations. The risk depends on the severity of preeclampsia as well as gestational age at onset in the index pregnancy. The recurrence rate is 65% if preeclampsia develops in the midtrimester and 20% if it develops at term. Sibai and associates[20] reviewed recurrence rates of preeclampsia and HELLP syndrome in patients who had pregnancies complicated by HELLP syndrome. Their findings noted that the recurrence risk of preeclampsia in the otherwise normotensive group was 19% and the risk of recurrence of HELLP syndrome was 3%. This is in contrast to a group of patients with underlying chronic hypertension who had recurrence rates of preeclampsia and HELLP syndrome of 75% and 5%, respectively. The rate of recurrence of eclampsia is approximately 1% to 2%.

Contraception

Women with hypertensive disease in pregnancy, whether preeclampsia or chronic hypertension, will seek advice regarding contraceptive methods postpartum. It is important to be familiar with options available to patients and be able to discuss potential risk factors. No contraindications exist with the use of barrier methods with regard to hypertension. There are no contraindications for hypertensive patients desiring to use an intrauterine device. The greatest concern in finding appropriate contraception for the hypertensive patient is with regard to hormonal contraception. Oral contraceptive pills are the most widely used reversible form of birth control in the United States. Combination oral contraceptives are known to elevate blood pressure minimally, increase clotting factors, and increase total cholesterol levels.[21] Once again, it is extremely important to be familiar with any coexisting disease in a hypertensive patient. Overall, the contraceptive choices afforded hypertensive patients are the same as in normotensive patients. The risks and benefits of contraception must be weighed and patients counseled accordingly. Avoiding the morbidity associated with pregnancy in some patients may be a benefit that outweighs the risk of contraceptive use.

References

1. American College of Obstetricians and Gynecologists: Chronic hypertension in pregnancy. ACOG Practice Bulletin no. 29. Obstet Gynecol 2001;98:177–185.
2. American College of Obstetricians and Gynecologists: Diagnosis and management of preeclampsia and eclampsia. ACOG Practice Bulletin no. 33. Obstet Gynecol 2002;99:159–167.
3. Report of the National High Blood Pressure Education Program Working Group on High Blood Pressure in Pregnancy. Am J Obstet Gynecol 2000;183:S1–S22.
4. Sibai BM: Diagnosis and management of gestational hypertension and preeclampsia. Obstet Gynecol 2003;102:181–192.
5. Sibai BM: Chronic hypertension in pregnancy. Obstet Gynecol 2002;100:369–377.
6. Sibai BM, Lindheimer M, Hauth J, et al: Risk factors for preeclampsia, abruptio placentae, and adverse neonatal outcomes among women with chronic hypertension. N Engl J Med 1998;339:667–671.
7. Rey E, Couturier A: The prognosis of pregnancy in women with chronic hypertension. Am J Obstet Gynecol 1994;171:410–416.
8. McCowan LM, Buist RG, North RA, Gamble G: Perinatal morbidity in chronic hypertension. Br J Obstet Gynaecol 1996;103:123–129.
9. Sibai BM, Abdella TN, Anderson GD: Pregnancy outcome in 211 patients with mild chronic hypertension. Obstet Gynecol 1983;61:571–576.
10. Sibai BM: Management of chronic hypertension in pregnancy. Obstet Gynecol 2002;100:369–377.
11. Sibai BM: Preeclampsia. Lancet 2005;365:785–799.
12. Sibai BM: Diagnosis, controversies, and management of the syndrome of hemolysis, elevated liver enzymes, and low platelet count. Obstet Gynecol 2004;103:981–991.
13. Dekker GA, Sibai BM: Etiology and pathogenesis of preeclampsia: Current concepts. Am J Obstet Gynecol 1998;179:1359–1375.
14. Levine RJ, Maynard SE, Qian C, et al: Circulating angiogenic factors and the risk of preeclampsia. N Engl J Med 2004;350:672–683.
15. Sibai BM: Prevention of preeclampsia: A big disappointment. Am J Obstet Gynecol 1998;179:1275–1278.
16. Witlin AG, Sibai BM: Magnesium sulfate therapy in preeclampsia and eclampsia. Obstet Gynecol 1998;92:883–889.
17. Livingston JC, Livingston LW, Ramsey R, et al: Magnesium sulfate in women with mild preeclampsia: A randomized controlled trial. Obstet Gynecol 2003;101:217–220.
18. Dekker GA, Sibai BM: Etiology and pathogenesis of preeclampsia: Current concepts. Am J Obstet Gynecol 1998;179:1359–1375.
19. Nisell H, Lintu H, Lunell NO, et al: Blood pressure and renal function seven years after pregnancy complicated by hypertension. Br J Obstet Gynaecol 1995;102:876–881.
20. Sibai BM, Ramadan MK, Chari RS, Friedman SA: Pregnancies complicated by HELLP syndrome (hemolysis, elevated liver enzymes, and low platelets): Subsequent pregnancy outcome and long-term prognosis. Am J Obstet Gynecol 1995;172(1 Pt 1):125–129
21. Repke JT: Contraception for the woman with hypertension. In Sibai BM (ed): Hypertensive Disorders in Women. Philadelphia: WB Saunders, 2001.

Further Reading

Burt VL, Whetton P, Rochella EJ, et al: Prevalence of hypertension in the US adult population: Results from the third national health and nutrition examination survey, 1988–1991. Hypertension 1995;23:305–313.

Sibai BM: Magnesium sulfate prophylaxis in preeclampsia. Lessons learned from recent trials. Am J Obstet Gynecol 2004;190:1520–1526.

Chapter 42

Renal Disease in Pregnancy

Mounira Habli and Baha M. Sibai

There has been marked improvement in maternal and perinatal outcome for pregnancies complicated by renal disease in the past 40 to 50 years. An understanding of the disease processes and improvements in obstetric care, with more successful and earlier intervention, have led to the improved outcomes. Renal disorders in pregnancy can range from asymptomatic bacteriuria (ASB) to end-stage renal disease requiring dialysis and transplantation, all being influenced by the physiologic changes of pregnancy. This chapter reviews the physiology of renal changes during pregnancy and provides a summary of renal disorders.

PHYSIOLOGIC CHANGES DURING PREGNANCY

Several renal physiologic changes occur during pregnancy. These changes include renal anatomy, hemodynamics, acid-base regulation, and metabolic regulation (e.g., water, mineral) (Table 42-1). Thus, tests of renal function in pregnancy must be interpreted in relation to the changes in plasma volume, glomerular filtration, and tubular reabsorption that normally occur with advancing gestation. Many of the commonly used tests of renal function yield lower results in pregnancy than in the nonpregnant state. Consequently, values that may be regarded as normal in the nonpregnant state may well indicate renal dysfunction in pregnancy.

RENAL DISEASE COMPLICATING PREGNANCY

Asymptomatic Bacteriuria, Urinary Tract Infections, and Acute Pyelonephritis

The prevalence of ASB in pregnancy is 4% to 7%.[1] The risk of ASB increases with increasing parity, lower socioeconomic status, increased age, sexual activity, sickle cell trait or disease, diabetes, and previous urinary tract infection (UTI). The diagnosis of ASB is based on a clean-catch voided urine culture revealing more than 100,000 colonies/mL of a single organism.[2] It is important to diagnose and treat ASB in pregnancy. Untreated ASB will develop into symptomatic UTI in as many as 40% of these patients.[3,4] Recognition of and therapy for ASB can eliminate 70% of acute UTIs in pregnancy. Women should be screened for bacteriuria at their first prenatal visit. Therapy for ASB should be continued for 3 to 7 days. The patient should have another culture performed 1 to 2 weeks after discontinuing therapy. The most commonly used agent in ASB and uncomplicated UTI is nitrofurantoin. ASB is associated with an adverse perinatal outcome. Evidence combined from multiple studies suggests that ASB is associated with both preterm delivery and low birth weight.[1]

UTIs are the most common medical complication of pregnancy. Acute cystitis occurs in 1.3%[5] and acute pyelonephritis in 1%[6] of pregnant women. The causal agents of UTIs in pregnancy are the same as those of acute uncomplicated UTI in nonpregnant women. *Escherichia coli* causes 80% to 90% of UTIs in pregnancy, and *Proteus mirabilis*, *Klebsiella pneumoniae*, *Staphylococcus saprophyticus*, and enterococci are the usual isolates from the remainder of patients with uncomplicated infections. In pregnancy, group B β-hemolytic streptococci are also potential urinary tract pathogens.[7] The treatment goals of UTI in pregnancy are to eradicate the infection with the shortest possible course of antibiotics and to maintain sterile urine for the remainder of pregnancy. A 3- to 7-day course of antibiotic therapy is recommended to treat ASB or uncomplicated acute UTI in pregnancy.

Pyelonephritis is the most common nonobstetric cause of hospitalization during pregnancy.[8] Acute pyelonephritis should be initially treated on an inpatient basis, using intravenous antibiotics. Empiric therapy should be begun as soon as the presumptive diagnosis is made. Therapy can be tailored to the specific organism after sensitivities have been obtained approximately 48 hours later.

Table 42-1 Physiologic Changes during Pregnancy

	Changes in Pregnancy	Mechansims
Renal anatomy	Increase in kidney size 1 cm in length Dilatation of the collecting system with a pelvicalceal diameter up to 2 cm is physiological hydronephrosis Increased GFR, urine formation, and urine flow Changes persist until 12 wk postpartum	Increase in renal vascular volume and kidney hypertrophy Estrogen and progesterone effects Mechanical obstruction of ureters (right > left)
Renal hemodynamics	GFR increases by 50%, then decreases by 20% in the last trimester RBF increase by 85% in second trimester Creatinine clearance increase by 50% to 150–200 mL/min No increase in glomerular capillary pressure	Increase in CO by 30%–40% Increase in renal vasodilation of both afferent and efferent arterioles secondary to EDRF/NO
Metabolic regulation	Water retention especially in late third trimester with transient diabetes insipidus Sodium retention Potassium balance maintained Calcium absorption from gastrointestinal increases Increase in urate clearance until 24 wk, then back to prepregnant state Increase in filtered glucose and protein and less efficient tubule reabsorption leads to renal glucosuria, proteinuria (not exceeding 300 mg/24 hr)	Secondary to high placental vasopressinase By increasing sodium reabsorption both in proximal and in distal tubules Progesterone plays a role in preventing kaliuresis High $1,25(OH)_2 D_3$ levels produced by kidney and placenta leading to hypercalciuria (>300 mg/day)
Acid-base regulation	Mild respiratory alkalosis compensated by metabolic acidosis	Increase in minute ventilation compensated by more bicarbonate excretion by kidneys
Hormonal changes	Increase in erythropoietin, renin, and vitamin D Increase in level of antinatriuretic hormones, especially mineralocorticoids, aldosterone, and desoxycorticosterone Increased serum atrial natriuretic peptide levels Decrease in parathyroid hormones	

$1,25 (OH)_2 D_3$ 1,25-dinydroxycholecalciferol; CO, cardiac output; EDRF/NO, endothelin-derived relaxing factor/nitric oxide; GFR, glomerular filtration rate; RBF, renal blood flow.
From Linheimer MD, Katz AI: Renal physiology and disease in pregnancy. In Seldin DW, Giebisch G (eds): The Kidney: Physiology and Pathophysiology, 3rd ed. Philadelphia: Lippincott Williams & Wilkins, 2000; Davison JM, Vollotton MB, Lindheimer MD: Plasma osmolality and urinal concentration and dilution during and after pregnancy: Evidence that lateral recumbency inhibits maximal urinary concentrating ability. Br J Obstet Gynaecol 1981;88:472; and Davison JM, Dunlop W: Changes in renal hemodynamics and tubular function induced by normal pregnancy. Semin Nephrol 1984;4:198.

Acute Renal Failure

Since the 1960s, the overall incidence of pregnancy-related acute renal failure (PR-ARF) has decreased from 1 per 3000 to 1 per 15,000 to 1 per 20,000. Similarly, the proportion of total cases of PR-ARF has decreased from 20% to 40% in the 1960s to 2% to 10% in the 1980s.[9–11]

PR-ARF ranges from serum creatinine of more than 0.8 mg/dL to dialysis requirement and urine output less than 400 mL in 24 hours. Conceptually, ARF has been described as a deterioration of renal function over a period of hours and days, resulting in the failure of the kidney to excrete nitrogenous waste products and to maintain fluid and electrolyte hemostasis.[12] The Acute Dialysis Quality Initiative developed a model for diagnosis of ARF based on creatinine, glomerular filtration rate, and urine output (Table 42-2).[8] ARF is divided into prerenal, intrarenal, and postrenal.[12] The cause of ARF in pregnancy could be due to either pregnancy-related conditions (such as preeclampsia, acute fatty liver, amniotic fluid embolism, and hypovolumic shock) or other causes related to reproductive age women. Thus, PR-ARF is treated based on the underlying cause. Thus, every PR-ARF patient should have a detailed history, physical examination, and the laboratory assessment including complete blood count, platelet count, blood urea nitrogen, creatinine level, electrolyte, glomerular filtration rate, urinanalysis, urine sodium concentration, urine osmolality, and fractional excretion of sodium. The main goal of treatment involves treatment of underlying disease, prevention of further damage, and supportive treatment until recovery. Management of PR-ARF begins with correction of the underlying causal factors by removal of renal toxins, proper dosing of medications, and prevention and treatment of infection because sepsis is the most common cause of mortality in ARF. Fluid resuscitation is the single most important intervention to restore and maintain renal perfusion. Pharmacologic

Table 42-2   Diagnostic Scheme for Acute Renal Failure

	GFR Criteria	Urine Output Criteria
Increase risk (RIFLE-R)	Increased serum creatinine × 1.5 or GFR decrease > 25%	UO <0.5 mL/kg/hr × 6 hr
Renal injury (RIFLE-I)	Increased serum creatinine × 2 or GFR decrease > 50%	UO <0.5 mL/kg/hr × 12 hr
Renal failure (RIFLE-F)	Increased serum creatinine × 3, GFR decrease 75% or serum creatinine ≥ 4 mg/dL in the setting of an acute increase ≥ 0.5 mg/dL)	UO <0.3 mL/kg/hr × 24 hr or anuria × 12 hr
Loss of renal function (RIFLE-L)	Persistent acute renal failure = complete loss of kidney function >4 wk	
End-stage kidney disease (RIFLE-E)	End-stage kidney disease (>3 mo)	

GFR, glomerular filtration rate; RIFLE, risk injury failure loss end-stage kidney disease; UO, urine output.
From Bellomo R: Defining, quantifying, and classifying acute renal failure. Crit Care Clin 2005;21:223–237.

measures as low-dose dopamine (no significant clinical benefit[13]), loop diuretics (controversial evidence, reserved for treatment of ARF in volume overload conditions to avoid renal replacement therapy.[14])

Other pharmacologic drugs such as calcium channel blockers, dopamine agonists, theophylline, N-acetylcysteine, and osmotic agents such as mannitol are controversial with no clear clinical benefit.[12] Complications of PR-ARF include anemia, hyperkalemia, and metabolic acidosis. Hyperkalemia can be treated with glucose and insulin or potassium-binding resins.[12] Anemia in ARF could be due to either hemolysis (uremia-induced red blood cell membrane fragility) or decreased hematopoiesis due to decreased erythropoietin levels.[15] Anemia is treated initially with transfusion and then if needed erythropoietin supplementation. Renal replacement therapy, including dialysis, is initiated if these measures are insufficient or there are volume overload, refractory hyperkalemia, metabolic acidosis, symptomatic uremia including pericarditis, neuropathy, and mental status changes. In PR-ARF, the most common problems that neonates face are related to prematurity. Adverse perinatal outcome is mainly related to altered uteroplacental hemodynamics. Thus, a multidisciplinary team approach including a neonatologist, nephrologist, and perinatologist is crucial to optimize the pregnancy outcome.

Underlying Renal Disease or Renal Insufficiency

The diagnosis of renal disease before pregnancy ranges between 0.03%[16] and 0.12%.[17] The prevalence of moderate to severe renal insufficiency ranges between 2 per 10,000[18] to 6 per 10,000.[19] In pregnancy, renal insufficiency could be mild (serum creatinine levels of 0.9–1.4 mg/dL), moderate (1.4–2.5 mg/dL), or severe (>2.5 mg/dL).[20,21] There are many different causes of chronic renal disease including diabetes, glomerulonephritis, hypertension, lupus nephritis, IgA nephropathy, and polycystic kidney disease. The natural history of renal disease during and after pregnancy depends mostly on the prepregnant renal function status and the presence or absence of hypertension.

EFFECT OF PREGNANCY ON RENAL DISEASE

The long-term effect of pregnancy on renal disease remains controversial. These patients may experience deterioration of renal function (increase in serum creatinine and worsening of proteinuria) and may be more prone to escalating hypertension. Early in pregnancy, an increase in glomerular filtration rate and a decrease in serum creatinine occur in all patients with renal disease except those with severe renal impairment.

The serum creatinine level begins to increase to and beyond prepregnancy levels during the second trimester.[22] It is not possible, however, to predict which patients with renal insufficiency will experience a permanent reduction in renal function. This deterioration occurs more frequently in women with diffuse glomerulonephritis. If renal function significantly worsens during gestation, termination of pregnancy may not reverse the process. Abortion therefore cannot be routinely recommended for patients who become pregnant and whose baseline serum creatinine level exceeds 1.5 mg/dL. Ideally, patients with chronic renal disease should be thoroughly counseled about the possible consequences of pregnancy before conception. Hypertension is the greatest threat in pregnancies complicated by preexisting renal disease. Approximately 50% of these patients will have worsening hypertension as pregnancy progresses, and diastolic blood pressures of 110 mm Hg or greater will develop in approximately 20% of cases.[23] Those patients with diffuse proliferative glomerulonephritis and nephrosclerosis are at greatest risk of developing severe hypertension. Blood pressure control is the cornerstone of successful treatment of chronic renal disease in pregnancy. Furthermore, worsening proteinuria is common and often reaches the nephrotic range.[23] Another important factor in determining development of fetal complications is maternal urea level. An increased urea level of more than 10 mmol/L is associated with polyhydramnios. A high maternal urea level leads to osmotic load in the fetus and polyuria. A maternal urea level greater than 20 to 25 mmol/L is associated with the risk of fetal death.

EFFECT OF RENAL DISEASE ON PREGNANCY

Although pregnancies complicated with chronic renal disease are at an increased risk of both maternal and perinatal morbidity, still more than 85% of women with chronic renal disease will have a surviving infant if renal function is well preserved (serum creatinine ≤ 1.4 mg/dL) and in whom hypertension is absent or well controlled. Morbidities associated with chronic renal disease include development of preeclampsia, end-stage renal disease, preterm delivery, anemia, chronic hypertension, growth restriction, and cesarean section (Table 42-3). Moreover, hypertension is an indicator of poor pregnancy outcome. A pregnant woman with minimal renal dysfunction and normal blood pressure has more than a 90% chance of successful pregnancy outcome.[24] Conversely, adverse obstetric outcomes range from 7% to 55% in the presence of both hypertension and renal dysfunction.

PREGNANCY OUTCOME BASED ON SEVERITY OF RENAL DISEASE

The severity of renal disease indirectly affects pregnancy outcome. Patients with mild renal insufficiency have a low complication rate (4.4%–22%) and no stillbirths.[20] The rate of complications is higher in pregnant women with moderate to severe renal insufficiency than in women with milder disease (see Table 42-3). Almost 50% of the pregnant women with a serum creatinine level of 1.4 mg/dL or more had an increase in serum creatinine during pregnancy to a mean of 2.5 mg/dL in the third trimester.[21] The risk of accelerated progression to end-stage renal disease is highest when the serum creatinine level is more than 2.0 mg/dL at the beginning of pregnancy.[21] Within 6 months after delivery, 23% of such women had progression to end-stage renal disease. Moreover, women with a serum creatinine level greater than 2.0 mg/dL should be counseled that they have a one in three chance of progressing to end-stage renal disease within 1 year postpartum.[25]

SPECIFIC PREEXISTING RENAL DISEASE IN PREGNANCY

Still, maternal and perinatal outcomes differ based on the cause of the preexisting disease. Diabetic nephropathy complicates 4% to 10% of pregnancies in women with diabetes. It is unclear whether diabetic nephropathy is accelerated by pregnancy. A few studies have shown that pregnancy has an adverse affect on diabetic nephropathy, increasing proteinuria.[26] Other studies have not observed any progression or development of nephropathy in women with diabetes.[27] Most studies involve a small number of patients and are observational. Women with diabetic nephropathy are at increased risk of adverse maternal and fetal outcome, especially preterm delivery, intrauterine growth restriction, preeclampsia, and hypertensive complications. The rates of preterm delivery at less than 34 weeks' gestation range from 16% to 31%,[26] and the rates of intrauterine growth restriction range from 9% to 22%.[28] In addition, the rate of preeclampsia may be as high as 50%.[26] It is very important to maintain the blood pressure at less than 130 mm Hg systolic and less than 80 mm Hg diastolic. Angiotensin-converting enzymes and angiotensin receptor blockers are antihypertensive agents that are renoprotective but should not be used in pregnancy. Calcium channel blockers seem to have no major adverse effects on the fetus and may be renoprotective.

Collagen vascular diseases are systemic disorders of unknown cause characterized by multiorgan inflammation and unpredictable remissions and exacerbations. Renal involvement is generally an unfavorable prognostic sign. Systemic lupus erythematosus is by far the most common collagen vascular disorder encountered in obstetric practice. The activity status at conception provides no guide to the course of lupus nephropathy. The prognosis is most favorable when patients are in remission at least 6 months before conception. Proteinuria may increase during pregnancy, and the serum creatinine level may either increase or not decrease normally. Exacerbations of lupus nephropathy are usually moderate and can easily be controlled by steroid therapy. However, the course of maternal lupus nephritis is especially poor when systemic lupus erythematosus (SLE) presents during pregnancy.[29] SLE with superimposed preeclampsia may present with signs and symptoms indistinguishable from a flare-up of lupus nephritis. Antibody assays may help to differentiate these conditions. Increasing titers of anti-DNA antibodies or decreasing levels of complement C3 or C4 are compatible with an exacerbation of SLE.[29] Patients with SLE in pregnancy should receive steroid therapy if clinical or immunological signs or symptoms of disease activity develop. Hypertension should be treated with antihypertensive agents. Bobrie and colleagues[29] favor routine administration of steroids postpartum to prevent a flare-up.

Table 42-3 Outcome in Pregnancy Complicated by Chronic Renal Disease

Author/Pregnancy Outcome	Preeclampsia	Anemia	Chronic Hypertension	Growth Restriction	Preterm Delivery	Cesarean Rate
Trevisan et al[19]	25%	48%	56%	—	60%	52%
Bar et al[21] (mostly mild renal insufficiency)	22%	—	—	13%	22%	24%
Jones et al[20]	—	—	—	37%	59%	59%

MANAGEMENT

Management should begin with prepregnancy counseling. Fertility is dependent on the degree of renal impairment. Women should be counseled about the possible deterioration of renal function during pregnancy and pregnancy-related complications such as preeclampsia and worsening hypertension. Fetal outcome should be discussed thoroughly including preterm delivery, growth restriction, and the possibility of a higher risk of fetal death, especially if there is severe renal disease or the patient is on dialysis. Factors that affect pregnancy outcome such as hypertension and the urea and serum creatinine level should be well controlled to optimize pregnancy outcome.

During pregnancy, management guidelines are based on observational and retrospective studies. The care of such high-risk pregnancies should entail a multidisciplinary approach at a tertiary center with closer surveillance and frequent visits. Maternal assessment should include serum creatinine and blood urea levels, electrolytes, albumin, cholesterol, complete blood count, platelet count, 24-hour urine collection, and urinalysis and urine culture as well as other laboratory assessments such as antinuclear antibody and complement levels if indicated. Proper control of blood pressure and the underlying cause of renal disease is crucial to improve pregnancy outcome. Prenatal visits every 2 weeks until 30 to 32 weeks and then weekly for the remainder of the pregnancy are preferable. As for fetal surveillance, we usually start at 30 to 32 weeks with weekly biophysical profiles and fetal growth assessment every 4 to 6 weeks. Uterine and umbilical Doppler flow can be used as of 24 weeks. This approach can change based on the severity of disease and other variables such as hypertension.

The role of renal biopsy during pregnancy is generally limited. The theoretical concerns are mainly the possible increased morbidity of the procedure in pregnancy. Dennis and colleagues[30] demonstrated complication rates of 1.6% to 4.4% including perirenal bleeding and perirenal hematoma and 17% gross hematuria. Some authors reported the following indications for renal biopsy in pregnancy: new-onset hematuria, proteinuria, or impaired renal function in the first or second trimester.[31] However, recent reviews suggest that the invasiveness of the procedure and complications should factor in the decision to perform a renal biopsy in pregnancy.

PREGNANCY IN WOMEN WITH END-STAGE RENAL DISEASE (DIALYSIS)

The medical literature reporting outcome of dialysis in pregnancy is limited to case reports and retrospective studies from the dialysis registry. Since the first case report of a successful pregnancy in a woman on dialysis in 1971[32] and an initial case series in the 1980s that suggested high rates of preterm birth, low birth weight, and refractory hypertension,[33] the overall prognosis for these patients has improved significantly. However, these pregnancies continue to be high risk, and outcomes remain quite variable. There is evidence to suggest that these improvements may be due to several modifications to the dialysis dose, frequency, and other variables[34-40] (Table 42-4). The goal of these adjustments is to improve the pregnancy outcome by having a less uremic fetal environment, more liberal maternal diet and fluid intake, a decrease in the amplitude of blood volume and fluid shifts, controlling hypertension, and lowering the risk of hypotension. These recommendations have significantly improved perinatal outcomes. Okundaye and colleagues[34] reported a 2.2% incidence of conception with a 45.6% spontaneous abortion rate, 40.2% surviving infants with 5.7% stillbirth rate, and 2.8% neonatal death. The average gestational age at delivery was 32.4 weeks in this series. Other reported fetal complications include polyhydramnios, intrauterine growth restriction, premature preterm rupture of membranes, and preterm deliveries. Historically, the standard dialysis treatment was hemodialysis. Most reported series suggest both peritoneal dialysis and hemodialysis with no major differences in morbidity. These reported series also suggest hemodialysis due to the ease of fluid control and fewer complications. Dialysis should be initiated as early as possible in pregnancy. To minimize solute and fluid shift changes, continuous renal replacement therapy was introduced.[34-40] There is no recommendation as yet with regard to continuous renal replacement therapy use. For fetal surveillance, we recommend weekly visits at the time of fetal viability (24 weeks), fetal ultrasound scan every 4 weeks for growth assessment, weekly amniotic fluid assessment if polyhydramnios is present, frequent Doppler evaluation of umbilical and uterine arteries, and a weekly biophysical profile beginning at 28 weeks of gestation.

PREGNANCY IN WOMEN WITH A RENAL ALLOGRAFT

In women of childbearing age with a functioning renal transplant, the pregnancy rate has recently improved from 2% to 5%.[41] However, many aspects must be carefully considered before a conscious decision can be made in such conditions, considering both sides, that is, on the maternal side, the influence that the pregnancy can have on renal graft outcome and maternal morbidity and, on the fetal side, the influence that the renal graft can have on fetal outcomes in both short and long term.

Maternal Effects

During pregnancy, hemodynamic, anatomical, and immunologic changes all exert an effect on the renal allograft. Both increased glomerular filtration rate and renal blood flow occur during normal pregnancy as well as in pregnancies complicated by a renal transplant and chronic renal disease.[42] It has been suggested that this glomerular hyperfiltration can cause progressive damage to the renal allograft and eventually to glomerular sclerosis.[43] The short-term effects of this can be seen as increased proteinuria, especially in the last 3 months of pregnancy, and they resolve 3 months postpartum.[43] Pregnancy, conversely, is a state of immunologic tolerance due to immunodepressant function of lymphocytes and fetal microchimerism in the mother. This raises the concern of acute rejection as well as long-term worsening of the renal allograft. There is consensus that acute rejection during pregnancy and for 3 months postdelivery is similar to nonpregnant transplant recipients.[44] The incidence ranges from 3% to 14.5%.[44] Risk factors for acute rejection are a high serum creatinine level at conception and changes in the immunosuppressive

Table 42-4   Modifications to Dialysis in Pregnancy

Dialysis Parameters	Specific Considerations
Indications	Severe refractory metabolic acidosis
	Retention of toxins
	Refractory hyperkalemia
	volume overload
Dialysis frequency and procedure	>20 hr/wk with 5–6 sessions/wk
	Should be initiated when serum creatinine is 3.4–5.0 mg/dL or GFR <20 mL/min
	A nonreusable biocompatible less teratogenic
	Smaller surface area dialyzer can decrease ultrafiltration rate during treatments
Urea, serum bicarbonate level, and electrolyte level	Maintain serum urea level <50 mg/dL
	Low bicarbonate dialysate (25 mEq/L) because serum bicarbonate level decreased from 24–30 mEq/L to 18–21 mEq/L
	Prevent hyperphosphatemia because it can affect fetal skeletal development
Anemia	Exogenous erythropoietin needed, because therapeutic doses are higher in pregnancy
	Observe for side effects of erythropoietin such as hypertension
	Target hemoglobin 10–11 g/dL, hematocrit 30%–35%
	Transfusion requirements may increase
	IV iron may be needed; this is monitored by transferrin level (should be maintained >30%)
Nutritional consideration	Proper weight gain for better outcome; recommend 1–1.25 kg total in first trimester and 0.3 to 0.5 kg/wk in second and third trimesters
	Need to increase supplementation of vitamins and folate because they are removed by dialysis
	Avoid hypercalcemia; calciferol doses must often be reduced
	Protein intake should be 1.8 g/kg/day
	Serum albumin and transferin used to evalute protein status
Hemodynamics	Avoid hypotension, fluid fluctuations, and volume changes to lessen the chance of fetal hypoperfusion
	Hypertension should be treated aggressively
	Maternal diastolic blood pressure should be maintained at 80–90 mm Hg
	Careful monitoring of maternal respiratory rate, oxygen saturation
Anticoagulation	Increased dose of heparin to prevent clotting of dialysis lines because pregnancy is a hypercoagulable state

Data from references 34–40.

drug level. Diagnosis could require a renal biopsy due to the resemblance to other diseases such as preeclampsia. High doses of steroids are the first-line treatment.

There are several medical problems in a pregnancy complicated by a renal transplant. In this population, hypertension and preeclampsia are four times more frequent than in the general population.[45] UTI is the most common complication during gestation in transplant recipients (19%–40%), particularly in women with chronic pyelonephritis or ureteral reflux as the primary cause of their renal disease.[46] Keep in mind that

UTI can be painless due to complete loss of nerve connection. This can lead to secondary complications such as rejection and papillary necrosis.[47] Thus, preventive measures such as monthly urine culture screening are recommended.

With all these changes, renal function progression in transplant recipients becomes a concern. Uncontrolled studies, mainly provided by international registries, demonstrated the persistent worsening of renal function in 15% of cases and graft loss within 2 years of pregnancy in 7% to 10% of women treated with cyclosporine and cyclosporine in emulsion and tacrolimus.[48,49] The majority of these studies suggested that at least two important criteria strongly affect long-term maternal renal prognosis: the serum creatinine level at conception and the interval between transplantation and conception.

Pregnancy does not have a detrimental effect on renal function if serum creatinine at conception is less than 1.5 mg/dL. However, patients with serum creatinine more than 2 mg/dL are at risk of renal impairment progression and will require dialysis within 2 years after birth.[45] Indeed, recipients with serum creatinine more than 2.5 mg/dL were three times more likely to have graft loss compared with patients with serum creatinine less than 1.5 mg/dL, as well as an increased rejection rate before (54 vs. 33%), during (13 vs. 2%), and after pregnancy (28 vs. 5%).[45] As to the interval between transplantation and conception, the important conclusion from the available studies is that the optimal interval for conception is more than 2 and less than 5 years post-transplantation. In fact, recipients who became pregnant less than 2 years after transplantation experienced more frequent rejections and long-term worsening in renal functionas well as worse fetal prognosis.[50] However, too long an interval (>5 years) can have a deleterious effect on pregnancy outcome because of older maternal age and renal function deterioration over time.[50] Thus, renal function, blood pressure, proteinuria, and adequate interval from transplantation to conception are the most important factors in predicting good maternal and graft outcomes.

Table 42-5 Recommendations for Management of Pregnancy in Kidney Transplant Recipients

Period	Recommendations
Preconception criteria for pregnancy	At least 2 yr after cadaver transplantation (1 yr after living donor transplantation) and <5 yr from transplantation in good general health
	Stable renal function with serum Cr at least <2 mg/dL (better if <1.5 mg/dL
	No recent episodes (or ongoing signs) of acute rejection
	BP ≤140/90 mm Hg on minimal medications
	Proteinuria < 500 mg/24 hr
	Normal graft ultrasound scan
	Recommended drugs: prednisone ≤15 mg/day, azathioprine ≤ 2 mg/kg/day, cyclosporine and tacrolimus at therapeutic levels, MMF and sirolimus are contraindicated and must be stopped 6 wk before conception
	Rubella vaccine should be administered before transplantation
During gestation	Performing monthly urine cultures and treating all asymptomatic infections
	Monitoring BP, proteinuria, and weight every 2–4 wk
	Changing hypertensive drugs to those tolerated during pregnancy, abolishing ACE inhibitors and angiotensin II receptor antagonists
	Looking at blood levels of immunosuppressive drugs, modifying doses according to pharmacokinetic changes during pregnancy
	Monitoring of most common viral infection is also recommended: titers of anti-CMV IgG and IgM every 3 mo, test for toxoplasma every 6 mo
Fetal surveillance	Growth scans every 2–4 wk as of 28 wk or as clinically indicated
	Nonstress test as of 30 wk or as clinically indicated
	Doppler flows as of 24 wk
Postpartum period	Vaginal delivery is recommended, but cesarean section is required in at least 50% of women
	Steroid dose must be increased in the perinatal period to avoid postpartum rejection
	Renal function, BP, proteinuria, fluid balance, and blood immunosuppressant levels should be closely monitored in the puerperium
	Breast-feeding is not recommended due to transfer of immunosuppressive drugs into breast milk
	Neonatal classic vaccinations should be delayed until after the first 6 mo of life in view of the potential risk of suboptimal immunological responses and adverse events

ACE, angiotensin-converting enzyme; BP, blood pressure; CMV, cytomegalovirus; Cr, creatinine; MMF, mycophenolate mofetil.
From Stratta P, Canavese C, Giacchino F, et al: Pregnancy in kidney transplantation: Satisfactory outcomes and harsh realities. J Nephrol 2003;16:792–806.

Another major concern is the impact of a renal transplant on maternal mortality. It is estimated that 10% of renal transplant patients die within 7 years of pregnancy and 50% within 15 years.

Fetal Effects

These pregnancies have several perinatal complications including intrauterine growth restriction (20%–30%), prematurity (40%–60%), perinatal mortality, neonatal death (10-fold more than general population), congenital malformations, and long-term developmental effects. As for long-term effects, there are few data on long-term effects on offspring and pediatric follow-up is scarce. Stanley and colleagues[51] reported during a follow-up period of 4 months to 12 years among 175 children of 133 women on steroids plus cyclosporine, 29 children (16%) had delayed development or at the age of 5 to 12 years, 10 (14%) needed educational support and eight (11%) required medication for attention-deficit/hyperactivity disorder.

Based on the described maternal and fetal outcomes, there should be a multidisciplinary team approach used in these pregnancies with very close follow-up before conception, during pregnancy, and in the postpartum period (Table 42-5). Cesarean delivery is only recommended for obstetric indications. However, studies have shown more frequent cesarean deliveries in women with a transplant, ranging between 25% and 80%.

All women of childbearing age with a renal transplant should have prepregnancy counseling. Generally, women with chronic renal disease should plan a pregnancy before the serum creatinine level reaches values greater than 2 mg/dL and with well-controlled blood pressure and minimal protein. If the serum creatinine is more than 2 mg/dL, women might consider delaying pregnancy until after transplantation. Post-transplantation, all women should be advised to use an effective contraceptive method for at least 1 year. Fertility and ovulation usually return to normal as of the first month after transplantation. The use of intrauterine devices is discouraged due to risk of infection. Low-dose birth control pills are recommended.

References

1. Harris RE, Thomas VL, Shelokov A: Asymptomatic bacteriuria in pregnancy: Antibody-coated bacteria renal function, and intrauterine growth retardation. Am J Obstet Gynecol 1976;126:20–25.
2. Kass E: Asymptomatic infections of the urinary tract. Trans Assoc Am Physicians 1956;69:56–64.
3. Savage W, Hajj S, Kass E: Demographic and prognostic characteristics of bacteriuria in pregnancy. Medicine (Baltimore) 1967;46:385–407.
4. Whalley P: Bacteriuria of pregnancy. Am J Obstet Gynecol 1967;97:723–738.
5. Gilstrap LC, Cunningham FG, Whalley PJ: Acute pyelonephritis in pregnancy: An anterospective study. Obstet Gynecol 1981;57:409–413.
6. Mead PJ, Harris RE: Incidence of group B beta-hemolytic streptococcus in antepartum urinary tract infections. Obstet Gynecol 1978;51:412–414.
7. Kass EH: The role of asymptomatic bacteriuria in the pathogenesis of pyelonephritis. In Quinn EL, Kass EH (eds): Biology of Pyelonephritis. Boston: Little, Brown, 1960, pp 399–412.
8. Plattner MS: Pyelonephritis in pregnancy. J Perinatol Neonat Nurs 1994;8:20–27.
9. Grunfeld J, Pertuiset N: Acute renal failure in pregnancy: 1987. Am J Kidney Dis 1987;9:359–362.
10. Stratta P, Canavese C, Dogliani M, et al: Pregnancy-related acute renal failure. Clin Nephrol 1989;32:14–20.
11. Turney J, Ellis C, Parsons F: Obstetric acute renal failure 1956–1987. Br J Obstet Gynaecol 1989;96:679–687.
12. Thadhani R, Pascual M, Bonventre J: Acute renal failure. N Engl J Med 1996;334:1448–1460.
13. Marik PE: Low-dose dopamine: A systematic review. Intensive Care Med 2002;28:877–873.
14. Uchino S, Doig S, Bellomo R, et al: Diuretics and mortality in acute renal failure. Crit Care Med 2004;32:1669–1677.
15. Hoste EA, De Waele JJ: Physiologic consequences of acute renal failure on the critically ill. Crit Care Clin 2005;21:251–260.
16. Fink JC, Schwartz SM, Benedetti TJ, Stehman-Breen CO: Increased risk of adverse maternal and infant outcomes among women with renal disease. Paediatr Perinat Epidemiol 1998;12:277–287.
17. Fischer MJ, Lehnerz SD, Hebert JR, Parikh CR: Kidney disease is an independent risk factor for adverse fetal and maternal outcomes in pregnancy. Am J Kidney Dis 2004;43:415–423.
18. Cunningham FG, Cox SM, Harstad TW, et al: Chronic renal disease and pregnancy outcome. Am J Obstet Gynecol 1990;163:453–459.
19. Trevisan G, Ramos JG, Martins-Costa S, Barros EJ: Pregnancy in patients with chronic renal insufficiency at Hospital de Clinicas of Porto Alegre, Brazil. Ren Fail 2004;26:29–34.
20. Jones DC, Hayslett JP: Outcome of pregnancy in women with moderate or severe renal insufficiency [published erratum appears in N Engl J Med 1997;336:739]. N Engl J Med 1996; 335:226–232.
21. Bar J, Orvieto R, Shalev Y, et al: Pregnancy outcome in women with primary renal disease. Isr Med Assoc J 2000;2:178–181.
22. Epstein FH: Pregnancy and renal disease. N Engl J Med 1996; 335:277–278.
23. Katz A, Davison J, Hayslett J, et al: Pregnancy in women with kidney disease. Kidney Int 1980;18:192–206.
24. Lindheimer MD, Katz AI: Gestation in women with kidney disease: Prognosis and management. Baillieres Clin Obstet Gynaecol 1994;8:387–404.
25. Davison JM: Renal disorders in pregnancy. Curr Opin Obstet Gynecol 2001;13:109–114.
26. Gordon M, Landon MB, Samuels P, et al: Perinatal outcome and long-term follow-up associated with modern management of diabetic nephropathy. Obstet Gynecol 1996;87:401–409.
27. Reece E, Coustan DR, Hayslett JP, et al: Diabetic nephropathy: Pregnancy performance and fetomaternal outcome. Am J Obstet Gynecol 1998;159:56–66.
28. Reece E, Leguizamon G, Homko C: Stringent control in diabetic nephropathy associated with optimization of pregnancy outcomes. J Matern Fetal Med 1998;7:213–216.
29. Bobrie G, Liote F, Houillier P, et al: Pregnancy in lupus nephritis and related disorders. Am J Kidney Dis 1987;9:339–343.
30. Dennis E, McIver F, Smythe C: Renal biopsy in pregnancy. Clin Obstet Gynecol 1968;11:473–486.
31. Schewitz L, Friedman I, Pollack V: Bleeding after renal biopsy in pregnancy. Obstet Gynecol 1965;26:295–304.
32. Confortini P, Galanti G, Ancona G, et al: Full term pregnancy and successful delivery in a patient on chronic haemodialysis. Proc Eur Dial Transplant Assoc 1971;8:74–78.
33. Anonymous: Successful pregnancies in women treated by dialysis and kidney transplantation. Report from the Registration Committee of the European Dialysis and Transplant Association. Br J Obstet Gynaecol 1980;87:839–845.
34. Okundaye I, Abrinko P, Hou S: Registry of pregnancy in dialysis patients. Am J Kidney Dis 1998;31:766–773.

35. Bagon JA, Vernaeve H, De Muylder X, et al: Pregnancy and dialysis. Am J Kidney Dis 1998;31:756–765.

36. Hull AR: More dialysis appears beneficial for pregnant ESRD patients (at least in Belgium). Am J Kidney Dis 1998;31:863–864.

37. Prasad S, Parkhurst D, Morton MR, et al: Increased delivery of haemodialysis assists successful pregnancy outcome in end-stage renal failure. Nephrology 2003;8:311–314.

38. Okundaye I, Hou S: Management of pregnancy in women undergoing continuous ambulatory peritoneal dialysis. Adv Perit Dial 1996;12:151–155.

39. Hou S: Pregnancy in women treated with peritoneal dialysis: Viewpoint 1996. Perit Dial Int 1996;16:442–443.

40. Chao A-S, Huang JY, Lien R, et al: Pregnancy in women who undergo long-term hemodialysis. Am J Obstet Gynecol 2002; 187:152–156.

41. Tan PK, Tan A, Koon TH, Vathsala A: Effect of pregnancy on renal graft function and maternal survival in renal transplant recipients. Transplant Proc 2002;34:1161–1163.

42. Davison JM: The effect of pregnancy on kidney function in renal allograft recipients. Kidney Int 1985;27:74–79.

43. Milne JE, Lindheimer MD, Davison JM: Glomerular heteroporous membrane modeling in third trimester and postpartum before and during amino acid infusion. Am J Physiol Renal Physiol 2002; 282:F170–F175.

44. EBPG Expert Group on Renal Transplantation: European best practice guidelines for renal transplantation. Section IV: Long-term management of the transplant recipient. IV 10. Pregnancy in renal transplant recipients. Nephrol Dial Transplant 2002;117(Suppl 4):1–67.

45. Armenti VT, Wilson GA, Radomski JS, et al: Report from the National Transplantation Pregnancy Registry (NTPR): Outcomes of pregnancy after transplantation. Clin Transpl 1999: 111–119.

46. Hou S: Pregnancy in organ transplant recipients. Med Clin North Am 1989;73:667–683.

47. Franz M, Horl WH: Common errors in diagnosis and management of urinary tract infection. II: Clinical management. Nephrol Dial Transplant 1999;14:2754–2762.

48. Ehrich JH, Loirat C, Davison JM, et al: Repeated successful pregnancies after kidney transplantation in 102 women (report by the EDTA Registry). Nephrol Dial Transplant 1996;11: 1314–1317.

49. Kainz A, Harabacz I, Cowlrick IS, et al: Analysis of 100 pregnancy outcomes in women treated systemically with tacrolimus. Transpl Int 2000;13(Suppl 1):S299–S300.

50. Armenti VT, Radomski JS, Moritz MJ, et al., National Transplantation Pregnancy Registry: Report from the National Transplantation Pregnancy Registry (NTPR): Outcomes of pregnancy after transplantation. Clin Transpl 2002;121–130.

51. Stanley CW, Gottlieb R, Zager R, et al: Developmental well-being in offspring of women receiving cyclosporine post-renal transplant. Transplant Proc 1999;31:241–242.

Further Reading

Bellomo R: Defining, quantifying, and classifying acute renal failure. Crit Care Clin 2005;21:223–237.

Board JA, Lee HM, Draper DA, Hume DM: Pregnancy following kidney homotransplantation from a non-twin. Report of a case with concurrent administration of azathioprine and prednisone. Obstet Gynecol 1967;29:318–323.

Dashe JS, Ramin SM, Cunningham FG: The long-term consequences of thrombotic microangiopathy (thrombotic thrombocytopenic purpura and hemolytic uremic syndrome) in pregnancy. Obstet Gynecol 1998;91:662–668.

Davison JM, Vallotton MB, Lindheimer MD: Plasma osmolality and urinal concentration and dilution during and after pregnancy: Evidence that lateral recumbency inhibits maximal urinary concentrating ability. Br J Obstet Gynaecol 1981;88:472–479.

Davison JM, Dunlop W: Changes in renal hemodynamics and tubular function induced by normal pregnancy. Semin Nephrol 1984;4:198–206.

Drakeley AJ, Le Roux PA, Anthony J, et al: Acute renal failure complicating severe preeclampsia requiring admission to an obstetric intensive care unit. Am J Obstet Gynecol 2002;186:253–256.

Norton CW, Kass EH: Bacteriuria of pregnancy: A critical appraisal. Annu Rev Med 1968;19:431–470.

Sibai BM, Ramadan MK: Acute renal failure in pregnancies complicated by hemolysis, elevated liver enzymes, and low platelets. Am J Obstet Gynecol 1993;168:1682–1690.

Sibai BM, Villar MA, Mabie BC: Acute renal failure in hypertensive disorders of pregnancy. Pregnancy outcome and remote prognosis in thirty-one consecutive cases. Am J Obstet Gynecol 1990;162:777–783.

Stratta P, Canavese C, Giacchino F, et al. Pregnancy in kidney transplantation: Satisfactory outcomes and harsh realities. J Nephrol 2003;16:792–806.

Toma H, Tanabe K, Tokumoto T, et al: Pregnancy in women receiving renal dialysis or transplantation in Japan: A nationwide survey. Nephrol Dial Transplant 1999;14:1511–1516.

PART VIII

Pediatric Nephrology

CONTENTS

Chapter 43

Management of Pediatric Kidney Disease

Nancy M. Rodig and Michael J.G. Somers

Although few children are afflicted with serious renal disease, a wide variety of nephrologic problems may present in childhood. Many of these same problems may also be found in adults, but in children, there are often significant differences in the etiology, the approach to diagnostic evaluation, and therapy. Moreover, the low incidence of pediatric renal disease has often precluded the execution of large controlled studies to provide evidence-based assessments of specific treatments. As a result, many therapies in children are either empiric or based on experiences drawn from treating adults. An additional distinguishing and important feature of the approach to therapy in the child is the need to consider the effect of any intervention on the child's ongoing physical and cognitive development. In this chapter, many of the more common renal conditions in children are discussed, with particular attention to the aspects of management or therapy most germane to the pediatric patient that may contrast with the approach to the adult patient with a similar problem.

PROTEINURIA

As a common and readily detected sign of renal disease, proteinuria often triggers a diagnostic evaluation for significant underlying renal pathology. As with adults, all children excrete a small amount of protein daily in their urine. Normal parameters are related to both size and age, and, as a general rule, children younger than 10 years of age rarely excrete more than 100 mg of urinary protein per day.[1] In older children and adolescents, urinary protein excretion can increase to as much as the 150 to 200 mg/day threshold considered normal in adults.[2] In most children, proteinuria is asymptomatic and detected as part of a general examination during which a random sample of urine is assayed by a qualitative colorimetric test strip. In urine samples in which a more precise estimation of protein excretion is needed, a urinary protein-to-creatinine ratio can prove more useful and has been demonstrated to be an accurate method for assessing daily protein excretion in children.[3] A ratio less than 0.5 in a child younger than 2 years old or less than 0.2 in an older child is considered normal. These ratios can be followed to assess changes in proteinuria over time and have, for the most part, replaced routine 24-hour urine collections, which are often cumbersome to collect and inaccurate in pediatric patients.

Isolated proteinuria is a relatively common finding in children. As reported in several studies, mass screening of schoolchildren for proteinuria points to a prevalence between 5% and 10%.[4,5] Proteinuria appears to be more common in adolescence than early childhood. Most proteinuria in childhood is transient and not indicative of renal disease. When nearly 9000 schoolchildren in Helsinki were followed for 1 year with intermittent urine samples, 10% were found to have proteinuria more than 1+ on urinary dipstick on an initial screen.[6] Only 2.5% were found to have persistent proteinuria on one of an additional three follow-up collections. Similarly, in a large survey done in pediatric office practice, only 10% of children initially found to have proteinuria on dipstick still manifested proteinuria 1 year later.[4] Such studies have called into question the utility of regular urinary screenings to detect early kidney disease because, in the vast majority of asymptomatic children, any detected abnormality tends to clear spontaneously.

Transient proteinuria often accompanies stress, acute febrile illness, or exercise. Such isolated proteinuria is thought to be most likely mediated by intrarenal hemodynamic changes, decreasing renal plasma flow out of proportion to glomerular filtration rate (GFR) and enhancing the concentration gradient of protein into Bowman's space.[7] There is no long-term residual renal damage with transient proteinuria, and these children do not require a diagnostic evaluation.

With persistent proteinuria, fixed proteinuria should be distinguished from orthostatic proteinuria. With fixed proteinuria, every urine sample has significant proteinuria; with orthostatic proteinuria, protein excretion is linked to body position. Thus, with orthostatic proteinuria, abnormally high rates of protein excretion occur while the child is upright or ambulatory and normal protein excretion ensues when the child is recumbent. The mechanism of orthostatic proteinuria is thought to arise from an enhanced renal sensitivity to the normal hemodynamic and hormonal alterations that occur with changes in position, resulting in enhanced glomerular protein permeability.[8]

Orthostatic proteinuria is quite common and accounts for as much as two thirds of pediatric proteinuria, especially in adolescents. Generally, in orthostatic proteinuria, excretion of urinary protein is less than 1 g/day.[5,6] Many children go on to clear their postural proteinuria with time, but some may always demonstrate orthostatic proteinuria. Most follow-up studies of individuals found to have postural proteinuria point to no increased incidence of long-term renal disease as long as the proteinuria is an isolated finding and not accompanied by hematuria, an active urinary sediment, or hypertension.[9] However, some patients with orthostatic proteinuria followed for more than 35 years did demonstrate late-onset renal insufficiency.[10]

With persistent nonorthostatic proteinuria, a diagnostic evaluation usually ensues to rule out any underlying glomerular or renal parenchymal disease. With increasing daily excretion of urinary protein of more than 1 g in the adolescent or more than 600 mg/m^2 in the younger child, there must be an increased index of clinical suspicion that there may be more serious ongoing renal disease, and these children often proceed to renal biopsy.[11]

In children with lower grade fixed isolated proteinuria, the majority exhibit no evidence of progressive renal disease. Most of these children demonstrate normal or nonspecific changes on renal biopsy. However, some children will have evidence of focal segmental glomerulosclerosis on renal biopsy.[12,13] These children often have higher levels of proteinuria that may exceed nephrotic range over time and nearly 50% progress to end-stage renal disease (ESRD). Thus, in children with any element of fixed proteinuria, there should be long-term follow-up to monitor the degree of proteinuria and to assess for the development of hematuria, hypertension, or renal insufficiency.

The diagnostic evaluation of the child with proteinuria is best done in phases (Box 43-1). The evaluation is focused on confirming and quantifying proteinuria, distinguishing fixed proteinuria from orthostatic proteinuria, and identifying whether the proteinuria is isolated or whether there are accompanying clinical signs or symptoms suggestive of increased likelihood of renal disease. The child who has proteinuria as part of the nephrotic syndrome should be considered separately because the evaluation, as well as the management and prognosis, varies.

NEPHROTIC SYNDROME

Because of the overwhelming preponderance of minimal change disease as the cause of nephrosis in the prepubertal child (Table 43-1), the initial evaluation and management of nephrotic syndrome in children differ from the approach for adults.[14] It is much less likely for children to undergo an extensive initial laboratory evaluation or a renal biopsy and much more likely for them to be placed on empiric steroid therapy. Moreover, the vast majority of children with nephrotic syndrome eventually outgrow this as a recurrent problem, with no long-term compromise of renal function.[15]

Nephrotic syndrome in children is characterized by massive proteinuria exceeding 50 mg/kg/day or 40 mg/m^2/hr. Serum albumin levels will be less than 2.5 g/dL and may often be profoundly depressed (<0.5 g/dL). Edema may be quite problematic, especially at presentation or during protracted relapses. Hyperlipidemia may also be quite pronounced, especially in light of normal pediatric cholesterol levels rarely exceeding 180 mg/dL.

In children younger than 16 years of age, the annual incidence of nephrotic syndrome is 2 per 100,000, with a cumulative prevalence of just less than 20 per 100,000.[16] Presentation in the first year of life is uncommon and especially in the first 3 months of life should raise the suspicion of congenital nephrotic syndrome, a condition quite unlike minimal change nephrosis both in its cause and long-term prognosis.[14] Typically, most children with nephrosis present between 2 and 6 years of age, and in younger children, there is up to a 2:1 ratio of affected boys to girls.[17] In older children and adolescents

---

Box 43-1 Diagnostic Evaluation of Asymptomatic Proteinuria in the Child

Phase 1
Reconfirm proteinuria in random urine sample
Microscopic urinalysis to assess for red or white blood cells, casts, or crystals
Focused history and physical examination: urinary tract infection, family history of renal disease, growth parameters, blood pressure, presence of edema or rash

Phase 2
Serum creatinine
Assess for postural proteinuria by comparing proteinuria in first morning urine sample with random void later in day
If postural proteinuria confirmed with normal renal function, no further evaluation. Child needs annual follow-up

Phase 3
Quantitate proteinuria with urinary protein-to-creatinine ratio or timed collection
Other blood work as clinically indicated: albumin, cholesterol, antinuclear antibody, serologies
Renal ultrasonography
Consider voiding cystourethrography if ultrasonography suggests reflux or scarring

Phase 4
Consider renal biopsy if active urinary sediment, significant microhematuria or macrohematuria, fixed proteinuria that is exacerbating or .600 mg/m^2/day, hypertension, renal insufficiency, or family history of end-stage renal disease

Table 43-1 Etiology of Nephrotic Syndrome in Children Who Had a Biopsy at Presentation

Histologic Category	Frequency (%)
Minimal change	77
Focal and segmental glomerulosclerosis	9
Membranoproliferative glomerulonephritis	7
Other or unclassified	5
Mesangial proliferative glomerulonephritis	2

Based on data from International Study of Kidney Disease in Children: Nephrotic syndrome in children: Prediction of histopathology from clinical and laboratory characteristics at time of diagnosis. Kidney Int 1981;13:159–165.

Table 43-2 Frequency of Clinical Characteristics in Pediatric Nephrosis at Presentation

Clinical Characteristic	Minimal Change (%)	Focal Sclerosis (%)
Age < 6 yr	80	50
Male gender	60	70
Hypertension	20	50
Microhematuria	25	50
Increased serum creatinine	30	40

Based on data from International Study of Kidney Disease in Children: Nephrotic syndrome in children: Prediction of histopathology from clinical and laboratory characteristics at time of diagnosis. Kidney Int 1981;13:159–165.

who present with nephrotic syndrome, this ratio is closer to 1:1.[18] There appear to be racial differences in the virulence of nephrotic syndrome in children. For instance, in North America, data suggest that African American and Hispanic children are more likely to have steroid-resistant disease that progresses to end-stage renal failure.[19]

Minimal Change Disease

The typical child with minimal change disease presents following a nonspecific viral illness. Many children are first brought to medical attention because of periorbital edema, and it is quite common to elicit a history that the child has been given diphenhydramine for "allergies," but the edema has not abated. Clinically, minimal change disease can be distinguished from nephritis or other chronic glomerulopathies by the absence of signs or symptoms consistent with glomerular inflammation. Thus, it is quite uncommon to see a child with minimal change disease present with macroscopic hematuria, severe hypertension, or azotemia.[14] Pertinent clinical characteristics and their frequency in minimal change disease are outlined in Table 43-2.

In a prepubertal child with nephrosis, normal blood pressure, nonnephrotic urinary sediment, and normal renal function, the presumed diagnosis is minimal change disease, and empiric steroid therapy is indicated. Most pediatric centers start such children on prednisone 60 mg/m²/day or its equivalent to a maximum dose of 80 mg/day. The steroid dose may be given in one total daily dose or divided according to local practice or parental preference. Most children with minimal change disease respond to steroid therapy within 2 weeks, and more than 90% of children who are steroid responsive respond by 4 weeks of daily steroid therapy.[20] Lack of response to oral steroids after 6 to 8 weeks of daily therapy should prompt reassessment of the treatment regimen and may call for renal biopsy.

Treatment lengths vary for the child who presents with presumed minimal change disease, but there is evidence to suggest that an initial 3- to 4-month steroid regimen combining daily and then alternate-day therapy may result in fewer relapses.[21] A typical regimen for a newly diagnosed case of pediatric nephrosis would be prednisone 60 mg/m²/day for

4 weeks. If remission has yet to be achieved, this dose would be continued for as much as an additional 4 weeks. If remission is achieved, then after 4 weeks of daily therapy, prednisone would be tapered to 40 mg/m² on alternate days for 1 to 2 months, and then the dose tapered by 10 mg/m² every 1 to 2 weeks over the next 1 to 2 months.

In relapses, daily steroid therapy at a dose of 60 mg/m²/day is often used until remission is induced, and then a tapering steroid course is initiated over weeks to months depending on the patient's individual history. With frequent relapses, long-term use of low-dose alternate-day therapy in the range of 10 to 15 mg/m² may actually reduce overall steroid burden by sustaining remission and minimizing exposure to daily high-dose steroid therapy.

Minimal change disease in children is a relapsing condition. Less than 20% of affected children have only one episode of nephrosis, whereas nearly 50% frequently relapse, with three or more relapses within 6 months of presentation.[22] Between 30% and 40% of children become steroid dependent, having relapses while still being treated with steroids or within 2 weeks of concluding steroid therapy. Sequelae of steroid therapy are common and include hypertension, loss of bone density, cataracts, gastritis, emotional lability, and increased susceptibility to infection. An adverse effect of chronic steroid use of particular concern in children is growth impairment. A child's somatic growth must be monitored quite closely and standardized growth charts used to assess growth velocity.

The development of significant steroid sequelae is the most common impetus for consideration of alternative drug therapy in minimal change disease. Most commonly, alkylating agents such as cyclophosphamide and chlorambucil are used. A daily dose of cyclophosphamide 2 to 3 mg/kg for 8 to 12 weeks to a cumulative dose of 168 mg/kg has proved quite effective.[23,24] Nearly 70% of steroid-sensitive children are in remission for at least 1 year and 40% remain in a sustained remission for at least 5 years.[23] Alkylating agents seem most efficacious in steroid-sensitive children who have frequent relapses but are somewhat less effective in inducing long-term remission in children with steroid-dependent disease.[25] Cyclophosphamide has also been shown to be effective in converting approximately one third of children with steroid-resistant disease to steroid responsiveness.[26,27] In steroid-sensitive children, these agents seem to work best if given while the child is in remission and on concomitant steroid therapy.

There are multiple toxicities associated with the use of alkylating agents. Acutely, bone marrow suppression is common, and patients must be monitored for leukopenia. Other acute toxicities include alopecia, gastrointestinal discomfort, and hemorrhagic cystitis. With chlorambucil, there is also a small risk of idiosyncratic seizures. Longer term complications include dose-related gonadal toxicity and concerns regarding future malignancies, although no direct data exist linking alkylating agent use in nephrotic children with increased rates of future malignancies.

In children with particularly recalcitrant minimal change disease, calcineurin inhibitors such as cyclosporine may induce remission.[28–30] An initial dose of 6 mg/kg/day divided into two doses often induces and sustains a remission, and most children with minimal change disease can be weaned off steroid therapy and steroid sequelae will improve. After a period of remission, cyclosporine may be tapered or discontinued. If relapses occur, the child may be placed back on steroids to see whether the nephrotic syndrome now follows a less relapsing and more steroid-sensitive course or, if necessary, placed back on cyclosporine therapy. Cyclosporine levels need to be monitored closely and changes in renal function carefully assessed. Some children on long-term cyclosporine therapy with increasing serum creatinine values may require interval renal biopsies to assess for histologic changes compatible with cyclosporine-induced nephrotoxicity. Interestingly, cyclosporine-associated arteriopathy seems to recede after cessation of cyclosporine in children with nephrotic syndrome, whereas tubulointerstitial changes and focal glomerular lesions do not regress.[31]

In an attempt to prolong remission and to spare overall steroid burden, multiple medications have been used as adjunctive therapy in minimal change disease. Levamisole, an anthelminthic immunostimulant, appears to be beneficial in maintaining remissions.[32,33] Levamisole is generally given orally concurrently with tapering doses of steroids over the course of many months to several years. Unlike the alkylating agents, levamisole does not seem to have as dramatic an effect on the natural history of minimal change disease, and children who had frequent relapses tend to begin to have relapses more frequently again after levamisole therapy is discontinued. Although widely used in parts of Europe and Asia, the drug has been employed less commonly in North America due to problems with its availability and clinician inexperience with its prescription. Adverse effects are rare with levamisole therapy but include agranulocytosis, liver function abnormalities, and an antineutrophil cytoplasmic antibody–positive vasculitis syndrome after protracted therapy.[34]

Azathioprine and, more recently, mycophenolate mofetil (MMF) have also been used as steroid-sparing agents. Although there is no indication that azathioprine is advantageous as monotherapy, its concurrent use with steroids may allow tapering of steroids to low enough doses to ameliorate or preclude steroid sequelae.[35] There have been several case reports or small series of children with minimal change disease treated with MMF. In the largest multicenter study, 32 children with frequently relapsing nephrotic syndrome were treated with MMF 600 mg/m^2 (maximal dose 1 g) twice daily for 6 months.[36] For the first 16 weeks of MMF therapy, steroids were also provided at 1 mg/kg on alternate days for the first 8 weeks and then 0.5 mg/kg on alternate days for weeks 9 to 16. Persistent remission was seen in 24 children (75%) during MMF therapy. After MMF was discontinued, eight children remained in a sustained remission off all therapy, with follow-up ranging from 18 to 30 months.

Most children with minimal change disease eventually outgrow their disease and by early adulthood are in long-term remission and considered cured. These children do not appear to be at increased risk of other renal disease or of developing functional renal impairment. Early follow-up studies identified that nearly 15% of affected children may continue to have relapses as adults.[15] Newer longitudinal data from two large pediatric centers point toward as many as one third of adults with a history of pediatric minimal change disease having at least one relapse of nephrosis as an adult.[37,38] Most often, the relapses are infrequent and continue to follow a steroid-sensitive pattern.

Focal Segmental Glomerulosclerosis

Approximately 10% to 15% of prepubertal children with nephrotic syndrome have focal segmental glomerulosclerosis (FSGS). This incidence increases to more than one third of affected adolescents.[39] The median age at onset of FSGS is 6 years, and, similar to minimal change disease, there seems to be a male gender predisposition in young children. Most affected children present acutely with nephrotic syndrome, but nearly one fourth can present initially with asymptomatic proteinuria. Children with FSGS are more likely to manifest microhematuria, hypertension, and renal insufficiency at presentation than children with minimal change disease[14] (see Table 43-2).

Almost all children with FSGS are likely to have the idiopathic or primary form. Renal biopsy reveals focal involvement, with some areas of the kidney appearing absolutely normal and other areas showing segmental capillary collapse, mesangial matrix proliferation, and frank sclerosis.[40] The same histology may be seen in secondary FSGS, in which focal glomerular disease arises as a result of a concomitant renal insult, a nephrotoxin, or systemic disease such as reflux nephropathy, heroin-induced nephropathy, or human immunodeficiency virus.[41]

The clinical course of idiopathic FSGS in children is often characterized by steroid-resistant disease. Although as many as one third of children with FSGS respond to an 8-week trial of oral steroids, many initial responders later go on to become steroid unresponsive.[42] With steroid-unresponsive disease, there are few data to suggest that an oral alkylating agent by itself is likely to have a beneficial effect; in fact, one study comparing alternate-day steroid therapy with alternate-day steroids and cyclophosphamide found equivalent remission rates.[43] Children who do show sensitivity to initial oral therapy with steroids or alkylating agents are more likely to have less aggressive disease and may follow a course with few relapses or with sustained remissions.[44,45]

In children with FSGS who do not respond to initial therapy, more aggressive immunosuppressive regimens have met with some success in inducing partial or complete remission. Unfortunately, evaluation of treatment efficacy and comparison of treatment approach have been complicated by the lack of randomized or well-controlled studies in children with this disease. Many clinicians now use a 10-week induction course of frequent pulse intravenous methylprednisolone and concomitant oral prednisone to achieve a remission and then attempt to maintain a remission with continued oral steroids and less frequent intravenous pulses.[46] Initial treatment failure or any improvement with relapse leads to reinduction and the addition of a 3-month course of oral cyclophosphamide. In some reports, nearly three fourths of children achieve a long-term partial or complete remission of their FSGS following this type of protocol.[47] Other reports have demonstrated considerably less long-term efficacy and have also raised the issues that black children may not respond as well to such treatment and that there may be serious clinical complications that arise related to the high-dose steroids and the potential for repeated courses of alkylating agents.[48,49]

Cyclosporine has also been shown capable of inducing a partial or complete remission in many children with FSGS.[50–52] Doses of 5 to 6 mg/kg in one single daily dose or divided into two equal daily doses have been used. Although this approach avoids many of the sequelae of therapy with high-dose steroids or alkylating agents, children with FSGS who respond to cyclosporine almost always have a relapse if cyclosporine therapy is withdrawn and thus remain cyclosporine dependent. As a result, some children treated with cyclosporine are at risk of developing long-term nephropathy due to chronic exposure to calcineurin inhibitors.[53] Consequently, attention to cyclosporine levels and serum creatinine must be part of the regular follow-up, and some patients may require intermittent renal biopsy to assess possible drug nephrotoxicity. There are data to suggest that children with FSGS who are treated with cyclosporine may have a less rapid progression to ESRD, with one trial demonstrating only one fourth of cyclosporine-treated patients progressing to ESRD within 5 years of diagnosis compared with more than three fourths of historical controls who had been steroid and cyclophosphamide resistant.[54]

In children resistant to cyclosporine, tacrolimus therapy may also be beneficial. In a report of 16 Canadian children with steroid- and cyclosporine-resistant nephrosis, 13 with confirmed FSGS on biopsy, 13 went into a complete remission and 2 went into a partial remission after a mean of 2 months on tacrolimus therapy.[55]

Many clinicians have begun to use angiotensin-converting enzyme (ACE) inhibitors or angiotensin receptor blockers as adjunctive therapy in children with FSGS.[56,57] These agents decrease glomerular filtration through their interaction with the homeostatic mechanisms involved with maintaining glomerular perfusion. As a result of the decrease in GFR, there is concomitantly less proteinuria. Although serum albumin levels may increase with the decreased proteinuria, they do not generally become normal in children with FSGS. However, the decreased proteinuria and the alteration in glomerular hemodynamics are thought to be beneficial in decreasing the rate of glomerulosclerosis.

Similar to the experience with minimal change disease, there are limited data as to the utility of therapy with MMF in FSGS.[58,59] Some reports point toward its efficacy in children with FSGS who have been unresponsive to oral steroids or a combination of oral steroids and alkylating agents. It is often used in combination with ACE inhibitors or angiotensin receptor blockers to see whether there is a synergistic effect on reducing proteinuria.

A multicenter trial of therapy in pediatric FSGS is now ongoing, comparing a regimen of cyclosporine, alternate-day steroids, and angiotensin blockade with a second regimen using MMF, alternate-day steroids, and angiotensin blockade. Other therapies reported successful in very small numbers of children include plasmapheresis and the use of the anti-CD 20 receptor monoclonal rituximab, but more data are needed to substantiate the efficacy of either approach. Unlike the uniformly excellent long-term prognosis seen in minimal change disease, a substantial number of children with FSGS manifest eventual renal insufficiency. Approximately one fourth of affected children reach ESRD as early as 5 years after disease onset.[60] Pediatric registry data confirm that FSGS is the most common glomerular disease leading to renal replacement therapy in children.[61]

In children undergoing renal transplantation for FSGS, recurrent disease may commonly be seen, often in the immediate postoperative period. Although recurrent disease can be treated successfully, generally using a combined approach of plasmapheresis and intensification of immunosuppression, there is accelerated graft loss in recurrent FSGS, and the usual graft survival advantage seen with kidneys donated from living donors is lost in children with FSGS who undergo transplantation.[62]

The cause of idiopathic FSGS in children is unknown. However, in many children with FSGS, a circulating lymphokine has been isolated that increases the albumin permeability of perfused rat glomeruli in vitro.[63] Some children with recurrent FSGS after renal transplantation appear to manifest more permeability in this assay, leading to speculation that they may have a more virulent circulating factor. The ability to induce a remission with the use of therapies aimed at immunomodulation and lymphokine removal, such as pheresis, also seems to support the role of some systemic factor in this disease.[64]

Recent genetic studies in children with FSGS point toward both an autosomal dominant and autosomal recessive mode of inheritance in some children with steroid-resistant disease.[65–68] These studies arose initially from the observation that although nephrotic syndrome is rare in the sibling of an affected child, in those cases of apparent familial nephrosis, steroid-unresponsive FSGS was the common lesion. Unlike idiopathic FSGS, this form of the disease is less likely to respond to any immunomodulatory therapy and also unlikely to recur in a renal allograft. As the molecular genetics of this condition continue to be discerned, it may lead to an ability to screen children with nephrotic syndrome and avoid exposure to unnecessary and potentially toxic drug therapies in children with certain genotypes. Currently, most pediatric nephrologists advise genetic screening for children with steroid-resistant FSGS or a family history of consanguinity or previously reported nephrosis.

Congenital Nephrotic Syndrome

Congenital nephrotic syndrome is a rare condition generally diagnosed in the initial months of life. Although prenatal diagnosis has been reported as a result of alterations in amniotic fluid volume and protein content, infants may also present with edema and the associated proteinuria and hypoalbuminemia are then discerned. The etiology of congenital nephrotic syndrome generally follows one of three subtypes: (1) related to intrauterine or congenital infection, (2) related to diffuse mesangial sclerosis (DMS) as part of Denys-Drash syndrome or as an isolated mutation in the *WT1* gene, or (3) related to a defect in the podocyte protein nephrin as part of a mutation in the *NPHS1* gene commonly referred to as Finnish-type congenital nephrotic syndrome (CNF). A recent review of 89 European children with infantile nephrosis (presentation at younger than 1 year of age) confirmed that genetic mutations can be detected in two thirds of affected families, and in the children with congenital nephrosis in this cohort, 85% had *NPHS1* mutations linked to CNF.[69]

History and physical examination often help guide the initial diagnostic evaluation, and renal biopsy can provide a definitive histologic diagnosis. Congenital infections such as syphilis can be excluded with negative TORCH titers (a panel antibody screen for toxoplasmosis, syphilis, rubella, cytomegalovirus, and herpesvirus) and the absence of early rash, jaundice, or hepatosplenomegaly in the infant. In the extremely rare instance of congenital infection, treatment of the underlying infection should lead to resolution of nephrosis. With other forms of congenital nephrotic syndrome, the long-term renal prognosis is guarded and most of these children inevitably progress to ESRD.

DMS may be isolated or related to Denys-Drash syndrome with associated pseudohermaphroditism and Wilms' tumor. Mutations in the *WT1* gene, a transcription factor that plays a key role in normal development and function of the urogenital tract, are associated with Denys-Drash syndrome.[70] Abnormalities in *WT1* are well described in Wilms' tumor and other urogenital anomalies, but its exact role as a mediator of glomerular pathology in DMS is unclear.

Detection and appropriate resection and follow-up of Wilms' tumor or other urogenital malignancy are critical components of the care of an infant with DMS due to Denys-Drash syndrome. Other therapy is aimed at management of the sequelae of nephrosis-range proteinuria and may involve frequent infusion of 25% albumin, intensive nutritional therapy, and other supportive care. Children with DMS may have slower progression of their renal insufficiency than children with CNF and may have less profound protein losses, making their management somewhat less complex and more open to options such as unilateral nephrectomy or the use of high-dose ACE inhibitors or prostaglandin inhibitors to decrease glomerular filtration and overall protein losses in the urine to more acceptable levels.[71]

Renal transplantation is the ultimate treatment for children with DMS. Most children do well after transplantation without disease recurrence.[72] Because of concerns regarding an incomplete Denys-Drash syndrome, even in children with apparently isolated DMS, bilateral nephrectomy at the time of transplantation or onset of ESRD is recommended.[73]

CNF is an autosomal recessive disorder most common in, but not exclusive to, people of Finnish heritage. It results from genetic mutations in the *NPHS1* gene that encodes for nephrin, an adhesion protein exclusively expressed in the podocyte and a main component of the slit diaphragm.[74] The exact mechanism of nephrosis due to nephrin anomalies remains unclear. If there is no family history of CNF, it may be suspected in an infant with congenital nephrotic syndrome and none of the manifestations of Denys-Drash syndrome. Infants with CNF are often born prematurely and have a large placenta, weighing more than 25% of the infant's birth weight.[73] There is often elevated maternal serum or amniotic fluid alpha fetoprotein in the absence of neural tube defects or other structural abnormalities.[75]

Infants with CNF are at significant risk of morbidity and mortality if not treated aggressively for the sequelae of their nephrosis (Box 43-2).[76] They must receive intravenous albumin and diuretics to manage edema and are at profound risk of sepsis and thrombosis due to loss of immunoglobulin and coagulation factors in the urine. Significant improvement in long-term outcome has been accomplished by intensive medical support through early infancy until the child reaches 6 to 9 months of age, at which point bilateral nephrectomy can be performed and peritoneal dialysis initiated for several months until the child reaches an appropriate size for renal transplantation. Some infants may need to be nephrectomized earlier in infancy if they have life-threatening infections, severe thrombotic events, or failure

---

Box 43-2 Management of Congenital Nephrotic Syndrome in Early Infancy

Infusion of 25% albumin at dose up to 2 g/kg/day; loop diuretic midway and at end of infusion

Supplemental oral loop or thiazide diuretics may be considered

Minimal caloric intake of 120 kcal/kg/day with 3–4 g/kg/day protein; increase caloric density for fluid restriction

Aggressive treatment of any fever; initiate broad-spectrum antibiotics while awaiting cultures; infusion of IV immunoglobulin 200–400 mg/kg/day during antibiotic therapy

Thyroid function tests monthly and initiation of thyroxine for increased thyroid-stimulating hormone

Long-term anticoagulation with coumadin or salicylate if any thrombotic complications

Early initiation of erythropoietin with doses two to three times normal

Consider therapeutic trial with captopril, gradually increasing dose to 5 mg/kg/day with or without concomitant indomethacin up to 4 mg/kg/day; response to therapy monitored with urinary protein-to-creatinine ratios

Consider early supplementation with activated vitamin D

Nephrectomies and initiation of peritoneal dialysis at 6–9 mo of age; consider earlier if any life-threatening complications of nephrosis such as sepsis, thrombosis, and severe failure to thrive

Based in part on recommendations and data outlined by Holmberg C, Antikainen M, Ronnholm K, et al: Management of congenital nephrotic syndrome of the Finnish type. Pediatr Nephrol 1995;9:87–93.

to thrive despite intensive therapy aimed at minimizing these complications.[77]

Long-term neurodevelopmental and renal allograft outcome is quite good in children with CNF managed in this fashion.[78] In a subset of children, there can be recurrent proteinuria within a year after renal transplantation that may progress and cause renal allograft loss.[79] This posttransplantation proteinuria appears to be related to the extent of the initial nephrin mutation and whether the child has immunologically encountered nephrin before renal transplantation. In the absence of native nephrin, as seen with some CNF mutations, there may be production of antinephrin antibodies and ensuing damage to the slit diaphragms and podocytes of the transplanted kidney.[80] Some children with recurrent proteinuria have been successfully treated with plasmapheresis or the addition of cyclophosphamide to their immunosuppressive regimen.[78]

HEMATURIA

Despite its rare association with malignancy or a renal condition that is progressive or requires treatment, the presence of blood in a child's urine sample often provokes significant anxiety and requires a thoughtful, cost-effective evaluation. The increased availability and use of very sensitive urinary dipsticks for screening has facilitated the identification of children with microhematuria.

In general pediatric practice, isolated microscopic hematuria is now a relatively frequent finding, with an overall prevalence rate of 1.5% of asymptomatic children screened. In a 5-year prospective study of hematuria in 12,000 schoolchildren between the ages of 6 and 12 years, the prevalence was as high as 3.3% when hematuria was defined as five or more erythrocytes per high-power microscopy field occurring in at least two of three consecutive urine samples.[81] Hematuria frequency increased steadily with advancing age and was found more often in girls. In a Finnish study of nearly 9000 healthy children, 4.2% had more than six erythrocytes per high-power microscopy field.[82] However, this number decreased to 1.1% when hematuria was defined as occurring in two or more specimens. Of note, the number of children with isolated microscopic hematuria in these studies is disproportionately large compared with the number of children who have serious functional kidney disease or a threatening anatomic anomaly, suggesting that the majority of children with microhematuria have benign or self-limited conditions.

Gross hematuria occurs far less frequently in children than microhematuria. The frequency of gross hematuria in a pediatric emergency department over a 24-month period was 0.13% of all patient encounters.[83] Urinary tract infection (UTI) was documented or suspected in 49% of these cases. The combined diagnoses of perineal irritation, meatal stenosis, and trauma accounted for an additional 25% of cases. Apparent glomerular disease accounted for only 9% of cases of gross hematuria. At the time of this study, it was not routine to screen for hypercalciuria in children. In a later study, 43% of children presenting with gross hematuria were found to be hypercalciuric.[84] Thus, it is likely that a significant number of these children may also have had excessive urinary calcium excretion.

Cause and Evaluation

The differential diagnosis of pediatric hematuria is large (Box 43-3). The ability to localize the source of hematuria greatly facilitates further evaluation. Urine that is tea- or cola-colored with concomitant proteinuria suggests glomerular pathology. Urine that is red or pink and is associated with clots or dysuria is most consistent with lower urinary tract

---

Box 43-3   Causes of Childhood Hematuria

Renal Parenchymal Disease
Glomerular
  Inherited
    Benign familial hematuria
    Alport's syndrome
  Primary
    IgA nephropathy
    Focal segmental glomerulosclerosis
    Membranoproliferative glomerulonephritis
    Membranous glomerulonephritis
  Systemic
    Hemolytic uremic syndrome
    Henoch-Schönlein purpura
    Systemic lupus erythematosus
    Wegener's granulomatosis
    Microscopic polyarteritis
    Goodpasture's syndrome
  Infectious
    Poststreptococcal glomerulonephritis
    Hepatitis B–associated glomerulonephritis
    Shunt nephritis
    Subacute bacterial endocarditis
Tubulointerstitial
  Inherited
    Polycystic kidney disease
    Juvenile nephronophthisis
    Cystinosis
    Oxalosis
    Tuberous sclerosis
  Acquired
    Hypercalciuria
    Nephrotoxic drugs
    Interstitial nephritis
    Renal transplant rejection

Vascular
Renal vein thrombosis
Renal artery thrombosis
Sickle cell disease

Urinary Tract Disorders
Nephrolithiasis
Urinary tract infection
Urethritis
Trauma

Coagulation Disorders
Anticoagulant use
Hemophilia
Thrombocytopenic purpura

bleeding. Phase-contrast microscopy allows assessment of urinary erythrocyte morphology and the presence of red cell casts is pathognomonic of glomerular hematuria. Hematuria in urine samples from a parent or sibling points to an inherited etiology. Crystalluria may connote abnormal solute excretion predisposing to nephrolithiasis.

The evaluation of hematuria begins with a careful history and physical examination. In infants, the history should include questions regarding birth asphyxia, umbilical vessel catheterization, and abnormalities detected on prenatal ultrasonography. In older children, the history should include questions regarding pain and accompanying voiding symptoms. If macroscopic hematuria exists, determining the timing of the visible hematuria during voiding is important. Gross hematuria at initiation of urination that subsequently clears suggests urethral irritation. Terminal gross hematuria suggests trigonitis. Urine that is persistently tea colored or brown is likely due to glomerulonephritis. In many children who are already independently toilet trained, there may be a significant delay between the onset of symptoms and evaluation because of the failure of the child to recognize the ramifications of hematuria.

As some causes of hematuria may be inherited, a thorough family history is invaluable. A family history of isolated microhematuria without progression to renal insufficiency would suggest benign familial hematuria (BFH). However, a family history of hematuria, proteinuria, and progressive renal failure with associated high-frequency sensorineural hearing loss or visual impairment would raise concern for a familial nephritis such as Alport's syndrome (AS). A family history of cystic kidney disease, IgA nephropathy, nephrolithiasis, coagulopathies, and sickle cell disease would also be significant.

Associated signs and symptoms often provide further etiologic clues. Dysuria, frequency, flank pain, and fever point to UTI. Radiating pain in the loin or groin is consistent with renal colic from nephrolithiasis. The presence of acute edema formation and hypertension would suggest glomerulonephritis. As glomerular disease can be part of a systemic illness, the presence of rash, abdominal pain, and joint inflammation may suggest Henoch-Schönlein purpura (HSP), systemic lupus erythematosus, or a vasculitis.

Laboratory and Radiographic Studies

If the child has at least five urinary erythrocytes per high-power microscopy field on at least two samples over a 2- to 3-week period, further investigation should proceed. Urine studies include culture and quantification of urinary calcium and creatinine. If there is a history of nephrolithiasis, quantification of urinary citrate, oxalate, and uric acid should also be considered. If the protein is greater than trace on the dipstick, especially in a dilute sample, then urinary protein and creatinine should also be quantified. Recommended serum studies include creatinine and C3 complement level to screen for renal insufficiency and chronic hypocomplementemic glomerulonephritis. When clinically appropriate, screening for systemic lupus erythematosus, hepatitis, or coagulopathies should be considered. Renal ultrasonography should be checked in all children younger than 7 years of age to rule out Wilms' tumor and in older children if there are concerns regarding structural anomalies or stones. Urine samples from parents and siblings should also be assessed for the presence of a familial hematuria.

In the absence of a history suggestive of lower urinary tract bleeding, cystoscopy is seldom indicated in the child with isolated microhematuria. Unlike adults, bladder malignancies are quite uncommon and sonography usually suffices as a screen to detect rare structural anomalies.

Benign Familial Hematuria and Alport's Syndrome

In children, the differential diagnosis of isolated microscopic hematuria often includes BFH and AS. The ability to distinguish between these two conditions is critical because it allows accurate prognosis, although this may be difficult as the microscopic examination of the urine and early glomerular basement membrane (GBM) changes may be identical.

The renal biopsy specimen in patients with BFH is normal by light microscopy and immunofluorescence. The abnormality in BFH is apparent by electron microscopy, which demonstrates thinning of the lamina densa of the GBM. Thinning of the GBM may also be the only abnormality seen in patients with early AS or in female carriers of X-linked AS. However, the GBM abnormalities in AS continue to evolve, resulting in areas of irregular thinning, thickening, splitting, and multilamination, clearly distinguishing AS from BFH.[85,86]

Whereas BFH is inherited in an autosomal dominant manner, AS is most often inherited in an X-linked pattern. An autosomal recessive form of AS accounts for 15% of cases, whereas the autosomal dominant form is quite rare.[85] Type IV collagen is the major structural component of the GBM, and mutations of this gene are the molecular basis for AS. X-linked AS has been attributed to mutations of the *COL4A5* gene, whereas the recessive and dominant forms are linked to mutations of the *COL4A3-COL4A4* locus.[85] Two families with BFH have had their disease linked to the *COL4A4* gene.[87,88] These reports suggest that these BFH patients may be carriers of autosomal recessive AS. Those patients who are heterozygous for certain *COL4A4-COL4A3* locus mutations have BFH, whereas patients who have homozygous or compound heterozygous mutations in the same locus develop autosomal recessive AS.

Clinical features and family history are critical in distinguishing between BFH and AS.[86,89] Unlike patients with AS who typically develop proteinuria and progressive renal failure, patients with BFH do not develop significant proteinuria and preserve renal function over time. In addition, patients with AS may have a family history of high-frequency sensorineural hearing loss and lenticonus. Although BFH can be distinguished from AS with some certainty based on clinical features and family history, without a confirmatory renal biopsy, it is a diagnosis of exclusion. Thus, in children with BFH as a putative diagnosis, regular follow-up must make sure that no concerning clinical or laboratory features, such as the development of proteinuria or decreasing renal function, evolve. In this event, a diagnostic renal biopsy should be performed.

Although patients with AS typically progress to ESRD as young adults, angiotensin blockade has been used with success to blunt the associated proteinuria and to slow down the loss of effective renal function, although there is significant variability among patients as to an efficacious dose.[90]

Idiopathic Hypercalciuria

Hypercalciuria is present in approximately 5% of healthy white children and is diagnosed in as many as 35% of children evaluated for hematuria.[84,91] Hypercalciuria may be secondary to hyperparathyroidism, metabolic acidosis, distal renal tubular acidosis, vitamin D intoxication, ketogenic diet, immobilization, and therapy with loop diuretics. Most children, however, have normocalcemic idiopathic hypercalciuria. The pathogenesis of idiopathic hypercalciuria is unknown and could be secondary to increased intestinal absorption, reduced renal tubular reabsorption, increased osseous resorption, or a combination of these factors.[92] A recent study demonstrated no major alterations of intestinal calcium absorption based on an oral strontium load test.[93]

Hypercalciuria exists when urinary calcium excretion exceeds 4 mg/kg/day. In young children, a 24-hour collection may be impractical and calcium excretion can be estimated by a spot-urine calcium-to-creatinine ratio. Urinary calcium-to-creatinine ratios vary with geographic area and age. The variation related to geography is likely determined by race, climate, exposure to sunlight, mineral content of drinking water, and nutritional habits.[94] The ratios are much higher in infants than in older children and adults. When children and adults were studied in the northeastern United States, the 95th percentile urinary calcium-to-creatinine ratios for infants and children younger than 7 months, 8 to 18 months, and 19 months to 6 years were 0.86, 0.6, and 0.42, respectively, whereas the 95th percentile for adults was 0.22.[95] When a child's urinary calcium-to-creatinine ratio is elevated based on the normative data for the population, a definitive diagnosis of hypercalciuria should be established with a 24-hour urinary collection when possible.

Presenting clinical features of hypercalciuria include microscopic hematuria, gross hematuria, frequency dysuria, abdominal or flank pain, and urolithiasis.[96] Although there is considerable clinical overlap, macroscopic hematuria and a family history of urolithiasis have been found to be more common in hypercalciuric patients. The reported incidence of documented urolithiasis at presentation varies depending on the population studied. In a report of the Southwest Pediatric Nephrology Study Group, all children with painless isolated hematuria and hypercalciuria underwent excretory urography or renal ultrasonography at presentation, and no child had urolithiasis at diagnosis.[84] In comparison, another study focused on children with hypercalciuria who presented with painless microhematuria, dysuria, recurrent abdominal or flank pain, and a family history of nephrolithiasis.[97] All children underwent renal ultrasonography at entry; 57% had microcalculi and 5% had urolithiasis.

The natural history of idiopathic hypercalciuria is persistent hematuria and possible urolithiasis. In a longitudinal study of 58 untreated children with hematuria and hypercalciuria, 40% continued to have hematuria and 70% had hypercalciuria at 1 year.[98] At 2 and 3 years, 21 children were available for study; 40% still had hematuria and 50% had hypercalciuria. During the follow-up period, 16% of children developed urolithiasis. Children who developed stones were older when initially evaluated and were more likely to present with macroscopic hematuria, and all had a family history of urolithiasis. In the Southwest Pediatric Nephrology Study Group study, 13% of hypercalciuric patients developed urolithiasis or stone-like episode over a follow-up period of as long as 4 years.[84] In addition to hematuria and urolithiasis, idiopathic hypercalciuria has been associated with UTIs in children.[99]

Hypercalciuria and hematuria clearly identify a group of children at high risk of subsequent urolithiasis. Conservative measures should be taken, including high fluid intake and a diet low in sodium. A restricted calcium diet is not recommended and may even predispose to increased stone formation.[100] If citrate excretion is found to be low, citrate supplementation should be provided, preferably as the potassium salt.[101] Children with idiopathic hypercalciuria associated with hypocitraturia may be at risk of reduced bone mineral density when compared with children with hypercalciuria and normal citrate excretion, although further studies are needed.[102] If conservative measures are unsuccessful, thiazide diuretics can be considered. Thiazides can predispose, however, to electrolyte abnormalities and increased total cholesterol and low-density lipoprotein. Decisions regarding the use of thiazides for idiopathic hypercalciuria should take into consideration the clinical circumstances of the individual case, such as personal or family history of urolithiasis.

GLOMERULONEPHRITIS

Glomerulonephritis is the leading cause of acquired chronic renal failure during childhood.[103] As with adults, glomerulonephritis may be a manifestation of systemic disease, such as vasculitis or lupus, or may be due to a primary renal process. Similarly, the clinical course may be acute with subsequent full recovery or may progress to renal insufficiency. Certain forms of glomerulonephritis, such as HSP nephritis, are seen more commonly in children. In other chronic forms of glomerulonephritis, such as membranoproliferative glomerulonephritis (MPGN) and IgA nephropathy, therapeutic approaches in children have often differed from those used in adults.

Henoch-Schönlein Purpura

HSP is a multisystem IgA-mediated vasculitis predominantly affecting the skin, joints, gastrointestinal tract, and kidneys. HSP and IgA nephropathy share many immunologic and pathologic features, although HSP is a systemic disease and IgA nephropathy is clinically confined to the kidneys. Despite great research efforts, the exact pathogenesis of HSP and IgA nephropathy remains unclear. Both enhanced IgA synthesis and decreased IgA clearance have been implicated.[104] Total serum IgA levels are increased in 40% to 50% of these patients. Patients who develop HSP nephropathy were found to have abnormal glycosylation of serum IgA, and it has been proposed that the abnormal glycosylation may contribute to the immune complex deposition.[105]

Histologically, both IgA nephropathy and HSP nephritis are characterized by mesangial proliferation and matrix expansion with varying degrees of epithelial cell crescent formation. Unlike IgA nephropathy, HSP nephritis may be associated with polymorphonuclear leukocyte infiltration of the glomerular tufts. Tubulointerstitial changes may be apparent but generally reflect the severity of the glomerular lesions. Immunofluorescence staining invariably reveals IgA in the mesangium, often with weaker staining for C3 and IgG. Deposits may also be seen segmentally in the capillary wall.

Although HSP can occur at any age, most cases affect children between the ages of 2 and 10 years[106–108] and children who present at an older age may have a worse prognosis than younger children.[109] Unlike HSP in adults, which affects men and women equally, boys are as much as two times more likely to develop HSP than girls.[110] The disease is somewhat more prevalent during the winter months and early spring. The onset is usually sudden, frequently preceded by an acute illness that often involves a mucosal upper respiratory tract infection.

The clinical manifestations of HSP are due to the small-vessel vasculitis of affected organs. Hallmark signs and symptoms are a nonthrombocytopenic purpuric rash, arthralgias or a nonerosive arthritis, abdominal pain, and nephritis. The rash is often the most distinctive feature of the disease and characteristically involves the buttocks and extensor surfaces of the lower extremities in a symmetric pattern. When skin biopsies are performed, the pathology reveals leukocytoclastic vasculitis. The rash can persist for weeks, with some patients having recurrent episodes of new lesions. Angioedema may be present and involves the eyelids, lips, and dorsa of the hands and feet.

Approximately two thirds of patients have arthralgias or arthritis. Ankles and knees are the most commonly affected joints. The arthritis is nonerosive and not deforming. Gastrointestinal symptoms occur in approximately two thirds of patients, and one study found that the abdominal symptoms preceded the rash in as many as 14% of patients. The most frequent abdominal symptoms are periumbilical pain, vomiting, diarrhea, and hematochezia. Surgical emergencies develop in approximately 5% of patients, with ileoileal intussusception being the most common.[111] The acute morbidity of HSP is usually related to severe gastrointestinal complications.

The exact prevalence of nephritis in children is unknown, although rates as high as 54% have been reported.[112,113] If nephritis is to develop, 90% of cases present within 6 weeks of diagnosis of HSP, and rarely do urinary abnormalities present later than 6 months. Therefore, if a child's urinalyses remain normal during the first 6 months after presentation, further screening for nephritis is generally not required.[114]

The long-term outlook for children with HSP depends on the extent of renal involvement, but the overall prognosis of HSP nephritis is good. In a longitudinal study of 270 patients with HSP, 1.1% developed chronic renal insufficiency.[112] Poor prognosis has been associated with the development of nephritic or nephrotic syndrome, initial renal insufficiency, and more than 50% crescent formation on biopsy.[114-117] Nephritis is manifested in the majority of children as microscopic hematuria with or without proteinuria, and these patients have a good long-term prognosis.[116] In one series, 33% of patients with HSP nephritis had nephritic features or a combined nephritic-nephrotic syndrome.[112] Long-term follow-up of a similar cohort of more severely affected patients found that 44% developed chronic hypertension or renal insufficiency.[116] The majority of children have mild nephritis, recover fully, and require no specific therapy.

Once HSP has developed, there are conflicting reports about the efficacy of early prednisone therapy to prevent significant nephritis.[117,118] More recently, two randomized, placebo-controlled studies have been published to determine the effect of 2- and 4-week courses of oral prednisone. The first study included 40 patients and reported no effect of early steroid therapy on the risk of renal involvement at 1 year.[119] The subsequent study included 171 patients who were followed for 6 months.[120] Early prednisone treatment was effective in decreasing abdominal and joint symptoms but did not prevent renal involvement. Therapy with prednisone appeared, however, to improve the course of the nephritis with resolution of renal symptoms in 61% of the treated patients compared with 34% of those who received placebo.

The optimal treatment of children with more extensive renal disease remains controversial. Numerous uncontrolled studies have shown benefit when patients are treated with steroids with or without other agents such as azathioprine, cyclophosphamide, and anticoagulants.[121-125] A randomized, controlled trial of 6 weeks of oral cyclophosphamide at 90 mg/m^2/day with mean follow-up of 6.9 years did not show a difference in outcome between the two groups.[126] Plasmapheresis has also been reported to improve prognosis in a small number of children with rapidly progressive HSP nephritis.[127,128] A recent retrospective analysis reviewed the course of 14 children with severe HSP nephritis and 2 children with IgA nephropathy who were treated with plasmapheresis and no steroids, immunomodulators, or antiplatelet agents.[129] One child with HSP was referred late and had a poor renal outcome. The remaining children with HSP who were referred early were doing well at 4 years (range, 1–7.5 years) with normal estimated GFR, no or mild proteinuria, and no need for antihypertensive agents. Well-designed, randomized, controlled studies are needed to better assess the outcomes of patients treated with various immunosuppressive regimens. ACE inhibitors should be given to patients with persistent proteinuria and glomerular scarring.

IgA Nephropathy

IgA nephropathy is the most common form of pediatric primary glomerulopathy. Initially considered a benign disease, long-term follow-up studies suggest that a significant proportion of adult patients progress to ESRD. Similarly, study of the natural history of IgA nephropathy diagnosed in childhood demonstrates progression in many patients. In a study of 103 American children diagnosed with IgA nephropathy before 18 years of age, ESRD developed in 6% of children by 5 years, 13% by 10 years, 18% by 15 years, and 30% by 20 years.[130] Similarly, a study in Japan found that 5% of children with IgA nephropathy developed chronic renal failure by 5 years after diagnosis and 11% by 15 years from onset.[131]

The clinical presentation of IgA nephropathy varies from asymptomatic hematuria to a mixed nephritic-nephrotic syndrome.[132] The presence of heavy proteinuria and more active urinary sediment indicates more severe glomerular changes. The incidence of macroscopic hematuria is higher in children than adults and often occurs in association with a mucosal infection of the upper respiratory tract. The interval between the precipitating illness and an episode of macroscopic hematuria is generally 1 to 2 days. Acute renal failure is sometimes seen in flares of IgA nephropathy, although it is usually reversible. However, a small subset of patients with significant crescentic changes have a rapidly progressive course to renal failure. Other histologic correlates with poor clinical outcome include diffuse mesangial proliferation, a high proportion of glomeruli with sclerosis or capsular adhesions, and moderate to severe tubulointerstitial disease.[133] Persistent hypertension and heavy proteinuria also predict a more progressive course.[134]

As the outcome of IgA nephropathy may be so variable, therapy remains challenging. Well-controlled studies are lacking, especially those focusing exclusively on children. Selecting the patients most likely to benefit from therapy is critical.

Patients with more severe histologic changes, heavy proteinuria, persistent hypertension, and decreased GFR at presentation should be considered for specific therapy. Studies assessing the benefit of tonsillectomy alone or in combination with other therapies have arrived at conflicting conclusions.[135-137] A regimen of alternate-day prednisone (40–60 mg/m^2) and daily azathioprine (2 mg/kg) for at least 1 year has been successful in children with severe IgA nephropathy.[138] Therapy resulted in significant decreases in proteinuria and improvement in biopsy results, most notably decreased cellular crescents. Benefits from corticosteroids, including decreased proteinuria and lower incidence of chronic renal failure, were also seen in another small cohort of children with risk factors for progressive IgA nephropathy.[139] A recent report of 181 Japanese children younger than 15 years old with biopsy-proven IgA nephropathy suggested efficacy of immunosuppressive therapy if there were proliferative changes on the renal biopsy specimen. After 7 years of follow-up, of those children with original histologic evidence of more aggressive disease, 50% had normal urinalyses and renal function and only 14% demonstrated loss of GFR.[140] The Japanese Pediatric IgA Nephropathy Treatment Study Group treated 78 children with IgA nephropathy with either a combination of prednisolone, azathioprine, heparin-warfarin, and dipyridamole (group 1) or heparin-warfarin and dipyridamole (group 2) for 2 years.[141] Children in group 1 showed decreased proteinuria and a tendency toward decreased progression of glomerulosclerosis compared with group 2. In a more recent report, this group compared combination therapy with prednisone alone, demonstrating significant increased efficacy in terms of clearing proteinuria and preventing further renal scarring with combination therapy.[142]

Use of fish oil and angiotensin blockade seems to decrease the loss of renal function in certain adult cohorts.[143-146] A recent report from the Southwest Pediatric Nephrology Study Group compared outcomes in 96 patients with IgA nephropathy, normal GFR, and 1.4 to 2.2 g/day of proteinuria who were treated with one of three regimens for 2 years: fish oil (4 g/day of ω-3 fatty acids), a tapering course of alternate-day oral prednisone (60 mg/m^2 on alternate days for 3 months, then 40 mg/m^2 for 9 months, then 30 mg/m^2 for 1 year), or a placebo.[147] Hypertensive children received concomitant angiotensin blockade. Among these groups, children receiving steroids or placebo did equally well, with only 9% in each group showing a decrease in GFR less than 60% of baseline. With children receiving fish oil, 19% showed such a decrease in GFR. None of these changes were, however, statistically significant.

Studies of ACE polymorphisms have demonstrated that genotypes leading to higher levels of ACE are associated with more progressive disease.[148,149] Angiotensin blockade remains a mainstay of therapy in IgA nephropathy when there is any significant proteinuria, and although there are not the same data as in adults, combination therapy with both ACE inhibitors and angiotensin receptor blockers is used in the hope of decreasing proteinuria and slowing progressive loss of GFR.

Postinfectious Glomerulonephritis

Postinfectious glomerulonephritis is the leading cause of acute glomerulonephritis in children and has been associated with a host of bacteria, viruses, and parasites. In children, group A β-hemolytic streptococci are the most frequently implicated organisms, and pyoderma and pharyngitis are the classic preceding illnesses. Streptococcal pharyngitis occurs most frequently in school-age children during the cooler months. The latent period from onset of pharyngitis to acute poststreptococcal glomerulonephritis (APSGN) is typically a few weeks. Streptococcal impetigo occurs more frequently in younger children during the warmer months, and APSGN after impetigo has a longer latent period of 2 to 6 weeks. Over the past two decades, the prevalence of APSGN has been decreasing in children in the United States and South America.[150,151]

In children who become symptomatic with APSGN, the clinical onset is typically abrupt. Approximately 85% of patients develop edema, as many as 80% have varying degrees of hypertension, as many as one third have gross hematuria, and oliguria is common.[152] Hypertension may be severe during the first week of clinical nephritis, with accompanying headaches, somnolence, or seizures, and should be aggressively treated. Generally, the clinical symptoms of APSGN begin to resolve within 1 to 2 weeks as evidenced by diuresis and normalization of blood pressure. The gross hematuria fades rapidly, but microscopic hematuria may persist for years. Proteinuria typically improves rapidly and resolves within 6 months. Recurrences are rare but have been reported.[153-155] More commonly, recurrence of gross hematuria should raise the suspicion for an underlying chronic glomerulonephritis such as IgA nephropathy, MPGN, or membranous glomerulonephritis.

Laboratory studies during a typical episode of APSGN reflect a nephritic process with activation of the alternative complement pathway. The urine sediment shows erythrocytes and leukocytes and may contain red cell casts. Proteinuria is found frequently but is rarely in the nephrotic range. GFR is often decreased, although severe azotemia is rare and should raise the concern for a rapidly progressive process. If azotemia is significant, electrolyte abnormalities including hyponatremia, hyperkalemia, and acidemia may be present. Serologic tests to document recent streptococcal infection are helpful but do not prove causation. When interpreting serologies, it is important to realize that antibiotic use may blunt the increase in titer and that a significant number of children are asymptomatic carriers of streptococci.[156-158] Serologic tests available include antibodies against streptolysin O and the streptozyme test. The streptozyme test assesses several antibodies including streptolysin O, antideoxyribonuclease B, and antihyaluronidase. Streptolysin O binds to lipids in the skin and results in blunting of the immune response in cases of streptococcal impetigo. The antideoxyribonuclease B titer is therefore more sensitive in detecting evidence of recent streptococcal skin infection.

The majority of patients have a low total hemolytic complement and a low C3 complement with a normal C4. The C3 level typically recovers in 6 to 8 weeks, although prolonged hypocomplementemia has been reported in as many as one fourth of patients.[159] If the C3 remains depressed after 3 months or the C4 is low, diagnostic considerations include chronic forms of nephritis such as MPGN and lupus nephritis. The possibility of a chronic form of glomerulonephritis warrants close surveillance, and a renal biopsy should be considered. Renal biopsy is generally not indicated in typical APSGN, but may be necessary if the diagnosis is in question or if the course is consistent with rapidly progressive glomerulonephritis. The biopsy shows diffuse endocapillary proliferation, predominant IgG and C3 deposition in the capillary loop on immunofluorescence, and subepithelial dense humps on electron microscopy.

The mainstay of therapy for APSGN is supportive care. Hospitalization is recommended if the child is hypertensive or has decreased creatinine clearance. Blood pressure should be checked regularly early in the illness, and if hypertension is present, diuretic therapy with concomitant salt and fluid restriction is considered. If needed, short-acting calcium channel blockers or hydralazine can also be used. In most cases, significant improvement in hypertension, edema, and azotemia is seen within 2 weeks. In children with more persistent hypertension that does not directly respond to diuretics or vasodilation, angiotensin blockade is often used, especially if there is concomitant proteinuria. In a cohort of children with postinfectious glomerulonephritis half of whom received enalapril therapy for 6 weeks after diagnosis, enalapril-treated children had significantly earlier decreases in blood pressure as well as better short-term echocardiographic parameters.[160]

In children whose course is consistent with rapidly progressive glomerulonephritis, an immediate renal biopsy for histologic diagnosis is warranted to guide any necessary therapeutic intervention. Intravenous methylprednisolone, with or without other agents such as cyclophosphamide, has been beneficial in the therapy of rapidly progressive glomerulonephritis of various causes in children.[161,162] With poststreptococcal glomerulonephritis, such immunomodulation including prednisone, azathioprine, and cyclophosphamide has not been shown to change the natural course of the disease, even with significant crescentic changes.[163]

In the absence of rapidly progressive disease, the prognosis for complete recovery is considered to be good even in the face of initial concerning clinical features such as renal insufficiency and significant histologic aberrations.[163] Several groups have studied the long-term prognosis of patients who initially recovered and found that 3.4% to 20% of patients developed mild residual symptoms, including proteinuria, hematuria, and hypertension.[164–166] Azotemia develops in less than 3% of patients.[167] Although outcomes are good overall, these results indicate the need for regular monitoring to detect late sequelae.

Membranoproliferative Glomerulonephritis

MPGN is a chronic glomerulonephritis characterized histologically by diffuse thickening of the GBM and endocapillary proliferation and subcategorized by the location of deposits on electron microscopy. Most MPGN in children is idiopathic, although occasional secondary cases of MPGN related to hepatitis virus or other infectious etiologies occur.

Either the classical or alternative complement pathways may be involved, resulting in a low serum C3 and, less commonly, a normal or low serum C4. Hypocomplementemia has been reported in as many as 95% of children at presentation.[168–171] In type 2 MPGN, also termed dense deposit disease, abnormal complement regulatory proteins such as aberrant factor H have been described in some patients, and these anomalies have been hypothesized to affect the alternative complement cascade and predispose to renal disease.[172] MPGN is primarily a disease of older children, adolescents, and young adults and is rarely reported in children younger than 6 years of age. MPGN was diagnosed in 7.5% of children referred to

tertiary centers for renal biopsy for evaluation of nephrotic syndrome.[14] At presentation, one third of children had macroscopic hematuria or hypertension, as many as two thirds had nephrosis, and one third had renal insufficiency.[168–171] The long-term renal prognosis in children with MPGN is guarded, and natural history studies suggest that as many as 50% progress to ESRD within 10 years of onset.[168]

The small number of affected children has hampered evaluation of putative therapies. Treatment regimens have included corticosteroids, alkylating agents, and anticoagulants. Corticosteroids have not proven beneficial in adults, although various combinations of aspirin, dipyridamole, and warfarin have resulted in diminished proteinuria and an inconsistent impact on maintaining the GFR.[172–175] In the pediatric population, corticosteroids have shown greater benefit.[176,177] In 71 children followed at a single center for an average of 7.7 years and mainly treated with alternate-day oral steroids, the cumulative renal survival was 82% at 10 years and 56% at 20 years after onset.[171]

The International Study of Kidney Disease in Children conducted a randomized, double-blind, placebo-controlled clinical trial in children with primary MPGN.[178] Criteria for enrollment included nephrosis-range proteinuria and normal renal function. Children received alternate-day oral prednisone or a lactulose placebo for a mean duration of 41 months. At 130 months, 61% of patients receiving prednisone showed stable renal function compared with only 12% of patients receiving placebo. Similarly, data from the Japanese school urinary screening program have shown efficacy to long-term steroid therapy, with 15 of 19 children receiving alternate-day steroids for 4 to 12 years manifesting normal urinary findings and complement levels, with the remaining members of this cohort having mild proteinuria alone.[179] Intravenous pulses of methylprednisolone followed by alternate-day oral prednisone have also been used in children, with improvement of hematuria, proteinuria, serum albumin, and creatinine clearance.[177] More recent data from a small cohort of children treated with either pulse intravenous steroids or oral steroids suggested greater benefit with pulse therapy. After an average follow-up of 5 years, only 1 of the 11 children receiving pulse therapy progressed to ESRD versus 4 of the 8 children on oral therapy.[180]

Although these studies support the use of corticosteroids in children with MPGN with nephrosis-range proteinuria, benefit of the same therapy in MPGN with nonnephrosis-range proteinuria is less clear. In a retrospective study of 39 children with MPGN, the outcome of the 11 nonnephrotic patients was excellent, with 100% renal survival at 10 years[170]; of these nonnephrotic patients, seven were untreated. In this report, the absence of nephrosis was predictive of a good long-term outcome, regardless of therapy, and suggests that a more tailored treatment approach in nonnephrotic children with MPGN may be useful.

Given the identification of complement pathway regulatory protein anomalies in some children with dense deposit disease, new approaches to its therapy have been proposed including plasma infusion or plasmapheresis and the use of specific monoclonal antibodies. These therapies are aimed at normalizing alternative pathway complement activity and, as further insight is gained into some of the genetic underpinnings of some forms of MPGN, other treatments are likely to be introduced.[172]

HEMOLYTIC UREMIC SYNDROME

Hemolytic uremic syndrome (HUS) is defined by the clinical triad of microangiopathic hemolytic anemia, thrombocytopenia, and acute renal failure. HUS is the cause of ESRD in approximately 3% of children who have received renal transplants and is a frequent cause of acute renal failure in children.[61,181] HUS can be broadly divided into typical forms associated with prodromal diarrhea (D+ HUS) and atypical cases distinguished by the absence of diarrhea (D− HUS). The majority of childhood cases of HUS include a diarrheal prodrome and are frequently due to infection with enterohemorrhagic Escherichia coli (EHEC).[182] Atypical HUS is a heterogeneous disorder accounting for approximately 10% of cases in children and generally carries a poorer prognosis. Atypical HUS may result from abnormalities in complement regulatory proteins or can be precipitated by numerous triggers, including drugs, malignancies, bone marrow transplantation, and nonenteric infections such as streptococcal pneumonia.

D+ Hemolytic Uremic Syndrome

Although outbreaks of diarrhea-associated HUS are dramatic and draw considerable public attention, only approximately 10% of cases in children arise from epidemics.[183,184] A variety of organisms have been implicated in the pathogenesis of HUS, including Shigella dysenteriae type 1, Salmonella, and Yersinia. The majority of cases, however, have been linked with EHEC, which produces a potent cytotoxin known as Shiga-like toxin or verotoxin. E. coli O157:H7 is the serotype isolated in more than 90% of EHEC infections in the United States.[182] EHEC may be carried in the intestines of asymptomatic cattle, and higher carriage rates are noted in the summer months and early fall, mimicking the seasonal variation of human disease that peaks from June through September.[185]

Ground beef, vegetables, unpasteurized milk or juice, and water all serve as possible vectors of disease via contamination with bovine feces. Rarely, child-to-child transmission also occurs via oral-fecal contamination.[186] Although children of all ages can be infected, the highest attack rate for E. coli O157:H7 infection occurs among children younger than 5 years of age.[187] Infected children may excrete the organism in stool for as long as 3 weeks. Approximately 10% to 15% of children who develop culture-confirmed E. coli O157:H7 gastroenteritis progress to HUS, and the risk of progressing to HUS may be increased with use of antimotility agents early in the course of colitis.[183,188]

Central to the pathogenesis of HUS is microvascular endothelial cell injury. Only a small inoculum of 50 to 100 EHEC organisms is required to colonize the intestine.[187] Once established, EHEC elaborates verotoxin leading to intestinal hemorrhagic and ulcerative lesions. With the integrity of the intestinal mucosa compromised, verotoxin gains access to the circulation and extraintestinal sites. Verotoxin is composed of one A subunit and five B subunits. The B subunits are required for binding of the toxin to the high-affinity glycolipid receptor glycosphingolipid globotriosyl ceramide, a protein especially expressed on renal microvascular endothelium. After binding, the A subunit is internalized and undergoes partial proteolysis to become an active enzyme capable of inactivating the 60S ribosome, thereby suppressing protein synthesis.[188]

During the acute phase of HUS, numerous proinflammatory cytokines are elaborated. Along with released bacterial products, these cytokines activate and promote adhesion of leukocytes and platelets to vascular endothelium. The pathogenic cascade results in swollen and detached endothelial cells, exposing the thrombogenic basement membrane and promoting microvascular thrombosis.

In D+ HUS, colitis typically precedes the development of the classic triad of HUS by several days.[182,189] The diarrhea may be bloody and associated with vomiting and severe abdominal pain and often resolves at the time microangiopathy becomes clinically apparent. Gastrointestinal complications include bowel wall necrosis, toxic megacolon, intussusception, and rectal prolapse.[189–191]

The severity of the acute nephritis varies widely. The clinical course ranges from microscopic hematuria and mild proteinuria without renal insufficiency to fulminant renal failure. In a retrospective review of D+ HUS in Utah over a 20-year period, 60% of children experienced anuria or oliguria lasting a median of 6 days (range, 1–32 days).[192] Dialysis was performed in 43% of cases. Hypertension was present in two thirds of children but was usually mild and resolved by the time of discharge. Severe disease, including oliguria for more than 14 days, anuria for more than a week, and extrarenal structural damage such as central nervous system infarct, occurred in one fourth of children and was found to be associated with age younger than 2 years, anuria during the diarrheal prodrome, and an elevated white blood cell count at presentation. With oliguria, metabolic derangements including metabolic acidosis, hyperkalemia, and dilutional hyponatremia can be seen.

The hematologic abnormalities reflect the microangiopathic process with microthrombi formation. Laboratory studies show decreasing hemoglobin, increased reticulocytes, and increased lactate dehydrogenase coupled with a blood smear demonstrating fragmented erythrocytes and schistocytes. Coagulation studies are generally normal, distinguishing HUS from sepsis and disseminated intravascular coagulation. The indirect and direct Coombs' test should be negative. Thrombocytopenia may be severe, although a small minority of patients have a normal platelet count. The degree of hemolysis and thrombocytopenia does not correlate with the degree of renal involvement. An increase in the platelet count is one of the first signs of recovery, denoting decreased microangiopathy.

Special mention of central nervous system involvement in HUS is warranted because this results in significant morbidity and is the most common cause of death in children.[193] As in other organs, the major insult to the central nervous system is thrombotic microangiopathy. The majority of children demonstrate some degree of encephalopathy as irritability and somnolence. Seizures and cerebral infarct occur in 10% and 4% of children, respectively, and predict a poorer prognosis.[192,194]

Essentially any organ can be affected by the microangiopathy of HUS to varying degrees. Pancreatitis occurs and can be associated with transient or permanent diabetes mellitus. Liver involvement results in hepatomegaly and elevated transaminases. Clinical involvement of the heart or lung is not usually apparent, although rare cases of severe myocardial suppression have been reported.[195]

The mainstay of therapy for D+ HUS is meticulous supportive care. As children often present after several days of gastrointestinal losses and poor oral intake, judicious fluid resuscitation with isotonic saline should be provided when indicated to ameliorate prerenal physiology. A recent prospective study of 29 children with *E. coli* O157:H7 associated HUS found that fluid management in the pre-HUS course could affect the renal outcome. The children whose renal failure was characterized by nonoligoanuria had received more intravenous fluid and sodium before microangiopathy developed compared with the children who developed oligoanuric renal failure. This suggests that early recognition and parenteral volume expansion during *E. coli* O157:H7 infections before the development of HUS may attenuate the renal outcome.[196] After the initial volume resuscitation, strict attention should be given to the patient's fluid status, with daily assessment of weight and accurate accounting of fluid input and urine output.

In the oligoanuric child, both intravenous and oral intake should match any measurable output and insensible water losses, estimated at 300 mL/m^2/day. The choice of replacement fluid can be guided by serum and urine electrolytes, with avoidance of potassium and phosphorus supplementation. If oligoanuria develops despite expansion of the intravascular volume, one or two doses of furosemide (1–3 mg/kg) are justified. Renal and bladder ultrasound scans should be performed in patients with progressive renal failure to rule out rare instances of urinary tract obstruction.

A large percentage of children with acute HUS will need renal replacement therapy. Indications for dialysis include clinically significant volume overload such as evolving pulmonary edema or congestive heart failure, progressive azotemia, hyperkalemia unresponsive to conservative therapy, and the need for blood product transfusions or nutritional support in the oligoanuric patient. Adequate nutritional support is imperative to reverse the catabolic state associated with the acute disease. Many patients are unable to tolerate enteral nutrition, necessitating the use of total parenteral nutrition.

Packed red blood cell transfusions should be provided for symptomatic anemia or vigorous hemolysis with a hematocrit decreasing to less than 16% to 20%. Directed transfusions from blood relatives should be avoided as this may sensitize the patient against a potential kidney donor should ESRD develop. In the setting of thrombotic microangiopathy, transfused platelets will be consumed quickly and not result in a sustained increase in the platelet count. Platelets should therefore be transfused only if the patient is actively bleeding with significant clinical sequelae or a surgical procedure is intended.

Hypertension is common in acute HUS. If there are prolonged episodes of blood pressure higher than the 95th percentile for a child's height and age, medical therapy should be considered. Vasodilatory agents such as hydralazine or calcium channel blockers are effective and are preferred over ACE inhibitors in the setting of fluctuating glomerular perfusion.

D$^+$ HUS is a potentially preventable disease. Ground beef should be cooked thoroughly and unpasteurized food products should be avoided. Children who are infected should be excluded from day care, and enteric precautions should be taken until stool cultures are negative. Antibiotic treatment of *E. coli* O157:H7 infection is not recommended as this has been shown to increase the risk of developing HUS.[197]

The renal prognosis of self-limited *E. coli* O157:H7 gastroenteritis appears to be excellent, without findings of hypertension, proteinuria, or decreased renal function 4 years after the acute illness.[194] Although the majority of children with D$^+$ HUS recover fully from the acute illness, the long-term renal prognosis is guarded. Acute mortality rates as high as 5% have been reported, and a small percentage of children remain dialysis dependent from disease onset.[192,198] Predictors of fatality at the time of hospital admission included oligoanuria, increased white blood cell count more than 20×10^9/L, and hematocrit more than 23%.[193] In a study of 140 cases of pediatric D$^+$ HUS over a 20-year period, after the acute HUS episode, half of the children went on to develop one or more abnormalities including hypertension, proteinuria, and chronic renal insufficiency.[192] ESRD had already developed in another 4% of patients. A study of 29 French children with a distant history of D$^+$ HUS also suggested significant long-term sequelae.[199] After 15 to 25 years of follow-up, only 35% had no renal abnormalities, whereas 41% had hypertension, significant proteinuria, or a slightly decreased GFR, 10% had chronic renal insufficiency, and 14% had already progressed to ESRD. The best indicator of prognosis was the extent of patchy cortical necrosis on a renal biopsy specimen obtained at the time of recovery from the acute HUS episode. These studies underscore the importance of long-term and regular follow-up of children after D$^+$ HUS.

In children with ESRD secondary to D$^+$ HUS, renal transplantation is generally quite successful. The North American Pediatric Renal Transplant Cooperative Study reviewed the data from 61 patients with all types of HUS who received 68 renal transplants.[200] HUS recurred in six (8.8%) allografts in five patients. Four of these patients had D$^-$ HUS. In all but one graft, the HUS recurred within 33 days. The time elapsed before transplantation and the use of cyclosporine did not seem to affect the risk of HUS recurrence. In support of this relatively low rate of recurrent disease in children undergoing transplantation after D$^+$ HUS, another review of 18 children in Argentina found no recurrences.[201]

Atypical or D$^-$ Hemolytic Uremic Syndrome

Atypical or D$^-$ HUS is distinguished by the absence of diarrheal prodrome and accounts for approximately 10% of HUS cases.[202] A heterogeneous disorder, a variety of triggers have been identified, including infection with *Streptococcus pneumoniae*, human immunodeficiency virus, malignancies, drugs such as cyclosporine and tacrolimus, and transplantation. Evidence of a pathologic role of the alternative pathway of complement has been identified, and an increasing number of genetic mutations associated with atypical HUS have been described.[203] Mutations of the complement regulatory proteins factor H, factor I, and membrane cofactor protein (MCP) have been found in approximately 50% of patients studied.[204] Factor H mutations are most commonly detected, occurring in approximately 25% to 30% of cases. The frequency of reported mutations of factor I and MCP are 5% to 13% and 10% to 15%, respectively.[204,205] The importance of genetic screening has been emphasized because the identification of specific mutations may predict the disease course or outcome after renal transplantation. In addition to genetic mutations, autoantibodies to factor H were found in three of 48 pediatric patients with atypical HUS. This resulted in an acquired factor H dysfunction in patients who had no genetic mutations and normal plasma antigenic levels.[206]

Given the heterogeneous nature of atypical HUS, the reported clinical presentation and outcome has varied. A single-center experience retrospectively compared the clinical features and outcome of 28 episodes of atypical HUS (22 children) with 266 cases of typical HUS (265 children).[202] Four patients with atypical disease demonstrated a recurrent course. The presence of prodromal features, other than the presence or absence of diarrhea, was similar in the two groups. Atypical HUS was significantly less likely to result in oliguria or anuria or to require dialysis. At follow-up, there was no statistically significant difference in the incidence of hypertension, decreased renal function, or proteinuria. Although there was no difference in the incidence of ESRD, two of the four patients with recurrent atypical HUS eventually developed ESRD. With the exception of the patients with a recurrent course, those with atypical HUS did not experience a worse outcome in this series.

A subsequent study compared the hospital course and short-term outcome of 24 children with atypical HUS with 145 children with typical HUS. Nearly 40% of the cases of atypical HUS followed a pneumococcal infection. The patients with atypical HUS required dialysis more often and had longer hospital admissions.[207] Although clinical characteristics vary, atypical HUS may carry a worse prognosis, which is most apparent in patients with recurrent disease.[208]

Although the clinical course of atypical HUS varies, the recently identified mutations in the complement regulatory proteins have allowed genotypic-phenotypic correlations.[209] The most severe prognosis is seen in those with mutations of factor H and factor I. Approximately 70% of patients with these mutations had onset before 1 year of age, whereas none of the patients with mutations of MCP had onset before the age of 1 year but typically presented in early childhood. Patients without an identified mutation may have onset at any age. Sixty percent of patients with factor H mutations reached ESRD or died within 1 year. The course of patients with factor I mutations was more variable, with half progressing to ESRD rapidly and half recovering. The clinical course of MCP mutation–associated HUS was more favorable. These patients had a relapsing course, although none reached ESRD at 1 year and complete recovery was common. The 5-year renal survival for mutations of factor H, factor I, MCP, and disease without detected mutation was 27%, 50%, 62%, and 68%, respectively.

In addition to meticulous supportive care as described for cases of typical HUS, plasma therapy may result in clinical improvement. Plasma therapy will likely be initiated before results of genetic testing are available, and approximately one third of patients will demonstrate a favorable response.[209] Mutation of the MCP results in reduced surface expression, and therefore patients with this mutation would not be predicted to have a response to plasma therapy. In patients with an identified MCP mutation, remission was achieved in approximately 90% of plasma-treated and plasma-untreated episodes.[205] If response to plasma therapy is evident, a gradual taper of therapy should be pursued with close monitoring of parameters. Complement inhibitor therapies may provide hope for the future.

When ESRD results and renal transplantation are to be considered, a full assessment of regulators of complement should be pursued, including determination of C3, complement factors H and I, MCP levels, ADAMTS-13 activity, and genetic testing of factor H, factor I, and MCP for specific mutations.[203] The overall success rate of renal transplantation has been poor, with only one third of grafts functioning at follow-up. Of note, vascular thrombosis has been a leading cause of graft failure, accounting for approximately 50% of graft loss in one pediatric series; post-transplantation HUS recurrence occurred in 53% of the whole group and in 80% of patients with factor H mutation.[209] Given the surface expression of MCP, it is predicted that recurrence should be of relatively low risk because the renal allograft should express normal MCP.

In patients who lose their initial graft to recurrence, they generally have a very poor chance of success with a second graft.[210] Of note, many centers do not recommend living-related donor transplantation because of the risk of recurrence. In addition, de novo disease in donors has been reported.[211] In cases of factor H mutations with recurrence of disease after transplantation, a small number of combined liver and renal transplantations have been pursued to restore normally functioning factor H that is synthesized in the liver. Initial reports of such procedures had poor outcomes with two of the three patients dying and the third left with neurological disability.[212] A more recent report of a combined liver-kidney transplant with preoperative plasma exchange was successful, although overall experience with combined transplantation is limited.[213]

HYPERTENSION

In marked contrast to the adult population, the prevalence of hypertension in children has historically been low (1%–3%) and its etiology less likely to be primary or essential and more likely to be due to an underlying renal anomaly.[214] Unlike adults, in whom normal blood pressure values have been established based on epidemiological assessment of end-organ damage, blood pressure parameters in children are based on screening data aimed at identifying the normal distribution of blood pressures in the pediatric population. In 2004, the National High Blood Pressure Education Program Working Group on Hypertension Control in Children and Adolescents updated blood pressure tables for children based on the screening of more than 60,000 children.[215] These data demonstrated that there are several clinical factors that affect blood pressure in children, particularly age, gender, and height. Blood pressure increases with age during childhood and reaches adult levels as the child becomes an adolescent. For any given age, boys tend to have somewhat higher normal blood pressures than girls. Heavier and taller children also have higher blood pressures than their more average-sized peers.

These tables statistically defined hypertension in relation to a sample group of children of the same age, gender, and height. Normal blood pressure is a preponderance of readings lower than the 90th percentile. Prehypertension or what used to be considered high-normal range is between the 90th and 95th percentiles. Children are considered hypertensive if blood pressure readings are higher than the 95th percentile persistently on at least three separate occasions. Stage I hypertension refers to readings between the 95th and 99th percentiles and stage II hypertension encompasses readings higher than the 99th percentile.

These tables serve as a resource for the clinician in determining whether a child should be considered hypertensive compared with his or her peers of a similar size. They also provide data for the 50th percentile to give clinicians a better sense of average readings for a child of any size and age. Blood pressure tends to decrease with repeated measurements due to accommodation; thus, although 5% of pediatric blood pressure readings are statistically in the hypertensive range by definition, a significantly smaller number of children will be persistently hypertensive.

Most children should have their blood pressure checked annually as part of their visit to the pediatrician. In addition, blood pressure should be assessed in any child hospitalized or in an emergency facility, not only because hypertension may complicate an acute illness but also because the detection of transient hypertension in children during stressful occasions may serve as a marker for the development of future hypertension. Abnormal blood pressure readings require follow-up. High-normal or marginally increased readings should prompt a repeat blood pressure in 3 to 6 months. Asymptomatic blood pressure readings as much as 10 mm Hg higher than normal require follow-up within 2 to 4 weeks. Higher blood pressure elevations demand speedier follow-up or, in the case of a child with potential symptomatic hypertension or complicating comorbid medical conditions, immediate attention.

Measuring blood pressure in children can be problematic. The cuff must be appropriately sized, with the width of the cuff's bladder equaling 40% of the mid-upper arm circumference or the cuff bladder encircling three fourths of the upper arm length as measured from the olecranon to the acromion.[216] Some surveys have estimated that as many as 50% of patients have their blood pressure measured with an incorrectly sized cuff.[217] Before blood pressure measurement, children should be inactive and acclimated to the examination room for at least 5 minutes. With auscultation, systolic blood pressure is the first Korotkoff sound (K1) and diastolic pressure in all children and adolescents is the fifth Korotkoff sound (K5) when all sounds disappear. In some small children, the diastolic pressure may be auscultated down to 0 mm Hg. Although this is not the true diastolic pressure, it does eliminate any concern of diastolic hypertension.

Small uncooperative children or older children suspected of anxiety-induced hypertension may be relaxed by allowing a parent or nurse to measure their blood pressure in a familiar setting, so that the reading is more representative of the child's usual blood pressure. Some facilities have access to ambulatory blood pressure monitors, small devices worn by the patient that measure and record blood pressure frequently. Advantages of ambulatory monitoring include the ability to record blood pressure during a child's usual daily routine and during sleep so as to determine whether hypertension exists, how often it occurs, how extensive it may be, and if the measured blood pressure manifests a normal circadian variation.[218]

The normative blood pressure tables are based on auscultation of blood pressure using a cuff on an upper extremity. In many clinical settings, oscillometry is used to measure blood pressure. Although adequate for screening, studies in children demonstrate that oscillometry regularly overestimates auscultated blood pressures, often averaging readings 5 to 10 mm Hg higher.[219,220]

Because an organic cause of hypertension is more common in a child, the diagnostic evaluation is slanted very much toward excluding renal parenchymal or vascular diseases. In fact, more than three fourths of nonobese hypertensive children can be found to have a renal etiology of their hypertension (Table 43-3).[221] The child's history is elicited with emphasis on potential renal insults or other medical conditions

Table 43-3 Cause of Hypertension in Children

Cause	Specific Diagnoses	Frequency (%)
Renal parenchymal disease	Acute or chronic glomerulonephritis, reflux nephropathy, cystic disease, hemolytic uremic syndrome	70
Renal vascular disease	Renal artery stenosis, vascular thrombosis	10
Primary hypertension		10
Cardiovascular disease	Aortic coarctation	5
Endocrine disease	Pheochromocytoma, hyperthyroidism, hyperaldosteronism, Cushing's disease	3
Central nervous system anomaly	Increased intracranial pressure	0.5
Medication effect	Sympathomimetics	0.01

suggesting a secondary cause of hypertension (Box 43-4). The physical examination includes careful general assessment for a unifying condition such as Williams or Turner's syndrome or a disorder such as tuberous sclerosis or neurofibromatosis that may have been overlooked and that commonly includes renally mediated hypertension. Four extremity blood pressures should be measured and a focused examination conducted for pertinent findings such as adenoma sebaceum, café-au-lait marks, abdominal bruits, retinal vessel abnormalities, peripheral pulse variations, and aberrant sexual characteristics.

Obesity significantly predisposes children to the development of hypertension. In one longitudinal study of cardiac disease and cardiac risk factors in nearly 10,000 children in the southern United States, obese children were shown to be much more likely to show evidence of the metabolic syndrome including hypertension and to mature into adults with hypertension and obesity.[222] In a survey of schoolchildren in

---

Box 43-4 Pertinent Medical History in Pediatric Hypertension

Birth history: prematurity, prolonged ventilation, umbilical catheter
Medical history: urinary tract infection, unexplained fevers, recent systemic infections, changes in appearance of urine
Family history: hypertension in first- and second-degree relatives, history of stroke or myocardial infarction, endocrine or neurocutaneous disease, renal disease
Medication history: decongestants, oral contraceptives, street drugs, chewing tobacco, cigarettes, ethanol
Review of systems: headache, palpitations, sweating, flushing, visual changes

Texas, the relative risk of hypertension was more than three times greater in obese than normal weight children.[223] The percentage of obese children is increasing and in some populations now approaches 25%.[224] With this epidemic of obesity in children, the likelihood of a child manifesting hypertension without a discernible organic cause other than obesity is increasing. Certainly a large population of obese and hypertensive children has profound public health implications, especially as these children mature and face the potential earlier onset of cardiovascular and renal complications from long-term obesity and hypertension.

A phased laboratory evaluation consists of some general studies in almost every hypertensive child and tailored follow-up studies that depend on these results and the child's history, physical findings, and overall level of clinical suspicion. Baseline screening tests should include a microscopic urinalysis of a freshly voided urine, serum electrolytes to rule out acidosis or hypokalemia, as seen in some of the mineralocorticoid-excess states, serum creatinine to assess renal function, and renal ultrasonography to assess renal anatomy.

In some children, screening tests will be normal and a diagnosis of primary hypertension strongly suspected. Although primary hypertension in children is often considered a diagnosis of exclusion, many children with primary hypertension follow a typical clinical profile: older child or adolescent, low-grade hypertension, cardiovascular reactivity with stress, high resting pulse rates, obesity, and a family history of primary hypertension.[225] In these children, no further diagnostic work-up is needed immediately; after a review of cardiac risk factors, the child's hypertension should be treated if necessary and followed with regular blood pressure checks and emphasis on adjunctive therapies for hypertension, such as weight reduction, exercise, and dietary counseling.

In children who do not meet the clinical profile for primary hypertension and who have otherwise unremarkable screening test results, further renal imaging with renal scintigraphy can be useful to determine whether there is any renal scarring. If this is negative and the patient is significantly hypertensive, renal arteriography should be performed to diagnose any renal vascular abnormalities. Noninvasive imaging of the renal vasculature with computed tomography or magnetic resonance angiography can be entertained with the caveat that children may be more likely than adults to have lesions in smaller segmental vessels that may be better appreciated by conventional arteriography. Ideally, any invasive arteriography should be performed by a physician experienced with transluminal angioplasty in children so that this technique can be performed at the same time if an appropriate lesion is identified.

Other laboratory evaluation is of low yield unless there are appropriate concerns from the child's history or physical evaluation. Random serum renin and aldosterone levels are rarely useful unless they are extremely skewed. For instance, in some families with a pedigree suggestive of glucocorticoid-remediable aldosteronism (difficult to treat, early-onset hypertension in many family members), a random plasma renin level should be nearly nonexistent, prompting more specific genetic testing. Similarly, in rare patients, there may be consideration of urinary catecholamine measurement or abdominal magnetic resonance imaging for a catecholamine-secreting tumor, but again this should be guided by individual signs and symptoms and any potential confounding variables such as

the coexistence of neurofibromatosis or a family history of pheochromocytoma.

Therapy for hypertension is tailored for two basic populations of children. If there is relatively mild hypertension, a cardiac echocardiogram should be considered to rule out left ventricular hypertrophy or other evidence of end-organ effect of sustained high blood pressure. In the absence of end-organ damage, nonpharmacologic therapy could be instituted involving weight reduction, exercise, and dietary counseling. If the blood pressure remains increased despite these interventions or if there is significantly increased blood pressure, then pharmacologic therapy should be instituted along with counseling about weight, diet, and exercise.

As with adults, drug therapy in pediatric hypertension involves selecting an initial therapeutic agent and then stepping up therapy if it proves inadequate. In general, an agent based on the underlying presumed physiology is chosen. A submaximal dose of the drug is begun and then titrated to a maximal dose as needed, aiming to decrease the blood pressure to at least the 90th percentile for age, gender, and height. If there is an inadequate response to the maximal dose of the first medication, a second medication is usually begun, also in a gradual fashion.

Many antihypertensive drugs have not been studied in children, although in the past 5 years an increasing number of antihypertensives have received U.S. Food and Drug Administration labeling for pediatric use after undergoing specific pediatric trials. As with most medications in children, dosing is based on body weight rather than standard dosing amounts and, in agents not studied specifically in children, dosing has largely arisen from clinical experience. Moreover, with the pediatric population, there can be limitations in the ability of the patient to take a medication: the drug may not be available in a liquid or crushable form if pills cannot be swallowed, and issues of palatability are often troublesome. Table 43-4 lists some of the more commonly used antihypertensive medications and their effective doses in children.

Rarely, children present with a hypertensive urgency or a hypertensive crisis. Often, these children have concomitant significant renal pathology, such as an acute nephritis or renal insufficiency. The initial aim of therapy is to decrease the blood pressure by approximately 30% over the first few hours of care to prevent or minimize end-organ or central nervous system damage. Table 43-5 lists medications and dosing guidelines that are often effective in treating hypertensive emergencies in children. After the child's blood pressure has been stabilized, it can then be returned more deliberately to an acceptable range by use of more routine antihypertensive medications. Treatment of a child with a hypertensive emergency is best accomplished in a pediatric intensive care unit by clinicians familiar with blood pressure management in children.

URINARY TRACT INFECTION AND VESICOURETERAL REFLUX

Unlike adults, in whom UTI and especially cystitis is more commonly encountered, UTI in children is infrequent, affecting 3% to 8% of girls and 1% to 2% of boys. Of more concern, however, is that as many as one half of girls and two thirds of boys with UTIs have accompanying high fever, suggestive of an upper tract UTI or pyelonephritis rather than simple

Table 43-4   Blood Pressure Medication in Children

	Initial Dose (mg/kg/day)	Maximal Dose (mg/kg/day)	Dosing Frequency
ACE Inhibitors			
Captopril (neonate)	0.03–0.15	2	bid/tid
Captopril (child)	1.5	6	bid/tid
Enalapril	0.15	Up to 40 mg/day total	qd/bid
Calcium Channel Blockers			
Nifedipine	0.25	3	XL or SR form bid
Amlodipine	0.1	0.4	qd/bid
Diuretics			
Hydrochlorothiazide	1	2–3	qd/bid
Furosemide	0.5–1.0	10	qd/bid
Spironolactone	1	3	bid/tid
Adrenergic Agents			
Atenolol (β-blocker)	0.5	2–3	qd/bid
Propranolol (β-blocker)	1	6–8	bid
Labetalol (αβ-blocker)	1	3	bid
Prazosin (α-blocker)	0.05–0.1	0.5	bid/tid
Vasodilators			
Hydralazine	0.5	10	tid/qid
Minoxidil	0.1–0.2	1	qd/bid
α-Agonist			
Clonidine	0.05–0.1 mg/day total	0.6 mg/day total	bid/tid, patch every week

ACE, angiotensin-converting enzyme; SR, sustained release; XL, extended release.

cystitis.[226] The propensity for upper tract infection in children stems in part from the association between UTI and vesico-ureteral reflux (VUR). In some series, as many as one half of children with UTI have VUR, whereas in children with no history of UTI, only 2% have VUR.[227]

The signs and symptoms of UTI and pyelonephritis may be far less specific in children than in adults. Infants and young children generally have fever, but their symptoms are otherwise often vague and include anorexia, lethargy, and irritability. In older children and adolescents, there is an increased likelihood of localizing symptoms such as dysuria, frequency, and flank pain. Because significant delay in the diagnosis and treatment of pyelonephritis in children has been associated with an increased likelihood of significant long-term renal damage, appropriate diagnostic and therapeutic interventions become all the more crucial.

The clinical diagnosis of pyelonephritis in children is usually based on finding bacteria and white blood cells in the urine of a febrile child. Gram stain of the urine and then subsequent urine culture confirms the diagnosis and helps to tailor therapy. Obtaining the best possible urine specimen for culture poses more problems in the pediatric patient than with adults. In toilet-trained children, meticulous attention to collecting a midstream urine sample is usually successful. In younger children and infants, a catheterized specimen or a suprapubic aspirate may be required. Urine collected from a bag taped to the child's perineum is easily contaminated and is only useful if there is ultimately no bacterial growth.

Most UTIs in children are caused by gram-negative bacteria of the family *Enterobacteriaceae*, such as *Escherichia*, *Klebsiella*, *Enterobacter*, and *Citrobacter*.[228] Less commonly, gram-positive bacteria may be pathogens, especially in patients with urinary tract malformations, voiding dysfunction, or instrumentation.

In the child with a febrile UTI, antibiotic therapy should be started quickly. In neonates and older infants and children with more complicated illness, hospitalization for parenteral therapy is warranted. Empiric therapy for hospitalized children is most often a third-generation cephalosporin or an aminoglycoside and ampicillin pending urine culture results. In older children with suspected pyelonephritis who do not appear toxic, therapy can commence on an ambulatory basis

Table 43-5   Medications for Hypertensive Emergencies in Children

	Mechanism	Dose	Onset	Duration
Hydralazine	Arteriolar dilator	0.15–0.25 mg/kg IV to maximum dose of 20 mg	5–15 min	3–8 hr
Labetalol	αβ-Blocker	Initial IV bolus 0.25 mg/kg; repeat every 15 min at increasing doses up to 1 mg/kg until effective or total dose of 4 mg/kg	5 min	2–6 hr
		Maintenance IV infusion: 1–3 mg/kg/hr		
Nifedipine	Calcium channel blocker	0.25–0.5 mg/kg oral or sublingual	10–20 min	3–6 hr
Diazoxide	Arteriolar dilator	Rapid IV bolus 1 mg/kg; repeat after 10–15 min if insufficient response; maximum dose 5 mg/kg	3–10 min	4–10 hr
Nitroprusside	Venous and arteriolar dilator	Start at 0.5 μg/kg/min IV	1–2 min	3–5 min

with an injection of a third-generation cephalosporin such as ceftriaxone and then transition to appropriate oral therapy to complete a 10- to 14-day course of therapy. In children with suspected cystitis, oral therapy may commence with a medication such as trimethoprim-sulfamethoxazole, nitrofurantoin, or cefixime that has antimicrobial coverage for the usual gram-negative organisms associated with UTI. Empiric antibiotic choice can be guided by Gram stain results and knowledge of community antibiotic sensitivity patterns for usual urinary pathogens. Ultimate oral therapy can be chosen after appropriate sensitivities are obtained from urine culture. In all children treated for UTI, a repeat urine culture should be obtained sometime after appropriate therapy has been initiated to document sterilization of the urinary tract. A short duration of oral therapy of 3 to 5 days in children with uncomplicated cystitis seems to be as effective as longer therapy, but most clinicians still treat febrile UTIs or smaller children with a longer duration of therapy.[229]

In any child with a first episode of febrile UTI, renal ultrasonography should be performed to assess urinary tract anatomy. In children older than age 7 years, a normal renal ultrasound scan may preclude further urinary tract imaging. In the younger child or the older child with sonographic abnormalities such as hydronephrosis or renal scarring, a voiding cystourethrogram (VCUG) should be obtained to exclude VUR. A VCUG may be performed at any time after the child is no longer symptomatic and the urine is sterile. If the child has completed the therapeutic course of antibiotics before a VCUG, prophylactic antibiotic therapy with once-daily trimethoprim-sulfamethoxazole or nitrofurantoin should be initiated until a VCUG is obtained.

If the diagnosis of pyelonephritis is in question, renal scintigraphy with technetium-labeled dimercaptosuccinic acid is a sensitive and specific test. Renal scintigraphy has been shown to be superior to intravenous pyelography, computed tomography, or ultrasonography in documenting renal cortical injury.[230] Its use is most helpful in children with chronic or recurrent infections to determine whether parenchymal scarring is occurring.

In children with VUR, higher grades of reflux and especially intrarenal reflux predispose to renal scarring. Less than 5% of children with grade I VUR manifest renal scars compared with 50% of children with grade V VUR.[231] In a series of 200 children followed for as long as 20 years after an episode of pyelonephritis, renal scarring was almost always associated with moderate to severe VUR.[232] Infants and young children appear more prone to developing renal scars with pyelonephritis. As children reach elementary school age, it becomes increasingly less common to see renal scarring, even in the presence of continued VUR.[233]

Most children with low-grade VUR (grades I–III) can be managed with nightly oral antibiotic prophylaxis and monitored with an annual VCUG or radionuclide cystogram to determine whether VUR has spontaneously resolved. In children with higher grade reflux, VUR is less likely to spontaneously resolve. All children younger than 1 year of age are usually managed initially with oral antibiotic prophylaxis. In children with persistent grade V VUR, ureteral reimplantation is generally recommended given its infrequent spontaneous resolution. In children with grade IV VUR, there seems to be no advantage of reimplantation over medical therapy in terms of preventing further renal scarring.[234] Over time, there is a decreasing incidence of VUR even in children with higher grades of reflux at presentation, leading many to favor medical therapy unless repeated breakthrough infection, poor compliance, or parental request favor surgical correction with ureteral reimplantation.[235,236] There is also increasing use of endoscopic correction of reflux with periureteral polymer injection of dextranomer/hyaluronic acid with good short- and longer term results.[237]

Because the risk of parenchymal scarring seems to decrease with age, the need for long-term antibiotic prophylaxis in VUR has been questioned in older children who have had a benign clinical course. One study of 51 children (mean age, 8 years) with persistent VUR but no history of voiding abnormalities or renal scarring demonstrated that prophylaxis could be stopped successfully with no long-term effect on renal scarring.[238] Studies are under way that look more systematically at the provision or withdrawal of prophylactic antibiotic therapy in children with VUR, and it is likely that prophylactic antibiotic therapy with VUR may become less widespread if more data accumulate suggesting that rapid therapy of any UTI in a child with VUR is as good a long-term strategy as daily antibiotics.

Children who develop extensive renal scarring have an increased incidence of proteinuria, hypertension, and renal insufficiency. The risk of developing these sequelae seems to be most closely linked to the severity of the scarring and the length of follow-up.[239] In children with significantly decreased renal reserve due to parenchymal scarring, there is the risk of hyperfiltration injury in remnant glomeruli and the development of secondary focal glomerulosclerosis and renal insufficiency. Such a consequence of chronic pyelonephritis or reflux nephropathy accounts for as many as 10% of the cases of pediatric ESRD.[61]

References

1. Miltenyi M: Urinary protein excretion in healthy children. Clin Nephrol 1979;12:216–221.
2. Peterson PA, Evrin P, Berggard I: Differentiation of glomerular, tubular and normal proteinuria: Determination of urinary excretions of beta-2 microglobulin, albumin and total protein. J Clin Invest 1968;48:1189–1198.
3. Houser M: Assessment of proteinuria using random urine samples. J Pediatr 1984;104:845–848.
4. Randolph MF, Greenfield M: Proteinuria: A six year study of normal infants, preschool and school-aged populations previously screened for urinary tract disease. Am J Dis Child 1967;114:631–638.
5. Wagner MA, Smith FG Jr, Tinglof BO, et al: Epidemiology of proteinuria. J Pediatr 1968;73:825–832.
6. Vehaskari VM, Rapola J: Isolated proteinuria: Analysis of a school-age population. J Pediatr 1982;104:661–668.
7. Brenner BM, Baylis C, Deen WM: Transport of molecules across renal glomerular capillaries. Physiol Rev 1976;56:502–534.
8. Kim M: Proteinuria. Clin Lab Med 1988;8:527–539.
9. Rytand DA, Sprieter S: Prognosis in postural (orthostatic) proteinuria. N Engl J Med 1981;305:618–621.
10. Martin-Arevalo DL, Yee J, Pugh J, et al: Fixed and reproducible orthostatic proteinuria: A 35 year follow-up study (abstract). J Am Soc Nephrol 1996;7:1323.
11. Vehaskari VM, Robson AM: Proteinuria. In Edelmann CM (ed): Pediatric Kidney Disease. Boston: Little, Brown, 1992, pp 531–551.
12. Yoshikawa N, Kitagawa K, Ohta K, et al: Asymptomatic constant isolated proteinuria in children. J Pediatr 1991;119:375–379.
13. Habib R: Proteinuria. In Royer P (ed): Pediatric Nephrology. Philadelphia: WB Saunders, 1974, pp 247–252.
14. International Study of Kidney Disease in Children: The nephrotic syndrome in children. Prediction of histopathology from clinical and laboratory characteristics at the time of diagnosis. Kidney Int 1978;13:159–165.
15. Trompeter RS, Hicks J, Lloyd BW, et al: Long term outcome for children with minimal change nephrotic syndrome. Lancet 1985;1:368–370.
16. Sclesinger ER, Sulz HA, Mosher WE, et al: The nephrotic syndrome. Its incidence and implications for the community. Am J Dis Child 1968;116:623–632.
17. White RHR, Glasgow EF, Mills RJ: Clinicopathological study of nephrotic syndrome in childhood. Lancet 1970;1:1353–1359.
18. Clark AG, Barratt TM: Steroid-responsive nephrotic syndrome. In Barratt TM, Avner ED, Harmon WE (eds): Pediatric Nephrology, 4th ed. Baltimore: Lippincott Williams & Wilkins, 1999, pp 731–747.
19. Ingulli E, Tejani A: Racial differences in the incidence and renal outcome of idiopathic focal segmental glomerulosclerosis in children. Pediatr Nephrol 1991;5:393–397.
20. Arbeitsgemeinschaft fur Padiatrische Nephrologie: Short versus standard prednisone therapy for initial treatment of idiopathic nephrotic syndrome in children. Lancet 1988;1:380–383.
21. Ehrich JH, Brodehl J: Long versus standard prednisone therapy for initial treatment of idiopathic nephrotic syndrome in children. Arbeitsgemeinschaft fur Padiatrische Nephrologie. Eur J Pediatr 1993;152:357–361.
22. Koskimies O, Vilska J, Rapola J, et al: Longterm outlook of primary nephrotic syndrome. Arch Dis Child 1982;57:544–548.
23. Barratt TM, Bercowsky A, Osofsky SG, et al: Cyclophosphamide treatment in steroid sensitive relapsing nephrotic syndrome of childhood. Lancet 1975;1:55–58.
24. Arbeitsgemeinschaft fur Padiatrische Nephrologie: Cyclophosphamide treatment of steroid dependent nephrotic syndrome: Comparison of eight week with 12 week course. Arch Dis Child 1987;62:1102–1106.
25. Garin EH, Pryor ND, Fennell RS, et al: Pattern of response to prednisone in idiopathic minimal lesion nephrotic syndrome as a criterion in selecting patients for cyclophosphamide therapy. J Pediatr 1978;92:304–308.
26. Siegel NJ, Gur A, Krassner LS: Minimal lesion nephrotic syndrome with early resistance to steroid therapy. J Pediatr 1975;87:377–380.
27. Bergstrand A, Bollgren I, Samuelson A: Idiopathic nephrotic syndrome of childhood. Cyclophosphamide induced conversion from steroid refractory to highly steroid sensitive disease. Clin Nephrol 1973;1:302–306.
28. Niaudet P, French Society of Pediatric Nephrology: Comparison of cyclosporin and chlorambucil in the treatment of steroid-dependent idiopathic nephrotic syndrome: A multicentre controlled trial. Pediatr Nephrol 1992;6:1–3.
29. Smoyer WE, Gregory MJ, Bajwa RS, et al: Quantitative morphometry of renal biopsies prior to cyclosporine in nephrotic syndrome. Pediatr Nephrol 1998;12:737–743.
30. Neuhaus TJ, Burger HR, Klingler M, et al: Long-term low-dose cyclosporin A in steroid dependent nephrotic syndrome of childhood. Eur J Pediatr 1992;151:775–778.
31. Hamahira K, Iijima K, Tanaka R, et al: Recovery from cyclosporine-associated arteriopathy in childhood nephrotic syndrome. Pediatr Nephrol 2001;16:723–727.
32. Bragga A, Sharma A, Srivastava RN: Levamisole therapy in corticosteroid-dependent nephrotic syndrome. Pediatr Nephrol 1997;11:415–417.
33. Tenbrock K, Muller-Berghaus J, Fuchshuber A, et al: Levamisole treatment in steroid-sensitive and steroid-resistant nephrotic syndrome. Pediatr Nephrol 1998;12:459–462.
34. Bragga A, Hari P: Levamisole-induced vasculitis. Pediatr Nephrol 2000;14:1057–1058.
35. Hiraoka M, Tsukahara H, Hori C, et al: Efficacy of long-term azathioprine for relapsing nephrotic syndrome. Pediatr Nephrol 2000;14:776–778.
36. Hogg RJ, Fitzgibbons L, Bruick J, et al: Mycophenolate mofetil in children with frequently relapsing nephrotic syndrome: A report from the Southwest Pediatric Nephrology Study Group. Clin J Am Soc Nephrol 2006;1:1173–1178.
37. Fakhouri F, Bocquet N, Taupin P, et al: Steroid-sensitive nephrotic syndrome: From childhood to adulthood. Am J Kidney Dis 2003;41:550–557.
38. Ruth EM, Kemper MJ, Leumann EP, et al: Children with steroid-sensitive nephrotic syndrome come of age: Long-term outcome. J Pediatr 2005;147:202–207.
39. Gulati S, Sural S, Sharma RK, et al: Spectrum of adolescent-onset nephrotic syndrome in Indian children. Pediatr Nephrol 2001;16:1045–1048.

40. Chesney RW, Novello AC: Forms of nephrotic syndrome more likely to progress to renal impairment. Pediatr Clin North Am 1987;34:609–627.

41. Niaudet P: Steroid resistant idiopathic nephrotic syndrome. In Avner ED, Harmon WE, Niaudet P (eds): Pediatric Nephrology, 5th ed. Philadelphia: Lippincott Williams & Wilkins, 2004, pp 557–573.

42. Tune BM, Lieberman E, Mendoza SA: Steroid-resistant nephrotic focal segmental glomerulosclerosis: A treatable disease. Pediatr Nephrol 1996;10:772–778.

43. Tarshish P, Tobin JN, Bernstein J, et al: Cyclophosphamide does not benefit patients with focal segmental glomerulosclerosis. A report of the International Study of Kidney Disease in Children. Pediatr Nephrol 1996;10:590–593.

44. Arbus GS, Poucell S, Bacheyie GS, et al: Focal segmental glomerulosclerosis with idiopathic nephrotic syndrome: Three types of clinical response. J Pediatr 1982;101:40–45.

45. Mongeau J-G, Corneille L, Rabitaille P, et al: Primary nephrosis in childhood associated with focal glomerular sclerosis: Is long-term prognosis that severe? Kidney Int 1981;20:743–746.

46. Mendoza SA, Reznik VM, Griswold W, et al: Treatment of steroid resistant focal segmental glomerulosclerosis with pulse methylprednisolone and oral alkylating agents. Pediatr Nephrol 1990;4:303–307.

47. Tune BM, Kirpekar R, Sibley RK, et al: Intravenous methylprednisolone and oral alkylating agent therapy of prednisone-resistant pediatric focal segmental glomerulosclerosis: A long-term follow-up. Clin Nephrol 1995;43:84–88.

48. Guillot AP, Kim MS: Pulse steroid therapy does not alter the course of focal glomerulosclerosis [abstract]. J Am Soc Nephrol 1993;4:276.

49. Waldo FB, Benfield MR, Kohaut EC: Methylprednisolone treatment of patients with steroid-resistant nephrotic syndrome. Pediatr Nephrol 1992;6:503–505.

50. Chishti AS, Sorof JM, Brewer ED, et al: Long-term treatment of focal segmental glomerulosclerosis in children with cyclosporine given as a single daily dose. Am J Kidney Dis 2001;38:754–760.

51. Singh A, Tejani C, Tejani A: One-center experience with cyclosporine in refractory nephrotic syndrome in children. Pediatr Nephrol 1992;13:26–32.

52. Lieberman KV, Tejani A: A randomized double-blind placebo-controlled trial of cyclosporine in steroid-resistant idiopathic focal segmental glomerulosclerosis in children. J Am Soc Nephrol 1996;7:56–63.

53. Gregory MJ, Smoyer WE, Sedman A, et al: Long-term cyclosporine therapy for pediatric nephrotic syndrome: A clinical and histologic analysis. J Am Soc Nephrol 1991;5:587–590.

54. Ingulli E, Singh A, Baqi N, et al: Aggressive, long-term cyclosporine therapy for steroid-resistant focal segmental glomerulosclerosis. J Am Soc Nephrol 1995;5:1820–1825.

55. Loeffler K, Gowrishankar M, Yiu V: Tacrolimus therapy in pediatric patients with treatment-resistant nephrotic syndrome. Pediatr Nephrol 2004;19:281–287.

56. Milliner DS, Morgenstern BZ: Angiotensin converting enzyme inhibitors for reduction of proteinuria in children with steroid resistant nephrotic syndrome. Pediatr Nephrol 1991;5:587–590.

57. Fitzwater DS, Brouhard BH, Cunningham RJ 3rd: Use of angiotensin converting inhibitors for the treatment of focal segmental glomerulosclerosis. Am J Dis Child 1990;144:522.

58. Briggs WA, Choi MJ, Scheel PJ Jr: Successful mycophenolate mofetil treatment of glomerular disease. Am J Kidney Dis 1998;31:364–365.

59. Chandra M, Susin M, Abitbil C: Remission of relapsing childhood nephrotic syndrome with mycophenolate mofetil. Pediatr Nephrol 2000;14:224–226.

60. Broyer M, Meyrier A, Niaudet P, et al: Minimal changes and focal segmental glomerulosclerosis. In Cameron S, Davison AM, Grunfield JP, et al (eds): Oxford Textbook of Clinical Nephrology. Oxford: Blackwell Scientific Publications, 1992, pp 298–339.

61. Smith JM, Stablein DM, Munoz R, et al: Contributions of the transplant registry: The 2006 annual report of the North American Pediatric Renal Trials and Collaborative Studies (NAPRTCS). Pediatr Transplant 2007;11:366–373.

62. Baum MA, Stablein DM, Panzarino VM, et al: Loss of living donor renal allograft survival advantage in children with focal segmental glomerulosclerosis. Kidney Int 2001;59:328–333.

63. Savin VJ, Sharma R, Sharma M, et al: Circulating factor associated with increased glomerular permeability to albumin in recurrent focal segmental glomerulosclerosis. N Engl J Med 1996;334:878–883.

64. Artero M, Sharma R, Savin V, et al: Plasmapheresis reduces proteinuria and serum capacity to injure glomeruli in patients with recurrent focal segmental glomerulosclerosis. Am J Kidney Dis 1994;23:574–581.

65. Mathis B, Kim S, Calabrese K, et al: A locus for inherited focal segmental glomerulosclerosis maps to chromosome 19q13. Kidney Int 1998;53:282–286.

66. Kaplan J, Kim S, North K, et al: Mutations in ACTN4, encoding alpha-actinin-4, cause familial focal segmental glomerulosclerosis. Nat Genet 2000;24:251–256.

67. Tsukaguchi H, Yager H, Dawborn J, et al: A locus for adolescent and adult onset familial focal segmental glomerulosclerosis on chromosome 1q25-31. J Am Soc Nephrol 2000;11:1674–1680.

68. Caridi G, Bartelli R, DiDuca M, et al: Prevalence, genetics, and clinical features of patients carrying podocin mutations in steroid-resistant nonfamilial focal segmental glomerulosclerosis. J Am Soc Nephrol 2001;12:2742–2746.

69. Hinkes BG, Mucha B, Vlangos CN, et al: Nephrotic syndrome in the first year of life: Two thirds of cases are caused by mutations in 4 genes (NPHS1, NPHS2, WT1, and LAMB2). Pediatrics 2007;119:e907–e919.

70. Little M, Wells CA: Clinical overview of WT1 gene mutations. Hum Mutat 1997;9:209–225.

71. Heaton PA, Smales O, Wong W: Congenital nephrotic syndrome responsive to captopril and indomethacin. Arch Dis Child 1999;81:174–175.

72. Habib R: Nephrotic syndrome in the 1st year of life. Pediatr Nephrol 1993;7:347–353.

73. Holmberg C, Tryyvason K, Kestila MK, et al: Congenital nephrotic syndrome. In Avner ED, Harmon WE, Niaudet P (eds): Pediatric Nephrology, 5th ed. Philadelphia: Lippincott Williams & Wilkins, 2004, pp 503–516.

74. Kestila M, Lenkkeri U, Lamerdin J, et al: Positionally cloned gene for a novel glomerular protein—nephrin—is mutated in congenital nephrotic syndrome. Mol Cell 1998;1:575–582.

75. Seppala M, Aula P, Rapola J, et al: Congenital nephrotic syndrome: Pre-natal diagnosis and genetic counseling by estimation of amniotic fluid and maternal serum alpha-fetoprotein. Lancet 1976;2:123–124.

76. Holmberg C, Antikainen M, Ronnholm K, et al: Management of congenital nephrotic syndrome of the Finnish type. Pediatr Nephrol 1995;9:87–93.

77. Kim MS, Primack W, Harmon WE: Congenital nephrotic syndrome: Preemptive bilateral nephrectomy and dialysis before renal transplantation. J Am Soc Nephrol 1992;3:260–263.

78. Holmberg C, Patrakka J, Laine J, et al: Post-transplant proteinuria in Finnish type nephrotic syndrome. In Cochat P (ed): Recurrence of the Disease in the Renal Graft. Paris: John Libby Eurotext, 2001, pp 35–38.

79. Lane J, Jalanko H, Holthofer H, et al: Post-transplantation nephrosis in congenital nephrotic syndrome of the Finnish type. Kidney Int 1993;44:867–874.

80. Patrakka J, Ruotsalainen V, Reponen P, et al: Recurrence of nephrotic syndrome in kidney grafts of patients with congenital nephrotic syndrome of the Finnish type: Role of nephrin. Transplantation 2002;73:394–403.

81. Dodge W, West E, Smith E, et al: Proteinuria and hematuria in schoolchildren: Epidemiology and early natural history. J Pediatr 1976;88:327–347.

82. Vehaskari V, Rapola J, Koskimies O, et al: Microscopic hematuria in schoolchildren: Epidemiology and clinicopathologic evaluation. J Pediatr 1979;95:676–684.

83. Ingelfinger J, Davis A, Grupe W: Frequency and etiology of gross hematuria in a general pediatric setting. Pediatrics 1977;59:557–561.

84. Stapleton F: Idiopathic hypercalciuria: Association with isolated hematuria and risk for urolithiasis in children. Kidney Int 1990;37:807–811.

85. Smeets H, Knoers V, van de Heuvel L, et al: Heredity disorders of the glomerular basement membrane. Pediatr Nephrol 1996;10:779–788.

86. Gubler MC, Heidet L, Antignac C: Inherited glomerular disease. In Avner ED, Harmon WE, Niaudet P (eds): Pediatric Nephrology, 5th ed. Philadelphia: Lippincott Williams & Wilkins, 2004, pp 517–542.

87. Ozen S, Ertoy D, Heidt L, et al: Benign familial hematuria associated with a novel COL4A4 mutation. Pediatr Nephrol 2001;16:874–877.

88. Lemmink H, Nillesen W, Mochizuki T, et al: Benign familial hematuria due to mutation of the type IV collagen alpha 4 gene. J Clin Invest 1996;98:1114–1118.

89. Pajari H, Kaariainen H, Muhohnen T, et al: Alport's syndrome in 78 patients: Epidemiological and clinical study. Acta Paediatr 1996;85:1300–1306.

90. Proesmans W, VanDyck M: Enalapril in children with Alport syndrome. Pediatr Nephrol 2004;19:271–275.

91. Stapleton F, Roy S, Noe N, et al: Hypercalciuria in children with hematuria. N Engl J Med 1984;310:1345–1348.

92. Ordonez F, Fernandez P, Rodriquez J, et al: Rat models of normocalcemic hypercalciuria of different pathogenic mechanisms. Pediatr Nephrol 1998;12:201–205.

93. Fernandez P, Santos F, Sotorrio P, et al: Strontium oral load test in children with idiopathic hypercalciuria. Pediatr Nephrol 2007;22:1303–1307.

94. So N, Osori A, Simon S, Alon U: Normal urinary calcium/creatinine ratios in African-American and Caucasian children. Pediatr Nephrol 2001;16:133–139.

95. Sargent JD, Stukel T, Kresel J, et al: Normal values for random urinary calcium to creatinine ratios in infancy. J Pediatr 1993;123:393–397.

96. Stapleton F: Hematuria associated with hypercalciuria and hyperuricosuria: A practical approach. Pediatr Nephrol 1994;8:756–761.

97. Polito C, La Manna A, Cioce F, et al: Clinical presentation and natural course of idiopathic hypercalciuria in children. Pediatr Nephrol 2000;15:211–214.

98. Garcia C, Miller L, Stapleton F: Natural history of hematuria associated with hypercalciuria in children. Am J Dis Child 1991;145:1204-1207.

99. Stojanovic VD, Milosevic BO, Djapic MB, et al: Idiopathic hypercalciuria associated with urinary tract infection in children. Pediatr Nephrol 2007;22:1291–1295.

100. Borghi L, Schianchi T, Meschi T, et al: Comparison of two diets for the prevention of recurrent stones in idiopathic hypercalciuria. N Engl J Med 2002;346:77–84.

101. Lemann J, Pleuss J, Gray R, et al: Potassium administration increases and potassium deprivation reduces urinary calcium excretion in healthy adults. Kidney Int 1991;39:973–983.

102. Penido MG, Lima EM, Souto MF, et al: Hypocitraturia: A risk factor for reduced bone mineral density in idiopathic hypercalciuria? Pediatr Nephrol 2006;21:74–90.

103. United States Renal Data Service: Pediatric end stage renal disease. Am J Kidney Dis 1994;24(Suppl 2):S112–S127.

104. Rai A, Nast C, Alder S: Henoch-Schonlein purpura nephritis. J Am Soc Nephrol 1999;10:2637–2644.

105. Allen A, Willis F, Beattie T, et al: Abnormal IgA glycosylation in Henoch-Schonlein purpura restricted to patents with clinical nephritis. Nephrol Dial Transplant 1998;13:930–934.

106. Meadow S, Glasgow E, White R, et al: Schönlein-Henoch nephritis. Q J Med 1972;41:241–258.

107. Cream J, Gumpel J, Peachey R: Schonlein-Henoch purpura in the adult. A study of 77 adults with anaphylactoid Schonlein-Henoch purpura. Q J Med 1970;39:461–484.

108. Balmelli C, Laux-End R, Di Rocco D, et al: Anaphylactoid purpura nephritis in childhood: Natural history and immunopathology. Adv Nephrol Necker Hosp 1976;6:183–228.

109. Shenoy M, Bradbury MG, Lewis MA, et al: Outcome of Henoch-Schonlein purpura nephritis treated with long-term immunosuppression. Pediatr Nephrol 2007;22:1717–1722.

110. Trapani S, Micheli A, Grisolia F, et al: Henoch Schonlein purpura in childhood: Epidemiological and clinical analysis of 150 cases over a 5-year period and review of literature. Semin Arthritis Rheum 2005;35:143–153.

111. Choong C, Beasley S: Intra-abdominal manifestations of Henoch-Schonlein purpura. J Paediatr Child Health 1998;34:405–409.

112. Stewart M, Savage J, Bell B, et al: Long term renal prognosis of Henoch-Schonlein purpura in an unselected childhood population. Eur J Pediatr 1988;147:113–115.

113. Calvino M, Llorca J, Garcia-Porrua C, et al: Henoch-Schonlein purpura in children from northwestern Spain. Medicine 2001;80:279–290.

114. Farine M, Poucell S, Geary D, et al: Prognostic significance of urinary findings and renal biopsies in children with Henoch-Schonlein nephritis. Clin Pediatr 1986;25:257–259.

115. Austin, H, Balow J: Henoch-Schonlein nephritis: Prognostic features and the challenge of therapy. Am J Kidney Dis 1983;2:512–520.

116. Goldstein A, White R, Akuse R, et al: Long-term follow-up of childhood Henoch-Schonlein nephritis. Lancet 1992;339:280–282.

117. Mollica F, LiVolti S, Garozzo R, et al: Effectiveness of early prednisone treatment in preventing the development of nephropathy in anaphylactoid purpura. Eur J Pediatr 1992;151:140–144.

118. Saulsbury F: Corticosteroid therapy does not prevent nephritis in Henoch-Schonlein purpura. Pediatr Nephrol 1993;7:69–71.

119. Huber AM, King J, McLaine P, et al: A randomized, placebo-controlled trial of prednisone in early Henoch Schonlein purpura. BMC Med 2004;2:7.

120. Ronkainen J, Koskimies O, Ala-Houhala M, et al: Early prednisone therapy in Henoch Schonlein purpura: A randomized, double-blind, placebo-controlled trial. J Pediatr 2006;149:241–247.

121. Flynn J, Smoyer W, Bunchman T, et al: Treatment of Henoch Schonlein purpura glomerulonephritis in children with high-dose corticosteroids plus oral cyclophosphamide. Am J Nephrol 2001;21:128–133.

122. Foster B, Bernard C, Drummond K, et al: Effective therapy for severe Henoch Schonlein purpura nephritis with prednisone and azathioprine: A clinical and histopathologic study. J Pediatr 2000;136:370–375.

123. Oner A, Tinaztepe K, Erdogan O: The effect of triple therapy on rapidly progressive type of Henoch-Schonlein nephritis. Pediatr Nephrol 1995;9:6–10.

124. Niaudet P, Habib R: Methylprednisolone pulse therapy in the treatment of severe forms of Schonlein-Henoch purpura nephritis. Pediatr Nephrol 1998;12:238–243.

125. Iijima K, Ito-Kariya S, Nakamura H, et al: Multiple combined therapy for severe Henoch-Schonlein nephritis in children. Pediatr Nephrol 1998;12:244–248.

126. Tarshish P, Bernstein J, Edelmann CM: Henoch-Schonlein purpura nephritis: Course of disease and efficacy of cyclophosphamide. Pediatr Nephrol 2004;19:51–56.

127. Hattori M, Ito K, Konomoto T, et al: Plasmapheresis as the sole therapy for rapidly progressive Henoch Schonlein purpura nephritis in children. Am J Kidney Dis 1999;33:427–433.

128. Schrarer K, Krmar R, Querfeld U, et al: Clinical outcome of Schonlein-Henoch purpura nephritis in children. Pediatr Nephrol 1999;13:816–823.

129. Shenoy M, Ogujanovic MV, Coulthard MG: Treating severe Henoch-Schonlein and IgA nephritis with plasmapheresis alone. Pediatr Nephrol 2007;22:1167–1171.

130. Wyatt R, Krichevsky S, Woodford S, et al: IgA nephropathy: Long-term prognosis for pediatric patients. J Pediatr 1995;127:913–919.

131. Yoshikawa N, Ito H, Yoshira S, et al: IgA nephropathy in children from Japan. Child Nephrol Urol 1989;9:191–199.

132. Yoshikawa N, Tanaka R, Iijima K: Pathophysiology and treatment of IgA nephropathy in children. Pediatr Nephrol 2001; 16:446–457.

133. Yoshikawa N, Ito H, Nakamura H: Prognostic indicators in childhood IgA nephropathy. Nephron 1992;60:60–67.

134. Hogg R, Silva F, Wyatt R, et al: Prognostic indicators in children with IgA nephropathy: Report of the Southwest Pediatric Nephrology Study Group. Pediatr Nephrol 1994;8:15–20.

135. Hotta O, Furuta T, Chiba S, et al: Regression of IgA nephropathy: A repeat biopsy study. Am J Kidney Dis 2002;39:493–502.

136. Hotta O, Miyazaki M, Furuta T, et al: Tonsillectomy and steroid pulse therapy significantly impact on clinical remission in patients with IgA nephropathy. Am J Kidney Dis 2001;38:736–743.

137. Rasche F, Schwarz A, Keller F: Tonsillectomy does not prevent a progressive course in IgA nephropathy. Clin Nephrol 1999;51: 147–152.

138. Andreoli S, Bergstein J: Treatment of severe IgA nephropathy in children. Pediatr Nephrol 1989;3:248–253.

139. Waldo F, Wyatt R, Kelly D: Treatment of IgA nephropathy in children: Efficacy of alternate-day oral prednisone. Pediatr Nephrol 1993;7:529–532.

140. Nozawa R, Suzuki J, Takahashi A, et al: Clinicopathological features and the prognosis of IgA nephropathy in Japanese children on long-term observation. Clin Nephrol 2005;64:171–179.

141. Yoshikawa N, Ito H, Sakai T: A controlled trial of combined therapy for newly diagnosed severe childhood IgA nephropathy. The Japanese Pediatric IgA Nephropathy Treatment Study Group. J Am Soc Nephrol 1999;10:101–109.

142. Yoshikawa N, Honda M, Iijima K, et al: Steroid treatment for severe childhood IgA nephropathy: A randomized, controlled trial. Clin J Am Soc Nephrol 2006;1:511–517.

143. Donadio J, Bergstralh E, Offord K, et al: A controlled trial of fish oil in IgA nephropathy. N Engl J Med 1994;331: 1194–1199.

144. Donadio J, Grande J, Bergstralh E, et al: The long-term outcome of patients with IgA nephropathy treated with fish oil in a controlled trial. J Am Soc Nephrol 1999;10:1772–1777.

145. Donadio J, Larson T, Bergstralh E, et al: A randomized trial of high-dose compared with low-dose omega-3 fatty acids in severe IgA nephropathy. J Am Soc Nephrol 2001;12:791–799.

146. Wolf G, Neilson E: Angiotensin II as a renal growth factor. J Am Soc Nephrol 1993;3:1531–1540.

147. Hogg RJ, Lee J, Nardelli N, et al: Clinical trial to evaluate omega-3 fatty acids and alternate day prednisone in patients with IgA nephropathy: Report from the Southwest Pediatric Nephrology Study Group. Clin J Am Soc Nephrol 2006;1:467–474.

148. Hunley T, Julian B, Phillips J, et al: Angiotensin converting enzyme gene polymorphism: Potential silencer motif and impact on progression in IgA nephropathy. Kidney Int 1996;49:571–577.

149. Stratta P, Canavese C, Ciconne G, et al: Angiotensin I-converting enzyme genotype significantly affects progression of IgA glomerulonephritis in an Italian population. Am J Kidney Dis 1999;33:1071–1079.

150. Cole B, Salinas-Madrigal L: Acute proliferative glomerulonephritis and crescentic glomerulonephritis. In Barrat T, Avner E, Harmon W (eds): Pediatric Nephrology, 4 ed. Baltimore: Lippincott Williams & Wilkins, 1999, pp 669–678.

151. Berrios X, Lagomarsino E, Solar E, et al: Post-streptococcal acute glomerulonephritis in Chile—20 years of experience. Pediatr Nephrol 2004;19:306–312.

152. Nissensona AR, Baraff L, Fine R, et al: Poststreptococcal acute glomerulonephritis: Fact and controversy. Ann Intern Med 1979;91:76–86.

153. Watanabe T, Yoshizawa N: Recurrence of acute poststreptococcal glomerulonephritis. Pediatr Nephrol 2001;16:598–600.

154. Velhote V, Saldanha L, Malheiro P, et al: Acute glomerulonephritis: Three episodes demonstrated by light and electron microscopy, and immunofluorescence studies. A case report. Clin Nephrol 1986;26:307–310.

155. Rosenberg H, Donoso P, Vial S, et al: Clinical and morphological recovery between two episodes of acute glomerulonephritis: A light and electron microscopy study with immunofluorescence. Clin Nephrol 1984;21:350–354.

156. Navaneeth B, Ray N, Chawda S, et al: Prevalence of beta hemolytic streptococci carrier rate among schoolchildren in Salem. Indian J Pediatr 2001;68:985–986.

157. Pichichero M, Marsocci S, Murphy M, et al: Incidence of streptococcal carriers in private pediatric practice. Arch Pediatr Adolesc Med 1999;153:624–628.

158. Begovac J, Bobinac E, Benic B, et al: Asymptomatic pharyngeal carriage of beta-hemolytic streptococci and streptococcal pharyngitis among patients at an urban hospital in Croatia. Eur J Epidemiol 1993;9:405–410.

159. Dedeoglu I, Springate J, Waz W, et al: Prolonged hypocomplementemia in poststreptococcal acute glomerulonephritis. Clin Nephrol 1996;46:302–305.

160. Jankauskiene A, Cerniauskiene V, Jakutovic M, et al: Enalapril influence on blood pressure and echocardiographic parameters in children with acute postinfectious glomerulonephritis. Medicine (Kaunas) 2005;41:1019–1025.

161. Bolton W, Sturgill B: Methylprednisolone therapy for acute crescentic rapidly progressive glomerulonephritis. Am J Nephrol 1989;9:368–375.

162. Kunis C, Kiss B, Williams G, et al: Intravenous "pulse" cyclophosphamide therapy of crescentic glomerulonephritis. Clin Nephrol 1992;37:1–7.

163. Roy S, Murphy WM, Arant BS. Poststreptococcal crescenteric glomerulonephritis in children: Comparison of quintuple therapy versus supportive care. J Pediatr 1981;98: 403–410.

164. Kasahaa T, Hayakawa H, Okubo S, et al: Prognosis of acute poststreptococcal glomerulonephritis (APSGN) is excellent in children, when adequately diagnosed. Pediatr Int 2001;43: 364–367.

165. Popovic-Rolovic M, Kosic M, Antic-Peco A, et al: Medium- and long-term prognosis of patients with acute poststreptococcal glomerulonephritis. Nephron 1991;58:393–399.

166. Clark G, White R, Glasgow E, et al: Poststreptococcal glomerulonephritis in children: Clinicopathological correlations and long-term prognosis. Pediatr Nephrol 1988;2:381–388.

167. Baldwin D, Gluck M, Schacht R, et al: The long-term course of poststreptococcal glomerulonephritis. Ann Intern Med 1974;80:342–358.

168. Cameron S, Turner R, Heaton J, et al: Idiopathic mesangiocapillary glomerulonephritis. Am J Med 1983;74:175–192.

169. Habib R, Kleinknecht C, Gubler M, et al: Idiopathic membranoproliferative glomerulonephritis in children. Report of 105 cases. Clin Nephrol 1973;1:194–214.

170. Somers M, Kertesz S, Rosen S, et al: Non-nephrotic children with membranoproliferative glomerulonephritis: Are steroids indicated? Pediatr Nephrol 1995;9:140–144.

171. Iitaka K, Ishidate T, Hojo M, et al: Idiopathic membranoproliferative glomerulonephritis in Japanese children. Pediatr Nephrol 1995;9:272–277.

172. Donadio J, Anderson C, Mitchell J, et al: Membranoproliferative glomerulonephritis: A prospective clinical trial of platelet-inhibitor therapy. N Engl J Med 1984;310:1421–1426.

173. Zimmerman S, Moorthy A, Dreher W, et al: Prospective trial of warfarin and dipyridamole in patients with membranoproliferative glomerulonephritis. Am J Med 1983;75:920–927.

174. Catran D, Cardella C, Roscoe J, et al: Results of a controlled drug trial in membranoproliferative glomerulonephritis. Kidney Int 1985;27:436–441.

175. Zauner I, Bohler J, Braun N, et al: Effect of aspirin and dipyridamole on proteinuria in idiopathic membranoproliferative glomerulonephritis: A multicentre prospective clinical trial. Nephrol Dial Transplant 1994;9:619–622.

176. McEnery P: Membranoproliferative glomerulonephritis: The Cincinnati experience. Cumulative renal survival from 1957 to 1989. J Pediatr 1990;116:S109–S114.

177. Bergstein J, Andreoli S: Response of type I membranoproliferative glomerulonephritis to pulse methylprednisone and alternate-day prednisone therapy. Pediatr Nephrol 1995;9:268–271.

178. Tarshish P, Bernstein J, Tobin J, et al: Treatment of mesangiocapillary glomerulonephritis with alternate-day prednisone: A report of the International Study of Kidney Disease in Children. Pediatr Nephrol 1992;6:123–130.

179. Yanagihara T, Hayakawa M, Yoshida J, et al: Long-term follow-up of diffuse membranoproliferative glomerulonephritis type 1. Pediatr Nephrol 2005;20:585–590.

180. Bahat E, Akkaya BK, Akman S, et al: Comparison of pulse and oral steroid in childhood membranoproliferative glomerulonephritis. J Nephrol 2007;20:234–245.

181. Quan A, Sullivan E, Alexander S: Recurrence of hemolytic uremic syndrome after renal transplantation in children (a report of the North American Pediatric Renal Transplant Cooperative Study). Transplantation 2001;72:742–745.

182. Seigler R: The hemolytic uremic syndrome. Pediatr Clin North Am 1995;42:1505–1529.

183. Brandt J, Fouser L, Watkins S, et al: *Escherichia coli* O157:H7-associated hemolytic-uremic syndrome after ingestion of contaminated hamburgers. J Pediatr 1994;125:519–526.

184. Seigler R: Hemolytic uremic syndrome in children. Curr Opin Pediatr 1995;7:159–163.

185. Hancock D, Besser T, Kinsel M, et al: The prevalence of *Escherichia coli* O157:H7 in dairy and beef cattle in Washington state. Epidemiol Infect 1994;113:199–207.

186. Belongia E, Osterholm M, Soler J, et al: Transmission of *Escherichia coli* O157:H7 infection in Minnesota child day-care facilities. JAMA 1993;269:883–888.

187. Kaplan B, Meyers K, Schulman S: The pathogenesis and treatment of hemolytic uremic syndrome. J Am Soc Nephrol 1998;9:1126–1133.

188. Moake J: Haemolytic-uraemic syndrome: Basic science. Lancet 1994;343:393–397.

189. Grodinsky S, Telmesani A, Robson W, et al: Gastrointestinal manifestations of hemolytic uremic syndrome: Recognition of pancreatitis. J Pediatr Gastroenterol Nutr 1990;11:518–524.

190. Brandt M, O'Regan S, Rousseau E, et al: Surgical complications of the hemolytic-uremic syndrome. J Pediatr Surg 1990;25:1109–1112.

191. Tochen M, Campbell J: Colitis in children with the hemolytic-uremic syndrome. J Pediatr Surg 1977;12:213–219.

192. Siegler R, Pavia A, Christofferson R, et al: A 20-year population-based study of postdiarrheal hemolytic uremic syndrome in Utah. Pediatrics 1994;94:35–40.

193. Oakes RS, Siegler RS, McReynolds MA, et al: Predictors of fatality in postdiarrheal hemolytic uremic syndrome. Pediatrics 2006;117:1656–1662.

194. Garg AX, Suri RS, Barrowman N, et al: Long-term renal prognosis of diarrhea-associated hemolytic uremic syndrome: A systematic review, meta-analysis, and meta-regression. JAMA 2003;290:1360–1370.

195. Tobias JD: Hemolytic-uremic syndrome and myocardial dysfunction in a 9 month old boy. Pediatr Anaesth 2007;17:584–587.

196. Ake JA, Jelacic S, Ciol MA, et al: Relative nephroprotection during *Escherichia coli* O157:H7 infections: Association with intravenous volume expansion. Pediatrics 2005;115:e673–e680.

197. Wong C, Jelacic S, Habeeb R, et al: The risk of the hemolytic-uremic syndrome after antibiotic treatment of *Escherichia coli* O157:H7 infections. N Engl J Med 2000;32:1930–1936.

198. Spizzirri F, Rahman R, Biblioni N, et al: Childhood hemolytic uremic syndrome in Argentina: Long-term follow-up and prognostic features. Pediatr Nephrol 1997;11:156–160.

199. Gagnadoux M, Habib R, Gubler M, et al: Long-term (15–25 years) outcome of childhood hemolytic-uremic syndrome. Clin Nephrol 1996;46:39–41.

200. Quan A, Sullivan E, Alexander S: Recurrence of hemolytic uremic syndrome after renal transplantation in children. A report of the North American Pediatric Renal Transplant Cooperative Study. Transplantation 2001;72:742–745.

201. Bassani C, Ferraris J, Gianantonio C, et al: Renal transplantation in patients with classical haemolytic-uraemic syndrome. Pediatr Nephrol 1991;5:607–611.

202. Siegler RL, Pavia AT, Hansen FL, et al: Atypical hemolytic-uremic syndrome: A comparison with postdiarrheal disease. J Pediatr 1996;128:505–511.

203. Kavanagh D, Richards A, Fremeaux-Bacchi V, et al: Screening for complement system abnormalities in patients with atypical hemolytic uremic syndrome. Clin J Am Soc Nephrol 2007;2:592–596.

204. Jokiranta TS, Zipfel PF, Fremeaux-Bacchi V, et al: Where next with atypical hemolytic uremic syndrome? Mol Immunol 2007;44:3889–3900.

205. Caprioli J, Noris M, Brioschi S, et al: Genetics of HUS: The impact of MCP, CFH, and IF mutations on clinical presentation, response to treatment, and outcome. Blood 2006;108:1267–1279.

206. Dragon-Durey MA, Loirat C, Clarec S, et al: Anti–factor H auto-antibodies associated with atypical hemolytic uremic syndrome. J Am Soc Nephrol 2005;16:555–563.

207. Constantinescu AR, Bitzan M, Weiss LS, et al: Non-enteropathic hemolytic uremic syndrome: Causes and short-term course. Am J Kidney Dis 2004;43:976–982.

208. Renaud C, Niaudet P, Gagnadoux MF, et al: Haemolytic uraemic syndrome: Prognostic factors in children over 3 years of age. Pediatr Nephrol 1995;9:24–29.

209. Sellier-Leclerc AL, Fremeaux-Bacchi V, Dragon-Durey MA, et al: Differential impact of complement mutations on clinical characteristics in atypical hemolytic uremic syndrome. J Am Soc Nephrol 2007;18:2392–2400.

210. Zimmerhackl LB, Scheiring J, Prufer F, et al: Renal transplantation in HUS patients with disorders of complement regulation. Pediatr Nephrol 2007;22:10–16.

211. Donne RL, Abbs I, Barany P, et al: Recurrence of hemolytic uremic syndrome after live related renal transplantation associated with subsequent de novo disease in the donor. Am J Kidney Dis 2002;40:E22.

212. Kavanagh D, Goodship THJ, Richards A: Atypical haemolytic uraemic syndrome. Br Med Bull 2006;77–78:5–22.

213. Saland JM, Emre SH, Shneider BL, et al: Favorable long-term outcome after liver-kidney transplant for recurrent hemolytic uremic syndrome associated with a factor H mutation. Am J Transplant 2006;6:1948–1952.

214. Sinaiko AR, Gomez-Marin O, Prineas RJ: Prevalence of significant hypertension in junior high school-aged children. The children and adolescent blood pressure program. J Pediatr 1989;114:664–669.

215. The fourth report on the diagnosis, evaluation, and treatment of high blood pressure in children and adolescents. Pediatrics 2004;114(Suppl):555–576.

216. National High Blood Pressure Education Program Working Group on Hypertension Control in Children and Adolescents: Update on the 1987 Task Force report on high blood pressure in children and adolescents: A working group report from the National High Blood Pressure Education Program. Pediatrics 1996;98:649–658.

217. Matoo TK: Arm cuff in the measurement of blood pressure. Am J Hypertens 2002;15:67S–68S.

218. Lurbe E, Redon J: Reproducibility and validity of ambulatory blood pressure monitoring in children. Am J Hypertens 2002;15:69S–73S.

219. Park MK, Menard SW, Yuan C: Comparison of auscultatory and oscillometric blood pressure. Arch Pediatr Adolesc Med 2001;155:50–53.

220. Podoll A, Grenier M, Croix B, et al: Inaccuracy in pediatric outpatient blood pressure measurement. Pediatrics 2007;119: e538–e543.

221. Swinford RD, Ingelfinger JR: Evaluation of hypertension in childhood diseases. In Barratt TM, Avner ED, Harmon WE (eds): Pediatric Nephrology, 4th ed. Baltimore: Lippincott Williams & Wilkins, 1999, pp 1007–1030.

222. Berenson GS. Obesity—a critical issue in preventive cardiology: The Bogalusa Heart Study. Prev Cardiol 2005;8:234–241.

223. Sorof JM, Lai D, Turner J, et al: Overweight, ethnicity, and the prevalence of hypertension in school-aged children. Pediatrics 2004;113:475–482.

224. Thompson DR, Obarzanek E, Franko DL, et al: Childhood overweight and cardiovascular disease risk factors: The National Heart, Lung, and Blood Institute Growth and Health Study. J Pediatr 2007;150:18–25.

225. Sadowski RH, Falkner B: Hypertension in pediatric patients. Am J Kidney Dis 1996;27:305–315.

226. Hellstrom AL, Hanson E, Hansson S, et al: Association between urinary symptoms at 7 years old and previous urinary tract infection. Arch Dis Child 1991;66:232–234.

227. Bailey RR: Vesicoureteral reflux in healthy infants and children. In Hodson J, Kincaid-Smith P (eds): Reflux Nephropathy. New York: Masson, 1979, pp 59–61.

228. Rushton HG: Urinary tract infections in children: Epidemiology, evaluation, and management. Pediatr Clin North Am 1997;44:1133–1169.

229. Michael M, Hodson EM, Craig JC, et al: Short compared with standard duration of antibiotic treatment for urinary tract infection: A systematic review of randomized controlled trials. Arch Dis Child 2002;87:118–123.

230. Lavocat MP, Granjon D, Allard D, et al: Imaging of pyelonephritis. Pediatr Radiol 1997;27:159–165.

231. Skoog SJ, Belman AB, Majd M: A nonsurgical approach to the management of primary vesicoureteral reflux. J Urol 1987;138:941–946.

232. Smellie JM, Normand JC, Katz G: Children with urinary infections: A comparison of those with and those without vesicoureteric reflux. Kidney Int 1981;20:717–722.

233. Olbing H, Claesson I, Ebel KD, et al: Renal scars and parenchymal thinning in children with vesicoureteral reflux: A 5-year report of the International Reflux Study in Children (European branch). J Urol 1992;148:1653–1656.

234. Tamminen-Mobius T, Bruner E, Ebel KD, et al: Cessation of vesicoureteral reflux for 5 years in infants and children allocated to medical treatment. J Urol 1992;148:1662–1666.

235. Smellie JM, Jodal U, Lax H, et al: Outcome at 10 years of severe vesicoureteric reflux managed medically: Report of the International Reflux Study in Children. J Pediatr 2001;199:656–663.

236. Wennerstrom M, Hansson S, Jodal U, et al: Disappearance of vesico-ureteric reflux in children. Arch Pediatr Adolesc Med 1998;152:879–883.

237. Wadie GM, Tirabassi MV, Courtney RA, et al: The deflux procedure reduces the incidence of urinary tract infections in patients with vesicoureteral reflux. J Laparoendosc Adv Surg Tech A 2007;17:353–359.

238. Cooper CS, Chung BI, Kirsch AJ, et al: The outcome of stopping prophylactic antibiotics in older children with vesicoureteral reflux. J Urol 2000;163:269–272.

239. Rushton HG: Vesicoureteral reflux and scarring. In Avner ED, Harmon WE, Niaudet P (eds): Pediatric Nephrology, 5th ed. Philadelphia: Lippincott Williams & Wilkins, 2004, pp 1027–1048.

Further Reading

Chang SL, Shortliffe LD: Pediatric urinary tract infections. Pediatr Clin North Am 2006;53:379–400.

Gipson DS, Chin H, Presler TP, et al: Differential risk of remission and ESRD in childhood FSGS. Pediatr Nephrol 2006;21:344–349.

Greenfield SP, Williot P, Kaplan D: Gross hematuria in children: A ten year review. Urology 2007;69:166–169.

Mattoo TK: Medical management of vesicoureteral reflux. Pediatr Nephrol 2007;22:1113–1120.

Mitsnefes M: Hypertension in children and adolescents. Pediatr Clin North Am 2006;53:493–512.

Seikaly MG: Hypertension in children: An update on treatment strategies. Curr Opin Pediatr 2007;19:170–177.

Sellier-Leclerc AL, Fremeaux-Bacchi V, Dragon-Durev MA, et al: Differential impact of complement mutations on clinical characteristics in atypical hemolytic uremic syndrome. J Am Soc Nephrol 2007;18:2392–2400.

Tryggvason K, Patrakka J, Wartiovaara J: Hereditary proteinuria syndromes and mechanisms of proteinuria. N Engl J Med 2006;354:1387–1401.

Zorc JJ, Kiddoo DA, Shaw KN: Diagnosis and management of pediatric urinary tract infections. Clin Microbiol Rev 2005;18:417–422.

Chapter 44

Management of End-Stage Renal Disease in Childhood and Adolescence

Joana E. Kist-van Holthe, David M. Briscoe, and Vikas R. Dharnidharka

The management of children and adolescents with end-stage renal disease (ESRD) differs from that for adults. Children have unique problems that are not only associated with renal failure itself but can also be related to current therapies. The optimal treatment of ESRD in a child is one that not only reverses the biochemical and hematologic abnormalities related to the disease but also achieves normal physiologic patterns of growth and neurodevelopment. Such a treatment facilitates maximal educational and vocational opportunities and optimizes the quality of life of the child.

ESRD occurs in one to three per million total population of children per year.[1,2] The most common diagnoses of ESRD in small children are noted in Table 44-1.[3] Chronic renal insufficiency in children is associated with many biochemical and hematologic abnormalities as well as hypertension, hyperparathyroidism, anemia, and growth retardation, all of which require specific therapeutic interventions. Indications for renal replacement therapy include hypervolemia, hyperkalemia, symptoms of uremia not responsive to conservative therapy, failure to thrive due to limitations in total caloric intake, severe refractory hypertension, growth retardation not responsive to growth hormone therapy, and delayed psychomotor development.[4] The Kidney Disease Outcomes Quality Initiative clinical practice guideline and Center for Medicare and Medicaid Services recommend initiation of renal replacement therapy at a glomerular filtration rate less than 15 mL/min/1.73 m^2.[5,6] All children can undergo dialysis therapy, although the mortality associated with dialysis can be especially high in infants. In older children, the mortality of dialysis is similar to that seen in adults.

Renal transplantation is a feasible treatment for ESRD and is widely recognized as the treatment of choice for all children.[7,8] In contrast to children on dialysis, children with a functioning renal transplant can have adequate growth, psychomotor development, and school achievements.[9-15] Absolute contraindications for renal transplantation are few but include active malignancy, active infection with hepatitis B or human immunodeficiency virus, severe multiorgan failure, and a positive direct cross-match within the previous 3 to 12 months.[4,8]

SPECIAL CLINICAL ISSUES IN CHILDREN WITH END-STAGE RENAL DISEASE

Nutrition

Inadequate nutrition in children with ESRD inevitably results in growth failure when caloric intake is less than 70% of the recommended dietary allowance.[16,17] Current recommendations are that children on dialysis should receive an energy intake that is at least 100% of the recommended dietary allowance (Table 44-2).[18,19] For infants on peritoneal dialysis, a slightly higher caloric intake (130%–140% recommended dietary allowance) and a high protein intake of 2.5 to 3 g/kg/day is needed for adequate growth.[19-22] Likewise for prepubertal and pubertal children receiving peritoneal dialysis, high protein intakes (1.5–2 g/kg/day) are advised to maintain physiologic growth patterns and to avoid protein malnutrition. The higher protein intake may result in a slightly higher blood

Table 44-1 Primary Diagnoses (%) of Children with End-Stage Renal Disease Who Received a Renal Allograft

Primary Diagnosis	Percent
Congenital abnormalities of the urinary tract	39.6
Obstructive uropathy	15.8
Aplastic/hypoplastic/dysplastic kidneys	15.9
Reflux nephropathy	5.2
Prune-belly syndrome	2.7
Glomerulonephritis	18.3
Focal segmental sclerosis	11.7
Membranoproliferative glomerulonephritis	2.7
Idiopathic crescentic glomerulonephritis	1.8
Membranous nephropathy	0.5
Systemic lupus erythematosus	1.6
Chronic glomerulonephritis	3.4
Medullary cystic/juvenile nephronophthisis	2.8
Hemolytic uremic syndrome	2.7
Congenital nephrotic syndrome	2.6
Polycystic kidney disease	2.9
Miscellaneous	27.7

Adapted from Smith JM, Stablein DM, Munoz R, et al: Contributions of the Transplant Registry: The 2006 Annual Report of the North American Pediatric Renal Trials and Collaborative Studies (NAPRTCS). Pediatr Transplant 2007;11:366–373.

urea nitrogen level, which needs to be treated with adequate and efficient dialysis. Urea kinetic modeling is thus an important tool for monitoring optimal protein intake and delivery of dialysis.[23]

The management of fluid intake can be difficult in children, especially those with minimal urine output. In these children, as just discussed, high-calorie nutrition must be administered. To achieve nutritional goals without problems of fluid overload, small volumes of high-calorie supplements containing additional glucose polymers and/or medium-chain triglycerides are required. Many infants and small children are treated through either nasogastric or gastrostomy tubes to ensure adequate intake because they may be unwilling or unable to consume the required amount of nutrition orally.[22,24,25] It is important to note that gastrostomy feeding is not contraindicated for children receiving peritoneal dialysis.[26] Several studies have documented that this nutritional strategy is effective, and long-term enteral nutrition may prevent or reverse weight loss and growth retardation in infants and young children. Furthermore, if growth failure has already occurred, adequate nutrition can result in catch-up growth if started before the age of 2 years.[22,27] In addition, aggressive nutritional therapy can contribute to favorable psychomotor development in infants who develop ESRD in early infancy.[15] Together these data suggest that provision of adequate nutrition is critical for effective treatment of ESRD in children.

Growth and Other Endocrine Disorders

Growth retardation is common in children with ESRD and occurs even with mild renal insufficiency. The correction of growth is of paramount importance in the treatment of ESRD in children. Growth is calculated as centimeters of growth per year and is measured frequently and plotted on a standard growth curve chart, as is typical for any normal child. As the glomerular filtration rate decreases, the rate of growth

Table 44-2 Recommend Daily Intakes for Energy,* Protein,* Calcium,† and Phosphorus† for Children with Renal Disease

Age (yr)	Energy RDA (g/kg)	Protein RDA (g/kg)	Protein Intake for Hemodialysis (g/kg)	Protein Intake for Peritoneal Dialysis (g/kg)	Calcium (mg)	Phosphorus (mg)
0–0.5	108	2.2	2.6	3.0	210	100
0.5–1	98	1.6	2.0	2.4	270	275
1–3	102	1.2	1.6	2.0	500	380
4–6	90	1.2	1.6	2.0	800	400
7–8	70	1.0	1.4	1.8	800	400
9–10	70	1.0	1.4	1.8	1300	1050
11–14 (M)	55	1.0	1.4	1.8	1300	1050
11–14 (F)	47	1.0	1.4	1.8	1300	1050
15–18 (M)	45	0.9	1.3	1.5	1300	1050
15–18 (F)	38	0.8	1.2	1.5	1300	1050

F, female; M, male; RDA, recommended dietary allowance for healthy children.
*From Clinical practice guidelines for nutrition in chronic renal failure: Pediatric guidelines. Am J Kidney Dis 2000;35:S105–S136.
†From Institute of Medicine: Dietary Reference Intakes for Calcium, Phosphorus, Magnesium, Vitamin D and Fluoride. Washington, DC: National Academy Press, 2000.

decreases; it is at this time that treatment must begin to correct any rate of decline in linear growth. If untreated, growth failure will be progressive and catch-up is difficult to achieve. Treatment involves ensuring that (1) recommended caloric and protein intakes are achieved, (2) metabolic disturbances (e.g., acidosis, hyponatremia) are normalized, and (3) parathyroid hormone (PTH), calcium intake, and phosphorus load are normalized to correct any problems related to renal osteodystrophy. These factors may all contribute to decreased linear growth. For children on dialysis, more efficient clearance can also improve growth.[28,29] If growth retardation occurs despite these treatment measures, growth hormone therapy is indicated.[30] Growth hormone therapy significantly accelerates short- and long-term growth.[31–33] Thus, the clinician must not wait until growth retardation has occurred but must maintain normal growth patterns with the use of growth hormone.[30] However, in a large study from Centers for Medicare and Medicaid Services, only 39% of children on hemodialysis with short stature received growth hormone.[34] Growth hormone therapy consists of 0.05 mg/kg or 4 U/m^2 injected subcutaneously as a daily dose (usually in the evening). The dose of growth hormone is adjusted to achieve normal growth patterns; some children require decreased dosing, whereas others require increased dosing. Children receiving growth hormone should be monitored regularly for response, including assessment of growth velocity and bone age. Nonetheless, final adult height was retarded in 57% of renal allograft recipients and therefore continues to be suboptimal.[35]

As discussed above, achievement of normal growth rates is a mainstay of therapy for children with chronic renal insufficiency either before or during dialysis as well as after transplantation. Renal transplantation alone was once thought to be a good treatment for growth retardation as catch-up growth could occur, whereas this was not possible on dialysis. However, recent reports of renal transplantation with regard to growth have been disappointing. Results of multicenter studies have demonstrated that catch-up growth after renal transplantation occurs in only 25% of children, predominantly young children. Indeed, even in this group, catch-up growth is seen in only 47% of children aged 0 to 5 years.[3,36] This implies that the treatment of growth retardation must begin before the initiation of renal replacement therapy, whether this therapy is dialysis or renal transplantation. After renal transplantation, growth hormone can be given to children and can improve final adult height, without adversely affecting renal function.[37–39] Also after renal transplantation, the use of alternate-day steroid dosing versus daily dosing can result in improved growth patterns without increased rejection or allograft loss.[40] To optimize growth, several centers in the United States are currently participating in a randomized, placebo-controlled, steroid-withdrawal trial to assess its potential for optimizing growth patterns without altering long-term graft function. The pilot study suggests that growth with steroid avoidance is not better than alternate-day steroid dosing; it is only promising in that other steroid side effects are avoided.[41,42]

In addition to its effects on growth, ESRD is also associated with other endocrine disorders. These are thought to be related to inappropriate circulating hormone concentrations or changed hormonal action at the target site. Children with ESRD have an average delay of puberty of 2.5 years and two thirds of adolescents with ESRD enter puberty beyond the normal range.[43] Furthermore, in children with ESRD, there is a marked decrease in tissue sensitivity to insulin, in glucose uptake, and in metabolic clearance of insulin that can lead to glucose intolerance.[44] Thyroid abnormalities have also been reported in association with ESRD. All these endocrine disorders should be managed according to standard therapeutic regimens to achieve normal patterns of hormonal homeostasis.

Renal Osteodystrophy

Renal osteodystrophy is an important problem in children with chronic renal failure. Its incidence increases as the glomerular filtration rate approaches 50% of normal. Once established, osteodystrophy leads to deceleration of linear growth, muscle weakness, and bone pain; when severe, it results in skeletal deformities such as bowing of lower extremities, fractures, and epiphyseal slipping. Renal osteodystrophy represents a spectrum of activity, from high-turnover to low-turnover bone disease. Renal osteodystrophy occurs in children due to a lack of 1,25-dihydroxyvitamin D_3, hypocalcemia, and hyperphosphatemia. A detailed review of the pathophysiology of renal osteodystrophy can be found in Chapter 69 and Martin and Slatopolsky.[45] All children with renal insufficiency (glomerular filtration rate < 70 mL/min/1.73 m^2) should be monitored by frequent assessment of serum calcium, phosphorus, alkaline phosphatase, and PTH and by occasional radiographs of the hand. Bone densitometry can also be used, but normal values are not known for children younger than 5 years of age.

The most common type of renal osteodystrophy seen in children is high-turnover bone disease, which is associated with high PTH levels and secondary hyperparathyroidism. In recent years, aggressive management of calcium, phosphorus, and PTH has led to a decreasing incidence of secondary hyperparathyroidism.[46]

Prevention of renal osteodystrophy consists of avoidance of hyperphosphatemia using phosphate restriction (80% of dietary reference intake; see Table 44-2) and/or calcium-containing phosphate binders (calcium carbonate or calcium acetate) or non–calcium-containing phosphate binders (sevelamer) taken with all meals (see Table 44-2). Serum phosphate levels should be maintained at normal levels for age.[47–49] Aluminum-containing phosphate binders should be avoided because the aluminum accumulates in bone and can lead to low-turnover aluminum bone disease. Furthermore, excess aluminum can lead to central nervous system dysfunction.[50] Optimal management also involves following PTH levels carefully, administration of active vitamin D_3, and assessment of biochemical response. Various active forms of vitamin D are used, preparations include 1α-hydroxyvitamin D_3 (alfacalcidol), and 1,25-dihydroxyvitamin D_3 (calcitriol).[49,51,52] The mode of administration of the active metabolite of vitamin D, oral or intravenous, has the same efficacy.[53] To avoid adynamic bone disease, plasma PTH should be maintained at a level two to four times above the upper limit of normal.[19,47–49,54] Hypercalcemia as a result of excessive vitamin D supplementation must be avoided because calcium deposits can form in various tissues, particularly if serum calcium $\times$ phosphate product exceeds 60 mg/100 mL or 5 mmol/L.[48,49]

Bone disease also occurs in children after renal transplantation. Steroid therapy has been shown to exacerbate preexisting bone disease; 70% of young children who received a renal transplant in childhood already have osteopenia. In a multiple regression analysis, it was found that the cumulative dose of steroids was inversely related to bone mineral density score. Steroids are associated with osteoporosis and avascular bone necrosis after transplantation.[55]

Anemia

The management of anemia in the pediatric population is similar to that in adults (discussed in Chapter 68). Most pediatric patients with ESRD (glomerular filtration rate < 30 mL/min) require erythropoietin therapy to maintain normal hematocrit. The use of erythropoietin has dramatically improved the outcome of dialysis and quality of life in children and has abolished the typical iron-overload syndromes that were associated with frequent transfusions as a result of dialysis anemia.[56–58]

Dosing recommendations when starting erythropoietin therapy for patients younger than 1 year are 350 U/kg per week; 275 U/kg/week for those 2 to 5 years; 250 U/kg/week for those 6 to 12 years; and 200 U/kg/week subcutaneously in one to three doses for those older than 12 years. For children on hemodialysis, intravenous administration is preferred because it is less painful.[59] Although infrequently performed, patients on peritoneal dialysis can have erythropoietin administered in the peritoneal dialysis fluid; however, the amount required to correct anemia is much higher.[60] Subsequently, the dose is titrated to achieve a hemoglobin concentration of 11 to 13 g/dL (6.8–8.1 mmol/L).[59] The median maintenance dose is age dependent and is higher for younger children. Children on hemodialysis generally require a higher dose than those on peritoneal dialysis therapy.[59] Iron deficiency is common in children receiving erythropoietin therapy and supplementation with oral (3 mg/kg/day in three doses) or intravenous iron (1 mg/kg/week, not to exceed 125 mg) is often necessary.[57,59,61–64] Serum iron levels should be maintained in the normal range, transferrin saturation at more than 20%, and serum ferritin levels greater than 100 ng/mL.[59] When starting therapy with erythropoietin, blood pressure and hemoglobin should be measured regularly.

Recently long-acting darbepoetin was proven to have a similar efficacy as erythropoeitin.[65] Two hundred units of erythropoietin is approximately equivalent to 0.5 μg darbepoetin. A starting dose of 0.5 μg/kg/week IV/SC effectively treats anemia in children with chronic renal failure. For many. this dose may be proportionally increased and injected less than once weekly.[66] However, darbepoetin generally produces an increased degree of pain at the injection site compared with most short-acting erythropoietins.[67] Darbepoetin can also be administered intraperitoneally starting with 0.45 μg/kg/week and increasing to a median of 0.63 to 0.79 μg/kg/week.[68]

Hypertension and Cardiovascular Disease

Although isolated blood pressure measurements are typically used in children with ESRD, it is recommended that 24-hour ambulatory blood pressure is monitored at intervals.[69,70] When evaluated by ambulatory blood pressure monitoring, 70% of peritoneal dialysis and 33% of hemodialysis patients were found to be hypertensive. In contrast, isolated blood pressure

measurements demonstrated hypertension in only 47% of peritoneal dialysis and 44% of hemodialysis patients.[69] Nevertheless, the primary goal of antihypertensive therapy is to decrease blood pressure to less than the 90th percentile for age, gender, and height.[71,72] Choice of medication depends on the likely cause of the hypertension. For instance, an angiotensin-converting inhibitor is a good choice for treatment of hypertension associated with renal insufficiency. In contrast, a vasodilator and/or β-blocker is the most usual choice for therapy in a dialysis patient in whom hypertension may be associated with fluid overload. Blood pressure increases can be marked and very difficult to control. Hypertension is a highly significant and independent predictor for the progression of chronic renal insufficiency in children.[73] Furthermore, cardiovascular issues were the cause of 20% to 25% of all deaths in children with ESRD. This proportion increases to more than 40% in long-term studies of children with ESRD starting in childhood.[74,75] It is thus most important to be aggressive and to lower blood pressure into the normal range in all children.

In children with hypertension, one should consider evaluation of cardiac function and structure with echocardiography at initial presentation and yearly thereafter.[76,77] Severe left ventricular hypertrophy is seen in almost half of all young dialysis patients.[78] Better control of blood pressure, anemia, and hypervolemia may be important in preventing left ventricular hypertrophy and improving long-term cardiac outcome. ESRD patients younger than 20 years of age rarely have evidence of coronary artery calcification, whereas patients aged 20 to 30 years are more likely to show disease.[79]

All children, regardless of symptoms, require assessment for cardiovascular disease and should be screened for traditional cardiovascular risk factors such as dyslipidemia and hypertension at initiation of dialysis and at regular intervals thereafter.[80] Assessment of dyslipidemia should consist of a fasting profile with total cholesterol, low-density lipoprotein (LDL) cholesterol, high-density lipoprotein (HDL) cholesterol, and triglycerides.[81] Hyperlipidemia is defined as lipid levels higher than the 95th percentile for age and gender. All children with dyslipidemia should follow the recommendations for therapeutic lifestyle changes, which involve a decrease in saturated fat intake, increase in fiber intake, and moderate physical activity. Kidney Disease Outcomes Quality Initiative guidelines recommend treatment with statins for adolescents if LDL cholesterol is more than 130 mg/dL (>3.36 mmol/L) and non-HDL cholesterol (total cholesterol − HDL) is more than 160 mg/dL (>4.14 mmol/L).[81] In the United States, atorvastatin (10–20 mg once daily) is the only drug approved by the U.S. Food and Drug Administration for use in children.

Neurodevelopmental Outcome, Psychosocial Adjustment, and Quality of Life

It is well established in the literature that neurodevelopmental delay, cognitive and motor abnormalities, cerebral cortical atrophy, and progressive encephalopathy are associated with chronic renal insufficiency in children, especially within the first year of life.[10,82] However, improvements in nutrition, elimination of aluminum binders from treatment regimens, psychomotor therapy, and access to play specialists have all been shown to improve cognitive function and long-term outcome.[15] Furthermore, early renal transplantation is known to be beneficial for normalization of neurodevelopmental outcome.[13,83]

Current data indicate that 77% of children on peritoneal dialysis and 46% on hemodialysis attend school full time.[84] Dialysis patients function below their age and grade levels in all areas. In contrast, transplant recipients achieve at or above the levels achieved by dialysis patients.[12] Data suggest that ESRD, not dialysis/transplant status, is still a risk factor for lower IQ and academic achievement. Cognitive development or low IQ is most notable in younger children and in children whose mothers/caregivers have lower educational levels.[85]

Last, it is important to note that children with chronic renal disease are at risk of psychosocial adjustment disturbances, as occurs with many chronic diseases. In addition, low self-esteem, anxiety, and depressed mood are more severe in children on dialysis.[86] Thus, most pediatrics centers involve psychologists and social workers in the treatment of children with ESRD.

Quality of life has increasingly been studied in children requiring renal replacement therapy. Not surprisingly, health-related quality-of-life scores were significantly lower than in healthy controls. Transplant recipients reported better physical and psychosocial health than dialysis patients. No difference was noted between hemodialysis and peritoneal dialysis patients for any quality-of-life domain.[87] Furthermore, caring for children on dialysis has significant adverse psychosocial effects on the caretakers. The prevalence of depression was significantly more common in parents of children treated for ESRD (28%) compared with parents of healthy children (5%).[88] In addition, prolonged dialysis during childhood may decrease the ability to gain high-skilled professions and social independence. Unemployment is twice as high in patients with childhood-onset ESRD compared with healthy persons, but more than twice as low compared with patients with adult-onset ESRD.[89]

Mortality of Children on Renal Replacement Therapy

There is a high mortality associated with dialysis therapy in children, especially young children.[90,91] Furthermore, it is clear that time on dialysis is associated with mortality. The most common causes of death in children are infection and cardiopulmonary disease.[92] In children younger than 2 years of age, it has been shown that ESRD associated with oliguria or anuria, multiorgan failure, and the presence of nonrenal disease, especially pulmonary disease and/or pulmonary hypoplasia, are all risk factors for mortality.[93] Long-term survival among children requiring renal replacement therapy in the Australia and New Zealand Dialysis and Transplant Registry was 79% at 10 years and 66% at 20 years. Overall, a trend toward improved survival was observed over the four decades of the study. In this cohort, the most common cause of death was cardiovascular disease (45%), and the second most common cause was infection (21%).[94]

In contrast, patient survival after transplantation is excellent. Overall patient survival at 1, 2, and 5 years after transplantation is 97.7%, 96.8% and 94.3%, respectively.[95] When patient survival is analyzed by age, it appears that younger children are more at risk of death after transplantation. Infants who receive cadaver donor transplants have a higher mortality than those who receive living donor renal transplants. Also, even in the youngest age groups, the mortality after renal transplantation is less than that seen with dialysis alone.[95]

DIALYSIS THERAPY

All children are candidates for peritoneal dialysis or hemodialysis. In general, the decision to perform either form of dialysis involves patient preference, distance from a pediatric hemodialysis center, and center bias. In young children, there is a preference for peritoneal dialysis because hemodialysis is associated with vascular access problems and also involves significant expertise on the part of personnel. Thus, peritoneal dialysis has become the more common treatment in many centers. Nearly 60% of the pediatric dialysis population are currently maintained on peritoneal dialysis.[92] Some reports suggest that younger children fare better with peritoneal dialysis, although data indicate that as long as efficiency is maintained, there are no significant therapeutic differences between peritoneal dialysis and hemodialysis.

Peritoneal Dialysis

Peritoneal dialysis is discussed in great detail in Chapters 81 to 83. Here, we focus on specific issues pertaining to peritoneal dialysis in childhood. Peritoneal dialysis is preferred for infants as it obviates the need for vascular access, which can be especially difficult in this group of children.[56] Another advantage of peritoneal dialysis over hemodialysis is that it requires less fluid restriction. As discussed earlier, this may be important for adequate administration of nutrition. Automated continuous cycler-assisted peritoneal dialysis at night is used most frequently in younger children.[56]

In older children and especially adolescents, compliance with dialysis prescription can be a problem and can thus affect dialysis efficiency. The requirement for a permanent intra-abdominal catheter can distort body image and its presence becomes unwanted. This can lead to treatment issues and puts parents in a compromising situation if they wish to be caregivers. Therefore, peritoneal dialysis in an adolescent needs careful monitoring. Hemodialysis has become the more common form of renal replacement therapy in this group because it provides adequate treatment and also enables assessment of compliance and adequacy.

Initiation of peritoneal dialysis in all children involves the use of a curled catheter, typically pointing downward and situated in the lower half of the abdomen.[96] In younger children with lax abdominal musculature, the catheter preferably has two cuffs to avoid leakage and infections. The catheter and cuff are typically allowed to heal for a minimum of 2 weeks before the initiation of dialysis to prevent leakage. Omentectomy during the insertion of the catheter is especially important in young children because it decreases the incidence of obstruction to 2% compared with 15% to 32% incidence in the absence of omentectomy (15%–32%).[97]

Dialysis Prescription

When prescribing peritoneal dialysis, volume input according to nutritional needs, residual urine output, and renal function must all be taken into account. In children, initial target peritoneal dialysis exchange volume of 1000 to 1200 mL/m^2 is used with a maximum of 1400 mL/m^2 and up to at least 8 L/m^2 per session.[98,99] In young children, eight to 10 exchanges are performed over 12 to 16 hours at night by an automated peritoneal dialysis cycler (continuous-cycling peritoneal dialysis). In older children, continuous ambulatory peritoneal dialysis is the usual mode of therapy, performed in a manner similar to that for adults. In addition to normalizing biochemical abnormalities, it must also be administered in a manner to facilitate growth. With all forms of peritoneal dialysis, ultrafiltration is adjusted to facilitate adequate volume intake according to nutritional needs. Typically, the ultrafiltration goal depends on analysis of the nutritional needs and the requirement for administration of volume.

Dialysis Adequacy

A peritoneal equilibration test can be used to study the transport capacity of the peritoneal membrane. Peritoneal equilibration test values for children have been calculated.[100,101] Warady and colleagues[101] found that the peritoneal membrane was stable in children over a mean interval of 20 months. However, peritonitis is a risk factor for peritoneal dialysis failure. Follow-up of peritoneal solute kinetics is recommended in patients with a history of peritonitis to permit early identification of patients at risk of dialysis failure.[102,103] Dialysis adequacy can be expressed as urea Kt/V, calculated as the ratio of 24-hour dialysate (+ urinary) urea clearance divided by total body water, where K is urea clearance (L/hr), t is time on dialysis (hours), and V is urea distribution volume and equals total body water volume (L). The target dialysis adequacy in children is a total weekly urea Kt/V of at least 1.8 to 2.0.[99,104] Higher values for weekly urea Kt/V as high as 2.75 to 3.1 can be achieved and have been correlated with improved clinical outcome.[19,105,106] However, a report from the Endstage Renal Disease Network of New England indicates that a urea Kt/V more than 2.75 may result in albumin loss and may thus hinder nutrition.[107]

Complications

Complications of peritoneal dialysis in children include exit-site/tunnel infections, peritonitis, catheter-related problems (leakage and blockage), and the development of hernias due to increased intra-abdominal pressure and relatively weak musculature. In one report, 11% of pediatric patients on peritoneal dialysis had an exit-site/tunnel infection at 1 month, 26% between 1 and 6 months, and 30% between 6 months and 1 year of follow-up.[108] Patients with tunnel infections have twice the risk of developing peritonitis and the need for access revision.

Peritonitis is the major complication of peritoneal dialysis in children. The mean occurrence of peritonitis has been reported to be once every 13.2 patient-months.[108] Peritonitis rates decrease with age and are significantly lower when catheters with two cuffs and downward-pointed exit sites are used.[56,84,109] There is no difference in peritonitis in children treated with curled or straight catheters. Overall, 25% of patients on peritoneal dialysis switch to hemodialysis, and in most patients, the switch is due to repeated infections.[56,108]

Hemodialysis

Improvements in technology have enabled pediatric centers to perform hemodialysis in infants and young children effectively and efficiently. Important advances relate to dialysis access catheters and lines, complex machines that allow control of low blood volume, the ability to exactly control ultrafiltration, and compatible dialysis membranes and the composition of dialysates.[110,111]

Overall, one third of children who are on dialysis use hemodialysis. Hemodialysis is the preferred dialysis modality for children older than 12 years of age, who comprise 64% of all children requiring dialysis.[56] In contrast, only 12% of children younger than 5 years of age receive hemodialysis.

Permanent access in the form of a fistula or graft is the preferred form of vascular access for pediatric patients on maintenance hemodialysis therapy.[5,112,113] However, in small children, surgical expertise in placing fistula or grafts may be limited and the use of percutaneous catheters may be unavoidable. In addition, many children on hemodialysis are taken to renal transplantation fairly quickly, thus further limiting the use of fistulas.

Dialysis Prescription

For all patients, the dialysis prescription is calculated by dialyzer type, blood flow, and dialysate flow. The duration of each treatment can be easily calculated to optimize urea clearance. In infants and small children, blood flow rates as low as 50 mL/min can be used such that the dialysis prescription can be calculated according to the ability of the patient to tolerate a given flow rate. In older children and adults, blood flow rates of 200 to 300 mL/min are frequently used. Knowledge of the clearance curve of the dialyzer is essential in estimating the total urea clearance at a given blood flow rate. Extracorporeal blood volume (dialyzer priming volume plus blood tubing volume) should be kept to less than 8 mL/kg (<10% of total blood volume) to avoid hemodynamic instability and hypoxemia. Routine determination of target dry weight, using noninvasive hematocrit monitoring, decreases both the risk of chronic fluid overload and the need for antihypertensive medication and does not lead to increased intra- or interdialytic symptomatology.[114] Adequate anticoagulation can be achieved with standard heparin dosing. To attain adequate clearance, three hemodialysis treatments are usually given each week. Although the optimal dialysis dose requirement for children remains uncertain, reports of longer duration and/or daily dialysis show that they are more effective for phosphate control and may improve growth than conventional hemodialysis. Therefore, longer duration and/or daily dialysis should be considered at least for some high-risk patients with cardiovascular impairment or to overcome the free diet of very uncompliant patients.[29,115,116] As in adults, nocturnal home hemodialysis is also feasible in selected children. However, the burden on the family is substantial, and home nocturnal hemodialysis requires support of a dedicated multidisciplinary team.[117]

Dialysis Adequacy

Adequate dialysis combined with adequate nutrition reduces mortality and promotes growth in children.[28,118] Urea kinetic modeling is used to assess dialysis adequacy and nutritional status.[23] Hemodialysis efficiency is expressed as Kt/V, where K is urea clearance (L/hr), t is session length (hours), and V is urea distribution volume and equals total body water volume (L). Goldstein and colleagues[119] found no difference between the results of a formal urea kinetic modeling technique for obtaining Kt/V and results obtained by using Daugirdas's[120] formula for the single-pool natural logarithm approximation equation for Kt/V. Thus, the ease with which Kt/V can be calculated using the natural logarithm supports its regular use in the monitoring of children on hemodialysis.[19,121] An appropriate goal is to achieve a single-pool Kt/V of 1.2, at least equal to that recommended for adults.[5] There is a controversy over whether higher Kt/V values are necessary for growing children.[5,19,28,122] The Kidney Disease Outcomes Quality Initiative guideline for hemodialysis adequacy advises that for young pediatric patients, prescription of higher dialysis doses and higher protein intakes at 150% of the recommended nutrient intake for age may be important.[5] In a large study from the Centers for Medicare and Medicaid Services in adolescents, more than 79% had a mean Kt/V more than 1.2.[123]

Complications

The most common complications of hemodialysis are clotting and infection of the hemodialysis catheter, arteriovenous fistula, or graft. Infection of the hemodialysis access site when using a catheter can easily lead to septicemia, which is the most frequent cause of death in children on hemodialysis.[56] Other complications, such as disequilibrium syndrome, hypotension, anaphylactic reactions, hemolysis, and hypoxemia, are discussed in detail in Chapter 80.

RENAL TRANSPLANTATION

Renal transplantation is the optimal treatment for ESRD in children because it offers the best hope for normalization of physiologic processes. Most important is the ability of renal transplantation to normalize growth and cognitive function and to enable a child to enjoy a relatively normal quality of life. Because of the mortality associated with dialysis therapy in young children and the risk/benefit ratio, the National Organ Allocation System in the United States has given preference to children on waiting lists to receive cadaver transplants.

In the United States, an approximately equal number of renal transplantations in children are performed with living and cadaver donors.[124] As a therapy, renal transplantation is very successful and, with current immunosuppressive regimens, 1- and 5-year graft survival rates are excellent: the 5-year graft survival rates are currently 85.1% for living related donor grafts and 76.1% for cadaver donors.[124] The projected half-life of renal transplants in pediatric recipients is equal to or even better than that in adult recipients.[125,126] However, as discussed later, rejection remains a major cause of graft loss in the first posttransplantation year.[124] Newer immunosuppressive agents have decreased the incidence of acute rejection and have improved 1-year graft survival rates, especially for recipients of cadaver donor transplants. The current 1-year graft survival rates for cadaver donor and living related donor transplants are approximately equal at 93.7% and 95.4%.[124] Most importantly, increased numbers of acute rejection episodes (more than two rejections, see "Chronic Rejection") has been found to correlate with a high risk of developing chronic rejection. Moreover, in the most recent era of immunosuppression, the decrease in acute rejection episodes in pediatric transplant recipients has been reported to decrease graft failures due to chronic rejection.[127] Interestingly, although the youngest recipients (younger than 2 years) have higher risks of early graft loss, their risk of later graft attrition is the lowest.[128]

Preparation for Pediatric Renal Transplantation

Every transplantation center has its own practices regarding the preparation of a child for renal transplantation. However, there are certain issues that have been recommended as key factors for consideration. These are reviewed and detailed elsewhere.[4] Of paramount importance is the evaluation of living donors who must be carefully examined by an independent advocate so that they are not put at risk. Living donor advocacy is such an important issue that it was recently reviewed and a national consensus was published.[129] Living donor advocacy is uniquely important in pediatrics because donors tend to be parents; they are highly motivated but are also the caregivers. Siblings can also feel pressure to donate. Thus, the concept of donor advocacy (that of being a separate individual from those in the transplant program) ensures that donors are treated in a fair manner.

Donor

If available, a living donor has clear advantages over a cadaver donor. Living donation ensures adequate transplantation preparation and optimizes elective transplantation, particularly for pediatric patients. Preemptive transplantation is much easier to accomplish and improves graft survival.[130] Furthermore, long-term survival of living donor renal allografts is superior to cadaver donor allografts. For details of selection and preparation of a living donor, see Chapter 85. Contrary to early reports, it has become clear that allografts from young cadaver donors (younger than 6 years of age) do not fare well in young recipients (due to higher thrombosis rates) and that the best donor for a young child is an adult donor. A cadaver donor for children should ideally be 20 to 40 years of age and not younger than 6 years of age because the youngest donors are associated with an increased risk of graft failure.[3] Thus, the best donor is an adult, whether living or dead (Table 44-3).

Recipient

An important aspect of renal transplantation is that success can also be determined by careful management of the recipient before transplantation. Most pediatric centers use a multispecialty team to ensure that hematologic, biochemical, neurological, and urologic parameters and potentially serious infections are corrected before transplantation. Many centers have adopted specific screening mechanisms, and some of the major considerations are reviewed in Box 44-1. Assessment of bladder function and correction of bladder dysfunction before transplantation is essential for patients in whom bladder disease or obstructive uropathy was the original cause of ESRD. Some patients may require bladder augmentation and/or medication to improve bladder function before transplantation. Transplantation into a dysfunctional bladder or the use of ileal loops or other forms of urinary drainage are not optimal for long-term success. Thus, it is important to have a pediatric urology team assess

Table 44-3 Relative Hazard of Individual Prognostic Risk Factors for Graft Failure by Donor source

	LIVING DONOR		DECEASED DONOR	
	RH	P	RH	P
Recipient age (>2 vs. 0–1)	1.13	NS	0.59	<.001
Previous transplantation	1.35	.006	1.43	<.001
No induction antibody administration	1.15	.035	1.09	NS
>5 lifetime transfusions	1.31	.003	1.28	<.001
No HLA-B matches	1.40	.008	1.16	.014
No HLA-DR matches	0.87	NS	1.14	.024
Black race	1.95	<.001	1.56	<.001
Previous dialysis	1.16	.052	1.23	.040
Cold storage time > 24 hr	—	—	1.14	.034
Transplant year	0.95	<.001	0.94	<.001
Native nephrectomy (no)	0.87	.051	0.96	NS
Gender (male)	0.87	.036	0.85	.005

HLA, human leukocyte antigen; RH, relative hazard.
From from Smith JM, Stablein DM, Munoz R, et al: Contributions of the Transplant Registry: The 2006 Annual Report of the North American Pediatric Renal Trials and Collaborative Studies (NAPRTCS). Pediatr Transplant 2007;11:366–373.

a child before transplantation and be involved with the entire transplantation process.

Prevention of infections, especially viral infections, involves analysis of patient status and the use of chemoprophylaxis. This is a high priority with all pediatric patients because they typically acquire these infections during childhood and are not immune to many viruses before transplantation.[131] Knowledge of titers of varicella-zoster virus, cytomegalovirus, Epstein-Barr virus, diphtheria, tetanus, poliovirus, measles, mumps, rubella, *Haemophilus influenzae* B, *Streptococcus pneumoniae*, hepatitis B, hepatitis C, and human immunodeficiency virus before transplantation is of paramount importance. Vaccination can prevent

morbidity and mortality after transplantation.[132,133] All live viral vaccines should be administered before transplantation as best as possible. Cytomegalovirus and Epstein-Barr virus prophylaxis must be considered for patients at high risk, that is, seronegative recipients receiving seropositive organs and patients who have received antilymphocyte antibodies.[134] Trimethoprim prophylaxis has reduced the incidence of *Pneumocystis carinii* pneumonia after transplantation from 3.7% to 0%.[134]

Bilateral native kidney nephrectomy before transplantation is currently performed in 24% of patients in the United States to avoid urinary tract infection in patients with reflux nephropathy, native kidney-related hypertension, and a steal

Box 44-1 Preparation of Pediatric Renal Transplant Recipient

Nutrition
Adjustment of caloric, protein, sodium, and potassium balance

Growth
Supply adequate nutrition, correct metabolic disturbances (e.g., acidosis, hyponatremia), renal osteodystrophy; consider growth hormone therapy

Renal Osteodystrophy
Phosphate binders, calcium supplement, active vitamin D_3

Anemia
Correct iron deficiency; consider erythropoietin

Infection Prevention
Check titers of DTP, MMR, Hib, VZV, pneumococcus, HBV, HCV, CMV, EBV, and HIV
Vaccinate if necessary (e.g., VZV, HBV, influenza); check tuberculosis status

Bladder Work-up
VCUG and bladder work

Psychosocial Status
Social work assessment

CMV, cytomegalovirus; DTP, diphtheria/tetanus/pertussis; EBV, Epstein-Barr virus; HBV, hepatitis B virus; HCV, hepatitis C virus; Hib, *Haemophilus influenzae* B; MMR, measles/mumps/rubella; VCUG, voiding cystourethrogram; VZV, varicella-zoster virus.

syndrome resulting in diminished blood flow through the allograft.[3] Most renal allografts are transplanted extraperitoneally into the retroperitoneal cavity, even when a large adult kidney is used for a small child recipient. This technique does not seem to affect surgical complication rates and has the advantage of fewer gastrointestinal complications.[135–138] However, occasionally adult-sized kidneys are transplanted intraperitoneally in small children. There are other issues that require consideration, but these are beyond the scope of this chapter and are discussed in detail elsewhere.[4]

Immunosuppressive Therapy

There are currently many immunosuppressive agents available to the transplantation physician. This has resulted in multiple protocols each with a center bias, such that therapy can be center dependent. Induction therapy, predominantly with anti–interleukin-2 receptor antibodies (anti-CD25: daclizumab, basiliximab) is followed by triple therapy, consisting of steroids, a calcineurin inhibitor, and an antiproliferative agent.[139] The calcineurin inhibitor tacrolimus is the primary immunosuppressant, with 63% of pediatric renal transplant recipients receiving the drug during the first month; 12% of recipients receive cyclosporine. Azathioprine has been replaced by mycophenolate mofetil, which is currently given to more than 90% of transplant recipients in the United States.[124] Approximately one third of patients who receive maintenance steroid therapy in the long-term receive alternate-day therapy to achieve better catch-up growth.[3,124,139,140]

The advent of new immunosuppressive agents has enabled therapy to be administered on an individual basis and based on risk. The newer more potent immunosuppressive agents and protocols that have been shown to limit acute rejection have provided tremendous advantages for the transplant recipient but they come at a price, which is the risk of infections and posttransplantation lymphoproliferative disease (PTLD). Posttransplantation infections have increased over time and now exceed acute rejection as the cause for hospitalization. In the first 24 months after transplantation, 52% of patients were hospitalized, 40% for infection and 23% for acute rejection[141] (see "Posttransplantation Infections"). Adverse effects of immunosuppressive therapy besides infection and malignancy include hypertension, hyperlipidemia, diabetes mellitus, osteoporosis, and, in the case of long-term steroid use, growth failure (see "Growth and Other Endocrine Disorders").[142]

Exciting new immunosuppressive drugs have been introduced into practice based on their ability to further decrease acute rejection. It is hoped that they will also improve long-term graft survival. The most exciting agents include alemtuzumab (anti-CD52), a newer anti–T-cell agent that has been introduced to limit acute rejection in the early posttransplantation period. Leflunomide, a promising immunosuppressive drug that inhibits de novo pyrimidine biosynthesis, also has antiviral activity, in particular against BK virus. Belatacept, an inhibitor of costimulation of T cells, is nonnephrotoxic, but in clinical studies, it was found that this agent is a potent immunosuppressive and thus its use may increase the risk of PTLD.[143]

A recent study evaluating the elimination of calcineurin inhibitors and conversion to a rapamycin (sirolimus)-based immunosuppressive regimen after pediatric living donor renal transplantation has had promising results.[144] Furthermore,

a strategy of lymphoid depletion with antithymocyte globulin and tacrolimus monotherapy appears safe and effective for pediatric kidney recipients.[145] Although new protocols are currently in clinical trials, the optimal immunosuppressive strategy for a given patient will likely be individualized in the future; risk stratification for each type of protocol for individual patients will be forthcoming.[146]

Posttransplantation Infections

Newer immunosuppressive agents have dramatically reduced the rates of acute graft rejection over the past decade but may have exacerbated the problem of posttransplantation infections. Posttransplantation infections currently exceed acute rejection as the cause of posttransplantation hospitalization and are the most frequent cause of mortality.[124,141] Younger children are at higher risk of hospitalization for infection, and there is an association with the use of anti–T-cell antibodies as induction therapy.[141]

Typical infections after renal transplantation are urinary tract infections, BK virus infections, and PTLD. Febrile urinary tract infection is a frequent (33%–36%) posttransplantation complication, especially in girls and in children with urinary tract malformation and neurogenic bladder.[147,148] Polyoma BK virus nephropathy is emerging as a significant early and late complication of renal transplantation, which may lead to renal dysfunction and graft loss.[149] Limited prospective studies screening for BK virus document the presence of viruria in 19% to 33% of patients and viremia in 5.6% to 13.4% of patients. Of the latter, nearly half have BK nephropathy on renal biopsy.[150–152] These findings support the routine screening of pediatric renal transplant recipients for BK virus. Treatment of BK nephropathy consists of a decrease in immunosuppression and/or treatment with cidovovir.[149]

The prevalence of Epstein-Barr virus–induced PTLD shows a significant increase per year and currently is 2.0%.[124] Cadaver donor source and white race are risk factors for PTLD.[153] In an analysis of PTLD after polyclonal antibody induction, only equine antithymocyte globulin was associated with a twofold higher risk of PTLD, whereas rabbit antithymocyte globulin and antilymphocyte globulin were not.[154] Recent North American Pediatric Renal Transplant Cooperative Study data show that tacrolimus and mycophenolate mofetil are not associated with increased risk of PTLD after pediatric kidney transplantation.[155] Treatment of PTLD consists of a decrease in immunosuppression, anti-CD20 antibody treatment (rituximab), and occasionally chemotherapy. Experimental data suggest that rapamycin (sirolimus) may inhibit the growth of Epstein-Barr virus–infected B cells and may be helpful in the treatment of PTLD.[156]

Causes of Graft Failure in Pediatric Recipients

The North American Pediatric Renal Transplant Cooperative Study, which includes data on more than 8990 transplantations, analyzes risk factors for graft loss after pediatric renal transplantation.[3,124,139,140,157] The most common cause of graft failure is chronic rejection.[124] Vascular thrombosis is also a major cause of graft failure, especially in young children, and accounts for approximately 12% of all pediatric renal allograft failures. Risk factors for vascular thrombosis include recipient age and cadaver donor age, especially donors younger than 6 years of age.[3,158] Long-term graft survival rates for teenage recipients are significantly lower compared with all age groups, including infants. Adolescents have a significantly higher incidence of late acute rejection episodes and higher rates of incomplete rejection reversal than any other age group.[159] Noncompliance among teenagers is well recognized.[128,159–161] Strategies to address noncompliance in adolescents must have a high priority.

Acute Rejection

With new immunosuppressive therapies, acute rejection episodes occur less frequently after pediatric transplantation. Indeed, acute rejection in 1987 at the beginning of the North American Pediatric Renal Transplant Cooperative Study was as high as 54% and 69% for living and cadaver donors, respectively, and has now decreased to 13% and 16% in the first posttransplantation year. It has become evident that more aggressive therapy, including the use of induction therapy regimens, and surveillance biopsies to establish a diagnosis of "silent" rejection are associated with improved short-term outcome.[162,163] Acute rejection is of special concern because of its relationship to the development of chronic rejection.[3] Even one episode of acute rejection increases the risk of developing chronic rejection. Thus, strategies that decrease acute rejection rates and improve short-term graft survival rates can translate into improved long-term survival.[127,164]

Chronic Rejection

Chronic rejection is characterized histologically by progressive fibrosis and mononuclear cell infiltration with interstitial cell atrophy. Chronic rejection can be diagnosed as early as 3 months after transplantation, and its presence in biopsy specimens 6 months posttransplantation is prognostic for long-term outcome.[165] Thus, early biopsy 3 to 6 months after transplantation can be evaluated for surrogate markers that may predict the ultimate development of chronic rejection.[165] Once established, chronic rejection is progressive and ultimately leads to graft failure. For pediatric patients receiving a renal allograft, chronic rejection is responsible for approximately 41% of graft losses.[124]

Understanding risk factors for chronic rejection in pediatric patients has been a major undertaking of the North American Pediatric Renal Transplant Cooperative Study. Preventing or minimizing risk factors has been proposed to have an impact on long-term graft survival. Risk factors for chronic rejection have been defined and are multifactorial. They include human leukocyte antigen mismatch, ischemia reperfusion injury, repeat transplantations, acute rejection, and other factors such as hypertension and hyperlipidemia. However, an extensive study established that acute rejection is the most important risk factor for the development of chronic rejection. Two or more acute rejection episodes increases the risk of chronic rejection fourfold, and late initial acute rejection increases the risk of chronic rejection by 3.6-fold.[127] These data are similar to those of studies performed in adults that also identified acute rejection as a harbinger of chronic rejection.[125] It is proposed that acute rejection establishes an immune reaction within the graft that facilitates positive feedback loops for immune inflammation and persistent graft injury and the production of cytokines and growth factors such as the fibrogenic cytokine transforming growth factor β.[166] Another possible etiology contributing to the development of chronic rejection is decreased renal mass leading to hyperfiltration, which has a damaging effect on the renal parenchyma and produces the characteristic histology of chronic rejection.[166]

Currently there is no specific therapy for chronic rejection, so efforts must be directed toward preventing major risk factors such as acute rejection. Aggressive induction therapy to prevent acute rejection has not translated into better long-term graft survival but is associated with increased risk of infections.[167] Other ideas include limiting calcineurin inhibitor–based immunosuppressive therapy, which is associated with progressive renal injury as a result of profound nephrotoxicity.[144,166]

SUMMARY

In this chapter, we discuss unique problems associated with the management of ESRD in children. We discuss strategies to understand and prevent malnutrition and growth retardation in children with ESRD. In addition, we review important issues for the optimization of neurodevelopment and cognitive function. Last, we review current available treatment options including peritoneal dialysis and hemodialysis and discuss renal transplantation as a successful therapeutic option. All these treatments are options for children with ESRD.

References

1. United States Renal Data System: USRDS 1996 Annual Data Report. Bethesda, MD: USRDS, 1996.
2. Broyer M, Chantler C, Donckerwolcke R, et al: The paediatric registry of the European Dialysis and Transplant Association: 20 years' experience. Pediatr Nephrol 1993;7:758–768.
3. Seikaly M, Ho PL, Emmett L, Tejani A: The 12th Annual Report of the North American Pediatric Renal Transplant Cooperative Study: Renal transplantation from 1987 through 1998. Pediatr Transplant 2001;5:215–231.
4. Davis ID, Bunchman TE, Grimm PC, et al: Pediatric renal transplantation: Indications and special considerations. A position paper from the Pediatric Committee of the American Society of Transplant Physicians. Pediatr Transplant 1998;2:117–129.
5. K/DOQI: Guidelines for Hemodialysis Adequacy, update 2006. Am J Kidney Dis 2006;48:S1–S276.
6. Seikaly MG, Loleh S, Rosenblum A, Browne R: Validation of the Center for Medicare and Medicaid Services algorithm for eligibility for dialysis. Pediatr Nephrol 2004;19:893–897.
7. Fine RN: Renal transplantation for children—the only realistic choice. Kidney Int Suppl 1985;17:S15–S7.
8. European best practice guidelines for renal transplantation. Section IV: Long-term management of the transplant recipient. IV.11 Paediatrics (specific problems). Nephrol Dial Transplant 2002;17(Suppl 4):55–58.
9. Mendley SR, Zelko FA: Improvement in specific aspects of neurocognitive performance in children after renal transplantation. Kidney Int 1999;56:318–323.
10. Rotundo A, Nevins TE, Lipton M, et al: Progressive encephalopathy in children with chronic renal insufficiency in infancy. Kidney Int 1982;21:486–491.
11. McGraw ME, Haka-Ikse K: Neurologic-developmental sequelae of chronic renal failure in infancy. J Pediatr 1985;106:579–583.
12. Lawry KW, Brouhard BH, Cunningham RJ: Cognitive functioning and school performance in children with renal failure. Pediatr Nephrol 1994;8:326–329.

13. Davis ID, Chang PN, Nevins TE: Successful renal transplantation accelerates development in young uremic children. Pediatrics 1990;86:594–600.

14. Kramer L, Madl C, Stockenhuber F, et al: Beneficial effect of renal transplantation on cognitive brain function. Kidney Int 1996;49: 833–838.

15. Warady BA, Belden B, Kohaut E. Neurodevelopmental outcome of children initiating peritoneal dialysis in early infancy. Pediatr Nephrol 1999;13:759–765.

16. Simmons JM, Wilson CJ, Potter DE, Holliday MA: Relation of calorie deficiency to growth failure in children on hemodialysis and the growth response to calorie supplementation. N Engl J Med 1971;285:653–656.

17. Betts PR, Magrath G: Growth pattern and dietary intake of children with chronic renal insufficiency. Br Med J 1974;2:189–193.

18. Clinical Practice Guidelines for Nutrition in Chronic Renal Failure: Pediatric Guidelines. Am J Kidney Disease 2000;35: S105–S136.

19. Warady BA, Alexander SR, Watkins S, et al: Optimal care of the pediatric end-stage renal disease patient on dialysis. Am J Kidney Dis 1999;33:567–583.

20. Geary DF, Ikse KH, Coulter P, Secker D: The role of nutrition in neurologic health and development of infants with chronic renal failure. Adv Perit Dial 1990;6:252–254.

21. Edefonti A, Picca M, Damiani B, et al: Dietary prescription based on estimated nitrogen balance during peritoneal dialysis. Pediatr Nephrol 1999;13:253–258.

22. Ledermann SE, Scanes ME, Fernando ON, et al: Long-term outcome of peritoneal dialysis in infants. J Pediatr 2000;136:24–29.

23. Harmon WE: Urea kinetic modeling to prescribe hemodialysis in children. In Nissenson AR, Fine RN (eds): Dialysis Therapy, 3rd ed. Philadelphia: Hanley & Belfus, 2002, pp 462–466.

24. Ellis EN, Yiu V, Harley F, et al: The impact of supplemental feeding in young children on dialysis: A report of the North American Pediatric Renal Transplant Cooperative Study. Pediatr Nephrol 2001;16:404–408.

25. Warady BA: Gastrostomy feedings in patients receiving peritoneal dialysis. Perit Dial Int 1999;19:204–206.

26. Ramage IJ, Harvey E, Geary DF, et al: Complications of gastrostomy feeding in children receiving peritoneal dialysis. Pediatr Nephrol 1999;13:249–252.

27. Kari JA, Gonzalez C, Ledermann SE, et al: Outcome and growth of infants with severe chronic renal failure. Kidney Int 2000;57: 1681–1687.

28. Tom A, McCauley L, Bell L, et al: Growth during maintenance hemodialysis: Impact of enhanced nutrition and clearance. J Pediatr 1999;134:464–471.

29. Fischbach M, Terzic J, Menouer S, et al: Intensified and daily hemodialysis in children might improve statural growth. Pediatr Nephrol 2006;21:1746–1752.

30. Mahan JD, Warady BA: Assessment and treatment of short stature in pediatric patients with chronic kidney disease: A consensus statement. Pediatr Nephrol 2006;21:917–930.

31. Tonshoff B, Mehis O, Heinrich U, et al: Growth-stimulating effects of recombinant human growth hormone in children with end-stage renal disease. J Pediatr 1990;116:561–566.

32. Hokken-Koelega AC, Stijnen T, de Muinck Keizer-Schrama SM, et al: Placebo-controlled, double-blind, cross-over trial of growth hormone treatment in prepubertal children with chronic renal failure. Lancet 1991;338:585–590.

33. Vimalachandra D, Hodson EM, Willis NS, et al: Growth hormone for children with chronic kidney disease. Cochrane Database Syst Rev 2006;3:CD003264.

34. Gorman G, Fivush B, Frankenfield D, et al: Short stature and growth hormone use in pediatric hemodialysis patients. Pediatr Nephrol 2005;20:1794–1800.

35. Fine RN, Ho M, Tejani A: The contribution of renal transplantation to final adult height: A report of the North American Pediatric Renal Transplant Cooperative Study (NAPRTCS). Pediatr Nephrol 2001;16:951–956.

36. Fine RN: Growth post renal-transplantation in children: Lessons from the North American Pediatric Renal Transplant Cooperative Study (NAPRTCS). Pediatr Transplant 1997;1:85–89.

37. Hokken-Koelega AC, Stijnen T, de Ridder MA, et al: Growth hormone treatment in growth-retarded adolescents after renal transplant. Lancet 1994;343:1313–1317.

38. Hokken-Koelega AC, Stijnen T, de Jong RC, et al: A placebo-controlled, double-blind trial of growth hormone treatment in prepubertal children after renal transplant. Kidney Int Suppl 1996;53:S128–S134.

39. Fine RN, Stablein D: Long-term use of recombinant human growth hormone in pediatric allograft recipients: A report of the NAPRTCS Transplant Registry. Pediatr Nephrol 2005;20:404–408.

40. Jabs K, Sullivan EK, Avner ED, Harmon WE: Alternate-day steroid dosing improves growth without adversely affecting graft survival or long-term graft function. A report of the North American Pediatric Renal Transplant Cooperative Study. Transplantation 1996;61:31–36.

41. Sarwal MM, Vidhun JR, Alexander SR, et al: Continued superior outcomes with modification and lengthened follow-up of a steroid-avoidance pilot with extended daclizumab induction in pediatric renal transplantation. Transplantation 2003;76: 1331–1339.

42. Sarwal MM, Yorgin PD, Alexander S, et al: Promising early outcomes with a novel, complete steroid avoidance immunosuppression protocol in pediatric renal transplantation. Transplantation 2001;72:13–21.

43. Scharer K: Growth and development of children with chronic renal failure. Study Group on Pubertal Development in Chronic Renal Failure. Acta Paediatr Scand Suppl 1990;366:90–92.

44. Mak RH, Haycock GB, Chantler C: Glucose intolerance in children with chronic renal failure. Kidney Int Suppl 1983;15: S22–S26.

45. Martin KJ GE, Slatopolsky E: Renal Osteodystrophy. In Brenner B (ed): The Kidney, 7th ed. Philadelphia: Saunders, 2004, pp 2255–2304.

46. Salusky IB, Ramirez JA, Oppenheim W, et al: Biochemical markers of renal osteodystrophy in pediatric patients undergoing CAPD/CCPD. Kidney Int 1994;45:253–258.

47. Rigden SP: The treatment of renal osteodystrophy. Pediatr Nephrol 1996;10:653–655.

48. K/DOQI: Clinical practice guideline for bone metabolism and disease in chronic kidney disease. Am J Kidney Dis 2005;46: S12–S100.

49. Klaus G, Watson A, Edefonti A, et al: Prevention and treatment of renal osteodystrophy in children on chronic renal failure: European guidelines. Pediatr Nephrol 2006;21:151–159.

50. Sedman A: Aluminum toxicity in childhood. Pediatr Nephrol 1992;6:383–393.

51. Hamdy NA, Kanis JA, Beneton MN, et al: Effect of alfacalcidol on natural course of renal bone disease in mild to moderate renal failure. Br Med J 1995;310:358–363.

52. Greenbaum LA, Grenda R, Qiu P, et al: Intravenous calcitriol for treatment of hyperparathyroidism in children on hemodialysis. Pediatr Nephrol 2005;20:622–630.

53. Ardissino G, Schmitt CP, Testa S, et al: Calcitriol pulse therapy is not more effective than daily calcitriol therapy in controlling secondary hyperparathyroidism in children with chronic renal failure. European Study Group on Vitamin D in Children with Renal Failure. Pediatr Nephrol 2000;14:664–668.

54. Salusky IB, Goodman WG: The management of renal osteodystrophy. Pediatr Nephrol 1996;10:651–653.

55. Boot AM, Nauta J, Hokken-Koelega AC, et al: Renal transplantation and osteoporosis. Arch Dis Child 1995;72:502–506.

56. Lerner GR, Warady BA, Sullivan EK, Alexander SR: Chronic dialysis in children and adolescents. The 1996 annual report of

the North American Pediatric Renal Transplant Cooperative Study. Pediatr Nephrol 1999;13:404–417.

57. Van Damme-Lombaerts R, Herman J: Erythropoietin treatment in children with renal failure. Pediatr Nephrol 1999;13:148–152.

58. Gerson A, Hwang W, Fiorenza J, et al: Anemia and health-related quality of life in adolescents with chronic kidney disease. Am J Kidney Dis 2004;44:1017–1023.

59. K/DOQI: Clinical practice recommendations for anemia in chronic kidney disease in children. Am J Kidney Dis 2006;47: S86–S108.

60. Jacobs C: Starting r-HuEPO in chronic renal failure: When, why, and how? Nephrol Dial Transplant 1995;10(Suppl 2):43–47.

61. Van Damme-Lombaerts R, Broyer M, Businger J, et al: A study of recombinant human erythropoietin in the treatment of anaemia of chronic renal failure in children on haemodialysis. Pediatr Nephrol 1994;8:338–342.

62. Greenbaum LA, Pan CG, Caley C, et al: Intravenous iron dextran and erythropoietin use in pediatric hemodialysis patients. Pediatr Nephrol 2000;14:908–911.

63. Tenbrock K, Muller-Berghaus J, Michalk D, Querfeld U: Intravenous iron treatment of renal anemia in children on hemodialysis. Pediatr Nephrol 1999;13:580–582.

64. Warady BA, Zobrist RH, Finan E: Sodium ferric gluconate complex maintenance therapy in children on hemodialysis. Pediatr Nephrol 2006;21:553–560.

65. Warady BA, Arar MY, Lerner G, et al: Darbepoetin alfa for the treatment of anemia in pediatric patients with chronic kidney disease. Pediatr Nephrol 2006;21:1144–1152.

66. Geary DF, Keating LE, Vigneux A, et al: Darbepoetin alfa (Aranesp) in children with chronic renal failure. Kidney Int 2005;68:1759–1765.

67. Schmitt CP, Nau B, Brummer C, et al: Increased injection pain with darbepoetin-alpha compared to epoetin-beta in paediatric dialysis patients. Nephrol Dial Transplant 2006;21:3520–3524.

68. Rijk Y, Raaijmakers R, van de Kar N, Schroder C: Intraperitoneal treatment with darbepoetin for children on peritoneal dialysis. Pediatr Nephrol 2007;22:436–440.

69. Lingens N, Soergel M, Loirat C, et al: Ambulatory blood pressure monitoring in pediatric patients treated by regular haemodialysis and peritoneal dialysis. Pediatr Nephrol 1995;9: 167–172.

70. Soergel M, Kirschstein M, Busch C, et al: Oscillometric twenty-four-hour ambulatory blood pressure values in healthy children and adolescents: A multicenter trial including 1141 subjects. J Pediatr 1997;130:178–184.

71. The fourth report on the diagnosis, evaluation, and treatment of high blood pressure in children and adolescents. Pediatrics 2004;114(2 Suppl):555–576.

72. K/DOQI: Clinical practice guidelines on hypertension and antihypertensive agents in chronic kidney disease. Am J Kidney Dis 2004;43:S1–S290.

73. Mitsnefes M, Ho PL, McEnery PT: Hypertension and progression of chronic renal insufficiency in children: A report of the North American Pediatric Renal Transplant Cooperative Study (NAPRTCS). J Am Soc Nephrol 2003;14:2618–2622.

74. Groothoff JW, Gruppen MP, Offringa M, et al: Mortality and causes of death of end-stage renal disease in children: A Dutch cohort study. Kidney Int 2002;61:621–629.

75. Parekh RS, Carroll CE, Wolfe RA, Port FK: Cardiovascular mortality in children and young adults with end-stage kidney disease. J Pediatr 2002;141:191–197.

76. United States Renal Data System: The USRDS 1998 Annual Report Pediatric ESRD. Am J Kidney Dis 1998;32:S98–S108.

77. United States Renal Data System:. The USRDS 1998 Annual Report Pediatric ESRD. Am J Kidney Dis 1998;32:S81–S88.

78. Mitsnefes MM, Daniels SR, Schwartz SM, et al: Severe left ventricular hypertrophy in pediatric dialysis: Prevalence and predictors. Pediatr Nephrol 2000;14:898–902.

79. Goodman WG, Goldin J, Kuizon BD, et al: Coronary-artery calcification in young adults with end-stage renal disease who are undergoing dialysis. N Engl J Med 2000;342:1478–1483.

80. K/DOQI: Clinical practice guidelines for cardiovascular disease in dialysis patients. Am J Kidney Dis 2005;45:S16–S153.

81. K/DOQI: Clinical practice guidelines for managing dyslipidemias in chronic kidney disease. Am J Kidney Dis 2003;41: S1–S58.

82. Gerson AC, Butler R, Moxey-Mims M, et al: Neurocognitive outcomes in children with chronic kidney disease: Current findings and contemporary endeavors. Ment Retard Dev Disabil Res Rev 2006;12:208–215.

83. Hulstijn-Dirkmaat GM, Damhuis IH, Jetten ML, et al: The cognitive development of pre-school children treated for chronic renal failure. Pediatr Nephrol 1995;9:464–469.

84. Warady BA, Hebert D, Sullivan EK, et al: Renal transplantation, chronic dialysis, and chronic renal insufficiency in children and adolescents. The 1995 Annual Report of the North American Pediatric Renal Transplant Cooperative Study. Pediatr Nephrol 1997;11:49–64.

85. Brouhard BH, Donaldson LA, Lawry KW, et al: Cognitive functioning in children on dialysis and post-transplantation. Pediatr Transplant 2000;4:261–267.

86. Garralda ME, Jameson RA, Reynolds JM, Postlethwaite RJ: Psychiatric adjustment in children with chronic renal failure. J Child Psychol Psychiatry 1988;29:79–90.

87. Goldstein SL, Graham N, Burwinkle T, et al: Health-related quality of life in pediatric patients with ESRD. Pediatr Nephrol 2006;21:846–850.

88. Tsai TC, Liu SI, Tsai JD, Chou LH: Psychosocial effects on caregivers for children on chronic peritoneal dialysis. Kidney Int 2006;70:1983–1987.

89. Groothoff JW, Grootenhuis MA, Offringa M, et al: Social consequences in adult life of end-stage renal disease in childhood. J Pediatr 2005;146:512–517.

90. The 2006 Annual Report of the North American Pediatric Renal Trials and Collaborative Studies (NAPRTCS): Available at: www.web.emmes.com/study/ped/annlrept/annlrept2006. pdf 2006. Accessed April 17, 2008.

91. Shroff R, Rees L, Trompeter R, et al: Long-term outcome of chronic dialysis in children. Pediatr Nephrol 2006;21: 257–264.

92. Neu AM, Ho PL, McDonald RA, Warady BA: Chronic dialysis in children and adolescents. The 2001 NAPRTCS Annual Report. Pediatr Nephrol 2002;17:656–663.

93. Wood EG, Hand M, Briscoe DM, et al: Risk factors for mortality in infants and young children on dialysis. Am J Kidney Dis 2001;37:573–579.

94. McDonald SP, Craig JC: Long-term survival of children with end-stage renal disease. N Engl J Med 2004;350:2654–2662.

95. Smith JM, Stablein DM, Munoz R, et al: Contributions of the Transplant Registry: The 2006 Annual Report of the North American Pediatric Renal Trials and Collaborative Studies (NAPRTCS). Pediatr Transplant 2007;11:366–373.

96. White CT, Gowrishankar M, Feber J, Yiu V: Clinical practice guidelines for pediatric peritoneal dialysis. Pediatr Nephrol 2006;21:1059–1066.

97. Reissman P, Lyass S, Shiloni E, et al: Placement of a peritoneal dialysis catheter with routine omentectomy—does it prevent obstruction of the catheter? Eur J Surg 1998;164:703–707.

98. Chadha V, Warady BA: What are the clinical correlates of adequate peritoneal dialysis? Semin Nephrol 2001;21:480–489.

99. Fischbach M, Stefanidis CJ, Watson AR: Guidelines by an ad hoc European committee on adequacy of the paediatric peritoneal dialysis prescription. Nephrol Dial Transplant 2002;17:380–385.

100. Twardowski ZJ, Nolph KD, Khanna R, et al: Peritoneal equilibration test. Perit Dial Int 1987;7:378–383.

101. Warady BA, Alexander SR, Hossli S, et al: Peritoneal membrane transport function in children receiving long-term dialysis. J Am Soc Nephrol 1996;7:2385–2391.

102. Andreoli SP, Leiser J, Warady BA, et al: Adverse effect of peritonitis on peritoneal membrane function in children on dialysis. Pediatr Nephrol 1999;13:1–6.

103. Warady BA, Fivush B, Andreoli SP, et al: Longitudinal evaluation of transport kinetics in children receiving peritoneal dialysis. Pediatr Nephrol 1999;13:571–576.

104. K/DOQI: Clinical practice guidelines for peritoneal dialysis, update 2006. Am J Kidney Dis 2006;48:S91–S97.

105. Schaefer F, Klaus G, Mehls O: Peritoneal transport properties and dialysis dose affect growth and nutritional status in children on chronic peritoneal dialysis. Mid- European Pediatric Peritoneal Dialysis Study Group. J Am Soc Nephrol 1999;10:1786–1792.

106. Holtta T, Ronnholm K, Jalanko H, Holmberg C: Clinical outcome of pediatric patients on peritoneal dialysis under adequacy control. Pediatr Nephrol 2000;14:889–897.

107. Brem AS, Lambert C, Hill C, et al: Outcome data on pediatric dialysis patients from the end-stage renal disease clinical indicators project. Am J Kidney Dis 2000;36:310–317.

108. Furth SL, Donaldson LA, Sullivan EK, Watkins SL: Peritoneal dialysis catheter infections and peritonitis in children: A report of the North American Pediatric Renal Transplant Cooperative Study. Pediatr Nephrol 2000;15:179–182.

109. Warady BA, Sullivan EK, Alexander SR: Lessons from the peritoneal dialysis patient database: A report of the North American Pediatric Renal Transplant Cooperative Study. Kidney Int Suppl 1996;53:S68–S71.

110. Fischbach M, Terzic J, Menouer S, et al: Hemodialysis in children: Principles and practice. Semin Nephrol 2001;21:470–479.

111. Bunchman TE: Pediatric hemodialysis: Lessons from the past, ideas for the future. Kidney Int Suppl 1996;53:S64–S7.

112. Bourquelot P, Cussenot O, Corbi P, et al: Microsurgical creation and follow-up of arteriovenous fistulae for chronic haemodialysis in children. Pediatr Nephrol 1990;4:156–159.

113. Gradman WS, Lerner G, Mentser M, et al: Experience with autogenous arteriovenous access for hemodialysis in children and adolescents. Ann Vasc Surg 2005;19:609–612.

114. Michael M, Brewer ED, Goldstein SL: Blood volume monitoring to achieve target weight in pediatric hemodialysis patients. Pediatr Nephrol 2004;19:432–437.

115. Fischbach M, Edefonti A, Schroder C, Watson A: Hemodialysis in children: General practical guidelines. Pediatr Nephrol 2005;20:1054–1066.

116. Fischbach M, Terzic J, Laugel V, et al: Daily on-line haemodiafiltration: A pilot trial in children. Nephrol Dial Transplant 2004;19:2360–2367.

117. Geary DF, Piva E, Tyrrell J, et al: Home nocturnal hemodialysis in children. J Pediatr 2005;147:383–387.

118. Innes A, Charra B, Burden RP, et al: The effect of long, slow haemodialysis on patient survival. Nephrol Dial Transplant 1999;14:919–922.

119. Goldstein SL, Sorof JM, Brewer ED: Natural logarithmic estimates of Kt/V in the pediatric hemodialysis population. Am J Kidney Dis 1999;33:518–522.

120. Daugirdas JT: Second generation logarithmic estimates of single-pool variable volume Kt/V: An analysis of error. J Am Soc Nephrol 1993;4:1205–1213.

121. Hingorani S, Watkins SL: Dialysis for end-stage renal disease. Curr Opin Pediatr 2000;12:140–145.

122. Gorman G, Furth S, Hwang W, et al: Clinical outcomes and dialysis adequacy in adolescent hemodialysis patients. Am J Kidney Dis 2006;47:285–293.

123. Frankenfield DL, Neu AM, Warady BA, et al: Adolescent hemodialysis: Results of the 2000 ESRD Clinical Performance Measures Project. Pediatr Nephrol 2002;17:10–15.

124. Smith JM Stablein DM, Munoz R, et al: Contributions of the Transplant Registry: The 2006 Annual Report of the North American Pediatric Renal Trials and Collaborative Studies (NAPRTCS). Pediatr Transplant 2007;11:366–373.

125. Hariharan S, Johnson CP, Bresnahan BA, et al: Improved graft survival after renal transplantation in the United States, 1988 to 1996. N Engl J Med 2000;342:605–612.

126. Cecka JM: The OPTN/UNOS renal transplant registry. Clin Transpl 2004:1–16.

127. Tejani A, Ho PL, Emmett L, Stablein DM: Reduction in acute rejections decreases chronic rejection graft failure in children: A report of the North American Pediatric Renal Transplant Cooperative Study (NAPRTCS). Am J Transplant 2002;2:142–147.

128. Cecka JM, Gjertson DW, Terasaki PI: Pediatric renal transplantation: A review of the UNOS data. United Network for Organ Sharing. Pediatr Transplant 1997;1:55–64.

129. Abecassis M, Adams M, Adams P, et al: Consensus statement on the live organ donor. JAMA 2000;284:2919–2926.

130. Vats AN, Donaldson L, Fine RN, Chavers BM: Pretransplant dialysis status and outcome of renal transplantation in North American children: A NAPRTCS Study. North American Pediatric Renal Transplant Cooperative Study. Transplantation 2000;69:1414–1419.

131. Dharnidharka VR, Harmon WE: Management of pediatric postrenal transplantation infections. Semin Nephrol 2001;21:521–531.

132. Furth SL, Neu AM, Sullivan EK, et al: Immunization practices in children with renal disease: A report of the North American Pediatric Renal Transplant Cooperative Study. Pediatr Nephrol 1997;11:443–446.

133. Webb NJ, Fitzpatrick MM, Hughes DA, et al: Immunisation against varicella in end stage and pre-end stage renal failure. Trans-Pennine Paediatric Nephrology Study Group. Arch Dis Child 2000;82:141–143.

134. Elinder CG, Andersson J, Bolinder G, Tyden G: Effectiveness of low-dose cotrimoxazole prophylaxis against Pneumocystis carinii pneumonia after renal and/or pancreas transplantation. Transpl Int 1992;5:81–84.

135. Healey PJ, McDonald R, Waldhausen JH, et al: Transplantation of adult living donor kidneys into infants and small children. Arch Surg 2000;135:1035–1041.

136. Nahas WC, Mazzucchi E, Scafuri AG, et al: Extraperitoneal access for kidney transplantation in children weighing 20 kg or less. J Urol 2000;164:475–478.

137. Tanabe K, Takahashi K, Kawaguchi H, et al: Surgical complications of pediatric kidney transplantation: A single center experience with the extraperitoneal technique. J Urol 1998;160:1212–1215.

138. Valdes R, Munoz R, Bracho E, et al: Surgical complications of renal transplantation in malnourished children. Transplant Proc 1994;26:50–51.

139. Elshihabi I, Chavers B, Donaldson L, et al: Continuing improvement in cadaver donor graft survival in North American children: The 1998 annual report of the North American Pediatric Renal Transplant Cooperative Study (NAPRTCS). Pediatr Transplant 2000;4:235–246.

140. McDonald R, Donaldson L, Emmett L, Tejani A: A decade of living donor transplantation in North American children: The 1998 annual report of the North American Pediatric Renal Transplant Cooperative Study (NAPRTCS). Pediatr Transplant 2000;4:221–234.

141. Dharnidharka VR, Stablein DM, Harmon WE: Post-transplant infections now exceed acute rejection as cause for hospitalization: A report of the NAPRTCS. Am J Transplant 2004;4:384–389.

142. Tejani A, Harmon WE: Clinical Transplantation. In Barratt TM, Avner ED, Harmon WE (eds): Pediatric Nephrology, 4th ed. Baltimore: Lippincott Williams & Wilkins, 1999, pp 1309–1337.

143. Vincenti F, Larsen C, Durrbach A, et al: Costimulation blockade with belatacept in renal transplantation. N Engl J Med 2005;353:770–781.

144. Harmon W, Meyers K, Ingelfinger J, et al: Safety and efficacy of a calcineurin inhibitor avoidance regimen in pediatric renal transplantation. J Am Soc Nephrol 2006;17:1735–1745.

145. Shapiro R, Ellis D, Tan HP, et al: Antilymphoid antibody preconditioning and tacrolimus monotherapy for pediatric kidney transplantation. J Pediatr 2006;148:813–818.

146. Sho M, Samsonov DV, Briscoe DM: Immunologic targets for currently available immunosuppressive agents: What is the optimal approach for children? Semin Nephrol 2001;21:508–520.

147. John U, Everding AS, Kuwertz-Broking E, et al: High prevalence of febrile urinary tract infections after paediatric renal transplantation. Nephrol Dial Transplant 2006;21:3269–3274.

148. Ranchin B, Chapuis F, Dawhara M, et al: Vesicoureteral reflux after kidney transplantation in children. Nephrol Dial Transplant 2000;15:1852–1858.

149. Hymes LC, Warshaw BL: Polyomavirus (BK) in pediatric renal transplants: Evaluation of viremic patients with and without BK associated nephritis. Pediatr Transplant 2006;10:920–922.

150. Alexander RT, Langlois V, Tellier R, et al: The prevalence of BK viremia and urinary viral shedding in a pediatric renal transplant population: A single-center retrospective analysis. Pediatr Transplant 2006;10:586–592.

151. Herman J, Van Ranst M, Snoeck R, et al: Polyomavirus infection in pediatric renal transplant recipients: Evaluation using a quantitative real-time PCR technique. Pediatr Transplant 2004;8:485–492.

152. Haysom L, Rosenberg AR, Kainer G, et al: BK viral infection in an Australian pediatric renal transplant population. Pediatr Transplant 2004;8:480–484.

153. Dharnidharka VR, Sullivan EK, Stablein DM, et al: Risk factors for posttransplant lymphoproliferative disorder (PTLD) in pediatric kidney transplantation: A report of the North American Pediatric Renal Transplant Cooperative Study (NAPRTCS). Transplantation 2001;71:1065–1068.

154. Dharnidharka VR, Stevens G: Risk for post-transplant lymphoproliferative disorder after polyclonal antibody induction in kidney transplantation. Pediatr Transplant 2005;9:622–626.

155. Dharnidharka VR, Ho PL, Stablein DM, et al: Mycophenolate, tacrolimus and post-transplant lymphoproliferative disorder: A report of the North American Pediatric Renal Transplant Cooperative Study. Pediatr Transplant 2002;6:396–399.

156. Majewski M, Korecka M, Kossev P, et al: The immunosuppressive macrolide RAD inhibits growth of human Epstein-Barr virus–transformed B lymphocytes in vitro and in vivo: A potential approach to prevention and treatment of posttransplant lymphoproliferative disorders. Proc Natl Acad Sci U S A 2000;97:4285–4290.

157. Benfield MR, McDonald R, Sullivan EK, et al: The 1997 Annual Renal Transplantation in Children Report of the North American Pediatric Renal Transplant Cooperative Study (NAPRTCS). Pediatr Transplant 1999;3:152–167.

158. Murphy BG, Hill CM, Middleton D, et al: Increased renal allograft thrombosis in CAPD patients. Nephrol Dial Transplant 1994;9:1166–1169.

159. Smith JM, Ho PL, McDonald RA: Renal transplant outcomes in adolescents: A report of the North American Pediatric Renal Transplant Cooperative Study. Pediatr Transplant 2002;6:493–499.

160. Meyers KE, Thomson PD, Weiland H: Noncompliance in children and adolescents after renal transplantation. Transplantation 1996;62:186–189.

161. Morgenstern BZ, Murphy M, Dayton J, et al: Noncompliance in a pediatric renal transplant population. Transplant Proc 1994;26:129.

162. Melter M, Briscoe DM: Challenges after pediatric transplantation. Semin Nephrol 2000;20:199–208.

163. Tejani AH, Stablein DM, Sullivan EK, et al: The impact of donor source, recipient age, pre-operative immunotherapy and induction therapy on early and late acute rejections in children: A report of the North American Pediatric Renal Transplant Cooperative Study (NAPRTCS). Pediatr Transplant 1998;2:318–324.

164. Tejani A, Sullivan EK: The impact of acute rejection on chronic rejection: A report of the North American Pediatric Renal Transplant Cooperative Study. Pediatr Transplant 2000;4:107–111.

165. Rush D, Somorjai R, Deslauriers R, et al: Subclinical rejection—a potential surrogate marker for chronic rejection—may be diagnosed by protocol biopsy or urine spectroscopy. Ann Transplant 2000;5:44–49.

166. Tejani A, Emmett L: Acute and chronic rejection. Semin Nephrol 2001;21:498–507.

167. Puliyanda DP, Stablein DM, Dharnidharka VR: Younger age and antibody induction increase the risk for infection in pediatric renal transplantation: A NAPRTCS report. Am J Transplant 2007;7:662–666.

Further Reading

Clinical Practice Guidelines for Nutrition in Chronic Renal Failure: Pediatric Guidelines. Am J Kidney Disease 2000;35:S105–S136.

Dharnidharka VR, Neu AM, Benfield M, et al: CME monograph. Issues in pediatric kidney transplantation. Ideon HealthCare, August 2005.

Fischbach M, Edefonti A, Schroder C, Watson A: Hemodialysis in children: General practical guidelines. Pediatr Nephrol 2005;20:1054–1066.

Fischbach M, Stefanidis CJ, Watson AR: Guidelines by an ad hoc European committee on adequacy of the paediatric peritoneal dialysis prescription. Nephrol Dial Transplant 2002;17:380–385.

K/DOQI: Clinical practice guideline for bone metabolism and disease in chronic kidney disease. Am J Kidney Dis 2005;46: S12–S100.

K/DOQI: Clinical practice recommendations for anemia in chronic kidney disease in children. Am J Kidney Dis 2006;47:S86–S108.

Klaus G, Watson A, Edefonti A, et al: Prevention and treatment of renal osteodystrophy in children on chronic renal failure: European guidelines. Pediatr Nephrol 2006;21:151–159.

Mahan JD, Warady BA: Assessment and treatment of short stature in pediatric patients with chronic kidney disease: A consensus statement. Pediatr Nephrol 2006;21:917–930.

Mitsnefes MM: Cardiovascular complications of pediatric chronic kidney disease. Pediatr Nephrol 2008;23:27–39.

Neu AM: Special issues in pediatric kidney transplantation. Adv Chronic Kidney Dis 2006;13:62–69.

The 2006 Annual Report of the North American Pediatric Renal Trials and Collaborative Studies (NAPRTCS). Available at: www .web.emmes.com/study/ped/annlrept/annlrept2006.pdf. Accessed April 17, 2008.

PART IX

Inherited Renal Disease

CONTENTS

Chapter 45

Renal Cystic Disorders

Arlene B. Chapman and Frederic F. Rahbari-Oskoui

Renal cystic disorders include a variety of genetic and acquired diseases, such as autosomal dominant polycystic kidney disease (ADPKD), autosomal recessive polycystic kidney disease, simple renal cysts, acquired cystic disease, von Hippel-Lindau disease, juvenile nephronophthisis/medullary cystic kidney disease, medullary sponge kidney, and tuberous sclerosis. We review ADPKD because of its high prevalence, the improved understanding of its pathogenesis and disease progression, and potential new therapies currently under clinical investigation.

AUTOSOMAL DOMINANT POLYCYSTIC KIDNEY DISEASE

ADPKD is a systemic disorder affecting 1 in 700 to 1000 individuals.[1] It is the most common inherited renal disorder, the fourth most common cause of end-stage renal disease (ESRD) after hypertension and diabetes and accounts for 2.5% of incident cases in the United States. Renal enlargement in ADPKD is progressive from birth; however, serum creatinine levels typically do not increase until the fourth or fifth decade of life. The majority of patients with ADPKD reach ESRD by the fifth decade of life.[2]

The Consortium for Radiologic Imaging Studies of Polycystic Kidney Disease was established by the National Institute of Diabetes and Digestive and Kidney Disease to determine whether change in renal and cyst volume measured by magnetic resonance imaging could be detected over a short period of time and whether structural measures correlate with a decline in renal function. A total of 243 patients with ADPKD underwent iothalamate glomerular filtration rate measurements and magnetic resonance imaging of the kidneys and the liver annually for 3 years. Age-adjusted renal ($R = 0.31$), cyst ($R = 0.36$), and percentage of cyst volume ($R = 0.35$) inversely correlated with the glomerular filtration rate[3] and larger renal volumes (>1500 mL; normal, 200 mL) demonstrated a significant decline in the glomerular filtration rate (approximately 5.2 mL/min/yr).[4] Polycystic kidney disease 1 (PKD1) patients demonstrated larger renal volumes than PKD2 patients, and renal volume increased at a similar rate. PKD2 individuals demonstrated fewer renal cysts than PKD1, accounting for the differences in renal size seen. These results have important design implications for clinical trials aimed at targeting new interventions in ADPKD before massive kidney enlargement has occurred.

ADPKD is a systemic disease characterized by the presence of renal, hepatic, pancreatic, and thyroid cysts, intracranial aneurysms (ICAs), inguinal and ventral hernias, and cardiac valvular abnormalities, mitral valve prolapse, and aortic insufficiency.[5] Renal manifestations of ADPKD include pain, gross hematuria, cyst hemorrhage, nephrolithiasis, infections, and a common early presence of hypertension. Table 45-1 lists the common manifestations and summarizes the recommended therapies.

Extrarenal Manifestations

Polycystic Liver Disease

Polycystic liver disease (PLD) (two or more liver cysts in an ADPKD individual) is a common manifestation of ADPKD, historically presenting later than renal cystic disease.[6,7] PLD occurs in the majority of both men and women, although more frequently and earlier in women. Magnetic resonance imaging of the liver in 243 participants in the Consortium for Radiologic Imaging Studies of Polycystic Kidney Disease cohort demonstrated liver cystic disease in 55% by age 25 and 94% by age of 45.[8]

Estrogen or progesterone exposure is associated with more frequent and severe PLD.[6,9,10] In a study of 11 patients, 1 year of postmenopausal estrogen therapy was associated with greater liver cyst growth compared with placebo-treated controls ($N = 8$).[11] Liver cyst growth can be massive, associated with significant pain, shortness of breath, early satiety, weakness, and fatigue. Although PLD can result in massive involvement of liver, noncystic liver parenchymal volume is increased with minimal loss of drug clearance and metabolism.[12] Rarely, massive PLD can be fatal secondary to inferior vena cava obstruction, infection, or Budd-Chiari syndrome or due to the development of end-stage liver disease with portal hypertension.[13]

Current approaches to the treatment of PLD have relied on medical, surgical, or radiological interventions. Attempts to avoid extensive estrogen exposure include minimizing use of

Table 45-1 Management of Complications of Autosomal Dominant Polycystic Kidney Disease

Complication	Frequency	Management
Extrarenal		
Hepatic cysts	83%	Minimize estrogen use, fenestration, decortication, resection, liver transplantation
Cholangiocarcinoma	Rare	
Congenital hepatic fibrosis	Rare	
Caroli's disease	Rare	
Budd-Chiari syndrome	Rare	
Hepatocellular carcinoma	Rare	
Pancreatic cysts	10%–11%	
Thyroid cysts	Rare	
Intracranial arterial aneurysms	5%–8%	MRA if positive family history; clip, coil, or inject if >5–10 mm
Intracranial arterial dolichoectasis	2%–3%	
Pineal cysts		
Mitral valve prolapse	20%–25%	
Aortic insufficiency	5%	
Hernias (inguinal and ventral)	15%	
Seminal vesicle cysts	40%	
Renal		
Multiple cysts	100%	
Infection	30%–50% lifetime risk	4–6 wk trimethoprim-sulfamethoxazole, fluoroquinolone for cyst infection; cyst decompression
Hypertension	60% (normal renal function), 90% (CKD)	ACE inhibitor
Hematuria	50% lifetime risk	
Pain (due to cyst size, infection, rupture, nephrolithiasis)		
Nephrolithiasis (uric acid and calcium oxalate)	20%	
Subnephrosis-range proteinuria	27%	
Decreased concentration ability	100%	

ACE, angiotensin-converting enzyme; CKD, chronic kidney disease; MRA, magnetic resonance angiography

oral contraceptives. When postmenopausal estrogen replacement therapy is indicated, administration of cutaneous estrogen patches should be considered to avoid higher biliary estradiol concentrations that occur with oral ingestion.

Surgical fenestration-resection or partial hepatic resection results in symptomatic improvement in those with massive PLD.[14] Laparoscopic liver cyst decortication is also available; its advantages include shorter recovery and smaller surgical incisions.[15] Both surgical procedures have marginal success for diffuse PLD where multiple small cysts predominate.[16] Postoperative complications include pleural effusions, ascites, lower extremity edema, hypertension, and infection. Finally, individuals have undergone either liver or combined liver-renal transplantation for massive PLD.[17]

Intracranial Aneurysms

ICAs occur more frequently in ADPKD (5%–8%) than in the general population (1%–2%).[18,19] Hypertensive strokes and subarachnoid hemorrhage are responsible for the majority (75%) of cerebrovascular deaths in ADPKD.[20] Dolichoectasia is found in increased frequency (3%)[21] and subarachnoid or pineal cysts are not uncommon in ADPKD. Saccular as opposed to fusiform dilations are the most frequent ICA in ADPKD, and ICAs are found in the anterior portion of the circle of Willis in 75%. Only a family history of ICA has been found to be associated with the presence of ICA in ADPKD.[19] Given the difficulty in obtaining an accurate family history of the cause of cerebrovascular events, when in doubt, a positive or suspicious family history should be assigned to the individual. ADPKD individuals with ICA rupture[19] are more often women, relatively young (mean age, 34 years), and with a higher frequency of family history of ICA (20%).[19] Neuroimaging demonstrates a new ICA in 12% of patients who have suffered a ruptured ICA.[22] ICAs cluster in less than 5% of ADPKD families and the 5′ position of mutations in PKD1 is more commonly associated with ICAs. Other genetic modifiers may also be responsible for ICA in ADPKD.[23]

Magnetic resonance angiography is the appropriate screening imaging modality for cerebral aneurysms and can identify ICAs as small as 3 mm. Four-vessel cerebral angiography is the gold standard for confirmation of questionable ICAs.[19] Given the relatively low frequency of ICA in ADPKD, it is only cost-effective to screen those at risk of ICA (a positive family history) or whose current occupation (e.g., airline pilot) or lifestyle (e.g., scuba diving) significantly increases the likelihood or consequences of rupture. In addition, for those individuals in whom knowledge of a positive or negative result would improve their quality of life, a screening test for the presence of an ICA is warranted. In 130 asymptomatic ADPKD individuals with initial negative magnetic resonance screening studies who underwent repeat imaging 3 to 15 years later (mean, 9.7 years), no ICAs were found. Therefore, repeat screening in asymptomatic ADPKD subjects should be after more than 10 years.

Mortality and morbidity associated with a ruptured ICA remain more than 50%. However, in the general population, 50% of ICAs remain intact throughout life. The risk of rupture of ICA is related to the size of the aneurysm, with risk of rupture for ICAs more than 10 mm increasing exponentially with an estimated rupture rate of one in 5 patient-years. Longitudinal imaging of asymptomatic ADPKD individuals with intact ICAs less than 5 mm demonstrate little or no change in size. Less reliable data also suggest that those less than 10 mm do not change; however, the number of individuals studied is small.[24,25]

The outcome of surgical interventions for intact ICAs is extremely good compared with those presenting with rupture. Rare surgical complications include death or cerebrovascular accident with permanent neurological sequelae. However, recovery from elective neurosurgery for ICAs is usually associated with significant neurocognitive dysfunction as well as mood and sleep disorders for 6 to 12 months. Therefore, the decision to undergo elective surgery, clipping, coiling, or injection of intact small ICAs should be done only after discussion with the neurosurgeon, neurologist, and nephrologist and should take into account the patient's expectations and general health.

Renal Manifestations

Infections

Lower and upper urinary tract infections are common (30%–50%) and may be associated with a faster rate of renal functional loss in ADPKD.[26] Differentiating upper and lower tract infections is important. Upper urinary tract infections may be due to pyelonephritis, nephrolithiasis, obstruction, or cyst infection. Differentiating among these conditions relies on laboratory and radiographic studies. Pyelonephritis and stone-related infections often have urinary abnormalities (leukocyturia and bacteriuria) and positive urine cultures as opposed to cyst infections. With cyst infections, blood cultures are more likely (50%) to be positive than urine cultures. The triad of localized pain, fever, and the presence of a complex cyst on an ultrasound scan, magnetic resonance imaging, or computed tomography (CT) are the diagnostic features of renal cyst infection. Nephrolithiasis can be identified using CT. Cyst calcifications must be ruled out. Complex cysts, either consolidated hemorrhagic or infected, can be identified more often by CT. If symptoms are present in the area of the complex cyst, empiric antibiotic coverage is warranted.

The majority of cysts are detached from the parent nephron resulting in inadequate intracystic drug levels for aminoglycosides, penicillins, or cephalosporins. In pharmacologic studies during elective surgical cyst reduction procedures, good intracystic antibiotic levels have been demonstrated with trimethoprim-sulfamethoxazole, fluoroquinolones, chloramphenicol, and vancomycin.[27]

Given that cysts are detached from their parent nephron, cyst infections are equivalent to abscesses and require prolonged therapy (4–6 weeks) to ensure successful treatment. In individuals with cysts larger than 5 cm, antibiotic therapy alone is often unsuccessful and percutaneous or surgical cyst decompression with parenteral antibiotic treatment may be necessary.[28] Early identification of cyst infection and prolonged treatment with antibiotics is the key to successful eradication of cyst infections in ADPKD. Failure to use this approach can result in pyelonephritis and loss of the kidney.

Perinephric abscesses and refractory infected cysts may need surgical drainage. Nephrectomy should be the treatment of last resort and can be performed by laparotomy or laparoscopy.[29] Indications for nephrectomy include gas-forming pyelonephritis, recurrent infections in pretransplantation setting, and staghorn calculi in a nonfunctioning kidney.

Hypertension

Sixty percent of ADPKD adults with normal renal function (mean age, 31 years) and 10% to 22% of children with ADPKD have hypertension.[1,30] The frequency of hypertension defined by ambulatory measures is approximately 33% in children when 24-hour ambulatory blood pressure monitors are used.[31] Hypertension early in ADPKD is usually mild and adequately controlled with one to two antihypertensive medications. Importantly, hypertension is a significant independent predictor of progression to renal failure in ADPKD.

The mechanisms responsible for the development of hypertension in ADPKD include activation of the renin-angiotensin-aldosterone system (RAAS).[32,33] Individuals with ADPKD with hypertension and normal renal function demonstrate larger kidney volumes compared with their age- and gender-matched ADPKD normotensive counterparts. This suggests that cyst growth and expansion lead to compression and stretch of renal arterioles and activation of the intrarenal RAAS similar to bilateral renal artery stenosis.[33] Relative improvement in effective renal plasma flow and a decline in filtration fraction occur in hypertensive patients with ADPKD undergoing single-dose or short-term therapy with angiotensin-converting enzyme (ACE) inhibitors compared with matched essential hypertensives.

Left ventricular hypertrophy is present in approximately 50% of hypertensive ADPKD individuals.[34] Increased left ventricular mass index is also present in normotensive ADPKD individuals compared with age-matched controls. Hypertensive and normotensive ADPKD patients have a higher myocardial performance index, a measure of right ventricular dysfunction.[35] The left ventricular mass index also correlates with both diurnal and nocturnal systolic blood pressure based on 24-hour ambulatory blood pressure monitoring in normotensive adults as well as in children with ADPKD and normal kidney function.[36,37]

Proteinuria in ADPKD is usually low grade (<1 g/day) and occurs in a minority (17%) of patients. However, proteinuria is more common in hypertensive versus normotensive ADPKD individuals and is related to the level of blood pressure control.[38] Proteinuria is more common in ADPKD children (27%) and is also related to blood pressure level.[39] Microalbuminuria is present in approximately 27% of adults with ADPKD and 34% of children with ADPKD and is also a predictor of poor renal outcome in ADPKD.

Hypertension is associated with a faster rate of progression to renal failure in ADPKD and is the most treatable risk factor associated with disease progression. Importantly, when other factors related to renal progression are taken into account, age, renal volume, proteinuria, and blood pressure level or hypertension status are important risk factors for progression to ESRD. Progression to ESRD in ADPKD has significantly slowed since 1980 with an increasing age at onset of ESRD of 4 to 10 years on average.[9] Better blood pressure control, being followed by a nephrologist, and increased use of ACE inhibitors have all been implicated as being responsible for the slowing of progression to renal failure. Long-term ACE inhibitor therapy (7 years) of hypertension in ADPKD has improved left ventricular mass index and decreased the frequency of left ventricular hypertrophy and albuminuria[40] with the greatest decrease in albuminuria found in those whose blood pressures were treated to less than 125/75 mm Hg. The improvement in the left ventricular mass index and frequency of left ventricular hypertrophy after treatment may not be specific to ACE inhibitors because rigorous (mean arterial pressure < 93 mm Hg) compared with moderate (mean arterial pressure 100–107 mm Hg) blood pressure control demonstrated beneficial effects. Although ACE inhibitors have renoprotective effects with regard to proteinuria, no clear benefit in slowing the rate of progression to renal failure has been demonstrated in ADPKD.[40–42] However, studies have been of short duration, using multiple simultaneous interventions (i.e., protein restriction and different blood pressure levels) and included patients with advanced renal disease. Importantly, observational studies demonstrate that the use of diuretics as opposed to ACE inhibitors are associated with faster progression to ESRD,[43] whereas β-blockers and ACE inhibitors demonstrate similar effects on the rate of renal progression.[44]

There is lack of data available regarding the benefit of angiotensin receptor blockers, alone or in combination with ACE inhibitors in ADPKD.[45] There is significant variability in the level of blockade of the RAAS by ACE inhibitors and the additional use of angiotensin receptor blockers may maximize the blockade of the RAAS. The COOPERATE study randomly assigned 366 patients with nondiabetic kidney disease to either trandolapril, losartan, or a combination of the two and found a 61% decrease in the composite endpoint of doubling of serum creatinine, ESRD, or death in the combination group versus the other groups.[45]

The PKD HALT network, a multicenter initiative funded by the National Institutes of Health, is currently investigating the role of dual blockade of the RAAS using lisinopril and telmisartan versus lisinopril alone in more than 1100 participants (HALT PKD trial). This trial includes those with chronic kidney disease types I, II, and III. The impact of dual blockade of the RAAS and the level of blood pressure control—120 to 130/70 to 80 mm Hg versus less than 110/75 mm Hg on total renal volume—is being evaluated in patients with chronic kidney disease I and II, whereas dual blockade of the RAAS is being evaluated in patients with CKD III with a composite endpoint of the time to a 50% reduction of baseline estimated glomerular filtration rate, ESRD, or death.

Kidney Pain in Autosomal Dominant Polycystic Kidney Disease

Kidney pain could be due to a variety of conditions such as chronic kidney pain, infections (cystic or parenchymal), nephrolithiasis, and cyst hemorrhage, and an accurate diagnosis is required before treatment. A thorough clinical history, physical examination, urinalysis and urine cultures, and imaging studies are usually sufficient to identify the cause of pain.

Chronic kidney pain is common and is associated with larger kidneys and increasing age. It can be unilateral or bilateral with varying intensity.[1] The presence of hematuria is possible, but painless hematuria is also common in ADPKD. Urine cultures are usually negative.

For mild pain, symptomatic relief with analgesics other than nonsteroidal anti-inflammatory drugs should be used. In cases of more severe and debilitating pain or occurrence of narcotic dependence, the possibility of intervention should be entertained. CT-guided cyst aspiration with or without sclerotherapy (with ethanol or tetracyclines) can be offered if only few large cysts are responsible for the pain.[46] Laparoscopic or open cyst reduction surgery is more complicated and is associated with more serious complications such as persistent postsurgical pain, leakage from the surgical site, ascites, and recurrent infections. It should be reserved for debilitating and refractory pain.[47] Infections have already been extensively discussed previously.

Cyst hemorrhage usually presents with sharp, acute pain without fever, but low-grade fever and leukocytosis can be present in some cases. Cyst hemorrhages can be confined to the cyst or communicate with the urinary (causing hematuria), perinephric, or retroperitoneal spaces. CT or MRI (especially when compared with previous studies) may confirm the diagnosis. Treatment is based on pain management. Prophylactic oral antibiotherapy for a week to avoid infections could be considered.

Nephrolithiasis occurs in approximately 20% of patients with ADPKD. The most common type of kidney stones are composed of uric acid (>50%) and the remainder of calcium oxalate (40%).[48] They usually present as acute-onset episodes of flank pain with microscopic hematuria. The imaging study of choice should be CT. Medical management should consider abundant water intake (almost a gallon per day), low-salt diet, citrate supplements in case of hypocitraturia, and allopurinol in case of hyperuricosuria. Cystoscopy and/or extracorporeal shock wave therapy should be considered if kidney stones are less than 2 mm. Kidney stones larger than 2 mm, particularly if they are associated with infection and obstruction, may require open surgical removal.[48] Table 45-2 summarizes differential diagnoses and treatment of kidney pain in ADPKD.

Table 45-2   Differential Diagnosis and Treatment of Kidney Pain in Autosomal Dominant Polycystic Kidney Disease

	Pain Characteristics	Associated Features	U/A	Cultures	Imaging	Treatment
Cyst hemorrhage	Sudden onset, localized, unilateral, sharp, improves after few days	Usually afebrile, nausea/vomiting, hematuria possible	±/Hematuria, cultures negative	Negative	CT or MRI	Analgescis, bed rest and hydration, compression on affected side; if shock: transfusions
Pyelonephritis	Uni-bilateral, progressive, diffuse ++	High-grade fever, nausea/vomiting, dysuria, sepsis	WBCs/pyuria, ± bacteria, ± hematuria	Urine positive, ± positive blood	Not indicated with positive cultures, CT or MRI	IV antibiotics with good urine concentration (4 wk), followed by PO treatment
Cyst infection	Unilateral, localized, subacute, sharp +++	Fever, nausea/vomiting	Usually bland	Urine negative, blood positive	CT or MRI, WBC tagging if uncertain	Cyst-penetrating antibiotics (4 wk minimum), longer recovery time
Nephrolithiasis	Unilateral, acute, sharp +++, paroxysmal, renal colic, radiation to pelvis or groin	Usually afebrile unless infection, nausea/vomiting	Hematuria common, crystals (uric acid and/or calcium oxalate)	Usually negative unless infected stone	Spiral CT, stone protocol	IV hydratation, analgesics, ureteroscopy, percutaneous nephrolithotomy, open surgery
Chronic renal pain	Diffuse, constant, variable intensity, positional in nature aggravated by inspiration, automobile, sudden impact	Afebrile	Usually bland, occasional hematuria	Negative	Usually negative	Analgesics, cyst aspiration ± sclerosis with ethanol or tetracyclines if few large cysts causing pain, cyst reduction

++, moderate; +++, severe; CT, computed tomography; MRI, magnetic resonance imaging; WBCs, white blood cells.

Therapeutic Modalities to Slow Disease Progression in Autosomal Dominant Polycystic Kidney Disease

The Modification of Diet in Renal Disease study, evaluating the role of protein restriction in the course of renal disease in 222 ADPKD patients with a baseline glomerular filtration rate between 25 and 55 mL/min, did not demonstrate benefit. At present, dietary protein restriction to less than 0.8 g/kg/day is not recommended in patients with ADPKD. Other approaches such as alkali therapy,[49] amiloride,[50,51] caffeine intake,[52] and cyst drainage[46,47] have been investigated in animal or in vitro models of PKD with evidence of benefit. There are, however, no data from randomized clinical trials on the efficacy of these agents. Better understanding of cellular and molecular mechanisms of cystogenesis has opened the way to new approaches to delay progression of ADPKD. Recently, testing for exciting new treatments has begun based on the understanding of the underlying pathophysiology of cyst growth in ADPKD as well as positive preclinical results in murine models of ADPKD.

Evidence suggests that increased intracellular cyclic adenosine monophosphate plays a significant role in proliferative and fluid secretion pathways in cyst formation and expansion in PKD.[53] The vasopressin V_2 receptor antagonist OPC-31260, which lowers renal epithelial cell intracellular cyclic adenosine monophosphate levels, has been evaluated in a transgenic model of PKD2 and demonstrated a significant decrease in renal and cyst enlargement and renal dysfunction. Renal cyclic adenosine monophosphate levels were decreased, with a decrease in cystic fluid collection.[54] Administration of the selective V_2 receptor antagonist tolvaptan (OPC-41061) also lowered renal cyclic adenosine monophosphate levels, decreased the severity of cyst formation, and resulted in lower kidney weights and cyst and fibrosis volumes in a model of autosomal recessive PKD, the PCK rat.[55]

Phase IIA studies of tolvaptan in adult patients with ADPKD and normal kidney function confirmed a dose-dependent response with increasing urine output and decreasing urine osmolality in 11 patients. In addition, the safety and tolerability of four escalating doses of oral tolvaptan were established in 27 individuals who maintained 24-hour urine osmolality less than 300 mOsm with an average daily urine output of 6 L after 5 days of treatment.[56] Phase IIB and III trials investigating the safety and efficacy of tolvaptan therapy targeting urinary concentration are currently ongoing. Increased water intake could mimic the results obtained by blocking vasopressin and associated pathways. A 3.5-fold increase in water intake in PCK rats by using a 5% glucose solution was associated with a significant decrease (>60%) in renal expression of arginine vasopressin V_2 receptors, B-Raf, phosphorylated extracellular signal–regulated kinase, and proliferating cell nuclear antigen–positive renal cells. High water intake ultimately decreased the kidney-to-body weight ratio 28.0% and improved renal function.[57]

Somatostatin C (octreotide) is a synthetic analogue of the natural hormone and has been successfully used in the treatment of multiple endocrine tumors.[58] Experimental data suggest that cyst fluid secretion in several animal models requires active chloride transport. Somatostatin C inhibits this phenomenon. The cyclic adenosine monophosphate pathway is also inhibited by somatostatin in one animal model of PKD.[59] In a pilot study comparing somatostatin with placebo

in patients with PKD, active therapy was associated with a smaller increase in cyst and total kidney volume after 6 months of treatment.[60]

Polycystin-1 functions by inducing the formation of a complex with tuberin and the Ser/Thr kinase mTOR thereby inhibiting mTOR activity. Rapamycin is an antiproliferative agent, which inhibits tubular epithelial cell proliferation through the mTOR pathway. Rapamycin reverses this inhibition and has been shown to inhibit cyst formation and renal failure in the Han:SPRD rat model of PKD1.[61] A clinical trial of rapamycin is currently ongoing in ADPKD patients.

The use of triptolide (the active diterpene in the traditional Chinese medicine Lei Gong Teng) in a murine model of ADPKD arrests cellular proliferation and attenuates overall cyst growth by induction of Ca^{2+} release through a polycystin 2–dependent mechanism.[62] Potential uses of this agent are being tested in preclinical models of PKD.

In summary, multiple pathways, selectively targeted based on the cell signaling or trafficking abnormalities defined in transgenic animal models of PKD and cell culture systems of PKD epithelia, provide a range of therapeutic options. In addition to the systemic and general renal benefits obtained from agents that inhibit the RAAS, targeted therapies for high-risk ADPKD individuals will be available to optimize therapy early, before the loss of renal function.

References

1. Gabow PA: Autosomal dominant polycystic kidney disease. N Engl J Med 1993;329:332–342.
2. United States Renal Data System: 2006 Annual Report Data. Bethesda, MD: NIH-NIDDK, 2006.
3. Chapman AB, Guay-Woodford LM, Grantham JJ, et al: Renal structure in early autosomal-dominant polycystic kidney disease (ADPKD): The Consortium for Radiologic Imaging Studies of Polycystic Kidney Disease (CRISP) cohort. Kidney Int 2003;64:1035–1045.
4. Grantham JJ, Torres VE, Chapman AB, et al, for the CRISP Investigators: Volume progression in polycystic kidney disease. N Engl J Med 2006;354:2122–2130.
5. Gabow PA: Autosomal dominant polycystic kidney disease—more than a renal disease. Am J Kidney Dis 1990;16:403–413.
6. Gabow PA, Johnson AM, Kaehny WD, et al: Risk factors for the development of hepatic cysts in autosomal dominant polycystic kidney disease. Hepatology 1990;11:1033–1037.
7. Ramos A, Torres VE, Holley KE, et al: The liver in autosomal dominant polycystic kidney disease. Implications for pathogenesis. Arch Pathol Lab Med 1990;114:180–184.
8. Bae KT, Zhu F, Chapman AB, et al: Magnetic resonance imaging evaluation of hepatic cysts in early autosomal-dominant polycystic kidney disease: The consortium for radiologic imaging studies of polycystic kidney disease cohort. Clin J Am Soc Nephrol 2006; 1:64–69.
9. Schrier RW, McFann KK, Johnson AM: Epidemiological study of kidney survival in autosomal dominant polycystic kidney disease. Kidney Int 2003;63:678–685.
10. Grunfeld JP, Bennett WM: Clinical aspects of autosomal dominant polycystic kidney disease. Curr Opin Nephrol Hypertens 1995;4:114–120.
11. Sherstha R, McKinley C, Russ P, et al: Postmenopausal estrogen therapy selectively stimulates hepatic enlargement in women with autosomal dominant polycystic kidney disease. Hepatology 1997;26:1282–1286.

12. Everson GT, Scherzinger A, Berger-Leff N, et al: Polycystic liver disease: Quantitation of parenchymal and cyst volumes from computed tomography images and clinical correlates of hepatic cysts. Hepatology 1988;8:1627–1634.

13. Nakanuma Y, Hoso M, Hayashi M, Hirai N: Adult polycystic liver presenting with progressive hepatic failure. J Clin Gastroenterol 1989;11:592–594.

14. Que F, Nagorney DM, Gross JB Jr, Torres VE: Liver resection and cyst fenestration in the treatment of severe polycystic liver disease. Gastroenterology 1995;108:487–494.

15. Katkhouda N, Hurwitz M, Gugenheim J, et al: Laparoscopic management of benign solid and cystic lesions of the liver. Ann Surg 1999;229:460–466.

16. Turnage RH, Eckhauser FE, Knol JA, Thompson NW: Therapeutic dilemmas in patients with symptomatic polycystic liver disease. Am Surg 1988;54:365–372.

17. Jeyarajah DR, Gonwa TA, Testa G, et al: Liver and kidney transplantation for polycystic disease. Transplantation 1998;66:529–532.

18. Chapman AB, Rubinstein D, Hughes R, et al: Intracranial aneurysms in autosomal dominant polycystic kidney disease. N Engl J Med 1992;327:916–920.

19. Investigators of the International Study of Unruptured Intracranial Cerebral Aneurysms: Unruptured intracranial aneurysms–risk of rupture and risks of surgical intervention. N Engl J Med 1998;339:1725–1733. Erratum in: N Engl J Med 1999;340:744.

20. Fick GM, Johnson AM, Hammond WS, Gabow PA: Causes of death in autosomal dominant polycystic kidney disease. J Am Soc Nephrol 1995;5:2048–2056.

21. Schievink WI, Torres VE, Wiebers DO, Huston J 3rd: Intracranial arterial dolichoectasia in autosomal dominant polycystic kidney disease. J Am Soc Nephrol 1997;8:1298–1303.

22. Belz MM, Fick-Brosnahan GM, Hughes RL, et al: Recurrence of intracranial aneurysms in autosomal-dominant polycystic kidney disease. Kidney Int 2003;63:1824–1830.

23. Rossetti S, Chauveau D, Kubly V, et al: Association of mutation position in polycystic kidney disease 1 (PKD1) gene and development of a vascular phenotype. Lancet 2003;361:2196–2201.

24. Huston J 3rd, Torres VE, Wiebers DO, Schievink WI: Follow-up of intracranial aneurysms in autosomal dominant polycystic kidney disease by magnetic resonance angiography. J Am Soc Nephrol 1996;7:2135–2141.

25. Gibbs GF, Huston J 3rd, Qian Q, et al: Follow-up of intracranial aneurysms in autosomal-dominant polycystic kidney disease. Kidney Int 2004;65:1621–1627.

26. Sklar AH, Caruana RJ, Lammers JE, Strauser GD: Renal infections in autosomal dominant polycystic kidney disease. Am J Kidney Dis 1987;10:81–88.

27. Bennett WM, Elzinga L, Pulliam JP, et al: Cyst fluid antibiotic concentrations in autosomal-dominant polycystic kidney disease. Am J Kidney Dis 1985;6:400–404.

28. Chapman AB, Thickman D, Gabow PA: Percutaneous cyst puncture in the treatment of cyst infection in autosomal dominant polycystic kidney disease. Am J Kidney Dis 1990;16:252–255.

29. Dunn MD, Portis AJ, Elbahnasy AM, et al: Laparoscopic nephrectomy in patients with end-stage renal disease and autosomal dominant polycystic kidney disease. Am J Kidney Dis 2000;35:720–725.

30. Tee JB, Acott PD, McLellan DH, Crocker JF: Phenotypic heterogeneity in pediatric autosomal dominant polycystic kidney disease at first presentation: A single-center, 20-year review. Am J Kidney Dis 2004;43:296–303.

31. Seeman T, Šikut M, Konrad M, et al: Blood pressure and renal function in autosomal dominant polycystic kidney disease. Pediatr Nephrol 1997;11:592–596.

32. Wang D, Strandgaard S: The pathogenesis of hypertension in autosomal dominant polycystic kidney disease. J Hypertens 1997;15:925–933.

33. Chapman AB, Johnson A, Gabow PA, Schrier RW: The renin-angiotensin-aldosterone system and autosomal dominant polycystic kidney disease. N Engl J Med 1990;323:1091–1096.

34. Chapman AB, Johnson AM, Rainguet S, et al: Left ventricular hypertrophy in autosomal dominant polycystic kidney disease. J Am Soc Nephrol 1997;8:1292–1297.

35. Oflaz H, Alisir S, Buyukaydin B, et al: Biventricular diastolic dysfunction in patients with autosomal-dominant polycystic kidney disease. Kidney Int 2005;68:2244–2249.

36. Valero FA, Martinez-Vea A, Bardaji A, et al: Ambulatory blood pressure and left ventricular mass in normotensive patients with autosomal dominant polycystic kidney disease. J Am Soc Nephrol 1999;10:1020–1026.

37. Zeier M, Geberth S, Schmidt KG, et al: Elevated blood pressure profile and left ventricular mass in children and young adults with autosomal dominant polycystic kidney disease. J Am Soc Nephrol 1993;3:1451–1457.

38. Chapman AB, Johnson AM, Gabow PA, Schrier RW: Overt proteinuria and microalbuminuria in autosomal dominant polycystic kidney disease. J Am Soc Nephrol 1994;5:1349–1354.

39. Sharp C, Johnson A, Gabow P: Factors relating to urinary protein excretion in children with autosomal dominant polycystic kidney disease. J Am Soc Nephrol 1998;9:1908–1914.

40. Ecder T, Chapman AB, Brosnahan GM, et al: Effect of antihypertensive therapy on renal function and urinary albumin excretion in hypertensive patients with autosomal dominant polycystic kidney disease. Am J Kidney Dis 2000;35:427–432.

41. Maschio G, Alberti D, Janin G, et al: Effect of the angiotensin-converting-enzyme inhibitor benazepril on the progression of chronic renal insufficiency. The Angiotensin-Converting-Enzyme Inhibition in Progressive Renal Insufficiency Study Group. N Engl J Med 1996;11;334:939–945.

42. Schrier R, McFann K, Johnson A, et al: Cardiac and renal effects of standard versus rigorous blood pressure control in autosomal-dominant polycystic kidney disease: Results of a seven-year prospective randomized study. J Am Soc Nephrol 2002;13:1733–1739.

43. Ecder T, Edelstein CL, Fick-Brosnahan GM, et al: Diuretics versus angiotensin-converting enzyme inhibitors in autosomal dominant polycystic kidney disease. Am J Nephrol 2001;21:98–103.

44. van Dijk MA, Breuning MH, Duiser R, et al: No effect of enalapril on progression in autosomal dominant polycystic kidney disease. Nephrol Dial Transplant 2003;18:2314–2320.

45. Nakao N, Yoshimura A, Morita H, et al: Combination treatment of angiotensin-II receptor blocker and angiotensin-converting-enzyme inhibitor in non-diabetic renal disease (COOPERATE): A randomized controlled trial. Lancet 2003;361:117–124.

46. Uemasu J, Fujihara M, Munemura C, et al: Cyst sclerotherapy with minocycline hydrochloride in patients with autosomal dominant polycystic kidney disease. Nephrol Dial Transplant 1996;11:843–846.

47. Elzinga LW, Barry JM, Torres VE, et al: Cyst decompression surgery for autosomal dominant polycystic kidney disease. J Am Soc Nephrol 1992;2:1219–1226.

48. Torres VE, Wilson DM, Hattery RR, Segura JW: Renal stone disease in autosomal dominant polycystic kidney disease. Am J Kidney Dis 1993;22:513–519.

49. Torres VE, Mujwid DK, Wilson DM, Holley KH: Renal cystic disease and ammoniagenesis in Han:SPRD rats. J Am Soc Nephrol 1994;5:1193–1200.

50. Grantham JJ, Uchic M, Cragoe EJ Jr, et al: Chemical modification of cell proliferation and fluid secretion in renal cysts. Kidney Int 1989;35:1379–1389.

51. Gardner KD Jr, Burnside JS, Skipper BJ, et al: On the probability that kidneys are different in autosomal dominant polycystic disease. Kidney Int 1992;42:1199–1206.

52. Belibi FA, Wallace DP, Yamaguchi T, et al: The effect of caffeine on renal epithelial cells from patients with autosomal dominant polycystic kidney disease. J Am Soc Nephrol 2002;13:2723–2729.

53. Grantham JJ: Lillian Jean Kaplan International Prize for advancement in the understanding of polycystic kidney disease. Understanding polycystic kidney disease: A systems biology approach. Kidney Int 2003;64:1157–1162.

54. Torres VE, Wang X, Qian Q, et al: Effective treatment of an orthologous model of autosomal dominant polycystic kidney disease. Nat Med 2004;10:363.

55. Wang X, Gattone V 2nd, Harris PC, Torres VE: Effectiveness of vasopressin V2 receptor antagonists OPC-31260 and OPC-41061 on polycystic kidney disease development in the PCK rat. J Am Soc Nephrol 2005;16:846–851.

56. Chapman AB, Torres VE, Grantham JJ, et al: A phase IIB pilot study of the safety and efficacy of tolvaptan, a vasopressin V2 receptor antagonist (V2RA), in patients with ADPKD. J Am Soc Nephrol 2006;16:68A.

57. Nagao S, Nishii K, Katsuyama M, et al: Increased water intake decreases progression of polycystic kidney disease in the PCK rat. J Am Soc Nephrol 2006;17:2220–2227.

58. Trendle MC, Moertel CG, Kvols LK: Incidence and morbidity of cholelithiasis in patients receiving chronic octreotide for metastatic carcinoid and malignant islet cell tumors. Cancer 1997;79:830–834.

59. Silva P, Stoff JS, Leone DR, Epstein FH: Mode of action of somatostatin to inhibit secretion by shark rectal gland. Am J Physiol 1985;249:R329–R334.

60. Ruggenenti P, Remuzzi A, Ondei P, et al: Safety and efficacy of long-acting somatostatin treatment in autosomal-dominant polycystic kidney disease. Kidney Int 2005;68:206–216.

61. Tao Y, Kim J, Schrier RW, Edelstein CL: Rapamycin markedly slows disease progression in a rat model of polycystic kidney disease. J Am Soc Nephrol 2005;16:46–51.

62. Leuenroth SJ, Okuhara D, Shotwell JD, et al: Triptolide is a traditional Chinese medicine-derived inhibitor of polycystic kidney disease. Proc Natl Acad Sci U S A 2007;104:4389–4394.

Further Reading

Arnold HL, Harrison SA: New advances in evaluation and management of patients with polycystic liver disease. Am J Gastroenterol. 2005;100:2569–2582.

Bisceglia M, Galliani CA, Senger C, et al: Renal cystic diseases: A review. Adv Anat Pathol 2006;13:26–56.

Chapman AB: Autosomal dominant polycystic kidney disease: Time for a change? J Am Soc Nephrol 2007;18:1399–1407.

Rossetti S, Consugar MB, Chapman AB, et al., CRISP Consortium: Comprehensive molecular diagnostics in autosomal dominant polycystic kidney disease. J Am Soc Nephrol 2007l;18:2143–2160.

Schrier RW, Belz MM, Johnson AM, et al: Repeat imaging for intracranial aneurysms in patients with autosomal dominant polycystic kidney disease with initially negative studies: A prospective ten-year follow-up. J Am Soc Nephrol 2004;15:1023–1028.

Torres VE, Harris PC, Pirson Y: Autosomal dominant polycystic kidney disease. Lancet 2007;369:1287–1301.

Chapter 46

Noncystic Hereditary Diseases of the Kidney

Russell W. Chesney

The techniques of gene cloning, chromosomal localization, and genomic evaluation have more clearly elucidated the pathogenesis and treatment strategies of many of the inherited renal disorders. This chapter reviews a number of clinical disorders that have as their basis a defect in some transport or metabolic function of the renal tubular epithelium. Using this model of inherited disorders of renal tubular transport, one is able to define conditions in which single or multiple substances are lost, in which inorganic ions or organic solutes are overly excreted, and in which the whole body pool of these substances is diminished due to excessive urinary losses. Conversely, sometimes metabolites are stored to excess, with toxic effects. The basic genetic and pathophysiologic mechanisms underlying these transport and metabolic defects are detailed elsewhere.[1-5] The intent of this chapter is to focus on current therapeutic approaches.

AMINOACIDURIAS

The aminoacidurias may be specific to a single amino acid or to a group of amino acids whose structure and charge are similar.[2,4] In recent years, virtually all amino acid transporters have been cloned.[5] The technique of amino acid analysis of urine or plasma permits diagnosis of these disorders, particularly the measurement of urinary clearance or fractional excretion. Several of the aminoacidurias, such as iminoglycinuria in which excessive amounts of L-proline, hydroxy-L-proline, and glycine are found in the urine, are benign traits requiring no treatment.[1] In dicarboxylic aminoaciduria, there are no apparent clinical features and hence no recommended therapy.[1]

Hartnup disease is an autosomal recessive disorder characterized by massive urinary losses and intestinal malabsorption of the neutral monoamino-monocarboxylic amino acids. Affected patients develop features of pellagra[2,4] because of inability to synthesize minimal concentrations of nicotinamide as a result of extensive bowel and urinary L-tryptophan losses. Thus, insufficient absorption and reabsorption of L-tryptophan results in niacin deficiency. Treatment consists of providing nicotinamide (40–150 mg/day) or an American diet containing leafy green vegetables. This effectively bypasses the need for tryptophan. With the provision of nicotinamide, the red scaly rash heals and neurologic problems improve.

Renal and urinary tract stones develop in cystinuria, an autosomal recessive disorder in which the poorly soluble disulfide amino acid is excreted into the urine in increased amounts.[6] Cystinuria is a relatively frequent cause of nephrolithiasis, found in 1 in 12,000 persons worldwide. The initial goal of therapy is to decrease the urinary concentration of cystine below its solubility limit and is generally accomplished by a forced high fluid intake. Unfortunately, this form of therapy requires strenuous compliance, with frequent ingestion of fluids and nocturnal awakening to empty the bladder and drink additional fluids. Patients should also receive oral alkali therapy because the solubility of cystine is pH dependent (urinary solubility of cystine increases sharply at pH values greater than 7.5). A suggested dose is 650 mg of sodium bicarbonate every 6 to 8 hours.

Should these more conservative measures fail, the next line of therapy is the thiol-containing agents. Oral D-penicillamine (dimethylcystine), a mercaptan that undergoes an in vivo disulfide exchange reaction with cystine, causing urinary excretion of a more readily soluble penicillamine-cystine mixed disulfide. In parallel, the concentration of cystine in the urine of a cystinuric subject actually decreases.[2,4] Treatment with oral D-penicillamine at 1 to 2 g/day in the adult and 30 mg/kg in the child is highly effective in decreasing urinary cystine excretion to less than 200 to 300 mg/day, but patient tolerance is poor and adverse effects are frequent.[6] Serious adverse effects that result in discontinuance of the drug occur in 30% to 50% of patients and include skin rash, membranous or linear IgG antiglomerular basement membrane antibody–induced

547

nephropathy, nausea, vomiting, impairment or loss of taste or smell, and pemphigus.[1]

Because of these serious adverse effects, other disulfide compounds have been used. Indeed, D-penicillamine should probably not be a first-line drug of choice. Most experience has been gained with 2-mercaptopropionylglycine (α-MPG, tiopronin), which is 1.5 times as effective as D-penicillamine in decreasing free cystine and in increasing the quantity of mixed disulfides appearing in the urine.[6] Tiopronin also results in adverse effects, including nausea, vomiting, and rash, but far less frequently than D-penicillamine. Development of the nephrotic syndrome is rare. The final dose of tiopronin needed to reduce urinary cystine varies from 100 to 200 mg/ day. Although patients may experience adverse effects, it is seldom necessary to discontinue therapy, and only 6% of patients receiving tiopronin because of D-penicillamine toxicity must stop taking it.[2,4]

Surgery for staghorn calculi or obstructing stones can potentially be avoided by the use of extracorporeal shock wave lithotripsy.[7] In ultrasonic lithotripsy, an ultrasound probe is passed up the ureter during cystoscopy; it is 97% effective in removing an obstructing calculus. Extracorporeal shock wave lithotripsy employs a totally external technique, with patients placed in a special bath, anesthetized, and then receiving thousands of precisely directed shock waves. The main drawbacks are hematuria, failure of stone passage, and mild to moderate obstruction and infection, although most patients pass the stone fragments with lesser symptoms of colic. Cystine stones are less effectively fragmented than are calcium oxalate stones.[7]

Hypercystinuria probably requires no treatment because patients do not excrete the same quantities of cystine as patients with classic cystinuria.[7]

GLYCOSURIAS

The renal glycosurias are a group of conditions in which excessive urinary excretion of glucose occurs in the absence of hyperglycemia. The glycosurias occur because of abnormal renal tubular reabsorption of glucose due to mutations in the two renal isoforms of the sodium-dependent glucose transporter. The clinical course of the primary renal glycosurias is benign because there is neither progressive renal deterioration nor serious metabolic derangement, and there is no specific therapy. It is important to distinguish the primary renal glycosurias from diabetes mellitus, which requires insulin or other hypoglycemic therapy.

CLASSIC PSEUDOHYPOALDOSTERONISM

Classic pseudohypoaldosteronism is a condition in which both renal tubular salt wasting and hyperkalemia are observed, despite normal renal and adrenal function.[2] The defect relates to abnormalities of the renal aldosterone or mineralocorticoid receptor, with an ultimate defect in the epithelial sodium channel.[4] Salt wasting does not respond to exogenous mineralocorticoids alone, so sodium chloride supplements must be provided. This hyperkalemic state occurs in infancy, and 24-hour Na^+ and Cl^- losses are as high as 10 to 15 mEq/kg, despite hypovolemia and hyponatremia. The administration of gluco-

corticoids, deoxycorticosterone acetate, or fluorinated glucocorticoids (which have extensive mineralocorticoid activity) do essentially nothing to reverse hyponatremia and hyperkalemia because of defective epithelial sodium channel or mineralocorticoid receptor. The most effective therapy is supplemental sodium chloride, with the dose based on the magnitude of measured urinary losses (mEq/kg/24 hr).[2,4] In infants, salt supplements normalize growth and correct serum Na^+ and Cl^- concentrations, despite the finding of persistently elevated plasma renin and aldosterone concentrations. A potassium-binding resin may be required to correct the concomitant hyperkalemia, and oral bicarbonate or citrate therapy is necessary to correct the acidosis. Patients can often have their salt supplements decreased or discontinued after infancy without effect, and they continue to grow at a normal rate.[2]

HEREDITARY PHOSPHATURIAS

Phosphorus is the most prevalent mineral anion found in bone (75%–85% of total body phosphate pool) and is also essential for numerous life processes.[1] Because phosphate is a key anion for important biologic systems, processes that affect the maintenance of phosphate homeostasis are important. The proximal tubule is the major site of regulation of phosphate homeostasis.[2] A number of clinically distinct phosphaturic syndromes have been defined,[1,4] all of which result in excess renal phosphate wasting and hypophosphatemic osteomalacia. If these conditions present during childhood, the result is incomplete mineralization and the radiographic appearance of rickets, with bowing of the lower extremities. Because the fundamental pathogenic mechanisms of the major phosphaturic syndromes differ, their treatment is also distinctly different (Table 46-1).

Primary or X-Linked Hypophosphatemic Rickets

This X-linked dominant disorder is the most common of the phosphaturic syndromes and involves a double renal tubular defect: (1) failure of Na^+/PO_4^{3-} cotransport across the brush border membrane of the proximal tubule and (2) reduction in the conversion of 25-hydroxyvitamin D_3 to 1,25-dihydroxyvitamin D_3 by proximal tubule cell mitochondria.[2,4] A defective phosphate regulatory protein (PHEX) that fails to degrade fibroblast growth factor 23 is the cause of this condition.

The current recommendation regarding the most appropriate form of treatment is a combination of oral 1,25-dihydroxyvitamin D_3 in as low a dose as possible (5–50 ng/day) plus oral phosphate supplements (70 mg/kg/day).[1,4,8] Although this therapy has been shown to improve calcium and phosphate retention, phosphate must be administered every 4 to 5 hours because the renal phosphate leak persists (see Table 46-1). Therapy is probably needed throughout the life of the patient. Not only will the rachitic growth plate lesion be improved but endosteal bone trabecular lesions will also improve, a change not apparent when using vitamin D_2 or D_3 alone. Oral phosphate can be administered as Joulie solution[8] or as neutral phosphate.[9] The latter is commercially available and far easier to use. This form of therapy should be given during childhood. Medical

Table 46-1 Features of Different Forms of Primary Hypophosphatemic Rickets

Condition	Pattern of Inheritance	Gene Defect	Associated Findings	Salient Clinical Features	Age Detected	Therapy
X-linked hypophosphatemic rickets (vitamin D dependent or familial)	X-linked dominant (rarely dominant or AR)	Defect in PHEX, a regulator of protein coded Xp22.1–22.2	Occasional parathyroid adenoma/hyperplasia	Bowing lower segment, short stature, no myopathy; more severe in males (lyon effect)	9–13 mo	Oral phosphate 70–100 mg/kg/day (4–5 times daily); oral 1,25-(OH)₂D₃ 5–50 ng/kg/day
Hypophosphatemic nonrachitic bone disease	AD or sporadic	FGF23	Glycinuria	No radiographic evidence of rickets; slight short stature may develop late	3 yr to adult	Oral phosphate and vitamin D; 1,25-(OH)₂ D₃ may heal osteomalacia
Hereditary hypophosphatemic rickets and hypercalciuria	AR; consanguinity frequent	Unknown	High plasma 1,25-(OH)₂ D₃; increased intestinal calcium absorption, hypercalciuria, low urine cAMP	Rickets, short stature, osteomalacia, equal sex distribution	Early child-hood	Oral phosphate (70–100 mg/kg/day)
Oncogenous rickets with phosphaturia	Sporadic or AD/AR	Presumed defect in phosphatonin activity; failure to degrade FGF23	Neurofibromatosis, polyostotic fibrous dysplasia, epidermal nevus syndrome	Rickets healed by removal of tumor where measured; serum 1,25-(OH)₂D₃ values are usually low	Birth onward	Oral phosphate and 1,25-(OH)₂D₃ reverse hypophosphatemia; surgery may be curative
Adult sporadic hypophosphatemic osteomalacia	Sporadic	Not relevant	Glycinuria	Severe bone pain, vertebral flattening, Looser-Milkman zones, severe myopathy/weakness	Adult	Oral phosphate and vitamin D (any form)

AD, autosomal dominant; AR, autosomal recessive; cAMP, cyclic adenosine monophosphate; FGF23, fibroblast growth factor 23; 1,25-(OH)₂D₃, 1,25-dihydroxyvitamin D₃; PHEX, phosphate-regulating gene on the X chromosome with homologies to endopeptidases.

noncompliance is a major problem, as are excessively loose stools due to oral sodium phosphate. Hydrochlorothiazide and amiloride may be used in some cases in which there appears to be resistance to the combination of vitamin D and phosphate supplementation in terms of calcium malabsorption and hypercalciuria.

No long-term studies have been reported that confirm the role of lifetime phosphorus supplementation in adults with this disorder. However, studies indicate that calcification of ligaments and joints (enthesopathy) can occur in untreated adult patients,[10] suggesting the need for therapy during adult life. Severely affected adults who continue to have osteodystrophy, stress fractures, and dental caries require prolonged treatment, yet those who are asymptomatic may not always need to continue treatment. Normal pregnancies have been reported both in mothers treated with vitamin D/phosphate supplementation and in those not treated. The concomitant use of recombinant human growth hormone, as an adjunct to standard therapy, probably improves growth.

Autosomal Dominant Hypophosphatemic Rickets

Hypophosphatemic nonrachitic bone disease is an autosomal dominant or possibly sporadic disorder in which hypophosphatemia is milder than in X-linked hypophosphatemia and rickets is absent.[1,4] Both the T_m PO_4/glomerular filtration rate in hypophosphatemic patients and serum 1,25-dihydroxycholecalciferol concentrations are normal. Therapy with vitamin D_2 and oral phosphate salts appears to improve bone mineralization; however, oral 1,25-dihydroxyvitamin D_3 can be used in place of vitamin D_2 or D_3.

Hereditary Hypophosphatemic Rickets with Hypercalciuria

This is a familial disorder that manifests as rickets, short stature, phosphaturia, hypercalciuria (8 mg/kg/24 hr), and augmented intestinal calcium and phosphate absorption.[11] Circulating 1,25-dihydroxyvitamin D_3 concentrations are two to five times normal compared with decreased concentrations in X-linked hypophosphatemic rickets and normal concentrations in hypophosphatemic bone disease. This disorder represents a renal phosphate leak that results in hypophosphatemia, which in turn stimulates 1,25-dihydroxyvitamin D_3 synthesis. Higher vitamin D metabolite concentrations lead to increased active intestinal calcium absorption, suppression of parathyroid hormone (PTH) secretion, and hypercalciuria. As 1,25-dihydroxyvitamin D_3 concentrations in plasma are elevated, vitamin D therapy is not indicated. Long-term oral phosphate alone reverses the biochemical features of this rare disorder.[11]

MAGNESURIAS

Magnesium depletion is an uncommon mineral disorder and is frequently overlooked because it usually arises within a complex clinical setting. Renal magnesium wasting may be part of a primary inherited disorder (Gitelman's syndrome),[12,13] a single defect in magnesium reabsorption,[14] or associated with several other clinical disorders.[2,4] Excessive urinary losses of magnesium can also be associated with diabetic ketoacidosis,

hyperaldosteronism, hypercalciuria (with concomitant use of loop diuretics), Gitelman's syndrome, and the use of several therapeutic agents such as cisplatin, aminoglycoside antibiotics, diuretics, and cyclosporine.[4] Hereditary isolated renal magnesium wasting is due to defects in three genes: a Na^+/K^+-ATPase subunit (a routing defect) and paracellin,[1] a protein located on the tight junction,[14] and transient receptor potential cation channels.[15] Gitelman's syndrome is discussed later.

A predominant feature of magnesium deficiency is hypocalcemia related to altered parathyroid gland function. Hypomagnesemia alters end-organ (bone) responsiveness to PTH[4] and hence contributes to hypocalcemia. Further, the provision of intravenous magnesium supplements to magnesium-deficient hypocalcemic patients has been shown to augment serum values of PTH.[4] Magnesium may also be an important factor in the action and/or metabolism of vitamin D in that some hypomagnesemic patients respond to 1α-vitamin D metabolites only after correction of serum magnesium values.[3,4] Serum concentrations of 1,25-dihydroxyvitamin D_3 are decreased in many magnesium-depleted patients.[4] Thus, the mineral abnormalities can include reduced serum concentrations of magnesium, calcium, 1,25-dihydroxyvitamin D_3, and PTH, all of which may be restored to normal by infusion or oral ingestion of magnesium. Therapy with magnesium oxide 1 to 5 g (50–250 mEq) in three divided doses daily causes the following changes: increased serum and urine magnesium and calcium, decreased serum phosphate, increased urine phosphate, and increased serum 1,25-dihydroxyvitamin D_3 and PTH.[16] Although the doses of oral magnesium required vary from one patient to the next, improved magnesium homeostasis can usually be achieved. Magnesium should be taken three to four times daily as magnesium oxide or magnesium pyrrolidine carboxylate because urinary magnesium losses occur continuously, and patients who have magnesium wasting will constantly lose this divalent ion.

Infants who have hypomagnesemic tetany should receive 0.4 to 0.8 mg/kg of a 50% solution of magnesium sulfate either intramuscularly or intravenously. Intravenous magnesium should be infused slowly with monitoring, and calcium gluconate or lactate should be on hand to reverse dysrhythmias. Finally, renal magnesium wasting can occur in conjunction with varying degrees of renal insufficiency,[16] and these patients may also require oral vitamin D analogues and calcium salts. A daily dose of 0.25 to 1.0 μg of 1,25-dihydroxyvitamin D_3 may be needed as well as calcium lactate, carbonate, or acetate.

FANCONI SYNDROME

Fanconi syndrome is a generalized disorder of proximal tubule function that can occur either as a primary disorder or as secondary to a number of inherited conditions.[1–4] Patients always show hyperexcretion of substances that are reabsorbed and diminished excretion of substances that are secreted.[1–3,5] The manifestations of Fanconi syndrome often vary depending on the underlying disorder. Tubular dysfunction typically involves glycosuria, phosphaturia, generalized aminoaciduria, proteinuria, polyuria, and proximal renal tubular acidosis. Other substances frequently excreted in increased quantities include uric acid, sodium, potassium, magnesium, citrate, and proteins of molecular mass less than 45,000 kd.[14] Because of phosphaturia, hypophosphatemia, and sometimes renal insufficiency, various bone disorders may be found, including rickets, osteomalacia, osteoporosis, and osteitis fibrosa.[17] Adult patients may have severe osteomalacia and may present with intense bone pain and muscle weakness.[1–3,5] Symptomatic hypokalemia is manifested by muscle weakness, growth failure, dehydration, unexplained fevers due to volume depletion, and profound metabolic acidosis.[17]

Therapy of Fanconi syndrome depends on the underlying cause. Symptomatic therapy includes large doses of oral alkali (sodium bicarbonate, often as much as 10–15 mEq/kg/day), phosphate supplements given four to five times daily (Table 46-2), a vitamin D analogue (usually calcitriol), adequate water, and adequate sodium and potassium replacement to correct volume depletion and signs of hypokalemia. Indomethacin may reduce urine volume.[17]

Patients with infantile nephropathic cystinosis have specific therapeutic needs. Cystine deposition within the cornea leads to photophobia, which may be improved with dark glasses, wetting solutions, and the use of cysteamine eyedrops that can dissolve cystine deposits.[17] The molecular defect in this disorder involves reduction in the rate of efflux of cystine, but not cysteine, from within a lysosomal compartment; the oxidized (-S-S-) form of this sulfur amino acid remains trapped, thus forming intralysomal cystine crystals. The defective gene encodes the lysosomal cystine transporter (cystinosin) and represents a defect in the endocytic pathway.[14,17] At least two cystine-depleting agents, cysteamine and pantethine (its precursor), can be used to deplete the lysosomes, creating mixed disulfides with cystine that are freely permeable across the lysosomal membrane. The reduced SH form is then free to exit the lysosome as well and thus intracellular cystine decreases.[14,17] The results of the Collaborative Cysteamine Study indicated that 98 patients receiving cysteamine showed a real slowing of the progression to renal failure and improved linear growth compared with more than 100 historic control cystinotic subjects.[18] A recent analysis of 88 patients followed for more than 10 years identified not only uremia but also hepatomegaly, splenomegaly, neurological disease, progressive ocular disease, and continuing poor growth despite a functioning renal allograft.[18] These results suggest the need for continuing cysteamine therapy, but this is only now being addressed by clinical trials. The drug Cystagon (cysteamine bitartrate) in capsule form has been approved by the U.S. Food and Drug Administration for

use in patients with cystinosis at a daily dose of 1.3 g/m². Patient compliance should be ensured by measuring leukocyte cystine content on a scheduled basis.[18]

Because of glandular cystine crystal deposition, hypothyroidism is universal in cystinosis, and therefore low-dose thyroxine is needed to prevent the clinical features of this endocrinopathy.[17] The dose of L-thyroxine is chosen by determining the amount needed to suppress thyroid-stimulating hormone levels to the normal range. Cystinotic patients have also been shown to lose massive amounts of carnitine and therefore have a deficiency of this acyl-transporting compound. Oral carnitine therapy may reverse muscle carnitine depletion and the histologic features of the deficiency.[17] Finally, recall that cystinosis is a lifelong disorder with continuing cystine deposition. The long-term involvement of organs other than the kidney is only now being appreciated since long-term survivors of renal transplantation became available for study.[19]

Lowe syndrome is an X-linked disorder that presents with cataracts, glaucoma, growth impairment, hypotonia, severe mental retardation, and features of Fanconi syndrome. It is caused by defective inositol polyphosphate 5′-phosphatase activity, presumably involving the phosphatidylinositol signaling pathway.[1] Treatment is directed at correcting the metabolic derangements of Fanconi syndrome. Renal dysfunction begins with tubular dysfunction but can progress to chronic renal failure. Tubular dysfunction eventually diminishes because of the decline in glomerular filtration rate. Patients with this syndrome usually die of infection or renal insufficiency but have a lifelong need for ophthalmologic evaluations. Most patients are boys, although girls with Lowe syndrome have been described due to chromosomal translocations.[1,4]

Patients with galactosemia, an autosomal recessive deficiency of galactose 1-phosphate uridyltransferase, develop a Fanconi syndrome that is totally reversible when patients are maintained on a galactose- and lactose-free diet.[1] This diet is a lifelong necessity.

Tyrosinosis is due to an autosomal recessive defect in fumarylacetoacetate fumaryl hydrolase, with the accumulation of succinylacetone and succinylacetoacetate, which in turn leads to hepatomegaly, cirrhosis, and full-blown Fanconi syndrome.[1,2] The disorder has a poor prognosis and usually results in death in children due to cirrhosis and/or hepatoblastomas. A low-tyrosine, low-phenylalanine diet can treat the Fanconi syndrome

Table 46-2 Phosphate Preparations for Therapy of Phosphaturic Syndromes and Fanconi Syndrome

Content	Constituents	Phosphate
K-Phos M.F.	Potassium acid phosphate, sodium acid phosphate	125.6 mg per tablet
K-Phos No. 2	Potassium acid phosphate, sodium acid phosphate	250 mg per tablet
K-Phos Neutral	Potassium acid phosphate, monobasic; sodium acid phosphate, monobasic/dibasic	250 mg per tablet
Neutra Phos	Potassium acid phosphate, monobasic; sodium acid phosphate, monobasic/dibasic	1 g/300 mL
Neutra Phos (capsules)	Potassium acid phosphate, monobasic; sodium acid phosphate, monobasic/dibasic	250 mg per capsule (dissolve in water)
Joulie solution*	Sodium phosphate, phosphoric acid	30.4 mg/mL

*Must be prepared by a pharmacist.

and prevent rickets but does not prevent cirrhosis. The definitive form of therapy is liver or liver-kidney transplantation.[20] Most authorities suggest liver-kidney transplantation.

Hereditary fructose intolerance is an autosomal recessive disorder caused by mutations in the aldolase B gene, resulting in decreased aldolase B activity in the liver, renal cortex, and small intestine and leading to accumulation of fructose 1-phosphate.[1,4] Diagnostic clues to this condition include an aversion to sweets, a lack of dental caries, and hepatomegaly. Development of Fanconi syndrome is temporally related to exposure to fructose, and treatment is directed at assiduously avoiding this sugar in the diet. As in galactosemia, development of Fanconi syndrome may occur within a few minutes to hours after ingestion of fructose and patients may become gravely ill with profound acidosis. Patients generally quickly recognize the advantage of avoiding fructose-containing foods.

Fanconi syndrome can be seen in certain children with an as yet untyped glycogen storage disease that is associated with hepatomegaly, massive glycosuria, glucose and galactose intolerance, and a mutation in the glucose transporter GLUT-4.[14,21] These patients are also profoundly growth retarded. Treatment consists of controlling the symptoms of Fanconi syndrome with sodium bicarbonate, phosphate, potassium chloride, and vitamin D, and patients tend to improve with age.

Wilson's disease is an autosomal recessive hepatocellular disorder of copper metabolism that presents with hepatomegaly and Fanconi syndrome. Copper deposits are noted in the brain, liver, and kidney.[1] Patients with Wilson's disease also have, in addition to proximal renal tubular acidosis, findings that can only be explained as distal renal tubular acidosis, and urinary calculi are common. Hypoparathyroidism has also been described in one patient with Wilson's disease, possibly related to copper deposits in the parathyroid gland.[1] Therapy for Wilson's disease consists of D-penicillamine, which can be

troublesome in some patients, as noted in the discussion on cystinuria. Whenever D-penicillamine cannot be used, triethylene tetramine dihydrochloride can be used without fear of the same allergic manifestations.[4]

When Fanconi syndrome appears in conjunction with the nephrotic syndrome, it is usually found in association with a familial pattern and focal segmental glomerulosclerosis. Tubular atrophy and interstitial fibrosis are prominent.[1] Treatment of this glomerulopathy is unsatisfactory, and features of Fanconi syndrome continue until renal failure ensues.

Finally, Fanconi syndrome is associated with mutations of the mitochondrial genome,[22] particularly if the respiratory chain is affected. Treatment is symptomatic, as described previously.

BARTTER SYNDROME

Bartter syndrome is characterized by hyperplasia of the juxtaglomerular apparatus, increased circulating angiotensin II concentrations, normal blood pressure with diminished pressor response to infused angiotensin II, hyperaldosteronism, hypokalemic alkalosis, and vasopressin-resistant polyuria.[2,4] This condition is heterogeneous, and most patients present in infancy or later childhood, although a presentation after the age of 40 has occurred.[4] The inheritance pattern is sporadic or autosomal recessive.

Recent progress in molecular biology has clarified certain aspects of this syndrome (Table 46-3).[14,23–25] The genetic mutations that underlie Bartter syndrome involve defects in (1) the luminal $Na^+/K^+/2Cl^-$ cotransporter (NKCC2), (2) the outwardly directed K^+ channel (ROMK), or (3) the Cl^- channel (ClCNKB). These transport proteins are all located in the thick ascending limb of the Henle's loop; NKCC2 and ROMK are in the luminal membrane and ClCNKB in the peritubular membrane.[25] Gitelman's syndrome is caused by a mutation in the

Table 46-3 Forms of Bartter Syndrome

Type	Defective Protein	Clinical Characteristics	Inheritance Mode	Location	Therapy
Bartter type I	Bumetamide-sensitive sodium-potassium-chloride cotransporter	APP, HMA, nephrocalcinosis	AR	TAL	KCl, indomethacin
Bartter type II	Potassium channel, ROMK1	APP, HMA, nephrocalcinosis	AR	TAL	KCl, indomethacin
Bartter syndrome	Calcium-sensing receptor	HMA, hypomagnesemia	AD	TAL	KCl, magnesium oxide
Bartter type III	Chloride channel kidney B	Growth retardation, hypercalciuria, HMA	AR	TAL	KCl, indomethacin
Bartter type IV	Barttin (regulates chloride channel kidney A and B)	APP, HMA, sensorineural deafness, developmental delay	AR contiguous gene deletion	TAL	KCl, indomethacin
Gitelman's syndrome	Thiazide-sensitive sodium-chloride cotransporter	HMA, hypocalciuria, hypomagnesemia, chondrocalcinosis (onset in late childhood or adolescence)	AR	Distal convoluted tubule	Magnesium oxide or Mg pyrrolidine (30 mmol/day)

APP, antenatal with polyhydramnios and prematurity; AR, autosomal recessive; HMA, hypokalemic metabolic alkalosis; ROMK, renal outer medulla potassium channel; TAL, thick ascending Henle's loop.

thiazide-sensitive Na^+/Cl^- cotransporter in the lumen of the distal convoluted tubule. Differences in the function of these four ion-transport systems help explain the clinical heterogeneity in Bartter and Gitelman's syndromes.

Children may present with growth failure as well as weakness, muscle cramps, polyuria, and abdominal pain; delayed or slowed mentation is seen in all children with Bartter syndrome. The laboratory features are also heterogeneous in that patients show variable degrees of increased urinary losses of potassium, sodium, chloride, magnesium, calcium, and kallikrein and increased production and excretion of prostaglandin E_2.[13] The differential diagnosis includes Fanconi syndrome, incomplete distal renal tubular acidosis, use of diuretics, abuse of laxatives, cyclical vomiting, chloride-deficient diets, and cystic fibrosis. Alkalosis is associated with administration of impermeable anions, mineralocorticoid excess, and primary renal magnesium wasting (Gitelman's syndrome).[25] Because of abnormalities in the concentration of prostaglandins in plasma and urine, it was once thought that the primary defect was one of prostaglandin metabolism[4]; this was before the roles of ion channels or transporters were understood.[13,25] Elevated prostaglandin levels could potentially explain vasodilation, the lack of responsiveness to pressors, the inhibition of chloride transport in Henle's loop, and potassium hyperexcretion and metabolic alkalosis. However, prostaglandin inhibition does not always correct the defect in these patients.[13] Recent studies suggest that at least five different pathogenetic mechanisms produce this syndrome.[24] Moreover, in disorders that mimic hereditary Bartter syndrome, such as bulimia, chronic diuretic abuse, and chloride-deficient formula-induced disease, the same plasma profile is evident.[1]

Therapy of Bartter syndrome is problematic.[4,24] Potassium supplementation is necessary, and large doses of potassium chloride may be required. Prostaglandin inhibitors have short-lived effects when used alone[24]; indomethacin has been used most often. Prostaglandin inhibition is an adjunct therapy that limits the need for potassium chloride supplements.[4,24]

In a subset of patients, the use of supplemental potassium chloride and treatment with a prostaglandin synthetase inhibitor may not fully correct hypokalemia, which should be the primary aim of therapy. In these cases, a potassium-sparing diuretic such as amiloride or triamterene in the usual doses can be useful.[1,4] If constantly applied, these therapeutic approaches usually result in improved growth and development in children and improved symptoms in adult patients with Bartter syndrome.

Patients with Gitelman's syndrome have renal magnesium wasting, hypokalemia, metabolic alkalosis, and hypocalciuria.[4,14,23] Some patients may have a tendency toward hypocalcemia,[23] and cramps may be common. If magnesium wasting is present, magnesium supplementation is clearly indicated. Supplementation with magnesium oxide or magnesium pyrrolidine carboxylate 30 mmol/day improves hypomagnesemia, sometimes corrects hypokalemia, and increases hypocalcemia.[23]

LIDDLE SYNDROME

Liddle syndrome is a rare familial cause of hypokalemia associated with failure to thrive, sodium retention, hypertension, and suppressed plasma levels of renin and aldosterone.[27] The specific transport defect is located in the cytoplasmic region of the β or γ subunit of the sodium channel or the amiloride-sensitive channel in the distal nephron segments.[26,27] Sodium reabsorption is excessive even with dietary salt excess. Therapy is aimed at reducing dietary salt intake and the use of amiloride.[27]

CHLORIDE SHUNT (GORDON'S) SYNDROME

The chloride shunt syndrome (type 2 pseudohypoaldosteronism) is almost a mirror image of Bartter syndrome. The principal metabolic derangement is a hyperkalemic, hyperchloremic metabolic acidosis.[28] The primary cause is a defect in WNK1 or WNK4 (serine/threonine kinases).[4] Clinical variants include Gordon's syndrome and Spitzer-Weinstein syndrome,[2] with hyperkalemia, hyperchloremia, normal glomerular filtration rate, and hypertension. The hypertension is associated with low plasma aldosterone and plasma renin activity; blood pressure is often normal in children. Muscular weakness may be a presenting symptom of this disorder, and hypercalciuria is sometimes present.

A similar syndrome of metabolic acidosis with hyperkalemia is also associated with short stature and has been called Spitzer-Weinstein syndrome.[29,30] Thiazide diuretics have been used in the management of both Gordon's syndrome and Spitzer-Weinstein syndrome, with varying results.

FAMILIAL MEDITERRANEAN FEVER

Familial Mediterranean fever (FMF) is a hereditary systemic disorder with recurrent bouts of polyserositis and fever. Mutations in the *MEFV* (Mediterranean fever) gene result in abnormal forms of the protein pyrin.[31] This protein, localized mainly in neutrophils, functions to inhibit the chemotactic factor C5a. Unimpeded chemotaxis promotes the release of inflammatory cytokines and factors including C-reactive protein, fibrinogen, interleukin-6, interleukin-1, tumor necrosis factor α, and interleukin-8.[31,32] The peritoneal fluids of FMF patients contain low levels of the inhibitor to C5a and interleukin-8.[33]

Episodes last from 2 to 4 days with severe peritonitis, pleuritis, arthritis, and other serosal sites associated with a rash and high fever. Certain individuals develop amyloidosis and the nephrotic syndrome. This amyloid kidney can lead to chronic renal failure and hence is of interest to nephrologists.[32,33]

The disease is far more common in people of Mediterranean origin with high carrier rates among Arabic, Turkish, Armenian, Ashkenazi Jewish, and Sephardic Jewish people, and especially Jewish people from North Africa. Many in the last group have a specific mutation of the *MEFV* gene that is associated with progression to renal failure and with more serious recurrent attacks of fever and serositis.[31–33]

The therapeutic goal for FMF is to effectively protect against FMF attacks and FMF-related amyloidosis, and colchicine is the drug of choice (Table 46-4).[34] Its mode of action is to block activation of neutrophils by binding β-tubulin and producing β-tubulin–colchicine complexes. These actions result in inhibition of assembly of microtubules and mitotic spindle formation. Ultimately, colchicine moderates chemokines and prostanoids and inhibition of adhesion molecules in neutrophils and endothelial cells.[32,34]

Table 46-4 Therapeutic Options in Familial Mediterranean Fever

Drug	Dose
Colchicine, PO	Children: 0.5–1.0 mg/day Adults: 1.0–2.0 mg/day
Colchicine, IV	1.0 mg/wk
Anti–TNF-α monoclonal antibodies	0.8 mg/kg/wk, IV infusion
Interferon alfa	3–10 million IU (variable), SC injection

TNF-α, tumor necrosis factor α.

The minimal dose in adults is 1.0 mg/day and 0.5 to 1 mg/day in children.[34,35] Careful trials in children show that a dose of 0.07 mg/kg/day or 1.9 mg/m² in children younger than 5 years of age and 0.03 ± 0.02 mg/kg/day or 1.16 mg/m² in older children is effective. The plasma half-life is prolonged in patients with liver or renal failure. The major side effects are gastrointestinal in nature; therefore, many patients are placed on lactose-free diets and with evaluation for *Helicobacter pylori* infection.[31,34]

Children pose an especially vexing therapeutic challenge because overdose can be associated with massive organ failure.[36] A salutary effect of colchicine is improvement in height and weight velocity in children receiving prophylactic doses of this drug.[37]

Approximately 10% to 15% of FMF patients fail to respond to colchicine prophylactic therapy. These patients pose a special problem, and several strategies are being explored. First, laboratories are trying to develop colchicine analogues with less toxicity and a more effective therapeutic profile.[34] Intravenous colchicine has been used to treat FMF patients unresponsive to the orally administered drug.[38] Patients were treated with weekly injections of 1 mg, and decreases occurred in the number and mean severity of abdominal attacks, the number of overall attacks, chest attacks, the erythrocyte sedimentation rate, and the number of analgesic tablets administered. Anti–tumor necrosis factor α monoclonal antibodies have also been used,[39,40] especially in patients with protracted attacks. A dose of etanercept 0.8 mg/kg/week was used.[40] Some studies have also examined the role of interferon alfa as a therapeutic agent.[41]

The patients who appear to require the keenest attention to preventing attacks and the development of amyloid renal disease are those patients from North Africa who are homozygous for the M694V mutation of the *MEFV* gene.[42] The risk of amyloidosis is greatest in males bearing polymorphism a/a in the *SAAI* gene.

FABRY'S DISEASE

Fabry's disease is a rare X-linked lysosomal storage disorder due to partial or complete deficiency of the lysosomal enzyme α-galactosidase. Although Fabry's disease mainly affects males and most female carriers are asymptomatic or have milder disease than males, some heterozygous females develop full-blown disease because of X-chromosomal inactivation.[43]

The deficiency of α-galactosidase leads to accumulation of the glycosphingolipid globotriaosylceramide in visceral organs and vascular endothelium, which results in crises of pain, paresthesias of the hands and feet, and corneal and lenticular opacities. The skin shows characteristic lesions called *angiokeratomas*.[44] This cutaneous manifestation with acroparesthesia should strongly suggest Fabry's disease. Neuropathy is another prominent feature,[45] with accumulation of globotriosylceramide in Schwann cells, dorsal root ganglia, and the central nervous system. Cardiac manifestations include premature coronary artery disease, myocardial infarctions, angina, and arrhythmias.[45–47]

The nephrologic aspects include proteinuria, Maltese crosses on microscopy of the urine, and features of the Fanconi syndrome.[46] The nephrologist may also notice the angiokeratomas, which represent vasodilatation from lipid-laden vascular endothelial cells in a typical "bathing suit" distribution. Renal failure usually occurs by the fourth to fifth decades of life. The kidney is enlarged due to accumulation of globotriosylceramide in every renal cell type, but especially in Henle's loop and distal tubule, with early loss of concentrating ability. A renal biopsy specimen usually reveals inclusion bodies in the cytoplasm with concentric lamellation that have an onion skin appearance under electron microscopy.[46–48]

Therapy of Fabry's disease is directed at early diagnosis and enzyme replacement therapy.[49,50] A major breakthrough is the cloning and development of agalsidase alfa and beta, which have now been infused into hundreds of patients around the world (Table 46-5). Although early results are encouraging, long-term follow-up is essential.[51] In one study involving 201 patients and infusion for as long as 4.7 years, enzyme replacement therapy was associated with a decrease in serum creatinine.[52] The slope of serum creatinine decrease was steep during the first year of therapy and then flattened. When enzyme replacement therapy was begun in childhood, salutary changes in neuropathy, anhidrosis, and the need for antineuropathic analgesics occurred.[50]

The plethora of clinical trials has led to the formation of an international panel of physicians with expertise in Fabry's disease that can develop guidelines for the recognition, evaluation, and surveillance of disease-associated morbidities.[53] A Cochrane-type analysis has looked at agalsidase alfa (from a human cell line) and beta (from a Chinese hamster ovary cell line). Eleven trials can be analyzed. No direct head-to-head comparisons of the alfa and beta forms have been performed. Compared with placebo, enzyme replacement therapy has positive effects on the heart, kidneys, and central nervous system as well as the quality of life.[54] The major side effects of therapy are mild to moderate infusion reactions and the development of IgG antibodies against agalsidase alfa.[50]

Table 46-5 Therapy of Fabry's Disease

Enzyme	Source	Dose of Infusion
Agalsidase-α	Human cell line	0.2 mg/kg (males); 1.0–2.0 mg/kg (females)
Agalsidase-β	Chinese hamster ovary cell line	0.2 mg/kg (males), 1.0–2.0 mg/kg (females)

Serial testing of cardiopulmonary exercise[55] revealed improvement after enzyme replacement therapy, but no change in coronary arterial microvasculature was found.[56] A placebo-controlled trial of agalsidase beta showed slowing of progression to primary clinical event (renal, cardiac, cerebrovascular, or death) in patients with advanced Fabry's disease on therapy.[57] Patients whose creatinine clearance was greater than 55 mL/min/1.73 m^2 had a greater treatment versus placebo than those with lower clearance values.[57] A dose of 1 mg/kg body weight was employed. A drawback to this therapy is an annual cost of US$240,000, which makes lifelong therapy problematic.[58]

Home infusion therapy with agalsidase alfa at 0.02 mg/kg in males and 1 to 2 mg/kg in females has been used successfully.[59] No infusion-related reaction, described in three of 30 patients, required hospitalization.

Alternative therapeutic strategies include inhibition of the multiple drug resistance protein 1 (MDR1) in a Fabry mouse model using cyclosporin A.[60] Cyclosporin A treatment depleted globotriaosylceramide from Fabry mouse liver. Other strategies include the development of chemical chaperones, chemicals that deplete sites of substrate storage, and stem-cell therapy.[58]

At present, the U.S. Food and Drug Administration has approved only agalsidase beta, whereas both the alfa and beta forms have been approved in Europe.

References

1. Scriver CR, Beaudet AL, Valle D, et al (eds): The Metabolic Basis of Inherited Disease, Vol IV, 8th ed. New York: McGraw-Hill, 2001, pp 4891–5240.
2. Chesney RW, Novello AC: Defects of renal tubular transport. In Massry SG, Glassock R (eds): Textbook of Nephrology, 4th ed. Baltimore: Lippincott Williams & Wilkins, 2001, pp 462–476.
3. Christensen EI, Gburek J: Protein reabsorption in renal proximal tubule-function and dysfunction in kidney pathophysiology. Pediatr Nephrol 2004;19:714–721.
4. Guay-Woodford LM, Sedor JR: Disorders of tubular transport. NephSAP 2007;6:40–53.
5. Malandro MS, Kilberg MS: Molecular biology of mammalian amino acid transporters. Annu Rev Biochem 1996;65:305–336.
6. Nicoletta JA, Lande MB: Medical evaluation and treatment of urolithiasis. Pediatr Clin North Am 2006;53:479–491.
7. Chesney RW: Cystinuria. In Glassock R (ed): Current Therapy in Nephrology and Hypertension, 5th ed. St Louis: BC Decker, 2000, pp 96–98.
8. Glorieux FH, Scriver CR, Reade TM, et al: Use of phosphate and vitamin D to prevent dwarfism and rickets in X-linked hypophosphatemia. N Engl J Med 1972;287:481–487.
9. Latta K, Hisano S, Chan JC: Therapeutics of X-linked hypophosphatemic rickets. Pediatr Nephrol 1993;7:744–748.
10. Polisson RP, Martinez S, Khoury M, et al: Calcification of entheses associated with X-linked hypophosphatemic osteomalacia. N Engl J Med 1985;313:1–6.
11. Tieder M, Modai D, Samuel R, et al: Hereditary hypophosphatemic rickets with hypercalciuria. N Engl J Med 1985;312:611–617.
12. Gitelman HJ, Graham JB, Welt LG: A new familial disorder characterized by hypokalemia and hypomagnesemia. Trans Assoc Am Physicians 1966;79:221–235.
13. Jentsch TJ: Chloride transport in the kidney: Lessons from human disease and knockout mice. J Am Soc Nephrol 2005;16:1549–1561.
14. Zelikovic I: Molecular pathophysiology of tubular transport disorders. Pediatr Nephrol 2001;16:919–935.
15. Schlingmann KP, Sassen MC, Weber S, et al: Novel TRPM6 mutations in 21 families with primary hypomagnesemia and secondary hypocalcemia. J Am Soc Nephrol 2005;16:3061–3069.
16. Zelikovic I, Dabbagh S, Friedman AL, et al: Severe renal osteodystrophy without elevated serum immunoreactive parathyroid hormone concentrations in hypomagnesemia due to renal magnesium wasting. Pediatrics 1987;79:403–409.
17. Gahl WA, Thoene JG, Schneider JA: Cystinosis. N Engl J Med 2002;347:111–121.
18. Schneider JA, Clark KF, Greene AA, et al: Recent advances in the treatment of cystinosis. J Inherit Metab Dis 1995;18:387–397.
19. Gahl WA, Balog JZ, Kleta R: Nephropathic cystinosis in adults: Natural history and effects of oral cysteamine therapy. Ann Intern Med 2007;147:242–250.
20. Cochat P, Guibaud P, Baverel G: [Renal involvement in type I tyrosinemia]. Arch Pediatr 1994;1:417–418.
21. Chesney RW, Kaplan BS, Teitel D, et al: Metabolic abnormalities in the idiopathic Fanconi syndrome: Studies of carbohydrate metabolism in two patients. Pediatrics 1981;67:113–118.
22. Niaudet P: Genetic forms of nephrotic syndrome. Pediatr Nephrol 2004;19:1313–1318.
23. Bettinelli A, Basilico E, Metta MG, et al: Magnesium supplementation in Gitelman syndrome. Pediatr Nephrol 1999;13:311–314.
24. Karolyi L, Ziegler A, Pollak M, et al: Gitelman's syndrome is genetically distinct from other forms of Bartter's syndrome. Pediatr Nephrol 1996;10:551–554.
25. Kleta R, Bockenhauer D: Bartter syndromes and other salt-losing tubulopathies. Nephron Physiol 2006;104:73–80.
26. Geller DS, Zhang J, Zennaro MC, et al: Autosomal dominant pseudohypoaldosteronism type 1: Mechanisms, evidence for neonatal lethality, and phenotypic expression in adults. J Am Soc Nephrol 2006;17:1429–1436.
27. Kamynina E, Debonneville C, Hirt RP, et al: Liddle's syndrome: A novel mouse Nedd4 isoform regulates the activity of the epithelial Na(+) channel. Kidney Int 2001;60:466–471.
28. Cope G, Golbang A, O'Shaughnessy KM: WNK kinases and the control of blood pressure. Pharmacol Ther 2005;106:221–231.
29. Spitzer A, Edelmann CM Jr., Goldberg LD, et al: Short stature, hyperkalemia and acidosis: A defect in renal transport of potassium. Kidney Int 1973;3:251–257.
30. Weinstein SF, Allan DM, Mendoza SA: Hyperkalemia, acidosis, and short stature associated with a defect in renal potassium excretion. J Pediatr 1974;85:355–358.
31. Meyerhoff J: Mediterranean fever, familial, 2006. Available at: www.emedicine.com/med/topic1410.htm. Accessed January 2007.
32. Toubi E, Gershoni-Baruch R, Kuten A: Cisplatin treatment triggers familial Mediterranean fever attacks. Tumori 2003;89:80–81.
33. Medlej-Hashim M, Loiselet J, Lefranc G, et al: [Familial Mediterranean fever (FMF): From diagnosis to treatment]. Sante 2004;14:261–266.
34. Cerquaglia C, Diaco M, Nucera G, et al: Pharmacological and clinical basis of treatment of familial Mediterranean fever (FMF) with colchicine or analogues: An update. Curr Drug Targets Inflamm Allergy 2005;4:117–124.
35. Ozkaya N, Yalcinkaya F: Colchicine treatment in children with familial Mediterranean fever. Clin Rheumatol 2003;22:314–317.
36. Rigante D, La Torraca I, Avallone L, et al: The pharmacologic basis of treatment with colchicine in children with familial Mediterranean fever. Eur Rev Med Pharmacol Sci 2006;10:173–178.
37. Zung A, Barash G, Zadik Z, et al: Familial Mediterranean fever and growth: Effect of disease severity and colchicine treatment. J Pediatr Endocrinol Metab 2006;19:155–160.

38. Lidar M, Kedem R, Langevitz P, et al: Intravenous colchicine for treatment of patients with familial Mediterranean fever unresponsive to oral colchicine. J Rheumatol 2003;30:2620–2623.

39. Metyas S, Arkfeld DG, Forrester DM, et al: Infliximab treatment of familial Mediterranean fever and its effect on secondary AA amyloidosis. J Clin Rheumatol 2004;10:134–137.

40. Sakallioglu O, Duzova A, Ozen S: Etanercept in the treatment of arthritis in a patient with familial Mediterranean fever. Clin Exp Rheumatol 2006;24:435–437.

41. Tunca M, Akar S, Soyturk M, et al: The effect of interferon alpha administration on acute attacks of familial Mediterranean fever: A double-blind, placebo-controlled trial. Clin Exp Rheumatol 2004;22:S37–S40.

42. Ben-Chetrit E: Familial Mediterranean fever (FMF) and renal AA amyloidosis—phenotype-genotype correlation, treatment and prognosis. J Nephrol 2003;16:431–434.

43. Lidove O, Bekri S, Goizet C, et al: [Fabry disease: Proposed guidelines for its diagnosis, treatment and follow-up]. Presse Med 2007;36:1084–1097.

44. Jansen T, Brokalaki E, Hillen U, et al: [Manifestation of Fabry disease in a heterozygous female patient. New perspectives using enzyme replacement therapy]. Dtsch Med Wochenschr 2006;131:1590–1593.

45. Schiffmann R: Neuropathy and Fabry disease: Pathogenesis and enzyme replacement therapy. Acta Neurol Belg 2006;106:61–65.

46. Fabry disease monograph [Genzyme Therapeutics], 2003. Available at: http://www.fabrycommunity.com/healthcare/about/fc_p_hc_fabry-disease-monograph.asp. Accessed January 2007.

47. Meroni M, Sessa A, Battini G, et al: Kidney involvement in Anderson-Fabry disease. In Sessa A, Conte F, Meroni M, et al (eds): Hereditary Kidney Diseases. Basel: Karger, 1997, pp 178–184.

48. Peters FPJ, Sommer A, Vermeulen A, et al: Fabry's disease: A multidisciplinary disorder. Postgrad Med J 1997;73:710–712.

49. Beck M, Ricci R, Widmer U, et al: Fabry disease: Overall effects of agalsidase alfa treatment. Eur J Clin Invest 2004;34:838–844.

50. Ries M, Clarke JT, Whybra C, et al: Enzyme-replacement therapy with agalsidase alfa in children with Fabry disease. Pediatrics 2006;118:924–932.

51. Hopkin RJ, Bissler J, Grabowski GA: Comparative evaluation of alpha-galactosidase A infusions for treatment of Fabry disease. Genet Med 2003;5:144–153.

52. Schwarting A, Dehout F, Feriozzi S, et al: Enzyme replacement therapy and renal function in 201 patients with Fabry disease. Clin Nephrol 2006;66:77–84.

53. Eng CM, Germain DP, Banikazemi M, et al: Fabry disease: Guidelines for the evaluation and management of multi-organ system involvement. Genet Med 2006;8:539–548.

54. Lidove O, Joly D, Barbey F, et al: Clinical results of enzyme replacement therapy in Fabry disease: A comprehensive review of the literature. Int J Clin Pract 2007;61:293–302.

55. Bierer G, Balfe D, Wilcox WR, et al: Improvement in serial cardiopulmonary exercise testing following enzyme replacement therapy in Fabry disease. J Inherit Metab Dis 2006;29:572–579.

56. Elliott PM, Kindler H, Shah JS, et al: Coronary microvascular dysfunction in male patients with Anderson-Fabry disease and the effect of treatment with alpha galactosidase A. Heart 2006;92:357–360.

57. Banikazemi M, Bultas J, Waldek S, et al: Agalsidase-beta therapy for advanced Fabry disease: A randomized trial. Ann Intern Med 2007;146:77–86.

58. Schiffmann R: Enzyme replacement in Fabry disease: The essence is in the kidney. Ann Intern Med 2007;146:142–144.

59. Linthorst GE, Vedder AC, Ormel EE, et al: Home treatment for Fabry disease: Practice guidelines based on 3 years experience in the Netherlands. Nephrol Dial Transplant 2006;21:355–360.

60. Mattocks M, Bagovich M, De Rosa M, et al: Treatment of neutral glycosphingolipid lysosomal storage diseases via inhibition of the ABC drug transporter, MDR1. Cyclosporin A can lower serum and liver globotriaosyl ceramide levels in the Fabry mouse model. FEBS J 2006;273:2064–2075.

Further Reading

Beck M, Ricci R, Widmer U, et al: Fabry disease: Overall effects of agalsidase alfa treatment. Eur J Clin Invest 2004;34:838–844.

Gahl WA, Thoene JG, Schneider JA: Cystinosis. N Engl J Med 2002;347:111–121.

Guay-Woodford LM, Sedor JR: Disorders of tubular transport. NephSAP 2007;6:40–53.

Kleta R, Bockenhauer D: Bartter syndromes and other salt-losing tubulopathies. Nephron Physiol 2006;104:73–80.

Meyerhoff J: Mediterranean fever, familial, 2006. Available at: http://www.emedicine.com/med/topic1410.htm. Accessed January 2007.

Scriver CR, Beaudet AL, Valle D, et al (eds): The Metabolic Basis of Inherited Disease, Vol IV, 8th ed. New York: McGraw Hill, 2001, pp 4891–5240.

Chapter 47

Prospects for Gene Therapy

Enyu Imai, Yoshitaka Isaka, and Yoshitsugu Takabatake

The primary goal of this chapter is to discuss prospects for gene therapy in the kidney. We briefly review general concepts of gene therapy and vectors for this purpose. We discuss specific considerations unique to the kidney that affect gene therapy approaches to renal diseases, based on current data from clinical trials and studies in experimental renal diseases.

DEFINITION OF GENE THERAPY AND GENERAL CONSIDERATIONS

Gene therapy is defined as the delivery of DNA or RNA coding a particular sequence into targeted nongermline cells by vectors to provide beneficial effects by inducing or inhibiting synthesis of a particular protein(s). Gene therapy can provide correction of cellular dysfunction by expressing a gene, the addition of a new function for a cell by transferring exogenous genes, and inhibition of unfavorable cellular action by introducing counteracting genes. Gene therapy targeting germline cells is ethically prohibited.

General considerations in designing gene therapy are delivery, expression, and safety. Delivery refers to the ability to introduce the gene of interest where it needs to affect the disease process. Gene therapy approaches can be divided into in vivo and ex vivo. In vivo gene therapy uses either viral or nonviral vectors for gene delivery and is treated as a drug to be administered with or without a specific delivery system. Localized gene delivery can be used for systemic delivery of the product (e.g., skeletal muscle is an ideal organ for producing secretory proteins for systemic delivery). Ex vivo gene therapy refers to the genetic modification of cells or organs by gene transfer outside the body and subsequent placement of genetically engineered tissue into a patient. The source of cells may be from patients or be generic human or animal cells appropriately altered genetically. Xenotransplantation is an attractive target for ex vivo gene therapy if rejection can be surmounted. If universal donor cells could be developed, the cost of ex vivo gene therapy would decrease and its application would expand dramatically.

Expression of a particular gene must be controllable. Given that overexpression of a therapeutic protein may cause harmful effects, regulation of transgene expression is an important issue to be considered. The issue of safety is an important problem not only for patients, but also for the population at large. Toxic effects of gene therapy include inflammation, injury, functional damage to the transduced organ, and induction of gene mutations that may cause cancer. These considerations must be examined in the context of the particular disease to be treated: its severity and clinical course, alternative treatment available, organs affected, and so forth. Consideration needs to be given to selecting patients at certain stages of disease, perhaps those with the worst prognosis, and to carefully weighing risks and benefits.

CONSIDERATIONS FOR APPLICATION TO RENAL DISEASE

The kidney is a complex organ whose function depends on its architecture, which is composed of glomeruli, tubules, vasculature, and interstitium. Consequently, it is not possible to introduce genes into all its various cell types by a single method. In principle, five routes to transfer genes by injection into the kidney exist whether by ex vivo or by in vivo methods: renal artery, renal vein, parenchyme, subcapsular region, and ureter in the retrograde direction.

VECTORS

Because excellent detailed articles exist on the vector for gene therapy, only a brief summary is provided. The advantage and disadvantage of various vector systems have been discussed extensively[1-3] and are subjects of intense ongoing investigation.

Viral Vectors

Retroviruses are well studied for ex vivo application because of their broad host range and their ability to give long-term expression through proviral integration into the host genome.

However, in vivo fragility and low titers limit in vivo applications, as does the requirement for cell division for DNA integration. In addition, human gene therapy trials using retroviral vector for X-linked severe combined immunodeficiency indicate that quasi-random integration of transgene can induce malignant transformation in transduced cells.[4]

Adenoviruses are DNA viruses that have a wide host range and survive robustly in the circulation. High titers of replication-deficient adenovirus can easily be generated, and the virus can infect nondividing cells. The duration of expression is largely limited by a T-cell response to low levels of adenoviral proteins and of the transgene itself produced in the transduced cells. The ideal vector would contain only the *cis* elements required for packaging, namely, the inverted terminal repeats and the packaging signal, and progress toward the construction of such a vector has been reported.[5] However, these advances do not circumvent the antibody response to adenoviral proteins, which precludes secondary infection with the same serotype, although not with a different serotype.[6] The nonspecific inflammatory response that can be produced even by empty vector may also limit the amount of adenovirus that can be delivered. However, adenoviral vectors have been used for treatment of cancer because of their efficiency of gene transfer and also because cellular toxicity and immunogenicity may enhance the antitumor effects.

Vectors based on recombinant adeno-associated virus (rAAV) have attracted much attention as potent gene delivery vehicles because of sustainable expression of the transgene and excellent preclinical safety.[7] AAV vectors package and deliver an inactive single-stranded DNA genome that is converted into active double-stranded DNA in the nucleus. A new rAAV designed using the serotype 5 AAV inverted terminal repeat has enhanced gene expression.[8] The AAV integrates at high frequency at a specific region on human chromosome 19 in a reaction that requires the AAV *rep* gene. After infection with helper viruses such as adenovirus or herpesvirus that provide factors necessary for replication, the virus can enter a lytic cycle. However, it appears that when rAAV is used as a gene delivery vehicle, most transgene expression results from extrachromosomal viral genomes that persist as double-stranded circular or linear episomes,[9] which decreases the risk of insertional mutagenesis. rAAV has drawn attention because of the potential for gene targeting through homologous recombination, which allows efficient, high-fidelity, nonmutagenic gene repair in a host cell.[7]

Lentivirus-based vectors are used for gene delivery into nondividing cells.[10] Vesicular stomatitis virus–pseudotyped lentiviral vectors can be delivered directly in vivo. Stable, long-term transgene expression has been observed without detectable pathologic consequence. Weak and localized but stable expression of transgene for 3 months was reported in the outer medulla and corticomedullary junction of the kidney after parenchymal or ureteral injections.[11]

Nonviral Vectors

Nonviral vectors for gene delivery include naked DNA or DNA in combination with liposomes or with pegylated (polyethylene glycol-conjugated) nanoparticles with multiple components.[12] Hydrodynamic delivery of plasmid DNA has been reported with successful expression of the transgene in kidney and liver. Maruyama and colleagues[13] reported that the rapid injection of naked DNA with large volume of saline into the vena cava induced potent gene transfer into the liver and kidney. Electroporation after hydrodynamic delivery of plasmid, small DNA, or small RNA provides an efficient gene transfer into the kidney.[14] To target cancer, pegylated nanoparticles with multiple components are the most promising nonviral vector for systemic delivery.[15] Such vectors are relatively nontoxic and nonimmunogenic, but generally the transduction efficiency in vivo is less than with viral vectors and the duration of the gene expression is relatively short. Repeated administration may be needed.

RNA Interference

The discovery of RNA interference (RNAi) has changed the strategy of gene therapy. RNAi is an endogenous mechanism for posttranscriptional gene regulation. Therapeutic RNAi, initiated by the introduction of double-stranded RNA into the cell, leads to the sequence-specific destruction of endogenous RNA.[16] Long endogenous or exogenous double-stranded RNAs are cleaved intracellularly by the protein Dicer, which contains RNase III domains, leading to the formation of small interfering RNAs (siRNAs) (21–23 nt long) with a symmetric 2 nt overhang at its 3′ end and a 5′ phosphate and 3′ hydroxy group. One strand of the siRNA duplex, termed the guide strand, is incorporated into a nuclease-containing multiprotein complex called the RNA-induced silencing complex, whereas the second, passenger strand is released and degraded. Once incorporated into RNA-induced silencing complex, the guide strand guides this complex to the target mRNA and induces endonucleolytic cleavage. This cleavage leads to the rapid degradation of the entire mRNA molecule due to the generation of its unprotected RNA ends, whereas the RNA-induced silencing complex is recovered for further cleavage cycles.

Novel therapeutics using RNAi are being actively developed partly by learning lessons from the setbacks experienced with antisense oligonucleotides and conventional DNA vectors. Indeed, a number of biotech companies are actively working in this area to make RNAi-based drugs a reality. Phase I clinical trials have already been initiated for age-related macular degeneration, a vascular-proliferative disorder of the retina using siRNA for vascular endothelial growth factor or vascular endothelial growth factor receptor and for respiratory syncytial virus infection.

Viral vectors expressing siRNA that have been intensively investigated for application to in vivo gene therapy in animal models include lentivirus,[17] adenovirus,[18] AAV,[19] and baculovirus.[20] Nonviral delivery of siRNAs or siRNA expression vectors has also been intensively studied. Chemical modifications, encapsulation of the siRNA in microparticles or liposomes, and/or binding siRNAs to particulate carriers have been developed to circumvent the shortcomings of the naked siRNAs. The goals of these approaches are (1) prolonged duration of the RNAi activity by stabilization, (2) improvement of the cellular tropism, (3) enhancement of the silencing activity, and/or (4) selective tissue delivery.

siRNAs are rather stable compared with single-stranded RNA in serum, but will still be degraded within a few hours due to the cleavage activity of an RNase. Therefore, the development of chemical modifications that make them resistant to RNase is the rational approach. These include the use of boranophosphate[21] and the phosphothioates 2'-deoxy, 2'-fluoro,[22] and 2'-O-Me, but it has yet to be fully elucidated which modification best increases the stability.

Another approach to increase the plasma stability and/ or direct the preferential uptake by the target cells is the use of envelope packaged siRNA. Various liposomes are reported to be efficient in vivo, including oligofectamine,[23] cationic 1,2 dioleoyl-3-trimethylammonium-propane (DOTAP) liposomes,[24] neutral 1,2-dioleoyl-sn-glycero-3-phosphatidylcholine (DOPC) liposomes,[25] and gelatin.[26] Urban-Klein and colleagues[27] demonstrated that the noncovalent complexation of siRNAs with low molecular weight polyethylenimine efficiently stabilizes siRNAs and in vivo systemic delivery of the polyethylenimine-complexed siRNAs targeting HER2 reduced tumor growth.

Several attempts have been directed at realizing specific tissue tropism by simple delivery (e.g., intravenous injection). Song and colleagues[28] developed an antibody-conjugated siRNA technique. First, the authors constructed a conjugate composed of an antibody against a cell surface receptor and a basic cellular protein protamine, and then this conjugate was noncovalently linked to siRNAs targeting the gene of interest. They injected an antibody against human immunodeficiency virus envelope glycoprotein pg160-protamine conjugate mixed with siRNAs targeting c-Myc, transformed 3T3 cell double minute 2 (MDM2), and vascular endothelial growth factor intravenously as well as intratumorally in a xenograft tumor mouse model. As a result, significant tumor growth retardation was observed by targeting pg160-positive cells. In another attempt, polyethylene glycol strands were conjugated to the outer surface of a liposome, and specific antibodies attached to these polyethylene glycol strands, creating a pegylated immunoliposome.[29] The authors successfully delivered this siRNA expression vector to an implanted brain tumor across the blood-brain barrier and the tumor cell membrane by conjugating it with a monoclonal antibody to a transferrin receptor.

Recently it has been reported that siRNAs and short hairpin RNAs (shRNAs) have broad and complicated effects beyond the selective silencing of target genes when introduced into cells. This is of critical importance because siRNAs are currently being explored for their potential therapeutic use.

High sequence specificity is the major characteristic of RNAi. However, several reports raise questions about its specificity. Jackson and colleagues[30] report in vitro silencing of nontargeted genes containing as few as 11 contiguous nucleotides of identity to the siRNA. These results demonstrate that siRNAs may cross-react with targets of limited sequence similarity. There is no doubt that siRNAs have advantages over conventional antisense oligonucleotides in their sequence specificity, but these off-target effects must always be kept in mind when exploring RNAi in clinical applications.

Another nonspecific effect that deserves attention is the interferon response, which is the first line of defense system activated by double-stranded RNA derived from viral infection. Activation of interferon responses results not only in the up-regulation of many interferon-related genes but also in inhibition of cellular protein synthesis and induction of apoptosis.

Because siRNAs and shRNAs are artificial orthologues of microRNAs, siRNA- and shRNA-mediated RNAi share the components used for the endogenous microRNA-induced gene activation. Therefore, it is possible that the transfections of siRNA or shRNA, especially at high doses, would interfere with normal cellular physiology that is mediated by micro-RNAs. Grimm and colleagues[19] systematically investigated the long-term effect of the introduction of shRNA based on AAV type 8 in adult mice after intravenous infusion. An evaluation of 49 distinct AAV/shRNA vectors, unique in length and sequence and directed against six targets, showed that 36 resulted in dose-dependent liver injury, with 23 ultimately causing death. Morbidity was associated with the down-regulation of liver-derived microRNAs, indicating possible competition of microRNAs with shRNAs for limiting cellular factors, including the nuclear exportin-5. They also found that the risk of oversaturating endogenous small RNA pathways can be minimized by optimizing shRNA dose and sequence.

APPLICATION TO KIDNEY DISEASES

Kidney Transplantation

The transplant kidney is an ideal setting for gene therapy. After the kidney is harvested from the donor, ex vivo gene therapy can be easily performed on the kidney and the surplus vector can be flushed out before transplantation, which reduces the harmful effects from inappropriate delivery to other organs. Gene products could be delivered for four purposes: (1) to reduce ischemia/reperfusion injury, (2) to decrease organ antigenicity for acute rejection, (3) to induce tolerance or block the effector arm of the immune system for chronic rejection, and (4) to improve organ preservation.

Candidate genes (given individually or in combination) might include donor major histocompatibility complex class I or II molecules,[31,32] cytotoxic T-lymphocyte antigen 4 immunoglobulin,[33–36] interleukin (IL)-4, IL-10,[37] Fas ligand,[38] galectin,[39] adenoviral E3 gene, soluble tumor necrosis factor receptor, IL-1 receptor antagonist, adhesion molecules, transforming growth factor β (TGF-β),[40] hepatocyte growth factor (HGF),[41,42] and catalase.[43] Inhibition of the following genes might provide beneficial effects: nuclear factor κB (NF-κB),[44] nitric oxide synthase,[45] and CD28.[36]

Acute rejection occurs as a consequence of T-cell activation. In this process, the engagement of T-cell receptor and alloantigens presented by major histocompatibility complex molecules is essential, and the activation of costimulator signals, such as CD28 and B7, is also important. Tomasoni and colleagues[35] injected an adenoviral vector encoding the chimeric fusion protein, cytotoxic T-lymphocyte antigen 4 immunoglobulin, ex vivo into the artery of Brown Norway rat kidneys, which were then transplanted into Lewis rats. The rats that received cytotoxic T-lymphocyte antigen 4 immunoglobulin gene therapy had inhibited T-cell activation and prolonged survival by 50 days. Azuma and colleagues[44] investigated whether transfection of NF-κB decoys into the donor kidney would prevent acute rejection and prolong graft survival. They introduced NF-κB decoy DNA into the transplant kidney by microbubble-mediated gene transfer. The NF-κB decoy improved renal function and histology of the transplant kidney by reducing expression of NF-κB–regulated cytokines and adhesion molecules. In the early phase of kidney transplantation, when the transplant kidney is exposed to insults by ischemia/reperfusion, high doses of the immunosuppressant HGF may afford protection against acute kidney injury and may enhance tubular cell regeneration. Isaka and colleagues[42] studied the renoprotective action of *HGF* gene transfer using a model of porcine kidney transplantation after 10 minutes of warm ischemia injury. The harvested right kidney was transfected with *HGF* gene injected via the renal artery with hydropressure followed by electroporation. After removing the left kidney, the genetically modified kidney was transplanted. The warm ischemia induced tubular injury in the control kidney, followed by tubulointerstitial fibrosis, whereas HGF-transfected kidneys showed no initial tubular damage and little fibrosis at 6 months posttransplantation.

Short-term outcome of clinical transplantation has improved remarkably with the development of better immunosuppressants, but the long-term outcome of transplantation has not. Benigni and colleagues[36] applied rAAV for cytotoxic T-lymphocyte antigen 4 immunoglobulin gene transfer to protect major histocompatibility complex–mismatched renal allografts from chronic rejection. The expression of the transgene lasted for 90 days, renal function was preserved, and glomerulosclerosis and interstitial fibrosis were ameliorated.

Additional problems specific to xenotransplantation are hyperacute rejection and acute rejection of the transplanted kidney, which are caused by antibody against alpha-1,3-galactosidase and complement-mediated hyperacute rejections. Ex vivo gene transfer of H-transferase[46] and CD59 or decay-accelerating factor[47] before transplantation may be worthy of consideration.

Renal Cancer (Renal Cell Carcinoma)

The most challenging issue for gene therapy in cancer is that of metastatic disease. Because localized renal cell carcinoma is an indication for surgical treatment, advanced renal cell carcinoma has been a target of gene therapy and has been confirmed to be a considerable success. Most of the cases of gene therapy for renal cell carcinoma use immunotherapy, which strengthens the immunity against cancer-specific antigens. IL-2 is a cytokine with potent immunomodulatory activities including activation of T cells and natural killer cells. The administration of IL-2 protein results in significant clinical benefits for patients with renal cell carcinoma.[48] Despite producing beneficial effects with some durable remissions, recombinant IL-2 therapy is often limited by potential life-threatening side effects, including pulmonary edema, hypertension, anemia, and organ dysfunction resulting from capillary leak syndrome. An alternative approach to IL-2 cancer immunotherapy would be an effective delivery of small amounts of IL-2 directly to the tumor microenvironment by gene therapy. This can be approached by direct injection of IL-2 gene into tumor cells for local secretion or by ex vivo introduction of IL-2 gene to tumor cells in culture. Galanis and colleagues[49] reported the effects of direct injection of leuvectin (a cationic lipid mixture with a plasmid vector containing the human IL-2 gene) into the tumors. They treated 14 patients with renal cell carcinoma, and two patients responded partially with a reduction in the size of tumor and two had regression of the injected lesion by more than 25%. Schmidt-Wolf and colleagues[50] also reported IL-2 immunotherapy by ex vivo gene transfer of IL-2 gene to autologous natural killer–like T lymphocytes. This report did not identify the patients but treated one patient with advanced renal cell carcinoma and eight patients with colon cancer with multiple metastasis. Six patients remained in progression, and three patients showed no change with treatment, suggesting that it is somewhat effective in some cases. Ongoing clinical trials for renal cell carcinoma are encouraging in that IL-2 gene therapy using nonviral vector systems can decrease the tumor burden.

Wittig and colleagues[51] reported immunotherapy by therapeutic vaccination with IL-7 and granulocyte/macrophage colony–stimulating factor (GM-CSF) gene-transfected tumor cells. The genetically modified autologous tumor cells expressing IL-7 and GM-CSF were introduced in patients, and in consequence, they showed the capability of autologous expression–modified and –immunomodulated tumor cell vaccines to stimulate a strong immune response in some patients with metastatic cancer even in the presence of a large tumor. In Japan, GM-CSF gene therapy for renal cell carcinoma is in progress, and a case of regression was observed but no conclusive result is reported yet.[52]

Glomerulonephritis and Renal Fibrosis

Gene therapy for experimental glomerulonephritis and interstitial fibrosis has been energetically tackled. For an effective molecular intervention, the choice of the target tissue or cells for gene transfer is crucial. Strategies for gene therapy can be divided into two categories: tissue- or organ-specific delivery and systemic delivery. It has been reported that growth factors and cytokines are involved in the progression of glomerular and tubulointerstitial diseases. Therefore, numerous DNA- or RNA-based biopharmaceuticals attempt to control disease progression by inhibiting these genes. The potential therapeutics include antisense oligonucleotides, decoys, ribozymes, DNAzymes, and siRNA. In this case, the therapeutic gene has to be delivered to the specific tissue or organ, for example, mesangial cells in glomerular diseases or interstitial fibroblasts in tubulointerstitial diseases. Conversely, several somatic tissues, such as skeletal muscle, can be used to introduce the foreign gene if the transgene product is secreted in plasma.

Recent understanding of the molecular pathogenesis has led to the identification of new therapeutic targets. One of these targets is TGF-β, which plays an important role in the progression of glomerulosclerosis and interstitial fibrosis.[53] The introduction of antisense oligonucleotides,[54,55] DNAzyme,[56] or siRNA[57] against TGF-β into glomerular mesangial cells[54,56,57] and interstitial fibroblasts[55] resulted in the suppression of TGF-β and of the consequent glomerular extracellular matrix expansion in rats with anti–Thy-1 glomerulonephritis and of the interstitial fibrosis in unilateral ureteral obstruction (UUO) (a model of acute tubulointerstitial fibrosis), respectively. Another target is early growth response gene 1 (*egr-1*), a transcription factor involved in mesangial cell proliferation and phenotypic alteration of myofibroblasts. The transfer of antisense oligonucleotides[58] and DNAzyme[59] against *egr-1* prevented *egr-1* expression and eventually inhibited mesangial proliferation in anti–Thy-1 glomerulonephritis and interstitial phenotypic alteration in UUO rats, respectively.

Double-stranded oligonucleotides containing a *cis* binding element for a particular transcription factor can act as a decoy and inhibit transactivation of the particular promoter coding the *cis* element. E2F decoy inhibits cell proliferation by mimicking the *cis* element of the promoter regions of dihydrofolate reductase, c-myc, cdc2 kinase, and proliferating cell nuclear antigen, whereas NF-κB decoy suppresses inflammatory genes including IL-1, IL-6, IL-8, intracellular cell adhesion molecule 1, vascular cell adhesion molecule, and endothelial leukocyte adhesion molecule. E2F decoy[60] and NF-κB decoy[61] successfully inhibit the mesangial proliferation and extracellular matrix expansion in experimental glomerulonephritis. The overexpression of inhibitory molecules in signal transduction has also been reported. The introduction of Smad-7 inhibited TGF-β action and suppressed renal fibrosis in the UUO model.[62,63] The inhibition of NF-κB by gene therapy of a truncated IκBα, a dominant negative-type molecule, reduced renal fibrosis in a protein-overload model.[64]

Skeletal muscle-targeted gene therapy for renal diseases is more practical and less invasive because it provides high efficiency and long-lasting gene expression compared with the kidney.[65] Inhibitory molecules against TGF-β were extensively studied for muscle-targeted gene therapy. The transduction of decorin,[66] a natural inhibitor against TGF-β, or the artificial soluble receptor for TGF-β[67] in muscle cells led to the competitive inhibition against glomerular TGF-β, which resulted in the amelioration of glomerulosclerosis. Gene therapy of the artificial soluble receptor for platelet-derived growth factor B[68] also inhibited glomerulosclerosis in anti–Thy-1 glomerulonephritis. Electroporation-mediated gene transfer into skeletal muscle with the soluble form interferon gamma receptor successfully induced the interferon gamma/Fc protein in the serum and ameliorated murine lupus nephritis model.[69] Intravenous administration of adenoviral vector coding for the adrenomedullin gene significantly improves the renal histology of streptozotocin-induced diabetic rats.[70]

HGF is a multifunctional cytokine that regulates mitosis, angiogenesis, morphogenesis, cell movement, and apoptosis.[71] As HGF acts against TGF-β and recombinant HGF administration suppresses renal fibrosis in the UUO model,[72] HGF gene therapy was examined in the UUO model. The transduction of HGF in the kidney suppressed renal fibrosis in the UUO model.[73,74] The introduction of plasmid coding 7ND, a dominant-negative type antagonist against membrane cofactor protein 1, into the kidney[75] attenuated the interstitial fibrosis in a protein-overload proteinuria model. Intraparenchymal injection of adenoviral vector encoding IL-10 suppresses proteinuria of focal segmental glomerulosclerosis in a mouse model.[76]

The therapeutic impact of siRNA or siRNA expression vectors targeting the kidney has been reported. For example, Hamar and colleagues[77] described the administration of siRNAs targeting Fas via the tail vein or renal vein of mice with ischemia-reperfusion injury. A single hydrodynamic injection of Fas siRNA decreased its mRNA and protein expression in the kidney fourfold. Kidneys from mice that received Fas siRNA 2 days earlier had less tubular damage and apoptosis. siRNA expression vector targeting Fas or caspase 8, transfected via the inferior vena cava[78] or targeting the C3 component of complement transfected via tail vein,[29] have also been reported to decrease ischemic-reperfusion injury. Kushibiki and colleagues[26] investigated the in vivo transfection efficiency of a plasmid DNA expressing TGF-β1 receptor type II siRNA with various cationized gelatins of nonviral carriers and evaluated the antifibrotic effect on a mouse model of UUO. The complex of a plasmid DNA with a biodegradable cationized gelatin prevented DNase digestion, decreasing the molecular size and making the net charge of the complex positive, which led to facilitated and stable gene expression. The injection of the complex of the plasmid DNA expressing TGF-β1 receptor type II siRNA and the cationized gelatin via the ureter of the UUO model mice led to the marked decrease in the TGF-β

receptor expression and the collagen content of mice kidney, and eventually suppressed the progression of renal interstitial fibrosis. Takabatake and colleagues[57] demonstrated that the injection of synthetic siRNAs or siRNA expression vector via the renal artery, followed by electroporation, could be an effective therapeutic approach to the glomeruli in which there is a central region of inflammatory response in the initiation and progression of various kidney diseases. RNAi targeting against TGF-β1 significantly suppressed TGF-β1 mRNA and protein expression, thereby ameliorating the progression of matrix expansion in experimental glomerulonephritis.

Genetically modified macrophage-like cells have been developed for the treatment of anti–glomerular basement membrane glomerulonephritis. Yokoo and colleagues[79] differentiated bone marrow cells into $CD11b^+CD18^+$ cells, which migrate into inflamed glomeruli. The genetically modified macrophage-like cells migrated into inflamed glomeruli in experimental anti–glomerular basement membrane antibody-induced glomerulonephritis and supplied the functional secretory protein, IL-1 receptor antagonist, into the inflamed glomeruli.[80] These results suggest that reconstitution of bone marrow for the continuous supply of anti-inflammatory cells may be a useful strategy for the treatment of chronic inflammation.

Renal Anemia

Erythropoietin (EPO), which is secreted from the kidney in response to hypoxia, is an essential stimulator of erythropoiesis. The shortage of EPO leads to anemia in most cases of advanced renal failure. EPO gene transcription is driven by a transcription factor, hypoxia inducible factor 2α, in tubulointerstitial fibroblasts, which are the responsive cells in EPO production.

Gene therapy for renal anemia has been a challenge for 15 years. Recombinant human EPO is commercially available for clinical use. However, demand for successful gene therapy still remains because recombinant human EPO is relatively expensive, and the treatment must last a long time.

A variety of methods have been reported for experimental EPO gene therapy. The simplest method is injection of plasmid encoding the EPO gene into skeletal muscle followed by electroporation.[81] Maruyama and colleagues[82] treated experimental renal anemia with gene therapy and showed increases in hematocrit in uremic rats. Long-term EPO gene expression was also achieved using a lentiviral vector.[83] Adenovirus-mediated EPO gene transfer also succeeded in long-term EPO delivery from skeletal muscle.[84] Transplantation of genetically modified fibroblasts succeeded in long-term supply of the EPO gene.[85] Rinsch and colleagues[86] used homozygous EPO SV40 T antigen (EPO-Tagh) transgenic mice, which have a target disruption in the 5′ untranslated region of the EPO gene that causes severe anemia by dramatically decreasing EPO expression. They demonstrated that the renal anemia of EPO-Tagh mice was corrected by implantation of encapsulated fibroblasts secreting EPO.

Inducible gene therapy of EPO by mifepristone administration has been reported.[87] Two plasmids encoding a gene switch responsive to mifepristone and an inducible transgene for EPO were introduced into skeletal muscle by electroporation. Intraperitoneal administration of mifepristone resulted in an increase in serum EPO, leading to an increase in hematocrit. A recent development in EPO gene therapy is the use of an inducible gene responsive to the degree of hypoxia. Binley and colleagues[88] developed an oxygen-regulated gene therapy strategy by using an AAV vector carrying the EPO gene driven by the Oxford Biomedica hypoxia response element (OBHRE) promoter, which responds to hypoxia by binding of hypoxia inducible factor 1α. They injected the AAV vector carrying OBHRE-EPO into hindlimb skeletal muscle of EPO-Tagh mice and observed an increase in the hematocrit from 20% to 50%. The hematocrit stabilized at normal levels and did not increase to the polycythemic range because the transactivation of OBHRE promoter was switched off by oxygenation of peripheral blood cells. The constant regulation persisted for at least 5 months. This result suggested that the OBHRE promoter gives rise to physiologically controlled regulation of EPO gene expression in an anemic mouse model. This approach for renal anemia may provide more physiologic and less expensive treatment than recombinant human EPO.

Meanwhile, human EPO gene therapy was reported from Israel. Lippin and colleagues[89] harvested subcutaneous dermal samples (dermal core, 30–35 × 1.5–2.5 mm) from 13 patients. The *EPO* gene was transfected into the dermal core by adenoviral vector, and the transfected dermal core was implanted into the forearm of 10 patients. The EPO level was increased on day 1 and persisted for 14 days. The EPO level was decreased on day 14, coincident with infiltration of CD8 T cells into the dermal core. This first human trial of gene therapy with EPO was successful, and no adverse event was observed.

Hemodialysis Vascular Access

The number of patients with end-stage renal disease has been increasing worldwide and is expected to reach 210 million by 2010. More than 140 million will be treated with hemodialysis. Vascular access is critical for good hemodialysis treatment and the creation of a good native arteriovenous fistula is a key to successful dialysis because arteriovenous fistulas have a relative low rate of infection and thrombosis.[90] Venous stenosis followed by thrombosis is caused by neointimal hyperplasia and vascular remodeling. Therefore, the ideal therapy for vascular stenosis is likely to be an intervention to block both adverse remodeling and neointimal hyperplasia. Gene therapy for neointimal hyperplasia in AVF has been proposed.[91] Inhibition of neointimal hyperplasia in experimental models has been achieved by gene therapy with endothelial nitric oxide synthase, cyclin-dependent kinase inhibitor p21[KIP1], GATA-6, GAX, HGF, and decoy of E2F.[92] A phase II trial of E2F decoy is currently in progress in arteriovenous grafts.[90]

References

1. Imai E, Isaka Y: Perspectives for gene therapy in renal disease. Intern Med 2004;43:85–96.
2. Kelley V, Sukhatme V: Gene transfer in the kidney. Am J Physiol 1999;276:F1–F9.
3. Kay M, Glorioso J, Naldini L: Viral vectors for gene therapy: The art of turning infectious agents into vehicles of therapeutics. Nat Med 2001;7:33–40.
4. Hacein-Bey-Abina S, von Kalle C, Schmidt M, et al: A serious adverse event after successful gene therapy for X-linked severe combined immunodeficiency. N Engl J Med 2003;348:255–256.
5. Kockanek S, Clemens P, Mitani K, et al: A new adenoviral vector: Replication of all viral coding sequences with 28kb of DNA independently expressing both full-length dystrophin and b-galactosidase. Proc Natl Acad Sci U S A 1996;93:5731–5736.
6. Mastrangeli A, Harvey B, Yao J, et al: "Sero-switch" adenovirus-mediated in vivo gene transfer: Circumvention of anti-adenovirus vector administration by changing the adenovirus serotype. Hum Gene Ther 1996;7:79–87.
7. Vasileva A, Jessberger R: Precise hit: Adeno-associated virus in gene targeting. Nat Rev Microbiol 2005;3:837–847.
8. Bec C, Douar A: Gene therapy progress and prospects vectorology: Design and production of expression cassettes. Gene Ther 2006;13:805–813.
9. Nakai H, Yant SR, Storm TA, et al: Extrachromosomal recombinant adeno-associated virus vector genomes are primarily responsible for stable liver transduction. J Virol 2001;75:6969–6976.
10. Naldini L, Blomer U, Gallay P, et al: In vivo gene delivery and stable transduction of nondividing cells by a lentiviral vector. Science 1996;272:263–267.
11. Gusella G, Fedorova E, Hanss B, et al: Lentiviral gene transduction of kidney. Hum Gene Ther 2002;13:407–414.
12. Li S, Huang L: Gene therapy progress and prospects: Non-viral gene therapy by systemic delivery. Gene Ther 2006;13:1313–1319.
13. Maruyama H, Higuchi N, Nishikawa Y, et al: Kidney-targeted naked DNA transfer by retrograde renal vein injection in rats. Hum Gene Ther 2002;13:455–468.
14. Tsujie M, Isaka Y, Nakamura H, et al: Electroporation-mediated gene transfer that targets glomeruli. J Am Soc Nephrol 2001;12:949–954.
15. Brannon-Peppas S, Blanchette J: Nanoparticle and targeted systems for cancer therapy. Adv Drug Deliv Rev 2004;56:1649–1659.
16. Elbashir S, Harborth J, Lendeckel W, et al: Duplexes of 21-nucleotide RNAs mediate RNA interference in cultured mammalian cells. Nature 2001;411:494–498.
17. Dittgen T, Nimmerjahn A, Komai S, et al: Lentivirus-based genetic manipulations of cortical neurons and their optical and electrophysiological monitoring in vivo. Proc Natl Acad Sci U S A 2004;101:18206–18211.
18. Xia H, Mao Q, Paulson H, Davidson B: siRNA-mediated gene silencing in vitro and in vivo. Nat Biotech 2002;20:1006–1010.
19. Grimm D, Streetz K, Jopling C, et al: Fatality in mice due to oversaturation of cellular microRNA/short hairpin RNA pathways. Nature 2006;441:537–541.
20. Ong S, Li F, Du J, et al: Hybrid cytomegalovirus enhancer-h1 promoter-based plasmid and baculovirus vectors mediate effective RNA interference. Gene Ther 2005;16:1404–1412.
21. Hall A, Wan J, Shaughnessy E, et al: RNA interference using boranophosphate siRNAs: Structure-activity relationships. Nucleic Acids Res 2004;32:5991–6000.
22. Layzer J, McCaffrey A, Tanner A, et al: In vivo activity of nuclease-resistant siRNAs. RNA 2004;10:766–771.
23. Flynn M, Casey D, Todryk S, Mahon B: Efficient delivery of small interfering RNA for inhibition of IL-12p40 expression in vivo. J Inflamm 2004;1:4.
24. Sorensen D, Leirdal M, Sioud M: Gene silencing by systemic delivery of synthetic siRNAs in adult mice. J Mol Biol 2004;327:761–766.
25. Landen CJ, Chavez-Reyes A, Bucana C, et al: Therapeutic EphA2 gene targeting in vivo using neutral liposomal small interfering RNA delivery. Cancer Res 2005;65:6910–6918.
26. Kushibiki T, Nagata-Nakajima N, Sugai M, et al: Enhanced antifibrotic activity of plasmid DNA expressing small interference RNA for TGF-b type II receptor for a mouse model of obstructive nephropathy by cationized gelatin prepared from different amine compounds. J Control Release 2006;110:610–617.

27. Urban-Klein B, Werth S, Abuharbeid S, et al: RNAi-mediated gene-targeting through systemic application of polyethylenimine (PEI)-complexed siRNA in vivo. Gene Ther 2005;12:461–466.

28. Song E, Zhu P, Lee S, et al: Antibody mediated in vivo delivery of small interfering RNAs via cell-surface receptors. Nat Biotech 2005;23:709–717.

29. Zhang Y, Boado RJ, Pardridge WM: In vivo knockdown of gene expression in brain cancer with intravenous RNAi in adult rats. J Gene Med 2003;5:1039–1045.

30. Jackson A, Bartz S, Schelter J, et al: Expression profiling reveals off-target gene regulation by RNAi. Nat Biotech 2003;21: 635–637.

31. Skyes M, Sachs D, Nienhuis A, et al: Specific prolongation of skin graft survival following retroviral transduction of bone marrow with an allogenic major histocompatibility complex gene. Transplantation 1993;55:197–202.

32. Madsen J, Superina R, Wood K, Morris P: Immunological unresponsiveness induced by recipient cells transfected with donor MHC genes. Nature 1988;332:161–164.

33. Baliga P, Chavin Y, Qin L: CTLA4Ig prolongs allograft survival while suppressing cell-mediated immunity. Transplantation 1994;58:1082–1090.

34. Lenschow D, Zeng Y, Thistlethwaite J: Long-term survival of xenogenic pancreatic islet graft induced by CTLA4Ig. Science 1992;257:789–792.

35. Tomasoni S, Azzollini N, Casiraghi F, et al: CTLA4Ig gene transfer prolongs survival and induced donor-specific tolerance in a rat renal allograft. J Am Soc Nephrol 2000;11:747–752.

36. Benigni A, Tomasoni S, Truka L, et al: Adeno-associated virus-mediated CTLA4Ig gene transfer protects MHC-mismatched renal allografts from chronic rejection. J Am Soc Nephrol 2006; 17:1665–1672.

37. Abramowicz D, Durez P, Gerard C, et al: Neonatal induction of transplantation tolerance in mice is associated with in vivo expression of IL-4 and -10 mRNAs. Transplant Proc 1993;25: 312–313.

38. Lau H, Yu M, Fontana A, Stockert CJ: Prevention of islet allograft rejection with engineered myoblasts expressing fas1 in mice. Science 1996;273:109–112.

39. Perillo N, Pace K, Sellhamer J, Baum L: Apoptosis of T cells mediated by galectin-1. Nature 1995;378:736–738.

40. Qin L, Chavin K, Ding Y, et al: Gene transfer for transplantation. Prolongation of allograft survival with transforming growth factor-b1. Ann Surg 1994;220:508–518.

41. Azuma H, Takahara S, Matsumoto K, et al: Hepatocyte growth factor prevents the development of chronic allograft nephropathy in rats. J Am Soc Nephrol 2001;12:1280–1292.

42. Isaka Y, Yamada K, Takabatake Y, et al: Electroporation-mediated HGF gene transfection protected the kidney against graft injury. Gene Ther 2005;12:815–820.

43. Erzurum S, Lemarchand P, Rosenfeld M, et al: Protection of human endothelial cells from oxidant by adenovirus-mediated transfer of the human catalase cDNA. Nucleic Acids Res 1993;21: 1607–1612.

44. Azuma H, Tomita N, Kaneda Y, et al: Transfection of NF kappaB-decoy oligodeoxynucleotides using efficient ultrasound-mediated gene transfer into donor kidneys prolonged survival of rat renal allografts. Gene Ther 2003;10:415–425.

45. Noiri E, Peresleni T, Miller F, Goligorsky M: In vivo targeting of inducible NO synthase with oligodeoxynucleotides protects rat kidney against ischemia. J Clin Invest 1996;97:2377–2383.

46. Sandrin M, Fodor W, Mouhtoutis E, et al: Enzymatic remodelling of the carbohydrate surface of a xenogenic cell substantially reduces human antibody binding and complement-mediated cytolysis. Nat Med 1995;1:1261–1267.

47. McCurry K, Kooyman D, Alvarado C, et al: Human complement regulatory proteins protect swine-to-primate cardiac xenografts from humoral injury. Nat Med 1995;1:423–427.

48. Rosenberg S, Lotze M, Muul L, et al: Observations on the systemic administration of autologous lymphokine-activated killer cells and recombinant interleukin-2 to patients with metastatic cancer. N Engl J Med 1985;313:1485–1492.

49. Galanis E, Hersh E, Stopeck A, et al: Immunotherapy of advanced malignancy by direct gene transfer of an interleukin-2 DNA/DMRIE/DOPE lipid complex: Phase I/II experience. J Clin Oncol 1999;17:3313–3323.

50. Schmidt-Wolf I, Finke S, Trojaneck B, et al: Phase I clinical study applying autologous immunological effector cells transfected with the interleukin-2 gene in patients with metastatic renal cancer, colorectal cancer and lymphoma. Br J Cancer 1999;81:1009–1016.

51. Wittig B, Marten A, Dorbic T, et al: Therapeutic vaccination against metastatic carcinoma by expression-modulated and immunomodified autologous tumor cells: A first clinical phase I/II trial. Hum Gene Ther 2001;12:267–278.

52. Kawai K, Tani K, Yamashita N, et al: Advanced renal cell carcinoma treated with granulocyte-macrophage colony-stimulating factor gene therapy: A clinical course of the first Japanese experience. Int J Urol 2002;9:462–466.

53. Border W, Noble N: Transforming growth factor beta in tissue fibrosis. N Engl J Med 1994;331:1286–1292.

54. Akagi Y, Isaka Y, Arai M, et al: Inhibition of TGF-beta 1 expression by antisense oligonucleotides suppressed extracellular matrix accumulation in experimental glomerulonephritis. Kidney Int 1996;50:148–155.

55. Isaka Y, Tsujie M, Ando Y, et al: Transforming growth factor-beta 1 antisense oligodeoxynucleotides block interstitial fibrosis in unilateral ureteral obstruction. Kidney Int 2000;58:1885–1892.

56. Isaka Y, Nakamura H, Mizui M, et al: DNAzyme for TGF-beta suppressed extracellular matrix accumulation in experimental glomerulonephritis. Kidney Int 2004;66:586–590.

57. Takabatake Y, Isaka Y, Mizui M, et al: Exploring RNA interference as a therapeutic strategy for renal disease. Gene Ther 2005; 12:965–973.

58. Carl M, Akagi Y, Weidner S, et al: Specific inhibition of Egr-1 prevents mesangial cell hypercellularity in experimental nephritis. Kidney Int 2003;63:1302–1312.

59. Nakamura H, Isaka Y, Tsujie M, et al: Introduction of DNA enzyme for Egr-1 into tubulointerstitial fibroblasts by electroporation reduced interstitial alpha-smooth muscle actin expression and fibrosis in unilateral ureteral obstruction (UUO) rats. Gene Ther 2002;9:495–502.

60. Maeshima Y, Kashihara N, Yasuda T, et al: Inhibition of mesangial cell proliferation by E2F decoy oligodeoxynucleotide in vitro and in vivo. J Clin Invest 1998;101:2589–2597.

61. Tomita N, Morishita R, Tomita S, et al: Transcription factor decoy for NFkappaB inhibits TNF-alpha-induced cytokine and adhesion molecule expression in vivo. Gene Ther 2000;7:1326–1332.

62. Lan HY Mu W, Tomita N, et al: Inhibition of renal fibrosis by gene transfer of inducible Smad7 using ultrasound-microbubble system in rat UUO model. J Am Soc Nephrol 2003;14:1535–1548.

63. Terada Y, Hanada S, Nakao A, et al: Gene transfer of Smad7 using electroporation of adenovirus prevents renal fibrosis in post-obstructed kidney. Kidney Int 2002;61(Suppl 1):94–98.

64. Takase O, Hirahashi J, Takayanagi A, et al: Gene transfer of truncated IkappaBalpha prevents tubulointerstitial injury. Kidney Int 2003;63:501–513.

65. Imai E, Isaka Y: New paradigm of gene therapy: Skeletal-muscle-targeting gene therapy for kidney disease. Nephron 1999;83: 296–300.

66. Isaka Y, Brees D, Ikegaya K, et al: Gene therapy by skeletal muscle expression of decorin prevents fibrotic disease in rat kidney. Nat Med 1996;2:418–423.

67. Isaka Y, Akagi Y, Ando Y, et al: Gene therapy by transforming growth factor-beta receptor-IgG Fc chimera suppressed extracellular matrix accumulation in experimental glomerulonephritis. Kidney Int 1999;55:465–475.

68. Nakamura H, Isaka Y, Tsujie M, et al: Electroporation-mediated PDGF receptor-IgG chimera gene transfer ameliorates experimental glomerulonephritis. Kidney Int 2001;59:2134–2145.

69. Lawson B, Prud'homme G, Chang Y, et al: Treatment of murine lupus with cDNA encoding IFN-gammaR/Fc. J Clin Invest 2000;106:207–215.

70. Dobrzynski E, Montanari D, Agata J, et al: Adrenomedullin improves cardiac function and prevents renal damage in streptozotocin-induced diabetic rats. Am J Physiol Endocrinol Metab 2002;283:E1291–1298.

71. Matsumoto K, Nakamura T: Hepatocyte growth factor: Renotropic role and potential therapeutics for renal diseases. Kidney Int 2001;59:2023–2038.

72. Mizuno S, Matsumoto K, Nakamura T: Hepatocyte growth factor suppresses interstitial fibrosis in a mouse model of obstructive nephropathy. Kidney Int 2001;59:1304–1314.

73. Gao X, Mae H, Ayabe N, et al: Hepatocyte growth factor gene therapy retards the progression of chronic obstructive nephropathy. Kidney Int 2002;62:1238–1248.

74. Yang J, Dai C, Liu Y: Hepatocyte growth factor gene therapy and angiotensin II blockade synergistically attenuate renal interstitial fibrosis. J Am Soc Nephrol 2002;13:2464–2477.

75. Shimizu H, Maruyama S, Yuzawa Y, et al: Anti-monocyte chemoattractant protein-1 gene therapy attenuates renal injury induced by protein-overload proteinuria. J Am Soc Nephrol 2003;14:1496–1505.

76. Choi Y, Kim Y, Park H, et al: Suppression of glomerulosclerosis by adenovirus-mediated IL-10 expression in the kidney. Gene Ther 2003;10:559–568.

77. Hamar P, Song E, Kokeny G, et al: Small interfering RNA targeting Fas protects mice against renal ischemia-reperfusion injury. Proc Natl Acad Sci U S A 2004;101:14883–14888.

78. Du C, Wang S, Diao H, et al: Increasing resistance of tubular epithelial cells to apoptosis by shRNA therapy ameliorates renal ischemia-reperfusion injury. Am J Transplant 2006;6:2256–2267.

79. Yokoo T, Ohashi T, Utsunomiya Y, et al: Prophylaxis of antibody-induced acute glomerulonephritis with genetically modified bone marrow-derived vehicle cells. Hum Gene Ther 1999;10:2673–2678.

80. Yokoo T, Ohashi T, Utsunomiya Y, et al: Genetically modified bone marrow continuously supplies anti-inflammatory cells and suppresses renal injury in mouse Goodpasture syndrome. Blood 2001;98:57–64.

81. Rizzuto G, Cappelletti M, Mennuni C, et al: Gene electrotransfer results in a high-level transduction of rat skeletal muscle and corrects anemia of renal failure. Hum Gene Ther 2000;11:891–900.

82. Maruyama H, Ataka K, Gejyo F, et al: Long-term production of erythropoietin after electroporation-mediated transfer of plasmid DNA into the muscles of normal and uremic rats. Gene Ther 2001;8:461–468.

83. Seppen J, Barry S, Harder B, et al: Lentivirus administration to rat muscle provides efficient sustained expression of erythropoietin. Blood 2001;98:594–596.

84. Osada S, Ebihara I, Setoguchi Y, et al: Gene therapy for renal anemia in mice with polycystic kidney using an adenovirus vector encoding the human erythropoietin gene. Kidney Int 1999;55:1234–1240.

85. Hamamori Y, Samal B, Tian J, Kedes L: Myoblast transfer of human erythropoietin gene in a mouse model of renal failure. J Clin Invest 1995;95:1808–1813.

86. Rinsch C, Dupraz P, Schneider B, et al: Delivery of erythropoietin by encapsulated myoblasts in a genetic model of severe anemia. Kidney Int 2002;62:1395–1401.

87. Terada Y, Tanaka H, Okado T, et al: Ligand-regulatable erythropoietin production by plasmid injection and in vivo electroporation. Kidney Int 2002;62:1966–1976.

88. Binley K, Askham Z, Iqball S, et al: Long-term reversal of chronic anemia using a hypoxia-regulated erythropoietin gene therapy. Blood 2002;100:2406–2413.

89. Lippin Y, Dranitzki-Elhalel M, Brill-Almon E, et al: Human erythropoietin therapy for patients with chronic renal failure. Blood 2005;106:2280–2286.

90. Roy-Chaudhury P, Sukhatme V, Cheung A: Hemodialysis vascular access dysfunction: A cellular and molecular viewpoint. J Am Soc Nephrol 2006;17:1112–1127.

91. Sukhatme V: Vascular access stenosis: Prospect for prevention and therapy. Kidney Int 1996;49:1161–1174.

92. Dzau V, Braun-Dullaeus R, Sedding D: Vascular proliferation and atherosclerosis: New perspectives and therapeutic strategies. Nat Med 2002;8:1249–1256.

Further Reading

Benigni A, Tomasoni S, Truka L, et al: Adeno-associated virus-mediated CTLA4Ig gene transfer protects MHC-mismatched renal allografts from chronic rejection. J Am Soc Nephrol 2006;17:1665–1672.

Elbashir S, Harborth J, Lendeckel W, et al: Duplexes of 21-nucleotide RNAs mediate RNA interference in cultured mammalian cells. Nature 2001;411:494–498.

Hamar P, Song E, Kokeny G, et al: Small interfering RNA targeting Fas protects mice against renal ischemia-reperfusion injury. Proc Natl Acad Sci U S A 2004;101:14883–14888.

Kay M, Glorioso J, Naldini L: Viral vectors for gene therapy: The art of turning infectious agents into vehicles of therapeutics. Nat Med 2001;7:33–40.

Lippin Y, Dranitzki-Elhalel M, Brill-Almon E, et al: Human erythropoietin therapy for patients with chronic renal failure. Blood 2005;106:2280–2286.

Matsumoto K, Nakamura T: Hepatocyte growth factor: Renotropic role and potential therapeutics for renal diseases. Kidney Int 2001;59:2023–2038.

Roy-Chaudhury P, Sukhatme V, Cheung A: Hemodialysis vascular access dysfunction: A cellular and molecular viewpoint. J Am Soc Nephrol 2006;17:1112–1127.

Song E, Zhu P, Lee S, et al: Antibody mediated in vivo delivery of small interfering RNAs via cell-surface receptors. Nat Biotech 2005;23:709–717.

Takabatake Y, Isaka Y, Mizui M, et al: Exploring RNA interference as a therapeutic strategy for renal disease. Gene Ther 2005;12:965–973.

Tomasoni S, Azzollini N, Casiraghi F, et al: CTLA4Ig gene transfer prolongs survival and induces donor-specific tolerance in a rat renal allograft. J Am Soc Nephrol 2000;11:747–752.

Vasileva A, Jessberger R: Precise hit: Adeno-associated virus in gene targeting. Nat Review Microbiol 2005;3:837–847.

Xia H, Mao Q, Paulson H, Davidson B: siRNA-mediated gene silencing in vitro and in vivo. Nat Biotech 2002;20:1006–1010.

PART X

Management of Essential Hypertension

CONTENTS

Chapter 48

Decisions for Management of High Blood Pressure: A Perspective

Lawrence R. Krakoff

Treatment of hypertension is a most important way for primary care practitioners and medical subspecialists to preserve their patients' health. This is a daily activity in offices and clinics and a cornerstone for prevention of both cardiovascular disease (CVD) and end-stage renal disease. The evidence provided by the abundance of randomized clinical trials of antihypertensive therapy fully supports antihypertensive drug treatment and its widespread application for lowering blood pressure in those at risk. These trials, taken individually or in aggregate via meta-analysis, demonstrate that, for both middle-aged and elderly hypertensive individuals, antihypertensive drug therapy is highly and predictably effective for preventing fatal and nonfatal cerebrovascular disease (stroke) and cardiac disease (myocardial infarction and heart failure).[1] Progression of renal disease by antihypertensive drug therapy is also well documented.[2] Thus, there is no longer doubt that antihypertensive therapy is beneficial.

Are there any decisions to be made by those who treat hypertension? Have choices become unnecessary because evidence-based guidelines have eliminated or decreased decision making? Decisions or choices imply a lack of certainty and are not automatic (as is the case for computer algorithms). Decisions in medicine can be considered choices made in "ignorance," which, in this setting, means incomplete information rather than a total lack of relevant facts. Despite the wealth of information now available, significant gaps remain that require careful thought and analysis for decisions. The lessons and limitations of recent trials and research reveal these gaps. They expose areas where certainty should yield to best judgment, that is, decision making. This chapter focuses on the set of decisions (and areas of uncertainty) that I consider are most important at present (Box 48-1).

- Decision 1: What is hypertension and who is hypertensive?
- Decision 2: Which blood pressures are most accurate and useful for diagnosis and treatment? When should supplemental pressures, ambulatory monitoring, or home blood pressures be used?

- Decision 3: How should those with prehypertension or high-normal pressures be managed: by lifestyle improvement alone or by drug treatment?
- Decision 4: Treatment of hypertension: should goals be based on blood pressure or on reversible global risk of future disease? Guidelines compared: Is there agreement?
- Decision 5: How should elderly hypertensive patients be treated?

These five sets of decisions imply that the strategies and decisions related to initiating, maintaining, and changing antihypertensive therapy, although often thought to be quite simple, in reality are often highly complex. Both simple and complex decisions rely on a successful synthesis of the clinical characteristics of each patient with evidence from appropriate clinical trials, knowledge of pathophysiology and pharmacology, and good sense. This chapter focuses on the evidence and rationale for decisions linked to the five issues listed.

DECISION 1: WHAT IS HYPERTENSION AND WHO IS HYPERTENSIVE?

Hypertension can now be defined in several ways. Guidelines use specific cutoff points for classification: 140/90 mm Hg has been selected by most guideline committees.[3–5] However, some suggest that any arterial pressure higher than that associated with the lowest epidemiologic risk of future cardiovascular problems (i.e., 120/80 mm Hg) should be considered hypertensive. A major problem with the latter definition is the lack of trial evidence to support it. A more useful definition is the baseline blood pressure that, when lowered by antihypertensive therapy in clinical trials, predicts benefit. This definition includes the results of trials enrolling patients with abundant target organ damage, diabetic nephropathy, or chronic renal disease in which antihypertensive drugs (angiotensin-converting enzyme inhibitors or angiotensin receptor blockers) were effective

Box 48-1   Factors to Be Assessed in Establishing Cardiovascular and Renal Risk Status

Related to Blood Pressure	**Nonpressure Risk Factors**	**Target Organ Damage Pathology**
Ambulatory and home blood pressures; for all ages, estimate of usual average pressures; consideration of abnormal diurnal pattern in selected patients	Best established: presence or absence of type 1 or 2 diabetes, history of smoking, lipid status (elevated LDL, low HDL cholesterol, metabolic syndrome cluster)	Cardiac: left ventricular enlargement, ischemia, previous MI or angina, abnormal stress test, impaired systolic function, arrhythmia
Age < 50 yr: diastolic pressure most important	Less well established but may be useful: plasma renin profile, triglyceride levels	Renal microalbuminura or proteinuria, decreased GFR, increased creatinine
Age 50–60 yr: both systolic and diastolic pressures equally important	Suggested by recent research: C-reactive protein, fibrinogen, lipoprotein(a), homocysteine	Peripheral vascular: Ankle-arm index, claudication, arterial bruits, aortic aneurysm
Age > 60 yr: systolic pressure and pulse pressure are more important		Cerebrovascular: history of TIA or stroke, carotid bruit
Age > 85 yr: increased risk of lower pressures, orthostatic hypotension, and low diastolic pressure; J-curve issue		

GFR, glomerular filtration rate; HDL, high-density lipoprotein; LDL, low-density lipoprotein; MI, myocardial infarction; TIA, transient ischemic attack.

when baseline pressures were less than 140/90 mm Hg and goals of treatment were less than 130/80 mm Hg. Thus, the definition of hypertension becomes contextual, related to other risk predictors for a patient rather than limited to a single cutoff point. For some older patients, hypertension may need to be defined as systolic pressures higher than 160 mm Hg and goals for treatment set higher than 140/90 mm Hg.[6] A context-based definition, related to likelihood of benefit from blood pressure lowering, can go higher or lower than the rigid 140 mm Hg systolic to benefit individuals within definable subgroups, but must be validated by trial evidence. Epidemiologic association between pressures higher than the optimal and risk that is not validated by therapeutic trials is a weak basis for clinical decisions.

Some suggest that hypertension is a high-risk state for CVD that is independent of high blood pressure. This implies that antihypertensive drug treatment might be beneficial for those with other risk factors and/or target organ damage irrespective of their baseline blood pressure.[7] Trying to separate hypertension from high blood pressure creates semantic confusion and ignores the abundant evidence that the major therapeutic effect of antihypertensive drugs for the high-risk group is their ability to decrease pressure, even when pretreatment pressures are in the high-normal range. This is consistent with the context-based definition. Some drugs classed as antihypertensive, however, have other actions that are beneficial for selected populations. Thus, β-blockers for coronary heart disease or angiotensin receptor blockers for diabetic nephropathy have added unique value apart from decreasing pressure. Furthermore, the cardiovascular pathology often associated with hypertension may occur in those with normal pressures but other risk factors and unknown etiologies. Thus, an attempt to separate hypertension from high blood pressure is confusing and unnecessary.[8]

DECISION 2: WHICH BLOOD PRESSURES ARE MOST ACCURATE AND USEFUL FOR DIAGNOSIS AND TREATMENT?

The measurement of blood pressure made at a single visit in the highly contrived atmosphere of a busy medical practice is insufficient for a diagnosis of normal pressure, prehypertension, or hypertension. Screening or clinic blood pressures are often inaccurate and misleading, especially when they are either not clearly normal (<120/80 mm Hg) or very high (>180/110 mm Hg). It is now evident from many studies of ambulatory and home pressure measurement (supplemental pressures) that the average pressure is best related to risk. This average requires several measurements for confidence. The distribution of blood pressures in a population approaches a normal bell shape. The various cut points for blood pressure that have been used to divide high-normal from hypertensive are all on the upper part of the down slope of these distributions. This implies that a large fraction of those with high-normal pressures (or the prehypertensives) may be falsely labeled as hypertensive, for a small measurement error (5–10 mm). It is less likely that a patient with hypertension will be falsely classified as normal or prehypertensive, but this remains a worrisome possibility, as some with normal clinic pressures have increased supplemental pressures (i.e., masked hypertension) because the clinic measurements give a false-negative diagnosis.[9] Only by accumulating enough measurements through supplemental pressures can an accurate classification be made for normal, prehypertension, or hypertension.

Ambulatory blood pressure monitoring has become a widespread and available technique as a result of its recognition for improved diagnostic accuracy. It is the gold standard for clinical diagnosis.[10–14] Self-recorded home blood pressures may be nearly as useful.[15,16] Home pressures can be valuable for determining average pretreatment pressures and assessing treatment effects for adjusting antihypertensive medication.[17]

The systolic pressure is clearly a major determinant of risk in middle-aged and elderly populations,[18,19] which is supported by results of clinical trials of antihypertensive therapy.[20] However, retrospective analysis of some databases has suggested that the simple arithmetic difference between systolic and diastolic pressures, the pulse pressure, may be a superior predictor of later CVD when compared with systolic pressure alone and that for equally high pulse pressures, a higher diastolic pressure confers less risk for older patients.[21] In treating older patients, an excessive decrease in diastolic pressure may be as harmful as an adverse effect of an overzealous decrease in systolic pressure.[22] However, reanalysis of age-related trends in the Framingham study indicates that for those younger than 50 years of age, diastolic pressure remains the better predictor of risk; between ages 50 and 59, both systolic and diastolic pressures are directly related to risk; and for ages older than 59 years, systolic and pulse pressures are the best predictors.[23] Thus, the age of the patient must be considered in determining whether the average systolic or diastolic pressure has the greatest clinical relevance. This is another example of a context-based definition. For the elderly, the risk of a low diastolic pressure needs greater emphasis for proper decisions in treatment.

DECISION 3: PREHYPERTENSION OR HIGH NORMAL PRESSURE?

The Joint National Committee on Prevention, Detection, Evaluation, and Treatment of High Blood Pressure Report 7 (JNC-7) provided a new classification for high arterial blood pressure: optimal blood pressure, prehypertension, and hypertension.[3] The novel feature of this advisory was the introduction of the term *prehypertension* to identify those with blood pressure higher than the optimal level (120/80 mm Hg), but lower than the hypertensive range (140/90 mm Hg). This classification is based only on clinic measurements, omitting supplemental pressures to reclassify patients more precisely should false-positive or false-negative assessments occur due to inaccurate or misleading clinic measurements.[9] Before the JNC-7, the term high-normal had been applied to those pressures near the hypertensive range, generally 130 to 139/80 to 89 mm Hg. The JNC-7 did not include an age-based classification. However, the rationale for recommending that *prehypertension* be used could be found in the high likelihood that those with this level of pressure in middle age would eventually become hypertensive as they age, as shown by the longitudinal Framingham study.[24] It is not surprising that retrospective assessments of population studies, such as the National Health and Nutrition Examination Survey, report that a large fraction (20%–30%) of the sample could be classified as prehypertensive.[25] The important factors contributing to the transition from prehypertension or high-normal pressure to hypertension, in addition to age, are the actual pressure level, overweight, and weight gain.[26] High salt intake may also contribute to this transition.[27] Increased C-reactive protein levels have also been identified as a predictor of future hypertension, but this finding may be related only to overweight.[28,29]

Long-term follow-up has revealed that prehypertension is associated with eventual rates of CVD that are intermediate between those with optimal pressure at baseline and those that are hypertensives.[30] As a group, prehypertensives tend to be overweight and have serum lipid abnormalities and type 2 diabetes or the metabolic syndrome, but smoking is less frequently a factor. Many prehypertensive individuals have a cluster of cardiovascular risk factors with high-normal blood pressure alone in only a small fraction. A schematic comparison of this relationship for prehypertension, compared with established hypertension, is given in Figure 48-1. Some risk calculations attribute all future risk of CVD in those who are prehypertensive to factors other than the blood pressure.[31] That conclusion clearly implies that interventions to decrease the risk should focus on lifestyle improvement through weight loss, improved nutrition, and increased exercise.

Is there any basis for treatments to lower blood pressure as a primary goal for management of prehypertension or should all attention be given to encouraging a favorable lifestyle that may have benefit whether or not pressure is lowered? What is the evidence to help clinicians make best decisions?

Many lifestyle interventions reduce blood pressure in short-term studies. Those best studied are weight loss, decreased diet salt with increased potassium, and increased exercise.[32] Changing the source of diet protein from a meat-based source to soy lowers pressure.[33] The Dietary Approaches to Stop Hypertension trial diet, a diet high in potassium, fruits, and vegetables combined with low fat and restricted salt intake, has been given much attention in this regard. However, over 18 months, this strategy has a relatively small effect on blood pressure but does reduce the transition from prehypertension to hypertension.[34] Bear in mind, however, that this event (new hypertension) occurred when the clinic systolic pressure could increase as little as 1 mm Hg (from 139 to 140 mm Hg between visits), a very artificial and unstable definition. In a population survey of middle-aged women, there is no correlation between ingestion of a Dietary Approaches to Stop Hypertension–like diet and either hypertension or cardiovascular mortality after adjustment for other risk factors.[35]

Do any lifestyle interventions impart a reduction in future CVD? Only diet salt reduction has been shown to cause a small, but significant, decrease in CVD events and mortality, in a combined analysis of two components from the Trial of Prevention of Hypertension. There was, over a 5- to 10-year follow-up period, a 25% decrease in relative risk of cardiovascular events and a 19% decrease in relative risk of death.[36] The absolute reductions were 1.5% for cardiovascular events and 0.3% for mortality. The numbers needed to treat, based on a 10-year follow-up with a 5% dropout rate per year, are 106 for one cardiovascular event and 528 for one death; these numbers are, however, compelling for an effective and safe population-based strategy.

There is a widespread consensus that the other lifestyle interventions, now favored by advisory groups, ought to be beneficial, yet no trial evidence has yet emerged to confirm this hope. Perhaps there should be more emphasis on a decrease in diet salt for those who are prehypertensive and equal emphasis on weight decrease and increased exercise for the entire population, regardless of their blood pressure, as those with optimal pressure may still be at risk due to overweight, lipid abnormalities, and high-normal blood glucose.

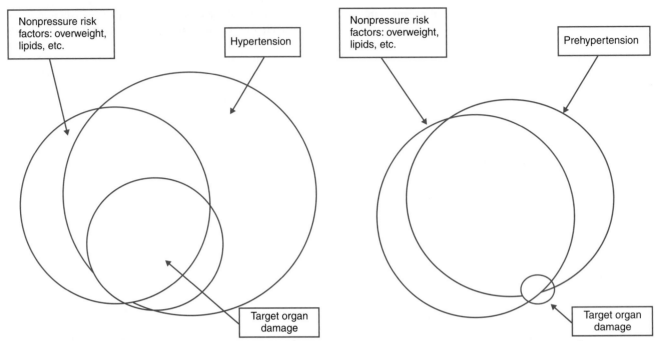

Figure 48-1 Comparison of the relationships between nonpressure risk factors and target organ damage in prehypertension or established hypertension (**A**) and high-normal blood pressure (**B**).

Many antihypertensive drugs lower pressure in hypertensive populations, and some appear to be beneficial in nonhypertensives who have abundant target organ damage (preexisting CVD) or diabetes. Candesartan, the angiotensin type I receptor blocker (ARB) decreased blood pressure significantly in a placebo-controlled, randomized trial of prehypertensives who were young with no CVD.[37] The design of the trial called for 2 years of active treatment combined with lifestyle advice followed by a 2-year phase in which the active drug was withdrawn and both groups were placed on placebo. In this second phase, a high fraction of those whose pressure had previously been lowered by the angiotensin receptor blocker returned to higher pressure levels and became hypertensive at nearly the same rate as those on placebo in both phases. There were too few CVD events in the trial for evidence that angiotensin receptor blocker treatment is effective for decreasing mortality or morbidity as a treatment for prehypertension or high-normal pressure.

What decisions should be made for the treatment of prehypertension? Should prehypertensives be treated differently from those with optimal pressure who are overweight or have other risk factors or should they be treated as if they already had hypertension? Should they be treated only for the risk factors that are present— obesity, lipid disorders, or high fasting glucose (prediabetes)—or by addition of antihypertensive drugs? Given the results of the Trial of Prevention of Hypertension follow-up observations, would a low-dose diuretic be the equivalent of low-salt diet for long-term benefit? Is the long-term risk of diabetes related to diuretics a concern?[38] Without better evidence, these decisions can be made as well with a coin toss or by theoretical reasoning so that the decision, for any given patient with prehypertension, is for each clinician to make. It is not yet time for guidelines to set the rules.

DECISION 4: TREATMENT OF HYPERTENSION: SHOULD GOALS BE BASED ON BLOOD PRESSURE OR ON REVERSIBLE GLOBAL RISK OF FUTURE DISEASE? GUIDELINES COMPARED: IS THERE AGREEMENT?

The factors that determine future cardiovascular disease for hypertensive patients can be divided into categories: (1) age alone, (2) average pressures, (3) non–pressure-related reversible risk factors, and (4) preexisting cardiovascular or renal pathology, that is, target organ damage such as left ventricular enlargement. For any given level of pressure, future risk of stroke, coronary heart disease, or renal failure varies over a wide range. However, the abundant evidence from clinical trials clearly supports drug treatment of established hypertension.

Guidelines for the diagnosis and treatment of hypertension emerged shortly after evidence from randomized clinical trials demonstrated the effectiveness of drug treatment for high blood pressure. The most recent advisory from the United States is JNC-7.[3] Guidelines have also been issued from a combined effort by the European Society of Hypertension with the European Society of Cardiology[4] and the British Hypertension Society.[5] Although these three guidelines share many features, there are differences with regard to diagnostic categories and recommendations for treatment. Prehypertension is defined only in the JNC-7 recommendation, whereas the other two guidelines retain the term *high-normal blood pressure* for those with clinic measurements of 130 to 139/85 to 89 mm Hg. For stage 1 hypertension, clinic pressures of 140 to 159/90 to 100 mm Hg, the JNC-7 advises drug treatment for all and favors starting with a thiazide-type diuretic. The European Society of Hypertension with the European Society of Cardiology and British Hypertension Society take a more restrained view using a global risk–based approach. For those with low risk and stage 1 hypertension, there is more emphasis on continued observation and patient preference. All guidelines recommend a favorable lifestyle change (smoking cessation, increased exercise, weight loss, and diet improvement) irrespective of the need for drug treatment.

For initiation of drug treatment, the British Hypertension Society guideline originally took age and ethnic status into account using the ABCD strategy. For those younger than 55 years and nonblack, initial treatment with either an angiotensin-converting enzyme inhibitor (A) or β-blocker (B) was initially suggested. For those 55 years and older and/or black, the recommended initial treatment is a calcium blocker (C) or a thiazide-type diuretic (D). Due to evidence that β-blockers are associated with increased incidence of diabetes and a lack of clear-cut effectiveness,[39] the B was dropped, resulting in the ACD strategy in a revision of the British Hypertension Society guideline.[40] The European Society of Hypertension with the European Society of Cardiology approach is less stringent in suggesting monotherapy with any selected class as the first step. Both age and risk status are included as bases for choice.

For definite hypertension, all three guidelines share the recognition that most patients will require two to three drugs for effective control (e.g., an angiotensin-converting enzyme inhibitor plus a diuretic or a calcium channel blocker). Goals for treatment are similar: lower than 140/90 for most patients and lower than 130/80 mm Hg for those with either diabetes or chronic renal disease. The guidelines also recommend drug treatment for definite hypertension from at least age 50 to age 80, due to the abundant trial evidence of this conclusion. For those older than 80 years of age, there is recognition that definitive trial evidence is lacking. The European Society of

Hypertension with the European Society of Cardiology and British Hypertension Society guidelines emphasize the need for individualization and recognize the risk of overtreatment and the need to screen for orthostatic hypotension in this age group to avoid syncope. Table 48-1 lists the main features for screening, classifying, and treatment for these three guidelines.

How should a clinician decide which guideline to use? Are the diagnosis and treatment of hypertension to be defined by national borders or are international standards more appropriate? One consideration for those nations with limited resources for health care is to favor the most cost-effective strategies with emphasis on high-risk groups for control of hypertension to minimize inefficient resource consumption.[41] The risk-based approach to choice of treatment will decrease or withhold drug treatment for those with the combination of stage 1 or grade 1 hypertension and low-risk profiles represented by less than a 10% to 15% likelihood of CVD over the next 10 years. All those with higher stages or higher risk will be given drug treatment. This strategy would decrease the number needed to treat for benefit of individual patients and should be cost-effective, a necessity for nations with limited funds for health care. The JNC-7 imperative to treat all stage 1 hypertensives with drug treatment irrespective of their overall risk profiles may lead to overtreatment with no benefit for many (a high number needed to treat), excess cost, adverse effect (diuretics are still a problem in this regard), and dilution of the effort to find and effectively treat those with high risk due to higher blood pressure or presence of other risk factors and/or target organ damage.

I suggest that those who manage hypertension be aware that experts who write guidelines have differing opinions due to lack of evidence and that treating physicians tailor the

Table 48-1 Comparison of the Guidelines for Detection of Hypertension and Goals for Treatment

Initial Classification	JNC-7	ESH-ECS	BHS
Prehypertension	120–139/80–89	Not used	Not used
High normal	No longer used	A: 130–139/85–89	130–139/85–89
Hypertension	Stage 1: 140+/90+ to 159/100; stage 2: > 159/100	B: 140–179/90–109; C: ≥180/≥110	Grade 1: 140–159/90–99 Grade 2: 160–179/100–109 Grade 3: ≥180/≥110
Isolated systolic hypertension	≥140/<90	≥140/<90	Grade 1: 140–159/<90 Grade 2: ≥160/<90
Goals for treatment	<140/90 nondiabetic	<140/90 nondiabetic	<140/85 nondiabetic
	<130/80 diabetes and chronic renal disease	<130/80 diabetes	<130/80 diabetes, renal disease, established cardiovascular disease
Initial treatment nondiabetics	Diuretic preferred	Any drug class	ACD* selection based on age and ethnic status (black-white)
Initial treatment diabetics	Two drugs, usually including ACEI or ARB	ACEI or ARB	Type I: ACE Type II: ARB

All blood pressures are given as mm Hg.
*AA, angiotensin-converting enzyme inhibitor for white patients and those younger than 55 years; CD, calcium blocker or diuretic for black or older patients.
ACEI, angiotensin-converting enzyme inhibitor; ARB, angiotensin II receptor blocker; BHS, British Hypertension Society guidelines for hypertension management, 2004 (BHS-IV)[5,40]; ESH-ECS, 2003 European Society of Hypertension–European Society of Cardiology guidelines for the management of arterial hypertension[4]; JNC-7, Seventh Report of the Joint National Committee on Prevention, Detection, Evaluation and Treatment of High Blood Pressure.[3]

guidelines to the patient rather than force the patient to fit into a guideline. This is particularly the case for those with prehypertension or high-normal pressure or low-risk stage 1 or grade 1 hypertensive patients.

DECISION 5: HOW SHOULD ELDERLY HYPERTENSIVE PATIENTS BE TREATED?

In developed countries, a larger fraction now survives longer than 80 years of age, with many alive in the 85- to 100-year range. Epidemiologic surveys project that more than 90% in this age range will be hypertensive according to current criteria, most with isolated systolic hypertension.[42] Antihypertensive drug treatment of hypertension in those as old as 80 years of age is effective for reduction in stroke and CVD and prevention of heart failure.[21] The evidence is less convincing with those older than 85 years of age. Furthermore, the trials have largely recruited healthy older groups, yet many of the old-old have other diseases leading to frailty, diminished mobility, and, all too often, dementia. Low diastolic pressures often occur in the elderly that might decrease to levels near or below the threshold for coronary perfusion with antihypertensive treatment, leading to higher mortality due to lower treatment pressures, the J-curve phenomenon.[22] Orthostatic hypotension is more likely in older patients, adding to risk of syncope and fractures.[43] Where then does antihypertensive drug treatment find its place in the complex balance of considerations for this group? Epidemiologic surveys of the very old suggest that those with the lowest blood pressure actually have the highest short-term mortality rates compared with those with higher (even hypertensive) pressures.[44,45] A meta-analysis of old-old subgroups selected from reports of larger trials found that active treatment does decrease the rate of stroke, but increases overall mortality.[46] A pilot trial of active treatment compared with placebo in hypertensives 85 years of age and older, found a similar pattern: reduced stroke and higher mortality.[47] A larger trial (the Hypertension in the Very Elderly Trial) will investigate the effect of antihypertensive treatment in the old-old on cardiovascular event rates, dementia, and fractures.[48,49] It is hoped that the results will be available in 2009.

The value of antihypertensive drug treatment in the old-old offers potential benefit and harm. This potential is conveyed in Figure 48-2, which portrays the likelihood of benefit versus harm in relation to age. Until additional trials coupled with careful observational studies are available, emphasis should be placed on thoughtful assessment of each individual patient to ponder reversible risk of cardiovascular disease, quality of life, likelihood of syncope (orthostatic hypotension) and patient's preferences. *Primum non nocere* should be balanced against the urge to write prescriptions in order to make the best decisions.

CONCLUSIONS

Physicians evaluate and treat patients one by one. The lessons learned from large epidemiologic and clinical trials need translation and individualized application for optimal decision making. It is recommended that physicians consider the views presented in this chapter to give attention to the

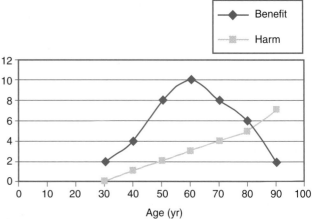

Figure 48-2   Schematic estimate of the relationship between benefit and harm of treatment of hypertension in relation to age. Based on trial evidence, benefit clearly exceeds harm when drug treatment is given to those 50 to 80 years of age and very likely for those between 40 and 50. With increasing frailty in the elderly, the presence of other diseases requiring medications, and the likelihood of drug interactions, the potential for harm increases and may cross the benefit line at ages 80 to 85.

following: (1) focus on the daily average pressure for diagnosis and treatment with recognition that age-based criteria for either systolic or diastolic pressure are relevant, (2) be aware of the limited or absent evidence of effective treatment of prehypertension or high-normal pressure, and (3) recognize that well-meaning guidelines differ among groups who are distant from the day-to-day challenges of patient care. Lowering blood pressure to compensate for other risk factors may be valuable in selected, but not all, cases.[4] Treating systolic hypertension in the elderly and especially the old-old is a multifaceted challenge that should combine realistic goals for treatment with principles of geriatric medicine.

Decisions (choices made in ignorance) are built into the practice of preventive medicine. The current abundance of evidence combined with useful guidelines has reduced, but not eliminated, the ignorance, so that the best decisions will require knowledge, thought, and wisdom.

References

1. Blood Pressure Lowering Treatment Trialists' Collaboration: Effects of different blood pressure-lowering regimens on major cardiovascular events in individuals with and without diabetes mellitus: Results of prospectively designed overviews of clinical trials. Arch Intern Med 2005;165:1410–1419.
2. Casas JP, Chua W, Loukogeorgakis S, et al: Effect of inhibitors of the renin-angiotensin system and other antihypertensive drugs on renal outcomes: Systematic review and meta-analysis. Lancet 2005;366:2026–2033.
3. Chobanian AV, Bakris GL, Black HR, et al: The seventh report of the Joint National Committee on Prevention, Detection, Evaluation and Treatment of High Blood Pressure: The JNC 7 Report. JAMA 2003;289:2560–2572.
4. Guidelines Committee: 2003 European Society of Hypertension–European Society of Cardiology guidelines for the management of arterial hypertension. J Hypertens 2003;21:1011–1053.

5. Williams B, Poulter NR, Brown MJ, et al: British Hypertension Society guidelines for hypertension management 2004 (BHS-IV): Summary. Br Med J 2004;328:634–640.

6. Chaudhry SJ, Krumholz HM, Foody JM: Systolic hypertension in older persons. JAMA 2004;292:1074–1080.

7. Giles TD, Berk BC, Black HR, et al: Expanding the definition and classification of hypertension. J Clin Hypertens 2005;7:505–512.

8. Krakoff LR: New definitions of hypertension. J Clin Hypertens 2006;8:282–283.

9. Marshall T: Misleading measurements: Modeling the effects of blood pressure misclassification in a United States population. Med Decis Making 2006;26:624–632.

10. Clement D, De Buyzere M, De Bacqer DA, et al: Prognostic value of ambulatory blood-pressure recordings in patients with treated hypertension. N Engl J Med 2003;348:2407–2415.

11. Dolan E, Stanton A, Thijs L, et al: Superiority of ambulatory over clinic blood pressure measurement in predicting mortality: The Dublin outcome study. Hypertension 2005;46:156–161.

12. Fagard RH, Staessen JA, Thijs L, et al: Relationship between ambulatory blood pressure and follow-up clinic blood pressure in elderly patients with systolic hypertension. J Hypertens 2004;22:81–87.

13. Hansen TW, Jeppesen J, Rasmussen S, et al: Ambulatory blood pressure and mortality. Hypertension 2005;45:499–504.

14. Kikuya M, Ohkubo T, Asayama K, et al: Ambulatory blood pressure and 10-year risk of cardiovascular and noncardiovascular mortality: The Ohasama study. Hypertension 2005;45:240–245.

15. Bobrie G, Chatellier G, Genes N, et al: Cardiovascular prognosis of "masked hypertension" detected by blood pressure self-measurement in elderly treated hypertensive patients. JAMA 2004;291:1342–1349.

16. Verberk WJ, Kroon AA, Kessels AG, de Leeuw PW: Home blood pressure measurement: A systematic review. J Am Coll Cardiol 2005;46:743–751.

17. Ho PM, Rumsfeld JS: Beyond inpatient and outpatient care: Alternative model for hypertension management. BMC Public Health 2006;6:257.

18. Izzo JL Jr, Levy D, Black HR: Importance of systolic blood pressure in older Americans. Hypertension 2000;35:1021–1024.

19. Sagie A, Larson MG, Levy D: The natural history of borderline isolated systolic hypertension. N Engl J Med 1993;329:1912–1917.

20. Mulrow CD, Cornell JA, Herrera CR, et al: Hypertension in the elderly. Implications and generalizability of randomized trials. JAMA 1994;272:1932–1938.

21. Staessen J, Gasowski J, Wang JG, et al: Risks of untreated and treated isolated systolic hypertension in the elderly: Meta-analysis of outcome trials. Lancet 2000;355:865–872.

22. Messerli FH, Mancia G, Conti CR, et al: Dogma disputed: Can aggressively lowering blood pressure in hypertensive patients with coronary artery disease be dangerous? Ann Intern Med 2006;144:884–893.

23. Franklin SS, Larson M, Kahn S, et al: Does the relation of blood pressure to coronary heart disease risk change with aging? The Framingham Heart Study. Circulation 2001;103:1245–1249.

24. Vasan RS, Levy D: Rates of progression to hypertension among non-hypertensive subjects: Implications for blood pressure screening. Eur Heart J 2004;23:1067–1070.

25. Greenlund KJ, Croft JB, Mensah GA: Prevalence of heart disease and stroke risk factors in persons with prehypertension in the United States, 1999–2000. Arch Intern Med 2004;164:2113–2118.

26. Leitschuh M, Cupples LA, Kannel W, et al: High-normal blood pressure progression to hypertension in the Framingham Heart Study. Hypertension 1991;17:22–27.

27. Intersalt Cooperative Research Group: Intersalt: An international study of electrolyte excretion and blood pressure. Results for 24 hour urinary sodium and potassium excretion. Br Med J 1988;297:319–328.

28. Lakoski SG, Herrington DM, Siscovick DM, Hulley SB: C-reactive protein concentration and incident hypertension in young adults: The CARDIA Study. Arch Intern Med 2006;166:345–349.

29. Sesso HD, Buring JE, Rifai N, et al: C-reactive protein and the risk of developing hypertension. JAMA 2003;290:2945–2951.

30. Hsia J, Margolis KL, Eaton CB, et al: Prehypertension and cardiovascular disease risk in the Women's Health Initiative. Circulation 2007;115:855–860.

31. Mainous AG III, Everett CJ, Liszka H, et al: Prehypertension and mortality in a nationally representative cohort. Am J Cardiol 2004;94:1496–1500.

32. Whelton PK, He J, Appel LJ, et al: Primary prevention of hypertension: Clinical and public health advisory from the National High Blood Pressure Education Program. JAMA 2002;288:1882–1888.

33. He J, Gu D, Wu X, et al: Effect of soybean protein on blood pressure: A randomized, controlled trial. Ann Intern Med 2005;143:1–9.

34. Elmer PJ, Obarzanek E, Vollmer WM, et al: Effects of comprehensive lifestyle modification on diet, weight, physical fitness, and blood pressure control: 18-month results of a randomized trial. Ann Intern Med 2006;144:485–495.

35. Folsom AR, Parker ED, Harnack LJ: Degree of concordance with DASH diet guidelines and incidence of hypertension and fatal cardiovascular disease. Am J Hypertens 2007;20:225–232.

36. Cook NR, Cutler JA, Obarzanek E, et al: Long term effects of dietary sodium reduction on cardiovascular disease outcomes: Observational follow-up of the trials of hypertension prevention (TOHP). Br Med J 2007;334:885.

37. Julius S, Nesbitt SD, Egan BM, et al: Feasibility of treating prehypertension with an angiotensin-receptor blocker. N Engl J Med 2006;354:1685–1697.

38. Elliott WJ, Meyer PM: Incident diabetes in clinical trials of antihypertensive drugs: A network meta-analysis. Lancet 2007;369:201–207.

39. Gress TW, Nieto J, Shahar E, et al, for the Atherosclerosis Risk in Communities Study: Hypertension and antihypertensive therapy as risk factors for type 2 diabetes. N Engl J Med 2000;342:905–912.

40. Sever P: New hypertension guidelines from the National Institute for Health and Clinical Excellence and the British Hypertension Society. J Renin Angiotensin Aldosterone Syst 2006;7:61–63.

41. Gaziano TA, Opie LH, Weinstein MC: Cardiovascular disease prevention with a multidrug regimen in the developing world: A cost-effectiveness analysis. Lancet 2006;368:679–686.

42. Vasan RS, Beiser A, Seshadri S, et al: Residual lifetime risk for developing hypertension in middle-aged women and men: The Framingham Heart Study. JAMA 2002;287:1003–1010.

43. Rutan GH, Hermanson B, Bild DE, et al: Orthostatic hypotension in older adults. The Cardiovascular Health Study. CHS Collaborative Research Group. Hypertension 1992;19:508–519.

44. Glynn RJ, Field TS, Rosner B, et al: Evidence for a positive linear relation between blood pressure and mortality in elderly people. Lancet 1995;345:825–829.

45. Rastas S, Pirttila T, Viramo P, et al: Association between blood pressure and survival over 9 years in a general population aged 85 and older. J Am Geriatr Soc 2006;54:912–918.

46. Gueyffier F, Bulpitt C, Boissel JP, et al: Antihypertensive drugs in very old people: A subgroup meta-analysis of randomized controlled trials. Lancet 1999;353:793–796.

47. Bulpitt CJ, Beckett NS, Cooke J, et al: Results of the pilot study for the Hypertension in the Very Elderly Trial. J Hypertens 2003;21:2409–2417.

48. Bulpitt CJ, Peters R, Staessen JA, et al: Fracture risk and the use of a diuretic (Indapamide SR) +/- perindopril: A substudy of the Hypertension in the Very Elderly Trial (HYVET). Trials 2006;7:33.

49. Peters R, Beckett N, Nunes M, et al: A substudy protocol of the Hypertension in the Very Elderly Trial assessing cognitive decline and dementia incidence (HYVET-COG): An ongoing randomised, double-blind, placebo-controlled trial. Drugs Aging 2006;23:83–92.

Further Reading

Blood Pressure Lowering Treatment Trialists' Collaboration: Effects of different blood pressure-lowering regimens on major cardiovascular events in individuals with and without diabetes mellitus: Results of prospectively designed overviews of clinical trials. Arch Intern Med 2005;165:1410–1419.

Chaudhry SJ, Krumholz HM, Foody JM: Systolic hypertension in older persons. JAMA 2004;292:1074–1080.

Cook NR, Cutler JA, Obarzanek E, et al: Long term effects of dietary sodium reduction on cardiovascular disease outcomes: Observational follow-up of the trials of hypertension prevention (TOHP). BMJ 2007;334:885.

Dolan E, Stanton A, Thijs L, et al: Superiority of ambulatory over clinic blood pressure measurement in predicting mortality: The Dublin outcome study. Hypertension 2005;46:156–161.

Greenlund KJ, Croft JB, Mensah GA: Prevalence of heart disease and stroke risk factors in persons with prehypertension in the United States, 1999–2000. Arch Intern Med 2004;164:2113–2118.

Ho PM, Rumsfeld JS: Beyond inpatient and outpatient care: Alternative model for hypertension management. BMC Public Health 2006;6:257.

Mainous AG, III, Everett CJ, Liszka H, et al: Prehypertension and mortality in a nationally representative cohort. Am J Cardiol 2004;94:1496–1500.

Marshall T: Misleading measurements: Modeling the effects of blood pressure misclassification in a United States population. Med Decis Making 2006;26:624–632.

Messerli FH, Mancia G, Conti CR, et al: Dogma disputed: Can aggressively lowering blood pressure in hypertensive patients with coronary artery disease be dangerous? Ann Intern Med 2006;144:884–893.

Rastas S, Pirttila T, Viramo P, et al: Association between blood pressure and survival over 9 years in a general population aged 85 and older. J Am Geriatr Soc 2006;54:912–918.

Chapter 49

Nonpharmacologic Treatment

Paul R. Conlin

There is a continuum of risk between blood pressure and cardiovascular events. Although 27% of the U.S. adult population has hypertension and often receives some form of pharmacological therapy,[1] many fewer are counseled about, or actually implement, nonpharmacologic treatments. However, the greatest impact of nonpharmacologic treatments may actually be in the large group of individuals with prehypertension. Nonpharmacologic interventions involving dietary and lifestyle changes, such as weight loss, sodium restriction, and changes in dietary patterns, either alone or in combination, may decrease the incidence and prevalence of hypertension. Clinicians do not place sufficient emphasis on these interventions because patient acceptance and adherence are often low.

The treatment of hypertension has evolved over the past 40 years. Research has generated changes in strategies, approaches, treatment options, and effects of nonpharmacologic treatment. However, what has remained constant is the recognition that lifestyle modifications are a cornerstone of treatment. Although clinical trials of nonpharmacologic treatments have not had sufficient power to show differences in cardiovascular events, implementing these interventions can be supported from cardiovascular risk reduction associated with their blood pressure effects per se.

This chapter summarizes the results of studies that evaluate the effects of nonpharmacologic treatments in prehypertensives and hypertensives. A summary of systolic blood pressure changes that may be anticipated with the interventions is shown in Table 49-1.

EFFECTS OF DIETARY PATTERNS

A diet that replaces animal products with vegetable products decreases blood pressure. However, it is unrealistic to assume that vegetarian diets would be widely accepted. Features of a vegetarian diet have been identified (e.g., higher fiber, potassium, and magnesium content and decreased fat content) that may affect blood pressure. Although each of these individual nutrients is associated with decreased blood pressure, trials that have tested the effects of such individual nutrients have seen only small blood pressure changes. This may be due to each nutrient by itself having a small effect so that only when all are consumed together is a clinically significant effect observed.

The Dietary Approaches to Stop Hypertension (DASH) trial[2] was designed to identify a diet that decreases blood pressure and is also palatable and acceptable to the general population. Individuals with a diastolic blood pressure of 80 to 95 mm Hg and a systolic blood pressure less than 160 mm Hg were randomized to receive one of three intervention diets. Participants were provided with all their meals for an 11-week period. After a 3-week run-in period on a control diet, participants were randomized to either continue with the control diet or receive (1) a diet rich in fruits and vegetables (fruits and vegetables diet) but otherwise similar to the control diet in fat and carbohydrate content or (2) a diet that combined the increased fruits and vegetables of the fruits and vegetables diet with increased low-fat dairy products and overall decreased total and saturated fat and cholesterol (DASH diet). All diets had similar sodium content (approximately 3 g/day). The diets and feeding protocols were designed to prevent significant weight change.

Participants randomized to the DASH diet had a significant decrease in blood pressure. The fruits and vegetables diet produced an intermediate effect. The DASH diet decreased blood pressure by −6/−3 mm Hg. The response was greater in African Americans (−7/−4 mm Hg systolic/diastolic) than in whites (−3/−0.5 mm Hg) and those with hypertension benefited the most (−12/−5 mm Hg).[3] By the end of the trial, 70% of participants who entered the study with hypertension had normal blood pressure (<140/90 mm Hg) if they ate the DASH diet compared with only 23% of those eating the control diet.[4] The DASH diet was well accepted and self-reported adherence with the diet was more than 90%.

Other dietary patterns that build on the components of the DASH diet may also be beneficial for blood pressure in individuals with prehypertension and hypertension. Evidence supporting favorable effects of protein and unsaturated fat intake on blood pressure led to the Optimal Macronutrient Intake Trial to Prevent Heart Disease (OMNI-Heart).[5] Three healthy dietary patterns were assessed: a carbohydrate-rich diet (similar to the DASH diet), a diet rich in protein (approximately one half from plant sources), and a diet rich in unsaturated fat (mostly monounsaturated fat). All the diets were enriched in vegetables, fiber, potassium, and other minerals, with decreased saturated fat and cholesterol. Participants consumed each of the

Table 49-1 Nonpharmacologic Treatments to Prevent and Manage Hypertension

Intervention	Approximate Systolic Blood Pressure Reduction (mm Hg)
Dietary patterns	
DASH	6–12
DASH with higher protein or monounsaturated fat intake	8–14
Individual micronutrients	
Potassium	4
Calcium	1
Magnesium	No change
Other dietary changes	
Restricting alcohol intake	3
Coffee consumption	+2
Cocoa consumption	1–3
Weight loss	5–20/10 kg
Exercise	7
Other lifestyle changes	
Smoking cessation	No change (short term)
Tai chi	No change
Transcendental meditation	3
Acupuncture	No change

DASH, Dietary Approaches to Stop Hypertension study.

diets for 6 weeks. Each diet significantly decreased blood pressure. However, the diets that substituted protein or unsaturated fat for carbohydrate (~10% of total calories) further decreased systolic blood pressure by as much as 4 mm Hg in hypertensive participants.

Each of these feeding studies was a short-term trial that assessed effects on blood pressure. Other epidemiologic studies have confirmed the favorable long-term effects of similar lifestyle modifications on cardiovascular disease outcomes. Modifying dietary fat intake for secondary prevention of coronary heart disease (CHD) was confirmed in the Lyon Diet Heart Study, which showed that a Mediterranean-type diet, enriched in linolenic acid but with decreased saturated fat, decreased CHD mortality by 70%.[6] Two large cohort studies, the Nurses' Health Study (>75,000 women) and the Health Professionals' Follow-up Study (>38,000 men), indicated that risk of ischemic stroke was decreased by 31%[7] and the risk of CHD was decreased by 20%[8] among individuals consuming the highest quintile for daily intake of fruits and vegetables (approximately five to six servings per day). In other analyses from the Nurses' Health Study, a dietary pattern similar to that of the DASH diet was associated with a 24% decreased risk of CHD over a 12-year period.[9] Higher fiber intake was associated with a 47% risk reduction for CHD events[10] and higher whole-grain intake with a 43% decrease in ischemic stroke.[11]

Thus, the DASH diet and similar dietary patterns studied in the OMNI-Heart Trial decrease blood pressure. Components of these dietary patterns are also associated with a decreased incidence of cardiovascular events. These findings provide abundant evidence that dietary patterns enriched in fruits and vegetables and low in saturated fat are an effective, well-tolerated, nonpharmacologic treatment for prehypertension and stage 1 hypertension.

EFFECTS OF INDIVIDUAL DIETARY MICRO- AND MACRONUTRIENTS

In an attempt to dissect the blood pressure effects of individual dietary nutrients, several studies have evaluated effects of mineral intake (i.e., potassium, calcium, and magnesium) and macronutrient intake (i.e., protein, carbohydrate, and fat).

Substantial evidence exists for an effect of higher potassium intake on blood pressure. A number of clinical trials and meta-analyses have confirmed that increased potassium intake is associated with lower blood pressure. Whelton and colleagues[12] showed that a net increase in potassium intake of 2 g/day (50 mmol/day) resulted in a significant decrease in blood pressure by −4/−3 mm Hg. Blood pressure effects in African Americans appear to be greater than those in whites.

Support for a small effect on blood pressure by increased calcium intake comes from a series of observational and interventional studies. Although increased calcium intake per se is associated with lower blood pressure, a meta-analyses of trials showed that the effects are modest, amounting to approximately 1 mm Hg or less for systolic and diastolic blood pressures.[13,14] Similarly, although there is an association between increased magnesium intake and lower blood pressure, an analysis of 20 trials did not show a significant effect on blood pressure.[15]

Increased potassium, calcium, and magnesium intake may be achieved through individual supplements or food intake. However, the preferred strategy is to increase such micronutrient intake from foods rather than nutritional supplements because the former would also provide other nutrients. For example, adhering to the DASH dietary pattern provides intake of these micronutrients at or near recommended levels, approximately 4.7 g/day of potassium, 0.5 g/day of magnesium, and 1.25 g/day of calcium, based on 2100 kcal/day.

Dietary intake of macronutrients, that is, carbohydrate, protein, and fat, may also affect blood pressure. However, in general the effects are less certain and likely complex. Probably the most consistent evidence is an inverse relationship between blood pressure and protein intake (primarily from plant sources).[16] However, in studies in which one macronutrient is altered, there is always a concomitant change in others, making it difficult to discern whether an effect is due to increases in one or decreases in another. In the OMNI-Heart Trial,[5] a carbohydrate-rich diet similar to the DASH diet decreased blood pressure significantly, but partial substitution of carbohydrate with protein or monounsaturated fat further decreased blood pressure. Thus, these findings are consistent with the hypothesis that substituting carbohydrate with either protein or monounsaturated fat decreases blood pressure further. However, it is unclear whether this is mediated by the increases in protein or unsaturated fat rather than decreases in carbohydrate intake.

EFFECTS OF DIETARY SODIUM RESTRICTION

Sodium restriction has been well documented to decrease blood pressure in normal and hypertensive individuals. Guidelines for the prevention and treatment of hypertension continue to advocate restriction of dietary sodium intake in the general population by limiting intake to no more than 2.3 g/day.[17] A discussion of the evidence and recommendations for reduced sodium intake are detailed in Chapter 50.

EFFECTS OF OTHER DIETARY CHANGES

There is ample evidence showing a direct relationship between alcohol intake and blood pressure. Some evidence suggests that not only the amount but also the pattern of alcohol intake affects blood pressure. Binge drinking has acute effects on blood pressure compared with similar amounts consumed in a distributed manner.[18] Although moderate alcohol intake is associated with favorable effects on CHD, this same relationship is not evident for the incidence of ischemic stroke. Possibly through its effects on blood pressure, increased alcohol intake is associated with higher risk.[19] Decreasing excess alcohol intake decreases blood pressure. Results from a meta-analysis of 15 trials showed that decreasing alcohol intake by approximately 75% resulted in a significant decrease in blood pressure ($-3/-2$ mm Hg).[20]

Coffee consumption has a complex relationship with blood pressure. Some evidence suggests a positive relationship, with intake of more than five cups per day associated with increased blood pressure ($+2/+1$ mm Hg).[21] One study suggested a direct relationship between coffee intake and incident hypertension[22]; another study showed a U-shaped relationship, with coffee abstainers and those with higher intake (more than six cups/day) having the lowest risk of hypertension.[23] However, studies of coffee intake have not adequately controlled for other lifestyle factors, such as stress, smoking, alcohol intake, and brewing methods that may produce more or less caffeine in the beverage. Coffee contains a mixture of substances that affect blood pressure. In a meta-analysis of studies evaluating coffee intake compared with caffeine per se, intake of caffeine tablets increased blood pressure by $+4/+2$ mm Hg, whereas coffee intake increased blood pressure by $+1/+0.5$ mm Hg.[24] In contrast, long-term green tea consumption has no significant short-term effects on blood pressure[25] but is associated with decreased risk of incident hypertension.[26]

Recently there has been much interest in the effects of cocoa consumption on blood pressure and endothelial function. Several short-term studies have investigated the effects of cocoa consumption on blood pressure. In a meta-analysis of five trials, cocoa drinkers had a $-5/-3$ mm Hg decrease in blood pressure compared with control groups over a median of 2 weeks, with the greatest effects seen in younger hypertensive individuals.[25] Although these early results are intriguing, most studies are of short duration and conducted in an unblinded manner. At present, it is unclear whether long-term increased cocoa consumption is effective in decreasing blood pressure. Because most forms of dietary cocoa are contained in high-fat or carbohydrate-rich foods, cocoa consumption should be approached with caution, with particular attention to calorie substitution for other calorie-dense portions of the typical diet.

EFFECTS OF WEIGHT LOSS

Weight loss as a lifestyle modification has long been advocated to decrease blood pressure and other cardiovascular risk factors. This has been explored in relationship to blood pressure in several recent trials.[27-32] In each, weight loss (particularly among obese participants) decreased blood pressure, prevented the development of hypertension, or potentiated the effects of antihypertensives.

The Trials of Hypertension Prevention phase I entailed an 18-month lifestyle modification in which individuals with high-normal blood pressure were randomized to weight loss, sodium restriction, or a control group.[29] Follow-up examinations (7 years after randomization) were conducted in 181 of the 208 participants studied at Johns Hopkins University.[30] During the original 18-month study, significant weight loss was achieved in the group randomized to the weight-loss intervention. This was associated with a significant decrease in blood pressure. However, after 7 years of follow-up, the weight-loss group did not differ from the other intervention groups in body weight or urinary sodium excretion. Despite this, the weight-loss group retained a decreased incidence of hypertension of 77%.

The Trials of Hypertension Prevention phase II study had a similar design but enrolled more patients and had 3 to 4 years of follow-up.[28,31] The group randomized to weight loss (595 individuals with high-normal blood pressure who were 110%–165% of ideal body weight) had a 2-kg weight difference at 3 years of follow-up. This modest weight loss was associated with a 19% decreased risk of developing hypertension; those with a sustained 4.5-kg weight loss had a 65% decreased risk.

In a substudy of the Hypertension Optimal Treatment study, obese hypertensive patients were randomly assigned to receive a weight-loss intervention, including individual and group counseling, or no intervention.[32] Those in the weight-loss group lost significantly more weight than the control group during the initial 6 months, but at 30 months of follow-up, there was no significant difference. Despite this, patients in the weight-loss group used fewer medications to achieve the same blood pressure.

These results show that weight-loss interventions may facilitate control of blood pressure and prevent the progression to hypertension or may control blood pressure with fewer antihypertensive medications, even without producing sustained weight loss.

EFFECTS OF EXERCISE

Exercise is frequently promoted as a tool to facilitate weight loss and decrease blood pressure. Indeed, exercise and weight loss together result in lower blood pressure than either alone.[33] The mechanisms that mediate decreasing of blood pressure with exercise likely include effects on the sympathetic nervous system, renin-angiotensin system, and endothelial function. These effects appear to be independent of changes in weight or body composition.

Several studies have evaluated the effects of moderate-intensity aerobic exercise or resistance training on blood pressure. Among individuals with high-normal or stage 1 hypertension, aerobic exercise decreases blood pressure significantly, although the effects tend to be smaller than those seen with moderate sodium restriction.[34] Among postmenopausal women[35] or elderly individuals,[36] low- to moderate-intensity aerobic exercise (e.g., walking) significantly decreases blood pressure. Among postmenopausal women, increased frequency of moderate physical activity is associated with a 30% decreased risk of mortality over 7 years.[37]

Meta-analyses have compared the effects of walking, aerobic exercise, and resistance exercise on blood pressure. One may conclude that regular aerobic exercise produces the greatest reduction in blood pressure ($-7/-6$ mm Hg)[38,39] compared with walking ($-3/-2$ mm Hg)[40] or resistance exercise ($-3/-3$ mm Hg).[41]

Thus, the optimal exercise program for decreasing blood pressure should include moderate-intensity aerobic exercise three to five times per week for 30 to 60 minutes per session. Resistance exercise has limited effects on blood pressure. There is no apparent age- or sex-related difference in the response to exercise. Weight loss is facilitated by exercise programs that expend 1255 to 2090 kJ/day. Exercise intensity and duration should be appropriate to the individual's abilities and concomitant medical conditions. In some cases, an assessment of cardiovascular risk may be appropriate before participation in a regular exercise program. As with most lifestyle modifications, the greatest effects on blood pressure occur in individuals with high-normal or stages 1 to 2 hypertension.

EFFECTS OF OTHER LIFESTYLE CHANGES

Smoking cessation clearly decreases cardiovascular risk. However, its effects on blood pressure are uncertain. Indeed, several studies have shown that former smokers have a significant risk of developing hypertension with longer duration of smoking cessation. Among former smokers who quit for more than 3 years, the relative risk of hypertension was 3.5.[42] Much of this increased risk of hypertension may relate to the weight gain that frequently occurs after smoking cessation.[43,44] Smoking is also associated with diffuse vascular changes including increased vascular stiffness and pulse wave velocity. Unlike the increasing risk of hypertension among former smokers, more than 10 years of smoking cessation reverses these vascular changes.[45]

Complementary and alternative medicine techniques to decrease blood pressure have been evaluated, although limitations and biases are present in many studies. In a systematic review of the health outcomes of tai chi, there appears to be some physiologic and psychological benefits.[46] However, specific studies of effects of tai chi on blood pressure have shown no benefit. In a study that directly compared tai chi with resistance training among healthy elderly participants over a 12-month period, tai chi had no significant effect on blood pressure.[47]

Stress reduction through transcendental meditation (TM) has varied effects on blood pressure. Results of a meta-analysis of randomized trials of TM revealed no convincing evidence of an effect of TM on blood pressure, with significant concerns about study methodologies and potential author bias. However, in a study of hypertensive African Americans, TM for 20 minutes twice daily decreased blood pressure $-3/-5$ mm Hg over 12 months.[48] A randomized trial of TM compared with health education in patients with CHD showed significant benefits in blood pressure ($-3/-2$ mm Hg) and insulin resistance over a 16-week period.[49] In a study of long-term follow-up of participants in trials of TM and other behavioral stress-reducing interventions, the TM group had a 23% decrease in all-cause mortality and a 30% decrease in cardiovascular mortality.[50] Thus, stress-reducing interventions such as TM may have beneficial effects among individuals with hypertension, but good-quality evidence is lacking.

Small studies and anecdotal evidence initially supported an effect of acupuncture on blood pressure in hypertensive patients.[51] However, the results of a randomized, controlled trial of acupuncture has now debunked that purported effect. The Stop Hypertension with Acupuncture Research Program study enrolled 192 participants with untreated hypertension, randomized to individualized or standardized acupuncture compared with sham acupuncture.[52] After a 10-week period, there was no significant difference between those receiving acupuncture compared with the sham control subjects. Thus, use of acupuncture to decrease blood pressure likely offers no significant clinical benefit.

EFFECTS OF COMBINED DIETARY AND NONPHARMACOLOGIC INTERVENTIONS

Although clinical trials have often studied the effects of single dietary or lifestyle interventions on blood pressure, guidelines and recommendations advocate combining multiple interventions. Those studies that have carefully evaluated such comprehensive lifestyle modifications have shown significant favorable effects on blood pressure.

The PREMIER study assessed the blood pressure effects of implementing all the major lifestyle modifications. This randomized trial was designed to assess the effects of multiple established lifestyle recommendations with or without the addition of the DASH diet.[53] Participants with prehypertension and stage 1 hypertension were studied. Compared with a control group that received advice about adopting such lifestyle changes, both groups that received the multiple behavioral interventions experienced significant weight loss, improved fitness, and decreased sodium intake, whereas the group that received counseling on the DASH diet also increased fruit, vegetable, and dairy intake over the 6 months of study. When compared with the advice-only group, the overall change in systolic blood pressure from the combined interventions including the DASH diet was -4 mm Hg. The prevalence of hypertension was decreased from 38% to 12% among those following the behavioral intervention that included the DASH diet. No participants had blood pressure less than 120/80 mm Hg at baseline, but this number increased to 35% in the group that received counseling on the DASH diet. More than 90% of study participants were followed for as long as 18 months to see whether the recommended lifestyle changes persisted and to assess their clinical effects. Blood pressure remained lower in the groups that received the multiple behavioral interventions with or without the DASH diet. The odds ratio for developing hypertension at 18 months was decreased by 23% among those following the DASH diet (see Table 49-2).[54]

This same approach has been applied to individuals with treated hypertension. In a study of overweight hypertensive patients taking a single antihypertensive medication, participants were randomized to a control group or to a group that received a weight-reducing version of the DASH diet with sodium restriction and a supervised moderate-intensity exercise program.[55] After 9 weeks, those in the intervention group had significant reductions in 24-hour ambulatory blood pres-

sure ($-10/-5$ mm Hg), weight (-5 kg), and cholesterol (-25 mg/dL).

The Trial of Nonpharmacologic Interventions in the Elderly (TONE) studied hypertensive patients between 60 and 80 years of age who were treated with one antihypertensive medication.[27] Overweight patients were randomized to either sodium restriction (<1.8 g/day), weight loss (at least 10 lb), combined weight loss and decreased sodium intake, or usual care, whereas normal-weight patients were assigned to sodium reduction or usual care. Those in the weight-loss group lost an average of 8 to 10 lb. Thirty-eight percent of those in the sodium-reduction group decreased their

Table 49-2 Following the Dietary Approaches to Stop Hypertension (DASH) Diet

Food Group	Daily Servings (Except as Noted)	Serving Sizes	Examples and Notes	Significance of Each Food Group to the DASH Eating Plan
Grain and grain products	7–8	1 slice bread 1 oz dry cereal* ½ cup cooked rice, pasta, or cereal	Whole wheat bread, English muffin, pita bread, bagel, cereals, grits, oatmeal, crackers, unsalted pretzels, popcorn	Major sources of energy and fiber
Vegetables	4–5	1 cup raw leafy vegetable ½ cup cooked vegetable 6 oz vegetable juice	Tomatoes, potatoes, carrots, green peas, squash, broccoli, turnip greens, collards, kale, spinach, artichokes, green beans, lima beans, sweet potatoes	Rich sources of potassium, magnesium, and fiber
Fruits	4–5	6 oz fruit juice 1 medium fruit ¼ cup dried fruit ½ cup fresh, frozen, or canned fruit	Apricots, bananas, dates, grapes, oranges, orange juice, grapefruit, grapefruit juice, mangoes, melons, peaches, pineapples, prunes, raisins, strawberries, tangerines	Important sources of potassium, magnesium, and fiber
Low-fat or fat-free dairy foods	2–3	8 oz skim milk 1 cup yogurt 1½ oz cheese	Fat-free (skim) or low-fat (1%) milk, fat-free or low-fat fat buttermilk, fat-free or low-fat regular or frozen yogurt, low-fat and fat-free cheese	Major sources of calcium and protein
Meats, poultry, and fish	≤2	3 oz cooked meats, poultry, or fish	Select only lean; trim away visible fats; broil, roast, or boil instead of frying; remove skin from poultry	Rich sources of protein and magnesium
Nuts, seeds, and dry beans	4–5 per week	⅓ cup or 1½ oz nuts 2 tbsp or ½ oz seeds ½ cup cooked dry beans	Almonds, filberts, mixed nuts, peanuts, walnuts, sunflower seeds, kidney beans, lentils, peas	Rich sources of energy, magnesium, potassium, protein, and fiber
Fats and oils†	2–3	1 tsp soft margarine 1 tbsp low-fat mayonnaise 2 tbsp light salad dressing 1 tsp vegetable oil	Soft margarine, low-fat mayonnaise, light salad dressing, vegetable oil (such as olive, corn, canola, and safflower)	DASH has 27% of calories as fat, including that in or added to foods

*Equals ½ to 1¼ cups, depending on cereal type. Check the product's nutrition label.
†Fat content changes serving counts for fats and oils; for example, 1 tbsp of regular salad dressing equals one serving; 1 tbsp of a low-fat dressing equals ½ serving; 1 tbsp of a fat-free dressing equals 0 servings.
The Dietary Approaches to Stop Hypertension (DASH) eating plan is based on a calorie intake of 2000 calories per day. The number of daily servings in a food group may vary based on the caloric needs of the individual.
From Facts about the DASH Diet (NIH publication 01-4082), Bethesda, MD: NHLBI Health Information Center, May 2001.

sodium intake to less than 1.8 g/day. After 30 months, 30% were off antihypertensive medications. The need for antihypertensive medications was decreased by 31% with sodium restriction, by 36% with weight loss, and by 53% with the combination of both.

CONCLUSION AND RECOMMENDATIONS

There is ample evidence showing favorable blood pressure effects with consumption of low-fat diets enriched in fruits and vegetables such as the DASH diet, sodium restriction, weight-loss interventions, restricting alcohol intake, and increased aerobic exercise. There is some evidence of favorable effects with relaxation techniques such as TM. There are no clear blood pressure benefits from restricting coffee intake and smoking cessation, although these and other lifestyle changes may have benefits for cardiovascular health that extend beyond blood pressure control.

The results of these studies have broad applicability. Although lifestyle modifications and nonpharmacologic treatments are difficult to sustain, a population-wide decrease in blood pressure to the same extent as was observed with the DASH diet would reduce the incidence of CHD by 15% and stroke by 27%.[17] The long-term effects on blood pressure of weight-loss interventions, with or without aerobic exercise, provide a strong case to continue advocating for obese individuals to receive weight management counseling. A secondary benefit of these lifestyle changes (2–3 kg weight loss) also includes a decreased incidence of type 2 diabetes mellitus, particularly in those with impaired glucose tolerance.[56]

The foods that comprise the DASH diet are readily available. The DASH diet is not expensive, but eating the DASH diet requires attention to food groups, caloric requirements, and the calorie content of foods (Table 49-2). The servings of fruits and vegetables (8–10 daily) are approximately twice the typical daily consumption of four servings by U.S. adults. Likewise, the three servings of dairy products are twice the typical daily U.S. consumption.[57] More detailed summaries of the findings of the DASH studies and some menus that employ the DASH diet have been published for lay audiences.[58,59]

Results from studies of lifestyle and dietary modifications are relevant to the care of patients with prehypertension and hypertension.[60] However, it is important to keep in mind a few points that have not been addressed:

1. Most studies have involved only short-term intervention periods. In some cases, it is not known whether such blood pressure changes are sustained over longer periods of time.
2. Some studies of dietary patterns provided foods to study participants and therefore facilitated adherence to the diet. When such dietary patterns are replicated in real life and individuals are responsible for purchasing and preparing their own foods, it is not known what level of adherence to the dietary pattern is necessary to produce the same effect.
3. Studies of dietary patterns did not assess the effects of individual components of the diets. Thus, one cannot conclude that specific food items and/or nutrients (e.g., potassium, magnesium, carbohydrate) produce the effects of the dietary pattern. It is very likely that an interaction of effects

from the various dietary constituents is responsible for the favorable effects.
4. Lifestyle changes have greater blood pressure effects in patients with hypertension than in those with prehypertension. However, individuals with higher levels of blood pressure (e.g., stage 2 hypertension) will likely require adjunctive therapy (i.e., antihypertensive medications) to fully control blood pressure.
5. The DASH dietary pattern is enriched in potassium, magnesium, and protein, which should be limited in patients with kidney disease. Therefore, this dietary pattern should be implemented with caution in such patients.

Patients can implement lifestyle modifications and nonpharmacologic treatments on their own. Such interventions involve minimal risk, may have a positive impact on quality of life, and may also be less expensive than antihypertensive medications. The long-term beneficial effects of eating a dietary pattern such as the DASH diet have been demonstrated. Clearly, the role of lifestyle modifications has been affirmed in both the prevention and treatment of hypertension.

References

1. Hyman DJ, Pavlik VN: Characteristics of patients with uncontrolled hypertension in the United States. N Engl J Med 2001; 345:479–486.
2. Appel LJ, Moore TJ, Obarzanek E, et al: A clinical trial of the effects of dietary patterns on blood pressure. N Engl J Med 1997;336:1117–1124.
3. Svetkey LP, Simons-Morton D, Vollmer WM, et al: Effects of dietary patterns on blood pressure: Subgroup analysis of the Dietary Approaches to Stop Hypertension (DASH) randomized clinical trial. Arch Intern Med 1999;159:285–293.
4. Conlin PR, Chow D, Miller ER, et al: The effect of dietary patterns on blood pressure control in hypertensive patients: Results from the Dietary Approaches to Stop Hypertension (DASH) Trial. Am J Hypertens 2000;13:949–955.
5. Appel LJ, Sacks FM, Carey V, et al: The effects of protein, monounsaturated fat, and carbohydrate intake on blood pressure and serum lipids: Results of the OmniHeart Randomized Trial. JAMA 2005;294:2455–2464.
6. de Lorgeril M, Salen P, Martin J-L, et al: Mediterranean diet, traditional risk factors, and the rate of cardiovascular complications after myocardial infarction: Final report of the Lyon Diet Heart Study. Circulation 1999;99:779–785.
7. Joshipura KJ, Ascherio A, Manson JE, et al: Fruit and vegetable intake in relation to risk of ischemic stroke. JAMA 1999;282: 1233–1239.
8. Joshipura KJ, Hu FB, Manson JE, et al: The effect of fruit and vegetable intake on risk for coronary heart disease. Ann Intern Med 2001;134:1106–1114.
9. Fung TT, Willet WC, Stampfer MJ, et al: Dietary patterns and the risk of coronary heart disease in women. Arch Intern Med 2001;161:1857–1862.
10. Wolk A, Manson JE, Stampfer MJ, et al: Long-term intake of dietary fiber and decreased risk of coronary heart disease among women. JAMA 1999;281:1998–2004.
11. Liu S, Manson JE, Stampfer MJ, et al: Whole grain consumption and risk of ischemic stroke in women: A prospective study. JAMA 2000;284:1534–1540.
12. Whelton PK, He J, Cutler JA, et al: Effects of oral potassium on blood pressure. Meta-analysis of randomized controlled clinical trials. JAMA 1997;277:1624–1632.

13. Allender PS, Cutler JA, Follmann D, et al: Dietary calcium and blood pressure: A meta-analysis of randomized clinical trials. Ann Inter Med 1996;124:825–831.

14. Bucher HC, Cook RJ, Guyatt GH, et al: Effects of dietary calcium supplementation on blood pressure: A meta-analysis of randomized controlled trials. JAMA 1996;275:1016–1022.

15. Jee SH, Miller ER, Guallar E, et al: The effect of magnesium supplementation on blood pressure: A meta-analysis of randomized clinical trials. Am J Hypertens 2002;15:691–696.

16. Obarzanek E, Velletri PA, Cutler JA: Dietary protein and blood pressure. JAMA 1996;275:1598–1603.

17. Chobanian AV, Bakris GL, Black HR, et al, for the Joint National Committee on Prevention, Detection, Evaluation, and Treatment of High Blood Pressure. National Heart, Lung, and Blood Institute; National High Blood Pressure Education Program Coordinating Committee: Seventh report of the Joint National Committee on Prevention, Detection, Evaluation, and Treatment of High Blood Pressure. Hypertension 2003;42:1206–1252.

18. Marques-Vidal P, Arveiler D, Evans A, et al: Different alcohol drinking and blood pressure relationships in France and Northern Ireland: The PRIME Study. Hypertension 2001;38:1361–1366.

19. Mukamal KJ, Asherio A, Mittleman MA, et al: Alcohol and risk for ischemic stroke in men: The role of drinking patterns and usual beverage. Ann Intern Med 2005;142:11–19.

20. Xin X, He J, Frontini MG, et al: Effects of alcohol reduction on blood pressure: A meta-analysis of randomized controlled trials. Hypertension 2001;38:1112–1117.

21. Jee SH, He J, Whelton PK, et al: The effects of chronic coffee drinking on blood pressure: A meta-analysis of controlled clinical trials. Hypertension 1999;33:647–652.

22. Uiterwaal CS, Verschuren WM, Bueno-de-Medquita HB, et al: Coffee intake and incidence of hypertension. Am J Clin Nutr 2007;85:718–723.

23. Klag MJ, Wang NY, Meoni LA, et al: Coffee intake and risk of hypertension: The Johns Hopkins precursors study. Arch Intern Med 2002;162:657–662.

24. Noordzij M, Uiterwaal CS, Arends LR, et al: Blood pressure response to chronic intake of coffee and caffeine: A meta-analysis of randomized controlled trials. J Hypertens 2005;23:921–928.

25. Taubert D, Roesen R, Schömig E: Effect of cocoa and tea intake on blood pressure: A meta-analysis. Arch Intern Med 2007;167:626–634.

26. Yang YC, Lu FH, Wu JS, et al: The protective effect of habitual tea consumption on hypertension. Arch Intern Med 2004;164:1534–1540.

27. Whelton PK, Appel LJ, Espeland MA, et al: Sodium reduction and weight loss in the treatment of hypertension in older persons: A randomized controlled trial of nonpharmacologic interventions in the elderly (TONE). JAMA 1998;279:839–846.

28. The Trials of Hypertension Prevention Collaborative Research Group: Effects of weight loss and sodium reduction intervention on blood pressure and hypertension incidence in overweight people with high-normal blood pressure: The Trials of Hypertension Prevention, Phase II. Arch Intern Med 1997;157:657–667.

29. Trials of Hypertension Prevention Collaborative Research Group: The effects of non-pharmacologic interventions on blood pressure of persons with high normal levels: Results of the Trials of Hypertension Prevention, Phase 1. JAMA 1992;267:1213–1220.

30. He J, Whelton PK, Appel LJ, et al: Long-term effects of weight loss and dietary sodium reduction on incidence of hypertension. Hypertension 2000;35:544–549.

31. Stevens VJ, Obarzanek E, Cook NR, et al: Long-term weight loss and changes in blood pressure: Results of the Trials of Hypertension Prevention, Phase II. Ann Intern Med 2001;134:72–74.

32. Jones DW, Miller ME, Wofford MR, et al: The effect of weight loss intervention on antihypertensive medication requirements in the Hypertension Optimal Treatment (HOT) Study. Am J Hypertens 1999;12:1175–1180.

33. Steffen PR, Sherwood A, Gullette EC, et al: Effects of exercise and weight loss on blood pressure during daily life. Med Sci Sports Exerc 2001;33:1635–1640.

34. Seals DR, Tanaka H, Clevenger CM, et al: Blood pressure reductions with exercise and sodium restriction in post-menopausal women with elevated systolic pressure: Role of arterial stiffness. J Am Coll Cardiol 2001;38:506–513.

35. Seals DR, Silverman HG, Reiling MJ, Davy KP: Effect of regular aerobic exercise on elevated blood pressure in postmenopausal women. Am J Cardiol 1997;80:49–55.

36. Ehsani AA: Exercise in patients with hypertension. Am J Geriatr Cardiol 2001;10:253–259.

37. Kushi LH, Fee RM, Folsom AR, et al: Physical activity and mortality in postmenopausal women. JAMA 1997;277:1287–1292.

38. Kelley G, McClellan P: Antihypertensive effects of aerobic exercise: A brief meta-analytic review of randomized controlled trials. Am J Hypertens 1994;7:115–119.

39. Fagard RH: Effects of exercise, diet, and their combination on blood pressure. J Hum Hyper 2005;19(Suppl):S20–S24.

40. Kelley GA, Kelley KS, Tran ZV: Walking and resting blood pressure in adults: A meta-analysis. Prev Med 2001;33:120–127.

41. Kelley GA, Kelley KS: Progressive resistance exercise and resting blood pressure: A meta-analysis of randomized controlled trials. Hypertension 2000;35:838–843.

42. Lee D-H, Myung-Hwa H, Jang-Rak K, Jacobs DR. Effects of smoking cessation on changes in blood pressure and incidence of hypertension: A 4 year follow-up study. Hypertension 2001;37:194–198.

43. Halmini JM, Giraudeau B, Vol S, et al: The risk of hypertension in men: Direct and indirect effects of chronic smoking. J Hypertens 2002;20:187–193.

44. John U, Meyer C, Hanke M, et al: Smoking status, obesity and hypertension in a general population sample: A cross-sectional study. Q J Med 2006;99:407–415.

45. Jatoi NA, Jerrard-Dunne P, Feely J, Mahmud A: Impact of smoking and smoking cessation on arterial stiffness and aortic wave reflection in hypertension. Hypertension 2007;49:981–985.

46. Wang C, Collet JP, Lau J: The effects of tai chi on health outcomes in patients with chronic conditions: A systematic review. Arch Intern Med 2004;164:493–501.

47. Thomas GN, Hong AW, Tomlinson B, et al: Effects of tai chi and resistance training on cardiovascular risk factors in elderly Chinese subjects: A 12 month longitudinal, randomized, controlled intervention study. Clin Endocrinol (Oxf) 2005;63:663–669.

48. Schneider RH, Alexander CN, Staggers F, et al: A randomized controlled trial of stress reduction in African Americans treated for hypertension over one year. Am J Hypertens 2005;18:88–98.

49. Paul-Labrador M, Polk D, Dwyer JH, et al: Effects of a randomized controlled trial of transcendental meditation on components of the metabolic syndrome in subjects with coronary artery disease. Arch Intern Med 2006;166:1218–1224.

50. Schneider RH, Alexander CN, Staggers F, et al: Long-term effects of stress reduction on mortality in persons > or = 55 years of age with systemic hypertension. Am J Cardiol 2005;95:1060–1064.

51. Yin C, Seo B, Park HJ, et al: Acupuncture, a promising adjunctive therapy for essential hypertension: A double-blind, randomized, controlled trial. Neurol Res 2007;29(Suppl 1):S98–S103.

52. Macklin EA, Wayne PM, Kalish LA, et al: Stop Hypertension with the Acupuncture Research Program (SHARP): Results of a randomized, controlled trial. Hypertension 2006;48:838–845.

53. Appel LJ, Champagne CM, Harsha DW, et al, for the Writing Group of the PREMIER Collaborative Research Group: Effects of comprehensive lifestyle modifications on blood pressure control: Main results of the PREMIER clinical trial. JAMA 2003; 289:2083–2093.

54. Elmer PJ, Obarzanek E, Vollmer WM, et al, for the PREMIER Collaborative Research Group: Effects of comprehensive lifestyle modifications on diet, weight, physical activity, and blood pressure control: 18 month results of a randomized trial. Ann Intern Med 2006;144:485–495.

55. Miller ER, Erlinger TP, Young DR, et al: Results of the Diet, Exercise, and Weight Loss Intervention Trial (DEW-IT). Hypertension 2002;40:612–618.

56. Tuomilehto J, Lindstrom J, Eriksson J, et al: Prevention of type 2 diabetes mellitus by changes in lifestyle among subjects with impaired glucose tolerance. N Engl J Med 2001;344: 1343–1350.

57. Cleveland LE, Goldman JD, Borrud LG: Data tables: Results from the USDA's 1994 Continuing Survey of Food Intakes by Individuals and the 1994 Diet and Health Knowledge Survey. Riverdale, MD: Food Surveys Research Group, 1996.

58. National Institutes of Health: Facts about the DASH Diet. Bethesda, MD: National Institutes of Health, NIH Publication no. 01-4082, 2001.

59. Moore TM, Pao-Hwa L, Karanja N, et al: The DASH Diet for Hypertension. New York: Free Press, 2001.

60. Appel LJ, Brands MW, Daniels SR, et al: Dietary approaches to prevent and treat hypertension: A scientific statement from the American Heart Association. Hypertension 2006;47: 296–308.

Further Reading

Appel LJ, Brands MW, Daniels SR, et al: Dietary approaches to prevent and treat hypertension: A scientific statement from the American Heart Association. Hypertension 2006;47:296–308.

Appel LJ, Champagne CM, Harsha DW, et al, for the Writing Group of the PREMIER Collaborative Research Group: Effects of comprehensive lifestyle modifications on blood pressure control: Main results of the PREMIER clinical trial. JAMA 2003;289:2083–2093.

Beyer FR, Dickinson HO, Nicolson DJ, et al: Combined calcium, magnesium and potassium supplementation for the management of primary hypertension in adults. Cochrane Database Syst Rev 2006;(3):CD004805.

Chobanian AV, Bakris GL, Black HR, et al for the Joint National Committee on Prevention, Detection, Evaluation, and Treatment of High Blood Pressure. National Heart, Lung, and Blood Institute; National High Blood Pressure Education Program Coordinating Committee. Seventh report of the Joint National Committee on Prevention,
Detection, Evaluation, and Treatment of High Blood Pressure. Hypertension 2003;42:1206–1252.

Dickinson HO, Mason JM, Nicolson DJ, et al: Lifestyle interventions to reduce raised blood pressure: A systematic review of randomized controlled trials. J Hypertens 2006;24:215–233.

Dickinson HO, Nicolson DJ, Campbell F, et al: Potassium supplementation for the management of primary hypertension in adults. Cochrane Database Syst Rev 2006;(3):CD004641.

National Institutes of Health: Facts about the DASH Diet. NIH Publication no. 03-4082. Bethesda, MD: National Institutes of Health, 2003.

Chapter 50

Dietary Salt Reduction

Francesco P. Cappuccio

CHAPTER CONTENTS

Cardiovascular diseases (CVDs) are the leading cause of mortality, morbidity, and disability worldwide.[1] Although CVDs are proportionally more relevant in developed countries, currently 70% of the total number of cardiovascular deaths occurs in developing countries. Globally, high blood pressure causes 7 million premature deaths per year.[1] In particular, hypertension affects approximately 1 billion individuals.[2] The burden of hypertension-related diseases is likely to increase as the population ages.[3] Overall, high blood pressure is the most important and independent risk factor for myocardial infarction, heart failure, stroke, and kidney disease. Accordingly, prevention and treatment of hypertension are increasingly regarded as a priority in both developed and developing countries.

Nonpharmacologic interventions, also termed lifestyle modifications, represent an essential approach to the primary prevention of high blood pressure and an important component of the treatment of hypertension. These lifestyle modifications are effective in decreasing blood pressure, increasing the efficacy of pharmacologic therapies, and decreasing the global risk of CVD. In this chapter, I evaluate the appropriateness of recommendations at a population level regarding the reduction of dietary salt intake, the different approaches to intervention needed to implement a successful strategy to prevent hypertension in developing and developed countries, and the recommendations to individuals to reduce dietary salt intake for the overall management of hypertension.

DEFINITIONS

Publications refer to sodium intake as either mass or millimolar amounts of sodium or mass of sodium chloride (salt) (1 g of sodium chloride = 17.1 millimolar amounts of sodium or 393.4 mg of sodium). In this chapter, the word *salt* is used to refer to sodium and sodium chloride intake. The term *reduction in dietary salt intake* implies the reduction in total sodium intake from all dietary sources including, for example, additives such as monosodium glutamate and preservatives.

EFFECT OF DECREASING DIETARY SALT INTAKE ON BLOOD PRESSURE AND CARDIOVASCULAR DISEASE

Animal studies, ecologic analyses, epidemiologic investigations, and clinical trials support a relationship between salt intake and blood pressure. The amount of dietary salt is an important determinant of blood pressure levels and of hypertension risk in both individuals and populations. This relationship is direct and progressive without an apparent threshold. Thus, the reduction in dietary salt intake is one of the most important and effective lifestyle modifications to decrease blood pressure and control hypertension.[4,5]

The importance of salt intake in determining blood pressure and the incidence of hypertension is well established. Furthermore, randomized, controlled clinical trials of moderate reductions in salt intake show a dose-dependent cause-and-effect relationship and a lack of threshold effect within usual levels of salt intake.[6] The effect is independent of age, sex, ethnic origin, baseline blood pressure, and body mass. Prospective studies[7–10] with one exception[11] also indicate that higher salt intake predicts the incidence of cardiovascular events. Finally, participants in randomized clinical trials of long-term moderate reduction in salt intake (e.g., ~2.5 g of salt reduction) show a 30% reduction in cardiovascular events 10 to 15 years later.[12]

That habitual salt intake could be associated with blood pressure levels was suggested several millennia ago, in the history of humankind, after the transition from food gathering to food producing with the addition of salt to preserve food and the consequent shift to a high-salt diet.[13]

More than 50 randomized clinical trials support a role for decreasing salt intake in the prevention and management of high blood pressure. In the largest of these trials, the Dietary Approaches to Stop Hypertension (DASH) trial,[14] salt reduction alone from a high to a low level was associated with a decrease in blood pressure of 8.3/4.4 mm Hg (systolic/diastolic) among hypertensive individuals and 5.6/2.8 mm Hg among normotensive individuals. Moreover, the combination of this amount of salt reduction and the DASH diet further decreased blood pressure by 11.5/5.7 mm Hg and 7.1/3.7 mm Hg, respectively, among those with and without hypertension. In subgroup analyses, significant effects of salt intake reduction on blood pressure levels were present in both genders and all racial and age groups, although they were more marked among African Americans, women, and those older than 45 years of age.[15]

Pooled estimates from meta-analyses of clinical trials on the effects of salt intake reduction on blood pressure levels indicate a decrease in blood pressure of 7.1/3.9 mm Hg in hypertensive individuals and 3.6/1.7 mm Hg in normotensive individuals per 100 mmol reduction of 24-hour urinary sodium excretion (~6 g of salt per day). For example, He and MacGregor[16] estimated blood pressure decreases of 5.0/2.7 mm Hg in hypertensives and 2.0/1.0 in normotensives for a median reduction in urinary sodium of 78 mmol/day. In the latest published meta-analysis of 40 randomized trials, an average decrease in urinary sodium excretion of 77 mmol/day was associated with a decrease in blood pressure levels of 2.5/2.0 mm Hg.[17] Blood pressure response was significantly greater in hypertensive than normotensive individuals (systolic: −5.2 vs. −1.3 mm Hg; diastolic: −3.7 vs. −1.1 mm Hg). Accordingly, findings from randomized clinical trials support a role for decreasing dietary salt intake in the primary prevention and management of hypertension.[18,19]

The response of blood pressure to dietary changes in salt intake, as to other environmental stimuli, may vary between individuals. This phenomenon has been termed salt sensitivity,[20] and it is likely to be due to the degree of response of the renin-angiotensin system.[21,22] The weaker the response of this system is to a change in sodium intake, the greater the response of the blood pressure will be. This phenomenon explains why the blood pressure–lowering effect of salt intake reduction is greater in hypertensive individuals, the elderly, and low-renin black populations. These groups are all characterized by weaker responses of the renin-angiotensin system to changes in the amount of salt ingested, showing a greater blood pressure decrease as a result of a decrease in dietary salt intake. Indeed, although a significant decrease in blood pressure induced by decreased salt intake has been observed in children and adolescents as well,[23] this response increases with age and is greatest in the elderly.[24] Furthermore, the blood pressure decrease observed in the elderly as a result of a dietary salt reduction may decrease the need for antihypertensive medication.[25] These observations are relevant to the prevention of hypertension-related diseases in developed countries, where the majority of strokes occur in the elderly and individuals with blood pressure levels below the treatment threshold for hypertension.[26] Nevertheless, several antihypertensive drugs blocking the renin-angiotensin system (e.g., angiotensin-converting enzyme inhibitors, β-blockers, angiotensin II receptor antagonists, and renin inhibitors) have an additive effect on blood pressure reduction in those patients already on a reduced salt diet[27] (see later).

Furthermore, people of black African origin show a greater blood pressure response when dietary salt intake is decreased.[14,22,28] For example, the efficacy of a moderate decrease in salt intake has recently been tested in two short-term trials in both urban and rural areas of West Africa (Nigeria and Ghana), where the prevalence of hypertension is increasing.[29,30] In both studies, a moderate decrease in salt intake was associated with a significant decrease in blood pressure. In areas such as sub-Saharan Africa, the prevalence of hypertension is increasing, the health care resources are scarce, and thus the identification of people with hypertension is still haphazard. The effectiveness of a decrease in salt intake at a population level might prove extremely important for policy makers.

Given the overwhelming evidence of the efficacy of decreasing dietary salt intake in the prevention and management of hypertension, the debate is currently based on issues regarding the long-term outcome benefits and thereafter the appropriateness of a population-wide strategy to reduce dietary salt intake. The major benefit of salt reduction is the lowering of blood pressure. It has been argued that the blood pressure decrease realistically achievable at a population level (i.e., 1–3 mm Hg in systolic blood pressure) is small, not clinically significant, and with long-term benefits remaining unclear.[31] However, a meta-analysis of 61 prospective studies estimated that even a decrease of 2 mm Hg in systolic blood pressure would determine a 10% decrease in stroke mortality and a 7% decrease in mortality from coronary heart disease or other cardiovascular causes, meaning a large number of premature deaths and disabilities would be avoided.[32] Other results corroborate these estimates and suggest that the benefits of such a small decrease in blood pressure, induced by reducing dietary salt intake, in the population would be almost immediate.[16] Finally, recent evidence from randomized clinical trials suggests a 30% decrease in CVD mortality after a moderate decrease in salt intake.[13] Moreover, although the principal benefit of decreasing dietary salt intake is a decrease in blood pressure, it is not the only one. There is a large body of evidence that supports other benefits: regression of left ventricular hypertrophy, reduction in proteinuria and glomerular hyperfiltration, reduction in bone mineral loss with age and osteoporosis, protection against stomach cancer, stroke, asthma attacks, and possibly cataracts.[33]

In light of the present evidence, decreasing dietary salt intake appears a plausible population-wide recommendation for the prevention and treatment of hypertension.[4,5] A decrease in dietary salt intake to no more than 6 g/day (2.3 g or <100 mmol of sodium) represents a reasonable goal at a population level given the current dietary patterns of high levels of salt intake worldwide. However, this decrease will be feasible in Western societies only if efforts are made by the food industry, manufacturers, and restaurants to decrease the amount of salt added to processed food.[34] In fact, in these societies, a large proportion of salt intake (75%–80%) comes from processed food and bread.[35] On the contrary, in developing countries where the prevalence of hypertension continues to increase, more traditional health promotion strategies would be applicable and nutritional education might have an important effect in these settings.[26,30,36] In the next sections, the issues pertaining to the implementation of public health strategies to reduce dietary salt intake in both developed and developing countries are more specifically addressed.

PUBLIC HEALTH STRATEGIES TO REDUCE SALT INTAKE IN DEVELOPED COUNTRIES

In developed countries, the estimated prevalence of hypertension is, on average, 28% in North America (Canada and the United States) and 44% in Western Europe.[37] Community-based intervention trials to decrease blood pressure by means of decreasing dietary salt intake are scanty. For example, a community-based intervention trial in Portugal over 2 years involved a whole town receiving a health education program to reduce salt intake, while another town was not given any advice and was used as a control.[38] The average blood pressure decreased by 3.6/5.0 mm Hg at 1 year and 5.0/5.1 mm Hg at 2 years in the former. In developed countries, the majority of an individual's salt intake is not added by the person but is already present in foods. Indeed, given that 75% to 80% of salt intake comes from salt added to bread and processed foods,[35] a population-wide strategy involving the food industry would be more effective in the long term. The North Karelia Project is a meaningful example to support this concept. The program was launched in 1972 in Finland to prevent noncommunicable diseases and, primarily, to decrease the mortality and morbidity from CVDs.[39] The interventions implemented during this trial were extensive: collaborations with the community, health services, and food industry were added to a mass media campaign. The results have been outstanding. Over 25 years, the age-adjusted mortality rate from CVDs among men aged 25 to 64 years decreased by 73%. These results clearly show that a comprehensive and collaborative program involving the food industry and health and community services is essential to successfully implement strategies of primary prevention of CVDs in developed countries.

A complementary approach to lower salt intake in developed countries may reside in the use of salt substitutes. The American Heart Association recommends the use of nonchloride salts of sodium because they do not increase blood pressure.[40]

In summary, in developed countries, comprehensive population strategies to reduce the average levels of salt intake are required. The expected benefits of a modest decrease in blood pressure across the whole population would be significant, especially on stroke, coronary heart disease, and all other cardiovascular conditions for which high blood pressure is a causative risk factor. The benefits would be greater in the elderly because they have a much higher stroke incidence (greater absolute risk); additionally, in this age group, most strokes occur at blood pressure levels not always requiring drug therapy (more stroke events attributable to the effect of blood pressure).

PUBLIC HEALTH STRATEGIES TO REDUCE SALT INTAKE IN DEVELOPING COUNTRIES

In developing countries, noncommunicable diseases are increasingly becoming an important threat to the health of populations.[1] Worldwide, stroke is second only to ischemic heart disease as a cause of death, and most of these deaths occur in developing countries.[41] For example, data from Tanzania suggest a high burden of stroke comparable with that observed in developed countries.[42] Likewise, in areas such as sub-Saharan Africa, the prevalence of hypertension is elevated and comparable with figures from developed regions.[2,36] Thus, preventing the impending epidemic of CVDs in these countries is critical as they are facing a rapid demographic change and already experiencing a double burden of disease, that is, communicable and noncommunicable. In the 30-year period from 2000 to 2030, the population of elderly persons is projected to double in many sub-Saharan African countries.

Salt consumption in developing countries is becoming more common as urbanization increases. However, interventions to decrease salt intake at a population level have not been extensively studied in these countries. The population approach to reduce salt consumption is particularly relevant in developing countries due to the cost-effectiveness of these measures.[43] Furthermore, in countries of sub-Saharan Africa where effective health care provision for chronic diseases is haphazard, a population strategy to limit salt consumption might prove extremely effective. It can be predicted that the same decrease in salt intake obtained with a behavioral intervention will be more effective in black African origin populations than in white populations due to the higher salt sensitivity of people of black African origin and because most of the salt ingested is added to food by the consumer, whereas processed food is used relatively rarely compared with in developed countries.[26] Two short-term trials in sub-Saharan Africa have confirmed that simple, cost-effective, and culturally adapted behavioral and educational interventions to decrease blood pressure can be successfully implemented.[29,30] Concerns about population-wide strategies to limit salt consumption in developing countries pertain to the perceived risk of counteracting worldwide policies directed at the prevention of iodine deficiency disorders through universal salt iodination. There is therefore an urgent need to consider alternative vehicles for the deliveries of iodine to populations.

In summary, in developing countries, which are experiencing an increasing burden of CVDs, multiple risk factor interventions and community-based programs of primary prevention should be encouraged. In particular, public health measures to promote dietary changes such as reduction in salt intake should be strongly recommended given that the prevalence of hypertension is likely to increase in these countries.

IMPORTANCE OF DIETARY PATTERNS

Diet plays a major role in the regulation of blood pressure and is one of the most important determinants of blood pressure levels in both individuals and populations. There are large variations in dietary patterns across populations that are likely to account for a considerable part of the observed differences in mean blood pressure levels, with populations consuming mostly plant-based diets having lower blood pressure than populations in industrialized countries. Additionally, even within industrialized countries, individuals consuming diets with increased intakes of fruits and vegetables and decreased intake of saturated fats tend to have, on average, lower blood pressure than individuals following more typical Western diets.[44]

DIETARY APPROACHES TO STOP HYPERTENSION (DASH) DIET

The Seventh Report of the Joint National Committee on Prevention, Detection, Evaluation, and Treatment of High Blood Pressure[4] and a recent scientific statement from the American Heart Association[5] emphasize the importance of adopting a dietary regimen resembling the so-called DASH diet as one major lifestyle modification to prevent and treat hypertension. The DASH dietary plan provides large intakes of fruits, vegetables, and low-fat dairy products; comprises whole grains, poultry, fish, and nuts; and has limited amounts of red meat, sweets, and sugar-containing beverages. Thus, compared with habitual diets of Western societies, the DASH dietary pattern provides higher intake of potassium, magnesium, calcium, fiber, and proteins and lower intake of total fat, saturated fat, and cholesterol.[45] The blood pressure–lowering effect of this diet is the result of the combined effects of these nutrients when consumed together in food rather than of the specific effect of a single nutrient. Indeed, the DASH trial was designed to test the effects on blood pressure of a change in dietary patterns rather than the effects of a change in a single nutrient, as generally tested in previous trials.[46] This trial was an 11-week feeding program including 459 adults with ($N = 133$) and without ($N = 326$) hypertension. For 3 weeks, participants followed a control diet that was low in fruits, vegetables, and dairy products. Then, for the next 8 weeks, participants were randomly allocated to three groups and each group was fed a different diet. One group was fed the same control diet, the second group a diet richer in fruits and vegetables but similar to the control diet for other nutrients, and the third group was fed the DASH diet, which is a diet rich in fruits and vegetables, low-fat or fat-free dairy products, and reduced saturated and total fat content—in other words, a high potassium, magnesium, calcium, fiber, and protein diet. The salt intake was held constant in the three groups. Overall, findings indicated a gradient in the decrease in blood pressure among the diets. The DASH diet significantly decreased blood pressure by 5.5/3.0 mm Hg, and the fruits and vegetables diet significantly decreased blood pressure by 2.8/1.1 mm Hg compared with the control diet. Among subjects with hypertension, the blood pressure decreases in the DASH diet group were more marked. Further subgroup analyses showed significant effects of the DASH diet in all major subgroups (e.g., sex, race, age, body mass index), although the effects were more marked among African Americans than in whites.[47]

In 2001, findings from a further trial in the same population testing the effects of the DASH diet in combination with decreased salt intake were published.[14] A total of 412 participants were randomly allocated to two dietary regimens, one following a control diet representative of the average diet in the United States and one following the DASH diet. Within these two dietary regimens, participants were randomly assigned to three decreasing levels of salt consumption, defined as high (~9 g of salt or 150 mmol or 3.5 g of sodium per day, reflecting typical consumption in the United States), intermediate (<6 g of salt or 100 mmol or 2.3 g of sodium per day, reflecting the upper limit of the current recommendations), and low (<3 g of salt or 50 mmol or 1.6 g of sodium per day). Each feeding period lasted 30 consecutive days. Overall, findings indicate that (1) the DASH diet lowers blood pressure independently of the level of salt intake; (2) the blood pressure–lowering effect of a decrease in salt intake occurs by decreasing the salt intake even to levels below the currently recommended limit (i.e., <6 g/day); (3) the effects of salt intake reduction are observed in all major subgroups; (4) greater lowering effects on blood pressure may derive from the combination of the two interventions than from adopting either the DASH diet or low-salt diet individually. In fact, the difference in systolic blood pressure between the DASH low-salt group and the control high-salt group was a substantial decrease of 7.1 mm Hg in participants

without hypertension and 11.5 mm Hg in participants with hypertension. The last finding resembles the effect of a single-drug therapy in hypertensive individuals. Thus, the combination of the DASH diet and decreased salt intake represents an alternative to drug therapy for individuals with mild hypertension and willing to comply with long-term dietary changes.

More recently, findings from the Optimal Macronutrient Intake Trial to Prevent Heart Disease (OmniHeart) have extended the observations derived from the DASH trial.[48]

ASSESSMENT OF HYPERTENSIVE PATIENTS

All hypertensive patients should have a thorough history and physical examination, but need only a limited number of routine investigations. It is beyond the scope of this chapter to discuss every detail of the clinical evaluation, but it is important to consider and document the following: the causes of secondary hypertension, contributory factors, complications of hypertension, CVD risk factors to allow the assessment of CVD risk, and contraindications to specific drugs. Routine investigation must include urine strip test for protein and blood, serum creatinine and electrolytes, blood glucose (ideally fasted), lipid profile (ideally fasted), and an electrocardiogram. A case should be made for the inclusion of 24-hour urinary collections for sodium, potassium, and creatinine to assess levels of sodium (salt) and potassium intake, given than more than 95% of the ingested salt and more than 80% of the ingested potassium are excreted in the urine daily. Chest radiograph, urine microscopy and culture, and an echocardiogram are not required routinely. An echocardiogram is valuable to confirm or refute the presence of target organ damage. When the clinical evaluation or results of these simple investigations suggest a need for further investigation, it may be best to refer for specialist advice if the additional investigations needed are difficult to arrange from general practice.

PRIMARY PREVENTION OF HYPERTENSION

Current approaches to the prevention of adverse cardiovascular sequelae due to hypertension are unsatisfactory because they require prolonged drug therapy for a large proportion of the adult population. Moreover, this strategy does not reduce the risk of treated hypertensive patients compared with that of the normotensive population.[49] A population strategy is therefore necessary to (1) prevent the increase in blood pressure with age and therefore decrease the prevalence of hypertension, (2) reduce the need for antihypertensive drug therapy, and (3) reduce CVD burden.

The following lifestyle modifications for the primary prevention of hypertension are consistent with those recently outlined by the U.S. National High BP Education Program and the British Hypertension Society: (1) maintain normal body weight for adults (e.g., body mass index 20–25 kg/m^2), (2) decrease dietary salt intake to less than 6 g/day (<100 mmol or <2.4 g of sodium per day), (3) engage in regular aerobic physical activity such as brisk walking (30 minutes per day, most days of the week), (4) limit alcohol consumption to no more than three units per day in men and no more than two units per day in women, (5) consume a diet rich in fruits and vegetables (e.g., at least five portions per day), and (6) consume a diet with reduced saturated and total fat content.

LIFESTYLE CHANGES IN ESTABLISHED HYPERTENSION

Recent controlled trials[5] have confirmed that lifestyle changes can lower blood pressure. Clear verbal and written advice on lifestyle measures and moderate decrease in dietary salt intake in particular (Box 50-1) should be provided for all hypertensive patients and also those with high-normal blood pressure or a strong family history. Effective lifestyle modification may lower blood pressure as much as a single blood pressure–lowering drug.[14] Combinations of two or more lifestyle modifications can achieve even better results. Lifestyle interventions reduce the need for drug therapy, can enhance the antihypertensive effects of drugs, reduce the need for multiple drug regimens, and can favorably influence overall CVD risk. Conversely, failure to adopt these measures may attenuate the response to antihypertensive drugs.

In patients with grade 1 (mild) hypertension, but no cardiovascular complications or target organ damage, the response to these measures should be observed during the first 4 to 6 months of evaluation. When drug therapy has to be introduced more urgently, for example, in patients with grade 3 (severe) hypertension, lifestyle measures should be instituted along with drug treatment. The initiation of drug treatment should never be delayed unnecessarily, especially in patients at higher levels of risk.

Weight reduction by calorie restriction is appropriate for the majority of hypertensive patients because most are overweight.[50] The blood pressure–lowering effect of weight reduction may be enhanced by a decrease in salt intake.[19] Salt reduction from an average of 10 to 5 g (5 g is ~1 teaspoon) daily lowers blood pressure by approximately 5/2 mm Hg, with greater blood pressure decreases in the elderly and in those with higher initial blood pressure levels. These effects are additive to the blood pressure–lowering effect of a healthy diet. As indicated earlier, all hypertensive patients should have clear verbal and written advice to reduce salt intake to less than 6 g/day (<100 mmol/day) (see Box 50-1). This will be achieved more effectively through dedicated sessions held by well-trained nurses or other health professionals outside the clinical consultation. In suitable cases, online resources aimed at increasing education and awareness about the salt content of food and how to read food labels and make an informed choice should be used. Many will already have stopped adding salt at the table and even when cooking, but few are aware of the large amount of salt in processed foods, such as bread (one slice contains on average of ~0.5 g of salt), some breakfast cereals, prepared meals, and flavor enhancers such as stock cubes or manufactured sauces. Patients and those who cook for patients should be provided with specific written advice.

THE NATIONAL INSTITUTE FOR CLINICAL EXCELLENCE–BRITISH HYPERTENSION SOCIETY ALGORITHM

Hypertension control remains suboptimal in the United Kingdom and around the world.[37] Most people require more than one drug to control blood pressure, and yet the majority of treated hypertensive patients continue to receive monotherapy.[37] The National Institute for Clinical Excellence and the British Hypertension Society have recently jointly published a treatment algorithm (ACD) designed to encourage improved blood pressure control (Fig. 50-1). The theory underpinning the ACD algorithm is that hypertension

---

Box 50-1   Practical Advice for Patients on How to Reduce Dietary Salt Intake

Target daily salt intake should not exceed 6 g/day

1. Never Add Salt to a Meal

Do Not
Use rock salt or sea salt
Add sauces

Instead
Use pepper, garlic, lemon, and herbs.

2. Do Not Add Salt When Cooking

Do Not
Use stock cubes, gravy browning, soy sauce, salted dry fish, curry powers, and prepared mustards

Instead
Try other flavorings: any herbs, spices, lemon or lime, vinegar, onions, garlic, ginger, and chilies.

3. Avoid Manufactured or Processed Foods with Added Salt

Food Labeling
Salt is sodium chloride. At present, most food labels only report sodium as grams per 100 g of food. To convert to salt, multiply by 2.5.
1 g of sodium per 100 g of food is the equivalent to the saltiness of seawater.

Beware
Most breads, many cereals
Ready-made soups and meals, processed meats, pizzas, Chinese take out

Ideally
Only choose food items with no more than 0.3 g of sodium per 100 g of food.

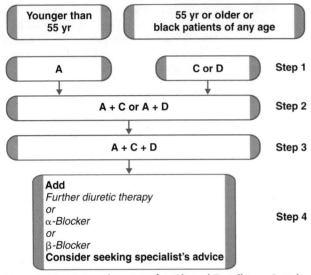

Figure 50-1 National Institute for Clinical Excellence–British Hypertension Society algorithm for the pharmacologic management of hypertension. A, angiotensin-converting enzyme inhibitors or angiotensin receptor blockers; C, calcium channel blockers; D, diuretics.

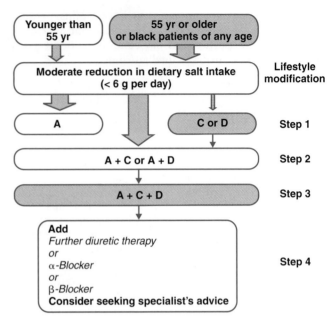

Figure 50-2 Modified National Institute for Clinical Excellence–British Hypertension Society algorithm with the inclusion of a moderate reduction in dietary salt intake as lifestyle modification step. The size of the arrow indicates the strength of the estimated effect. A, angiotensin-converting enzyme inhibitors or angiotensin receptor blockers; C, calcium channel blockers; D, diuretics.

can be broadly classified as high renin or low renin and is, therefore, best initially treated by one of two categories of antihypertensive drug, that is, those that inhibit (angiotensin-converting enzyme inhibitors, angiotensin receptor blockers, renin inhibitors, or β-blockers) and those that do not inhibit (calcium channel blockers or diuretics) the renin-angiotensin system. Renin profiling studies have demonstrated that younger people (younger than 55 years) and whites tend to have higher renin levels relative to older people (older than 55 years) or the black population (of African descent). Thus, the drugs that reduce blood pressure at least in part by suppressing the renin-angiotensin system at one point or another are generally more effective as initial blood pressure–lowering therapy in younger white patients. In contrast, calcium channel blockers and diuretics are less effective as initial blood pressure–lowering therapy in these patients and are better used as first-line treatment in older whites or the black population of any age.[51] The detailed analysis of this algorithm is beyond the scope of this chapter. However, it is important to consider the use of a moderate dietary salt reduction in the overall therapeutic framework. A moderate reduction in dietary salt intake is effective in lowering blood pressure on its own but is also additive to pharmacologic treatment and can be as effective as a low-dose thiazide diuretic. Furthermore, based on the underlying principles informing the ACD algorithm, a moderate decrease in dietary salt intake can be added to the algorithm, emphasizing its additive blood pressure–lowering effect to drug classes that predominantly block the renin-angiotensin system (such as angiotensin-converting enzyme inhibitors, angiotensin receptor blockers, renin inhibitors, β-blockers), with less predicted additive effect to thiazide and thiazide-like diuretics, dihydropyridine calcium channel blockers, and α-blockers (Fig. 50-2). Furthermore, a moderate decrease in dietary salt intake is more effective in low renin hypertension as seen in people of black African origin, in the elderly, and in many cases of type 2 diabetes and metabolic

syndrome whether or not associated with hyperfiltration or microalbuminuria.

CONCLUSIONS

Extensive and consistent evidence provides the scientific basis for clinical and public health strategies directed at long-term lifestyle modifications to prevent and reduce the burden of disease related to high blood pressure in both individuals and populations. In the clinical setting, a comprehensive lifestyle intervention, including a moderate reduction in dietary salt intake, represents a cost-effective therapeutic option among nonhypertensive individuals with above-optimal blood pressure levels as well as among hypertensive individuals who are not receiving medication therapy but who comply with long-term lifestyle changes. In addition, a moderate decrease in dietary salt intake is an essential adjuvant therapy in hypertensive individuals who are already pharmacologically treated. In the public health arena, there is an urgent need to develop and implement population-wide strategies aimed at substantial societal changes to tackle the current epidemic of hypertension in both developed and developing countries. However, these changes will be realistic only if collaborative initiatives are implemented at multiple levels: government, manufacturers, health care providers, researchers, and the general public.[34] In the clinical setting, there is the need to provide specific and targeted advice on how to effectively reduce dietary salt intake and to provide support to patients to sustain the decreases by monitoring compliance through regular assessment of salt intake with 24-hour urine collections.

References

1. World Health Organization: The World Health Report 2002. Reducing Risks, Promoting Healthy Life. Geneva: World Health Organization, 2002.
2. Kearney PM, Whelton M, Reynolds K, et al: Global burden of hypertension: Analysis of worldwide data. Lancet 2005;365: 217–223.
3. Vasan RS, Beiser A, Seshadri S, et al: Residual lifetime risk for developing hypertension in middle-aged women and men: The Framingham Heart Study. JAMA 2002;287:1003–1010.
4. Chobanian AV, Bakris GL, Black HR, et al, for the National Heart, Lung, and Blood Institute Joint National Committee on Prevention, Detection, Evaluation, and Treatment of High Blood Pressure; National High Blood Pressure Education Program Coordinating Committee: The Seventh Report of the Joint National Committee on Prevention, Detection, Evaluation, and Treatment of High Blood Pressure: The JNC 7 report. JAMA 2003;289:2560–2572.
5. Appel LJ, Brands MW, Daniels SR, et al: Dietary approaches to prevent and treat hypertension: A scientific statement from the American Heart Association. Hypertension 2006;47:296–308.
6. He FJ, MacGregor GA: How far should salt intake be reduced? Hypertension 2003;42:1093–1099.
7. Sasaki S, Zhang XH, Kesteloot H: Dietary sodium, potassium, saturated fat, alcohol and stroke mortality. Stroke 1995;26: 783–789.
8. He J, Ogden LG, Vupputuri S, et al: Dietary sodium intake and subsequent risk of cardiovascular disease in overweight adults. JAMA 1999;282:2027–2034.
9. Tuomilehto J, Jousilahti P, Rastenyte D, et al: Urinary sodium excretion and cardiovascular mortality in Finland: A prospective study. Lancet 2001;357:848–851.
10. Nagata C, Takasuka N, Shimizu N, Shimizu H: Sodium intake and risk of death from stroke in Japanese men and women. Stroke 2004;35:1543–1547.
11. Cohen HW, Hailpern SM, Fang J, Alderman MH: Sodium intake and mortality in the NHANES II follow-up study. Am J Med 2006;119:275.e7–e14.
12. Cook NR, Cutler JA, Obarzanek E, et al: Long term effects of dietary sodium reduction on cardiovascular disease outcomes: Observational follow-up of trials of hypertension prevention. Br Med J 2007;334:885.
13. Ruskin A: Classics in arterial hypertension. Springfield, IL: Charles C Thomas, 1956.
14. Sacks FM, Svetkey LP, Vollmer WM, et al: Effects on blood pressure of reduced dietary sodium and the Dietary Approaches to Stop Hypertension (DASH) diet. DASH–Sodium Collaborative Research Group. N Engl J Med 2001;344:3–10.
15. Vollmer WM, Sacks FM, Ard J, et al: Effects of diet and sodium intake on blood pressure: Subgroup analysis of the DASH-sodium trial. Ann Intern Med 2001;135:1019–1028.
16. He FJ, MacGregor GA: Effect of modest salt reduction on blood pressure: A meta-analysis of randomized trials: Implications for public health. J Hum Hypertens 2002;16:761–770.
17. Geleijnse JM, Kok FJ, Grobbee DE, et al: Blood pressure response to changes in sodium and potassium intake: A meta-regression analysis of randomised trials. J Hum Hypertens 2003;17:471–480.
18. The Trials of Hypertension Prevention Collaborative Research Group: Effects of weight loss and sodium reduction intervention on blood pressure and hypertension incidence in overweight people with high-normal blood pressure: The Trials of Hypertension Prevention, phase II. Arch Intern Med 1997;157:657–667.
19. Whelton PK, Appel LJ, Espeland MA, et al: Sodium reduction and weight loss in the treatment of hypertension in older persons: A randomized controlled trial of nonpharmacologic interventions in the elderly (TONE). TONE Collaborative Research Group. JAMA 1998;279:839–846.
20. Weinberger MH, Miller JZ, Luft FC, et al: Definitions and characteristics of sodium sensitivity and blood pressure resistance. Hypertension 1986;8:II127–II134.
21. Cappuccio FP, Markandu ND, Sagnella GA, MacGregor GA: Sodium restriction lowers high blood pressure through a decreased response of the renin system—direct evidence using saralasin. J Hypertens 1985;3:243–247.
22. He FJ, Markandu ND, Sagnella GA, MacGregor GA: Importance of the renin system in determining blood pressure fall with salt restriction in black and white hypertensives. Hypertension 1998;32:820–824.
23. Simons-Morton DG, Obarzanek E. Diet and blood pressure in children and adolescents. Pediatr Nephrol 1997;11:244–249.
24. Cappuccio FP, Markandu ND, Carney C, et al: Double-blind randomised trial of modest salt restriction in older people. Lancet 1997;350:850–854.
25. Wofford MR, Hall JE: Pathophysiology and treatment of obesity hypertension. Curr Pharm Dis 2004;10:3621–3637.
26. Cappuccio FP: Salt and blood pressure. Issues for population-based prevention and public health strategies. Public Health Med 2000;2:57–61.
27. Cappuccio FP, Siani A: Nonpharmacologic treatment of hypertension. In Crawford MH, DiMarco JP, Paulus WJ (eds): Cardiology. Philadelphia: Mosby, 2004, pp 523–532.
28. Poulter N, Cappuccio FP, Chaturvedi N, Cruickshank K: High Blood Pressure and the African-Caribbean Community in the UK. Birmingham: MediNews Ltd., 1996, pp 1–47.
29. Adeyemo AA, Prewitt TE, Luke A, et al: The feasibility of implementing a dietary sodium reduction intervention among free-living normotensive individuals in south west Nigeria. Ethn Dis 2002;12:207–212.
30. Cappuccio FP, Kerry SM, Micah FB, et al: A community programme to reduce salt intake and blood pressure in Ghana (ISRCTN 88789643). BMC Public Health 2006;6:13.
31. Hooper L, Bartlett C, Davey Smith G, Ebrahim S: Systematic review of long term effects of advice to reduce dietary salt in adults. Br Med J 2002;325:628–632.
32. Prospective Studies Collaboration: Age-specific relevance of usual blood pressure to vascular mortality: A meta-analysis of individual data for one million adults in 61 prospective studies. Lancet 2002;360:1903–1913.
33. Cappuccio FP, MacGregor GA: Dietary salt restriction: Benefits for cardiovascular disease and beyond. Curr Opin Nephrol Hypertens 1997;6:477–482.
34. Cappuccio FP: Salt and cardiovascular disease. Br Med J 2007; 334:859–860.
35. Mattes RD, Donnelly D: Relative contributions of dietary sodium sources. J Am Coll Nutr 1991;10:383–393.
36. Cappuccio FP, Micah FB, Emmett L, et al: Prevalence, detection, management and control of hypertension in Ashanti, West Africa. Hypertension 2004;43:1017–1022.
37. Wolf-Maier K, Cooper RS, Banegas JR, et al: Hypertension prevalence and blood pressure levels in 6 European countries, Canada, and the United States. JAMA 2003;289: 2363–2369.
38. Forte JG, Miguel JM, Miguel MJ, et al: Salt and blood pressure: A community trial. J Hum Hypertens 1989;3:179–184.
39. Puska P, Pirjo P, Ulla U: Influencing public nutrition for noncommunicable disease prevention: From community intervention to national programme—experiences from Finland. Public Health Nutr 2002;5:245–251.
40. Kotchen TA, McCarron DA: Dietary electrolytes and blood pressure: A statement for healthcare professionals from the American Heart Association Nutrition Committee. Circulation 1998;98:613–617.
41. Lopez AD, Mathers CD, Ezzati M, et al: Global and regional burden of disease and risk factors, 2001: Systematic analysis of population health data. Lancet 2006;367:1747–1757.

42. Walker RW, McLarty DG, Kitange HM, et al: Stroke mortality in urban and rural Tanzania. Lancet 2000;355:1684–1687.

43. Murray CJ, Lauer JA, Hutubessy RC, et al: Effectiveness and costs of interventions to lower systolic blood pressure and cholesterol: A global and regional analysis on reduction of cardiovascular-disease risk. Lancet 2003;361:717–725.

44. Berkow SE, Barnard ND: Blood pressure regulation and vegetarian diets. Nutr Rev 2005;63:1–8.

45. Karanja NM, Obarzanek E, Lin PH, et al: Descriptive characteristics of the dietary patterns used in the Dietary Approaches to Stop Hypertension Trial: DASH Collaborative Research Group. J Am Diet Assoc 1999;99:S19–S27.

46. Appel LJ, Moore TJ, Obarzanek E, et al: A clinical trial of the effects of dietary patterns on blood pressure: DASH Collaborative Research Group. N Engl J Med 1997;336:1117–1124.

47. Svetkey LP, Simons-Morton D, Vollmer WM, et al: Effects of dietary patterns on blood pressure: Subgroup analysis of the Dietary Approaches to Stop Hypertension (DASH) randomized clinical trial. Arch Intern Med 1999;159:285–293.

48. Appel LJ, Sacks FM, Carey V, et al: Effects of protein, monounsaturated fat, and carbohydrate intake on blood pressure and serum lipids: Results from the OmniHeart randomized trial. JAMA 2005;294:2455–2464.

49. Andersson OK, Almgren T, Persson B, et al: Survival in treated hypertension: Follow up study after two decades. Br Med J 1998;317:167–171.

50. Poulter NR, Zographos D, Mattin R, et al: Concomitant risk factors in hypertensives: A survey of risk factors for cardiovascular disease amongst hypertensives in English general practices. Blood Pressure 1996;5:209–215.

51. Cappuccio FP, MacGregor GA: Combination therapy in hypertension. In Laragh JH, Brenner BM (eds): Hypertension: Pathophysiology, Diagnosis and Management, 2nd ed. New York: Raven Press, 1995, pp 2969–2983.

Further Reading

Adshead SAM: Salt and Civilization. London: MacMillan Academic & Professional Ltd., 1992.

Cappuccio FP: Calcium and magnesium supplementation. In Whelton PK, He J, Louis GT (eds): Lifestyle Modification for the Prevention and Treatment of Hypertension. New York and Basel: Marcel Dekker, 2003, pp 227–242.

Cappuccio FP, Gomez G: Lifestyle modifications and value of non-drug therapy. In Battegay EJ, Lip GYH, Bakris GL (eds): Hypertension: Principles and Practice. New York: Taylor & Francis, 2005, pp 383–403.

Cappuccio FP, Siani A: Nonpharmacologic treatment of hypertension. In Crawford MH, Di Marco JP, Paulus WJ (eds): Cardiology. Philadelphia: Mosby, 2004, pp 523–532.

Stranges S, Cappuccio FP: Non-pharmacological management of hypertension. In Lip GYH, Hall JH (eds): Comprehensive Hypertension. Philadelphia: Elsevier, 2007, pp 1–56.

Williams B, Poulter NR, Brown MJ, et al: Guidelines for management of hypertension: Report of the Fourth Working Party of the British Hypertension Society, 2004—BHS IV. J Hum Hypertens 2004;18:139–185.

World Health Organization: Reducing Salt Intake in Populations: Report of a WHO Forum and Technical Meeting. Geneva: World Health Organization, 2007.

Chapter 51

Diuretics and β-Blockers

Andrew Hall, Hamish Dobbie, Giovambattista Capasso, and Robert Unwin

The original large-scale trials that established the benefit of lowering blood pressure (BP) in reducing cardiovascular mortality in uncomplicated hypertension were based largely on the use of β-blockers and diuretics. Until recently both have remained first-line treatments. However, since the last edition of this book, the situation has changed. The role of β-blockers has been questioned because of growing evidence of adverse metabolic effects (such as glucose intolerance) and recognition that β-blockers may be inferior to other first-line treatments in reducing the risk of stroke. These conclusions are controversial; moreover, newer β-blockers may redress these concerns. Yet thiazide diuretics retain their position as an excellent, inexpensive first-line therapy. Debate continues as to whether they are superior to other first-line options, such as angiotensin-converting enzyme (ACE) inhibitors. Diuretic therapy for patients with normal renal function is usually based on thiazides. Loop diuretics are not effective antihypertensive therapy because of their short duration of action and the postdiuretic renal salt retention that occurs unless they are given two or three times daily with restriction of dietary salt intake; however, they are used to control fluid retention and hypertension and in patients with renal failure who are refractory to thiazides.

RANDOMIZED TRIALS OF DIURETIC OR β-BLOCKER TREATMENT AGAINST PLACEBO

Although the place of β-blockers as first-line therapy has recently been called into question,[1] the original studies established that these drugs lower BP and reduce the risk of stroke. The results of randomized trials comparing diuretics or β-blockers with placebo are discussed extensively in the meta-analysis and review by Psaty and colleagues.[2] The 18 trials identified included 48,220 patients followed for an average of 5 years. The earlier trials were conducted mainly in middle-aged adults given higher doses of diuretics or β-blockers, whereas trials from the late 1980s were mainly in older adults given lower doses. High-dose diuretics, low-dose diuretics, and β-blockers *all* reduced the risk of stroke, with relative risks (RR) in the meta-analysis of 0.49, 0.66, and 0.71, respectively. The risk of coronary artery disease (CAD) was reduced in the low-dose diuretic trials (RR, 0.72), but not in the high-dose diuretic trials or in the β-blocker trials. These results are surprising in view of the proven benefits of β-blockers in secondary prevention of CAD. It is not clear if this difference in the rate of coronary events is due to differences in the patient groups included in these trials or to real biologic differences in these therapies, including their metabolic side effects (see "Adverse Effects of Diuretics and β-Blockers" in this chapter). Cardiovascular mortality was significantly reduced with high-dose and low-dose diuretic therapy, but not with β-blockers. There was a trend toward reduced overall mortality for all therapies, but in no case did this reach statistical significance.

In a 22-year follow-up of hypertensive men identified and treated in the 1970s, a significant excess of deaths due to cardiovascular disease and stroke has been shown, despite apparently adequate control of their BP.[3] This suggests that even patients adequately treated with current therapies do not return to the cardiovascular risk of the general population. An overview and meta-analysis of drug treatment of hypertension concluded that even over the short term (a few years), effective treatment of hypertension reduces the risk of stroke in treated patients by almost exactly the amount expected from epidemiologic studies.[4] However, the reduction in risk of CAD, although clinically and statistically significant, is less than might have been expected from the observed fall in BP. It has been suggested that this failure of predominantly diuretic-based treatments to reverse the increased mortality associated with hypertension may be due to the adverse metabolic effects of diuretics.[5] Hypertension often occurs in the setting of the *metabolic syndrome,* which is associated with a number of risk factors for cardiovascular disease, such as insulin resistance, glucose intolerance, hypertriglyceridemia, and central obesity, which are not addressed by lowering BP alone.

RANDOMIZED TRIALS OF DIURETICS OR β-BLOCKERS AGAINST OTHER ANTIHYPERTENSIVE TREATMENTS

General agreement concerning the benefits of treatment of hypertension in middle-aged and elderly persons now exists. Further placebo-controlled trials are probably no longer ethically justified. Therefore, recent trials have compared one therapy with another.

The established dogma has been that β-blockers, diuretics, ACE inhibitors, and calcium channel blockers (CCBs) are equally effective in lowering BP. The choice of therapy should be tailored to the individual patient according to the side effect profile and the specific indications or contraindications of one other agent. Thiazides and β-blockers have often been used as first-line treatment because of their low cost. However, two recent developments have questioned this approach.

First, a large meta-analysis of trials comparing β-blockers with other therapies published in the *Lancet* in 2005[1] concluded that β-blockers were associated with an increased risk of stroke of approximately 16% (although β-blockers did reduce the risk when compared with placebo). There was a nonsignificant trend toward increased mortality. The authors argued that β-blockers could no longer be recommended as first-line treatment for hypertension in the absence of other specific indications, such as secondary prevention of CAD. They suggested possible reasons for this difference, including the adverse metabolic and hemodynamic effects of β-blockers. Most antihypertensive agents act by decreasing systemic vascular resistance (SVR). However, β-blockers can increase SVR by allowing unopposed activation of vascular smooth muscle α-adrenergic receptors. They can also reduce cardiac output. Newer vasodilating β-blockers have been developed to address these concerns, although outcome data for these β-blockers are limited.

These new findings remain controversial. A subsequent meta-analysis of the β-blocker trials subdivided them into those involving younger or older (>60 years) patients. The authors concluded that the increased risk of stroke with β-blocker therapy only applied to the older age group.[6] This result may be explained by differences in the underlying pathophysiology in the two groups, with hypertension in younger patients believed to be due to an increase in cardiac output (*hyperdynamic circulation*), whereas hypertension in the elderly is due to an increase in SVR. The guidelines have begun to change. In 2004, The British Hypertension Society did not recommend β-blockers as first-line therapy for uncomplicated hypertension, because of the risk of developing diabetes.[7] Moreover, the Canadian Hypertension Education Program recommends that β-blockers should only be first line treatment in patients younger than 60 years of age,[8] in accordance with the meta-analysis referred to previously.

Unlike β-blockers, thiazide diuretics have retained their position as recommended first-line therapy for hypertension. In the second major recent development, it was suggested that thiazides may actually be superior to other first-line therapies. This finding derives from the ALLHAT study, which compared a thiazide diuretic (chlorthalidone) with either an ACE inhibitor (lisinopril), a CCB (amlodopine), or an α-adrenoreceptor blocker.[9] The last arm of the study was halted early due to an increase in the risk of heart failure. When compared with the ACE inhibitor or the CCB, the thiazide diuretic had a better outcome in heart failure (vs. amlodopine) and stroke (vs. lisinopril). The Joint National Committee on Prevention, Detection, Evaluation, and Treatment of High BP now recommends thiazides as first-line treatment for uncomplicated hypertension.[10] However, this view has been challenged,[11] and it was not endorsed in the 2003 guidelines issued jointly by the European Society of Hypertension and the European Society of Cardiology.[12]

ADVERSE EFFECTS OF DIURETICS AND β-BLOCKERS

Hypokalemia

Thiazide diuretics reduce serum potassium concentration in a dose-dependent fashion. In the Multiple Risk Factor Intervention Trial, in a subgroup of patients with abnormal electrocardiograms at baseline, there was an increase in the risk of death due to CAD in those patients randomized to high-dose thiazide diuretics.[13] However, in patients with normal electrocardiograms, there was a lower mortality in this group. In the Systolic Hypertension in the Elderly Program (SHEP) trial, patients randomized to diuretics had significantly lower serum potassium levels than those on placebo (average reduction, 0.36 mmol/L), and significantly more of them were clearly hypokalemic (7.2% vs. 1%).[14] Hypokalemic patients had higher event rates, similar to those seen in patients on placebo. A case-control study reported that patients on high-dose diuretics were at increased risk of cardiac arrest.[15] The lowest risk of all was in patients taking thiazides in combination with a potassium-sparing diuretic. A recent meta-analysis of trials involving thiazide diuretics also suggested that an inverse relationship exists between hypokalemia and hyperglycemia,[16] providing an additional mechanism for the association of thiazide usage with the development of glucose intolerance and diabetes.

It is clearly important to measure serum potassium in patients taking thiazide diuretics and, if necessary, to correct hypokalemia. However, the increasing use of treatment combinations to lower BP with agents such as ACE inhibitors, which can raise serum potassium concentrations, and the low doses of thiazides currently recommended, make hypokalemia with thiazide diuretic treatment less common. This can be easily prevented by combined therapy with a thiazide and a distal-acting potassium-sparing diuretic.

Dyslipidemia

Diuretics cause modest adverse changes in serum lipids in short-term studies. A meta-analysis concluded that thiazides caused a significant increase in total and low-density lipoprotein cholesterol but no change in high-density lipoprotein cholesterol.[17] These changes were more marked in patients on higher doses of diuretic. However, in longer-term studies these effects do not persist beyond about 1 year.[18,19] In the Treatment Of Mild Hypertension Study (TOMHS), no difference was seen in serum lipids between the placebo and diuretic groups after the first year.[18] In the Multicentre Isradipine Diuretic Atherosclerosis Study (MIDAS), the difference in lipids noted in the first year between patients treated with thiazides or CCBs disappeared by the third year. The ALLHAT study reported that after 4 years of treatment thiazide diuretics increased total cholesterol when compared with an ACE inhibitor or a CCB,[9] although this did not translate into any worsening of outcome. A longer follow-up period may be required to evaluate this potentially adverse, but small, metabolic effect of diuretics.

The effects of both thiazides and β-blockers on serum lipids appear small and of little clinical significance.[20] The widespread use of statins in hypertensive patients may counteract any detrimental effect of a small rise in serum lipids. Carvedilol, a newer third-generation β-blocker, does not cause significant changes in serum cholesterol.[21]

Insulin Resistance/Diabetes

Diuretics and β-blockers can impair glucose tolerance. The ALLHAT study[9] reported an increased incidence of diabetes in the group taking a thiazide diuretic compared with either lisinopril or amlodipine. However, this did not translate into any observed worsening of outcomes over the 8 years of the study. Hyperglycemia has been related to hypokalemia in patients taking diuretics.[16] Other studies have not detected any increase in diabetes in patients on thiazides.[22,23]

One prospective study of middle-aged patients found no increased risk of diabetes with thiazide diuretics, CCBs, or ACE inhibitors,[22] but a 28% increased risk in patients taking β-blockers. However, because the study was not randomized, differences in patient selection for these drug classes cannot be ruled out. An increased risk of diabetes with β-blockers compared with other antihypertensives may be due to the protective effects of ACE inhibitors[24] and CCBs[25] rather than to any adverse effects of β-blockers.

Suggested mechanisms of β-blocker-induced diabetes include systemic vasoconstriction with reduced tissue glucose uptake, impaired insulin secretion from the pancreas, weight gain, and increased hepatic gluconeogenesis (for review, see Sarafidis and Bakris[26]). In the United Kingdom Prospective Diabetes Study (UKPDS 38), diabetic patients randomized to a β-blocker-based regimen had as much cardiovascular disease protection as those receiving ACE inhibitors, perhaps reflecting the high incidence of CAD in the diabetic population and the protective effects of β-blockers.[27] Carvedilol, a newer vasodilating and antioxidant β-blocker, has shown promise that may translate into additional benefit. In a controlled trial (GEMINI) involving diabetic hypertensive patients random-

ized to carvedilol or metoprolol, with similar control of BP, carvedilol was associated with better insulin sensitivity.[28] Longer-term trials are required to see if this translates into better morbidity and mortality outcomes.

A recent "network meta-analysis" examined the risk of diabetes associated with antihypertensive drugs.[29] Only angiotensin receptor blockers were associated with a significantly reduced risk of developing diabetes, and only diuretics with a significantly increased risk. However, the numbers of new diabetics were small, and the absolute differences in the incidence of new-onset diabetes were less than 5%. Thus, this may only be a factor in high-risk groups such as the obese.

Hyperuricemia

Diuretics raise serum urate levels by decreasing renal secretion and increasing reabsorption. Gout is one of the few contraindications to thiazide therapy. Hyperuricemia per se is associated with cardiovascular disease.[30] However, in the Framingham cohort urate level was not found to be a significant predictor once allowance had been made for other risk factors.[31] Urate production may be toxic, perhaps through the generation of free radicals,[32] but the association with CV risk may not be causal.[31] Among patients in the SHEP trial,[33] the baseline serum urate level did predict subsequent events. Relative risk for the highest versus the lowest quintile of serum urate was only 1.32. Baseline urate levels did not affect the demonstrable benefits of active treatment in this trial. However, treatment with a thiazide increased serum urate by a median of 0.06 mmol/L. After dividing patients into two groups according to the increase in serum urate level, those with a small change in serum urate (<0.06 mmol/L) had a highly significant reduction in event rates on treatment, whereas those with a larger increase in urate had no decrease in event rates on active treatment.

These data suggest that patients' cardiovascular risk can be stratified according to their serum urate response to thiazides. However, there is no direct evidence that the increases in urate observed in patients taking thiazides are harmful per se. Moreover, thiazides have similar effects to β-blockers and ACE inhibitors (which do not affect serum urate) on the risk of cardiac death.

Sexual Dysfunction

A high incidence of impotence was reported in the Medical Research Council trial of mild hypertension, leading to the withdrawal of 12.6% of male patients in the diuretic arm, compared with 6.3% in the β-blocker arm and 1.3% in the placebo arm.[34] The incidence of this adverse effect seems to be lower in more recent trials, although whether this relates to the lower doses of diuretics used or the older patients studied in more recent trials is not clear. A review of trials involving β-blockers found overall a small increased risk of sexual dysfunction and fatigue, with no increased risk of depressive symptoms (another side effect previously associated with β-blockers).[35]

The incidence of sexual dysfunction is increased in men with hypertension, whether they are on treatment or not. The incidence of complete erectile dysfunction was 15% in those with treated hypertension and 14% in those with untreated hypertension in a population sample of American men in whom the overall incidence of impotence was 9.6%.[36] A post hoc subanalysis of patients in trials of sildenafil who were taking antihypertensives concluded that sildenafil was as effective in these patients as in those not on antihypertensives and was no more likely to cause adverse effects.[37] Whether antihypertensive treatment causes sexual dysfunction in women is less clear, although most investigators have reported no significant problems. Prisant and colleagues[38] concluded that only high-dose diuretics consistently cause sexual dysfunction.

Increased Risk of Cancer

An association of diuretic use with renal or colonic cancers has been noted.[39] Case-control studies have suggested an increased risk of renal cell carcinoma. However, the largest of these studies found that the excess risk associated with being hypertensive was larger than that associated with any drug exposure. The risk associated with diuretics disappeared once adjusted for the risk associated with hypertension itself.[40] A more recent case-control study of women with breast cancer reported an association with both hypertension and diuretic usage.[41] However, this was most pronounced in women with a high body mass index (a recognized risk factor), perhaps indicating that the link may be more with shared metabolic risk factors in hypertension and cancer (including diet), rather than any causal relationship.

No clinical trial of diuretics and β-blockers has demonstrated an increased risk of cancer in treated patients, although, because most trials are followed up for less than 5 years and many patients take antihypertensive medication for decades, this issue is still an open question. In a cohort of hypertensive men treated for longer than 2 decades with therapy based on these agents, there was no increase in cancer mortality.[3] At present, the proven benefit of BP reduction outweighs the unproven, and rather poorly defined, risk of cancer.

Effects on Bone

Thiazide diuretics reduce urinary calcium excretion and are thought to reduce postmenopausal bone loss. Numerous case-control studies have demonstrated a reduction in risk of fractures in patients taking thiazides.[42] Hypertension itself has been suggested as a risk factor for bone mineral loss[43] (and is also associated with renal stone disease). A recent randomized, controlled trial demonstrated that thiazides slow cortical bone loss in postmenopausal women, although the effect was small[44]; a recent extension to this trial has shown that the effect persists for at least 4 years.[45]

Studies in mice have suggested that β-blockers can increase bone mass,[46] but human studies have failed to show any significant association; at present β-blockers are not indicated for the treatment of osteoporosis.[47]

Chronic Obstructive Pulmonary Disease and Bronchospasm

β-Blockers have traditionally been withheld from patients with chronic obstructive pulmonary disease (COPD) because of the risk of provoking bronchospasm by blocking β$_2$-adrenergic receptors in the lung, even with more selective β$_1$-blockers. However, a Cochrane database systematic review of trials comparing cardioselective (β$_1$-adrenergic receptor-specific) β-blockers with

placebo found no adverse respiratory effects and concluded that these drugs need not be withheld in COPD patients who have a valid indication for β-blocker therapy, such as CAD or heart failure.[48]

DIURETIC AND β-BLOCKER USE IN SPECIFIC GROUPS OF PATIENTS

Elderly Patients

The evidence for the benefits of drug treatment of isolated systolic hypertension in elderly patients is now very strong.[14,49,50] The most dramatic reductions are in risk of stroke, both ischemic and hemorrhagic,[51] but there are also reductions in the risk of CAD and heart failure. Elderly patients also benefit from the treatment of diastolic hypertension.[52] There is still some uncertainty about the treatment of patients over age 80, although a subgroup meta-analysis of patients over this age included in the trials of the past 20 years concluded that they too can benefit from treatment.[53] Thiazide diuretics are well tolerated in the elderly and are of proven effectiveness.[52] A systematic review of the risk of falls in elderly patients on antihypertensive drugs found a modestly increased risk with diuretics (odds ratio, 1.08) and nonsignificant differences for β-blockers (perhaps surprisingly) and other classes of antihypertensive drugs.[54] However, none of the studies was randomized and the effects were small. The presence or absence of postural hypotension should always be determined in elderly patients before commencing antihypertensive therapy.

Because of their high absolute risk of stroke and cardiovascular events, elderly patients have much to gain from effective BP control. In older patients, a low-dose thiazide is the preferred treatment. An appropriate second or additional treatment is a CCB. β-Blockers seem to be less well tolerated by older patients; because they are apparently less effective in preventing stroke in older age groups, they should probably be avoided, unless there is a specific indication (e.g., angina or post–myocardial infarction [MI]).[55]

Black Patients

There is considerable evidence that black people have higher rates of hypertension.[56] They also have higher risks of stroke and renal failure, although (at least in the UK) not of CAD.[57] Black patients are more likely to have salt-sensitive hypertension and are less likely to have high renin levels.[58] Hypertensive black men have a larger BP response to hydrochlorothiazide than to propranolol, whereas there is no significant difference in responses in white men.[59] Studies have usually found that black patients respond well to diuretics[19] but require higher doses of ACE inhibitors to achieve a given level of BP control. A trial from South Africa[60] concluded that in black patients, CCBs were more effective as monotherapy than either diuretics or ACE inhibitors; however, these patients were younger than those in most other published studies. A systematic review of hypertension treatment in blacks has concluded that β-blockers are less efficacious than either diuretics or CCBs. However, there is no difference in outcome if BP is lowered to the same level by using combinations of drugs that contain a β-blocker.[61] Current UK and U.S. guidelines recommend using thiazides as the preferred treatment in black patients.

Patients with Cardiovascular Disease

In patients who have suffered an MI, prescription of a β-blocker reduces mortality by approximately 20%.[62] This also applies to diabetic patients.[63] ACE inhibitors also benefit this group of patients. Many patients should be taking both drugs, as well as aspirin.[64] The Heart Outcomes Prevention Evaluation (HOPE) study showed that the ACE inhibitor ramipril reduced the risk of death, MI, and stroke, each by approximately 20% in patients at high vascular risk.[65] Although 80% of patients in this trial had previously suffered an MI, only 40% were on a β-blocker. Patients in the HOPE study had acceptable control of BP at study entry, and the investigators concluded that the effects of ACE inhibition were not due to BP reduction; this has been vigorously challenged.

Although there is clear evidence for the use of β-blockers in patients who have suffered an MI, the evidence is less good for the use of these agents in patients with hypertension and stable CAD but no history of a major cardiac event. Although β-blockers are an effective treatment for the symptoms of angina, as with other antianginals, outcome data are lacking. In the INVEST trial, which looked specifically at patients with hypertension and CAD, no significant difference was observed between either a verapamil/trandolapril-based or atenolol/hydrochlorothiazide-based strategy,[25] suggesting that treatment of BP per se may be more important than the choice of antihypertensive agent.

In the PROGRESS perindopril-based trial of secondary prevention of stroke, a lower risk of subsequent stroke was recorded among actively treated patients, although subgroup analysis found that only those treated with both an ACE inhibitor and a thiazide diuretic had significant benefit.[66] As previously mentioned, β-blockers are not thought to be suitable first-line agents in the prevention of stroke.

Patients with Heart Failure

β-Blockers are negatively inotropic and can worsen or precipitate heart failure, especially at high doses. For this reason, heart failure was long considered a contraindication to β-blocker therapy. However, trials have shown that closely supervised β-blocker treatment is associated with reduced mortality in patients with moderate[67,68] and severe heart failure. This is partly due to a reduction in the incidence of sudden death. Trials have used the cardioselective β-blockers bisoprolol and metoprolol and the nonselective αβ-blocker carvedilol. It remains unclear whether these have the same benefit. A head-to-head comparison showed a greater improvement in left ventricular ejection fraction with carvedilol but a greater increase in exercise capacity with metoprolol.[68] A more recent study compared nebivolol (another vasodilating β-blocker) with placebo in patients over age 70 and found a reduction in all-cause mortality.[69] Further trials are needed to establish whether newer β-blockers are superior to older agents.

The most appropriate strategy, based on currently published data, is to treat with both ACE inhibitors and β-blockers, if tolerated, and to aim for a BP target of 130/70 mm Hg or less.

Diuretics can be added to control fluid retention, although there is no evidence that this alters outcome.

Patients with Left Ventricular Hypertrophy

Left ventricular hypertrophy (LVH) is an independent risk factor for cardiovascular events and sudden cardiac death.[70] Patients with hypertension often have LVH. In the Framingham Heart Study of persons older than age 40, less than 1% had an ECG suggesting LVH, but 15.5% of men and 21% of women had LVH on echocardiography.[70] Some of the newer antihypertensives may be better at inducing regression of LVH than diuretics or β-blockers. A meta-analysis of randomized studies concluded that ACE inhibitors are more effective at reducing LVH than β-blockers, CCBs, or diuretics.[71] However, direct head-to-head trial evidence suggests that diuretics are as effective as other drugs in inducing regression of LVH, although β-blockers seem less effective. In the LIFE study of patients with diabetes and hypertension (with echocardiographic evidence of LVH), losartan reduced cardiovascular morbidity and mortality compared with atenolol.[72] In the Veterans Study,[73] hydrochlorothiazide was at least as effective as any other drug in reversing LVH. In the TOMHS trial, diuretic treatment was superior to any other drug.[74]

Patients with Hypertension in Pregnancy

The treatment of hypertension in pregnancy is an especially difficult area. There remains disagreement as to the most appropriate treatment strategy (see Chapter 41). β-Blockers have been widely used in treating hypertension in pregnancy, particularly in the United States. A Cochrane review of trials of β-blockers for the treatment of mild-to-moderate hypertension in pregnancy concluded that although β-blockers lower BP when compared with placebo, no benefit to either the mother or baby has been demonstrated. In addition, the authors found a trend toward small-for-gestational-age infants and no advantages over other established drugs such as methyldopa.[75]

Diuretics have not been widely used in pregnancy-associated hypertension because of concerns about contraction of the circulating volume. However, they can be safely continued during pregnancy in those taking them for hypertension before conception.[76]

Patients with Chronic Kidney Disease

The goal of treatment in patients with hypertension and chronic kidney disease (CKD) is twofold: first, to reduce the rate of decline of renal function, and, second, to reduce mortality from cardiovascular disease (for which CKD is a significant and independent risk factor). Generally, very few studies have examined the treatment of hypertension in CKD patients. Guidelines extrapolate data from studies on patients with normal renal function.

In patients with significant proteinuria, ACE inhibitors are generally thought to be the agents of choice,[77] particularly in diabetic patients with renal disease.[78] A meta-analysis reported that regimens containing ACE inhibitors are more effective in slowing the progression of renal disease than those without, but for the subset of patients with proteinuria less than 0.5 g/day, no definite advantage of ACE inhibitors is evident.[79] This is probably because the rate of decline of renal function in patients with minimal proteinuria is very slow.

A recent meta-analysis of trials published in 2005 challenged this view, concluding that in patients with proteinuric CKD, ACE inhibitors provide only a very small benefit in comparison with other drug classes, and that any additional benefits observed in placebo-controlled trials are due only to a greater reduction in BP rather than any class-specific effect.[80] This view remains controversial, but it does highlight the paucity of data on the treatment of hypertension in CKD and the need on more trials to determine which agents should be first-line. In support of this, UKPDS 38 found no differences between patients randomized to captopril or atenolol as their first antihypertensive agent, again suggesting that tight control of BP is much more important than the agent used to achieve it.[27]

In practice, patients with renal disease often require multiple drugs for BP control. In the REIN follow-up study, 77% of patients required antihypertensives in addition to ramipril to keep their diastolic BP below 90 mm Hg.[81] The majority of patients are currently undertreated. For dialysis patients, adjustment of circulating volume is a key nonpharmacologic factor in BP control. Water-soluble β-blockers such as atenolol can accumulate in renal failure; doses should be reduced. This recommendation does not apply to lipid-soluble drugs such as metoprolol. In addition, β-blockers can worsen hyperkalemia by causing a shift of potassium from the intracellular to extracellular compartment. In a subset analysis of the ALLHAT study in patients with CKD Stage 3 (glomerular filtration rate, 30–59 mL/min), thiazide diuretics appeared equivalent to either ACE inhibitors or CCBs in reducing the rate of decline of renal function.[9] For more advanced stages of CKD, thiazides are less effective natriuretic agents, and loop diuretics are more commonly used.

Patients Outside the Developed World

The vast majority of patients in trials of hypertension have come from Western Europe, North America, Australia, and New Zealand. One major exception is the Sys-China trial, which demonstrated significant benefits for stroke risk and reduced mortality when older Chinese patients with isolated systolic hypertension were treated.[82] The Global Burden of Disease Study attempted to look at premature mortality and disability worldwide. This study found that in 1990 ischemic heart disease was the fifth leading cause of disability-adjusted life years lost and that cerebrovascular disease was the sixth leading cause.[83] Projections for 2020 are that cardiovascular disease will be the leading cause of disability-adjusted life years lost and cerebrovascular disease will be the fourth leading cause.[84] The overall burden of cerebrovascular and cardiovascular disease worldwide is projected to almost double by 2020 from what it was in 1990, with the biggest increase occurring in the developing world.

Evidence from Africa indicates that urbanization leads to a significant increase in the incidence of hypertension.[85] Very high age-adjusted rates of stroke are seen in sub-Saharan Africa.[86] Because other cardiovascular risk factors are largely absent in this population, these high rates have been attributed to untreated hypertension. The countries of Eastern Europe are also suffering an epidemic of cardiovascular disease.[87,88] Clearly, a great need exists for effective and inexpensive treatment of hypertension in these populations. In view of their low cost and documented effectiveness, thiazides and

β-blockers are the drugs of choice, although outcome trials in these populations are urgently needed. Sadly, a World Health Organization study of 10,000 patients with either CAD or cerebrovascular disease in middle- to low-income countries found that many modifiable cardiovascular risk factors were still not being addressed.[89]

CONCLUSIONS AND TREATMENT ALGORITHM

Several epidemiologic studies in Europe and the United States have shown that many patients known to be hypertensive have poorly controlled BP, either because they are not on treatment or because their treatment is inadequate.[90] These findings have been confirmed in a study of 24-hour BP control.[91] It is becoming increasingly clear that a significant proportion of all patients requiring treatment for hypertension need a combination of drugs to bring their BP down to a desirable level.[55] At present, guidelines from the British Hypertension Society and the US Joint National Committee on Prevention, Detection, Evaluation and Treatment of High BP recommend thiazide diuretics as first-line agents for the treatment of hypertension. The latter committee goes further, currently recommending thiazides over other agents in the absence of any other specific indications. β-Blockers have lost their place as first-line treatment because of more recent concerns over metabolic side effects and possibly reduced efficacy in reducing stroke, particularly in an aging population. This view has been endorsed by a recent Cochrane systematic review.[92] Perhaps with time, newer vasodilating β-blockers may be shown to address these concerns. In certain cases, such as secondary prevention of CAD and heart failure, β-blockers are still indicated as first-line antihypertensive therapy.

A low starting dose of a thiazide diuretic or β-blocker (e.g., hydrochlorothiazide 12.5 mg, bendrofluazide 1.25 mg, or atenolol 25 mg) should always be used initially. If after 4 weeks the BP is not adequately controlled, these doses can be doubled. Little further gain in BP control is seen by increasing doses beyond these levels, and there is also good evidence that more adverse side effects will occur.[93] Patients receiving diuretics should have their serum potassium level checked within the first month of treatment and at least annually thereafter. Significant hypokalemia is not common on low-dose thiazide diuretics; its occurrence should raise the possibility of an underlying endocrine abnormality such as primary aldosteronism. Patients who become hypokalemic should have the serum potassium level corrected. No clear evidence exists on whether oral potassium supplementation or the addition of a potassium-sparing diuretic is the better way to do this, although both have been shown to be effective.[94] Our practice is to add amiloride or spironolactone (the latter may be more beneficial in patients with CKD or heart failure[95]).

Patients in whom BP control is still poor after 3 months of treatment require a change of therapy. In practice, most patients need a combination of antihypertensive drugs to reach their target BP.[55] Monotherapy is rarely successful. We recommend adding another agent sooner rather than later and before the maximum dose of the starting agent has been reached.

Some of the commonly used diuretics and β-blockers in hypertension are listed in Tables 51-1 and 51-2. An algorithm for the use of diuretics or β-blockers in the treatment of hypertension is shown in Figure 51-1.

Table 51-1 Diuretics for the Treatment of Hypertension

	Initial Daily Dose (mg)	Maximum Daily Dose (mg)
Hydrochlorothiazide	12.5	50
Bendroflumethiazide	1.25	5
Chlorthalidone	25	50
Trichloromethiazide	2	4
Amiloride	5	10
Spironolactone	25	100

Table 51-2 β-Blockers for the Treatment of Hypertension*

	Initial Dose	Maximum Dose
Atenolol	25 mg once daily	100 mg once daily
Metoprolol†	50 mg once daily	100 mg twice daily
Propranolol†	40 mg twice daily	80 mg three times daily
Bisoprolol	2.5 mg once daily	10 mg once daily
Carvedilol†	12.5 mg once daily	25 mg twice daily
Nebivolol	2.5 mg once daily	10 mg once daily

*Low doses of β-blockers are appropriate for the treatment of hypertension, as discussed in the text. Higher doses (if tolerated) are of proven benefit in the treatment of heart failure and should be employed in this situation.
†A sustained-release preparation is available for once-daily dosing.

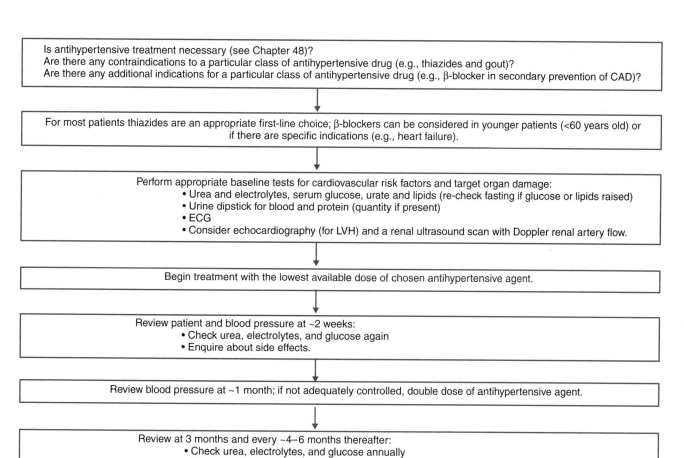

Is antihypertensive treatment necessary (see Chapter 48)?
Are there any contraindications to a particular class of antihypertensive drug (e.g., thiazides and gout)?
Are there any additional indications for a particular class of antihypertensive drug (e.g., β-blocker in secondary prevention of CAD)?

For most patients thiazides are an appropriate first-line choice; β-blockers can be considered in younger patients (<60 years old) or if there are specific indications (e.g., heart failure).

Perform appropriate baseline tests for cardiovascular risk factors and target organ damage:
• Urea and electrolytes, serum glucose, urate and lipids (re-check fasting if glucose or lipids raised)
• Urine dipstick for blood and protein (quantity if present)
• ECG
• Consider echocardiography (for LVH) and a renal ultrasound scan with Doppler renal artery flow.

Begin treatment with the lowest available dose of chosen antihypertensive agent.

Review patient and blood pressure at ~2 weeks:
• Check urea, electrolytes, and glucose again
• Enquire about side effects.

Review blood pressure at ~1 month; if not adequately controlled, double dose of antihypertensive agent.

Review at 3 months and every ~4–6 months thereafter:
• Check urea, electrolytes, and glucose annually
• If hypokalemic on thiazides, evaluate for hyperaldosteronism and add amiloride or spironolactone
• If blood pressure is still not controlled, add a different class of antihypertensive agent.

Figure 51-1 Algorithm for the use of thiazides or β-blockers in the treatment of hypertension.

References

1. Lindholm LH, Carlberg B, Samuelsson O: Should beta blockers remain first choice in the treatment of primary hypertension? A meta-analysis. Lancet 2005;366:1545–1553.

2. Psaty BM, Smith NL, Siscovick DS, et al: Health outcomes associated with antihypertensive therapies used as first-line agents. A systematic review and meta-analysis. JAMA 1997;277:739–745.

3. Andersson OK, Almgren T, Persson B, et al: Survival in treated hypertension: Follow up study after two decades. BMJ 1998; 317:167–171.

4. Collins R, Peto R, MacMahon S, et al: Blood pressure, stroke, and coronary heart disease. Part 2, Short-term reductions in blood pressure: Overview of randomised drug trials in their epidemiological context. Lancet 1990;335:827–838.

5. Kaplan NM: How bad are diuretic-induced hypokalemia and hypercholesterolemia? Arch Intern Med 1989;149:2649.

6. Khan N, McAlister FA: Re-examining the efficacy of beta-blockers for the treatment of hypertension: A meta-analysis. CMAJ 2006; 174:1737–1742.

7. Williams B, Poulter NR, Brown MJ, et al: Guidelines for management of hypertension: Report of the fourth working party of the British Hypertension Society, 2004—BHS IV. J Hum Hypertens 2004;18:139–185.

8. Khan NA, McAlister FA, Rabkin SW, et al: The 2006 Canadian Hypertension Education Program recommendations for the management of hypertension: Part II—Therapy. Can J Cardiol 2006;22:583–593.

9. The Antihypertensive and Lipid-Lowering Treatment to Prevent Heart Attack Trial (ALLHAT): Major outcomes in high-risk hypertensive patients randomized to angiotensin-converting enzyme inhibitor or calcium channel blocker vs diuretic. JAMA 2002;288: 2981–2997.

10. Chobanian AV, Bakris GL, Black HR, et al: Seventh report of the Joint National Committee on Prevention, Detection, Evaluation, and Treatment of High Blood Pressure. Hypertension 2003;42: 1206–1252.

11. Hebert LA, Rovin BH, Hebert CJ: The design of ALLHAT may have biased the study's outcome in favor of the diuretic cohort. Nat Clin Pract Nephrol 2007;3:60–61.

12. 2003 European Society of Hypertension—European Society of Cardiology guidelines for the management of arterial hypertension. J Hypertens 2003;21:1011–1053.

13. Multiple Risk Factor Intervention Trial Research Group: Risk factor changes and mortality results. JAMA 1982;248: 1465–1477.

14. SHEP Cooperative Research Group: Prevention of stroke by antihypertensive drug treatment in older persons with isolated systolic hypertension. Final results of the Systolic Hypertension in the Elderly Program (SHEP). JAMA 1991;265:3255–3264.

15. Siscovick DS, Raghunathan TE, Psaty BM, et al: Diuretic therapy for hypertension and the risk of primary cardiac arrest. N Engl J Med 1994;330:1852–1857.

16. Zillich AJ, Garg J, Basu S, et al: Thiazide diuretics, potassium, and the development of diabetes: A quantitative review. Hypertension 2006;48:219–224.

17. Kasiske BL, Ma JZ, Kalil RS, Louis TA: Effects of antihypertensive therapy on serum lipids. Ann Intern Med 1995;122: 133–141.

18. Grimm RH, Jr., Flack JM, Grandits GA, et al, for the Treatment of Mild Hypertension Study (TOMHS) Research Group: Long-term effects on plasma lipids of diet and drugs to treat hypertension. JAMA 1996;275:1549–1556.

19. Materson BJ, Reda DJ, Cushman WC, et al, for the Department of Veterans Affairs Cooperative Study Group on Antihypertensive Agents: Single-drug therapy for hypertension in men. A comparison of six antihypertensive agents with placebo. N Engl J Med 1993;328:914–921.

20. Weir MR, Moser M: Diuretics and beta-blockers: Is there a risk for dyslipidemia? Am Heart J 2000;139:174–183.

21. Seguchi H, Nakamura H, Aosaki N, et al: Effects of carvedilol on serum lipids in hypertensive and normotensive subjects. Eur J Clin Pharmacol 1990;38(Suppl 2):S139–S142.

22. Gress TW, Nieto FJ, Shahar E, et al: Hypertension and antihypertensive therapy as risk factors for type 2 diabetes mellitus. Atherosclerosis Risk in Communities Study. N Engl J Med 2000;342:905–912.

23. Savage PJ, Pressel SL, Curb JD, et al, for the SHEP Cooperative Research Group: Influence of long-term, low-dose, diuretic-based, antihypertensive therapy on glucose, lipid, uric acid, and potassium levels in older men and women with isolated systolic hypertension: The Systolic Hypertension in the Elderly Program. Arch Intern Med 1998;158:741–751.

24. Hansson L, Lindholm LH, Niskanen L, et al: Effect of angiotensin-converting-enzyme inhibition compared with conventional therapy on cardiovascular morbidity and mortality in hypertension: The Captopril Prevention Project (CAPPP) randomised trial. Lancet 1999;353:611–616.

25. Pepine CJ, Handberg EM, Cooper-DeHoff RM, et al: A calcium antagonist vs a non-calcium antagonist hypertension treatment strategy for patients with coronary artery disease. The International Verapamil-Trandolapril Study (INVEST): A randomized controlled trial. JAMA 2003;290:2805–2816.

26. Sarafidis PA, Bakris GL: Antihypertensive treatment with beta-blockers and the spectrum of glycaemic control. QJM 2006;99: 431–436.

27. UK Prospective Diabetes Study Group: Tight blood pressure control and risk of macrovascular and microvascular complications in type 2 diabetes: UKPDS 38. BMJ 1998;317:703–713.

28. Bakris GL, Fonseca V, Katholi RE, et al: Metabolic effects of carvedilol vs metoprolol in patients with type 2 diabetes mellitus and hypertension: A randomized controlled trial. JAMA 2004; 292:2227–2236.

29. Elliott WJ, Meyer PM: Incident diabetes in clinical trials of antihypertensive drugs: A network meta-analysis. Lancet 2007;369: 201–207.

30. Alderman MH, Cohen H, Madhavan S, Kivlighn S: Serum uric acid and cardiovascular events in successfully treated hypertensive patients. Hypertension 1999;34:144–150.

31. Culleton BF, Larson MG, Kannel WB, Levy D: Serum uric acid and risk for cardiovascular disease and death: The Framingham Heart Study. Ann Intern Med 1999;131:7–13.

32. McCord JM: Oxygen-derived free radicals in postischemic tissue injury. N Engl J Med 1985;312:159–163.

33. Franse LV, Pahor M, Di BM, et al: Serum uric acid, diuretic treatment and risk of cardiovascular events in the Systolic Hypertension in the Elderly Program (SHEP). J Hypertens 2000;18:1149–1154.

34. Medical Research Council (MRC) Working Party: MRC trial of treatment of mild hypertension: Principal results. BMJ (Clin Res Ed) 1985;291:97–104.

35. Ko DT, Hebert PR, Coffey CS, et al: Beta-blocker therapy and symptoms of depression, fatigue, and sexual dysfunction. JAMA 2002;288:351–357.

36. Feldman HA, Goldstein I, Hatzichristou DG, et al: Impotence and its medical and psychosocial correlates: Results of the Massachusetts Male Aging Study. J Urol 1994;151:54–61.

37. Kloner RA, Brown M, Prisant LM, Collins M, for the Sildenafil Study Group: Effect of sildenafil in patients with erectile dysfunction taking antihypertensive therapy. Am J Hypertens 2001;14:70–73.

38. Prisant LM, Carr AA, Bottini PB, et al: Sexual dysfunction with antihypertensive drugs. Arch Intern Med 1994;154:730–736.

39. Grossman E, Messerli FH, Goldbourt U: Does diuretic therapy increase the risk of renal cell carcinoma? Am J Cardiol 1999;83: 1090–1093.

40. McLaughlin JK, Chow WH, Mandel JS, et al: International renal-cell cancer study. VIII. Role of diuretics, other anti-hypertensive medications and hypertension. Int J Cancer 1995;63:216–221.

41. Largent JA, McEligot AJ, Ziogas A, et al: Hypertension, diuretics and breast cancer risk. J Hum Hypertens 2006;20:727–732.

42. Ray WA, Griffin MR, Downey W, Melton LJ III: Long-term use of thiazide diuretics and risk of hip fracture. Lancet 1989;1:687–690.

43. Cappuccio FP, Meilahn E, Zmuda JM, Cauley JA, for the Study of Osteoporotic Fractures Research Group: High blood pressure and bone-mineral loss in elderly white women: A prospective study. Lancet 1999;354:971–975.

44. Reid IR, Ames RW, Orr-Walker BJ, et al: Hydrochlorothiazide reduces loss of cortical bone in normal postmenopausal women: A randomized controlled trial. Am J Med 2000;109:362–370.

45. Bolland MJ, Ames RW, Horne AM, et al: The effect of treatment with a thiazide diuretic for 4 years on bone density in normal postmenopausal women. Osteoporos Int 2006;18:479–486.

46. Takeda S, Elefteriou F, Levasseur R, et al: Leptin regulates bone formation via the sympathetic nervous system. Cell 2002;111:305–317.

47. Reid IR, Gamble GD, Grey AB, et al: β-Blocker use, BMD, and fractures in the study of osteoporotic fractures. J Bone Miner Res 2005;20:613–618.

48. Salpeter S, Ormiston T, Salpeter E: Cardioselective beta-blockers for chronic obstructive pulmonary disease. Cochrane Database Syst Rev 2005;(4)CD003566.

49. Staessen JA, Fagard R, Thijs L, et al, for the Systolic Hypertension in Europe (Syst-Eur) Trial Investigators: Randomised double-blind comparison of placebo and active treatment for older patients with isolated systolic hypertension. Lancet 1997;350:757–764.

50. Staessen JA, Gasowski J, Wang JG, et al: Risks of untreated and treated isolated systolic hypertension in the elderly: Meta-analysis of outcome trials. Lancet 2000;355:865–872.

51. Perry HM, Jr., Davis BR, Price TR, et al: Effect of treating isolated systolic hypertension on the risk of developing various types and subtypes of stroke: The Systolic Hypertension in the Elderly Program (SHEP). JAMA 2000;284:465–471.

52. Medical Research Council (MRC) Working Party: MRC trial of treatment of hypertension in older adults: Principal results. BMJ 1992;304:405–412.

53. Pahor M, Psaty BM, Alderman MH, et al: Health outcomes associated with calcium antagonists compared with other first-line antihypertensive therapies: A meta-analysis of randomised controlled trials. Lancet 2000;356:1949–1954.

54. Leipzig RM, Cumming RG, Tinetti ME: Drugs and falls in older people: A systematic review and meta-analysis: II. Cardiac and analgesic drugs. J Am Geriatr Soc 1999;47:40–50.

55. Morgan TO, Anderson AI, MacInnis RJ: ACE inhibitors, beta-blockers, calcium blockers, and diuretics for the control of systolic hypertension. Am J Hypertens 2001;14:241–247.

56. Cooper RS, Liao Y, Rotimi C: Is hypertension more severe among U.S. blacks, or is severe hypertension more common? Ann Epidemiol 1996;6:173–180.

57. Wild S, McKeigue P: Cross sectional analysis of mortality by country of birth in England and Wales, 1970–92. BMJ 1997;314:705–710.

58. Preston RA, Materson BJ, Reda DJ, et al, for the Department of Veterans Affairs Cooperative Study Group on Antihypertensive Agents: Age-race subgroup compared with renin profile as predictors of blood pressure response to antihypertensive therapy. JAMA 1998;280:1168–1172.

59. Veterans Administration Cooperative Study Group on Antihypertensive Agents: Comparison of propranolol and hydrochlorothiazide for the initial treatment of hypertension. I. Results of short-term titration with emphasis on racial differences in response. JAMA 1982;248:1996–2003.

60. Sareli P, Radevski IV, Valtchanova ZP, et al: Efficacy of different drug classes used to initiate antihypertensive treatment in black subjects: Results of a randomized trial in Johannesburg, South Africa. Arch Intern Med 2001;161:965–971.

61. Brewster LM, van Montfrans GA, Kleijnen J: Systematic review: Antihypertensive drug therapy in black patients. Ann Intern Med 2004;141:614–627.

62. Yusuf S, Wittes J, Friedman L: Overview of results of randomized clinical trials in heart disease. I. Treatments following myocardial infarction. JAMA 1988;260:2088–2093.

63. Chen J, Marciniak TA, Radford MJ, et al: Beta-blocker therapy for secondary prevention of myocardial infarction in elderly diabetic patients. Results from the National Cooperative Cardiovascular Project. J Am Coll Cardiol 1999;34:1388–1394.

64. Mehta RH, Eagle KA: Secondary prevention in acute myocardial infarction. BMJ 1998;316:838–842.

65. Yusuf S, Sleight P, Pogue J, et al, for the Heart Outcomes Prevention Evaluation Study Investigators: Effects of an angiotensin-converting-enzyme inhibitor, ramipril, on cardiovascular events in high-risk patients. N Engl J Med 2000;342:145–153.

66. Randomised trial of a perindopril-based blood-pressure-lowering regimen among 6,105 individuals with previous stroke or transient ischaemic attack. Lancet 2001;358:1033–1041.

67. Effect of metoprolol CR/XL in chronic heart failure: Metoprolol CR/XL Randomised Intervention Trial in Congestive Heart Failure (MERIT-HF). Lancet 1999;353:2001–2007.

68. Metra M, Giubbini R, Nodari S, et al: Differential effects of beta-blockers in patients with heart failure: A prospective, randomized, double-blind comparison of the long-term effects of metoprolol versus carvedilol. Circulation 2000;102:546–551.

69. Flather MD, Shibata MC, Coats AJ, et al: Randomized trial to determine the effect of nebivolol on mortality and cardiovascular hospital admission in elderly patients with heart failure (SENIORS). Eur Heart J 2005;26:215–225.

70. Levy D, Garrison RJ, Savage DD, et al: Prognostic implications of echocardiographically determined left ventricular mass in the Framingham Heart Study. N Engl J Med 1990;322:1561–1566.

71. Schmieder RE, Martus P, Klingbeil A: Reversal of left ventricular hypertrophy in essential hypertension. A meta-analysis of randomized double-blind studies. JAMA 1996;275:1507–1513.

72. Lindholm LH, Ibsen H, Dahlof B, et al: Cardiovascular morbidity and mortality in patients with diabetes in the Losartan Intervention For Endpoint reduction in hypertension study (LIFE): A randomised trial against atenolol. Lancet 2002;359:1004–1010.

73. Gottdiener JS, Reda DJ, Massie BM, et al, for the Department of Veterans Affairs Cooperative Study Group on Antihypertensive Agents: Effect of single-drug therapy on reduction of left ventricular mass in mild to moderate hypertension: Comparison of six antihypertensive agents. Circulation;95:2007–2014.

74. Liebson PR, Grandits GA, Dianzumba S, et al: Comparison of five antihypertensive monotherapies and placebo for change in left ventricular mass in patients receiving nutritional-hygienic therapy in the Treatment of Mild Hypertension Study (TOMHS). Circulation 1995;91:698–706.

75. Magee LA, Duley L: Oral beta-blockers for mild to moderate hypertension during pregnancy. Cochrane Database Syst Rev 2003;(3):CD002863.

76. Report of the National High Blood Pressure Education Program Working Group on High Blood Pressure in Pregnancy. Am J Obstet Gynecol 2000;183:S1–S22.

77. The GISEN Group (Gruppo Italiano di Studi Epidemiologici in Nefrologia): Randomised placebo-controlled trial of effect of ramipril on decline in glomerular filtration rate and risk of terminal renal failure in proteinuric, non-diabetic nephropathy. Lancet 1997;349:1857–1863.

78. The EUCLID Study Group: Randomised placebo-controlled trial of lisinopril in normotensive patients with insulin-dependent

diabetes and normoalbuminuria or microalbuminuria. Lancet 1997;349:1787–1792.

79. Jafar TH, Schmid CH, Landa M, et al: Angiotensin-converting enzyme inhibitors and progression of nondiabetic renal disease. A meta-analysis of patient-level data. Ann Intern Med 2001;135: 73–87.

80. Casas JP, Chua W, Loukogeorgakis S, et al: Effect of inhibitors of the renin-angiotensin system and other antihypertensive drugs on renal outcomes: Systematic review and meta-analysis. Lancet 2005;366:2026–2033.

81. Ruggenenti P, Perna A, Gherardi G, et al, for Gruppo Italiano di Studi Epidemiologici in Nefrologia (GISEN): Renal function and requirement for dialysis in chronic nephropathy patients on long-term ramipril: REIN (Ramipril Efficacy in Nephropathy) follow-up trial. Lancet 1998;352:1252–1256.

82. Liu L, Wang JG, Gong L, et al, for the Systolic Hypertension in China (Syst-China) Collaborative Group: Comparison of active treatment and placebo in older Chinese patients with isolated systolic hypertension. J Hypertens 1998;16:1823–1829.

83. Murray CJ, Lopez AD: Global mortality, disability, and the contribution of risk factors: Global Burden of Disease Study. Lancet 1997;349:1436–1442.

84. Murray CJ, Lopez AD: Alternative projections of mortality and disability by cause 1990–2020: Global Burden of Disease Study. Lancet 1997;349:1498–1504.

85. Poulter NR, Khaw KT, Hopwood BE, et al: The Kenyan Luo migration study: Observations on the initiation of a rise in blood pressure. BMJ 1990;300:967–972.

86. Walker RW, McLarty DG, Kitange HM, et al: Stroke mortality in urban and rural Tanzania. Adult Morbidity and Mortality Project. Lancet 2000;355:1684–1687.

87. Notzon FC, Komarov YM, Ermakov SP, et al: Causes of declining life expectancy in Russia. JAMA 1998;279:793–800.

88. Sarti C, Rastenyte D, Cepaitis Z, Tuomilehto J: International trends in mortality from stroke, 1968 to 1994. Stroke 2000;31: 1588–1601.

89. The World Health Report 1999. The Double Burden: Emerging Epidemics and Persistent Problems. Geneva: WHO, 1999. Available at: http://www.who.int/whr/1999/en/whr99_ch2_en.pdf. Accessed May 7, 2008.

90. Hyman DJ, Pavlik VN: Characteristics of patients with uncontrolled hypertension in the United States. N Engl J Med 2001; 345:479–486.

91. Mancia G, Sega R, Milesi C, et al: Blood-pressure control in the hypertensive population. Lancet 1997;349:454–457.

92. Wiysonge C, Bradley H, Mayosi B, et al: Beta-blockers for hypertension. Cochrane Database Syst Rev 2007;(1):CD002003.

93. Carlsen JE, Kober L, Torp-Pedersen C, Johansen P: Relation between dose of bendrofluazide, antihypertensive effect, and adverse biochemical effects. BMJ 1990;300:975–978.

94. Schnaper HW, Freis ED, Friedman RG, et al: Potassium restoration in hypertensive patients made hypokalemic by hydrochlorothiazide. Arch Intern Med 1989;149:2677–2681.

95. Bianchi S, Bigazzi R, Campese VM: Long-term effects of spironolactone on proteinuria and kidney function in patients with chronic kidney disease. Kidney Int 2006;70:2116-2123.

Further Reading

Chobanian AV, Bakris GL, Black HR et al: Seventh report of the Joint National Committee on Prevention, Detection, Evaluation, and Treatment of High Blood Pressure. Hypertension 2003;42:1206–1252.

Khan N, McAlister FA: Re-examining the efficacy of beta-blockers for the treatment of hypertension: A meta-analysis. CMAJ 2006;174:1737–1742.

Lindholm LH, Carlberg B, Samuelsson O: Should beta blockers remain first choice in the treatment of primary hypertension? A meta-analysis. Lancet 2005;366:1545–1553.

The Antihypertensive and Lipid-Lowering Treatment to Prevent Heart Attack Trial (ALLHAT): Major outcomes in high-risk hypertensive patients randomized to angiotensin-converting enzyme inhibitor or calcium channel blocker vs diuretic. JAMA 2002;288:2981–2997.

2003 European Society of Hypertension–European Society of Cardiology guidelines for the management of arterial hypertension. J Hypertens 2003;21:1011–1053.

Williams B, Poulter NR, Brown MJ, et al: Guidelines for management of hypertension: Report of the fourth working party of the British Hypertension Society, 2004-BHS IV. J Hum Hypertens 2004;18:139–185.

Wiysonge C, Bradley H, Mayosi B, et al: Beta-blockers for hypertension. Cochrane Database Syst Rev 2007;(1):CD002003.

Chapter 52

ACE Inhibitors, Angiotensin Receptor Blockers, Mineralocorticoid Receptor Antagonists, and Renin Antagonists

Norman K. Hollenberg

When pharmacologic interruption of the renin-angiotensin system first became possible through the development of angiotensin-converting enzyme (ACE) inhibitors, even the wildest enthusiast could not have predicted the evolution of this field.[1,2] Agents that block the renin system were thought by many at that time to hold promise only in a small patient population, those with hypertension associated with elevated plasma renin activity. This group of patients is important, because it includes those with accelerated hypertension and those in whom hypertension tends to be difficult to treat, but these processes are relatively uncommon. This class of drug was therefore perceived to occupy an important but rather small niche.

That niche has grown and, indeed, continues to grow. The introduction of ACE inhibitors was marked by early success in patients with extremely high blood pressure (BP) resistant to the effects of triple-drug regimens. A series of studies over the past two decades has identified a much broader range of efficacy for ACE inhibitors, indicating that these drugs are also remarkably helpful in patients with advanced heart failure, those with a large anterior myocardial infarction, and those at risk of diabetic nephropathy, other forms of nephropathy, and (in the HOPE study) the consequences of atherosclerosis.[2] ACE inhibitors have gradually emerged, therefore, as the leading class for the treatment not only of those complicated patients initially described, but also of the patient with mild-to-moderate essential hypertension who is free of any identifiable target organ damage and who is at rather low risk. Although this chapter lies in a section entitled Management of Essential Hypertension, and there are separate and relevant chapters on drug dosing and renal failure, prevention of progressive renal failure, cardiovascular complications, control of cardiovascular risk factors in hypertension, and individualization of pharmacologic therapy, as well as on management of diabetic nephropathy, IgA nephropathy, and other forms of

glomerulonephritis, and clinical trials in nephrology and hypertension—with inevitable overlap—it is necessary to touch on many of these subjects in this chapter. Because the drugs are not the subject of any other individual chapter, greater emphasis will be given to their pharmacology and to their handling in patients who have lost kidney function.

Despite their remarkable record of success, it is important to recognize that ACE inhibition was not the product of a planned pharmacologic approach, but rather was an accidental byproduct of snake venom toxicology. A pharmacologist examining the renin cascade would first have chosen two alternative points as candidates for blockade.[3] In principle, blockade of a system is most effective at the rate-limiting step: in the renin cascade, the interaction between renin and its substrate, angiotensinogen. Renin inhibitors were developed and were efficacious, but poor bioavailability and cost of synthesis brought development programs to a halt for more than a decade. With the development of aliskiren, the first clinically approved renin inhibitor, we have a new tool, as is discussed under Pharmacology of Direct Renin Inhibition in this chapter. Blockade at the level of the angiotensin II receptor is also attractive, especially if non-ACE-dependent pathways for angiotensin II generation exist. Evidence for such pathways (especially in the kidney) in the intact human is growing,[3] which makes blockade of the renin system at the level of the angiotensin II receptor an important therapeutic step.

Another factor shapes use of these agents. The angiotensin II antagonists are products of imidazole chemistry, and imidazole derivatives have a wide range of pharmacologic activity.[4] Thus, no one could have anticipated how remarkably well tolerated this class of agents is. In study after study, AT_1 receptor blockers compare favorably with placebo in frequency of adverse reactions,[1,5] a statement that could never have been made about antihypertensive agents in the past.

PHARMACOLOGY OF THE ACE INHIBITORS

Angiotensin-converting enzyme is a widely distributed zinc metallopeptidase that represents the final enzymatic step in the lysis of angiotensin I to produce angiotensin II. There are three main ACE isoforms: somatic ACE, plasma ACE, and testicular ACE. Somatic ACE is attached to the cell membrane and has an extracellular region that consists of two homologous domains,[6,7] each of which contains an active catalytic site. Testicular ACE, conversely, has only one catalytically active site. Plasma ACE is thought to be derived from the somatic ACE but lacks the transmembrane domain and intracellular portion. Like somatic ACE, plasma ACE contains two active sites. The presence of two catalytic sites in somatic ACE, each capable of converting angiotensin I to angiotensin II and displaying different kinetics, has raised the interesting possibility that ACE inhibitors could differ in their affinity for the two sites. The C-terminal site accounts for approximately 75% of total ACE[7] and is largely responsible for the conversion of angiotensin I to angiotensin II. It has been suggested that the N-terminal site has greater responsibility for the metabolism of other peptide substrates.[8]

ACE inhibitors interact differently with ACE-active sites, depending on their structure.[9,10] Lisinopril, for example, shows affinity for only one binding site on both somatic and testicular ACE, suggesting that it binds only the C-terminal active site of ACE. Conversely, cilazaprilat has affinity for the two binding sites on somatic ACE. These findings suggest that the two active sites of somatic ACE have different structural requirements. Although of interest, at the moment there are no compelling data to indicate a functional or therapeutic implication for these findings.

ACE generally functions as a carboxyl-dipeptide hydrolase, which includes many substrates, not only angiotensin I and bradykinin, but also a wide range of peptides, including enkephalins, substance P, and the beta chain of insulin.[11] Clearly there are consequences to the broad range of peptide substrates degraded by ACE for the specificity of ACE inhibitor function. A number of studies in animal models, not yet supported by information from studies in humans, have suggested that bradykinin might play a role in the tissue-sparing effects of ACE inhibitors. Conversely, it is thought that the same mechanism might underlie the cough so often induced by ACE inhibitors, which represents their main drawback.[11]

The first early effective ACE inhibitor, captopril, is a sulfhydryl-containing compound, which is relatively rapid in onset and short acting.[11] Thereafter, all of the ACE inhibitors that have been developed are longer-acting and, with the exception of lisinopril and captopril, undergo metabolic conversion into an active diacid form. There is no evidence that this conversion is ever rate-limiting. The ACE inhibitors are structurally heterogeneous in both their primary binding sites to the ACE receptor and in the side chains capable of binding ACE. The sulfhydryl group in captopril was replaced by a carboxyl group in most of the remaining ACE inhibitors, with the exception of a phosphinyl group in fosinopril. Although there are a number of claims that these substitutions have functional significance—for example, the reduced frequency of cough claimed for fosinopril and free-radical scavenging for the sulfhydryl group on captopril—in fact,

Table 52-1 Clinical Pharmacology of ACE Inhibitors

Drug	Elimination Route	Serum Half-life (hr)	Effect of Food	Protein Binding (%)
Benazepril	Renal, some biliary	10–11	None	>95
Captopril	Renal, as disulfides	<2	Reduced	25–30
Enalapril	Renal	11	None	50
Fosinopril	Renal = hepatic	11	None	95
Lisinopril	Renal	13	None	10
Moexipril	Renal, some biliary	2–9	Reduced	50
Perindopril	Renal	7	None	60
Quinapril	Renal > hepatic	2	Reduced	97
Ramipril	Renal	13–17	Reduced	73
Trandolapril	Renal > hepatic	16–24	None	80–94

clinically meaningful difference remains to be proved. Indeed, beyond the frequency of dosing and handling of these agents in the patient with renal failure, there are few persuasive differences.

For all of the ACE inhibitors, with the exception of fosinopril and trandolapril, the diazo-form is excreted primarily via renal clearance, involving both filtration and tubular secretion.[11,12] In the case of fosinopril and trandolapril, excretion is more balanced, and hepatic excretion rises with a reduction in renal function (Table 52-1).

Although there are many claims that ACE inhibitors differ in functionally important ways, such as tissue penetration and action on endothelial function, in fact the available evidence for such differences is not persuasive; neither is there clear evidence that these differences have therapeutic implications. Most of the impetus for such claims has come from industry. Quantitatively important differences in duration of action and in metabolism have implications for use in the patient with renal failure.

PHARMACOLOGY OF THE ANGIOTENSIN RECEPTOR BLOCKERS

The first antagonists to angiotensin II and its receptor were peptide analogs of angiotensin II, developed as a byproduct of analyses of the structural requirements for binding of angiotensin II to its receptor and the synthesis of many structural analogs of angiotensin II.[1,5] The most widely studied angiotensin receptor blocker (ARB), saralasin, is an octapeptide that differs from angiotensin II in structure at the eighth amino acid, where alanine is the residue, and at the first amino acid, where sarcosine—an amino acid that does not occur in mammals—was employed to slow the degradation of the molecule. Because saralasin could only be given intravenously, was a partial agonist, and was very expensive to manufacture, it never developed a major role in therapy or diagnostics.

In 1982, an unanticipated advance was made through the application of high throughput screening in the laboratory of Takeda in Japan.[13] They identified a series of imidazole derivatives that bound specifically to the angiotensin II receptor. Structure action work at Dupont Laboratories led to the development of losartan, the first of a new class of nonpeptide, clinically effective ARBs.[14] Most of the antihypertensive action of losartan in vivo involves conversion of the parent compound to EXP-3174, the carboxylic acid metabolite of losartan.[15] Further structural modifications led to the identification of valsartan, irbesartan, candesartan, and telmisartan.[5] All are biphenyl tetrazoles. Investigators at SmithKline Beecham pursued an alternative pathway from the original Takeda compound to produce eprosartan, which is a nonbiphenyl, nontetrazole compound.[16]

One clear difference among the available agents involves structure. All of the currently marketed AT_1 receptor antagonists, with the exception of eprosartan, are biphenyl tetrazoles.[4,5] Eprosartan also differs from all of the other marketed drugs in its interaction with the AT_1 receptor. Eprosartan is a pure competitive antagonist, the action of which is surmountable by sufficiently high angiotensin II concentration.[17] Valsartan, irbesartan, candesartan, telmisartan, and the active metabolite of losartan, EXP-3174, all show noncompetitive kinetics, which suggests a nonequilibrium relation to the receptor.[18] When the binding is sufficiently tight, equilibrium conditions required to show competitive antagonism are not in place, and the kinetics become insurmountable. In the case of losartan, the parent molecule is a weak competitive antagonist, and virtually all of the blockade after the first several hours depends on the 15% that is converted to a much more potent nonequilibrium antagonist, EXP-3174. One clinically relevant byproduct of the tight binding is the very long duration of action of the nonequilibrium ARBs. The half-life in plasma poorly predicts the duration of the blockade because of the long sojourn of the blocker on the receptor.

The available angiotensin II receptor blockers differ from one another in their oral bioavailability, metabolism, and elimination.[1,5] Candesartan cilexetil is a true prodrug, the active agent being candesartan, which is freed from the complex during passage through the gut wall. Losartan is an active agent, a very weak competitive antagonist, with an active metabolite (EXP-3174) that is substantially more potent and long acting. Bioavailability ranges from approximately 25% for valsartan to 80% for irbesartan (Table 52-2). The absorption of neither candesartan nor irbesartan is influenced by food, whereas valsartan and losartan do show interference with absorption by food. With the exception of candesartan, which has a 60% renal route of elimination, for most of the agents the primary excretion is biliary (see Table 52-2). Only one of the agents, losartan, has a tubular action that leads to increased uric acid excretion.

The angiotensin II receptors are divided into AT_1 and AT_2 subtypes, characterized both pharmacologically and by cloning. All of the clinically important, well-defined actions of angiotensin on the kidney are mediated via the AT_1 receptor. Studies in animal models where AT_2 receptor

Table 52-2 *Clinical Pharmacology of Angiotensin Receptor Blockers*

Drug	Elimination Route	Effect of Food	Protein Binding (%)	Uricosuric
Candesartan	Renal (60%)	No	99	No
Eprosartan	Biliary (70%)	No	90	No
Irbesartan	Biliary (99%)	No	90	No
Losartan	Biliary (90%)	Yes	98	Yes
EXP-3174	Renal (50%)	—	99	Yes
Telmesartan	Biliary (99%)	No	99	No
Valsartan	Biliary (70%)	Yes	95	No

competitive antagonists are available has suggested that the renal actions supported by the AT_2 receptor are opposite to those of the AT_1 receptor, including vasodilation, natriuresis, and growth inhibition.[19] The AT_2 receptor is prominent during embryogenesis, in the kidney and elsewhere, but becomes rapidly and progressively more sparse after birth. Any discussion of the role played by the AT_2 receptor in humans is speculative, because there are no direct data available from studies in humans. Species difference in the contribution of the renin-angiotensin system to renal control mechanisms is discussed in Renal Actions of Renin-Angiotensin System Blockers in this chapter, and may well be relevant. For example, there is a single AT_1 receptor and responsible gene in humans and two AT_1 receptor isoforms in the rat.[20]

PHARMACOLOGY OF DIRECT RENIN INHIBITION

Although renin inhibition has long been recognized as a preferred site for blockade of the renin-angiotensin system because renin is the rate-limiting step in the cascade, until recently the development of renin inhibitors has been limited by poor bioavailability, limited efficacy, and substantial cost.[21-23] The aid of molecular modeling and x-ray structure analysis has brought about significant improvement in the design of potent and selective inhibitors of renin. The result has been the development of aliskiren, the first orally effective direct renin inhibitor approved for use in humans. Significant improvement in binding has resulted from the recognition of compounds that optimize the interaction of the molecule with elements of the active site. Although aliskiren has limited bioavailability, with some 2% to 3% of an oral dose being absorbed, its affinity for the receptor is profound, with an IC50 of 0.6 nmol/L. Thus, the limited plasma concentrations achieved are more than adequate to produce complete inhibition of renin.

The importance of the direct renin inhibitor has been enhanced by the recent recognition of a functional role for prorenin at the tissue level in the pathogenesis of a number of clinical problems. Data are available, for example, to indicate that prorenin acting on a special renin receptor found in the glomerular mesangium and in arteries contributes to the pathogenesis of diabetic nephropathy and retinopathy.[24-25]

Aliskiren is very long acting, with a half-life of approximately 40 hours after ingestion, and is extremely hypophilic.[21-23]

The usual doses employed in humans, 150 and 300 mg, are well tolerated and appear to be largely free of important adverse effects. Frequent diarrhea limits the use of doses of 600 mg or more.

Although the BP effects of aliskiren are similar to the responses to ACE inhibitors and ARBs in double-blind studies,[21-23] there is evidence at the tissue level that aliskiren may have effects that go beyond what can be achieved with an ACE inhibitor or an ARB.[26] These effects include an especially prominent influence on the kidney.[26]

RENAL ACTIONS OF RENIN-ANGIOTENSIN SYSTEM BLOCKERS

The renal response to blocking the renin-angiotensin system with any of the three classes of blocker that have been studied depends on three factors. The first is the actions of angiotensin II on the kidney in the setting of the study. Thus, for example, salt intake is a major determinant of the response to blocking the renin system, because salt intake influences the production and action of angiotensin II on the kidney. Second, the completeness of blockade induced by the agent is a crucial factor. In many studies, a somewhat arbitrary dose of a blocker has been employed, often much less than the optimal dose for blockade. The third major factor involves additional actions of the pharmacologic agent employed. Achieving an overall synthesis of the data is further complicated by the important species differences both in the renin-angiotensin system pathways and in the additional effects of the agents used to block the system.[20] Moreover, in protocols performed in animals, anesthesia is often used, which further modifies both the state of the renin-angiotensin system and the condition of the kidney.[21]

Shortly after the first ACE inhibitor, the peptide teprotide, became available, studies in dogs and rabbits made it clear that when the renin system was activated by a low-salt diet, the administration of the ACE inhibitor would lead to striking and consistent renal vasodilation and natriuresis, with little or no change in glomerular filtration rate.[3] In studies performed in trained animals that could be studied without anesthesia, it became apparent that the responses were much smaller when the animals were studied on a high-salt diet to suppress the renin-angiotensin system. The angiotensin II receptor blocker available at that time, saralasin, was a partial agonist with substantial angiotensin-like activity—especially when the dose was pushed. When used properly, saralasin revealed a qualitatively similar, albeit smaller, renal vasodilator response as that seen with the ACE inhibitor. Essentially identical findings were found with teprotide, captopril, and saralasin in humans.[27]

The striking influence of salt intake on the renal vasodilator response to ACE inhibition, recognized early, supported a dominant role for the angiotensin II mechanism.[20] If the renal vasodilator response induced by ACE inhibitors in humans included a substantial component due to bradykinin, prostaglandins, nitric oxide, or some other vasodilator pathway, several conclusions follow. First, if alternative vasodilator pathways were engaged, the vasodilation should have been associated with blunting of the renal vascular response to angiotensin II. Conversely, if the vasodilator response reflected a reduction in angiotensin II formation, enhancement of the renal vascular response to angiotensin II would be expected. Because such enhancement was found, it seemed likely that the other vasodilator pathways were less important.

A second consequence would have been that the renal vasodilator response to renin inhibition would have been substantially less than the response to ACE inhibition. In fact, in humans the renal vasodilator response to two renin inhibitors exceeded expectations from earlier experience with ACE inhibition.[3] Because of the notorious risk of employing historical controls, a coded, double-blind study was performed in which volunteers received an ACE inhibitor, a renin inhibitor, or placebo during the same week. The response was unambiguous: Renin inhibition induced a substantially larger renal vasodilator response than did ACE inhibition. That left no room for ACE inhibition-induced activation of renal vasodilator pathways, but did not provide an explanation for why the response to renin inhibition was substantially larger. In this case, the angiotensin II receptor blocker provided a "tie breaker." If the renin inhibitor indeed operated via the renin-angiotensin system cascade, one would anticipate a similar or larger renal vasodilator response to the angiotensin II antagonist in studies performed with an identical protocol. This is precisely what was found. Three angiotensin II receptor blockers—eprosartan, irbesartan, and candesartan—induced a renal vasodilator response that matched or slightly exceeded the response to renin inhibition in healthy humans in balance on a low-salt diet.[20] All of the studies were performed at the top of the relationship between drug dose and renal vascular response.

From this observation, a series of conclusions is reasonable. The renal hemodynamic response to ACE inhibition has systematically underestimated the contribution of angiotensin II to renal vascular tone in humans. The effectiveness of renin inhibition suggests that this response represents interruption of primarily renin-dependent but non-ACE-dependent pathways, probably involving chymase. From quantitative considerations—response to ACE inhibition was 90 to 100 mL/min/1.73 m^2 in this model as opposed to the 140 to 150 mL/min/1.73 m^2 induced by renin inhibition or angiotensin II receptor blockers—it follows that 30% to 40% of angiotensin-dependent renal vascular tone reflects angiotensin generated via a non-ACE-dependent pathway.[3] That percentage is higher when the renin system is suppressed by a high-salt diet in healthy humans.[22]

In more recent studies in an identical model, aliskiren has led to a response substantially larger than ever seen with an ACE inhibitor or an ARB, averaging at peak dose approximately 200 mL/min/1.73m^2.[26] Given the specificity of renin inhibition, it is unlikely that a nonrenin pathway is involved. A more likely explanation is that the direct renin inhibitor is also interfering with pathways involving prorenin.[24,25]

Several important species differences merit discussion.[20] The first involves pathways for non-ACE generation. In humans and other primates the enzyme chymase has a single substrate, angiotensin I, and a single product, angiotensin II. Indeed, it should have been called *angiotensin-converting enzyme,* but that name was subsumed for another enzyme in the 1950s. The primate separated from other mammals in phylogeny millions of years ago. Since that time, there have been ample opportunities for shifts in metabolic pathways. In the rat and rabbit, chymase does not have angiotensin I as its substrate, but rather has angiotensin II as its substrate and degradation products of angiotensin II as its product. Thus, the action of chymase in humans and in small animals is opposite. One would anticipate that ACE inhibitors and angiotensin II receptor blockers would have similar actions. In these small creatures, they do.

A second major species-dependent difference involves the mechanism by which ACE inhibition influences the renal blood supply. In rats and dogs, considerable evidence indicates that bradykinin and other vasodilator pathways make a substantial contribution to the renal vasodilator response to ACE inhibition. Conversely, in the rabbit and humans, available evidence suggests that the dominant action, by far, involves a reduction in angiotensin II production with little evidence of activation of these alternative pathways.[28] The biochemical explanation underlying these differences is not yet available.

RENIN-ANGIOTENSIN SYSTEM BLOCKADE AND THE NATURAL HISTORY OF RENAL INJURY

Opinion will vary as to the first observation that pointed to a specific renal action of ACE inhibitors, especially their potential for preserving renal function. One can argue that this was first recognized in 1979, in a description of maintenance of renal function with BP control during captopril treatment of two patients with unequivocal scleroderma renal crisis.[24] Because this process is characterized by a rapidly progressive downhill course, with no exceptions in the literature, it was clear that something special had happened. The outcome did raise debate on whether it was BP control, which was improved with ACE inhibition, that led to improvement of the renal course or whether ACE inhibition offered other renal protective qualities.

In 1985, studies in animal models and in patients with proteinuria led to the first discussion of the possibility that ACE inhibition might be renal protective and to discussions of a possible ambitious therapeutic trial in patients with type 1 diabetes mellitus. The decision to focus on the patient with type 1 diabetes mellitus had nothing to do with the special role of ACE inhibitor therapy in diabetes, but rather recognized that these patients represent a very attractive target for establishing a principle. The disease course is relatively predictable based on renal function and level of proteinuria; the patient population is relatively homogeneous and young, so that the natural history of nephropathy is less likely to be complicated by cardiovascular events. Thus, one could isolate a specific renal influence and thereby establish a principle. In part because the study was planned as a collaboration between a corporate sponsor and the National Institutes of Health, several years were required before the study was launched, and the data did not become available until late 1993.[27] During that time, a large literature had accrued both in animal models and in humans, reported as a meta-analysis of 100 clinical studies performed during that time. With the 1993 publication, policy changed; for the first time, a regulatory agency approved a drug for a specific renal protective indication. Since that time, studies on ACE inhibition have been extended to studies in patients with type 2 diabetes mellitus and nondiabetic renal disease.[26]

What of the ARBs? Until recently, their potential utility in preventing the progression of renal disease was a construct. The outcome predicted depended on whether one thought that non-ACE angiotensin II generation (in which case, the ARBs would be better) or the non-angiotensin-dependent actions of ACE inhibition (in which case, the ACE inhibitors would be better) was quantitatively important. In 2001, three studies appeared in a single issue of the New England Journal of Medicine.[27,29–32] In patients with type 2 diabetes mellitus and nephropathy, both irbesartan and losartan reduced the frequency of progression to a renal endpoint—doubling serum creatinine, need for dialysis, or death—by approximately 20%. The study in which irbesartan was employed included three limbs: irbesartan in one limb, placebo addon in the second limb, and amlodipine addon in the third limb. Amlodipine proved to be essentially identical to placebo. Perhaps the most exciting finding was in the third study, in which two doses of irbesartan were employed in patients with type 2 diabetes mellitus and microalbuminuria to assess the frequency with which the patients would move on to frank proteinuria.[31] The results were extraordinarily striking. The 150-mg irbesartan dose reduced the frequency of progression from about 15% to about 10%. An increase in the irbesartan dose to 300 mg reduced the frequency of progression further, to about 5%. Overall, at the highest dose, the protective effect was a 70% reduction, much the largest reduction in risk induced by blockade of the renin-angiotensin system in any clinical condition. The important message seems to be that it is better, indeed far better, to treat early.

RENIN SYSTEM BLOCKADE AND NEPHROPATHY: WHY DO THE NEWSPAPERS SAY THERE IS A CONTROVERSY?

Recently, the special role of the renin-angiotensin system in determining the progression of renal disease was called into question. The first challenge came from the Antihypertensive and Lipid-Lowering Treatment to Prevent Heart Attack Trial (ALLHAT),[33] and the second came from a recent meta-analysis on this subject.[34] The third challenge arose from an epidemiological study in Canada. In the last study, they claimed not only that ACE inhibitors were not protective, but moreover that they may have contributed to the development of end-stage renal disease (ESRD).[35] Here we discuss each in turn.[36]

ALLHAT was not designed specifically to address the issue of kidney disease, but with the massive number of patients enrolled, in fact it is the largest study on diabetes yet reported. Had nephrologists designed such a study, surely they would have insisted on better renal evaluation, measurement of proteinuria, and more regular follow-up. However, it must be accepted that the likelihood that the investigators missed ESRD is small. ALLHAT found that patients who were treated with the ACE inhibitor lisinopril did not show the anticipated protection from renal injury. Patients who were treated with a diuretic did as well as lisinopril-treated patients. The authors of a report emphasized their failure to confirm the value of renin system blockade: The premise, not stated, was that the earlier studies were "wrong" and that ALLHAT—presumably by virtue of the fact that it was big—provided the correct answer.

But, did it? One of the fundamentals of therapeutics is dose.[37] Each of the major clinical trials that led to approval used a very substantial dose of the ACE inhibitor or the ARB. Indeed, in one of these important studies, the experimental design involved identifying the relationship between dose and response. Whereas 150 mg/day of irbesartan was effective, it was substantially less effective than 300 mg/day of irbesartan.[31]

In ALLHAT, they initiated lisinopril treatment with a daily dose of 10 mg. Few would choose to use 10 mg of lisinopril in the average patient. Experts do not hesitate to titrate upward. Conversely, the physicians involved in ALLHAT were often reluctant to update drug dose. Information on which drug dose the patient received was not given in the original article but has appeared recently in response to a letter to the editor.[38,39] More than 50% of the patients randomly assigned to lisinopril either were taking no ACE inhibitor or had remained at the lowest dosage level in year 1, year 3, and year 5. Only a little more than one third received the top dose. From this study, we can conclude firmly only that an inadequate dose of ACE inhibitor is not better than other antihypertensive agents. Surely, if we did not already know that, we at least so suspected.

The second source of confusion and one that received substantial attention in the lay press is a recent meta-analysis[34] that concluded that there was little or no advantage to renin-system blockade in preventing nephropathy. In view of the fact that the meta-analysis involved more than 73,000 patients who were culled from 127 studies, they were confident that their conclusion was correct. Thus, the predecessors must have been wrong.

The large studies that led to regulatory approval shared a number of features. All were big enough to have the necessary power. In each the dose of drug was adequate to the task. Finally, in each, follow-up was sufficiently long that an endpoint could be achieved. A useful meta-analysis would have required that all three criteria be met. Regretfully, this meta-analysis did not. Adding small, poor studies to large, excellent studies does not improve the information yield. The problems of many of the studies were that the drug doses were too low and follow-up was too short.

The third challenge to a contribution of the renin system to ESRD came from an epidemiologic study in Canada. The authors, using a database that provides information on clinically relevant events, concluded not only that ACE inhibition did not protect patients from ESRD, but that in fact ACE inhibition promoted ESRD.[35] The authors treated the groups as though the individual patients were randomly assigned to drug therapy. Nowhere in their article does it indicate the possibility that patients who were at greater risk for ESRD received captopril and other ACE inhibitors preferentially because of that risk. Proteinuria is an important driving force in clinical decision making, and proteinuria was not listed in their database. By the early to the mid-1980s, there was already substantial interest in the possibility that ACE inhibition might improve the natural history of renal disease.[40]

For all of these reasons, the use of the term *controversial* is inappropriate.

USE OF THESE AGENTS IN THE PATIENT WITH RENAL FAILURE

ACE inhibitors are used in the patient who has lost renal excretory function for two reasons: to control hypertension and to retard the progression of renal injury. There is much less clinical experience with the ARBs, but the goal of their use is the same, and preliminary data indicate that their efficacy is probably similar to that of ACE inhibitors. ACE inhibitors are effective antihypertensive agents in most patients with renal insufficiency, but their use is complicated by their tendency to increase azotemia in certain patients. This is especially likely to occur in the patient who has been treated aggressively with restriction of salt intake or diuretic therapy, and their use may be difficult to manage in the patient who is already very azotemic. Too often physicians are tempted to discontinue ACE inhibitor therapy because of an abrupt rise in serum creatinine during initiation of treatment.[11] Whenever possible, generally when the patient is free of symptoms of azotemia, it is worthwhile to maintain ACE inhibitor therapy. In the Collaborative Study Group Trial of captopril in patients with type 1 diabetes mellitus, the patients who were already azotemic at baseline showed the greatest benefit from captopril treatment,[25] and most showed increased azotemia during initial therapy.

In such patients, it is important to be aware of the possibility of drug accumulation during treatment because of renal excretion.[12] Although not entirely predictable, in general, dosage modification is not required with the use of fosinopril, trandolapril, or quinipril. With the use of perindopril, benazepril, enalapril, lisinopril, and ramipril, a 50% to 75% reduction in dose is recommended. In the case of captopril, the dose should be reduced by 50% to 75% and administered only once daily.

In general, the principles for the use of ARBs are the same, although only candesartan is more than 50% excreted by the kidney, and there is little information to suggest that dose adjustment is crucial in the patient with renal failure for any of these agents.[5]

Another consideration in the use of drugs that block the renin-angiotensin system in the patient with renal failure involves potential hyperkalemia.[11,12] The patient at greatest risk has diabetes mellitus, mild to moderate azotemia, and evidence of hyporeninemic hypoaldosteronism, such as a high baseline serum potassium concentration. In addition, often evidence of metabolic acidosis that is more severe than expected for the degree of renal failure is present. Such patients should be treated cautiously and seen within 48 hours of beginning ACE inhibitor therapy for repeat serum potassium and creatinine measurement because they can develop a life-threatening rise in serum potassium. The use of cyclooxygenase inhibitors in such patients can precipitate hyporeninemic hypoaldosteronism; patients should be cautioned about their use.

For reasons that are not entirely clear, the ARBs appear to cause less hyperkalemia than do ACE inhibitors.[1,5,41] Because a close correlation was found between the uricosuric effect and kaliuretic effect when losartan was used, it was initially believed that the potassium effect of losartan reflected a tubular action rather than angiotensin receptor blockade. This explanation has been called into question by the recent observation that valsartan, which has no tubular action, also appears to spare potassium.[29] In the patient in whom hyperkalemia is an important threat, the uses of one of these two ARBs in place of an ACE inhibitor should be considered.

Goal BP for such patients is the subject of substantial debate, remains controversial, and is addressed in greater detail elsewhere. Most advisory groups now recommend a goal of less than 130/80 mm Hg in patients at risk of progression to ESRD, and it will not be surprising to find groups recommending systolic BPs of 120 mm Hg or lower—if only we can find a way to get down to those BP levels.

ALDOSTERONE ANTAGONISTS

The first aldosterone antagonist, spironolactone, was introduced in 1959, well before ACE inhibitors were developed. The agent, a 17-spirolactone steroid, was an unanticipated byproduct of progesterone chemistry and pharmacology. It was quickly shown to be a specific competitive antagonist of aldosterone at the receptor level and was developed as a potassium-sparing diuretic. Because of a substantial frequency of side effects, it was of limited therapeutic interest until about 10 years ago when interest in a specific interruption of aldosterone production or action began to grow, arising from three major sources. The first involves a series of studies in the heart and kidney that indicated that aldosterone leads to substantial fibrosis and tissue injury via a mechanism that could be interrupted by an aldosterone antagonist.[42-44] Indeed, in some studies, a substantial portion of the tissue sparing provided by ACE inhibition involved reduction in plasma aldosterone concentration.

The second line of investigation leading to renewed interest in blockade of aldosterone effects was the RALES Trial in patients with advanced heart failure. In this study, the addition of spironolactone in very low doses—averaging 25 mg a day—reduced cardiovascular event rate by a striking 30%.[45] Because the doses were very low, the agent was well tolerated, but the doses are probably too low to have a major influence on BP or electrolyte homeostasis. Thus, another mechanism must be sought.

The third reason for a renewal of interest in aldosterone antagonists as a therapeutic area involved the development of a new aldosterone antagonist, eplerenone, which is much better tolerated than spironolactone. Eplerenone doses producing a substantial influence on BP and electrolyte homeostasis, comparable to the top of the spironolactone dose-response (believed to be about 150 mg daily) had little or no effect on libido, gynecomastia, or breast pain and tenderness.

Epstein and colleagues recently reported compelling results in a study with eplerenone in patients with type 2 diabetes mellitus.[46] The 268 patients enrolled were randomized into three equal-sized groups, each of which was maintained on enalapril, 20 mg/day. In one third a placebo was added for 12 weeks; in a second group eplerenone was added at 50 mg/day; in a third group eplerenone was added at 100 mg/day. By week 12, proteinuria was reduced by 7.4% in the placebo group, by 41% in the eplerenone 50 mg group, and by 48.4% in the eplerenone 100 mg group. The frequency of hyperkalemia was not different in any of the three treatment groups. These striking results suggest that we should be more involved in blocking aldosterone in such patients. DelVecchio and co-workers[47] recently reviewed eight small studies in patients with proteinuria treated with an aldosterone antagonist. Results in all studies are in striking accord of those of Epstein and colleagues.

MECHANISMS AND PHARMACOLOGY OF ALDOSTERONE ANTAGONISTS

Although until recently most attention had focused on the distal tubules in the nephron, in fact aldosterone receptors are found in many tissues. Spironolactone acts as a competitive inhibitor of aldosterone binding to its receptor. Spironolactone is extensively metabolized in humans, and at least some of the metabolites—

especially canrenone—have anti-aldosterone activities, but the dominant effect appears to be due to the parent compound.

In part because it was developed in the 1950s, the pharmacokinetics of spironolactone have not been well worked out. Concomitant food intake enhances bioavailability by increasing the absorption of spironolactone and decreasing the first-pass effect.[48,49] A gradual onset of diuretic action is seen, requiring 3 days to reach its maximum, and the diuretic response persists for 2 or 3 days.[49] It is unlikely that the tissue-sparing effect involves sodium or potassium handling, and little is known about the kinetics of that action.

The most troubling adverse effect of spironolactone has been gynecomastia. This adverse effect is dose sensitive. In a systematic comparison of spironolactone doses of 100, 200, and 400 mg/day, the 200- and 400-mg/day doses were associated with a striking increase of gynecomastia and no greater antihypertensive effect than that associated with 100 mg/day.[50,51] In general, spironolactone has much more often been used in combination with a thiazide diuretic, as much for the potassium-sparing effect as for the primary diuretic action.

The adverse effect of greatest concern is hyperkalemia. The risk of hyperkalemia was found to be greatly increased in patients with renal insufficiency and in those in whom there was simultaneous exposure to potassium supplements.[49,50] In one large survey, 8.6% of patients taking spironolactone developed hyperkalemia. The frequency was only 2.8% in those with a normal blood urea nitrogen in that study and rose to 42.1% in those in whom blood urea nitrogen exceeded 50 mg/dL.[38]

At least in part because of the interaction between azotemia and hyperkalemia, few studies have been performed in patients with renal failure. Glomerular filtration rate has been shown to be stable over 3 months of spironolactone therapy.[52]

Substantially less has been published on eplerenone, which is not yet marketed for hypertension. Presumably many of the issues addressed in this review will become available in the medical literature before long.

OPTIMIZATION OF RENIN SYSTEM BLOCKADE

It is now about three decades since the introduction of renin-system blockade with the advent of the ACE inhibitor captopril. The first two decades or so involved large studies designed to ascertain when blocking the renin system provided benefit. The past several years have seen a shift in emphasis to address the issue of optimization of renin system blockade. The addition of aldosterone antagonists to an ACE inhibitor or ARB represents one approach to doing so. The use of combinations of ACE inhibitors and ARBs represents a second approach. Although there have been dozens of reports on such combinations in the patient with proteinuria, the literature is not very useful, because the issue of dose has not been addressed directly.[53]

As an alternative, very high-dose ARBs have received recent attention.[54] These studies take advantage of the fact that angiotensin receptor blockers are so well tolerated that very high doses can be employed. In fact, there is a very clear benefit to using very high doses of ARBs in the patient with proteinuria. The drugs employed have included irbesartan (to 900 mg), valsartan (to 640 mg), and candesartan (to 96 mg).

Renin inhibition clearly will join these three other approaches to optimization of treatment. We have a lot of work to do. The next 10 years should prove to be very interesting.

Acknowledgments

I am grateful to Ms. Diana Capone for her assistance in the preparation and submission of this chapter.

References

1. Burnier M, Brunner HR: Angiotensin II receptor antagonists. Lancet 2000;355:637–645.
2. Epstein M, Williams G, Weinberger M, et al, for the Heart Outcome Prevention Evaluation (HOPE) Study Investigators: Effects of an angiotensin-converting enzyme inhibitor, ramipril, on death from cardiovascular causes, myocardial infarction and stroke in high risk patients. New Engl J Med 2000;342:145–153.
3. Hollenberg NK, Fisher NDL, Price DA: Pathways for angiotensin II generation in intact human tissue. Evidence from comparative pharmacological interruption of the renin system. Hypertension 1998;32:387–392.
4. Nickerson M, Hollenberg NK: Blockade of alpha-adrenergic receptors. In Root W (ed): Physiological Pharmacology. New York: Academic Press, 1967, pp 243–305.
5. Ruddy MC, Kostis JB: Angiotensin II receptor antagonist. In Oparil S, Weber MA (eds): Hypertension: A Companion to Brenner and Rector's The Kidney. Philadelphia: WB Saunders, 1999, pp 621–637.
6. Perich RB, Jackson B, Rogerson FM, et al: Two binding sites on angiotensin converting enzyme: Evidence from radioligand binding studies. Molecular Pharmacol 1992;42:286–293.
7. Wei L, Alhenc-Gelas F, Corvol P, Clauser E: The two homologous domains of human angiotensin I-converting enzyme are both catalytically active. J Biol Chem 1991;266:9002–9008.
8. Ehlers MRW, Riordan JF: Angiotensin-converting enzyme: Zinc and inhibitor binding stoichiometries of the somatic and testis isozymes. Biochemistry 1991;30:7118–7126.
9. Wei L, Clauser E, Alhenc-Gelas F, Corvol P: The two homologous domains of human angiotensin I-converting enzyme interact differently with competitive inhibitors. J Biol Chem 1992;267:13398–13405.
10. Perich RB, Jackson B, Attwood MR, et al: Angiotensin-converting enzyme inhibitors act at two different binding sites on angiotensin-converting enzyme. Pharma Pharmacol Let 1991;1:41–43.
11. Sica DA, Todd W, Gehr B: Angiotensin-converting enzyme inhibitors. In Oparil S, Weber M (eds): Hypertension: A Companion to Brenner and Rector's The Kidney. Philadelphia, WB Saunders, 1999, pp 599–609.
12. Wilcox CS: Management of hypertension in patients with renal disease. In Smith TW (ed): Cardiovascular Therapeutics: A Companion to Braunwald's Heart Disease. Philadelphia: WB Saunders, 1996, pp 538–545.
13. Furakawa Y, Kishimoto S, Nishikawa K: Hypotensive imidazole derivatives and hypotensive imidazole 5-acetic acid derivatives. Patents issued to Takeda Chemical Industries, Ltd., on 20 July 1982, and 19 October 1992, respectively. U.S. Patents 4,340,598 and 4,355,040, Osaka, Japan, 1982 and 1992.
14. Wexler RR, Greenlee WJ, Irvin JD, et al: Nonpeptide angiotensin II receptor antagonists: The next generation in antihypertensive therapy. J Med Chem 1996;39:626–656.
15. Wong PC, Price WA, Chiu AT, et al: Nonpeptide angiotensin antagonists. IX: Pharmacology of EXP-3174: an active metabolite of DuP 753, an orally active antihypertensive agent. J Pharmacol Exp Ther 1990;255:211–217.
16. Keenan RM, Weinstock J, Finkelstein JA, et al: Potent nonpeptide angiotensin II receptor antagonists. 1-(carboxybenzyl)imidazole-5-acrylic acids. J Med Chem 1993;36:1880–1892.
17. Edwards RM, Aiyar N, Ohlstein EH, et al: Pharmacological characterization of the nonpeptide angiotensin II receptor antagonist, SK&F 108566. J Pharmacol Exp Ther 1992;260:175–181.
18. Vauquelin G, Fierens F, Vanderheyden P: Distinction between surmountable and insurmountable angiotensin II AT$_1$ receptor antagonists. In Epstein M, Brunner HR (eds): Angiotensin II Receptor Antagonists. Philadelphia: Hanley & Belfus, 2001, pp 105–118.
19. Navar LG, Harrison-Bernard LM, Imig JD, Mitchell KD: Renal actions of angiotensin II and AT$_1$ receptor blockers. In Epstein M, Brunner HR (eds): Angiotensin II Receptor Antagonists. Philadelphia: Hanley & Belfus, 2001, pp 189–214.
20. Hollenberg NK: Arthur C. Corcoran Lecture. Implications of species difference for clinical investigation: Studies on the renin-angiotensin system. Hypertension 2000;35:150–154.
21. Azizi M, Webb R, Nussberger J, Hollenberg NK: Renin inhibition with aliskiren: Where are we now, and where are we going? J Hypertension 2006;24:243–256.
22. Staessen JA, Yan L, Richart T: Oral renin inhibitors. Lancet 2006;368:1449–1456.
23. Tice CM: Renin inhibitors. Ann Rep Med Chem 2006;41:155–167.
24. Nguyen G, Burckle CA, Sraer J-D: Renin/prorenin-receptor biochemistry and functional significance. Curr Htn Reports 2004;6:129–132.
25. Danser AH, Batenburg WW, van Esch JHM: Prorenin and the (pro)renin receptor—an update. Nephrol Dial Transplant 2007;22:1288–1292.
26. Fisher NDL, Hollenberg NK: Unprecedented renal responses to direct blockade of the renin-angiotensin system with Aliskiren, a novel renin inhibitor. Circulation 2008, in press.
27. Lewis EJ, Hunsicker LG, Bain RP, Rohde RD for the Collaborative Study Group: The effect of angiotensin-converting enzyme inhibition on diabetic nephropathy. N Engl J Med 1993;329:1456–1462.
28. Lansang MC, Hollenberg NK: ACE inhibition and the kidney: Species variation in the mechanisms responsible for the renal hemodynamic response. JRAAS 2000;1:119–124.
29. Giatras I, Lau J, Levey AS for the Angiotensin-Converting Enzyme Inhibition and Progressive Renal Disease Study Group: Effect of angiotensin-converting enzyme inhibitors on the progression of nondiabetic renal disease: A meta analysis of randomized trials. Ann Intern Med 1997;127:337–345.
30. Lewis EJ, Hunsicker LG, Clarke WR, et al, for the Collaborative Study Group: Renoprotective effect of the angiotensin-receptor antagonist irbesartan in patients with nephropathy due to type 2 diabetes. N Engl J Med 2001;345:851–860.
31. Parving H-H, Lehnert H, Brochner-Mortensen J, et al, for the Irbesartan in Patients with Type 2 Diabetes and Microalbuminuria Study Group: The effect of irbesartan on the development of diabetic nephropathy in patients with type 2 diabetes. N Engl J Med 2001;345:870–878.
32. Brenner BM, Cooper ME, DeZeeuw D, et al, for the RENAAL Study Investigators: Effects of losartan on renal and cardiovascular outcomes in patients with type 2 diabetes and nephropathy. N Engl J Med 2001;345:861–869.
33. The Antihypertensive and Lipid-Lowering Treatment to Prevent Heart Attack Trial (ALLHAT): Major outcomes in high risk hypertensive patients randomized to Angiotensin-converting enzyme inhibitor or calcium channel blocker vs diuretic. JAMA 2002;288:2981–2997.
34. Casas JP, Chua W, Loukageorgakis S, et al: Effect of inhibitors of the renin-angiotensin system and other antihypertensive drugs on renal outcomes. Systematic review and meta-analysis. Lancet 2005;366:2026–2033.

35. Suissa S, Hutchinson T, Brophy JM, Kezouh A: ACE inhibitor use and the long-term risk of renal failure in diabetes. Kidney Int 2006;69:913–919.
36. Hollenberg NK, Epstein M: Renin angiotensin system blockade and nephropathy: Why is it being called into question, and should it be? Clin J Am Soc Nephrol 2006;1:1046–1048.
37. Hollenberg NK: Is there a pharmacologic basis for combination renin axis blockade? Kidney Int 2005;68:2901–2903.
38. Hollenberg NK: Omission of drug dose information [Letter]. Arch Intern Med 2006;166:368.
39. Rahman M, Pressel SL, Davis BR: Reply to letter to the editor: Omission of drug dose information. Arch Intern Med 2006;166: 368–369.
40. Hollenberg NK, Raij L: Angiotensin-converting enzyme inhibition and renal protection. An assessment of implications for therapy. Arch Intern Med 1993;153:2426–2435.
41. Bakris GL, Siomos M, Richardson D, et al: ACE inhibition or angiotensin receptor blockade: Impact on potassium in renal failure. Kidney Int 2000;58:2084–2092.
42. Brilla CG, Weber KT: Mineralocorticoid excess, dietary sodium and myocardial fibrosis. J Lab Clin Med 1992;120:893–901.
43. Greene EL, Kren S, Hostetter TH: Role of aldosterone in the remnant kidney model in the rat. J Clin Invest 1996;98:1063–1068.
44. Rocha R, Stier CT, Kifor I, et al: Aldosterone: A mediator of myocardial necrosis and renal arteriopathy. Endocrinology 2000;141:3871–3878.
45. Pitt B, Zannad F, Remme WJ, et al: The effect of spironolactone on morbidity and mortality in patients with severe heart failure. Randomized aldactone evaluation study investigators [See Comments]. N Engl J Med 1999;341:709–717.
46. Epstein M, Williams G, Weinberger M, et al: Selective aldosterone blockade with eplerenone reduces albuminuria in patients with type 2 diabetes. CJASN 2006;1:940–951.
47. Del Vecchio L, Procaccio M, Vigano S, Cusi D: Mechanisms of disease: The role of aldosterone in kidney damage and clinical benefits of its blockade. Nature Clin Pract Nephrol 2007;3:42–49.
48. Overdiek JWPM, Merkus FWHM: Influence of food on the bioavailability of spironolactone. Clin Pharmacol Ther 1986;40:531.
49. Shackelton CR, Wong NLM, Sutton RAL: Distal (potassium-sparing) diuretics. In Dirks JH, Sutton RAL (eds): Diuretics, Physiology, Pharmacology and Clinical Use. Philadelphia: WB Saunders, 1986, pp 117–134.
50. Schrijver G, Weinberger MH: Hydrochlorothiazide and spironolactone in hypertension. Clin Pharmacol Ther 1979;25:33–49.
51. Greenblatt DJ, Koch-Weser J: Adverse reactions to spironolactone: A report from the Boston Collaborative Drug Surveillance Program. JAMA 1973;225:40–43.
52. Roos JC, Dorhout Mees EJ, Koomans HA, Boer P: Intrarenal sodium handling during chronic spironolactone treatment. Nephron 1984;38:226–232.
53. Fernandez-Juarez G, Barrio V, de Vinuesa SG, et al: Dual blockade of the renin-angiotensin system in the progression of renal disease: The need for more clinical trials. J Am Soc Nephrol Suppl 2006;17:250–254.
54. Hollenberg NK, Parving H-H, Viberti G, et al: Albuminuria responses to high-dose valsartan in type 2 diabetes mellitus. J Hypertension 2007;25:1921–1926.

Further Reading

Azizi M, Webb R, Nussberger J, Hollenberg NK: Renin inhibition with aliskiren: Where are we now, and where are we going? J Hypertension 2006;24:243–256.

Beckerman B: Selective aldosterone blockade with eplerenone reduces albuminuria in patients with type 2 diabetes. CJASN 2006;1:940–951.

Burnier M, Brunner HR: Angiotensin II receptor antagonists. Lancet 2000;355:637–645.

Danser AH, Batenburg WW, van Esch JHM: Prorenin and the (pro)renin receptor—an update. Nephrol Dial Transplant 2007; 22:1288–1292.

Epstein M, Williams G, Weinberger M, et al, for The Heart Outcome Prevention Evaluation (HOPE) Study Investigators: Effects of an angiotensin-converting enzyme inhibitor, ramipril, on death from cardiovascular causes, myocardial infarction and stroke in high risk patients. New Engl J Med 2000;342:145–153.

Hollenberg NK, Epstein M: Renin Angiotensin system blockade and nephropathy: Why is it being called into question, and should it be? Clin J Am Soc Nephrol 2006;1:1046–1048.

Hollenberg NK, Fisher NDL, Price DA: Pathways for angiotensin II generation in intact human tissue. Evidence from comparative pharmacological interruption of the renin system. Hypertension 1998;32:387–392.

Navar LG, Harrison-Bernard LM, Imig JD, Mitchell KD: Renal actions of angiotensin II and AT_1 receptor blockers. In M Epstein and HR Brunner (eds): Angiotensin II Receptor Antagonists. Philadelphia: Hanley & Belfus, 2001, pp 189–214.

Chapter 53

Calcium Channel Blockers

Douglas G. Shemin and Lance D. Dworkin

Calcium channel blockers (CCBs) were developed in the 1960s, introduced for clinical practice in the 1980s, and are widely used for the treatment of hypertension, angina, and cardiac arrhythmias. They are structurally heterogeneous but share the universal property of blocking the transmembrane flow of calcium ions through voltage-derived channels (L-type channels) in vascular and nonvascular smooth muscle.[1] Blockade of these channels results in smooth muscle relaxation, decreased peripheral vascular resistance, dilation of coronary arteries, and a decrease in myocardial contractility.

CLINICAL PHARMACOLOGY

Calcium channel blockers can be divided into two classes based on differences in structure and function: dihydropyridines and nondihydropyridines. Dihydropyridines block L-type channels relatively selectively in peripheral vascular tissue and act primarily by dilating resistance vessels. Nondihydropyridines block L-type channels in both vascular and cardiac tissue and therefore affect cardiac function and the atrioventricular (AV) node in addition to causing vasodilation. They decrease heart rate and prevent reflex tachycardia. Only nondihydropyridine agents decrease glomerular protein and albumin sieving and decrease renal protein excretion.[1]

Most CCBs currently in use are dihydropyridines. In the United States, commercially available dihydropyridines include amlodipine, felodipine, isradipine, nicardipine, nifedipine, nimodipine, nisoldipine, and nitrendipine. The two nondihydropyridines are verapamil, a phenylalkylamine, and diltiazem, a benzothiapine (Table 53-1). Barnidipine, lacidipine, lercanidipine, and manidipine, all dihydropyridines, are not commercially available in the United States. Nimodopine, a dihydropyridine, is approved for use as a cerbral vasodilator but not for hypertension.

The newer agents and formulations of most CCBs have a relatively long half-life and time to peak effect, either because the intrisinc half-life is long, as in the case of amlodipine, or because drug delivery has been manipulated. Immediate-release, relatively short-acting preparations of diltiazem, verapimil, nifedipine, and nicardipine are also available. Diltiazem, nicardipine, and verapamil are available in intravenous formulations. Because of the potential risks of short-acting agents, only the long-acting preparations are recommended for use in hypertension, although the short-acting nondihydropyridine agents can be used to decrease AV nodal conduction in arrhythmias or atrial tachycardia.

Calcium channel blockers are primarily metabolized in the liver. Dose adjustment generally is not required even in end-stage renal disease (ESRD),[2] although there have been reports of toxicity with long-acting verapamil in patients with ESRD.[3,4]

Clinical studies of CCBs in hypertensive patients have examined their use in four settings: controlling hypertension, reducing cardiovascular morbidity and mortality, preventing progression of kidney disease, and treating hypertension associated with ESRD.

EFFICACY IN TREATMENT FOR ESSENTIAL HYPERTENSION

In short-term studies single-agent therapy with CCBs yields results at lowering of blood pressure (BP) similar to those seen with other antihypertensive agents. In the VA cooperative study, hypertensive patients were randomized to placebo or one of six agents as monotherapy. Those randomized to diltiazem had the highest rate of success compared to those given hydrochlorothiazide, atenolol, captopril, clonidine, or

Table 53-1 Calcium Channel Blockers: Recommended Doses for Hypertension

	U.S. Trade Name	Half-life (hr) (Normal/ESRD)	Dosage	Comment
Amlodipine	Norvasc	35–50/50	Initial: 2.5 mg/day Maintenance: 2.5–10 mg/day	Dihydropyridine Combinations with benazepril and atorvtastatin available Dosage adjustment for liver disease
Barnidipine		24/24		Dihydropyridine Not in use in the U.S.
Diltiazem	Dilacor, Cardizem, Cartia, Tiazac	2–8/2–8	Initial: 120–180 mg/day Maintenance: 120–360 mg/day	Benzothiazepine Greater potential than dihydropyridines to cause AV nodal dysfunction and impaired LV function Dosage adjustment for liver disease Comes in long-acting (CD, XR, LA) formulations for once-daily dosing
Felodipine	Plendil	10–14/21	5–10 mg/day	Dihydropyridine; combination with enalapril available
Isradipine	Dynacirc	2–5/10–12	Initial: 5 mg/day Maintenance: 5–10 mg/day	Dihydropyridine Comes in long-acting (CR) formulation
Lacidipine		12/12		Dihydropyridine Not in use in the U.S.
Lercanidipine		8–10/8–10		Dihydropyridine. Not in use in the U.S.
Manidipine		4–6/4–6		Dihydropyridine Not in use in the U.S.
Nicardipine	Cardene	5/5–8	Initial: 60 mg/day Maintenance: 60–120 mg/day IV: 1–15 mg/hr	Dihydropyridine Comes in long-acting (SR) preparations Can be given parenterally as continuous infusion in malignant hypertension
Nifedipine	Adalat, Procardia	4–6/6–8	Initial: 30–60 mg SR/day Maintenance: 30–90 mg SR/day	Dihydropyridine Comes in long-acting (CC, XL) preparations
Nimodopine	Nimotop	1–3/20–24	60 mg q4h for 21 days	Dihydropyridine Not approved for hypertension Used to treat neurological deficits due to cerebral artery spasm in patients with subarachnoid hemorrhage
Nisoldipine	Sular	6–8/7–10	Initial: 20 mg/day Maintenance: 10–40 mg/day	Dihydropyridine Dosage adjustment for liver disease
Nitrendipine		4–6/4–6	Initial: 10 mg/day Maintenance: 10–40 mg/day	Dihydropyridine
Verapamil	Calan, Covera, Isoptin, Verelan	3–7/3–7	180–480 mg/day	Phenylalkylamine Greater potential than dihydropyridines to cause AV nodal dysfunction or LV dysfunction Comes in long-acting (SR, HS, PM) preparations Combination with trandolapril available

AV, atrioventricular; LV, ventricular.

prazosin.[5] In the Treatment Of Mild Hypertension Study (TOMHS), amlodipine was as effective as chlorthalidone, acebutolol, doxazosin, or enalapril in hypertensive men and women.[6] In the German HANE study, nitrendipine was equivalent in BP lowering to hydrochlorothiazide, atenolol, or enalapril.[7]

PREVENTION OF CARDIOVASCULAR MORBIDITY AND MORTALITY

Table 53-2 lists the major prospective, randomized clinical trials in which cardiovascular outcomes were compared in hypertensive patients randomly assigned to receive a CCB or to another antihypertensive agent. In general, CCBs are as, or marginally less, effective than other agents, particularly when they are prescribed as sole agents. In the FACET study (Fosinopril versus Amlodipine Cardiovascular Events Randomized Trial), hypertensive diabetics were randomly assigned to receive fosinopril or amlodipine; the rate of cardiovascular morbid and mortal events was greater in the amlodipine group.[8] In the Verapamil in Hypertension and Atherosclerosis Study (VHAS), there was no difference in outcome between patients randomly assigned to receive verapamil or a diuretic.[9] In the STOP-2 trial, elderly patients with hypertension were randomly assigned to a calcium channel blocker (isradipine or felodipine), an angiotensin-converting enzyme (ACE) inhibitor, or conventional therapy with diuretics and β-blockers. CCBs were equivalent to ACE inhibitors and conventional therapies in preventing most cardiovascular morbidity, but were inferior to ACE

inhibitors in preventing congestive heart failure or myocardial infarction (MI).[10] In the Intervention as a Goal in Hypertension Treatment (INSIGHT) trial, in patients randomly assigned to long-acting nifedipine, a trend was seen toward a lower risk of stroke compared to those receiving a diuretic, but the risk of fatal MI, congestive heart failure, or any cardiovascular mortality was significantly increased.[11] In the Appropriate Blood Pressure Control in Diabetes (ABCD) trial, subjects with diabetes and hypertension were randomly assigned to receive nisoldipine or enalapril. The study was stopped prematurely because of an increase in the risk of nonfatal MI in the nisoldipine group.[12] However, there was no significant difference in overall mortality, and the original assessment of relative risk was lowered when additional patient safety data became available.[13] In the Multicenter Isradipine Diuretic Atherosclerosis Study (MIDAS), patients were randomly assigned to isradipine or hydrochlorothiazide.[14] Some adverse cardiovascular effects, such as the development of angina, occurred more commonly in the isradipine group. In the huge Antihypertensive and Lipid Lowering treatment to prevent Heart Attack Trial (ALLHAT), patients were randomly assigned to amlodipine, a diuretic, or an ACE inhibitor. The primary endpoints of fatal coronary disease or nonfatal MI did not differ in the amlodipine-treated group, but patients receiving amlodipine were significantly more likely to have heart failure than the diuretic-treated group.[15] In the Controlled ONset Verapamil INvestigation of Cardiovascular Endpoints (CONVINCE) trial, patients were randomly assigned to extended-release verapamil or a β-blocker/hydrochlorothiazide combination; most cardiovascular endpoints were equivalent in the two

Table 53-2   Summary of Studies of Calcium Channel Blockers in Prevention of Cardiovascular Disease in Hypertensive Patients

Study and Reference	Patients (N)	Drugs Studied	CV Morbidity*	CV Mortality*	Stroke*
FACET[8]	380	Amlodipine vs. ACE inhibitor		2.04 (1.05–3.84)	2.56 (0.81–8.33)
VHAS[9]	498	Verapamil vs. diuretic	Lower event rate		
STOP-2[10]	6614	Isradipine/felodipine vs. diuretic/β-blocker vs. ACE inhibitor	0.99 (0.87–1.12)	0.97 (0.80–1.17)	0.88 (0.73–1.06)
INSIGHT[11]	6321	Nifedipine vs. diuretic	1.11 (0.90–1.36)	3.22 (1.18–8.80)	0.87 (0.61–1.26)
ABCD[12]	470	Nisoldipine vs. ACE inhibitor	3.3 (1.5–7.1)	NS	
MIDAS[14]	883	Isradipine vs. diuretic	1.78 (0.94–3.38)		2.00 (0.50–7.93)
ALLHAT[15]	33,357	Amlodipine vs. diuretic	0.98 (0.90–1.07)		
CONVINCE[16]	8241	Verapamil vs. β-blocker vs. diuretic		1.08 (0.93–1.26)	1.15 (0.90–1.48)
VALUE[17]	15,245	Amlodipine vs. ARB		1.04 (0.90–1.16)	0.98 (0.72–1.19)
IDNT[19]	1715	Amlodipine vs. ARB	1.11 (0.91–1.35)	0.74 (0.48–1.12)	0.64 (0.35–1.19)
CAMELOT[20]	1991	Amlodipine vs. ACE inhibitor	0.81 (0.63–1.04)	1.07 (0.31–3.70)	0.76 (0.26–2.20)
SYST-EUR[22]	4695	Nitrendipine vs. placebo	0.69 (0.55–0.86)	0.73 (0.52–1.02)	0.58 (0.40–0.83)
NORDIL[23]	10,881	Diltiazem vs. β- blocker	1.04 (0.91–1.18)	1.11 (0.87–1.43)	0.80 (0.65–0.99)
INVEST[25]	22,576	Verapamil vs. β- blocker	1.03 (0.93–1.14)	0.98 (0.90–1.07)	0.89 (0.70–1.12)
ASCOT[26]	19,257	Amlodipine vs. β- blocker		0.89 (0.81–0.99)	0.77 (0.66–0.99)

*Data presented are for relative risk of those randomized to calcium channel blockade (95% confidence intervals).
ACE, angiotensin-converting enzyme; ARB, angiotensin receptor blocker; CV, cardiovascular.

groups, but there was a higher risk of hemorrhage in the verapamil group.[16] In the NICS-EH (National Intervention Cooperative Study in Elderly Hypertensives; nicardipine vs. diuretic), the CAMELOT (Comparison of AMlodipine vs Enalapril to Limit Occurrences of Thrombosis; amlodipine vs. enalapril), the VALUE (Valsartan Antihypertensive Long-term Use Evaluation trial; amlodipine vs. valsartan), and the IDNT (Irbesartan Diabetic Nephropathy Trial; irbesartan vs. amlodipine), cardiovascular events were similar in CCB-treated groups and comparison groups.[17–20] In a recent meta-analysis of more than 150,000 patients in 29 trials,[21] comparing therapies based on different categories of antihypertensive drugs, CCB-based therapy was superior to placebo in preventing stroke and coronary heart disease and inferior to diuretic/β-blocker therapy and ACE inhibitor therapy in preventing heart failure.

On the other hand, a number of clinical trials have shown improved cardiovascular outcomes in patients randomly assigned to CCBs, especially in prevention of cerebrovascular disease. In the SYST-EUR study, elderly patients with hypertension were randomly assigned to nitrendipine or placebo; ACE inhibitors and diuretics were added to both groups to decrease the systolic BP equivalently. The risk of cardiovascular events and stroke was lower in the nitrendipine group.[22] In the Nordic Diltiazem (NORDIL) study, patients were randomly assigned to diltiazem or to a β-blocker and diuretic; there was a lower risk of stroke in the diltiazem group.[23] A large meta-analysis of more than 100,000 patients in 13 trials demonstrated a 10% lower risk of stroke in patients randomly assigned to CCBs; this benefit was greatest with dihydropyridines.[24]

A number of studies support the use of CCBs in prevention of cardiovascular disease when these agents are used in combination with other antihypertensive agents to achieve low BP targets. In the International Verapamil-Trandolapril Study (INVEST), patients were randomly assigned to verapamil or a β-blocker; an ACE inhibitor and diuretic were added to both groups to achieve JNC-VI blood pressure targets; the verapamil- and β-blocker-treated groups had similar outcomes.[25] In the Anglo-Scandinavian Cardiac Outcomes Trial (ASCOT), patients were randomized to amlodipine with the subsequent addition of an ACE inhibitor, or to a β-blocker with the subsequent addition of a diuretic. Patients randomly assigned to the amlodipine/ACE inhibitor arm had lower rates of cardiovascular morbidity and all-cause mortality.[26] Finally, in the Hypertension Optimal Treatment (HOT) trial, patients with hypertension were randomized to three different diastolic BP goals, from less than 80 mm Hg to 90 mm Hg. Felodipine was given to every patient; other agents were added to reach the specific BP target. Patients whose diastolic BP fell below 85 mm Hg benefited from the use of a CCB; this effect was greater in diabetics.[27]

The rate of cardiovascular effects in the HOT trial was lower than reported in previous studies; along with the other studies discussed here, this suggests that CCBs do improve cardiovascular outcomes, but this effect is greatest when low BP targets are achieved and CCBs are used in conjunction with other agents, especially ACE inhibitors. The question of which combination of antihypertensive therapy is optimal will hopefully be addressed by the Avoiding Cardiovascular events through COMBination Therapy

in Patients Living with Systolic Hypertension (ACCOMPLISH) trial,[28] which randomizes 11,000 hypertensive patients to an ACE inhibitor/diuretic (benazepril/hydrochlorothiazide) versus ACE inhibitor/calcium channel blocker (benazepril/amlodipine) combination. Study results should be available by 2009.

PREVENTION OF PROGRESSION OF CHRONIC KIDNEY DISEASE

Calcium channel blockers modulate the progression of chronic kidney disease (CKD) by a number of mechanisms, including alterations in renal hemodynamics and renal growth, and by direct effects on the production and/or responses to cytokines, growth factors, and vasoconstrictor substances by glomerular or tubular cells. CCBs tend to have a protective effect on renal progression in experimental models, but the results are inconsistent. Explanations for these divergent findings are not always apparent; findings have been attributed to differences in the animal model, the drug or dose administered, variability in systemic or intraglomerular pressure, and other factors. A detailed discussion of these data is beyond the scope of this chapter; the reader is referred to some recent comprehensive reviews.[29–32]

The effects of CCBs on progression of renal disease in humans has been examined in several randomized, prospective clinical trials. A discussion of these trials follows, divided into three categories: (1) studies examining the development of renal disease in hypertensive patients with normal renal function, (2) studies in patients with CKD in which CCBs were compared to drugs that block the renin-angiotensin-aldosterone system, and (3) studies in patients with CKD in which CCBs were added to drugs that block the renin-angiotensin-aldosterone system.

Studies Examining the Effect of Calcium Channel Blockers on the Development of Kidney Disease

The ALLHAT study excluded patients with a serum creatinine level above 2.0 mg/dL. There was no difference in the incidence of either a 50% decrease in the glomerular filtration rate (GFR) or the development of ESRD in patients who were randomly assigned to chlorthalidone, amlodipine, or lisinopril.[33]

The BEergamo NEphrologic Diabetic Complications Trial (BENEDICT)[34] randomly assigned hypertensive diabetics with normal kidney function and normoalbuminuira to the ACE inhibitor trandolapril, long-acting verapamil, a combination of the two, or placebo, with additional agents given to reduce BP to less than 130/80 mm Hg. The group receiving ACE inhibitors had a significantly lower risk of microalbuminuria, even when the BP was not controlled to the target range.

A meta-analysis of 16 trials of the effect of various antihypertensive agents on the development of diabetic nephropathy, defined as the development of microalbuminuria, in diabetic patients with normoalbuminura, showed that there was a 42% lower risk of development of microalbuminuria in patients given ACE inhibitors rather than CCBs in clinical trials. The effect of CCBs compared to β-blockers or other antihypertensive agents on the development of renal disease was not examined.[35]

Studies Comparing Calcium Channel Blockers to Blockers of the Renin-Angiotensin-Aldosterone System on Progression of Kidney Disease

Most comparison studies evaluating the progression of renal disease have compared CCBs to ACE inhibitors. Zucchelli and colleagues studied 121 patients with hypertension and CKD[36]; patients were observed for 1 year on standard therapy and then randomly assigned to captopril or long-acting nifedipine. The mean BP dropped by more than 20 mm Hg in both groups; mean protein excretion did not significantly decline, and the rate of renal functional decline was slowed significantly, but was similar in both groups. The study concluded that ACE inhibitors and CCBs have similar renal protective effects when hypertension is aggressively treated.

Velussi and colleagues[37] studied 44 patients with hypertension and type 2 diabetes mellitus; they had microalbuminuria or no proteinuria and all had normal renal function. They were randomly assigned to the ACE inhibitor cilazopril or to amlodipine. Blood pressure was lowered aggressively. The GFR stabilized after an initial decline, and protein excretion declined comparably in both groups. In another relatively small study, Bakris and colleagues[38] compared treatment with diltiazem or verapamil to the ACE inhibitor lisinopril or the β-blocker atenolol in 52 patients with type 2 diabetes mellitus and diabetic nephropathy. The decline of the creatinine clearance was modest and similar in patients receiving lisinopril or one of the CCBs, and proteinuria was reduced similarly by all three agents.

The dihydropyridine CCB nisoldipine was compared to the ACE inhibitor enalapril, examining its effects on the rate of change in creatinine clearance in 470 hypertensive diabetic subjects, in the ABCD trial.[12] The study was stopped prematurely because of an increase in nonfatal MI in the nisoldipine group. The renal endpoint data were subsequently analyzed, and there was little difference between the two groups. The enalapril-treated patients had an initial decline in proteinuria, but there was no difference in proteinuria, or in progression of proteinuria, between the groups by the end of the study; changes in renal function were equivalent.

The Modification of Diet in Renal Disease (MDRD) study examined the effect of a low BP target on progression of nondiabetic CKD.[39] Post hoc subset analysis suggested that African Americans with hypertensive nephropathy specifically benefited from a low BP target, but the number of subjects was insufficient. The African American Study of Kidney Disease and Hypertension (AASK) was launched to address this question.[40] Participants were 1094 African Americans with hypertension and presumed nephrosclerosis, with GFR between 20 and 63 mL/min/1.73 m^2. Subjects were randomized to a usual (102–107 mm Hg) or low (92 mm Hg) mean BP goal and to one of three antihypertensive agents as preferred therapy: the β-blocker metoprolol, the ACE inhibitor ramipril, or amlodipine. Additional agents were used to attain the target BP. The primary endpoint of the study was the rate of change in GFR. The amlodipine intervention was discontinued prematurely because of an apparent increase in the rate of decline of the GFR in proteinuric patients randomized to this group. A final analysis failed to confirm a significant difference in the rate of decline in GFR. However, significantly more subjects assigned to the amlodipine group had a reduction in GFR of at least 50%, developed ESRD, or died during the study compared to the subjects assigned to ramipril, and the risk of development of new-onset glucose intolerance was more common in subjects assigned to amlodipine.[40] There were no significant differences in the rate of decline in GFR between those randomly assigned to the ACE inhibitor or the β-blocker, or between those randomized to the normal or low BP goal.

In the Irbesartan Diabetic Nephropathy Trial (IDNT), Lewis and colleagues examined the BP-independent capacity of the angotensin receptor blocker irbesartan and amlodipine to slow progression of kidney disease in patients with type 2 diabetes mellitus and nephropathy.[19] Subjects were randomly assigned to receive irbesartan, amlodipine, or placebo, and BP was treated aggressively in all groups to an average value of 142/77 mm Hg. The risk of reaching the primary endpoint (doubling of serum creatinine, development of ESRD, or death) was reduced by 23% in patients receiving irbesartan compared to those receiving amlodipine or placebo. Primary outcomes were not significantly different in patients receiving amlodipine and placebo (the "placebo arm" were receiving diuretics, β-blockers, and other agents and had similar BPs as the other groups). The risk of doubling of serum creatinine was 37% lower in the irbesartan group, whose urine protein excretion was also substantially lower.

Studies in Which Calcium Channel Blockers Were Combined with Blockers of the Renin-Angiotensin-Aldosterone System to Prevent Progression of Kidney Disease

Bakris and colleagues[41] randomly assigned 37 patients with hypertension and diabetic nephropathy to receive the ACE inhibitor trandolapril, the CCB verapamil, or both drugs in combination. Blood pressure was reduced in all three groups to less than 140/90 mm Hg; virtually all patients needed the addition of a diuretic to achieve this goal. Protein excretion was reduced somewhat in the verapamil group and to a greater extent in the trandolapril group, but to the greatest extent (a drop of 62%) in the group receiving combination therapy.

The Ramipril Efficacy in Nephropathy (REIN) Study[42] randomized patients with nondiabetic CKD (GFR 20–70 mL/min, >1 g proteinuria/24 hr) to either the ACE inhibitor ramipril or to placebo. Antihypertensive agents, including CCBs, were given to lower the diastolic BP to less than 90 mm Hg. Patients randomly assigned to ramipril had significant decreases in proteinuria and in the rate of decrease of GFR. In a subsequent report Ruggenenti and colleagues described a subset of 117 patients in the study given CCBs.[43] Subjects in the placebo group (not receiving an ACE inhibitor) who received a CCB had an increase in protein excretion and a more rapid decline in the GFR. However, if the BP was well controlled or if the patients received an ACE inhibitor, proteinuria declined and renal progression was slowed.

A similar outcome was observed in patients with type 2 diabetes mellitus in the Reduction of Endpoints in NIDDM (RENAAL) trial,[44] which enrolled 1500 patients with type 2 diabetes and nephropathy and randomly assigned them to receive the angiotensin receptor blocker losartan or placebo; BP was treated to a goal BP of 140/90 mm Hg or less; subjects received other antihypertensive agents to achieve this goal. Losartan administration reduced the number of patients who doubled their serum creatinine level or reached ESRD, compared to the patients who received placebo. More than 85% of patients in both arms received CCBs, and more than 60%

received dihydropyridine CCBs. This study showed that simultaneous therapy with CCBs does not detract from the beneficial effects of losartan.

Table 53-3 summarizes clinical trials examining the effects of CCBs on the progression of CKD.

Table 53-3 Summary of Long-term Randomized Clinical Trials Examining the Effects of Calcium Channel Blockers on Progression of Chronic Kidney Disease

Ref.	Renal Disease	Patients (N)	Duration	Drugs	Effect on Proteinuria	Effect on GFR Decline
ABCD[12]	Hypertensive NIDDM	470	5 yr	Nisoldipine vs. enalapril	No change	Stable in patients with microalbuminuria Annual rate of decline 5–6 mL/min in patients with overt albuminuria
ALLHAT[15]	Hypertensives with serum creatinine < 2.0 mg/dL	33,357	6 yr	Amlodipine vs. chlorthalidone vs. lisinopril	Not measured	No differences between groups in decline of GFR
IDNT[19]	NIDDM with nephropathy	1715	2.6 yr	Amlodipine vs. irbesartan vs. placebo	Declined by 6%, similar to placebo, inferior to losartan	Decline similar to placebo, inferior to irbesartan
BENEDICT[34]	Hypertensives with normal GFR	1204	3.6 yr	Verapamil vs. trandolapril vs. combination	Lower rate of microalbuminuria in trandolapril groups	Not measured
Zucchelli et al[36]	Nondiabetic	121	3 yr	Nifedipine vs. captopril	Declined if MAP < 100 mm Hg	50% reduction in rate of decline compared to baseline
Velussi et al[37]	NIDDM	44	3 yr	Amlodipine vs. cilazapril	Declined	Annual rate of decline 2 mL/min
Bakris et al[38]	Hypertensive NIDDM	52	63 mo	Diltiazem or verapamil vs. lisinopril vs. atenolol	Decreased	Annual rate of decline 1.44 mL/min on CCBs
AASK[40]	African-Americans with hypertensive nephrosclerosis	653	3 yr	Amlodipine vs. ramipril	Increased	Annual rate of decline 3.22 mL/min for all Faster with baseline proteinuria or GFR < 40 mL/min
Bakris[41]	NIDDM with nephropathy	37	1 yr	Verapamil vs. trandolapril vs combination	Declined by 27% on verapamil alone, 62% on combination therapy	GFR unchanged
REIN[43]	Nondiabetic nephropathies	117	18 mo	Various dihydropyridines ± ramipril	Increased by 20%, but not in patients on ACE inhibitor and good BP control	30% faster than non-CCBs, but not in patients on ACE inhibitors with good BP control
RENAAL[44]	NIDDM with nephropathy	1513	3.4 yr	Various CCBs ± losartan	No adverse impact on beneficial response to ARB	No adverse impact on beneficial response to ARB

ACE, angiotensin-converting enzyme; ARB, angiotensin receptor blockers; BP, blood pressure; CCBs, calcium channel blockers; GFR, glomerular filtration rate; MAP, mean arterial pressure; NIDDM, non–insulin-dependent diabetes mellitus.

USE IN END-STAGE RENAL DISEASE AND RENAL TRANSPLANTATION

Hypertension is prevalent in ESRD requiring dialysis. More than 70% of these patients receive antihypertensive therapy.[45] See Chapter 60 for a detailed discussion of therapy of dialysis-associated hypertension. CCBs are commonly used in this population because of the lack of efficacy of diuretics as urine output declines, as well as the toxicity of angiotensin-aldosterone blockers as renal function declines and hyperkalemia becomes problematic. The United States Renal Data System (USRDS) Dialysis Morbidity and Mortality Study (DMMS) Wave 2 reported that CCBs were by far the most commonly prescribed class of antihypertensive agent in a cohort of almost 3000 hemodialysis patients.[46] Of these, 54% were prescribed a dihydropyridine agent and 18% a nondihydropyridine agent; CCBs were used more than twice as often as ACE inhibitors, which were the next most commonly used drug class.[46] In a survey from 2003, CCBs were used in 61% of patients; they were still the most common class of antihypertensive agent used.[47]

Very little data is available on cardiovascular outcomes in patients prescribed one or another class of antihypertensive agent, and such data that exists is observational or retrospective. In the USRDS DMMS study, the use of both dihydropyridine and nondihydropyridine CCBs was associated with a lower risk of all-cause mortality and cardiovascular mortality.[21] This conflicts with the findings of an earlier study,[48] which observed that hemodialysis patients prescribed β-blockers had a mortality advantage over those prescribed CCBs. In contradiction, Kestenbaum and colleagues[49] reported that the prescription of a CCB in a prospective cohort study of 4000 hemodialysis patients was associated with decreased overall and cardiovascular mortality, even when adjusted for other comorbidities. In this study, 25% of patients used ACE inhibitors and none used angiotensin receptor blockers. Kestenbaum's observations were confirmed in a smaller prospective observational study of 188 hemodialysis patients; patients taking CCBs had a significantly lower mortality rate after adjustment for age and smoking status.[50] In the Dialysis Outcomes and Practice Patterns Study (DOPPS), in 2500 U.S. patients with arteriovenous grafts and fistulae for dialysis access, the use of CCBs for hypertension was associated with an improved arteriovenous graft patency rate.[47]

The dose of dihydropyridine CCBs does not need to be changed in patients with chronic kidney failure or those treated with dialysis. Although the recommended dose of nondihydropyridine agents is also unchanged in chronic kidney failure,[2] there have been case reports[3,4] of dangerous junctional bradycardias in patients with ESRD treated with long-acting verapamil.

Hypertension complicating renal transplant is discussed in Chapter 59. Many centers avoid renin-angiotensin-aldosterone blockers out of concern that they may exacerbate azotemia with concomitant calcineurin inhibitor therapy and may delay a diagnosis of rejection if azotemia is attributed to their use. Consequently, CCBs are widely prescribed. In a series of more than 600 hypertensive renal transplant recipients, CCBs were prescribed to more than 40% of subjects.[51]

In the 1990s, when cyclosporine-based immunosuppression was used extensively, CCBs, especially dihydropyridines, were recommended as the agents of choice in renal transplant patients because of their ability to reverse cyclosporine-induced vasoconstriction.[52] Calcium channel blockers also were reputed to be mildly immunosuppressive, because of the relationship between intracellular calcium levels and T cell activation. In a study over a 2-year period of 154 renal transplant recipients receiving cyclosporine who were randomly assigned to receive nifedipine or the ACE inhibitor lisinopril, patients treated with nifedipine had BPs equal to those treated with lisinopril, but a lower serum creatinine level. It is possible that the worse renal function in the lisinopril group was due to renal hemodynamic effects.[53] A meta-analysis of 21 studies showed no clear evidence that CCBs had independent effects on preventing renal transplant rejection.[54] However, a report of an observational cohort of more than 600 hypertensive renal transplant recipients concluded that patients prescribed a CCB for hypertension had a reduced renal graft survival and a higher mortality.[51] In a recent study of 60 renal transplant patients prospectively randomized to amlodipine or the angiotensin receptor blocker losartan,[55] BP control and renal function were equivalent at 1 year after transplant. This study reported that amlodipine use was often associated with edema.

The controversy over whether renin-angiotensin-aldosterone blockers or CCBs are optimal for transplant hypertension may have been resolved by a study of 200 French renal transplant recipients randomly assigned to amlodipine, the ACE inhibitor enalapril, or a combination of enalapril and amlodipine.[56] There was a higher degree of BP control in the combination group. The creatinine clearance was lowest in the enalapril group and was unchanged in the combination group, suggesting that amlodipine mitigated adverse renal hemodynamic changes due to the ACE inhibitor. This study suggests that combination therapy with a CCB may be ideal for this population.

Dihydropyridine CCBs have no significant drug interactions with immunosuppressive agents used in renal transplantation. Verapamil and diltiazem decrease the clearance of cyclosporine and, to a lesser extent, tacrolimus and may contibute to high plasma levels of cyclosporine and tacrolimus unless the dose is decreased.[2]

SAFETY

Short-acting CCBs were anecdotally linked to a number of serious acute cardiovascular morbid events beginning in the 1980s. This was especially true for nifedipine administered sublingually for severe hypertension, perhaps because of reflex activation of the adrenergic system induced by sudden changes in BP. The use of short-acting CCBs for the treatment of hypertension is not recommended and has largely been abandoned.[30] In addition, a series of observational studies has described an increased risk of cardiovascular morbidity associated with the use of CCBs; for example, the Nurses Health Study of more than 14,000 women reported that those taking a CCB had an increased risk of death or MI.[57] A meta-analysis of 16 observational trials noted a dose-dependent link between nifedipine and cardiovascular mortality. Most of these studies included a large group of heterogeneous patients, and the choice of antihypertensive agent was not controlled. Differences in patient characteristics may explain the different outcomes. For example, in the Nurses Health Study, CCBs were more likely to be used in women with underlying heart disease. In addition, a number of studies did not differentiate between long-acting and the more risky short-acting CCBs.

A few population-based studies in the 1990s reported a higher risk of cancer and gastrointestinal bleeding in patients taking CCBs.[58,59] However, this observation was subsequently refuted by other observational studies, and a subcommittee of the World Health Organization and the International Society of Hypertension that formally reviewed the issue found no relationship between the use of CCBs and the risk of cancer or bleeding.[60]

Calcium channel blockers generally are not associated with drug-drug interactions, aside from the obvious ones—for example, hypotension when combined with another antihypertensive agent or AV nodal dysfunction when diltiazem or verapamil are combined with a β-blocker or digoxin. An important exception is with the nondihydropyridine agents verapamil and diltiazem, which inhibit hepatic oxidation of statins, cyclosporine, carbamazepine, and quinidine, thereby increasing their blood levels.[2]

Most adverse effects associated with CCBs are relatively minor. They include dose-dependent dizziness, hypotension, and tachycardia with dihydropyridines and bradycardia and AV nodal dysfunction with nondihydropyridines. The most common side effect is peripheral edema, which is attributed to greater arteriolar than venular dilation that increases intracapillary pressure.[61] More common with dihydropyridines, this effect is dose dependent,[61] and is reduced if the treatment is combined with an ACE inhibitor.[62] Symptoms of gastrointestinal reflux and constipation[2] are more common with CCB use.

CONCLUSIONS

Calcium channel blockers are effective and generally well tolerated antihypertensive agents. Their long duration of action and favorable adverse effect profile are benefits, and they are very widely prescribed. In observational studies, 30% to 40% of patients with hypertension are prescribed a CCB,[63] and the prevalence of their use is increasing.[64]

When used as monotherapy, CCBs seem to be equal or superior to agents of other classes in decreasing BP. Although data is not completely consistent, when used as monotherapy, they are no better, and may be worse, than alternative agents, especially β-blockers, ACE inhibitors, and diuretics, in decreasing cardiovascular morbidity and mortality, with the possible exception of the beneficial effect of dihydropyridine agents on decreasing the risk of stroke. However, they do effectively decrease cardiovascular morbidity when used in combination with other agents, such as ACE inhibitors, while aggressive BP goals are targeted.

Calcium channel blockers as monotherapy probably do not increase the risk of developing renal disease in nondiabetic hypertensive subjects, but may be inferior to agents blocking the renin-angiotensin-aldosterone system, especially ACE inhibitors, in preventing the development of renal disease in diabetics. When used as initial therapy or as monotherapy, dihydropyridine CCBs seem to be inferior to ACE inhibitors and angiotensin receptor blockers in preventing progression of kidney disease, especially in diabetics. Most studies have been done with dihydropyridine CCBs. Data is scantier with nondihydropyridine CCBs, and it is possible that nondihydropyridine agents may be as protective as

renin-angiotensin-aldosterone blockers. When used in combination with ACE inhibitors or angiotensin receptor blockers, CCBs do not detract from the renal protective actions of these agents and might have an additive beneficial effect on decreasing the rate of progression of kidney disease if they further lower the BP.

Calcium channel blockers are widely used in patients with ESRD. There is evidence that they may be associated with a survival benefit, but most of this data comes from studies with low rates of use of ACE inhibitors or angiotensin receptor blockers. CCBs are effective in renal transplant recipients as antihypertensive agents, especially with the concomitant use of cyclosporine. They do not seem to have an independent effect on renal transplant function.

In summary, CCBs for patients with uncomplicated hypertension may be used as initial therapy or monotherapy, or added therapy to achieve a BP target of less than 140/90 mm Hg. They should not be used as initial therapy or monotherapy in patients at increased risk for cardiovascular disease, in those with renal disease or diabetes, or in those who are at risk for renal disease progression. They can be selected as second-, third-, or fourth-line agents to achieve a BP target of less than 130/80 mm Hg. Their widespread use continues because it is difficult to achieve a low BP target without them.

References

1. Abernethy DR, Schwart JB: Calcium antagonist drugs. N Engl J Med 1999;341:1447–1457.
2. Sica DA, Prisant LM: Pharmacologic and therapeutic considerations in hypertension therapy with calcium channel blockers: Focus on verapamil. J Clin Hypertens 2007;9(S2):1–22.
3. Pritza DR, Bierman MH, Hammeke MD: Acute toxic effects of sustained release verapamil in chronic renal failure. Arch Intern Med 1991;151:2081–2084.
4. Vazquez C, Huelmos A, Alegria E, et al: Verapamil deleterious effects in chronic kidney failure. Nephron 1996;72:461–464.
5. Materson BJ, Reda DJ, Cushman WC: Single drug therapy for hypertension in men. N Engl J Med 1993;328:914–921.
6. Neaton JD, Grimm RH, Prineas RJ: Treatment Of Mild Hypertension Study: Final results. JAMA 1993;270:713–724.
7. Philipp T, Anlauf M, Distler A, et al: Randomized, double blind, multicenter controlled comparison of hydrochlorthiazide, atenolol, nitrendipine, and enalapril in antihypertensive treatment: The results of the HANE study. BMJ 1997;315:154–159.
8. Tatti P, Pahor M, Byington RP: Outcome results of the Fosinopril versus Amlodipine Cardiovascular Events randomized Trial (FACET) in patients with hypertension and NIDDM. Diabetes Care 1998;21:597–603.
9. Zanchetti A, Rosei EA, Dal Palu C, et al: The Verapamil in Hypertension and Atherosclerosis Study (VHAS): Results of long term randomized treatment with either verapamil or chlorthalidone on carotid intima-media thickness. J Hypertens 1998;16:1667–1676.
10. Hansson L, Lindholm LH, Ekblom T, et al: Randomized trial of old and new antihypertensive drugs in elderly patients: Cardiovascular disease and morbidity. The Swedish Trial in Old Patients with Hypertension 2 study. Lancet 1999;354:1751–1756.
11. Brown MJ, Palmer CR, Castaigne A, et al: Morbidity and mortality in patients randomized to double blind treatment with a long acting calcium channel blocker or diuretic in the International Nifedipine GITS Study: Intervention as a Goal in Hypertension Treatment (INSIGHT). Lancet 2000;356:366–372.

12. Estacio RO, Jeffers BW, Hiatt WR, et al: The effect of nisoldipine as compared to enalapril on cardiovascular outcomes in patients with non-insulin dependent diabetes and hypertension. N Engl J Med 1998;338:645–652.

13. Schrier RW, Estacio RO: Additional follow-up from the ABCD trial in patients with type 2 diabetes and hypertension. N Engl J Med 2000;343:1969.

14. Borhani NO, Mercuri M, Borhani PA, et al: Final outcome results of the Multicenter Isradipine Diuretic Atherosclerosis Study (MIDAS): A randomized placebo controlled trial. JAMA 1996;276:785–791.

15. ALLHAT Officers and Coordinators for the ALLHAT Collaborative Research Group: Major outcomes in high-risk hypertensive patients randomized to angiotensin-converting enzyme inhibitor or calcium channel blocker vs diuretic: The Antihypertensive and Lipid Lowering treatment to prevent Heart Attack Trial (ALLHAT). JAMA 2002;288:2981–2997.

16. Black HR, Elliott WJ, Grandis G, et al: Principal results of the Controlled ONset Verapamil INVestigation of Cardiovascular End points (CONVINCE) Trial. JAMA 2003;289:207–2082.

17. Julius S, Kjedsen SE, Weber M, et al: Outcomes in hypertensive patients at high cardiovascular risk treated with regimens based on valsartan or amlodipine: The VALUE randomised trial. Lancet 2004;363:2022–2031.

18. Kuwajima I, Kuramoto K, Ogihara T, et al: Tolerability and safety of a calcium channel blocker in comparison with a diuretic in the treatment of elderly patients with hypertension: Secondary analysis of the NICS-EH. Hypertension Res 2001;24:475–480.

19. Lewis EJ, Hunsicker LG, Clarke WR, et al: Renoprotecive effect of the angiotensin-receptor antagonist irbesartan in patients with nephropathy due to type 2 diabetes. N Engl J Med 2001;345:851–860.

20. Nissen SE, Tuzcu EM, Libby P, et al: Effect of antihypertensive agents on cardiovascular events in patients with coronary disease and normal blood pressure. JAMA 2004;292:2217–2226.

21. Blood Pressure Lowering Treatment Trialists' Collaboration: Effects of different blood pressure lowering regimens on major cardiovascular events in individuals with and without diabetes mellitus. Arch Intern Med 2005;165:1410–1419.

22. Staessen JA, Fagard R, Thijs L, et al: Randomized double blind comparison of placebo and active treatment for elderly patients with isolated systolic hypertension. Lancet 1997;350:757–764.

23. Hansson L, Hedner T, Lund-Johansen P, et al: Randomised trial of the effects of calcium antagonists compared with diuretics and beta blockers on cardiovascular morbidity and mortality in hypertension: The Nordic Diltiazem (NORDIL) Study. Lancet 2000;356:359–365.

24. Angeli F, Verdecchia P, Reboldi GP: Calcium channel blockade to prevent stroke in hypertension. Am J Hypertens 2004;17:817–822.

25. Pepine CJ, Handberg EM, Cooper-deHoff RM, et al: A calcium antagonist vs a non-calcium antagonist hypertension treatment strategy for patients with coronary artery disease: The International Verapamil-Trandolapril Study (INVEST): A randomized clinical trial. JAMA 2003;290:2805–2816.

26. Dahlof B, Sever PS, Poulter NR, et al: Prevention of cardiovascular events with an antihypertensive regimen of amlodipine adding perindopril as required versus atenolol adding bendroflumethiazide as required, in the Anglo-Scandinavian Cardiac Outcomes Trial—Blood Pressure Lowering arm (ASCOT-BPLA): A multicenter randomised conrolled trial. Lancet 2005;366:895–906.

27. Hansson L, Zanchetti A, Carruthers SG, et al: Effects of intensive blood pressure lowering and low dose aspirin in patients with hypertension: Principal results of the Hypertension Optimal Treatment (HOT) randomized trial. Lancet 1998;351:1755–1762.

28. Jamerson KA: The first hypertension trial comparing the effects of two fixed-dose combination therapy regimens on cardiovascular events: Avoiding Cardiovascular events through COMbination therapy in Patients Living with Systolic Hypertension (ACCOMPLISH). J Clin Hypertension 2003;5(S3):29–35.

29. Epstein M: Calcium antagonists and renal disease. Kidney Int 1998;54:1771–1784.

30. Griffin KA, Bidani AK: Calcium channel blockers and the progression of renal disease. Curr Hypertens Rep 1999;1:436–445.

31. Kloke HJ, Branten AJ, Hysmanns FT, et al: Antihypertensive treatment of patients with proteinuric renal diseases: Risks or benefits of calcium channel blockers? Kidney Int 1998;53:1559–1573.

32. Weir M, Dworkin LD: Antihypertensive drugs, dietary salt, and renal protection: How low should you go and with which therapy? Am J Kidney Dis 1998;32:1–22.

33. Rahman M, Pressel S, Davis BR, et al: Renal outcomes in high risk hypertensive patients treated with an angiotensin converting enzyme inhibitor or a calcium channel blocker or a diuretic. Arch Intern Med 2005;165:936–946.

34. Ruggenenti P, Fassi A, Ilieva AP, et al: Preventing microalbuminuria in type 2 diabetes. N Engl J Med 2004;351:1941–1951.

35. Strippoli GF, Craig M, Schena FP, et al: Antihypertensive agents for primary prevention of diabetic nephropathy. J Am Soc Nephrol 2005;16:3081–3091.

36. Zucchelli P, Zuccala A, Borghi M, et al: Long-term comparison between captopril and nifedipine in the progression of renal insufficiency. Kidney Int 1992;42:452–458.

37. Velussi M, Brocco E, Frigato F, et al: Effects of cilazapril and amlodipine on kidney function in hypertensive NIDDM patients. Diabetes 1996;45:216–222.

38. Bakris GL, Copley JB, Vicknair N, et al: Calcium channel blockers versus other antihypertensive therapies on progression of NIDDM associated nephropathy. Kidney Int 1996;50:1641–1650.

39. Klahr S, Levey AS, Beck GJ, et al: The effects of dietary protein restriction and blood pressure control on the progression of kidney disease. N Engl J Med 1994;330:877–884.

40. Wright JT, Bakris G, Greene T, et al: Effect of blood pressure lowering and antihypertensive drug class on progression of hypertensive kidney disease: Results from the AASK trial. JAMA 2002;288:2421–2431.

41. Bakris GL, Weir M, DeQuattro V, et al: Effects of an ACE inhibitor/calcium antagonist combination on proteinuria in diabetic nephropathy. Kidney Int 1998;54:1283–1289.

42. Gisen Group: Randomized placebo-controlled trial of effect of ramipril on decline in glomerular filtration rate and risk of terminal renal failure in proteinuric, nondiabetic nephropathy. Lancet 1997;349:1857–1863.

43. Ruggenenti P, Perna A, Benini R, et al: Effects of dihydropyridine calcium channel blockers, angiotensin-converting enzyme inhibition, and blood pressure control on chronic, nondiabetic nephropathies. J Am Soc Nephrol 1998;9:2096–2101.

44. Brenner BM, Cooper ME, de Zeeuw D, et al: Effects of losartan on renal and cardiovascular outcomes in patients with type 2 diabetes and nephropathy. N Engl J Med 2001;345:861–869.

45. Rocco MV, Yan G, Heyka RJ, et al: Risk factors for hypertension in chronic hemodialysis patients: Baseline data from the HEMO study. Am J Nephrol 2001;21:280–288.

46. Griffith TF, Chua BS, Allen AS, et al: Characteristics of treated hypertension in incident hemodialysis and peritoneal dialysis patients. Am J Kidney Dis 2003;42:1260–1269.

47. Andreucci VE, Fissell RB, Bragg-Greshan JL, et al: Dialysis outcomes and practice patterns study (DOPPS) and medications in hemodialysis patients. Am J Kidney Dis 2004;44 (S2):S61–S67.

48. Foley RN, Herzog CA, Collins AJ: Blood pressure and long-term mortality in United States hemodialysis patients: USRDS Waves 3 and 4. Kidney Int 2002;62:1784–1790.

49. Kestenbaum B, Gillen DL, Sherrard DJ, et al: Calcium channel blocker use and mortality among patients with end stage renal disease. Kidney Int 2002;61:2157–2162.

50. Tepel M, van der Gier M, Park A, et al: Association of calcium channel blockers and mortality in hemodialysis patients. Clin Sci 2002;103:511–515.

51. Tutone VK, Mark PB, Stewart GA, et al: Hypertension, antihypertensive agents, and outcomes following renal transplantation. Clin Transplant 2005;19:181–192.

52. Weir M: Therapeuic benefits of calcium channel blockers in cyclosporine treated organ transplant recipients: Blood pressure control and immunosuppression. Am J Med 1991;90(S5A): 32S–36S.

53. Midtvedt K, Hartmann A, Foss A, et al: Sustained improvement of renal graft function for 2 years in hypertensive renal transplant recipients treated with nifedipine as compared to lisinopril. Transplantation 2001;72:1787–1792.

54. Ladefoged SD, Andersen CB: Calcium channel blockers in kidney transplantation. Clin Transplant 1994;8:128–133.

55. Formica RN, Friedman AL, Lorber MI, et al: A randomized trial comparing losartan with amlodipine as initial therapy for hypertension in the early post-transplant period. Nephr Dial Transplant 2006;12:1389–1394.

56. Halimi JM, Girardeau B, Buchler M, et al: Enalapril-amlodipine combination in cyclosporine-treated renal transplant recipients: A prospective randomized trial. Clin Transplant 2007;21:277–284.

57. Michels K, Rosner B, Manson J: Prospective study of calcium channel blocker use, cardiovascular disease, and total mortality in hypertensive women. Circulation 1998;97:1540–1548.

58. Pahor M, Guralnik JM, Corti M, et al: Calcium channel blockade and incidence of cancer in aged populations. Lancet 1996;348:493–497.

59. Pahor M, Guralnik JM, Furberg C, et al: Risk of gastrointestinal hemorrhage with calcium antagonists in hypertensive patients over 67 years old. Lancet 1996;347:1061–1065.

60. Ad Hoc subcommittee of the World Health Organization/ International Society of Hypertension Liaison Committee: Effects of calcium antagonists on the risks of coronary heart disease, cancer, and bleeding. J Hypertens 1997;15:105–115.

61. Messerli FH, Grossman E: Pedal edema—not all dihydropyridine calcium antagonists are created equal. Am J Hypertens 2002;15:1019–1020.

62. Messerli FH, Oparil S, Feng Z: Comparison of efficacy and side effects of combination therapy of angiotensin-converting enzyme inhibitor (benazepril) with calcium antagonist (either nifedipine or amlodipine) versus high dose calcium antagonist monotherapy for systemic hypertension. J Am Coll Cardiol 2000;86:1182–1187.

63. Lloyd-Jones DM, Evans JC, Levy D: Hypertension in adults across the age spectrum. JAMA 2005;294:466–472.

64. Manolio TA, Cutler JA, Furberg CD, et al: Trends in pharmacologic management of hypertension in the United States. Arch Intern Med 1995;155:829–837.

Further Reading

Angeli F, Verdecchia P, Reboldi GP: Calcium channel blockade to prevent stroke in hypertension. Am J Hypertens 2004;17:817–822

Opie LH: Calcium channel blockers in hypertension: Reappraisal after new trials and major meta-analyses. Am J Hypertens 2001;14:1074–1081.

Segura J, Garcia-Donaire JA, Ruilope LM: Calcium channel blockers and renal protection: insights from the latest clinical trials. J Am Soc Nephrol 2005;16:S64–S66.

Sica DA, Prisant LM: Pharmacologic and therapeutic considerations in hypertension therapy with calcium channel blockers: Focus on verapamil. J Clin Hypertens 2007;9(Suppl 2):1–22.

Staessen JA, Wang JG, Thijs L: Calcium-channel blockade and cardiovascular prognosis: Recent evidence from clinical outcome trials. Am J Hypertens 2002;15:85S–95S.

Chapter 54

Individualization of Pharmacologic Therapy

Norman M. Kaplan

All of the nondrug and drug therapies described in the preceding chapters can reduce the cardiovascular and renal consequences of hypertension.[1] Most, if not all, of this benefit derives from their ability to lower the blood pressure (BP).[2]

Faced with this large number of possible choices, what should the prudent practitioner do? In this age of evidence-based medicine, the number of choices can be reduced by deletion of modalities that have been shown to have no benefit (e.g., acupuncture) or that have not yet been tested for meaningful outcomes (e.g., direct renin inhibitors). Even so, there are many choices and they need to be carefully adapted to each patient. This is *individualized therapy.*

To be sure, all drugs approved for use in the treatment of hypertension will, in moderate doses, lower elevated BP by approximately 10% in about two thirds of patients. This uniformity of response is inherent in the approval process: Each drug must have been shown to lower BP significantly when compared to placebo and to have an efficacy equal to other antihypertensive drugs. Doses are chosen to provide significant but not excessive lowering of BP so that patients will tolerate them and achieve a demonstrable effect.

When comparisons between various antihypertensive drugs are made, they almost always demonstrate similar antihypertensive efficacy.[3] However, individual patients show considerable differences in their response to one drug or another. Some of this variability can be accounted for by patient characteristics, including age and race, which in turn could be mediated by differences in activity of the renin-angiotensin system. In a Veterans Administration cooperative 1-year trial, 1292 men were randomly given one of six drugs from each major class; overall, and in the black patients, the calcium channel blocker (CCB) was most effective, but the angiotensin-converting enzyme (ACE) inhibitor was best in younger whites.[4] Similarly, in a randomized, crossover trial of elderly patients with isolated systolic hypertension given a representative of four major classes (ACE inhibitor, β-blocker, CCB, and diuretic) each for 1 month, diuretics or CCBs were more effective than β-blockers or ACE inhibitors.[5] In a similarly designed trial of younger patients with combined systolic and diastolic hypertension, the ACE inhibitor or β-blocker was more effective than the CCB or diuretic.[6]

A general pattern emerges from these various comparative trials.[7] Younger and white patients, who have higher renin levels, respond better to drugs that work in large part by blocking the renin-angiotensin system. Conversely, older and black patients, who tend to have lower renin levels, respond better to diuretics and CCBs, which work in ways independent of initial renin levels. As portrayed in the algorithm presented by the British Hypertension Society (Fig. 54-1),[8] this separation can be used to decide on the first choice. However, the U.S. Seventh Joint National Committee algorithm recommends a low-dose thiazide diuretic for initial therapy for almost all patients.[9]

In clinical practice, the decision for first drug is less relevant now that two or more drugs are generally used to adequately control BP in most patients to below 140/90 mm Hg.[10,11] This is even more the case for higher-risk patients, including those with diabetes or chronic renal disease who have been found to do better with BP below 130/80 mm Hg.[1]

Fortunately all members of the major classes of drugs except CCBs are marketed with a low-dose thiazide diuretic. Therefore, the choice could easily be the diuretic first, followed by a combination of a diuretic plus a renin-angiotensin inhibitor (i.e., β-blocker, ACE inhibitor, or angiotensin receptor blocker [ARB]).

Combinations of a CCB, in particular the now generic amlodipine, with either an ACE inhibitor or an ARB will become more widely marketed and may logically be used, along with a diuretic, for the third level of therapy.

COMPELLING INDICATIONS

Most hypertensive patients have one or more coexisting conditions for which one class of antihypertensive drugs is either indicated or contraindicated (Table 54-1). Even though overall and cardiovascular mortality is similar with equal degrees of BP reduction by any drug, it is logical to choose an antihypertensive agent that has been shown to also improve a coexisting condition. Examples that have been strongly documented include β-blockers and ACE inhibitors post-myocardial infarction[12] and either ACE inhibitors or ARBs with heavy proteinuria.[13]

AVOIDANCE OF DIABETES

As obesity grows, the need to avoid diabetes increases. Antihypertensives differ in their propensity to provoke diabetes.[14] High doses of diuretic and β-blockers are the worst; ACE

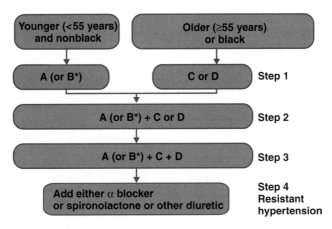

A: ACE inhibitor or angiotensin receptor blocker
B: β blocker
C: Calcium channel blocker
D: Diuretic (thiazide and thiazide-like)

*Combination therapy involving B and D may induce more new
onset diabetes compared with other combination therapies

Figure 54-1 An algorithm for initial and subsequent choices of antihypertensive therapy. (Modified from Williams B, Poulter NR, Brown MJ, et al: British Hypertension Society guidelines for hypertension management, 2004 [BHS-IV]: Summary. BMJ 2004;238:634–640.)

Table 54-1 Guidelines for Selecting Drug Treatment of Hypertension

Class of Drug	Compelling Indications	Possible Indications	Compelling Contraindications	Possible Contraindications
Diuretics	Heart failure Elderly patients Systolic hypertension	Diabetes	Gout	Dyslipidemia
β-Blockers	Angina After myocardial infarction Tachyarrhythmias	Heart failure Pregnancy Diabetes	Asthma and COPD Heart block	Dyslipidemia Athletes and physically active patients Peripheral vascular disease
ACE inhibitors or angiotensin receptor blockers	Heart failure Left ventricular dysfunction After myocardial infarction Diabetic nephropathy		Pregnancy Hyperkalemia Bilateral renal artery stenosis	
Calcium channel blockers	Angina Elderly patients Systolic hypertension	Peripheral vascular disease	Heart block	Congestive heart failure
α-Blockers	Prostatic hypertrophy	Glucose intolerance Dyslipidemia		Orthostatic hypotension

From Guidelines Subcommittee: 1999 World Health Organization—International Society of Hypertension guidelines for the management of hypertension. J Hypertens 1999;17:151.

inhibitors and ARBs are the best. Part of the difference may relate to the length of time that patients have been exposed to the metabolic influences of the various agents. However, there is a measurable influence of the various agents on insulin sensitivity, so these differences are almost certainly real. Therefore, an obese patient with a family history of diabetes and a borderline elevated blood sugar level should be given an ACE inhibitor or an ARB.

If the results of two ongoing trials comparing the ARB telmisartan to an ACE inhibitor confirm the experimental and limited clinical evidence of this drug's significant PPAR gamma agonist activity, telmisartan may become the ARB of choice.[15]

THE FALL OF β-BLOCKERS

A meta-analysis on the degree of *primary* prevention of heart attacks and stroke by the various classes of antihypertensives[16] corroborates a previous warning about the lesser effectiveness of β-blockers.[17] The degree of protection against heart attack was the same with β-blockers as with other drugs, but there was a 16% higher incidence of stroke with β-blockers.

This lesser protection against stroke has been attributed to a lesser fall in central BP with β-blockers despite equal efficacy on peripheral BP. The adverse effects on lipids and insulin sensitivity may also be involved.

β-Blockers are vital for *secondary* protection, but they should not be used in the absence of a compelling indication (see Table 54-1).

THE RISE OF ALDOSTERONE RECEPTOR BLOCKERS

In the British Hypertension Society algorithm (see Fig. 54-1), spironolactone is shown as a fourth choice, to be added to those who are not controlled on three drugs.[8] This later positioning may rapidly change as the efficacy and safety of low doses of spironolactone are increasingly recognized.[18] In the study by Chapman and colleagues,[18] as well as in most other recently published studies, spironolactone has been used primarily in resistant patients. However, there is a good reason to use it much earlier, particularly since a potassium-sparing agent is useful to prevent diuretic-induced potassium wastage, which, in turn, has been closely correlated with worsening of glucose tolerance.[19]

Both currently available aldosterone antagonists, spironolactone and eplerenone, are now generic. This will save the patient money but will prevent effective marketing of the agents by pharmaceutical companies, so physicians may not use them as often as they should. When an aldosterone antagonist is added to an ACE inhibitor or ARB in patients with any degree of renal impairment, close monitoring of serum potassium is needed to identify hyperkalemia.

CONCLUSION

More than 50 years after the advent of effective oral antihypertensive drugs, more choices are available, but they are often not provided in the most effective and least bothersome manner. The principles of individualization reviewed in this chapter should be useful guidelines to do better.

References

1. Kaplan NM: Treatment of hypertension: Drug therapy. In Kaplan NM (ed): Kaplan's Clinical Hypertension, 9th ed. Philadelphia: Lippincott Williams & Wilkins, 2006, pp 217–310.
2. Staessen JA, Wang JG, Thijs L: Cardiovascular prevention and blood pressure reduction: A quantitative overview updated until 1 March 2003. J Hypertens 2003;21:1055–1076.
3. Neaton J, Grimm RH Jr, Prineas RJ, et al: Treatment Of Mild Hypertension Study (TOMHS). JAMA 1993;270:713–724.
4. Materson BJ, Reda DJ, Cushman WC: Department of Veterans Affairs single-drug therapy of hypertension study. Am J Hypertens 1995;8:189–192.
5. Morgan TO, Anderson AI, MacInnis RJ: ACE inhibitors, beta-blockers, calcium blockers, and diuretics for the control of systolic hypertension. Am J Hypertens 2001;14:241–247.
6. Dickerson JE, Hingorani AD, Ashby MJ, et al: Optimization of antihypertensive treatment by crossover rotation of four major classes. Lancet 1999;353:2008–2013.
7. Donnelly R, Elliott HL, Meredith PA: Antihypertensive drugs: Individualized analysis and clinical relevance of kinetic-dynamic relationships. Pharmacol Ther 1992;53:67–79.
8. Williams B, Poulter NR, Brown MJ, et al: British Hypertension Society guidelines for hypertension management 2004 (BHS-IV): Summary. BMJ 2004;328:634–640.
9. Joint National Committee: The seventh report of the Joint National Committee on detection, evaluation, and treatment of high blood pressure. JAMA 2003;289:2560–2572.
10. Major outcomes in high-risk hypertensive patients randomized to angiotension-converting enzyme inhibitor or calcium channel blocker vs diuretic: The Antihypertensive and Lipid-Lowering Treatment to prevent Heart Attack Trial (ALLHAT). JAMA 2002;288:2981–2997.
11. Dahlof B, Sever PS, Poulter NR, et al, for the ASCOT Investigators: Prevention of cardiovascular events with an antihypertensive regimen adding perindopril versus atenolol adding bendroflumethiazide as required, in the Anglo-Scandinavian Cardiac Outcomes Trial–Blood Pressure Lowering Arm (ASCOT–BPLA): A multicenter randomized controlled trial. Lancet 2005;366: 895–906.
12. McDonald MA, Simpson SH, Ezekowitz JA, et al: Angiotensin receptor blockers and risk of myocardial infarction: Systematic review. BMJ 2005;331:873.
13. Brenner BM, Cooper ME, de Zeeuw D, et al: Effects of losartan on renal and cardiovascular outcomes in patients with type 2 diabetes and nephropathy. N Eng J Med 2001;345:861–869.
14. Elliott WJ, Meyer PM: Incident diabetes in clinical trials of antihypertensive drugs: A network meta-analysis. Lancet 2007;369: 201–207.
15. Pravenec M, Kurtz TW: Molecular genetics of experimental hypertension and the metabolic syndrome: From gene pathways to new therapies. Hypertension 2007;49(5):941–952.
16. Lindholm LH, Carlberg B, Samuelsson O: Should beta-blockers remain first choice in the treatment of primary hypertension? A meta-analysis. Lancet 2005;366:1545–1553.
17. Messerli FH, Grossman E, Goldbourt U: Are β-blockers efficacious as first-line therapy for hypertension in the elderly? JAMA 1998;279:1903–1907.
18. Chapman N, Dobson J, Wilson S, et al: Effect of spironolactone on blood pressure in subjects with resistant hypertension. Hypertension 2007;49:839–845.
19. Zillich AJ, Garg J, Basu S, et al: Thiazide diuretics, potassium, and the development of diabetes: A quantitative review. Hypertension 2006;48:219–224.

Further Reading

Dahlof B, Sever PS, Poulter NR, et al, for the ASCOT Investigators: Prevention of cardiovascular events with an antihypertensive regimen adding perindopril versus atenolol adding bendroflumethiazide as required, in the Anglo-Scandinavian Cardiac Outcomes Trial–Blood Pressure Lowering Arm (ASCOT–BPLA): A multicenter randomized controlled trial. Lancet 2005;366:895–906.
Julius S, Nesbitt SD, Egan BM, for the Trial of Preventing Hypertension (TROPHY) Study Investigators: Feasibility of treating prehypertension with an angiotensin-receptor blocker. N Engl J Med 2006;354:1685–1697.

Kaplan NM: Kaplan's Clinical Hypertension, 9 ed. Philadelphia: Lippincott Williams & Wilkins, 2006.

Kripalani S, Yao X, Haynes RB: Interventions to enhance medication adherence in chronic medical conditions: A systematic review. Arch Intern Med. 2007;167:540–550.

Lindholm LH, Carlberg B, Samuelsson O: Beta blockers in primary hypertension: Do age and type of beta-blocker matter? J Hypertens 2006;24:2143–2145.

Mochizuki S, Dahlof B, Shimizu M, et al: Valsartan in a Japanese population with hypertension and other cardiovascular disease (Jikei Heart Study): A randomised, open-label, blinded endpoint morbidity-mortality study. Lancet 2007;369:1431–1439.

Oh BH, Mitchell J, Herron JR, et al: Aliskiren, an oral renin inhibitor, provides dose-dependent efficacy and sustained 24-hour blood pressure control in patients with hypertension. J Am Coll Cardiol 2007;49:1157–1163.

Ong KL, Cheung BM, Man YB: Prevalence, awareness, treatment, and control of hypertension among United States adults 1999–2004. Hypertension 2007;49:69–75.

Staessen JA, Wang JG, Thijs L: Cardiovascular prevention and blood pressure reduction: A quantitative overview updated until 1 March 2003. J Hypertens 2003;21:1055–1076.

Wang YR, Alexander GC, Stafford RS: Outpatient hypertension treatment, treatment intensification, and control in Western Europe and the United States. Arch Intern Med 2007;167:141–147.

Hypertensive Emergencies

Samuel J. Mann

The term *hypertensive emergency* covers many clinical situations, with the degree of urgency determined by either the severity or acuteness of onset of blood pressure (BP) elevation or the presence of a critical underlying medical condition (e.g., acute aortic dissection) when even modest degrees of BP elevation may require immediate treatment.

True hypertensive "emergencies" (Box 55-1) require lowering of BP within minutes. The drug employed should act immediately and be predictably effective. In contrast, more gradual lowering of BP, over 30 minutes to hours, is appropriate in treating medical "urgencies" (Box 55-2). Rapidly acting drugs requiring intra-arterial monitoring are not necessary.

Rapid lowering of BP greatly increases the risk of unwanted adverse effects that can exceed benefits, particularly in the elderly and in patients in whom urgent treatment is not needed. Patients with severe, but asymptomatic, BP elevations usually do not require urgent therapy to lower BP.

NATURAL HISTORY OF UNTREATED SEVERE HYPERTENSION

Accelerated or Malignant Hypertension

The classic hypertensive crisis of accelerated or malignant hypertension is characterized by severe elevation of arterial pressure (usually with diastolic pressure > 140 mm Hg) and vascular damage manifested by retinal hemorrhages and exudates.[1] The term accelerated signifies the absence, and malignant the presence, of papilledema. The pathogenesis, management, and prognosis of accelerated and malignant hypertension are similar.[2]

The syndrome usually occurs as an accelerated phase of preexisting hypertension.[3] Severe and inadequately treated essential hypertension, particularly in smokers,[2] is the most common antecedent. Renovascular and renal parenchymal disorders, as well as primary hyperaldosteronism, are also associated with hypertensive crises.[4]

Why some individuals with hypertension proceed to an accelerated phase is not clear. A vicious cycle has been postulated whereby vascular damage from severe hypertension causes renal ischemia, which stimulates renin secretion and angiotensin-mediated vasoconstriction, which in turn worsens renal ischemia and further activates the renin-angiotensin system.[3] Elevations of plasma renin activity and serum aldosterone concentration are commonly found. Moreover, angiotensin-converting enzyme (ACE) inhibitors usually lower BP.[2]

Hypertensive Encephalopathy

Hypertensive encephalopathy is characterized by a reversible alteration in neurological function during a severe or abrupt BP elevation. Manifestations include headache, altered mental status, visual impairment, nausea, and seizures.[5] Focal neurological signs can occur.[5] Although frequently a complication of

Hypertension associated with acute myocardial ischemia
　or infarct
Hypertensive encephalopathy
Hypertension associated with intracranial hemorrhage
Hypertension associated with stroke
Hypertension associated with pulmonary edema
Adrenergic crisis
Dissecting aortic aneurysm
Eclampsia
Perioperative hypertension
Severe epistaxis

Box 55-2　Hypertensive Urgencies

Hypertension associated with left ventricular failure
Accelerated or malignant hypertension
Hypertension associated with angina
Perioperative hypertension
Preeclampsia
Acute glomerulonephritis
Scleroderma renal crisis

malignant hypertension, hypertensive encephalopathy can result from an acute, albeit less severe, BP elevation from other causes, such as acute glomerulonephritis, preeclampsia, clonidine withdrawal, cocaine, or monoamine oxidase (MAO) inhibitor/tyramine interaction. The risk of encephalopathy or hemorrhage may be present at relatively modest BP elevation in patients without preexisting hypertension who lack protective vascular thickening.

Encephalopathy is ascribed by some to cerebral ischemia as a result of luminal narrowing and spasm[2] and even occlusion[5] and by others to a breakdown (or failure) of autoregulation at high systemic pressures, leading to localized hyperperfusion and edema.[5,6] Cerebral edema is a constant finding.[2] Pathologic findings suggest that both may occur because patients can have cerebral microinfarctions, petechial hemorrhages, and edema.[2]

Magnetic resonance imaging or computed tomography of the brains of patients with hypertensive encephalopathy show white matter edema in the posterior regions of the cerebral hemispheres, brain stem, or cerebellum.[7] This disorder, named *reversible posterior leukoencephalopathy,* can occur without severe BP elevation.[8] It has been associated with preeclampsia, hemolytic uremic syndrome, and drugs such as erythropoietin, tacrolimus, and interferon-alfa.[8] It requires urgent BP lowering. Radiologic recovery occurs within days; complete clinical recovery, within weeks.

TREATMENT OF HYPERTENSIVE EMERGENCIES

General Considerations

Two initial decisions that must be made are how quickly and by how much to lower BP. Normalization of BP can cause

complications that are sometimes irreversible, particularly in patients with cerebrovascular or coronary artery disease. Unintended hypotension exaggerates this risk. Therefore, rapid normalization of BP should not generally be the goal of acute management.

The choice of antihypertensive agents should take into consideration the following factors.

Age

Elderly patients are at greater risk for adverse effects of acute BP lowering. Known or occult coronary and cerebrovascular disease, together with reduced autoregulatory capacity, predispose to hypoperfusion as BP is lowered. Often an increased sensitivity to the pharmacologic effect of drugs is present; this should prompt the use of lower doses, selection of a higher target BP, and careful monitoring in elderly patients.

Volume Status

Severe hypertension, particularly in the malignant phase, is often accompanied by vasoconstriction that reduces the intravascular volume.[2,9] This volume constriction may be exaggerated by nausea, vomiting, reduced oral intake, or prior use of diuretics. Potent vasodilators can cause a precipitous fall in BP in patients with reduced vascular volume that may require 1 to 2 L of crystalloid infusion initially. Therefore, diuretics should usually be withheld until sodium retention induced by administration of a vasodilator is evident. In contrast, patients with volume overload, such as hypertension associated with left ventricular failure, renal parenchymal disease, acute glomerulonephritis, or iatrogenic volume overload, require diuretics.

Concurrent Antihypertensive Treatment

Antihypertensive medications taken before presentation may have blocked compensatory mechanisms sufficiently to lead to a drastic reduction in BP in response to the drug given acutely. Therefore, short-acting parenteral drugs should be considered.

Duration of Hypertension

Autoregulation of cerebral blood flow is impaired in chronic hypertension.[10] Therefore, rapid normalization of BP can produce cerebral ischemia. Localized areas of ischemia may occur in malignant hypertension. Thus, cerebral ischemia can occur at a BP level that is close to normal, even in the absence of large-vessel cerebrovascular disease.

Underlying Medical Conditions

As described in Drugs for Hypertensive Emergencies in this chapter, central nervous system depressant drugs such as clonidine, methyldopa, and reserpine should be avoided in patients requiring neurological monitoring. Drugs that increase myocardial oxygen consumption or cardiac contractility should be avoided in patients with myocardial ischemia or dissecting aortic aneurysm. Other specific examples are considered later in this chapter.

Oral Versus Parenteral Agents

Oral agents are not always safer than those administered parenterally. Oral captopril and short-acting nifedipine can lower BP precipitously, whereas agents with short half-lives that are infused intravenously can be titrated more accurately.

Predictability of Response

A universally effective agent should be employed in true emergencies. Intravenous nitroprusside and labetalol are more predictably effective than enalaprilat, which is effective in only about 60% of hypertensive urgencies.[11,12] An ACE inhibitor seems better suited in hypertensive urgencies, in which the initial BP response can help to predict the response to subsequent treatment with an oral ACE inhibitor or an angiotensin receptor blocker (ARB). ACE inhibitors have a unique therapeutic advantage in hypertensive urgencies associated with congestive heart failure.

Cost

Treatment with oral labetalol, captopril, or other agents that do not require intra-arterial monitoring in an intensive care unit reduces costs. Agents such as nitroprusside should be reserved for true emergencies.

Drugs for Hypertensive Emergencies

Drugs for the treatment of hypertensive emergencies are outlined in Table 55-1.

Sodium Nitroprusside

Sodium nitroprusside provides rapid onset and offset of action, ease of titration, and almost universal effectiveness. It is an arterial and venous dilator that reduces myocardial oxygen requirement and is highly suitable for patients with coronary artery disease. Adverse effects are attributed to both the rapidity of BP lowering and toxic effects. The risk of unintended hypotension mandates intra-arterial monitoring in an intensive care unit. Computer-controlled infusion facilitates BP control.[13]

Thiocyanate toxicity causes blurred vision, tinnitus, confusion, and seizures. It occurs only rarely at infusion rates below 3 μg/kg/min for up to 72 hours, except in patients with renal insufficiency. Blood thiocyanate levels should be monitored during high-dose or prolonged treatment. Cyanide accumulation can occur when the infusion rate is above 2 μg/kg/min, and concern about undiagnosed and hazardous cyanide toxicity has been raised.[14] Thiosulfate infusion (150–200 mg/kg over 15 minutes) can prevent or treat cyanide toxicity.[15,16] However, because the frequency of cyanide toxicity is unclear and because thiosulfate infusion can cause thiocyanate accumulation, particularly in patients with reduced renal function, the use of prophylactic thiosulfate infusion remains controversial.

Labetalol

Labetalol, a combination α- and β-receptor blocker, is usually effective, can be given intravenously for a rapid onset, has a sustained effect, is of low toxicity, and does not require intra-arterial monitoring. However, the use of large initial boluses (1–2 mg/kg) has been associated with precipitous falls in BP.[2] An initial bolus of 10 to 20 mg or an infusion of 1 to 2 mg/min can lower blood pressure within 15 minutes.[2] If an initial bolus does not lower blood pressure, repeat boluses of 20 to 40 mg can be administered at 10-minute intervals, up to a maximum cumulative dose of 300 mg.

Labetalol reduces peripheral resistance without reflex stimulation of cardiac output. Because of its β-blocking effect, it can cause deterioration in patients with preexisting left ventricular dysfunction.[2] It is useful in the treatment of hyperadrenergic states, including hypertension after coronary artery bypass graft (CABG), and clonidine withdrawal.[2] However, in patients with pheochromocytoma, it is generally preferable to first establish α-blockade and then add a β-blocker because of the risk of a paradoxical pressor response associated with β-blockade.

Diazoxide

Diazoxide is an arterial vasodilator. It fell into disfavor because of reports of precipitous falls in BP resulting in cerebral and coronary complications after administration of 300 mg as a rapid bolus.[2] However, the use of repeated smaller (e.g., 50 mg) boluses or a continuous infusion appears safer.[2]

Diazoxide is almost universally effective. Its sustained effect obviates the need for minute-to-minute monitoring once BP reduction has been achieved. A precipitous fall in BP is unlikely to occur beyond 5 minutes after administration, enabling repeated boluses to be given as frequently as every 5 to 10 minutes.[2] The sustained action is undesirable when BP lowering may cause clinical deterioration.

Because of reflex increases in cardiac rate, contractility, and output, diazoxide should not be used in patients with coronary disease or dissecting aneurysm. Adjunctive treatment with a diuretic and sympatholytic agent is generally required. The drug may cause hyperglycemia by inhibiting insulin release. Monitoring of blood glucose is advisable.[2]

Nitroglycerin

Intravenous nitroglycerin reduces BP, afterload, left ventricular filling pressures, and myocardial oxygen consumption. For an equivalent degree of BP reduction, it reduces myocardial oxygen consumption more and preserves coronary perfusion better than nitroprusside. Thus, it is favored for coronary insufficiency.[16] It is also suitable in treating perioperative hypertension, including that following CABG.[16] Nitroprusside is more effective in patients with severe hypertension.

Phentolamine

Phentolamine is a nonselective α-adrenergic blocker. It is most effective in situations of catecholamine excess, such as pheochromocytoma. It can be useful in diagnosing a pheochromocytoma but can lower BP precipitously. A test dose of 0.5 to 1 mg infused in 1 minute is generally advised, followed by infusion at 1 mg/min or more. The absence of a dramatic response virtually rules out the diagnosis.

Trimethaphan Camsylate

Trimethaphan is a rapidly acting, titratable, ganglionic blocking agent. It is rarely used because of adverse effects resulting from autonomic blockade and rare unpredictable reactions that include respiratory arrest. Because it impairs pupillary reflexes, it is contraindicated in patients requiring neurological monitoring. Its use requires intra-arterial monitoring of BP in an intensive care unit. It is more difficult to achieve stable BP with trimethaphan than with nitroprusside.

Its use has been generally limited to the following special situations: (1) hypertension associated with dissecting aortic aneurysm, for which blockade of a sympathetically mediated increase in ejection velocity is advantageous; (2) nitroprusside

Table 55-1 Drugs for the Treatment of Hypertensive Emergencies or Urgencies

	Method of Administration	Dosage Range	Precautions and Initial Dose or Interval	Onset	Duration	Adverse Effects
Direct Vasodilators						
Sodium nitroprusside*	IV infusion	0.3–0.5 µg/kg/min	0.5–10 µg/kg/min	Immediate	2–3 min	Shield infusate from light Thionate toxicity
Diazoxide	IV bolus	50–100 mg	50–100 mg at 5- to 10-min intervals to maximum 600 mg	1–2 min	3–15 hr	Hypotension: hyperglyce-mia, fluid retention, reflex tachycardia
Hydralazine	IV infusion IV bolus IM	10 mg/min 10 mg 10–25 mg	10–30 min 10–50 mg at 10- to 20-min intervals 10–50 mg at 20- to 30-min intervals	5–10 min 10–20 min	2–6 hr 2–6 hr	Reflex tachycardia
Nitroglycerin	IV infusion	5 µg/min	5–100 µg/min	2–3 min	3–5 min	Tachyphylaxis
ACE Inhibitors						
Captopril	Oral	6.25–50 mg	12.5–50 mg at 30- to 45-min intervals	10–15 min	2–6 hr	Hypotension; renal failure (if bilateral renal artery stenosis)
Enalaprilat	IV bolus	0.625 mg	0.625–2.5 mg	10–15 min	2–6 hr	Hypotension; renal failure (if bilateral renal artery stenosis)
Dopamine Antagonist						
Fenoldopam	IV infusion	0.03–0.1 µg/kg/min	0.1–1.6 µg/kg/min	5 min	15 min	Increased intraocular pressure

Continued

Table 55-1 Drugs for the Treatment of Hypertensive Emergencies or Urgencies—cont'd

	Method of Administration	Dosage Range	Precautions and Initial Dose or Interval	Onset	Duration	Adverse Effects
α-Adrenergic Blockers						
Phentolamine	IV infusion	0.5–1 mg bolus or 1 mg/min	1–5 mg/min	1–2 min	15–60 min	Hypotension; tachycardia
Labetalol	IV bolus	10–20 mg	20–80 mg at 5- to 10-min intervals	5 min	2–6 hr	Hypotension
	IV infusion	0.5 mg/min	0.5–2 mg/min	5–30 min	2–6 hr	
Prazosin	Oral	1 mg	1–2 mg at 1-hr intervals	15–60 min	2–6 hr	Hypotension
Calcium Channel Blocker						
Nicardipine	IV infusion	5 mg/hr	5–15 mg/hr	5–20 min	1–4 hr	Tachycardia, headache
Ganglionic Blocker						
Trimethaphan	IV infusion	0.5 mg/min	0.5–5 mg/min	1–5 min	5–10 min	Urine retention, ileus; respiratory arrest
Sympatholytic Agents						
Clonidine	*Oral	0.1–0.2 mg	0.05–0.1 mg	1–2 hr	8–12 hr	Drowsiness
Methyldopa	IV	250 mg	250–500 mg at 4- to 8-hr intervals	1–2 hr	8–12 hr	Drowsiness

*Preferred drug for true emergency.
Adapted from Mann SJ, Atlas SA: Hypertensive emergencies. In Laragh JH, Brenner BM (eds): Hypertension: Pathophysiology, Diagnosis and Management, 2nd ed. New York: Raven Press, 1995, pp. 3009–3022.

resistance or toxicity; and (3) absence of alternative effective therapy.

New Agents

Fenoldopam

Fenoldopam is a vasodilator, a dopamine (D_1) receptor agonist that increases cardiac output, heart rate, and renal sodium excretion and preserves glomerular filtration rate.[17,18] Its antihypertensive effect is comparable to that of nitroprusside, but is slower in onset.[17] The dose can be titrated every 15 minutes. In comparison to nitroprusside, fenoldopam offers the advantages of lack of toxicity, a lower likelihood of hypotension, and lack of need for intra-arterial BP monitoring or shielding of the infusion line from light.[19]

Fenoldopam can substitute for nitroprusside in most hypertensive urgencies. The most common adverse effects are headache and increase in heart rate.[19] Because fenoldopam increases intraocular pressure, it is contraindicated in patients with glaucoma.

Urapidil

Urapidil is a combination α_1-adrenergic blocker and central serotonin antagonist at $5HT_{1A}$ receptors that prevents reflex tachycardia.[20] Urapidil lowers BP in hypertensive urgencies, although the onset of effect and time to BP target is slower than with nitroprusside.[21] It requires further study.

Drugs for Hypertensive Urgencies

ACE Inhibitors

Captopril is most effective in patients with an activated renin-angiotensin system, such as those with accelerated or malignant hypertension, scleroderma, and other forms of renal vasculitis.[2] The antihypertensive response is exacerbated by volume depletion,[2] which can lead to hypotension requiring aggressive intravenous fluid replacement. Conversely, the BP response is small or absent in volume-expanded patients. The acute BP response is usually predictive of the chronic response. Thus, nonresponders can be switched to a different class of drug (Fig. 55-1). Patients with elevated plasma renin activity are much more likely to respond than patients with lower renin activity.[22] Enalaprilat is the bioactive form of the prodrug enalapril that acts within 5 minutes when given intravenously.[23] Doses higher than 0.625 mg increase the duration, but not the magnitude, of the initial response.[9,23] However, because enalaprilat is not universally effective, it is generally not a preferred drug in the treatment of true emergencies.

Direct Vasodilators

Intravenous hydralazine has been used for rapid reduction of BP in urgent situations, particularly preeclampsia. However, in a true emergency, more universally effective agents are preferable. Minoxidil may be effective within 4 hours of oral administration at doses of 5 to 20 mg. However, marked sodium retention and tachycardia require the addition of a diuretic and adrenergic blocker and discourage its more widespread use. Sympathetically mediated increases in cardiac contractility and heart rate associated with both of these drugs contraindicate their use in patients with coronary insufficiency or dissecting aortic aneurysm. Isosorbide dinitrate, given either by sublingual or aerosol route, is an alternative to intravenous agents.[24]

Calcium Channel Blockers

Nifedipine

Short-acting nifedipine causes a rapid fall in BP that can cause coronary or cerebrovascular events, even at a "normal" BP.[25] Consequently, its use in hypertensive urgencies is no longer recommended, particularly in elderly patients and those with suspected coronary or cerebrovascular disease. Reflex sympathetic discharge and tachycardia are the basis for contraindications to its use in patients with coronary insufficiency or dissecting aortic aneurysm. The use of nondihydropyridine calcium channel blockers in hypertensive emergencies is less well studied.

Nicardipine

Nicardipine is a dihydropyridine calcium channel blocker. A continuous infusion of nicardipine requires fewer dose adjustments, is associated with fewer adverse effects, and appears equally effective to nitroprusside.[26,27] The infusion rate can be increased at 5- to 15-minute intervals. The mean time to response is 12 minutes.[28] It is selective for vascular tissue and actually increases cardiac output.[28] It causes less headache and tachycardia than nitroprusside.[28]

Adrenergic Blocking Agents

Labetalol

Intravenous labetalol can be used in hypertensive urgencies. Oral labetalol, at doses of 100 to 400 mg, can lower BP within 1 to 3 hours.[2] A second dose can be administered after 3 to 4 hours.

Other β-Receptor Blockers

Intravenous propranolol, metoprolol, and esmolol have little acute BP-lowering effect but minimize reflex cardiac stimulation. They are useful in combination with vasodilators such as nitroprusside, in patients with acute aortic dissection or coronary insufficiency, and in combination with phentolamine in patients with pheochromocytoma.

Sympatholytic Agents

Clonidine lowers BP with a maximal response within 2 to 4 hours and little risk of a precipitous fall. However, the acute response and dosage do not predict the long-term response. Prolonged treatment with clonidine causes bothersome adverse effects (i.e., drowsiness, dry mouth, impotence, and constipation).

MANAGEMENT OF SPECIFIC CONDITIONS

Table 55-2 lists recommended agents.

Accelerated or Malignant Hypertension

Unless complicated by encephalopathy, symptomatic coronary insufficiency, or severe congestive heart failure, malignant hypertension is a medical urgency that does not require intravenous drugs, such as nitroprusside. A target diastolic BP of 100 to 110 mm Hg or higher is recommended during the first 24 to 48 hours of treatment. When time allows, the

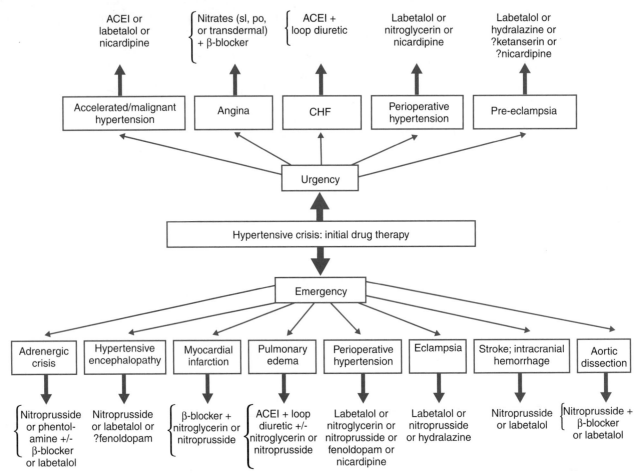

Figure 55-1 Algorithm for approach to treatment of hypertensive crises. ACE, angiotensin-converting enzyme.

response to a rapidly acting ACE inhibitor such as oral capto-pril or intravenous enalaprilat can provide useful diagnostic and therapeutic information. A different agent should be given if there is no response within 30 minutes.

Hypertensive Encephalopathy

The risk of imminent brain damage necessitates rapid lowering of BP. Treatment ameliorates the signs and symptoms of encephalopathy rapidly,[5] but if BP falls below the autoregulatory limit, cerebral ischemia can worsen.[29] Therefore, drugs with a rapid offset of effect, such as nitroprusside, are recommended. If the neurological status deteriorates, the BP should be allowed to rise and other diagnoses, such as cerebrovascular accident, head injury, or other cerebral pathologic processes, should be considered as a contributory factor.

The mean BP in patients known to be hypertensive should generally be reduced during the first hour by a maximum of 20%, or to a diastolic BP of 100 to 110 mm Hg, although even higher target BPs may be advisable in selected patients. In previously normotensive patients, rapid normalization of BP is less hazardous.

Cerebrovascular Accident

Blood pressure elevation commonly accompanies thrombotic stroke.[30] Increased sympathetic tone and intracranial pressure may contribute. Whether BP elevation has the beneficial effect of increasing flow through partially occluded, stenotic, or collateral vessels or a harmful effect by aggravating local edema formation is hotly debated.

Although there is agreement that mild BP elevation during an acute thrombotic stroke should not be treated, the need to treat acute and severe BP elevation is more controversial. An acute fall in BP might reduce cerebral blood flow and exacerbate the neurological deficit, particularly in the elderly, in which cerebral autoregulation is impaired. A recent meta-analysis of 32 trials concluded that there is still inadequate evidence to evaluate the effect of BP lowering on outcome.[31] Recent guidelines for management of hypertension in acute stroke are presented in Table 55-3.[32] Patients in whom thrombolytic therapy has been given or is being considered require intervention if systolic BP is higher than 180 mm Hg, or diastolic pressure is higher than 110 mm Hg.[32]

Antihypertensive treatment in patients with hemorrhagic infarction after thrombotic stroke should follow the preceding guidelines. Stroke due to hypertensive hemorrhage may be treated more aggressively. However, this requires careful differentiation between hemorrhagic stroke and hemorrhagic infarction after thrombotic stroke.

Subarachnoid Hemorrhage

The best management of hypertension during subarachnoid hemorrhage is controversial. An abrupt reduction in BP might prevent rebleeding and reduce edema but could reduce cerebral

Table 55-2   Drugs of Choice

	Drugs	Relative Contraindications
Hypertensive encephalopathy	Nitroprusside, labetalol IV	Centrally acting sympatholytic agents
Malignant hypertension	ACE inhibitor, labetalol IV, clonidine, ? fenoldopam	
Hypertension associated with:		
Intracranial hemorrhage	Nitroprusside, labetalol IV	Diazoxide, nifedipine
Stroke	Nitroprusside, labetalol IV	Diazoxide, nifedipine
Left ventricular failure		
Pulmonary edema	ACE inhibitor + loop diuretic ± nitroprusside or nitroglycerin	β-Blocker, verapamil
Congestive heart failure	ACE inhibitor + loop diuretic	β-Blocker, verapamil
Coronary insufficiency		
Acute myocardial infarction	Nitroglycerin ± β-blocker Nitroprusside ± β-blocker	Diazoxide, hydralazine
Unstable angina	Nitrates (sublingual, oral, or transdermal) ± β-blocker, or as for myocardial infarction	Diazoxide, hydralazine
Adrenergic crisis	Nitroprusside, phentolamine ± β-blocker, ? IV labetalol	β-Blocker monotherapy
Dissecting aortic aneurysm	Nitroprusside + β-blocker; labetalol	Diazoxide, hydralazine, nifedipine
Perioperative hypertension	Nitroprusside, nitroglycerin, labetalol; fenoldopam, nicardipine	

Adapted from Mann SJ, Atlas SA: Hypertensive emergencies. In Laragh JH, Brenner BM (eds): Hypertension: Pathophysiology, Diagnosis and Management, 2nd ed. New York: Raven Press, 1995, pp 3009–3022.

perfusion, particularly in patients with chronic hypertension or increased intracranial pressure. Although mortality and rebleeding are higher in patients presenting with a systolic pressure exceeding 160 mm Hg,[33] the effect of BP lowering on mortality is uncertain.

It seems reasonable to treat acutely and severely elevated BP with rapidly acting and easily titratable drugs. However, there is less evidence of benefit in patients with mildly elevated BP, or those with chronic hypertension. Nimodipine improves neurological outcome, likely by reducing cerebral vasospasm.[34] However, nicardipine, although also reducing vasospasm, does not affect the long-term outcome.[35] Treatment according to the guidelines for hypertension after stroke (see Table 55-3) is recommended, although definitive studies do not exist.

Hypertension Associated with Left Ventricular Failure

Left ventricular failure increases catecholamines and angiotensin II. The resultant elevation of peripheral vascular resistance can impair left ventricular performance. Consequently, vasodilators, including nitrates and ACE inhibitors, can improve cardiac output dramatically.

Acute pulmonary edema generally requires parenteral therapy. Either nitroglycerin or nitroprusside can be used initially, although nitroprusside is more effective. Administration of

oral captopril or intravenous enalaprilat, often with a loop diuretic, assists weaning from parenteral therapy.

Hypertension Associated with Myocardial Infarction or Coronary Ischemia

The goal of acute antihypertensive therapy is to reduce myocardial oxygen demand and increase myocardial blood supply. Intravenous nitroglycerin is ideal because it reduces myocardial oxygen consumption more than nitroprusside and sustains regional blood flow distal to a stenosis. β-Blockers generally have little acute antihypertensive effect but can reduce heart rate and oxygen consumption. The combined effects of β-blockers and nitrates are advantageous. The use of short-acting nifedipine can aggravate ischemia and is contraindicated.

Dissecting Aortic Aneurysm

Acute BP reduction reduces the distending forces on the damaged aorta. However, arterial vasodilators, such as hydralazine, diazoxide, and nifedipine, which cause a reflex increase in the rate and velocity of left ventricular ejection, are contraindicated because they can increase endothelial shear force. Nitroprusside combined with a β-blocker has replaced trimethaphan as the treatment of choice for immediate reduction in

Table 55-3 Approach to Elevated Blood Pressure in Acute Ischemic Stroke: AHA and American Stroke Association Guidelines

Blood Pressure	Intervention
Not Eligible for Thrombolytic Therapy	
SBP < 220 mm Hg or DBP < 120 mm Hg	Observe unless other indications for urgent BP lowering
SBP > 220 mm Hg or DBP 121–140 mm Hg	Labetalol 10–20 mg IV; repeat or double q10min (max dose 300 mg) OR nicardipine 5 mg/hr IV infusion; titrate by 2.5 mg/hr q5min (max 15 mg/hr) Aim for 10%–15% BP reduction
DBP > 140 mm Hg	Nitroprusside, starting with 0.5 mg/kg/min infusion Aim for 10%–15% BP reduction

Blood Pressure	Intervention
Eligible for Thrombolytic Therapy *Pretreatment*	
SBP > 185 mm Hg or DBP > 110 mm Hg	Labetalol 10–20 mg IV, may repeat 1 time; nitropaste 1–2 inches
During/After Treatment	
1. BP monitoring	Monitor q15min for 2 hr, then q30min for 6 hr, then q1h for 16 hr
2. DBP > 140 mm Hg	Nitroprusside, as above
3. SBP > 230 mm Hg or DBP 121–140 mm Hg	Labetalol as above, or 10-mg bolus followed by drip at 2–8 mg/min If ineffective, consider nitroprusside OR nicardipine as above
4. SBP 180–230 mm Hg or DBP 105–120 mm Hg	Labetalol as above, or 10-mg bolus followed by drip at 2–8 mg/min

DBP, diastolic blood pressure; SBP, systolic blood pressure
Adapted from Adams H, Adams R, del Zoppo G, Goldstein LB: Guidelines for the early management of patients with ischemic stroke. 2005 Guidelines Update. A scientific statement from the Stroke Council of the American Heart Association/American Stroke Association. Stroke 2005;36:916–921.

BP. Thereafter, intravenous labetalol can serve as a bridge to oral α- plus β-blockade.

Adrenergic Crises

Increased catecholamine and sympathetic tone mediate the acute hypertension complicating clonidine withdrawal, pheochromocytoma, cocaine abuse, MAO inhibitor/tyramine interaction, and use of sympathomimetics such as phenyl-propanolamine. Acute BP elevation is largely due to α-mediated vasoconstriction.

Although the use of phentolamine is logical, nitroprusside is equally effective and more familiar. However, if adjunctive therapy with β-blockers is indicated (e.g., because of severe tachycardia or ventricular ectopy), establishment of α-blockade (with phentolamine or perhaps prazosin) should be accomplished first. β-Blockade, in the absence of prior α-blockade, can produce an undesired pressor effect due to unopposed α tone and loss of β-mediated vasodilation. Intravenous labetalol appears effective, but further experience with its use in pheochromocytoma is needed. If time allows, oral clonidine is an effective alternative for hypertension caused by clonidine withdrawal.

Preeclampsia

Hypertensive crises near the end of pregnancy are traditionally treated with parenteral hydralazine or labetalol. A recent trial found intravenous hydralazine and intravenous labetalol to be equally effective.[36] Magnesium sulfate can also lower BP but is indicated specifically to prevent convulsions.

Recent trials have examined the role of newer agents. Although the selective serotonin ($5HT_{2A}$)-receptor antagonist ketanserin is as effective as hydralazine[37] and nicardipine is as effective as labetalol,[38] their roles in clinical practice remain to be established.

Postoperative Hypertension

Postoperative hypertension is characterized by increased sympathetic tone and vascular resistance. Pain and overhydration contribute to blood pressure elevation. Nonspecific vasodilators, including intravenous nitroglycerin and nitroprusside, are effective,[39] but nitroglycerin is preferred after CABG. Isradipine,[40] nicardipine,[41] fenoldopam[17,19] and, in patients with preserved left ventricular function, labetalol[42] provide alternatives. Fenoldopam used after CABG achieves BP control as rapidly as nitroprusside.[28] After carotid endarterectomy, nicardipine controls BP elevation within 10 minutes in most patients.[43] Nicardipine resembles labetalol in its rapid onset and slow offset of action, and is an alternative to labetalol, particularly in patients in whom a β-blocker is contraindicated.

Postoperative hypertension is often a consequence of overzealous hydration, in which case an intravenous loop diuretic merits consideration.

Renal Failure

First and foremost in treatment of hypertension in the setting of renal failure is the need to increase sodium excretion. Furosemide doses up to 80 to 240 mg are required in those unresponsive to thiazides. Adding a thiazide diuretic such as metolazone to a loop diuretic further promotes sodium excretion and lowers BP. Aggressive volume control often increases serum creatinine. If it is not extreme, it is not a contraindication to continued diuretic therapy.

The renin-angiotensin system frequently contributes to hypertension in patients with renal failure. Thus, ACE inhibitors or ARBs are usually effective. Excretion of ACE inhibitors is reduced in renal insufficiency, and dosage should be reduced, with the exception of fosinopril. Dosage and excretion of ARBs is not altered in renal insufficiency. Combining an ACE inhibitor with an ARB is less effective than combining either agent with a drug from a different class. Other agents, including calcium channel blockers, β-blockers, and α-blockers, are also effective, but studies provide little guidance as to which to choose. Erythropoietin can precipitate hypertensive crisis, especially if the hematocrit rises abruptly; phlebotomy has been reported to be helpful in management.[44]

The majority of patients requiring hemodialysis have hypertension.[45] All classes of antihypertensive agents except diuretics can lower BP,[46] but hypertension remains uncontrolled in 62%.[46] Prominent reasons for this include failure to achieve dry weight, interdialytic weight gain, inadequate medication, and withholding of medication before dialysis.[46] If hypotension during dialysis prevents attainment of dry weight, withholding of antihypertensive agents such as ACE inhibitors, calcium channel blockers, or α-blockers on the day of dialysis can be helpful. For further discussion, see Chapter 60.

The blood levels of renally excreted agents such as atenolol persist longer in patients with renal failure, and lower dosage is usually sufficient.[47] Because atenolol is dializable, it should be given after dialysis.[47]

"Severe" Hypertension

Severe hypertension usually does not constitute an emergency or urgency. If a patient presents with a BP of 180–220/110–130 mm Hg but is asymptomatic, without retinal hemorrhages or exudates or renal insufficiency, prescription of oral agents with close follow-up is appropriate.

The low probability of controlling severe hypertension with a single agent provides a rationale for ACE inhibitor/diuretic and ARB/diuretic combinations. A diuretic should nearly always be a component of any multidrug regimen. Failure to control hypertension is frequently due to inadequate diuretic dosage. Addition of a potassium-sparing diuretic such as spironolactone, eplerenone, or amiloride or, in patients with renal insufficiency, substitution of a loop diuretic, can enhance control of BP and blood volume.

CONCLUSIONS

Hypertensive "crises" can be viewed as a spectrum, from nonurgent, to urgent, to truly emergent. Most instances of severe but asymptomatic hypertension need not be treated urgently unless required by underlying conditions. Hypertensive urgencies can be treated with oral or intravenous agents, whereas true emergencies require short-acting intravenous agents such as sodium nitroprusside. The treatment of accelerated or malignant hypertension is usually sufficiently urgent to preclude the use of agents that can help identify pathogenetic mechanisms and guide subsequent treatment (see Fig. 55-1). Therapeutic restraint, particularly in patients with severe but asymptomatic BP elevation, is required to avoid complications from unnecessary and overzealous lowering of BP.

References

1. Kincaid-Smith P: Malignant hypertension: Mechanisms and management. Pharmacol Ther 1980;9:245–269.
2. Mann SJ, Atlas SA: Hypertensive emergencies. In Laragh JH, Brenner BM (eds): Hypertension: Pathophysiology, Diagnosis and Management, 2nd ed. New York, Raven Press, 1995, pp 3009–3022.
3. Kincaid-Smith P: Understanding malignant hypertension. Aust NZ J Med 1981;11(Suppl 1):64–68.
4. Labinson PT, White WB, Tendler BE, Mansoor GA: Primary hyperaldosteronism associated with hypertensive emergencies. Am J Hypertens 2006;19:623–627.
5. Chester EM, Agamanolis DP, Banker BQ: Hypertensive encephalopathy: A clinicopathologic study of 20 cases. Neurology 1978;28:928–939.
6. Johansson B, Strandgaard S, Lassen NA: On the pathogenesis of hypertensive encephalopathy. The hypertensive "breakthrough" of autoregulation of cerebral blood flow with forced vasodilatation, flow increase, and blood-brain-barrier damage. Circ Res 1974;34/35(Suppl 1):I167–I171.
7. Hinchey J, Chaves C, Appignani B, et al: A reversible posterior leukoencephalopathy syndrome. N Engl J Med 1996;334:494–500.
8. Mirza A: Posterior reversible encephalopathy syndrome: A variant of hypertensive encephalopathy. J Clin Neurosci 2006;13:590–595.
9. Kincaid-Smith P, McMichael J, Murphy EA: The clinical course and pathology of hypertension with papilledema. Q J Med 1958;27:117–154.
10. Strandgaard S, Olesen J, Skinhoj E, et al: Autoregulation of brain circulation in severe arterial hypertension. BMJ 1973;1:507–510.
11. Huey J, Thomas P, Hendricks DR, et al: Clinical evaluation of intravenous labetalol in the treatment of hypertensive urgency. Am J Hypertens 1988;1:284S–289S.
12. Hirschl MM, Binder M, Bur A, et al: Clinical evaluation of different doses of intravenous enalaprilat in patients with hypertensive crisis. Arch Intern Med 1995;155:2217–2223.
13. Chitwood WR Jr, Cosgrove DH III, Lust RM: Multicenter trial of automated nitroprusside infusion for postoperative hypertension. Titrator Multicenter Study Group. Ann Thorac Surg 1992;54:517–522.
14. Robin ED, McCauley R: Nitroprusside-related cyanide poisoning: Time (long past due) for urgent, effective interventions. Chest 1992;102:1842–1845.
15. Friederich JA, Butterworth JF: Sodium nitroprusside: twenty years and counting. Anesth Analg 1995;81:152–162.
16. Fremes SE, Weisel RD, Mickle DAG: A comparison of nitroglycerin and nitroprusside: I. Treatment of post-operative hypertension. Ann Thorac Surg 1985;39:53–60.
17. Oparil S, Aronson S, Deeb GM, Taylor A: Fenoldopam: A new parenteral antihypertensive: Consensus roundtable on the management of perioperative hypertension and hypertensive crises. Am J Hypertens 1999;12:653–664.
18. Murphy MB, Murray C, Shorten GD. Fenoldopam—a selective peripheral dopamine-receptor agonist for the treatment of severe hypertension. N Engl J Med 2001;345:1548–1557.
19. Frishman WH: Fenoldopam: A new dopamine agonist for the treatment of hypertensive urgencies and emergencies. J Clin Pharmacol 1998;38:2–13.
20. Hirschl MM: Guidelines for the drug treatment of hypertensive crises. Drugs 1995;50:991–1000.
21. Hirschl MM, Binder M, Bur A, et al: Safety and efficacy of urapidil and sodium nitroprusside in the treatment of hypertensive emergencies. Intensive Care Med 1997;23:885–888.
22. Hirschl MM, Binder M, Bur A, et al: Impact of the renin-angiotensin-aldosterone system on blood pressure response to intravenous enalaprilat in patients with hypertensive crises. J Hum Hypertens 1997;11:177–183.
23. Dipette DJ, Ferraro JC, Evans RR, et al: Enalaprilat, an intravenous angiotensin-converting enzyme inhibitor in hypertensive crises. Clin Pharmacol Ther 1985;38:199–204.
24. Rodriguez-Lopez L, Lozano-Nuevo JJ, Trejo-Orozco N: Comparison between isosorbide dinitrate in aerosol and in tablet for the treatment of hypertensive emergencies. Angiology 2001;52:131–135.

25. Grossman E, Messerli FH, Grodzicki T, Kowey P: Should a moratorium be placed on sublingual nifedipine capsules given for hypertensive emergencies and pseudoemergencies? JAMA 1996; 276:1328–1331.

26. Neutel JM, Smith DHG, Wallin D, et al: A comparison of intravenous nicardipine and sodium nitroprusside in the immediate treatment of severe hypertension. Am J Hypertens 1994;7: 623–628.

27. Habib GB, Dunbar LM, Rodrigues R, et al: Evaluation of the efficacy and safety of oral nicardipine in treatment of urgent hypertension: A multicenter, randomized, double-blind, parallel, placebo-controlled clinical trial. Am Heart J 1995;129:917–923.

28. Erstad BL, Barletta JF: Treatment of hypertension in the perioperative patient. Ann Pharmacother 2000;34:66–79.

29. Strandgaard S, Paulson OB: Cerebral autoregulation. Stroke 1984; 15:413–415.

30. Wallace JD, Levy LL: Blood pressure after stroke. JAMA 1981;246: 2177–2180.

31. The Blood Pressure in Acute Stroke Collaboration: Vasoactive drugs for acute stroke. Cochrane Database Syst Rev 2000;(4): CD002839.

32. Adams H, Adams R, del Zoppo G, Goldstein LB: Guidelines for the early management of patients with ischemic stroke. 2005 Guidelines Update. A scientific statement from the Stroke Council of the American Heart Association/American Stroke Association. Stroke 2005. 36:916–921.

33. Nibbelink DW: Antihypertensive and antifibrinolytic therapy following subarachnoid hemorrhage from ruptured intracranial aneurysm. In Sahs AL, Nibbelink DW, Torner JC (eds): Aneurysmal Subarachnoid Hemorrhage: Report of the Cooperative Study. Baltimore: Urban and Schwartzenberg, 1981, pp 287–296.

34. Wong MCW, Haley EC Jr: Calcium antagonists: Stroke therapy coming of age. Stroke 1990;21:494–501.

35. Haley EC Jr, Kassell NF, Torner JC, et al: A randomized controlled trial of high dose intravenous nicardipine in aneurysmal subarachnoid hemorrhage. A report of the Cooperative Aneurysm Study. J Neurosurg 1993;78:537–547.

36. Vigil-DeGracia P, Lasso M, Ruiz E, et al, for the HYLA treatment study: Severe hypertension in pregnancy: Hydralazine or labetalol. A randomized clinical trial. Eur J Obstet Gynecol 2006;128:157–162.

37. Bolte AC, Eyck JV, Kanhai HH, et al: Ketanserin versus dihydralazine in the management of severe early-onset preeclampsia: Maternal outcome. Am J Obstet Gynecol 1999;180:371–377.

38. Elatrous S, Nouira S, Ouanes Besbes L, et al: Short-term treatment of severe hypertension of pregnancy: Prospective comparison of nicardipine and labetalol. Intensive Care Med 2002; 28:1281–1286.

39. Hackman BB, Griffin B, Mills M, et al: Comparative effects of fenoldopam mesylate and nitroprusside on left ventricular performance in severe systemic hypertension. Am J Cardiol 1992;69:918–922.

40. Ruegg PC, David D, Loria Y: Isradipine for the treatment of hypertension following coronary artery bypass graft surgery: A randomized trial versus sodium nitroprusside. Eur J Anaesthesiol 1992;9:293–305.

41. Halpern NA, Goldberg M, Neely C, et al: Postoperative hypertension: A multicenter, prospective, randomized comparison between intravenous nicardipine and sodium nitroprusside. Crit Care Med 1992;20:1637–1643.

42. Cruise CJ, Skrobik Y, Webster RE, et al: Intravenous labetalol versus sodium nitroprusside for treatment of hypertension post coronary bypass surgery. Anesthesiology 1989;71:835–839.

43. Dorman T, Thompson DA, Breslow MJ, et al: Nicardipine versus nitroprusside for breakthrough hypertension following carotid endarterectomy. J Clin Anesth 2001;13:16–19.

44. Fahal IH, Yaqoob M, Ahmad R: Phlebotomy for erythropoietin-induced malignant hypertension. Nephron 1992;61:214–216.

45. Salem MM: Hypertension in the hemodialysis population: A survey of 649 patients. Am J Kidney Dis 1995;26:461–468.

46. Rahman M, Dixit A, Donley V, et al: Factors associated with inadequate blood pressure control in hypertensive hemodialysis patients. Am J Kidney Dis 1999;33:498–506.

47. Agarwal R: Strategies and feasibility of hypertension control in a prevalent hemodialysis cohort. Clin Nephrol 2000;53:344–353.

Further Reading

Adams H, Adams R, del Zoppo G, Goldstein LB: Guidelines for the early management of patients with ischemic stroke. 2005 Guidelines Update. A scientific statement from the Stroke Council of the American Heart Association/American Stroke Association. Stroke 2005;36:916–921.

Agarwal R: Strategies and feasibility of hypertension control in a prevalent hemodialysis cohort. Clin Nephrol 2000;53:344–353.

The Blood Pressure in Acute Stroke Collaboration: Vasoactive drugs for acute stroke. Cochrane Database Syst Rev 2000;(4): CD002839.

Labinson PT, White WB, Tendler BE, Mansoor GA: Primary hyperaldosteronism associated with hypertensive emergencies. Am J Hypertens 2006;19:623–627.

Mirza A: Posterior reversible encephalopathy syndrome: A variant of hypertensive encephalopathy. J Clin Neurosci 2006;13:590–595.

Murphy MB, Murray C, Shorten GD: Fenoldopam—a selective peripheral dopamine-receptor agonist for the treatment of severe hypertension. N Engl J Med 2001;345:1548–1557.

Rahman M, Dixit A, Donley V, et al: Factors associated with inadequate blood pressure control in hypertensive hemodialysis patients. Am J Kidney Dis 1999;33:498–506.

Chapter 56

Management of Associated Cardiovascular Risk in Essential Hypertension

Vasilios Papademetriou

Hypertension is a major contributor to cardiovascular disease (CVD). Whereas some CVD endpoints, such as encephalopathy, hemorrhagic stroke, and acute renal failure, may be directly attributable to elevated blood pressure (BP), the most common consequence of chronic hypertension is progressive atherosclerosis. Hypertension plays a significant and independent role in atherogenesis, but its impact is greatly exaggerated by the presence of other risk factors. It seems that there is a threshold of BP required for the development of atherosclerosis. Lesions do not appear in normally low-pressure vascular beds, such as the pulmonary vasculature, but do appear in patients with pulmonary hypertension. Veins do not develop atherosclerosis until they are utilized as grafts in the systemic circulation. Animal experiments demonstrate that the development of atherosclerosis can be altered by manipulation of BP.[1,2]

In the Framingham Heart Study, the risk of ischemic heart disease over a 10-year period was greatly influenced by other risk factors, as shown in Figure 56-1.[3,4] The presence of other CVD risk factors is important for other reasons: (1) they influence the decision to treat, how aggressively to treat, and with what agents; (2) they affect the response to hypertension therapy; and (3) they influence the expected benefit on CVD endpoints (Box 56-1).

INFLUENCE OF DYSLIPIDEMIAS

A synergistic interaction between the risk for CVD events, systolic BP, and low-density lipoprotein (LDL) cholesterol has been shown. High-density lipoprotein (HDL) cholesterol enhances the removal of oxidized LDL from the tissues. An inverse relationship exists between HDL cholesterol and systolic BP.[5,6] The interaction of LDL and HDL cholesterol and BP is shown in Figure 56-2. Several large randomized trials in patients with and without preexisting CVD have demonstrated conclusively that lowering of LDL cholesterol substantially reduces the risk of myocardial infarction (MI) and coronary events.[6–10] Although epidemiologic observations have not detected a relationship between LDL and stroke, post hoc analysis has concluded that lowering LDL cholesterol also apparently lowers stroke incidence.[11] Women, minorities, diabetic patients, and the elderly have been underrepresented in these trials. Three prominent primary prevention trials are the Helsinki Heart Study,[12] the West of Scotland Coronary Prevention Study (WOSCOPS),[9] and the Air Force/Texas Coronary Atherosclerosis Prevention Study (AFCAPS/TexCAPS).[13]

The upper age limit for enrollment in the Helsinki Heart Study[12] was 55 years. The baseline LDL cholesterol averaged 270 mg/dL. This study demonstrated a 34% reduction in combined CVD events with the fibric acid derivative gemfibrozil. WOSCOPS was also limited to middle-aged men, with an upper age limit of 64 years and mean baseline LDL cholesterol of 272 mg/dL. This study also demonstrated a reduction of combined coronary events, CVD death, nonfatal MI, and all cardiovascular deaths by nearly one third, using pravastatin as the lipid-lowering intervention. The AFCAPS/TexCAPS included a lower risk but more representative population: the average age was 58 years, but 21% were older than age 65, 15% were women, 3% blacks, and 7% Hispanics. The average LDL cholesterol at baseline was 150 mg/dL. Treatment with lovastatin reduced the risk of coronary events, MI, and revascularization, but the number of participants in the subgroups was too small to allow definitive conclusions.

Three major secondary prevention trials established the benefit of lipid-lowering therapy in patients with known CVD. Although these studies also focused primarily on middle-aged men, they included women and patients older than age 65; they also included patients with LDL cholesterol from the high-normal range (110 mg/dL) and the very high range (232 mg/dL). The Scandinavian Simvastatin Survival Study (4S) included patients with established CVD and LDL cholesterol of 174 to 232 mg/dL (average, 188 mg/dL), of whom 19% were women and 23% were older than age 65.[7] In this study, simvastatin resulted in a significant reduction in total mortality, coronary events, CVD deaths, revascularization procedures, and strokes. The Cholesterol And Recurrent Events (CARE) trial included post-MI patients with LDL cholesterol of 116 to 174 mg/dL (mean, 139 mg/dL), of whom 14% were women and 31% were older than age 65. In this study, treatment with pravastatin resulted in a 24% risk reduction of fatal coronary events and nonfatal MI and a 25% reduction in the need for revascularization.[10,14] The Long-term

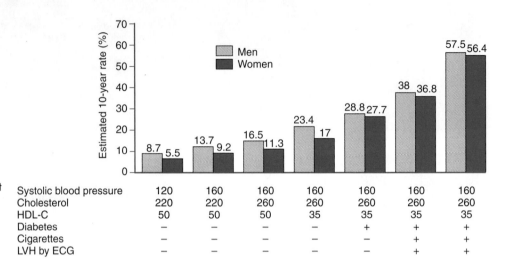

Figure 56-1 Estimated risk of ischemic heart disease over 10 years according to various combinations of risk factors for men and women. HDL, high-density lipoprotein; LVH, left ventricular hypertrophy. (From Anderson KM, Wilson PWF, Odell PM, et al: An updated coronary risk profile. Statement for health professionals. Circulation 1991;83:357–363.)

Box 56-1   Cardiovascular Risk Factors That May Interact with Hypertension

Major Risk Factors	Emerging Risk Factors
High LDL cholesterol (>130 mg/dL)	High lipoprotein (a) level
	High homocysteine level
Low HDL cholesterol (<40 mg/dL)	High-sensitivity CRP
	Prothrombotic factors
Cigarette smoking	Proinflammatory factors
Diabetes mellitus	Impaired fasting glucose
Physical activity	Subclinical atherosclerosis
Obesity	High uric acid
	Vascular calcification

CRP, C-reactive protein; HDL, high-density lipoprotein; LDL, low-density lipoprotein.

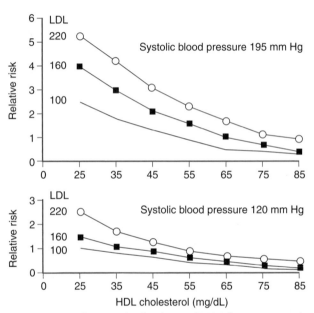

Figure 56-2 Relative risk of ischemic heart disease according to high-density lipoprotein cholesterol (HDL), low-density lipoprotein cholesterol (LDL), and systolic blood pressure in the Framingham Study. All subjects were men ages 50 to 70 years. (From Gordon T, Kannel WB, Castelli WP, et al: Lipoproteins, cardiovascular disease, and death: The Framingham Study. Arch Intern Med 1981;252:1123–1131.)

Intervention with Pravastatin in Ischemic Disease (LIPID) study included patients with a broad range of serum cholesterol levels (155–271 mg/dL).[15] Average LDL at baseline was 150 mg/dL. Of the patients in this study, 17% were women and 39% were older than age 65. This study also demonstrated that treatment with pravastatin reduced the risk of major cardiovascular events, including stroke, by about 25%.

In a recent meta-analysis, LaRosa and colleagues[16] examined the data from the five large trials that used statins as the lipid-lowering intervention (i.e., 4S, WOSCOPS, CARE, AFCAPS/TexCAPS, LIPID), with primary focus on risk reduction in women and the elderly. Collectively, these trials included 30,817 patients, of whom 13% were women and 29% were older than age 65. The overall proportional risk reduction for major cardiovascular events was similar in men and women, in younger and older patients, and in patients with or without hypertension. However, the effect on coronary deaths remained unclear. Overall, only two of the studies (4S and LIPID) showed significant reduction in coronary deaths, whereas the subgroups of women and the elderly were too small for definitive conclusions.

More recent studies have shed light on the optimal level of LDL cholesterol according to the risk of the patient. The lipid-lowering trial ALLHAT randomized 10,000 patients with hypertension and mild LDL cholesterol elevation to pravastatin or placebo. Unfortunately, during the course of the trial more than 25% of the control patients received therapy with other statins. The end result was a small difference in LDL cholesterol of 11%, which resulted in a nonsignificant 9% reduction on fatal/nonfatal MI.[17] In a recent meta-analysis, Cannon and colleagues[18] presented four recently published clinical trials comparing moderate to aggressive LDL cholesterol reduction with statin therapy (Table 56-1). Two studies addressed high-risk patients with stable coronary artery disease (CAD),[19,20]

Table 56-1   Summary of Major Features of Intensive Versus Moderate Lipid-Lowering Trials

Trial	Enrollment	Population Studied	Treatments	LDL Achieved	Duration of Follow-up	Result
Secondary Prevention in Stable Patients						
TNT	10,001	History of MI or angina and coronary revascularization, LDL-C 130–250 mg/dL	Atorvastatin 10 mg vs. 80 mg	101 vs. 77 mg/dL	Median 4.9 years	HR 0.78 for major cardiac events (P < .001)
IDEAL	8888	History of MI meeting national guideline recommendations for cholesterol lowering	Simvastatin 20 mg vs. atorvastatin 80 mg	104 mg/dL vs. 81 mg/dL	Median 4.8 years	HR 0.89 death/MI/ cardiac arrest (P = .07)
Secondary Prevention Following Acute Coronary Syndrome						
A to Z	4497	Acute coronary syndrome	Simvastatin placebo/20 mg vs. 40/80 mg	81 mg/dL vs. 66 mg/dL	Median 2.0 years	HR 0.89 for CV death/MI/stroke/ ACS (P = .14)
PROVE IT—TIMI 22	4162	Acute coronary syndrome	Pravastatin 40 mg vs. Atorvastatin 80 mg	95 mg/dL vs. 62 mg/dL	Median 2.0 years	HR 0.84 for death/ MI/UA/revascularization/stroke (P = .005)

A to Z, Aggrastat to Zocor; ACS, acute coronary syndrome; CV, cardiovascular; IDEAL, Incremental Decrease in End Points Through Aggressive Lipid Lowering; LDL-C, LDL cholesterol; MI, myocardial infarction; PROVE IT, Pravastatin or Atorvastatin Evaluation and Infection Therapy; TNT, Treating to New Targets; UA, unstable angina.
From Cannon CP, Steinberg BA, Murphy SA, et al: Meta-analysis of cardiovascular outcomes trials comparing intensive versus moderate statin therapy. J Am Coll Cardiol 2006;48:438–445.

and two studies addressed patients with acute coronary syndrome.[21,22] These studies demonstrated that lower LDL cholesterol is better. The revised guidelines currently recommend LDL of less than 70 mg/dL in very high-risk patients. Whether there is benefit at even lower levels has not been yet established. These results are applicable to hypertensive and normotensive high-risk patients.

Role of Low HDL Cholesterol

Considerable epidemiologic data demonstrate that low HDL cholesterol is a major risk factor for CVD and stroke.[23–26] Low HDL cholesterol is the most common lipid abnormality in men with CVD in the United States. Furthermore, low HDL cholesterol better distinguishes populations with CAD from those without. The Veterans Administration High-density lipoprotein cholesterol Intervention Trial (VA-HIT) established substantial benefits of interventions to raise low HDL cholesterol. The VA-HIT included 2531 men with known CAD, low HDL cholesterol, and fairly normal LDL cholesterol. Approximately 45% were also hypertensive. Patients were randomized to receive gemfibrozil (600 mg bid) or placebo. At baseline, the average total cholesterol was 175 mg/dL, triglycerides 162 mg/dL, LDL cholesterol 111 mg/dL, and HDL cholesterol 32 mg/dL. After 1 year of treatment and throughout the study, therapy with gemfibrozil reduced triglycerides by 31% and increased HDL cholesterol by 6%. No change in LDL cholesterol or total cholesterol was noted.

Over a median follow-up of 5.1 years, gemfibrozil therapy resulted in a significant 22% reduction in the primary endpoint of nonfatal MI and CVD death and a 31% reduction in atherothrombotic strokes.[27] Further extensive analysis of the data demonstrated that the reduction in the primary endpoint was significantly related with on-therapy changes in HDL cholesterol but not LDL cholesterol or triglycerides.[28] The benefits observed were similar among all subgroups analyzed, including hypertensive and diabetic patients. Thus, this study established for the first time that raising HDL cholesterol in patients with CVD and no other major lipid abnormality is beneficial. This was true even though the change in HDL cholesterol was only 6%.

Greater increases in HDL cholesterol can be achieved with niacin. Increases of up to 30% have been noted with daily doses of 3 g. However, several problems have limited the widespread use of niacin. Short-acting preparations need to be administered three times a day with food and/or aspirin to avoid flushing and gastrointestinal symptoms. Slow-release preparations are well tolerated but are associated with substantial hepatotoxicity.[29] A recently developed intermediate-release niacin (Niaspan) given at night with a snack is well tolerated and is devoid of hepatotoxicity. Changes in lipid profile noted with this intermediate-release preparation are similar to those seen with short-acting niacin and include up to 30% increase in HDL cholesterol, 15% reduction in triglycerides, 20% reduction in LDL cholesterol, and 28% reduction in lipoprotein (a) [Lp(a)]. These lipid improvements may confer substantial improvements in CVD outcomes, particularly when combined with a statin.[30]

More than 30 years ago, the Coronary Drug Project examined the effect of niacin on prevention of CVD.[31] Over a 6.2-year follow-up, the study demonstrated that niacin-treated patients experienced 26% fewer MIs and 24% fewer strokes; need for cardiovascular surgery was reduced by 47%. After 15 years of follow-up the study still continued to show 11% lower total mortality in the niacin-treated patients ($P <$ .0004).[32] Interest in HDL continued unabated; the recently developed cholesteryl ester transfer protein (CETP) inhibitors entered clinical testing. The first to be evaluated extensively in humans was torcetrapib, whose use has been associated with substantial increases in HDL. Torcetrapib was evaluated in recent trials, of which the largest is the ILLUSTRATE.[33] Patients were treated with atorvastatin 10 to 40 mg as needed to reduce LDL cholesterol to close to 100 mg/dL. After 4 to 6 weeks of therapy, patients were randomized to either continue atorvastatin or to have 60 mg of torcetrapib added to the regimen. The primary endpoint for the study was average reduction in atheroma volume as measured by intravascular ultrasound. After 2 years of treatment, torcetrapib resulted in a 58% increase in HDL cholesterol and a further 12% reduction in LDL cholesterol, but no change in atheroma volume was noted. Overall adverse events were more freqent in the torcetrapib group. Systolic BP increased on average by 4.6 mm Hg, and a trend toward an increase in cardiovascular events was noted. The study was terminated prematurely and torcetrapib withdrawn from further testing. The future of CETP inhibitors remains uncertain.

Cholesterol and Blood Pressure Regulation

Therapy with a statin attenuates the onset and progression of hypertension and renal disease in Dahl salt-sensitive rats.[34] More recent data demonstrate a similar effect of long-term treatment with lovastatin in spontaneously hypertensive rats.[35] The mechanism by which statin therapy attenuates the development of hypertension may not be directly related to lipid lowering. Treatment shifts the relation between renal perfusion pressure and sodium excretion toward a lower BP. This effect has been attributed to the ability of statins to prevent vascular hypertrophy, thus improving pressure natriuresis. The effect of statins is largely related to their ability to inhibit synthesis of mevalonate, a precursor of isoprenoids,[36] and not to reduction of LDL cholesterol. A review of the literature suggests that a reduction of plasma cholesterol in humans is associated with a significant 3 to 5 mm Hg reduction in diastolic BP.[37] Statin therapy resulted in the greatest reduction of BP, and patients with the highest cholesterol benefited the most. In the Brisighella Heart Study, more than 1500 hyperlipidemic patients were randomly treated with either a statin or other lipid-lowering therapy (fibrates or cholestyramine) for 5 years.[38] Changes in lipid profile and BP were assessed every 6 months. Lipid lowering was associated with a significant reduction of both systolic and diastolic BP (10–15 mm Hg) only among hypertensive patients in the higher two quartiles. There was only a weak correlation between changes in total cholesterol and blood pressure ($R = 0.16, P < 0.044$).

Glorioso and colleagues[39] conducted a double-blind, crossover study of patients with untreated hypertension and hypercholesterolemia. Participants were randomly assigned to either pravastatin or placebo. Pravastatin resulted in a significant reduction of systolic, diastolic, and pulse pressure and blunted the cold pressor response. This study also found that the effect of statin therapy on BP was largely independent of the effects on LDL and total cholesterol.

More impressive data have been published recently from studies using 24-hour ambulatory blood pressure measurements. This more reliable methodology for assessment of BP changes has less variability, higher reproducibility, and no placebo effect compared to standard BP measurements. The four such studies suggest that statin therapy can reduce BP by an average of 6–7/5–6 mm Hg, particularly in patients in whom hypertension is not well controlled.[40–43]

These data strongly suggest that treatment of hyperlipidemic hypertensive patients with a statin may result in better regulation of BP. The most plausible mechanism is a vasodilatory effect due to improvement in endothelial dysfunction. Increased cholesterol contributes to reduced arterial compliance[44] and increased BP. Reduction in cholesterol with statins can therefore contribute to improved arterial compliance and BP regulation and also may contribute to up-regulation of nitric oxide.[45]

SMOKING AND HYPERTENSION

Epidemiologic data indicate that smoking and hypertension are additive major CVD risk factors. Approximately 30% of the U.S. population and 35% of hypertensive patients smoke.[46] The relative risk for death attributable to hypertension in participants in the Medical Research Council (MRC) Hypertension Trial was 1.9 for men smokers and 1.7 for women smokers, as opposed to 1.3 and 1.2 in nonsmoking men and women, respectively. The acute short-term effects of smoking on BP are related to nicotine, carbon monoxide, and other constituents of tobacco smoke. Heart rate and BP increase within 1 minute of smoking and rise about 30% during the first 10 minutes. The effects of nicotine are maintained for several minutes after smoking has ceased. The half-life of nicotine is more than 2 hours. Thus, heavy smokers may maintain elevated heart rates and BPs for most of their waking hours.[47] Several studies have suggested that infrequent and moderate smokers may have lower BP than nonsmokers.[48] However, in most of these studies, patients abstained from smoking before BP determination. The lower BP found in smokers persists after adjustments are made for body weight.[48] A recent study examined the effect of smoking cessation on BP and the incidence of hypertension in 8170 healthy male employees of a steel manufacturing company.[49] Mildly hypertensive patients were excluded from this analysis. Adjustments were made for baseline age, body mass index, cigarette smoking, alcohol consumption, exercise, family history of hypertension, systolic BP, and change in body mass index over the follow-up period of 4 years. The adjusted relative risks of hypertension in those who had quit smoking for less than 1 year, 1 to 3 years, and more than 3 years were 0.6, 1.5, and 3.5, respectively, compared with nonsmokers. The trends were similar among those who lost or gained weight during the follow-up period. The mechanism by which long-term smoking lowers BP or prevents hypertension and by which smoking cessation increases the frequency of hypertension is not clear, but it should not distract from the well-known harmful effects of cigarette smoking.

Cigarette smoking increases the risk of MI, ischemic heart disease, sudden death, stroke, and peripheral arterial disease; worsens outcomes after percutaneous vascular procedures and bypass surgery; and worsens complications of hypertension.[50]

Cigarette smokers may not derive the expected benefits from hypertension control. In the MRC trial β-blocker therapy in smokers was less effective in preventing strokes than thiazide diuretics.[51] In the Heart Attack Primary Prevention in Hypertension (HAPPHY) trial, β-blockers failed to improve coronary morbidity in smokers.[52] It is important, therefore, to inform patients of the importance of smoking cessation and encourage them to stop smoking at every visit. Smoking cessation is an important intervention in reducing CVD risk in patients with hypertension. Use of various smoking deterrents may be helpful. Pharmacotherapy for smoking cessation is a cost-effective intervention and it should be offered to all consenting smokers.

DIABETES IN PATIENTS WITH HYPERTENSION

Diabetes and hypertension commonly coexist. In the United States, more than 60% of diabetics have hypertension and approximately 20% of hypertensives have diabetes.[53] Diabetics are two to three times more likely to have hypertension than nondiabetics. The incidence is even higher among African Americans. Diabetes is the most common cause of end-stage renal disease and a major contributor to CVD.[54] Even mild elevations of BP in diabetics increase the risk of CVD and renal disease dramatically. It is therefore of the utmost importance to control both BP and blood glucose tightly in diabetics with hypertension.

Aggressive treatment of BP in diabetics has been largely ignored, although it may confer greater reduction of CVD events than glycemic control. The goal for BP reduction has been set at lower levels in diabetics, mostly because studies have shown continued benefit with lower BP. The Appropriate Blood Pressure Control in Diabetes (ABCD)[55] and the Hypertension Optimal Treatment (HOT)[56] trials indicated that aggressive reduction of diastolic BP to below 80 mm Hg provides greater reduction in CVD events. Similarly, the UK Prospective Diabetes Study (UKPDS) demonstrated that tight control of BP had greater impact on CVD events than tight glycemic control.[57] The impact on CVD events included a 44% reduction in strokes, a 24% reduction in diabetes-associated endpoints, and a 32% reduction in deaths. For every 10-mm Hg reduction in systolic BP, there was an associated risk reduction of 12% for any complication related to diabetes.[58] For these reasons, the recommended target BP in patients with diabetes is lower than 130/80 mm Hg. Angiotensin-converting enzyme inhibitors and angiotensin receptor blockers provide better vascular and renal protection, although most patients require combinations of three to four drugs to achieve target BP control.

The UKPDS study compared the effects of intensive blood glucose control with conventional treatment on microvascular and macrovascular complications of diabetes over 10 years in more than 4000 patients.[59,60] Average glycosylated hemoglobin (HbA$_{1c}$) was reduced to 7% in the intensively treated group and to 7.9% in the conventional group. This difference resulted in a 12% reduction in diabetes-related endpoints, a 10% reduction in deaths, and a 25% reduction in microvascular complications. There was minimal reduction in macrovascular disease. For every 1% reduction in HbA$_{1c}$, there was a 21% reduction in any endpoint related to diabetes, a 21% reduction in deaths, a 14% reduction in MIs, and a 37% reduction in microvascular complications. There was no threshold for any of the endpoints.

These observations suggest that aggressive glycemic and BP control is important in patients with diabetes and hypertension.

Whether lower levels of BP and HbA$_{1c}$ confer better benefits for prevention of cardiovascular outcomes in diabetics has not been yet defined. The Action to Control Cardiovascular Risk in Diabetes (ACCORD), an ongoing study, targets HbA$_{1c}$ less than 6.0% and systolic BP lower than 120 mm Hg as compared to recommended levels, in 10,000 patients with type 2 diabetes mellitus. Recently the glycemic arm of the study was discontinued prematurely because an interim analysis showed increased mortality and cardiovascular morbidity in patients randomized to tight glycemic control.

DIET, WEIGHT LOSS, AND EXERCISE IN PATIENTS WITH HYPERTENSION

Epidemiologic studies have consistently shown a substantial correlation between hypertension, excess body weight, and physical inactivity. Although all three variables are independently associated with increased CVD risk,[61-63] their coexistence increases the risk for complications cumulatively. Guidelines for the management of hypertension recommend lifestyle changes for nonpharmacologic treatment of hypertension.[61,64] Dietary changes are effective even without weight loss. The DASH study showed that a combination diet of fruits and vegetables low in saturated fats reduces BP in patients in the high-normal BP range. This diet was more effective in African Americans and in patients with established hypertension.[65] There is roughly a 1-mm Hg reduction in diastolic BP for every kilogram of weight loss in obese subjects. The World Health Organization/International Society of Hypertension guidelines recommend at least 5 kg of weight loss to induce BP reduction.[64]

Numerous observational studies have shown an inverse relationship between physical activity and BP.[66,67] We identified 12 prospective, randomized trials completed in the past 10 years.[68] Significant reduction in resting BP was reported with aerobic exercise in 10 of these studies. The average BP reduction was 8.7/7.0 mm Hg in the exercise group, compared with 3.8/1.3 mm Hg in the controls despite body weight remaining unchanged. An important observation is that low- to moderate-intensity exercise may be more effective in lowering BP than high-intensity exercise. Exercise appears safe and effective in improving hypertension in treated patients with severe hypertension and left ventricular hypertrophy. In a study of 46 African Americans with severe hypertension, we found that regular aerobic exercise for 30 to 60 minutes at least three times per week resulted in significant reduction of BP despite a decrease in antihypertensive medication of 30% to 40%. The body weight in the exercise and control groups and the BP in the controls remained unchanged at 32 weeks.[68] Blumenthal and colleagues[69] studied 134 patients with stage 1 hypertension. They compared the effect of aerobic exercise alone with weight management, including exercise. Aerobic exercise was more effective and reduced BP by 7/5 mm Hg.

These data indicate that diet, weight reduction, and exercise can reduce BP independently. However, reductions are modest. A combination can be more effective. Their feasibility and application in clinical practice remains to be demonstrated.

EMERGING CARDIOVASCULAR RISK FACTORS

New CVD risk factors have emerged in recent years. These have been associated with a high risk for coronary atherosclerosis, CVD complications, and cardiac death. These new risk factors include Lp(a), homocysteine, inflammatory markers, high triglycerides, coronary calcifications, high uric acid, and others. Extensive coverage of these risk factors is beyond the scope of this chapter. In general, clinical associations have been well established with all these factors, but interventional data conclusively demonstrating benefit is lacking in most instances. Figure 56-3 demonstrates the relative predictive value of many of these emerging risk factors derived from the Women's Health Study.

Lipoprotein (a)

Lipoprotein (a) resembles LDL but contains a highly glycosylated protein, apolipoprotein A. Elevated Lp(a) has been associated with CAD in most but not all studies. Some studies suggest gender differences in the prognostic significance of Lp(a). In a large cohort study, 4967 men and 4968 women free of atherosclerosis were followed for up to 14 years. There was a significant increase in the adjusted hazards ratio for CAD with increased Lp(a) (1.9 for women, 1.6 for men), but the association with cerebrovascular disease was less certain.[70] Lp(a) can be reduced significantly with niacin (up to 30% reduction), but the clinical importance of such an intervention has not been demonstrated.

Homocysteine

Homocysteinemia is an independent predictor of CAD, MI, and peripheral vascular disease. One recent study examined the association of homocysteine levels with recurrent events in 110 young patients (<56 years old) who had suffered a prior MI. Over a 7-year follow-up, patients with normal homocysteine levels had significantly fewer combined events

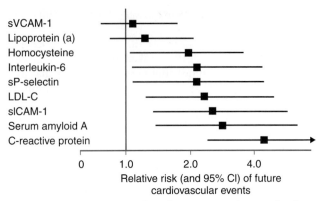

Figure 56-4 Prognostic value of various cardiovascular biomarkers in healthy women in the Women's Health Study. The combination of high-sensitivity CRP with the total cholesterol: high-density lipoprotein cholesterol (TC:HDL-C) ratio provided a stronger predictor than either CRP or TC:HDL-C alone. Relative risks and 95% confidence interval (CI) are shown for individuals in the top versus the bottom quartile for each factor. sICAM-1 indicates soluble intracellular adhesion molecule-1; and sVCAM-1, soluble vascular adhesion molecule-1. Top versus the bottom quartile, after adjustment for age and smoking. (From Willerson JT, Ridker PM: Inflammation as a cardiovascular factor. Circulation 2004;109[Suppl]:II2–II10.)

(26% vs. 72%), lower mortality (1.6% vs. 6%), lower morbidity (14% vs. 36%), and less need for revascularization (18% vs. 48%).[71] Other studies, however, failed to demonstrate any benefit with drug therapy to reduce homocysteine. Definite interventional data with treatment to reduce homocysteine (vitamin B$_6$, vitamin B$_{12}$, or folic acid) is lacking. Similar deficiencies exist for all other emerging CVD risk factors.

C-Reactive Protein

Low-grade inflammation occurs in the vasculature in response to injury, lipid oxidation, and perhaps infection. All cardiovascular risk factors, including hypertension, diabetes, and smoking, are amplified by mild modification and oxidation of LDL cholesterol. Oxidation of LDL leads to inflammation, recruitment of monocytes, and production of

Figure 56-3 Multivariable-adjusted relative risks of cardiovascular disease according to levels of high-sensitivity C-reactive protein (hs-CRP) and categories of low-density lipoprotein cholesterol (LDL-C). hs-CRP levels add prognostic information at all levels of LDL-C and at all levels of the Framingham Risk Score. (From Willerson JT, Ridker PM: Inflammation as a cardiovascular factor. Circulation 2004; 109[Suppl]:II2–II10.)

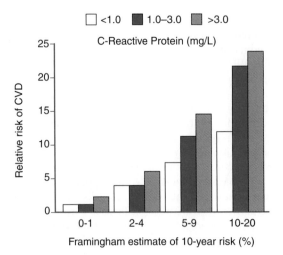

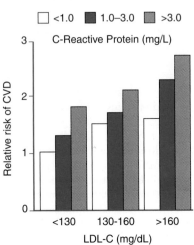

inflammatory markers that initiate the atherosclerotic process. Observational and experimental data have consistently shown a strong association between inflammatory markers and risk of cardiovascular events. Of all markers of inflammation the most reliable, reproducible, and widely available marker is currently high-sensitivity C-reactive protein (hs-CRP). It has been shown in many large trials to be a strong predictor of MI and stroke. Among 28,263 apparently healthy postmenopausal women[72] monitored prospectively in the Women's Health Study, hs-CRP was the strongest predictor of cardiovascular events, outperforming homocysteine, LP(a), and LDL cholesterol (Fig. 56-4; see also Fig. 56-3). CRP is drastically reduced with good management of high cholesterol and treatment of hypertension.

References

1. Dustan HP: Role of hypertension and its control: Experimental aspects. Prog Biochem Pharmacol 1983;19:177–191.
2. Tobian LJ: Interrelationships of sodium volume, CNS and hypertension. Prog Biochem Pharmacol 1983;19:208–229.
3. Kannel WB, Sorlie P: Hypertension in Framingham. In Paul O (ed): Epidemiology and Control of Hypertension. Chicago: Symposia Specialists, 1993.
4. Anderson KM, Wilson PWF, Odell PM, et al: An updated coronary risk profile. Statement for health professionals. Circulation 1991;83:357–363.
5. Kannel WB, Castelli WP, Gordon T: Cholesterol in the prediction of atherosclerotic disease. New perspectives based on the Framingham Study. Ann Intern Med 1979;90:85–91.
6. Gordon T, Kannel WB, Castelli WP, et al: Lipoproteins, cardiovascular disease, and death: The Framingham Study. Arch Intern Med 1981;252:1123–1131.
7. Scandinavian Simvastatin Survival Study Group. Randomized trial of cholesterol lowering in 4444 patients with coronary heart disease: The Scandinavian Simvastatin Survival Study. Lancet 1994;344:1383–1389.
8. Miettinen TA, Pyorala K, Olsson AG, et al: Cholesterol-lowering therapy in women and elderly patients with myocardial infarction or angina pectoris. Circulation 1997;96:4211–4218.
9. Shepherd J, Cobbe SM, Ford I, et al: Prevention of coronary heart disease with pravastatin in men with hypercholesterolemia. N Engl J Med 1995;333:1301–1307.
10. Sacks FM, Pfeffer MA, Moye LA, et al: The effect of pravastatin on coronary events after myocardial infarction in patients with average cholesterol levels. N Engl J Med 1996;335:1001–1009.
11. Prospective Studies Collaboration: Cholesterol, diastolic blood pressure and stroke: 13,000 strokes in 450,000 people in 45 prospective cohorts. Lancet 1995;346:1647–1653.
12. Cholesterol Treatment Trialists' Collaboration: Protocol for a prospective collaborative overview of all current and planned randomized trials of cholesterol treatment regimens. Am J Cardiol 1995;75:1130–1134.
13. Downs JR, Clearfield M, Weis S, et al: Primary prevention of acute coronary events with lovastatin in men and women with average cholesterol levels: Results of AFCAPS/TexCAPS. JAMA 1998;279:1615–1622.
14. Lewis SJ, Sacks FM, Mitchell JS, et al: Effect of pravastatin on cardiovascular events in women after myocardial infarction. J Am Coll Cardiol 1998;32:140–146.
15. Long-term Intervention With Pravastatin in Ischaemic Disease (LIPID) Study Group: Prevention of cardiovascular events and death with pravastatin in patients with coronary heart disease and a broad range of initial cholesterol levels. N Engl J Med 1998;339:1349–1357.
16. LaRosa JC, He J, Vupputuris S: Effect of statins on risk of coronary disease. JAMA 1999;282:2340–2346.
17. ALLHAT Officers and Coordinators for the ALLHAT Collaborative Research Group: The Antihypertensive and Lipid-Lowering treatment to prevent Heart Attack Trial (ALLHAT-LLT). JAMA 2002;288:2998–3007.
18. Cannon CP, Steinberg BA, Murphy SA, et al: Meta-analysis of cardiovascular outcomes trials comparing intensive versus moderate statin therapy. J Am Coll Cardiol 2006;48:438–445.
19. Waters DD, Guyton JR, Herrington DM, et al, for the TNT Steering Committee Members and Investigators: Treating to New Targets (TNT) Study: Does lowering low-density lipoprotein cholesterol levels below currently recommended guidelines yield incremental clinical benefit? Am J Cardiol 2004;93:154–158.
20. Pedersen TR, Faergeman O, Kastelein JJ, et al: High-dose atorvastatin vs. usual-dose simvastatin for secondary prevention after myocardial infarction: The IDEAL study: A randomized controlled trial. JAMA 2005;294:2437–2445.
21. Wiviott SD, de Lemos JA, Cannon CP, et al: A tale of two trials: A comparison of the post-acute coronary syndrome lipid-lowering trials A to Z and PROVE IT-TIMI 22. Circulation 2006;113:1406–1414.
22. Ray KK, Cannon CP, McCabe CH, et al: Early and late benefits of high-dose atorvastatin in patients with acute coronary syndromes: Results of the PROVE IT-TIMI 22 trial. J Am Coll Cardiol 2005;46:1405–1410.
23. Gordon DJ, Probstfield JL, Garrison RJ, et al: High-density lipoprotein cholesterol and cardiovascular disease: Four prospective American studies. Circulation 1989;79:8–15.
24. Tanne D, Yaari S, Goldbourt U: High-density lipoprotein cholesterol and risk of ischemic stroke mortality: A 21-year follow-up of 8586 men from the Israeli Ischemic Heart Disease Study. Stroke 1997;28:83–87.
25. Wannamethee S, Shaper AG, Ebrahim S: HDL-cholesterol, total cholesterol, and the risk of stroke in middle-aged British men. Stroke 2000;31:1882–1888.
26. Rubins HB, Robins SJ, Collins D, et al: Gemfibrozil for the secondary prevention of coronary heart disease in men with low levels of high-density lipoprotein cholesterol. N Engl J Med 1999;341:410–418.
27. Rubins HB, Robins SJ, Collins D, et al: Gemfibrozil for the secondary prevention of coronary heart disease in men with low levels of high-density lipoprotein cholesterol. Veterans Affairs High-Density Lipoprotein Cholesterol Intervention Trial Study Group. N Engl J Med 1999;341:410–418.
28. Robins SJ, Collins D, Wittes JT, et al, for the VA-HIT Study Group: Relation of gemfibrozil treatment and lipid levels with major coronary events. VA-HIT: A randomized controlled trial. JAMA 2001;285:1585–1591.
29. Golberg A, Alagona P, Capuzzi DM, et al: Multiple-dose efficacy and safety of an extended-release form of niacin in the management of hyperlipidemia. Am J Cardiol 2000;85:1100–1105.
30. Brown G, Zhao XO, Chait A, et al: Simvastatin and niacin, antioxidant vitamins, or the combination for the prevention of coronary disease. N Engl J Med 2001;345:1583–1592.
31. Clofibrate and niacin in coronary heart disease. JAMA 1975;231:360–381.
32. Canner PL, Berge KG, Wenger NK, et al: Fifteen year mortality in Coronary Drug Project patients: Long-term benefit with niacin. J Am Coll Cardiol 1986;8:1245–1255.
33. Nissen SE, Tardif JC, Nicolls SJ, et al: The effect of torcetrapib on the progression of coronary atherosclerosis The ILLUSTRATE study. N Engl J Med 2007;356:1304–1316.
34. O'Donnell MP, Kasiske BL, Katz SA, et al: Lovastatin but not enalapril reduces glomerular injury in Dahl salt-sensitive rats. Hypertension 1992;20:651–658.
35. Wilson TW, Alonso-Galicia M, Roman RJ: Effects of lipid-lowering agents in the Dahl salt-sensitive rat. Hypertension 1998;31:225–231.

36. Jiang J, Roman RJ: Lovastatin prevents development of hypertension in spontaneously hypertensive rats. Hypertension 1997;30:968–974.

37. Goode GK, Miller JP, Heagerty AM: Hyperlipidemia, hypertension, and coronary heart disease. Lancet 1995;345:362–364.

38. Borghi C, Gaddi A, Ambrosini E, et al: Improved blood pressure control in hypertensive patients treated with statins. J Am Coll Cardiol 2001;37(Suppl A):233A–234A.

39. Glorioso N, Troffa C, Filigheddu F, et al: Effect of the HMG-CoA reductase inhibitors on blood pressure in patients with essential hypertension and primary hypercholesterolemia. Hypertension 1999;34:1281–1286.

40. Abetel G, Poget PN, Bonnabry JP: Hypotensive effect of an inhibitor of cholesterol synthesis (fluvastatin). A pilot study. Schweiz Med Wochenschr 1998;128:272–277.

41. Magen E, Visckoper R, Mishal J, et al: Resistant arterial hypertension and hyperlipidemia: Atorvastatin, not vitamin C, for blood pressure control. Isr Med Assoc J 2004;6:742–746.

42. Kanbay M, Yildirir A, Bosbas H, et al: Statin therapy helps to control blood pressure levels in hypertensive patients. Ren Fail 2005;27:297–303.

43. Terzoli L, Mircoli L, Raco R, Ferrari AU: Lowering of elevated ambulatory blood pressure by HMG-CoA reductase inhibitors. J Cardiovasc Pharmacol 2005;46:310–315.

44. Lewis TV, Cooper BA, Dart AM, et al: Responses to endothelium-dependent agonists in subcutaneous arteries excised from hypercholesterolaemic men. Br J Pharmacol 1998;124:222–228.

45. Kaesemeyer WH, Caldwell RB, Huang J, et al: Pravastatin sodium activates endothelial nitric oxide synthase independent of its cholesterol-lowering actions. J Am Coll Cardiol 1999;33:234–241.

46. De Cesaris R, Ranieri G, Filitti V, et al: Cardiovascular effects of cigarette smoking. Cardiology 1992;81:233–237.

47. Groppelli A, Giorgi DM, Omboni S, et al: Persistent blood pressure increase induced by heavy smoking. J Hypertens 1992;10:495–499.

48. Green MS, Jucha E, Lz Y: Blood pressure in smokers and nonsmokers: Epidemiologic findings. Am Heart J 1986;111:932–940.

49. Savdie E, Grosslight GM, Adena MA: Relation of alcohol and cigarette consumption to blood pressure and serum creatinine levels. J Chron Dis 1984;37:617–623.

50. Duk-Hee L, Myung-Hwa H, Jang-Rak K, et al: Effects of smoking cessation on changes in blood pressure and incidence of hypertension. Hypertension 2001;37:194–198.

51. Dollery C, Brennan PJ: The Medical Research Council Hypertension Trial: The smoking patient. Am Heart J 1988;115:276–281.

52. Wilhelmsen L, Berglund G, Elmfeldt D, et al: Beta-blockers versus diuretics in hypertensive men: Results from the HAPPHY trial. J Hypertens 1987;5:561–570.

53. Bloomgarden ZT: Perspective on the news: Cardiovascular disease in type 2 diabetes. Diabetes Care 1999;22:1739–1744.

54. American Diabetes Association: National Diabetes Fact Sheet. Alexandria, VA: American Diabetes Association, December 1997.

55. Estacio RO, Jeffers BW, Hiatt WR, et al: The effect of nisoldipine as compared with enalapril on cardiovascular outcomes in patients with non-insulin-dependent diabetes and hypertension. N Engl J Med 1998;338:645–652.

56. Hansson L, Zanchetti A, Carruthers G, et al: Effects of intensive blood-pressure lowering and low-dose aspirin in patients with hypertension: Principal results of the Hypertension Optimal Treatment (HOT) randomized trial. Lancet 1998;351:1755–1762.

57. UK Prospective Diabetes Study Group (UKPDS): Tight blood pressure control and risk of macrovascular and microvascular complications in type 2 diabetes (UKPDS 38). BMJ 1998;317:703–713.

58. Adler AI, Stratton IM, Neil HA, et al: Association of systolic blood pressure with macrovascular and microvascular complications of type 2 diabetes (UKPDS 36): Prospective observational study. BMJ 2000;321:412–419.

59. UK Prospective Diabetes Study (UKPDS) Group: Intensive blood-glucose control with sulphonylureas or insulin compared with conventional treatment and risk of complications in patients with type 2 diabetes (UKPDS 33). Lancet 1998;352:837–853.

60. Straton IM, Adler AI, Neil AW, et al: Association of glycaemia with macrovascular and microvascular complications of type 2 diabetes (UKPDS 35): Prospective observational study. BMJ 2000;321:405–412.

61. Joint National Committee: The Sixth Report of the Joint National Committee on Prevention, Detection, Evaluation, and Treatment of High Blood Pressure. Arch Intern Med 1997;157:2413–2446.

62. Eckel RH: Obesity and heart disease: A statement for healthcare professionals from the Nutrition Committee, American Heart Association. Circulation 1997;96:3248–3250.

63. Appel LJ, Moore TJ, Obarzanek E, et al: A clinical trial of dietary patterns on blood pressure. N Engl J Med 1997;336:1117–1124.

64. Guidelines Subcommittee: 1999 World Health Organization/International Society of Hypertension Guidelines for the Management of Hypertension. J Hypertens 1999;17:151–183.

65. Svetky LP, Simons-Morton D, Vollmer WM, et al: Effects of dietary patterns on blood pressure: Subgroup analysis of the Dietary Approaches to Stop Hypertension (DASH) randomized clinical trial. Arch Intern Med 1999;159:285–293.

66. Hickey N, Mulcahy R, Bourke GJ, et al: Study of coronary risk factors related to physical activity in 15,171 men. BMJ 1975;3:507–509.

67. Miall WE, Oldham PD: Factors influencing arterial blood pressure in the general population. Clin Sci 1958;17:409–444.

68. Papademetriou V, Kokkinos P: The role of exercise in the control of hypertension and cardiovascular risk. Curr Opin Nephrol Hypertens 1996;5:459–462.

69. Blumenthal JA, Sherwood A, Gullette ECD, et al: Exercise and weight loss reduce blood pressure in men and women with mild hypertension: Effects on cardiovascular, metabolic, and hemodynamic functioning. Arch Intern Med 2000;160:1947–1958.

70. Nguyen TT, Ellefson RD, Hodge DO, et al: Predictive value of electrophoretically detected lipoprotein (a) for coronary heart disease and cerebrovascular disease in a community-based cohort of 9936 men and women. Circulation 1997;96:1390–1397.

71. Reis RP, Azinheira J, Reis HP, et al: Prognostic significance of blood homocysteine after myocardial infarction. Rev Port Cardiol 2000;19:581–585.

72. Ridker PM: Role of inflammation biomarkers in prediction of coronary heart disease. Lancet 2001;342:836–843.

Further Reading

Ballantyne C, Arroll B, Shepherd J: Lipids and CVD management: Towards a global concensus. Eur Heart J 2005. 26:2224–2231.

Barzilay JI, Cuttler JA, Davis BR: Antihypertensive therapy and risk of diabetes mellitus. Curr Opin Nephr Hypertens. 2007;16:256–260.

Calabro P, Yeh ETH:The pleotropic effects of statins. Curr Opin Cardiol 2006;20:541–546.

Fruchart JC, Nierman MC, Stroes ESG, et al: New risk factors for atherosclerosis and patient risk assessment. Circulation 2004;109(Suppl III):15–19.

McDonald KC, Blackwell JC: What lifestyle changes should we recommend for the patient with newly diagnosed hypertension? J Family Pract 2006;55:991–993.

Nissen SE, Tardif JC, Nicholls SJ, et al: Effect of torsetrapib on the progression of coronary atherosclerosis. N Engl J Med 2007;356:1304–1316.

Tonstad S, Johnston JA: Cardiovascular risks associated with smoking. A review for clinicians. Eur J Cardiovasc Prev Rehabil 2006;13: 507–513.

Wiviott SD, Cannon CP: The safety and efficacy of achieving very low LDL-cholesterol concentrations with high dose statin therapy. Curr Opin Lipidol 2006;17:626–630.

Wild SH, Byrne CD: Risk factors for diabetes and coronary heart disease. BMJ 2006;333:1009–1011.

Willerson JT, Ridker PM: Inflammation as a cardiovascular factor. Circulation 2004;109 (Suppl):II2 –II10.

PART XI

Management of Secondary Hypertension

CONTENTS

Chapter 57

Medical Management of Patients with Renal Artery Stenosis

Lance D. Dworkin and Christopher S. Wilcox

The effects of medical treatment on the control of blood pressure (BP) and on stabilization or improvement of renal function in trials of patients with renovascular disease have been reviewed comprehensively.[1–7] The indications for, and expected outcomes from, angioplasty and surgery for renal artery stenosis are reviewed in Chapter 58.

Renal artery stenosis (RAS) is defined as a narrowing of one or both renal arteries or their branches (usually by more than 70% to 80% to be functionally significant).[8] It can be caused by either malformation of the renal arteries, the most common type being fibromuscular dysplasia, or by atherosclerotic disease. These two conditions occur in different settings and have distinct clinical consequences and treatment. However, atherosclerosis is about three times more common. In the Medicare population the incidence of clinically manifest atherosclerotic RAS is 0.5% overall and 5.5% in those with chronic kidney disease (CKD).[9] This value undoubtedly underestimates the true incidence of RAS because patients are often asymptomatic (approximately 7% in one community-based screening study).[10] Interest in this diagnosis is spurred by the belief that hemodynamically significant RAS is a major cause of hypertension and CKD in affected patients. However, although RAS is common, the prevalence of *renovascular hypertension,* defined as hypertension caused by RAS, is unknown. No test reliably identifies hypertension that is improved or cured after correction of RAS.

Fibromuscular dysplasia is rarely associated with kidney failure, but impaired renal function is common in patients with atherosclerotic disease. The term *ischemic nephropathy* is often applied to individuals with atherosclerotic RAS and abnormal kidney function. However, in the absence of complete occlusion, there is little evidence that stenosis of the main renal artery actually causes renal failure or that renal ischemia causes progressive loss of renal function. Therefore, this condition is better referred to as *azotemic renovascular disease.* Regardless of whether hypertension and CKD are a direct consequence of the renovascular lesion, it is important to diagnose atherosclerotic RAS because clinical outcomes are significantly worse in such patients. It is essential to understand the natural history of untreated subjects and the underlying pathophysiology to plan for rational therapy.

NATURAL HISTORY OF UNTREATED PATIENTS

Fibromuscular dysplasia has numerous subtypes. The most common is medial fibroplasia, which is not normally progressive. Thus, the aim of therapy is to improve or cure hypertension rather than to prevent azotemic renovascular disease. Approximately half of carefully selected patients may be cured of hypertension by percutaneous transluminal renal angioplasty (PTRA) or reconstructive surgery.[11] In contrast, cure of hypertension after correction of RAS due to atherosclerosis occurs in less than 20% of patients.[12] Studies with duplex ultrasound measurements over 5 years reported progression of atherosclerotic RAS in more than one third of patients and complete occlusion in 3% to 15%.[13] Contemporary studies indicate that less than 10% to 15% of patients with RAS treated medically develop intractable hypertension, progressive renal insufficiency, or total arterial occlusion.[13–15] In fact, in contrast to early studies, which suggested that RAS was a frequent cause of end-stage renal disease (ESRD), patients with untreated RAS often have stable kidney function for many years; progression to ESRD is relatively uncommon.[16] Numerous observational studies[1,2] have shown that, after intervention with PTRA and stenting (PTRA-S) or reconstructive surgery, approximately 25% of patients have a worthwhile improvement in glomerular filtration rate (GFR) matched by a reduction in serum creatinine concentration and blood urea nitrogen (BUN), approximately 50% have a stable GFR, and approximately 20% have a deterioration in GFR. Outcomes in the three small prospective, randomized studies reported to date were inconclusive. In the Dutch Renal Artery Stenosis Intervention Cooperative (DRASTIC) trial, the largest study, the creatinine clearance was unchanged at 1 year both in patients treated medically and in those who were revascularized.[14] A recent comprehensive review of published series and trials concluded that available evidence fails to demonstrate that revascularization or medical therapy is the treatment of choice for atherosclerotic RAS.[5] Weak data suggest that mortality and cardiovascular event rates are similar for medically treated and revascularized patients. There is also a trend toward lower BP with angioplasty in patients with bilateral disease. However, this trend is based on very few patients, the data are more than 10 years old, and medical therapy has evolved significantly in that time. No study to date has compared aggressive medical therapy with revascularization. All of the studies in the review suffer from serious methodologic weakness. One observation that continues to drive clinical practice is that some patients appear to benefit either because of improvement in BP control or in kidney function. However, others deteriorate, either because of—or despite—the intervention. Published studies fail to adequately assess adverse events associated with revascularization.

These considerations give rise to the following suggestions regarding the choice of medical therapy or intervention:

1. Medical therapy is appropriate for patients with fibromuscular disease because it is not progressive and does not lead to significant loss of renal function. On the other hand, rates of cure of hypertension after intervention are high, and complications of PTRA-S (such as atheroembolism) are quite uncommon. Therefore, most patients with troublesome hypertension are offered an intervention, but this can be preceded by a prolonged trial of medical therapy.

2. Few patients with atherosclerotic RAS will benefit from intervention (see Chapter 58). It is reasonable to use medical therapy alone for atherosclerotic RAS, regardless of the level of kidney function, the presence of resistant hypertension, or episodes of congestive heart failure.

3. Whether or not an intervention is performed, all patients with RAS require intensive medical therapy to reduce the risk of adverse cardiovascular and renal events. This includes tight control of BP, administration of an antiplatelet agent, and treatment of any associated dyslipidemia, diabetes, or CKD.

4. In patients with resistant hypertension and atherosclerotic RAS, revascularization may be associated with a reduction in the number of medications needed to control BP, but almost all patients will continue to require some antihypertensive medications.

5. The small risk of progression to ESRD in patients with RAS is not predictably reduced by intervention. Nevertheless, it is reasonable to offer intervention to patients with progressive renal insufficiency and bilateral high-grade stenosis or high-grade unilateral stenosis to a solitary functioning kidney. Revascularization is unlikely to improve kidney function if the kidney distal to the stenosis is less than 7 to 8 cm in length or if the patient has impaired function in the setting of unilateral RAS. A renal biopsy in selected patients may help predict the response to revascularization.

PATHOPHYSIOLOGIC BASIS FOR THERAPY

Animal models provide some insight into what may be anticipated from medical therapy. The two-kidney, one-clip (2K,1C) Goldblatt rat model of unilateral RAS is characterized by an early rise in BP and plasma renin activity. Hypertension initially is entirely dependent on angiotensin II. It can be rapidly restored to normal by an angiotensin converting enzyme (ACE) inhibitor or an angiotensin receptor blocker (ARB). After 2 to 12 months, the BP increases further, and many rats perish from malignant hypertension. The remainder develop normal-renin hypertension complicated by vascular and renal damage. At this stage, acute administration of an ACE inhibitor or ARB does little to the BP. However, prolonged administration over 3 days can restore BP to a nearly normal level.[17]

The one-kidney, one-clip (1K,1C) Goldblatt model of bilateral RAS or stenosis of a single or dominant kidney is characterized by an early rise in BP. The plasma renin activity increases only if fluid retention is prevented. The hypertension depends on the combined effects of salt intake and angiotensin II.[18]

Human renovascular disease usually has components of both models. Therefore, therapy directed at an overactive renin-angiotensin system on the one hand, and inappropriate renal salt and water retention on the other, is usually required for full control of hypertension, but carries risks of adverse changes in renal function, as described in Chapter 52.

The role of angiotensin II in maintaining BP and renal hemodynamics in Goldblatt hypertension has been studied with the use of ARBs and ACE inhibitors.[18–20] As shown in Figure 57-1, compared with spontaneously hypertensive rats, an ACE inhibitor causes a larger fall in mean arterial pressure in 2K,1C Goldblatt rats.[19,20] The GFR and excretion of fluid and sodium ions increase with the ACE inhibitor in the contralateral kidney, but decrease in the postclipped kidney. There is an increase in renal blood flow (RBF) at the contralateral kidney but variable changes at the poststenotic kidney, according to how the BP falls. The filtration fraction falls quite sharply.

The renal microvessels downstream from a functionally significant RAS are under two dominant influences (Fig. 57-2). One is renal autoregulation—vasodilation, especially of the afferent but also of the efferent arterioles—that maintains RBF. The second is the release of renin from the juxtaglomerular cells in the afferent arteriole in response to decreased stretch and decreased sodium chloride delivery to the macula densa[21] (see Fig. 57-2). The ensuing increase in the generation of angiotensin I from angiotensinogen, and the action of ACE, increase the interstitial generation of angiotensin II in the kidney. Angiotensin II acts on angiotensin type 1 (AT$_1$) receptors to preferentially constrict the efferent arterioles, thereby maintaining a reasonable pressure for ultrafiltration at the glomerular capillaries despite a fall in mean arterial pressure. Therefore, an ACE inhibitor or an ARB may prevent an increase in efferent arteriolar resistance, leading to a fall in the pressure for ultrafiltration with a consequent fall in the GFR. However, RBF may be maintained because of a reduction in overall renal vascular resistance. These effects have been confirmed in studies of split renal function in patients with unilateral RAS.[22,23]

A recent study compared responses to an ACE inhibitor and an ARB in 1K,1C Goldblatt hypertensive rats.[24] Both lowered

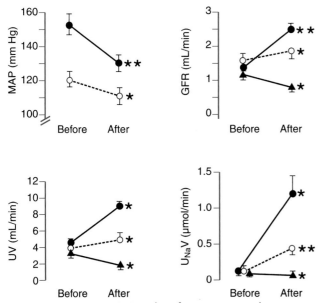

Figure 57-1 Mean ± SEM values for mean arterial pressure (MAP), renal excretion of fluid and sodium (UV, $U_{Na}V$), and glomerular filtration rate (GFR) in anesthetized rats. Data are shown for spontaneously hypertensive rats (*open symbols and broken lines*) and for rats with Goldblatt two-kidney, one-clip hypertension (*solid symbols and lines*) for the contralateral kidney (*solid circles*); and postclipped kidney (*solid triangles*). Each panel shows values before and after administration of an angiotensin converting enzyme inhibitor, compared to before *P < .05; **P < .01. (Drawn from data from Huang WC, Ploth DW, Bell PD, et al: Bilateral renal function responses to converting enzyme inhibitor (SQ 20,881) in two-kidney, one clip Goldblatt hypertensive rats. Hypertension 1981;3:285–293.)

the BP similarly, but the fall in GFR was greater with the ACE inhibitor, perhaps due to accumulation of bradykinin and its effects on the bradykinin type 2 receptor. A current study has contrasted the acute effects of an ACE inhibitor (enalaprilat) with an ARB (candesartan) in rats with early 2K,1C hypertension.[25] Whereas the ACE inhibitor reduced renal cortical blood flow and oxygen tension and actually increased the renal vascular resistance, the ARB did not cause these perturbations. Of interest was the finding that blockade of angiotensin type 2 (AT_2) receptors produced effects similar to those of the ACE inhibitor on renal hemodynamics and oxygenation. The authors concluded that angiotensin II can have a paradoxical effect by its action on AT_2 receptors in the poststenotic kidney, maintaining blood flow and oxygenation. Further analysis in this model demonstrated that these beneficial effects of AT_2 receptors in the postclipped kidney are due to generation of nitric oxide from nitric oxide synthase. Although these results have yet to be confirmed clinically, they suggest the possibility of some advantage of ARBs over ACE inhibitors in patients with renovascular disease who experience a reduction in GFR during treatment.

Calcium channel blockers (CCBs) administered to animals with angiotensin-induced hypertension reduce BP and renal vascular resistance substantially. However, in contrast to ACE inhibitors and ARBs, CCBs increase the GFR.[26] This is attributed to a preferential effect on vasodilation of afferent—rather than efferent—arterioles because of selective distribution of voltage-gated calcium channels to the afferent arteriole[27] (see Fig. 57-2). These effects of CCBs have been confirmed in studies of split renal function in patients with renovascular hypertension.[22]

ACE inhibitors and CCBs should have contrasting effects on glomerular hemodynamics in the clipped kidney. Two studies compared therapy with ACE inhibitors and CCBs in Goldblatt hypertensive rats over 5 to 6 weeks.[28,29] ACE inhibitor

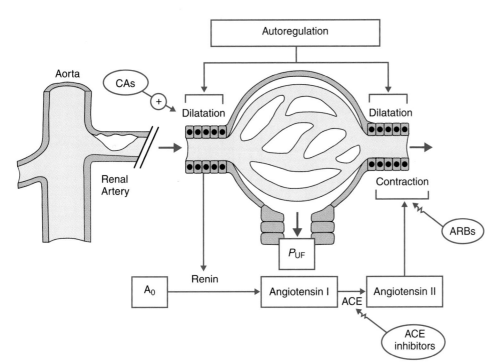

Figure 57-2 Diagrammatic representation of factors affecting the pressure for ultrafiltration (P_{Uf}) in the glomerulus downstream from a functional renal artery stenosis. Autoregulation leads to vasodilation of the afferent and efferent arterioles. Afferent arteriolar vasodilation is further enhanced by a calcium antagonist (CA). Renin release from the afferent arteriole acts on angiotensinogen (A_0) to form angiotensin I, which, after action by angiotensin-converting enzyme (ACE), forms angiotensin II. Angiotensin II preferentially constricts the efferent arteriole. ACE inhibitors or angiotensin receptor blockers prevent these effects of angiotensin II on type 1 receptors and reduce the P_{Uf}.

therapy prevented glomerular hypertrophy and glomerular sclerosis in the contralateral kidney, whereas CCB therapy worsened these changes.[28] Only the ACE inhibitor reduced proteinuria from the clipped kidney.[29] Interestingly, the CCB worsened the lesions in the clipped kidney to the same extent as the ACE inhibitor.[29] These data suggest the possibility of a trade-off: ACE inhibitor therapy may reduce the GFR, and perhaps enhance irreversible atrophy in the poststenotic kidney, but may improve function in the contralateral kidney through better antihypertensive action, better control of glomerular capillary hypertension, and prevention of the fibrotic and sclerotic effects of angiotensin II. The role of ARBs and CCBs in therapy is not yet clear.

Further insight into potential therapeutic differences between ACE inhibitors and ARBs on the one hand, and vasodilators or CCBs on the other, comes from longer-term studies. In the 2K,1C model, both minoxidil, a vasodilator, and enalapril, an ACE inhibitor, compared with no treatment, reduced the BP, although the ACE inhibitor was more effective (Fig. 57-3). After 1 year, the postclipped kidney of the ACE inhibitor–treated rats was atrophic and had no residual function, but that of the minoxidil-treated rats that survived retained some residual GFR. This led to the concept of *pharmacologic nephrectomy* with ACE inhibitors.[30] This adverse effect of ACE inhibitors was, however, offset by two benefits. First, there was a significant increase in the GFR of the contralateral kidney with the ACE inhibitor, but not with the vasodilator. This resulted in an overall GFR of animals treated with an ACE inhibitor that was better preserved than those treated with minoxidil. Second, the 1-year survival was 15% in untreated rats, 48% in minoxidil-treated rats, and 84% in ACE inhibitor–treated rats. This study poses very elegantly the clinical dilemma: can a loss of GFR, with potential structural atrophy of the postclipped kidney during ACE inhibitor therapy, be considered a reasonable trade-off for improved function of the contralateral kidney, overall better BP control, and better cardiovascular survival? These issues are discussed in this chapter in the context of data from human subjects with renovascular disease (see "Specific Agents," in this chapter).

Clinical studies have shown that there is a critical level of vascular occlusion beyond which the RBF and GFR fall with any further reduction in BP because the renal perfusion pressure is below autoregulatory limits.[31,32] Revascularization can restore the ability of such kidneys to tolerate a reduction of BP to normal levels. The report of the Joint National Commission (JNC)[33] explicitly recognizes the potential for BP reduction to slow renal disease progression. It sets reduced goals (<130/75 mm Hg) for BP reduction in azotemic patients with proteinuria. However, a reduction of systemic pressures in patients with critical renal artery stenosis can cause a sharp fall in GFR, regardless of the type of antihypertensive agent used. Hence, chronic azotemic renovascular disease must be considered before vigorous BP reduction to low target goals is undertaken in patients with renal disease.

Atherosclerotic Renal Artery Stenosis, Comorbidities, and Clinical Outcomes

Atherosclerotic RAS is closely associated with hypertension, CKD, and vascular disease in other beds, including coronary artery disease, cerebrovascular disease, and peripheral vascular disease. Kalra and colleagues[9] performed a retrospective analysis of patients with renal vascular disease in the U.S. Medicare population using a random sample of Medicare patients without RAS as controls. Results shown in Table 57-1 demonstrate a markedly greater prevalence and relative risk of CKD and other vascular disease in patients with RAS. Somewhat surprising, several other conditions thought to be highly associated with atherosclerotic RAS were in fact not more common than in controls. Thus, although quite prevalent, both congestive heart failure and diabetes mellitus had relative risks of 1 or less in patients with RAS after adjusting for other known risk factors and comorbidities.

Patients with RAS have worse outcomes from cardiovascular disease. In a large group of patients in whom renal arteriography was performed at the time of cardiac catheterization,

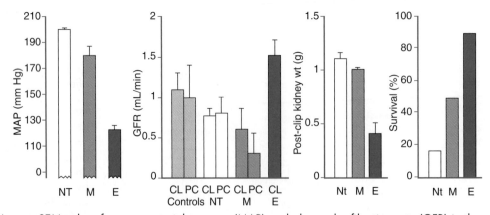

Figure 57-3 Mean ± SEM values for mean arterial pressure (MAP) and glomerular filtration rate (GFR) in the contralateral (CL) and postclipped (PC) kidneys, the weight of the PC kidney, and number of animals surviving for control (Cont), and two-kidney, one-clip Goldblatt hypertensive rats given for 1 year either no treatment (NT), a vasodilator (minoxidil, M), or an angiotensin-converting enzyme inhibitor (enalapril, E). (Drawn from data by Jackson B, Franze L, Sumithran E, Johnston CI: Pharmacologic nephrectomy with chronic angiotensin converting enzyme inhibitor treatment in renovascular hypertension in the rat. J Lab Clin Med 1990;115:21–27.

Table 57-1 Prevalence and Relative Risk of Hypertension, Chronic Kidney Disease, Other Vascular Disease, Congestive Heart Failure, and Diabetes in Medicare Patients with Atherosclerotic RAS

Comorbid Condition	No RAS N = 1,085,250 (%)	With RAS N = 5875 (%)	Adjusted Odds Ratio	P Value
Hypertension	53.4	90.8	4.31 (3.93–4.73)	<.0001
Chronic kidney disease	2.3	24.6	4.61 (4.27–4.98)	<.0001
Coronary artery disease	24.9	66.8	2.45 (2.30–2.61)	<.0001
CVA or TIA	12.0	36.9	1.58 (1.49–1.67)	<.0001
Peripheral vascular disease	12.7	56.0	3.96 (3.74–4.20)	<.0001
Aortic aneurysm	0.5	6.4	3.38 (3.00–3.81)	<.0001
Congestive heart failure	13.6	37.6	1.01 (0.94–1.07)	.9
Diabetes mellitus	17.9	32.5	0.89 (0.84–0.95)	.0001

CVA, cerebrovascular accident; TIA, transient ischemic attack
Adjusted odds ratio was calculated using a multiple logistic regression model that included multiple variables, including all those shown in the first column. Data from Kalra PA, Guo H, Kausz AT, et al: Atherosclerotic renovascular disease in United States patients aged 67 years or older: Risk factors, revascularization, and prognosis. Kidney Int 2005;68:293–301.

those with RAS had a much higher incidence of adverse cardiovascular events.[34] Furthermore, there was a direct correlation between the degree of stenosis and survival. Patients with renal artery narrowings greater than 95% had only about a 40% 4-year survival, as compared to 80% in those with normal arteries. These findings were independent of whether the patients underwent revascularization. In a cohort of almost 900 patients older than age 65 followed prospectively, the presence of RAS detected by duplex ultrasonography was associated with 1.96 (95% confidence interval, 1.00–3.83; $P = .05$) increased risk of an adverse coronary event after adjusting for demographics, prevalent cardiovascular disease, and traditional cardiovascular risk factors. The explanation for the increased risk of cardiovascular events in RAS is uncertain but may relate to concomitant atherosclerosis in other vascular beds.[35–41] Alternatively, neuroendocrine systems activated by renal ischemia may lead to deleterious cardiovascular and renal outcomes. Angiotensin II has direct adverse effects on multiple tissues[42–50] that may persist even when BP is controlled.[51] Renal dysfunction itself is associated with increased rates of cardiovascular events[52–55] and cardiovascular mortality.[56,57] This is particularly true for patients with RAS.[58,59] Renal ischemia may lead to neuroendocrine activation, hypertension, and renal insufficiency, which may accelerate atherosclerosis and promote thrombosis, renal dysfunction, and left ventricular hypertrophy. These may hasten the onset of congestive heart failure, myocardial infarction, stroke, progressive renal insufficiency, and ultimately death. Therefore, clinical outcomes may depend on the extent to which specific pathways, such as the renin-angiotensin-aldosterone system, are interrupted, and on preserving kidney function, which requires drug therapy and sometimes intervention.

Treatment has the following aims: (1) to control BP to recommended targets, (2) to improve or preserve kidney function, and (3) to treat common comorbidities and prevent adverse cardiovascular events.

OUTCOMES AND GOALS OF MEDICAL THERAPY

Three controlled trials and many observational trials have compared the outcomes of patients treated medically with those treated by intervention.[5,6,14,60] In contrast, no controlled trials have examined specific medical therapies for renovascular disease. Consequently, the optimal medical management of patients with RAS has not been established. Nevertheless, extrapolations of data from other populations suggest that standard medical interventions should produce significant reductions in cardiovascular event rates. By analogy to patients with vascular disease in other beds, medical therapy should include BP control to standard targets with a regimen that includes an agent that inhibits the renin-angiotensin-aldosterone system if tolerated. Cholesterol management to the low target recommended for patients with vascular disease, antiplatelet therapy, tight glycemic control in diabetic patients, smoking cessation, and treatment of the complications of CKD, including anemia and secondary hyperparathyroidism, are recommended.

Hypertension

The optimal target BP for patients with RAS has not been established. However, by extension from other populations, a BP of no more than 140/90 mm Hg is suggested for patients without other comorbidities, and no more than 130/80 mm Hg for those with diabetes, or with CKD and proteinuria above 1 g/day.

Three groups performed controlled trials in which patients were randomized to receive medical therapy or intervention with PTRA.[14,60] Blood pressure was measured with automated devices. Each group concluded that patients randomized to intervention had a similar reduction in BP as those randomized to medical therapy, although those receiving the intervention required on average about one less antihypertensive drug.[14,60] Apparently, modern antihypertensive drug therapy given under protocol conditions is effective in controlling hypertension in the majority of patients with renovascular disease. These trials were relatively short-term (6–12 months). They provide no compelling evidence for intervention to control BP. However, it has yet to be determined whether these conclusions will hold over a longer period, whether reductions in BP achieved by medical therapy versus revascularization are equally effective in preventing adverse cardiovascular and renal events, and whether the choice of antihypertensive agent will influence the outcome.

Specific Agents

No controlled trials have been performed in patients with renovascular disease comparing classes of antihypertensive agents.

Angiotensin-Converting Enzyme Inhibitors and Angiotensin Receptor Blockers

Three groups measured the BP of patients with renovascular hypertension during steady-state treatment with an ACE inhibitor and compared it with BP recorded after intervention by PTRA or reconstructive surgery.[61] There was a close correlation between the systolic and diastolic BP achieved by these two forms of treatment. This implies that medical therapy with an ACE inhibitor is generally as effective in controlling hypertension as interventions. When these agents are given to patients with essential hypertension, they normally increase the GFR and block the sodium and fluid retention that normally accompanies a fall in BP. On the other hand, they can cause a sharp fall in GFR in some patients with chronic renal failure due to polycystic kidney disease[62] or nephrosclerosis[63] when given with salt-depleting therapy. When given to patients with renovascular hypertension, they can reduce the GFR in the poststenotic kidney.[22,64–67] There may be unacceptable worsening of azotemia if these drugs are given to patients with bilateral RAS or stenosis of a single or dominant kidney. Although many cases of acute renal failure have been reported, the risk is relatively low; renal function usually returns to baseline with cessation of the inciting drug. In patients with hypertension and CKD with or without RAS, a sharp fall in BP produced by any antihypertensive drug may be associated with a significant decline in GFR, at least in the first few weeks or months of treatment.[31,68] Even the effects of angiotensin II on enhancing efferent arteriolar resistance cannot maintain the pressure for ultrafiltration of the glomerular capillaries in the presence of a tight stenosis and a sharp fall in arterial pressure.

Van de Ven and colleagues[69] studied 108 patients at high risk for renovascular disease. All patients received a 2-week course of ACE inhibitor therapy. This increased the serum creatinine level by more than 20% in all 52 patients with severe bilateral RAS when volume retention was prevented by diuretic therapy. These authors proposed that a reversible increase in serum creatinine could be used as a safe clinical test for bilateral renovascular disease. These interesting results also show that caution is needed when using ACE inhibitors in patients with bilateral RAS and azotemia, especially during diuretic therapy.

Long-term studies over 6 to 24 months in a small number of patients with renovascular disease have shown that ACE inhibitor therapy is effective in reducing or normalizing BP and does not lead (in the group as a whole) to a progressive deterioration in renal function or to a decrease in size of the poststenotic kidney.[70,71] In a worldwide study of 269 patients treated with captopril, 40% were azotemic before therapy; a similar fraction had either a solitary kidney or advanced bilateral renovascular disease.[72] Even within this latter group, clinically significant renal failure during captopril therapy developed in only 12%. Overall, there was good control of BP.

In another study, 75 patients with renovascular hypertension were randomized to triple therapy (hydrochlorothiazide, β-blocker, and hydralazine) or to an ACE inhibitor and a diuretic. Antihypertensive control was clearly better in the group given an ACE inhibitor plus diuretic; some 80% of this group maintained their GFR over a mean follow-up period of 7.5 months. However, 10 patients—mostly with very high-grade RAS—had a deterioration of renal function.[73]

In a 4-year study of patients with renovascular hypertension, Losito and colleagues[74] found a cumulative survival of only 60%. Cerebrovascular and cardiovascular disease caused 92% of these deaths. A multivariate analysis identified treatment with ACE inhibitors as the only factor associated with significantly better survival. Their observational data highlights once more the dilemma facing physicians using medical therapy for renovascular disease. Do the benefits from better control of hypertension and prevention of associated cardiovascular disease with ACE inhibitors or ARBs outweigh the possibility of a reduction in the GFR of the poststenotic kidney?

An important issue is whether a reduction in the GFR of a poststenotic kidney during long-term ACE inhibitor treatment for RAS leads to irreversible renal atrophy, as in the animal model.[30] In a study of split renal function in six patients with RAS, Miyamori and colleagues[75] reported the individual kidney responses to 1 week and 1 year of captopril therapy (Fig. 57-4). After 1 week, the GFR of the poststenotic kidney was reduced, but renal plasma flow to the two kidneys was maintained or increased. These changes remained stable over 1 year. This study is reassuring because it shows that progressive loss of GFR leading to renal atrophy is quite unlikely in RAS patients treated with ACE inhibitors. However, this conclusion may not hold for patients with high-grade RAS.

Another potentially important consideration is the effects of renin-angiotensin-aldosterone system blockade on the nonstenotic kidney in patients with unilateral RAS. Clinical and experimental data in patients with hypertension and CKD from other causes suggest that ACE inhibitors and ARBs often improve renal outcomes, and these data may be relevant to effects on the nonstenotic kidney in patients with unilateral RAS. Theoretically, reducing the glomerular pressure with these drugs should be associated with better preservation of structure and function in the nonstenotic kidney and, therefore, equivalent or better long-term preservation of total kidney function. The use of ACE inhibitors and ARBs in hypertension is discussed in Chapter 52.

Diuretics

Renovascular disease is a high-renin state. It has been considered resistant to diuretic therapy. However, there are good reasons for selecting a diuretic with dietary salt restriction as a first-line therapy for many patients. The poststenotic kidney has sharply reduced perfusion pressure, which is a powerful stimulus for salt and water retention. The contralateral kidney, although perfused at high pressure, is under the influence of unusually high levels of circulating angiotensin II and aldoste-

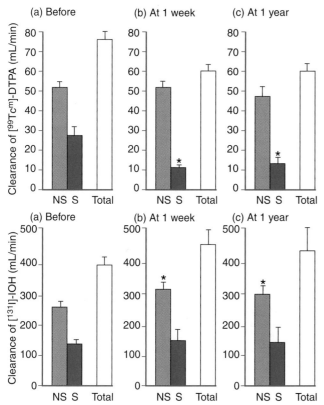

Figure 57-4 Mean ± SEM values from four patients with unilateral renal artery stenosis studied (a) before, (b) 1 week after, and (c) 1 year after starting therapy with captopril. Using split renal function for glomerular filtration rate and effective renal plasma flow, data were obtained for the overall function (Total) and individual functions in the nonstenotic (NS) and stenotic (S) kidneys. Compared with before *P < .05. (After Miyamori I, Yasuhara S, Takeda Y, et al: Effects of converting enzyme inhibition on split renal function in renovascular hypertension. Hypertension 1986;8:415–421.)

rone. Its pressure natriuresis mechanism is also reset to favor salt retention. Moreover, the contralateral kidney may be damaged by nephrosclerosis or may develop a stenosis of its artery, which will leave no normal kidney to regulate salt balance. Severe and unpredictable episodes of primary renal salt and fluid retention can occur, leading to overflow flash pulmonary edema.[76] Diuretics and salt restriction enhance the antihypertensive response to all other medical therapies, except perhaps CCBs. For these reasons, dietary salt should be restricted and a diuretic used at an early stage in most treatment regimens. Because diuretics cause a further stimulation of plasma renin activity, with enhancement of angiotensin II and aldosterone, additional measures to combat renin secretion or inhibit its effects are usually necessary. Renin secretion can be inhibited by a β-blocker, and the effects of angiotensin II and aldosterone blunted by an ACE inhibitor, ARB, spironolactone, or eplerenone.

Dietary salt restriction and diuretics have little effect on the GFR of normal subjects.[77] However, in patients with renal disease and hypertension, such treatment often reduces the GFR—at least initially.[78] Therefore, some increase in serum creatinine and BUN after initiating diuretic therapy should be anticipated. Diuretic therapy for hypertension is discussed in Chapter 51.

β-Blockers

β-Blockers are most effective in patients with high-renin hypertension. Thus, these are a rational treatment for renovascular hypertension. Moreover, β-blockers inhibit renin secretion powerfully,[79] so it is rational to combine β-blockers with diuretics to prevent the further rise in plasma renin activity that would otherwise occur. β-Blockers are strongly indicated in patients with angina or with prior myocardial infarction. β-Blocker therapy for hypertension is discussed in Chapter 51.

Central Agents and α-Blockers

Central agents such as clonidine, or peripheral α- and β-blockers such as labetalol or carvedilol, are effective in hypertension that is associated with increased sympathetic drive. During renovascular or renal parenchymal hypertension, there is increased neural input from the affected kidney, which engages a central sympathetic drive that maintains the hypertension.[80] Therefore, the use of these agents is rational, and usually effective as adjunctive treatment for more severe forms of renovascular disease. Comparison of the short-term response to clonidine and an ACE inhibitor in patients with renovascular disease shows that both agents reduce the BP, although the ACE inhibitor is more effective.[64] However, the ACE inhibitor reduces the GFR in the poststenotic kidney, whereas this remains stable with clonidine.

Calcium Channel Blockers

Calcium channel blockers reverse the hypertension and renal vasoconstriction associated with prolonged angiotensin II infusion and selectively vasodilate the afferent arteriole.[26] They should, therefore, be ideal for patients with renovascular disease by controlling hypertension without compromising GFR in the poststenotic kidney, which is prevented from barotrauma by the upstream stenosis. Moreover, they have mild natriuretic actions and can blunt the aldosterone response to angiotensin II.[81] Their role in treatment is not yet clear. The effects of CCBs seen in animal models are confirmed in acute studies of patients with renovascular disease. In studies of patients with RAS[65] or postrenal transplant stenosis,[66] the GFR in the poststenotic kidney is reduced by ACE inhibitors but unchanged by CCBs. During longer-term studies in patients with unilateral RAS, both ACE inhibitors and CCBs reduce the blood pressure and increase the RBF in the contralateral kidney.[22] The total GFR is not affected significantly by either treatment, but the GFR of the poststenotic kidney is reduced by 54% during ACE inhibitor therapy, compared to only 21% during CCB therapy. Hence, there can be a relative sparing of the GFR of the poststenotic kidney with a CCB. Therefore, CCBs are indicated in patients with renovascular hypertension when renal function is already compromised or has been unacceptably reduced by an ACE inhibitor or ARB. Moreover, CCBs can be used in azotemia without modification of the dosage. Further study is needed on the role of CCBs in long-term management of patients with renovascular disease. CCB therapy for hypertension is discussed in Chapter 53.

Renal Function

In general, trials that have compared an intervention by PTRA alone or combined with stenting (PTRA-S) with medical therapy have failed to show statistically significant differences in renal function at follow-up.[1,2] On the other hand, case series[82] describe patients with global renal ischemia and progressive renal impairment in whom renal function is stabilized or improved after PTRA-S, suggesting that patients with documented progression of renal insufficiency may benefit from revascularization. In a large case series of patients with RAS and elevated levels of serum creatinine who underwent surgical revascularization and were followed for at least 3 years, 25% had an improvement in kidney function, it was unchanged in about half, and 20% experienced a significant worsening in function. Without a control group for comparison, it is unclear how patients would have fared if they had been treated medically. However, improvements in kidney function are rarely seen in medically treated patients. Nevertheless, for the group as a whole, there was little net benefit of revascularization on kidney function.

To date, only one controlled trial, by van Jaarsveld and colleagues,[14] has compared the renal function of patients randomized to medical therapy or PTRA, examining approximately 100 patients over 1 year. At completion there were no differences in creatinine clearance between the two groups, leading to the conclusion that there was no clear benefit of PTRA over medical therapy. However, closer inspection highlights problems with this study that make it difficult to interpret. Some 44% of the patients randomized to medical therapy were subsequently referred for PTRA during the 1 year of study because they were felt not to have responded adequately to medical therapy. These crossover patients were nevertheless analyzed with the medical treatment group, thereby very seriously confounding the interpretation of the results. Of concern, 12% of patients in the medical treatment group suffered complete occlusion of a renal artery, and twice as many suffered a significant decline in renal function, as indicated by a doubling of serum creatinine level or a need for hemodialysis. This trial included patients with refractory hypertension and an RAS of more than 50%. Recent studies show clearly that a narrowing of 75% to 80% is required to produce renovascular disease.[8] Thus, many patients in this study may not have had functional renovascular disease and therefore could not have benefited from therapy. However, similar outcomes for renal function after treatment with medical therapy or interventions lead to the conclusion that medical therapy is an acceptable choice for patients with RAS and CKD, at least in the short term. Medical therapy is less expensive and less likely to produce serious short-term adverse effects, such as atheroembolic disease or contrast nephropathy.[60]

Many patients with RAS have renal insufficiency that may progress over time. Elevation in serum creatinine is a relatively insensitive marker for reductions in GFR in elderly patients. A formula such as the one derived from the Modification of Diet in Renal Disease (MDRD) study should be used to estimate GFR more accurately in affected patients. If renal functional impairment is present, practitioners should follow the guidelines established by the National Kidney Foundation Kidney Disease Quality Initiatives (DOQI). Treatment of hypertension, diabetes, and lipid disorders are specifically addressed elsewhere in this chapter. Dietary modifications and vitamin supplements, as outlined in the DOQI guidelines, may be needed as GFR declines. Anemia commonly develops as renal disease progresses, even before the need for renal replacement therapy. This should be treated with erythropoeitin or a related analogue when the hemoglobin falls below approximately 11 g/dL.[83] Many patients also require either oral or parenteral iron supplements once therapy with erythropoeitin is initiated.

COMMON COMORBIDITIES AND ADVERSE CARDIOVASCULAR EVENTS

Dyslipidemia

Data suggest that therapy that reduces low-density lipoprotein (LDL) cholesterol reduces total mortality, cardiovascular mortality, major cardiovascular events, and strokes in persons with established coronary artery disease. No specific evidence exists for treatment of LDL cholesterol in patients with RAS. However, according to the established guidelines, RAS should be considered a coronary artery disease equivalent for cardiovascular risk. Therefore, as in patients with established coronary artery disease, an LDL cholesterol below 70 mg/dL is the goal of therapy.[84,85] This goal should be accompanied by therapeutic lifestyle changes, including diet and exercise. However, if these measures fail, patients should be started on one or more lipid-lowering medications, including statins, nicotinic acids, or fibrates (see Chapters 56 and 63).

Diabetes Mellitus

Of the patients with atherosclerotic RAS, approximately 20% to 30% will have diabetes, predominantly type 2 diabetes. In addition to controlling BP to a lower target than recommended in hypertensive patients without diabetes, evidence-based guidelines regarding glucose control should be followed (see Chapter 28). Clear evidence suggests that tight glucose control to an HbA$_{1c}$ of less than 7% is associated with reductions in microvascular and macrovascular complications in both type 1 and type 2 diabetes.[86,87] Additionally, medical nutrition therapy, multidisciplinary foot care (particularly for patients with peripheral vascular disease), eye care to prevent and treat diabetic retinopathy, and physical activity are recommended.

Smoking

Smoking is common among patients with RAS. Cessation is an important, but underemphasized, component of therapy for these patients. Smoking triggers vascular spasm, reduces the anti-ischemic and antihypertensive effects of β-blockers, and increases mortality after acute myocardial infarction. Smoking may accelerate the course of RAS by promotion of atherosclerosis and cholesterol emboli. Smoking worsens atherosclerotic disease in normotensive, nondiabetic, elderly patients with normal GFR. This is associated with a lower renal plasma flow, which likely results from ischemic nephropathy.[88] Smoking cessation reduces progression of vascular disease and the rates of reinfarction and death within 1 year after quitting. Unfortunately, many patients who quit smoking relapse within 6 to 12 months. Practitioners treating patients with RAS should adopt an aggressive approach to encourage and assist patients in smoking cessation (see Chapter 56).

Antiplatelet Agents

The long-term use of aspirin in patients with hypertension and those who have had a myocardial infarction is associated with a significant reduction in subsequent cardiovascular events and mortality.[89] In a meta-analysis of randomized, controlled trials in patients 1 week to 7 years after a myocardial infarction, those receiving aspirin experienced a 13% reduction in mortality, a

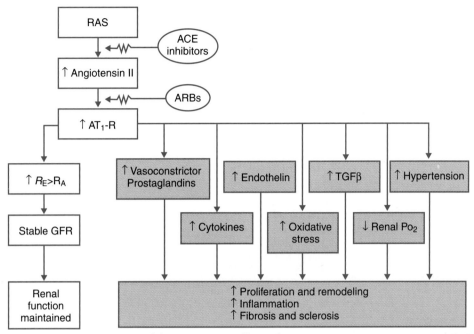

Figure 57-5 A diagrammatic representation of the contrasting effects of angiotensin-converting enzyme (ACE) inhibitor or angiotensin receptor blocker (ARB) therapy in patients with renovascular disease. Such therapy reduces the glomerular filtration rate (GFR) due to the effect of angiotensin II, increasing resistance of the efferent arteriole (R_E) compared to the afferent arteriole (R_A) of the poststenotic kidney. However, it counteracts many of the adverse mediators generated in response to angiotensin II action on type 1 receptors (AT_1-R) in blood vessels and kidneys. These include endothelin, vasoconstrictor prostaglandins, transforming growth factor-β (TGF-β), and numerous cytokines, as well as physiologic changes related to hypertension, hypoxia, and oxidative stress.

31% reduction in nonfatal reinfarction, and a 42% decline in nonfatal stroke.[90] Although these trials involved the use of aspirin in doses ranging from 300 to 1500 mg/day, a trial of 75 mg/day in patients with hypertension demonstrated a significant 15% reduction in cardiovascular events.[91] This suggests that, even though there are no direct data in patients with RAS, long-term administration of aspirin in a dose as low as 75 mg/day is effective and should be recommended to patients with RAS. Thienopyridines such as clopidogrel or ticlopidine may also be useful for the prevention of cardiovascular events, either as alternatives or in addition to aspirin.

CONCLUSIONS AND RECOMMENDATIONS

Although the studies are small and suffer from methodologic flaws, controlled clinical trials in patients with RAS have not shown any particular benefit of intervention over medical management for short-term changes in BP or renal function.[14,60] Therefore, medical management is a reasonable choice for most patients with newly diagnosed renovascular disease. It is important to recognize that patients with atherosclerotic RAS are a high-risk group with poor outcomes, primarily due to adverse cardiovascular events. Therefore, regardless of whether an intervention is performed, all patients with atherosclerotic RAS require multifaceted medical intervention aimed at reducing their cardiovascular risk.

No long-term comparisons have been made between specific antihypertensive drugs in patients with renovascular disease. Therefore, definite, evidence-based recommendations cannot be made. Nevertheless, as in other forms of hypertension, many patients benefit from a reduction in dietary salt intake and a low dose of diuretic. A reasonable goal for daily dietary salt intake is 100 mmol. The level of sodium intake can be assessed from the level of sodium excretion in a 24-hour urine collection. Data from a variety of studies in other settings suggest that blocking the renin-angiotensin-aldosterone system is beneficial both to slow progression of chronic renal disease and reduce cardiovascular risk. Case series suggest that ACE inhibitors or ARBs can be safely administered to patients with hypertension and RAS, often produce marked declines in BP, and may even improve clinical outcomes. Therefore, it is suggested that these drugs be included in the antihypertensive regimen for such patients. The small risk of severe acute renal failure in patients with bilateral high-grade RAS developing during renin system intervention mandates that serum creatinine, and serum potassium should be closely monitored after initiation of an ACE inhibitor or an ARB in this population. An early adverse change in renal function is not necessarily grounds to discontinue treatment. In any patient with an abrupt fall in BP, there may be a temporary decline in GFR with a rise of serum creatinine and BUN. This usually amounts to no more than a 20% to 30% increase, peaks in 3 to 7 days, and returns to baseline over the following few weeks or months of therapy. The trade-off hypothesis for beneficial and adverse effects of therapy in patients with renovascular hypertension is summarized in Figure 57-5.

Additional therapies depend on the clinical circumstances, concurrent disease, and identified cardiovascular risk factors

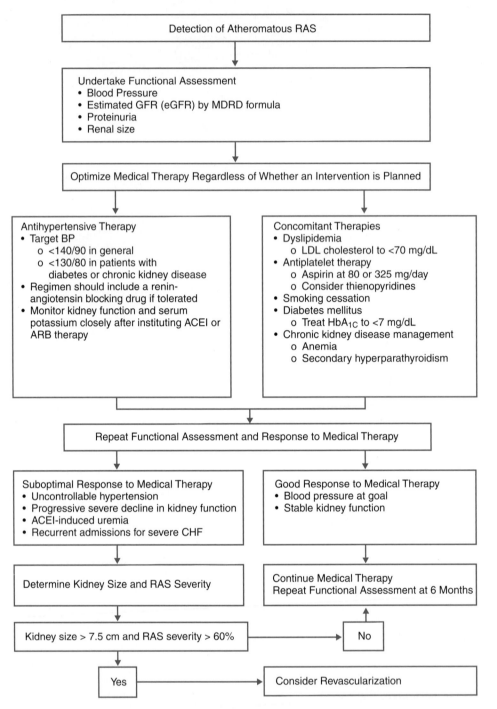

Figure 57-6 An algorithm for the approach to medical management of patients with renovascular disease. ACEI, angiotensin-converting enzyme inhibitor; ARB, angiotensin receptor blocker; BP, blood pressure; CHF, congestive heart failure; GFR, glomerular filtration rate; LDL, low-density lipoprotein; MDRD, Modification of Diet in Renal Disease; RAS, renal artery stenosis.

(see Chapter 56). All patients require a lipid profile with correction of any identified increases in LDL cholesterol and lipoprotein(a) with appropriate use of statins, slow-release nicotinic acid, or other treatments (see Chapter 63). A low target for LDL cholesterol, such as 70 mg/dL, is indicated because the cardiovascular risk for patients with peripheral vascular disease or RAS is roughly equivalent to those with documented coronary artery disease. Consideration should be given to all patients for lifelong therapy with aspirin, at least in low doses (e.g., 80 mg once daily). The use of high-dose aspirin or other antiplatelet agents should also be considered. If the patient is a current smoker, a therapeutic antismoking program must be a high priority. Other rational recommendations include three to four periods of exercise of 20 to 30 minutes each week, a diet to limit intake of saturated fats and salt and, if necessary, a lower body weight.

Nontraditional cardiovascular risk factors have been identified in patients with renal insufficiency.[92] These include hyperhomocysteinemia, oxidative stress, and nitric oxide deficiency related to accumulation of asymmetric dimethyl arginine[93,94] (see Chapters 56, 64, and 65). The complications of chronic renal disease or diabetes, if present, should be treated according to published guidelines.

Patients who are established on medical therapy who do not have evidence of functional deterioration can often be managed by continued therapy under close medical supervision with regular quantitative assessments, as indicated in Figure 57-6. Those who receive intervention with PTRA, PTRA-S, or reconstructive surgery also require close follow-up using similar quantitative measures, because there is approximately a 20% rate of restenosis, even in those treated by stenting, and a significant probability of developing a stenosis in the contralateral kidney.

A group of patients exists who either cannot be controlled adequately by medical therapy or who experience dangerous complications, such as recurrent flash pulmonary edema. Others have less to lose from a failed intervention, namely those who are already receiving dialysis therapy or are very close to ESRD. These patients may benefit from an intervention with PTRA, PTRA-S, or reconstructive surgery. (This is discussed further in Chapter 58.)

The individual steps in the algorithm shown in Figure 57-6 have not been subjected to properly controlled clinical trials. Therefore, they represent only an attempt at providing rational advice.

References

1. Textor SC, Wilcox CS: Ischemic nephropathy/azotemic renovascular disease. Semin Nephrol 2000;20:489–502.
2. Textor SC, Wilcox CS: Renal artery stenosis: A common, treatable cause of renal failure? Annu Rev Med 2001;52:421–442.
3. Textor SC: Epidemiology and clinical presentation. Semin Nephrol 2000;20:426–431.
4. Levin A, Linas S, Luft FC, et al: Controversies in renal artery stenosis: A review by the American Society of Nephrology Advisory Group on Hypertension. Am J Nephrol 2007;27:212–220.
5. Balk E, Raman G, Chung M, et al: Effectiveness of management strategies for renal artery stenosis: A systematic review. Ann Intern Med 2006;145:901–912.
6. Dworkin LD, Jamerson KA: Is renal artery stenting the correct treatment of renal artery stenosis? Case against angioplasty and stenting of atherosclerotic renal artery stenosis. Circulation 2007;115:271–276.
7. Dworkin LD: Controversial treatment of atherosclerotic renal vascular disease: The cardiovascular outcomes in renal atherosclerotic lesions trial. Hypertension 2006;48:350–356.
8. Simon G: What is critical renal artery stenosis? Implications for treatment. Am J Hypertens 2000;13:1189–1193.
9. Kalra PA, Guo H, Kausz AT, et al: Atherosclerotic renovascular disease in United States patients aged 67 years or older: Risk factors, revascularization, and prognosis. Kidney Int 2005;68:293–301.
10. Hansen KJ, Edwards MS, Craven TE, et al: Prevalence of renovascular disease in the elderly: A population-based study. J Vasc Surg 2002;36:443–451.
11. Davidson RA, Barri Y, Wilcox CS: Predictors of cure of hypertension in fibromuscular renovascular disease. Am J Kidney Dis 1996;28:334–338.
12. Barri YM, Davidson RA, Senler S, et al: Prediction of cure of hypertension in atherosclerotic renal artery stenosis. South Med J 1996;89:679–683.
13. Caps MT, Zierler RE, Polissar NL, et al: Risk of atrophy in kidneys with atherosclerotic renal artery stenosis. Kidney Int 1998;53:735–742.
14. van Jaarsveld BC, Krijnen P, Pieterman H, et al: The effect of balloon angioplasty on hypertension in atherosclerotic renal-artery stenosis. Dutch Renal Artery Stenosis Intervention Cooperative (DRASTIC) Study Group. N Engl J Med 2000;342:1007–1014.
15. Chabova V, Schirger A, Stanson AW, et al: Outcomes of atherosclerotic renal artery stenosis managed without revascularization. Mayo Clin Proc 2000;75:437–444.
16. Leertouwer TC, Pattynama PM, van den Berg-Huysmans A: Incidental renal artery stenosis in peripheral vascular disease: A case for treatment? Kidney Int 2001;59:1480–1483.
17. Wilcox CS, Cardozo J, Welch WJ: AT1 and TxA2/PGH2 receptors maintain hypertension throughout 2K,1C Goldblatt hypertension in the rat. Am J Physiol 1996;271(4 Pt 2):R891–R896.
18. Ploth DW: Angiotensin-dependent renal mechanisms in two-kidney, one-clip renal vascular hypertension. Am J Physiol 1983;245:F131–F141.
19. Huang WC, Ploth DW, Bell PD, et al: Bilateral renal function responses to converting enzyme inhibitor (SQ 20,881) in two-kidney, one clip Goldblatt hypertensive rats. Hypertension 1981;3:285–293.
20. Huang WC, Ploth DW, Navar LG: Angiotensin-mediated alterations in nephron function in Goldblatt hypertensive rats. Am J Physiol 1982;243:F553–F560.
21. Welch WJ: The pathophysiology of renin release in renovascular hypertension. Semin Nephrol 2000;20:394–401.
22. Miyamori I, Yasuhara S, Matsubara T, et al: Comparative effects of captopril and nifedipine on split renal function in renovascular hypertension. Am J Hypertens 1988;1(4 Pt 1):359–363.
23. Mimran A, Ribstein J, DuCailar G: Converting enzyme inhibitors and renal function in essential and renovascular hypertension. Am J Hypertens 1991;4(1 Pt 2):7S–14S.
24. Demeilliers B, Jover B, Mimran A: Contrasting renal effects of chronic administrations of enalapril and losartan on one-kidney, one clip hypertensive rats. J Hypertens 1998;16:1023–1029.
25. Palm F, Connors S, Welch W, Wilcox C: Angiotensin (Ang) II AT-2-receptor-induced nitric oxide (NO) release sustains blood perfusion and oxygen availability in the post-clip kidney of two-kidney, one clip hypertensive (2K1C) rats. FASEB J 2007;(A497):595.
26. Huelsemann JL, Sterzel RB, McKenzie DE, Wilcox CS: Effects of a calcium entry blocker on blood pressure and renal function during angiotensin-induced hypertension. Hypertension 1985;7(3 Pt 1):374–379.
27. Carmines PK, Navar LG: Disparate effects of Ca channel blockade on afferent and efferent arteriolar responses to ANG II. Am J Physiol 1989;256(6 Pt 2):F1015–F1020.
28. Wenzel UO, Troschau G, Schoeppe W, et al: Adverse effect of the calcium channel blocker nitrendipine on nephrosclerosis in rats with renovascular hypertension. Hypertension 1992;20:233–241.
29. Veniant M, Heudes D, Clozel JP, et al: Calcium blockade versus ACE inhibition in clipped and unclipped kidneys of 2K-1C rats. Kidney Int 1994;46:421–429.
30. Jackson B, Franze L, Sumithran E, Johnston CI: Pharmacologic nephrectomy with chronic angiotensin converting enzyme inhibitor treatment in renovascular hypertension in the rat. J Lab Clin Med 1990;115:21–27.
31. Textor SC, Novick AC, Tarazi RC, et al: Critical perfusion pressure for renal function in patients with bilateral atherosclerotic renal vascular disease. Ann Intern Med 1985;102:308–314.
32. Textor SC, Smith-Powell L: Post-stenotic arterial pressures, renal haemodynamics and sodium excretion during graded pressure reduction in conscious rats with one- and two-kidney coarctation hypertension. J Hypertens 1988;6:311–319.
33. Joint National Committee (JNC): The 6th Report of the Joint National Committee on Prevention, Detection, Evaluation and Treatment of High Blood Pressure. National Institutes of Health. Arch Intern Med 1997;157:2413–2446.
34. Conlon PJ, Little MA, Pieper K, Mark DB: Severity of renal vascular disease predicts mortality in patients undergoing coronary angiography. Kidney Int 2001;60:1490–1497.
35. Roberts J, Moses C, Wilkins R: Autopsy studies in atherosclerosis. I. Distribution and severity of atherosclerosis in patients dying with morphologic evidence of atherosclerotic catastrophe. Circulation 1959;20:511–519.

36. Roberts J, Wilkins R, Moses C: Autopsy studies in atherosclerosis. II. Distribution and severity of atherosclerosis in patients dying with morphologic evidence of atherosclerotic catastrophe. Circulation 1959;20:520–556.

37. Rossi GP, Rossi A, Zanin L, et al: Excess prevalence of extracranial carotid artery lesions in renovascular hypertension. Am J Hypertens 1992;5:8–15.

38. Horvath JS, Waugh RC, Tiller DJ, Duggin GG: The detection of renovascular hypertension: A study of 490 patients by renal angiography. Q J Med 1982;51:139–146.

39. Iglesias JI, Hamburger RJ, Feldman L, Kaufman JS: The natural history of incidental renal artery stenosis in patients with aortoiliac vascular disease. Am J Med 2000;109:642–647.

40. Uzu T, Inoue T, Fujii T, et al: Prevalence and predictors of renal artery stenosis in patients with myocardial infarction. Am J Kidney Dis 1997;29:733–738.

41. Missouris CG, Belli AM, MacGregor GA: "Apparent" heart failure: A syndrome caused by renal artery stenoses. Heart 2000;83:152–155.

42. Korner PI: Cardiovascular hypertrophy and hypertension: Causes and consequences. Blood Press Suppl 1995;2:6–16.

43. Wahlander H, Isgaard J, Jennische E, Friberg P: Left ventricular insulin-like growth factor I increases in early renal hypertension. Hypertension 1992;19:25–32.

44. Losito A, Fagugli RM, Zampi I, et al: Comparison of target organ damage in renovascular and essential hypertension. Am J Hypertens 1996;9:1062–1067.

45. de Simone G, Devereux RB, Camargo MJ, et al: In vivo left ventricular anatomy in rats with two-kidney, one clip and one-kidney, one clip renovascular hypertension. J Hypertens 1992;10:725–732.

46. Gavras H, Lever AF, Brown JJ, et al: Acute renal failure, tubular necrosis, and myocardial infarction induced in the rabbit by intravenous angiotensin II. Lancet 1971;2:19–22.

47. Yamazaki T, Shiojima I, Komuro I, et al: Involvement of the renin-angiotensin system in the development of left ventricular hypertrophy and dysfunction. J Hypertens 1994;12(10 Suppl):S153–S157.

48. Hocher B, George I, Rebstock J, et al: Endothelin system-dependent cardiac remodeling in renovascular hypertension. Hypertension 1999;33:816–822.

49. Robertson AL Jr, Khairallah PA: Angiotensin II: Rapid localization in nuclei of smooth and cardiac muscle. Science 1971;172:1138–1139.

50. Ehmke H, Faulhaber J, Munter K, et al: Chronic ETA receptor blockade attenuates cardiac hypertrophy independently of blood pressure effects in renovascular hypertensive rats. Hypertension 1999;33:954–960.

51. Phillips PA: Interaction between endothelin and angiotensin II. Clin Exp Pharmacol Physiol 1999;26:517–518.

52. Parfrey PS, Foley RN: The clinical epidemiology of cardiac disease in chronic renal failure. J Am Soc Nephrol 1999;10:1606–1615.

53. Shulman NB, Ford CE, Hall WD, et al: Prognostic value of serum creatinine and effect of treatment of hypertension on renal function. Results from the hypertension detection and follow-up program. The Hypertension Detection and Follow-up Program Cooperative Group. Hypertension 1989;13(5 Suppl):I80–I93.

54. Culleton BF, Larson MG, Wilson PW, et al: Cardiovascular disease and mortality in a community-based cohort with mild renal insufficiency. Kidney Int 1999;56:2214–2219.

55. Mann JF, Gerstein HC, Pogue J, et al: Renal insufficiency as a predictor of cardiovascular outcomes and the impact of ramipril: The HOPE randomized trial. Ann Intern Med 2001;134:629–636.

56. Al Suwaidi J, Reddan DN, Williams K, et al: Prognostic implications of abnormalities in renal function in patients with acute coronary syndromes. Circulation 2002;106:974–980.

57. McCullough PA, Soman SS, Shah SS, et al: Risks associated with renal dysfunction in patients in the coronary care unit. J Am Coll Cardiol 2000;36:679–684.

58. Johansson M, Herlitz H, Jensen G, et al: Increased cardiovascular mortality in hypertensive patients with renal artery stenosis. Relation to sympathetic activation, renal function and treatment regimens. J Hypertens 1999;17(12 Pt 1):1743–1750.

59. Dorros G, Jaff M, Mathiak L, et al: Four-year follow-up of Palmaz-Schatz stent revascularization as treatment for atherosclerotic renal artery stenosis. Circulation 1998;98:642–647.

60. Plouin PF, Chatellier G, Darne B, Raynaud A: Blood pressure outcome of angioplasty in atherosclerotic renal artery stenosis: A randomized trial. Essai Multicentrique Medicaments vs Angioplastie (EMMA) Study Group. Hypertension 1998;31:823–829.

61. Wilcox CS: Use of angiotensin-converting-enzyme inhibitors for diagnosing renovascular hypertension. Kidney Int 1993;44:1379–1390.

62. Chapman AB, Gabow PA, Schrier RW: Reversible renal failure associated with angiotensin-converting enzyme inhibitors in polycystic kidney disease. Ann Intern Med 1991;115:769–773.

63. Toto RD, Mitchell HC, Lee HC, et al: Reversible renal insufficiency due to angiotensin converting enzyme inhibitors in hypertensive nephrosclerosis. Ann Intern Med 1991;115:513–519.

64. Wilcox CS, Smith TB, Frederickson ED, et al: The captopril glomerular filtration rate renogram in renovascular hypertension. Clin Nucl Med 1989;14:1–7.

65. Ribstein J, Mourad G, Mimran A: Contrasting acute effects of captopril and nifedipine on renal function in renovascular hypertension. Am J Hypertens 1988;1(3 Pt 1):239–244.

66. Mourad G, Ribstein J, Argiles A, et al: Contrasting effects of acute angiotensin converting enzyme inhibitors and calcium antagonists in transplant renal artery stenosis. Nephrol Dial Transplant 1989;4:66–70.

67. Textor SC, Tarazi RC, Novick AC, et al: Regulation of renal hemodynamics and glomerular filtration in patients with renovascular hypertension during converting enzyme inhibition with captopril. Am J Med 1984;76(5B):29–37.

68. Textor SC, Novick AC, Steinmuller DR, Streem SB: Renal failure limiting antihypertensive therapy as an indication for renal revascularization. A case report. Arch Intern Med 1983;143:2208–2211.

69. van de Ven PJ, Beutler JJ, Kaatee R, et al: Angiotensin converting enzyme inhibitor–induced renal dysfunction in atherosclerotic renovascular disease. Kidney Int 1998;53:986–993.

70. Arzilli F, Giovannetti R, Meola M, et al: ACE-inhibition vs. surgical treatment in the outcome of ischemic kidney of renovascular patients: A one year follow-up. High Blood Press 1992;1:47–50.

71. Fyhrquist F, Gronhagen-Riska C, Tikkanen I, Junggren IL: Long-term monotherapy with lisinopril in renovascular hypertension. J Cardiovasc Pharmacol 1987;9(Suppl 3):S61–S65.

72. Hollenberg NK: Medical therapy for renovascular hypertension: A review. Am J Hypertens 1988;1(4 Pt 2):338S–343S.

73. Franklin SS, Smith RD: Comparison of effects of enalapril plus hydrochlorothiazide versus standard triple therapy on renal function in renovascular hypertension. Am J Med 1985;79(3C):14–23.

74. Losito A, Gaburri M, Errico R, et al: Survival of patients with renovascular disease and ACE inhibition. Clin Nephrol 1999;52:339–343.

75. Miyamori I, Yasuhara S, Takeda Y, et al: Effects of converting enzyme inhibition on split renal function in renovascular hypertension. Hypertension 1986;8:415–421.

76. Pickering TG, Herman L, Devereux RB, et al: Recurrent pulmonary oedema in hypertension due to bilateral renal artery stenosis: Treatment by angioplasty or surgical revascularisation. Lancet 1988;2:551–552.

77. Wilcox CS, Mitch WE, Kelly RA, et al: Response of the kidney to furosemide. I. Effects of salt intake and renal compensation. J Lab Clin Med 1983;102:450–458.

78. Cianciaruso B, Bellizzi V, Minutolo R, et al: Renal adaptation to dietary sodium restriction in moderate renal failure resulting from chronic glomerular disease. J Am Soc Nephrol 1996;7: 306–313.

79. Wilcox CS, Lewis PS, Peart WS, et al: Renal function, body fluid volumes, renin, aldosterone, and noradrenaline during treatment of hypertension with pindolol. J Cardiovasc Pharmacol 1981;3:598–611.

80. Converse RL Jr, Jacobsen TN, Toto RD, et al: Sympathetic overactivity in patients with chronic renal failure. N Engl J Med 1992;327:1912–1918.

81. Wilcox CS, Loon NR, Ameer B, Limacher MC: Renal and hemodynamic responses to bumetanide in hypertension: Effects of nitrendipine. Kidney Int 1989;36:719–725.

82. Korsakas S, Mohaupt MG, Dinkel HP, et al: Delay of dialysis in end-stage renal failure: Prospective study on percutaneous renal artery interventions. Kidney Int 2004;65:251–258.

83. UK Prospective Diabetes Study (UKPDS): Intensive blood-glucose control with sulphonylureas or insulin compared with conventional treatment and risk of complications in patients with type 2 diabetes. Lancet 1998;352:837–853.

84. Nissen SE, Nicholls SJ, Sipahi I, et al: Effect of very high-intensity statin therapy on regression of coronary atherosclerosis: The ASTEROID trial. JAMA 2006;295:1556–1565.

85. Ray KK, Cannon CP, McCabe CH, et al: Early and late benefits of high-dose atorvastatin in patients with acute coronary syndromes: results from the PROVE IT–TIMI 22 trial. J Am Coll Cardiol 2005;46:1405–1410.

86. American Diabetes Association: Clinical practice recommendations. Diabetes Care 2002;I:S1–S147.

87. Reichard P, Nilsson BY, Rosenqvist U: The effect of long-term intensified insulin treatment on the development of microvascular complications of diabetes mellitus. N Engl J Med 1993;329:304–309.

88. Collins A: Anemia management prior to dialysis: Cardiovascular and cost-benefit observations. Nephrol Dial Transplant 2003(Suppl 2):II2–II6.

89. Baggio B, Budakovic A, Casara D, et al: Renal involvement in subjects with peripheral atherosclerosis. J Nephrol 2001;14: 286–292.

90. Hennekens CH, Dyken ML, Fuster V: Aspirin as a therapeutic agent in cardiovascular disease: a statement for healthcare professionals from the American Heart Association. Circulation 1997;96:2751–2753.

91. Antithromotic Trialists' Collaboration: Collaborative meta-analysis of randomized trials of antiplatelet therapy for prevention of death, myocardial infarction, and stroke in high risk patients. BMJ 2002;324:71–86.

92. Kitiyakara C, Gonin J, Massy Z, Wilcox CS: Non-traditional cardiovascular disease risk factors in end-stage renal disease: Oxidate stress and hyperhomocysteinemia. Curr Opin Nephrol Hypertens 2000;9:477–487.

93. Kielstein JT, Boger RH, Bode-Boger SM, et al: Asymmetric dimethylarginine plasma concentrations differ in patients with end-stage renal disease: Relationship to treatment method and atherosclerotic disease. J Am Soc Nephrol 1999;10:594–600.

94. Miyazaki H, Matsuoka H, Cooke JP, et al: Endogenous nitric oxide synthase inhibitor: A novel marker of atherosclerosis. Circulation 1999;99:1141–1146.

Further Reading

Balk E, Raman G, Chung M, et al: Effectiveness of management strategies for renal artery stenosis: A systematic review. Ann Intern Med 2006;145:901–912.

Cooper CJ, Murphy TP: Is renal artery stenting the correct treatment of renal artery stenosis? The case for renal artery stenting for treatment of renal artery stenosis. Circulation 2007;115: 263–269.

Dworkin LD, Jamerson K: The case against angioplasty and stenting of atherosclerotic renal artery stenosis. Circulation 2007;115:271–276.

Dworkin LD: Controversial treatment of renal artery stenosis. Hypertension 2006;48:350–356.

Garovic VD, Textor SC: Renovascular hypertension and ischemic nephropathy. Circulation 2005;112:1362–1374.

Levin A, Linas S, Luft FC, Chapman AB, Textor S: Controversies in renal artery stenosis: A review by the American Society of Nephrology Advisory Group on Hypertension. Am J Nephrol 2007;27:212–220.

Textor SC: Renovascular disease: Epidemiology and clinical presentation. Semin Nephrol 2000;20:426–431.

Chapter 58

Renovascular Hypertension and Ischemic Nephropathy: Angioplasty and Stenting

Stephen C. Textor and Michael McKusick

Few problems in nephrology are more controversial than decisions about when to undertake revascularization for renal artery stenosis (RAS). Technical advances related to endovascular stenting have led to widespread application of these procedures in the United States over the past decade. Minor degrees of stenosis may be detected "incidentally" in many patients with atherosclerosis elsewhere. These are often of minimal significance. However, high-grade RAS can lead to renovascular hypertension, which remains one of the most common secondary causes of hypertension. More severe lesions can produce critical loss of renal perfusion in the form of *ischemic nephropathy,* a potentially treatable form of progressive renal failure (Box 58-1). Advances in detection and imaging of RAS, in medical therapy of hypertension, and in endovascular methods, including vascular stents, make this a rapidly evolving field. With the use of endovascular stents, restoring the renal circulation becomes a realistic possibility for patients with ostial lesions, who were previously considered at unacceptable risk for major surgical procedures.

At the same time, application of endovascular procedures has expanded the range of clinicians caring for patients with refractory hypertension and declining kidney function. During the era of surgical reconstruction of renal arteries, the clinical care of refractory hypertension fell mainly to internists specializing in hypertension and kidney disease, who worked quite closely with vascular surgeons. Renal revascularization was applied cautiously because of the morbidity associated with aortic surgery and only after major efforts to ensure clinical benefit. As awareness of atherosclerotic renal artery disease has grown and noninvasive imaging has become more widely applied, general internists and cardiologists now address these problems. The finding that renal artery lesions commonly occur with other atherosclerotic disease has prompted some centers to perform aortic and renal angiography along with coronary angiography.[1,2] Renal arterial lesions that are detected are frequently treated with endovascular stents. During the years between 1996 and 2000 the number of Medicare claims for renal artery stenting rose from 7660 to 18,520. This was mainly due to procedures performed by interventional cardiologists[3] (Fig. 58-1A). Recent guidelines proposed by interventional groups reinforce these practices, even while acknowledging the limited outcomes data to support this approach.[4,5] This practice continues to expand. One stent manufacturer (Boston Scientific, personal communication) indicated that more than 60,000 procedures were undertaken during 2005. Whether these procedures produce objective clinical benefits is questionable, according to evidence of published studies of randomized, controlled trials.[6] For this reason, the U.S. Centers for Medicare & Medicaid Services (CMS) is reviewing reimbursement criteria for renal artery stenting with a stated goal to limit Medicare reimbursement for this procedure. Several prospective trials are in progress in the United States and elsewhere to better define the natural history and need for intervention in the current era of cardiovascular risk reduction. The National Heart, Lung, and Blood Institute (NHLBI) is funding a randomized, prospective trial of intensive medical therapy with and without stenting—the Cardiovascular Outcomes of Renal Atherosclerotic Lesions (CORAL) trial, which is scheduled for completion in 2011.[7]

The purpose of angioplasty with or without stenting is to restore blood flow and perfusion pressure to the kidney beyond a stenotic lesion. Ultimately, these procedures are intended to improve blood pressure (BP) control and to reduce the risks of hypertension—in principle, to "cure" renovascular hypertension—and to salvage kidney function beyond a "critical" RAS. Although these goals seem quite reasonable, it remains difficult to identify individual patients who have the greatest likelihood of achieving them. Nephrologists recognize that invasive renal vascular procedures present hazards even in the best of circumstances. Complications from atheroemboli,

Box 58-1 Clinical syndromes of renal artery stenosis

Asymptomatic
Incidental renal artery stenosis
Easily treated hypertension

Symptomatic
Treatment-resistant hypertension
Bilateral disease/solitary function kidney
Progressive renal failure in treated hypertension
Renal failure limiting antihypertensive therapy
Pulmonary vascular congestion: "flash" pulmonary edema
End-stage renal disease

vessel dissection, contrast toxicity, and other adverse events sometimes worsen renal function and aggravate hypertension, such that renovascular procedures cannot be undertaken casually. Moreover, these proceedings entail considerable expense. Hence, the risks and benefits for each patient's situation require careful consideration. The goal of this chapter is to summarize our current state of knowledge regarding patient selection, technical features, outcomes, and hazards of renal artery angioplasty and stenting in the current era.

DEMOGRAPHICS OF RENOVASCULAR DISEASE

Patients with fibromuscular diseases of the renal arteries are more commonly young and female than those with atherosclerosis. The former constitute 16% to 20% of patients with renovascular lesions referred for vascular procedures, at least for refractory hypertension. It should be emphasized that patients with fibromuscular disease usually have normal renal function

and are at low risk for progressive occlusive disease and renal functional loss.[8] Such patients are sometimes detected as a result of developing hypertension during pregnancy or at an early age. Most often patients with fibromuscular disease have normal-appearing aortic vessels and are at low risk for complications of vascular manipulation. As a result, the potential risks of angioplasty are low and the benefits of improved BP more likely to offer long-term advantage. As a result, revascularization is often recommended for these patients.[9]

The advancing age of the U.S. population is associated with the rising prevalence of RAS from atherosclerosis.[10] Whether the true prevalence is increasing is not known. What is certain, however, is that the mean age of reported series of renal revascularization has increased by more than 15 years from the 1970s.[11] The median age of treated patients is now 71 years (see Fig. 58-1B). As a result, patients with atherosclerosis have a longer background history of hypertension and a greater risk of comorbid disease (including diabetes, peripheral vascular disease, coronary disease, and carotid disease). Atherosclerosis is a systemic disease. Thus, it is not surprising that some degree of atherosclerosis affects the kidney in 30% to 50% of individuals when atherosclerosis is detected elsewhere (e.g., during coronary or lower extremity angiography).[12] The benefits and goals of renal revascularization must be weighed in the context of "competing" risk from other cardiovascular diseases. These competing risks can offset the benefits of restoring the renal circulation in marginal cases.

RISKS OF DISEASE PROGRESSION

One of the compelling reasons to restore renal artery patency is the potential for untreated lesions to progress to total occlusion and functional loss of the entire kidney. Such arguments have led to speculation that unsuspected renal artery

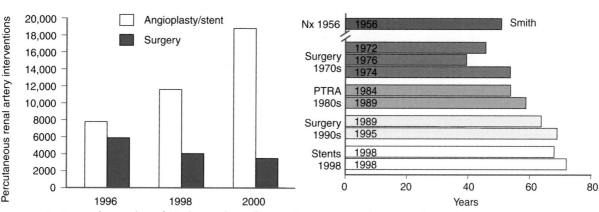

Figure 58-1 **A,** Rise in the number of Medicare claims for renal artery revascularization during the years 1996–2000, corresponding to widespread application of endovascular stents. The largest rise in procedures came from interventional cardiologists (2.4-fold increase). (From Murphy TP, Soares G, Kim M: Increase in utilization of percutaneous renal artery interventions by Medicare beneficiaries 1996–2000. Am J Roentgenol 2004;183:561–568.) **B,** Mean ages of selected series of surgical or endovascular intervention for renal artery stenosis. Early data, including unilateral nephrectomy, are included as a reference point. The techniques available have changed, with a marked increase in the use of angioplasty and stenting in recent years. The ages and associated comorbid disease risks have increased considerably during this period. Reasons for the change in demographics include changes in survival from coronary disease and stroke, changes in medical therapy, and the ability to intervene safely in patients considered at unacceptable risk in the past (see text). PTRA, percutaneous transluminal renal angioplasty.

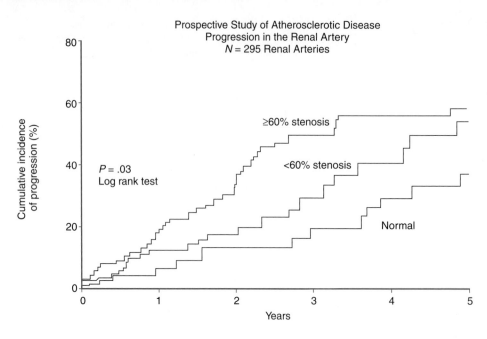

Figure 58-2 Rates of progressive vascular disease, as evidenced by increased flow velocities in 295 arteries measured prospectively at 6-month intervals between 1990 and 1997. The probability of disease progression was related to the initial severity of stenosis, but remarkably few proceeded to total occlusion (9/295 vessels, or 3%). Estimates of change in vessel characteristics are higher than the number demonstrating clinical progression in the form of either intractable hypertension or renal dysfunction (see text). (From Caps MT, Perissinotto C, Zierler RE, et al: Prospective study of atherosclerotic disease progression in the renal artery. Circulation 1998;98: 2866–2872.)

occlusive disease may account for up to 14% to 20% of patients, particularly whites, reaching end-stage renal disease (ESRD).[13] Doppler ultrasound studies conducted between 1990 and 1997 confirm that stenotic lesions can progress, as evidenced by increases in blood flow velocities over time (Fig. 58-2).[14] The likelihood of progression is directly related to the severity of the initial stenosis. Remarkably, total occlusion was observed in only 9 of 295 vessels (3%). This is a lower frequency than had been reported in earlier angiographic series.

Whether progressive vascular stenosis by Doppler ultrasonography translates into clinical progression is less clear. Reports from The Netherlands of high-grade renal artery disease discovered incidentally suggest that none resulted in renal failure during follow-up periods of 8 to 10 years.[15] Serial measurements of kidney size during Doppler ultrasound measurements identify loss of kidney volume as less frequent than a change in renal hemodynamics[16] (Fig. 58-3). Follow-up studies of patients with incidental high-grade RAS (>70% lumen affected), who were managed without revascularization during

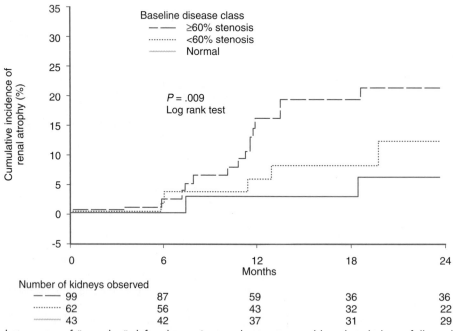

Figure 58-3 Cumulative rates of "atrophy," defined as a 1-cm reduction in renal length in kidneys followed prospectively by Doppler ultrasonography between 1990 and 1997. The likelihood of loss of size was less than that for measurable progression of flow velocities; atrophy was infrequently associated with a rise in creatinine. Predictors of atrophy included peak systolic velocity above 400 cm/sec. (From Caps MT, Zierler RE, Polissar NL, et al: Risk of atrophy in kidneys with atherosclerotic renal artery stenosis. Kidney Int 1998;53:735–742.)

1989–1993 in the United States, indicate that only 10% to 15% come to revascularization based on progressive renal dysfunction or uncontrollable hypertension.[17] Recent population-based studies indicate that 6.8% of individuals older than age 65 have more than 60% renal artery stenosis but that rates of progression appear to be approximately between 0.5% and 1.3% per year.[18] During an 8-year follow-up, just 4% progressed to "significant" stenosis. These observations are supported by follow-up of 40 patients with high-grade RAS treated with "aggressive" medical therapy, only 6 of whom later went on to revascularization on clinical grounds.[19] The hazard of RAS is different for patients with unilateral disease (one kidney affected by stenosis, the other without stenosis) compared to those with bilateral disease (usually identified as high-grade stenosis to both kidneys or stenosis to a solitary functioning kidney).[20] In the former, vascular progression, even to the loss of one kidney, is buffered by a "spare" contralateral kidney. Therefore, the change in renal function associated with unilateral disease is usually minor. Moreover, both kidneys are rarely affected to the same degree. Many clinical reports focus on tracking the "reciprocal creatinine" or other estimates of glomerular filtration rate (GFR) over time.[21] Although this method is time-honored with regard to monitoring progression of parenchymal kidney diseases such as diabetic nephropathy, it has only limited relevance to tracking the decline in function associated with renovascular disease. Cases have been observed in which slope has changed from negative to zero with complete occlusion of one renal artery, a change that might wrongly have been attributed to a benefit of "successful" stenting as proposed by some interventional guidelines.[22] Presumably, improved function of the other kidney must have offset loss of negligible function in the thrombosed kidney.

In the instance of RAS to the entire renal mass, however, progressive loss of blood supply does threaten renal function overall, making renal failure and circulatory congestion, or "flash" pulmonary edema, genuine concerns.[23] Understanding the true magnitude of progression risk for the individual patient is crucial to identifying the risk-benefit ratio regarding angioplasty and stenting. It is likely that current levels of disease progression will continue to fall. This may reflect more intense efforts at BP control, smoking cessation, and lipid lowering.

DIAGNOSTIC CONSIDERATIONS IN RENAL ARTERY DISEASE

Physicians in the United States are encouraged to obtain basic information regarding kidney function and cardiovascular risk and to follow recommendations of the Joint National Commission (JNC) to minimize testing and focus on BP reduction.[24] With the widespread application of effective antihypertensive medications, including agents that interrupt the renin-angiotensin system, such as angiotensin-converting enzyme (ACE) inhibitors and angiotensin receptor blockers (ARBs), many individuals with RAS are treated effectively and are never detected (see Chapter 48 and Chapter 52 regarding recommendations for medical therapy). Thus, many patients considered candidates for renal revascularization have been treated for hypertension for a long time. Consideration for revascularization often begins as they develop recognizable syndromes of progressive renovascular disease, as summarized in Box 58-1. Most of these include a combination of

resistance to antihypertensive therapy and deterioration of renal function. Often, these signal more severe stenoses or the development of bilateral disease.

Diagnostic studies now focus primarily on establishing whether high-grade RAS is present, whether it affects both kidneys or the entire functioning renal mass, and whether it is amenable to endovascular repair or is associated with more widespread aortic disease, such as an abdominal aortic aneurysm. Biochemical studies to determine renin release or lateralization are less commonly performed. In many centers, angiography is reserved until these issues are resolved, with the intention of undertaking endovascular repair at the same sitting if needed. As a result, most individuals undergo some form of vascular staging, which may consist of Doppler ultrasonography, captopril renography, and magnetic resonance angiography (MRA) or computed tomographic angiography (CTA). The last two now produce excellent images, including localization of the site of lesions and associated aortic disease (Fig. 58-4). CTA has the disadvantage of requiring iodinated contrast and carries a risk of contrast nephrotoxicity, particularly in patients with preexisting impairment of kidney function or diabetes.[25] Although gadolinium contrast carries little or no nephrotoxic risk at the doses used for MRA, recent reports of nephrogenic systemic fibrosis have led the U.S. Food and Drug Administration (FDA) to express concern that gadolinium-based contrast may be a contributory factor. This rare condition, a disabling fibrotic process that restricts movement of skin, joints, and muscles,[26] has been reported to date only in patients with reduced GFR (<30 mL/min/1.73 m^2),

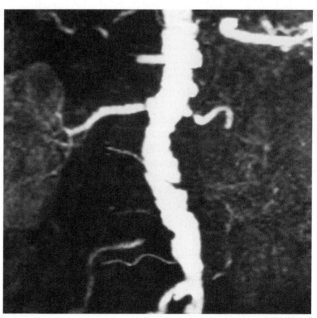

Figure 58-4 Magnetic resonance angiogram in an 81-year-old woman with deteriorating renal function and accelerated hypertension. This study illustrates extensive aortic disease associated with high-grade stenoses of both renal arteries and a delayed nephrogram in the left kidney. Although these images can be obtained with little risk of nephrotoxicity, recent concerns about the potential for gadolinium-based contrast to produce nephrogenic systemic fibrosis limit its use to subjects with estimated glomerular filtration rate above 30 mL/min/1.73 m^2 (see text).

often in those with hepatorenal syndrome in and around the period of liver transplantation. Until now, no treatment for nephrogenic systemic fibrosis has proven effective; it appears to be irreversible. The FDA has offered an "alert" regarding the need to limit procedures in patients with estimated GFR (eGFR) less than 30 mL/min, attempt to avoid them in patients with eGFR less than 15 mL/min, and inform patients of the potential risks. There is a pressing need to improve alternative methods for imaging the renal vasculature in patients with reduced GFR.

Predictors of a favorable response to renal revascularization remain elusive. Recent progression of hypertension despite therapy or recent loss of GFR remain among the most valuable features. Some authors argue that demonstration of elevated resistive index on Doppler ultrasonography portends intrinsic fibrosis and small-vessel disease in the kidney that will not improve after stenting.[27] Other reports challenge this observation.[28,29]

RENAL ANGIOPLASTY AND STENTING

Goals of Renal Angioplasty and Stenting

The goals of correcting RAS include improving BP and preserving renal function. These goals for clinical success differ from the goal of technical success, restoring vessel patency.

Angioplasty alone for fibromuscular disease can open the renal arteries with excellent results.[30] This disease often affects the midportion segments of the renal artery and may comprise "webs" with partial obstructive effects in series. Individuals with fibromuscular disease often have normal kidney function and may derive more clinical benefit than patients with parenchymal renal disease. Occasionally, fibromuscular disease and atherosclerosis may coexist and must be addressed separately in the same patient.

Atherosclerosis commonly affects the proximal portion of the renal artery, particularly at the ostium. It may represent extension of an aortic plaque into the renal artery. Such lesions typically do not respond well to balloon angioplasty alone and tend to recoil immediately after dilation. For that reason, stents have been employed to maintain vessel patency for ostial lesions. Randomized, prospective studies indicate that stents unquestionably improve primary patency rates for ostial renal artery stenoses.[31] Although in the United States stents are approved by the FDA for use in the renal arteries only for *failed angioplasty,* interventional radiologists and cardiologists now commonly employ them for "primary" stenting of atherosclerotic lesions.

The role of distal embolic protection devices in the renal artery is unclear. Although these devices are approved for use in specific coronary artery procedures and are commonly used in carotid stenting, the anatomy of the renal arteries differs in some respects from those vessels. Whereas atheroemboli represent a major concern for the success of renal artery stenting, experimental studies indicate that embolic phenomena can occur at any stage of the procedure, including the initial passage of the guidewire, inflation of the balloon, and expansion of the stent. Clinical studies indicate that embolic phenomena can develop in subsequent days or weeks. Initial reports indicate that embolic protection devices can, in fact, capture embolic debris, but whether they improve long-term

results is not yet known. Initial experience in CORAL using a protection device led to enough adverse events that its use was discontinued.

Techniques of Renal Angioplasty and Stenting

Renal arteriography with angioplasty and stent placement should be performed in a peripheral vascular suite with digital subtraction capability by an individual who is properly trained and skilled in percutaneous vascular intervention. In general, these procedures are done under conscious intravenous sedation from a transfemoral approach. For patients with chronic renal insufficiency, especially those who are diabetic, an alternative to iodinated contrast material for arteriography should be considered. Although image quality may not be as good, carbon dioxide or gadolinium provide sufficient enhancement for diagnostic imaging and intervention and lack the nephrotoxicity of iodine. However, as noted above, the potential for gadolinium to predispose to nephrogenic systemic fibrosis favors avoiding this agent when the eGFR is lower than 30 mL/min/1.73 ml^2.

The tools for endovascular therapy have improved.[32] Equipment manufacturers now provide a wide variety of smaller catheters (commonly 0.014 mm) and an array of low-profile systems. The interventionist can now safely open even the most severely stenosed renal artery arising from a tortuous, ulcerated aorta. Digital imaging systems with high-quality fluoroscopy, excellent image acquisition, and accurate stenosis assessment programs provide physicians maximum flexibility in treating patients with atheromatous disease in all vascular beds. The proliferation of these systems in cardiology catheterization laboratories, radiology angiography suites, and surgical operating rooms testifies to the broad acceptance of endovascular therapy for occlusive arterial disease by both the public and the majority of practitioners.

Patients with fibromuscular dysplasia are treated with balloon angioplasty alone. Atheromatous disease is now treated almost universally with balloon-expandable stents. Present placement planning has been simplified by the three-dimensional angiographic images generated via CTA and MRA. It is now common in most experienced centers to have such studies available before catheterization as part of a thorough workup to determine eligibility and suitability for invasive treatment.

Femoral access for stent placement is preferred for most patients. Some patients with severe inferior angled renal arteries may be better approached from the brachial artery. If a patient has adequate prior imaging of the aorta, it is not necessary to do an aortic flush. Direct baseline imaging of the renal artery is performed with a guide catheter chosen to fit the anatomy. The image intensifier is angled to produce a tangential view of the origin of the renal artery from the aorta. Confirming the degree of stenosis with imaging software is recommended, because simple visual estimates (the "eyeball" technique) overestimate the severity.[32] Intravenous heparin is administered to achieve an activated clotting time of 225 to 300 seconds. Using a 0.014-mm wire, the stenosis is crossed and the wire advanced only as far as needed to gain purchase for catheter manipulation. If filter wire protection is desired, the wire can be positioned at this time. Some practitioners measure pressure gradients routinely as well, a practice recommended for borderline lesions. In general, a 20 mm Hg systolic or 10 mm Hg mean gradient is considered significant.[32] Most lesions do not require predilatation when using low-profile, premounted stents. The stent should be sized so that it completely covers the lesion and extends slightly into the abdominal aorta. The diameter should be such that the stent does not overexpand the natural diameter of the vessel. The balloon-mounted stent should be positioned across the lesion and checked with small contrast injections to allow for adjustment. Balloon expansion is done slowly while holding the system steady. The stent is allowed to "dog bone" slightly and can be adjusted for optimal positioning. Slow, gradual balloon inflation with a steady hand on the guide catheter, balloon, and wire can avoid movement of the stent during deployment.

After stent placement, careful imaging is important to confirm stent position and expansion and to identify renal artery branches. A nephrogram should be visualized. This step allows one to determine if additional stent expansion is needed. Documenting preservation of renal parenchyma or identifying embolic complications or peripheral branch dissections is helpful for immediate postprocedure management.

The presence of multiple renal arteries can complicate therapy. These arteries tend to be smaller caliber vessels that can originate from awkward locations. The likelihood of restenosis or technical failure is greater in smaller vessels.[33] It is our opinion that stenting arteries smaller than 4 mm in diameter should be avoided. Early renal artery bifurcations also can pose a technical challenge. They may require multiple stents with coordinated junctions (*kissing stents*). In patients with difficult anatomy, having two interventional operators with experience working together has proven to be useful.

After stent placement, patients are placed on an antiplatelet regimen (usually clopidogrel) for 6 to 8 weeks and evaluated with Doppler ultrasonography. Because renal artery stent restenosis is common, careful follow-up is needed to allow for timely re-intervention if in-stent hyperplasia occurs.

Embolic Protection Devices

The effect of renal artery stent placement on renal function remains ambiguous, in part because no randomized, prospective studies compare medical therapy directly with stent placement. Perhaps just as important, observational cohort studies from patients with reduced GFR indicate that renal function after stent placement sometimes improves (~25%), sometimes remains stable (no clinically important change, ~50%), but sometimes worsens (18%–24%).[34,35] For some of those patients with functional deterioration, local and systemic embolization play a role. In patients with low functional reserve, even small amounts of microembolic particles may cause further losses in glomerular filtration. Investigators have explored the renal artery application of filtration devices designed for coronary and cerebral vascular procedures.

Walker and associates reported that particles as large as 3 mm in diameter could be aspirated from guide catheters placed into renal arteries during intervention.[36] Angiographers have observed atheromatous debris welling out of a backbleeding catheter hub in patients with advanced atherosclerosis. Hiramoto and colleagues reported that manipulating a 0.018-mm guidewire across an ex vivo aortorenal atheroma could release thousands of tiny particles and that stent expansion was associated with further embolic particle

release.[37] It is likely that nearly any vascular manipulation releases some embolic debris. Remarkably, overt clinical manifestations remain uncommon.

Although distal microembolization during renal artery stent placement undoubtedly occurs, its true prevalence is not known. Many patients appear to have sufficient renal functional reserve to mask the effect of microembolization. For those with preexisting renal insufficiency, the clinical effects of atheroemboli can be significant. In a prospective series of 95 cases with acute renal failure developing from atheroemboli, 37% of patients required dialysis, 24% progressed to ESRD, and mortality was 38%.[38] Krishnamurthi and colleagues reported a decreased 5-year survival in patients with renal biopsy-proven atheroembolus (54%) as opposed to those without (85%) after open renal revascularization.[39] There is no treatment for atheroembolism. Prevention is the only solution.

Currently available embolic protection devices are basically either balloon occluders or filters. A device developed for renal intervention (Angiogard, Cordis Corp, Warren, N.J.) was used in the CORAL trial, but its use was discontinued. Operator experience indicated many limitations, and it was considered uneconomical. Because of the variability of renal artery anatomy, not all cases will be suitable for embolic protection device use. Our experience is that effective use of these devices requires experience because improper use can result in significant complications.

Few published reports examine renal protection devices. Holden and associates achieved improved or stabilized renal function in 95% of 37 patients with renal insufficiency using the Angioguard device.[40] Embolic debris was demonstrated in 65% of cases. Henry and colleagues reported results in 105 poorly controlled hypertensive patients in which they used both balloon occlusion and filter types of protection devices during stent placement[41]; 39 of these patients had a serum creatinine of 1.5 mg/dL or greater. Particulate debris was captured in more than 80% of cases. At 6 months, only 1 of 91 patients who had moderate renal insufficiency had a deterioration in renal function, whereas 21 with renal insufficiency had improved renal function and 69 patients had stable function. At 2 years (75 patients), only 2 patients had deteriorations in renal function (3%). These results suggest a significant benefit to using a renal protection device as opposed to stenting without protection, based on historical comparisons.

Conversely, Cooper and colleagues reported their experience to the 2007 American College of Cardiology Innovation in Intervention Summit on a multicenter trial in which 100 patients undergoing renal artery stent placement were randomized to the use of an Angioguard device or double-blinded use of a glycoprotein IIb/IIIa inhibitor (abciximab) in a 2×2 factorial design (C. Cooper, personal communication). There was no benefit to renal function in the patients treated with the filter alone. Only patients who had both filter wire use and received abciximab had any improvement in renal function after stent placement.

Although distal protection during stent placement seems reasonable, much more work needs to be done. Optimal patient selection needs to be defined. Randomized trials are essential. An easily deployed device designed specifically for the renal arteries is required before this technology can be established for renal artery revascularization.

Outcomes of Renal Artery Angioplasty and Stenting

Endovascular procedures are evaluated by considering the benefits on BP control and renal function in comparison with complications.

Fibromuscular Disease

"Technical success" exceeds 90% in fibromuscular disease (Fig. 58-5). These lesions are made more complicated if they extend into segmental branches. Occasionally fibromuscular disease is associated with aneurysmal dilation, which does not benefit from angioplasty. Dilation of dysplastic webs occasionally leads to arterial dissection or occlusion of the small segmental vessels.

Blood Pressure Outcomes

Clinical effectiveness of intervention for fibromuscular disease is high. Some patients need no further antihypertensive medications (Table 58-1),[8,42,43] and many others are considered "improved." As a result, many authors consider balloon angioplasty as standard therapy for fibromuscular disease. As noted by Aurell and Jensen, Ramsay and Waller,[42,44] and others, reported response rates to percutaneous transluminal renal angioplasty (PTRA) differ widely between studies and between different time periods. This may be the case for several reasons that are worth emphasizing:

1. Target BP levels are changing, generally to lower levels. Earlier studies used criteria of achieved BPs lower than 160/95 mm Hg, or simply diastolic pressure lower than 90 mm Hg, whereas more recent targets seek to achieve BP levels lower than 140/90 mm Hg. Consequently, fewer patients remain medication-free or are considered "cured."
2. Standards for measuring BP and administering antihypertensive therapy are highly variable. Therefore, interpretation of "benefit" is inconsistent.
3. Patient selection varies among studies, including such factors as duration of hypertension and urgency of intervention.

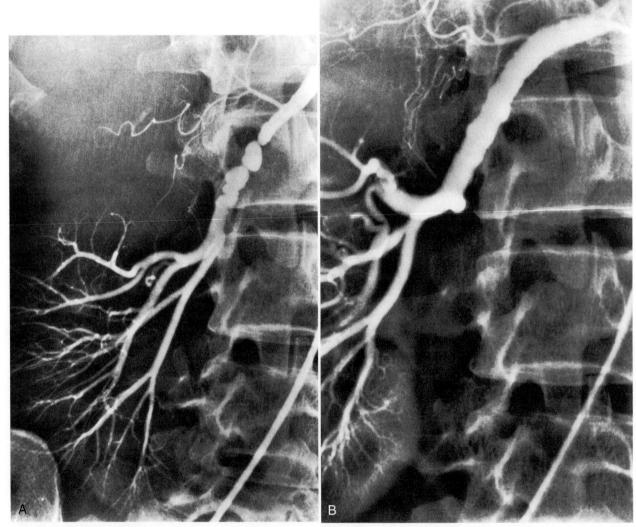

Figure 58-5 **A,** Focal fibromuscular disease in the midportion of the right renal artery in a 42-year-old female. Note that distal vessels are well preserved with normal renal function but severe hypertension. **B,** This lesion was dilated successfully using percutaneous transluminal renal angioplasty with an excellent technical result and clinical outcome.

Table 58-1 Results of Percutaneous Transluminal Angioplasty of the Renal Arteries in Patients with Fibromuscular Renovascular Disease and Hypertension

Study	Year	Patients (N)	Technical Success Rate (%)	EFFECT ON BLOOD PRESSURE			Months of Follow-up (mean range)	Complication Rate (%)
				Cured (%)	Improved (%)	Unimproved (%)		
Sos et al	1983	31	87	59	34	7	16 (4–40)	6
Baert et al	1990	22	83	58	21	21	26 (6–72)	NR
Tegmeyer et al	1991	66	100	39	59	2	39 (1–121)	13
Bonelli et al	1995	105	89	22	63	15	43 (0–168)	11 (major)
Jensen et al	1995	30	97	39	47	14	12 (NR)	3 (major) 12 (minor)
Davidson et al	1996	23	100	52	22	26	NR	13
Klow et al	1998	49	98	26	44	30	9 (1–96)	0
Birrer et al	2002	27	100		74*	26	10 (NR)	7.4
Surowiec et al	2003	14	95		79*	21	NR	28.5
De Fraissinette et al	2003	70	94	14	74	12	39 (1–204)	11

*The percentage shown is the total for cured and improved.
Summary of published series for PTRA (percutaneous transluminal renal angioplasty) for fibromuscular diseases between 1983 and 2003. Recent series emphasize the potential for high rates of technical success, with improved blood pressure control in 74% to 88% of subjects. Nonetheless, 12% to 26% of patients have little blood pressure response, and complication rates range between 7% and 28%. Patients with fibromuscular disease are at less risk for systemic emboli than those with aortic atherosclerotic disease.
NR, not reported.
Reproduced from Slovut DP, Olin JW: Current concepts: Fibromuscular dysplasia. N Engl J Med 2004;350:1862–1871 with permission.

Renal Function Outcomes

Most patients with isolated fibromuscular disease have normal renal function. Medial fibroplasia is the most common variant of fibromuscular disease and rarely progresses to renal insufficiency. Hence, there is little justification for undertaking balloon dilation of these lesions for preservation of renal function alone.

Atherosclerotic Disease

The results of PTRA with or without stents for atherosclerosis are more ambiguous and merit close consideration. A recent review of the field commissioned by the U.S. Agency for Healthcare Research and Quality (AHRQ) concluded that ". . . the evidence is not sufficiently robust to determine the comparative effectiveness of angioplasty (with or without stenting) and medical treatment alone. . ."[6]

Blood Pressure Outcomes

Many reports are limited to retrospective observations of BP before and at intervals after a procedure, without standardization of conditions or antihypertensive therapy. Several summaries have been published comprising more than 1000 people subjected to PTRA and stenting. Some of these are summarized in Tables 58-2A and B. Lack of standard medical therapy has led to reports of reduced "number of medications" with little regard for differences between medication regimens. This point deserves emphasis because three prospective, randomized controlled trials comparing medical therapy of atherosclerotic renal artery disease with PTRA, in which therapy and BP measurement were standardized, found only minor BP benefits from PTRA (Table 58-3).[45–47] These

Table 58-2A Outcomes of PTRA and Stenting

Blood Pressure	ATHEROSCLEROTIC DISEASE		
	"Cured"	Improved	Failed
Stent (N = 678)	20%	49%	31%
PTRA (N = 644)	10%	53%	37%
Renal Function	"Improved"	Stable	Worse
Stent (N = 678)	30%	38%	32%
PTRA (N = 674)	38%	49%	21%
Surgery (N = 733)	25%–30%	45%–50%	20%–25%

Summary of published outcomes of PTRA (angioplasty) and stenting for atherosclerotic renal artery stenosis. Interpretation of these reports must be considered in the context of highly variable definitions of "cure" and "improved" blood pressure responses, which lead to high variability between reports[42–44] (see text). Results in patients with atherosclerotic disease generally are worse than in those with fibromuscular disease. The results with PTRA and stents are adapted from a recent "meta-analysis" of published series.[56]

studies were small and limited by patient selection, but they underscore the effectiveness of current drug regimens and the relative infrequency of "cure" in patients with atherosclerosis. They excluded many patients with progressive renal dysfunction, accelerated hypertensive disease, or recent cardiovascular events.

The DRASTIC study (Dutch RAS Intervention Cooperative Study Group) included 106 patients with relatively resistant hypertension, randomized to either medical therapy or PTRA. The lack of difference in BP after 1 year between patients treated with PTRA and those treated medically led the authors to conclude that "angioplasty has little advantage over antihypertensive drug therapy."[47] This study was analyzed under "intention to treat" statistical rules, in which 22/50 patients assigned to medical therapy (44%) crossed over to the PTRA arm due to uncontrolled BP at 3 months. Some might argue that this group provides compelling evidence of medical treatment failures and the benefit of the renal revascularization for such individuals.

The ambiguity of these recent studies highlights changes in medical practice. In the era before potent antihypertensives, renovascular hypertension commonly presented as refractory to treatment, with accelerated or malignant-phase manifestations. Reports from emergency departments suggested that nearly 30% of hypertensive emergencies in white people were derived from individuals with renovascular hypertension. Some of these were refractory to therapy with the agents then available; the patients suffered recurrent episodes of malignant hypertension, sometimes requiring bilateral nephrectomy as a lifesaving measure.[48] With the introduction of more effective and tolerable antihypertensive regimens, particularly those capable of blocking activation of the renin-angiotensin system, an inability to control BP is a far less frequent motivation for renal revascularization. What must be considered in each case is whether the limits of antihypertensive therapy have been reached and whether progressive occlusive disease poses a hazard for the individual patient.

Renal Function Outcomes

Some authors argue that the primary motivation for renal revascularization is now "preservation of renal function."[49] This premise is based on the potential for progressive loss of renal function beyond critical levels of RAS and the possibility of restoring blood flow with effective procedures. Dramatic proof of this concept is available from case studies of individual patients with advanced renal insufficiency regaining viable kidney function after successful PTRA or surgery.[50,51] In some instances, this has meant that they no longer require dialysis therapy. Few experiences are more rewarding to nephrologists. Even when advanced renal dysfunction is not present, it is sometimes prudent to revascularize the kidney to protect it from future progressive vascular occlusion. An example of this is illustrated in Figures 58-6 and 58-7.

However, this argument is tempered by review of renal functional outcomes in several recent series, summarized in Table 58-1. Remarkably, group mean measures of renal function, as reflected by serum creatinine levels, are rarely changed by renal revascularization, with either surgery or PTRA. However, mean values obscure several distinctly different outcomes.[34] Some patients experience major improvements in renal function (20%–25%). Most have no detectable change in function (50%). Unfortunately, the first group is

Table 58-2B   Effects of Renal Artery Revascularization versus Medical Treatment Alone on Clinical Outcomes

Outcomes	Strength of Evidence	STUDIES (PARTICIPANTS), N			Conclusion
		Randomized Trials	Other Comparative Studies	Cohort Studies	
Death	Weak	1 (55)	4 (381)	30 (4646)	No large difference in mortality up to about 5 yr between revascularization and medical treatment.
Kidney function	Acceptable	2 (103)	7 (428)	34 (4916)	No substantial difference in kidney function; improvements were reported in cohort studies only among patients receiving revascularization.
Blood pressure	Acceptable	2 (103)	8 (597)	34 (4275)	Some evidence that blood pressure may be lowered more after angioplasty than with medical treatment alone, particularly among patients with bilateral disease (range, no difference to 26/10 mm Hg lower after angioplasty); cure of hypertension was reported in cohort studies only among patients receiving revascularization.
Cardiovascular events	Weak	1 (55)	1 (52)	3 (560)	No large differences found in comparative studies up to about 4 yr.
Adverse events	Weak	2 (103)	4 (323)	31 (4906)	Evidence does not support meaningful conclusions about relative adverse events or complications from angioplasty compared with medical treatment.

Summary of randomized trials, comparative studies, and observational cohort studies with more than 5000 patients reviewed as part of an Agency for Healthcare Research and Quality (AHRQ) report on comparative effectiveness strategies for renal artery stenosis.[6]

Table 58-3   Three Randomized, Prospective Studies Comparing Medical Therapy and PTRA (with and without Stents)

Study	Number of Subjects	Features	Outcome
Webster et al[45]	N = 55 Unilateral = 27	Run-in medical therapy	No difference in BP, renal function, survival ?Crossover?
Plouin et al[46]	N = 49 All unilateral	Multicenter Ambulatory BP monitoring at 6 months No ACE inhibitors	No difference in BP Slightly fewer meds in PTRA group, more complications Crossover in medical therapy: 7/26 (27%)
Van Jaarsveld[47]	N = 106	Multicenter, office and automated BP measurement, lateralization studies (scan, renal vein renin)	No difference in BP at 12 mos Crossover in medical therapy: 22/50

Summary of three recent prospective, randomized, controlled trials comparing medical therapy to PTRA in atherosclerotic RAS. These series were limited to selected groups of patients, but had the benefit of careful prospective use of antihypertensive medications, standardized BP measurement, and definitions of outcomes. The results of these trials are less dramatic than those of observational reports.[45-47]
ACE, angiotensin-converting enzyme; BP, blood pressure; PTRA, percutaneous transluminal renal angioplasty.

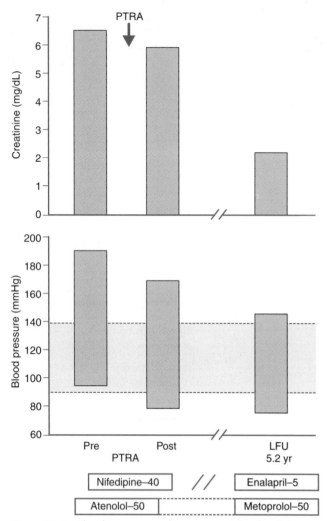

Figure 58-6 Blood pressure and serum creatinine levels in a patient with bilateral renal artery stenosis treated with percutaneous transluminal renal angioplasty. Blood pressure control improved during more than 5 years of follow-up, although medication was still required, including an angiotensin-converting enzyme inhibitor. Most importantly, far advanced renal dysfunction (serum creatinine above 6 mg/dL) improved, avoiding need for renal replacement therapy. Although not uniformly observed, such cases establish the concept that angioplasty and stenting can provide major clinical benefits in selected cases. (Adapted from Textor SC, Wilcox CS: Ischemic nephropathy/azotemic renovascular disease. Semin Nephrol 2000;20:489–502.)

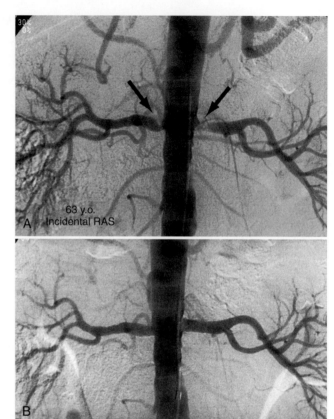

Figure 58-7 **A,** Bilateral ostial atherosclerotic disease in a 63-year-old male first detected incidentally, then later associated with accelerated hypertension. **B,** Post-stent films indicate excellent vessel patency despite their proximal location, which would previously have made them unlikely to remain patent after percutaneous transluminal renal angioplasty alone.

offset by a substantial fraction (15%–22%) who rapidly lose renal function.

Results in the latter group remain the Achilles heel of general application of renal revascularization, whether achieved by endovascular stenting or surgery. Nearly one in five subjects with advanced chronic kidney disease will lose additional renal function, sometimes drastically, as a result of the procedure. The precise reasons for this are not well understood. It is agreed that atheroemboli commonly develop within the renal parenchyma, sometimes producing irreversible renal injury.[52] Importantly, adverse renal outcomes may only unfold days or weeks after the procedure. Patients who follow this course

have a far worse prognosis for renal and patient survival.[38,53] Hence, the clinician must weigh the potential hazards of an adverse outcome of renal revascularization against the true potential for disease progression or adverse events from uncontrolled hypertension.

It has been difficult to predict who will gain from renal revascularization procedures. Greatly advanced renal dysfunction (serum creatinine > 3 mg/dL) is an adverse sign, as are small kidneys (<7 cm in length). Recent studies using Doppler "resistive index" suggest that high vascular resistance within the poststenotic kidney is an adverse sign.[27] The duration and rapidity of onset of renal dysfunction appear to be relevant, although these are difficult to quantify. Some individuals appear to have preserved renal parenchyma via capsular arteries and have been successfully restored to viable renal function after years on dialysis, although this is rare.

Complications of Angioplasty and Stenting

Procedure-related complications from PTRA with stenting (PTRA-S) are common, usually clinically insignificant, and directly proportional to the experience and skill of the operator.[54] Complications include events related to catheter insertion and aortoiliac manipulation, guidewire and catheter negotiation of

Box 58-2 Complications of percutaneous transluminal renal angioplasty and stenting

Most Common
Groin hematoma
Contrast toxicity
Renal artery dissection
Segmental infarction/thrombosis

Most Severe
Cholesterol embolism
Cerebral hemorrhage
Bowel infarction

Vascular Events
Iliac artery dissection
Aortic dissection
Peripheral atheroemboli

Miscellaneous
Sepsis
Stent migration
Perinephric hematoma

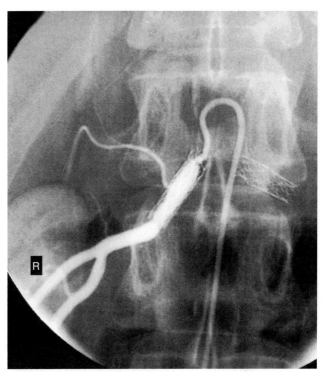

Figure 58-8 Angiogram demonstrating development of restenosis within an endovascular stent and development of a stenotic lesion at the distal portion of the stent. The latter may relate to movement of the kidney relative to a fixed stent. Such lesions may account for worsening hypertension and declining renal function and require repeat intervention. Rates of restenosis currently appear to be in the 14% to 20% range within the first year.

the renal artery and branches, balloon angioplasty and stent placement itself, and adverse effects of contrast material on renal function (Box 58-2).

Groin hematoma after renal PTRA-S occurs in at least 20% of patients. False aneurysms of the common femoral artery occur far less frequently and are now readily treated with ultrasound compression or thrombin injection. More serious is cholesterol or atheromatous embolization of either the lower extremities or kidneys, which can occur in as many as 10% of patients.[55] This can lead to a permanent reduction in renal function or even death.

Review of data from the Mayo Clinic in Rochester, Minn., during a 3-year period (1997–2000) indicates an overall major complication rate of 7.5% per attempted procedure in 140 consecutive patients. No deaths were directly attributable to PTRA-S. Complications included renal artery rupture in 2%, partial kidney infarction in 2.7%, transient or permanent elevation of serum creatinine of 20% or more in 9.5%, procedure-induced requirement of hemodialysis in 2.7%, and blood transfusion in 2.7%.

As serious as these complications were, it is noteworthy that none of these patients required open surgical rescue. Stents allowed endovascular treatment of renal artery rupture or wire perforation and renal artery dissection. Renal artery stent placement is probably safer than balloon angioplasty alone. These data are supported by observations from a meta-analysis comparing 678 patients after renal artery stent placement and 644 patients treated with PTRA alone. The authors concluded that technical success, vessel patency, and restenosis were improved by the use of stents. Remarkably, clinical outcomes in the short term (6–15 months) were no different between the PTRA-S and PTRA groups.[56]

Restenosis

Although implantable metallic stents have expanded the population of patients eligible for PTRA or PTRA-S intervention, restenosis rates remain substantial (Fig. 58-8). A meta-analysis of 14 published series reporting on a total of 678 patients revealed

an angiographically proven restenosis rate of 17% (range, 0%–39%) during a follow-up period of 6 to 29 months.[56] Restenosis is related to renal artery size. Henry and colleagues[57] reported restenosis in 17.6% of stents 5 mm in diameter or less, whereas those 6 mm or larger had a 10.2% rate. This should limit the use of these devices in patients with multiple small renal arteries or severely atrophic kidneys. Studies of coated stents in the renal arteries have been disappointing,[58] further tempering the enthusiasm for stent placement in "incidental" lesions of marginal clinical significance, in which the probability of requiring reintervention for restenosis may exceed the probability of progressive disease needing intervention at all.[17]

Periodic Doppler ultrasonography is useful to evaluate instent stenosis.[59] The decision to redilate should be based on the clinical response to the initial intervention. Secondary patency rates are well over 85% and usually do not require additional stent placement. However, the costs of additional intervention are not trivial.

Selection of Patients for Percutaneous Transluminal Renal Angioplasty and Stenting

Selection for endovascular renal revascularization involves a considered judgment of risks and benefits for each patient. With current medical regimens using effective antihypertensive drugs and intensive measures to reduce cardiovascular risk, many individuals with RAS can be managed indefinitely without renal revascularization. There is sufficient ambiguity as to the benefits of vascular intervention that several randomized, prospective trials (including CORAL, ASTRAL, NITER, and STAR) are in progress to better define these issues. The current issues are summarized in recent debates in the cardiology literature and position papers from nephrologists.[60–63] Until results from such trials are available, clinicians will continue to apply their best judgment to individual cases.

Several points merit re-emphasis in this regard: Patients with unilateral renovascular disease with reasonable BP control and stable kidney function may gain little from vascular procedures; most will continue to need antihypertensive ther-

apy. Every effort should be directed to medical management, including limiting atherosclerosis by statins and providing meticulous control of BP and other risk factors, including cessation of smoking.

Patients with bilateral disease (or stenosis to a solitary functioning kidney) face particular risks for both deterioration of renal function and unsatisfactory BP control with medical management alone.[17] Studies that most consistently indicate benefits to renal function after endovascular stenting are limited to patients with stenosis affecting the entire functioning renal mass.[64] Although many individuals with bilateral disease can be managed without clinical evidence of progression, they

Management of Renovascular Hypertension and Ischemic Nephropathy

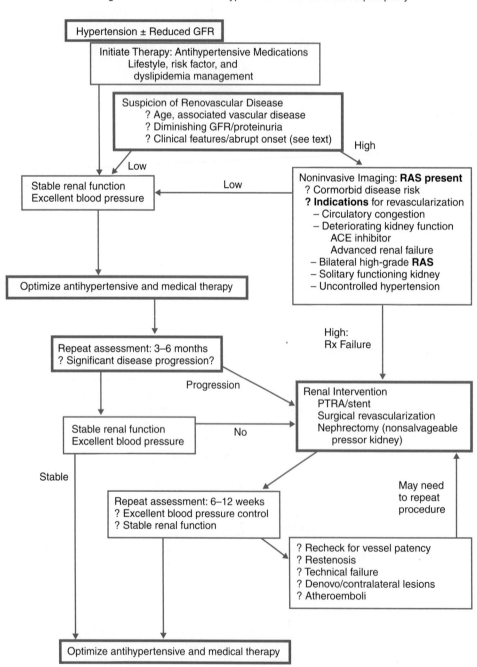

Figure 58-9 Algorithm for an approach to the management of patient with renal artery stenosis.

may have more to gain from successful renal revascularization than other groups, although this has not been proven.

Many patients fall between these limits, with relatively stable BP and kidney function, but at risk for progressive disease and extensive comorbid risk factors. They merit close follow-up and reconsideration based on demonstrated vascular progression. RAS is analogous to other vascular lesions, such as an abdominal aneurysm or carotid stenoses, both of which may exist for many years without posing a true hazard. Evidence of progression may be the critical determinant of who will gain the most from angioplasty or stenting in the kidney also.

SUMMARY

The endovascular techniques of angioplasty and stenting offer effective alternatives for restoring renal blood flow to a wide group of patients. Interventional procedures should be considered for patients with progressive hypertension or loss of renal parenchymal function due to renal artery lesions. There is a potential for recurrence (restenosis) and for serious adverse effects, although these are not common. Clinicians must balance the potential for benefit against the potential for adverse effects. An algorithm for the approach to management is presented in Figure 58-9.

References

1. Harding MB, Smith LR, Himmelstein SI, et al: Renal artery stenosis: Prevalence and associated risk factors in patients undergoing routine cardiac catheterization. J Am Soc Nephrol 1992;2: 1608–1616.
2. Khosla S, Kunjummen B, Manda R, et al: Prevalence of renal artery stenosis requiring revascularization in patients intially referred for coronary angiography. Catheteriz Cardiovasc Interven 2003;58:400–403.
3. Murphy TP, Soares G, Kim M: Increase in utilization of percutaneous renal artery inteventions by Medicare beneficiaries 1996–2000. Am J Roentgenol 2004;183:561–568.
4. Hirsch AT, Haskal ZJ, Hertzer NR, et al: ACC/AHA guidelines for the management of patients with peripheral arterial disease (lower extremity, renal, mesenteric, and abdominal aortic): A collaborative report from the American Associations for Vascular Surgery, Society for Vascular Surgery, Society for Cardiovascular Angiography and Interventions, Society for Vascular Medicine and Biology, Society of Interventional Radiology, and the ACC/AHA Task Force on Practice Guidelines. J Vasc Interv Radiol 2006;17:1383–1397.
5. White CJ, Jaff MR, Haskal ZJ, et al: Indications for renal arteriography at the time of coronary arteriography. Circulation 2006;114:1892–1895.
6. Balk E, Raman G, Chung M, et al: Effectiveness of management strategies for renal artery stenosis: A systematic review. Ann Intern Med 2006;145:901–912.
7. Cooper CJ, Murphy TP, Matsumoto A, et al: Stent revascularization for the prevention of cardiovascular and renal events among patients with renal artery stenosis and systolic hypertension: rationale and design of the CORAL trial. Am Heart J 2006;152:59–66.
8. Slovut DP, Olin JW: Current concepts: Fibromuscular dysplasia. N Engl J Med 2004;350:1862–1871.
9. Garovic V, Textor SC: Renovascular hypertension and ischemic nephropathy. Circulation 2005;112:1362–1374.
10. Schneider E, Guralnik J: The aging of America: Impact on health care costs. JAMA 1990;263:2335–2340.

11. Textor SC: Renovascular hypertension and ischemic nephropathy. In Brenner BM (ed): Brenner and Rector's The Kidney. Philadelphia: WB Saunders, 2004, pp 2065–2108.
12. Jaff MR, Olin JW: Atherosclerotic stenosis of the renal arteries. Tex Heart Inst J 1998;25:34–39.
13. Scoble JE: The epidemiology and clinical manifestations of atherosclerotic renal disease. In Novick AC, Scoble J, Hamilton G (eds). Renal Vascular Disease. London: WB Saunders, 1996, pp 303–314.
14. Caps MT, Perissinotto C, Zierler RE, et al: Prospective study of atherosclerotic disease progression in the renal artery. Circulation 1998;98:2866–2872.
15. Leertouwer TC, Pattynama PMT, van den Berg-Huysmans A: Incidental renal artery stenosis in peripheral vascular disease: A case for treatment? Kidney Int 2001;59:1480–1483.
16. Caps MT, Zierler RE, Polissar NL, et al: Risk of atrophy in kidneys with atherosclerotic renal artery stenosis. Kidney Int 1998;53: 735–742.
17. Chabova V, Schirger A, Stanson AW, et al: Outcomes of atherosclerotic renal artery stenosis managed without revascularization. Mayo Clin Proc 2000;75:437–444.
18. Pearce JD, Craven BL, Craven TE, et al: Progression of atherosclerotic renovascular disease: A prospective, population-based study. J Vasc Surg 2006;44:955–963.
19. Hanzel G, Balon H, Wong O, et al: Prospective evaluation of aggressive medical therapy for atherosclerotic renal artery stenosis, with renal artery stenting reserved for previously injured heart, brain or kidney. Am J Cardiol 2005;96:1322–1327.
20. Bloch MJ, Trost DW, Pickering TG, et al: Prevention of recurrent pulmonary edema in patients with bilateral renovascular disease through renal artery stent placement. Am J Hyper 1999;12:1–7.
21. Harden PN, Macleod MJ, Rodger RS, et al: Effect of renal-artery stenting on progression of renovascular renal failure. Lancet 1997;349:1133–1136.
22. Rundback JH, Sacks D, Kent KC, et al: Guidelines for reporting of renal artery revascularization in clinical trials. Circulation 2002;106:1572–1585.
23. Hricik DE, Browning PJ, Kopelman R, et al: Captopril-induced functional renal insufficiency in patients with bilateral renal-artery stenosis or renal-artery stenosis in a solitary kidney. N Engl J Med 1983;308:377–381.
24. Chobanian AV, Bakris GL, Black HR, et al: Seventh Report of the Joint National Committee on Prevention, Detection, Evaluation, and Treatment of High Blood Pressure (Complete Version). Hypertension 2003;42:1206–1252.
25. McCullough PA, Stacul F, Becker CR, et al: Contrast-induced nephropathy (CIN) Consensus Working Panel: Executive summary. Rev Cardiovas Med 2006;7:177–197.
26. Marckmann P, Skov L, Rossen K, et al: Nephrogenic systemic fibrosis: Suspected causative role of gadodiamide used for contrast-enhanced magnetic resonance imaging. J Am Soc Nephrol 2006;17:2359–2362.
27. Radermacher J, Chavan A, Bleck J, et al: Use of Doppler ultrasonography to predict the outcome of therapy for renal-artery stenosis. N Engl J Med 2001;344:410–417.
28. Zeller T, Frank U, Muller C, et al: Predictors of improved renal function after percutaneous stent-supported angioplasty of severe atherosclerotic ostial renal artery stenosis. Circulation 2003;108: 2244–2249.
29. Bardelli M, Veglio F, Arosio E, et al: New intrarenal echo-Doppler velocimetric indices for the diagnosis of renal artery stenosis. Kidney Int 2006;69:580–587.
30. Tegtmeyer CJ, Selby JB, Hartwell GD, et al: Results and complications of angioplasty in fibromuscular disease. Circulation 1991;83(Suppl):I155–I161.
31. van de Ven PJ, Kaatee R, Beutler JJ, et al: Arterial stenting and balloon angioplasty in ostial atherosclerotic renovascular disease: A randomised trial. Lancet 1999;353:282–286.

32. White CJ: Catheter-based therapy for atheroscerotic renal artery stenosis. Circulation 2006;113:1464–1473.

33. Zeller T, Rastan A, Kliem M, et al: Impact of carbon coating on the restenosis rate after stenting of atherosclerotic renal artery stenosis. J Endovasc Ther 2005;12:605–611.

34. Textor SC, Wilcox CS: Renal artery stenosis: A common, treatable cause of renal failure? Annu Rev Med 2001;52:421–442.

35. Ramos F, Kotliar C, Alvarez D, et al: Renal function and outcome of PTRA and stenting for atherosclerotic renal artery stenosis. Kidney Int 2003;63:276–282.

36. Walker C, Kowalski J, Knan M, et al: Proximal protection before distal protection: Preventing large atheroemboli during renal intervention. Am J Cardiol 2002;90:28.

37. Hiramoto J, Hansen KJ, Pan XM, et al: Atheroemboli during renal artery angioplasty: An ex-vivo study. J Vasc Surg 2005;41:1026–1030.

38. Scolari F, Ravani P, Pola A, et al: Predictors of renal and patient outcomes in atherembolic renal disease: A prospective study. J Am Soc Nephrol 2003;14:1584–1590.

39. Krishnamurthi V, Novick AC, Myles JL: Atheroembolic renal disease: Effect on morbidity and survival after revascularization for atherosclerotic renal artery stenosis. J Urol 1999;161:1093–1096.

40. Holden A, Hill A, Jaff MR, Pilmore H: Renal artery stent revascularization with embolic protection in patients with ischemic nephropathy. Kidney Int 2007;70:948–955.

41. Henry M, Klonaris C, Henry I, et al: Protected renal stenting with the PercuSurge Guardwire device: A pilot study. J Endovasc Ther 2001;8:227–237.

42. Aurell M, Jensen G: Treatment of renovascular hypertension. Nephron 1997;75:373–383.

43. Bonelli FS, McKusick MA, Textor SC, et al: Renal artery angioplasty: Technical results and clinical outcome in 320 patients. Mayo Clinic Proc 1995;70:1041–1052.

44. Ramsay LE, Waller PC: Blood pressure response to percutaneous transluminal angioplasty for renovascular hypertension: An overview of published series. BMJ 1990;300:569–572.

45. Webster J, Marshall F, Abdalla M, et al: Randomised comparison of percutaneous angioplasty vs. continued medical therapy for hypertensive patients with atheromatous renal artery stenosis. J Hum Hypertens 1998;12:329–335.

46. Plouin PF, Chatellier G, Darne B, Raynaud A: Blood pressure outcome of angioplasty in atherosclerotic renal artery stenosis: A randomized trial. Hypertension 1998;31:822–829.

47. van Jaarsveld BC, Krijnen P, Pieterman H, et al: The effect of balloon angioplasty on hypertension in atherosclerotic renal-artery stenosis. N Engl J Med 2000;342:1007–1014.

48. Bennett AH, Lazarus JM: Bilateral nephrectomy performed on an emergency basis for life-threatening malignant hypertension. Surg Gyn Obstet 1973;137:451–452.

49. Pohl MA: Renal artery stenosis, renal vascular hypertension and ischemic nephropathy. In Schrier RW, Gottschalk CW (eds): Diseases of the Kidney. Boston: Little Brown, 1997, pp 1367–1423.

50. Kaylor WM, Novick AC, Ziegelbaum M, Vidt DG: Reversal of end stage renal failure with surgical revascularization in patients with atherosclerotic renal artery occlusion. J Urol 1989;141:486–488.

51. Hansen KJ, Thomason RB, Craven TE, et al: Surgical management of dialysis-dependent ischemic nephropathy. J Vasc Surg 1995;21:197–209.

52. Meyrier A, Hill GW, Simon P: Ischemic renal diseases: New insights into old entities. Kidney Int 1998;54:2–13.

53. Theriault J, Agharazzi M, Dumont M, et al: Atheroembolic renal failure requiring dialysis: Potential for renal recovery? A review of 43 cases. Nephron 2003;94:c11–c18.

54. Palmaz JC: The current status of vascular intervention in ischemic nephropathy. J Vasc Intervent Radiol 1998;9:539–543.

55. Beek FJ, Kaatee R, Beutler JJ, et al: Complications during renal artery stent placement for atherosclerotic ostial stenosis. Cardiovasc Intervent Radiol 1997;20:184–190.

56. Leertouwer TC, Gussenhoven EJ, Bosch JP, et al: Stent placement for renal arterial stenosis: Where do we stand? A meta-analysis. Radiology 2000;21:78–85.

57. Henry M, Amor M, Henry I, et al: Stents in the treatment of renal artery stenosis: Long-term follow-up. J Endovasc Surg 1999;6:42–51.

58. Zeller T, Rastan A, Rothenpieler U, Muller C: Restenosis after stenting of atherosclerotic renal artery stenosis: Is there a rationale for the use of drug-eluting stents? Catheteriz Cardiovasc Interven 2006;68:125–130.

59. Tullis MJ, Zierler RE, Glickerman DJ, et al: Results of percutaneous transluminal angioplasty for atherosclerotic renal artery stenosis: A follow-up study with duplex ultrasonography. J Vasc Surg 1997;25:46–54.

60. Cooper CJ, Murphy TP: Is renal artery stenting the correct treatment of renal artery stenosis? The case for renal artery stenting of renal artery stenosis. Circulation 2007;115:263–269.

61. Dworkin LD, Jamerson KA: Is renal artery stenting the correct treatment of renal artery stenosis? Case against angioplasty and stenting of renal artery stenosis. Circulation 2007;115:271–276.

62. Srivastava S, Beevers DG: Angioplasty for atheromatous renal artery stenosis: Current knowledge and trial results awaited. J Hum Hypertens 2007;21:507–508.

63. Levin A, Linas SL, Luft FC, et al: Controversies in renal artery stenosis: A review by the American Society of Nephrology Advisory Group on Hypertension. Am J Nephrol 2007;27:212–220.

64. Watson PS, Hadjipetrou P, Cox SV, et al: Effect of renal artery stenting on renal function and size in patients with atherosclerotic renovascular disease. Circulation 2001;102:1671–1677.

Further Reading

Balk E, Raman G, Chung M, et al: Effectiveness of management strategies for renal artery stenosis: a systematic review. Ann Intern Med 2006;145:901–912.

Cooper CJ, Murphy TP, Matsumoto A, et al: Stent revascularization for the prevention of cardiovascular and renal events among patients with renal artery stenosis and systolic hypertension: rationale and design of the CORAL trial. Am Heart J 2006;152:59–66.

De Bruyne B, Manoharan G, Pijls NHJ, et al: Assessment of renal artery stenosis severity by pressure gradient measurements. J Am Coll Cardiol 2006;48:1851–1855.

Hanzel G, Balon H, Wong O, et al: Prospective evaluation of aggressive medical therapy for atherosclerotic renal artery stenosis, with renal artery stenting reserved for previously injured heart, brain or kidney. Am J Cardiol 2005;96:1322–1327.

Henry M, Henry I, Klonaris C, et al: Clinical review: The role of embolic-protection devices in renal angioplasty and stenting. Vasc Dis Manage 2007;4:99–111.

Khosla S, Ahmed A, Siddiqui M, et al: Safety of angiotensin-converting enzyme inhibitors in patients with bilateral renal artery stenosis following successful renal artery stent revascularization. Am J Ther 2006;13:306–308.

Krumme B, Hollenbeck M: Doppler sonography in renal artery stenosis—does the Resistive Index predict the success of intervention? Nephrol Dial Transplant 2007;22:692–696.

Mistry S, Ives N, Harding J, et al: Angioplasty and STent for Renal Artery Lesions (ASTRAL) trial: Rationale, methods and results so far. J Hum Hypertens 2007;21:511–515.

Rocha-Singh K, Jaff MR, Rosenfield K, for the ASPIRE-2 Trial Investigators: Evaluation of the safety and effectiveness of renal artery stenting after unsuccessful balloon angioplasty: The ASPIRE-2 study. J Am Coll Cardiol 2005;46:776–783.

Wierema TKA, Kroon AA, deLeeuw PW: Poor performance of diagnostic tests for atherosclerotic renal artery stenosis—discrepancies between stenosis and renal function. Nephrol Dial Transplant 2007;22:689–692.

Chapter 59

Hypertension in Renal Transplant Recipients

John J. Curtis and Robert S. Gaston

Management of hypertension is a common challenge for physicians involved in the care of renal allograft recipients. Hypertension may appear at any time after engraftment, and ultimately afflicts 75% to 80% of patients in the current era of immunosuppressive therapy.[1] Advances in therapeutics for transplantation patients have reduced graft loss due to rejection.[2] Current recipients are older and have more comorbid disease. The most common cause of transplant failure is death with a functioning allograft, and the most common cause of death is cardiovascular disease. The risk of cardiovascular mortality in transplant recipients greatly exceeds that of the general population.[1] Clearly hypertension is a significant risk factor for accelerated atherosclerosis and premature coronary disease, and the impact of hypertension and other variables on cardiovascular risk is exaggerated in transplant recipients.[3,4] In addition, hypertension increases the risk of allograft failure and may accelerate deterioration of graft function.[5,6] Thus, the primary objectives for management of posttransplant hypertension include reducing cardiovascular morbidity and mortality and preserving allograft function.

CLINICAL FEATURES

Whereas more than 90% of cases of hypertension in the general population are *essential* hypertension, most cases of posttransplant hypertension have an evident cause. Although age, sex, and race predispose patients to essential hypertension, they do not significantly influence development of post-transplant hypertension. The nature of a recipient's original renal disease is of little importance. Posttransplant hypertension is usually mild to moderate in severity.[7]

In the past, hypertension was noted most frequently in renal transplant recipients with retained native kidneys or with a cadaveric organ. However, under current immunosuppressive protocols, the impact of calcineurin inhibitor therapy with cyclosporine or tacrolimus overrides the influence of other factors.[8] Definable causes of posttransplant hypertension may be grouped conveniently as either intrinsic or extrinsic to the allograft (Box 59-1). Several pathogenic factors often coexist. Some causes are amenable to specific diagnosis and correction; others are relatively fixed, needing long-term antihypertensive therapy. Virtually all posttransplant hypertension is related to impaired renal allograft function.

APPROACH TO THE PATIENT WITH HYPERTENSION AFTER RENAL TRANSPLANTATION

The initial challenge is to identify correctable causes. Immediately after transplantation, delayed graft function (with sodium and volume excess) may be the main cause of elevated blood pressure (BP). Inadequately controlled postoperative pain may contribute. Thereafter, new or worsening hypertension may represent the onset of acute rejection. Alternatively, because plasma levels of cyclosporine and tacrolimus are usually kept highest during the early post-transplant period, a dose-dependent elevation in BP often results. Six months after transplant, acute rejection becomes less likely; in the recipient with de novo or worsening hypertension, other causes should be considered. These include toxicity from calcineurin inhibitors, recurrent disease, chronic rejection, or transplant renal artery stenosis (TRAS). Finally, retained native kidneys may contribute to hypertension at any time.[7]

Initial studies should document allograft function (Fig. 59-1) with serum creatinine levels, 24-hour urinary protein excretion, and a reliable estimate of glomerular filtration rate (GFR) or renal plasma flow (RPF). Control of extracellular volume should be optimized. If allograft dysfunction is present, renal biopsy may distinguish specific causes.

Immunosuppressants play a major role in the pathogenesis of posttransplant hypertension. Thus, antirejection therapy may need reassessment. Calcineurin inhibitors (either cyclosporine or tacrolimus) remain the cornerstone of current immunosuppressive regimens. Although recent data indicate that hypertension is slightly less common with tacrolimus, both agents are nephrotoxic and—particularly at high blood levels—elevate BP.[9] The dose of cyclosporine or tacrolimus should be optimized. Excessive reduction of the dose to reduce BP may increase the risk of acute rejection. When given in combination with cyclosporine, the immunosuppressant sirolimus

Box 59-1   Causes of Posttransplant Hypertension

Intrinsic
Delayed graft function
Acute rejection
Chronic rejection
Cyclosporine nephropathy (chronic)
Recurrent primary renal disease

Extrinsic
Native kidneys
Immunosuppression
- Cyclosporine
- Tacrolimus
- Corticosteroids
Transplant renal artery stenosis
Hypercalcemia

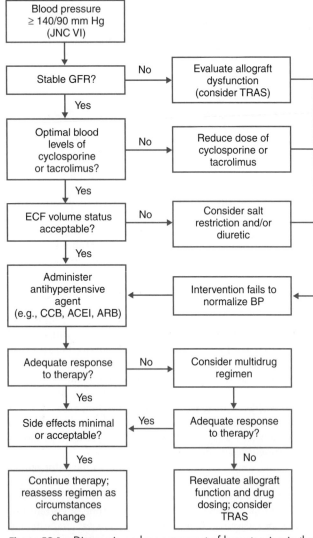

Figure 59-1   Diagnosis and management of hypertension in the renal allograft recipient. ACEI, angiotensin-converting enzyme inhibitor; ARB, angiotensin receptor blocker; BP, blood pressure; CCB, calcium channel blocker; ECF, extracellular fluid; GFR, glomerular filtration rate; JNC VI, Sixth Report of the Joint National Committee[20]; TRAS, transplant renal artery stenosis.

may potentiate hypertension, but independently it does not appear to cause high BP in transplant recipients.[10] Although corticosteroids clearly contribute to hypertension, the influence of prednisone at a maintenance dose of 5 to 10 mg/day on BP seems minimal, and withdrawal of steroids remains controversial.[11] Azathioprine and mycophenolate mofetil seemingly have no adverse effect on BP.

Late onset of hypertension, particularly in a previously stable recipient, is suggestive of TRAS. Administration of an angiotensin-converting enzyme (ACE) inhibitor or an angiotensin receptor blocker (ARB) may help to screen for hemodynamically significant stenosis because a low dose of an ACE inhibitor often causes an immediate and marked decline in GFR in TRAS. Such patients often demonstrate TRAS at angiography. Although radionuclide scanning and Doppler imaging may be useful adjuncts, magnetic resonance angiography has greatly simplified evaluation for TRAS. Use of conventional angiography and its risks can now be limited to patients with a high chance of benefiting from angioplasty or surgery.

Improvement in surgical experience and techniques has decreased the incidence of TRAS, which is now rarely seen but was once claimed to have an incidence of nearly 25%. Because TRAS can be treated and outcomes are excellent, the search for this now rare vascular complication should not be neglected. The most obvious clues are refractory hypertension and increasing serum creatinine level. Recently investigators have pointed to a history of acute rejection or delayed graft function and cytomegalovirus infection as other important clues to consider.[12,13] Although technical causes of TRAS have lessened, the incidence of stenosis of the aortoiliac segment proximal to the graft may be increasing with older transplant recipients. Such lesions can also be diagnosed via Doppler ultrasonography and respond well to intervention.[14]

Outcomes from various radiologic and surgical forms of treatment of TRAS are good, with lowering of BP and return of serum creatinine to baseline values. Restenosis is common after angioplasty, less frequent after stent placement, and much less frequent after surgical intervention, but the risk varies in reverse order and depends on the expertise of the center.

CALCINEURIN INHIBITORS AND HYPERTENSION

The introduction of the calcineurin inhibitors (CNIs) cyclosporine and tacrolimus dramatically reduced acute rejection for transplant recipients. Long-term graft survival, free of rejection, became more common. However, both agents cause hypertension. Before the introduction of these agents, the incidence of posttransplant hypertension was approximately 50%, but with these agents it is 90% or greater. It has been suggested that a lower incidence of hypertension is seen with tacrolimus than with cyclosporine. However, these reports are inconsistent; lower doses are now given, and different methods of monitoring BP are used. Moreover, the drug manufacturer sponsors many of the studies. For example, a recent large study comparison suggested that low-dose tacrolimus resulted in better BP control than cyclosporine,[15] whereas a large, controlled trial with cyclosporine C2 monitoring did not report differences in the incidence or severity of hypertension between the two agents.[16] Although most transplant centers in the United States have switched from cyclosporine to tacrolimus as their primary CNI, there does not seem to have been an improvement in either the incidence or prevalence of hypertension comparable to the 50% seen before routine use of CNIs.

The mechanisms of CNI-induced hypertension have not been identified with certainty. Sodium retention due to preglomerular vasoconstriction, sympathetic nerve stimulation, and direct effects of CNI on arterial vessels have all been documented. Controlling hypertension in patients treated with a CNI is difficult. Patients remain on multiple drug therapy. Suggested methods of treatment include using calcium channel blockers to reverse preglomerular vasoconstriction,[17] switching from cyclosporine to tacrolimus,[18]and minimizing the dose or withdrawing CNIs altogether.[19] The latter seems to have the best effect on CNI-induced hypertension but carries the risk of acute rejection.

MANAGEMENT

Normalization of BP (<140/90 mm Hg) has always been the goal of treatment for hypertensive transplant recipients with stable allograft function or those with chronic rejection. However, recent recommendations from the Joint National Committee (JNC)[20] and the World Health Organization/International Society of Hypertension[21] suggest a more aggressive target. A recent Task Force endorsed target BPs lower than 130/85 mm Hg for patients without proteinuria and 125/75 mm Hg for those excreting more than 1 g of urinary protein per day.[1]

Blood pressure may fluctuate considerably in the transplant recipient because of use of varying doses of steroids and CNIs and changes in GFR, requiring vigilance by the physician and continuous reevaluation of treatment. Although the Sixth Report of the JNC emphasizes the role of "lifestyle modifications" in treating hypertension (including smoking cessation, weight loss, limited sodium intake, and exercise), renal transplant recipients will generally require additional pharmacologic therapy to achieve adequate BP control.[1,20]

Calcium Channel Blockers

Calcium channel blockers (CCBs) effectively reduce BP in most patients. They attenuate both cyclosporine- and endothelin-induced vasoconstriction.[22] These agents can prevent the acute deterioration in RPF and GFR that may accompany elevated cyclosporine blood levels. Theoretically, their other benefits include enhancement of immunosuppression, prevention of delayed graft function, and improvement of GFR in cyclosporine-treated allograft recipients.[23]

Currently available CCBs differ in their effects on the metabolism of cyclosporine and tacrolimus, and on blood levels of the immunosuppressant sirolimus.[10] Verapamil, diltiazem, and the dihydropyridine nicardipine reduce the hepatic metabolism of cyclosporine, thereby increasing its blood level by 40% to 50%. Although some investigators have found this interaction beneficial, it clearly complicates immunosuppressive management. Dosages of the CCB and of the immunosuppressant must be altered concurrently. Other investigators prefer nifedipine or isradipine, which have little effect on blood levels of cyclosporine or tacrolimus. Amlodipine has an intermediate effect on cyclosporine metabolism, and the dose does not usually need adjustment.[24]

Calcium channel blockers are generally well tolerated. However, they may cause peripheral edema and can exacerbate cyclosporine-induced gingival hyperplasia. A retrospective study reported an increased risk of cardiac mortality in renal transplant recipients receiving dihydropyridine CCBs.[3] The implications of this observation remain unclear.

Angiotensin-Converting Enzyme Inhibitors and Angiotensin Receptor Blockers

Use of ACE inhibitors and ARBs to treat hypertension in transplant recipients is becoming increasingly common.[25,26] These agents effectively reduce BP and exert a salutary impact on renal hemodynamics. However, their use in cyclosporine-treated patients has been associated with acute renal failure, hyperkalemia, and anemia. A theoretical basis for avoiding ACE inhibitors and ARBs in such patients is the physiologic similarity between TRAS and cyclosporine-induced afferent arteriolar vasoconstriction. Because angiotensin II is critical for maintaining glomerular perfusion in both situations, inhibition of its effect in the postglomerular circulation might adversely affect GFR. Indeed, in a recent crossover study comparing amlodipine with losartan, there was a similar efficacy in BP reduction but an increase in GFR with amlodipine versus a slight (though not statistically significant) decline with the ARB.[25] However, only losartan significantly reduced proteinuria and plasma levels of transforming growth factor-β_1 (TGF-β_1). These effects may be beneficial in preserving renal function and reducing risk of cardiovascular disease.

Although therapy with these agents must be introduced cautiously, paying close attention to renal function, potassium levels, and blood counts, the vast majority of transplant recipients tolerate ACE inhibitors and ARBs quite well. In some of the 10% to15% of patients who develop anemia while receiving these drugs, we have at times prescribed recombinant erythropoietin to continue what appears to be beneficial therapy. Post-transplant erythrocytosis, a late complication seen most often in stable recipients with well-functioning grafts, resolves with ACE inhibitor or ARB therapy in most patients.[27]

Diuretics

Diuretics are an important therapeutic option because of the volume expansion and salt sensitivity that often accompany post-transplant hypertension. Although salt restriction may pose less of a medical risk, it is rarely adequate to achieve or enhance BP control in this population. Diuretics are a useful adjunct for those who respond to a CCB or another vasodilator with suboptimal BP control or worsening edema. In this setting, a loop diuretic (furosemide or bumetanide) may be required to achieve adequate natriuresis. Thiazides increase the risk of hyperuricemia and hypercalcemia but may also be effective. Given the predisposition of transplant recipients to hyperkalemia, there is little role for potassium-sparing agents.

Other Agents

There appear to be no distinct advantages or disadvantages associated with use of other antihypertensive agents (described extensively elsewhere in Part XI: Management of Secondary Hypertension in this book.

Refractory Posttransplant Hypertension

Transplant recipients with refractory hypertension, or those who require more than three drugs to normalize BP, should undergo evaluation for TRAS. When TRAS is demonstrated, it appears that surgical repair offers the best hope for both immediate and long-term cures (92% and 82%, respectively). However, angioplasty may be successful in as many as three quarters of patients, with long-lasting remissions in 40% to 50%. Most transplant physicians would thus offer angioplasty as a first intervention, particularly for those patients with lesions removed from the vascular anastomosis. Proximal lesions or stenoses at the vascular anastomosis may more frequently require surgical intervention.

When TRAS is excluded in the patient with well-preserved allograft function and no evidence of rejection, bilateral native kidney nephrectomy is an option for intractable hypertension. In experienced hands this substantial operation can be performed safely and—for most patients—will improve control of posttransplant hypertension. Unfortunately, no diagnostic study accurately predicts who will benefit from surgery. With the currently available medical therapies, native kidney nephrectomy is rarely indicated.

References

1. Levey AS, Beto JA, Coronado BE, et al: Controlling the epidemic of cardiovascular disease in chronic renal disease: What do we know? What do we need to learn? Where do we go from here? Am J Kidney Dis 1998;32:853–906.
2. U.S. Renal Data System: USRDS 2000. Excerpts from the United States Renal Data System Annual Data Report: 2000. Am J Kidney Dis 2000;36(Suppl 2):S15–S181.
3. Kasiske BL, Chakkera HA, Roel J: Explained and unexplained ischemic heart disease risk after renal transplantation. J Am Soc Nephrol 2000;11:1735–1743.
4. Massy ZA, Kasiske BL: Post-transplant hyperlipidemia: Mechanisms and management. J Am Soc Nephrol 1996;7:971–977.
5. Brazy PC, Pirsch JD, Belzer FO: Factors affecting renal allograft function in long-term recipients. Am J Kidney Dis 1992;19:558–566.
6. Sanders CE, Curtis JJ: Role of hypertension in chronic allograft dysfunction. Kidney Int 1995;48(Suppl 52):S43–S47.
7. Gaston RS, Curtis JJ: Hypertension following renal transplantation. In Massry SG, Glassock RJ (eds): Textbook of Nephrology. Philadelphia: Lippincott Williams & Wilkins, 2001, pp 1677–1681.
8. Curtis JJ, Luke RG, Jones P: Hypertension in cyclosporin-treated renal transplant recipients is sodium-dependent. Am J Med 1988;85:134–138.
9. Ligtenberg G, Hene RJ, Blankestijn PJ, et al: Cardiovascular risk factors in renal transplant patients: Cyclosporin versus tacrolimus. J Am Soc Nephrol 2001;12:368–373.
10. Saunders RN, Metcalfe MS, Nicholson ML: Rapamycin in transplantation: A review of the evidence. Kidney Int 2001;59:3–16.
11. Steroid Withdrawal Study Group: Prednisone withdrawal in kidney transplant recipients on cyclosporin and mycophenolate mofetil—a prospective randomized study. Transplantation 1999;68:1865–1874.
12. Yu LX, Xiong HY, Fu SJ, Liu XY: Retrospective study of the risk factors of transplant renal artery stenosis. J South Med Univ 2006;26:1160–1162.
13. Audard V, Matignon M, Hemery F, et al: Risk factors and long-term outcome of transplant renal artery stenosis in adult recipients after treatment by percutaneous transluminal angioplasty. Am J Transplant 2006;6:95–99.
14. Voiculescu A, Schmitz M, Hollenbeck M, et al: Management of arterial stenosis affecting kidney graft perfusion: A single-centre study in 53 patients. Am J Transplant 2005;5:1731–1738.
15. Kobashigawa JA, Patel J, Furukawa H, et al: Five-year results of a randomized, single-center study of tacrolimus vs. microemulsion cyclosporine in heart transplant patients. J Heart Lung Transplant 2006;25:434–439.
16. Vincenti F, Friman S, Scheuermann E, et al: Results of an international, randomized trial comparing glucose metabolism disorders and outcome with cyclosporine versus tacrolimus. Am J Transplant 2007;7:1506–1514.
17. Baroletti SA, Gabardi S, Magee CC, Milford EL: Calcium channel blockers as the treatment of choice for hypertension in renal transplant recipients: Fact or fiction. Pharmacotherapy 2003;23:788–801.
18. Hohage H, Welling U, Zeh M, et al: Switching immunosuppression from cyclosporine to tacrolimus improves long-term kidney function: A 6-year study. Transplant Proc 2005;37:1898–1899.
19. Mulay AV, Hussain N, Fergusson D, Knoll GA: Calcineurin inhibitor withdrawal from sirolimus-based therapy in kidney transplantation: A systematic review of randomized trials. Am J Transplant 2005;5:1748–1756.
20. JNC: Sixth Report of the Joint National Committee on Prevention, Detection, Evaluation, and Treatment of High Pressure. Arch Intern Med 1997;157:2413–2446.
21. World Health Organization/International Society of Hypertension Committee: World Health Organization/International Society of Hypertension 1999. Guidelines for the Management of Hypertension. J Hypertens 1999;17:151–183.
22. Ruggenenti P, Perico N, Mosconi L, et al: Calcium channel blockers protect transplant patients from cyclosporin-induced daily renal hypoperfusion. Kidney Int 1993;43:706–711.
23. Weir MR: Therapeutic benefits of calcium channel blockers in cyclosporin-treated organ transplant recipients: Blood pressure control and immunosuppression. Am J Med 1991;90(Suppl 5A):32S–36S.
24. Pesavento TE, Jones PA, Julian BA, et al: Amlodipine increases cyclosporin levels in hypertensive renal transplants: Results of a prospective study. J Am Soc Nephrol 1996;7:831–835.
25. Inigo P, Campistol JM, Lario S, et al: Effects of losartan and amlodipine on intrarenal hemodynamics and TGF-β_1 plasma levels in a crossover trial in renal transplant recipients. J Am Soc Nephrol 2001;12:822–827.
26. Mourad G, Ribstein J, Mimran A: Converting-enzyme inhibition versus calcium antagonist in cyclosporin-treated renal transplants. Kidney Int 1993;43:419–425.
27. Gaston RS, Julian BA, Curtis JJ: Posttransplant erythrocytosis: an enigma revisited. Am J Kidney Dis 1994;24:1–11.

Further Reading

Barri YM: Hypertension and kidney disease: A deadly connection. Curr Cardiol Rep 2006;8:411–417.

Beecroft JR, Rajan DK, Clark TW, et al: Transplant renal artery stenosis: Outcome after percutaneous intervention. J Vasc Interv Radiol 2004;15:1407–1413.

Castillo-Lugo JA, Vergne-Marini P: Hypertension in kidney transplantation. Semin Nephrol 2005;25:252–260.

El-Amm JM, Haririan A, Crook ED: The effects of blood pressure and lipid control on kidney allograft outcome. Am J Cardiovasc Drugs 2006;6:1–7.

Kasiske BL, Anjum S, Shah R, et al: Hypertension after kidney transplantation. Am J Kidney Dis 2004;43:1071–1081.

Ojo AO: Cardiovascular complications after renal transplantation and their prevention. Transplantation 2006;82:603.

Textor SC: Hypertension after renal transplantation. J Hum Hypertens 2004;18:835–836.

Tutone VK, Mark PB, Stewart GA, et al: Hypertension, antihypertensive agents and outcomes following renal transplantation. Clin Transplant 2005;19:181–192.

Weir MR: Blood pressure management in the kidney transplant recipient. Adv Chronic Kidney Dis 2004;11:172–183.

Chapter 60

Management of Hypertension in Patients Receiving Dialysis

Pouneh Nouri and Christopher S. Wilcox

Hypertension is an increasingly common cause of end-stage renal disease (ESRD).[1] The prevalence of hypertension increases with declining renal function. When renal disease reaches end-stage, approximately 80% to 90% of patients suffer from significant hypertension. Diseases that predominantly affect the renal interstitium may produce a salt-losing state, with normotension or even episodes of hypotension and hypovolemia, whereas the more common arterial and glomerular diseases almost invariably cause hypertension. In a meta-analysis by Thompson and Pickering,[2] it was shown that ambulatory blood pressure monitoring (ABPM) for 44 hours and home blood pressure (BP) monitoring over a 1-week period are superior to the routine method of intermittent measurements of BP in the hemodialysis center in predicting end-organ damage and interdialytic BP control. Loss of the nocturnal decline in ABPM has been linked to left ventricular hypertrophy (LVH), adverse cardiovascular outcomes, and all-cause mortality in patients with ESRD.[2]

Blood pressure control usually improves after initiation of dialysis therapy. Nevertheless, more than 75% of people receiving outpatient hemodialysis are also receiving antihypertensive drug therapy. Cheigh and colleagues[3] reported adequate control in only 15% of their patients monitored with ABPM over 48 hours despite widespread use of antihypertensive agents. The U.S. Renal Data System (USRDS) analyzed predialysis BP data on 5369 patients; even with antihypertensive therapy 63% of patients were hypertensive, which was classified as mild in 27%, moderate in 25%, and severe in 11%.[4] Multivariate analysis showed that higher BP was associated with greater intradialytic weight gain, noncompliance with the dialysis regimen, and younger age. This last surprising finding perhaps reflects the observation that patients with congestive heart failure (CHF) or coronary artery disease (CAD) are generally older and have low BP.

Dialysis patients are more prone to accelerated atherosclerosis, independent of comorbid conditions or age.[5]

Longitudinal observations in the general population have concluded that atherosclerosis is retarded by control of BP, which also appears to increase life expectancy. Cardiovascular disease and cerebrovascular disease are the major causes of mortality in the ESRD population. Among patients receiving hemodialysis or peritoneal dialysis, the rates of cardiovascular disease (CVD) mortality are 3 to 20 times higher than in age-matched subjects.[5] CVD is the primary cause of mortality and morbidity in the ESRD population, and is present in as many as 50% to 60% of ESRD patients. Some 28% of hemodialysis patients die each year, and CVD accounts for 45% of this alarming mortality. LVH occurs in 75%, CAD in 40%, and cardiac chamber dilation and CHF in 40% of dialysis patients. ESRD is associated with a 2- to 10-fold increased risk of cardiovascular events.[6] It is difficult to assess the importance of hypertension for CVD risk in ESRD. Remarkably, despite the very high prevalence of CVD and of hypertension in the dialysis population, the largest studies have shown an inverse relationship between BP and total cardiovascular death in these patients.[7-9] Closer examination of the data provides some insight into this paradox. First, the overall relationship between relative risk and BP is U-shaped (Fig. 60-1).[7,8] Patients with a predialysis systolic BP below 120 mm Hg (>10%) and the relatively few (>5%) who have dialysis-resistant, severe hypertension with a postdialysis systolic BP above 180 mm Hg both are at increased risk. However, there is no trend for increased risk among the many patients with moderate hypertension, or even among the 10% with severe predialysis hypertension. The sharply increased risk among those with low BP may relate to the high proportion of these patients who have CHF and CAD. Whereas in the general population CHF presents with fluid overload, in the dialysis population these symptoms are managed by fluid removal at dialysis. Consequently, many dialysis patients with CHF are not recognized, and their predominant finding is hypotension.

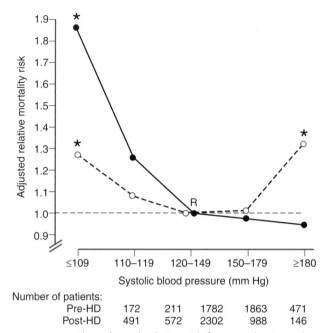

Number of patients:

	≤109	110–119	120–149	150–179	≥180
Pre-HD	172	211	1782	1863	471
Post-HD	491	572	2302	988	146

Figure 60-1 The adjusted relative risk for mortality in end-stage renal disease patients established on maintenance hemodialysis as a function of systolic blood pressure, measured predialysis *(solid circles and continuous lines)* or postdialysis *(open circles and broken lines)*. Compared to reference values at systolic blood pressure 120 to 149 mm Hg; *P < 0.06. Data are from 4500 patients. (Drawn from Port FK, Hulbert-Shearon TE, Wolfe RA, et al: Predialysis blood pressure and mortality risk in a national sample of maintenance hemodialysis patients. Am J Kidney Dis 1999;33:507–517.)

During the first 2 years of hemodialysis, low systolic BP is associated with a sharp increase in mortality.[7] During more prolonged follow-up, increased mortality is apparent in those with a high systolic BP. This suggests that those with low BP are at risk for early death from CHF and CAD. If this group is excluded, and later deaths are examined, hypertension is seen to enhance cardiovascular death modestly. These results are probably influenced by the very high prevalence of prolonged hypertension and atherosclerosis in this population before they begin receiving hemodialysis. This presumably contributes to the greatly increased risk of CVD in those receiving hemodialysis even at a normal BP level. An analysis of 1053 patients on peritoneal dialysis from USRDS related systolic BP lower than 111 mm Hg with higher all-cause and cardiovascular mortality and related systolic BP higher than 120 mm Hg with fewer hospital days during the mean follow-up of 2 years.[10]

As anticipated, cerebrovascular death is predicted by predialysis hypertension.[8] A Japanese study found that death from cerebral hemorrhage and the size of the intracerebral hematoma are positively related to BP in dialysis patients.[11] This confirms the very close association between incident BP and the occurrence and severity of cerebral hemorrhage in the general population.

No controlled interventional trials assess whether CVD is reduced by controlling hypertension in the hemodialysis population. Several lines of evidence from retrospective analyses support the benefit of angiotensin-converting enzyme (ACE) inhibitors in ESRD patients.[12,13] The FOSinopril In DIALysis

(FOSIDIAL) study evaluated the effect of reducing BP by the ACE inhibitor fosinopril on cardiovascular events in ESRD patients with LVH. Some 400 ESRD patients were randomized to fosinopril or placebo and followed for 2 years. Although the BP was significantly lower in the fosinopril group, there were no statistically significant benefits.[14] Good control of BP can cause regression of LVH in patients with ESRD, as in those with essential hypertension. Indeed, a controlled trial of ACE inhibitor therapy in normotensive hemodialysis patients over 2 years demonstrated regression of LVH in the treatment group, without a change in the control group.[15]

Sleep apnea is common in hemodialysis patients. In these patients nocturnal oxygen desaturation is related to "nondipper" BP status and predicts LVH.[16] Because nocturnal BP is not routinely assessed, the high incidence of "nondipping" may confound the relationship between BP measured during the day at dialysis sessions and CVD mortality. Indeed, in a small study of 48-hour ABPM in hemodialysis patients, this measure of BP was shown to be a much better predictor of LVH than predialysis BP.[17] Another study has reported a significant correlation between predialysis hypertension and cerebral atrophy in hemodialysis patients.[18]

These complex data suggest that low BP is a very serious prognostic sign in hemodialysis patients. Such patients should be urgently tested for occult CHF and CAD. Severe hypertension that is resistant to dialysis-induced fluid loss is also an established risk for CVD. Failure to detect a relationship between death from CVD and more modest elevations of BP may arise from a failure to detect nocturnal hypertension accompanying sleep apnea, the irreversible effect of pre-ESRD hypertension and atherosclerosis, and confounding effects due to early cardiovascular deaths from low BP. At this time, it seems reasonable to treat hypertension in patients receiving hemodialysis. Patients benefit from ABPM to assess their true BP burden and to diagnose and assess the effects of therapy on nocturnal hypertension or "nondipper" status.

PATHOPHYSIOLOGY

The pathophysiology of hypertension in renal failure has been reviewed[19] and is summarized in Figure 60-2. Blood pressure is a reflection of cardiac output and total peripheral resistance. A third factor that determines systolic BP and pulse pressure, and becomes important in patients with decreased arterial compliance, is the reflection of the systolic pressure wave retrograde from the resistance vessels.[20] In the elderly, in diabetic patients, and in those with advanced atherosclerosis and vascular calcification, this pressure wave travels sufficiently fast to reach the ascending aorta during systole, thereby accentuating the systolic BP and widening the pulse pressure. Many different factors interact in patients with ESRD to produce hypertension.

Salt and Fluid Retention

A reduction in renal function, associated with a fall in the glomerular filtration rate (GFR), restricts the excretion of salt (NaCl) and fluid. Early in renal failure, there is generally an increase in cardiac output with a relatively low total peripheral resistance that may partly be a response to the development of anemia. With further declines in the GFR, total peripheral resistance begins to increase, reflecting an autoregulatory response

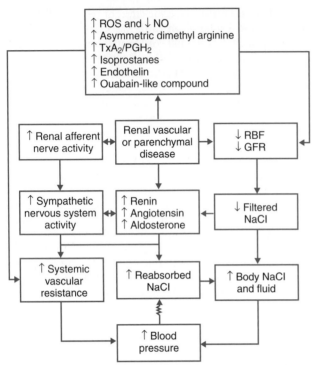

Figure 60-2 Some pathophysiologic mechanisms identified in patients, or animal models, that can increase blood pressure in chronic renal insufficiency. BP, blood pressure; GFR, glomerular filtration rate; NO, nitric oxide; PGH_2, prostaglandin H_2; RBF, renal blood flow; ROS, reactive oxygen species; TxA_2, thromboxane A_2. For full explanation, see text.

to a sustained increase in cardiac output. This phenomenon is known as *total body autoregulation*. However, activation of specific vasoconstrictor mechanisms and inhibition of vasodilator mechanisms can override this autoregulatory response.

Most studies of body fluid volumes in patients with renal insufficiency have shown an expansion of plasma, extracellular and intracellular fluid volumes, and of total body sodium and water.[21] Prolonged expansion of extracellular fluid (ECF) volume may be the major factor underlying hypertension in ESRD. As the GFR declines, the fraction of patients with salt-sensitive hypertension increases exponentially. Scrupulous control of ECF volume by fluid removal at dialysis and restriction of salt and fluid intake between dialysis treatments can reverse hypertension in many patients. In a multivariate analysis of a large USRDS database, large intradialytic weight gain and noncompliance with the dialysis regimen were significant determinants of hypertension.[4] These effects were most pronounced in those without CHF and with established hypertension. In a study conducted over 1 year, patients who were switched from conventional (three times per week) dialysis to dialysis six times per week had a significant reduction in BP, despite using fewer antihypertensive drugs.[22] Survival rate in this selected group of compliant and motivated patients was excellent. Another small study compared extended standard hemodialysis (three sessions of 4.5 to 5 hours per week) with a slower ultrafiltration rate with short daily hemodialysis (six sessions of 2 hours per week). Daily hemodialysis produced better BP control in a group of older hypertensive patients with other cardiovascular morbidities.[23] Another small study reported similar BP levels among patients receiving conventional

dialysis or high-flux dialysis for a shorter time.[24] These data suggest that a more frequent dialysis and good control of salt and fluid intake between treatments can maintain a more normal level of ECF and can moderate hypertension. Indeed, hypertension is remarkably rare in patients receiving daily overnight hemodialysis.[25]

Another technique to reduce thirst and thereby reduce the ECF volume is to reduce the dialysate sodium concentration. However, this can cause hypotension, dizziness, fatigue, and cramp. Another method is to use a variable sodium dialysis in which the dialysate [Na] is reduced exponentially from 155 to 135 mmol/L over 3 hours and maintained at this level for the last hour. A crossover study of this technique reported that it is tolerated, reduces intradialytic weight gain and the need for antihypertensives, and lowers BP.[26] Further study in larger groups is needed to evaluate this simple technique.

Structural Changes and Endothelial Dysfunction

Hypertension in patients with ESRD is associated with functional and morphologic changes in the resistance vessels. Vasodilation is limited by an increase of the media-to-lumen ratio in arterioles. There are increased levels of asymmetrical dimethyl arginine (ADMA, an endogenous nitric oxide synthase inhibitor), and endothelin, and diminished endothelium-dependent vasodilation in patients on dialysis. The impaired endothelial control of vascular smooth muscle tone is particularly important in those who are prone to intradialytic hypertension, whose inappropriately increased peripheral vascular resistance is not related to sympathetic stimulation or renin activation but correlates with the balance between nitric oxide metabolites and endothelin-1.[27]

Endogenous Na⁺/K⁺-Adenosine Triphosphatase Inhibitor

A ouabain-like factor has been extracted from uremic serum that might be an endogenous natriuretic substance that can inhibit Na^+/K^+-adenosine triphosphatase (ATPase) in renal tubules, thus promoting salt excretion.[28] Elevated levels, as seen in uremia, could cause more generalized inhibition of Na^+/K^+-ATPase, leading to increased intracellular sodium in vascular smooth muscle cells, diminished Na^+/Ca^{2+} exchange, and increased intracellular calcium concentration, thereby increasing vascular tone. Inhibition of Na^+/K^+-ATPase activity at synaptic neuronal clefts could reduce norepinephrine uptake, prolong activation of vascular smooth muscle cells, and further enhance vasoconstriction.

Renin-Angiotensin-Aldosterone System

Renin, angiotensin, and aldosterone are important in the pathogenesis of hypertension in most patients with chronic renal failure. In selected patients with intractable hypertension, BP control improves after bilateral nephrectomy and correlates with the prenephrectomy levels of plasma renin activity (PRA). Although PRA is normal or mildly elevated in most dialysis-dependent patients, the PRA is inappropriately high for the expansion of ECF volume and the high BP. Moreover, tissue angiotensin II may be important in patients in whom hypertension responds to ACE inhibitors yet the PRA is normal.

Angiotensin II may potentiate vascular and cardiac hypertrophy both as a vasoconstrictor and by trophic actions.

Sympathetic Nervous System

The sympathetic nervous system is implicated in the pathogenesis of hypertension in patients with ESRD. Total autonomic blockade, or selective inhibition of norepinephrine with debrisoquine, reduces total peripheral resistance and BP. However, plasma norepinephrine levels are variously reported as low, normal, or high, perhaps reflecting the complex nature of catecholamine release, reuptake, metabolism, and excretion in chronic renal failure. Converse and associates[29] made direct recordings of postganglionic sympathetic nerve activity using implanted microelectrodes. They reported that the frequency of sympathetic nerve discharge was nearly three times greater in patients receiving hemodialysis than in normal subjects. Interestingly, after bilateral nephrectomy, BP and peripheral vascular resistance were lowered, and normal rates of sympathetic nerve discharge were seen. These investigators concluded that chronic renal failure activates the sympathetic nervous system via afferent nerve signals arising in the failing kidney.

These studies demonstrate the complexity of the underlying pathophysiology of hypertension in ESRD. They provide a rational basis for using therapies aimed at reducing ECF volume, for using calcium channel blockers (CCBs) and therapies that interrupt the renin-angiotensin-aldosterone system or the sympathetic nervous system.

BLOOD PRESSURE GOALS

Values for lying and standing BP and heart rate should be obtained before and after dialysis treatment. Ideally, BP should be monitored periodically between hemodialysis sessions by 48-hour ABPM because casual measures do not reflect interdialytic BP control and cannot assess "nondipper" status.

The ideal target level for BP is controversial. Studies are lacking on BP goals that are safe and effective in minimizing cardiovascular events in ESRD. However, the Modification of Diet in Renal Disease (MDRD) study demonstrated that it was both feasible and safe, at least under protocol conditions, to have a reduced BP goal of approximately 120/75 mm Hg in patients with moderate or severe chronic kidney disease.[30] However, this study used a selected group that was free of recent cardiovascular or cerebrovascular disease.

We recommend a target predialysis systolic BP of 130 mm Hg in uncomplicated ESRD patients. This is based on experience gained by the MDRD, results from normal subjects in the epidemiologic study by MacMahon and Rodgers,[31] and hypertensive subjects in a trial by Hansson and colleagues[32] in which morbidity and mortality increased with BP levels above this target. It seems probable that many patients who have end-organ damage or LVH, and those with diabetes, would benefit from a lower systolic BP goal of 120 mm Hg. However, some elderly patients will not tolerate this lower BP and require a target of 140/90 mm Hg. Moreover, lower BPs are dangerous for patients who have recently sustained a stroke or an episode of coronary ischemia or myocardial infarction. It is important also to evaluate postdialysis BP in the standing position (or seated for those patients who cannot stand). A

reasonable goal is a systolic postdialysis BP of 110 mm Hg or above. It is preferable to assess BP intermittently with ABPM to assess the full BP burden and diurnal variation.

NONPHARMACOLOGIC TREATMENT

The first step in nonpharmacologic treatment is to set and to achieve a true target *dry weight*, defined as the weight at which intravascular volume is optimal. Weight above the target is accompanied by fluid overload, edema, and hypertension, whereas weight below target is accompanied by fatigue, orthostatic dizziness, hypotension during or between dialysis, excessive thirst, and cramps.[33]

The dry weight must be maintained by a combination of scrupulous attention to salt and water restriction between treatments and effective dialytic fluid removal. Some studies suggest that when this goal is achieved, 85% of hemodialysis patients no longer need antihypertensive medication. In practice, this ideal is rarely achieved. Generally, daily salt restriction to 2 g and daily fluid restriction to 1.0 to 1.25 L produces a tolerable interdialytic weight gain of 2 to 3 kg.

It is advisable to remove fluid gradually during initiation of dialysis over 6 to 8 weeks to achieve the target weight and to prevent hypotension and severe cramps. Overuse of antihypertensives at this time can complicate the removal of fluid because of severe falls in BP. Therefore, a stepwise withdrawal of antihypertensive agents is recommended as body weight is reduced toward the target dry weight. Some hemodialysis patients who do not tolerate removal of fluid by conventional ultrafiltration respond to sequential hemofiltration and hemodialysis, or to treatment with isolated ultrafiltration on consecutive days until the target dry weight is achieved. Others respond to a variable sodium bath regimen.[26]

Patients treated by continuous ambulatory peritoneal dialysis (CAPD) generally have better control of BP, probably because of the continuous and smooth ultrafiltration of fluid. Because daily NaCl and fluid losses are greater in CAPD, restriction of salt and water can be less stringent.

Other nonpharmacologic measures that help to control hypertension include reduction of body weight, regular exercise, avoidance of drugs causing hypertension (e.g., over-the-counter nasal decongestants and nonsteroidal anti-inflammatory drugs), and stress reduction. It is critical to tackle other cardiovascular risk factors, including smoking, dyslipidemia, and coagulopathy states (see Chapter 57).

PHARMACOLOGIC MANAGEMENT

Diuretics

Diuretics are reviewed in Chapters 33 and 51. Thiazide diuretics are generally ineffective when the GFR falls below 20 to 40 mL/min. Increasing dosage of loop diuretics is required in proportion to the reduction in GFR; they become ineffective when the GFR falls below 5 mL/min. An increase in urine output can be achieved in some hemodialysis patients by loop diuretics, reducing the interdialytic weight gain. However, because of the high doses needed in patients with ESRD (e.g., 100–250 mg of furosemide), plasma levels will be elevated and the likelihood of ototoxicity increased. Moreover, in a study of

CAPD patients with residual renal function, loop diuretics did not influence the rate of loss of renal function or the outcome.[34] Diuretics are often withdrawn as dialysis is initiated. However, in a study of 16,420 hemodialysis patients from the Dialysis Outcomes and Practice Patterns Study (DOPPS), diuretic use was associated with lesser interdialytic weight gain and lower odds of hyperkalemia. Patients with residual renal function who received diuretic therapy were almost twice as likely to retain renal function after 1 year in this study. Moreover, this group had a 7% lower all-cause mortality and a 14% lower cardiac-specific mortality risk.[35] It is important to emphasize that this is an observational study and does not prove that diuretics were the cause of these better outcomes.

Calcium Channel Blockers

These agents (Table 60-1) are reviewed in Chapter 53. They inhibit voltage-dependent Ca^{2+} channels in vascular smooth muscle cells and, to some extent, in cardiac cells. Three classes of chemical compounds and eight agents are currently approved for use in the United States.

These agents are readily absorbed after oral administration. No dosage adjustments of CCBs are required in dialysis patients because they are metabolized extensively in the liver, are not renally excreted, and are not significantly removed by hemodialysis or CAPD.

Calcium channel blockers are among the most frequently prescribed antihypertensive drugs in ESRD patients. Their antihypertensive efficacy, unlike all other classes of agents, is relatively well preserved in patients with volume expansion.

Calcium channel blockers are generally well tolerated in dialysis patients. Minor adverse effects relate to vasodilation and include dizziness, intradialytic hypotension (more marked in patients with high interdialytic weight gain), headache, flushing, and edema. Less common effects are nausea, constipation, skin rash, somnolence, and transient abnormalities in liver function tests. Studies in hypertensive patients without ESRD have implicated short-acting CCBs in increased cardiovascular morbidity and mortality. Short-acting agents are not recommended even for hypertensive urgencies. Verapamil and diltiazem have negative inotropic and chronotropic actions. Therefore, they should be used with great caution in patients with poor cardiac function or in those receiving β-blockers.

Because of their efficacy, their safety in renal failure, their removal by metabolism, and a low profile of adverse effects, long-acting CCBs are appropriate for hypertension in dialysis patients. They have added benefits in patients with ischemic heart disease, dilated cardiomyopathy, peripheral vascular disease, Raynaud's phenomenon, and vascular headaches. Further information is needed about their risk-benefit ratio for this group of patients.

β-Blockers

β-Blockers (Table 60-2) are reviewed in Chapter 51. They block renin release and initially reduce cardiac output, central adrenergic drive, and norepinephrine release. In patients with essential hypertension, cardiac output returns toward pretreatment levels over the first 1 or 2 months of therapy, and any fall in BP is due to a reduction in peripheral resistance. It

Table 60-1   Calcium Channel Blockers

Agent	Daily Dose in ESRD (mg)	Dose Modification in ESRD	Special Adverse Effects	REMOVAL WITH DIALYSIS	
				HD	PD
Phenylalkylamine					
Verapamil SR	120–240 max 480 qid	None	Bradycardia, constipation	N	U
Benzodiazepam					
Diltiazem CD	120–360 qid	None	Bradycardia	N	U
Dihydropyridines					
Amlodipine	5–10 qid	None		N	U
Bepridil	200–400 qd	None	Prolonged Q–T, torsades de pointes, agranulocytosis	U	U
Felodipine	5–20 qid	None	Tachyarrhythmia	N	U
Isradipine	2.5–10 bid	None		N	U
Nicardipine SR	30–60 bid	None		N	U
Nifedipine XL	30–120 qid	None	Tachycardia	N	N
Nisoldipine	20–50 qid	None		U	U

CD, controlled diffusion; ESRD, end-stage renal disease; HD, hemodialysis; N, not dialyzed; PD, peritoneal dialysis; Q–T, interval on EEG; SR, slow release; XL, extended length; U, unknown.

Table 60-2   β-Blockers

Agent	ISA/CS/ α+β	Daily Dose in ESRD (mg)	Dose Modification in ESRD	Special Adverse Effects	REMOVAL WITH DIALYSIS	
					HD	PD
Acebutolol	+/+/0*	NR			Y	U
Atenolol	0/+/0	NR			Y	Y
Betaxolol	0/+/0	NR			N	N
Bisoprolol	0/+/0	NR			N	N
Carvedilol	0/0/+	6.25–12.5 bid		Orthostasis	N	N
Carvedilol CR	0/0/+	10, 20, 40, 80		Bradycardia, dizziness, shortness of breath	N	N
Labetalol	0/0/+	200–600 tid	None	Orthostasis	N	N
Metoprolol	0/+/0	50–100 bid	Additional dose post-HD		Y	U
Nadolol	0/0/0	NR			Y	U
Nebivolol	0/0/0	1.25, 2.5, 5, 10, 20		Bradycardia	U	U
Pindolol	+/0/0	NR			Y	N
Propanolol	0/0/0	80–160 bid	Additional dose post-HD		N	N
Sotalol	0/0/0	NR		Torsades de pointes	Y	N
Timolol	0/0/0	10 bid		Hypotension	U	U

+, present; 0, not present at therapeutic doses; *, drug has active metabolites.
α+β, alpha- and beta-blocking activity; CS, cardioselectivity; ESRD, end-stage renal disease; HD, hemodialysis; ISA, intrinsic sympathomimetic activity; N, no; NR, not recommended for initial therapy in ESRD because the drug is cumulative and, if used, needs careful monitoring and dose reduction; PD, peritoneal dialysis; U, unknown; Y, yes.

is not known if similar changes occur in hemodialysis patients. Labetalol and carvedilol also block α-adrenergic receptors, which significantly increases their antihypertensive efficacy, and carvedilol is an antioxidant drug. Moreover, these additional actions maintain cardiac output.

β-Blockers are either predominantly lipid-soluble (*lipophilic*) or water-soluble (*hydrophilic*). Lipophilic β-blockers such as propranolol or metoprolol are metabolized extensively in the liver and have a short duration of action. However, the metabolites may be active and may be hydrophilic, as in the case of acebutolol. Hydrophilic β-blockers such as atenolol and nadolol are long-acting, are excreted by the kidneys, and are removed during hemodialysis or CAPD. They accumulate in patients with renal failure. Therefore, nadolol, atenolol, acebutolol, and sotalol must be used with extra caution in patients with ESRD. Some noncompliant or confused patients may not be able to manage a daily intake of antihypertensives. For them, a dose of long-acting atenolol after hemodialysis provides a measure of BP control between dialysis. Nebivolol is a relatively new lipophilic β-blocker approved for hypertension that is devoid of intrinsic sympathomimetic or membrane-stabilizing activity. Its unique

properties are nitric oxide-mediated vasodilation, which appears to protect left ventricular function. It requires study in hemodialysis patients.

β-Blockers produce a spectrum of dose-dependent adverse effects. They can increase insulin resistance and dyslipidemia, which are correlates of cardiovascular mortality. However, these effects are less obvious with cardioselective agents such as metoprolol or those with intrinsic sympathomimetic activity such as pindolol. Other adverse effects include hyperkalemia, bradycardia, Raynaud's phenomenon, and central nervous system effects, including nightmares and sleep disturbance, fatigue, and depression. β-Blockers may exaggerate cardiac failure in poorly compensated patients or produce bronchospasm in patients with asthma; they may mask the symptoms of hypoglycemia in patients with diabetes.

β-Blockers can be used as antihypertensive agents in patients with ESRD. Antihypertensive efficacy in essential hypertension is greater in white than in black patients, in young than in old, and in those with high plasma renin levels. Therefore, they are most effective in ESRD patients who are maintained at a low target weight. Their beneficial effect on cardiovascular morbidity and mortality, on symptomatic angina, and on preventing death in patients who have had a myocardial infarction have not been studied in ESRD. However, because of the experience with these drugs in other areas, they are our preferred treatment for ESRD patients with these conditions, even in a patient without significant hypertension.

An important finding in patients on hemodialysis with dilated cardiomyopathy is that after 1 year of treatment with carvedilol their left ventricular ejection fraction increased by 39%, and their left ventricular systolic anad diastolic volumes decreased by 16% and 6%, respectively, compared with those treated with placebo. Remarkably, by the end of the second year of the trial, 49% fewer patients in the carvedilol group died compared with those receiving placebo.[36] These are some of the most positive clinical trial data in patients with ESRD. Although they require confirmation, these findings provide a strong rationale for the use of slow-release carvedilol in the many hemodialysis patients with dilated cardiomyopathy.

ACE Inhibitors

ACE inhibitors (Table 60-3) are reviewed in Chapter 52. They lower BP by reducing peripheral vascular resistance. They not only inhibit conversion of angiotensin I to angiotensin II in the circulation and tissues, but also inhibit bradykinin degradation by blocking kinase II. The increased bradykinin levels stimulate nitric oxide and prostaglandin synthesis. ACE inhibitors reset the baroreflex and dampen the sympathetic nervous system so that heart rate does not normally change.

ACE inhibitors are divided into three broad groups: sulfhydryl-containing (captopril), dicarboxyl-containing (lisinopril, benazepril, quinapril, ramipril, spirapril, perindopril, enalapril, and cilazapril), and phosphorus-containing (fosinopril). Only captopril and lisinopril are active drugs; the others are prodrugs that are converted in vivo to active compounds.

Absorption of captopril is markedly affected by food. It should be taken 1 hour before meals. The active form of most ACE inhibitors and their metabolites is largely excreted by the kidneys. However, another important route of elimination for fosinopril, spirapril, and benazepril is by hepatic metabolism. In renal failure, this compensates for lack of renal excretion and prevents substantial accumulation of these agents. Quinapril is tightly bound to tissue angiotensin-converting enzyme, which prevents major accumulation in ESRD. Therefore, only modest dose reduction is required.

ACE inhibitors are generally well tolerated. Common adverse effects include cough in 5% to 20%. Serious hyperkalemia can occur but is uncommon in hemodialysis patients. Other adverse effects are quite rare but include skin rashes, angioedema, abnormal taste, neutropenia, and hepatotoxicity. Anaphylactoid reactions have been reported in patients on ACE inhibitors treated with the high-flux dialysis membrane AN69. Therefore, this membrane should be avoided in patients receiving ACE inhibitors.

ACE inhibitors (or β-blockers) are particularly effective in treating hypertension that is resistant to dialysis, in which high levels of plasma renin activity are encountered. In contrast, they have little antihypertensive action in patients who are overloaded with fluid and salt and in those who have very low levels of plasma renin activity. Other beneficial actions of ACE inhibitors in treating essential hypertension include an increase in large artery compliance, reduction in LVH, and improvement in insulin resistance. These drugs can moderate the excessive thirst that plagues some patients with ESRD. A

Table 60-3   Angiotensin-Converting Enzyme Inhibitors

Agent	Daily Dose in ESRD (mg)	Dose Modification in ESRD	REMOVAL WITH DIALYSIS	
			HD	PD
Benazepril	2.5–20 qid	50%–75% dose reduction	N	U
Captopril	12.5–25 qid	50% dose reduction, and once-daily dosing; additional dose post-HD	Y	N
Enalapril	2.5–10 bid	50% dose reduction, and additional dose post-HD	Y	N
Fosinopril*	10–40 qid	Additional dose post-HD	Y	N
Lisinopril	2.5–20 qid	50%–75% dose reduction, and additional dose post-HD	Y	N
Moexipril	7.5–15 qid		U	U
Quinapril*	10–40 qid	0–25% dose reduction, and additional dose post-HD	Y	N
Ramipril	2.5–10 qid	50%–75% dose reduction, and additional dose post- HD	Y	N
Spirapril*	3–6 qid	None	U	U
Trandolapril	1–3 qid	50% dose reduction	U	U

*Preferred agents in end-stage renal disease (ESRD) because major modifications of dose are not required.
HD, hemodialysis; N, no; PD, peritoneal dialysis; U, unknown; Y, yes.

controlled trial of fosinopril in 400 hemodialysis patients with LVH failed to detect statistically significant benefit.[14]

Angiotensin II Receptor Blockers

These drugs (Table 60-4) are reviewed in Chapter 52. They act by blocking the binding of angiotensin II to its type 1 receptors (AT_1). The role of angiotensin II type 2 receptors (AT_2) is unclear, and no therapeutic AT_2 receptor antagonists are available. Angiotensin receptor blockers (ARBs) reduce BP and inhibit the effects of angiotensin II on the kidney, sympathetic nervous system, and aldosterone secretion.

Losartan is readily absorbed. It has a bioavailability of 33%, and is metabolized in the liver to active metabolites. Losartan and its metabolite have plasma half-lives of 2 hours and 6 to 9 hours, respectively. Only 4% to 7% is excreted through the kidneys. Thus, accumulation in renal failure is not likely. The safety and efficacy of losartan in ESRD has been established in a controlled study.[37] Unlike an ACE inhibitor, losartan does not produce cough or angioedema, but it has other adverse effects that are similar to those of ACE inhibitors and may also cause headache, lightheadedness, and gastrointestinal prob-

lems. Other ARBs appear well tolerated and are effective in patients with ESRD. Because none is excreted significantly in an active form by the kidney, they do not accumulate in hemodialysis patients.

Centrally Acting Drugs

These agents (Table 60-5) reduce BP by activating α_2-adrenergic receptors and imidazoline-preferring receptors in the brain. This reduces sympathetic outflow and thus reduces peripheral vascular resistance.

Centrally acting drugs are well absorbed after oral administration. Methyldopa is metabolized to α-methylnorepinephrine, which is the active compound in the brain. The active metabolites of methyldopa and 50% of the dose of clonidine and guanfacine are excreted by the kidneys. Therefore, these drugs accumulate modestly in ESRD.

Sedation and dry mouth are dose-dependent adverse effects that usually improve after several weeks of treatment. Sexual dysfunction with decreased libido is common. Bradycardia, especially in patients with sinoatrial nodal disease, may necessitate discontinuation of treatment.

Clonidine has been used extensively in ESRD and is an effective antihypertensive. A clonidine transdermal patch is particularly beneficial when compliance is a problem. It provides useful background antihypertensive action in patients undergoing hemodialysis.

Adrenergic Blocking Agents

These agents (Table 60-6) antagonize the action of catecholamines at postjunctional α_1-receptors, thereby inhibiting vasoconstriction. This results in dilation of arterial (resistance) and venous (capacitance) vessels that reduce peripheral vascular resistance and BP. Cardiac output and heart rate are not usually affected.

These drugs are well absorbed, metabolized extensively in the liver, and excreted in the bile. Very small amounts are excreted unchanged in urine. They do not accumulate in ESRD.

Short-acting adrenergic blocking agents can cause a first-dose phenomenon, in which marked hypotension and

Table 60-4 Angiotensin Receptor Blockers

Agent	Daily Dose in ESRD (mg)	Removal with HD	Removal with PD
Candesartan	8–32	N	N
Eprosartan	400–800	N	N
Irbesartan	150–300	N	N
Losartan	25–100	N	N
Telmisartan	40–80	N	N
Valsartan	80–320	N	N

None of these agents requires major dose reductions in HD patients. ESRD, end-stage renal disease; HD, hemodialysis; PD, peritoneal dialysis.

Table 60-5 Centrally Acting Agents

Agent	Daily Dose in ESRD (mg)	Dose Modification in ESRD	Special Adverse Effects	REMOVAL WITH DIALYSIS HD	REMOVAL WITH DIALYSIS PD
Methyldopa	250–500 qid	Increase dose interval to once-daily dosing; additional dose of 250 mg post-HD	Hepatotoxicity, HUS, Coombs-positive hemolytic anemia, LE-like syndrome, retroperitoneal fibrosis, pancreatitis, bone marrow suppression	Y	Y
Clonidine	0.1–0.3 bid	25%–50% dose reduction, and bid dosing	Contact dermatitis with patch	N	N
Guanfacine	0.5–1.5 qid	25%–50% dose reduction		N	N

ESRD, end-stage renal disease; HD, hemodialysis; HUS, hemolyticuremic syndrome; LE, lupus erythematosus; N, no; PD, peritoneal dialysis. Y, yes.

Table 60-6   Adrenergic Blocking Agents

Agent	Daily Dose in ESRD (Mg)	Dose Modification in ESRD	REMOVAL WITH DIALYSIS	
			HD	PD
Doxazosin	1–16 qid	None	N	N
Prazosin	1–15 bid	None	N	N
Terazosin	1–20 qid	None	U	U

ESRD, end-stage renal disease; HD, hemodialysis; N, no; PD, peritoneal dialysis; U, unknown.

syncope occur 30 to 90 minutes after taking the medication. Other adverse effects, such as headache, dizziness, drowsiness, and nausea, are usually transient. However, their use in ESRD can exacerbate hypotension during dialysis-induced fluid removal. Therefore, they require careful monitoring and are not the drugs of first choice for these patients.

Nonspecific Vasodilators

These drugs (Table 60-7) lower BP by acting directly on vascular smooth muscle cells. Minoxidil produces vasodilation through its metabolite, which activates ATP-dependent potassium channels in vascular smooth muscle cells, thereby increasing cellular potassium ion influx. This leads to cell membrane hyperpolarization, exit of calcium ions, and vasodilation. Minoxidil is readily absorbed and metabolized in the liver. Only 10% to 20% is excreted unchanged in urine.

Minoxidil remains an important agent for short-term treatment of severe and refractory hypertension in ESRD (see Fig. 60-3) despite an adverse-effect profile that includes pericardial effusion, hypertrichosis, tachycardia, sympathetic excitation, and postural hypotension. It is contraindicated in patients with diastolic dysfunction and severe LVH, in whom it can cause cardiac failure. It can induce nonspecific T-wave changes, rashes, Stevens-Johnson syndrome, glucose intolerance, formation of antinuclear antibodies, and thrombocytopenia.

Hydralazine is also a direct vasodilator, but its mechanism of action is not well understood. It causes quite marked tachycardia due to reflex sympathetic activation. It is well absorbed and is inactivated by acetylation in the liver and bowel. The rate of acetylation is genetically determined. The

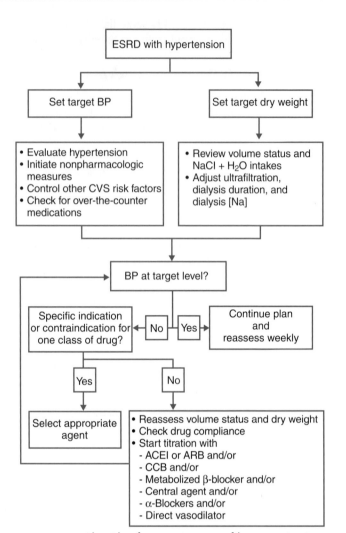

Figure 60-3   Algorithm for management of hypertension in hemodialysis patients. ACEI, angiotensin-converting enzyme inhibitor; BP, blood pressure; CCB, calcium channel blocker; CVS, cardiovascular system; ESRD, end-stage renal disease.

drug is excreted hepatically, but its metabolite is excreted primarily by the kidneys. It has a longer duration of action in patients with ESRD. Adverse effects include headache, flushing, hypotension, palpitations, tachycardia, dizziness, and angina pectoris. Other important, but less common, reactions include drug-induced lupus, hemolytic anemia, serum

Table 60-7   Vasodilators

Agent	Daily Dose in ESRD (mg)	Dose Modification in ESRD	Special Adverse Effects	REMOVAL WITH DIALYSIS	
				HD	PD
Hydralazine	25–50 bid	bid dosing	Lupuslike syndrome	N	N
Minoxidil	5–30 bid	Additional dose post-HD	Pericardial effusion	Y	Y
Nitroprusside	0.25–8 μg/kg/min	Not be used for more than 36–72 hr	Thiocyanate toxicity	Y	Y

ESRD, end-stage renal disease; HD, hemodialysis; N, no; PD, peritoneal dialysis; Y, yes.

sickness, and vasculitis. The use of hydralazine in ESRD has diminished with the advent of more effective agents that have fewer adverse effects.

Sodium nitroprusside is a nitrovasodilator with considerable value in hypertensive emergencies. It is converted in smooth muscle to nitric oxide, which activates guanyl cyclase, providing cyclic guanosine monophosphate, which leads to vasorelaxation. It is used parenterally in hypertensive emergencies (see Chapter 55). The thiocyanate produced during its metabolism is excreted solely through the kidneys and accumulates in patients with ESRD, in whom it causes lactic acidosis, central nervous system disturbance, seizures, and coma.

OVERVIEW OF HYPERTENSION MANAGEMENT IN ESRD

Our approach to hypertension management is reviewed in Figure 60-3. The first step toward controlling hypertension in ESRD is fluid management. Removal of salt and water with dialysis should be complemented by educating patients about restriction of their salt and water intake. If medications are required, they should be tailored according to the needs of each patient and their own associated medical conditions (see Chapter 56). BP control is improved by judicious use of ABPM to review control of arterial pressure and to make appropriate adjustment of treatment. Long-term studies of BP control in dialysis populations and the relative importance of different agents, in particular the role of ACE inhibitors and ARBs, are urgently required.

References

1. U.S. Renal Data System: 1999 Annual Data Report. Bethesda, Md.: National Institutes of Health, National Institute of Diabetes and Digestive and Kidney Diseases, 1999.
2. Thompson AM, Pickering TG: The role of ambulatory blood pressure monitoring in chronic and end stage renal disease. Kidney Int 2006;70:1000–1007.
3. Cheigh JS, Milite C, Sullivan JF, et al: Hypertension is not adequately controlled in hemodialysis patients. Am J Kidney Dis 1992;19:453–459.
4. Rahman M, Fu P, Sehgal AR, et al: Interdialytic weight gain, compliance with dialysis regimen, and age are independent predictors of blood pressure in hemodialysis patients. Am J Kidney Dis 2000;35:257–265.
5. Foley RN, Parfrey PS, Sarnak MJ: Clinical epidemiology of cardiovascular disease in chronic renal disease. Am J Kidney Dis 1998;32:S112–S119.
6. U.S. Renal Data System: 2004 Annual Data Report: Atlas of End-Stage Renal Disease in the United States. Bethesda, Md.: National Institutes of Health, National Institute of Diabetes and Digestive and Kidney Diseases, 2004.
7. Mazzuchi N, Carbonell E, Fernández-Cean J: Importance of blood-pressure control in hemodialysis patient survival. Kidney Int 2000;58:2147–2154.
8. Port FK, Hulbert-Shearon TE, Wolfe RA, et al: Predialysis blood pressure and mortality risk in a national sample of maintenance hemodialysis patients. Am J Kidney Dis 1999;33:507–517.
9. Zager PG, Nikolic J, Brown RH, et al: "U" curve association of blood pressure and mortality in hemodialysis patients. Kidney Int 1998;54:561–569.
10. Goldfarb-Rumyantzef AS, Baird BC, Leypoldt JK, Cheung AK: The association between BP and mortality in patients on chronic peritoneal dialysis. Nephrol Dial Transplant 2005;20:1693–1701.
11. Kawamura M, Fijimoto S, Hisanaga S, et al: Incidence, outcome, and risk factors of cerebrovascular events in patients undergoing maintenance hemodialysis. Am J Kidney Dis 1998;31:991–996.
12. Efrati S, Zaidenstein R, Dishy V, et al: ACE inhibitors and survival of hemodialysis patients. Am J Kidney Dis 2002;40:1023–1029.
13. McCullough PA, Sandberg KR, Yee J, et al: Mortality benefit of angiotensin-converting enzyme inhibitors after cardiac event in patients with end stage renal disease. J Renin Angiotensin Aldosterone Syst 2002;3:188–191.
14. Zannad F, Kessler M, Lehert P, et al: Prevention of cardiovascular events in end stage renal disease: Results of a randomized trial of fosinopril and implications for future studies. Kidney Int 2006;70:1318–1324.
15. Cannella G, Paoletti E, Delfino R, et al: Prolonged therapy with ACE inhibitors induces the regression of left ventricular hypertrophy of dialysed uremic patients independently from hypotensive effects. Am J Kidney Dis 1997;5:659–664.
16. Zoccali C, Benedetto FA, Tripepi G, et al: Nocturnal hypoxemia, night-day arterial pressure changes and left ventricular geometry in dialysis patients. Kidney Int 1998;53:1078–1084.
17. Cannella G, Paoletti E, Ravera G, et al: Inadequate diagnosis and therapy of arterial hypertension as causes of left ventricular hypertrophy in uremic dialysis patients. Kidney Int 2000;58:260–268.
18. Savazzi GM, Cusmano F, Bergamaschi E, et al: Hypertension as an etiopathological factor in the development of cerebral atrophy in hemodialysed patients. Nephron 1998;81:17–24.
19. Wilcox CS: Management of hypertension in patients with renal disease. In Smith TS (ed): Cardiovascular Therapeutics. Cambridge, UK: WB Saunders, 1996, pp 538–545.
20. O'Rourke MF, Kelly RP: Wave reflection in the systemic circulation and its implications in ventricular function. J Hypertens 1993;11:327–337.
21. Mitch WE, Wilcox CS: Disorders of body fluids, sodium and potassium in chronic renal failure. Am J Med 1982;72:536–550.
22. Woods JD, Port FK, Orzol S, et al: Clinical and biochemical correlates of starting "daily" hemodialysis. Kidney Int 1999;55:2467–2476.
23. Fagugli RM, Pasini P, Pasticci F, et al: Effects of short daily hemodialysis and extended standard hemodialysis on blood pressure and cardiac hypertrophy. A comparative study. J Nephrol 2006;19(1):77–83.
24. Velasquez MT, von Albertini B, Lew SQ, et al: Equal levels of blood-pressure control in ESRD patients receiving high-efficiency hemodialysis and conventional hemodialysis. Am J Kidney Dis 1998;31:618–623.
25. Charra B, Calemard E, Ruffet M, et al: Survival as an index of adequacy of dialysis. Kidney Int 1992;41:1286–1291.
26. Flanigan MJ, Khairullah QT, Lim VS: Dialysate sodium delivery can alter chronic blood pressure management. Am J Kidney Dis 1997;29:383–391.
27. Chou Kj, Lee PT, Chiou CW, et al: Physiological changes during hemodialysis in patients with intradialysis hypertension. Kidney Int 2006;69:1833–1838.
28. Huang BS, Veerasingham SJ, Leenen FH: Brain "ouabain," Ang II, and sympathoexcitation by chronic central sodium loading in rats. Am J Physiol 1998;274:H1269–H1276.
29. Converse RL Jr, Jacobsen TN, Toto RD, et al: Sympathetic overactivity in patients with chronic renal failure. N Engl J Med 1992;327:1912–1918.
30. Klahr S, Levey AS, Beck GJ, et al: The effects of dietary protein restriction and blood-pressure control on the progression of chronic renal disease. N Engl J Med 1994;330:877–884.
31. MacMahon S, Rodgers A: The effects of blood pressure reduction in older patients: An overview of five randomized controlled trials in elderly hypertensives. Clin Exp Hypertens 1993;15:967–978.

32. Hansson L, Zanchetti A, Carruthers SG, et al: Effects of intensive blood-pressure lowering and low-dose aspirin in patients with hypertension: Principal results of the Hypertension Optimal Treatment (HOT) randomised trial. Lancet 1998;351: 1755–1762.

33. Mailloux LU, Fields S, Campese VM: Hypertension in chronic dialysis patients. In Nissenson AR, Fine RN (eds): Dialysis Therapy. Philadelphia: Hanley & Belfus, 2000, pp 341–352.

34. Medcalf JF, Harris KP, Walls J: Role of diuretics in the preservation of residual renal function in patients on continuous ambulatory peritoneal dialysis. Kidney Int 2001;59:1128–1133.

35. Bragg-Gresham JL, Fissell RB, Mason NA, et al: Diuretic use, residual renal function, and mortality among hemodialysis patients in the Dialysis Outcomes and Practice Pattern Study (DOPPS). Am J Kidney Dis 2007;49:426–431.

36. Cice G, Ferrara L, D'Andrea A, et al: Carvedilol increases two-year survival in dialysis patients with dilated cardiomyopathy: a prospective, placebo-controlled trial. J Am Coll Cardiol 2003;41:1438–1444.

37. Shahinfar S, Simpson RL, Carides AD, et al: Safety of losartan in hypertensive patients with thiazide-induced hyperuricemia. Kidney Int 1999;56:1879–1885.

Further Reading

Bishu K, Gricz KM, Chewaka S, Agarwal R: Appropriateness of antihypertensive drug therapy in hemodialysis patients. Clin J Am So Nephrol 2006;1:820–824.

Copley JB: Optimizing hypertension control in patients with multiple cardiovascular risk factors. J Clin Hyperten 2006;10(Suppl 3): 2–4.

Dasselaar JJ, Huisman RM, de Jong PE, et al: Effects of relative blood volume-controlled hemodialysis on blood pressure and volume status in hypertensive patients. Am Soc Artif Intern Org J 2007;53(3):357–364.

Inrig JK, Patel UD, Gillespie BS, et al: Relationship between interdialytic weight gain and blood pressure among prevalent hemodialysis patients. Am J Kidney Dis 2007;50(1):108–118.

Resistant hypertension: Current diagnosis, treatment, and management strategies. J Clin Hyperten 2007;1(Suppl 1):1–32.

Chapter 61

Adrenal Disorders

Emmanuel L. Bravo

ADRENOCORTICAL DISORDERS

The adrenal cortex can cause hypertension through overproduction of 11-deoxycorticosterone (DOC), aldosterone, or cortisol. DOC and aldosterone are mineralocorticoids that produce hypertension primarily through salt and water retention. Cortisol is a glucocorticoid that can cause hypertension, in part by exerting a mineralocorticoid effect because of incomplete metabolism at target sites. The adrenal medulla can cause hypertension by overproduction of catecholamines from a pheochromocytoma.

Hypertensive Syndromes Due to Excess Production of 11-Deoxycorticosterone

Congenital adrenocortical disorders due to enzyme deficiency of either 11β-hydroxylase[1] or 17α-hydroxylase[2] reduce production of cortisol, leading to uninhibited secretion of corticotropin, which drives the zona fasciculata to increase production of DOC. In both 11β- and 17α-hydroxylase deficiency, physiologic replacement doses of dexamethasone 0.5–0.75 mg/day) decrease DOC production by inhibiting corticotropin release, resulting in normalization of arterial blood pressure (BP) and serum potassium concentration.

In generalized glucocorticoid resistance, cortisol secretion remains corticotropin-dependent but is reset to a higher than normal level.[3] There is a corticotropin-dependent increase in mineralocorticoids (primarily DOC) and adrenal androgens. Because there is no peripheral resistance to these hormones, they produce their clinical effects of hypertension and hypokalemia (together with signs of excess androgens). Two strategies are used to treat generalized glucocorticoid resistance. The first employs large doses of dexamethasone (i.e., supraphysiological amounts) to suppress corticotropin secretion. The second employs mineralocorticoid or androgen antagonists.

Hypertensive Syndromes Due to Excess Production of Aldosterone

Primary Aldosteronism

The therapeutic goals in all patients with excessive aldosterone production are threefold: first, to control BP; second, to correct hypokalemia, which is often associated with cardiac arrhythmias;

and third, to normalize plasma aldosterone concentration or block aldosterone activity with a mineralocorticoid receptor antagonist. Increasing evidence indicates that prolonged elevations of circulating aldosterone contribute to cardiac injury[4] and progressive renal disease.[5]

Medical therapy (Table 61-1) is indicated in patients with adrenal hyperplasia, in those with adenoma who are poor surgical risks, and in those with bilateral adrenal adenomas. Total bilateral adrenalectomy has no place in the management of primary aldosteronism because adrenal insufficiency may be more difficult to treat than hypertension caused by aldosteronism. The hypertension associated with primary aldosteronism is salt and water dependent and is best treated by sustained salt and water depletion (Fig. 61-1).[6]

An approach to medical management of patients with primary aldosteronism is illustrated in Figure 61-2.[7] An aldosterone receptor antagonist is given first to correct the hypokalemia. Prompt normalization of serum potassium occurs within 1 to 2 weeks without any change in BP. Thereafter, addition of a diuretic promptly reduces BP with maintenance of serum potassium at normal values. The usual doses of diuretics are hydrochlorothiazide 25 to 50 mg/day or furosemide 80 to 160 mg/day in combination with either spironolactone 100 to 200 mg/day or amiloride 10 to 20 mg/day.

In cases in which BP is not yet at goal after 6 to 8 weeks on maximal doses of the drug combination, addition of a β-blocker or a vasodilator may be necessary. For those patients who refuse surgery or are not surgical candidates, long-term administration of a mineralocorticoid receptor antagonist is an effective alternative. In our study of 24 patients treated medically for at least 5 years,[8] systolic and diastolic BP decreased from a mean of 175/106 to 129/79 mm Hg and serum potassium increased from a mean of 3.0 to 4.3 mEq/L. There was no evidence of malignant transformation in any of the patients. Five tumors increased in size by at least 0.5 cm while maintaining their benign characteristics (as determined by computed tomography scan).

Placebo-controlled, randomized trials evaluating the relative efficacy of different drugs in the management of primary aldosteronism are not available. Spironolactone is highly efficacious and has always been the drug of choice. In addition, it is readily available and inexpensive. However, it is associated with undesirable side effects. Because it also blocks androgen and progesterone receptors, its chronic use often results in

Table 61-1 Drugs for the Medical Management of Primary Aldosteronism

Drug Class*	RECOMMENDED DOSES	
	Initial	Maximal
Mineralocorticoid Receptor Antagonists (Mineralocorticoid Dependent)		
Spironolactone	12.5–50 mg bid	75–100 mg bid
Eplerenone[†]	25–50 mg bid	100 mg bid
Decrease Epithelial Sodium Channels (Mineralocorticoid Independent)		
Amiloride	5–10 mg bid	20 mg bid
Triamterene	37.5–50 mg bid	100 mg bid

*Antihypertensive response can be enhanced with concomitant use of either hydrochlorothiazide (25–50 mg/day) or furosemide (80–160 mg/day).
[†]Doses are approximate. No published data of its use in primary aldosteronism exist.

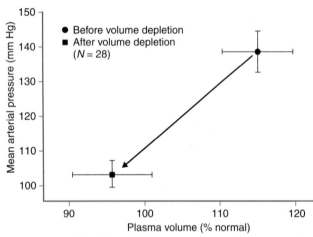

Figure 61-1 The effect of adequate volume depletion on the blood pressure of patients with primary aldosteronism and resistant hypertension. Spironolactone (200 mg/day) and hydrochlorothiazide (50–100 mg/day) were added to current therapy. Blood pressure and plasma volume values were those obtained after 8 to 12 weeks of continued therapy. Mean arterial pressure (MAP) was significantly reduced in all. For the group as a whole, it fell from 138±2 to 103±9 (SEM) mm Hg (P < .01). Associated with reduction in MAP were decreases in plasma volume (from 114±3 to 97±2 [SEM]% normal) (P < .01). (From Bravo EL: Primary aldosteronism. Issues in diagnosis and management. Endocrinol Metab Clin North Am 1994;23:271–283.)

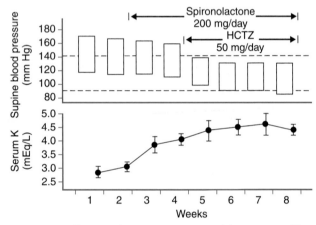

Figure 61-2 Diuretic therapy in primary aldosteronism. The effect of spironolactone combined with hydrochlorothiazide (HCTZ) on blood pressure and serum potassium concentrations in patients with aldosterone-producing tumors. (From Bravo EL, Dustan HP, Tarazi RC: Spironolactone as a nonspecific treatment for primary aldosteronism. Circulation 1973;48:491–498. By permission from the American Heart Association, Inc.)

impotence, decreased libido, and gynecomastia in males and menstrual irregularities and breast engorgement or enlargement in females. These adverse events had no relationship to dose in one long-term study[8] but were found to be dose-dependent in another study.[9]

Eplerenone is a highly selective mineralocorticoid receptor antagonist with none of the endocrine side effects of spironolactone. However, it has only 75% of the activity of spironolactone and has been approved only for the treatment of uncomplicated essential hypertension[10] and for heart failure after acute myocardial infarction.[11] Its efficacy in patients with primary aldosteronism has not been reported.

Potassium-sparing diuretics (amiloride, triamterene) decrease epithelial sodium channel activity in the renal collecting duct and can increase serum potassium values. Neither are effective antihypertensive agents by themselves. A diuretic should be added to achieve good BP control. These drugs do not block mineralocorticoid receptors, and persistence of elevated plasma aldosterone concentrations could lead to deleterious effects on the heart.[12] For this reason, they should not be used as first-line drugs in the management of patients with primary aldosteronism.

Agents that block transmembrane calcium flux and inhibit in vitro aldosterone production induced by angiotensin II, corticotropin, and potassium[13] are potent direct arteriolar vasodilators and, in some studies, are reported to have natriuretic properties.[14] For these reasons, calcium channel blockers should be ideally suited for treating the hypertension associated with excessive aldosterone production. In a study by Bravo and colleagues,[15] nifedipine (30–80 mg/day) was given for at least 4 weeks to 8 hypertensive patients with solitary adenomas, followed by the addition of spironolactone (100–200 mg/day) for 4 weeks, after which nifedipine was discontinued and patients remained on spironolactone alone. During the fourth week of each phase of the study, weekly averages of supine home BP, plasma volume, plasma renin activity (PRA), plasma aldosterone concentration, and serum electrolyte levels were assessed. Nifedipine decreased blood pressure, but not to normal levels (157/97±4/4 mm Hg [SE]), and did not alter plasma volume, PRA, aldosterone, or serum potassium concentration. Spironolactone normalized BP (122/80±5/3 mm Hg) and serum potassium concentration, reduced plasma volume, and increased PRA and plasma aldosterone concentration. Nifedipine plus spironolactone did not result in greater antihypertensive effect than spironolactone alone. These results suggest that nifedipine is not as efficacious as spironolactone in the treatment of primary aldosteronism.

Surgical excision of an aldosterone-producing adenoma normalizes BP and the biochemical defects in most patients. Surgery renders arterial pressure easier to control with medications. Neither the duration and severity of hypertension, nor the degree of target organ involvement, has any relationship to the arterial pressure response after surgery.[16] One year postoperatively, approximately 70% of patients are normotensive, but 5 years postoperatively, only 53% remain normotensive. The restoration of normal potassium homeostasis is permanent.

Patients undergoing surgery should receive drug treatment for at least 8 to 10 weeks both to decrease BP and to correct metabolic abnormalities. These patients have significant potassium deficiency that must be corrected preoperatively because hypokalemia increases the risk of cardiac arrhythmias during anesthesia. Prolonged control of BP (at least 3 months before surgery) permits the use of intravenous fluids during surgery without producing hypertension and decreases morbidity. Administration of antihypertensive medications should normally be continued until surgery. Glucocorticoid administration is not needed before surgery. After removal of an aldosterone-producing adenoma, selective hypoaldosteronism usually occurs, even in patients whose PRA has been stimulated with chronic diuretic therapy.[17] Potassium supplementation, therefore, should be given cautiously, and serum potassium values should be monitored closely. Residual mineralocorticoid activity is often sufficient to prevent excessive renal retention of potassium provided that sodium intake is adequate (i.e., at least 150 mEq/day). If hyperkalemia does occur, furosemide in doses of 80 to 160 mg/day should be started. Treatment with fludrocortisone is not usually necessary, but if it is required, 0.1 mg/day may be used as the initial dose with liberalized salt intake. Abnormalities in aldosterone production can persist for as long as 3 months after tumor removal.

Glucocorticoid-Remediable Aldosteronism

Glucocorticoid-remediable aldosteronism is an inherited autosomal disorder that mimics primary aldosteronism.[18] It is caused by a genetic mutation that results in a chimeric gene product fusing nucleotide sequences of the 11β-hydroxylase and aldosterone synthase genes.[19] The structure of the duplicated gene contains 5′ regulatory sequences conferring the corticotropin responsiveness of 11β-hydroxylase fused to more distal coding sequences of the aldosterone synthase gene. This hybrid gene is regulated by corticotropin and has aldosterone synthase activity. It dictates ectopic expression of aldosterone synthase activity in the corticotropin-regulated zona fasciculata, which normally produces cortisol.[19]

No controlled studies of treatment of glucocorticoid-remediable aldosteronism have been reported. The suppression of corticotropin with exogenous glucocorticoid should correct all glucocorticoid-remediable aldosteronism abnormalities. However, this may cause complications of glucocorticoid administration. Moreover, patients may become mineralocorticoid-insufficient when therapy is initiated before the renin-angiotensin axis recovers fully. Additional treatment modalities include mineralocorticoid receptor blockade with spironolactone or inhibition of the mineralocorticoid-sensitive distal tubule sodium channel with amiloride.

Activation of Mineralocorticoid Receptors by Decreased Metabolism of Cortisol at Target Sites

Mineralocorticoid receptors in the distal nephron have equal affinity for their two ligands—aldosterone and cortisol—but are protected from activation by cortisol by 11β-hydroxysteroid dehydrogenase (11β-OHSD), which converts cortisol to the inactive cortisone.[20] The 11,18-hemiacetal structure of aldosterone protects it from the action of 11β-OHSD. Consequently, aldosterone gains access to the receptors. When this mechanism fails within the kidney, cortisol increases sufficiently to activate mineralocorticoid receptors,[21] resulting in antinatriuresis and kaliuresis, thereby producing hypertension and hypokalemia. A genetic disorder of the syndrome of apparent mineralocorticoid excess[22] or prolonged ingestion of licorice or licorice-like compounds (such as carbenoxolone) both cause defects in the 11β-OHSD enzyme type 2, which is the kidney isoform.[23] Such patients have clinical features similar to those with primary aldosteronism but have low aldosterone production. The features are reversed by spironolactone or dexamethasone but are exacerbated by administration of physiological doses of cortisol.

In patients with Cushing's phenomenon associated with ectopic corticotropin secretion, cortisol secretion may be so high that it exceeds the metabolic capacity of 11β-OHSD enzyme type 2,[24] resulting in severe hypokalemic metabolic alkalosis and hypertension. The initial goal of therapy is blockade of the mineralocorticoid effects of cortisol to normalize serum potassium concentration and to control BP. The ultimate goal is to reduce plasma cortisol concentrations by resection of the ectopic source of corticotropin. If the ectopic sources of corticotropin cannot be localized, bilateral adrenalectomy is performed. If the patient is not a surgical candidate, cortisol production can be reduced with adrenocortical enzyme inhibitors, such as ketoconazole, metyrapone, aminoglutethimide, and etomidate.[25]

PHEOCHROMOCYTOMA

The aim of management of pheochromocytoma (Box 61-1) is to prevent hypertensive crises and complications mediated by catecholamine-induced α-adrenergic receptor stimulation and to diminish postoperative hypotension. The use of α-blockers is advocated for control of BP. Phenoxybenzamine

Box 61-1 Suggested Approach to Preoperative Management of Patients with Pheochromocytoma

1. Start with doxazosin, 2 mg once daily. Increase by 2 mg every third day up to a total of 10 mg once daily.
2. Add a calcium channel blocker (amlodipine preferred) if blood pressure is not yet at goal.
3. Add β-blocker for persistent tachycardia or signs and symptoms of ischemic heart disease.
4. Other measures:
   - No diuretics unless deemed essential
   - High salt intake (10–12 g NaCl/day)
5. Therapeutic goals:
   - Supine BP < 140/90 mm Hg
   - No cardiac arrhythmias
   - No orthostatic hypotension
   - Completely asymptomatic for at least 6–8 weeks before surgery
   - Continue all medications on day of surgery

hydrochloride (Dibenzyline, 10–20 mg tid to qid) is given in increasing doses until the BP is controlled and symptomatic paroxysms are prevented. Theoretically, phenoxybenzamine should permit vascular volume repletion, block α-adrenergic receptors noncompetitively, and disable the effects of released catecholamines.[26] Its blockade of presynaptic α_2-adrenergic receptors produces significant tachycardia, which requires concomitant β-adrenergic blockade. It may prolong BP reduction after removal of the tumor because it decreases receptor number and synthesis. Total elimination of cardiovascular disturbances is seldom achieved despite adequate α-blockade. Significant elevations of BP are to be anticipated during manipulation of the tumor.[27]

Other α-adrenergic antagonists may circumvent some of the disadvantages of phenoxybenzamine. Doxazosin is a selective postsynaptic α_1-adrenergic receptor antagonist that does not produce tachycardia and has a shorter duration of action, thereby allowing more rapid adjustment of dosage and decreasing the duration of postoperative hypotension. It has been reported to be as potent as phenoxybenzamine with fewer adverse effects.[28] The initial dose of doxazosin is 2 mg once daily, increased as needed at increments of 2 mg every 3 days up to a total dose of 10 mg. No β-adrenergic blockade is required unless tachycardia is present. Labetalol is an α- and β-adrenergic blocker. It was reported to be effective in the control of BP and clinical manifestations associated with pheochromocytoma.[29] The initial dosage is 100 mg 4 times daily, increased stepwise to a maximum of 800 to 1600 mg/day. However, its safety has been questioned because it occasionally precipitates hypertensive crises.

Calcium channel blockers have also been successful in controlling BP in patients with pheochromocytoma.[30] These agents have the advantage of not producing overshoot hypotension or orthostatic hypotension and therefore may be used safely in patients who are normotensive but who have occasional episodes of paroxysmal hypertension. They are useful agents in managing cardiovascular complications because they may also prevent catecholamine-induced coronary vasospasm and myocarditis.[31] They have none of the complications associated with chronic use of α-adrenergic blockers. In

doses of 40 to 60 mg/day, nifedipine normalizes basal BP in hypertensive patients and prevents the hypertensive response to provocative challenge. Verapamil and diltiazem produce similar results.[32] It is likely that they reduce arterial pressure by inhibiting norepinephrine-mediated transmembrane calcium influx in vascular smooth muscle and not by decreasing catecholamine synthesis in tumors.

Doxazosin combined with a calcium channel blocker is often sufficient to control the signs and symptoms. A β-blocker may be added if there is persistent tachycardia. Patients should be advised to maintain a high salt intake (10–12 g NaCl/day). Diuretics should be discontinued unless they are deemed necessary. Hypertensive crises may be managed with intravenous phentolamine mesylate (Regitine) or sodium nitroprusside. Nifedipine, 10 mg orally or sublingually, has been used successfully.

Patients with pheochromocytoma have a high plasma volume requirement, both during and after surgery. The expansion of the intravascular volume approximately 12 hours before operation, with generous replacement of blood lost during the procedure, greatly reduces the frequency and severity of postoperative hypotension. Persistence of hypotension may be caused by hemorrhage, sudden increases in venous capacitance, inadequate volume repletion, or residual effects of preoperative α-blockade. Fluids should be administered first, keeping in mind that these patients require large amounts of volume after tumor resection. Pressor agents are not usually effective in the presence of persistent hypovolemia. It is often difficult to withdraw vasopressors once they have been started.

Until recently, a pheochromocytoma was removed only through an open approach. With technological advances and experience in minimally invasive techniques, the tumor can now be removed safely and successfully with laparoscopic surgery. In a recent study,[33] 14 patients who underwent laparoscopic surgery for pheochromocytoma were compared with 20 patients who underwent the traditional open approach. The intraoperative hemodynamic values during laparoscopic surgery (adrenalectomy) were comparable to those during open surgery. However, in patients undergoing laparoscopy, intraoperative hypotension was less severe (mean lowest BP, 98/57 mm Hg vs. 80/50 mm Hg, $P = .05$) and hypotensive episodes were less frequent (median, 0 vs. 2 episodes, $P = .005$). The median estimated blood loss was 100 mL (range, 100–200 mL) in the laparoscopy group and 400 mL (range, 150–1500 mL) in the open group ($P = .0001$). Surgery time was not different (196 ± 69 min for open vs. 177 ± 59 min for laparoscopy). Patients who underwent laparoscopy recovered quicker. The time to ambulation was 1.5 versus 4 days ($P = .002$). They resumed oral food intake sooner (median, 1 vs. 3.5 days, $P = .001$) and required fewer days in hospital (median, 3 vs. 7.5 days, $P = .001$). This study indicates that laparoscopic removal of pheochromocytoma is not only safe, but also has marked advantages over the open approach. Patients have faster recovery, shorter hospitalization, and better cosmetic outcome.

References

1. White PC, Speiser PW: Steroid 11 β-hydroxylase deficiency and related disorders. Endocrinol Metab Clin N Am 1994;23:325–339.
2. Biglieri EG, Herron MA, Brust N: 17-hydroxylation deficiency in man. J Clin Invest 1966;45:1946–1954.

3. Malchoff CD, Malchoff DM: Glucocorticoid resistance in humans. Trends Endo Metab 1995;6:89–94.

4. Milliez P, Girerd X, Plouin PF, et al: Evidence for an increased rate of cardiovascular events in patients with primary aldosteronism. J Am Coll Cardiol 2005;45:1243–1248.

5. Rossi GP, Bernini G, Desideri G, et al: Renal damage in primary aldosteronism. Results of the PAPY study. Hypertension 2006; 48:232–238.

6. Bravo EL, Fouad-Tarazi FM, Tarazi RC, et al: Clinical implications of primary aldosteronism with resistant hypertension. Hypertension 1988;11(2 Pt 2):I207–I211.

7. Bravo EL, Dustan HP, Tarazi RC: Spironolactone as a nonspecific treatment for primary aldosteronism. Circulation 1973;48: 491–498.

8. Ghose RP, Hall PM, Bravo EL: Medical management of aldosterone-producing adenomas. Ann Intern Med 1999;131: 105–108.

9. Lim PO, Young WF, MacDonald TU: A review of the medical treatment of primary aldosteronism. J Hypertens 2001;19:353–361.

10. Burgess ED, Lacourciere Y, Ruilope-Urioste LU, et al: Long term safety and efficacy of the selective aldosterone blocker eplerenone in patients with essential hypertension. Clin Ther 2003; 25:2388–2404.

11. Pitt B, Remme W, Zannad F, et al: Eplerenone, a selective aldosterone blocker, in patients with left ventricular dysfunction after myocardial infarction. N Engl J Med 2003;238:1309–1322.

12. Griffing GT, Cole AG, Aurecchia SA, et al: Amiloride in primary aldosteronism. Clin Pharmacol Ther 1982;31:56–61.

13. Schiffrin EL, Lis M, Gutkowska J, Genest J: Role of Ca2+ in response of adrenal glomerulosa cells to angiotensin II, ACTH, K+ and ouabain. Am J Physiol 1981;241:E42–E46.

14. Kiowski W, Bertel O, Erne P, et al: Hemodynamic and reflex responses to acute and chronic antihypertensive therapy with the calcium entry blocker nifedipine. Hypertension 1983;5(2 Pt 2): I70–I74.

15. Bravo EL, Fouad FM, Tarazi RC: Calcium channel blockade with nifedipine in primary aldosteronism. Hypertension 1986; 8(Suppl I):I-191–I-194.

16. Bravo EL: Pheochromocytoma and mineralocorticoid hypertension. In Glassock RJ (ed): Current Therapy in Nephrology and Hypertension, 4th ed. St. Louis: Mosby-Year Book, 1998, p 330.

17. Bravo EL, Dustan HP, Tarazi RC: Selective hypoaldosteronism despite prolonged pre- and postoperative hyperreninemia in primary aldosteronism. J Clin Endocrinol Metab 1975;41: 611–617.

18. Lifton RP, Dluhy RG, Powers M, et al: A chimaeric 11 β-hydroxylase/aldosterone synthase gene causes glucocorticoid-remediable aldosteronism and human hypertension. Nature 1992;355:262–265.

19. Lifton RP, Dluhy RG, Powers M, et al: Hereditary hypertension caused by chimaeric gene duplications and ectopic expression of aldosterone synthase. Nat Genet 1992;2:66–74.

20. Edwards CR, Stewart PM, Burt D, et al: Localisation of 11 β-hydroxysteroid dehydrogenase—tissue specific protector of the mineralocorticoid receptor. Lancet 1988;2:986–989.

21. Funder JW, Pearce PT, Smith R, et al: Mineralocorticoid action: Target tissue specificity is enzyme, not receptor, mediated. Science 1988;242:583–585.

22. Stewart PM, Corrie JE, Shackleton CH, Edwards CR: Syndrome of apparent mineralocorticoid excess. A defect in the cortisol-cortisone shuffle. J Clin Invest 1988;82:340–349.

23. Funder JW: 11β-Hydroxysteroid dehydrogenase: New answers, new questions. Eur J Endocrinol 1996;134:267–268.

24. Ulick S, Wang JZ, Blumenfeld JD, Pickering TG: Cortisol inactivation overload: A mechanism of mineralocorticoid hypertension in the ectopic adrenocorticotropin syndrome. J Clin Endocrinol Metab 1992;74:961–962.

25. Orth DN, Liddle GW: Results of treatment of 108 patients with Cushing's syndrome. N Engl J Med 1971;285:243–247.

26. Hoffman BB: Catecholamines, sympathomimetic drugs, and adrenergic receptor antagonists. In Hardman JG, Lombard LE (eds): The Pharmacological Basis of Therapeutics, 10th ed. Philadelphia: McGraw-Hill, 2001, p 215.

27. Stenstrom G, Haljamae H, Tisell LE: Influence of pre-operative treatment with phenoxybenzamine on the incidence of adverse cardiovascular reactions during anaesthesia and surgery for phaeochromocytoma. Acta Anaesthesiol Scand 1985;29:797–803.

28. Prys-Roberts C: Pheochromocytoma—recent progress in its management. Br J Anaesth 2000;85:44–59.

29. Oates JA, Brown NJ: Antihypertensive agents and the drug therapy of hypertension. In Hardman JG, Lombard LE (eds): Goodman & Gillman's The Pharmacological Basis of Therapeutics. Philadelphia: McGraw-Hill, 2001, p 871.

30. Serfas D, Shoback DM, Lorell BH: Phaeochromocytoma and hypertrophic cardiomyopathy: Apparent suppression of symptoms and noradrenaline secretion by calcium-channel blockade. Lancet 1983;2:711–713.

31. Van Vliet PD, Burchell HB, Titus JL: Focal myocarditis associated with pheochromocytoma. N Engl J Med 1966;274:1102–1108.

32. Bravo EL: Secondary hypertension: Adrenal and nervous systems. In Hollenberg NK (ed): Atlas of Heart Diseases, 3rd ed. Philadelphia: Current Medicine, 2001, p 118.

33. Sprung J, O'Hara JF Jr, Gill IS, et al: Anesthetic aspects of laparoscopic and open adrenalectomy for pheochromocytoma. Urology 2000;55:339–343.

Further Reading

Bravo EL, Tagle R: Pheochromocytoma: State-of-the-art and future prospects. Endocrin Rev 2003;24:539–553.

Sechi LA, Novello M, Lapenna R, et al: Long term renal outcomes in patients with primary aldosteronism. JAMA 2006;295:2638–2645.

Torpy DJ, Ilias N, Nieman LK: Association of hypertension and hypokalemia with Cushing's syndrome caused by ectopic ACTH secretion. A series of 58 cases. Ann N Y Acad Sci 2002;1970: 134–144.

White PC, Mune T, Agarwal AK: 11β-hydroxysteroid dehydrogenase and the syndrome of apparent mineralocorticoid excess. Endocrinol Rev 1997;18:135–156.

Young WF: Renaissance of a syndrome. Clin Endocrinol (Oxf) 2007;66:607–618.

PART XII

Chronic Renal Failure and Its Systemic Manifestations

CONTENTS

Chapter 62

Prevention of Progressive Renal Failure

Maarten W. Taal

Despite substantial advances in medical science over the past 50 to 60 years, there are as yet few effective treatments for specific renal diseases. Consequently, many cases progress to chronic renal failure and the population of patients requiring renal replacement therapy continues to grow rapidly. In the United States alone 335,963 people were receiving chronic dialysis and 136,136 had a functioning renal transplant at the end of 2004, resulting in annual Medicare costs of $20.1 billion.[1] Moreover, the mortality rate on dialysis remains as high as 20% to 25% per annum,[1] and there is a worldwide shortage of organs for transplantation. The publication of a classification system for chronic kidney disease (CKD) by the Kidney Disease Outcomes Quality Initiative (K/DOQI)[2] and subsequent epidemiologic studies based on that classification have drawn attention to the fact that up to 17% of the U.S. population may suffer from CKD.[3] There is thus an urgent need to identify undiagnosed cases and to minimize the risk of progression. It has been appreciated for several decades that substantial loss of functioning nephrons due to kidney disease of any etiology provokes a common syndrome characterized by systemic hypertension, proteinuria, and a progressive decline in glomerular filtration rate (GFR), the rate of which depends more on individual patient characteristics than specific disease etiology.[4,5] These observations suggest that CKD progresses via a common pathway of mechanisms and that therapeutic interventions that inhibit this pathway may be successful in slowing the rate of progression of CKD irrespective of the initiating cause. We review experimental and clinical evidence in support of this hypothesis and discuss how interventions based on an understanding of common pathway mechanisms may be combined into a comprehensive strategy for achieving maximal renoprotection.

MECHANISMS UNDERLYING CHRONIC KIDNEY DISEASE PROGRESSION

Glomerular Hemodynamic Factors

When rats are subjected to surgical ablation of five sixths of their renal mass, they develop hypertension, proteinuria, and a progressive loss of GFR, features similar to those of human CKD. Brenner and colleagues, using micropuncture techniques, measured the glomerular capillary hydraulic pressure (P_{GC}) and GFR in single nephrons (single nephron GFR; SNGFR) and showed that when nephrons were lost, remaining glomeruli underwent hemodynamic adaptations resulting in substantial increases in SNGFR (glomerular hyperfiltration) and P_{GC} (glomerular capillary hypertension).[6] The presence of structural injury to glomerular cells as early as 1 week after five sixths nephrectomy suggests that these hemodynamic changes provoke glomerular damage that results in a further loss of nephrons, thereby establishing a vicious cycle of progressive renal injury.[7] Support for this hypothesis was provided by experimental studies showing that renoprotective interventions were associated with attenuation of the glomerular hemodynamic changes.

Low-protein diet feeding was associated with normalization of SNGFR and P_{GC} as well as substantial protection from progressive glomerular injury.[6] Treatment with an angiotensin-converting enzyme (ACE) inhibitor had little effect on SNGFR but did normalize P_{GC} and afforded renoprotection, suggesting that P_{GC} rather than SNGFR was the critical determinant of glomerular injury in the remnant kidney.[8] Treatment with a combination of hydralazine, hydrochlorothiazide, and reserpine resulted in a similar lowering of systemic blood pressure to that seen with ACE inhibitor treatment but did not lower P_{GC} or prevent glomerulosclerosis.[9] Micropuncture studies in a rodent model of diabetic nephropathy confirmed that glomerular hypertension and hyperfiltration are present. The importance of these hemodynamic factors in the complex pathogenesis of diabetic nephropathy was confirmed by experimental studies showing that normalization of P_{GC} by low-protein diet or treatment with an ACE inhibitor resulted in the prevention of progressive renal injury despite persistent chronic hyperglycemia.[10,11]

Angiotensin II

Angiotensin II has been identified as an important mediator of the glomerular hemodynamic changes associated with progressive renal injury. Experimental studies have revealed several nonhemodynamic effects of angiotensin II that may also be important in CKD progression. These include loss of glomerular size permselectivity resulting in proteinuria, mesangial cell proliferation and induction of transforming growth factor-β (TGF-β) expression, stimulation of plasminogen activator inhibitor-1 production by endothelial and vascular smooth muscle cells, macrophage activation, and increased phagocytosis, as well as induction of cytokine expression and fibrogenic effects via aldosterone.[12] Angiotensin II has thus emerged as a central mediator in the pathogenesis of progressive renal injury and is therefore a logical target for interventions to slow CKD progression (Fig. 62-1).

Tubulointerstitial Fibrosis

In CKD, progressive glomerulosclerosis is accompanied by tubulointerstitial fibrosis, the extent of which correlates closely with prognosis.[13] Several mechanisms have been proposed to link glomerular and tubulointerstitial damage. These include adverse effects of the abnormal filtration of plasma proteins that provoke proinflammatory and profibrotic responses when absorbed by renal tubule cells,[14] downstream effects of cytokines filtered or produced by injured glomeruli,[15] misdirection of protein-rich glomerular filtrate into the interstitium,[16] epithelial to mesenchymal transition of tubule cells to form interstitial myofibroblasts,[17] and reduced perfusion of peritubular capillaries resulting in hypoxia.[18] Mechanisms that may contribute to progressive renal injury are discussed further in the sections that follow and are summarized in Figure 62-1.

INTERVENTIONS FOR SLOWING THE RATE OF CKD PROGRESSION

Antihypertensive Therapy

Optimal Blood Pressure

The treatment of systemic hypertension was the first intervention shown to significantly slow the rate of CKD progression, and it remains fundamental to renoprotective strategies. Among insulin-dependent diabetic patients with diabetic nephropathy, the initiation of antihypertensive therapy resulted in marked reductions in rates of GFR decline,[19,20] implying that hypertension, an almost universal consequence of impaired renal function, also contributes to the progression of CKD. Similar observations were reported among patients with nondiabetic forms of CKD.[21–23] Uncertainty remains, however, about how much blood pressure (BP) lowering is required to achieve optimal renoprotection.

The Modification of Diet in Renal Disease (MDRD) study sought to resolve this issue by evaluating whether lower than previously recommended BP targets afforded greater

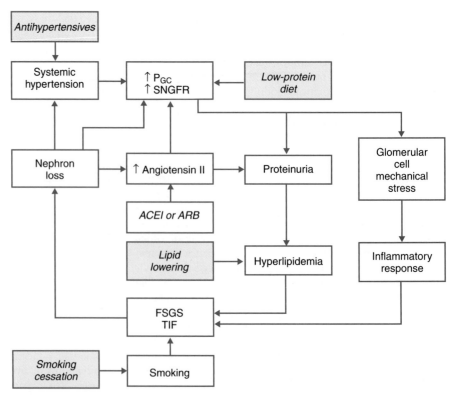

Figure 62-1 Schema depicting the proposed mechanisms resulting in a common pathway of progressive nephron loss in chronic kidney disease and illustrating the actions of different interventions (*in italics*) in interrupting this pathway. ACEI, angiotensin-converting enzyme inhibitor; AngII, angiotensin II; ARB, angiotensin receptor blocker; FSGS, focal and segmental glomerulosclerosis; P_{GC}, glomerular capillary hydraulic pressure; SNGFR, single nephron glomerular filtration rate; TIF, tubulointerstitial fibrosis.

renoprotection than "usual" BP control among patients with predominantly nondiabetic CKD. Patients were randomized to a target mean arterial pressure (MAP) of 107 mm Hg (equivalent to BP of 140/90 mm Hg) or 92 mm Hg (equivalent to BP of 125/75 mm Hg). Whereas primary analysis did not show any overall difference in rate of GFR decline between these groups, patients randomized to the low BP group evidenced an early rapid decrease in GFR, likely due to associated renal hemodynamic effects, that obscured a later significantly slower rate of GFR decline than that observed in the "usual" BP target group. Baseline proteinuria more than 1 g/day was associated with more rapid GFR decline in usual versus low BP groups.[24] Secondary analysis revealed significant correlations between the rate of GFR decline and achieved blood pressure, an effect that was also more marked among those with greater baseline proteinuria. The authors conclude by recommending a BP goal of lower than 125/75 mm Hg (MAP = 92 mm Hg) for CKD patients with more than 1 g/day of proteinuria, and a goal of lower than 130/80 mm Hg (MAP = 98 mm Hg) for those with proteinuria of 0.25 to 1 g/day.[25] Subsequent follow-up of MDRD patients suggests that the benefits of lower blood pressure may become evident only over a longer period; after a mean of 6.6 years the risk of end-stage renal disease (ESRD) (adjusted hazard ratio [HR], 0.68; 95% confidence interval [95% CI], 0.57–0.82) was lower and that of a combined endpoint of ESRD or death (adjusted HR, 0.77; 95% CI, 0.65–0.91) was lower in patients randomized to the low BP target even though treatment and BP data were not available beyond the 2.2 years of the original trial.[26] Unfortunately, these results are confounded by the random use of ACE inhibitor treatment in the study. Consequently, it remains unclear whether the level of blood pressure attained is critically important in CKD patients receiving an ACE inhibitor or angiotensin receptor blocker (ARB). However, among patients with type 1 diabetes and established nephropathy receiving ACE inhibitor treatment, randomization to a low (MAP = 92 mm Hg) versus "usual" (MAP = 100–107 mm Hg) target blood pressure was associated with significantly lower levels of proteinuria after 2 years but no significant difference in the loss of GFR.[27] Secondary analysis of data from the Irbesartan Diabetic Nephropathy Trial (IDNT) revealed greater renoprotection among patients who achieved lower BP targets; an achieved systolic blood pressure higher than 149 mm Hg was associated with a 2.2-fold higher risk of developing ESRD or a doubling of serum creatinine versus an achieved systolic blood pressure lower than 134 mm Hg, independent of ARB treatment.[28]

Other studies have failed to find additional benefit associated with lower BP targets. For example, intensive BP control was not associated with significantly improved preservation of renal function among patients with autosomal dominant polycystic kidney disease, but the authors point out that the study may not have had adequate statistical power to detect a difference.[29] In the African American Study of Kidney Disease and Hypertension (AASK), no significant difference in the rate of GFR decline was observed between patients randomized to MAP goals of no more than 92 mm Hg compared to those assigned to MAP goals of 102 to 107 mm Hg. One possible explanation for the lack of a benefit is that these patients generally had low baseline levels of proteinuria (mean urine protein, 0.38–0.63 g/day).[30] In the Ramipril Efficacy in Nephropathy 2 (REIN-2) trial, additional BP reduction (<130/80 mm Hg versus diastolic BP < 90 mm Hg irrespective of systolic BP) with a nondihydropyridine

calcium channel blocker (CCB) plus ACE inhibitor treatment in patients with nondiabetic CKD did not yield additional renoprotection.[31] However, the degree of additional BP reduction (4.1/2.8 mm Hg) may have been insufficient or the specific antihypertensive agent may have been ineffective.

Two additional pieces of evidence support a lower BP target; a meta-analysis of 11 randomized trials that included 1860 patients revealed that the lowest risk of progression of nondiabetic CKD was associated with an achieved systolic blood pressure of 110 to 129 mm Hg, independent of ACE inhibitor treatment.[32] Secondly, results from several clinical trials that included diabetic and nondiabetic CKD revealed a slower rate of CKD progression in patients achieving the lowest blood pressures.[33] Two recent reports raise a note of caution. They suggest that excessive lowering of blood pressure may be associated with adverse effects. In the same meta-analysis, an achieved systolic blood pressure lower than 110 mm Hg was associated with an increased risk of CKD progression (relative risk [RR], 2.48; 95% CI, 1.07–5.77),[32] and in the IDNT an achieved systolic blood pressure lower than 120 mm Hg was associated with increased all-cause mortality and no further improvement in renal outcomes.[28]

In summary, results from randomized trials comparing "low" and "usual" BP targets among CKD patients have not yielded unequivocal results, but the overall picture suggests that lower BP targets are associated with more effective renoprotection, particularly among those with significant proteinuria. These observations have led to a consensus that blood pressure should be lowered to less than 130/80 mm Hg in all patients with CKD[33,34] and, for patients with more than 1 g/day of proteinuria, a blood pressure of less than 125/75 mm Hg should be achieved. Potentially dangerous hypotension, particularly in patients with autonomic neuropathy, labile blood pressure, or atherosclerosis with decreased vascular compliance, should be avoided.

Antihypertensive Drugs

Data from the Antihypertensive and Lipid-Lowering Treatment to Prevent Heart Attack Trial (ALLHAT) have been misinterpreted to imply that the choice of antihypertensive drug does not affect renal outcomes in patients with CKD. ALLHAT was designed to investigate the effect of antihypertensive drugs on cardiovascular outcomes in patients with hypertension and at least one cardiovascular risk factor; they found no significant difference in the incidence of the primary outcome of fatal ischemic heart disease or nonfatal myocardial infarction among patients randomized to treatment with a thiazide diuretic, a CCB, or an ACE inhibitor.[35] In a post hoc analysis there was also no difference found in the secondary outcome of ESRD or more than 50% decrease in GFR. Notably, patients with serum creatinine levels higher than 2 mg/dL were specifically excluded from the analysis, resulting in only a minority of patients (5662 of 33,357) having CKD (estimated GFR, <60 mL/min/1.73 m^2), and there was no assessment of proteinuria.[36] In contrast to the ALLHAT results, a large body of evidence supports the use of ACE inhibitors or ARBs as first-line antihypertensive therapy in patients with CKD (see "Pharmacologic Inhibition of the Renin-Angiotensin System" in this chapter).

Nevertheless, dietary salt restriction and diuretics are important antihypertensive therapies in the treatment of CKD. Studies have demonstrated that high dietary sodium intake may abrogate the antiproteinuric effect of ACE inhibitor treatment but that addition of a thiazide diuretic restores the antiproteinuric effect despite ongoing high sodium intake.[37] Addition of a thiazide diuretic to ARB treatment was found to reduce blood pressure and proteinuria in patients with IgA nephropathy.[38] We recommend dietary salt restriction with a thiazide diuretic as second-line antihypertensive therapy for patients with stage 1 to 3 CKD who are not achieving adequate BP control with an ACE inhibitor or ARB alone. With more advanced CKD, a loop diuretic should be used to reduce extracellular volume and blood pressure.

There is concern that the dihydropyridine class of CCBs may adversely affect the progression of CKD. In experimental studies dihydropyridine CCB treatment allowed greater transmission of systemic blood pressure to the renal microcirculation and was associated with more rapid progression of renal injury when compared to ACE inhibitor treatment in the five sixths nephrectomy model.[39] Whereas one relatively small study found no difference between the renoprotective effects of the dihydropyridine CCB nifedipine and the ACE inhibitor captopril,[40] but two larger studies have reported adverse outcomes associated with the use of dihydropyridine CCBs. A secondary analysis of data from REIN-2 found that treatment with the dihydropyridine CCBs nifedipine and amlodipine was associated with higher levels of proteinuria and more rapid GFR decline than other antihypertensives in patients who failed to achieve a MAP less than 100 mm Hg and were not receiving an ACE inhibitor.[41] In AASK,[42] patients with CKD and hypertension were randomized to treatment with an ACE inhibitor, the dihydropyridine CCB amlodipine, or a β-blocker and diuretic in combination. Amlodipine therapy was stopped prematurely due to identification of a more rapid decline in GFR compared to patients receiving the β-blocker or ACE inhibitor, particularly in the presence of proteinuria higher than 1 g/day. As discussed previously, the REIN-2 study found no additional renoprotection when a dihydropyridine CCB was added to ACE inhibitor treatment in patients with nondiabetic CKD.[31]

In contrast, nondihydropyridine CCBs lower P_{GC}, reduce proteinuria, and afford renoprotection in experimental studies. In one clinical study, the combination of ACE inhibitor and nondihydropyridine CCB treatment resulted in greater reduction of proteinuria than either treatment alone in patients with type 2 diabetes and overt nephropathy.[43] A meta-analysis of data from 28 randomized, clinical trials in hypertensive patients with proteinuria found a 2% increase in proteinuria with dihydropyridine CCB treatment versus a 30% reduction with nondihydropyridine CCB treatment despite similar effects on blood pressure.[44] Consequently, we recommend that dihydropyridine CCBs should be avoided in patients with CKD unless they are required as combination therapy with other antihypertensives to achieve the targets for BP control outlined in this chapter and used in combination with ACE inhibitor or ARB treatment. If possible nondihydropyridine CCBs should be used in preference to dihydropyridine CCBs.

Pharmacologic Inhibition of the Renin-Angiotensin System

A large number of published clinical trials and meta-analyses provide clear evidence to support the use of pharmacologic inhibitors of the renin-angiotensin system as an essential component of any strategy aiming to achieve maximal renoprotection in patients with CKD (summarized in Table 62-1).

Angiotensin-Converting Enzyme Inhibitors

Diabetic Nephropathy

In 1993, the Captopril Collaborative Study Group demonstrated specific renoprotection attributable to ACE inhibitor treatment in human CKD for the first time.[45] In this study, 409 patients with type 1 diabetes and established nephropathy (proteinuria > 0.5 g/day; serum creatinine < 2.5 mg/dL) were randomized to receive captopril or placebo to achieve a BP goal of less than 140/90 mm Hg. After median follow-up of 3 years, captopril treatment was associated with a 50% reduction in the risk of the combined endpoint of death, dialysis, and renal transplantation and a 48% reduction in the risk of a doubling of serum creatinine level. Renoprotection was not attributable simply to the antihypertensive effects of ACE inhibitors because BP control was not statistically different between the groups. Subsequently, investigators evaluated whether ACE inhibitor would also benefit type 1 diabetic patients with microalbuminuria. A meta-analysis of 12 studies, including 689 patients with type 1 diabetes followed for at least a year, found that ACE inhibitor treatment was associated with a significant reduction in the risk of progression to overt nephropathy (odds ratio, 0.38) and three times the incidence of complete normalization of microalbuminuria.[46] Another study showed that ACE inhibitors prevented progression to overt nephropathy over 8 years and was associated with preservation of a normal GFR.[47] Finally, a subgroup analysis of the EUCLID study found that ACE inhibitor treatment reduced albuminuria by 12.7% among normotensive, normoalbuminuric type 1 diabetic patients; this trend was not statistically significant and was associated with a lower blood pressure.[48]

Data on the renoprotective effects of ACE inhibitors in patients with type 2 diabetes are conflicting because studies have included relatively small numbers of patients and only one[49] was able to show a greater reduction in GFR decline associated with ACE inhibitors versus other antihypertensives.[50-52] In contrast, the diabetic subgroup analysis of the Heart Outcomes Prevention Evaluation (HOPE) study revealed beneficial effects of ACE inhibitor treatment in decreasing microalbuminuria[53-55] and reducing the number of patients progressing from microalbuminuria to overt proteinuria among type 2 diabetic patients (risk reduction, 24%–67%).[56-58] The HOPE study also revealed a 25% reduction in the combined primary endpoint of myocardial infarction, stroke, or cardiovascular death in ramipril-treated type 2 diabetic patients who had risk factors for cardiovascular disease. Finally, a beneficial role for ACE inhibitor treatment in primary prevention of nephropathy among 156 normotensive, normoalbuminuric type 2 diabetic patients has been reported, noting a 12.5% absolute risk reduction for microalbuminuria.[59,60] Another study has reported similar benefit among 1204 hypertensive normoalbuminuric type 2 diabetic patients (estimated acceleration factor, 0.39 for trandolapril + verapamil versus placebo and 0.47 for trandolapril versus placebo; $P = .01$ for both).[60] On the other hand, one relatively large study found no renoprotective benefit of ACE inhibitor over β-blocker treatment among hypertensive type 2 diabetic patients with normoalbuminuria or microalbuminuria.[61] Regarding meta-analyses, one included only studies of type 2 diabetes and concluded there was a statistically significant reduction in albuminuria associated with ACE

Table 62-1   Summary of Studies Showing the Renoprotective Effects of Angiotensin-Converting Enzyme Inhibitors and Angiotensin Receptor Blockers in Diabetic and Nondiabetic Chronic Kidney Disease

CKD Type	Trial Outcome	Ref.
Angiotensin-Converting Enzyme Inhibitors (ACEIs)		
Type 1 DM + CKD	50% ↓ risk of dialysis, transplant, or death	45
Type 1 DM + μA	↓ Risk of overt nephropathy (OR = 0.38)	46, 47
Type 1 DM + NA	12.7% ↓ in albuminuria (NS)	48
Type 2 DM + CKD	Benefit in only one study	49–52
Type 2 DM + μA	24%–67% ↓ risk of overt nephropathy	53–58
Type 2 DM + NA	12.5% ↓ risk of developing μA	59, 60
Nondiabetic CKD	↓ Creatinine doubling/ESRD (RR = 0.52)	66–69
Advanced CKD	43% ↓ risk of creatinine doubling, ESRD or death	70
Angiotensin Receptor Blockers (ARBs)		
Type 2 DM + μA	↓ Risk of overt nephropathy (HR = 0.30)	76
Type 2 DM + CKD	25%–37% ↓ risk of creatinine doubling	
	23%–28% ↓ risk of ESRD	74, 75
Combination ACEI and ARB		
Type 2 DM + μA	↓ BP and ↓ albuminuria vs. ACEI or ARB	90
Nondiabetic CKD	HR for ESRD 0.38–0.40 vs. ACEI or ARB	89
All CKD (meta-analysis)	Mean 440mg/day less proteinuria vs. ACEI	94

CKD, chronic kidney disease; ESRD end-stage renal disease; HR hazard ratio; μA, microalbuminuria; NA, normoalbuminuria; OR odds ratio; RR, risk ratio.

inhibitor treatment versus placebo.[62] A second, larger analysis combined data from studies of type 1 and type 2 diabetes and reported weak evidence that ACE inhibitors were associated with a reduced risk of doubling of serum creatinine (RR, 0.60; 95% CI, 0.34–1.05) or incidence of ESRD (RR, 0.64; 95% CI, 0.40–1.03) even though there was stronger evidence of reduced risk of progression of microalbuminuria to macroalbuminuria (RR, 0.45; 95% CI, 0.28–0.71). All-cause mortality was significantly reduced in patients receiving ACE inhibitors (RR, 0.79; 95% CI, 0.63–0.99).[63] Finally, a meta-analysis of 16 trials that assessed the effect of ACE inhibitors on reducing the risk of microalbuminuria in type 1 and type 2 diabetes found a significantly lower risk of developing microalbuminuria versus placebo (RR, 0.60; 95% CI, 0.43–0.84) or CCB treatment (RR, 0.58; 95% CI, 0.40–0.84).[64]

Consequently, we recommend ACE inhibitor treatment for all type 1 diabetic patients with microalbuminuria or overt nephropathy. Insufficient data exist to support the use of ACE inhibitors in normoalbuminuric type 1 diabetic patients, but it seems reasonable to recommend ACE inhibitors for those with elevated blood pressure. There is no clear evidence of specific benefit associated with ACE inhibitors in slowing the progression of established nephropathy in type 2 diabetic patients, but this may be due to the lack of adequately powered studies. The

evidence does support the recommendation to use ACE inhibitors to reduce progression to overt nephropathy in type 2 diabetic patients with microalbuminuria or to prevent microalbuminuria from developing in patients with hypertension. Finally, cardiovascular disease is the most common cause of morbidity and mortality among type 2 diabetic patients, and ACE inhibitors should be considered to reduce cardiovascular risk in these patients.

Nondiabetic CKD

Regarding renoprotection in nondiabetic CKD, an early study reported a 53% reduction in the risk of reaching the combined endpoint of doubling of serum creatinine level or incidence of ESRD associated with ACE inhibitor treatment. However, blood pressure was lower among patients receiving an ACE inhibitor versus placebo, making it impossible to separate the beneficial effects of lowering blood pressure from any unique effects of ACE inhibitor treatment.[65] In the REIN study of 352 patients with nondiabetic CKD randomized to either ACE inhibitor or placebo, blood pressures were similar in the two groups. Among patients with at least 3 g/day of proteinuria at baseline, the study was stopped early because the rate of decline in GFR was significantly slower in patients receiving the ACE inhibitor (0.53 vs. 0.88 mL/min/mo).[66] There also was a significant reduction in the risk of the combined endpoint of a doubling of serum creatinine or ESRD with ACE inhibitor treatment (risk ratio = 1.91 for the placebo group). When REIN patients who had received placebo were switched to an ACE inhibitor, there was a significant reduction in the rate of decline in GFR. Patients continuing ACE inhibitor treatment had a further reduction in the rate of GFR decline. Notably, patients who received ACE inhibitors from the start had a significantly lower risk of reaching ESRD than those subsequently switched to ACE inhibitors (RR for placebo group, 1.86; 95% CI, 1.07–3.26); over 36 to 54 months of follow-up, none of the patients who received ACE inhibitors from the start reached ESRD.[67,68] When 186 REIN patients with less than 3 g/day of proteinuria were followed for a median of 31 months after randomization, similar results were seen. ACE inhibitor treatment significantly reduced the incidence of ESRD (RR for placebo group, 2.72; 95% CI, 1.22–6.08), particularly among those with a baseline GFR of less than 45 mL/min.[69] Even in advanced stages of CKD (244 patients with a serum creatinine of 3.1–5.0 mg/dL at baseline randomly assigned to ACE inhibitor treatment), ACE inhibitors are associated with a 52% reduction in proteinuria and a 43% reduction in the risk of the primary endpoint (doubling of serum creatinine, ESRD, or death).[70] A meta-analysis of 11 studies that included 1860 patients with nondiabetic CKD confirmed these findings[71]; ACE inhibitor treatment was associated with significantly lower risks of reaching ESRD (RR, 0.69; 95% CI, 0.51–0.94) or the combined endpoint of a doubling in serum creatinine or ESRD (RR, 0.70; 95% CI, 0.55–0.88). Thus, the renoprotective effects of ACE inhibitors are mediated by factors in addition to their antihypertensive and antiproteinuric effects, and benefits of their use were greater in patients with higher levels of baseline proteinuria but not in those patients with less than 0.5 g/day of proteinuria. Even in patients with autosomal dominant polycystic kidney disease, ACE inhibitor treatment reduced proteinuria, but the overall evidence of slowing CKD progression was inconclusive and limited to those with higher levels of proteinuria.[72]

In addition to the renoprotective benefits of ACE inhibitor treatment, the HOPE study revealed substantial reductions in overall (RR, 0.84) and cardiovascular mortality (RR, 0.74) in patients receiving an ACE inhibitor versus placebo among 9297 patients at increased risk of cardiovascular disease.[73] Although the HOPE study did not include large numbers of patients with nondiabetic CKD, cardiovascular disease remains the single largest cause of morbidity and mortality in this population, and the HOPE study results provide a further rationale for the use of ACE inhibitor therapy in patients with CKD.

In light of these trials regarding renoprotection and the probable reduction in cardiovascular risk, we recommend ACE inhibitor treatment for all patients with CKD and proteinuria more than 0.5 g/day unless there are specific contraindications.

Angiotensin Receptor Blockers

Angiotensin receptor blockers inhibit the renin-angiotensin system by blocking angiotensin II subtype 1 (AT_1) receptors.[12] Despite differences in their effects on the renin-angiotensin system, experimental studies have found that ACE inhibitor and ARB treatment produce similar changes in glomerular hemodynamics and afford equivalent renoprotection in a variety of experimental CKD models.[12]

The simultaneous publication of three large randomized studies clearly established a role for ARB therapy in achieving renoprotection in patients with type 2 diabetes. In the Reduction of Endpoints in NIDDM with Angiotensin II Antagonist Losartan (RENAAL) Trial, 1513 patients with overt diabetic nephropathy were randomized to ARB treatment or placebo and followed for a mean of 3.4 years.[74] ARB treatment was associated with significant, 25% reduction in the incidence of a doubling of baseline serum creatinine and ESRD (RR reduction = 28%). In the IDNT, 1715 patients with overt diabetic nephropathy were randomized to treatment with ARB, amlodipine, or placebo.[75] After a mean of 2.6 years, ARB treatment was associated with a 33% lower risk of doubling of serum creatinine versus placebo and a 37% reduction versus amlodipine. Although not statistically significant, the ARB was associated with a 23% reduction in the risk of ESRD versus placebo and amlodipine. Because achieved blood pressure between groups was closely matched in both of these trials, the additional renoprotective effects of ARB treatment cannot be attributed merely to their antihypertensive effects. A third study examined the renoprotective effects of an ARB (irbesartan) in 590 type 2 diabetic patients with hypertension and microalbuminuria.[76] Patients were randomized to irbesartan at two different doses (300 or 150 mg/day) or placebo. After 2 years there were significant differences in the incidence of overt proteinuria (5.2% vs. 9.7% vs. 14.9%); the higher dose of irbesartan was also associated with substantial reduction in the risk of overt nephropathy (HR, 0.30; 95% CI, 0.14–0.61 vs. placebo). The practical implication of this dose-dependent effect is that when ARBs are used to treat diabetic microalbuminuria, the dose should be titrated to the maximum antihypertensive dose.

A meta-analysis has confirmed the results of individual trials by showing a significant reduction in the risk of ESRD (RR, 0.78; 95% CI, 0.67–0.91) and doubling of serum creatinine (RR, 0.79; 95% CI, 0.67–0.93) as well as a reduction in risk of progression from microalbuminuria to macroalbuminuria (RR, 0.49; 95% CI, 0.32–0.75) among diabetic patients treated with ARB versus placebo.[63] Interestingly, there was no reduction in all cause mortality. In summary, clear evidence of the renoprotective effects of ACE inhibitor in type 2 diabetic patients with overt nephropathy is lacking, but there is sufficient evidence to support the use of ARB treatment to achieve renoprotection in these patients. ARB treatment is also effective in preventing progression from microalbuminuria to overt diabetic nephropathy. Preliminary results show that doses of ARB higher than the recommended maximum may result in greater lowering of proteinuria without a further reduction in blood pressure,[77,78] but further trials are required before this can be recommended.

ACE Inhibitor versus ARB Treatment

Strict application of available evidence would result in a recommendation for ACE inhibitor treatment to achieve renoprotection in patients with type 1 diabetes and microalbuminuria or overt diabetic nephropathy, type 2 diabetes with hypertension or microalbuminuria, and nondiabetic CKD with proteinuria greater than 0.5 g/day. ARBs would be indicated for patients with type 2 diabetes and microalbuminuria or overt nephropathy. It should be noted, however, that no adequate placebo-controlled trials of ARB treatment in patients with type 1 diabetes or in those with nondiabetic nephropathy have been conducted, and few studies have directly compared ACE inhibitor and ARB treatment in patients with CKD. The only substantial trial was conducted in a mixed group of type 2 diabetic patients with microalbuminuria as well as macroalbuminuria and was designed to assess noninferiority. There was no significant difference between ACE inhibitor and ARB treatment in the primary outcome—namely, a change in GFR—or in the secondary outcome of decreasing the urine albumin-to-creatinine ratio.[79] A meta-analysis of small trials comparing ACE inhibitor and ARB treatment in patients with diabetic CKD reported similar benefits with respect to incidence of ESRD, doubling of creatinine, and progression of microalbuminuria to macroalbuminuria.[80] Most national and international guidelines therefore recommend ACE inhibitor or ARB treatment for all forms of diabetic and nondiabetic CKD and leave the choice to individual physicians. One advantage of ARBs over ACE inhibitors is their more favorable adverse-effect profile. In clinical trials, ARBs have been reported to have adverse-effect profiles similar to placebo[81,82]; in particular, they are not associated with the cough that may occur in up to 20% of patients receiving an ACE inhibitor. Among patients converted from ACE inhibitor to ARB therapy, recurrence of a cough was significantly lower than in patients rechallenged with an ACE inhibitor.[83,84] In choosing between ACE inhibitor and ARB therapy for patients with type 2 diabetes and diabetic nephropathy, physicians have to consider evidence of proven renoprotection for ARB treatment versus a mortality benefit associated with ACE inhibitor treatment (in patients without established diabetic nephropathy).

One meta-analysis has called into question the value of renin-angiotensin system inhibition for renoprotection. Trials of ACE inhibitor and ARB treatment were pooled; when all studies of diabetic and nondiabetic CKD were considered, the analysis found a benefit in reducing the risk of ESRD (RR, 0.87; 95% CI, 0.75–0.99) and urine albumin excretion (mean, −15.7mg/day; 95% CI, −24.7 to −6.7 mg/day) but no significant benefit in reducing the risk of doubling of serum creatinine (RR, 0.71; 95% CI, 0.49–1.04). When diabetic and nondiabetic studies were considered separately, no significant benefits were evident with respect to incidence of ESRD or doubling of creatinine, but the benefit for albuminuria reduction persisted. The authors concluded that any renoprotective effects of ACE inhibitor or ARB therapy result only from their antihypertensive effects.[85] These conclusions have been rejected by many nephrologists because of principal weaknesses: inclusion of data from the very large ALLHAT study, in which only a minority of patients (5662 of 33,357) actually had CKD[36]; heterogeneity across trials, invalidating a pooling method; and lack of patient-level data.[86]

Combination ACE Inhibitor and ARB Treatment

The added antihypertensive effects of combination therapy with ACE inhibitors and ARBs have made it difficult to separate the benefits of additional BP lowering from benefits directly attributable to dual blockade of the renin-angiotensin system. Two studies have reported an additional reduction in proteinuria and blood pressure in patients receiving combination versus monotherapy.[87,88] One large study revealed additional renoprotective benefit with combination therapy in the absence of additional BP lowering: In the COOPERATE study, 263 patients with nondiabetic CKD were randomized to treatment with trandolapril or losartan or a combination of both.[89] In a unique study design, hypertension was intensively controlled with drugs other than renin-angiotensin system inhibitors before initiating the trial medication. If patients became hypotensive after adding the study medication, the dose of other antihypertensives was reduced. Combination therapy was associated with

significantly greater reductions in proteinuria (−75.6% vs. −44.3% with ACE inhibitor and −42.1% with ARB treatment) and a lower incidence of the primary endpoint (doubling of serum creatinine or ESRD; HR, 0.38; 95% CI, 0.18–0.63 vs. ACE inhibitor and HR, 0.40; 95% CI, 0.17–0.69 vs. ARB). Studies of diabetic CKD patients have been small or limited to microalbuminuria. The Candesartan And Lisinopril Microalbuminuria (CALM) study included 199 patients with type 2 diabetes, hypertension, and microalbuminuria, randomized first to ACE inhibitor or ARB therapy and then, after 12 weeks, to combination therapy or continued monotherapy. Combination therapy afforded greater reductions in blood pressure and albuminuria, but the incidence of macroalbuminuria and preservation of renal function were not reported.[90] Small studies have uncovered an additional BP lowering and proteinuria reduction when ARB treatment was added to patients with type 1 diabetes[91] or type 2 diabetes[92] but with persistent proteinuria and hypertension despite ACE inhibitor treatment. Two meta-analyses have confirmed the findings of the above individual trials; one analysis reported a small additional reduction in blood pressure with combination therapy that was largely attributable to the use of submaximal doses of ACE inhibitor or short-acting ACE inhibitors. Combination therapy in several studies was associated with additional reduction of proteinuria that was independent of blood pressure.[93] The other analysis found a significant additional reduction in proteinuria with combination therapy versus monotherapy that was evident in patients with diabetic and nondiabetic CKD (weighted mean difference, 440 mg/day; 95% CI, 289–591 vs. ACE inhibitor alone).[94]

In summary, combination ACE inhibitor and ARB therapy seems to reduce blood pressure and proteinuria to a greater extent than monotherapy. Whether this effect is attributable to additional BP lowering that could be achieved by other antihypertensive agents remains unanswered, but the COOPERATE study suggests there is a unique benefit attributable to dual blockade of the renin-angiotensin system. Further studies are required to confirm the long-term benefits of combination therapy with respect to preservation of renal function in other groups of CKD patients, but we recommend that the combination should be considered in CKD patients who have not achieved therapeutic goals for BP and proteinuria reduction with ACE inhibitor or ARB monotherapy.

Safety Considerations

Despite the clear trial evidence of renoprotection by ACE inhibitors and ARBs, many physicians remain reluctant to prescribe these drugs because of concerns about a potential rise in serum creatinine or potassium level. It should be noted, however, that the incidence of these complications in published trials is low. Discontinuation of therapy due to uncontrolled hyperkalemia has been reported in only 0 to 4% of patients, and the overall incidence of hyperkalemia was not different in ACE inhibitor– versus non–ACE inhibitor-treated patients when data from 6 studies were combined.[95] The discontinuation of potassium supplements, avoidance of potassium-sparing diuretics, and dietary advice to avoid high-potassium foods may all help to reduce the incidence of hyperkalemia. Similarly, a progressive rise in serum creatinine rarely occurs in patients unless there is bilateral renal artery stenosis (in this case, ACE inhibitor and ARB treatment is contraindicated). It is important to appreciate that an initial increase in serum creatinine level probably results from the renal hemodynamic effects of ACE inhibitors or ARBs and may predict greater renoprotective efficacy.[96] Provided that the increase in serum creatinine is less than 30% and that it is not progressive, an initial rise should not be an indication for discontinuing ACE inhibitor therapy. Patients with compromised renal perfusion due to intravascular volume depletion, for example, are most likely to exhibit a serious decline in renal function after the introduction of ACE inhibitor or ARB therapy. It is therefore important to ensure adequate hydration, omit or reduce diuretics for 48 to 72 hours, and avoid nonsteroidal anti-inflammatory drugs before starting an ACE inhibitor in CKD patients. In addition, the ACE inhibitor or ARB should be started at a low dose and titrated upward with repeated monitoring. Figure 62-2 is an algorithm to facilitate the safe initiation of ACE inhibitor or ARB treatment in patients with CKD.

Proteinuria as a Therapeutic Target

Proteinuria has traditionally been regarded as a marker of glomerular filtration barrier integrity, and the extent of proteinuria has been used as an indicator of glomerular disease severity. Indeed, the severity of proteinuria at baseline is the most important independent predictor of renal outcomes in randomized trials of patients with diabetic nephropathy[97,98] and nondiabetic CKD.[66,99,100] It has also been proposed that proteinuria per se contributes to progressive renal injury[14];

therefore, proteinuria reduction should be viewed as a therapeutic goal. For example, results from the MDRD showed that a reduction in proteinuria, independent of blood pressure, was associated with slower progression of CKD; the degree of benefit achieved through blood pressure lowering depended on the extent of baseline proteinuria.[25]

Other studies have observed that the percentage reduction in proteinuria after initiation of ACE inhibitor or ARB treatment and the absolute level of proteinuria are independent predictors of the subsequent rate of decline in GFR among patients with diabetic nephropathy[97,98] and nondiabetic CKD.[100,101] A meta-analysis of data from 1860 patients with nondiabetic CKD confirmed these findings and showed that during antihypertensive treatment, the achieved level of proteinuria was a powerful predictor of the combined endpoint of doubling of baseline serum creatinine level or onset of ESRD (RR, 5.56; 95% CI, 3.87–7.98 for each 1 g/day increase in achieved level of proteinuria).[102] One prospective study has reported improved preservation of GFR when ACE inhibitor or ARB therapy was titrated to the maximum antiproteinuric dose.[103] Whether or not proteinuria contributes directly to renal injury, the strong association between the degree of proteinuria reduction and renoprotection in clinical studies implies that minimization of proteinuria should be regarded as an important independent therapeutic goal in renoprotective strategies.

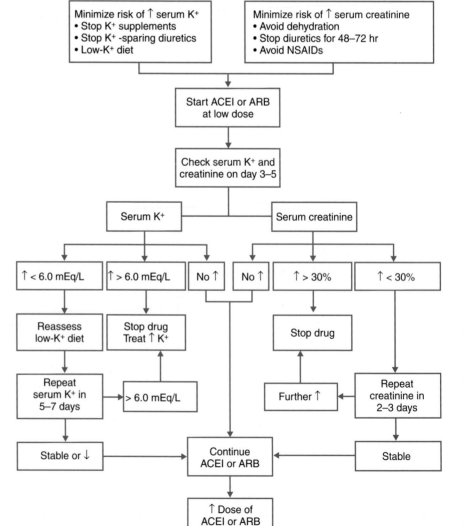

Figure 62-2 An algorithm for the safe initiation of ACE inhibitor or ARB treatment in patients with CKD. K^+, potassium; NSAID, nonsteroidal anti-inflammatory drugs.

Dietary Interventions

Weight Loss

Obesity has been shown in experimental models to cause glomerular hypertension and hyperfiltration, factors that are central to mechanisms of CKD progression.[104] In humans as well, obesity is associated with glomerular hyperfiltration and albuminuria, both of which are reversed by weight loss.[105] Epidemiologic studies have identified obesity as a risk factor for CKD[106,107]; in one study, obesity was an independent risk factor for progression of CKD (IgA nephropathy).[108] Large interventional studies of weight loss in patients with CKD are lacking, but based on the above data it seems reasonable to recommend weight loss in obese patients with CKD.

Sodium Restriction

In the general population high dietary sodium intake is associated with hypertension, and sodium restriction produces a significant reduction in blood pressure.[109] One observational study among patients with CKD reported that those who restricted their sodium intake to less than 100 mmol/day evidenced a lower rate of decline in GFR versus those with a high sodium intake (>200 mmol/day); there was no increase in proteinuria despite having lower creatinine clearance and higher levels of proteinuria at baseline. BP control was similar between the groups.[110] Several other small studies have sought to investigate the effect of dietary sodium intake on CKD progression. A recent systematic review of 16 studies concluded that marked heterogeneity between the studies precluded meta-analysis.[111] Nevertheless, there was a general trend for increasing sodium intake to be associated with worsening albuminuria. Only two reports indicated no benefit from reducing dietary sodium, and both were of low methodologic quality. High dietary sodium intake has also been shown to negate the antiproteinuric effects of ACE inhibitor treatment,[37] as well as the antihypertensive response. Long-term randomized trials are required to define the role of sodium restriction in renoprotective strategies, but even the incomplete evidence available supports a recommendation for moderate dietary sodium restriction (<100 mmol/day) in patients with CKD.

Protein Restriction

Based on the notion that reducing the excretory burden on the kidneys would slow the rate of progressive injury, dietary protein restriction was among the first interventions proposed to slow CKD progression. Experimental studies showed that a low-protein diet normalized glomerular hemodynamics in the remnant kidney model[6] and resulted in effective long-term renoprotection.[112] Unfortunately, clinical studies to date have failed to provide unambiguous evidence to support the use of protein restriction in human CKD.

In the MDRD study 585 patients with mostly nondiabetic CKD (GFR = 25–55 mL/min/1.73 m^2) were randomized to "usual" (1.3 g/kg/day) or "low" (0.58 g/kg/day) protein diet in study A, and 255 patients with GFR = 13–24 mL/min/1.73 m^2 to "low" (0.58 g/kg/day) or "very low" (0.28 g/kg/day) protein diet (study B). After a mean of 2.2 years' follow-up there was no difference in the rate of GFR decline in study A, and only a trend toward slower decline in the "very low" protein group in study B.[24] Further analysis, however, revealed that the desired protein intake was not achieved in the randomized groups; when data were analyzed according to

achieved dietary protein intake, a reduction in protein intake of 0.2 g/kg/day correlated with a 1.15 mL/min/year reduction in the rate of GFR decline, equivalent to a 29% reduction in mean rate of GFR decline, implying a 41% prolongation in renal survival.[113] Several factors have been identified that may account for the inconclusive results of the MDRD study, including the generally slow rate of decline in GFR (4 mL/min/year or less), short follow-up, high proportion of patients with adult polycystic kidney disease, and random use of ACE inhibitors in the different groups. Evidence supporting a renoprotective effect of low-protein diet was provided by meta-analyses of randomized studies.[114] Among 1413 patients with nondiabetic CKD from 5 studies (including those from study A of the MDRD), low-protein diet was associated with a relative risk of 0.67 (95% CI, 0.50–0.89) for ESRD or death. Similarly, among 108 type 1 diabetic patients from five studies, low-protein diet significantly slowed the increase in albuminuria or the decline in GFR/creatinine clearance (RR 0.56; 95% CI, 0.40–0.77). Unfortunately, long-term follow-up of the MDRD study A cohort has also proved inconclusive.[115] Small studies suggest that the antiproteinuric effects of dietary protein restriction are additive to those of ACE inhibitor treatment,[116] but large long-term studies are required to evaluate this further. Although no single study has yet provided conclusive evidence of the renoprotective effect of dietary protein restriction in humans, we believe that sufficient evidence exists to consider moderate protein restriction of 0.6 g/kg/day in patients with CKD and evidence of progression. In addition to possible renoprotective effects, dietary protein restriction results in reduced sodium, phosphate and acid intake, all of which are beneficial for CKD patients.[117] The decision to institute dietary protein restriction should be individualized; it should be avoided in patients with low serum albumin due to severe nephrotic syndrome or malnutrition. Fortunately, Medicare will pay for dietician visits for CKD patients in the United States.

Treatment of Dyslipidemia

Chronic kidney disease is commonly associated with abnormalities of plasma lipids: elevated levels of the triglyceride-rich lipoproteins very low-density lipoprotein and low-density lipoprotein, and reduced levels of high-density lipoprotein.[118] In addition to placing CKD patients at increased risk of cardiovascular disease, these lipid abnormalities may also accelerate the progression of CKD. In the MDRD study, low serum high-density lipoprotein cholesterol was an independent predictor of more rapid decline in GFR[99]; in another study elevated triglyceride-rich apolipoprotein B-containing lipoprotein correlated significantly with the rate of deterioration of renal function.[119] Hypercholesterolemia has been associated with more rapid progression among patients with diabetic[120–122] and nondiabetic CKD.[123] Mechanisms offered to explain why hyperlipidemia might contribute to CKD progression include stimulation of mesangial cell proliferation, cytokine expression, and extracellular matrix synthesis[124,125]; oxidation of LDL to form reactive oxygen species[126]; and elevations in P_{GC}.[127] In experimental studies, treatment of hyperlipidemia has resulted in attenuation of renal injury in a variety of models of CKD.[128,129] Results from large randomized trials of lipid-lowering therapy in CKD patients have not been reported, but a meta-analysis of 12 small studies that included both diabetic and nondiabetic CKD found that lipid-lowering therapy significantly reduced the rate of decline in GFR (mean reduction, 1.9 mL/min/year).[130] Several secondary analyses of data from clinical trials also suggest that lipid-lowering therapy may slow CKD progression; these results should be interpreted with caution. Among patients with a history of myocardial infarction, pravastatin slowed the rate of GFR decline in patients with estimated GFR values less than 40 mL/min/1.73 m², particularly in patients with proteinuria.[131] Similarly, in the Heart Protection Study, patients with previous cardiovascular disease or diabetes who were randomized to simvastatin treatment had a smaller increase in serum creatinine compared to those who received placebo.[132] In an open-label study, atorvastatin treatment of CKD patients with proteinuria and hypercholesterolemia was associated with preservation of creatinine clearance, whereas those receiving placebo evidenced a significant decline.[133] On the other hand, lipid lowering with fibrates has not been associated with preservation of renal function,[134,135] although one study did show reduced progression to microalbuminuria among type 2 diabetic patients receiving fenofibrate.[136] This suggests that some of the renoprotective effects observed above may be due to other, pleiotropic effects of "statins." Pending the results of trials in CKD patients, these results, plus the fact that CKD patients are at substantially increased risk for cardiovascular disease, support a policy of active dietary and drug intervention to correct dyslipidemia to the levels recommended for other patients at high cardiovascular risk (low-density lipoprotein cholesterol < 100 mg/dL).[137]

Smoking Cessation

Smoking has been identified as a risk factor for the development of microalbuminuria, overt proteinuria, and CKD progression in type 1 and 2 diabetes.[138–141] Smoking is also a risk factor for progression in a variety of forms of nondiabetic CKD: Among patients with adult polycystic kidney disease or IgA nephropathy, smokers had a substantially increased risk of progression to ESRD versus nonsmokers[142]; among patients with lupus nephritis,[143] the median time to ESRD was almost halved in smokers versus nonsmokers; patients with a primary glomerulonephritis and serum creatinine higher than 1.7 mg/dL were significantly more likely to be smokers than those with normal creatinine[144]; and smoking was the most powerful predictor of a rise in serum creatinine level among patients with severe essential hypertension.[145] Epidemiologic studies have identified smoking as a risk factor for albuminuria,[146,147] renal impairment,[106,148,149] and ESRD.[150] Proposed mechanisms whereby smoking may exacerbate renal injury include sympathetic nervous system activation, glomerular capillary hypertension, endothelial cell injury, and direct tubulotoxicity.[151] Although prospective studies showing renoprotective benefit from smoking cessation are lacking, these reports suggest that the kidney is another organ that is adversely affected by smoking. The well-established benefits of smoking cessation for prevention of lung and cardiovascular disease as well as malignancy mandate that all patients with CKD should be counseled to stop smoking and assisted in achieving this goal.

Control of Hyperglycemia

The role of glycemic control in diabetic renoprotection is discussed more fully in Chapter 28. Randomized trials have provided unequivocal evidence that tight glycemic control significantly reduces the risk of developing microalbuminuria or overt nephropathy among patients with type 1 diabetes[152] and type 2 diabetes.[153] Unfortunately the benefits of improved glycemic control in those who already have microalbuminuria are not well established. Only two of five small randomized studies have demonstrated a reduction in progression to overt nephropathy with "tight" versus "normal" glycemic control among type 1 diabetic patients with microalbuminuria.[154–158] On the other hand, there is evidence of histologic reversal of diabetic glomerulopathy lesions in type 1 diabetic patients with normoalbuminuria or microalbuminuria after pancreatic transplantation.[159] No data are available to assess the renoprotective effect of tight glycemic control among diabetic patients with established nephropathy. Despite the fact that glycemic control has not been proven to prevent progression of diabetic nephropathy, these patients are also at risk of developing other microvascular and macrovascular complications. We recommend tight glycemic control (target HBA_{1C} < 7.0%) in all patients, regardless of the severity of diabetic nephropathy.

Monitoring

Regular monitoring is essential to facilitate optimization of therapeutic interventions for slowing CKD progression. Serum creatinine provides a relatively insensitive estimate of GFR, but a plot of values of the reciprocal of serum creatinine (1/Scr) versus time for an individual patient yields a linear relationship.[4,5] This means that changes in creatinine clearance or GFR are also declining linearly with time; hence, the plot can be used to evaluate changes in progression of CKD.[5,24] Alternatively, renal function is assessed using estimated GFR derived from a serum creatinine measurement using the 4-variable MDRD equation.[160] Like 1/Scr, sequential values of estimated GFR can be plotted, with the goal of reducing the rate of GFR decline to less than 1 mL/min/year, a rate associated with normal aging. Many laboratories now facilitate this by reporting the estimated GFR with every serum creatinine measurement. As noted, an alternative method of monitoring progression is to plot 1/Scr. As discussed, proteinuria should be assessed after each change in therapy, with the goal of reducing it to less than 0.5 g/day. The use of urine protein-to-creatinine ratio measurements, which correlate well with 24-hour urinary protein excretion, allows frequent monitoring with minimal inconvenience to the patient.[161] Finally, blood pressure should be assessed at each examination and controlled to a level lower than 130/80 mm Hg. In some patients, particularly those affected by "white coat" hypertension, the use of home or ambulatory monitoring may be indicated.

Future Therapies

Currently available renoprotective therapies have in general achieved a slowing in the rate of progression of CKD, but relatively few patients have achieved complete cessation of progression and still fewer have evidenced a reversal of renal injury. Clearly, there is a need for more effective treatments. Novel renoprotective interventions are currently being investigated in experimental studies and clinical trials.

Drugs with Hemodynamic Effects

Endothelins are potent vasoconstrictor peptides that are upregulated in experimental models of CKD and could contribute to the glomerular hemodynamic changes that are central to CKD progression. In experimental diabetes, selective endothelin type A (ET_A) receptor antagonists, as well as combined ET_A/ET_B antagonists, ameliorate hypertension, renal vasoconstriction, proteinuria, and renal damage in experimental diabetes.[162] Recent evidence suggests that ET_A blockade also exerts anti-inflammatory effects that contribute to renoprotection.[163] Vasopeptidase inhibitors are molecules that simultaneously inhibit both angiotensin-converting enzyme and neutral endopeptidase. This latter ecto-enzyme is localized principally in the brush border membrane of renal tubule cells and catabolizes several vasodilator molecules, including the natriuretic peptides, adrenomedullin, and bradykinin. Thus, vasopeptidase inhibitor treatment is associated with reduced production of the vasoconstrictor angiotensin II and accumulation of the above vasodilators. Vasopeptidase inhibitors are effective antihypertensive agents in both low and high renin states.[164] In experimental models, vasopeptidase inhibitors produced a greater lowering of P_{GC} than an ACE inhibitor and more effective renoprotection despite equivalent control of systemic blood pressure.[165,166] Orally active inhibitors of renin are currently undergoing clinical trials and offer a novel pharmacologic intervention for inhibiting the renin-angiotensin system. Preliminary clinical evidence indicates that renin inhibitors are effective as antihypertensives,[167] but further studies are required to evaluate renoprotective benefits, as well as effects when combined with other renin-angiotensin system inhibitors.

Antiproteinuric and Antifibrotic Therapies

Recent insights into the role of proteinuria and fibrosis in CKD progression have prompted the development of several new therapies. For example, albuminuria can be reduced by preserving the integrity of the glomerular filtration barrier. In an experimental model of diabetes, glycosaminoglycan treatment has been shown to prevent the loss of glomerular basement membrane charge selectivity and to inhibit development of proteinuria. Treatment with sulodexide, an orally available glycosaminoglycan, reduced albuminuria among patients with type 1 or type 2 diabetes and microalbuminuria or microalbuminuria[168] and is currently being evaluated in clinical trials. Aldosterone has been identified as an important mediator of progressive renal injury via hemodynamic and profibrotic actions. Treatment with spironolactone and other aldosterone antagonists has produced renoprotective effects in experimental[169] and small clinical studies.[170] Further studies are required to evaluate the risk-benefit of this strategy in view of hyperkalemia, especially when a renin-angiotensin system inhibitor is combined with an aldosterone antagonist. Perfinidone is an orally active antifibrotic agent with evidence of renoprotective benefits in several experimental models of CKD. Importantly, these effects were additive to those of ARB treatment in one study,[171] and clinical trials of perfinidone are underway. Hepatocyte growth factor is up-regulated in experimental models of CKD and appears to exert multiple antifibrotic effects. Treatment with heptocyte growth factor prevents renal injury in several models; importantly, it was associated with reduced interstitial fibrosis in rats with established renal injury after five sixths nephrectomy.[172] Bone morphogenetic protein-7 has emerged as an endogenous antagonist of TGF-β; it also inhibits the epithelial to mesenchymal transition involved in interstitial fibrosis. Bone morphogenetic protein-7 treatment reduced interstitial fibrosis in the unilateral ureteral obstruction model[173] and ameliorated glomerulosclerosis as well

as interstitial fibrosis in an experimental model of diabetic nephropathy.[174]

A STRATEGY FOR MAXIMAL RENOPROTECTION

We have considered a variety of interventions that have been shown to slow the rate of progression of CKD. At best, however, each intervention slows the rate of progression by approximately 50%. Therefore, we suggest that for maximal long-term renoprotection, a comprehensive strategy employing multiple elements directed at different aspects of the pathogenesis of progressive renal injury is required (see Fig. 62-1). Once treatments have been introduced, frequent monitoring of blood pressure, proteinuria, and GFR is essential so therapy can be escalated to achieve established therapeutic goals (Table 62-2). Our approach is analogous to that applied in modern chemotherapeutic strategies for cancer; multiple agents are used and treatment is directed toward correcting all signs of disease activity until the patient is said to be in "remission." Importantly, data from a small number of patients suggest that if remission is maintained in the long term, some recovery of renal function or "regression" of renal disease may be achieved.[68] Limited data already indicate that significant improvements in renoprotection can be achieved with a combination strategy. Among 160 type 2 diabetic patients with microalbuminuria, a combined approach of intensive therapy resulted in a marked reduction in the risk of overt nephropathy (odds ratio, 0.27).[175] Similarly, 9 of 13 patients with resistant nephrotic range proteinuria and CKD referred to a "remission clinic" achieved reduction of proteinuria to less than 1 g/day and stabilization of renal function after application of a similar intensive therapy protocol.[95] These recommendations are based on currently available

Table 62-2 A Comprehensive Strategy and Therapeutic Goals for Achieving Maximal Renoprotection in Patients with Chronic Kidney Disease

Intervention	Goal
1. ACEI or ARB treatment (consider combination therapy if goals not achieved with monotherapy)	Proteinuria < 0.5 g/day GFR decline < 1 mL/min/year
2. Additional antihypertensive therapy	< 125/75 mm Hg if proteinuria > 1 g/day < 130/80 mm Hg if proteinuria < 1 g/day
3. Weight loss if obese	
4. Dietary sodium restriction	<100 mmol/day
5. Dietary protein restriction	0.6 g/kg/day
6. Tight glycemic control	HBA_{1C} < 7.0%
7. Smoking cessation	
8. Lipid lowering therapy	LDL cholesterol < 100mg/dL

ACE inhibitor, angiotensin-converting enzyme inhibitor: ARB, angiotensin receptor blocker; BP, blood pressure; GFR, glomerular filtration rate; HBA_{1c}, hemoglobin A_{1c}.

interventions and the monitoring methods already widely used, so a comprehensive approach to renoprotection is an achievable goal for all patients with CKD. Although it has been argued that there is a need for new renoprotective agents, it is also true that these available therapies have not yet been applied to all patients with CKD.[176] If widely implemented, a comprehensive renoprotective strategy may not only delay the need for dialysis in many patients, but may also substantially reduce the number of CKD patients progressing to ESRD. Recent reports of a small decline in the incidence of new patients starting dialysis therapy in the United States indicate that such strategies are starting to yield a benefit.[1]

References

1. U.S. Renal Data System: 2006 Annual Data Report: Atlas of Chronic Kidney Disease and End-Stage Renal Disease in the United States. Bethesda, MD: National Institutes of Health, National Institute of Diabetes and Digestive and Kidney Diseases, 2006.

2. Kidney Disease Outcomes Quality Initiative: K/DOQI clinical practice guidelines for chronic kidney disease: Evaluation, classification, and stratification. Am J Kidney Dis 2002;39:S1–S266.

3. Centers for Disease Control and Prevention: Prevalence of chronic kidney disease and associated risk factors—United States, 1999–2004. MMWR 2007. 56:161–165.

4. Mitch WE, Walser M, Buffington GA, et al: A simple method for estimating progression of chronic renal failure. Lancet 1976;2:1326–1328.

5. Maroni BJ, Mitch WE: Role of nutrition in prevention of the progression of renal disease. Ann Rev Nutr 1997;17:435–455.

6. Brenner BM, Meyer TW, Hostetter TH: Dietary protein intake and the progressive nature of kidney disease: The role of hemodynamically mediated glomerular injury in the pathogenesis of progressive glomerular sclerosis in aging, renal ablation, and intrinsic renal disease. N Engl J Med 1982;307:652–659.

7. Hostetter TH, Olson JL, Rennke HG, et al: Hyperfiltration in remnant nephrons: A potentially adverse response to renal ablation. J Am Soc Nephrol 2001;12:1315–1325.

8. Anderson S, Meyer TW, Rennke HG, et al: Control of glomerular hypertension limits glomerular injury in rats with reduced renal mass. J Clin Invest 1985;76:612–619.

9. Anderson S, Rennke HG, Brenner BM: Therapeutic advantage of converting enzyme inhibitors in arresting progressive renal disease associated with systemic hypertension in the rat. J Clin Invest 1986;77:1993–2000.

10. Zatz R, Meyer TW, Rennke HG, et al: Predominance of hemodynamic rather than metabolic factors in the pathogenesis of diabetic glomerulopathy. Proc Natl Acad Sci U S A 1985;82:5963–5967.

11. Zatz R, Dunn BR, Meyer TW, et al: Prevention of diabetic glomerulopathy by pharmacological amelioration of glomerular capillary hypertension. J Clin Invest 1986. 77:1925–1930.

12. Taal MW, Brenner BM: Renoprotective benefits of RAS inhibition: From ACEI to angiotensin II antagonists. Kidney Int 2000;57:1803–1817.

13. D'Amico G, Ferrario F, Rastaldi MP: Tubulointerstitial damage in glomerular diseases: Its role in the progression of renal damage. Am J Kidney Dis 1995;26:124–132.

14. Abbate M, Zoja C, Remuzzi G: How does proteinuria cause progressive renal damage? J Am Soc Nephrol 2006;17:2974–2984.

15. Hirschberg R, Wang S: Proteinuria and growth factors in the development of tubulointerstitial injury and scarring in kidney disease. Curr Opin Nephrol Hypertens 2005. 14:43–52.

16. Kriz W, LeHir M: Pathways to nephron loss starting from glomerular diseases—insights from animal models. Kidney Int 2005; 67:404–419.

17. Zeisberg M, Kalluri R: The role of epithelial-to-mesenchymal transition in renal fibrosis. J Mol Med 2004;82:175–181.

18. Norman JT, Fine LG: Intrarenal oxygenation in chronic renal failure. Clin Exp Pharmacol Physiol 2006;33:989–996.

19. Mogensen CE: Progression of nephropathy in long-term diabetics with proteinuria and effect of initial anti-hypertensive treatment. Scand J Clin Lab Invest 1976;36:383–388.

20. Parving HH, Andersen AR, Smidt UM, et al: Early aggressive antihypertensive treatment reduces rate of decline in kidney function in diabetic nephropathy. Lancet 1983;1:1175–1179.

21. Bergstrom J, Alvestrand A, Bucht H, et al: Progression of chronic renal failure in man is retarded with more frequent clinical follow-ups and better blood pressure control. Clin Nephrol 1986;25:1–6.

22. Brazy PC, Fitzwilliam JF: Progressive renal disease: Role of race and antihypertensive medications. Kidney Int 1990. 37:1113–1119.

23. Kes P, Ratkovic-Gusic I: The role of arterial hypertension in progression of renal failure. Kidney Int 1996;55(Suppl):S72–S74.

24. Klahr S, Levey AS, Beck GJ, et al, for the MDRD Study Group: The effects of dietary protein restriction and blood-pressure control on the progression of chronic renal disease. Modification of Diet in Renal Disease (MDRD) Study Group. N Engl J Med 1994;330:877–884.

25. Peterson JC, Adler S, Burkart JM, et al: Blood pressure control, proteinuria, and the progression of renal disease. The Modification of Diet in Renal Disease (MDRD) Study. Ann Intern Med 1995;123:754–762.

26. Sarnak MJ, Greene T, Wang X, et al: The effect of a lower target blood pressure on the progression of kidney disease: Long-term follow-up of the Modification of Diet in Renal Disease Study. Ann Intern Med 2005;142:342–351.

27. Lewis JB, Berl T, Bain RP, et al: Effect of intensive blood pressure control on the course of type 1 diabetic nephropathy. Am J Kidney Dis 1999;34:809–817.

28. Pohl MA, Blumenthal S, Cordonnier DJ, et al: Independent and additive impact of blood pressure control and angiotensin II receptor blockade on renal outcomes in the Irbesartan Diabetic Nephropathy Trial: Clinical implications and limitations. J Am Soc Nephrol 2005;16:3027–3037.

29. Schrier R, McFann K, Johnson A, et al: Cardiac and renal effects of standard versus rigorous blood pressure control in autosomal-dominant polycystic kidney disease: Results of a seven-year prospective randomized study. J Am Soc Nephrol 2002;13:1733–1739.

30. Wright JT Jr, Bakris G, Greene T, et al: Effect of blood pressure lowering and antihypertensive drug class on progression of hypertensive kidney disease: Results from the AASK trial. JAMA 2002;288:2421–2431.

31. Ruggenenti P, Perna A, Loriga G, et al: Blood-pressure control for renoprotection in patients with non-diabetic chronic renal disease (REIN-2): Multicentre, randomised controlled trial. Lancet 2005;365:939–946.

32. Jafar TH, Stark PC, Schmid CH, et al: Progression of chronic kidney disease: The role of blood pressure control, proteinuria, and angiotensin-converting enzyme inhibition: A patient-level meta-analysis. Ann Intern Med 2003;139:244–252.

33. Bakris GL, Williams M, Dworkin L, et al: Preserving renal function in adults with hypertension and diabetes: A consensus approach. National Kidney Foundation Hypertension and Diabetes Executive Committees Working Group. Am J Kidney Dis 2000;36:646–661.

34. Li PK, Weening JJ, Dirks J, et al: A report with consensus statements of the International Society of Nephrology 2004 Consensus Workshop on Prevention of Progression of Renal Disease, Hong Kong, 29 June 2004. Kidney Int 2005;94(Suppl):S2–S7.

35. ALLHAT: Major outcomes in high-risk hypertensive patients randomized to angiotensin-converting enzyme inhibitor or calcium channel blocker vs. diuretic: The Antihypertensive and Lipid-Lowering Treatment to Prevent Heart Attack Trial (ALLHAT). JAMA 2002;288:2981–2997.

36. Rahman M, Pressel S, Davis BR, et al: Renal outcomes in high-risk hypertensive patients treated with an angiotensin-converting enzyme inhibitor or a calcium channel blocker vs a diuretic: A report from the Antihypertensive and Lipid-Lowering Treatment to PreventHeart Attack Trial (ALLHAT). Arch Intern Med 2005;165:936–946.

37. Buter H, Hemmelder MH, Navis G, et al: The blunting of the antiproteinuric efficacy of ACE inhibition by high sodium intake can be restored by hydrochlorothiazide. Nephrol Dial Transplant 1998;13:1682–1685.

38. Uzu T, Harada T, Namba T, et al: Thiazide diuretics enhance nocturnal blood pressure fall and reduce proteinuria in immunoglobulin A nephropathy treated with angiotensin II modulators. J Hypertens 2005;23:861–865.

39. Griffin KA, Picken MM, Bidani AK: Deleterious effects of calcium channel blockade on pressure transmission and glomerular injury in rat remnant kidneys. J Clin Invest 1995. 96:793–800.

40. Zucchelli P, Zuccala A, Borghi M, et al: Long-term comparison between captopril and nifedipine in the progression of renal insufficiency. Kidney Int 1992;42:452–458.

41. Ruggenenti P, Perna A, Benini R, et al: Effects of dihydropyridine calcium channel blockers, angiotensin-converting enzyme inhibition, and blood pressure control on chronic, nondiabetic nephropathies. Gruppo Italiano di Studi Epidemiologici in Nefrologia (GISEN). J Am Soc Nephrol 1998;9:2096–2101.

42. Agodoa LY, Appel L, Bakris GL, et al: Effect of ramipril vs. amlodipine on renal outcomes in hypertensive nephrosclerosis: A randomized controlled trial. JAMA 2001. 285:2719–2728.

43. Bakris GL, Weir MR, DeQuattro V, et al: Effects of an ACE inhibitor/calcium antagonist combination on proteinuria in diabetic nephropathy. Kidney Int 1998;54:1283–1289.

44. Bakris GL, Weir MR, Secic M, et al: Differential effects of calcium antagonist subclasses on markers of nephropathy progression. Kidney Int 2004;65:1991–2002.

45. Lewis EJ, Hunsicker LG, Bain RP, et al: The effect of angiotensin-converting-enzyme inhibition on diabetic nephropathy. N Engl J Med 1993;329:1456–1462.

46. The ACE Inhibitors in Diabetic Nephropathy Trialist Group: Should all patients with type 1 diabetes mellitus and microalbuminuria receive angiotensin-converting enzyme inhibitors? A meta-analysis of individual patient data. Ann Intern Med 2001; 134:370–379.

47. Mathiesen ER, Hommel E, Hansen HP, et al: Randomised controlled trial of long term efficacy of captopril on preservation of kidney function in normotensive patients with insulin dependent diabetes and microalbuminuria. BMJ 1999;319:24–25.

48. The EUCLID Study Group: Randomised placebo-controlled trial of lisinopril in normotensive patients with insulin-dependent diabetes and normoalbuminuria or microalbuminuria. Lancet 1997;349:1787–1792.

49. Bakris GL, Copley JB, Vicknair N, et al: Calcium channel blockers versus other antihypertensive therapies on progression of NIDDM associated nephropathy. Kidney Int 1996;50: 1641–1650.

50. Lebovitz HE, Wiegmann TB, Cnaan A, et al: Renal protective effects of enalapril in hypertensive NIDDM: Role of baseline albuminuria. Kidney Int 1994;45(Suppl):S150–S155.

51. Nielsen FS, Rossing P, Gall MA, et al: Long-term effect of lisinopril and atenolol on kidney function in hypertensive NIDDM subjects with diabetic nephropathy. Diabetes 1997;46:1182–1188.

52. Fogari R, Zoppi A, Corradi L, et al: Long-term effects of ramipril and nitrendipine on albuminuria in hypertensive patients with type II diabetes and impaired renal function. J Hum Hypertension 1999;13:47–53.

53. Sano T, Kawamura T, Matsumae H, et al: Effects of long-term enalapril treatment on persistent micro-albuminuria in well-controlled hypertensive and normotensive NIDDM patients. Diabetes Care 1994;17:420–424.

54. Trevisan R, Tiengo A: Effect of low-dose ramipril on microalbuminuria in normotensive or mild hypertensive non-insulin-dependent diabetic patients. North-East Italy Microalbuminuria Study Group. Am J Hypertension 1995;8:876–883.

55. Agardh CD, Garcia-Puig J, Charbonnel B, et al: Greater reduction of urinary albumin excretion in hypertensive type II diabetic patients with incipient nephropathy by lisinopril than by nifedipine. J Hum Hypertens 1996;10:185–192.

56. Ravid M, Lang R, Rachmani R, et al: Long-term renoprotective effect of angiotensin-converting enzyme inhibition in non-insulin-dependent diabetes mellitus. A 7-year follow-up study. Arch Intern Med 1996;156:286–289.

57. Ahmad J, Siddiqui MA, Ahmad H: Effective postponement of diabetic nephropathy with enalapril in normotensive type 2 diabetic patients with microalbuminuria. Diabetes Care 1997;20: 1576–1581.

58. Andersen S, Tarnow L, Rossing P, et al: Renoprotective effects of angiotensin II receptor blockade in type 1 diabetic patients with diabetic nephropathy. Kidney Int 2000;57:601–606.

59. Ravid M, Brosh D, Levi Z, et al: Use of enalapril to attenuate decline in renal function in normotensive, normoalbuminuric patients with type 2 diabetes mellitus. A randomized, controlled trial. Ann Intern Med 1998;128(12 Pt 1):982–988.

60. Ruggenenti P, Fassi A, Ilieva AP, et al: Preventing microalbuminuria in type 2 diabetes. New Engl J Med 2004;351:1941–1951.

61. UK Prospective Diabetes Study (UKPDS) Group: Efficacy of atenolol and captopril in reducing risk of macrovascular and microvascular complications in type 2 diabetes. BMJ 1998;317: 713–720.

62. Hamilton RA, Kane MP, Demers J: Angiotensin-converting enzyme inhibitors and type 2 diabetic nephropathy: A meta-analysis. Pharmacotherapy 2003;23:909–915.

63. Strippoli GFM, Craig M, Deeks JJ, et al: Effects of angiotensin converting enzyme inhibitors and angiotensin II receptor antagonists on mortality and renal outcomes in diabetic nephropathy: Systematic review. BMJ 2004;329:828–831.

64. Strippoli GF, Craig M, Schena FP, et al: Antihypertensive agents for primary prevention of diabetic nephropathy. J Am Soc Nephrol 2005;16:3081–3091.

65. Maschio G, Alberti D, Janin G, et al, for the Angiotensin-Converting-Enzyme Inhibition in Progressive Renal Insufficiency Study Group: Effect of angiotensin-converting-enzyme inhibitor benazepril on the progression of chronic renal insufficiency. N Eng J Med 1996;334:939–945.

66. Gruppo Italiano di Studi Epidemiologici in Nefrologia (GISEN): Randomised placebo-controlled trial of effect of ramipril on decline in glomerular filtration rate and risk of terminal renal failure in proteinuric, non-diabetic nephropathy. Lancet 1997;349:1857–1863.

67. Ruggenenti P, Perna A, Gherardi G, et al: Renal function and requirement for dialysis in chronic nephropathy patients on long-term ramipril: REIN follow-up trial. Lancet 1998;352: 1252–1256.

68. Ruggenenti P, Perna A, Benini R, et al, for the Investigators of the GISEN Group: In chronic nephropathies prolonged ACE inhibition can induce remission: Dynamics of time-dependent changes in GFR. Gruppo Italiano Studi Epidemiologici in Nefrologia. J Am Soc Nephrol 1999;10:997–1006.

69. Ruggenenti P, Perna A, Gherardi G, et al: Renoprotective properties of ACE-inhibition in non-diabetic nephropathies with non-nephrotic proteinuria. Lancet 1999;354:359–364.

70. Hou FF, Zhang X, Zhang GH, et al: Efficacy and safety of benazepril for advanced chronic renal insufficiency. N Eng J Med 2006; 354:131–140.

71. Jafar TH, Schmid CH, Landa M, et al: Angiotensin-converting enzyme inhibitors and progression of nondiabetic renal disease. A meta-analysis of patient-level data. Ann Intern Med 2001;135: 73–87.

72. Jafar TH, Stark PC, Schmid CH, et al: The effect of angiotensin-converting-enzyme inhibitors on progression of advanced polycystic kidney disease. Kidney Int 2005;67:265–271.

73. The Heart Outcomes Prevention Evaluation Study Investigators: Effects of an angiotensin-converting-enzyme inhibitor, ramipril on cardiovascular events in high-risk patients. N Engl J Med 2000; 342:145–153.

74. Brenner BM, Cooper ME, de Zeeuw D, et al: Effects of losartan on renal and cardiovascular outcomes in patients with type 2 diabetes and nephropathy. N Engl J Med 2001;345:861–869.

75. Lewis EJ, Hunsicker LG, Clarke WR, et al: Renoprotective effect of the angiotensin-receptor antagonist irbesartan in patients with nephropathy due to type 2 diabetes. N Engl J Med 2001; 345:851–860.

76. Parving HH, Lehnert H, Brochner-Mortensen J, et al: The effect of irbesartan on the development of diabetic nephropathy in patients with type 2 diabetes. N Engl J Med 2001;345:870–878.

77. Rossing K, Schjoedt KJ, Jensen BR, et al: Enhanced renoprotective effects of ultrahigh doses of irbesartan in patients with type 2 diabetes and microalbuminuria. Kidney Int 2005;68:1190–1198.

78. Schmieder RE, Klingbeil AU, Fleischmann EH, et al: Additional antiproteinuric effect of ultrahigh dose candesartan: A double-blind, randomized, prospective study. J Am Soc Nephrol 2005; 16:3038–3045.

79. Barnett AH, Bain SC, Bouter P, et al: Angiotensin-receptor blockade versus converting-enzyme inhibition in type 2 diabetes and nephropathy. N Engl J Med 2004;351:1952–1961.

80. Strippoli GF, Bonifati C, Craig M, et al: Angiotensin converting enzyme inhibitors and angiotensin II receptor antagonists for preventing the progression of diabetic kidney disease. Cochrane Database Syst Rev 2006:(4):CD006257.

81. Goldberg AI, Dunlay MC, Sweet CS: Safety and tolerability of losartan potassium, an angiotensin II receptor antagonist, compared with hydrochlorothiazide, atenolol, felodipine ER, and angiotensin-converting enzyme inhibitors for the treatment of systemic hypertension. Am J Cardiol 1995;75:793–795.

82. Weber M: Clinical safety and tolerability of losartan. Clin Ther 1997;19:604–616.

83. Lacourciere Y, Brunner H, Irwin R, et al, for the Losartan Cough Study Group: Effects of modulators of the renin-angiotensin-aldosterone system on cough. J Hypertens 1994;12:1387–1393.

84. Benz J, Oshrain C, Henry D, et al: Valsartan, a new angiotensin II receptor antagonist: A double-blind study comparing the incidence of cough with lisinopril and hydrochlorothiazide. J Clin Pharmacol 1997;37:101–107.

85. Casas JP, Chua W, Loukogeorgakis S, et al: Effect of inhibitors of the renin-angiotensin system and other antihypertensive drugs on renal outcomes: Systematic review and meta-analysis. Lancet 2005;366:2026–2033.

86. Mann JF, McClellan WM, Kunz R, et al: Progression of renal disease—can we forget about inhibition of the renin-angiotensin system? Nephrol Dial Transplant 2006;2006: 2348–2351.

87. Ruilope LM, Aldigier JC, Ponticelli C, et al, for the European Group for the Investigation of Valsartan in Chronic Renal Disease: Safety of the combination of valsartan and benazepril in patients with chronic renal disease. J Hypertension 2000;18: 89–95.

88. Kincaid-Smith P, Fairley K, Packham D: Randomized controlled crossover study of the effect on proteinuria and blood pressure of adding an angiotensin II receptor antagonist to an angiotensin converting enzyme inhibitor in normotensive patients with chronic renal disease and proteinuria. Nephrol Dial Transplant 2002;17:597–601.

89. Nakao N, Yoshimura A, Morita H, et al: Combination treatment of angiotensin-II receptor blocker and angiotensin-converting-enzyme inhibitor in non-diabetic renal disease (COOPERATE): A randomised controlled trial. Lancet 2003;361:117–124.

90. Mogensen CE, Noltham S, Tikkanen I, et al: Randomised controlled trial of dual blockade of renin-angiotensin system in patients with hypertension, microalbuminuria, and non-insulin dependent diabetes: The Candesartan And Lisinopril Microalbuminuria (CALM) study. BMJ 2000;321:1440–1444.

91. Jacobsen P, Andersen S, Rossing K, et al: Dual blockade of the renin-angiotensin system in type 1 patients with diabetic nephropathy. Nephrol Dial Transplant 2002;17:1019–1024.

92. Rossing K, Christensen PK, Jensen BR, et al: Dual blockade of the renin-angiotensin system in diabetic nephropathy. Diabetes Care 2002;25:95–100.

93. Doulton TW, He FJ, MacGregor GA: Systematic review of combined angiotensin-converting enzyme inhibition and angiotensin receptor blockade in hypertension. Hypertension 2005;45:880–886.

94. MacKinnon M, Shurraw S, Akbari A, et al: Combination therapy with an angiotensin receptor blocker and an ACE inhibitor in proteinuric renal disease: A systematic review of the efficacy and safety data. Am J Kidney Dis 2006;48:8–20.

95. Ruggenenti P, Schieppati A, Remuzzi G: Progression, remission, regression of chronic renal diseases. Lancet 2001;357:1601–1608.

96. Bakris GL, Weir MR: Angiotensin-converting enzyme inhibitor-associated elevations in serum creatinine: Is this a cause for concern? Arch Int Med 2000;160:685–93.

97. de Zeeuw D, Remuzzi G, Parving HH, et al: Proteinuria, a target for renoprotection in patients with type 2 diabetic nephropathy: Lessons from RENAAL. Kidney Int 2004;65:2309–2320.

98. Atkins RC, Briganti EM, Lewis JB, et al: Proteinuria reduction and progression to renal failure in patients with type 2 diabetes mellitus and overt nephropathy. Am J Kidney Dis 2005;45:281–287.

99. Hunsicker LG, Adler S, Caggiulia A, et al: Predictors of progression of renal disease in the Modification of Diet in Renal Disease Study. Kidney Int 1997;51:1908–1919.

100. Lea J, Greene T, Hebert L, et al: The relationship between magnitude of proteinuria reduction and risk of end-stage renal disease: Results of the African American study of kidney disease and hypertension. Arch Intern Med 2005;165:947–953.

101. Ruggenenti P, Perna A, Remuzzi G: Retarding progression of chronic renal disease: The neglected issue of residual proteinuria. Kidney Int 2003;63:2254–2261.

102. Jafar TH, Stark PC, Schmid CH, et al: Proteinuria as a modifiable risk factor for the progression of non-diabetic renal disease. Kidney Int 2001;60:1131–1140.

103. Hou FF, Xie D, Zhang X, et al: Renoprotection of optimal antiproteinuric doses (ROAD) study: A randomized controlled study of benazepril and losartan in chronic renal insufficiency. J Am Soc Nephrol 2007;18:1889–1898.

104. Schmitz PG, O'Donnell MP, Kasiske BL, et al: Renal injury in obese Zucker rats: Glomerular hemodynamic alterations and effects of enalapril. Am J Physiol 1992;263:F496–F502.

105. Chagnac A, Weinstein T, Herman M, et al: The effects of weight loss on renal function in patients with severe obesity. J Am Soc Nephrol 2003;14:1480–1486.

106. Fox CS, Larson MG, Leip EP, et al: Predictors of new-onset kidney disease in a community-based population. JAMA 2004;291: 844–850.

107. Gelber RP, Kurth T, Kausz AT, et al: Association between body mass index and CKD in apparently healthy men. Am J Kidney Dis 2005;46:871–880.

108. Bonnet F, Deprele C, Sassolas A, et al: Excessive body weight as a new independent risk factor for clinical and pathological progression in primary IgA nephritis. Am J Kidney Dis 2001;37: 720–727.

109. Sacks FM, Svetkey LP, Vollmer WM, et al, for the DASH—Sodium Collaborative Research Group: Effects on blood pressure of reduced dietary sodium and the Dietary Approaches to Stop Hypertension (DASH) diet. N Engl J Med 2001;344:3–10.

110. Cianciaruso B, Bellizzi V, Minutolo R, et al: Salt intake and renal outcome in patients with progressive renal disease. Miner Electrolyte Metab 1998;24:296–301.

111. Jones-Burton C, Mishra SI, Fink JC, et al: An in-depth review of the evidence linking dietary salt intake and progression of chronic kidney disease. Am J Nephrol 2006;26:268–275. Epub 9 June 2006.

112. Hostetter TH, Meyer TW, Rennke HG, et al: Chronic effects of dietary protein in the rat with intact and reduced renal mass. Kidney Int 1986;30:509–517.

113. Levey AS, Adler S, Caggiula AW, et al: Effects of dietary protein restriction on the progression of advanced renal disease in the Modification of Diet in Renal Disease Study. Am J Kidney Dis 1996;27:652–663.

114. Fouque D, Laville M, Boissel JP: Low protein diets for chronic renal failure in non-diabetic adults. Cochrane Database Syst Rev 2006;(2):CD001892.

115. Levey AS, Greene T, Sarnak MJ, et al: Effect of dietary protein restriction on the progression of kidney disease: Long-term follow-up of the Modification of Diet in Renal Disease (MDRD) Study. Am J Kidney Dis 2006;48:879–888.

116. Gansevoort RT, de Zeeuw D, de Jong PE: Additive antiproteinuric effect of ACE inhibition and a low-protein diet in human renal disease. Nephrol Dial Transplant 1995;10:497–504.

117. Mitch WE: Beneficial responses to modified diets in treating patients with chronic kidney disease. Kidney Int 2005;(Suppl): S133–S135.

118. Monzani G, Bergesio F, Ciuti R, et al: Lipoprotein abnormalities in chronic renal failure and dialysis patients. Blood Purif 1996;14:262–272.

119. Samuelsson O, Attman PO, Knight-Gibson C, et al: Complex apolipoprotein B-containing lipoprotein particles are associated with a higher rate of progression of human chronic renal insufficiency. J Am Soc Nephrol 1998;9:1482–1488.

120. Krolewski AS, Warram JH, Christlieb AR: Hypercholesterolemia— a determinant of renal function loss and deaths in IDDM patients with nephropathy. Kidney Int 1994;45 (Suppl): S125–S131.

121. Ravid M, Brosh D, Ravid-Safran D, et al: Main risk factors for nephropathy in type 2 diabetes mellitus are plasma cholesterol levels, mean blood pressure, and hyperglycemia. Arch Intern Med 1998;158:998–1004.

122. Mulec H, Johnson S-A, Bjorck S: Relation between serum cholesterol and diabetic nephropathy. Lancet 1990;335:1537–1538.

123. Maschio G, Oldrizzi L, Rugiu C, et al: Serum lipids in patients with chronic renal failure on long-term, protein-restricted diets. Am J Med 1989;87:51N–54N.

124. Grone EF, Abboud HE, Hohne M, et al: Actions of lipoproteins in cultured human mesangial cells: Modulation by mitogenic vasoconstrictors. Am J Physiol 1992;263:F686–F696.

125. Rovin BH, Tan LC: LDL stimulates mesangial fibronectin production and chemoattractant expression. Kidney Int 1993;43:218–225.

126. Wheeler DC, Chana RS, Topley N, et al: Oxidation of low density lipoprotein by mesangial cells may promote glomerular injury. Kidney Int 1994;45:1628–1636.

127. Kasiske B, O'Donnell MP, Schmitz PG, et al: Renal injury of diet-induced hypercholesterolemia in rats. Kidney Int 1990;37:880–891.

128. Kasiske BL, O'Donnel MP, Garvis WJ, et al: Pharmacologic treatment of hyperlipidemia reduces injury in rat 5/6 nephrectomy model of chronic renal failure. Circ Res 1988;62:367–374.

129. O'Donell MP, Kasiske BL, Kim Y, et al: Lovastatin retards the progression of established glomerular disease in obese Zucker rats. Am J Kidney Dis 1993;22:83–89.

130. Fried LF, Orchard TJ, Kasiske BL: Effect of lipid reduction on the progression of renal disease: A meta-analysis. Kidney Int 2001;59:260–269.

131. Tonelli M, Moye L, Sacks FM, et al: Effect of pravastatin on loss of renal function in people with moderate chronic renal insufficiency and cardiovascular disease. J Am Soc Nephrol 2003;14:1605–1613.

132. Collins R, Armitage J, Parish S, et al: MRC/BHF Heart Protection Study of cholesterol-lowering with simvastatin in 5963 people with diabetes: A randomised placebo-controlled trial. Lancet 2005;361:2005–2016.

133. Bianchi S, Bigazzi R, Caiazza A, et al: A controlled, prospective study of the effects of atorvastatin on proteinuria and progression of kidney disease. Am J Kidney Dis 2003;41:565–570.

134. Manttari M, Tiula E, Alikoski T, et al: Effects of hypertension and dyslipidemia on the decline in renal function. Hypertension 1995;26:670–675.

135. Tonelli M, Collins D, Robins S, et al: Effect of gemfibrozil on change in renal function in men with moderate chronic renal insufficiency and coronary disease. Am J Kidney Dis 2004;44:832–839.

136. Ansquer JC, Foucher C, Rattier S, et al: Fenofibrate reduces progression to microalbuminuria over 3 years in a placebo-controlled study in type 2 diabetes: Results from the Diabetes Atherosclerosis Intervention Study (DAIS). Am J Kidney Dis 2005;45:485–493.

137. National Cholesterol Education Program: Executive Summary of The Third Report of The National Cholesterol Education Program Expert Panel on Detection, Evaluation, and Treatment of High Blood Cholesterol In Adults (Adult Treatment Panel III). JAMA 2001;285:2486–2497.

138. Chase HP, Garg SK, Marshall G, et al: Cigarette smoking increases the risk of albuminuria among subjects with type I diabetes. JAMA 1991;265:614–617.

139. McKenna K, Thompson C: Microalbuminuria: A marker to increased renal and cardiovascular risk in diabetes mellitus. Scot Med J 1997;42:99–104.

140. Muhlhauser I, Overmann H, Bender R, et al: Predictors of mortality and end-stage diabetic complications in patients with Type 1 diabetes mellitus on intensified insulin therapy. Diabetic Med 2000;17:727–734.

141. Orth SR, Schroeder T, Ritz E, et al: Effects of smoking on renal function in patients with type 1 and type 2 diabetes mellitus. Nephrol Dial Transplant 2005;20:2414–2419.

142. Orth SR, Stockmann A, Conradt C, et al: Smoking as a risk factor for end-stage renal failure in men with primary renal disease. Kidney Int 1998;54:926–931.

143. Ward MM, Studenski S: Clinical prognostic factors in lupus nephritis. The importance of hypertension and smoking. Arch Intern Med 1992;152:2082–2088.

144. Stengel B, Couchoud C, Cenee S, et al: Age, blood pressure and smoking effects on chronic renal failure in primary glomerular nephropathies. Kidney Int 2000;57:2519–2526.

145. Regalado M, Yang S, Wesson DE: Cigarette smoking is associated with augmented progression of renal insufficiency in severe essential hypertension. Am J Kidney Dis 2000;35:687–694.

146. Halimi JM, Giraudeau B, Vol S, et al: Effects of current smoking and smoking discontinuation on renal function and proteinuria in the general population. Kidney Int 2000;58:1285–1292.

147. Pinto-Sietsma SJ, Mulder J, Janssen WM, et al: Smoking is related to albuminuria and abnormal renal function in nondiabetic persons. Ann Intern Med 2000;133:585–591.

148. Bleyer AJ, Shemanski LR, Burke GL, et al: Tobacco, hypertension, and vascular disease: Risk factors for renal functional decline in an older population. Kidney Int 2000. 57:2072–2079.

149. Goetz FC, Jacobs DR Jr, Chavers B, et al: Risk factors for kidney damage in the adult population of Wadena, Minnesota. A prospective study. Am J Epidemiol 1997;145:91–102.

150. Haroun MK, Jaar BG, Hoffman SC, et al: Risk factors for chronic kidney disease: A prospective study of 23,534 men and women in Washington County, Maryland. J Am Soc Nephrol 2003;14:2934–2941.

151. Orth SR, Ritz E: The renal risks of smoking: An update. Curr Opin Nephrol Hypertens 2002;11:483–488.

152. The Diabetes Control and Complications Research Group: The effect of intensive treatment of diabetes on the development and progression of long-term complications in insulin-dependent diabetes mellitus. N Engl J Med 1993;329:977–386.

153. UK Prospective Diabetes Study (UKPDS) Group: Intensive blood-glucose control with sulphonylureas or insulin compared with conventional treatment and risk of complications in patients with type 2 diabetes (UKPDS 33). Lancet 1998;352:837–853.

154. Feldt-Rasmussen B, Mathiesen ER, Deckert T: Effect of two years of strict metabolic control on progression of incipient nephropathy in insulin-dependent diabetes. Lancet 1986;2:1300–1304.

155. Reichard P, Nilsson BY, Rosenqvist U: The effect of long-term intensified insulin treatment on the development of microvascular complications of diabetes mellitus. New Engl J Med 1993;329:304–309.

156. Bangstad HJ, Osterby R, Dahl-Jorgensen K, et al: Improvement of blood glucose control in IDDM patients retards the progression of morphological changes in early diabetic nephropathy. Diabetologia 1994;37:483–490.

157. Microalbuminuria Collaborative Study Group, United Kingdom: Intensive therapy and progression to clinical albuminuria in patients with insulin dependent diabetes mellitus and microalbuminuria. BMJ 1995;311:973–977.

158. The Diabetes Control and Complications Research Group: Effect of intensive therapy on the development and progression of diabetic nephropathy in the Diabetes Control and Complications Trial. Kidney Int 1995;47:1703–1720.

159. Fioretto P, Steffes MW, Sutherland DE, et al: Reversal of lesions of diabetic nephropathy after pancreas transplantation. New Engl J Med 1998;339:69–75.

160. Levey AS, Coresh J, Greene T, et al: Using standardized serum creatinine values in the modification of diet in renal disease study equation for estimating glomerular filtration rate. Ann Intern Med 2006;145:247–254.

161. Gaspari F, Perico N, Remuzzi G: Timed urine collections are not needed to measure urine protein excretion in clinical practice. Am J Kidney Dis 2006;47:1–7.

162. Ding SS, Qiu C, Hess P, et al: Chronic endothelin receptor blockade prevents both early hyperfiltration and late overt diabetic nephropathy in the rat. J Cardiovasc Pharmacol 2003;42:48–54.

163. Sasser JM, Sullivan JC, Hobbs JL, et al: Endothelin A receptor blockade reduces diabetic renal injury via an anti-inflammatory mechanism. J Am Soc Nephrol 2007;18:143–154. Epub 13 December 2006.

164. Weber M: Emerging treatments for hypertension: Potential role for vasopeptidase inhibition. Am J Hypertens 1999;12:139S–147S.

165. Taal MW, Nenov VD, Wong W, et al: Vasopeptidase inhibition affords greater renoprotection than angiotensin-converting enzyme inhibition alone. J Am Soc Nephrol 2001;12:2051–2059.

166. Benigni A, Zoja C, Zatelli C, et al: Vasopeptidase inhibitor restores the balance of vasoactive hormones in progressive nephropathy. Kidney Int 2004;66:1959–1965.

167. Oh BH, Mitchell J, Herron JR, et al: Aliskiren, an oral renin inhibitor, provides dose-dependent efficacy and sustained 24-hour blood pressure control in patients with hypertension. J Am Coll Cardiol 2007;49:1157–1163.

168. Gambaro G, Kinalska I, Oksa A, et al: Oral sulodexide reduces albuminuria in microalbuminuric and macroalbuminuric type 1 and type 2 diabetic patients: The DiNAS randomized trial. J Am Soc Nephrol 2002;13:1615–1625.

169. Aldigier JC, Kanjanbuch T, Ma LJ, et al: Regression of existing glomerulosclerosis by inhibition of aldosterone. J Am Soc Nephrol 2005;16:3306–3314.

170. Ponda MP, Hostetter TH: Aldosterone antagonism in chronic kidney disease. Clin J Am Soc Nephrol 2006;1:668–677.

171. Leh S, Vaagnes O, Margolin SB, et al: Pirfenidone and candesartan ameliorate morphological damage in mild chronic anti-GBM nephritis in rats. Nephrol Dial Transplant 2005;20:71–82. Epub 23 November 2004.

172. Dworkin LD, Gong R, Tolbert E, et al: Hepatocyte growth factor ameliorates progression of interstitial fibrosis in rats with established renal injury. Kidney Int 2004;65:409–419.

173. Hruska KA, Guo G, Wozniak M, et al: Osteogenic protein-1 prevents renal fibrogenesis associated with ureteral obstruction. Am J Physiol Renal Physiol 2000;279:F130–F143.

174. Sugimoto H, Grahovac G, Zeisberg M, Kalluri R: Renal fibrosis and glomerulosclerosis in a new mouse model of diabetic nephropathy and its regression by BMP-7 and advanced glycation end-product inhibitors. Diabetes 2007;56:1825–1833.

175. Gaede P, Vedel P, Parving HH, et al: Intensified multifactorial intervention in patients with type 2 diabetes mellitus and microalbuminuria: The Steno type 2 randomised study. Lancet 1999;353:617–622.

176. McClellan WM, Knight DF, Karp H, et al: Early detection and treatment of renal disease in hospitalized diabetic and hypertensive patients: Important differences between practice and published guidelines. Am J Kidney Dis 1997;29:368–375.

Further Reading

Kidney Disease: Improving Global Outcomes. www.kdigo.org.

Levey AS, Eckardt KU, Tsukamoto Y, et al: Definition and classification of chronic kidney disease: A position statement from Kidney Disease: Improving Global Outcomes (KDIGO). Kidney Int 2005;67:2089–2100.

Meguid El Nahas A, Bello AK: Chronic kidney disease: The global challenge. Lancet 2005;365:331–340.

National Kidney Foundation Kidney: Disease Outcomes Quality Initiative. www.kidney.org/professionals/KDOQI.

Ruggenenti P, Remuzzi G: Kidney failure stabilizes after a two-decade increase: Impact on global (renal and cardiovascular) health. Clin J Am Soc Nephrol 2007;2:146–150.

Taal MW, Brenner BM: Predicting initiation and progression of chronic kidney disease: Developing renal risk scores. Kidney Int 2006;70:1694–1705.

Chapter 63

Cholesterol Management in Patients with Chronic Kidney Disease

Robert D. Toto, Gloria Lena Vega, and Scott M. Grundy

In the past few decades, several important clinical trials have documented that lowering of serum cholesterol reduces the risk for development of myocardial infarction and other complications of coronary artery disease (CAD). These trials have added strength to national recommendations for detection and treatment of high serum cholesterol levels. In the United States, the most recent guidelines on the clinical management of elevated serum cholesterol have been published by the National Cholesterol Education Program (NCEP) as the Adult Treatment Panel III (ATP III) report.[1] The report did not provide specific advice on treating lipid disorders in patients with chronic kidney disease (CKD). However, the general framework of the guidelines may apply to many CKD patients who are at increased risk for CHD. We review the general features of the ATP III report, but it must be pointed out that clinical judgment is required when determining therapies for patients with complex medical conditions such as CKD using the ATP III guidelines. We do not attempt to provide "hard and fast" rules for management of lipid disorders in patients with CKD but instead review available information about the nature of lipid disorders in different types of CKD and outline areas for potential intervention.

Many CKD patients are at increased risk for major cardiovascular events, either because they already have established atherosclerotic disease or because they have risk factors for CAD. In addition, CKD by itself probably imparts a higher risk independent of the usual cardiovascular risk factors.[2,3] The extent of incremental risk likely depends on the type of CKD. Regardless, patients with most forms of CKD commonly have multiple cardiovascular risk factors. Among these are a variety of abnormalities in plasma lipoproteins. For these reasons, physicians who care for CKD patients often are faced with the need to make decisions whether to intervene in a given patient's lipid disorder and, if so, how.

SUMMARY OF ATP III GUIDELINES AS RELATED TO CKD

Low-Density Lipoprotein Cholesterol: The Primary Target of Therapy

There are several classes of lipoproteins, such as low-density lipoproteins (LDL), very low-density lipoproteins (VLDL), high-density lipoproteins (HDL), and lipoprotein(a) [Lp(a)]. Of these, elevated serum LDL has the most robust relationship to CAD.[1,4] LDL is usually identified in clinical practice as LDL cholesterol. The ATP III report recognizes it as the primary target of lipid-lowering therapy and provides a detailed listing of evidence supporting that concept. Recent clinical trials[5–9] have documented that LDL-lowering therapy will reduce the risk for developing CAD by about one third. The Treat to New Targets (TNT) trial, performed in more than 10,000 patients with stable CAD, revealed that intensive LDL cholesterol lowering to obtain levels below 100 mg/dL (mean, 77 mg/dL) using high-dose (80 mg daily) versus low-dose (10 mg daily) atorvastatin was associated with improved cardiovascular outcome.[10] Other lipoproteins are potential secondary targets of therapy. For example, many CKD patients have a lipoprotein abnormality called *atherogenic dyslipidemia*.[1] This disorder is characterized by raised serum triglyceride, small LDL particles, and low HDL cholesterol levels. It seems likely that LDL cholesterol should be the primary target of therapy in CKD patients, but the question of whether to intervene in those with atherogenic dyslipidemia is an important issue. Table 63-1 summarizes the ATP III classification of lipids, lipoproteins, and atherogenic dyslipidemia.

Table 63-1   ATP III LDL Cholesterol Goals and Cutpoints for Therapeutic Lifestyle Changes and Drug Therapy in Different Risk Categories and Proposed Modifications Based on Recent Clinical Trial Evidence

Risk Category	LDL Cholesterol Goal (Non-HDL Cholesterol Goals)*	Initiate TLC Based on LDL Cholesterol (or Non-HDL Cholesterol) Levels	Consider Drug Therapy Using LDL Cholesterol or (Non-HDL Cholesterol) Levels
High risk: CAD* or CAD risk equivalents[†] (10-year risk ≥20%)	<100 mg/dL (Optional goal: 70 mg/dL)	≥100 mg/dL[¶]	≥100 mg/dL (<100 mg/dL: consider drug options)**
Moderately high risk: 2+ risk factors[‡] (10-year risk 10%–20%)[‖]	<130 mg/dL	>130 mg/dL[¶]	>130 mg/dL (100–129 mg/dL: consider drug options)[††]
Moderate risk: 2+ risk factors[‡] (10-year risk ≤ 10%)[‖]	<130 mg/dL	≥130 mg/dL	≥160 mg/dL
Lower risk: 0–1 risk factor[§]	<160 mg/dL	≥160 mg/dL	≥190 mg/dL (160–189 mg/dL: LDL-lowering drug optional)

*Non-HDL cholesterol = VLDL cholesterol + LDL cholesterol; non-HDL cholesterol is about 30 mg/dL higher than LDL goal.
[†]CHD risk equivalents include clinical manifestations of noncoronary forms of atherosclerotic disease (peripheral arterial disease, abdominal aortic aneurysm, and carotid artery disease transient ischemic attacks or stroke of carotid origin or 50% obstruction of a carotid artery), diabetes, and two risk factors with 10-year risk for hard CHD of 20%.
[‡]Risk factors include cigarette smoking, hypertension (BP 140/90 mm Hg or antihypertensive medication), low HDL cholesterol (40 mg/dL), family history of premature CHD (CHD in male first-degree relative 55 years of age; CHD in female first-degree relative 65 years of age), and age (men 45 years, women 55 years).
[§]Almost all people with no risk factors or one risk factor have a 10-year risk of 10%, and 10-year risk assessment in people with no risk factors or one risk factor thus is not necessary.
[¶]Any person at high risk or moderately high risk who has lifestyle-related factors (e.g., obesity, physical inactivity, elevated triglyceride, low HDL-C, or metabolic syndrome) is a candidate for therapeutic lifestyle changes to modify these risk factors regardless of LDL-C level.
[‖]Electronic 10-year risk calculators are available at www.nhlbi.nih.gov/guidelines/cholesterol.
**When LDL-lowering drug therapy is employed, it is advised that the intensity of therapy be sufficient to achieve at least a 30% to 40% reduction in LDL-C levels.
[††]For moderately high-risk persons, when LDL-C level is 100–129 mg/dL, at baseline or on lifestyle therapy, initiation of an LDL-lowering drug to achieve an LDL-C level of 100 mg/dL is a therapeutic option on the basis of available clinical trial results.
ATP III, Adult Treatment Panel III report; HDL, high-density lipoprotein; LDL, low-density lipoprotein; TLC, therapeutic lifestyle changes.

Risk Assessment: First Step in Risk Management

The ATP III report indicates that the intensity of risk-reduction therapy should be adjusted to the patient's absolute risk. An assessment of risk depends on identifying medical conditions that impart higher risk and risk factors for cardiovascular disease. Several forms of CKD may increase the risk for CAD independent of the major risk factors; nonetheless, CKD patients often have multiple, major risk factors (Box 63-1), including the emerging risk factors that are common in patients with CAD (Box 63-2). Some CKD patients will have a constellation of risk factors, called the *metabolic syndrome* (Box 63-3). This condition includes several borderline risk factors that when combined confer higher risk. In patients without CAD, the ATP III report recommends that risk assessment be carried out using the Framingham risk algorithm.[11] In patients with CKD, however, Framingham scores may not accurately predict future cardiovascular events, and the presence of multiple risk factors likely raises the risk for major cardiovascular events in patients with CKD even more than suggested by Framingham scoring.

High-Risk Conditions: Established CAD and Risk Equivalents

Conditions at highest risk deserve the most intensive lipid-lowering therapy. The ATP III report recognizes three categories of high-risk patients: (1) very high risk, defined as the presence of established atherosclerotic cardiovascular disease and one or more of the following: multiple risk factors (especially diabetes), severe and poorly controlled risk factors (e.g., cigarette smoking), metabolic syndrome (especially high triglycerides ≥ 200 mg/dL and non-HDL cholesterol > 130 mg/dL with low HDL cholesterol ≤ 40 mg/dL) and acute coronary syndromes; (2) high risk, defined as those with established CAD; and (3) those with CAD risk-equivalents. According to the ATP III report, LDL

Box 63-1   Categorical Classification of Major Risk Factors

Cigarette smoking (any smoking in past year)
Hypertension (blood pressure ≥ 140/90 mm Hg or on antihypertensive medication)
High LDL cholesterol (≥ 160 mg/dL)*
Low HDL cholesterol (<40 mg/dL)[†]
High plasma glucose (≥ 126 mg/dL)[‡]
Family history of premature coronary artery disease (in male first-degree relative < 55 years; in female first-degree relative < 65 years)
Age (men ≥ 50 years; women ≥ 55 years)

*High LDL cholesterol is not included in the "risk factor" count in ATP III because it is the target of therapy based on other risk factors.
[†]HDL cholesterol > 60 mg/dL counts as a "negative" risk factor; its presence removes one risk factor from the total count.
[‡]High plasma glucose is not included in the "risk factor" count in ATP III because its presence identifies a patient as having diabetes, which is counted as a CAD risk-equivalent.

Box 63-2 Emerging Risk Factors

Lipid Risk Factors
Lipoprotein(a)
Apolipoproteins (CIII, B, AI)
Small lipoprotein particles (small LDL, small HDL)

Inflammatory Markers
High-sensitivity C-reactive protein
Cytokines
Fibrinogen

Prothrombotic Markers
Plasminogen activator inhibitor-1
Fibrinogen
Homocysteine

Box 63-3 Risk Factors of Metabolic Syndrome

Atherogenic dyslipidemia
    Elevated triglycerides ($\geq$50 mg/dL)
    Small LDL particles
    Elevated non-HDL cholesterol ($\geq$30 mg/dL)
    Low HDL cholesterol (<40 mg/dL in men; <50 mg/dL
    in women)
High-normal blood pressure (120–139/80–89 mm Hg)
Insulin resistance
± Impaired fasting glucose (110–126 mg/dL)
Proinflammatory*
Prothrombotic state†

---

*Indicated by one or more of elevated high-sensitivity C-reactive protein (hs-CRP) (> 3.0 mg/L), homocysteine ($\geq$15 mmol/L) or lipoprotein(a) [Lp(a)] ($\geq$30 mg/dL), and fibrinogen. Elevated hs-CRP appears to be the most reliable indicator of proinflammatory state. Lp(a) can be elevated on a genetic basis.
†Indicated by elevated plasminogen activator inhibitor-1, fibrinogen, or clotting factor VIIc.

cholesterol in very high risk patients should be lowered to the optimal level of less than 70 mg/dL; in high-risk patients, it should be lowered to less than 100 mg/dL (see Table 63-1). Many CKD patients will fall into one of these categories, particularly those with diabetic nephropathy or patients with nondiabetic CKD and heavy proteinuria (see Primary Nephrotic Syndrome in this chapter). The conditions that define established CAD are (1) history of acute coronary syndromes (unstable angina or myocardial infarction), (2) history of angina pectoris, and (3) history of coronary artery procedures (coronary angioplasty or coronary artery bypass grafting).

Any patient with CKD who has one of these forms of established CAD can be considered at high risk for future events. These patients, therefore, are candidates for intensive lowering of LDL cholesterol to a goal of less than 100 mg/dL (in very high risk patients, the goal is <70 mg/dL).

Lipid-lowering therapy is not the only intervention for patients with established CAD. The American Heart Association has published general guidelines for risk reduction in patients with CAD or other atherosclerotic diseases.[12] These guidelines, summarized in Box 63-4, include smoking cessation, blood pressure regulation, physical activity as part of a program of cardiac rehabilitation, weight loss in overweight patients, appropriate antiplatelet therapy, and cardioprotective drugs (β-blockers and angiotensin-converting enzyme inhibitors). A large body of data supports benefits from each of these regimens.[12] Particular attention should be given to using a full range of risk-reduction modalities in patients with CKD who also have established CAD.

Patients with CAD risk-equivalents have one of the following: (1) a noncoronary form of atherosclerotic disease (peripheral arterial disease, carotid artery disease [carotid transient ischemic attacks], carotid stroke, >50% obstruction of carotid artery) or abdominal aortic aneurysm; (2) diabetes mellitus; or (3) multiple risk factors, with 10-year risk for CAD higher than 10% (based on Framingham risk scoring).

Some investigators speculate that various forms of CKD constitute a CAD risk-equivalent similar to the presence of diabetes.[13] Certainly a sizable fraction of CKD patients will have diabetes, warranting their inclusion in the category of CAD risk-equivalent. Whether kidney disease per se without diabetes or noncoronary forms of atherosclerosis confers a high-risk status probably depends on the type of CKD. Two questions must be considered: (1) What is the absolute risk for patients with various forms of CKD? and (2) How effective is LDL-lowering in reducing major coronary events in such patients? For both questions, the literature is limited and generalizations are difficult, so clinical judgment is required to determine if it is appropriate to classify particular patients as CAD risk-equivalents. Framingham risk scoring probably underestimates the 10-year risk for CAD patients with CKD and therefore is of limited value in assessing absolute 10-year risk. Observational studies from large numbers of unselected clinic patients suggest that the presence of stage 3 to 5 CKD is an independent risk factor for cardiovascular morbidity and all-cause mortality.[14] It also is estimated that the 10-year CAD incidence among CKD patients is in the range of 20% based on Framingham risk score. Although the ATP III report does not consider the presence of CKD as a CAD equivalent, it seems reasonable to assume that most CKD patients with several major risk factors belong in the category of CAD risk-equivalents. The National Kidney Foundation guidelines for treatment of dyslipidemia in CKD recommend lowering LDL cholesterol into the optimal range (<100 mg/dL).[15] Standard doses of statin are recommended as first-line therapy in patients in whom this drug class is effective and generally well tolerated. For patients at very high risk, higher doses of statins or combining statins with cholesterol absorption inhibitors such as ezetimibe may be desirable. Cholesterol absorption inhibitors are generally better tolerated than bile acid resins or nicotinic acid derivatives, albeit more expensive.

For patients with established CAD or CAD risk-equivalents, the ATP III report recommends starting LDL-lowering drug therapy simultaneously with dietary therapy when LDL cholesterol levels are higher than 130 mg/dL. If baseline (or on-treatment) LDL cholesterol levels are in the range of 100 to 129 mg/dL, dietary therapy can be intensified first before starting (or intensifying) LDL-lowering drugs; in some cases, the LDL goal may be achieved without the need for starting (or changing) drug therapy.

Box 63-4 Risk Reduction Strategy in Patients with Coronary and Other Vascular Disease (Modified from American Heart Association Recommendations)

Smoking
Goal to stop tobacco use altogether
Encourage patient and family to stop smoking
Provide counseling and use cessation programs as appropriate

Hypertension
Blood pressure goal < 130/85 mm Hg
Modify life habits to lower blood pressure (weight control, exercise, alcohol moderation, moderate sodium restriction)
Add blood pressure medication if needed to achieve blood pressure goal (consider ACE inhibitors and β-blockers for concomitant benefits)

Physical Activity
Minimum goal of 30 min three or four times per week
Assess overall risk to guide prescription
Encourage use of cardiac rehabilitation programs for patients with CAD (when available)
Encourage moderate intensity exercise

Weight Management
Goal to achieve desirable body weight
Provide counseling and use of professional dietitian as appropriate

Antiplatelet Agents/Anticoagulants
Start aspirin 80–325 mg/day if not contraindicated

β-Blockers
Start and continue for 6 mo minimum in high-risk patients (arrhythmia, LV dysfunction, include ischemia)

ACE Inhibitors
Start early in stable high-risk patients (anterior MI, previous MI, Killip class II: S₃ gallop, radiographic CHF)

ACE, angiotensin-converting enzyme; CAD, coronary heart disease; CHF, congestive heart failure; LV, left ventricular; MI, myocardial infarction.

Low-Density Lipoprotein-Lowering Therapies

Two modalities of LDL-lowering therapy are recognized in the ATP III report: therapeutic lifestyle changes and drug therapy. Therapeutic lifestyle changes go beyond LDL lowering by dietary therapy to achieve maximal risk reduction. The changes include (1) maximal reduction of saturated fats and cholesterol, (2) adding LDL-lowering adjuncts (plant stanol or sterols or increased viscous fiber), (3) weight reduction (in overweight or obese patients), and (4) increased physical activity.

When therapeutic lifestyle changes are recommended, dietary saturated fatty acids should be reduced to less than 7% of total energy intake, and dietary cholesterol to less than 200 mg/day. Physicians are advised to seek consultation from a registered dietitian or other qualified nutritional profes-

sional to provide patients with appropriate medical nutrition therapy. In the United States, Medicare pays for dietary consultation for CAD patients. A cholesterol-lowering diet is only one component of medical nutrition therapy for CKD patients. Adding LDL-lowering adjuncts can provide another 10% to 15% reduction in LDL cholesterol levels; these include plant stanols or sterols (2 g/day) and increased viscous fiber (10–25 g/day). Medical nutrition therapy should include calorie restriction in overweight patients. To match the patient's clinical needs, the physician should prescribe regular physical activity. Several drugs are available for LDL lowering (Table 63-2). The statins, bile acid sequestrants, and cholesterol absorption inhibitors mainly lower LDL. Fibrates and nicotinic acid can moderately reduce LDL levels, but they are used primarily for treatment of atherogenic dyslipidemia. The use of these drugs is considered for each category of CKD discussed.

Atherogenic Dyslipidemia and the Metabolic Syndrome

Atherogenic dyslipidemia is common in CKD patients and represents a potential secondary target of lipid-lowering therapy. It consists of raised blood levels of triglycerides, small LDL particles, and low HDL cholesterol levels. In some patients, weight reduction and increased physical activity may help normalize levels of triglyceride and HDL, but in some forms of CKD, atherogenic dyslipidemia results mainly from metabolic defects secondary to the kidney disease.[16–18] The standard drugs for treatment of atherogenic dyslipidemia are fibrates and nicotinic acid. Unfortunately, both types of drugs can cause adverse effects that may be accentuated in CKD patients. For example, when fibrates are combined with statins, there is an increased risk for severe myopathy. This adverse effect is particularly dangerous in CKD patients because it may result in myoglobinuria and acute tubular necrosis.

In patients with atherogenic dyslipidemia, the primary target of therapy is still LDL. Nonetheless, the ATP III guidelines note that elevated VLDL cholesterol and triglycerides may contribute substantially to the risk for CAD. For this reason, the ATP III report identifies LDL plus VLDL cholesterol (also called *non-HDL cholesterol*) as a secondary target of therapy in patients with raised triglyceride levels. The goal for reduction of non-HDL cholesterol is a level 30 mg/dL higher than for LDL cholesterol. For example, with an LDL cholesterol goal of less than 100 mg/dL, the non-HDL cholesterol goal would be less than 130 mg/dL.

Some CKD patients have elements of the metabolic syndrome (see Box 63-3). Obesity is prevalent in patients with diabetic or nondiabetic forms of CKD and has been associated with increased risk for the development of kidney disease in the general population.[19,20] The ATP III report criteria for a clinical diagnosis of the metabolic syndrome are shown in Table 63-3. Patients with three of the five abnormalities shown in this table are diagnosed as having the metabolic syndrome. If a patient with CKD also has the metabolic syndrome, more intensive treatment of serum lipids seems warranted. Dietary intervention and aerobic exercise are recommended in the ATP III report for those without kidney disease. The literature is limited on the benefits of weight loss in obese CKD patients, but it seems prudent to apply the ATP III recommendations to these patients as well.

Table 63-2 Drugs for Lipid Management

Drug Class	Drugs and Daily Doses	Lipid/Lipoprotein Effects	Adverse Effects	Contraindications	Clinical Trial Results
Bile acid sequestrants	Cholestyramine 4–16 g Colestipol 5–20 g	LDL C: 15%–30% HDL C: 3%–5% TG: No change or increase	Gastrointestinal distress, constipation, decreased absorption of other drugs	Absolute: dysbetalipoproteinemia, TG > 400 mg/dL Relative: TG > 200 mg/dL	Reduced major coronary events and CAD deaths
HMG-CoA reductase inhibitors (statins)*	Lovastatin 20–80 mg Pravastatin 20–40 mg Simvastatin 20–80 mg Fluvastatin 20–80 mg Atorvastatin 10–80 mg Rosuvastatin 5–20 mg	LDL C: 18%–55% HDL C: 5%–15% TG: 7%–30%	Myopathy, increased liver enzymes	Absolute: active or chronic liver disease Relative: concomitant use of certain drugs†	Reduced major coronary events, CAD deaths, need for coronary procedures, stroke, and total mortality
Cholesterol absorption inhibitor	Ezetimibe 10–20 mg	LDL: 20%–30%	No increase in myopathy	Absolute: None	
Nicotinic acid	Immediate-release crystalline 1.5–3 g Extended-release Niaspan 1–2 g Sustained-release 1–2 g	LDL C: 5%–25% HDL C: 15%–35% TG: 20%–50%	Flushing, hyperglycemia, hyperuricemia (gout), upper gastrointestinal distress, hepatotoxicity	Absolute: chronic liver disease, severe gout Relative: diabetes, hyperuricemia, peptic ulcer disease	Reduced major coronary events and (possibly) total mortality
Fibric acid derivatives	Gemfibrozil 600 mg bid Fenofibrate 200 mg Clofibrate 1000 mg bid	LDL C: 5%–20% HDL C: 10%–20% TG: 10%–50%	Dyspepsia, gallstones, myopathy (may be increased in patients with high TG)	Absolute: severe renal disease, severe hepatic disease Relative: severe renal disease	Reduced major coronary events, increased non-CAD mortality (in 2 of 5 clinical trials)

*Standard starting doses of statins are lovastatin (40 mg), pravastatin (40 mg), simvastatin (20 mg), fluvastatin (40 mg), and atorvastatin (10 mg).
†Cyclosporine, gemfibrozil (or niacin), macrolide antibiotics, various antifungal agents and cytochrome P450 inhibitors.
CAD, coronary artery disease; HDL, high-density lipoproteins; HMG-CoA, α-hydroxy-γ-methylglutaryl coenzyme A; LDL, low-density lipoproteins; TG, triglycerides.

Table 63-3 Clinical Diagnosis of the Metabolic Syndrome (based on any three of the following)

Risk Factor	Defining Level
Abdominal obesity (waist circumference)*,†	
Men	>102 cm (>40 inches)
Women	>88 cm (>35 inches)
Triglycerides	≥150 mg/dL
HDL cholesterol	
Men	<40 mg/dL
Women	<50 mg/dL
Blood pressure	≥130/≥85 mm Hg
Fasting glucose	≥110 mg/dL

*Overweight and obesity are associated with insulin resistance and the metabolic syndrome. However, the presence of abdominal obesity is more highly correlated than elevated body mass index with metabolic risk factors. Therefore, the simple measure of waist circumference is recommended to identify the body weight component of the metabolic syndrome.

†Some male patients can develop multiple metabolic risk factors when the waist circumference is only marginally increased (e.g., 94–102 cm; 37–39 inches). Such patients may have a strong genetic contribution to insulin resistance. They should benefit from changes in life habits, similarly to men with categorical increases in waist circumference.

AREAS FOR POTENTIAL INTERVENTION

Primary Nephrotic Syndrome

Hyperlipidemia is a typical feature of the nephrotic syndrome. In most patients, serum LDL cholesterol levels are raised[21-24]; in some cases, VLDL cholesterol and VLDL triglycerides are increased as well.[18,23] The mechanisms causing nephrotic hyperlipidemia are not fully understood and appear to be multiple. Hepatic overproduction of lipoproteins is related to depletion of serum albumin in in vivo and in vitro studies.[25,26] Research in humans,[18,23] as well as in experimental animals,[27,28] indicates that catabolism of VLDL can be impaired, accentuating the high circulating triglyceride levels. Removal of LDL via LDL receptors also may be delayed,[18] raising LDL cholesterol levels further. Nephrotic patients apparently have increased serum levels of cholesterol ester transport protein[29] This abnormality could account for the high content of cholesterol in LDL particles.[23] In short, a single mechanism probably cannot explain nephrotic hyperlipidemia.

Prolonged severe hyperlipidemia in patients with an irreversible nephrotic syndrome almost certainly promotes coronary atherosclerosis and predisposes to premature CAD.[30-33] For such patients, application of the NCEP guidelines[1] for primary prevention seems appropriate. If LDL cholesterol levels exceed 100 mg/dL (or non-HDL cholesterol exceeds 220 mg/dL), cholesterol-lowering drugs can be employed in most patients. The goal of therapy for primary prevention is to reduce LDL cholesterol levels to less than 100 mg/dL (non-HDL cholesterol to < 130 mg/dL).

Several studies[23,34-36] have demonstrated that hyperlipidemia in the nephrotic syndrome is responsive to statin drugs.

Statins lower both LDL cholesterol and VLDL cholesterol levels. Bile acid sequestrants also reduce LDL levels and enhance LDL lowering when given in combination with statins.[37] Even when triglycerides and cholesterol are high in nephrotic patients, statins are the preferred therapy because of their ability to lower levels of VLDL remnants as well as LDL.[23,38] Nicotinic acid also reduces triglyceride levels[39] and may have additive effects with statins. The combination of statins plus fibrates has received little attention for patients with the nephrotic syndrome. Finally, it has been reported that LDL-pheresis can be used successfully to lower LDL in nephrotic patients with severe hypercholesterolemia.[40,41]

Recommendations

In patients with the nephrotic syndrome, LDL is the primary target of therapy (Fig. 63-1). Statins are first-line therapy and at moderate doses can be used safely in most patients. There is little experience with high-dose statins. In nephrotic patients with severe hypercholesterolemia, it may not be possible to reduce LDL cholesterol to the near-optimal or optimal levels shown in Table 63-1. The LDL lowering that can be achieved with statin therapy nonetheless can be enhanced by adding a bile acid sequestrant. Statins also lower VLDL remnants and thus remain the preferred therapy in patients with combined elevations of LDL cholesterol and triglycerides. Addition of

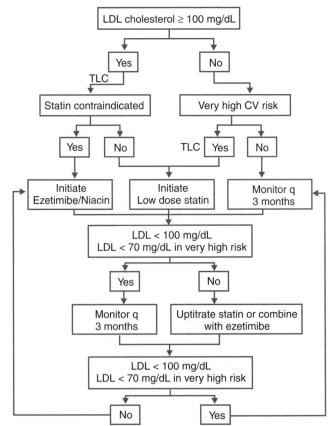

Figure 63-1 Management of hypercholesterolemia in chronic kidney disease. Very high risk ≥ 20% risk of MI in 10 years, coronary artery disease equivalent. TLC, therapeutic lifestyle changes; include low fat, low transfat diet, aerobic exercise 30 to 45 min 4 times/week, weight loss for overweight.

nicotinic acid to statin therapy can be considered for patients with combined hyperlipidemia. The combination of statin plus fibrate, however, should be used with caution; it may be contraindicated because of the increased risk of severe myopathy, rhabdomyolysis, and acute kidney disease.

Diabetic Nephropathy

One cause of the nephrotic syndrome in patients with type 1 or 2 diabetes is diabetic nephropathy. Lipid disorders are more common in patients with type 2 than type 1 diabetes. Diabetic dyslipidemia is essentially identical to atherogenic dyslipidemia (see Table 63-1).[1] When the nephrotic syndrome is present in patients with diabetes, LDL cholesterol levels are raised, and VLDL elevations are accentuated, causing combined hyperlipidemia.[42] In patients with type 1 diabetes, the development of the nephrotic syndrome apparently produces a lipoprotein pattern resembling that of the primary nephrotic syndrome (i.e., a predominance of hypercholesterolemia).[43]

Patients with diabetes are at high risk for CAD even before developing nephropathy.[1,4] The high-risk status is due to at least two factors: metabolic risk factors that are especially common in type 2 diabetes,[44] and hyperglycemia, which appears to accelerate atherogenesis. Because of the high risk for major coronary events, the ATP III report designated diabetes as a CAD risk-equivalent. This designation was partly due to a high risk for future coronary events, but there were other reasons: once patients with diabetes develop CAD, they have a poorer prognosis for survival compared to nondiabetics with CAD.[45] Identifying a CAD risk-equivalent for a diabetic patient leads to treatment until the LDL cholesterol goal of less than 100 mg/dL is reached. Because many patients with diabetes also have elevated triglycerides, a non-HDL cholesterol goal of less than 130 mg/dL is indicated.[46] These goals are independent of established CAD. The use of cholesterol-lowering drugs to achieve LDL cholesterol goals in patients with diabetes is supported in secondary prevention trials by the favorable outcomes of statin therapy.[47,48]

Available evidence indicates that the onset of nephropathy in patients with diabetes enhances CAD risk.[45] To lower cholesterol levels, combining a fibric acid derivative with a statin could be used, but there is an increased risk for myopathy. Therefore, prudence favors the use of a statin alone for most patients with diabetic nephropathy.

Recommendations

When a patient with diabetes also has CKD, that patient should be designated as having a CAD risk-equivalent, even if established CAD is not present. Regardless, the LDL cholesterol goal is less than 100 mg/dL and the non-HDL cholesterol goal is less than 130 mg/dL. To achieve these goals, LDL-lowering drugs are usually required; a statin is preferred (see Table 63-2). An alternative would be to combine a statin with a cholesterol absorption inhibitor, such as ezetimibe, because the combination is as effective as high-dose statin treatment. The combination may also be used for patients who cannot tolerate a high dose of a statin (e.g., patients receiving a fibrate or cyclosporine). A recent multicenter trial demonstrated that relatively low doses of extended-release nicotinic acid are well tolerated in patients with diabetes,[49] but for patients treated with a statin, lower doses of nicotinic acid are required to prevent worsening of diabetes.

CKD Not Requiring Dialysis

It is uncertain whether CKD before institution of dialysis independently raises CAD risk beyond that associated with major risk factors. Therefore, full attention should be given to modifying existing cardiovascular risk factors, such as cigarette smoking, hypertension, high LDL cholesterol, and low HDL cholesterol levels (see Box 63-1). Many CKD patients exhibit hypertriglyceridemia[3,17] because of an underlying defect in the catabolism of VLDL triglycerides.[50] The result is an accumulation of VLDL remnants.[17] Some investigators speculate that remnant lipoproteins are particularly atherogenic[51] and should be treated independent of LDL cholesterol levels. This is an attractive hypothesis, although evidence that therapeutic reduction of VLDL levels will reduce CAD risk is lacking from clinical trials. Meta-analyses from clinical trials conducted exclusively in patients with early and later stages of CKD and post hoc analyses from clinical trials that included participants with early stages of CKD demonstrated that long-term treatment with statins was associated with reduction in risk for major coronary events.[13,52-55] These studies suggest but do not prove that statin therapy is beneficial in patients with early and late stage CKD. Regardless, there are no definitive clinical trials demonstrating a benefit of cholesterol lowering in those with stages 4 and 5 CKD.

Recommendations

If a patient with CKD but not requiring dialysis has multiple CAD risk factors but no clinically manifested atherosclerotic disease, the LDL cholesterol target goal is less than 100 mg/dL (non-HDL cholesterol < 130 mg/dL).[1,15] For untreated patients with LDL cholesterol (or non-HDL cholesterol) levels above the target for high-risk primary prevention, the preferred drug is a statin. If non-HDL cholesterol levels are maintained below the target without statin therapy but hypertriglyceridemia is present, a fibric acid derivative can be used.[56-58] The dose of fibric acid derivative should be adjusted down as recommended in the package insert to reduce the risk for myopathy. In general, it is not appropriate to use a statin in combination with a fibric acid derivative in patients with CKD because of the increased danger of rhabdomyolysis and acute kidney disease.[59]

CKD with Dialysis Treatment

The risk of acute coronary events and CAD death goes up dramatically in patients treated by hemodialysis or peritoneal dialysis.[60] The mechanisms underlying this increase in risk are poorly understood. Two pathologic factors acting at the level of coronary arteries likely play a role: coronary plaques may become more fragile and prone to erosion or rupture, and a hypercoagulable state may exist, which will increase the size of any newly formed thrombus. These two abnormalities could increase both the frequency and size of myocardial infarction. It is almost certain that hemodialysis patients have an absolute risk for major coronary events that is sufficiently high to justify classification as a CAD risk-equivalent. To date, however, no clinical trials have documented how much LDL-lowering therapy reduces the risk. Nonetheless, reduction of LDL cholesterol (and non-HDL cholesterol) levels may help to stabilize coronary plaques and reduce the high frequency of acute coronary syndromes in this population.

The major lipoprotein abnormality in dialysis patients with CKD is a high VLDL level, reflected as an increase in VLDL cholesterol and triglycerides.[61–63] This abnormality results mainly from defective catabolism of VLDL particles.[61] In patients treated with peritoneal dialysis, high VLDL triglyceride levels are particularly common, probably from both hepatic overproduction of VLDL triglycerides due to a high carbohydrate content in dialysis fluid and from defective clearance of VLDL due to loss of kidney function. VLDL remnants in dialysis patients may be unusually atherogenic; if so, efforts to reduce VLDL levels would be warranted. Unfortunately, no clinical trials have investigated whether lowering of serum VLDL levels in dialysis patients will reduce risk for major coronary events. Considering the high absolute risk for CAD in these patients, however, it is reasonable to institute therapy to decrease VLDL levels as part of an overall regimen to control cardiovascular risk factors.

Recommendations

Because dialysis patients are at higher risk for CAD, reduction of LDL cholesterol into the optimal range seems warranted; a recent study[64] suggested that statin therapy reduces total mortality in patients with end-stage renal disease. In the 4-D study, which included approximately 1200 type 2 diabetic patients treated by maintenance hemodialysis, atorvastatin (20 mg once daily) failed to exert an overall cardiovascular mortality benefit, although cardiac morbidity was significantly reduced. In this study, the achieved mean plasma LDL cholesterol level in those assigned to 20 mg of atorvastatin was 77 mg/dL.[65] Even so, patients on dialysis are probably at higher risk for myopathy with statin therapy because of kidney dysfunction combined with multiple medications.[66–68] Based on currently available data, administration of a statin starting with a low dose and titrating upward to achieve the goals included in the ATP III report is a reasonable approach.[65,69] Two large-scale ongoing clinical trials are designed to determine whether cholesterol-lowering agents, including statins and ezetimibe, can reduce cardiovascular morbidity and mortality among CKD patients, including those on hemodialysis. The results of these trials should provide additional information that will modify guidelines for therapy.[70–72]

Many patients on dialysis have elevated triglyceride levels, and statin therapy can reduce levels of VLDL as well as LDL. An alternative approach is to reduce VLDL levels with a fibric acid derivative instead of with a statin.[16,73,74] Fibrates may in fact be more widely used in clinical practice than statins, because of the high frequency of elevated triglyceride levels. Even so, it is uncertain whether reduction of VLDL levels by fibric acid derivatives gives as great a decrease in CAD risk as statins. A recent report[64] found no benefit from fibrate therapy in patients with end-stage renal disease.

CKD Post–Kidney Transplant

Cardiovascular disease appears to be a major cause of death in postkidney transplant patients[60] compared to dialysis patients. A different set of factors may be responsible for this increased CAD risk. Post-transplant, the patients are more likely than dialysis patients to have high cholesterol levels, seemingly related to the use of immunosuppressive agents.[75,76] The ALERT study demonstrated a trend for reducing cardiovascular morbidity and mortality among postkidney transplant patients treated with fluvastatin. This trend was not statistically significant, although there were fewer cardiac events, including nonfatal myocardial infarctions, in the fluvastatin-treated group.[77]

Recommendations

The aim of therapy in postkidney transplant patients is to reduce LDL cholesterol levels to target goals (i.e., to <100 mg/dL) in patients with established CAD and CAD risk-equivalents.[15] Parallel reductions of non-HDL cholesterol levels are recommended for patients with hypertriglyceridemia. If drug therapy to lower serum cholesterol levels is required for post-transplant patients, statins appear to be the preferred agents.[75,76] Certainly they are more effective than fibric acid derivatives for lowering LDL and VLDL cholesterol levels. Nevertheless, it must be kept in mind that the combination of a statin with cyclosporine is accompanied by increased risk for severe myopathy.

References

1. Grundy SM, Cleeman JI, Merz CN, et al: Implications of recent clinical trials for the National Cholesterol Education Program Adult Treatment Panel III guidelines. Circulation 2004;110:227–239.
2. Gupta R, Birnbaum Y, Uretsky BF: The renal patient with coronary artery disease: Current concepts and dilemmas. J Am Coll Cardiol 2004;44:1343–1353.
3. Kwan BC, Kronenberg F, Beddhu S, Cheung AK: Lipoprotein metabolism and lipid management in CKD. J Am Soc Nephrol 2007;18:1246–1261.
4. Grundy SM: United States Cholesterol Guidelines 2001: Expanded scope of intensive low-density lipoprotein-lowering therapy. Am J Cardiol 2001;88:23J–27J.
5. LIPID Study Group: Prevention of cardiovascular events and death with pravastatin in patients with coronary heart disease and a broad range of initial cholesterol levels. The Long-Term Intervention with Pravastatin in Ischaemic Disease (LIPID) Study. N Engl J Med 1998;339:1349–1357.
6. Downs JR, Clearfield M, Weis S, et al: Primary prevention of acute coronary events with lovastatin in men and women with average cholesterol levels: Results of AFCAPS/TexCAPS. Air Force/Texas Coronary Atherosclerosis Prevention Study. JAMA 1998;279:1615–1622.
7. Sacks F, Pfeffer M, Moye L, et al: The effect of pravastatin on coronary events after myocardial infarction in patients with average cholesterol levels. N Engl J Med 1996;335:1001–1009.
8. Scandinavian Simvistatin Survival Study Group: Randomized trial of cholesterol lowering in 4444 patients with coronary heart disease. Lancet 1994;344:1383–1389.
9. Shepherd J, Cobbe SM, Ford I, et al, for the West of Scotland Coronary Prevention Study Group: Prevention of coronary heart disease with pravastatin in men with hypercholesterolemia. N Engl J Med 1995;333:1301–1307.
10. LaRosa JC, Grundy SM, Waters DD, et al: Intensive lipid lowering with atorvastatin in patients with stable coronary disease. N Engl J Med 2005;352:1425–1435.
11. Grundy SM, Gostino Sr RB, Mosca L, et al: Cardiovascular risk assessment based on US cohort studies: Findings from a National Heart, Lung, and Blood institute workshop. Circulation 2001;104:491–496.
12. Smith SC Jr, Blair SN, Bonow RO, et al: AHA/ACC Guidelines for Preventing Heart Attack and Death in Patients With Atherosclerotic Cardiovascular Disease: 2001 update. A statement for healthcare professionals from the American Heart Association and the American College of Cardiology. J Am Coll Cardiol 2001;38:1581–1583.

13. Tonelli M: Should CKD be a coronary heart disease risk equivalent? Am J Kidney Dis 2007;49:8–11.
14. Go AS, Chertow GM, Fan D, et al: CKD and the risks of death, cardiovascular events, and hospitalization. N Engl J Med 2004;351:1296–1305.
15. Kasiske B, Cosio FG, Beto J, et al: Clinical practice guidelines for managing dyslipidemias in kidney transplant patients: A report from the Managing Dyslipidemias in CKD Work Group of the National Kidney Foundation Kidney Disease Outcomes Quality Initiative. Am J Transplant 2004;4(Suppl 7):13–53.
16. Elisaf MS, Dardamanis MA, Papagalanis ND, Siamopoulos KC: Lipid abnormalities in chronic uremic patients. Response to treatment with gemfibrozil. Scand J Urol Nephrol 1993;27:101–108.
17. Nestel PJ, Fidge NH, Tan MH: Increased lipoprotein-remnant formation in chronic renal failure. N Engl J Med 1982;307:329–333.
18. Vega GL, Toto RD, Grundy S: Metabolism of low-density lipoproteins in nephrotic dyslipidemia: Comparison of hypercholesterolemia alone and combined hyperlipidemia. Kidney Int 1995;47:579–586.
19. Chen J, Muntner P, Hamm LL, et al: The metabolic syndrome and CKD in U.S. adults. Ann Intern Med 2004;140:167–174.
20. Hsu CY, McCulloch CE, Iribarren C, et al: Body mass index and risk for end-stage renal disease. Ann Intern Med 2006;144:21–28.
21. Baxter JH: Hyperlipoproteinemia in nephrosis. Arch Intern Med 1962;109:742–757.
22. Joven J, Villabona C, Vilella E, et al: Abnormalities of lipoprotein metabolism in patients with the nephrotic syndrome. N Engl J Med 1990;323:579–584.
23. Vega GL, Grundy SM: Lovastatin therapy in nephrotic hyperlipidemia: Effects on lipoprotein metabolism. Kidney Int 1988;33:1160–1168.
24. Warwick GL, Caslake MJ, Boulton-Jones JM, et al: Low-density lipoprotein metabolism in the nephrotic syndrome. Metabolism 1990;39:187–192.
25. Davis RA, Englhorn SCD, Weinstein DB, Steinberg D: Very low density lipoprotein secretion by cultured rat hepatocytes. J Biol Chem 1980;5:2039–2045.
26. Marsh JB, Drabkin DL: Experimental reconsturction of metabolic pattern of lipid nephrosis: Key role of hepatic protein synthesis. Metabolism 1960;9:946–955.
27. Furukawa S, Hirano T, Mamo JCL, et al: Catabolic defect of triglyceride is associated with abnormal very-low-density lipoprotein in experimental nephrosis. Metabolism 1990;39:101–107.
28. Garber DW, Gottlieb BA, Marsh JB, Sparks CE: Catabolism of very low density lipoproteins in experimental nephrosis. J Clin Invest 1984;74:1375–1383.
29. Moulin P, Appel G, Ginsberg H, Tall A: Increased concentration of plasma cholesteryl ester transfer protein in nephrotic syndrome: Role in dyslipidemia. J Lipid Res 1992;33:1817–1822.
30. Alexander JH, Schapel GJ, Edwards KDG: Increased incidence of coronary heart disease associated with combined elevation of serum triglyceride and cholesterol concentrations in the nephrotic syndrome in man. Med J Aust 1974;2:119–122.
31. Berlyne GM, Mallick NP: Ischaemic heart-disease as a complication of nephrotic syndrome. Lancet 1969;2:399–400.
32. Mallick NP, Short CD: The nephrotic syndrome and ischaemic heart disease. Nephron 1981;27:54–57.
33. Ordonez JD, Hiatt RA, Killebrew EJ, Fireman BH: The increased risk of coronary heart disease associated with nephrotic syndrome. Kidney Int 1993;44:638–642.
34. Biesenbach G, Zazgornik J: Lovastatin in the treatment of hypercholesterolemia in nephrotic syndrome due to diabetic nephropathy state IV-V. Clin Nephrol 1992;37:274–279.
35. Kasiske BL, Velosa JA, Halstenson CE, et al: The effects of lovastatin in hyperlipidemic patients with the nephrotic syndrome. Am J Kidney Dis 1990;15:8–15.
36. Toto RD, Grundy SM, Vega GL: Pravastatin treatment of very low density, intermediate density and low density lipoproteins in hypercholesterolemia and combined hyperlipidemia secondary to the nephrotic syndrome. Am J Nephrol 2000;20:12–17.
37. Rabelink AJ, Hene RJ, Erkelens DW, et al: Effects of simvastatin and cholestyramine on lipoprotein profile in hyperlipidaemia of nephrotic syndrome. Lancet 1988;2:1335–1338.
38. Massy ZA, Ma JZ, Louis TA, Kasiske BL: Lipid-lowering therapy in patients with renal disease. Kidney Int 1995;48:188–198.
39. Martin-Jadraque R, Tato F, Mostaza JM, et al: Effectiveness of low-dose crystalline nicotinic acid in men with low high-density lipoprotein cholesterol levels. Arch Intern Med 1996;156:1081–1088.
40. Muso E, Mune M, Fujii Y, et al, for the Kansai-FGS-Apheresis Treatment (K-FLAT) Study Group: Low density lipoprotein apheresis therapy for steroid-resistant nephrotic syndrome. Kidney Int 1999;71(Suppl):S122–S125.
41. Stenvinkel P, Alvestrand A, Angelin B, Eriksson M: LDL-apheresis in patients with nephrotic syndrome: Effects on serum albumin and urinary albumin excretion. Eur J Clin Invest 2000;30:866–870.
42. Ravid M, Neumann L, Lishner M: Plasma lipids and the progression of nephropathy in diabetes mellitus type II: Effect of ACE inhibitors. Kidney Int 1995;47:907–910.
43. Borch-Johnsen K, Kreiner S: Proteinuria: Value as predictor of cardiovascular mortality in insulin dependent diabetes mellitus. BMJ (Clin Res Ed) 1987;294:1651–1654.
44. Bierman EL: George Lyman Duff Memorial Lecture. Atherogenesis in diabetes. Arterioscler Thromb 1992;12:647–656.
45. Wingard R, Barrett-Connor E: Heart disease and diabetes. In Diabetes in America. Bethesda, MD: National Institutes of Health/NIDDK, 1995.
46. Garg A, Grundy S: Management of dyslipidemia in NIDDM. Diabetes Care 1990;13:153–169.
47. Goldberg RB, Mellies MJ, Sacks FM, et al, for the CARE Investigators: Cardiovascular events and their reduction with pravastatin in diabetic and glucose-intolerant myocardial infarction survivors with average cholesterol levels: Subgroup analyses in the cholesterol and recurrent events (CARE) trial. Circulation 1998;98:2513–2519.
48. Pyorala K, Pedersen TR, Kjekshus J, et al: Cholesterol lowering with simvastatin improves prognosis of diabetic patients with coronary heart disease. A subgroup analysis of the Scandinavian Simvastatin Survival Study (4S). Diabetes Care 1997;20:614–620.
49. Grundy SM, Vega GL, McGovern ME, et al: Efficacy, safety, and tolerability of once-daily niacin for the treatment of dyslipidemia associated with type 2 diabetes: Results of the Assessment of Diabetes Control and Evaluation of the Efficacy of Niaspan Trial. Arch Intern Med 2002;162:1568–1576.
50. Sanfellipo M, Grundy S Henderson L: Transport of very low density lipoprotein triglyceride (VLDL-TG): Comparison of hemodialysis and hemofiltration. Kidney Int 1979;16:878–886.
51. Havel RJ: Triglyceride-rich lipoproteins and atherosclerosis—new perspectives. Am J Clin Nutr 1994;59:795–796.
52. Colhoun HM, Szarek M, DeMicco DA, et al: Atorvastatin reduces the risk of major cardiovascular events in patients with diabetes and impaired renal function in the Collaborative Atorvastatin Diabetes Study (CARDS). American Diabetes Association 67th Scientific Sessions, 22–26 June 2007, Chicago.
53. Holdaas H, Wanner C, Abletshauser C, et al: The effect of fluvastatin on cardiac outcomes in patients with moderate to severe renal insufficiency: A pooled analysis of double-blind, randomized trials. Int J Cardiol 2007;117:64–74.
54. Navaneethan SD, Pansini F, Strippoli GF: Statins in patients with CKD: Evidence from systematic reviews and randomized clinical trials. PLoS Med 2006;3:e123.

55. Tonelli M: Do statins protect the kidney as well as the heart? Nephrol Dial Transplant 2006;21:3005–3006.

56. Norbeck HE, Anderson P: Treatment of uremic hypertriglyceridaemia with bezafibrate. Atherosclerosis 1982;44:125–136.

57. Pasternack A, Vattinen T, Solakivi T, et al: Normalization of lipoprotein lipase and hepatic lipase by gemfibrozil results in correction of lipoprotein abnormalities in chronic renal failure. Clin Nephrol 1987;27:163–168.

58. Williams AJ, Baker F, Walls J: The short term effects of bezafibrate on the hypertriglyceridaemia of moderate to severe uraemia. Br J Clin Pharmacol 1984;18:361–367.

59. Liu J, Kalantarinia K, Rosner MH: Management of lipid abnormalities associated with end-stage renal disease. Semin Dial 2006; 19:391–401.

60. U.S. Renal Data System: 2001 Annual Data Report: Atlas of End-Stage Renal Disease in the United States. Bethesda, MD: National Institutes of Health, National Institute of Diabetes and Digestive and Kidney Diseases, 2001.

61. Sanfelippo M, Grundy SM, Henderson L: Transport of very-low density lipoprotein triglyceride (VLDL-TG) metabolism. Circulation 1979;13:11a–74a.

62. Cattran DC, Steiner G, Fento SSA, Ampil M: Dialysis hyperlipemia: Response to dietary manipulations. Clin Nephrol 1980;13: 177–182.

63. Sanfelippo M, Grundy S, Henderson L: Response of plasma triglycerides to dietary change in patients on hemodialysis. Kidney Int 1978;14:180–186.

64. Seliger L, Weiss N, Gillen DK, et al: HMG-CoA reducatease inhibitors are associated with reduced mortality in ESRD patients. Kidney Int 2002;61:297–304.

65. Wanner C, Krane V, Marz W, et al: Randomized controlled trial on the efficacy and safety of atorvastatin in patients with type 2 diabetes on hemodialysis (4D study): Demographic and baseline characteristics. Kidney Blood Press Res 2004;27:259–266.

66. Malyszko J, Malyszko JS, Hryszko T, Mysliwiec M: Effects of long-term treatment with simvastatin on some hemostatic parameters in continuous ambulatory peritoneal dialysis patients. Am J Nephrol 2001;21:373–377.

67. Nishizawa Y, Shoji T, Tabata T, et al: Effects of lipid-lowering drugs on intermediate-density lipoprotein in uremic patients. Kidney Int 1999;71(Suppl):S134–S136.

68. Wanner C, Krane V, Metzger T, Quaschning T: Lipid changes and statins in chronic renal insufficiency and dialysis. J Nephrol 2001;14(Suppl 4):S76–S80.

69. Baber U, Toto RD, de Lemos JA: Statins and cardiovascular risk reduction in patients with CKD and end-stage renal failure. Am Heart J 2007;153:471–477.

70. Baigent C, Landray M, Warren M: Statin therapy in kidney disease populations: Potential benefits beyond lipid lowering and the need for clinical trials. Curr Opin Nephrol Hypertens 2004;13: 601–605.

71. Baigent C, Landry M: Study of Heart and Renal Protection (SHARP). Kidney Int 2003;(Suppl):S207–S210.

72. Fellstrom B, Holdaas H, Jardine AG, et al: Effect of rosuvastatin on outcomes in chronic haemodialysis patients: Baseline data from the AURORA study. Kidney Blood Press Res 2007;30:314–322.

73. De Guilio S, Boulu R, Drueke T, et al: Clofibrate treatment of hyperlipidemia in chronic renal failure. Clin Nephrol 1977; 8:509.

74. Sherrard DJ, Goldberg AB, Haas LB, Brunzell JD: Chronic clofibrate therapy in maintenance hemodialysis patients. Nephron 1980;25:219–221.

75. Cheung AK, DeVault GA Jr, Gregory MC: A prospective study on treatment of hypercholesterolemia with lovastatin in renal transplant patients receiving cyclosporine. J Am Soc Nephrol 1993;3:1884–1891.

76. Yoshimura N, Ohmori Y, Tsuji T, Oka T: Effect of pravastatin on renal transplant recipients treated with cyclosporine—4-year follow-up. Transplant Proc 1994;26:2632–2633.

77. Holdaas H, Fellstrom B, Jardine AG, et al: Effect of fluvastatin on cardiac outcomes in renal transplant recipients: A multicentre, randomised, placebo-controlled trial. Lancet 2003;361: 2024–2031.

Further Reading

Grundy SM, Cleeman JI, Merz CN, et al: Implications of recent clinical trials for the National Cholesterol Education Program Adult Treatment Panel III guidelines. Circulation 2004;110:227–239.

Praga M, Morales E: Obesity, proteinuria and progression of renal failure. Curr Opin Nephrol Hypertens 2006;15:481–486.

Vaziri ND: Dyslipidemia of chronic renal failure: The nature, mechanisms, and potential consequences. Am J Physiol Renal Physiol 2006;290:F262–F272.

Wanner C, Krane V, Marz W, et al: Atorvastatin in patients with type 2 diabetes mellitus undergoing hemodialysis. N Engl J Med 2005;353:238–248.

Chapter 64

Hyperhomocysteinemia

Joyce M. Gonin and Christopher S. Wilcox

Homocysteine is a sulfa-containing amino acid that circulates in oxidized, reduced, and complex forms. About 75% is bound to albumin, and routine assays measure total homocysteine (i.e., free plus bound homocysteine, or tHcy).[1,2] Homocysteine is manufactured in all cells, including erythrocytes. Consequently, it leaks into plasma in blood samples. Blood samples, therefore, must be cooled to 4°C, centrifuged, and the plasma separated rapidly to avoid artificially high plasma tHcy values. Reported normal values vary widely between laboratories but average 6 to 10 μmol/L. Hyperhomocysteinemia implies a value more than two standard deviations above normal; this is typically 12 to 16 μmol/L.

More than 90% of patients with end-stage renal disease (ESRD) receiving hemodialysis or continuous ambulatory peritoneal dialysis have hyperhomocysteinemia. Plasma levels of tHcy appear to be elevated to a similar degree in patients treated by either continuous ambulatory peritoneal dialysis or hemodialysis.[3–5] After renal transplantation, tHcy levels fall, but less than anticipated from the improvement in renal function.[6]

Very severe hyperhomocysteinemia (>100 μmol/L) occurs as a genetic metabolic defect and is associated with early and severe atherosclerosis. Mild hyperhomocysteinemia (12–20 μmol/L) occurs in otherwise normal people, often as a manifestation of vitamin B deficiency. Patients with ESRD usually have moderate hyperhomocysteinemia (20–100 μmol/L). Conflicting data exist regarding the relationship between hyperhomocysteinemia and cardiovascular disease. In retrospective and cross-sectional studies of the general population, a consistently strong relationship is seen between homocysteine concentrations and cardiovascular events.[7] This finding, however, is not confirmed in all prospective studies.[8] Five retrospective[9–12] and three prospective studies[13–15] concur that tHcy is an independent risk factor for the development of cardiovascular disease in patients with ESRD. Two recent reports have contradictory results, suggesting that the highest incidence of cardiovascular events is associated with the lowest quartile for homocysteine concentrations.[16,17] A subsequent study revealed that this phenomenon applied only to individuals with chronic inflammation and malnutrition, as defined by low serum albumin and high C-reactive protein values.[18]

The major determinant of tHcy in patients with chronic kidney disease is an increase in the serum creatinine concentration or a reduction in the glomerular filtration rate.[19] Among patients with ESRD, malnutrition, low serum albumin concentration,[20] and high-flux hemodialysis[21] predict lower levels of tHcy. The polymorphism status for 5,10-methylene tetrahydrofolate reductase (MTHFR) has a relatively minor effect on tHcy levels in ESRD patients.[22]

The mechanism causing hyperhomocysteinemia in ESRD remains obscure.[2] Therapy is empiric and remains highly unsatisfactory. Because no effective treatment has been devised to normalize tHcy in ESRD patients, it has not been possible to establish whether reversal of hyperhomocysteinemia reverses the associated risk of cardiovascular disease. Three large randomized trials are being conducted in patients with chronic kidney disease to evaluate the effect of treatment of hyperhomocysteinemia on cardiovascular outcome. The FAVORIT study will examine the effect of lowering homocysteine in 4000 renal transplant patients. Available data suggest that treatment with folic acid can normalize homocysteine in this population.[23] The Atherosclerosis and Folic Acid Supplementation Trial (ASFAST) will evaluate the effect of folic acid on cardiovascular outcome and endothelial function in 315 predialysis and dialysis patients.[24] The Homocysteinemia in Kidney and End State Renal Disease Study (HOST) is a U.S. Veterans Administration-industry funded study initiated in 2001 to assess the effects of 4 years of a daily regimen of folic acid, pyridoxine, and vitamin B_{12} on vascular outcomes.

METABOLISM

Homocysteine is metabolized to methionine via the remethylation pathway. Alternatively, it may be metabolized by transsulfuration (Fig. 64-1).[1] Two hypotheses have been proposed to explain hyperhomocysteinemia in renal failure: homocysteine metabolism and excretion by the kidneys may be impaired or extrarenal homocysteine metabolism is impaired. Homocysteine transsulfuration and remethylation enzymes are present in the kidney; a study in the rat showed that homocysteine is taken up and metabolized by the kidney.[25] However, two studies in humans with normal renal function did not find a significant arteriovenous difference in homocysteine concentration across the kidney.[26,27] Whole-body sulfur amino acid metabolism studied using a stable isotope method has demonstrated that total remethylation and transmethylation flux are decreased in ESRD patients, whereas the transsulfuration rate was similar to controls.[28–30] ESRD patients do fail to up-regulate the transsulfuration pathway in response to hyperhomocysteinemia.[31]

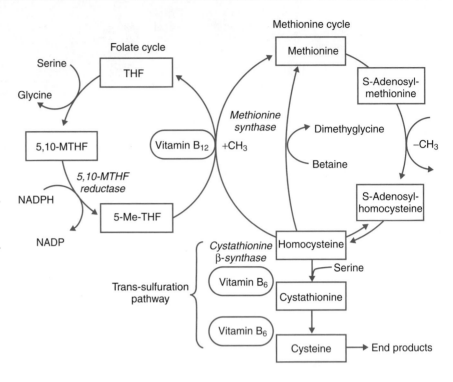

Figure 64-1 A diagrammatic representation of the pathways for methionine and homocysteine metabolism. 5,10-MTHF, 5,10-methyltetrahydrofolate; 5-Me-THF, 5-methyltetrahydrofolate; THF, tetrahydrofolate. (Reproduced from Kitiyakara C, Gonin J, Massy Z, et al: Nontraditional cardiovascular disease risk factors in end-stage renal disease: Oxidative stress and hyperhomocysteinemia. Curr Opin Nephrol 2001;9:477–487.)

Remethylation via methionine synthase depends on the active form of folate, 5-methyltetrahydrofolate (5-Me-THF), and the active form of vitamin B_{12}. The transsulfuration pathway is initiated by cystathionine β-synthase, which catalyzes the conjugation of homocysteine and serine to form cystathionine. This is a vitamin B_6-dependent pathway. Therefore, folate, vitamins B_{12} and B_6, or their active metabolites are essential for homocysteine metabolism. Indeed, defects in these three vitamins account for most cases of mild hyperhomocysteinemia in the general population.[32]

B vitamins are water-soluble and are removed significantly during dialysis. Therefore, dialysis patients normally receive a water-soluble multivitamin. One widely used capsule, Nephrocap, contains folic acid 1 mg, vitamin B_6 10 mg, and vitamin B_{12} 6 μg. Such a prescription should maintain plasma vitamin levels in the normal range for most dialysis patients.[33] There is a strong inverse relationship between the log of plasma folate concentration and the log of plasma tHcy concentration in both healthy adults and those with ESRD. However, the relationship is shifted to higher plasma levels of homocysteine in patients with ESRD.[10] This has prompted the hypothesis that ESRD is a state of folate- and B vitamin-resistance, requiring supranormal doses of these vitamins to reverse the defect.

PHARMACOLOGIC THERAPY

Prospective trials in patients with ESRD have evaluated the effects on hyperhomocysteinemia of folic acid (or its derivatives), vitamins B_6 and B_{12}, serine, and betaine.

The efficacy of supplementation with B vitamins in patients with ESRD has been the subject of 18 prospective clinical trials.[4,5,16,22,34–48] Despite this wealth of information, there are no firm conclusions about the role of vitamin supplementation in doses above those routinely recommended (folic acid 1 mg, vitamin B_6 10–50 mg, and vitamin B_{12} 5–50 μg daily).

Even though no consistent conclusions can be drawn from these trials, some trends are apparent:

1. All trials except two[44–46] report a statistically significant reduction in tHcy with folate supplementation. However, those two negative trials are among only three trials that were placebo-controlled,[34,44–46] and both used very high doses of folic acid (30 or 60 mg daily)[45,46] or of a folate metabolite (intravenous leucovorin 100 mg, three times per week).[44,46] The majority of fully controlled trials have failed to show any detectable reduction in tHcy even with massive supplemental doses of folic acid. The reason for the modest reductions seen in most uncontrolled trials is not yet clear but may relate to better compliance with vitamin replacement therapy.

2. Larger decreases in tHcy usually occur during active treatment, in part because routine vitamin supplementation is withdrawn before the trial starts, suggesting that the baseline tHcy level is what has been changed. In fact, participants in the two negative trials,[44–46] as well as those from some positive trials,[4,34,37,39,42] were studied while maintaining the standard of care prescription with folate. In some studies, the routine vitamin supplement was withdrawn before the trial.[5,35,36,40] On the whole, participants in these trials had the highest pretreatment values for tHcy, probably reflecting some B-vitamin deficiency caused by dialytic losses. Consequently, these patients generally had the most robust responses to folate therapy (Fig. 64-2A). Clearly, these trials are severely flawed; it has been known for many years that B-vitamin deficiency develops quite rapidly in hemodialysis patients if they are not provided with a routine supplement to replace dialysis losses.

3. There is no clear benefit from additional supplementation of vitamins B_6 and B_{12} over responses that are achieved with folic acid alone. This issue was studied specifically in

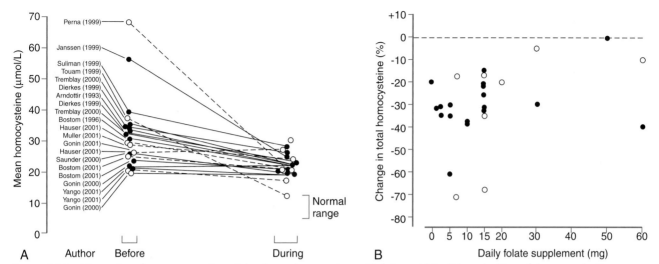

Figure 64-2   Mean data from prospective trials of supplementation with folic acid (*solid symbols*), or folate metabolites or analogues (*open symbols*) given with or without other treatments, such as vitamins B$_6$ and B$_{12}$. **A,** Mean total homocysteine (tHcy) for trial subjects before and during folate supplementation; the *shaded area* represents the normal range. **B,** Relationship between the mean fractional change of plasma tHcy concentration during therapy and the daily dose of folate or folate metabolite or analogue used.

one controlled trial in which groups of hemodialysis patients received either placebo, folic acid 30 mg or 60 mg, vitamins B$_6$ and B$_{12}$, or all three treatments together. There was no significant difference in any group relative to the placebo control.[45,46]

4. Although there are substantial, and largely unexplained, variations in the values for plasma tHcy before supplementation, all trials report mean values during supplementation of 12 to 27 μmol/L (see Fig. 64-2A).

5. The trials that used folate metabolites (5 Me-THF)[35,39,41] or folinic acid (leucovorin)[37,40,42,44,46–48] produced similar results to folic acid. Indeed, within-trial comparisons of folic acid and its metabolic derivatives have shown no significant differences.[37,39,41,42]

6. In only two trials were the values for tHcy normalized in the majority of patients. Touam and colleagues[40] supplemented patients with a single postdialysis injection of folinic acid (50 mg) given once weekly and 250 mg of vitamin B$_6$ after each dialysis session. They reported normalization of total plasma homocysteine levels. However, a subsequent study found no benefit of equimolar folinic acid over folic acid.[42] In a small study by Gonella and colleagues,[48] 89% of patients on hemodiafiltration treated with folinic acid and vitamins B$_6$ and B$_{12}$ for 4 months had normalized homocysteine values. This may reflect the process of hemodiafiltration as compared to routine hemodialysis.

7. Supplementation with serine alone or in addition to folate metabolites produces no further fall in tHcy.[44,46]

8. No relationship is apparent between the fractional change in tHcy concentration during therapy and the daily dose of folate (or metabolite) that is given as a supplement (see Fig. 64-2B). For example, one trial reported that compared to no vitamin supplements, supplementation with folic acid 1 mg daily reduced tHcy levels by 32%; an increase to 10 mg daily produced no further change.[36] The highest doses of folic acid (60 mg daily) or folinic acid (100 mg/day intravenously three times per week) tested have been reported to reduce tHcy by 38%[22] or to have no significant effect whatsoever.[44–46] The

complete absence of a relationship between the dose of folic acid delivered and the change in tHcy among the numerous trials summarized in Figure 64-2B refutes the hypothesis that hemodialysis patients have resistance to the effects of folic acid on tHcy. They also cast very serious doubt about the effectiveness of folic acid, above a routine replacement dose of 1 mg daily.

9. Several studies have suggested that intravenous vitamin B$_{12}$, when added to high-dose folic acid and pyridoxine, may achieve a reduction of homocysteine of 32% to 50%.[49–52] It has been suggested that inhibition of methionine synthase in uremia contributes to hyperhomocysteinemia in ESRD patients and that pharmacologic concentrations of vitamin B$_{12}$ given intravenously may increase methionine synthase activity via a post-translational mechanism.[53] These conditions require validation in formal trials.

An alternative approach to the lowering of homocysteine in ESRD is the administration of acetylcysteine, a thiol-containing antioxidant. Scholze and associates showed that a single dose of intravenous acetylcysteine given during a dialysis session lowered tHcy from 20 mmol/L to 2.2 mmol/L, compared to a reduction from 19.8 mmol/L to 11.9 mmol/L with placebo. Although tHcy rebounded after dialysis, it remained significantly lower in the treated group 2 days later.[54] In another randomized, controlled trial, 1200 mg of acetylcysteine was given orally twice a day for 4 weeks to patients with ESRD. The tHcy was lowered by 19% compared to 8% in the placebo group. Unfortunately, this difference was not statistically significant,[55] which casts doubt on the efficacy of oral acetylcysteine in these patients.

These reports lead to the following conclusions:

1. Presently there is no rational justification for recommending more than routine vitamin supplementation with a daily dose of folic acid (1 mg), vitamin B$_6$ (10–50 mg), and vitamin B$_{12}$ (5–50 g) in ESRD patients.

2. There is no benefit from active folate metabolites or folate analogues over folic acid itself.

3. Intravenous vitamin B_{12} may be more beneficial than oral vitamin B_{12}, but this requires validation before routine recommendation.

4. The potential benefits of N-acetylcysteine remain unproven.

5. There must be powerful, uncontrolled, and presently unrecognized factors in the studies to account for the high degree of variability reported in responses to vitamin supplementation.

Figure 64-2A demonstrates that ESRD patients should normally be able to achieve a predialysis tHcy concentration of less than 30 μmol/L. Patients with higher values require assessment to ensure that they have been prescribed, and are indeed receiving, the routine vitamin supplement. If this does not explain the above-average plasma level of tHcy, the plasma levels of folate, vitamin B_{12}, and vitamin B_6 should be assessed to ensure that they are within the normal range. Occasionally, patients present with very high values for tHcy due to unrecognized concurrent disease, such as pernicious anemia or hypothyroidism, or because of concurrent therapy with antifolate drugs such as methotrexate. An algorithm for evaluation and treatment of hyperhomocysteinemia in renal disease is presented in Figure 64-3.

Clearly, the present state of knowledge concerning hyperhomocysteinemia in patients with ESRD is highly unsatisfactory. On the one hand, hyperhomocysteinemia is almost universal in these patients and is a powerful predictor of associated or future development of cardiovascular disease. On the other, treatment is generally ineffective in normalizing hyperhomocysteinemia, and available clinical trials are so discordant that strong conclusions concerning the need for more than routine supplementation with folate and B vitamins are not warranted. Therapeutic advances may have to await the outcome of scientific studies that disclose the mechanism of hyperhomocysteinemia in ESRD and evaluate whether reductions in tHcy, or prolonged supplementation with high doses of B vitamins, indeed have beneficial effects in reducing cardiovascular disease in patients with ESRD.

References

1. Kitiyakara C, Gonin J, Massy Z, et al: Non-traditional cardiovascular disease risk factors in end-stage renal disease: Oxidative stress and hyperhomocysteinemia. Curr Opin Nephrol 2001;9: 477–487.
2. Friedman AN, Bostom AG, Selhub J, et al: The kidney and homocysteine metabolism. J Am Soc Nephrol 2001;12:2181–2189.
3. Vychytil A, Fodinger M, Wolfl G, et al: Major determinants of hyperhomocysteinemia in peritoneal dialysis patients. Kidney Int 1998;53:1775–1782.
4. Arnadottir M, Brattstrom L, Simonsen O, et al: The effect of high-dose pyridoxine and folic acid supplementation on serum lipid and plasma homocysteine concentrations in dialysis patients. Clin Nephrol 1993;40:236–240.
5. Janssen MJ, van Guldener C, de Jong GM, et al: Folic acid treatment of hyperhomocysteinemia in dialysis patients. Miner Electrolyte Metab 1996;22:110–114.
6. Arnadottir M, Hultberg B, Wahlberg J, et al: Serum homocysteine concentration before and after renal transplantation. Kidney Int 1998;54:1380–1384.
7. Moat SJ, Doshi SN, Lang D, et al: Treatment of coronary heart disease with folic acid: Is there a future? Am J Physiol Heart Circ Physiol 2004;287:H1–H7.
8. Danish J, Lewington S: Plasma homocysteine and coronary heart disease: Systematic review of published epidemilological studies. J Cardiovasc Risk 1998;5:229–232.
9. Robinson K, Gupta A, Dennis V, et al: Hyperhomocysteinemia confers an independent increased risk of atherosclerosis in end-stage renal disease and is closely linked to plasma folate and pyridoxine concentrations. Circulation 1996;94:2743–2748.
10. Dennis VW, Robinson K: Homocysteinemia and vascular disease in end-stage renal disease. Kidney Int 1996;50:S11–S17.
11. Manns BJ, Burgess ED, Hyndman ME, et al: Hyperhomocyst(e)inemia and the prevalence of atherosclerotic vascular disease in patients with end-stage renal disease. Am J Kidney Dis 1999;34:669–677.
12. Bachmann J, Tepel M, Zidek W, et al: Hyperhomocysteinemia and the risk for vascular disease in hemodialysis patients. J Am Soc Nephrol 1995;6:121–125.
13. Ducloux D, Motte G, Challier B, et al: Serum homocysteine and cardiovascular disease occurrence in chronic, stable renal transplant recipients: A prospective study. J Am Soc Nephrol 2000; 11:134–137.
14. Moustapha A, Naso A, Nahlawi M, et al: Prospective study of hyperhomocysteinemia as an adverse cardiovascular risk factor in end-stage renal disease. Circulation 1998;97:138–141.
15. Buccianti G, Baragetti I, Bamonti F, et al: Plasma homocysteine levels and cardiovascular mortality in patients with end-stage renal disease. J Nephrol 2004;17:405–410.
16. Wrone EM, Horenberger JM, Zehnder JL, et al: Randomized trial of folic acid for the prevention of cardiovascular events in end-stage renal disease. J Am Soc Nephrol 2004;15:420–426.

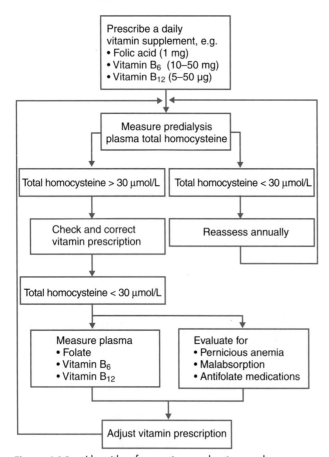

Figure 64-3 Algorithm for routine evaluation and management of hyperhomocysteinemia in patients with end-stage renal disease. tHcy, total homocysteine.

17. Kalanter-Zadeh K, Block B, Humphreys MH, et al: A low rather than a high, total plasma homocysteine is an indicator of poor outcome in hemodialysis patients. J Am Soc Nephrol 20004;15:442–453.

18. Ducloux D, Klein A, Kazory A, et al: Impact of malnutrition-inflammation on the association between homocysteine and mortality. Kidney Int 2006;69:331–335.

19. Wollesen F, Brattstrom L, Refsum H, et al: Plasma homocysteine and cysteine in relation to glomerular filtration rate in diabetes mellitus. Kidney Int 1999;55:1028–1035.

20. Suliman ME, Qureshi AR, Barany P, et al: Hyperhomocysteinemia, nutritional status, and cardiovascular disease in hemodialysis patients. Kidney Int 2000;57:1727–1735.

21. van Tellingen A, Grooteman MP, Bartels PC, et al: Long-term reduction of plasma homocysteine levels by super-flux dialyzers in hemodialysis patients. Kidney Int 2001;59:342–347.

22. Sunder Plassmann G, Födinger M, Buchmayer H, et al: Effect of high-dose folic acid therapy on hyperhomocysteinemia in hemodialysis patients: Results of the Vienna Multicenter study. J Am Soc Nephrol 2000;11:1106–1116.

23. Marucci R, Zanacci M, Bertoni E, et al: Vitamin supplementation reduces the progression of atherosclerosis in hyperhomocysteinemic renal-transplant recipients. Transplantation 2003; 75:1551–1555.

24. Zoungas S, Branley P, Kerr PG, et al; Atherosclerosis and Folic Acid Supplementation Trial in chronic renal failure: Baseline results. Nephrology 2004;9:130–141.

25. House JD, Brosman ME, Brosnan JT: Renal uptake and excretion of homocysteine in rats with acute hyperhomocysteinemia. Kidney Int 1998;54:1601–1607.

26. van Guldener C, Donker AJ, Jakobs C, et al: No net renal extraction of homocysteine in fasting humans. Kidney Int 1998;54:166–169.

27. Garibotto G, Sofia A, Saffioti S, et al: Interorgan exchange of aminothiols in humans. Am J Physiol Endocrinol Metab 2003;284:E757–E763.

28. van Guldener C, Kulik W, Berger R. et al: Homocysteine and methionine metabolism in ESRD: A stable isotope study. Kidney Int 1999;56:1064–1071.

29. Stam F, van Guldener C, ter Wee PM, et al: Homocysteine clearance and methylation flux rates in health and end-stage renal disease: Association with S-adenosylhomocysteine. Am J Physiol Renal Physiol 2004;287:F215–F223.

30. Stam F, van Guldener C, ter Wee PM, et al: Effect of folic acid on methionine and homocysteine metabolism in end-stage renal disease. Kidney Int 2005;67:259–264.

31. Guttormsen AB, Ueland PM, Svarstad E, et al: Kinetic basis of hyperhomocysteinemia in patients with chronic renal failure. Kidney Int 1997;52:495–502.

32. Hoogeveen EK, Kostense PJ, Jager A, et al: Serum homocysteine level and protein intake are related to risk of microalbuminuria: The Hoorn Study. Kidney Int 1998;54:203–209.

33. Descombes E, Hanck AB, Fellay G: Water soluble vitamins in chronic hemodialysis patients and need for supplementation. Kidney Int 1993;43:1319–1328.

34. Bostom AG, Shemin D, Lapane KL, et al: High dose B-vitamin treatment of hyperhomocysteinemia in dialysis patients. Kidney Int 1996;49:147–152.

35. Perna AF, Ingrosso D, De Santo NG, et al: Metabolic consequences of folate-induced reduction of hyperhomocysteinemia in uremia. J Am Soc Nephrol 1997;8:1899–1905.

36. Tremblay R, Bonnardeaux A, Geadah D, et al: Hyperhomocysteinemia in hemodialysis patients: Effects of 12-month supplementation with hydrosoluble vitamins. Kidney Int 2000;58: 851–858.

37. Hauser AC, Hagen W, Rehak PH, et al: Efficacy of folinic versus folic acid for the corrections of hyperhomocysteinemia in hemodialysis patients. Am J Kidney Dis 2001;37:758–765.

38. Dierkes J, Domrose U, Ambrosch A, et al: Response of hyperhomocysteinemia to folic acid supplementation in patients with end-stage renal disease. Clin Nephrol 1999;51:108–115.

39. Bostom AG, Shemin D, Gohh RY, et al: Treatment of hyperhomocysteinemia in hemodialysis patients and renal transplant recipients. Kidney Int 2001;59:S246–S252.

40. Touam M, Zingraff J, Jungers P, et al: Effective correction of hyperhomocysteinemia in hemodialysis patients by intravenous folinic acid and pyridoxine therapy. Kidney Int 1999;56:2292–2296.

41. Bostom A, Shemin D, Bagley P, et al: Controlled comaprison of L-5-methyltetrathydrofolate versus folic acid for the treatment of hyperhomocysteinemia in hemodialysis patients. Circulation 2000;101:2829–2832.

42. Yango A, Shemin D, Hsu N, et al: L-folinic acid versus folic acid for the treatment of hyperhomocysteinemia in hemodialysis patients. (Rapid communication.) Kidney Int 2001;59:324–327.

43. Suliman ME, Filho JCD, Barany P, et al: Effects of high-dose folic acid and pyridoxine on plasma and erythrocyte sulfur amino acids in hemodialysis patients. J Am Soc Nephrol 1999;10:1287–1296.

44. Gonin JM, Nguyen HT, Michels AM, et al: Evaluation of folinic acid and serine in hyperhomocysteinemia in ESRD: A prospective placebo-controlled randomized study. J Am Soc Nephrol 2001;12:356A.

45. Gonin, JM, Sarna A, Loya A, et al: A double-blind, controlled study of folate and vitamin therapy for hyperhomocysteinemia in hemodialysis (abstract). J Am Soc Nephrol 2000;11:269A.

46. Gonin JM, Nguyen H, Gonin R, et al: Controlled trials of very high dose folic acid, vitamins B12 and B6, intravenous folinic acid and serine for treatment of hyperhomocysteinemia in ESRD. J Nephrol 2003;16:522–534.

47. Mueller TF, Mueller N, Moser R, et al: Effect of oral substitution of reduced folates on homocysteine, neopterin, and lipid levels in patients treated with hemodialysis (abstract). J Am Soc Nephrol 2001;12:360A–361A.

48. Gonella M, Calabrese G, Mengozzi A, et al: The achievement of normal homocysteinemia in regular extracorporeal dialysis patients. J Nephrol 2004;17:411–413.

49. Elian KM, Hoffer LJ: Hydroxycobalamin reduces hyperhomocysteinemia in end-stage renal disease. Metabolism 2002;51: 881–886.

50. Koyama K, Usami T, Takeuchi O, et al: Efficacy of methylcobalamin on lowering total homocysteine plasma concentrations in haemodialysis patients receiving high-dose folic acid supplementation. Nephrol Dial Transplant 2002;17:916–922.

51. Hoffer LJ, Saboohi F, Golden M, et al: Cobalamin dose regimen for maximum homocysteine reduction in end-stage renal disease. Metabolism 2005;54:835–840.

52. Hoffer LJ, Djahangirian O, Bourgouin PE, et al: Comparative effects of hydroxycobalamin and cyanocobalamin on plasma homocysteine concentrations in end-stage renal disease. Metabolism 2005;54:1362–1367.

53. Oltean S, Banerjee R: Nutritional modulation of gene expression and homocysteine utilization by vitamin B_{12}. J Biol Chem 2003;278:20778–20784.

54. Scholze A, Rinder C, Beige J, et al: Acetylcysteine reduces plasma homocysteine concentration and improves pulse pressure and endothelial function in patients with end-stage renal failure. Circulation 2004;109:369–374.

55. Friedman AN, Bostom AG, Laliberty P, et al: The effect of n-acetylcysteine on plasma total homocysteine levels in hemodialysis: A randomized, controlled study. Am J Kidney Dis 2003;41:442–446.

Further Reading

De Bree A, Verschuren WMM, Kromhout D, et al: Homocysteine determinants and the evidence to what extent homocysteine determines the risk of coronary heart disease. Pharmacol Rev 2002;54:599–618.

De Vriese AS, Verbeke F, Schrijvers BF, Lameire NH: Is folate a promising agent in the prevention and treatment of cardiovascular disease in patients with renal failure? Kidney Int 2002;61:1199–1209.

Gonin JM: Folic acid supplementation to prevent adverse events in individuals with chronic kidney disease and end stage renal disease. Curr Opin Nephrol Hypertens 2005;14:277–281.

Ingrosso D, Cimmino A, Perna AF, et al: Folate treatment and unbalanced methylation and changes of allelic expression induced by hyperhomocystinaemia in patients with uraemia. Lancet 2003;36:1693–1699.

Liu CS, Chiang HC, Chen HW: Methylenetetrahydrofolate reductase polymorphism determines the plasma homocysteine-lowering effect of large-dose folic acid supplementation in patients with cardiovascular disease Nutrition 2004;20:974–978.

Moat SJ, Doshi SN, Lang D, et al: Treatment of coronary heart disease with folic acid: Is there a future? Am J Physiol Heart Circ Physiol 2004;287:H1–H7.

Chapter 65

Antioxidant Therapy in Chronic Kidney Disease

Shakil Aslam

Reactive oxygen species (ROS) include superoxide anions, hydroxyl anions, and hydrogen peroxide. Superoxide anion is the primary ROS, and it interacts with other molecules to generate secondary ROS, including reactive nitrogen species. ROS are produced as a by-product during oxygen metabolism. In physiologic concentrations ROS act as signaling molecules and play an important role in the regulation of renal and vascular functions.[1-5] In vascular endothelial cells, ROS regulate vascular tone, oxygen sensing, cell growth and proliferation, apoptosis, and inflammatory responses. Because of their highly reactive nature, the generation and elimination of ROS are very tightly regulated. Loss of this regulation with increased ROS accumulation leads to oxidative stress (OS), which causes vascular dysfunction by several mechanisms: Superoxide anion reduces the bioavailability of vasodilator nitric oxide and forms peroxynitrite, which inactivates prostacyclin synthase.[6] This reaction reduces the production of vasodilator and antiplatelet prostacyclins. By oxidizing low-density lipoprotein, ROS facilitates its uptake by macrophages via the scavenger receptor CD36, resulting in foam cell formation, an early event in atherosclerosis.[7]

An important interaction also occurs between OS and the production of methylated arginines that include asymmetric dimethylarginine (ADMA).[8] Asymmetric dimethylarginine is an endogenous inhibitor of endothelial nitric oxide synthase, and its levels are universally elevated in patients with chronic kidney disease (CKD).[9] OS increases the plasma levels of ADMA by inhibiting the activity of dimethylarginine dimethylaminohydrolase, the major enzyme responsible for ADMA metabolism. OS also up-regulates the expression of protein arginine methyltransferases, the enzymes that methylate arginine residues on proteins.[8,10] Plasma ADMA levels predict the presence of cardiovascular disease (CVD) and all-cause mortality in the normal population and in patients with CKD.[11]

In a remnant kidney model of CKD, the advanced oxidation protein products accelerated renal fibrosis, suggesting a deleterious effect of OS on CKD progression.[12] OS is highly prevalent in all stages of CKD[13-15] and therefore represents a logical therapeutic target.

STUDIES IN THE GENERAL POPULATION

Despite the compelling clinical and experimental data, large randomized, controlled studies in the general population using antioxidant vitamins that include vitamin C and vitamin E (α-tocopherol) failed to show an improvement in the primary or secondary cardiovascular endpoints (or in overall mortality).[16-18] Even in patients with mild to moderate renal insufficiency, treatment with 400 IU of vitamin E in the HOPE study had no beneficial effect on cardiovascular endpoints or proteinuria in a group of high-risk patients.[19] Before attempting to interpret these studies, their limitations must be noted: First, none of these studies actually measured any parameters of OS; the effectiveness of the antioxidant intervention in these studies is not known, partly due to the lack of an easily measurable, standardized, and widely available marker of OS for clinical use.[20] This is complicated by the fact that none of the available markers of OS have been prospectively shown to predict adverse cardiovascular outcome or mortality. Second, the optimum dose of vitamin E is not known. The doses used in the cited studies failed to reduce urinary 8-isoprostanes, a marker of lipid peroxidation, in healthy smokers.[21] A dose of 300 mg/day (equivalent to 660 IU/day) of synthetic vitamin E given to 10 healthy subjects failed to increase plasma total antioxidant activity despite a 30% rise in plasma levels.[22] Third, the bioavailability of vitamin E is highly variable and is regulated by α-tocopherol transfer protein. Genetic factors account for up 22% of the total variance in serum α-tocopherol levels.[23] Furthermore, serum α-tocopherol concentrations correlate poorly with dietary intake. Increased serum levels are seen with rising serum lipid levels, whereas smoking decreases the α-tocopherol bioavailability.[24] The attainment of an effective plasma level can only be ensured by measuring serum α-tocopherol levels, and this was not done in large trials. Establishing the relationship between a reduction in oxidative stress parameters (if any) and plasma levels of α-tocopherol in properly controlled dose-response studies in a group of subjects with oxidative stress is needed but absent. Last, several antihypertensive agents exhibit clinically significant antioxidant properties, and some of their apparent blood pressure-independent beneficial effects in CVD seen in large clinical trials may in fact be due to antioxidant properties. Therefore, interventional studies to test the antioxidant hypothesis should not be limited to testing vitamins and their analogues.

STUDIES IN PATIENTS WITH CHRONIC KIDNEY DISEASE

Most studies of CKD patients have been carried out in dialysis-dependent patients. They can be divided into two main categories: studies that used systemic vitamin E and studies that used vitamin E-coated hemodialysis membranes. Among the latter (Table 65-1), only two studies used reasonable surrogate clinical endpoints of CVD, namely the progression of aortic calcification[25] and changes in carotid intimal thickness.[26] The remainder used biochemical parameters of OS or immunologic parameters related to inflammatory responses to the hemodialysis membrane exposure, which is a measure of membrane biocompatibility.[27-29] Exposure of the patient's blood to an artificial membrane (and possibly back-diffusion of pyrogens or endotoxins in the dialysate) elicits a strong cellular immunologic response, manifested by leukopenia, complement activation, and production of free oxygen radicals by the activated white blood cells.[30] The hemodialysis procedure itself can contribute to OS and endothelial dysfunction.[31] To ameliorate hemodialysis-induced OS, many manufacturers offer vitamin E-coated dialyzers. In these dialyzers α-tocopherol is bonded to a cellulose- or polysulfone-based membrane. The membrane has other

modifications that affect its function and biocompatibility.[32] The inner surface of the hollow fiber is bound, via an acrylic polymer, to a complement-inhibiting fluororesin polymer and to an oleyl alcohol chain that inhibits platelet aggregation. The oleyl alcohol chain itself is bonded to α-tocopherol by hydrophobic-hydrophobic bonds. These modifications decrease the number of hydroxyl groups in the cellulose membrane and thereby increase its biocompatibility. Several studies have shown a beneficial effect of vitamin E-coated dialyzers on various parameters of OS and immunologic reaction to hemodialysis. Most of these studies, however, are small, unblinded, and poorly controlled; a critical flaw is that most have used less biocompatible membranes as controls. Furthermore, the clinical relevance of the measured biomarkers in these studies is not known. Although the concept of vitamin E-coated membranes is interesting, larger randomized, controlled studies with hard clinical endpoints are needed to prove their utility; current evidence does not support their use in routine clinical practice at present.

Table 65-2 lists studies that have examined systemic antioxidant agents, including N-acetylcysteine, α-tocopherol, and antihypertensive agents with antioxidant activity. The Secondary Prevention with Antioxidants of Cardiovascular disease in End-stage renal disease (SPACE) trial randomized 196 high-risk hemodialysis patients who had underlying CVD to either 800 IU/day of α-tocopherol or a placebo for a median follow-up of 519 days. The patients treated with α-tocopherol had a 54% relative-risk reduction in the primary endpoint of new cardiovascular events and acute myocardial infarction; the difference was statistically significant, but there was no difference in fatal myocardial infarction, CVD mortality, and all-cause

Table 65-1   Selected Studies of Vitamin E-Coated Hemodialysis Membranes

Year	Control Membrane	N	Duration	Study Design	Outcome
2006	Polysynthane	20	2 mo	Randomized	↓OS parameters and cytokines[43] greater ↓ with IV vitamin C
2005	PS	31	18 mo	RCT, crossover	↓OxLDL, MDA-LDL, ADMA[44]
2004	PS and hemophane	14	3 mo	Crossover	↓ Monocyte CD40, CD86; ↑lectin-induced T-cell proliferation[45]
2003	Cellulose	34	1 yr	Randomized	↓Carotid IMT, RBC viscosity, erythropoietin requirement[26]
2002	CA	8	6 mo	Randomized	↓Jun N-terminal kinase activation[46]
2002	Cellulose	10	3 mo	Randomized, crossover	↓Leukopenia, LDL oxidation, LDL, PMN superoxide generation[47]
2001	AN*	16	2 mo	Randomized, crossover	↓Intradialytic elastase, vitamin C oxidation; ↑basal vitamin C[48]
2000	Cellulose	7	10 wk	Randomized, crossover	↓Neutropenia, C3a, PMN activation, MPO[49]
2000	Various	110	2-9 mo	Randomized, crossover Cross-sectional	↓Leukocyte DNA 8-oH2dG, granulocyte ROS generation[50]
1999	Cellulose	50	2 yr	Randomized	↓LDL oxidation, MDA, % increase in aortic calcification[25]

*Synthetic biocompatible membrane.
ADMA, asymmetric dimethylarginine; AN, acylonitrile and metalylsulfonate copolymer; CA, cellulose acetate; IMT, intimal media thickness; IV, Intravenous; LDL, low-density lipoprotein; MDA, malondialdehyde; MPO, myeloperoxidase; OS, oxidative stress; OxLDL, oxidized LDL; PMN, polymorphonuclear leukocytes; PS, polysulfone; RBC, red blood cell; RCT, randomized controlled trial; ROS, reactive oxygen species; 8-oH2dG, 8-hydroxy, 2′deoxyguanosine.

Table 65-2   Selected Studies of Systemic Antioxidant Therapy in ESRD Patients

Year	N	Intervention	Duration	Study Design	Outcome
2006	19	Valsartan and amlo-dipine	6 wk	Randomized, double-blind, crossover	↓ OS parameters, ADMA, SDMA both drugs[41]
2006	29	α-Tocopherol 400 mg	5 wk	Randomized	No effect on CRP, ICAM-1, E-selectin, PAPP-A[51]
2006	47	α-Tocopherol 300 mg daily	20 wk	Randomized, placebo-controlled	↓ EOF, LPO[52]
2005	44	Atorvastatin ± α-tocopherol 800 IU	12 wk	Randomized, double-blind, placebo-controlled	↓ In vitro LDL oxidizability; no effect on oxLDL[53]
2003	134	N-Acetylcysteine 1200 mg daily	14.5 mo	Randomized, placebo-controlled	↓ Composite CVD events; no effect on mortality[34]
2002	196	α-Tocopherol 800 IU daily	519 days	Randomized, placebo-controlled	↓ MI, CVD events; no effect on mortality[33]
2000	22	α-Tocopherol 1200 IU daily	1 dose	Randomized, crossover	↓ IV iron-induced LPO[54]
1985	30	α-Tocopherol 600 mg daily	30 days	Randomized	↑ Hematocrit[55]
1984	35	α-Tocopherol 400 IU daily	20 wk	Randomized, placebo-controlled	No effect on hematocrit[56]

ADMA, asymmetric dimethylarginine; CRP, C-reactive protein; CVD, cardiovascular disease; EOF, erythrocyte osmotic fragility; ESRD, end-stage renal disease; ICAM-1, intercellular adhesion molecule-1; IV, intravenous; LPO, lipid peroxidation; MI, myocardial infarction; OS, oxidative stress; oxLDL, oxidized LDL; PAPP-A, pregnancy-associated plasma protein-A; RCT, randomized controlled trial; SDMA, symmetric dimethylarginine.

mortality among the treatment groups.[33] The second trial randomized 134 hemodialysis patients to receive either a reduced thiol-containing compound N-acetylcysteine or a placebo.[34] After a median follow-up of 14.5 months, the group treated with N-acetylcysteine had a statistically significant, 40% relative-risk reduction in the primary endpoint of cardiovascular events. There was, however, no difference in CVD mortality or death from any cause. The effects of these interventions on parameters of oxidative stress were not measured in either of these studies. Although these studies are encouraging because they demonstrate that either of two chemically dissimilar drugs that may be antioxidants do in fact reduce new myocardial infarctions, the results are presently inadequate to warrant the widespread use of antioxidant therapy in this patient population. Larger randomized studies will be needed to determine the true extent of any beneficial effect of such interventions, not only on reducing cardiovascular events, but also on decreasing overall mortality.

Antagonists of the renin-angiotensin-aldosterone system reduce oxidative stress in animal models of hypertension.[35] Moreover, some widely used antihypertensive drugs have a biochemical configuration that confers a direct antioxidant effect in vitro, including amlodipine,[36] carvedilol,[37] and hydralazine.[38] None of these have been widely studied as antioxidant strategies in CKD patients. The renin-angiotensin-aldosterone system antagonists block angiotensin II-induced superoxide generation by nicotinamide adenine dinucleotide phosphate oxidase.[39] The dihydropyridine calcium channel blocker amlodipine scavenges superoxide by donating two extractable protons in its dihydropyridine ring.[40] The angiotensin receptor blocker valsartan and amlodipine reduces OS in patients on hemodialy-

sis independent of the blood pressure-lowering effects of these drugs.[41] This reduction in OS is associated with a parallel reduction in plasma levels of ADMA and symmetric dimethylarginine; this suggests a strong link between OS and methylarginine metabolism. Because ADMA is one of the strongest predictors of CVD and mortality, it represents a novel therapeutic target for further studies with clinical endpoints.

SUMMARY

Oxidative stress is highly prevalent at all stages of CKD. It may contribute to the very high CVD mortality and the progressive deterioration in renal function. End-stage renal disease patients on maintenance hemodialysis are exposed to a multitude of unique stimuli that exacerbate OS. Although large randomized trials in the general population using α-tocopherol have been disappointing, this type of therapeutic intervention may be more relevant to CKD patients, who have high levels of OS. Given the complexity of OS, no single intervention may be adequate to address the many contributing mechanisms. Multiple agents administered systemically or modifications of the dialysis procedure may be needed to establish benefit. Novel agents, such as superoxide dismutase and glutathione peroxidase mimetics, should be explored because they exhibit strong antioxidant activity in experimental models of OS.[42] Large randomized controlled trials with CVD and overall mortality as endpoints are needed to confirm the beneficial effects of antioxidant therapy seen in small trials. It is my opinion that the strength of current evidence does not support the use of antioxidant therapy in patients with CKD.

References

1. Cai H, Li Z, Dikalov S, et al: NAD(P)H oxidase-derived hydrogen peroxide mediates endothelial nitric oxide production in response to angiotensin II. J Biol Chem 2002;277:48311–48317.
2. Felty Q, Xiong WC, Sun D, et al: Estrogen-induced mitochondrial reactive oxygen species as signal-transducing messengers. Biochemistry 2005;44:6900–6909.
3. Waypa GB, Marks JD, Mack MM, et al: Mitochondrial reactive oxygen species trigger calcium increases during hypoxia in pulmonary arterial myocytes. Circ Res 2002;91:719–726.
4. Wilcox CS: Oxidative stress and nitric oxide deficiency in the kidney: A critical link to hypertension? Am J Physiol Regul Integr Comp Physiol 2005;289:R913–R935.
5. Gill PS, Wilcox CS: NADPH oxidases in the kidney. Antioxid Redox Signal 2006;8:1597–1607.
6. Zou M, Martin C, Ullrich V: Tyrosine nitration as a mechanism of selective inactivation of prostacyclin synthase by peroxynitrite. Biol Chem 1997;378:707–713.
7. Podrez EA, Poliakov E, Shen Z, et al: A novel family of atherogenic oxidized phospholipids promotes macrophage foam cell formation via the scavenger receptor CD36 and is enriched in atherosclerotic lesions. J Biol Chem 2002;277:38517–38523.
8. Sydow K, Munzel T: ADMA and oxidative stress. Atherosclerosis 2003;4(Suppl):41–51.
9. Vallance P, Leone A, Calver A, et al: Accumulation of an endogenous inhibitor of nitric oxide synthesis in chronic renal failure. Lancet 1992;339:572–575.
10. Leiper J, Vallance P: New tricks from an old dog: Nitric oxide–independent effects of dimethylarginine dimethylaminohydrolase. Arterioscler Thromb Vasc Biol 2006;26:1419–1420.
11. Valkonen VP, Paiva H, Salonen JT, et al: Risk of acute coronary events and serum concentration of asymmetrical dimethylarginine. Lancet 2001;358:2127–2128.
12. Li HY, Hou FF, Zhang X, et al: Advanced oxidation protein products accelerate renal fibrosis in a remnant kidney model. J Am Soc Nephrol 2007;18:528–538.
13. Ikizler TA, Morrow JD, Roberts LJ, et al: Plasma F_2-isoprostane levels are elevated in chronic hemodialysis patients. Clin Nephrol 2002;58:190–197.
14. Oberg BP, McMenamin E, Lucas FL, et al: Increased prevalence of oxidant stress and inflammation in patients with moderate to severe chronic kidney disease. Kidney Int 2004;65:1009–1016.
15. Modlinger PS, Wilcox CS, Aslam S: Nitric oxide, oxidative stress, and progression of chronic renal failure. Semin Nephrol 2004;24:354–365.
16. GISSI-Prevenzione Investigators: Dietary supplementation with n-3 polyunsaturated fatty acids and vitamin E after myocardial infarction: Results of the GISSI-Prevenzione trial. Lancet 1999;354:447–455.
17. MRC/BHF Heart Protection Study: Study of antioxidant vitamin supplementation in 20,536 high-risk individuals: A randomised placebo-controlled trial. Lancet 2002;360:23–33.
18. Lonn EM, Yusuf S, Dzavik V, et al: Effects of ramipril and vitamin E on atherosclerosis: The Study to Evaluate Carotid Ultrasound changes in patients treated with Ramipril and vitamin E (SECURE). Circulation 2001;103:919–925.
19. Mann JF, Lonn EM, Yi Q, et al: Effects of vitamin E on cardiovascular outcomes in people with mild-to-moderate renal insufficiency: Results of the HOPE Study. Kidney Int 2004;65:1375–1380.
20. Dikalov S, Griendling KK, Harrison DG: Measurement of reactive oxygen species in cardiovascular studies. Hypertension 2007;49:717–727.
21. Patrignani P, Panara MR, Tacconelli S, et al: Effects of vitamin E supplementation on F_2-isoprostane and thromboxane biosynthesis in healthy cigarette smokers. Circulation 2000102:539–545.
22. Violi F, Micheletta F, Iuliano L: Antioxidant strategy for cardiovascular disease. Lancet 2001;357:1704.
23. Gueguen S, Leroy P, Gueguen R, et al: Genetic and environmental contributions to serum retinol and α-tocopherol concentrations: The Stanislas Family Study. Am J Clin Nutr 2005;81:1034–1044.
24. Munro LH, Burton G, Kelly FJ: Plasma RRR-α-tocopherol concentrations are lower in smokers than in non-smokers after ingestion of a similar oral load of this antioxidant vitamin. Clin Sci (Lond) 1997;92:87–93.
25. Mune M, Yukawa S, Kishino M, et al: Effect of vitamin E on lipid metabolism and atherosclerosis in ESRD patients. Kidney Int 1999;71(Suppl):S126–S129.
26. Kobayashi S, Moriya H, Aso K, et al: Vitamin E-bonded hemodialyzer improves atherosclerosis associated with a rheological improvement of circulating red blood cells. Kidney Int 2003;63:1881–1887.
27. Cheung AK, Leypoldt JK: The hemodialysis membranes: A historical perspective, current state and future prospect. Semin Nephrol 1997;17:196–213.
28. Gutierrez A, Alvestrand A, Bergstrom J, et al: Biocompatibility of hemodialysis membranes: A study in healthy subjects. Blood Purif 1994;12:95–105.
29. Hakim RM: Clinical sequelae of complement activation in hemodialysis. Clin Nephrol 1986;26(Suppl 1):S9–S12.
30. Chenoweth DE, Cheung AK, Henderson LW: Anaphylatoxin formation during hemodialysis: Effects of different dialyzer membranes. Kidney Int 1983;24:764–769.
31. Miyazaki H, Matsuoka H, Itabe H, et al: Hemodialysis impairs endothelial function via oxidative stress: Effects of vitamin E-coated dialyzer. Circulation 2000;101:1002–1006.
32. Sasaki M, Hosoya N, Saruhashi M: Vitamin E modified cellulose membrane. Artif Organs 2000;24:779–789.
33. Boaz M, Smetana S, Weinstein T, et al: Secondary prevention with antioxidants of cardiovascular disease in endstage renal disease (SPACE): Randomised placebo-controlled trial. Lancet 2000;356:1213–1218.
34. Tepel M, van der Giet M, Statz M, et al: The antioxidant acetylcysteine reduces cardiovascular events in patients with end-stage renal failure: A randomized, controlled trial. Circulation 2003;107:992–995.
35. Welch WJ, Wilcox CS: AT_1 receptor antagonist combats oxidative stress and restores nitric oxide signaling in the SHR. Kidney Int 2001;59:1257–1263.
36. Muda P, Kampus P, Zilmer M, et al: Effect of antihypertensive treatment with candesartan or amlodipine on glutathione and its redox status, homocysteine and vitamin concentrations in patients with essential hypertension. J Hypertens 2005;23:105–112.
37. Dandona P, Ghanim H, Brooks DP: Antioxidant activity of carvedilol in cardiovascular disease. J Hypertens 2007;25:731–741.
38. Daiber A, Mulsch A, Hink U, et al: The oxidative stress concept of nitrate tolerance and the antioxidant properties of hydralazine. Am J Cardiol 2005;96:25–36.
39. Chabrashvili T, Kitiyakara C, Blau J, et al: Effects of ANG II type 1 and 2 receptors on oxidative stress, renal NADPH oxidase, and SOD expression. Am J Physiol Regul Integr Comp Physiol 2003;285:R117–R124.
40. Mason RP, Walter MF, Trumbore MW, et al: Membrane antioxidant effects of the charged dihydropyridine calcium antagonist amlodipine. J Mol Cell Cardiol 1999;31:275–281.
41. Aslam S, Santha T, Leone A, et al: Effects of amlodipine and valsartan on oxidative stress and plasma methylarginines in endstage renal disease patients on hemodialysis. Kidney Int 2006;70:2109–2115.

42. Schnackenberg CG, Wilcox CS: Two-week administration of tempol attenuates both hypertension and renal excretion of 8-Iso prostaglandin f2(. Hypertension 1999;33:424–428.

43. Yang CC, Hsu SP, Wu MS, et al: Effects of vitamin C infusion and vitamin E-coated membrane on hemodialysis-induced oxidative stress. Kidney Int 2006;69:706–714.

44. Morimoto H, Nakao K, Fukuoka K, et al: Long-term use of vitamin E-coated polysulfone membrane reduces oxidative stress markers in haemodialysis patients. Nephrol Dial Transplant 2005;20:2775–2782.

45. Betjes MG, Hoekstra FM, Klepper M, et al: Vitamin E-coated dialyzer membranes downregulate expression of monocyte adhesion and co-stimulatory molecules. Blood Purif 2004;22:510–517.

46. Pertosa G, Grandaliano G, Soccio M, et al: Vitamin E-modified filters modulate *Jun* N-terminal kinase activation in peripheral blood mononuclear cells. Kidney Int 2002;62:602–610.

47. Tsuruoka S, Kawaguchi A, Nishiki K, et al: Vitamin E-bonded hemodialyzer improves neutrophil function and oxidative stress in patients with end-stage renal failure. Am J Kidney Dis 2002;39:127–133.

48. Clermont G, Lecour S, Cabanne JF, et al: Vitamin E-coated dialyzer reduces oxidative stress in hemodialysis patients. Free Radic Biol Med 2001;31:233–241.

49. Omata M, Higuchi C, Demura R, et al: Reduction of neutrophil activation by vitamin E modified dialyzer membranes. Nephron 2000;85:221–231.

50. Tarng DC, Huang TP, Liu TY, et al: Effect of vitamin E-bonded membrane on the 8-hydroxy 2′-deoxyguanosine level in leukocyte DNA of hemodialysis patients. Kidney Int 2000;58:790–799.

51. Hodkova M, Dusilova-Sulkova S, Kalousova M, et al: Influence of oral vitamin E therapy on micro-inflammation and cardiovascular disease markers in chronic hemodialysis patients. Ren Fail 2006;28:395–399.

52. Uzum A, Toprak O, Gumustas MK, et al: Effect of vitamin E therapy on oxidative stress and erythrocyte osmotic fragility in patients on peritoneal dialysis and hemodialysis. J Nephrol 2006;19:739–745.

53. Diepeveen SH, Verhoeven GW, Van Der PJ, et al: Effects of atorvastatin and vitamin E on lipoproteins and oxidative stress in dialysis patients: A randomized, controlled trial. J Intern Med 2005;257:438–445.

54. Roob JM, Khoschsorur G, Tiran A, et al: Vitamin E attenuates oxidative stress induced by intravenous iron in patients on hemodialysis. J Am Soc Nephrol 2000;11:539–549.

55. Ono K: Effects of large dose vitamin E supplementation on anemia in hemodialysis patients. Nephron 1985;40:440–445.

56. Sinsakul V, Drake JR, Leavitt JN Jr, et al: Lack of effect of vitamin E therapy on the anemia of patients receiving hemodialysis. Am J Clin Nutr 1984;39:223–226.

Further Reading

Dikalov S, Griendling KK, Harrison DG: Measurement of reactive oxygen species in cardiovascular studies. Hypertension 2007;49:717–727.

Gordon CA, Himmelfarb J: Antioxidant therapy in uremia: Evidence-based medicine? Semin Dial 2004;17:327–332.

Leiper J, Vallance P: New tricks from an old dog: Nitric oxide-independent effects of dimethylarginine dimethylaminohydrolase. Arterioscler Thromb Vasc Biol 2006;26:1419–1420.

Modlinger PS, Wilcox CS, Aslam S: Nitric oxide, oxidative stress, and progression of chronic renal failure. Semin Nephrol 2004;24:354–365.

Wilcox CS: Oxidative stress and nitric oxide deficiency in the kidney: A critical link to hypertension? Am J Physiol Regul Integr Comp Physiol 2005;289:R913–R935.

Chapter 66

Nutritional Therapy of Patients with Chronic Kidney Disease and Its Impact on Progressive Renal Insufficiency

Tahsin Masud and William E. Mitch

CHAPTER CONTENTS

The cost of care for patients with chronic kidney disease (CKD) and end-stage renal disease (ESRD) is a huge economic burden. In 2004, CKD and ESRD patients together consumed 23.7% of Medicare expenses, although they accounted for only 5.7% and 1.1% of the Medicare population, respectively.[1] There are now 385,000 people in the United States with a diagnosis of ESRD, but 19.2 million Americans are living with some form of CKD, constituting 11% of the adult U.S. population. For this reason the Centers for Disease Control has labeled CKD as a "public health disease that needs a public health action plan."[2] It is not only about the numbers: CKD patients have premature morbidity, a poor quality of life, and higher mortality. Therefore, we believe all methods should be used to slow the progression of renal disease and delay the onset of dialysis for CKD patients. The available methods include maintaining stringent control of blood pressure, use of angiotensin-converting enzyme inhibitors and angiotensin receptor blockers, maintaining glycemic control, targeting cardiovascular risk factors, and using controlled-protein diets to preserve the nutritional status of these patients. Before discussing the nutritional requirements of patients with CKD and the role of low-protein diets in the progression of renal disease, we clarify the commonly misunderstood term malnutrition in renal patients.

MALNUTRITION IN RENAL DISEASE

Malnutrition refers to abnormalities caused by an insufficient or imbalanced diet; hence, it should be cured simply by increasing dietary protein. Abundant evidence shows that patients with CKD, including those treated by peritoneal dialysis or hemodialysis, have decreased body weight and subnormal values of serum proteins.[3–5] The mechanisms for these abnormalities are complex and have not been fully identified, but assigning their cause to protein-energy malnutrition alone is misleading because they frequently cannot be overcome simply by supplying more food or altering the composition of the diet. Studies of rodents with experimental uremia and investigations of patients with kidney failure have suggested several other mechanisms that can account for fatigue, loss of lean body mass, and low serum proteins, the abnormalities mistakenly assigned to malnutrition (Fig. 66-1).[6]

Hypoalbuminemia and Inflammation

A low serum albumin level is clinically important because it is the strongest independent predictor of total and cardiovascular mortality in ESRD patients.[4,5] Much has been made of low serum albumin being an index of malnutrition, yet there are several other causes besides malnutrition for low serum albumin and loss of protein stores in renal patients.[6] The serum albumin concentration is influenced by age, fluid overload, capillary leakage, and inflammation in addition to the amount of dietary protein consumed.[7,8] Regarding its clinical relevance, there is a strong association between the severity of atherosclerosis, a low serum albumin level, and high C-reactive protein level in CKD patients.[9] In incident dialysis patients studied prospectively, malnutrition assessed by means of Subjective Global Assessment is best predicted by levels of C-reactive protein and interleukin-6 but not by serum albumin.[10] In this

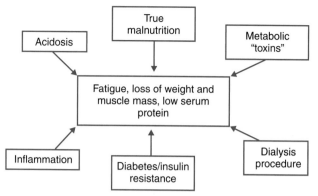

Figure 66-1   Factors leading to the fatigue, loss of lean body mass, and low serum proteins associated with loss of kidney function.

study, low serum albumin predicted mortality and a high interleukin-6 was the most reliable predictor of the presence of cardiovascular disease.[10] In dialysis patients, albumin generation and serum albumin levels are negatively correlated with markers of inflammation, including C-reactive protein, fibrinogen, and interleukin-6.[11] Contact of blood with "foreign" surfaces, such as the hemodialyzer membrane or peritoneal dialysate, activates several humoral and cellular pathways, with higher levels of C-reactive protein and other pro-inflammatory cytokines.[11,12] The common thread in inflammatory conditions that cause loss of muscle mass is activation of protein breakdown. This has been demonstrated repeatedly in models of sepsis and inflammatory conditions.[13] These findings suggest that inflammation, mediated by pro-inflammatory cytokines, causes hypoalbuminemia, loss of lean body mass, and the development of cardiovascular disease in CKD patients. In summary, a normal or low serum albumin concentration may not accurately reflect total albumin mass and should not be used as the sole indicator of protein stores.

Metabolic Acidosis

Metabolic acidosis is common in kidney failure; it acts to stimulate the irreversible destruction of the essential, branched-chain amino acids and accelerates the degradation of protein, especially of muscles.[14,15] Moreover, metabolic acidosis can cause endocrine abnormalities, including insulin resistance, decreased serum leptin level, and inflammation, among patients with CKD.[16] Correction of acidosis in patients treated by chronic ambulatory peritoneal dialysis suppresses the ubiquitin-proteasome proteolytic system and leads to gain of body weight.[17] Evidence also indicates that acidosis contributes to the low level of serum albumin in dialysis patients.[18,19] Therefore, metabolic acidosis in CKD patients should be corrected because it contributes substantially to the abnormalities presumed to be caused by malnutrition.

Insulin Resistance

Because diabetes is a common cause of CKD and uremia causes resistance to the hypoglycemic action of insulin, it is likely that diabetes or insulin resistance causes abnormalities similar to those caused by malnutrition.[20] Experimentally, acute diabetes mellitus causes rapid loss of body weight and

muscle mass due to activation of the ubiquitin-proteasome proteolytic system in muscle.[21] These catabolic responses are rapidly reversed by insulin but are independent of the acidosis of acute diabetes.[22]

Another potential cause of ESRD-associated abnormalities in weight, muscle mass, and serum proteins is the hodgepodge of accumulated waste products and metabolic abnormalities caused by the loss of kidney function. Again, this mechanism is not directly connected to an inadequate diet. In fact, the contrary is true because an excess of protein-rich foods only increases the accumulation of waste products such as phosphates, acid, and nitrogen-containing products.[23] To date, no cause-and-effect association has been demonstrated between the accumulation of nitrogen-containing waste products and a specific syndrome, despite intriguing investigations about links between unidentified "middle molecules" and depressed appetite.[24]

In summary, there are several adverse consequences of CKD, including the constellation of signs and symptoms glossed over as malnutrition. However, assigning these abnormalities to protein-energy malnutrition alone is misleading because these cannot be overcome by simply supplying more food.

ASSESSMENT OF NUTRITIONAL STATUS IN RENAL DISEASES

Because loss of lean body mass is a serious concern for patients with CKD, it is important to use longitudinal assessments of nutritional status to recognize substrate deficiencies early. No single method of assessment has been validated to accurately evaluate variables that affect nutritional status, so a number of indices are needed to define the nutritional status of patients (Box 66-1).

There must be a medical history for the type of renal disease and comorbid conditions, plus a physical examination. The dietary history should include the amount and patterns of nutrient intake, and a dietitian should obtain information about socioeconomic circumstances that could interfere with dietary needs. The energy level, appetite, physical activity, use of medications, and the use of dietary and herbal supplements, alcohol, and illicit drugs must also be documented.[25]

The most common methods for estimating intake in patients with renal disease are dietary recalls, dietary diaries, and determination of protein equivalent of nitrogen appearance (PNA). The dietary recall (usually obtained for the previous 24 hr) is a simple, rapid method of obtaining a crude assessment of dietary intake.[26] Dietary diaries are written reports of foods consumed during a specified length of time (i.e., 3–7 days). However, the validity and reliability of dietary interviews and diaries depend on the patient's ability to provide accurate data and the ability of the dietitian to conduct detailed and probing interviews.

Protein Equivalent of Nitrogen Appearance

This method for estimating protein intake is based on the concept that ingested nitrogen is equal to total nitrogen excretion if there is no change in body nitrogen pool. Ingested protein plus the products arising from endogenous protein are metabolized to several nitrogenous products (e.g., urea,

Box 66-1 Categories of Nutritional Assessment in Chronic Kidney Disease Patients

Clinical
Medical history
Physical examination
Psychosocial history
Dietary history
  Diet history
  Appetite assessment
  Food habits and patterns
  Dietary nutrient intake
  Food intake records and dietary recall
Protein equivalent of total nitrogen appearance (PNA)
Biochemical measurements
  Serum albumin, serum prealbumin, serum transferrin
  Serum bicarbonate, serum potassium, serum glucose
  Serum creatinine, urea nitrogen, calcium and phosphorus
  Serum cholesterol
Subjective Global Assessment (SGA)
Body composition
Anthropometric measurements
Creatinine kinetics
Bioelectrical impedance
Dual energy x-ray absorptiometry (DEXA)
Near infrared interactance
Total body nitrogen, total body potassium

Categories shown in italics are not routinely recommended.

Box 66-2 Estimation of Protein Intake for a Patient Prescribed a Diet Containing 1 g protein/kg/day

A patient weighs 70 kg and the 24-hr urinary collection contains: volume 2400 mL, creatinine 1100 mg, protein 7 g, urea nitrogen 7.9 g

Nitrogen balance (B_N) = nitrogen intake (IN) − urea nitrogen appearance (U) − nonurea nitrogen excretion (NUN)*

$$B_N = IN - U - NUN$$

If the patient is in steady state and is compliant, nitrogen input equals output, therefore:

$$IN = U + NUN$$
$$= 7.9 \text{ g N/day} +$$
$$(70 \text{ kg} \times 0.031 \text{ g N/kg/day} +$$
$$7 \text{ g urinary protein} \times 0.16)$$
$$= 7.9 \text{ g N/day} + (2.17 \text{ g N/kg/day} +$$
$$1.12 \text{ g N/kg/day})$$
$$= 11.19 \text{ g N/day}$$

Assuming that protein is 16% nitrogen (i.e. conversion factor is 1/0.16 = 6/25), the patient is eating:
11.19 × 6.25 = 70 g protein/day

*Nitrogen in feces, urine creatinine, uric acid, other unmeasured nitrogen-containing compounds, and urinary protein > 5 g.

amino acids, peptides, urate, and creatinine). If nitrogen balance is neutral (neither catabolism nor anabolism), the nitrogenous products that are removed from the body through urine, stool, and skin plus any change in the body's urea nitrogen pool are equal to the nitrogen intake. Because urea is the principal nitrogen waste product, protein intake in stable CKD patients can be estimated from the urea appearance rate in urine.[27,28] The urea nitrogen appearance rate (i.e., urine urea excretion plus accumulation) parallels protein intake, but nonurea nitrogen excretion (i.e., the nitrogen in feces and urinary creatinine, uric acid, ammonia, peptides, and so forth) does not vary substantially with dietary protein; it averages 0.031 g N/kg daily.

In the steady state (when blood urea nitrogen and weight are constant), the urea nitrogen appearance equals urinary urea nitrogen excretion. Consequently, nitrogen intake equals urinary urea nitrogen plus 0.031 g N/kg. To convert grams of nitrogen into its protein equivalent (PNA), multiply it by 6.25, because proteins on average consist of 16% nitrogen. This method of estimating protein intake can be used for assessment of compliance with a prescribed diet, as illustrated by the example in Box 66-2.

There are important limitations in interpreting urea-derived estimates of dietary protein intake. First, in catabolic states (e.g., acidosis, infection), endogenous protein breakdown can increase urea appearance so PNA will exceed protein intake estimates. Conversely, when a patient becomes anabolic, PNA will underestimate actual protein intake. Second, day-to-day variations in protein intake are reflected rapidly by the PNA, so a single measurement may not tell us about average

protein intake over the month. Finally, protein nitrogen appearance may not accurately estimate intake at extremes of protein intake. This is due to increased nitrogen losses through unmeasured pathways of excretion at higher protein intake and greater endogenous protein catabolism at lower protein intake.[29] Regardless, this method is much more accurate and reproducible than dietary history or recall methods.

Biochemical Values and Nutritional Assessment

Serum levels of albumin and prealbumin are often used as biochemical markers to assess visceral protein stores, to monitor the adequacy of responses to a nutritional intervention, and to identify patients who are at risk for complications or are responding poorly to medical/surgical treatment. However, there is substantial evidence that a low serum albumin level in CKD patients is generally due to inflammation rather than decreased dietary protein.[30] When comparative analysis of predictors of outcome in ESRD was studied, no significant difference in serum albumin levels was found between malnourished and well-nourished ESRD patients.[31] The serum prealbumin concentration also reflects its role as a negative acute-phase reactant; it is influenced by inflammation and is thus considered to be no more sensitive or accurate than serum albumin as a marker of visceral protein stores.[26]

Serum transferrin concentration is frequently reduced in renal failure independent of malnutrition, perhaps due to fluctuation in iron stores. Serum transferrin rises in iron deficiency, in pregnancy, and in the early phases of acute hepatitis; it decreases with certain chronic infections, liver diseases, cancer, and iron loading. In summary, no single serum protein measurement is ideal for detecting protein malnutrition.

Low serum bicarbonate levels in CKD patients usually reflect development of metabolic acidosis. In CKD and dialysis patients a low serum bicarbonate is also indicative of the amount of protein intake, because metabolism of amino acids, particularly cysteine and methionine, generates protons. As noted, metabolic acidosis affects nutrition by stimulating protein catabolism, and correction of acidosis decreases whole-body protein degradation.[32] The serum creatinine level in CKD patients is reflective of the estimated glomerular filtration rate (GFR), but in ESRD patients it may have some nutritional significance as a reflection of muscle mass and a decrease in meat in the diet. Likewise, a low serum potassium level in CKD patients is mostly due to the use of diuretics, whereas in ESRD patients this finding should raise the suspicion of a poor nutritional intake.

Anthropometrics are used to assess adipose stores and lean body mass. This series of noninvasive, inexpensive measurements, which include body weight, percent of usual weight, skeletal frame size, body mass index, body fat, and fat-free mass, can be determined reliably.[33] A decline in anthropometric measurements can detect a loss of lean body mass during long-term evaluations. The key is to have consistency in the measurements, preferably by having them performed by a single individual. Unfortunately, very little data are available on how closely subnormal anthropometric values correlate with an adverse clinical outcome in CKD patients, and the techniques have been used only for research purposes. Cross-sectional studies of large groups of patients do show a linkage between large body size and reduced risk of mortality in hemodialysis patients.[34,35] Body size is best estimated by body mass index, a measure of body fat based on height and weight that applies to both adult men and women. On the other hand, increased body mass index has been shown to be an independent risk factor for appearance of proteinuria, poor control of hypertension, adverse cardiovascular and mortality outcomes, and the progression of CKD.[36–39]

Subjective Global Assessment

Subjective Global Assessment is a nutritional assessment technique based on evaluating subjective and objective patient information, including medical history and physical examination, gastrointestinal symptoms, body weight patterns, and patient functional capacity, plus the presence of comorbid conditions that could affect nutritional requirements. The patient is assigned to one of the three nutritional status groups: (A) well nourished, (B) mildly to moderately malnourished, or (C) severely malnourished. The Subjective Global Assessment method was developed for hospitalized patients but has been used to assess nutritional status and predict increased risk of morbidity and mortality in CKD and ESRD patients.[40–42] Limitations of the Subjective Global Assessment include a heavy reliance on subjective judgment; it may not identify functional impairment due to malnutrition, and it also does not identify the type or amount of nutritional support needed to provide repletion of lost body protein stores. In summary, no single parameter has been defined to evaluate the variables that affect the nutritional status of CKD patients. Consequently, we recommend a complete nutritional evaluation using all the categories listed in Box 66-1.

MANAGEMENT OF NUTRITIONAL ISSUES IN CHRONIC KIDNEY DISEASE

The goals of dietary therapy for patients with CKD are to diminish the accumulation of nitrogenous wastes and limit the metabolic disturbances characteristic of uremia, to prevent malnutrition, and to slow the progression of renal failure. Protein-restricted diets improve uremic symptoms because they reduce the levels of uremic toxins, most of which result from the metabolism of protein. A low-protein diet also ameliorates specific complications of CKD, including metabolic acidosis, renal osteodystrophy, hyperkalemia, and hypertension, because a diet that is restricted in protein is invariably restricted in the quantities of sulfates, phosphates, potassium, and sodium eaten each day.[43,44] These considerations explain why dietary protein restriction has been used for decades to treat chronically uremic patients. However, there are some fundamental concerns regarding use of low-protein diets in CKD patients: (1) Do they change the progression of renal failure? (2) Are low-protein diets safe? and (3) Does delaying the start of renal replacement therapy affect patient outcomes?

Low-Protein Diets and Progression of Chronic Renal Failure

A number of studies have examined the influence of dietary protein restriction on the progression of renal disease, but many of these reports suffer from problems in design, differences in measurement of efficacy, a limited sample size, the type of diet, and degree of compliance with the diet.

The randomized, controlled trials that have enrolled only insulin-dependent diabetes patients have shown improved preservation of kidney function in patients assigned to a low-protein diet when compared to patients eating unrestricted amounts of dietary protein.[45–48] The number of diabetic patients studied in these trials was generally small, and the duration of follow-up was short. To examine this question in a larger number of patients, meta-analyses have been used; their results conclude that there is a significant benefit from low-protein diets in preserving the renal function of diabetic patients.[49–51]

Trials enrolling nondiabetic and noninsulin-dependent diabetic CKD patients in a randomized fashion have not consistently demonstrated that dietary protein restriction slows progression, at least when analyzed according to the prescribed diet. In the largest trial to address this question, the Modification of Diet in Renal Disease (MDRD), patients were randomized to protein intakes of 1.3 and 0.6 g/kg per day, with or without aggressive blood pressure control; when renal failure was more advanced, protein intake was 0.6 g protein/kg/day or 0.28 g/kg/day supplemented with ketoacids.[52] The intention-to-treat analysis of the results (i.e., the outcome regardless of whether patients did or did not ingest the prescribed diet) did not demonstrate a statistically significant benefit of the low-protein diet on the rate of loss of GFR. However, when the results were analyzed according to the degree of compliance with the low-protein diet, significant slowing of the loss of GFR was seen, as well as a substantial delay until patients reached the stage of disease when dialysis was required.[53] Similarly, all the other randomized trials (Table 66-1) studying the effect of protein restriction on the progression of renal disease suffered from significant

Table 66-1   Randomized Controlled Trials of Effect of Protein-restricted Diets on the Progression of Renal Failure

Ref.	Patients (N)	Mean Follow-up (mo)	Prescribed Protein for Randomized Groups (g/kg/day)	Actual Protein Intake (g/kg/day)	Outcome of Trial
Jungers et al[120]	14	9	0.6 vs. 0.4 + KA	0.7 vs. 0.4 + KA	Time to dialysis longer and mean slope of 1/S$_{Cr}$ lower in KA group
Bergström et al[121]	16	12–24	Unrestricted vs. 0.4 + EAA	0.86 vs. 0.65	Slope of 1/S$_{Cr}$ and drop in CrCl similar
Ihle et al[122]	64	18	Unrestricted vs. 0.4	>0.75 vs. 0.4	Significantly less decrease in GFR and progression to end-stage in low-protein group
Rosman et al[123]	239	48	Unrestricted vs. 0.4–0.6	No data available	Renal survival better in low-protein group after 2 yr but no difference after 4 yr
Locatelli et al[124]	456	24	1.0 vs. 0.6	0.9 vs. 0.78	No difference in renal survival
William et al[125]	95	19	>0.8 vs. 0.6	1.0–1.14 vs. 0.69	Rate of fall of CrCl and 1/S$_{Cr}$ similar
Klahr et al[52] Study A	585	26	1.3 vs. 0.58	1.1 vs. 0.77	The intention-to-treat analysis revealed no difference in GFR decline; when analyzed by degree of compliance low-protein group has significant slowing in GFR
Study B	255	26	0.58 vs. 0.28 + KA	0.73 vs. 0.48	No difference in slowing of GFR; on secondary analysis lower protein intake caused slower mean decline in GFR but no independent effect of KA
D'Amico et al[126]	128	27	1.0 vs. 0.6	1.1 vs. 0.8	Low-protein group had significant lower risk of progression

CrCl, creatinine clearance; EAA, essential amino acids; GFR, glomerular filtration rate; KA, ketoacids; S$_{Cr}$, serum creatinine.

differences in the prescribed and actual protein intake, thus confounding the interpretation of results.

Other shortcomings of the MDRD trial explain why this study did not find a slowing of loss of the renal function in CKD patients eating low-protein diets. First, the criteria for entering the MDRD study did not include a requirement that patients were, in fact, losing renal function; approximately 15% of the Study A control group had no evidence of progressive loss of GFR. This factor would increase the number of patients required to demonstrate a benefit from dietary manipulations. Second, the overall rate of loss of renal function in this study was slower than predicted.

Third, a disproportionate number of patients (~20%) had polycystic kidney disease. These patients are known to benefit minimally from dietary restriction, at least in terms of slowing progression of renal insufficiency, and so including these patients in the study might have obscured a benefit of the dietary manipulation. Fourth, patients in the MDRD study were not controlled for angiotensin-converting enzyme inhibitor therapy. Because these drugs can slow the loss of kidney function, their random use would make it more difficult to detect any benefit of eating a low-protein diet on preserving residual kidney function. Finally, the MDRD study lasted an average of only 2.2 years. This is important because the patients with modest CKD (Study A) had an initial rapid loss of GFR just after initiation of the low-protein diet followed by a slower loss of GFR. The long-term (up to 6 years) follow-up of patients after completion of the MDRD trial failed to show conclusive benefit of dietary protein restriction on progression of renal insufficiency.[54] However, the patients were not given dietary protein targets nor was there any measurement of protein intake. It is difficult to make any decision about the impact of a diet with such information.

In summary, the evidence to date has not settled the debate as to whether a low-protein diet is effective in slowing the loss of residual renal function in a large proportion of CKD patients. A recent meta-analysis of low-protein trials in nondiabetic CKD favors the reduction of renal death by 31% as compared with higher or unrestricted protein intake.[33]

Are Low-Protein Diets Safe?

Nonacidotic patients with CKD are remarkably efficient in adapting to dietary protein restriction. Goodship and associates showed that such patients reduce rates of amino acid oxidation and protein degradation in the same fashion as normal adults when their protein diet is restricted from 1.0 to 0.6 g/kg/day.[55] The same adaptive metabolic responses are activated when the diet is restricted to only 0.3 g/kg/day and a supplement of essential amino acids or their nitrogen-free analogues (ketoacids) is given. Such a dietary regimen maintains both neutral nitrogen balance and indices of adequate nutrition over 1 year of observation.[56] The supplement is required when the diet is so restricted to meet the requirements for essential amino acids.

The finding that dialysis patients often have low levels of serum proteins and evidence of malnutrition has led some to suggest that low-protein diets should be used cautiously or avoided in CKD patients and that early start of dialysis therapy should be considered.[57,58] It is true that if CKD patients are not properly instructed and supervised, there may well be a spontaneous decrease in protein intake and deterioration of some nutritional indices. On the other hand, hypoalbuminemia in these patients can be linked as much to evidence of inflammation as it is to dietary inadequacy. In fact, CKD patients treated with low-protein diets were found to have an increase in serum protein concentrations at the initiation of dietary therapy.[59,60] A low-protein diet is also associated with improved survival of CKD patients who subsequently began dialysis.[61] Finally, there is abundant evidence that with proper implementation, a low-protein diet yields neutral nitrogen balance and maintenance of normal serum proteins and anthropometric indices during long-term therapy.[56,62,63] Once on dialysis, patients treated with supplemented very low-protein diet rapidly increase their protein intake and gain in lean body mass.[64] In 5-year follow-up after initiation of renal replacement therapy, these patients revealed low mortality, correlating with age of the subject but not to nutritional parameters at the end of supplemented very low-protein diet therapy.[59]

Does Delaying the Start of Renal Replacement Therapy Affect Patient Outcomes?

The Kidney Disease Outcomes Quality Initiative (K/DOQI) guidelines for initiation of dialysis were appropriately updated in 2006, shifting the focus from relying solely on a specific level of

GFR to include other factors, such as nutrition; acid-base and bone metabolism; homeostasis of potassium, sodium, and volume; and quality-of-life considerations.[65] Observational studies clearly indicate that patients with comorbidities are sent to dialysis therapy at a higher level of estimated GFR.[65,66] The concerns about protein malnutrition in patients with delayed start of dialysis are unfounded. On the contrary, abundant evidence demonstrates that protein malnutrition is common in dialysis patients, suggesting that dialysis therapy could itself be a contributing factor to malnutrition.[67–71] Finally, those studies reporting a negative impact of low residual renal function on survival at the start of dialysis therapy are flawed by failure to take into account *lead-time bias,* the effect whereby measuring survival from the start of dialysis increases apparent survival of those who begin dialysis with more residual renal function (i.e., earlier in the course of the disease) than those who start dialysis with less residual renal function.[72] When CKD patients were followed from an estimated creatinine clearance of 20 mL/min, and divided into early and late start groups by the median estimated creatinine clearance (8.3 mL/min) for all patients at the initiation of dialysis, there was no benefit of survival from earlier initiation of dialysis.[73] More recently, Beddhu and colleagues examined data from the Dialysis Morbidity and Mortality Study, Wave 2, to evaluate if beginning dialysis at higher levels of creatinine clearance or GFR (estimated from the MDRD formula) would improve mortality.[74] They found an increase in mortality for each 5 mL/min increase in GFR at the initiation of dialysis. The authors concluded that there is insufficient evidence to advocate early initiation of dialysis. This observation is supported by another recent cross-sectional study that showed 2-year survival was determined by premorbid conditions rather than the timing of initiation of dialysis.[75] This argument is further strengthened by another recent study of patients age 70 years or older with very advanced CKD (GFR, 5–7 mL/min) but no uremic symptoms, when randomly assigned to initiate dialysis or supplemented very low-protein diet had similar 1-year mortality with fewer hospitalizations.[76]

In summary, no substantial evidence demonstrates improved survival with early initiation of dialysis in ESRD, nor is it associated with a better health-related quality of life.[77] The results of clinical trials evaluating the effect of low-protein diets on the progression of CKD to date have not settled whether such diets will be effective in slowing the loss of residual renal function in a large proportion of patients. When properly applied, these diets do not lead to malnutrition, even in patients with advanced renal insufficiency.[56,59,63] For these reasons, we recommend nutritional consultation be offered to all patients with moderate CKD, along with management of other important risk factors that affect progression of renal disease, such as optimal control of blood pressure, use of drugs blocking angiotensin II responses, treatment for hyperglycemia, and treatment for dyslipidemia. This wholesome approach requires education of the patient and interaction with a skilled dietitian who monitors intake of protein and calories and performs periodic assessment of the nutritional status of the patient.

Dietary Protein Prescription for Chronic Kidney Disease Patients

The optimum level of protein intake for patients with moderate to advanced CKD cannot be deduced from published trials. In western societies typical protein intake by healthy individuals is 1 to 2 g/kg/day, well above the World Health Organization recommended daily protein allowance of 0.8 g/kg/day (minimum daily requirement is 0.6 g/kg/day).[78] In response to a decrease in the amount of protein eaten, healthy subjects can and will activate the following adaptive mechanisms to promote neutral nitrogen balance: (1) amino acid oxidation is suppressed, allowing more efficient utilization of dietary essential amino acids; (2) as dietary protein intake approaches 0.6 g/kg/day, another adaptive response is activated, suppression of protein degradation, along with increasing protein synthesis. The increase in protein synthesis is of less magnitude than the limitation of protein degradation. Notably, patients with uncomplicated CKD will activate the same metabolic responses to dietary protein restriction, even if the patient is eating only approximately 0.3 g protein/kg/day plus a supplement with nitrogen-free analogues of essential amino acids (ketoacids).[56,62] Similar responses are activated in CKD patients with the nephrotic syndrome. In these patients, however, the degree of suppression of amino acid oxidation is pro-portional to the net protein intake (the amount of dietary protein minus the urinary loss of protein).[79] These critical adaptive responses, which act to maintain protein balance, can be impaired by factors that are commonly present in CKD patients, such as metabolic acidosis, inflammation, and infection. Based on these findings, we support the K/DOQI recommendations that patients with advanced renal disease (GFR < 25 mL/min), with or without symptoms attributable to uremia or with uncontrolled progressive renal insufficiency, be treated with a well-planned low-protein diet providing 0.6 g protein/kg/day[26] (Table 66-2). For individuals who will not accept such a diet or who are unable to maintain adequate protein-energy intake with such a diet, an intake can be increased up to 0.8 g protein/kg/day. Further increment in protein intake will not only generate more urea, but will also contribute to metabolic acidosis and renal osteodystrophy through hyperphosphatemia. At least 50% of the protein intake for all of these patients should be of high biologic value. The diet should be designed by a nutritionist with an interest in the implementation of diets for CKD patients to take advantage of

Table 66-2 Recommended Nutrient Intake in Chronic Kidney Disease Patients

Nutrient	Daily Recommendations
Protein*	
GFR (mL/min/1.73m^2)	Amount of protein (g/kg of ideal body weight)
>50	No restriction recommended
25–50	0.6–0.75 controlled
<25	0.6 or 0.3 plus supplementation†
Renal transplant recipient	
Early phase or acute rejection	1.3
Stable phase	As CKD
Nephrotic patient	0.8 +1 g of protein/g of proteinuria
Energy	(kcal/kg of ideal body weight)
<60 yr old	≥35
>60 yr old	30–35
Carbohydrates	35% of nonprotein calories
Fat	Polyunsaturated-to-saturated ratio of 2:1
Phosphorus	800–1000 mg
	No restriction in transplant recipient if serum phosphorus is normal
Calcium	Should not exceed 2.5 g (dietary + calcium-based binders)
Potassium	Individualized
Sodium and Water	As tolerated, to maintain body weight and blood pressure

*At least 50% of proteins should be of high biological value.
†Mixture of essential amino acids and ketoacids.[52]

the patient's food preferences and to ensure an adequate intake of calories and vitamins.

Energy Requirements

It is important to monitor energy intake because a diet containing too few calories will compromise the patient's ability to achieve nitrogen balance and lead to loss of muscle mass. It has been shown that a diet providing about 35 kcal/kg/day is necessary to maintain neutral nitrogen balance in patients with CKD.[80] Energy requirements for healthy CKD patients are not different from those for healthy adults.[81,82] Unfortunately, there is no simple method of estimating calorie intake, so the clinician must rely on repeated measurements of weight and muscle mass plus input from the dietitian.

Bicarbonate Therapy

To date there has been only one published randomized, controlled trial of use of oral bicarbonate in patients with mild to moderate CKD.[83] Maintaining serum bicarbonate and 22 to 26 mmol/L results in attenuation of rise in blood urea nitrogen and parathyroid hormone compared to those given placebo. Correction of metabolic acidosis in CKD patients results in improved measures of nutritional status, such as Subjective Global Assessment and PNA, and reduced hospitalization rates.[84,85] We recommend that predialysis patients or dialysis patients should have stabilized serum bicarbonate levels above 22 mmol/L.

Dietary Phosphorus

The increased incidence and severity of vascular calcification in uremia is attributed to the abnormalities of mineral metabolism, which are common in CKD patients, especially those on dialysis. Cross-sectional studies in patients with advanced CKD have clearly shown that the presence of arterial calcification is associated with adverse clinical outcomes, including myocardial infarction, congestive heart failure, endocarditis, valvular heart disease, and death.[86,87] Vascular calcification is more common and severe in diabetic patients with stage 3 to 5 CKD compared to diabetics with an early stage or no CKD.[88–90] For CKD patients on dialysis an association between elevated serum phosphorus, calcium-phosphorus product (Ca × P), or elevated parathyroid hormone and the risk for all-cause mortality and cardiovascular disease is clearly established.[91–93] These findings highlight the importance of controlling mineral metabolism from the early stages of CKD. When kidney function declines by 20% to 25%, phosphate retention develops; this plays a major role in causing secondary hyperparathyroidism even without detectable elevation of serum phosphorus levels. Thus, dietary counselling for reduced phosphorus intake should be instituted in patients with CKD who approach stage 3, limiting the intake of high-phosphorus foods, mainly dairy products and protein-rich foods. The recommended phosphorus intake for patients with hyperphosphatemia irrespective of the stage of CKD is 800 to 1000 mg/day.[94] For patients who in spite of dietary phosphorus restriction cannot control serum phosphorus levels, phosphate binders are required. For patients who have a high serum calcium-phosphorus product, the initial choice should be a noncalcium-containing phos-

phorus binder. If necessary, aluminum hydroxide should be used for only brief periods (especially in dialysis patients) to reduce the risk of aluminum toxicity. When serum calcium is low, calcium-based phosphate binders (carbonate or acetate) are effective and inexpensive.

Dietary Calcium

Biochemical measurements are not reflective of calcium nutritional status in subjects with normal kidney function nor in patients with CKD.[94] The major indirect measures of calcium nutritional adequacy are skeletal health assessed by risk of fractures, bone mass measurements, and desirable rates of calcium retention. Based on these surrogate markers, the recommended adequate intakes of calcium in healthy adults is about 1.3 g/day, with a tolerable upper level of 2.5 g/day.[95] In CKD patients decreased intestinal calcium absorption is thought to be linked to vitamin D deficiency; because an excess of phosphates in intestinal secretions will bind calcium, the CKD patient requires a higher intake of elemental calcium. Still the total should not exceed 2500 mg/day, including both dietary sources and calcium from phosphate binders.[96] As CKD progresses and patients are also prescribed vitamin D analogues to control secondary hyperparathyroidism, there is risk for developing hypercalcemia or elevated serum calcium-phosphorus product (Ca × P); thus, calcium-based drugs should not be the phosphate binders of choice. Again, dietary education is critical because dietary indiscretion, even by patients who are compliant with phosphate binders, leads to a rise in the calcium-phosphorus product, increasing the likelihood of spontaneous precipitation of calcium and phosphorus throughout the body.

Sodium

Control of blood pressure should be a part of any strategy directed at slowing the progression of CKD.[52] It is easy to achieve a recommended 2-g sodium diet when dietary protein is restricted; it will potentiate the efficacy of antihypertensive medicines.[43,97] Moreover, in edematous states, it is difficult if not impossible to achieve a net loss of sodium (and hence, extracellular volume) with diuretics unless dietary sodium is restricted.

Trace Elements and Vitamin Requirements

In uremia, there are significant alterations in blood and tissue concentrations of trace elements and vitamins. These derangements are due to a decrease in glomerular filtration, impaired tubular function, and protein binding of micronutrients. In addition, an inadequate diet or altered gastrointestinal absorption in patients with advanced uremia may limit the absorption of trace elements and vitamins. The water-soluble vitamin requirements for CKD patients are not different from those for healthy adults.[98] Pharmacologic doses of folic acid have been recommended for lowering plasma homocysteine levels, but whether this decreases cardiovascular risk in renal patients is yet to be established. Results of the two ongoing multicenter clinical trials are expected to provide more conclusive evidence as to whether lowering homocysteine levels in CKD patients with folic acid or vitamin B reduces the risk of cardiovascular disease.[99,100] Current expert opinion suggests that it is prudent to supplement rather than risk the deficiency, especially when supplementation is safe at the recommended level.[101] Serum levels of 25-hydroxyvitamin D, as a measure of body stores of vitamin D, are decreased in patients with stage 4 or higher CKD as compared to the general population.[102] In these patients, 25-hydroxyvitamin D insufficiency (<30 ng/mL) increases risks for secondary hyperparathyroidism, increased prevalence of vertebral fracture, and insulin resistance; it also has a possible role in the progression of renal disease.[102–104] We recommend measuring 25-hydroxyvitamin D level in all patients with stage 3 or higher CKD, irrespective of serum parathyroid hormone levels. For those patients with serum 25-hydroxyvitamin D insufficiency, supplementation with an oral vitamin D, such as ergocalciferol 50,000 IU every month for 6 months, is recommended. For more severe 25-hydroxyvitamin D deficiency (<15 ng/mL), the same dose should be given weekly for the first 3 months.[94] Vitamin C intake should be limited to 100 mg/day, because higher doses of supplementation can lead to tissue deposition of oxalate crystals, hastening renal insufficiency and increasing the risk of myocardial infarction, shunt failure, and muscle weakness in dialysis patients.[105] Vitamin A and retinol-binding protein plasma levels are increased in renal patients, so vitamin A–containing multivitamin preparations for kidney disease patients should be avoided. There is no evidence that vitamin E reduces the risk of cardiovascular events and routine supplementation is not recommended.[106]

In summary, the daily requirements for most trace elements and vitamins in renal patients are quite similar to those of healthy adults.[98] Patients with CKD who do not have a good appetite are advised to take B-complex vitamin, along with folic acid. Some of the common prescription brands with this combination include Nephro-Vite, Nephrocaps, and Nephroplex.

NUTRITIONAL ISSUES IN RENAL TRANSPLANT PATIENTS

A successful renal transplant into a patient with ESRD restores near-normal renal function and is expected to correct the nutritional abnormalities arising from uremia. The renal transplant recipient typically experiences a marked improvement of appetite, leading to weight gain. Nevertheless, these patients face many nutritional challenges that demand close dietary monitoring. The commonly prescribed immunosuppressives (i.e., corticosteroids, calcineurin inhibitors, and sirolimus) are known to induce metabolic adverse effects, such as protein hypercatabolism, hyperlipidemia, glucose intolerance, hyperkalemia, hypophosphatemia, hypomagnesemia, and obesity. The nutritional status after transplant is also determined by preexisting medical conditions, such as protein losses, renal osteodystrophy, hyperlipidemia, and cardiovascular disease. Moreover, these patients suffer from declining renal function due to recurrent acute or chronic rejection, varying degrees of proteinuria, hypertension, and poorly controlled diabetes. In the early postrenal transplant period the nutritional challenge is to counter the metabolic effects of protein hypercatabolism, hyperlipidemia, and hyperglycemia. For the stable transplant recipient, the nutritional status should be optimized, including weight gain, obesity control, and lipid control. With a failing graft, nutritional management is similar to that recommended for advanced CKD.

Dietary Protein and Calorie Prescription for Renal Transplant Patients

Soon after transplantation, there is a marked increase in amino acid and protein catabolism due to the use of large doses of steroids plus surgery-related stresses. Patients with preexisting malnutrition are at risk for poor wound healing and susceptibility to infection. Based on these concerns, a dietary protein intake of 1.3 g/kg body weight/day is recommended for the early postrenal transplant patient.[107] However, these recommendations are based on only a few nitrogen balance studies. The optimum dietary protein intake for transplant patients on maintenance immunosuppressive therapy is not well established. Transplant recipients have been shown to maintain neutral nitrogen balance on a low-protein intake of 0.6 g/kg/day as long as their energy intake is maintained at least 28 kcal/kg/day.[108] Results of a 12-year follow-up on renal function in transplant recipients consuming protein intake of 0.8 g/kg/day compared to those with protein intake of 1.4 g/kg/day showed those with the lower protein intake maintained unchanged renal function, whereas patients with the higher protein intake lost more than 40% of excretory efficiency.[109] Based on limited available data, it is reasonable to recommend protein intake of 0.8 g/kg/day along with minimal energy intake of 30 to 35 kcal/kg/day for stable renal transplant patients. Those patients with progressive graft failure should have a more stringent protein intake of 0.6 g/kg/day, because there is evidence that a low-protein diet is also associated with a reduction in proteinuria and decreased activity of the renin-angiotensin system.[110] During an acute rejection episode requiring treatment with high doses of corticosteroids, protein catabolism increases, yielding high blood urea nitrogen levels. Protein restriction in such patients can lead to severe negative nitrogen balance, so increasing protein intake to 1.2 g/kg/day is appropriate.

Obesity, defined as body mass index of more than 30 kg/m² or more than 130% ideal body weight, is present in 12% to 40% of recipients within 1 year after renal transplant.[111,112] Obesity is associated with decreased graft survival and increased prevalence of cardiovascular disease after transplantation.[113,114] For stable transplant recipients who require weight reduction, a caloric intake of 25 kcal/kg/day along with appropriate dietary and lifestyle measures, including an exercise program, should be recommended. Weight reduction diets in obese, hyperlipidemic transplant recipients cause a modest reduction in cholesterol levels, although statin drugs are usually required.[115] The American Heart Association one-step diet is a reasonable initial approach for hyperlipidemic renal transplant patients. This diet, consisting of less than 300 mg of cholesterol per day (with a goal of <250 mg/day), 30% total calories as fat, 50% as carbohydrate, and 20% as protein, is easily attainable and is familiar to renal dietitians.[116]

Dietary Phosphorus and Calcium after Renal Transplantation

Transient hypercalcemia and low-normal serum phosphorus levels can be observed after a successful kidney transplant. These biochemical changes are due to persistent hyperparathyroidism, improved parathyroid hormone sensitivity, and recently described non-parathyroid hormone humoral factor.[117,118] A phosphaturic action of steroids must also be considered; an increase in serum phosphorus levels after reduction of steroid doses has been reported.[119]

The major improvement over a patient's pretransplant renal diet is the liberalization of dietary phosphorus. Nevertheless, oral phosphate supplements are required for periods of up to 1 year after renal transplant. In the absence of hypercalcemia, calcium intake through diet and supplements should be limited to about 1000 to 1500 mg/day.

In summary, a successful renal transplant allows greater dietary freedom and resultant weight gain. Immunosuppressive medications contribute to the protein hypercatabolism, hyperlipidemia, hyperglycemia, and propensity toward weight gain. Protein requirements during the early phase are similar to the requirements of healthy adults. As GFR declines with failing graft, protein restrictions similar to those for CKD patients are re-instituted. Further, maintenance of optimal body weight, along with changes in lifestyle measures, including an exercise program, should be part of nutritional management in all renal transplant recipients.

References

1. U.S. Renal Data System: Excerpts from the USRDS 2006 Annual Data Report. Am J Kidney Dis 2006;49(Suppl 1):S1–S296.
2. Schoolwerth AC, Engelgau MM, Hostetter TH, et al: Chronic kidney disease: A public health problem that needs a public health action plan. Prev Chronic Dis [serial online]. 2006;3:A57.
3. U.S. Renal Data Systems: Excerpts from the USRDS 2002 Annual Data Report. Am J Kidney Dis 2002;4(Suppl 2)1:S1–S260.
4. Lowrie EG, Lew NL: Death risk in hemodialysis patients: The predictive value of commonly measured variables and an evaluation of death rate differences between facilities. Am J Kidney Dis 1990;15:458–482.
5. Avram MM, Goldwasser P, Erroa M, Fein PA: Predictors of survival in continuous ambulatory peritoneal dialysis patients: The importance of prealbumin and other nutritional and metabolic markers. Am J Kidney Dis 1994;23:91–98.
6. Mitch WE: Malnutrition: a frequent misdiagnosis for hemodialysis patients. J Clin Invest 2002;110:437–439.
7. Bergstrom J, Lindholm B, Lacson E Jr, et al: What are the causes and consequences of the chronic inflammatory state in chronic dialysis patients? Semin Dial 2000;13:163–175.
8. Kaysen GA: Biological basis of hypoalbuminemia in ESRD. J Am Soc Nephrol 1998;9:2368–2376.
9. Stenvinkel P, Heimburger O, Paultre F, et al: Strong association between malnutrition, inflammation, and atherosclerosis in chronic renal failure. Kidney Int 1999;55:1899–1911.
10. Honda H, Qureshi AR, Heimburger O, et al: Serum albumin, C-reactive protein, interleukin 6, and fetuin (as predictors of malnutrition, cardiovascular disease, and mortality in patients with ESRD. Am J Kidney Dis 2006;47:139–148.
11. Caglar K, Peng Y, Pupim LB, et al: Inflammatory signals associated with hemodialysis. Kidney Int 2002;62:1408–1416.
12. Qureshi AR, Alvestrand A, Divino-Filho JC, et al: Inflammation, malnutrition, and cardiac disease as predictors of mortality in hemodialysis patients. J Am Soc Nephrol 2002;13(Suppl 1):S28–S36.
13. Goodman MN: Tumor necrosis factor induces skeletal muscle protein breakdown in rats. Am J Physiol 1991;260:E727–E730.
14. Hara Y, May RC, Kelly RA, Mitch WE: Acidosis, not azotemia, stimulates branched-chain, amino acid catabolism in uremic rats. Kidney Int 1987;32:808–814.
15. May RC, Bailey JL, Mitch WE, et al: Glucocorticoids and acidosis stimulate protein and amino acid catabolism in vivo. Kidney Int 1996;49:679–683.
16. Kalantar-Zadeh K, Mehrotra R, Fouque D, Kopple JD: Metabolic acidosis and malnutrition-inflammation complex syndrome in chronic renal failure. Semin Dial 2004;17:455–465.
17. Pickering WP, Price SR, Bircher G, et al: Nutrition in CAPD: Serum bicarbonate and the ubiquitin-proteasome system in muscle. Kidney Int 2002;61:1286–1292.
18. Movilli E, Zani R, Carli O, et al: Correction of metabolic acidosis increases serum albumin concentrations and decreases kinetically evaluated protein intake in haemodialysis patients: A prospective study. Nephrol Dial Transplant 1998;13:1719–1722.
19. Ballmer PE, McNurlan MA, Hulter HN, et al: Chronic metabolic acidosis decreases albumin synthesis and induces negative nitrogen balance in humans. J Clin Invest 1995;95:39–45.
20. DeFronzo RA, Tobin JD, Rowe JW, Andres R: Glucose intolerance in uremia. Quantification of pancreatic beta cell sensitivity to glucose and tissue sensitivity to insulin. J Clin Invest 1978; 62:425–435.
21. Price SR, Bailey JL, Wang X, et al: Muscle wasting in insulinopenic rats results from activation of the ATP-dependent, ubiquitin-proteasome proteolytic pathway by a mechanism including gene transcription. J Clin Invest 1996;98:1703–1708.
22. Mitch WE, Bailey JL, Wang X, et al: Evaluation of signals activating ubiquitin-proteasome proteolysis in a model of muscle wasting. Am J Physiol 1999;276:C1132–C1138.
23. Hakim RM, Lazarus JM: Biochemical parameters in chronic renal failure. Am J Kidney Dis 1988;11:238–247.
24. Anderstam B, Mamoun AH, Sodersten P, Bergstrom J: Middle-sized molecule fractions isolated from uremic ultrafiltrate and normal urine inhibit ingestive behavior in the rat. J Am Soc Nephrol 1996;7:2453–2460.
25. Umeakunne K: Approaches to Succcessful Nutrition Intervention in Renal Disease, 4th ed. Philadelphia: Lippincott Williams and Wilkins, 2002.
26. National Kidney Foundation: K/DOQI clinical practice guidelines for nutrition in chronic renal failure. Am J Kidney Dis 2000;35:S1–S140.
27. Maroni BJ, Steinman TI, Mitch WE: A method for estimating nitrogen intake of patients with chronic renal failure. Kidney Int 1985;27:58–65.
28. Masud T, Manatunga A, Cotsonis G, Mitch WE: The precision of estimating protein intake of patients with chronic renal failure. Kidney Int 2002;62:1750–1756.
29. Panzetta G, Tessitore N, Faccini G, Maschio G: The protein catabolic rate as a measure of protein intake in dialysis patients: Usefulness and limits. Nephrol Dial Transplant 1990;5(Suppl 1):125–127.
30. Kaysen GA, Dubin JA, Muller HG, et al: Inflammation and reduced albumin synthesis associated with stable decline in serum albumin in hemodialysis patients. Kidney Int 2004;65: 1408–1415.
31. Stenvinkel P, Barany P, Chung SH, et al: A comparative analysis of nutritional parameters as predictors of outcome in male and female ESRD patients. Nephrol Dial Transplant 2002;17: 1266–1274.
32. Graham KA, Reaich D, Channon SM, et al: Correction of acidosis in hemodialysis decreases whole-body protein degradation. J Am Soc Nephrol 1997;8:632–637.
33. Fouque D, Laville M, Boissel JP: Low protein diets for chronic kidney disease in nondiabetic adults. Cochrane Database Syst Rev 2006;(2):CD001892.
34. Port FK, Ashby VB, Dhingra RK, et al: Dialysis dose and body mass index are strongly associated with survival in hemodialysis patients. J Am Soc Nephrol 2002;13:1061–1066.
35. Leavey SF, McCullough K, Hecking E, et al: Body mass index and mortality in "healthier" as compared with "sicker" haemodialysis

patients: Results from the Dialysis Outcomes and Practice Patterns Study (DOPPS). Nephrol Dial Transplant 2001;16:2386–2394.

36. Tozawa M, Iseki K, Iseki C, et al: Influence of smoking and obesity on the development of proteinuria. Kidney Int 2002;62:956–962.

37. Reisin E, Abel R, Modan M, et al: Effect of weight loss without salt restriction on the reduction of blood pressure in overweight hypertensive patients. N Engl J Med 1978;298:1–6.

38. Poirier P, Giles TD, Bray GA, et al: Obesity and cardiovascular disease: Pathophysiology, evaluation, and effect of weight loss. Arterioscler Thromb Vasc Biol 2006;26:968–976.

39. Bonnet F, Deprele C, Sassolas A, et al: Excessive body weight as a new independent risk factor for clinical and pathological progression in primary IgA nephritis. Am J Kidney Dis 2001;37:720–727.

40. Lawson JA, Lazarus R, Kelly JJ: Prevalence and prognostic significance of malnutrition in chronic renal insufficiency. J Ren Nutr 2001;11:16–22.

41. Steiber AL, Kalantar-Zadeh K, Secker D, et al: Subjective Global Assessment in chronic kidney disease: A review. J Ren Nutr 2004;14:191–200.

42. Cooper BA, Bartlett LH, Aslani A, et al: Validity of subjective global assessment as a nutritional marker in end-stage renal disease. Am J Kidney Dis 2002;40:126–132.

43. Weir MR: Is it the low-protein diet or simply the salt restriction? Kidney Int 2007;71:188–190.

44. Bellizzi V, Di Iorio BR, De Nicola L, et al: Very low protein diet supplemented with ketoanalogs improves blood pressure control in chronic kidney disease. Kidney Int 2007;71:245–251.

45. Brouhard BH, LaGrone L: Effect of dietary protein restriction on functional renal reserve in diabetic nephropathy. Am J Med 1990;89:427–431.

46. Zeller K, Whittaker E, Sullivan L, et al: Effect of restricting dietary protein on the progression of renal failure in patients with insulin-dependent diabetes mellitus. N Engl J Med 1991;324:78–84.

47. Dullaart RP, Beusekamp BJ, Meijer S, et al: Long-term effects of protein-restricted diet on albuminuria and renal function in IDDM patients without clinical nephropathy and hypertension. Diabetes Care 1993;16:483–492.

48. Raal FJ, Kalk WJ, Lawson M, et al: Effect of moderate dietary protein restriction on the progression of overt diabetic nephropathy: A 6-month prospective study. Am J Clin Nutr 1994;60:579–585.

49. Fouque D, Laville M, Boissel JP, et al: Controlled low protein diets in chronic renal insufficiency: Meta-analysis. BMJ 1992;304:216–220.

50. Pedrini MT, Levey AS, Lau J, et al: The effect of dietary protein restriction on the progression of diabetic and nondiabetic renal diseases: A meta-analysis. Ann Intern Med 1996;124:627–632.

51. Fouque D, Wang P, Laville M, Boissel JP: Low protein diets delay end-stage renal disease in non-diabetic adults with chronic renal failure. Nephrol Dial Transplant 2000;15:1986–1992.

52. Klahr S, Levey AS, Beck GJ, et al for the MDRD Study Group: The effects of dietary protein restriction and blood-pressure control on the progression of chronic renal disease. Modification of Diet in Renal Disease Study Group. N Engl J Med 1994;330:877–884.

53. Levey AS, Adler S, Caggiula AW, et al: Effects of dietary protein restriction on the progression of advanced renal disease in the Modification of Diet in Renal Disease Study. Am J Kidney Dis 1996;27:652–663.

54. Levey AS, Greene T, Sarnak MJ, et al: Effect of dietary protein restriction on the progression of kidney disease: Long-term follow-up of the Modification of Diet in Renal Disease (MDRD) Study. Am J Kidney Dis 2006;48:879–888.

55. Goodship TH, Mitch WE, Hoerr RA, et al: Adaptation to low-protein diets in renal failure: Leucine turnover and nitrogen balance. J Am Soc Nephrol 1990;1:66–75.

56. Tom K, Young VR, Chapman T, et al: Long-term adaptive responses to dietary protein restriction in chronic renal failure. Am J Physiol 1995;268:E668–E677.

57. Ikizler TA, Greene JH, Wingard RL, et al: Spontaneous dietary protein intake during progression of chronic renal failure. J Am Soc Nephrol 1995;6:1386–1391.

58. Hakim RM, Lazarus JM: Initiation of dialysis. J Am Soc Nephrol 1995;6:1319–1328.

59. Aparicio M, Chauveau P, De Precigout V, et al: Nutrition and outcome on renal replacement therapy of patients with chronic renal failure treated by a supplemented very low protein diet. J Am Soc Nephrol 2000;11:708–716.

60. Walser M: Does prolonged protein restriction preceding dialysis lead to protein malnutrition at the onset of dialysis? Kidney Int 1993;44:1139–1144.

61. Coresh J, Walser M, Hill S: Survival on dialysis among chronic renal failure patients treated with a supplemented low-protein diet before dialysis. J Am Soc Nephrol 1995;6:1379–1385.

62. Masud T, Young VR, Chapman T, Maroni BJ: Adaptive responses to very low protein diets: The first comparison of keto-acids to essential amino acids. Kidney Int 1994;45:1182–1192.

63. Bernhard J, Beaufrere B, Laville M, Fouque D: Adaptive response to a low-protein diet in predialysis chronic renal failure patients. J Am Soc Nephrol 2001;12:1249–1254.

64. Vendrely B, Chauveau P, Barthe N, et al: Nutrition in hemodialysis patients previously on a supplemented very low protein diet. Kidney Int 2003;63:1491–1498.

65. National Kidney Foundation: K/DOQI clinical practice guidelines and clinical practice recommendations for anemia in chronic kidney disease. Am J Kidney Dis 2006;47:S11–S145.

66. U.S. Renal Data System: Excerpts from the USRDS 2005 Annual Data Report. Am J Kidney Dis 2005;47:S1–S286.

67. Cianciaruso B, Brunori G, Kopple JD, et al: Cross-sectional comparison of malnutrition in continuous ambulatory peritoneal dialysis and hemodialysis patients. Am J Kidney Dis 1995;26:475–486.

68. Tai TW, Chan AM, Cochran CC, et al: Renal dietitians' perspective: Identification, prevalence, and intervention for malnutrition in dialysis patients in Texas. J Ren Nutr 1998;8:188–198.

69. Enia G, Sicuso C, Alati G, Zoccali C: Subjective global assessment of nutrition in dialysis patients. Nephrol Dial Transplant 1993;8:1094–1098.

70. Rocco MV, Paranandi L, Burrowes JD, et al: Nutritional status in the HEMO Study cohort at baseline. Hemodialysis. Am J Kidney Dis 2002;39:245–256.

71. Mancini A, Grandaliano G, Magarelli P, Allegretti A: Nutritional status in hemodialysis patients and bioimpedance vector analysis. J Ren Nutr 2003;13:199–204.

72. Korevaar JC, Jansen MA, Dekker FW, et al: When to initiate dialysis: Effect of proposed US guidelines on survival. Lancet 2001;358:1046–1050.

73. Traynor JP, Simpson K, Geddes CC, et al: Early initiation of dialysis fails to prolong survival in patients with end-stage renal failure. Nephrol Dial Transplant 2004;19:1009; author reply 1010.

74. Beddhu S, Samore MH, Roberts MS, et al: Impact of timing of initiation of dialysis on mortality. J Am Soc Nephrol 2003;14:2305–2312.

75. Wilson B, Harwood L, Locking-Cusolito H, et al: Optimal timing of initiation of chronic hemodialysis? Hemodial Int 2007;11:263–269.

76. Brunori G, Viola BF, Parrinello G, et al: Efficacy and safety of a very-low-protein diet when postponing dialysis in the elderly: A prospective randomized multicenter controlled study. Am J Kidney Dis 2007;49:569–580.

77. Korevaar JC, Jansen MA, Dekker FW, et al: Evaluation of DOQI guidelines: Early start of dialysis treatment is not associated with better health-related quality of life. National Kidney Foundation/Dialysis Outcomes Quality Initiative. Am J Kidney Dis 2002;39:108–115.

78. FAO/WHO/UNO: Energy and Protein Requirements. World Health Organization Technical Report Series 724. 1985;6.1.2: 1–206.

79. Maroni BJ, Staffeld C, Young VR, et al: Mechanisms permitting nephrotic patients to achieve nitrogen equilibrium with a protein-restricted diet. J Clin Invest 1997;99:2479–2487.

80. Kopple JD, Monteon FJ, Shaib JK: Effect of energy intake on nitrogen metabolism in nondialyzed patients with chronic renal failure. Kidney Int 1986;29:734–742.

81. Monteon FJ, Laidlaw SA, Shaib JK, Kopple JD: Energy expenditure in patients with chronic renal failure. Kidney Int 1986;30: 741–747.

82. Schneeweiss B, Graninger W, Stockenhuber F, et al: Energy metabolism in acute and chronic renal failure. Am J Clin Nutr 1990;52:596–601.

83. Mathur RP, Dash SC, Gupta N, et al: Effects of correction of metabolic acidosis on blood urea and bone metabolism in patients with mild to moderate chronic kidney disease: A prospective randomized single blind controlled trial. Ren Fail 2006;28:1–5.

84. Stein A, Moorhouse J, Iles-Smith H, et al: Role of an improvement in acid-base status and nutrition in CAPD patients. Kidney Int 1997;52:1089–1095.

85. Szeto CC, Wong TY, Chow KM, et al: Oral sodium bicarbonate for the treatment of metabolic acidosis in peritoneal dialysis patients: A randomized placebo-control trial. J Am Soc Nephrol 2003;14:2119–2126.

86. Dellegrottaglie S, Saran R, Rajagopalan S: Vascular calcification in patients with renal failure: Culprit or innocent bystander? Cardiol Clin 2005;23:373–384.

87. Blacher J, Guerin AP, Pannier B, et al: Arterial calcifications, arterial stiffness, and cardiovascular risk in end-stage renal disease. Hypertension 2001;38:938–942.

88. Kramer H, Toto R, Peshock R, et al: Association between chronic kidney disease and coronary artery calcification: The Dallas Heart Study. J Am Soc Nephrol 2005;16:507–513.

89. Qunibi WY, Abouzahr F, Mizani MR, et al: Cardiovascular calcification in Hispanic Americans (HA) with chronic kidney disease (CKD) due to type 2 diabetes. Kidney Int 2005;68: 271–277.

90. Merjanian R, Budoff M, Adler S, et al: Coronary artery, aortic wall, and valvular calcification in nondialyzed individuals with type 2 diabetes and renal disease. Kidney Int 2003;64:263–271.

91. Block GA, Klassen PS, Lazarus JM, et al: Mineral metabolism, mortality, and morbidity in maintenance hemodialysis. J Am Soc Nephrol 2004;15:2208–2218.

92. Ganesh SK, Stack AG, Levin NW, et al: Association of elevated serum PO_4, Ca × PO_4 product, and parathyroid hormone with cardiac mortality risk in chronic hemodialysis patients. J Am Soc Nephrol 2001;12:2131–2138.

93. Block GA, Port FK: Re-evaluation of risks associated with hyperphosphatemia and hyperparathyroidism in dialysis patients: Recommendations for a change in management. Am J Kidney Dis 2000;35:1226–1237.

94. National Kidney Foundation: K/DOQI clinical practice guidelines for bone metabolism and disease in chronic kidney disease. Am J Kidney Dis 2003;42:S1–S201.

95. Dietary References Intakes: Calcium, Phosphorus, Magnesium, Vitamin D_3 and Fluoride. Institute of Medicine. Washington, DC: National Academy Press, 2000.

96. Clinical practice guidelines for bone metabolism and disease in children with chronic kidney disease. Am J Kidney Dis 2005; 46:1–121.

97. Mitch WE, Wilcox CS: Disorders of body fluids, sodium and potassium in chronic renal failure. Am J Med 1982;72:536–550.

98. Masud T: Handbook of Nutrition and Kidney, 5th ed. Philadelphia: Lippincott, Williams & Wilkins, 2002.

99. The Folic Acid for Vascular Outcome Reduction In Transplantation (FAVORIT). Bethesda, MD: National Institute of Diabetes & Digestive & Kidney Diseases, 2004. Available at www .niddk.nih.gov/patient/favorit/favorit.htm

100. Homocysteine-lowering trials for prevention of cardiovascular events: A review of the design and power of the large randomized trials. Am Heart J 2006;151:282–287.

101. National Kidney Foundation: K/DOQI clinical practice guidelines for cardiovascular disease in dialysis patients. Am J Kidney Dis 2005;45:S1–S153.

102. Chonchol M, Scragg R: 25-Hydroxyvitamin D, insulin resistance, and kidney function in the Third National Health and Nutrition Examination Survey. Kidney Int 2007;71:134–139.

103. Remuzzi A: Vitamin D, insulin resistance, and renal disease. Kidney Int 2007;71:96–98.

104. Kuhlmann A, Haas CS, Gross ML, et al: 1,25-Dihydroxyvitamin D_3 decreases podocyte loss and podocyte hypertrophy in the subtotally nephrectomized rat. Am J Physiol Renal Physiol 2004; 286:F526–F533.

105. Bohm V, Tiroke K, Schneider S, et al: Vitamin C status of patients with chronic renal failure, dialysis patients and patients after renal transplantation. Int J Vitam Nutr Res 1997;67: 262–266.

106. Lonn E, Bosch J, Yusuf S, et al: Effects of long-term vitamin E supplementation on cardiovascular events and cancer: A randomized controlled trial. JAMA 2005;293:1338–1347.

107. Bertolatus J: Nutritional Requirements of Renal Transplant Patients, 5th ed. Philadelphia: Lippincott Williams &Wilkins, 2002.

108. Windus DW, Lacson S, Delmez JA: The short-term effects of a low-protein diet in stable renal transplant recipients. Am J Kidney Dis 1991;17:693–699.

109. Bernardi A, Biasia F, Pati T, et al: Long-term protein intake control in kidney transplant recipients: Effect in kidney graft function and in nutritional status. Am J Kidney Dis 2003;41: S146–152.

110. Salahudeen AK, Hostetter TH, Raatz SK, Rosenberg ME: Effects of dietary protein in patients with chronic renal transplant rejection. Kidney Int 1992;41:183–190.

111. Armstrong KA, Campbell SB, Hawley CM, et al: Impact of obesity on renal transplant outcomes. Nephrology (Carlton) 2005;10:405–413.

112. Baum CL, Thielke K, Westin E, et al: Predictors of weight gain and cardiovascular risk in a cohort of racially diverse kidney transplant recipients. Nutrition 2002;18:139–146.

113. Meier-Kriesche HU, Arndorfer JA, Kaplan B: The impact of body mass index on renal transplant outcomes: A significant independent risk factor for graft failure and patient death. Transplantation 2002;73:70–74.

114. European best practice guidelines for renal transplantation. Section IV: Long-term management of the transplant recipient. IV.5.1. Cardiovascular risks. Cardiovascular disease after renal transplantation. Nephrol Dial Transplant 2002;17(Suppl 4):24– 25.

115. Zaffari D, Losekann A, Santos AF, et al: Effectiveness of diet in hyperlipidemia in renal transplant patients. Transplant Proc 2004;36:889–890.

116. Moore RA, Callahan MF, Cody M, et al: The effect of the American Heart Association step one diet on hyperlipidemia following renal transplantation. Transplantation 1990;49: 60–62.

117. Ghanekar H, Welch BJ, Moe OW, Sakhaee K: Post-renal transplantation hypophosphatemia: A review and novel insights. Curr Opin Nephrol Hypertens 2006;15:97–104.

118. Reinhardt W, Bartelworth H, Jockenhovel F, et al: Sequential changes of biochemical bone parameters after kidney transplantation. Nephrol Dial Transplant 1998;13:436–442.
119. Higgins RM, Richardson AJ, Endre ZH, et al: Hypophosphataemia after renal transplantation: Relationship to immunosuppressive drug therapy and effects on muscle detected by 31P nuclear magnetic resonance spectroscopy. Nephrol Dial Transplant 1990;5:62–68.
120. Jungers P, Chauveau P, Ployard F, et al: Comparison of ketoacids and low protein diet on advanced chronic renal failure progression. Kidney Int 1987;22(Suppl):S67–S71.
121. Bergström J, Alvestrand A, Bucht H, Gutierrez A: Stockholm clinical study on progression of chronic renal failure—an interim report. Kidney Int 1989;27(Suppl):S110–S114.
122. Ihle BU, Becker GJ, Whitworth JA, et al: The effect of protein restriction on the progression of renal insufficiency. N Engl J Med 1989;321:1773–1777.
123. Rosman JB, Langer K, Brandl M, et al: Protein-restricted diets in chronic renal failure: A four year follow-up shows limited indications. Kidney Int 1989;27(Suppl):S96–S102.
124. Locatelli F, Alberti D, Graziani G, et al: Prospective, randomised, multicentre trial of effect of protein restriction on progression of chronic renal insufficiency. Northern Italian Cooperative Study Group. Lancet 1991;337:1299–1304.
125. Williams PS, Stevens ME, Fass G, et al: Failure of dietary protein and phosphate restriction to retard the rate of progression of chronic renal failure: A prospective, randomized, controlled trial. Q J Med 1991;81:837–855.
126. D'Amico G, Gentile MG, Fellin G, et al: Effect of dietary protein restriction on the progression of renal failure: A prospective randomized trial. Nephrol Dial Transplant 1994;9:1590–1594.

Further Reading

Fouque D, Laville M, Boissel JP: Low protein diets for chronic kidney disease in nondiabetic adults. Cochrane Database Syst Rev 2006;(2):CD001892.
Masud T, Manatunga A, Cotsonis G, Mitch WE: The precision of estimating protein intake of patients with chronic renal failure. Kidney Int 2004;62:1750–1756.
Levey AS, Greene T, Sarnak M: Effect of dietary protein restriction on the progression of kidney disease: Long-term follow-up of the Modification of Diet I Renal Disease (MDRD) study. Am J Kidney Dis 2006;48:879–888.
Mitch WE, Remuzzi G: Diets for patients with chronic kidney disease: still worth prescribing. J Am Soc Nephrol 2004;15:234–237.
National Kidney Foundation: K/DOQI clinical practice guidelines for nutrition in chronic renal failure. Am J Kidney Dis 2000;35:S1–S140.

Chapter 67

Iron and Erythropoietin-Related Therapies

Steven Fishbane

Anemia is a common problem for chronic kidney disease (CKD) patients. It may occur relatively early in the course of CKD and cause significant symptoms such as dyspnea and fatigue. By end-stage renal disease (ESRD) the majority of patients have significant anemia. Anemia is associated with important medical complications such as cardiac hypertrophy and an increased risk of death.[1] The clinician's task is to recognize the presence of anemia, to conduct an appropriate diagnostic evaluation, and to initiate treatment and monitor its effectiveness.

PATHOPHYSIOLOGY

The anemia of CKD is multifactorial in origin, but erythropoietin deficiency is the most important etiologic factor.[2] Erythropoietin is a glycoprotein hormone produced in renal peritubular cells. It stimulates erythropoietic progenitor cells in the bone marrow. Its greatest effect is on erythroid colony-forming units, cells that bear the highest concentration of erythropoietin receptors of any erythroid precursor.[3] When erythropoietin is not present, these cells rapidly undergo necrosis and apoptosis. Erythropoietin facilitates the survival of and increases the colony-forming units erythroid that are maturing into precursors of erythrocytes, including the first circulating form, the reticulocyte.

Under normoxic conditions, erythropoietin is produced at low, relatively continuous levels. When tissue hypoxia is present, erythropoietin production is greatly increased, with serum concentrations increasing 100- to 1000-fold. Hypoxemia or anemia may stimulate erythropoietin production; the presence of tissue hypoxia is sensed by the recently identified hypoxia inducible factor-1 (HIF) complex.[4] One component of this dimeric compound, HIF-1α, is rapidly degraded under normoxic conditions. When hypoxia is present, dimerization with HIF-1β occurs, yielding a HIF-1 complex that stimulates the activation of more than 90 oxygen-sensitive genes including erythropoietin.

Serum erythropoietin levels tend to be elevated by CKD, but are still insufficient for the degree of anemia present.[5,6] Some degree of response to anemia is maintained, at least until the late stages of CKD, but when creatinine clearance is less than 40 mL/min, the hemoglobin (Hgb) and serum erythropoietin concentrations become somewhat dissociated. Even in dialysis patients, however, a small erythropoietic response remains. In certain renal diseases, such as polycystic kidney disease, erythropoietin production may be somewhat preserved.

After the classic experiments of Eschbach and Adamson, the primary role of erythropoietin deficiency became clear. However, the relative importance of erythropoietic inhibitors remains controversial.[7] Both the beneficial effect of dialysis on improving anemia and the demonstration of a shortened erythrocyte half-life in ESRD suggest that there is at least some contribution of circulating inhibitors of erythropoietic responses to the anemia of kidney disease.

DEFINING ANEMIA IN CHRONIC KIDNEY DISEASE

The absolute Hgb level that defines anemia in CKD has been determined by the National Kidney Foundation's Kidney Disease Outcome Quality Initiative anemia guidelines as a level of less than 13.5 for men and 12.0 for women.[8] Periodic measurement of Hgb, to screen for anemia, is necessary for managing patients with CKD. The Kidney Disease Outcome Quality Initiative guidelines recommend testing at least once per year, but the decision to test for anemia first requires that CKD has been recognized, and this can sometimes prove problematic. For example, in older adults with mildly elevated serum creatinine, a clinician may fail to appreciate that there has been a substantial loss of renal function. Specifically, a 70-year-old woman with a serum creatinine level of 1.5 mg/dL has a creatinine clearance less than 50 mL/min, yet this level of serum creatinine may obscure the diagnosis. Failure to diagnose CKD and recognize the associated anemia is a missed opportunity to improve the patient's life through treatment.

IMPACT OF ANEMIA IN CHRONIC KIDNEY DISEASE

The primary adverse effect of anemia in CKD is the development of unpleasant symptoms such as fatigue and dyspnea that impair the individual's quality of life.[9] Symptoms are due to the direct as well as the compensatory biologic effects of anemia. Decreased erythrocyte mass results in decreased oxygen-carrying capacity to the body's tissues and organs. The reduction in oxygen delivery leads to compensatory changes such as increased cardiac output and vasodilation. This increases tissue perfusion and partially offsets the reduction in blood oxygen-carrying capacity, but there is a cost: increased cardiac work leading to cardiac hypertrophy and increased risk of cardiovascular disease.

The reduction in quality of life from anemia has been well documented. Treatment for anemia in CKD patients results in partial recovery, rehabilitation, and restoration of well-being.[9–12] There is general improvement in quality of life on partial to full correction of anemia. In an early study, Delano[10] treated 37 hemodialysis patients with epoetin to achieve partial correction of anemia. The mean hematocrit increased from 19.8% before therapy to 31.5% after therapy, and there was an improved sense of well-being in 84% of patients, with improvements in appetite (81%), sexual function (62%), socializing (70%), and sleep (68%).

Anemia in CKD has also been associated with left ventricular hypertrophy, an increase in the risk of hospitalization, and mortality.[13–17] It is unclear whether the relationship to mortality and hospitalization risk is causal as treatment studies have generally not demonstrated these benefits in outcomes.[18–21] In contrast, the relationship to left ventricular hypertrophy is more likely to be causal, given the increased workload of the heart when anemia is present. Levin and colleagues[22] found the association to be strong; each 1-g/dL decrease in Hgb was associated with a 6% increase in risk of left ventricular hypertrophy (LVH).[22] The prevalence of LVH increases in relation to lower levels of kidney function, reaching 74% at the initiation of hemodialysis.[23] Despite the clear association between anemia and LVH in CKD, treatment studies have generally not found a decrease in LVH with erythropoietin treatment.[20,21,24]

EVALUATION OF ANEMIA IN CHRONIC KIDNEY DISEASE

The intensity of the ensuing evaluation and treatment depends to an extent on the significance of symptoms. The clinician must ask directed questions of the patient related to energy, fatigue, shortness of breath, chest pain, and other symptoms. Symptoms may develop gradually, and the patient may partially compensate with restrictions in activities. To avoid this misdiagnosis, questions should probe changes in activity level, and the patient should be asked to compare current capabilities to previous abilities.

The diagnostic evaluation should be based on the premise that although most anemia in CKD proves to be due to erythropoietin deficiency, other causes of anemia may be present

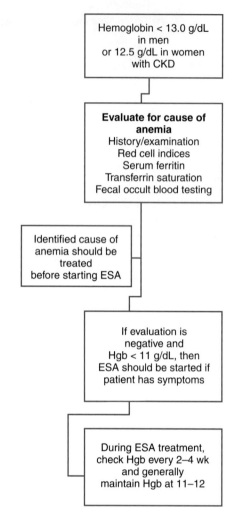

Figure 67-1 Algorithm for anemia evaluation in chronic kidney disease (CKD). ESA, erythropoiesis-stimulating agent; TSAT, transferrin saturation.

(Fig. 67-1). One of the most common management errors is to falsely assume that erythropoietin deficiency is causing anemia and to miss an important diagnosis such as gastrointestinal bleeding or vitamin B_{12} deficiency. In summary, any cause of anemia present in the age-related normal population of adults can cause anemia in CKD patients.

Because the diagnosis of erythropoietin deficiency is one of exclusion, the evaluation should focus on excluding other causes of anemia with an appropriate history, examination, and laboratory testing. The complete blood count should be reviewed for any related problems in the leukocyte or platelet cell lines. Red blood cell indices should be examined, and the anemia classified as microcytic, normocytic, or macrocytic. The anemia of kidney disease usually results in a normocytic erythrocyte classification. If microcytosis is present, then iron deficiency, thalassemia, and myelodysplasia should be considered. With macrocytosis, folic acid and vitamin B_{12} deficiency must be excluded. Fecal blood testing should be performed to evaluate for occult gastrointestinal bleeding. Serum ferritin and transferrin saturation should be measured to exclude iron deficiency. When there are appropriate clinical problems, multiple myeloma should be considered.

If the initial diagnostic evaluation is unrevealing, then a diagnosis of renal anemia due to erythropoietin deficiency is most likely. There is no utility in measuring serum erythropoietin because the deficiency is relative, not absolute (serum erythropoietin levels are generally higher in CKD patients compared with adults without kidney disease). However, the serum level is insufficient for the degree of anemia present, indicating that there is a relative deficiency. When ESRD is present, erythropoietin levels are substantially decreased, and overt erythropoietin deficiency is present.

TREATMENT OF THE ANEMIA OF CHRONIC KIDNEY DISEASE

General Concepts

After other causes of anemia have been excluded, treatment should be considered. Until recently, erythropoietin therapy involved only the administration of recombinant human erythropoietin. However, there are drugs currently in development that increase erythropoiesis without being erythropoietin analogues. Consequently, the preferred acronym is therapy with erythropoiesis-stimulating agents (ESAs).

The established benefits of ESA treatment are avoidance of blood transfusion and improvement in quality of life. However, the literature does not support an evidence-based Hgb level at which treatment should be initiated. The Kidney Disease Outcome Quality Initiative 2007 anemia update recommends that treatment of anemia should be individualized based on a patient's clinical characteristics.[25] If a patient has a decreased Hgb but no decrement in his or her quality of life, there is no pressing need to initiate ESA treatment. For example, if the Hgb is 10.2 g/dL, but there are no symptoms present and the patient is highly active, then treatment should not be initiated. In contrast, if symptoms are present, then treatment should be started when Hgb is less than 11 g/dL. Furthermore, if the patient has symptoms such as fatigue and dyspnea or feels cold despite Hgb levels higher than 12 g/dL, then treatment can be initiated (but the ESA costs may not be reimbursed). However, the latter clinical condition is unusual, and ESA treatment should not be used to increase Hgb to more than 13 g/dL because of the increased risk of adverse outcomes (see later).

Treatment with Erythropoiesis-Stimulating Agents

Because an adequate supply of iron is required for an optimal response to ESA, iron deficiency must be treated before initiating ESA therapy. Once the patient is iron replete, ESA dosing should begin. Unfortunately, there have been few studies that compare different strategies of initiating ESA treatment. A reasonable approach is to correct anemia in a gradual, gentle manner, avoiding overshoot of the Hgb to more than 12 to 13 g/dL. Specifically, an increase in Hgb of 1 g/dL per month will improve symptoms while reducing the risk of complications such as uncontrolled hypertension.

For patients with CKD, ESA treatment is often inconvenient and requires extra office visits, so a goal of therapy should be to avoid excessively frequent drug administration. In our clinic, we usually initiate treatment with either epoetin alfa or darbepoetin alfa, with injections once every 1 to 2 weeks (Table 67-1). Some patients may require more frequent injections, but most patients will have a beneficial response with this approach. For hemodialysis patients, ESAs are often administered intravenously three times weekly because of the convenience of readily available intravenous access. However, there is no pharmacologic or medical reason for such frequent injections and less frequent injections can be effective in achieving the desired Hgb level.

The ability to extend dosing intervals may vary with the ESA; darbepoetin alfa has differences in its sialic acid composition that prolong its serum half-life compared with epoetin alfa.[26] However, the lack of comparative studies between epoetin alfa and darbepoetin alfa makes it difficult to differentiate between the drugs with respect to extended dosing intervals in nondialysis CKD. Studies for each drug have suggested that the dose interval can be extended to once monthly in selected patients.[27,28] A drug currently in development, CERA (continuous erythropoietin receptor activator), has a serum half-life 5 to 16 times as long as that of epoetin alfa and has been found to maintain stable Hgb levels with monthly dosing.[29]

When initiating ESA treatment, Hgb and iron stores should be assessed every month. Monthly iron testing during ESA treatment initiation is necessary due to the rapid transfer of iron from storage tissues to the erythron as Hgb levels increase. Many patients will develop iron deficiency during this period, resulting in diminished response to ESA therapy. This is particularly true for hemodialysis patients, in whom iron stores are also challenged by repeated blood loss. Obviously, if the Hgb is increasing too slowly or rapidly, then the ESA dose should be decreased accordingly.

The treatment target published in the Kidney Disease Outcome Quality Initiative anemia guidelines is an Hgb level of 11 or 12 g/dL. As with all clinical practice guidelines, clinical judgment must be used when applying this recommendation in the context of an individual patient. The guidelines recommend not targeting Hgb levels greater than 13 g/dL. With the Hgb level in this range, the clinician must assess the patient's

Table 67-1 Erythropoiesis-Stimulating Agent Treatment for Patients with Chronic Kidney Disease

	IV Half-life	FDA Label Dose	FDA Label Dose Interval	Comments on Actual Clinical Practice
Epoetin alfa	8 hr	50–100 U/kg	tid	Often converted to once-weekly or less frequent administration
Darbepoetin alfa	25 hr	0.45 µg/kg	Once weekly	Often given every 2 wk or less frequently
CERA placeholder	134 hr			

CERA, continuous erythropoietin receptor activator.

symptoms; if fatigue or dyspnea persists, then cardiovascular, pulmonary, or other causes of symptoms should be pursued.

Complications of Erythropoiesis-Stimulating Agent Treatment

The primary complication found during treatment with ESAs is the development or worsening of hypertension.[30] It is likely that this occurs in 20% to 30% of patients treated.[31] The mechanism has not been fully elucidated but may relate to loss of the compensatory vasodilatation that should occur with anemia.[32] Because hypertension is a cardiovascular risk factor and there is a high prevalence of cardiac disease among CKD patients, avoiding uncontrolled hypertension is critically important. Furthermore, in CKD patients who are in the predialysis stage of their disease, hypertension plays a central role in determining progression of kidney disease (see Chapters 60 and 62).

There does not appear to be significant differences between the risk of hypertension with different ESAs, but with all ESAs, avoidance of excessively rapid increases in Hgb is important. An overshoot to Hgb levels of more than 13 g/dL will increase the risk of cardiovascular diseases. If blood pressure increases during therapy, then the antihypertensive drug regimen should be adjusted accordingly. If severe hypertension develops, then the ESA should be temporarily held. It is rare for permanent cessation of therapy to be required.

Other complications of ESA treatment are rare. Seizures and encephalopathy were reported during early trials of epoetin alfa, probably related to hypertension and excessively aggressive treatment.[33–35] These complications rarely occur with appropriate monitoring. Pure red cell aplasia, a condition detected by severely diminished erythropoiesis due to the development of antierythropoietin antibodies, was reported in Europe, peaking in 2002.[36–38] Cases outside of Europe were extremely rare. The majority of cases occurred with subcutaneous injection of epoetin alfa, and the patients lost all response to ESAs, becoming transfusion dependent. The cause of this problem was determined to be a change in the manufacturing practice, and correction of the problem has essentially eliminated pure red cell aplasia.

The Risk of Mortality with Higher Hemoglobin Levels

In March 2007, the U.S. Food and Drug Administration revised prescribing instructions for ESAs to include substantially higher levels of warnings related to safety. This followed the publication of two studies, the Cardiovascular Risk Reduction by Early Anemia Treatment with Epoetin Beta (CREATE) and Correction of Hemoglobin and Outcomes in Renal Insufficiency (CHOIR); both studies uncovered strong trends for increased risk of death with ESA treatment designed to achieve higher Hgb targets.[24,39] Three published studies, CHOIR, CREATE, and the Normal Hematocrit Cardiac Trial, included 3268 hemodialysis and nondialysis CKD patients. Each study revealed a trend for an increased risk of death from 21% to 48% with higher Hgb targets (P values of .07, .08, and .14, respectively).[18,24,39] Taken together, these studies and related results from studies of cancer patients have created strong and consistent evidence that indicates that using ESAs to target Hgb levels greater than 13 g/L is

harmful. Accordingly, the 2007 update to the Kidney Disease Outcome Quality Initiative anemia guidelines warns against targeting Hgb greater than 13 g/dL.[25]

Suboptimal Responses to Erythropoiesis-Stimulating Agent Treatment

The response of an individual patient to ESA treatment is highly variable. Approximately 10% to 20% of patients have significant degrees of hyporesponsiveness.[40,41] The definition used for hyporesponsiveness varies but operationally is defined as difficulty maintaining Hgb levels greater than 10 to 11 g/dL. In some patients, the Hgb level can be maintained only with very high doses of ESAs (e.g., epoetin alfa doses greater than 36,000 U/kg in a hemodialysis patient).

When ESA hyporesponsiveness is present, the underlying reason should be sought. The most frequent and therapeutically important cause is iron deficiency.[42] In hemodialysis patients, repeated losses of blood in dialysis lines and filters, frequent blood testing, surgery, and access bleeding cause iron deficiency. The incidence of iron deficiency in CKD patients is not clear, but it probably occurs less frequently than in hemodialysis patients.

Diagnosis of iron deficiency in CKD patients has been primarily based on the use of two tests: serum ferritin and transferrin saturation. Serum ferritin is a reflection of iron storage but can be greatly affected by other factors such as inflammation, infection, and nutritional status.[43,44] These noniron effects dilute the ability of serum ferritin to diagnose iron deficiency in CKD accurately. In fact, the sensitivity of serum ferritin (100–200 ng/mL) as an index of true iron deficiency in patients on hemodialysis has usually been found to be less than 50%.[45–47] Transferrin saturation is calculated as serum iron divided by total iron binding capacity (closely related to the serum transferrin concentration). It is a reflection of the small but important pool of circulating iron. It is a more sensitive marker of iron status in CKD patients than serum ferritin, but it is less specific. Therefore, the characteristics of these tests result in a difficult clinical paradox: the serum ferritin level is often very high, concomitant with a low level of transferrin saturation. These divergent data leave the clinician with a diagnostic and therapeutic dilemma, one that is currently difficult to unravel.

Treatment with iron is frequently necessary for patients treated by hemodialysis (Fig. 67-2). A series of studies has found that oral iron has no demonstrable efficacy in these patients. In contrast, intravenous iron treatment is highly effective and in studies in which the Hgb level has been maintained within a target range, intravenous iron treatment can reduce the ESA dose requirements by 25% to 75%.[48–56] In clinical practice, this translates into the ability to achieve Hgb levels greater than 11 g/dL more consistently.

There are currently three intravenous iron drugs that are widely available (Table 67-2). Iron dextran is highly effective but associated with occasional anaphylactic reactions.[57,58] Ferric gluconate and iron sucrose are nondextran forms of iron that probably have a much lower risk of anaphylaxis. In hemodialysis patients, a typical treatment strategy is to administer 1000 mg when iron deficiency develops. The treatment regimen is to give divided doses of 50 to 125 mg at successive hemodialysis treatments. An alternative approach to treatment is the periodic and regular administration of smaller doses of

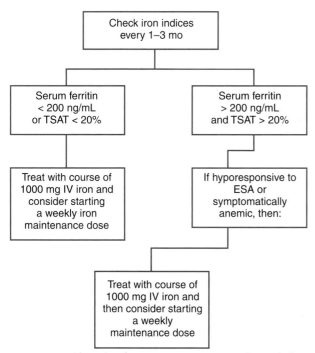

Figure 67-2 Algorithm for iron management in hemodialysis.

intravenous iron (e.g., iron sucrose 50 mg/wk). It is unclear which of these approaches is more effective.

In undialyzed CKD patients or those treated by peritoneal dialysis, iron deficiency probably occurs less frequently than in hemodialysis patients, but the efficacy of oral iron in these groups of patients has not been established as no studies comparing oral iron treatment with placebo or no iron treatment have been published. Still, we recommend assessing iron stores regularly because most patients treated with ESAs generally require iron supplements to support increased erythropoiesis adequately. A generic oral iron supplement may be sufficient for most patients.

The role of intravenous iron in nondialysis CKD or peritoneal dialysis patients has not been established. In nondialysis CKD patients, there have been four randomized, controlled trials comparing intravenous iron with oral iron treatment.[59–62] Two of the four showed no significant difference in efficacy between the groups. The other two studies found superior efficacy for intravenous iron. In the latter studies, there was only a modest degree of benefit. Intravenous iron treatment is inconvenient in nondialysis CKD patients, and occasionally severe hypotension occurs. When these considerations are balanced against only a modest benefit of intravenous iron, it appears clear that intravenous iron should be reserved only for nondialysis CKD patients with severe iron deficiency.

Other causes of ESA hyporesponsiveness include the presence of inflammation, infection, hyperparathyroidism, excessive blood loss, and superimposed hematologic diseases such as megaloblastic anemia and myelodysplasia.[41] Of these, inflammation may be the most important. A number of reports indicate that inflammation, usually signified by elevated C-reactive protein levels, is strongly associated with decreased ESA responsiveness.[44,63] The mechanisms by which inflammation hinders response to ESA treatment are multifactorial. One important component is a reduction in iron utilization and availability. When inflammation is present, the hepatic protein hepcidin blocks entry of iron from intestinal absorption and release of stored iron in tissues into the circulation.[64] The effect is that less iron is available for erythropoiesis. Although the cause of inflammation is often not clear, when present, as indicated by elevated CRP levels, an evaluation for occult infection should be conducted. Nassar and colleagues[65] have reported that infections in unused arteriovenous grafts may be a common cause of inflammation and ESA hyporesponsiveness. They found that removal of the infected graft led to a significant improvement in ESA response.

Table 67-2 Intravenous Iron Drugs

	Need for Test Dose	Indications	IV Push Administration
Iron dextran	Yes	General iron deficiency anemia	Yes
Sodium ferric gluconate	No	Iron deficiency in chronic hemodialysis	Yes
Iron sucrose	No	Iron deficiency in chronic kidney disease: dialysis and predialysis	Yes
Ferumoxytol placeholder			

References

1. Levin A: Prevalence of cardiovascular damage in early renal disease. Nephrol Dial Transplant 2001;16(Suppl 2):7–11.
2. Segal GM, Eschbach JW, Egrie JC, et al: The anemia of end-stage renal disease: Hematopoietic progenitor cell response. Kidney Int 1988;33:983–988.
3. Jelkmann W: Molecular biology of erythropoietin. Intern Med 2004;43:649–659.
4. Fandrey J: Oxygen-dependent and tissue-specific regulation of erythropoietin gene expression. Am J Physiol Regul Integr Comp Physiol 2004;286:R977–R988.
5. McGonigle RJ, Wallin JD, Shadduck RK, Fisher JW: Erythropoietin deficiency and inhibition of erythropoiesis in renal insufficiency. Kidney Int 1984;25:437–444.
6. Radtke HW, Claussner A, Erbes PM, et al: Serum erythropoietin concentration in chronic renal failure: Relationship to degree of anemia and excretory renal function. Blood 1979;54:877–884.
7. Delwiche F, Segal GM, Eschbach JW, Adamson JW: Hematopoietic inhibitors in chronic renal failure: Lack of in vitro specificity. Kidney Int 1986;29:641–648.
8. KDOQI; National Kidney Foundation: KDOQI clinical practice guidelines and clinical practice recommendations for anemia in chronic kidney disease. Am J Kidney Dis 2006;47(5 Suppl 3): S11–S145.
9. Moreno F, Lopez Gomez JM, Sanz-Guajardo D, et al: Quality of life in dialysis patients. A Spanish multicentre study. Spanish Cooperative Renal Patients Quality of Life Study Group. Nephrol Dial Transplant 1996;11(Suppl 2):125–129.

10. Delano BG: Improvements in quality of life following treatment with r-HuEPO in anemic hemodialysis patients. Am J Kidney Dis 1989;14(2 Suppl 1):14–18.

11. Moreno F, Sanz-Guajardo D, Lopez Gomez JM, et al: Increasing the hematocrit has a beneficial effect on quality of life and is safe in selected hemodialysis patients. Spanish Cooperative Renal Patients Quality of Life Study Group of the Spanish Society of Nephrology. J Am Soc Nephrol 2000;11:335–342.

12. Association between recombinant human erythropoietin and quality of life and exercise capacity of patients receiving haemodialysis. Canadian Erythropoietin Study Group. BMJ 1990;300:573–578.

13. Ma JZ, Ebben J, Xia H, Collins AJ: Hematocrit level and associated mortality in hemodialysis patients. J Am Soc Nephrol 1999;10:610–619.

14. Locatelli F, Pisoni RL, Combe C, et al: Anaemia in haemodialysis patients of five European countries: Association with morbidity and mortality in the Dialysis Outcomes and Practice Patterns Study (DOPPS). Nephrol Dial Transplant 2004;19:121–132.

15. Levin A, Djurdev O, Duncan J, et al: Hemoglobin levels prior to therapy predict survival in chronic kidney disease patients [abstract]. J Am Soc Nephrol 2002;13:461.

16. Sandgren PE, Murray AM, Herzog CA, et al: Anemia and new-onset congestive heart failure in the general Medicare population. J Card Fail 2005;11:99–105.

17. Sarnak MJ, Levey AS: Cardiovascular disease and chronic renal disease: A new paradigm. Am J Kidney Dis 2000;35(4 Suppl 1):S117–S131.

18. Besarab A, Bolton WK, Browne JK, et al: The effects of normal as compared with low hematocrit values in patients with cardiac disease who are receiving hemodialysis and epoetin. N Engl J Med 1998;339:584–590.

19. Furuland H, Linde T, Ahlmen J, et al: A randomized controlled trial of haemoglobin normalization with epoetin alfa in pre-dialysis and dialysis patients. Nephrol Dial Transplant 2003;18:353–361.

20. Parfrey PS, Foley RN, Wittreich BH, et al: Double-blind comparison of full and partial anemia correction in incident hemodialysis patients without symptomatic heart disease. J Am Soc Nephrol 2005;16:2180–2189.

21. Roger SD, McMahon LP, Clarkson A, et al: Effects of early and late intervention with epoetin alpha on left ventricular mass among patients with chronic kidney disease (stage 3 or 4): Results of a randomized clinical trial. J Am Soc Nephrol 2004;15:148–156.

22. Levin A, Thompson CR, Ethier J, et al: Left ventricular mass index increase in early renal disease: Impact of decline in hemoglobin. Am J Kidney Dis 1999;34:125–134.

23. Foley RN, Parfrey PS, Harnett JD, et al: Clinical and echocardiographic disease in patients starting end-stage renal disease therapy. Kidney Int 1995;47:186–192.

24. Drueke TB, Locatelli F, Clyne N, et al, for the CREATE Investigators: Normalization of hemoglobin level in patients with chronic kidney disease and anemia. N Engl J Med 2006;355:2071–2084.

25. KDOQI Clinical Practice Guideline and Clinical Practice Recommendations for anemia in chronic kidney disease: 2007 update of hemoglobin target. Am J Kidney Dis 2007;50:471–530.

26. Macdougall IC: Optimizing the use of erythropoietic agents—pharmacokinetic and pharmacodynamic considerations. Nephrol Dial Transplant 2002;17(Suppl 5):66–70.

27. Provenzano R, Bhaduri S, Singh AK; PROMPT Study Group: Extended epoetin alfa dosing as maintenance treatment for the anemia of chronic kidney disease: The PROMPT study. Clin Nephrol 2005;64:113–123.

28. Agarwal A, Silver MR, Walczyk M, et al: Once-monthly darbepoetin alfa for maintaining hemoglobin levels in older patients with chronic kidney disease. J Am Med Dir Assoc 2007;8:83–90.

29. Macdougall IC: CERA (continuous erythropoietin receptor activator): A new erythropoiesis-stimulating agent for the treatment of anemia. Curr Hematol Rep 2005;4:436–440.

30. Brunkhorst R, Nonnast-Daniel B, Koch KM, Frei U: Hypertension as a possible complication of recombinant human erythropoietin therapy. Contrib Nephrol 1991;88:118–125.

31. Buckner FS, Eschbach JW, Haley NR, et al: Hypertension following erythropoietin therapy in anemic hemodialysis patients. Am J Hypertens 1990;3:947–955.

32. Baskin S, Lasker N: Erythropoietin-associated hypertension. N Engl J Med 1990;323:999–1000.

33. Beccari M: Seizures in dialysis patients treated with recombinant erythropoietin. Review of the literature and guidelines for prevention. Int J Artif Organs 1994;17:5–13.

34. Brown AL, Tucker B, Baker LR, Raine AE: Seizures related to blood transfusion and erythropoietin treatment in patients undergoing dialysis. BMJ 1989;299:1258–1259.

35. Edmunds ME, Walls J, Tucker B, et al: Seizures in haemodialysis patients treated with recombinant human erythropoietin. Nephrol Dial Transplant 1989;4:1065–1069.

36. Rossert J, for the Pure Red Cell Aplasia Global Scientific Advisory Board (GSAB): Erythropoietin-induced, antibody-mediated pure red cell aplasia. Eur J Clin Invest 2005;35(Suppl 3):95–99.

37. Kharagjitsingh AV, Korevaar JC, Vandenbroucke JP, et al, for the NECOSAD Study Group: Incidence of recombinant erythropoietin (EPO) hyporesponse, EPO-associated antibodies, and pure red cell aplasia in dialysis patients. Kidney Int 2005;68:1215–1222.

38. Carson KR, Evens AM, Bennett CL, Luminari S: Clinical characteristics of erythropoietin-associated pure red cell aplasia. Best Pract Res Clin Haematol 2005;18:467–472.

39. Singh AK, Szczech L, Tang KL, et al, for the CHOIR Investigators: Correction of anemia with epoetin alfa in chronic kidney disease. N Engl J Med 2006;355:2085–2098.

40. Rossert J, Gassmann-Mayer C, Frei D, McClellan W: Prevalence and predictors of epoetin hyporesponsiveness in chronic kidney disease patients. Nephrol Dial Transplant 2007;22:794–800.

41. Fishbane S, Maesaka JK: Iron management in end-stage renal disease. Am J Kidney Dis 1997;29:319–333.

42. Van Wyck DB: Iron management during recombinant human erythropoietin therapy. Am J Kidney Dis 1989;14(2 Suppl 1):9–13.

43. Kalantar-Zadeh K, Rodriguez RA, Humphreys MH: Association between serum ferritin and measures of inflammation, nutrition and iron in haemodialysis patients. Nephrol Dial Transplant 2004;19:141–149.

44. Kalantar-Zadeh K, McAllister CJ, Lehn RS, et al: Effect of malnutrition-inflammation complex syndrome on EPO hyporesponsiveness in maintenance hemodialysis patients. Am J Kidney Dis 2003;42:761–773.

45. Fishbane S, Kowalski EA, Imbriano LJ, Maesaka JK: The evaluation of iron status in hemodialysis patients. J Am Soc Nephrol 1996;7:2654–2657.

46. Kalantar-Zadeh K, Hoffken B, Wunsch H, et al: Diagnosis of iron deficiency anemia in renal failure patients during the post-erythropoietin era. Am J Kidney Dis 1995;26:292–299.

47. Tessitore N, Solero GP, Lippi G, et al: The role of iron status markers in predicting response to intravenous iron in haemodialysis patients on maintenance erythropoietin. Nephrol Dial Transplant 2001;16:1416–1423.

48. Macdougall IC, Tucker B, Thompson J, et al: A randomized controlled study of iron supplementation in patients treated with erythropoietin. Kidney Int 1996;50:1694–1699.

49. Markowitz GS, Kahn GA, Feingold RE, et al: An evaluation of the effectiveness of oral iron therapy in hemodialysis patients receiving recombinant human erythropoietin. Clin Nephrol 1997;48:34–40.

50. Fudin R, Jaichenko J, Shostak A, et al: Correction of uremic iron deficiency anemia in hemodialyzed patients: A prospective study. Nephron 1998;79:299–305.

51. Besarab A, Amin N, Ahsan M, et al: Optimization of epoetin therapy with intravenous iron therapy in hemodialysis patients. J Am Soc Nephrol 2000;11:530-538.

52. DeVita MV, Frumkin D, Mittal S, et al: Targeting higher ferritin concentrations with intravenous iron dextran lowers erythropoietin requirement in hemodialysis patients. Clin Nephrol 2003;60:335–340.

53. Taylor JE, Peat N, Porter C, Morgan AG: Regular low-dose intravenous iron therapy improves response to erythropoietin in haemodialysis patients. Nephrol Dial Transplant 1996;11:1079–1083.

54. Sunder-Plassmann G, Horl WH: Importance of iron supply for erythropoietin therapy. Nephrol Dial Transplant 1995;10:2070–2076.

55. Sepandj F, Jindal K, West M, Hirsch D: Economic appraisal of maintenance parenteral iron administration in treatment of anaemia in chronic haemodialysis patients. Nephrol Dial Transplant 1996;11:319–322.

56. Fishbane S, Frei GL, Maesaka J: Reduction in recombinant human erythropoietin doses by the use of chronic intravenous iron supplementation. Am J Kidney Dis 1995;26:41–46.

57. Fishbane S, Ungureanu VD, Maesaka JK, et al: The safety of intravenous iron dextran in hemodialysis patients. Am J Kidney Dis 1996;28:529–534.

58. Hamstra RD, Block MH, Schocket AL: Intravenous iron dextran in clinical medicine. JAMA 1980;243:1726–1731.

59. Aggarwal HK, Nand N, Singh S, et al: Comparison of oral versus intravenous iron therapy in predialysis patients of chronic renal failure receiving recombinant human erythropoietin. J Assoc Physicians India 2003;51:170–174.

60. Stoves J, Inglis H, Newstead CG: A randomized study of oral vs intravenous iron supplementation in patients with progressive renal insufficiency treated with erythropoietin. Nephrol Dial Transplant 2001;16:967–974.

61. Charytan C, Qunibi W, Bailie GR, for the Venofer Clinical Studies Group: Comparison of intravenous iron sucrose to oral iron in the treatment of anemic patients with chronic kidney disease not on dialysis. Nephron Clin Pract 2005;100:c55–c62.

62. Van Wyck DB, Roppolo M, Martinez CO, et al., for the United States Iron Sucrose (Venofer) Clinical Trials Group: A randomized, controlled trial comparing IV iron sucrose to oral iron in anemic patients with nondialysis-dependent CKD. Kidney Int 2005;68:2846–2856.

63. Gunnell J, Yeun JY, Depner TA, Kaysen GA: Acute-phase response predicts erythropoietin resistance in hemodialysis and peritoneal dialysis patients. Am J Kidney Dis 1999;33:63–72.

64. Ganz T: Molecular control of iron transport. J Am Soc Nephrol 2007;18:394–400.

65. Nassar GM, Fishbane S, Ayus JC: Occult infection of old non-functioning arteriovenous grafts: A novel cause of erythropoietin resistance and chronic inflammation in hemodialysis patients. Kidney Int Suppl 2002;80:49–54.

Further Reading

Hsu C, McCulloch C, Curhan G: Epidemiology of anemia associated with chronic renal insufficiency among adults in the United States: Results from the Third National Health and Nutrition Examination Survey. J Am Soc Nephrol 2002;13:504–510.

Astor B, Muntner P, Levin A, et al: Association of kidney function with anemia. Arch Intern Med 2002;162:1401–1408.

El-Achkar TM, Ohmit SE, McCullough PA, et al: Higher prevalence of anemia with diabetes mellitus in moderate kidney insufficiency: The Kidney Early Evaluation Program. Kidney Int 2005;67:1483–1488.

Fandrey J: Oxygen-dependent and tissue-specific regulation of erythropoietin gene expression. Am J Physiol Regul Integr Comp Physiol 2004;286:R977–R988.

Fishbane S: Iron supplementation in renal anemia. Semin Nephrol 2006;26:319–324.

Hsu C, McCulloch C, Curhan G: Epidemiology of anemia associated with chronic renal insufficiency among adults in the United States: Results from the Third National Health and Nutrition Examination Survey. J Am Soc Nephrol 2002;13:504–510.

Jelkmann W: Molecular biology of erythropoietin. Intern Med 2004;43:649–659.

KDOQI; National Kidney Foundation: KDOQI Clinical Practice Guidelines and Clinical Practice Recommendations for Anemia in Chronic Kidney Disease. Am J Kidney Dis 2006;47(5 Suppl 3):S11–S145.

Ling B, Walczyk M, Agarwal A, et al: Darbepoetin alfa administered once monthly maintains hemoglobin concentrations in patients with chronic kidney disease. Clin Nephrol 2005;63:327–334.

Provenzano R, Bhaduri S, Singh AK; PROMPT Study Group: Extended epoetin alfa dosing as maintenance treatment for the anemia of chronic kidney disease: The PROMPT study. Clin Nephrol 2005;64:113–123.

Roberts TL, Foley RN, Weinhandl ED, et al: Anaemia and mortality in haemodialysis patients: Interaction of propensity score for predicted anaemia and actual haemoglobin levels. Nephrol Dial Transplant 2006;21:1652–1662.

Treatment of Anemia and Bleeding in Chronic Kidney Disease

Giuseppe Remuzzi, Luigi Minetti, and Arrigo Schieppati

Anemia, defined by the World Health Organization as a hemoglobin (Hb) level less than 13 g/dL in males and postmenopausal females and less than 12 g/dL in premenopausal females,[1] is present virtually in all patients with chronic kidney disease (CKD), including patients with impaired renal function, renal transplant recipients with allograft dysfunction, and those treated with long-term dialysis.[2–4]

The prevalence of anemia in CKD depends in part on the study population and in part on the level of Hb defined as constituting anemia. In a Canadian multicenter cohort study of patients referred to nephrology services, the prevalence of anemia was 25% in patients with creatinine clearance greater than 50 mL/min and increased stepwise to 87% when creatinine clearance was less than 25 mL/min.[5] In another cross-sectional study of adult patients with CKD, the mean level of Hb was 12.8 ± 1.5 in patients with CKD stage 1 and 2, 12.4 ± 1.6 in CKD stage 3, 12.0 ± 1.6 in CKD stage 4, and 10.9 ± 1.6 g/dL in CKD stage 5.[6] The Kidney Disease Outcome and Quality Initiative (K/DOQI) clinical practice guidelines and clinical practice recommendations for anemia in chronic kidney disease concluded that there is a definite trend toward lower Hb levels at lower levels of glomerular filtration rate.[7]

The anemia of renal failure is characterized by normocytic and normochromic red blood cells, a low reticulocyte count for the degree of anemia, and a hypoplastic erythroid series in the bone marrow with normal leukopoiesis and megakaryocytopoiesis.[8] The red cell mass and its adaptation to changes in oxygen need depend on erythropoietin. Both the oxygen sensor and the site of synthesis of erythropoietin (peritubular capillary endothelial cells) are in the renal cortex.[9] Erythropoietin is detectable in blood after bilateral nephrectomy, consistent with experimental findings that approximately 10% is produced by the liver. Erythropoietin stimulates proliferation and maturation of erythroid colony-forming units. It decreases programmed cell death, or apoptosis of erythroid progenitor cells in the bone marrow by binding to a receptor on the surface of erythroid cells, promoting a cascade of events starting by activation of JAK2 tyrosine kinase. There also is cell proliferation.[10]

Human erythropoietin was purified in 1977, and its molecular structure was characterized in 1986 as a sialylglycoprotein composed of 165 amino acids. Its plasma level normally ranges between 15 and 25 mU/mL but may increase 100-fold in anemia. Erythropoietin production in CKD patients is diminished, but the erythropoietin-Hb feedback still operates, although at a lower set point.

In addition to the hypoproliferative, normochromic, and normocytic anemia in CKD, there is a hemolytic component. Red cell half-life is reduced to approximately one half to two thirds of normal, possibly due to uremic toxins. The anemia of CKD can also be related to iron and folate deficiency, blood loss from repeated venipuncture or blood left in the dialyzer and tubing during dialysis, hyperparathyroidism, and aluminum toxicity.

The anemia of CKD has been associated with fatigue, decreased mental capacity, erectile dysfunction, altered menstrual cycles, immunodepression, a bleeding tendency, and, most importantly, cardiovascular complications.[11–15] Thus, anemia is indirectly responsible for decreased quality of life in CKD patients.

THERAPY FOR ANEMIA

Initial Evaluation

The correction of anemia in CKD patients is aimed at relieving symptoms, improving the quality of life, and possibly increasing patient survival (Box 68-1). In the opinion of the Anemia Working Group who constructed the revised K/DOQI guidelines, all CKD patients should be tested for Hb levels at least yearly; more frequent measurements are indicated in selected patients.[7] The K/DOQI guidelines conclude that evaluation of anemia should be considered for Hb less than

Box 68-1 Anemia Evaluation in Patients with Chronic Kidney Disease

Who must be evaluated for renal anemia
  All patients with chronic kidney disease
When
  Hemoglobin concentration
    <13.5 g/dL in adult males
    <12.0 g/dL in adult females
What must be evaluated
  Red blood cell indices: MCV, mean corpuscular hemo-globin, reticulocyte count
  Iron status: serum iron, ferritin, transferrin saturation, hypochromic red blood cells (if test is available)
  Assessment of occult gastrointestinal blood loss, serum vitamin B_{12} folate; tests for hemolysis; hematological evaluation if there is clinical suspicion of other causes of anemia

MCV, mean corpuscular volume.

13.5 g/dL in adult males and less than 12 g/dL in adult females. The European Best Practice Guidelines[16] have slightly different Hb cutoff levels. The treatment targets are based on Hb rather than hematocrit (Hct) levels because the stability of stored sample is greater and there is less variability with automated analyzers.[17]

In addition to Hb, the initial evaluation should include red blood cell (RBC) indices and a reticulocyte count as well as serum iron, total iron binding capacity, transferrin saturation, and serum ferritin.

Additional evaluations are warranted if there is a suspicion of occult blood loss from the gastrointestinal tract; the stool occult blood test is simple and inexpensive and should be included whenever there is iron deficiency.[18] Determination of folate and vitamin B_{12} levels is not recommended unless there is an obvious cause of deficiency. Determination of plasma erythropoietin concentration is not recommended in European and American guidelines (see Chapter 67).

Choice of Erythropoiesis-Stimulating Agents

The efficacy of the first erythropoiesis-stimulating agent (ESA), human recombinant erythropoietin (rhEPO) in reversing the anemia of uremia was established in the United States and in Europe and rhEPO quickly became available for clinical use.[2] There are two forms of rhEPO, epoetin alfa and epoetin beta, produced from genomic DNA and complementary DNA, respectively; they differ in their oligosaccharide components. Experimental and clinical findings suggest their pharmacological activity and other biological effects are similar. Epoetin alfa has an average half-life of 4 to 13 hours after IV administration and approximately 24 hours after SC injection (the maximum level is only approximately 10% of that achieved by the same IV dose). The kinetics of epoetin beta are similar to those of epoetin alfa. Both preparations appear to be eliminated primarily by nonrenal mechanisms. Darbepoetin alfa or novel erythropoiesis-stimulating protein is a molecule that stimulates erythropoiesis by the same mechanisms as rhEPO.[19] It has an elimination half-life two or three times longer than rhEPO; the mean

half-life of darbepoetin is 49 hours when given subcutaneously and 21 hours when given intravenously. Therefore, it requires less frequent dosing. It is as effective and safe as rhEPO in the anemia of CKD. Interestingly, ESA therapy brings red cell survival back to normal associated with increased erythrocyte elasticity and deformability as well as the antioxidant enzymatic system of red blood cells. ESA treatment aims to make blood transfusions unnecessary, to prevent the consequences of anemia, and to improve rehabilitation and the quality of life.

Target Hemoglobin

The complexity of establishing a target level for Hb has been recently highlighted.[20] In 2001, the K/DOQI anemia guidelines recommended a Hb target level of 11.0 to 12.0 g/dL in CKD patients.[21] Observational studies have shown that mortality rates were lower in hemodialysis (HD) patients who have Hb values close to 11 to 12 g/dL compared with HD patients with lower levels. Results from randomized, controlled trials comparing Hb targets suggest that partial correction of anemia to levels of approximately 11 to 12 g/dL leads to an improved quality of life.[22] Finally, limited evidence suggests that partial correction of anemia to levels of 11 to 12 g/dL is associated with partialregression of left ventricular hypertrophy.[23–26] The 2006 K/DOQI anemia guidelines confirm the recommendation that the lower limit for Hb level for patients with CKD should be 11 g/dL, but this is still lower than the normal range of Hb according to the World Health Organization definition of anemia.[27] The issue of risks and benefits with the upper limit of Hb correction has been addressed. A study of more than 1200 HD patients with significant cardiac disease had to be discontinued because of a trend toward higher mortality in the group targeted with an Hct of 42%. The difference between the treated and control groups did not reach statistical significance.[28] Recently, two studies involving a large population of patients were published in the *New England Journal of Medicine*, the Cardiovascular Risk Reduction by Early Anemia Treatment with Epoetin Beta (CREATE)[29] trial and the Correction of Hemoglobin and Outcomes in Renal Insufficiency (CHOIR).[30] Results of the CREATE trial showed that in CKD patients with an estimated glomerular filtration rate of 15 to 35 mL/min, the correction of anemia to a normal Hb range of 13.0 to 15.0 g/dL did not decrease the incidence of cardiovascular events when compared with partial correction of anemia (Hb value of 10.5–11.5 g/dL). The most surprising finding of this study was that a high target Hb level did not ameliorate left ventricular hypertrophy.

In the CHOIR trial, an Hb target of 13.5 g/dL versus 11.3 g/dL was associated with increased risk of death, myocardial infarction, and hospitalization for congestive heart failure and stroke; there was no improvement in the quality of life.

There are ongoing multicenter trials of complete versus partial correction of anemia in CKD patients. While waiting for publication of these trials, the available evidence suggests caution in treating the anemia of CKD patients.[31] A target Hb value between 11 and 12 g/dL, as suggested by K/DOQI anemia guidelines, should be considered the goal of ESA therapy.

Dose and Route of Administration

The safe and effective rate of increase in Hb level is 1 to 2 g/dL per month. The recommended initial SC dose for adults is 80 to 120 U/kg per week, typically given in two to three doses of 6000 U/week. The recommended IV regimen is 120 to 180 U/kg per week, typically given as 9000 U/week in three divided doses.

Starting doses of 100 U/kg three times weekly by IV injection increase Hb levels in 90% of patients, whereas a dose of 50 U/kg produces target Hb levels in 70% of patients. An increase of more than 3 g/dL in 4 weeks should be avoided because of the potential exacerbation of hypertension.[32] Doses exceeding 300 U/kg usually do not elicit more vigorous erythropoietic response. The Hb and Hct should be monitored every 1 to 2 weeks until the target Hb is reached and then every 2 to 4 weeks. If the increase in Hct is less than 2% in 4 weeks, the rhEPO dose should be increased by 50%; if it is more than 8%, the rhEPO should be decreased by 25%. It takes 4 weeks to assess the response to a change in dose and an increase in dose should not exceed 30 U/kg three times per week. When the Hb or Hct value is near the target, the dose should be decreased by approximately 25 U/kg three times per week to avoid overshooting the target; the dose is then down-titrated gradually.

Regarding the route of administration, the average rhEPO dose needed to maintain an Hct of 33% was lower when administered subcutaneously. In the maintenance phase of anemia treatment, the median IV dose necessary to keep Hb at approximately 12 g/dL is approximately 75 U/kg three times per week, but limits are wide; some patients need 25 U/kg three times per week and others more than 200 U/kg three times per week. Subcutaneous ESA maintenance doses can be substantially lower; patients on continuous ambulatory peritoneal dialysis have been effectively managed with SC doses of ESA less than 40 U/kg three times per week. The suggested initial dose of darbepoetin is 0.45 μg/kg once weekly (SC or IV). To change from rhEPO to darbepoetin, the rhEPO dose can be divided by 200 to obtain the darbepoetin dose.

An alarming side effect of ESA can be the development of anti-EPO antibodies and pure red cell bone marrow aplasia (PRCA).[33] There have been more than 200 reported cases of PRCA, and virtually all cases occurred in CKD patients who received a particular epoetin alfa product, Eprex, in single-use syringes.[34] The underlying cause may have been organic compounds acting as adjuvants because changes in storage and handling and discontinuation of SC administration of Eprex have led to a sharp decline in the incidence of anti-EPO antibody–mediated PRCA in CKD patients. Fortunately, EPO-related PRCA is extremely rare given the widespread use of EPO.

Iron Supplementation

Iron deficiency is frequent in CKD patients and is the main cause of hyporesponsiveness to ESA.[35] Therefore, iron status should be monitored before and after beginning ESA therapy and at regular intervals (usually every 2–3 months). Iron stores are most accurately assessed by staining the bone marrow for hemosiderin, but this is expensive, and generally the iron status is assessed from serum iron and ferritin and transferrin saturation. Ferritin is secreted by the reticuloendothelial cells in proportion to the intracellular iron concentration.[36] A ferritin level less than 100 ng/mL indicates iron deficiency (<50 ng/mL indicates absolute iron deficiency); a serum level greater than 600 ng/mL reflects iron overload. When the level is greater than 300 ng/mL, iron supplementation is generally not needed

(see Chapter 67), but iron deficiency can develop with ESA therapy because of consumption of iron deposits. Iron is also required when the transferrin saturation is less than 20%. Inadequate iron stores will prevent a vigorous response to ESA, and this can be a therapeutic problem despite a normal serum ferritin level; this condition is called functional iron deficiency. In this case, the developing RBCs are hypochromic. A quantitative assessment of the amount of Hb in newly released RBCs can be made by measuring the percentage of circulating red cells that are hypochromic, defined as a mean erythrocyte Hb concentration less than 28 g/dL. When the hypochromic cells exceed 10% (the normal range is <2.5% of circulating RBCs) in patients without a hemoglobinopathy or inflammatory disease, functional iron deficiency is present. More sophisticated tests for iron deficiency include determination of serum transferrin receptor concentrations and measurement of free erythrocytic protoporphyrin. The serum transferrin receptor concentration is measured with monoclonal antibodies; it increases with the severity of iron store depletion. The percentage of hypochromic RBCs is a better marker for assessing iron availability for Hb synthesis than transferrin saturation, but the test is not universally available, whereas ferritin and transferrin saturation are widely available and used to monitor iron status.

Iron supplements are given to keep serum ferritin greater than 100 ng/mL, transferrin saturation greater than 20%, and hypochromic red cells less than 10%. HD patients usually require 150 mg of iron to achieve a 1-g/dL increase in Hb. This requirement is difficult to achieve by oral medications, and IV iron administration is preferred. During correction of the anemia, 1000 mg of iron given over 6 to 12 weeks should ensure adequate supplementation.

There are three forms of iron that can be given intravenously: iron dextran, sodium ferric gluconate, and iron sucrose. The European Best Practice Guidelines[37] suggested that the first choice should be iron sucrose; the second choice is ferric gluconate, and iron dextran is not generally recommended because of the risk of serious adverse reactions. All IV iron formulations have been associated with vasoactive reactions and hypotension, but the rate of adverse reactions with IV iron dextran is reportedly 0.6% to 0.7% of patients. Therefore, a test dose is recommended before IV iron dextran is administered. Unfortunately, a successful test does not exclude a subsequent reaction on its administration.[37] The K/DOQI anemia guidelines strongly recommend that IV iron dextran be administered only by trained personnel and that proper emergency medications be readily available.[38] A test dose is not recommended before giving other iron preparations.

The protocol for IV iron dextran or iron gluconate in HD patients with absolute iron deficiency is 100 mg of iron dextran or 125 mg of iron gluconate during each dialysis for 10 or 8 doses, respectively. For maintenance iron therapy and for treating and preventing functional iron deficiency, the recommendation is 25 to 100 mg of IV iron dextran every week for 10 weeks or 31.25 to 125 mg of iron gluconate every week for 8 weeks (responses are evaluated by an increase in transferrin saturation and serum ferritin).[38]

The ideal route of iron administration for pre-HD CKD and for peritoneal dialysis patients is not established. A daily oral dose of approximately 200 mg of elemental iron is appropriate for most patients (approximately one sixth will be absorbed). Commercial oral iron preparations differ in their content of elemental iron; a 325-mg tablet provides 107 mg of ferrous fumarate, 65 mg of ferrous sulfate, or 39 mg of ferrous gluconate. When ferritin has a downward trend during oral iron supplementation, IV iron dextran may be necessary.

Side Effects

The incidences (per patient-year) of some adverse events are 0.75 for hypertension, 0.25 for clotted vascular access, 0.11 for hyperkalemia, and 0.048 for seizures. The association with seizures not related to hypertension is questionable because seizures can occur in patients not receiving ESA (0.05–0.10 per patient-year). Still, the rate of seizures appears to be higher during the first 90 days of ESA therapy, and strict control of the rate of the Hb increase (<1.5 g/dL every 4 weeks) and close monitoring of blood pressure are warranted. Hyperkalemia presumably reflects less efficient dialysis because the higher Hct decreases the plasma that can be treated and reflects poor dietary compliance with avoiding potassium-rich foods (it has been proposed that decreased dietary compliance is attributable to an improved sense of well-being). The aggravation or appearance of hypertension in patients during ESA therapy has been attributed to increased whole-blood viscosity, reversal of hypoxia-dependent peripheral vasodilatation, and activation or enhancement of vascular responsiveness to vasoactive agents. Other suggested mechanisms include a functionally or structurally decreased cross-sectional area of the peripheral vascular bed, normalization of cardiac output, and an increase in RBC mass with minimal decrease in plasma volume. Risk factors for developing or worsening of hypertension in dialysis patients include preexisting hypertension, rapid correction of anemia, and high doses of ESA. Notably, IV administration of ESA and "nondipper" conditions were not identified as risk factors. Increases in blood pressure are generally reported during the first 90 days of therapy. In most cases, hypertension is controlled by reducing dry body weight, starting or increasing antihypertensive therapy, and reducing the dose of ESA. No patient should be excluded from ESA treatment because of increased risk of hypertension.

Causes of an Inadequate Response in Addition to Iron Deficiency

When iron stores are repleted, more than 95% of patients will respond to ESA treatment by attaining the target Hb within 3 to 6 months. An inadequate response to ESA is defined as a failure to attain the target Hb in 6 months despite maximum ESA doses and adequate iron stores. Maximum rhEPO doses are 300 U/kg/week SC and 450 U/kg/week IV. A blunted or absent response may be due not only to iron deficiency but also to aluminum overload, underlying infectious, inflammatory or malignant diseases, gastrointestinal or other sources of blood loss, underlying hematologic disease, severe hyperparathyroidism, folate or vitamin B_{12} deficiency, the presence of circulating inhibitors of erythropoiesis, and down-regulation of erythropoietin receptors on the surface of committed cells.[39]

In HD patients, aluminum overload may provoke microcytic anemia even though iron stores are normal. Aluminum and iron share common pathways for intestinal absorption, transport in the plasma, binding to transferrin, and uptake into cells. Iron-depleted rats are more susceptible to aluminum accumulation, and this may influence patient responses as well. In HD patients, it is suggested that transferrin-bound aluminum may interfere with the insertion of iron into proto-

porphyrin to form heme. For example, a high plasma aluminum is related to a smaller erythropoietic response to ESA plus higher levels of protoporphyrin in red cells. Ferrochelatase activity and erythropoietic responses were not correlated. Fortunately, aluminum accumulation is becoming less common with increased use of deionizers and decreased use of aluminum-containing phosphate binders; aluminum in bone biopsy samples has an incidence of less than 5%. If suspected, aluminium toxicity should be documented with serum aluminum greater than 50 ng/mL and an increase in serum aluminum greater than 175 ng/mL after the deferoxamine (an aluminum-binding agent) challenge of a single IV dose of 500 to 1000 mg. Chelation treatment with IV deferoxamine can improve aluminum-induced microcytic anemia; it could also restore responsiveness to ESA.[38]

Erythropoiesis is negatively regulated by several macrophage-derived cytokines, including tumor necrosis factor α, interleukin-1, interleukin-6, and tumor growth factor β. These cytokines are all elevated in inflammatory processes and exert inhibitory effects on the erythroid progenitor cells, the targets of ESA. Cytokines may also impair iron metabolism by sequestering iron inside the macrophages. Characteristically, the anemia of chronic infectious and inflammatory diseases has a low reticulocyte count for the degree of anemia, and RBCs are often microcytic or hypochromic despite normal or increased levels of serum ferritin.[40–44] Does this kind of anemia respond to ESA? There is evidence that ESA can overcome the inhibition of erythropoiesis caused by inflammatory cytokines in chronic disease. Unrecognized infection or subtle inflammation can contribute to the anemia of uremia, and this is a diagnostic and therapeutic challenge; the anemia may be resistant to ESA at usual doses but responds, at least partially, to high doses.

HD patients with severe hyperparathyroidism need significantly more ESA.[45] Vitamin B_{12}/folate deficiency is no longer considered a problem for ESA therapy. Some commonly used drugs may influence erythropoiesis: Angiotensin-converting enzyme inhibitors can inhibit erythropoietin production and adversely affect erythropoiesis.[46,47]

BLEEDING IN CHRONIC KIDNEY DISEASE PATIENTS

An increased tendency to bleed as a major feature of uremia has been known for centuries.[48,49] Ecchymoses, epistaxis, and gastrointestinal bleeding are common, and subdural hematomas occur in 5% to 15% of HD adults. Hemopericardium and subcapsular hematoma of the liver occur but fortunately are less frequent than bleeding manifestations. The bleeding tendency increases the risk of surgery or invasive procedures in dialysis patients. Although the pathogenesis of uremic bleeding is multifactorial, the central factor is altered platelet function and an altered platelet-endothelium interaction.[50,51] The best measure of the platelet–vessel wall interaction is the bleeding time, a simple method tested by making a small incision of the skin (usually in forearm) and measuring the time from the first drop of blood to the last oozing of blood from the cut.[52] A normal bleeding time is 1 to 7 minutes, and the key to interpretation is to carefully standardize the technique; untrained personnel account for the substantial variation in the bleeding time. A prolonged bleeding time is a feature of uremic patients, but the prolongation does not correlate with retained metabolites including urea, creatinine, phenol, phenolic acids, and guanidinosuccinic acid; it is correlated with the Hct value.[53] Notably, the platelet count and other coagulation parameters (partial thromboplastin time, prothrombin time, fibrinogen) are not altered in uremia (see Box 68-1).

von Willebrand's factor (vWF) is an adhesion molecule that promotes platelet adhesion and aggregation to subendothelial collagen through an interaction with GPIb/IX receptors. This initiates a sequence of events resulting in the production of thromboxane A_2, a potent platelet-aggregating agent. In uremia, vWF is functionally defective and thromboxane A_2 formation is impaired.[54,55] Conversely, vascular synthesis of the antiaggregating prostaglandin I_2 is enhanced in uremia, tipping the balance in favor of reduced platelet aggregation.

The anemia of uremia has consequences for the rheology of platelets because they flow in the midstream, away from the endothelium, thereby decreasing the chance of platelet–vessel wall interaction.[56] Platelet dysfunction is potentiated by the use of aspirin and other nonsteroidal anti-inflammatory drugs. Such drugs should be prescribed for uremic patients only cautiously.[57] The pathogenesis of uremic bleeding is reviewed in references 50 and 51.

Therapy for Bleeding in Uremic Patients

Dialysis

HD shortens the prolonged bleeding time of uremic patients and partially corrects platelet dysfunction and the abnormal platelet-endothelial interaction. Unfortunately, removal of uremic toxins by HD is not enough to correct fully the hemostatic defects of uremia.[58] Moreover, the need for heparin administration to prevent clotting of the dialyzer suggests that HD (or at least heparin) should be avoided during active bleeding. It has been suggested that peritoneal dialysis is more effective in patients with uremic bleeding than HD, and tests of platelet function suggest this is the case, but controlled studies of clinical responses are lacking. Several methods have been proposed to minimize blood loss during HD in bleeding patients. These include regional heparinization and the use of low molecular weight heparins, prostacyclin, or no anticoagulation at all. The method of choice at our center involves frequent flushes of saline through the dialyzer at intervals but no heparin. This approach gives the best results when used in association with hemodiafiltration. The method is used after major surgery or trauma in HD patients (Table 68-1).

Correction of Anemia

Anemia has a major adverse influence on the bleeding time and bleeding tendency of uremic patients. An initial study of six uremic patients demonstrated that RBC transfusions shortened the bleeding time and controlled abnormal bleeding. This was subsequently confirmed in a larger group of patients.[56]

Relieving uremic anemia by ESA can also improve the hemostatic defects and normalize the bleeding time. Therefore, correction of the anemia, either by acute RBC transfusion or the use of ESA, is currently a major overall strategy for preventing and controlling abnormal bleeding in uremia.[59]

Cryoprecipitate and Desmopressin

Cryoprecipitate contains coagulation factor VIII, vWF, fibrinogen, and fibronectin. It has been used in uremic patients with very long bleeding times that were resistant to blood transfusions or HD or both.[60] In six uremic patients treated by infusing 10 units of cryoprecipitate, there was normalization or significant shortening of the bleeding time. Surgical procedures were undertaken in a few patients without excessive blood loss. The effect, however, was delayed (the nadir of

Table 68-1 Therapeutic Strategies for Uremic Bleeding

Treatment	Indication	Dose	EFFECT		
			Start	Peak	End
Blood or RBCs	Prophylaxis of bleeding in high-risk patients	According to the severity of anemia	Hct = 28%–32%		Relate to RBC life span
Recombinant human erythropoietin	Prophylaxis of bleeding in high-risk patients with anemia	80–120 U/kg IV	Hct = 28%–32%		
Cryoprecipitate*	Acute bleeding episodes	10 bags	1 hr	4–12 hr	24–36 hr
Desmopressin†	Acute bleeding episodes	0.3 µg/kg IV‡	1 hr	2–4 hr	6–8 hr
		0.3 µg/kg SC			
		3.0 µg/kg intranasal			
Conjugated estrogens	Major surgery or when long-lasting effect is required	0.6 mg/kg/day IV infusion for 5 consecutive days	6 hr	5–7 days	21–30 days

*Its use is not recommended because there is no uniformly observed favorable effect.
†It loses efficacy when administered repeatedly.
‡Added to 50 mL saline and infused over 30 minutes.
Hct, hematocrit; RBCs, red blood cells.

bleeding time occurred at 4–6 hours after the infusion) and was transient, lasting no longer than 24 to 36 hours. Cryoprecipitate infusion did not improve defects of platelet aggregation, even though blood levels of factor VIII and vWF, which were normal or high before infusion, increased. Notably, the use of cryoprecipitate carries a risk of transmitting viral diseases such as hepatitis and acquired immunodeficiency syndrome.

Desmopressin

Desmopressin, 1-deamino-8-D-arginine vasopressin (DDAVP), a synthetic derivative of antidiuretic hormone, was introduced in the late 1970s to control abnormal bleeding in patients with von Willebrand's disease and mild hemophilia A.[60] DDAVP acts by increasing the release of vWF multimers from endothelial stores. DDAVP has been studied in uremic patients as a potentially safer alternative to cryoprecipitate.[61,62] An open-label, controlled trial showed that DDAVP at a dose of 0.4 μg/kg IV shortened the prolonged bleeding times of CKD patients.[63]

This result was confirmed in a randomized, placebo-controlled, double-blind, crossover trial carried out in 12 uremic patients with a history of abnormal bleeding and prolonged bleeding times. The patients were infused with DDAVP 0.3 μg/kg IV in 50 mL saline, and the bleeding time was normalized in nine patients within 1 hour of infusion, decreased to less than 10 minutes at 2 hours and 4 hours, and returned to baseline by 8 hours (Box 68-2). There were no significant changes in platelet adhesion or aggregation, residual prothrombin, serum thromboxane B_2, or platelet cyclic adenosine phosphate, but the level of vWF increased above the elevated baseline values. DDAVP was well tolerated and caused no change in Hct or plasma osmolality. The effectiveness of DDAVP in shortening bleeding time and/or controlling abnormal bleeding associated with invasive procedures (biopsies and major surgery) in CKD patients has been substantiated by studies in which the drug was given intravenously, subcutaneously, or intranasally. Repeated

infusions during major surgery are associated with tachyphylaxis, probably due to depletion of vWF stores in endothelial cells. Although remarkably free of serious side effects, DDAVP is reported to cause a mild to moderate decrease in the platelet count, facial flushing, mild transient headache, nausea, abdominal cramps, mild tachycardia, water retention, and hyponatremia. There also is a single report of a patient who suffered a stroke immediately after infusion of DDAVP.

Based on the currently available results, it appears that DDAVP (0.3 μg/kg either IV or SC or as 3 μg/kg intranasally) is useful for treating acute bleeding and preventing abnormal bleeding that could occur with surgery or invasive procedures; DDAVP seems preferable to cryoprecipitate because of variations in clinical response and the risk of transmitting viral disease. The authors do not use cryoprecipitate.

Conjugated Estrogens

In an initial report, six uremic adults with a bleeding tendency and prolonged bleeding time were given conjugated estrogens (orally in one patient, intravenously in the other five) for a total dose of 30 to 75 mg over 2 to 5 days.[64] Bleeding times shortened in all patients within 2 to 5 days of starting treatment; it became normal in four patients and remained normal for 3 to 10 days after discontinuation of the drug. In a subsequent placebo-controlled, double-blind, crossover trial, conjugated estrogens were administered to six uremic patients with anemia and prolonged bleeding times. The dose was 0.6 mg/kg in 50 mL of saline and was infused intravenously over 40 minutes per day for 5 days (see Box 68-2). The bleeding time shortened within hours of the first infusion, and the effect lasted as long as 14 days (or 9 days after the last infusion). No changes were noted in levels of or the multimeric structure of vWF. No serious side effects were observed.[65]

A dose-finding study showed that 0.3 mg estrogens/kg had no significant effect on bleeding time, but there was a clear response to a cumulative dose. The effect of a single infusion of 0.6 mg/kg disappeared within 72 hours, but four or five infusions given at 24 hours apart resulted in marked shortening of the bleeding time and this effect was maintained for 14 days. Oral estrogens are also useful. Abnormal bleeding was corrected with regimens of 0.6 mg/kg/day IV for 5 days plus 60 mg/day PO for 5 days. Results from a small, placebo-controlled trial of four uremic patients indicate that conjugated estrogens given orally at a dose of 50 mg/day may markedly shorten the prolonged bleeding time after an average of 7 days of treatment; the dose may also control abnormal bleeding.[66] In addition to transient hot flushes (rare), minor side effects of conjugated estrogen include nausea, vomiting, loss of libido, and gynecomastia; these problems may limit prolonged use, particularly in men. The risks of malignancy and thromboembolic complications with intermittent high-dose conjugated estrogens are unknown. A recent review offers an evidence-based approach to current recommendations for uremic bleeding.[67]

Thrombotic Complications

Even though uremia is associated with a bleeding tendency, thrombotic occlusion of the dialysis vascular access is a frequent complication. Approximately 0.5 to 0.8 episodes of fistula thrombosis occur per patient per year. The cause of vascular

---

Box 68-2 Treatment of Renal Anemia with Erythropoiesis-Stimulating Agents

Choice of ESA erythropoiesis-stimulating agent: epoetin alfa, epoetin beta, darbepoetin.

The three erythropoiesis-stimulating agents are to be considered equivalent

Route of administration: subcutaneous administration is recommended, although in HD patients, intravenous route is preferred for practical reasons

Starting dose
Epoetin
80–120 U/kg/wk SC in two or three doses
120–180 U/kg/wk IV in two or three doses
Darbepoetin
0.45 μg/kg administered once weekly
Target hemoglobin: 11–12 g/dL
Desired hemoglobin increase rate: 0.3–0.5 g/wk
Interval to dose change: 4–6 wk
Dose change: Up-titration or down-titration by 25% of initial dose

Table 68-2 Summary of Relative Effects of Treatments of Uremic Bleeding

	Prevention of Platelet Dysfunction	In Acute Bleeding	Reduce Bleeding Time	Normalize Bleeding Time
Dialysis	+	−	++	+
Correction of anemia	+	+/−*	++	+
Cryoprecipitate	−	++	++	+
Desmopressin	−	+++	+++	++
Conjugated estrogens	−	+	++	+

*Correction of anemia in acute bleeding is achievable with red blood cell transfusion.
−, ineffective; +, moderately effective; ++, effective; +++ very effective.
Modified from Hedges SJ, Dehoney SB, Hooper JS, et al: Evidence-based treatment recommendations for uremic bleeding. Nat Clin Pract Nephrol 2007; 3:138–153.

access thrombosis is a stenotic lesion in the venous end of the anastomosis in approximately 75% of all cases. Other causes include sustained hypotension, excessive fistula compression, and a high Hct. Treatment of and prophylaxis against vascular access thrombosis are very important issues as the life of dialysis patients depends on the availability of a functioning vascular access, and this complication causes hospitalization and significant costs.[68,69] There are pharmacologic approaches to preventing clotting of the dialysis access, but no study has formally compared the efficacy of surgical thrombectomy with pharmacologic thrombolysis. Beathard[70] reported that thrombolysis is safe and as effective as surgical therapy in treating thrombosed dialysis access grafts. Because it preserves vascular access sites and yields long-term patency rates superior to those for surgical thrombectomy, it should be regarded as the treatment of choice. Thrombolysis is often the only choice for permanent catheters. Urokinase and tissue plasminogen activator are the agents most often employed successfully.[71,72]

The efficacy of prophylaxis using antiplatelet drugs in prolonging the patency of vascular grafts has been assessed in clinical trials, but the results are inconclusive. A randomized, double-blind trial in 44 patients found that aspirin 160 mg/day was better than placebo in preventing shunt thrombosis in uremic patients. It reduced the incidence of thrombi from 0.46 to 0.16 per patient per month ($P < .005$).[73] Other reports conclude that even low doses of aspirin also prolong the bleeding time, and occasional patients given aspirin will develop severe gastrointestinal bleeding. A meta-analysis of nine trials comprising 418 patients indicated that antiplatelet treatment (essentially aspirin alone or aspirin plus dipyridamole) reduced the risk of vascular occlusions by 70%.[74] The mean duration of these trials, however, was only 2 months. The absolute benefit of antiplatelet therapy appeared greater in patients with an arteriovenous shunt compared with results in patients with fistulas.

Few clinical studies have tested the effect of the antiplatelet agent ticlopidine in preventing the primary occlusion of arteriovenous fistulas. There appears to be a decreased incidence of thrombosis in treated patients.[75] All these studies, however, were small in size and of short duration.

A ticlopidine analogue, clopidogrel, was evaluated in a randomized, controlled trial to prevent graft thrombosis. The study was stopped early because of an excessive risk of bleeding in the active treatment group.[76]

There are few uncontrolled studies that have examined the effectiveness of systemic anticoagulation with warfarin in pre-venting occlusion of permanent central venous catheters (placed for purposes other than dialysis). Results of these studies suggest that low, fixed-dose warfarin may reduce the risk of venous thrombosis. It is not known whether this result can be extrapolated to HD permanent catheters (Table 68-2).

References

1. World Health Organization: Nutritional Anaemias: Report of a WHO Scientific Group. Geneva, Switzerland: World Health Organization, 1968.
2. Eschbach JW, Adamson JW: Anemia of end-stage renal disease (ESRD). Kidney Int 1985;28:1–5.
3. Astor BC, Muntner P, Levin A, et al: Association of kidney function with anemia: The Third National Health and Nutrition Examination Survey (1988–1994). Arch Intern Med 2002;162:1401–1408.
4. Hsu CY, McCulloch CE, Curhan GC: Epidemiology of anemia associated with chronic renal insufficiency among adults in the United States: Results from the Third National Health and Nutrition Examination Survey. J Am Soc Nephrol 2002;13:504–510.
5. Levin A, Thompson CR, Ethier J, et al: Left ventricular mass index increase in early renal disease: Impact of decline in hemoglobin. Am J Kidney Dis 1999;34:125–134.
6. Hsu CY, Bates DW, Kuperman GJ, Curhan GC: Relationship between hematocrit and renal function in men and women. Kidney Int 2001;59:725–723.
7. KDOQI, National Kidney Foundation: Clinical practice guidelines and clinical practice recommendations for anemia in chronic kidney disease in adults. 1.1. Identifying patients and initiating evaluation. Am J Kidney Dis 2006;47(Suppl 3): S17–S27.
8. Eschbach JW: Erythropoietin 1991—an overview. Am J Kidney Dis 1991;18:3–9.
9. Donnelly S: Why is erythropoietin made in the kidney? The kidney functions as a critmeter. Am J Kidney Dis 2001;38:415–425.
10. Fisher JW: Erythropoietin: Physiology and pharmacology update. Exp Biol Med 2003;228:1–14.
11. Perlman RL, Finkelstein FO, Liu L, et al: Quality of life in chronic kidney disease (CKD): A cross-sectional analysis in the Renal Research Institute-CKD study. Am J Kidney Dis 2005; 45:658–666.
12. Jones M, Ibels L, Schenkel B, Zagari M: Impact of epoetin alfa on clinical end points in patients with chronic renal failure: A meta-analysis. Kidney Int 2004;65:757–767.
13. Ross SD, Fahrbach K, Frame D, et al: The effect of anemia treatment on selected health-related quality-of-life domains: A systematic review. Clin Ther 2003;25:1786–1805.
14. Levin A: Anemia and left ventricular hypertrophy in chronic kidney disease populations: A review of the current state of knowledge. Kidney Int Suppl 2002;80:35–38.

15. Besarab A, Bolton WK, Browne JK, et al: The effects of normal as compared with low hematocrit values in patients with cardiac disease who are receiving hemodialysis and epoetin. N Engl J Med 1998;339:584–590.

16. Locatelli F, Aljama P, Bárány P, et al: Revised European best practice guidelines for the management of anaemia in patients with chronic renal failure. Section I. Anaemia evaluation. Nephrol Dial Transplant 2004;19(Suppl 2):ii2–ii5.

17. KDOQI, National Kidney Foundation: Clinical practice guidelines and clinical practice recommendations for anemia in chronic kidney disease in adults. 1.2. Identifying patients and initiating evaluation. Am J Kidney Dis 2006;47(Suppl 3):S28–S32.

18. Akmal M, Sawelson S, Karubian F, Gadallah M: The prevalence and significance of occult blood loss in patients with predialysis advanced chronic renal failure (CRF), or receiving dialytic therapy. Clin Nephrol 1994;42:198–202.

19. Macdougall IC, Padhi D, Jang G: Pharmacology of darbepoetin alfa. Nephrol Dial Transplant 2007;22(Suppl)4:iv2–iv9.

20. Ingelfinger JR: Through the looking glass: Anemia guidelines, vested interests and distortion. Clin J Am Soc Nephrol 2007;2:415–417.

21. National Kidney Foundation–Dialysis Outcomes Quality Initiative (NKF-DOQI): Clinical practice guidelines for anemia in chronic kidney disease, 2000. II. Target hemoglobin/hematocrit. Am J Kidney Dis 2001;37(Suppl):S190–S193.

22. Canadian Erythropoietin Study Group: Association between recombinant human erythropoietin and quality of life and exercise capacity of patients receiving haemodialysis. BMJ 1990; 300:573–578.

23. Silverberg DS, Wexler D, Blum M, et al: Aggressive therapy of congestive heart failure and associated chronic renal failure with medications and correction of anemia stops or slows the progression of both diseases. Perit Dial Int 2001;21(Suppl 3): S236–S240.

24. Silverberg DS, Wexler D, Blum M, et al: The effect of correction of anaemia in diabetics and non-diabetics with severe resistant congestive heart failure and chronic renal failure by subcutaneous erythropoietin and intravenous iron. Nephrol Dial Transplant 2003;18:141–146.

25. Silverberg DS, Wexler D, Blum M, et al: The use of subcutaneous erythropoietin and intravenous iron for the treatment of the anemia of severe, resistant congestive heart failure improves cardiac and renal function and functional cardiac class, and markedly reduces hospitalizations. J Am Coll Cardiol 2000;35:1737–1744.

26. London GM, Pannier B, Guerin AP, et al: Alterations of left ventricular hypertrophy in and survival of patients receiving hemodialysis: Follow-up of an interventional study. J Am Soc Nephrol 2001;12:2759–2767.

27. KDOQI, National Kidney Foundation: Clinical practice guidelines and clinical practice recommendations for anemia in chronic kidney disease in adults. 2.1. Hemoglobin range. Am J Kidney Dis 2006;47(Suppl 3):S33–S53.

28. Besarab A, Bolton WK, Browne JK, et al: The effects of normal as compared with low hematocrit values in patients with cardiac disease who are receiving hemodialysis and epoetin. N Engl J Med 1998;339:584–590.

29. Drueke TB, Locatelli F, Clyne N, et al, for the CREATE Investigators: Normalization of hemoglobin level in patients with chronic kidney disease and anemia. N Engl J Med 2006;355:2071–2084.

30. Singh AK, Szczech L, Tang KL, et al, for the CHOIR Investigators: Correction of anemia with epoetin alfa in chronic kidney disease. N Engl J Med 2006;355:2085–2098.

31. Remuzzi G, Ingelfinger JR: Correction of anemia—payoffs and problems. N Engl J Med 2006;355:2144–2146.

32. Patterson P, Allon M: Prospective evaluation of an anemia treatment algorithm in hemodialysis patients. Am J Kidney Dis 1998;32:635–641.

33. Casadevall N, Nataf J, Viron B, et al: Pure red-cell aplasia and antierythropoietin antibodies in patients treated with recombinant erythropoietin. N Engl J Med 2002;346:469–475.

34. Bennett CL, Cournoyer D, Carson KR, et al: Long-term outcome of individuals with pure red cell aplasia and antierythropoietin antibodies in patients treated with recombinant epoetin: A follow-up report from the Research on Adverse Drug Events and Reports (RADAR) Project. Blood 2005;106:3343–3347.

35. Horl WH: Clinical aspects of iron use in the anemia of kidney disease. J Am Soc Nephrol 2007;18:382–393.

36. Horl WH, Macdougall IC, Rossert J, Schaefer RM: OPTA-therapy with iron and erythropoiesis-stimulating agents in chronic kidney disease. Nephrol Dial Transplant 2007;22(Suppl 3):iii2–iii6.

37. Revised European best practice guidelines for the management of anaemia in patients with chronic renal failure: Section III. Treatment of renal anemia. Nephrol Dial Transplant 2004;19(Suppl 2):ii16–ii31.

38. KDOQI, National Kidney Foundation: Clinical Practice Guidelines and Clinical Practice Recommendations for Anemia in Chronic Kidney Disease in Adults. 3.2. Using iron agents. Am J Kidney Dis 2006;47(Suppl 3): S58–S70.

39. Macdougall IC: Poor response to erythropoietin; practical guidelines on investigation and management. Nephrol Dial Transplant 1995;10:607.

40. Goicoechea M, Martin J, De Sequera P, et al: Role of cytokines in the response to erythropoietin in hemodialysis patients. Kidney Int 1998;54:1337.

41. Gunnell J, Yeun JY, Depner TA, Kaysen GA: Acute-phase response predicts erythropoietin resistance in hemodialysis and peritoneal dialysis patients. Am J Kidney Dis 1999;33:63.

42. Lopez-Gomez JM, Perez-Flores I, Jofre R, et al: Presence of a failed kidney transplant in patients who are on hemodialysis is associated with chronic inflammatory state and erythropoietin resistance. J Am Soc Nephrol 2004;15:2494–2501.

43. Nassar GM, Fishbane S, Ayus JC: Occult infection of old nonfunctioning arteriovenous grafts: A novel cause of erythropoietin resistance and chronic inflammation in hemodialysis patients. Kidney Int 2002. 61(Suppl 80):49–54.

44. Roberts TL, Obrador GT, St Peter WL, et al: Relationship among catheter insertions, vascular access infections, and anemia management in hemodialysis patients. Kidney Int 2004; 66:2429–2436.

45. Rao DS, Shih MS, Mohini R: Effect of serum parathyroid hormone and bone marrow fibrosis on the response to erythropoietin in uremia. N Engl J Med 1993;328:171–175.

46. Albitar S, Genin R, Fen-Chong M, et al. High dose enalapril impairs the response to erythropoietin treatment in haemodialysis patients. Nephrol Dial Transplant 1998;13:1206–1210.

47. Schwarzbeck A, Wittenmeier KW, Hällfritzsch U: Anaemia in dialysis patients as a side-effect of sartanes. Lancet 1998; 352:286.

48. Rath CE, Mailliard JA, Schreiner GE: Bleeding tendency in uremia. N Engl J Med 1957;257:808–811.

49. Noris M, Remuzzi G: Uremic bleeding: Closing the circle after 30 years of controversies? Blood 1999;94:2569–2574.

50. Boccardo P, Remuzzi G, Galbusera M: Platelet dysfunction in renal failure. Semin Thromb Hemost 2004;30:579–589.

51. Kaw D, Malhotra D: Platelet dysfunction and end-stage renal disease. Semin Dial 2006;19:317–322.

52. Steiner RW, Coggins C, Carvalho ACA: Bleeding time in uremia: A useful test to assess clinical bleeding. Am J Hematol 1979;7:107–117.

53. Fernandez F, Goudable C, Sie P, et al: Low haematocrit and prolonged bleeding time in uraemic patients: Effect of red cell transfusion. Br J Haematol 1985;59:139–148.

54. Escolar G, Cases A, Bastida E, et al: Uremic platelets have a functional defect affecting the interaction of von Willebrand factor with glycoprotein IIb-IIIa. Blood 1990;76:1336–1340.

55. Gawaz MP, Dobos G, Spath M, et al: Impaired function of platelet membrane glycoprotein IIb-IIIa in end-stage renal disease. J Am Soc Nephrol 1994;5:36–46.

56. Livio M, Gotti E, Marchesi D, et al: Uraemic bleeding: Role of anemia and beneficial effect of red cell transfusions. Lancet 1982;2:1013–1015.

57. Gaspari F, Vigano G, Orisio S, et al: Aspirin prolongs bleeding time in uremia by a mechanism distinct from cyclooxygenase inhibition. J Clin Invest 1987;79:1788–1797.

58. Di Minno G, Martinez J, McKean ML, et al: Platelet dysfunction in uremia. Multifaceted defect partially corrected by dialysis. Am J Med 1985;79:552–559.

59. Viganò G, Benigni A, Mendogni D, et al: Recombinant human erythropoietin to correct uremic bleeding. Am J Kidney Dis 1991;18:44–49.

60. Janson PA, Jubelirer SJ, Weinstein MJ, et al: Treatment of the bleeding tendency in uremia with cryoprecipitate. N Engl J Med 1980;303:1318–1322.

61. Mannucci PM, Ruggeri ZM, Pareti FI, et al: 1-Deamino-8-d-arginine vasopressin: A new pharmacologic approach to the management of haemophilia and von Willebrand's diseases. Lancet 1977;1:869–872.

62. Watson AJ, Keogh JA: Effect of 1-deamino-8-d-arginine vasopressin on the prolonged bleeding time in chronic renal failure. Nephron 1982;32:49–52.

63. Mannucci PM, Remuzzi G, Pusineri F, et al: Deamino-8-d-arginine vasopressin shortens the bleeding time in uremia. N Engl J Med 1983;308:8–12.

64. Livio M, Mannucci PM, Viganò G, et al: Conjugated estrogens for the management of bleeding associated with renal failure. N Engl J Med 1986;315:731–735.

65. Viganò G, Gaspari F, Locatelli M, et al: Dose-effect and pharmacokinetics of estrogens given to correct bleeding time in uremia. Kidney Int 1988;34:853–858.

66. Shemin D, Elnour M, Amarantes B, et al: Oral estrogens decrease bleeding time and improve clinical bleeding in patients with renal failure. Am J Med 1990;89:436–440.

67. Hedges SJ, Dehoney SB, Hooper JS, et al: Evidence-based treatment recommendations for uremic bleeding. Nat Clin Pract Nephrol 2007;3:138–153.

68. Choudhury D: Vascular access thrombosis and prophylaxis. Semin Dial 2006;19:335–371.

69. Schwab SJ: Thrombotic complications of chronic hemodialysis vascular access. Fistulas and grafts. In Rose BD (ed): UpToDate. Waltham, MA: UpToDate, 2006.

70. Beathard GA: Mechanical versus pharmacological thrombolysis for the treatment of thrombosed dialysis access grafts. Kidney Int 1994;45:1401–1406.

71. Brunner MC, Matalon TA, Patel SK, et al: Ultrarapid urokinase in hemodialysis access occlusion. J Vasc Intervent Radiol 1991;2:503–506.

72. Ahmed A, Shapiro WB, Porush JG: The use of tissue plasminogen activator to declot arteriovenous accesses in hemodialysis patients. Am J Kidney Dis 1993;21:38–43.

73. Harter HR, Burch JW, Majerus PW, et al: Prevention of thrombosis in patients on hemodialysis by low dose aspirin. N Engl J Med 1979;301:577–579.

74. Antiplatelet Trialists' Collaboration: Collaborative overview of randomized trials of antiplatelet therapy. II: Maintenance of vascular graft of arterial patency by antiplatelet therapy. BMJ 1994;308:159–168.

75. Sreedhara R, Himmelfarb J, Lazarus JM, et al: Anti-platelet therapy in graft thrombosis: Results of a prospective, randomized, double-blind study. Kidney Int 1994;45:1477–1483.

76. Kaufman JS, O'Connor TZ, Zhang JH, Cronin RE: Randomized controlled trial of clopidogrel plus aspirin to prevent hemodialysis access graft thrombosis. J Am Soc Nephrol 2003;14:2313–2321.

Further Reading

Boccardo P, Remuzzi G, Galbusera M: Platelet dysfunction in renal failure. Semin Thromb Hemost 2004;30:579–589.

Choudhury D: Vascular access thrombosis and prophylaxis. Sem Dial 2006;19:335–371.

Fisher JW: Erythropoietin: Physiology and pharmacology update. Exp Biol Med 2003;228:1–14.

Hedges SJ, Dehoney SB, Hooper JS, et al: Evidence-based treatment recommendations for uremic bleeding. Nat Clin Pract Nephrol 2007;3:138–153.

Horl WH: Clinical aspects of iron use in the anemia of kidney disease. J Am Soc Nephrol 2007;18:382–393.

KDOQI, National Kidney Foundation: Clinical practice guidelines and clinical practice recommendations for anemia in chronic kidney disease in adults. Am J Kidney Dis 2006;47(Suppl 3):S16–S85.

Locatelli F, Aljama P, Bárány P, et al; European Best Practice Guidelines Working Group: Revised European Best Practice Guidelines for the management of anaemia in patients with chronic renal failure. nephrol dial transplant 2004;19(Suppl 2):ii1–ii47.

Chapter 69

Calcium, Phosphorus, Renal Bone Disease, and Calciphylaxis

Rizwan A. Qazi and Kevin J. Martin

A 40-year-old dialysis patient is 87 times more likely to suffer a hip fracture than a healthy control,[1] and a 25-year-old dialysis patient is more than 100 times more likely to suffer a cardiovascular event than a healthy control.[2] Chronic kidney disease (CKD)–mineral and bone disorder is implicated in the pathogenesis of both outcomes. Renal osteodystrophy was first described in 1943 and has many names. With the introduction of the new classification of CKD (CKD staging) and the Kidney Disease Outcome and Quality Initiative (K/DOQI) guidelines in 2003, more and more patients are being referred to nephrologists for management of CKD and its related mineral and bone disorder.[3] With loss of glomerular filtration, there is phosphorus retention, a decrease in calcitriol, and other factors that stimulate parathyroid (PTH) secretion and growth of the parathyroid glands. Even with normal serum calcium and phosphorus concentrations, patients with CKD stage 3 or 4 can still have an elevated PTH level. Levels of serum calcium and phosphorus are maintained within normal range in these patients because there is secondary hyperparathyroidism (HPT).[3-6] It should be diagnosed and dealt with early to preserve bone health; for diagnosis, the K/DOQI guidelines recommend measuring serum calcium, phosphorus, and intact PTH in all patients with CKD stages 3, 4, and 5 at regular intervals. There is strong evidence that the driving force for all these abnormalities is phosphate retention, which is a direct result of decreased excretion of phosphates by the damaged kidney. Treatment is based on decreasing phosphate

accumulation by decreasing phosphate intake. Phosphate retention increases PTH and decreases calcitriol directly and also indirectly by increasing the concentration of fibroblast growth factor-23.[7] Decreased levels of calcitriol lead to an additional stimulus of PTH. Hence, serum phosphorus must be kept within the target range by restricting the diet and limiting phosphate absorption from the intestine.

RENAL OSTEODYSTROPHY

Renal osteodystrophy occurs in CKD–mineral and bone disorder.[8] It should be emphasized that renal osteodystrophy is a qualitative disorder of bone in CKD patients. Dual x-ray absorptiometry scans or other imaging modalities are quantitative tests of bone mineral content and are not very helpful in determining the pathologic bone turnover states associated with various stages of CKD. Serum markers of bone metabolism such as alkaline phosphate, PTH, and osteocalcin are good predictive markers of the different types of bone turnover disease, but the definitive diagnosis can only be made by bone biopsy. This is true because bone is in a constant state of remodeling and is a buffer for calcium and other minerals; if serum calcium decreases, then PTH increases to release calcium from the bone. Conversely with a high calcium intake, calcium is deposited in bone. The iliac crest is the usual site of bone biopsy for assessment of bone, but before the biopsy, a patient should receive different types of tetracycline at 30 days and again at 4 days before biopsy to evaluate the amount and type of the bone formed during the time interval of administering the two tetracycline labels. Symptoms of renal osteodystrophy are nonspecific and may even be absent. They include pain and stiffness in joints, spontaneous tendon rupture, a predisposition to fractures, and proximal muscle weakness. A similar set of symptoms may be seen in both the low- and high-turnover type of skeletal abnormality.

High-Turnover Bone Disease

Calcium and phosphorus levels are disturbed with advancing kidney disease causing secondary HPT and parathyroid hyperplasia. The increase in PTH has skeletal and extraskeletal manifestations, as outlined in Figure 69-1. One skeletal abnormality is high-turnover bone disease, which is associated with increased levels of intact PTH in serum. Other signs of ongoing bone reabsorption are increases in serum phosphorus, alkaline phosphate, and osteocalcin. Secondary HPT can be present with serum calcium levels that are increased, normal, or low, but when PTH is high, it inhibits osteoclast apoptosis, causing increased bone resorption. At the same time, osteoblasts are stimulated to replace resorption areas with rapid bone formation, resulting in replacement of the normal lamellar bone with structurally inferior woven bone. There is fibrosis and sometimes cyst formation, hence yielding the name osteitis fibrosa cystica. Parathyroid hyperplasia and high-turnover bone disease are more recognized in patients

with CKD stage 5 but can be present at any stage of CKD. Treatment of this disorder is effective control of serum PTH using therapy as outlined later in the chapter.

Low-Turnover Bone Disease

There are two kinds of low-turnover bone disease: osteomalacia and adynamic bone disease. In both, PTH is typically not elevated,[9,10] but other serum bone markers like alkaline phosphatase and osteocalcin are in the normal range. Serum calcium may be normal or increased in patients with adynamic bone disease because of the lack of buffering capacity in bone when an oral calcium load is given.[11] In osteomalacia, there is usually aluminum deposition at the mineralization front, which blocks mineralization of osteoid. Osteomalacia is typically symptomatic, whereas adynamic bone disease is not. Adynamic bone disease is due to paucity of both osteoclasts and osteoblasts and is more prevalent in peritoneal dialysis patients than in hemodialysis patients. The disease can also occur in CKD (predialysis) patients.[12] Treatment options include avoiding oversuppression of PTH, which occurs with excessive doses of active vitamin D sterols or calcimimetic agents. Other factors have been implicated, including excessive oral calcium from high doses of calcium-containing phosphate binders.[13] If present, an evaluation for aluminum toxicity by history, examination, and blood tests should be done, and if aluminum toxicity is confirmed, then treatment involves deferoxamine 5 mg/kg/wk post-dialysis or intraperitoneally. The duration of therapy is typically 6 months to a year. Adverse effects associated with therapy include hearing loss, retinal damage, and infection with mucormycosis. Once-weekly dosing is associated with fewer adverse effects compared with administration three times per week.

PREVENTION OF PHOSPHORUS RETENTION AND HYPERPHOSPHATEMIA

Several large retrospective studies of patients on hemodialysis showed that patients with elevated phosphorus or calcium $\times$ phosphorus product had an increase in mortality[14,15]; 39% of dialysis patients had hyperphosphatemia. Those with serum phosphorus greater than 6.5 mg/dL had a 27% increase in mortality after adjustment for other comorbid conditions. The goal should be to maintain serum phosphorus in all stages of CKD at levels recommended by the K/DOQI guidelines (Table 69-1). The available options for decreasing phosphorus accumulation in patients at all stages of CKD include (1) decreasing dietary phosphorus intake, (2) preventing the absorption of phosphorus with phosphorus binders, and (3) enhancing the removal of phosphorus by dialysis. It can be more complicated with severe secondary HPT because some compliant patients can develop hyperphosphatemia due to mobilization of phosphorus from bone.

Dietary Phosphorus Restriction

Dietary phosphorus restriction should always be the first step in treating CKD–bone and mineral disease, especially in predialysis patients.[16–18] The phosphorus intake of normal adults is 1.0 to 1.8 g/day with the variation depending primarily on consumption of meat and dairy products. Poultry,

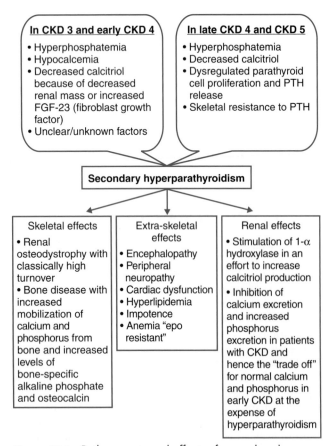

Figure 69-1 Pathogenesis and effects of secondary hyperparathyroidism in chronic kidney disease (CKD).

Table 69-1   Goals and Therapeutic Options for Chronic Kidney Disease–Mineral and Bone Disorder

Therapeutic Options	TARGETS			CKD stages
	Phosphorus	Calcium	PTH	
Restrict dietary phosphorus Correct low 25-dihydroxy vitamin D levels Phosphate binders, e.g., calcium acetate or calcium carbonate with meals Avoid oversuppression of PTH Avoid hypercalcemia	2.7–4.6 mg/dL (0.87–1.49 mmol/L)	Normal range for laboratory, e.g., 8.4–10.3 mg/dL	35–70 pg/mL	CKD 3: GFR 30–59 mL/min/1.73 m²
All the above treatments Aggressive control of phosphorus with diet and binders (use of sevelamer HCl and lanthanum carbonate as phosphate binders is not FDA approved for use in patients with CKD stages 3 and 4. Consider active vitamin D sterol if above not sufficient (e.g., calcitriol 0.5 μg PO on M/W/F or 0.25 μg every day or paricalcitol or doxercalciferol; paricalcitol is preferred)	2.7–4.6 mg/dL (0.87–1.49 mmol/L)	Normal range for laboratory, e.g., 8.4–10.3 mg/dL	70–110 pg/mL	CKD 4: GFR 15–29 mL/min/1.73 m²
Dietary phosphate restriction but liberalize protein intake to 1.0–1.2 g/kg Use vitamin D sterols with hemodialysis, e.g., paricalcitol 4 μg IV with hemodialysis. For peritoneal dialysis, administer PO every day or higher dose three times/week Use of noncalcium-based phosphate binders if hypercalcemia or any signs of vascular calcification, e.g., sevelamer 1600 mg with meals and large snacks Adequate dialysis to target kt/v. Consider cinacalcet to keep PTH at target if vitamin D sterol not adequate. Monitor serum calcium. PTX when, despite the above-mentioned options, PTH is very high, e.g., PTH > 1000 pg/mL and calcium or phosphorus limit other therapies	3.5–5.5 mg/dL (1.13–1.78 mmol/L)	Normal range for laboratory (preferably towards the lower half)	150–300 pg/mL	CKD 5: GFR < 15 mL/min/1.73 m²

CKD, chronic kidney disease; FDA, U.S. Food and Drug Administration; GFR, glomerular filtration rate; M/W/F, Monday/Wednesday/Friday; PTH, parathyroid hormone; PTX, parathyroidectomy.

fish, liver, most soft drinks (especially colas), whole-grain breads, and some cereals, nuts, and legumes are rich in phosphorus. With elimination of dairy products and limiting the diet to 60 g of protein per day, the dietary intake of phosphorus is 750 to 1000 mg/day. Once a patient is on maintenance dialysis and dietary protein increases, the phosphorus may be increased. The National Cooperative Dialysis Study suggested that with commencement of dialysis therapy, a patient should eat at least 0.8 to 1.0 g/day of protein, which would increase daily phosphorus intake to a range of 920 to 1200 mg/day. Therefore, it can be difficult to achieve a balance between nutritional demands and limiting phosphorus intake in dialysis patients. In contrast, restriction of dietary phosphorus intake can be the sole measure needed to avoid phosphate retention in patients at the predialysis stage of CKD.

Phosphate Binders

Phosphate binders are broadly divided into calcium based (calcium carbonate, calcium acetate) and noncalcium based (sevelamer hydrochloride, lanthanum carbonate, aluminum hydroxide, and magnesium carbonate).

Calcium-Based Phosphate Binders

The use of calcium-based phosphate binders is limited to a total calcium intake of 2 g of elemental calcium per day because vascular calcification is present in many CKD patients, and hypercalcemia from calcium-based phosphate binders is a factor contributing to the progression of vascular calcification.[3] Because the average daily intake of elemental calcium is 500 mg with meals, 1500 mg of elemental calcium can be taken as calcium-based binders. It should be pointed out, however, that calcium-based binders have been associated with progression of vascular calcification even at a dose of 1100 mg of elemental calcium per day.[19] The two types of calcium-based phosphate binders routinely used are calcium acetate and calcium carbonate: calcium acetate is available as 667-mg tablets providing 167 mg of elemental calcium per tablet and calcium carbonate is available in several sizes (tablets of 500 mg of calcium carbonate contain 200 mg of elemental calcium). The usual starting dose of these binders is one to two tablets with meals. Consequently, the 2-g limit of elemental calcium per day is exceeded if a patient takes approximately nine 667-mg calcium acetate tablets or seven 500-mg calcium carbonate tablets daily. It should be emphasized that calcium-based phosphate binders do not necessarily cause hypercalcemia if they are used judiciously.

Another important observation is that a sizable number of patients with CKD stage 4 or 5 have vascular calcification evident on plain radiographs, echocardiograms, or computed tomography scans. These patients will develop progressive vascular calcification irrespective of the type of binders used. However, calcium-based binders appear to aggravate and accelerate the vascular calcification, so calcium-based phosphate binders for these patients should be avoided. Patients who have no evidence of calcification when they begin dialysis will likely never develop calcification, and it seems reasonable to use calcium-based phosphate binders in these patients, but the 2 g/day limit should not be exceeded. Serum calcium must be monitored during the therapy to avoid hypercalcemia. Note that some patients will also be taking vitamin D therapy. Vitamin D avidly stimulates the adsorption of calcium and phosphorus from the gut. Another caveat is that calcium ingested when the stomach is empty or between meals can facilitate calcium absorption. For this reason, calcium-based binders should only be taken with meals. K/DOQI guidelines recommend using non–calcium-based phosphate binders in patients on dialysis if the serum PTH is less than 150 pg/mL and if there is evidence of vascular calcification or hypercalcemia. With other CKD patients, phosphate binders should be determined by patient preference, compliance, comorbid illnesses, side effects, cost, and the ability to control serum phosphorus levels while avoiding hypercalcemia (and limiting the total calcium intake).

Sevelamer Hydrochloride

Sevelamer hydrochloride is a non–calcium-based phosphate binder.[20] The usual effective dose is 2 to 8 g/day, given in divided doses with meals and with large snacks. Sevelamer is available as 400- and 800-mg tablets. It can be used in combination with other calcium- and non–calcium-based phosphate binders and active vitamin D sterols. Since its approval by the U.S. Food and Drug Administration in 1998, sevelamer has been used across the United States for CKD stage 5 patients on hemodialysis and peritoneal dialysis; it has not been approved for use in predialysis CKD patients. The binder is unique because it also lowers total cholesterol levels, principally by sequestering bile salts and lowering low-density lipoprotein levels.[21] The efficacy of this phosphate binder was compared with calcium-containing phosphate binders in a randomized, controlled year-long study. Both treatments reached target levels of serum phosphorus and the calcium × phosphorus products, but sevelamer treatment was associated

with less hypercalcemia and less oversuppression of PTH levels. In addition, the calcium-containing phosphate binders (both calcium acetate and calcium carbonate), but not sevelamer, led to progressive calcification of coronary arteries and the aorta.[19] The average amount of elemental calcium associated with vascular calcification was only 1.1 g/day, which is far less than the recommended K/DOQI maximum of 1.5 g/day. Treatment with sevelamer has also been associated with a survival benefit compared with the use of calcium-containing phosphate binders. The adverse side effects of sevelamer are gastrointestinal distress, bloating, and flatulence, and there are case reports of intestinal obstruction.

Lanthanum Carbonate

Lanthanum is a heavy metal ion, and lanthanum carbonate is an effective phosphate binder.[22] Unlike sevelamer hydrochloride, which is nonabsorbable by the intestines, a small amount of lanthanum is absorbed, and over a period of time, lanthanum can be found in various body tissues including bones and liver. To date, no adverse outcomes from this accumulation have been identified. The advantage of lanthanum carbonate is that it is chewable, which may improve compliance. In 2005, it was approved by the U.S. Food and Drug Administration for use in hemodialysis patients with CKD stage 5. The usual starting dose is 750 mg to 1 g, to be taken with meals or with meals and snacks. Lanthanum carbonate can be taken in combination with calcium- and noncalcium-based phosphate binders and vitamin D sterols.

Aluminum Hydroxide and Aluminum Carbonate

Aluminum is a very potent phosphate binder, yet it is potentially toxic. It was widely used around the world until the mid-1980s, when it was identified as a cause of a fatal neurological syndrome (seizures, dyspraxia, abnormal electroencephalogram); later, it also was implicated in causing fractures, myopathy, and microcytic anemia. The routine use of aluminum-based phosphate binder is not recommended because of these toxicities and because it can cause osteomalacia.[23] However, a course of aluminum hydroxide for a few days can be used to bring the serum phosphorus down acutely when the phosphorus or calcium phosphorus product in the serum is very high and traditional methods alone are insufficient to correct the abnormality.

Magnesium Carbonate

Magnesium carbonate is an effective phosphate binder but causes hypermagnesemia in renal failure patients. Hypermagnesemia can be treated with low- or magnesium-free dialysates. This poses a difficult logistic problem for outpatient dialysis units.

Vitamin D Deficiency

Vitamin D deficiency is prevalent in the general population and especially in patients with CKD. K/DOQI guidelines recommend measuring 25(OH) vitamin D levels and if low, correcting the level for patients with CKD stages 3, 4, and 5. The measurements should be made annually in CKD 3 and quarterly in CKD 4 and 5 patients. The level of 25-dihydroxyvitamin D (25-OH-D) considered normal is a value greater than 30 ng/mL. If there is severe vitamin D deficiency, a patient should be treated with weekly doses of 50,000 units of oral ergocalciferol for 12 weeks followed by the same dose given monthly for another 6 months. Milder degrees of deficiency can be treated with monthly oral doses of 50,000 units. CKD patients, especially those with heavy proteinuria, can develop vitamin D deficiency because of urinary losses of vitamin D binding protein. Consequently, 25-OH-D levels should be checked in these patients at regular intervals. There is evidence that repletion of a low 25-OH-D level in vitamin D–deficient CKD patient decreases PTH,[24] especially in CKD stage 3 patients. Even if there is no beneficial effect on PTH levels, we recommend measuring 25-OH-D in all patients with CKD stages 3, 4, and 5 with or without preexisting secondary HPT; vitamin D should be replaced if the plasma levels are low. Vitamin D deficiency should be considered as an independent condition with adverse outcomes that include aggravating secondary HPT, depressing the immune system, increasing cancer prevalence, and decreasing overall survival.

Use of Active Vitamin D Sterols

Some patients with CKD stage 3 or 4 and the majority of patients with CKD stage 5 will continue to have PTH levels above the goal even after bringing serum calcium, serum phosphorus, and 25-OH-D levels into the target range. These are the patients who will benefit from one of the many available active vitamin D sterols.

Calcitriol

Calcitriol is available as a pill or an intravenous (IV) formulation. Oral calcitriol effectively decreases PTH levels, decreases bone resorption, improves endosteal fibrosis and mineralization, and to some extent helps in the bone pains associated with renal osteodystrophy. Calcitriol has a direct inhibiting effect on PTH synthesis. In predialysis patients (CKD stages 3 and 4), the usual starting dose is 0.25 μg every day or every other day. In dialysis patients, the dose can be titrated upward. The unfavorable effects associated with calcitriol are hypercalcemia and hyperphosphatemia, mainly due to increased intestinal absorption of calcium and phosphorus. Intravenous calcitriol is given to hemodialysis patients and is associated with less hypercalcemia and a more profound decrease in PTH levels. The usual starting dose of intravenous calcitriol is 0.5 to 1.0 μg per dialysis session, and it can be increased to 4 μg or more if hypercalcemia does not occur. Hypercalcemia with oral or intravenous calcitriol requires a decrease in the dose by 25% to 50% and rechecking calcium and PTH levels.

Paricalcitol

Paricalcitol or 19-nor-1,25(OH)$_2$D$_2$ is a vitamin D analogue that decreases PTH secretion while minimizing hypercalcemia and hyperphosphatemia.[25,26] It does not appear to induce the vitamin D receptor in the intestine and hence does not promote calcium or phosphorus absorption from gut. Paricalcitol is available in oral and intravenous formulations; oral capsules are available as 1, 2, and 4 μg. The usual starting dose is 1 μg every day or 2 μg every other day in CKD stages 3 and 4 patients; the dose is titrated upward in CKD stage 5 patients treated by hemodialysis or peritoneal dialysis. Hemodialysis patients are usually treated with intravenous formulation, and the starting dose of intravenous paricalcitol is 0.04 to 0.1 μg/kg IV per dialysis session; it is increased as required. In retrospective studies, paricalcitol appears to have a potential survival advantage over calcitriol in patients with CKD stage 5.[27] Overall, paricalcitol is safe and effective in dialysis patients with secondary HPT and causes fewer changes in serum calcium and phosphorus levels than calcitriol.

Doxercalciferol

Doxercalciferol is a vitamin D$_2$ derivative, 1-(OH)-D$_2$, and must undergo 25-hydroxylation in the liver to become biologically active. In a randomized study of doxercalciferol 4 μg/day or 4 μg three times per week was effective in decreasing the PTH to the K/DOQI target range. However, the serum calcium increased from 8.8 mg/dL to 9.5 mg/dL along with a significant incidence of hyperphosphatemia.[28] Other studies have also revealed significant hypercalcemia that is associated with doxercalciferol, so there is little evidence of selectivity of action of doxercalciferol (i.e., PTH suppression without inducing hypercalcemia or hyperphosphatemia).[29]

Dialysis Adequacy

For hemodialysis patients with CKD stage 5, a single hemodialysis treatment can remove approximately 800 mg of phosphorus from the blood. Initially, there is a sharp gradient for phosphorus removal with increased removal in the first half of hemodialysis; removal decreases during the second half of the treatment because phosphorus is predominantly stored in the intracellular compartment and is not rapidly mobilized. Hence, a single session of dialysis, no matter how long, can only remove a limited amount of phosphorus. Emerging data from patients treated by daily hemodialysis indicate that they have far better serum phosphorus control with far fewer oral phosphate binders than patients treated with hemodialysis three times per week.[30] For hemodialysis patients, dialysis adequacy must be ensured and recirculation in the dialysis access excluded to be sure dialysis helps decrease the uremic and phosphorus burden of CKD patients.

Calcimimetic Agents

Calcimimetic agents are the newest addition to the armamentarium for treating secondary HPT. The available drug is cinacalcet hydrochloride in 30-, 60-, and 90-mg tablets.[31] The usual starting dose is 30 mg and is titrated upward depending on the PTH level. The maximum dose is 180 mg, but most patients will respond well to 90 or 120 mg. Two things must be kept in mind about calcimimetic agents: First, the drug is very effective in lowering PTH and is akin to chemical parathyroidectomy, and, second, the drug can cause significant hypocalcemia so serum calcium must be monitored.

Calcimimetic agents stimulate the calcium-sensing receptor so the parathyroid gland senses a higher ionized calcium, which decreases the secretion of PTH. A high concentration of calcium-sensing receptor is present in parathyroid cell membrane, the kidney, bone, brain, and lungs, and small changes in the extracellular ionized calcium level will activate this receptor. In fact, decreased secretion of PTH by parathyroid cells occurs within seconds of increasing blood ionized calcium. However, the calcium-sensing receptor is also sensitive to magnesium, trivalent elements, and gadolinium. Consequently, stimulation of the calcium-sensing receptor in the kidney increases urinary calcium and magnesium. Interestingly, concomitant treatment with vitamin D sterols often given to hemodialysis patients not only acts to decrease PTH but also helps by ameliorating the hypocalcemic effects of calcimimetic drugs. Currently, cinacalcet hydrochloride is not approved for treating patients with CKD stages 3 and 4.

Parathyroidectomy

Parathyroidectomy (PTX) for secondary HPT is indicated only if it is severe despite adequate medical management. There is no absolute PTH value signifying the need for PTX, but the presence of persistently elevated intact PTH levels greater than 1000 pg/mL plus high serum calcium $\times$ phosphorus products (typically >55 mg^2/dL^2) despite therapy and physical problems such as bony aches and pains or fractures suggests consideration of surgical PTX. It was recommended to perform a bone biopsy before performing a PTX because some of the CKD patients will have adynamic bone disease, and removing the parathyroid gland in such patients would prove catastrophic. A routine bone biopsy before PTX is no longer recommended because aluminum is rarely used as a phosphate binder. Because the exact location of all parathyroid glands in the neck is not consistent, a sestamibi nuclear scan can help locate the glands before surgery. Most experienced surgeons do not require a routine preoperative sestamibi scan. If a patient has persistent secondary HPT after renal transplantation or if a parathyroid adenoma is suspected, then sestamibi scan can help locate the culprit gland. The different surgical procedures are (1) subtotal PTX, (2) total PTX with autotransplantation of parathyroid tissue in the forearm, and (3) total PTX without autotransplantation. The number of surgical PTXs in the United States decreased between 1992 and 1998, but then steadily increased to the previous level in 2002. This probably reflects changes in the indications for PTX.

Postparathyroidectomy Management

PTX is usually performed as an inpatient surgery because of the immediate postoperative development of hungry bone syndrome. With chronic and severe secondary HPT, patients who undergo PTX can develop rapid recalcification of bones that have been demineralized by secondary HPT. This constitutes the hungry bone syndrome because serum calcium and phosphorus decrease sharply due to uptake into the bones. It requires a prompt and meticulous treatment plan. Postoperative management of such patients includes a concentrated calcium gluconate solution, usually prepared as 20 or 40 g of calcium gluconate dissolved in 1000 mL of 5% dextrose in water and administered at 20 to 30 mL/hr and adjusted by ± 5 mL/hr depending on serum calcium levels measured approximately every 6 hours. As soon as the patient is able to take oral medications, oral calcitriol 0.5 to 2.0 µg/day is given along with calcium carbonate 1 to 3 g/day on an empty stomach and at night to maximize intestinal calcium absorption. The calcium gluconate drip must not be stopped abruptly when there is a single high or normal reading for calcium because the bones may take up calcium very slowly Removing the calcium infusion can precipitate tetany and prove fatal. Once the calcium gluconate drip is discontinued and the patient is taking a stable dose of oral calcium and calcitriol, outpatient therapy is planned and the patient is instructed to contact the physicians if perioral numbness or tingling develops. This could indicate incipient tetany. Other laboratory abnormalities associated with postoperative PTX are hypophosphatemia, hypomagnesemia, and hyperkalemia; the first two require repletion because these minerals are also being taken up by the hungry bone and the latter requires standard therapy for hyperkalemia.

PERSISTENT SECONDARY HYPERPARATHYROIDISM AFTER RENAL TRANSPLANTATION

Persistent secondary HPT after renal transplantation is a frequent occurrence and rarely needs therapy. The usual recommendation is to wait as long as 1 year to let the parathyroid levels come back into the normal range. If therapy is needed, there are three ways to deal with the problem: (1) use bisphosphonates to block the osteoclastic effects of a persistently high PTH and wait for the serum PTH levels to normalize, (2) use calcimimetic agents to bring PTH levels into the normal range, and (3) surgically remove parathyroid gland tissue. In patients with persistent secondary HPT, a 24-hour urine specimen should be collected to measure calcium, phosphorus, and sodium excretion. If a patient is hypercalciuric (>200 mg/dL) while eating a normal salt diet, then the patient is most likely to benefit from bisphosphonates.[32] Conversely, if calcium excretion is low, then cinacalcet can be considered while serum calcium is measured at regular intervals.[33]

CALCIPHYLAXIS

Calciphylaxis is a rare but devastating disorder. Its pathogenesis is poorly understood, and emergency PTX was once considered to be definitive therapy for calciphylaxis. Subsequent reports of poor outcomes after PTX and the presence of calciphylaxis in patients who have had a PTX have changed this practice.[34] Calciphylaxis is synonymous with calcific uremic arteriopathy and obliterative calcific vasculopathy, but none of these terms describes the abnormality adequately. Calciphylaxis involves mural calcification, endovascular fibrosis, and thrombosis of small arterioles, venules, and capillaries, so an arteriopathy label is incomplete. Unfortunately, both calciphylaxis and calcific uremic arteriopathy are used to describe the disorder.

Risk factors associated with the development of calciphylaxis are obesity, female gender, white race, high serum calcium and phosphorus levels, a high serum PTH and calcium $\times$ phosphorus product, and coumadin treatment. Whether local trauma is a risk factor for calciphylaxis is not clear; in rodent models of calciphylaxis, sensitization with high calcium, phosphorus, and PTH levels followed by local trauma is usually required before the animal develops characteristic nonhealing ulcers. Moreover, many patients will report local trauma before developing the typical nonhealing ulcer.

The clinical features of calciphylaxis include painful subcutaneous nodules and dense plaques with an erythematous or violaceous color that progresses to necrotizing, nonhealing ulcers. A common site of involvement is the medial aspects of thighs, lower abdomen, and lower extremities. The diagnosis is based on characteristic nonhealing lesions. A bone scan is a modern way to diagnose and monitor the progression/regression of the disease. A skin biopsy should not be performed because nonhealing wounds can develop and progress to large gaping wounds requiring multiple débridements. This is particularly worrisome because the major morbidity and mortality are wound infection and sepsis. There is no definitive therapy for calciphylaxis/calcific uremic arteriopathy, and the prognosis is generally poor with a 1-year mortality rate as high as 85%. Therapeutic options include the following possibilities.

Daily Dialysis

Daily dialysis for a few weeks using a low calcium bath (2 mEq/L) can help reduce serum phosphorus and mobilize deposited calcium while correcting uremia.

Sodium Thiosulfate

There are case reports of using sodium thiosulfate (STS) with apparent healing of the ulcers.[35,36] STS is an antidote for cyanide and cisplatin toxicity and has antioxidant properties. The solubility of calcium thiosulfate in aqueous solutions can mobilize calcium from ectopic sources. The success of removing ectopic calcium is monitored by changes in bone scans. Investigators have given 25 g of STS/1.73 m^2 over 60 minutes after each dialysis session for 35 to 92 weeks. Intraperitoneal instillation of STS can also be used to treat calciphylaxis in peritoneal dialysis patients. Adverse effects associated with STS are nausea, vomiting, and metabolic acidosis.

Parathyroidectomy

PTX should not be considered in treating calciphylaxis because of poor healing. However, if serum PTH levels are very high despite medical management, then PTX could be a valid therapy.

Phosphate Regulation

Noncalcium-based phosphate binders should be used to cause a negative phosphate balance. Active vitamin D sterols should be avoided because they can increase calcium and phosphate absorption from the gut leading to hypercalcemia and hyperphosphatemia to aggravate the disorder. Daily dialysis helps decrease serum phosphorus to the K/DOQI target of 3.5 to 5.5 mg/dL. Dietary phosphorus restriction must be strictly followed because lowering serum phosphorus is probably the most important aspect in the treatment of this disorder.[37]

Pain Management

The pain associated with calciphylaxis/calcific uremic arteriopathy is considered to arise from the combination of ischemic and neuropathic pain. Pain control is often a challenge with options including nonsteroidal anti-inflammatory drugs (ketorolac), narcotics (fentanyl), ketamine, and in some severe cases even spinal anesthesia. In studies of STS, most patients reported marked pain relief within days of initiating STS therapy.

Wound Care and Antibiotics

Although wound débridement might seem tempting, it is important not to be aggressive with débridement as it can increase the size of wound and the potential for infection. Close attention should be given to appropriate antibiotics; the cause of death in these patients is usually sepsis from polymicrobial-resistant wound infection.

Other

There is evidence of osteoblastic transformation of vascular smooth muscle in CKD patients. The presence of bone matrix protein in blood vessels when there is calciphylaxis suggests that bisphosphonates will help. There is a case report that the first-generation bisphosphonate, etidronate disodium, given at 200 mg/day for 14 days led to dramatic improvement in skin ulceration.[38] Other therapeutic modalities that have had apparent success are cinacalcet hydrochloride (30–60 mg/day), and hyperbaric oxygen.[39,40] Further studies are needed to determine the most useful treatment in these patients.

References

1. Alem AM, Sherrard DJ, Gillen DL, et al: Increased risk of hip fracture among patients with end-stage renal disease. Kidney Int 2000;58:396–399.
2. Foley RN, Parfrey PS, Sarnak MJ: Clinical epidemiology of cardiovascular disease in chronic renal disease. Am J Kidney Dis 1998;32(Suppl):S112–S119.
3. KDOQI clinical practice guidelines for bone metabolism and disease in chronic kidney disease. Am J Kidney Dis 2003;42(Suppl): S1–S201.
4. Levin A, Bakris GL, Molitch M, et al: Prevalence of abnormal serum vitamin D, PTH, calcium, and phosphorus in patients with chronic kidney disease: Results of the study to evaluate early kidney disease. Kidney Int 2007;71:31–38.
5. Martinez I, Saracho R, Montenegro J, Llach F: The importance of dietary calcium and phosphorus in the secondary hyperparathyroidism of patients with early renal failure. Am J Kidney Dis 1997;29:496–502.
6. Slatopolsky E, Bricker NS: The role of phosphorus restriction in the prevention of secondary hyperparathyroidism in chronic renal disease. Kidney Int 1973;4:141–145.
7. Gutierrez O, Isakova T, Rhee E, et al: Fibroblast growth factor-23 mitigates hyperphosphatemia but accentuates calcitriol deficiency in chronic kidney disease. J Am Soc Nephrol 2005;16:2205–2215.
8. Moe S, Drueke T, Cunningham J, et al: Definition, evaluation, and classification of renal osteodystrophy: A position statement from Kidney Disease: Improving Global Outcomes (KDIGO). Kidney Int 2006;69:1945–1953.
9. Qi Q, Monier-Faugere MC, Geng Z, Malluche HH: Predictive value of serum parathyroid hormone levels for bone turnover in patients on chronic maintenance dialysis. Am J Kidney Dis 1995;26:622–631.
10. Wang M, Hercz G, Sherrard DJ, et al: Relationship between intact 1-84 parathyroid hormone and bone histomorphometric parameters in dialysis patients without aluminum toxicity. Am J Kidney Dis 1995;26:836–844.
11. Kurz P, Monier-Faugere MC, Bognar B, et al: Evidence for abnormal calcium homeostasis in patients with adynamic bone disease. Kidney Int 1994;46:855–861.
12. Coen G, Ballanti P, Bonucci E, et al: Renal osteodystrophy in predialysis and hemodialysis patients: Comparison of histologic patterns and diagnostic predictivity of intact PTH. Nephron 2002;91:103–111.
13. Couttenye MM, D'Haese PC, Verschoren WJ, et al: Low bone turnover in patients with renal failure. Kidney Int 1999;56: S70–S76.

14. Block GA, Hulbert-Shearon TE, Levin NW, Port FK: Association of serum phosphorus and calcium × phosphate product with mortality risk in chronic hemodialysis patients: A national study. Am J Kidney Dis 1998;31:607–617.

15. Block GA, Klassen PS, Lazarus JM, et al: Mineral metabolism, mortality, and morbidity in maintenance hemodialysis. J Am Soc Nephrol 2004;15:2208–2218.

16. Combe C, Aparicio M: Phosphorus and protein restriction and parathyroid function in chronic renal failure. Kidney Int 1994;46: 1381–1386.

17. Slatopolsky E, Brown A, Dusso A: Role of phosphorus in the pathogenesis of secondary hyperparathyroidism. Am J Kidney Dis 2001;37:S54–S57.

18. Slatopolsky E, Finch J, Denda M, et al: Phosphorus restriction prevents parathyroid gland growth. High phosphorus directly stimulates PTH secretion in vitro. J Clin Invest 1996;97:2534–2540.

19. Chertow GM, Burke SK, Raggi P: Sevelamer attenuates the progression of coronary and aortic calcification in hemodialysis patients. Kidney Int 2002;62:245–252.

20. Chertow GM, Dillon M, Burke SK, et al: A randomized trial of sevelamer hydrochloride (RenaGel) with and without supplemental calcium. Strategies for the control of hyperphosphatemia and hyperparathyroidism in hemodialysis patients. Clin Nephrol 1999;51:18–26.

21. Wilkes BM, Reiner D, Kern M, Burke S: Simultaneous lowering of serum phosphate and LDL-cholesterol by sevelamer hydrochloride (RenaGel) in dialysis patients. Clin Nephrol 1998;50: 381–386.

22. Finn WF: Lanthanum carbonate versus standard therapy for the treatment of hyperphosphatemia: Safety and efficacy in chronic maintenance hemodialysis patients. Clin Nephrol 2006;65: 191–202.

23. Sherrard DJ, Andress DL: Aluminum-related osteodystrophy. Adv Intern Med 1989;34:307–323.

24. Al-Aly Z, Qazi R, Gonzalez EA, et al: Changes in serum 25-hydroxyvitamin D and plasma intact PTH levels following treatment with ergocalciferol in patients with CKD. Am J Kidney Dis 2007;50:59–68.

25. Martin KJ, González EA, Gellens M, et al: 19-Nor-1-alpha-25-dihydroxyvitamin D2 (paricalcitol) safely and effectively reduces the levels of intact PTH in patients on hemodialysis. J Am Soc Nephrol 1998;9:1427–1432.

26. Slatopolsky E, Finch J, Ritter C, et al: A new analog of calcitriol, 19-nor-1,25-(OH)2D2, suppresses parathyroid hormone secretion in uremic rats in the absence of hypercalcemia. Am J Kidney Dis 1995;26:852–860.

27. Teng M, Wolf M, Lowrie E, et al: Survival of patients undergoing hemodialysis with paricalcitol or calcitriol therapy. N Engl J Med 2003;349:446–456.

28. Maung HM, Elangovan L, Frazao JM, et al: Efficacy and side effects of intermittent intravenous and oral doxercalciferol (1-alpha-hydroxyvitamin D₂) in dialysis patients with secondary hyperparathyroidism: a sequential comparison. Am J Kidney Dis 2001; 37:532–543.

29. Martin KJ, Gonzalez EA: Vitamin D analogs: Actions and role in the treatment of secondary hyperparathyroidism. Semin Nephrol 2004;24:456–459.

30. Mucsi I, Hercz G, Uldall R, et al: Control of serum phosphate without any phosphate binders in patients treated with nocturnal hemodialysis. Kidney Int 1998;53:1399–1404.

31. Block GA, Martin KJ, de Francisco AL, et al: Cinacalcet for secondary hyperparathyroidism in patients receiving hemodialysis. N Engl J Med 2004;350:1516–1525.

32. Fan SL, Almond MK, Ball E, et al: Pamidronate therapy as prevention of bone loss following renal transplantation. Kidney Int 2000;57:684–690.

33. Serra AL, Schwarz AA, Wick FH, et al: Successful treatment of hypercalcemia with cinacalcet in renal transplant recipients with persistent hyperparathyroidism. Nephrol Dial Transplant 2005;20:1315–1319.

34. Budisavljevic MN, Cheek D, Ploth DW: Calciphylaxis in chronic renal failure. J Am Soc Nephrol 1996;7:978–982.

35. Cicone JS, Petronis JB, Embert CD, Spector DA: Successful treatment of calciphylaxis with intravenous sodium thiosulfate. Am J Kidney Dis 2004;43:1104–1108.

36. Mataic D, Bastani B: Intraperitoneal sodium thiosulfate for the treatment of calciphylaxis. Ren Fail 2006;28:361–363.

37. Mazhar AR, Johnson RJ, Gillen D, et al: Risk factors and mortality associated with calciphylaxis in end-stage renal disease. Kidney Int 2001;60:324–332.

38. Shiraishi N, Kitamura K, Miyoshi T, et al: Successful treatment of a patient with severe calcific uremic arteriolopathy (calciphylaxis) by etidronate disodium. Am J Kidney Dis 2006;48:151–154.

39. Basile C, Montanaro A, Masi M, et al: Hyperbaric oxygen therapy for calcific uremic arteriolopathy: A case series. J Nephrol 2002;15:676–680.

40. Velasco N, MacGregor MS, Innes A, MacKay IG: Successful treatment of calciphylaxis with cinacalcet—an alternative to parathyroidectomy? Nephrol Dial Transplant 2006;21:1999–2004.

Further Reading

Block GA, Klassen PS, Lazarus JM, et al: Mineral metabolism, mortality, and morbidity in maintenance hemodialysis. J Am Soc Nephrol 2004;15:2208–2218.

Block GA, Raggi P, Bellasi A, et al: Mortality effect of coronary calcification and phosphate binder choice in incident hemodialysis patients. Kidney Int 2007;71:438–441.

Coyne D, Acharya M, Qiu P, et al: Paricalcitol capsule for the treatment of secondary hyperparathyroidism in stages 3 and 4 CKD. Am J Kidney Dis 2006;47:263–276.

Martin KJ, Gonzalez EA: Metabolic bone disease in chronic kidney disease. J Am Soc Nephrol 2007;18:875–885.

Martin KJ, Gonzalez EA. Vitamin D analogs: Actions and role in the treatment of secondary hyperparathyroidism. Semin Nephrol 2004;24:456–459.

Moe S, Drueke T, Cunningham J, et al: Definition, evaluation, and classification of renal osteodystrophy: a position statement from Kidney Disease: Improving Global Outcomes (KDIGO). Kidney Int 2006;69:1945–1953.

Moe SM, Chertow GM, Coburn JW, et al: Achieving NKF-K/DOQI bone metabolism and disease treatment goals with cinacalcet HCl. Kidney Int 2005;67:760–771.

Chapter 70

Cardiovascular Complications of End-Stage Renal Disease

Eberhard Ritz and Christoph Wanner

BACKGROUND

In patients with end-stage renal disease before (chronic kidney disease [CKD] stages 4 and 5) and after the start of dialysis treatment (stage 5D), angina pectoris, myocardial infarction, dysrhythmia, heart failure, stroke, and peripheral vascular disease are markedly more frequent than in the background population. The risk of death in dialysis patients is 15 times higher than in the background population. Age is a very prominent risk factor with a 3% risk increase per year in patients between 60 and 80 years old.[1] The cardiovascular risk (Box 70-1) starts to increase even in the earliest stages of CKD and increases exponentially with progressive loss of glomerular filtration rate (GFR).[2]

TREATMENT GOALS FOR UREMIC PATIENTS

In the distant past, it had appeared plausible that one should aim in uremic patients and in dialysis patients for the same treatment target values (Table 70-1) as in the general population. For a number of interventions, however, it has recently been suggested, unfortunately usually based on observational evidence, that targets for patients with end-stage renal disease should be different from those recommended in the general population, for example hemoglobin (Hb), parathyroid hormone (PTH), and blood pressure. Little controlled prospective evidence is available for patients with CKD, mainly because in the past patients with renal disease had deliberately been excluded from major cardiovascular intervention trials.

Further complexity has been created by some intervention trials documenting that mechanistically plausible interventions that had effectively improved cardiovascular outcome in nonrenal patients failed to yield significant benefit or yielded only marginal nonsignificant improvement in patients with end-stage renal disease, for example, lowering of low-density lipoprotein cholesterol with statins in patients with type 2 diabetes on hemodialysis,[3] lowering homocysteine concentrations with folate,[4] and administration of angiotensin-converting enzyme (ACE) inhibitors in dialysis patients.[5]

The absence of intervention trials with information on the efficacy and safety of treatments makes it often difficult to make definite statements so that recommendations and guidelines for patients with end-stage renal disease are mainly based on expert opinion or low-grade evidence from observational data. The absence of controlled evidence has led to definite deficits in the prescription of treatments particularly for cardiovascular disease, as suggested by comparisons of the use of aspirin, statins, β-blockers, ACE inhibitors or AT_1 receptor blockers in renal patients compared with nonrenal controls. Such deficit is deplorable because, conversely, observational data suggest that risk reduction by intervention in this extremely high-risk population may be particularly rewarding. As a result, there remains a need for intervention trials to provide convincing evidence; the Cochrane group has shown that among several specialties in internal medicine, nephrology was the one where the least number of controlled trials had been performed.[6]

Healthy Lifestyle

A healthy lifestyle is routinely recommended to end-stage renal disease patients.

Smoking

Smoking accelerates the progression of renal disease and increases the cardiovascular risk substantially by a factor of as much as 10-fold,[7,8] both in diabetic and nondiabetic patients.[8,9] There are conflicting reports whether smoking aggravates the cardiovascular risk in patients on dialysis, but analogy to nonrenal patients suggests that this assumption is

Box 70-1 Cardiovascular Risk Factors and Cardiovascular Events for Uremic Patients

---

Risk Factors
Smoking, glycemia, lack of exercise
Dyslipidemia
Anemia
Hyperphosphatemia
Lifestyle changes (metabolic syndrome)
Additional cardiovascular risk factors (obstructive sleep apnea, depression)
Dialysis modality

Cardiovascular Disease
Coronary heart disease
Sudden death
Heart failure

---

sensible. The proportion of smokers with early stages of CKD who stop smoking is disappointingly low, in our experience approximately 15%, although with the onset of ESRD, many smokers stop smoking.

The smoker with renal disease (and his or her partner) should be given advice, possibly nicotine replacement therapy or bupropion, but there is not sufficient safety information available to recommend nortriptyline, varencilline, rimonabant, or monoamine and selective serotonin reuptake inhibitors.

Normoglycemia

There is increasing (although not uniform) evidence that near-normal blood glucose levels as assessed by HbA1c or glycated albumin[10,11] are associated with decreased cardiovascular events and improved survival of diabetic patients on dialysis,[12] although the relationship is confounded by several factors.[13] For several reasons, HbA1c is not a perfect reflection of glycemic control, mainly because of the confounding influence of erythrocyte half-life and the measurement of carbamylated Hb in some assays.

Physical Exercise

Physical exercise has been shown to have beneficial metabolic and psychological effects,[14–17] but in today's elderly dialysis population, this intervention is, unfortunately, very difficult to implement.

Obesity

Among further lifestyle changes, weight reduction is an important issue for which there is currently no definite answer available. The presence of metabolic syndrome[18] and obesity[19] increases the risk of CKD and end-stage renal disease.[20,21] It would, therefore, appear rational to decrease the risk by weight reduction. Against this, one has to balance the recent observation that—for partially unclear reasons—survival on dialysis is better for those with a high body mass index, even in the range of morbid obesity.[22] However, when adequately corrected for duration of follow-up using an adequate control group, the effect of a high body mass index on better survival dissolves. Due to wasting, it is not advisable to recommend weight reduction in those with far advanced CKD, for example, CKD stage 4 or 5.[23]

Blood Pressure

In patients on long slow dialysis protocols, it has been shown that impressive survival rates are achieved with dialysis schedules resulting in normalization of blood pressure, primarily by low dietary salt intake, ultrafiltration to achieve dry weight, and prolonged dialysis sessions (8 hours).[24] Furthermore, a correlation was noted between blood pressure values (mostly in the normotensive range) and survival in the dialysis centers practicing long slow dialysis (e.g., Tassin[25]]. Strict normotension by decreased dietary salt intake and aggressive ultrafiltration has even led to reversal of left ventricular (LV) hypertrophy without antihypertensive medication.[26]

Similarly, impressive blood pressure control with less need for antihypertensives has recently been achieved by protocols with daily short dialysis[27,28] or daily nocturnal dialysis schedules,[29] which are not universally available, however. Improved blood pressure control is presumably the combined result of better control of hypervolemia, the potential removal of pressor agents (e.g., asymmetric dimethyl L-arginine), and a decrease in sympathetic overactivity.[30] There is a large trial ongoing to evaluate the clinical value of this modality.

The situation is much less clear in patients on the usual schedule of three times weekly short dialysis sessions (3 × 3–3 × 5 hr/wk). Initial analyses showed that high blood pressure values[31,32] were associated with no or minor increase in risk, whereas the risk was highest in patients with low blood pressure. This finding is now commonly interpreted as the result of reverse causality, that is, reversal of the normal blood pressure–survival relationship because of the presence of heart disease or autonomic dysfunction. In the 4D study in patients with type 2 diabetes receiving hemodialysis,[3] we found no correlation whatsoever between blood pressure and short-term patient survival.

Episodes of hypotension during dialysis carry a particularly adverse prognosis: Once blood pressure decreases below the threshold of coronary autoregulation of approximately 95 mm Hg systolic, the risk of cardiovascular death is significantly increased.[33]

In almost all studies, correct assessment of the impact of blood pressure on target organs is rendered difficult because of the absence of ambulatory blood pressure measurements. Because the circadian blood pressure profile is abnormal and particularly because nighttime blood pressure values tend to be high, the blood pressure burden on target organs is underestimated by the office blood pressure.

A further confounder is the situation that brachial artery blood pressure may markedly underestimate central (aortic) blood pressure to which the target organs are exposed (heart, brain, kidney).[34]

The frequently present high blood pressure amplitude is the result of increased aortic stiffness. Aortic stiffness, indirectly assessed by pulse wave velocity, is an independent predictor of adverse cardiovascular outcome.[35] A high blood pressure amplitude implies a low diastolic blood pressure, which exposes the patient to the risk of coronary underperfusion because coronary flow occurs only during diastole.

Recommended Blood Pressure in Dialysis Patients

Which blood pressure should one aim for? Little well-documented long-term evidence is available, but the following strategy appears sensible for patients on the usual dialysis schedules of three times for 3 to 5 hours per week.

Table 70-1   Basis for Treatment Targets in Uremic Patients According to Current Kidney Disease Outcome and Quality Initiative Guidelines

Parameter	Target/Goal	Evidence
Smoking	Cessation	Observational, strong opinion, no pharmacotherapy studies[1]
Physical activity	30 min/day, moderate intensity	Observational for hospitalizations and death[1] Intervention for surrogate outcomes (clinical chemistry)[1]
Healthy weight	Uremia (BMI < 18.5 kg/m^2 avoid)	Observational[2]
	Diabetes and CKD stage 1–4 (BMI 18.5–24.9 kg/m^2)	Observational[3]
Glycemia	Normoglycemia[3]	
	Preprandial capillary plasma glucose 90–130 mg/dL (5.0–7.2 mmol/L)	
	Peak postprandial capillary plasma glucose 4 < 180 mg/dL (10.0 mmol/L)	
	Hb$_{Alc}$ < 7%	Observational[3]
		One observational study[4]
Blood pressure	Pre-dialysis < 140/90 mm Hg	Interventional, post hoc observational[5]
	Post-dialysis < 130/80 mm Hg	Observational (avoid hypotension)[5]
LDL cholesterol	<100 mg/dL (mmol/L)	CKD stage 4–5D observational retrospective[3,6]
		CKD stage 1–3 meta-analysis of RCTs post hoc = observational[1,3]
	<70 mg/dL (mmol/L) (option)	CKD stage 1–4 KDOQI opinion[3]
Hemoglobin	Normalization	Observational, opinion[7]
	11–12 g/dL	Interventional[8]
	>13 g/dL, avoid	Interventional[8]
S-phosphorus	3.5–5.5 mg/dL (1.10–1.80 mmol/L)	Observational[9]

1. KDOQI clinical practice guidelines for cardiovascular disease in dialysis patients. Am J Kidney Dis 2005;45(Suppl 3):S1–S153.
2. de Mutsert R, Snijder MB, van der Sman-de Beer F, et al: Association between body mass index and mortality is similar in the hemodialysis population and the general population at high age and equal duration of follow-up. J Am Soc Nephrol 2007;18: 967–974.
3. KDOQI clinical practice guidelines and clinical practice recommendations for diabetes and chronic kidney disease. Am J Kidney Dis 2007;49(Suppl 2):S12–S154.
4. Foley RN, Parfrey PS, Harnett JD, et al: Impact of hypertension on cardiomyopathy, morbidity and mortality in end-stage renal disease. Kidney Int 1996;49:1379–1385.
5. KDOQI clinical practice guidelines on hypertension and antihypertensive agents in chronic kidney disease. Am J Kidney Dis 2004;43(Suppl 1):S1–S290.
6. National Kidney Foundation: K/DOQI clinical practice guidelines for managing dyslipidemias in chronic kidney disease. Am J Kidney Dis 2003;41(Suppl 3):S1–S92.
7. KDOQI clinical practice guidelines and clinical practice recommendations for anemia in chronic kidney disease: 2007 update of hemoglobin target. Am J Kidney Dis 2007;50:471–530.
8. KDOQI clinical practice guidelines and clinical practice recommendations for anemia in chronic kidney disease. Am J Kidney Dis 2006;47(Suppl 3):S11–S145.
9. National Kidney Foundation: KDOQI clinical practice guidelines for bone metabolism and disease in chronic kidney disease. Am J Kidney Dis 2003;42(Suppl 3):S1–S201.

BMI, body mass index; CKD, chronic kidney disease; Hb$_{Alc}$, hemoglobin Alc; KDOQI, Kidney Disease Outcome and Quality Initiative; RCTs, randomized, controlled trials.

In low-risk relatively young patients with potentially long life expectancy, one should aim for normotension according to Joint National Committee on Detection, Evaluation, and Treatment of High Blood Pressure.

In contrast, standards may have to be relaxed in the elderly polymorbid patient with poor ultrafiltration tolerance and predisposition to intradialytic hypotension, which by itself is a predictor of and contributor to an adverse cardiovascular outcome.

Dietary salt restriction, as originally recommended by Scribner and colleagues[36,37] is certainly the most neglected and underused aspect of dialysis patient management.[38]

Reduction of dietary salt intake, combined with modest lowering of dialysate sodium concentration (~135 mmol/L) and effective ultrafiltration, normalized blood pressure not only in centers with long slow dialysis but also centers with 3 × 5 hr/week dialysis.[26,39]

Why is salt intake so important for blood pressure control? Ingestion of 9 g of salt by an anuric patient increases the osmotic pressure, which forces the patient to drink 1 L of water to maintain osmolality. Although some salt is stored in a non-osmotic form,[40] daily intake of the usual amount of 13 to 14 g of salt in the Western diet increases body weight by 1.5 kg/day and causes hypervolemia, the most potent cause of hypertension in anuric patients. Furthermore, salt intake increases the plasma concentration of endogenous digitaloids,[41] which increase blood pressure.[42] Such blood pressure increase can be reversed by ouabain antagonists in experimental studies[43] documenting their causal role. In experimental studies, a salt-induced increase in the concentration of cardiotonic steroids reproduced the features of uremic cardiomyopathy.[44]

The majority of dialysis patients require antihypertensive therapy. Are there differences between the different antihypertensive agents?

There is recent controlled evidence from a small study in dialyzed patients with heart failure that the β-blocker carvedilol reduces cardiac mortality by approximately 50%.[45] In dialysis patients, the use of β-blockers was also associated with less onset of heart failure.[46] Furthermore, observational studies documented less mortality in dialysis patients treated with β-blockers.[33,47]

Recent preliminary studies suggest that angiotensin-receptor blockers on top of alternative antihypertensive medication improve survival of dialysis patients, although the study sizes were quite limited. The effect of ACE inhibitors examined in one study on elderly dialysis patients failed to document a statistically significant benefit, but showed a tendency for some improvement of outcomes.[5]

Calcium channel blockers are very effective in dialyzed patients and in some analyses of the most frequently used antihypertensive drug.[48]

In contrast to the dialyzed patient, the situation is entirely different in the patient with CKD. There is consensus that high blood pressure, particularly systolic blood pressure, is the key factor that promotes progressive loss of renal function. There has been much discussion concerning whether it is more important to lower blood pressure or to block the renin-angiotensin system (RAS).[49] There is no doubt that lowering blood pressure per se is of overriding importance, as illustrated by one striking comparison: Before the availability of antihypertensive treatment, the patient with diabetic nephropathy lost approximately 10 mL/min/1.73 m² GFR per year. In the RENAAL (Reduction of Endpoints in NIDDM with the Angiotensin II Antagonist Losartan) trial, the rate of loss of the estimated GFR was 5.24 mL/min/1.73 m² per year in the placebo arm and 4.4 mL/min/1.73 m² per year in the Losartan arm (Bakris, personal communication), illustrating the respective relative potencies for these two interventions. Controlled prospective evidence for this statement is somewhat weak, however. The Modification of Diet in Renal Disease study compared routine (target 107 mm Hg mean arterial pressure) and intensified (target 91 mm Hg mean arterial pressure) lowering of blood pressure. Intensified blood pressure lowering was associated with a GFR loss of

1.9 mL/min/1.73 m² compared with 3.4 mL/min/1.73 m², but this was not statistically significant.[50] In the long-term follow-up observation, the difference in the occurrence of end-stage renal disease was significant but small.[51]

Based on a number of observations, current guidelines recommend in patients with CKD a lower target blood pressure than in essential hypertension; most recommend 130/80 mm Hg. Such low blood pressure target is justified not only by the consideration of renal protection but also because of the high cardiovascular risk of CKD patients: Lewington and colleagues[52] had shown in individuals without renal disease that if systolic blood pressure was lowered by 20 mm Hg, the rate of cardiovascular events was lowered by 50%.

A specific benefit from blockade of the RAS using ACE inhibitors or angiotensin receptor blockers has been documented in a series of head-on comparisons between RAS blockade and blood pressure lowering without RAS blockade. Even in studies, for example, the Ramipril Effect in Nephropathy study, in which blood pressure values in the ACE inhibitor and non-ACE inhibitor arms were identical, a benefit, that is, less decrease in GFR, was seen with RAS blockade,[53] and this has been confirmed by a meta-analysis of further controlled trials.[54,55]

The beneficial effect of RAS blockade is particularly pronounced in patients with proteinuric renal disease and less certain in patients with CKD and proteinuria less than 1 g/24 hr.[56] One difficulty in interpretation relates to the fact that office blood pressure measurements are a poor reflection of the 24-hour blood pressure profile and may also substantially underestimate the level of central blood pressure (to which heart and kidney are exposed).

One drawback of RAS blockade is the phenomenon of escape, that is, gradual return of proteinuria to baseline values despite treatment after several years of RAS blockade. Modern approaches include dose escalation of ACE inhibitors and/or angiotensin receptor blockers, combination of ACE inhibitors and angiotensin receptor blockers.[57] Currently further approaches, for example, mineralocorticoid receptor blockade (which in patients with impaired renal function carries the substantial risk of hyperkalemia and is not advisable in such patients) and renin blockers are under investigation

When lowering blood pressure, one caveat is the J-curve phenomenon. At low diastolic pressures, coronary perfusion is endangered as recently shown in the INVEST (International Verapamil SR/Trandolapril) study.[58] Because of the high frequency of coronary heart disease, it is advisable to not lower diastolic pressure to values less than approximately 70 mm Hg.

The single most neglected aspect of antihypertensive treatment is decreasing the dietary salt intake and adequate diuretic treatment. The current discussions of which antihypertensive drug reduces progression of renal disease best is entirely academic because mostly three to six antihypertensive classes are necessary to achieve the target blood pressure.[59]

Lipid Abnormalities

Two decades ago, Degoulet and colleagues[60] made the counterintuitive observation that, in dialysis patients, the lower serum cholesterol is, the higher the mortality rate.[60] This observation has since been amply confirmed and does of course not imply that in end-stage renal disease high cholesterol is protective. Rather it is explained by so-called reverse causality, that is, confounding the relationship between serum cholesterol and cardiovascular death by factors such as inflammation. This interpretation gains credence from the study of Liu and colleagues[61] that documented that in CKD patients with high C-reactive protein low low-density lipoprotein cholesterol was associated with a high mortality rate, whereas in CKD patients with low C-reactive protein, the usual continuous positive relationship between serum cholesterol and cardiovascular risk was observed.

The contribution of lipids to the elevation of cardiovascular risk in renal patients cannot be fully assessed by routine laboratory measurements, particularly not by total cholesterol and low-density lipoprotein cholesterol. In CKD the typical constellation is low HDL cholesterol and high triglycerides. A number of further atherogenic lipid abnormalities are not measured routinely,[62–64] for example, accumulation of remnants (chylomicrons, intermediate-density lipoprotein, small dense low-density lipoprotein); inflammatory high-density lipoprotein; covalent modification of apo-lipoproteins by carbamylation, glycation, and oxidation; increased lipoprotein(a).

In view of the strikingly increased cardiovascular risk in renal patients,[65] the question arises whether statin treatment is indicated in CKD patients even when cholesterol values are not frankly increased, that is, whether CKD (analogous to diabetes) should be considered a coronary equivalent with a 10-year mortality of more than 20%.[66] Controlled information on this point is currently not available, but post hoc analyses of study participants with a decreased estimated GFR in the trials on cardiovascular disease showed that statins reduced cardiovascular events in patients with CKD stages 2 and 3.[67] There is no information available on patients with CKD stage 4.

In patients on dialysis, observational studies had suggested a lower mortality rate in patients on statins,[68] but in diabetic patients on hemodialysis, the prospective controlled 4D study failed to show significant benefit for a composite cardiovascular endpoint, although a trend of benefit was seen for adjudicated cardiovascular death, nonfatal myocardial infarction, bypass, percutaneous transluminal coronary angiography, which was less frequent by 18% per 1 mmol/L lower low-density lipoprotein cholesterol, exactly what had been seen for coronary death in trials on nonrenal patients.[69]

The prevailing opinion is currently that statin treatment should be started early in CKD and not stopped when patients go on dialysis, but the data do not justify de novo start of statin treatment for primary prevention in dialysis patients without clinical evidence of coronary heart disease. It is our opinion, however, that dialysis patients with established coronary heart disease should receive statins, although admittedly definite evidence on this point is currently lacking.

Anemia

In CKD, anemia is mainly the result of reduced plasma erythropoietin concentration, although additional factors such as chronic microinflammation, gastrointestinal blood loss, and iron deficiency play a role; in dialysis patients, blood loss through the dialysis procedure, blood sampling for laboratory investigation, etc. may further contribute. In the past, it was thought that anemia usually appears at an estimated GFR of approximately 30 mL/min, but more recent studies show that anemia may appear much earlier,[70] particularly in diabetic patients.[71] In observational studies, Hb and hematocrit are powerful predictors of mortality and adverse events.[72] This appeared plausible because the circulatory adaptation to anemia is maladaptive, that is, vasodilatation, increased venous return, cardiac enlargement, and increased cardiac output.[73] It had therefore been widely anticipated that correction of anemia including normalization of Hb values was beneficial.

Undoubtedly, in the past, several small studies suggested that correction of severe anemia with Hb 7 to 10 g/dL did not improve only the quality of life, but also objective surrogate parameters such as LV hypertrophy.[74] It was therefore extrapolated that normalization of Hb was a promising goal. For several reasons, this concept has recently been questioned. In the study of Besarab and colleagues,[75] dialysis patients with cardiac disease were randomized to erythropoietin treatment with the goal of achieving predialytic target hematocrit values of 42% versus 30%. The study was prematurely stopped when an excess of adverse events was seen in the high hematocrit patients. This was primarily because of more frequent thromboses of the vascular access. In a prospective study of dialysis patients with concentric LV hypertrophy or LV dilatation, the changes in the cavity volume index were similar in both targets in patients with LV dilatation, whereas in patients with an initially normal LV volume, an inverse relationship was seen between the change in the LV volume index and the mean Hb level, potentially implying that normalization of Hb was better in preventing than in reversing LV dilatation.[76] With respect to LV hypertrophy no significant effect of full Hb correction was seen in nondiabetic incident hemodialysis[77] and diabetic patients with CKD.[78] Furthermore, in the CREATE (Cardiovascular Risk Reduction with Early Anemia Treatment with Epoetin Beta) study, patients with advanced CKD and anemia were randomized to achieve an Hb of 10.5 to 11.5 g/dL and 13 to 15 g/dL, respectively.[79] There was no difference in cardiovascular outcomes and a suggestive shortening of the time to the start of dialysis, but the quality of life was significantly better in patients with a higher Hb. More recently, in the CHOIR (Correction of Hemoglobin and Outcomes in Renal Insufficiency) study, increased rates of cardiovascular events were observed in the arm with higher target hematocrit values.[80] As a result, much concern has been raised whether normalizing Hb is safe.[81] The definite answer will have to wait until the results of the ongoing TREAT (Trial to Reduce Cardiovascular Events with Aranesp) study in diabetic patients with CKD, in which normalization and incomplete normalization with erythropoietin beta are compared, are available.[82]

At the same time, it appears that current recommendations (European Renal Association guidelines) go the middle road between the undoubted adverse effects of Hb less than 10g/dL on surrogate markers such as LV hypertrophy,[74] on the one hand, and a potential (although currently not proven) cardiovascular risk of normalization of Hb.[81] Indeed, theoretically, mechanisms are conceivable regarding how renal failure may promote adverse effects of Hb normalization: Experimental work points to the importance of normal endothelial function to prevent adverse effects of erythropoietin and endothelial function is frequently disturbed in uremia.[83]

Calcium Phosphate Metabolism

In the past, the only known adverse effects of hyperparathyroidism and abnormal plasma concentrations of calcium and phosphate were bone disease and soft-tissue calcification. The treatment target was normalization of the PTH concentration by administration of active vitamin D (1,25-dihydroxychole-calciferol or its congeners) to prevent bone disease and to lower plasma phosphate by oral phosphate binders, mainly oral calcium carbonate or acetate.

It was recently recognized that both low- and high-turnover bone disease promote vascular calcification including coronary calcification[84] and that vascular calcification is closely related to adverse cardiovascular events as a result of arterial stiffening, increased blood pressure amplitude with decreased diastolic blood pressure, decreased coronary perfusion, and other factors.[85] The targets for treating abnormal mineral metabolism have therefore been broadened to include reduction of cardiovascular risk. The term CKD–metabolic bone disease has been coined to emphasize the link between metabolic bone disease and cardiovascular complications of CKD.[86]

Hyperparathyroidism has an impact on survival as illustrated by improved long-term survival after parathyroidectomy,[87,88] but, conversely, low immunoreactive PTH concentrations are associated with low bone turnover and increased risk of vascular calcification.[84]

Treatment of elevated immunoreactive PTH includes reduction of plasma phosphate, administration of active vitamin D (1,25-dihydroxycholecalciferol or its congeners) at doses that avoid hypercalcemia and/or hyperphosphatemia, the calcium receptor agonist (calcimimetic) cinacalcet,[89] and parathyroidectomy.[90]

Improved achievement of treatment targets with cinacalcet has been documented,[91] but evidence of a positive effect on hard endpoints is still lacking.

The rationale for the administration of active vitamin D (i.e., 1,25-dihydroxycholecalciferol or its congeners) may go beyond the inhibition of elevated immunoreactive PTH concentrations. Several observational studies on dialysis patients documented better survival of patients given active vitamin D, particularly the congener paricalcitol, independent of immunoreactive PTH, plasma calcium, and phosphate.[92,93] Although prospective controlled evidence is still lacking, an explanation for this unexpected finding may be the fact that active vitamin D inhibits renin secretion in the juxtaglomerular apparatus[94] and exerts PTH independent effects on the heart.[94–96]

It has been well documented that hyperphosphatemia affects patient survival[97] so that currently serum phosphate concentrations of 5.5 mg/dL are recommended as a therapeutic target, which is admittedly difficult to achieve with current dialysis schedules. Even lower serum phosphate values are associated with a higher risk of cardiovascular events in CKD patients[98] and even in coronary patients without CKD.[99]

The recognition that a positive calcium balance facilitates vascular calcification, including coronary calcification, has led to the introduction of noncalcium-containing phosphate binders for the prophylaxis of hyperphosphatemia. Although the phosphate binder sevelamer decreased vascular calcification,[100] thus far, despite suggestive trends,[101] definite evidence that it also decreases hard cardiovascular endpoints is absent. The latter is also true for lanthanum carbonate.

Currently used phosphate binders include calcium acetate or calcium or magnesium carbonate, lanthanum carbonate,[102] sevelamer,[100] and inhibition of intestinal phosphate absorption by nicotinamide.[103]

Finally, it was only recently recognized that patients with CKD tend to have low 25(OH) vitamin D_3 concentrations,[104] which has been shown to be related to a number of functions unrelated to mineral metabolism, for example, impaired infection control (specifically tuberculosis), impaired insulin secretion and insulin sensitivity, and altered immune response. It has therefore been recommended to normalize 25(OH)D concentrations by administration of native vitamin D_3 (or D_2) to achieve a target 25-dihydroxyvitamin D of 30 ng/mL.

Dialysis Modality

Uremia is a state of intoxication by retention not only of urea, but also the number of more or less hypothetical low molecular weight, water-soluble substances, which are not very effectively removed with current dialysis strategies.[105] There has been much recent interest in strategies to modify the dialysis procedure.

On the one hand, the relative value of removal of urea (Kt/V) versus hypothetical higher molecular weight substances was assessed in the HEMO (Hemodialysis) Study, which failed to provide a clear-cut result,[106] although the currently unpublished results of the European MPO (Membrane Permeability Outcomes) trial show that high-flux membranes improve hard endpoints in dialysis patients.

Even more spectacular are observations on dialysis procedures other than the routinely used 3 × 3 to 3 × 5-hours per week schedule, for example, daily short-term dialysis (2–3 hours), on the one hand[28,107] and daily nighttime dialysis.[29] Such modified schedules reduced hypertension and permitted reduction or omission of antihypertensive agents, facilitated phosphate removal, improved anemia, and decreased or eliminated the use of erythropoietin, improved sleep and sleep apnea syndrome as well as many other facets of the uremic syndrome. Ongoing controlled trials will provide information on the true real-life value of these alternative procedures.

CORONARY ARTERY DISEASE

Coronary artery disease is extremely common in the population of uremic patients. Its morphology differs from that of nonuremic individuals by the high prevalence of calcification[108] and higher degree of inflammatory changes and intraplaque hemorrhage.[109] Myocardial infarction accounts for approximately 9% of deaths of patients on dialysis, which, as a percentage of total death, appears low, but compared with absolute rates in the general population, it is high. The prognosis of myocardial infarction in dialysis patients is abysmal.[110] Observational studies suggest, despite higher perioperative risk, superior long-term survival with coronary artery bypass graft compared with percutaneous transluminal angioplasty with stent placement.[111] It is important that even minor reductions in renal function accelerate atherogenesis in experimental models[112] and that in observational studies, the risk of coronary heart disease increases progressively with decreasing GFR.[113] Unfortunately, patients with CKD tend to be undertreated with respect to interventions such as aspirin, β-blockers, and statins, although undertreatment alone does not fully account for the more adverse prognosis of coronary heart disease in CKD patients.

In patients with end-stage renal disease, the symptomatology of CHD is frequently atypical (dyspnea without precordial pain) and the exercise electrocardiogram usually cannot be performed because of muscular weakness. The best option is to perform coronarography if there is a high suspicion of coronary heart disease (particularly before renal transplantation) and if intervention by percutaneous transluminal angioplasty or bypass surgery is possible.

SUDDEN DEATH

Sudden death is the most common modality of death in dialysis patients.[114] In contrast to the general population, it occurs most frequently at night (patients are found dead in bed). Pathogenetic factors include myocardial fibrosis, repolarization disturbances, electrolyte changes, and possibly medication-induced QT prolongation. There is no documented prophylaxis, but medications causing QT prolongation should be avoided.[115] Although there is no formal proof, β-blockers are apparently helpful.[114]

HEART FAILURE

Heart failure is common in dialysis patients and is found in as many as 50% of patients if sophisticated techniques are used. Structural heart disease is common (aortic and mitral valve calcification/stenosis, coronary heart disease, cardiac hypertrophy and fibrosis, cardiac underperfusion because of microvessel disease). The role of endogenous cardiotonic digitaloids in the genesis of hypertension and organ damage of uremia had been postulated by Ahmad and colleagues[116] and was recently documented in the genesis of uremic cardiomyopathy by Kennedy and colleagues.[44]

A major correctable factor is overhydration by volume control (see earlier). Impressive results have been obtained by the prophylactic administration of β-blockers,[46] particularly carvedilol in trials involving a limited number of patients.

References

1. Sarnak MJ, Levey AS: Cardiovascular disease and chronic renal disease: A new paradigm. Am J Kidney Dis 2000;35(4 Suppl 1):S117–S131.
2. Van Biesen W, De Bacquer D, Verbeke F, et al: The glomerular filtration rate in an apparently healthy population and its relation with cardiovascular mortality during 10 years. Eur Heart J 2007;28:478–483.
3. Wanner C, Krane V, März W, et al, for the German Diabetes and Dialysis Study Investigators: Atorvastatin in patients with type 2 diabetes mellitus undergoing hemodialysis. N Engl J Med 2005;353:238–248.
4. Jamison RL, Hartigan P, Kaufman JS, et al, for the Veterans Affairs Site Investigators: Effect of homocysteine lowering on mortality and vascular disease in advanced chronic kidney disease and end-stage renal disease: A randomized controlled trial. JAMA 2007;298:1163–1170.
5. Zannad F, Kessler M, Lehert P, et al: Prevention of cardiovascular events in end-stage renal disease: Results of a randomized trial of fosinopril and implications for future studies. Kidney Int 2006;70:1318–1324.
6. Strippoli GF, Craig JC, Schena FP: The number, quality, and coverage of randomized controlled trials in nephrology. J Am Soc Nephrol 2004;15:411–419.
7. Muntner P, He J, Astor BC, et al: Traditional and nontraditional risk factors predict coronary heart disease in chronic kidney disease: Results from the atherosclerosis risk in communities study. J Am Soc Nephrol 2005;16:529–538.
8. Orth SR, Ritz E: The renal risks of smoking: An update. Curr Opin Nephrol Hypertens 2002;11:483–488.
9. Orth SR, Ritz E, Schrier RW: The renal risks of smoking. Kidney Int 1997;51:1669–1677.
10. Okada T, Nakao T, Matsumoto H, et al: Association between markers of glycemic control, cardiovascular complications and survival in type 2 diabetic patients with end-stage renal disease. Intern Med 2007;46:807–814.
11. Inaba M, Okuno S, Kumeda Y, et al: Glycated albumin is a better glycemic indicator than glycated hemoglobin values in hemodialysis patients with diabetes: Effect of anemia and erythropoietin injection. J Am Soc Nephrol 2007;18:896–903.
12. Oomichi T, Emoto M, Tabata T, et al: Impact of glycemic control on survival of diabetic patients on chronic regular hemodialysis: A 7-year observational study. Diabetes Care 2006;29:1496–1500.
13. Kalantar-Zadeh K, Kopple JD, Regidor DL, et al: A1C and survival in maintenance hemodialysis patients. Diabetes Care 2007;30:1049–1055.
14. Pupim LB, Flakoll PJ, Ikizler TA: Exercise improves albumin fractional synthetic rate in chronic hemodialysis patients. Eur J Clin Nutr 2007;61:686–689.
15. Kopple JD, Cohen AH, Wang H, et al: Effect of exercise on mRNA levels for growth factors in skeletal muscle of hemodialysis patients. J Ren Nutr 2006;16:312–324.
16. Cheema BS, Singh MA: Exercise training in patients receiving maintenance hemodialysis: A systematic review of clinical trials. Am J Nephrol 2005;25:352–364.
17. Parsons TL, Toffelmire EB, King-VanVlack CE: Exercise training during hemodialysis improves dialysis efficacy and physical performance. Arch Phys Med Rehabil 2006;87:680–687.
18. Chen J, Muntner P, Hamm LL, et al: The metabolic syndrome and chronic kidney disease in U.S. adults. Ann Intern Med 2004;140:167–174.
19. Ejerblad E, Fored CM, Lindblad P, et al: Obesity and risk for chronic renal failure. J Am Soc Nephrol 2006;17:1695–1702.
20. Hsu CY, McCulloch CE, Iribarren C, et al: Body mass index and risk for end-stage renal disease. Ann Intern Med 2006;144:21–28.
21. Iseki, K., Ikemiya Y, Kinjo K, et al: Body mass index and the risk of development of end-stage renal disease in a screened cohort. Kidney Int 2004;65:1870–1876.
22. Leavey SF, McCullough K, Hecking E, et al: Body mass index and mortality in 'healthier' as compared with 'sicker' haemodialysis patients: Results from the Dialysis Outcomes and Practice Patterns Study (DOPPS). Nephrol Dial Transplant 2001;16:2386–2394.
23. Kwan BC, Murtaugh MA, Beddhu S: Associations of body size with metabolic syndrome and mortality in moderate chronic kidney disease. Clin J Am Soc Nephrol 2007;2:992–998.
24. Charra B, Chazot C, Jean G, et al: Long 3 × 8 hr dialysis: A three-decade summary. J Nephrol 2003;16(Suppl 7):S64–S69.
25. Charra B, Calemard E, Ruffet M, et al: Survival as an index of adequacy of dialysis. Kidney Int 1992;41:1286–1291.
26. Ozkahya M, Ok E, Cirit M, et al: Regression of left ventricular hypertrophy in haemodialysis patients by ultrafiltration and reduced salt intake without antihypertensive drugs. Nephrol Dial Transplant 1998;13:1489–1493.
27. Kooistra MP: Frequent prolonged home haemodialysis: Three old concepts, one modern solution. Nephrol Dial Transplant 2003;18:16–19.
28. Kooistra MP, Vos J, Koomans H, Vos P: Daily home haemodialysis in The Netherlands: Effects on metabolic control,

haemodynamics, and quality of life. Nephrol Dial Transplant 1998;13:2853–2860.

29. Pierratos A, McFarlane P, Chan CT: Quotidian dialysis—update 2005. Curr Opin Nephrol Hypertens 2005;14:119–124.

30. Zilch O, Vos PF, Oey PL, et al: Sympathetic hyperactivity in haemodialysis patients is reduced by short daily haemodialysis. J Hypertens 2007;25:1285–1289.

31. Zager PG, Nikolic J, Brown RH, et al: "U" curve association of blood pressure and mortality in hemodialysis patients. Medical Directors of Dialysis Clinic, Inc. Kidney Int 1998;54:561–569.

32. Port FK, Hulbert-Shearon TE, Wolfe RA, et al: Predialysis blood pressure and mortality risk in a national sample of maintenance hemodialysis patients. Am J Kidney Dis 1999;33:507–517.

33. Koch M, Thomas B, Tschöpe W, Ritz E: Survival and predictors of death in dialysed diabetic patients. Diabetologia 1993;36:1113–1117.

34. Williams B, Lacy PS, Thom SM, et al: Differential impact of blood pressure-lowering drugs on central aortic pressure and clinical outcomes: Principal results of the Conduit Artery Function Evaluation (CAFE) study. Circulation 2006;113:1213–1225.

35. London GM, Marchais SJ, Guerin AP, Pannier B: Arterial stiffness: Pathophysiology and clinical impact. Clin Exp Hypertens 2004;26:689–699.

36. Scribner BH, Buri R, Caner JE, et al: The treatment of chronic uremia by means of intermittent hemodialysis: A preliminary report. 1960. J Am Soc Nephrol 1998;9:719–726.

37. Fishbane SA, Scribner BH: Blood pressure control in dialysis patients. Semin Dial 2002;15:144–145.

38. Ritz E, Dikow R, Morath C, Schwenger V: Salt—a potential 'uremic toxin'? Blood Purif 2006;24:63–66.

39. Krautzig S, Janssen U, Koch KM, et al: Dietary salt restriction and reduction of dialysate sodium to control hypertension in maintenance haemodialysis patients. Nephrol Dial Transplant 1998;13:552–553.

40. Titze J, Shakibaei M, Schafflhuber M, et al: Glycosaminoglycan polymerization may enable osmotically inactive Na+ storage in the skin. Am J Physiol Heart Circ Physiol 2004;287:H203–H208.

41. Bagrov AY, Fedorova OV, Dmitrieva RI, et al: Plasma marinobufagenin-like and ouabain-like immunoreactivity during saline volume expansion in anesthetized dogs. Cardiovasc Res 1996;31:296–305.

42. Schoner W, Scheiner-Bobis G: Endogenous and exogenous cardiac glycosides: Their roles in hypertension, salt metabolism, and cell growth. Am J Physiol Cell Physiol 2007;293:C509–C536.

43. Ferrari P, Ferrandi M, Valentini G, Bianchi G: Rostafuroxin: An ouabain antagonist that corrects renal and vascular Na+-K+-ATPase alterations in ouabain and adducin-dependent hypertension. Am J Physiol Regul Integr Comp Physiol 2006;290:R529–R535.

44. Kennedy DJ, Vetteth S, Periyasamy SM, et al: Central role for the cardiotonic steroid marinobufagenin in the pathogenesis of experimental uremic cardiomyopathy. Hypertension 2006;47:488–495.

45. Cice G, Ferrara L, D'Andrea A, et al: Carvedilol increases two-year survival in dialysis patients with dilated cardiomyopathy: A prospective, placebo-controlled trial. J Am Coll Cardiol 2003;41:1438–1444.

46. Abbott KC, Trespalacios FC, Agodoa LY, et al: Beta-blocker use in long-term dialysis patients: Association with hospitalized heart failure and mortality. Arch Intern Med 2004;164:2465–2471.

47. Foley RN, Herzog CA, Collins AJ: Blood pressure and long-term mortality in United States hemodialysis patients: USRDS Waves 3 and 4 Study. Kidney Int 2002;62:1784–1790.

48. Ishani A, Herzog CA, Collins AJ, Foley RN: Cardiac medications and their association with cardiovascular events in incident dialysis patients: Cause or effect? Kidney Int 2004;65:1017–1025.

49. Ruggenenti P, Perna A, Loriga G, et al, for the REIN-2 Study Group: Blood-pressure control for renoprotection in patients with non-diabetic chronic renal disease (REIN-2): Multicentre, randomised controlled trial. Lancet 2005;365:939–946.

50. Klahr S, Levey AS, Beck GJ, et al: The effects of dietary protein restriction and blood-pressure control on the progression of chronic renal disease. Modification of Diet in Renal Disease Study Group. N Engl J Med 1994;330:877–884.

51. Sarnak MJ, Greene T, Wang X, et al: The effect of a lower target blood pressure on the progression of kidney disease: Long-term follow-up of the modification of diet in renal disease study. Ann Intern Med 2005;142:342–351.

52. Lewington S, Clarke R, Qizilbash N, et al, for the Prospective Studies Collaboration: Age-specific relevance of usual blood pressure to vascular mortality: A meta-analysis of individual data for one million adults in 61 prospective studies. Lancet 2002;360:1903–1913.

53. Ruggenenti P, Perna A, Gherardi G, et al: Renoprotective properties of ACE-inhibition in non-diabetic nephropathies with non-nephrotic proteinuria. Lancet 1999;354:359–364.

54. Jafar TH, Schmid CH, Landa M, et al: Angiotensin-converting enzyme inhibitors and progression of nondiabetic renal disease. A meta-analysis of patient-level data. Ann Intern Med 2001;135:73–87.

55. Jafar TH, Stark PC, Schmid CH, et al, for the AIPRD Study Group: Progression of chronic kidney disease: The role of blood pressure control, proteinuria, and angiotensin-converting enzyme inhibition: A patient-level meta-analysis. Ann Intern Med 2003;139:244–252.

56. Peterson JC, Adler S, Burkart JM, et al: Blood pressure control, proteinuria, and the progression of renal disease. The Modification of Diet in Renal Disease Study. Ann Intern Med 1995;123:754–762.

57. Kunz R, Friedrich C, Wolbers M, Mann JF: Meta-analysis: Effect of monotherapy and combination therapy with inhibitors of the renin angiotensin system on proteinuria in renal disease. Ann Intern Med 2008;148:30–48.

58. Messerli FH, Mancia G, Conti CR, et al: Dogma disputed: Can aggressively lowering blood pressure in hypertensive patients with coronary artery disease be dangerous? Ann Intern Med 2006;144:884–893.

59. Schwenger V, Ritz E: Audit of antihypertensive treatment in patients with renal failure. Nephrol Dial Transplant 1998;13:3091–3095.

60. Degoulet P, Legrain M, Réach I, et al: Mortality risk factors in patients treated by chronic hemodialysis. Report of the Diaphane collaborative study. Nephron 1982;31:103–110.

61. Liu Y, Coresh J, Eustace JA, et al: Association between cholesterol level and mortality in dialysis patients: Role of inflammation and malnutrition. JAMA 2004;291:451–459.

62. Wanner C, Krane V: Uremia-specific alterations in lipid metabolism. Blood Purif 2002;20:451–453.

63. Ritz E, Wanner C: Lipid changes and statins in chronic renal insufficiency. J Am Soc Nephrol 2006;17(3 Suppl 3):S226–S230.

64. Wanner C, Krane V: Non-high-density lipoprotein cholesterol: A target of lipid-lowering in dialysis patients. Am J Kidney Dis 2003;41(3 Suppl 1):S72–S75.

65. Go AS, Chertow GM, Fan D, et al: Chronic kidney disease and the risks of death, cardiovascular events, and hospitalization. N Engl J Med 2004;351:1296–1305.

66. Hyre AD, Fox CS, Astor BC, et al: The impact of reclassifying moderate CKD as a coronary heart disease risk equivalent on the number of US adults recommended lipid-lowering treatment. Am J Kidney Dis 2007;49:37–45.

67. Tonelli M, Isles C, Curhan GC, et al: Effect of pravastatin on cardiovascular events in people with chronic kidney disease. Circulation 2004;110:1557–1563.

68. Seliger SL, Weiss NS, Gillen DL, et al: HMG-CoA reductase inhibitors are associated with reduced mortality in ESRD patients. Kidney Int 2002;61:297–304.

69. Baigent C, Keech A, Kearney PM, et al, for the Cholesterol Treatment Trialists' (CTT) Collaborators: Efficacy and safety of cholesterol-lowering treatment: Prospective meta-analysis of data from 90,056 participants in 14 randomised trials of statins. Lancet 2005;366:1267–1278.

70. Astor BC, Muntner P, Levin A, et al: Association of kidney function with anemia: The Third National Health and Nutrition Examination Survey (1988–1994). Arch Intern Med 2002;162:1401–1408.

71. Joss N, Patel R, Paterson K, et al: Anaemia is common and predicts mortality in diabetic nephropathy. Q J Med 2007;100:641–647.

72. Ofsthun N, Labrecque J, Lacson E, et al: The effects of higher hemoglobin levels on mortality and hospitalization in hemodialysis patients. Kidney Int 2003;63:1908–1914.

73. Macdougall IC, Lewis NP, Saunders MJ, et al: Long-term cardiorespiratory effects of amelioration of renal anaemia by erythropoietin. Lancet 1990;335:489–493.

74. Ayus JC, Go AS, Valderrabano F, et al, for the Spanish Group for the Study of the Anemia and Left Ventricular Hypertrophy in Pre-dialysis Patients: Effects of erythropoietin on left ventricular hypertrophy in adults with severe chronic renal failure and hemoglobin <10 g/dL. Kidney Int 2005;68:788–795.

75. Besarab A, Bolton WK, Browne JK, et al: The effects of normal as compared with low hematocrit values in patients with cardiac disease who are receiving hemodialysis and epoetin. N Engl J Med, 1998;339:584–590.

76. Foley RN, Parfrey PS, Morgan J, et al: Effect of hemoglobin levels in hemodialysis patients with asymptomatic cardiomyopathy. Kidney Int 2000;58:1325–1335.

77. Parfrey PS, Foley RN, Wittreich BH, et al: Double-blind comparison of full and partial anemia correction in incident hemodialysis patients without symptomatic heart disease. J Am Soc Nephrol 2005;16:2180–2189.

78. Ritz E, Laville M, Bilous RW, et al: Target level for hemoglobin correction in patients with diabetes and CKD: Primary results of the Anemia Correction in Diabetes (ACORD) Study. Am J Kidney Dis 2007;49:194–207.

79. Drüeke TB, Locatelli F, Clyne N, et al, for the CREATE Investigators: Normalization of hemoglobin level in patients with chronic kidney disease and anemia. N Engl J Med 2006;355:2071–2084.

80. Singh AK, Szczech L, Tang KL, et al, for the CHOIR Investigators: Correction of anemia with epoetin alfa in chronic kidney disease. N Engl J Med 2006;355:2085–2098.

81. Remuzzi G, Ingelfinger JR: Correction of anemia—payoffs and problems. N Engl J Med 2006;355:2144–2146.

82. Pfeffer MA: An ongoing study of anemia correction in chronic kidney disease. N Engl J Med 2007;356:959–961.

83. d'Uscio LV, Smith LA, Santhanam AV, et al: Essential role of endothelial nitric oxide synthase in vascular effects of erythropoietin. Hypertension 2007;49:1142–1148.

84. London GM, Marchais SJ, Guerin AP: Arterial calcifications and bone histomorphometry in end-stage renal disease. J Am Soc Nephrol 2004;15:1943–1951.

85. London GM: Cardiovascular calcifications in uremic patients: Clinical impact on cardiovascular function. J Am Soc Nephrol 2003;14(9 Suppl 4):S305–S309.

86. Moe SM, Drüeke T, Lameire N, Eknoyan G: Chronic kidney disease-mineral-bone disorder: A new paradigm. Adv Chronic Kidney Dis 2007;14:3–12.

87. Foley RN, Li S, Liu J, et al: The fall and rise of parathyroidectomy in U.S. hemodialysis patients, 1992 to 2002. J Am Soc Nephrol 2005;16:210–218.

88. Kestenbaum B, Andress DL, Schwartz SM, et al: Survival following parathyroidectomy among United States dialysis patients. Kidney Int 2004;66:2010–2016.

89. Block GA, Martin KJ, de Francisco AL, et al: Cinacalcet for secondary hyperparathyroidism in patients receiving hemodialysis. N Engl J Med 2004;350:1516–1525.

90. de Francisco AL, Fresnedo GF, Rodrigo E, et al: Parathyroidectomy in dialysis patients. Kidney Int Suppl 2002;80:161–166.

91. Moe SM, Chertow GM, Coburn JW, et al: Achieving NKF-K/DOQI bone metabolism and disease treatment goals with cinacalcet HCl. Kidney Int 2005;67:760–771.

92. Teng M, Wolf M, Ofsthun MN, et al: Activated injectable vitamin D and hemodialysis survival: A historical cohort study. J Am Soc Nephrol 2005;16:1115–1125.

93. Teng M, Wolf M, Lowrie E, et al: Survival of patients undergoing hemodialysis with paricalcitol or calcitriol therapy. N Engl J Med 2003;349:446–456.

94. Li YC, Kong J, Wei M, et al: 1,25-Dihydroxyvitamin D(3) is a negative endocrine regulator of the renin-angiotensin system. J Clin Invest 2002;110:229–238.

95. Park CW, Oh YS, Shin YS, et al: Intravenous calcitriol regresses myocardial hypertrophy in hemodialysis patients with secondary hyperparathyroidism. Am J Kidney Dis 1999;33:73–81.

96. Xiang W, Kong J, Chen S, et al: Cardiac hypertrophy in vitamin D receptor knockout mice: Role of the systemic and cardiac renin-angiotensin systems. Am J Physiol Endocrinol Metab 2005;288:E125–E132.

97. Block GA, Hulbert-Shearon TE, Levin NW, Port FK: Association of serum phosphorus and calcium × phosphate product with mortality risk in chronic hemodialysis patients: A national study. Am J Kidney Dis 1998;31:607–617.

98. Kestenbaum B, Sampson JN, Rudser KD, et al: Serum phosphate levels and mortality risk among people with chronic kidney disease. J Am Soc Nephrol 2005;16:520–528.

99. Tonelli M, Sacks F, Pfeffer M, et al: Relation between serum phosphate level and cardiovascular event rate in people with coronary disease. Circulation 2005;112:2627–2633.

100. Chertow GM, Burke SK, Raggi P: Sevelamer attenuates the progression of coronary and aortic calcification in hemodialysis patients. Kidney Int 2002;62:245–252.

101. Suki WN, Dialysis Clinical Outcomes Revisited Investigators: Effects of sevelamer and calcium-based phosphate binders on mortality in hemodialysis patients. Kidney Int 2007;72:1130–1137.

102. Albaaj F, Hutchison AJ: Lanthanum carbonate (Fosrenol): A novel agent for the treatment of hyperphosphataemia in renal failure and dialysis patients. Int J Clin Pract 2005;59:1091–1096.

103. Takahashi Y, Tanaka A, Nakamura T, et al: Nicotinamide suppresses hyperphosphatemia in hemodialysis patients. Kidney Int 2004;65:1099–1104.

104. LaClair RE, Hellman RN, Karp SL, et al: Prevalence of calcidiol deficiency in CKD: A cross-sectional study across latitudes in the United States. Am J Kidney Dis 2005;45:1026–1033.

105. Meyer TW, Hostetter TH: Uremia. N Engl J Med 2007;357:1316–1325.

106. Eknoyan G, Beck GJ, Cheung AK, et al, for the Hemodialysis (HEMO) Study Group: Effect of dialysis dose and membrane flux in maintenance hemodialysis. N Engl J Med 2002;347:2010–2019.

107. Fagugli RM, Pasini P, Pasticci F, et al: Effects of short daily hemodialysis and extended standard hemodialysis on blood pressure and cardiac hypertrophy: A comparative study. J Nephrol 2006;19:77–83.

108. Schwarz U, Buzello M, Ritz E, et al: Morphology of coronary atherosclerotic lesions in patients with end-stage renal failure. Nephrol Dial Transplant 2000;15:218–223.

109. Gross ML, Meyer HP, Ziebart H, et al: Calcification of coronary intima and media: Immunohistochemistry, backscatter imaging, and x-ray analysis in renal and nonrenal patients. Clin J Am Soc Nephrol 2007;2:121–134.

110. Herzog CA, Ma JZ, Collins AJ: Poor long-term survival after acute myocardial infarction among patients on long-term dialysis. N Engl J Med 1998;339:799–805.

111. Herzog CA, Ma JZ, Collins AJ: Comparative survival of dialysis patients in the United States after coronary angioplasty, coronary

artery stenting, and coronary artery bypass surgery and impact of diabetes. Circulation 2002;106:2207–2211.

112. Buzello M, Törnig J, Faulhaber J, et al: The apolipoprotein e knockout mouse: A model documenting accelerated atherogenesis in uremia. J Am Soc Nephrol 2003;14:311–316.

113. Bursztyn M, Motro M, Grossman E, Shemesh J: Accelerated coronary artery calcification in mildly reduced renal function of high-risk hypertensives: A 3-year prospective observation. J Hypertens 2003;21:1953–1959.

114. Ritz E, Wanner C: The challenge of sudden death in dialysis patients. Clin J Am Soc Nephrol 2008;3:920–929.

115. Gussak I, Gussak HM: Sudden cardiac death in nephrology: Focus on acquired long QT syndrome. Nephrol Dial Transplant 2007;22:12–14.

116. Ahmad S, Kenny, M, Scribner BH: Hypertension and a digoxin-like substance in the plasma of dialysis patients: Possible marker for a natriuretic hormone. Clin Physiol Biochem 1986;4:210–216.

Further Reading

Sarnak MJ Levey AS: Cardiovascular disease and chronic renal disease: A new paradigm. Am J Kidney Dis 2000;35(4 Suppl 1): S117–S131.

Tonelli M, Pfeffer MA: Kidney disease and cardiovascular risk. Annu Rev Med 2007;58:123–139.

Vassalotti JA, Stevens LA, Levey AS: Testing for chronic kidney disease: A position statement from the National Kidney Foundation. Am J Kidney Dis 2007;50:169–180.

Chapter 71

Treatment of Erectile Dysfunction in Chronic Kidney Disease

Aaron C. Lentz, Manish P. Patel, J. Eric Derksen, and Culley C. Carson III

In men with chronic kidney disease (CKD), quality of life is significantly affected by erectile dysfunction (ED).[1] The cause is often multifactorial. Uremia, medications, associated comorbid conditions, physiologic changes with dialysis, and the causative pathophysiology leading to the patient's CKD should be considered before initiating treatment (Box 71-1).

INCIDENCE

Is the incidence of ED greater than in normal men? Masters and Johnson[2] reported that the incidence of ED in normal men younger than the age of 50 years was less than 5%. The Massachusetts Male Aging Study reported that 5% of men at age 40 years have complete ED; and this increases to 50% among men aged 70.[3] Rodger and colleagues[4] reported on 100 uremic men with a significantly higher prevalence. In a current study, Rosas and colleagues[5] found that 82% of patients on hemodialysis had ED. ED was much more prevalent in the dialysis patients older than 50 years (63% in those younger than 50 compared with 90% in those older than 50).

Karacan[6] observed that rapid eye movement sleep was associated with penile tumescence, using a nocturnal penile tumescence (NPT) monitor. If psychological factors predominate, the NPT results should not be affected. Thus, these studies showed that organic disturbances or pharmacologic alteration of physiology correlated with altered NPT and impotence. Karacan reported that 50% of patients on hemodialysis had abnormal NPT.

CAUSES OF ERECTILE DYSFUNCTION IN CHRONIC KIDNEY DISEASE: AN OVERVIEW

Physiologic factors in the evaluation of ED include alterations in venous and arterial flow patterns, altered smooth muscle tone, hormonal aberrations, neurogenic abnormalities, and structural damage secondary to infection, trauma, or associated diseases. In addition, chronic fatigue, depression, and psychosocial stress may result from chronic indolent illnesses that can contribute as psychological components of ED.[7]

PHYSIOLOGIC ALTERATIONS IN CHRONIC KIDNEY DISEASE PREDISPOSING TO ERECTILE DYSFUNCTION

In evaluation of a patient with CKD who presents with erectile problems, several physiologic processes must be considered: endocrine abnormalities, neurological compromise, vascular

Box 71-1 Causes of Erectile Dysfunction in Men with Chronic Renal Failure

Anatomic (Trauma, Pelvic Surgery, Renal Transplant, Vasculitis, Penile Surgery, Arteriovenous Malformations)
Structural
Tunica albuginea
Corpora cavernosa
Corpora spongiosum/glans penis

Vascular
Arterial compromise
Veno-occlusive dysfunction

Neurological
Autonomic innervation
Somatic innervation

Physiologic
Endocrine
Abnormal testosterone metabolism and excretion
Stimulation of pituitary function
Elevated prolactin
Elevated parathyroid hormone
Diabetes mellitus

Neurogenic
Autonomic dysfunction
Supratentorial lesions (tumor, Alzheimer's disease, Parkinson's disease, trauma)
Infratentorial lesions
   Suprasacral
   Sacral
Peripheral somatic nervous system deterioration

Vascular
Arterial blood flow obstruction
Venous occlusive incompetence

Other
Pharmacologic causes
Hypoxia
Comorbid disease states (hypertension, diabetes mellitus, smoking, anemia, Paget's disease, Dupuytren's contracture, liver failure)
Pelvic radiation
Peyronie's disease
Psychosocial concerns

insufficiency, venous incompetence, pharmacologic manipulations, psychological disturbances, and associated chronic diseases (such as hypertension, diabetes mellitus, anemia, and electrolyte abnormalities).

ENDOCRINE ABNORMALITIES

CKD leads to abnormal hormonal balances throughout the hypothalamic-pituitary-gonadal axis. Semen quality is also affected and correlates with decreased testosterone levels.[8] The decrease in serum testosterone results from increased elimination, with maintained testicular hormone-binding capacity. Not all patients, however, have abnormal serum testosterone levels. Thus patients with CKD are likely to have a deficiency in hormone production and secretion as the primary mechanism for their hypogonadism, as well as an element of end-organ failure. Interestingly, giving exogenous testosterone to CKD patients with diminished levels of circulating testosterone does not improve erectile function or fertility.[9]

Men with CKD have abnormal secretion of luteinizing hormone, follicle-stimulating hormone, and prolactin. Luteinizing hormone levels are generally increased in response to low testosterone levels and because of a decrease in the metabolic clearance of luteinizing hormone.[10] Follicle-stimulating hormone is also elevated in those men with suboptimal spermatogenesis. The increase in serum luteinizing hormone and follicle-stimulating hormone correlates well with the pituitary response to hypothalamic stimulation by gonadotropin-releasing hormone, which is preserved in the CKD patient. Thus, if the luteinizing hormone response to low testosterone levels is inadequate, a pituitary abnormality may be present.

The frequently elevated prolactin levels in men with CKD may cause sexual dysfunction. Medications that induce hyperprolactinemia include methyldopa, digoxin, cimetidine, and metoclopramide. Patients with hyperprolactinemia often have ED. Once the hyperprolactinemia is treated, erectile function improves, as does fertility.

Diabetes mellitus is a common cause of ED. The autonomic and sensory neuropathic dysfunction resulting in ED is not amenable to medical therapy. This is especially difficult for the young patient who has adequate vascular and venous function but insufficient neurological ability to produce a sufficient erectile response.[10]

Secondary hyperparathyroidism is a common manifestation of CKD. Massry and associates[11] suggested in 1977 that the excess blood levels of parathyroid hormone in uremic patients might contribute, at least partly, to the disturbance in hormones of the hypothalamic-pituitary-gonadal axis and in the genesis of the impotence of uremia.

NEUROGENIC ALTERATIONS

In the flaccid state and during detumescence, sympathetic neural activity predominates. Norepinephrine activates postsynaptic α_{1a}, α_{1b}, and α_{1b} receptors, and its activity is modulated by presynaptic α_2 receptors (Fig. 71-1).[12] Erections are mediated through the parasympathetic system via acetylcholine. Activation of muscarinic receptors liberates nitric oxide, which relaxes smooth muscle and causes erection. There are also nonadrenergic, noncholinergic neurons that release nitric oxide (Fig. 71-2). Nitric oxide increases cyclic guanosine monophosphate production, which relaxes cavernous smooth muscle.[13]

In studies of 12 CKD patients with ED, an abnormal Valsalva maneuver correlated with abnormal NPT and diminished ability to achieve erections suitable for intercourse.[14] Peripheral neuropathy in CKD is frequent. Evaluation of patients with suspected neurogenic causes of impotency must rely on clinical judgment.[14]

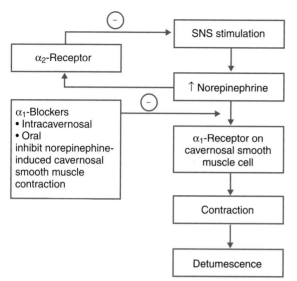

Figure 71-1 Sympathetic nervous system (SNS) effect on cavernosal smooth muscle.

VASCULAR COMPROMISE

Sexual stimulation releases nitric oxide, which relaxes smooth muscle and dilates the arterioles, thus increasing blood flow. Blood trapped in the expanding sinusoids compresses the venous system, increasing the pressure within the cavernosal bodies to approximately 100 mm Hg. Contraction of the ischiocavernosus muscle further increases pressure in the penis leading to a rigid erection.

Acceleration of atherosclerosis leads to vasculogenic ED by occluding large vessels and their arterial tributaries. Therefore, regardless of age, vasculogenic ED occurs even in younger men with CKD. Kaufman and colleagues[15] reported that 78% of impotent CKD patients had significant occlusive disease of the cavernosal artery.

Techniques to identify venous outflow abnormalities in ED include dynamic infusion studies, pharmacocavernosometry, and pharmacocavernosography.[16] In a series by Kaufman and colleagues,[15] 90% of CKD patients had venous occlusive incompetence.

MEDICINAL AGENTS IMPLICATED IN ERECTILE DYSFUNCTION

Medications frequently associated with ED are listed in Box 71-2. Reductions in libido are seen with centrally acting agents like clonidine and reserpine, as well as drugs that increase prolactin levels. ED has been associated with virtually all antihypertensive agents. Calcium channel blockers, angiotensin-converting enzyme inhibitors, angiotensin receptor blockers, and α-adrenergic antagonists are least likely to cause iatrogenic ED. Conversely, β-blockers, sympatholytics, and vasodilators are strongly associated.[17] These drugs, if causing ED, may be changed to α-adrenergic blocking agents such as terazosin, prazosin, or doxazosin, or angiotensin-converting enzyme inhibitors and calcium channel blockers.

ANEMIA AND DIMINISHED OXYGEN DELIVERY

Low partial pressure of oxygen (P_{O_2}) causes impotency by impairing cavernosal nitric oxide synthesis. Kim and colleagues[13] found decreased nitric oxide synthesis and elevated

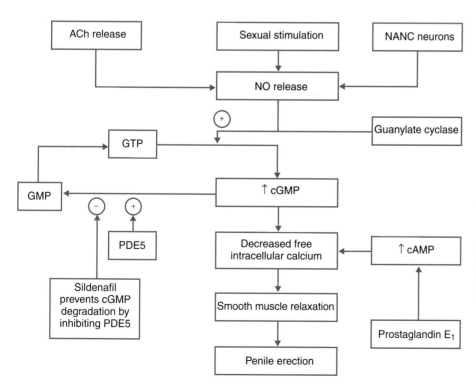

Figure 71-2 Nitric oxide (NO)–related neurogenic alterations. The primary pathway is cyclic guanosine monophosphate (cGMP) mediated, whereas cyclic adenosine monophosphate (cAMP) acts secondarily. Both decrease intracellular calcium, thus causing relaxation of smooth muscle. ACh, acetylcholine; GTP, guanosine triphosphate; NANC, nonadrenergic, noncholinergic; PDE5, phosphodiesterase-5.

Box 71-2   Medications Associated with Sexual Dysfunction

Antihypertensive Agents
Sympatholytics
Methyldopa
Clonidine
Reserpine
Guanethidine

β-Adrenergic Antagonists
Propranolol
Pindolol
Atenolol
Metoprolol
Labetalol

Vasodilators
Hydralazine

Diuretics
Thiazides
Spironolactone

Other Agents
Cimetidine
Digoxin
Clofibrate
Metoclopramide

Antidepressants
Tricyclics
Serotonin reuptake inhibitors

Box 71-3   Evaluation of Erectile Dysfunction in Men with Chronic Kidney Disease

Physical examination
General examination
  Genitourinary examination: testicles, scrotum, phallus, meatus, prepuce, and glans
  Digital rectal examination
  Neurological examination: S2 to S4 sensation, bulbo-cavernosus reflex, anal wink, anal tone, and peno-scrotal sensation
Laboratory evaluation to assess general and specific causes of erectile dysfunction
  Serum testosterone
  Luteinizing hormone
  Follicle-stimulating hormone
  Prolactin
  Complete blood count
  Serum glucose or hemoglobin A_{1C} and baseline electrolytes
  Lipid profile
  White men older than 50 years and black men younger than 40 years should have a prostate-specific antigen test
Further referral to a urologist if considering:
  Doppler screening studies
  Color Doppler ultrasonography for flow
  Pharmacocavernosography
  Pharmacocavernosometry
  Dynamic infusion studies
  Nocturnal penile tumescence studies
  Biothesiometry
  Injection therapy
  Surgical therapy

smooth muscle tone in patients with low Po_2 at the corpora cavernosa. Luscher and colleagues[18] found increased endothelium-derived contracting factors, which could further increase smooth muscle tone and inhibit erection. Finally, metabolites that inhibit nitric oxide synthase accumulation of CKD patients possibly contribute to ED.

EVALUATION OF ERECTILE DYSFUNCTION IN MEN WITH CHRONIC KIDNEY DISEASE

ED in men with CKD should proceed systematically as outlined in Box 71-3. The use of NPT monitors can identify patients with a true organic cause of their ED whose vascular problems are suggested. Doppler screening studies, pharmacocavernosometry, pharmacocavernosography, dynamic infusion studies, and color Doppler response studies may be helpful. Finally, hormonal studies, including testosterone, luteinizing hormone, follicle-stimulating hormone, and prolactin, should be obtained. These may be supplemented by serum glucose, hemoglobin A_{1C}, lipid profile, and thyroid function studies.

TREATMENT OPTIONS

Treatment options for ED are reviewed in Box 71-4.

Medical Management of Erectile Dysfunction

Hormone Regulation

Patients who have low testosterone levels may respond to replacement therapy, which normally improves libido without a significant impact on potency or fertility. Data on the effects of testosterone replacement in end-stage renal disease are scant. There have been several small studies suggesting that testosterone therapy does not improve erectile function in the majority of hemodialysis patients for which it was prescribed.[19–21] Effective replacements include injectable preparations, transdermal delivery systems, or sustained-release products. However, 100 to 200 mg of testosterone weekly by injection produces only small and variable responses in erectile function.[22]

Clomiphene citrate, which is a partial agonist of the estrogen receptor, increases secretion of gonadotropins and increases plasma testosterone in CKD. One study that found increased testosterone levels from the hypogonadal range to the high end of normal range in five uremic men using clomiphene citrate reported uniform increases in libido and sexual function.[23]

If hyperprolactinemia is found, chromophobic tumors of the anterior pituitary must be excluded because men may present with ED or decreased libido. Methyldopa and reserpine interfere with dopamine secretion and therefore lead to

Box 71-4 Treatment Options in Men with Chronic Kidney Disease and Impotence

Medical
Medications
Hormone replacement therapy
Oral medications to improve arterial flow
Intracavernosal injection therapy
Transurethral therapy
Dopaminergic agonists
Erythropoietin

Devices
Vacuum constriction device
Constriction bands

Surgical
Revascularization techniques
Penile prosthetic devices

Psychiatric
Posttransplantation

Other Issues
Adjust medications where appropriate
Control comorbid disease states
Evaluate for psychosocial stresses
Discuss expectations with patient
Routinely evaluate efficacy of therapy and patient satisfaction
Realize the changing patterns of erectile dysfunction and need to change therapy or modality
Consider early referral to a urologist

hyperprolactinemia. If these causes are excluded, dopaminergic agonists may be of benefit.[24,25] Bromocriptine (1.25–5.0 mg/day) and lisuride hydrogen maleate (0.05–0.2 mg/day) decrease prolactin and increase testosterone. Bromocriptine can induce hypotension, nausea, vertigo, and dizziness, side effects that are intolerable to many patients. These side effects are less prominent with lisuride hydrogen maleate.

For patients with symptomatic secondary hyperparathyroidism, it was recently found that sexual function of male patients can be improved by parathyroidectomy and autotransplantation. The report also demonstrated a decrease in the levels of prolactin in association with decreasing levels of calcium, phosphorus, and immunoreactive parathyroid hormone.[26]

Phosphodiesterase Inhibitors

Since 1998, the U.S. Food and Drug Administration has approved three selective type 5-phosphodiesterase inhibitors (PDE-5Is): sildenafil (Viagra, Pfizer), tadalafil (Cialis, Lilly), and vardenafil (Levitra, Bayer). Each of the three PDE-5I registration programs involved more than 2000 patients. In the United States, sildenafil was approved in 1998 and both vardenafil and tadalafil were approved in 2003.

Erectile function depends on the neuronal pathways (nonadrenergic, noncholinergic neurons) and release of nitric oxide.[27,28] PDE-5Is inhibit the breakdown of cyclic guanosine monophosphate, thereby allowing continued relaxation of smooth muscle in the corpus cavernosum.[29] All three drugs in this class have similar pharmacokinetic and pharmacodynamic profiles, and each is effective for patients with ED of all ages, severities, and causes.

In patients with CKD, sildenafil has the longest patient experience and the most robust data confirming its activity, safety, and tolerability. The best results in the initial human trials were obtained with 100 mg of sildenafil; however, as many as 24% of men responded effectively on the 50-mg dose schedule. Also significant was the increase in frequency of intercourse, with those receiving sildenafil making on average 5.9 successful attempts per month compared with 1.5 in those receiving placebo.[30] Sildenafil studies in patients on dialysis show a good response rate (66.7%–80%). The majority of sildenafil responders had success with the 50-mg tablets.[31,32] Sildenafil has been shown to be effective in patients with difficult-to-treat ED and the Sildenafil Diabetes Study Group[33] showed that 56% of men with ED and diabetes mellitus who received sildenafil (25–100 mg) treatment for 12 weeks reported improved erections, in contrast to 10% of patients receiving placebo ($P < .001$).

Sildenafil given to transplant recipients does not perturb plasma levels and has a 60% satisfactory response rate.[34] The most commonly reported side effects are headache (16%), flushing (10%), and dyspepsia (7%).[35] Hypotensive side effects occur particularly with concomitant nitrate administration. It is unclear how long the patient must wait until nitrates can be safely administered. Sildenafil decreases systolic and diastolic blood pressures by 10 and 7 mm Hg, respectively. Nitrate use leads to a synergistic increase in cyclic guanosine monophosphate levels, which can cause excessive hypotension and occasionally ischemic cardiac events or strokes.[28] Sildenafil can be safely administered in CKD if there is no serious cardiac disease. Sildenafil is primarily metabolized in the liver, but there is some renal excretion; lower doses are recommended initially (25 mg) in CKD patients.

In vitro studies have shown that the potency of vardenafil in inhibiting PDE-5 purified from the human corpus cavernosum tissue was approximately 25 times greater than that of sildenafil and 48 times greater than that of tadalafil.[36] In a study by Hellstrom and colleagues,[37] many patients returned to normal erectile function after treatment with vardenafil. For example, 89% of patients with mild ED at baseline return to normal function after treatment with 10 mg of vardenafil. Forty percent of patients with severe ED at baseline returned to normal function after treatment with 20 mg of vardenafil, compared with only 4% who received placebo. There is limited evidence that a small percentage of sildenafil nonresponders can be salvaged with vardenafil.[38] A starting dose of 5 mg of vardenafil should be used in men with severe renal impairment.[39]

Recent double-blind, placebo-controlled, multicenter trials have assessed the efficacy and safety of tadalafil in the treatment of ED. Significant improvements from baseline in the International Index of Erectile Function erectile frequency domain score, successful penetration attempts, successful intercourse, and overall satisfaction compared with placebo have been reported with an on-demand schedule of the drug.[40–42] Tadalafil has a terminal half-life of 17.5 hours, which is consistent with a broad window of clinical responsiveness.[42,43] Tadalafil enhances erectile frequency in men with ED for as long as 36 hours. Thus, tadalafil may be associated with less planning or pressure to have sexual intercourse after dosing. Unlike sildenafil and vardenafil, meal intake has no effect on the absorption of tadalafil.

The cytochrome P-450 system is the chief metabolic pathway for sildenafil, vardenafil, and tadalafil. All three agents are substrates for the cytochrome P-450 pathway P3A4, and concomitant administration of P3A4 inhibitors such as ritonavir, indinavir, ketoconazole, and erythromycin can increase plasma levels of the PDE-5Is.[44-46] Because these drugs potentiate the vasodilator/hypotensive effects of nitric oxide, treatment with any PDE-5I is contraindicated in patients taking organic nitrates.[44-46] According to United States prescribing information, coadministration of α-blockers with sildenafil, vardenafil, and tadalafil is listed as a precaution.[44-46] None of the three agents are dangerously associated with prolongation of the corrected QT interval on the electrocardiogram.

The recent advent of vardenafil, which has the highest in vitro potency of all available PDE-5Is, and tadalafil, which has a prolonged half-life that may enable couples to have sexual activity with less planning, represent further advances. However, although there are clear pharmacokinetic differences among these agents, the data on preference trials, head-to-head clinical trials, and selection trials are few.[47]

Intracavernosal Injection Therapy

Alprostadil (Caverject, Edex), an exogenous form of prostaglandin E_1, administered by intracavernosal injection is the only approved agent. Alprostadil causes smooth muscle relaxation, vasodilation, and inhibition of platelet aggregation. Approximately 96% of alprostadil is locally metabolized within 60 minutes. No change in peripheral blood levels occurs because of extensive pulmonary metabolism.[48] Linet and Neff[49] concluded that alprostadil produced full erections in 70% to 80% of patients. Side effects include pain (17%), hematoma or ecchymosis (1.5%), and priapism or prolonged erection (1.3%).

Other agents used alone or in combination with prostaglandin E_1 include papaverine and phentolamine mesylate (Regitine, CIBA Pharmaceuticals). Papaverine inhibits phosphodiesterase, leading to increases in cyclic adenosine monophosphate, elevated nitric oxide, and eventual relaxation of cavernosal smooth muscle and arterial dilation. Kapoor and colleagues[50] reported on the use of papaverine in men with spinal cord injuries, who obtained satisfactory erections capable of successful penetration in 98%. Papaverine, however, causes priapism and fibrosis in as many as 35% and 33% of men, respectively, with an increased incidence in young and neurogenic patients.[51]

Phentolamine mesylate is a competitive nonselective α-adrenergic receptor antagonist. It has been used in combination with papaverine to increase blood flow. Side effects include hypotension, reflex tachycardia, and nasal congestion.

These agents can be used successfully in CKD patients with vascular compromise, diabetic microangiopathy, moderate atherosclerosis, and partial arterial dysphasia, although higher doses may be necessary. Patients with venous occlusive disease may also benefit from increased engorgement of the corpora, leading to increased compression of the tunica albuginea and therefore occlusion of the emissary veins. It is interesting to note that patients with neurogenic and hormonal causes also do well with this therapy (as do older patients), without increased side effects. Long-term use of these injection therapies is effective, with few complications in transplant recipients.[52] No major complications on transplanted kidneys have been noted. The only contraindications to therapy are sickle cell anemia, severe psychiatric disorders, severe venous incompetence, and severe systemic disease.

Transurethral Suppositories

The transurethral delivery system, medicated urethral system for erection (MUSE), allows for delivery of alprostadril to the corpora by direct venous communication.[53] The mechanism of action of alprostadil has been discussed earlier. Success has been variable.

Erythropoietin, Anemia, and Erectile Dysfunction

The treatment of anemia with recombinant human erythropoietin in men with CKD improves sexual performance and elevates levels of follicle-stimulating hormone and testosterone.[54]

Devices

Vacuum Constriction Devices and Constriction Bands

Vacuum constriction devices work by engorging the penis with blood by negative pressure. A constriction band is placed at the base of the penis for no longer than 30 minutes to avoid injury. These devices have local side effects such as pain from the constriction band, entrapment of ejaculation by the constriction band, cold and dusky penis, numbness of the penis, and local irritation. Many men use these devices, but they can be difficult for men with a short penis or an extensive suprapubic fat pad. In those who need pharmacologic manipulation for an adequate erection but who have evidence of venous incompetence, a constriction band alone may be used to sustain rigidity of the penis that is suitable for intercourse.

Surgical Treatment of Erectile Dysfunction

Vascular Procedures for Erectile Dysfunction

As most patients with renal failure have small-vessel disease, the use of revascularization techniques and venous occlusive surgery is not commonly employed. These judgments are best left to the urologist.

Penile Prostheses

Implantation of a penile prosthesis is safe and usually successful, with low morbidity. Renal transplant recipients commonly benefit from the device.[55] Such procedures should be performed after renal transplantation, if possible, because many men have improved sexual function, fertility, and potency after transplantation surgery. In immunocompromised patients, the risks of implanting an artificial device include prosthetic infection.[56] Cuellar and Sklar[57] examined their own cohort of 46 patients who had undergone pelvic organ transplantation before placement of a penile prosthesis. The risk of infection after insertion of penile prostheses in patients with a pelvic organ transplant was similar to that in nontransplant patients.

IMPROVEMENT IN ERECTILE DYSFUNCTION AFTER RENAL TRANSPLANTATION

After renal transplantation, patients report improved erectile function and libido. Testosterone levels return to normal within 2 to 3 months, as do luteinizing hormone, follicle-stimulating hormone, and prolactin. Sperm counts normalize in 9 to 16 months. Patients who receive human chorionic gonadotropin stimulation show improved responses with higher testosterone levels. Salvatierra and colleagues[58] found pretransplantation potency to be 22% while on dialysis; however, after renal transplantation, 84% of men resumed levels of potency comparable with those of a time before the onset of uremia. Posttransplantation psychological disturbances, except for anxiety, appear to diminish.

Although data are limited, studies evaluating commonly used immunosuppressive agents such as cyclosporine, azathioprine, tacrolimus, and prednisone suggest that these agents do not have significant effects on the sex hormone profiles of renal transplant patients.[59–62] Sirolimus, a new immunosuppressive, has been found to lower total testosterone and increase luteinizing hormone and follicle-stimulating hormone in renal transplant recipients; however, this has not proven to result in a change in sexual function.[63]

It is important to remember that a significant proportion of men after transplantation will continue to have ED despite normalization of hormone values and improved physiology.[64] Many of these patients suffer from vasculogenic ED. These patients should be evaluated in a way similar to that for pretransplant recipients; treatment plans should be generated for their specific needs.

CONCLUSIONS

ED includes a vast array of organic, anatomic and psychosocial elements, which make evaluation and treatment complex. However, a practitioner who observes a good history, physical examination, and laboratory evaluation can provide a great service to the quality of life of his or her patient with CKD. The physician must address the topic and make the patient feel comfortable with his changing physiology and anatomy. Renal transplantation has the potential to normalize hormone profiles and subdue some of the physiologic changes, although it may not solve the problem in men because of associated comorbid conditions. Psychological, medical, and surgical therapies can be highly effective in correctly evaluated patients. A multidisciplinary approach to care should be employed that involves the primary care physician, a nephrologist, urologist, psychiatrist, and psychologist.

References

1. Patel MP, Carson CC: The epidemiology, anatomy, physiology, and treatment of erectile dysfunction in chronic renal failure patients. Adv Ren Replace Ther 1999;6:296–309.
2. Masters WH, Johnson VF: Human sexual inadequacy. Boston: Little, Brown, 1990, pp 88–101.
3. Feldman HA, Goldstein I, Hatzichristou DG, et al: Impotence and its medical and psychosocial correlates: Results of the Massachusetts Male Aging Study. Urology 1994;151:54–61.
4. Rodger KS, Fletcher K, Dewar JH, et al: Prevalence and pathogenesis of impotence in 100 uremic men. Uremia Invest 1984;8:89–96.
5. Rosas SE, et al: Prevalence and determinants of erectile dysfunction in hemodialysis patients. Kidney Int 2001;59:2259–2266.
6. Karacan I: NPT/rigidometry. In Kirby RS, Carson CC, Webster GD (eds): Impotence: Diagnosis and Management of Erectile Dysfunction. Boston: Butterworth Heinemann, 1991, pp 62–71.
7. Carson CC, Kirby R, Goldstein I: Textbook of Erectile Dysfunction. New York: Taylor and Francis, 1999, pp 551–562.
8. Copolla A, Cuomo C: Pituitary testicular evaluation in patients with chronic renal insufficiency in hemodialysis treatment. Minerva Med 1990;81:461–465.
9. Holdsworth S, Atkins RC, de Krettsker DM: The pituitary testicular axis in men with chronic renal failure. N Engl J Med 1977;296:1245–1251.
10. Brindley GS: Neurophysiology. In Kirby RS, Carson CC, Webster GD (eds): Impotence: Diagnosis and Management of Erectile Dysfunction. Boston: Butterworth, Heinemann, 1991, p 27.
11. Massry SG, Goldstein DA, Procci WR, et al: Impotence in patients with uremia: A possible role for parathyroid hormone. Nephron 1977;19:305–310.
12. Traish AM, Netsuwan N, Daley J, et al: A heterogeneous population of alpha-1 receptors mediates contraction of human corpus cavernosum smooth muscle to norepinephrine. J Urol 1995;153:222–227.
13. Kim N, Vardi Y, Padma-Nathan H, et al: Oxygen tension regulates the nitric oxide pathway. Physiological role in penile erection. J Clin Invest 1993;91:437–442.
14. Campese VM, Procci WR, Levitan D, et al: Autonomic nervous system dysfunction and impotence in uremia. Am J Nephrol 1982;2:140–143.
15. Kaufman J, Hatzichristou D, Mulhall J, et al: Impotence and chronic renal failure: A study of the hemodynamic pathophysiology. Urology 1994;151:612–618.
16. Carson CC: Impotence: New diagnostic modalities. Urol Annu 1992;6:229–311.
17. Brock GB, Lue TF: Drug-induced male sexual dysfunction. An update. Drug Saf 1993;8:414–426.
18. Luscher TF, Borelungeri M, Duhi Y, et al: Endothelium-derived contracting factors. Hypertension 1992;14:117–126.
19. Barton C, Mirahmadi M, Vaziri N: Effects of long-term testosterone administration on pituitary-testicular axis in end-stage renal failure. Nephron 1982;31:61–64.
20. Coevorden AV, Stolear J, Dhaene M, et al: Effect of chronic oral testosterone undecanoate administration on the pituitary-testicular axis of hemodialyzed male patients. Clin Nephrol 1986;26:48–54.
21. Lawrence I, Price D, Howlett T, et al: Correcting impotence in the male dialysis patient: Experience with testosterone replacement and vacuum tumescence therapy. Am J Kidney Dis 1998;31:313–319.
22. Lim VS: Reproductive function in patients with renal insufficiency. Am J Kidney Dis 1987;4:363–370.
23. Lim VS, Fang VS: Restoration of plasma testosterone levels in uremic men with clomiphene citrate. J Clin Endocrinol Metab 1976;43:1370–1374.
24. Ruilope L, Garcia-Robles R, Paya C, et al: Influence of lisuride and dopaminergic agonist on the sexual function of male patients with chronic renal failure. Am J Kidney Dis 1985;3:182–187.
25. Muir JW, Besser GM, Edwards CW, et al: Bromocriptine improves reduced libido and potency in men receiving maintenance hemodialysis. Clin Nephrol 1983;20:308–314.
26. Chou FF, Lee CH, Shu K, et al: Improvement of sexual function in male patients after parathyroidectomy for secondary hyperparathyroidism. J Am Coll Surg 2001;193:486–492.
27. Zusman RM, Morales A, Classer DB, et al: Overall cardiovascular profile of sildenafil citrate. Am Cardiol 1999;83:35–44.
28. Chuang AT, Strauss ID, Murphy RA, et al: Sildenafil, a type 5 cyclic GMP-dependent relaxation in rabbit corpus cavernosum smooth muscle in vitro. J Urol 1998;160:257–261.

29. Boolell M, Allen MJ, Ballard SA, et al: Sildenafil: An orally active type 5 cyclic CMP-specific phosphodiesterase inhibitor for the treatment of penile erectile dysfunction. Int J Impot Res 1996;8:47–52.

30. Goldstein I, Lue TF, Padma-Nathan H, et al: Oral sildenafil in the treatment of erectile dysfunction. N Engl J Med 1998;338:1397–1404.

31. Chen J, Mabjeesh NJ, Greenstein A, et al: Clinical efficacy of sildenafil in patients on chronic dialysis. J Urol 2001;165:819–821.

32. Rosas SE, Wasserstein A, Kobrin S, et al: Preliminary observations of sildenafil treatment for erectile dysfunction in dialysis patients. Am J Kidney Dis 2001;37:134–137.

33. Rendell MS, Raifer J, Wicker PA, et al: Sildenafil for treatment of erectile dysfunction in men with diabetes: A randomized controlled trial. Sildenafil Diabetes Study Group. JAMA 1999;281:421–426.

34. Prieto Castro R, Anglada Curado FJ, Regueiro Lopez JC, et al: Treatment with sildenafil citrate in renal transplant patients with erectile dysfunction. Br J Urol 2001;88:241–243.

35. Morales A, Gingell C, Collins M, et al: Clinical safety of oral sildenafil citrate (Viagra) in the treatment of erectile dysfunction. Int J Impot Res 1998;10:69–73.

36. Gbekor E, Bethell S, Fawcett L, et al: Selectivity of sildenafil and other phosphodiesterase type 5 (PDE5) inhibitors against all human phosphodiesterase families. Eur Urol 2002;1 (Suppl 1):63.

37. Hellstrom WJG, Gittelman M, Karlin G, et al: Vardenafil for treatment of men with erectile dysfunction: Efficacy and safety in a randomized, double-blind, placebo-controlled trial. J Androl 2002;23:763–771.

38. Brisson TE, Broderick GA, Thiel DD, et al: Vardenafil rescue rates of sildenafil nonresponders: Objective assessment of 327 patients with erectile dysfunction. Urology 2006;68:397–401.

39. Klotz T, Bauer RJ, Rohde G: Effect of renal impairment on the single-dose pharmacokinetics of vardenafil 20 mg, a selective PDE5 inhibitor for the treatment of erectile dysfunction. Pharmacotherapy 2002;22:418.

40. Padma-Nathan H, Rosen RC, Shabsigh R, et al: Cialis (IC351) provides prompt response and extended period of responsiveness in the treatment of men with erectile dysfunction (ED). J Urol 2001;165(Suppl):A293.

41. Padma-Nathan H, McMurray CG, Pullman WE, et al: On demand IC351 (Cialis) enhances erectile function in patients with erectile dysfunction. Int J Impot Res 2001;13:2–9.

42. Brock GB, McMahon CG, Chen KK, et al: Efficacy and safety of tadalafil for the treatment of erectile dysfunction: Results of integrated analyses. J Urol 2002;168:1332–1336.

43. Porst H, Padma-Nathan H, Giuliano F, et al: Efficacy of tadalafil for the treatment of erectile dysfunction at 24 and 36 hours after dosing: A randomized controlled trial. Urology 2003;62:121–125.

44. Pfizer: Sildenafil citrate (Viagra). U.S. prescribing information 2007. Available at www.pfizer.com/download/uspi_viagra.pdf. Accessed May 25, 2007.

45. Lilly ICOS LLC: Tadalafil (Cialis). U.S. prescribing information 2007. Available at pi.lilly.com/us/cialis-pi.pdf. Accessed May, 25, 2007

46. Bayer: Vardenafil hydrochloride (Levitra). U.S. prescribing information 2007. Available at www.univgraph.com/bayer/inserts/levitra.pdf. Accessed May 25, 2007.

47. Carson CC: PDE5 inhibitors: Are there differences? Can J Urol 2006;13(Suppl 1):34–39.

48. van Able H, Peskar BA, Sticht G, et al: Pharmacokinetics of vasoactive substances administered into the human corpus cavernosum. J Urol 1994;151:1227–1235.

49. Linet OI, Neff LL: Intracavernous prostaglandin E1 in erectile dysfunction. Clin Invest 1994;72:139–143.

50. Kapoor VK, Chahal AS, Jyoti SP, et al: Intracavernous papaverine for impotence in spinal cord injured patients. Paraplegia 1993;31:6757–6764.

51. Barada JH, McKimmy RM: Vasoactive pharmacotherapy. In Bennett AH (ed): Impotence. Philadelphia: WB Saunders, 1994, p 229.

52. Rodriguez Antolin A, Morales JM, Andres A, et al: Treatment of erectile impotence in renal transplant patients with intracavernosal vasoactive drugs. Transplant Proc 1992;24:105–112.

53. Padma-Nathan H, Bennett A, Gesundheit N, et al: Treatment of erectile dysfunction by the medicated urethral system for erection. J Urol 1995;153:975–984.

54. Imagawa A, Kawanish N, Numata A: Is erythropoietin effective for impotence in dialysis patients? Nephron 1990;54:95–109.

55. Kabalin JN, Kessler R: Successful implantation of penile prosthesis in organ transplant patients. Urology 1989;33:282–284.

56. Carson CC: Diagnosis, treatment and prevention of penile prosthesis infection. Int J Impot Res 2003;15(Suppl 5):139–146.

57. Cuellar DC, Sklar GN: Penile prosthesis in the organ transplant recipient. Urology 2001;57:138–141.

58. Salvatierra O, Fortmann JL, Belzer FO: Sexual function in males before and after renal transplantation. Scand J Urol Nephrol 1992;26:181–186.

59. Haberman J, Karwa G, Greenstein SM, et al: Male fertility in cyclosporin-treated renal transplant patients. J Urol 1991;145:294–296.

60. Hilbrands LB, Hoitsma AJ, Koene RA: The effect of immunosuppressive drugs on quality of life after renal transplantation. Transplantation 1995;59:1263–1270.

61. Shield CF, McGrath MM, Goss TF: Assessment of health-related quality of life in kidney transplant patients receiving tacrolimus (FK 506)-based vs. cyclosporine-based immunosuppression. Transplantation 1997;64:1738–1743.

62. Handelsman DJ, McDowell FW, Caterson ID, et al: Testicular function after renal transplantation: Comparison of cyclosporin A with azathioprine and prednisone combination regimes. Clin Nephrol 1984;22:144–148.

63. Lee S, Coco M, Greenstein SM, et al: The effect of sirolimus on sex hormone levels of male renal transplant recipients. Clin Transpl 2005;19:162–167.

64. Reinberg N, Bumgardner CL, Aliabadi H: Urological aspects after renal transplantation. J Urol 1991;143:1087–1094.

Further Reading

Ayub W, Fletcher S: End-stage renal disease and erectile dysfunction. Is there any hope? Nephrol Dial Transplant 2000;15:1525–1528.

Cerqueira J, Moraes M, Glina S: Erectile dysfunction: Prevalence and associated variables in patients with chronic renal failure. Int J Impot Res 2002;14:65–71.

Johansen K: Testosterone metabolism and replacement therapy in patients with end-stage renal disease. Semin Dial 2004;17:202–208.

Lasaponara F, Paradiso M, Milan MGL, et al: Erectile dysfunction after kidney transplantation: Our 22 years of experience. Transplant Proc 2004;36:502–504.

Palmer B: Sexual dysfunction in uremia. J Am Soc Nephrol 1999;10:1381–1388.

Tejada IS, Angulo J, Cellek S, et al: Pathophysiology of erectile dysfunction. J Sexual Med 2005;2:26–39.

Chapter 72

Treatment of Sleep Disorders in Patients with Renal Dysfunction

Suraj Kapa, Elizabeth H. Nora, Eddie L. Greene, and Virend K. Somers

Patients with chronic kidney disease (CKD) have a greater incidence of sleep-disordered breathing than the general population. Sleep-related disorders in this population can include insomnia,[1] nocturnal myoclonus, obstructive sleep apnea (OSA), and restless legs syndrome. A high prevalence of untreated sleep disorders results in diminished quality of life secondary to symptoms including but not limited to irritability, excessive snoring, daytime somnolence, and decreased concentration. Studies on the relationship between poor sleep quality and renal dysfunction have suggested a high correlation between the two, although the precise pathophysiologic relationship remains to be elucidated.[2]

We focus on OSA with special attention to (1) some of the available effective treatments, (2) benefits of treatment in improving quality-of-life issues associated with OSA, and (3) the association between OSA and common comorbid conditions in CKD, in particular, hypertension and cardiovascular disease.[3,4] Unfortunately, identifying patients with CKD and OSA may be made more difficult due to the overlap in symptoms between OSA and uremia. However, recognition of these symptoms and their underlying cause can afford patients the benefit of symptom-improving treatment. It can also have beneficial therapeutic implications related to other comorbidities.

SLEEP APNEA

Sleep apnea may be separated into central sleep apnea and OSA, although overlap between the two often exists. The severity of the OSA syndrome is defined by the number of apneic or hypopneic episodes per hour during sleep as well as the presence of symptoms. Apnea is defined as more than 10 seconds without airflow plus associated desaturation or arousal from sleep. Hypopnea is defined by a more than 50% reduction in airflow over the same period of time. The presence and severity of OSA may be partly defined by the apnea-hypopnea index (AHI) or by the number of apneic or hypopneic episodes per hour of sleep. When the AHI is greater than 15, patients are considered to have moderate to severe sleep apnea. However, even when the AHI is 15 or more and there is associated daytime sleepiness, OSA can be pathologic. The AHI may point toward a diagnosis of sleep apnea but not whether the cause is primarily central or due to obstruction to air flow.

PREVALENCE AND DIAGNOSIS OF OBSTRUCTIVE SLEEP APNEA

It is estimated that as many as one in four Americans may be at risk of OSA.[5] In CKD patients, the prevalence ranges from 16.4%[6] to 66%.[7] However, most reports have concentrated on patients treated by hemodialysis so the prevalence may be less in CKD patients who are not being treated with dialysis. A recent study of dialysis-independent patients concluded that patients with more severe renal dysfunction had higher AHI values.[8] Other studies have suggested that the quality of sleep as assessed by a survey is most diminished in the early stages of renal dysfunction and that there is no correlation with the severity of renal dysfunction.[2] There does appear to be a strong association between OSA and CKD, even based on the lowest estimate of the prevalence of OSA. Given the association and the potential for effective treatment, OSA evaluation of patients with renal dysfunction is warranted. This may be achieved by asking questions about sleep habits (snoring or apneas noted by the patient or the patient's bed partner), the quality of sleep (is the patient refreshed after a night's sleep), and daytime symptoms (daytime somnolence, irritability, decreased concentration, frequent falling asleep during performance of activities). Another means of identifying CKD patients who may have concomitant OSA is by observation during dialysis. Witnessed episodes of snoring or apnea/hypopnea or frequent or prompt falling asleep during dialysis should raise suspicions about undiagnosed OSA.

In patients who have signs suggestive of OSA, the initial screening may be achieved via overnight pulse oximetry to record the magnitude and number of periods of oxygen desaturation. Obstructive patterns with nocturnal desaturation are usually associated with sawtooth patterns in the oxygen saturation tracing. However, the actual diagnosis of OSA is best achieved via polysomnography, during which oxygen saturation, heart rate (electrocardiogram), and sleep stages by an electroencephalogram in addition to limb movements, changes in body position, airflow, and respiratory effort are monitored. Use of polysomnography helps to determine, first, the presence of sleep apnea, second, whether it is of central or obstructive origin, and, third, the type and efficacy of treatment.

PATHOPHYSIOLOGY

Patients with CKD and OSA do not necessarily follow the typical profile of OSA. For example, end-stage renal disease patients with OSA are not consistently obese.[7,9] This finding suggests that there may be other mechanisms at play in the evolution of OSA.[10,11] In addition to obesity, sleep apnea and other sleep disturbances may result from a combination of uremia, metabolic derangements, hematologic abnormalities, neuropathies, and fluid imbalances.

Uremia

Uremia may cause symptoms similar to those of sleep apnea, including somnolence, decreased ability to concentrate, and confusion. Uremia may also affect the central respiratory drive as well as airway muscle tone.[10,12,13] A possible role for uremia in OSA is supported by one recent study that suggests that the AHI score correlates with the urea concentration in diabetic and nondiabetic CKD patients who are not by treated by dialysis.[8]

Metabolic Derangements

CKD is associated with the development of chronic metabolic acidosis. Metabolic acidosis can affect the chemoreflex drive, which in turn affects respiratory drive. For this reason, chronic metabolic acidosis can lead to a decreased apneic threshold resulting in worsening frequency or number of apneic episodes.

Hematologic Abnormalities

In CKD and end-state renal disease patients with anemia, full correction of the anemia with erythropoietin is associated with improvement in arousals from sleep, sleep fragmentation, and daytime alertness.[14] This suggests that treatment of the underlying anemia may improve quality of life secondary to sleep disturbances in these patients.

Neuropathies

Neuropathies can occur in CKD secondary to the underlying cause of the renal failure (e.g., diabetes) or to metabolic derangements. Neuropathy can affect the normal neurologic input to the respiratory system, resulting in periodic breathing via effects on the respiratory drive.

Volume Overload

Volume overload may lead to edema of the upper airway, which can contribute to a mechanical obstruction of normal airflow. Reduction in the radius of the airway would result in exponentially increasing resistance to airflow. This resistance, in combination with other risk factors, can cause worsening or more frequent apnea or hypopnea. The role for fluid overload in OSA is supported by evidence that dialysis can help reduce apnea severity.

TREATMENT OF CHRONIC KIDNEY DISEASE: EFFECTS ON OBSTRUCTIVE SLEEP APNEA

Treatment of CKD may possibly alternate sleep apnea and thus may result in an improvement of quality of life. Case reports and results from formal studies suggest that effective dialysis[12] or kidney transplantation[15] can improve sleep apnea. For example, Hanly and Pierratos[9] suggest that nocturnal hemodialysis may attenuate sleep apnea. They studied 14 patients and 57% (8 of 14 patients) had OSA. Patients began an intensive program of daily nocturnal hemodialysis, and there was a significant reduction in their apnea/hypopnea index from 46 ± 19/hr to 9 ± 9/hr. In contrast, an earlier small study of 11 long-term hemodialysis patients did not show any reduction in sleep apnea with standard daytime hemodialysis.[6] There was no difference in their apneic episodes on the nights after dialysis compared with the nights during the interval between dialysis treatments. Sabbatini and colleagues[1] examined a series of 694 surveyed hemodialysis patients and concluded that the prevalence of insomnia was still very high, but the incidence of OSA was not determined. Tang and colleagues[16] also suggest that nocturnal peritoneal dialysis may have a therapeutic edge over continuous ambulatory peritoneal dialysis in treating sleep apnea based on their study of 46 stable patients with documented sleep apnea using the overnight polysomnography method. The prevalence of sleep apnea was reported to be 4.2% during the treatment with nocturnal peritoneal dialysis but 33.3% when patients were treated with continuous dialysis. The change in AHI was substantial: AHI was 3.4 during nocturnal dialysis and 14.0 during continuous dialysis.

These studies suggest there can be potential benefit for CKD patients with sleep apnea, but it should be recognized that there is a higher prevalence of sleep apnea among hemodialysis patients compared with the general population. Specifically, nocturnal dialysis appears to have a benefit over conventional dialysis. It is possible that any improvement in sleep apnea may be related to improved control of uremia, but the mechanism has not been defined.[17] In future studies, it would be important to relate the degree of improvement in metabolic, uremic, and volume parameters to changes in sleep apnea indices to clarify how treatment of uremia might improve sleep apnea.

TREATMENT OF OBSTRUCTIVE SLEEP APNEA: EFFECTS ON RENAL FUNCTION

Although the evidence suggests that OSA may improve after successful treatment of uremia, it is unclear whether treatment of OSA will improve renal function. OSA is a known risk factor for hypertension[18,19] by mechanisms that include increasing pressor and sympathetic activation responses to repetitive nocturnal hypoxemic episodes.[20] In this case, treatment of OSA could improve OSA-mediated pressor stress and the increased filtration that causes maladaptive architectural changes and proteinuria and kidney damage. Some reports suggest that proteinuria is associated with sleep apnea.[21–23] Other studies with a small number of patients indicated that proteinuria disappeared with treatment of OSA.[24] Kinebuchi and colleagues[25] suggest that continuous positive airway pressure (CPAP) can ameliorate glomerular hyperfiltration in sleep apnea patients. More recent reports, however, suggest that clinically significant proteinuria cannot be directly attributed to OSA alone.[26,27] Further studies are necessary to elucidate any potential etiological role in the association of sleep apnea and a decrease in renal function.

METHODS OF TREATING OBSTRUCTIVE SLEEP APNEA

Treatment of OSA can improve the quality of life for CKD patients. The mainstay of treatment for OSA is to use CPAP when patients are sleeping.[28] However, there are other treatment options for patients who cannot tolerate CPAP.[29] Methods to improve sleep apnea include weight loss, position changes in bed, (e.g., lying on one's back can worsen obstructive physiology), and avoiding alcohol. In some patients with OSA, mandibular devices, such as the anterior mandibular positioner, may be useful to prevent posterior displacement of the tongue during sleep and thereby alleviate obstruction of the airway. These devices are sometimes uncomfortable and generally are effective in patients with only mild to moderate airway obstruction. Patients with OSA associated with CKD appear to have a combination of central and obstructive components, making these devices less useful. They are not as effective as nasal CPAP in comparison studies.[30] The benefits of anterior mandibular positioner treatment is that it is sometimes more tolerable than CPAP and is more portable.

In patients with obesity, weight loss may require surgical intervention and gastric bypass. Gastric bypass is not a benign procedure, and for CKD patients, in whom obesity does not appear to have as common an association with OSA, this option may be useful for only a subset of patients. One report, however, concluded that gastric bypass in obese CKD patients may lead to a decrease in comorbid conditions.[31]

In patients with OSA secondary to craniofacial abnormalities, ear, nose, and throat procedures may prove beneficial; again, these procedures will not relieve the central nervous system causes of sleep apnea. The most widely used surgery is uvulopalatopharyngoplasty, but it is not very effective in decreasing the AHI over the long term, even in patients with pure OSA.[32] Other ear, nose, and throat procedures include geniohyoid advancement with hyoid resuspension, maxillomandibular advancement, tongue suspension via the repose system, or base-of-tongue somnoplasty. It is difficult to assess which patients will benefit from these invasive procedures; they probably should be reserved for patients in whom less-invasive treatments fail.[32]

CPAP works by directly applying Poiseuille's law to maintain an open airway via positive pressure; the pressure prevents collapse or obstruction during inspiration. In patients who can tolerate CPAP, it is highly effective, but many patients will have difficulty sleeping with a mask on their face or with the noise of the machine. Some patients may also experience claustrophobia or suffocation from the mask, drying of their mucosa, or nasal congestion. As a result, CPAP may be useful for only a subset of CKD patients. Before giving up, a smaller mask that covers only the nose should be tried because it relieves some of the complaints of claustrophobia and mucosal drying. Another option is an Adams Circuit, which uses a prong in each nostril with applied positive pressure (these options may not be as effective for mouth breathers). Typically, CPAP settings are titrated to each patient's needs based on symptoms and polysomnographic findings. There are machines capable of autotitrating CPAP to adapt settings over the course of the night automatically.

A last resort for treatment of OSA consists of tracheostomy. This is considered definitive treatment but should be used only in patients with OSA that is refractory to CPAP and who have significant complications, such as cardiac arrhythmias. It is used as a last resort.

The benefits of other treatment modalities, such as nocturnal hemodialysis, are still controversial but can be tried. Likewise, vigorous treatment of uremia should always be tried. Future studies of the effects of hemodialysis on sleep apnea should be directed at understanding the pathophysiology of the disorder. This is the first step for designing effective treatment strategies.

References

1. Sabbatini M, Minale B, Crispo A, et al: Insomnia in maintenance haemodialysis patients. Nephrol Dial Transplant 2002;17:852–856.
2. Iliescu EA, Yeates KE, Holland DC: Quality of sleep in patients with chronic kidney disease. Nephrol Dial Transplant 2004;19:95–99.
3. De Oliveira Rodriguez CJ, Marson O, Tufic S, et al: Relationship among end-stage renal disease, hypertension, and sleep apnea in nondiabetic dialysis patients. Am J Hypertens 2005;18:152–157.
4. Zoccali C, Mallamaci F, Tripepi G: Nocturnal hypoxemia: A neglected cardiovascular risk factor in end-stage renal disease? Blood Purif 2002;20:120–123.
5. Hiestand DM, Britz P, Goldman M, Phillips B: Prevalence of symptoms and risk of sleep apnea in the US population: Results from the National Sleep Foundation Sleep in America 2005 poll. Chest 2006;130:780–786.
6. Mendelson WB, Wadhwa NK, Greenberg HE, et al: Effects of hemodialysis on sleep apnea syndrome in end-stage renal disease. Clin Nephrol 1990;33:247–251.
7. Kuhlmann U, Becker HF, Birkhahn M, et al: Sleep apnea in patients with end-stage renal disease and objective results. Clin Nephrol 2000;53:460–466.
8. Markou N, Kanakaki M, Myrianthefs P, et al: Sleep-disordered breathing in nondialyzed patients with chronic renal failure. Lung 2006;184:43–49.
9. Hanly PJ, Pierratos A: Improvement of sleep apnea in patients with chronic renal failure who undergo nocturnal hemodialysis. N Engl J Med 2001;344:102–107.
10. Fletcher EC: Obstructive sleep apnea and the kidney. J Am Soc Nephrol 1993;4:1111–1121.
11. Novak M, Mendelssohn D, Shapiro CM, et al: Diagnosis and management of sleep apnea syndrome and restless legs syndrome in dialysis patients. Semin Dial 2006;19:210–216.
12. Fein AM, Niederman MS, Imbriano L, et al: Reversal of sleep apnea in uremia by dialysis. Arch Intern Med 1987;147:1355–1356.

13. De Santo NG, Cirillo M, Perna A, et al: The heart in uremia: Role of hypertension, hypotension, and sleep apnea. Am J Kidney Dis 2001;38:S38–S46.

14. Benz RL, Pressman MR, Hovick ET, et al: A preliminary study of the effects of correction of anemia with recombinant human erythropoietin therapy on sleep, sleep disorders, and daytime sleepiness in hemodialysis patients (The SLEEPO study). Am J Kidney Dis 1999;34:1089–1095.

15. Auckley DH, Schmidt-Nowara W, Brown LK: Reversal of sleep apnea hypopnea syndrome in end-stage renal disease after kidney transplantation. Am J Kidney Dis 1999;34:739–744.

16. Tang SC, Lam B, Ku PP, et al: Alleviation of sleep apnea in patients with chronic renal failure by nocturnal cycler-assisted peritoneal dialysis compared with conventional continuous ambulatory peritoneal dialysis. J Am Soc Nephrol 2006;17:2607–2616.

17. Perl J, Unruh ML, Chan CT: Sleep disorders in end-stage renal disease: 'Markers of inadequate dialysis'? Kidney Int 2006;70:1687–1693.

18. Van Meerhaeghe A, Moscariello A, Velkeniers B: Obstructive sleep apnoea-hypopnoea syndrome and arterial hypertension. Acta Cardiol 2006;61:95–102.

19. Weiss JW, Liu MD, Huang J: Physiological basis for a causal relationship of obstructive sleep apnoea to hypertension. Exp Physiol 2007;92:21–26.

20. Somers VK, Dyken ME, Clary MP, et al: Sympathetic neural mechanisms in obstructive sleep apnea. J Clin Invest 1995;96:1897–1904.

21. Chaudhary BA, Sklar AH, Chaudhary TK, et al: Sleep apnea, proteinuria, and nephrotic syndrome. Sleep 1988;11:69–74.

22. Sklar AH, Chaudhary BA, Harp R: Nocturnal urinary protein excretion rates in patients with sleep apnea. Nephron 1989;51:35–38.

23. Iliescu EA, Lam M, Pater J, et al: Do patients with obstructive sleep apnea have clinically significant proteinuria? Clin Nephrol 2001;55:196–204.

24. Sklar AH, Chaudhary BA: Reversible proteinuria in obstructive sleep apnea syndrome. Arch Intern Med 1988;148:87–89.

25. Kinebuchi S, Kazama JJ, Satoh M, et al: Short-term use of continuous positive airway pressure ameliorates glomerular hyperfiltration in patients with obstructive sleep apnoea syndrome. Clin Sci (Lond) 2004;107:317–322.

26. Mello P, Franger M, Boujaoude Z, et al: Night and day proteinuria in patients with sleep apnea. Am J Kidney Dis 2004;44:636–641.

27. Casserly LF, Chow N, Ali S, et al: Proteinuria in obstructive sleep apnea. Kidney Int 2001;60:1484–1489.

28. Basner RC: Continuous positive airway pressure for obstructive sleep apnea. N Engl J Med 2007;356:1751–1758.

29. Cistulli PA, Grunstein RR: Medical devices for the diagnosis and treatment of obstructive sleep apnea. Expert Rev Med Devices 2005;2:749–763.

30. Ferguson KA, Ono T, Lowe AA, et al: A short-term controlled trial of an adjustable oral appliance for the treatment of mild to moderate obstructive sleep apnea. Thorax 1997;52:362–368.

31. Alexander JW, Goodman H: Gastric bypass in chronic renal failure and renal transplant. Nutr Clin Pract 2007;22:16–21.

32. Loube DI: Technologic advances in the treatment of obstructive sleep apnea syndrome. Chest 1999;116:1426–1433.

Further Reading

Chakravorty I, Shastry M, Farrington K: Sleep apnoea in end-stage renal disease: A short review of mechanisms and potential benefit from its treatment. Nephrol Dial Transplant 2007;22:28–31.

Fletcher EC: Obstructive sleep apnea and the kidney. J Am Soc Nephrol 1993;4:1111–1121.

Hanly PJ, Pierratos A: Improvement of sleep apnea in patients with chronic renal failure who undergo nocturnal hemodialysis. N Engl J Med 2001;344:102–107.

Parker KP: Sleep disturbances in dialysis patients. Sleep Med Rev 2003;7:13128–143.

Perl J, Unruh ML, Chan CT. Sleep disorders in end-stage renal disease: 'Markers of inadequate dialysis'? Kidney Int. 2006;70:1687–1693.

Zoccali C, Mallamaci F, Tripepi G: Sleep apnea in renal patients. J Am Soc Nephrol 2001;12:2854–2859.

Neuropsychiatric Complications and Psychopharmacology of End-Stage Renal Disease

Adam M. Mirot, Edward G. Tessier, Michael J. Germain, and Lewis M. Cohen

CHAPTER CONTENTS

Neuropsychiatric disorders are common in patients with end stage renal disease (ESRD). They include "hardware" disorders that are primarily neurological in their presentation and "software" disorders that would more often be in the clinical province of the psychiatrist. This chapter is intended to help the treating nephrologist recognize, classify, and initiate treatment for commonly encountered, ESRD-associated neuropsychiatric issues. The following are several essential clinical points that should be kept in mind while reading the chapter.

1. A large array of pathologic processes associated with chronic kidney disease (CKD) can cause neuropsychiatric disorders in ESRD patients In addition, many commonly used nonpsychiatric medications are psychoactive and can produce iatrogenic complications. When confronted by mental status changes, look to the disease itself and to the unintended side effects of its treatment.

2. Treatment of neuropsychiatric disorders in ESRD patients favors a selected subset of the psychotropic agents used in non-ESRD patients, with dosing and titration adjusted for the altered pharmacokinetics of renal failure. The ESRD population is elderly, has multiple comorbidities, has often lost protein stores, and is prone to marked fluid and electrolyte shifts. These problems often translate into lower starting points and slower titration toward standard, non-ESRD target doses.

3. Drug absorption may be impaired by gastric fluid alkalinization.

4. Volume of drug distribution may be increased by edema and ascites, necessitating larger initial doses of some hydrophilic medications. Conversely, dehydration and muscle wasting may decrease the apparent volume of distribution, with the opposite effect on dosage requirements.

5. Most psychotropic medications are preferentially protein-bound. In the protein-deficient/uremic ESRD state, the free fraction of drug is often increased, boosting both therapeutic and toxic effects.

6. Nevertheless, standard psychotropic drugs can in general be used safely in ESRD patients. Most are lipophilic and easily penetrate the blood-brain barrier. Most are not removed by dialysis and are dependent on hepatic metabolism and enterohepatic elimination.

7. Research data to support clinical conventions in the employment of psychotropic drugs is far from solid, and future double-blind psychopharmacologic trials are sorely needed to assess pharmacologic measures in CKD patients.

8. Pharmacotherapy is not a substitute for skilled individual and family psychotherapy. Most counseling is provided by renal social workers, and their availability is a legally mandated requirement for dialysis programs. It is also advisable to have backup by consulting psychiatrists and a good working relationship with local hospital-based mental health units.

Figure 73-1 is a general clinical algorithm to direct treatment of common neuropsychiatric issues in the ESRD patient. Box 73-1 describes common neuropsychiatric syndrome etiologies. Table 73-1 describes commonly used neuropsychiatric drugs. Finally, several timely and helpful references are recommended to the interested nephrologist.

PRIMARY NEUROLOGICAL PROBLEMS AND THEIR MANAGEMENT

Patients with CKD frequently suffer from neurological symptoms. For elderly dialysis patients, central nervous system disorders rank prominently as a cause of hospitalization.[1] Chances of

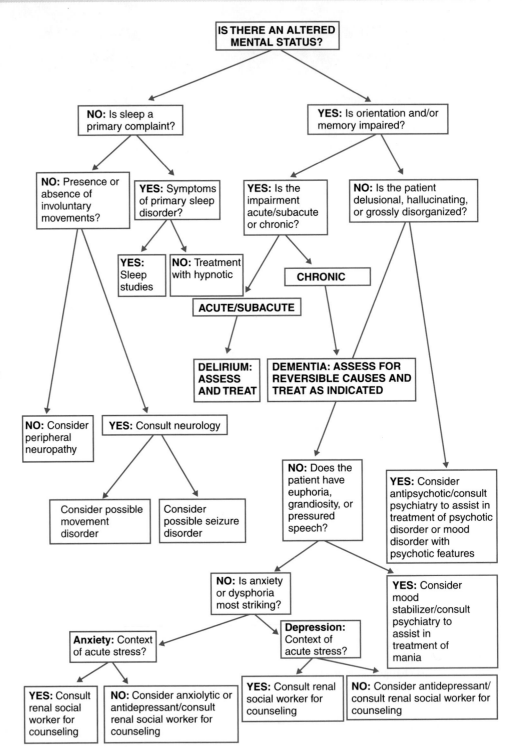

Figure 73-1 Algorithm to direct treatment of common neuropsychiatric issues in the patient with end-stage renal disease.

neurological problems increase parallel to the decline in renal function, classically appearing late in its course.[2,3] Causative factors include medication side effects, primary effects of the uremia itself, iatrogenic dialysis and transplantation pharmacotherapy effects, other comorbid conditions, and electrolyte disturbances. There is a multiplicity of chemical species on the list of possible uremic toxins, including homocysteine, β_2-microglobulin, glycosylated end products of metabolism, carbamylated proteins, myo-inositol, so-called middle molecules, indoles, phenols, parathyroid hormone, transketolase products, electrolytes, trace minerals, and water.[3] Subtle deficits in cogni-

tive function on neuropsychological testing can be found in CKD patients with moderate renal impairment and in adequately dialyzed patients as well as in uremic patients. As renal failure supervenes, delirium becomes apparent with confusion, lethargy, and progression to coma.[4] Seizures can occur in severe neuropathic states. If the alteration in mental status is solely due to uremia, encephalopathy may respond to dialysis. Paradoxically, dialysis itself, particularly in the first session or in patients with predisposing vulnerabilities of age, metabolism, or comorbid central nervous system disease can result in a disequilibrium syndrome that may progress to coma or status epilepticus.[3]

Box 73-1   Etiology of Neuropsychiatric Syndromes in Chronic Renal Disease

1. Common drugs leading to neuropsychiatric effects
   a. Psychotropic drugs
   b. Narcotics
   c. Illicit drugs
   d. Metoclopramide
   e. Antiseizure medications
   f. Cardiac medications, such as digoxin and amiodarone
   g. Transplant medications: calcineurin inhibitors, rapamycin, prednisone
2. Uremia
   a. Inadequate dialysis
   b. Glomerular filtration rate <12
3. Dialysis related
   a. Disequilibrium syndrome
   b. Dialysis dementia
4. Metabolic disturbance
   a. Hypoxemia
   b. Hypo- and hyperglycemia
   c. Sepsis
   d. Malignant hypertension
5. Structural neurological lesions
   a. Subdural hematoma
   b. Multi-infarct dementia
   c. Cerebral vascular accident
6. Electrolyte disturbances
   a. Hyper- and hypocalcemia
   b. Hypophosphatemia
   c. Hypermagnesemia
   d. Hyper- and hyponatremia
7. Anemia
8. Hyperparathyroidism
9. Heavy metal intoxications
   a. Lead
   b. Aluminum (dialysis dementia)
   c. Mercury
   d. Cadmium
10. Vitamin and mineral deficiencies
    a. Carnitine
    b. Zinc
11. Miscellaneous
    a. Hyper- and hypothyroidism
    b. Normal pressure hydrocephalus
    c. Sleep apnea
    d. Central pontine myelonolysis

Peripheral Neuropathies

The peripheral nervous system is vulnerable to uremia, with 65% prevalence of peripheral neuropathy in ESRD patients beginning dialysis; cranial neuropathies, including uremic amaurosis, have been described, and autonomic neuropathies are common.[3,5,6] Large nerve fibers are most frequently involved, with attendant impaired nerve conduction and dysautonomia, and patients may present with sensory or motor peripheral neuropathy as prominent aspects of their subjective illness burden. There is evidence that sensory neurons are in a state of axonal depolarization in predialytic CKD patients, with an increase in refractoriness of the affected nerves correlating with hyperkalemia.[6] In addition, the arteriovenous fistula used for hemodialysis may cause focal neuropathy as the result of a "steal syndrome." Carpal tunnel syndrome may be caused by the accumulation of β_2-microglobulin with resultant amyloidosis. Treatment options range from the prophylactic to the symptomatic. Dialysis itself leads to improvement in peripheral nerve excitability, with normalization of resting membrane potential after treatment.[7] Fistula-related neuropathy can be addressed by banding or tying off the offending vessel, whereas carpal tunnel syndrome may be helped by more intense dialysis with large surface area dialyzers to promote β_2-microglobulin clearance, by daily hemodialysis, wrist splints, or surgery.[3] Postural hypotension is addressed with compression stockings and/or midodrine, whereas sertraline, 50 mg predialysis, may prevent intradialytic hypotension. Metoclopramide can be prescribed as symptomatic treatment for gastroparesis and other neuropathic bowel motility disorders. Antidepressants and anticonvulsants are commonly used to treat polyneuropathic discomfort. Low-dose tricyclics can be effective, but the prescriber must be concerned about potential cardiac effects, given the common pairing of cardiac disease and CKD. In addition, tricyclics can promote confusion, worsen constipation, and lower the seizure threshold. It is worth knowing that desipramine and protriptyline substantially depend on renal elimination and can accumulate in patients with CKD or ESRD and that these drugs are not dialyzable. Of the commonly used anticonvulsants, gabapentin is renally excreted in unchanged form, and its dose must be decreased in tandem with a decrease in creatinine clearance. Posthemodialysis doses are also necessary with gabapentin. Carbamazepine and free valproic acid are subject to variable pharmacokinetics in renal failure, necessitating close monitoring of levels. Duloxetine is coming into wider use for diabetic neuropathy, but is contraindicated in renal failure because it is eliminated by the kidney.

Seizures

Seizures, including generalized tonic-clonic, partial motor, partial complex, and absence episodes are common in patients with CKD, particularly among those requiring dialysis (among whom the incidence has been estimated at 2%–10%), and nonconvulsive status epilepticus may be unrecognized.[8–10] Seizures may be predialytic as a result of uremia or be intra- or postdialytic in context of changes in hemodynamics and abrupt shifts in electrolytes.[11] Blood

Text continued on p. 809

Table 73-1 Neuropsychiatric Drugs with Comments on Likely Effects for Patients with Renal Failure

Drugs	Active Metabolites	Neurologic/ Psychiatric Adverse Reaction	Typical Adult Dose	$t_{1/2}$	Adult Dose in ESRD	$t_{1/2}$ in ESRD	Removed by Dialysis?	Comment	Ref.
Antidepressants (SSRIs)									
Escitalopram (Lexapro)	(S+)Desmethylcitalopram (SDMC) (S+)Didesmethylcitalopram	Insomnia Somnolence	10–20 mg/day	22–32 hr SDMC: 59 hrs	10 mg/day (20 w/ caution)	Likely similar to normal renal function	H: no	ESRD likely has minimal impact on escitalopram (similar to citalopram)	89,90
Citalopram (Celexa)	Desmethylcitalopram Didesmethylcitalopram Citalopram-N-oxide	Anxiety Agitation Hallucinations Somnolence	20–60 mg/day	33–37 hr	10–40 mg/day	43–49 hr	H: no	ESRD has minimal impact on citalopram kinetics	27,89
Fluoxetine (Prozac, Sarafem)	Norfluoxetine: NF	Anxiety Agitation Asthenia Insomnia Somnolence	20 mg/day	1–4 days NF 7–15 days	20 mg/day	1.8 days	H: no	No significant differences in fluoxetine and NF levels in renal failure Case report of venous thrombosis	22,28,91
Fluvoxamine (Luvox)	No active metabolites	Anxiety Agitation Asthenia Insomnia Somnolence	50–300 mg/day	15–22 hr	50–300 mg/day	Similar to normal renal function	H: no to modest (levels decreased by 22%)	No significant differences in renal failure; manufacturer recommends lower initial doses	28,29,92
Paroxetine (Paxil)	No active metabolites	Anxiety Agitation Asthenia Insomnia Somnolence	20–60 mg/day	17.3–25.1 hr	10–30 mg/day	10.9–54.8 hr	H: unknown	Increased AUC for paroxetine in ESRD (? related to metabolite that is inhibitor of CYP2D6); Reduced dose recommended; 10 mg effective in ESRD[104]	28,30,93

Drug	Side Effects	Dose	Half-Life	Dialyzability	Comments	References
Sertraline (Zoloft)	Anxiety Agitation Insomnia Somnolence	50–200 mg/day	24 hr		Minimal changes in kinetics in ESRD. Conflicting data on benefit in hemodialysis-related hypotension	31, 32, 94–97
Desmethylsertraline		50–200 mg/day	42–96 hr	H: minimal		
Antidepressants (Tricyclic)						
Amitriptyline (Elavil)	Sleep disturbance Confusion Delirium Hallucinations Paranoia Forgetfulness Asthenia	25 mg q8h (10–25 mg/hs for neuropathic pain)	32–40 hr		Elevated conjugated metabolites observed in renal failure; probably no difference in dosing. Use of therapeutic drug monitoring (TDM) with level of 75–175 ng/mL may guide therapy if used for depression	28, 98, 99, 102
Nortriptyline Hydroxyamitriptyline Hydroxynortriptyline		25 mg q8–12h	Active metabolites likely prolonged	H: no CAPD: no		
Clomipramine (Anafranil)		25–250 mg/day	19–37 hr DMC 54–77 hr		Few data in ESRD	28
Desmethylclopramine (DMC)		No data	No data			
Desipramine (Norpramin)	Sleep disturbance Confusion Delirium Depression Forgetfulness Hallucinations Paranoia	100–200 mg/day	12–54 hr 2OHD: 22 hr		Effective in small trial for depression. Use of TDM with level of 100–160 ng/mL may guide therapy if used for depression. Unconjugated amine and OH metabolites not removed by dialysis	28, 99, 100
2-Hydroxydesipramine (2OHD)		75–125 mg/day	Active metabolites likely prolonged	H: no CAPD: no		

Continued

Table 73-1 Neuropsychiatric Drugs with Comments on Likely Effects for Patients with Renal Failure—cont'd

Drugs	Active Metabolites	Neurologic/ Psychiatric Adverse Reaction	Typical Adult Dose	t$_{1/2}$	Adult Dose in ESRD	t$_{1/2}$ in ESRD	Removed by Dialysis?	Comment	Ref.
Doxepin (Sinequan)	Desmethyldoxepine (DMD)	Dizziness Somnolence	25 mg q8h	8–25 hr DMD: 30–80 hr	25 mg q8h	10–30 hr	H: no CAPD: no	Few data in ESRD	28
Imipramine (Tofranil)	Desipramine	Sleep disturbance Confusion Delirium Hallucinations Paranoia Forgetfulness	25 mg q8h	6–20 hr See Desipramine	25 mg q8h	See Desipramine	H: no CAPD: no	See Desipramine TDM with levels ≥200 ng/mL may guide therapy if used for depression	28,99
Nortriptyline (Aventil, Pamelor)	10-Hydroxynortriptyline E 10-hydroxynortriptyline Z 10-hydroxynortriptyline	Asthenia Somnolence	25 mg q6–8h	18–93 hr	25 mg q6–8h	15–66 hr Active metabolites likely	H: no CAPD: no	Use of TDM with level of 50–150 ng/mL may guide therapy if used for depression	28,33, 98, 99, 101, 102, 113
Antidepressants (Other)									
Bupropion (Wellbutrin, Zyban)	Hydroxybupropion (HB) Threobupropion (TB)	Hallucinations Insomnia Agitation Headache Seizures	100 mg q8h	10–21 hr	Limited data; use only with caution. ? Reduce to 1/3 of usual dose. SR may be less epileptogenic	HB: elevated TB: elevated	H: minimal	Risk of seizures with elevated levels of bupropion or metabolities. Use of TDM of bupropion (level 10–50 µg/L), HB (<1200 µg/L), and TB < 400 µg/L may guide therapy to avoid toxicity	28, 114

Drug	Metabolite	Side effects	Dose	Half-life	ESRD dose	ESRD pharmacokinetics	Dialyzability	Comments	References
Duloxetine (Cymbalta)	4-Hydroxy-D-glucuronide (4OHD) 5-Hydroxy-D-sulfate (5OHD) 6-Hydroxy-D-sulfate (6OHD) (See comments)	Dizziness Insomnia Somnolence Suicidal ideation	20–60 mg/day (often in divided dose)	12 hr	Not recommended	AUC: Duloxetine: ↑100% 4OHD: ↑700%–900% 5OHD: ↑700%–900% 6OHD: ↑700%–900%		Pharmacologic activity of metabolites may be minimal	105,106
Maprotiline (Ludiomil)	Desmethylmaprotiline Maprotiline-N-oxide	Asthenia Headache Somnolence	75–150 mg/day	48–51 hr	37.5–100 mg/day	Minimal data		May have more cardiovascular risk in ESRD. Elevated seizure risk of concern	107,108
Mirtazapine (Remeron)	Demethylmirtazapine (DMM)	Somnolence Dizziness Asthenia	15–45 mg/day	20–40 hr DMM 25 hr	7.5–22.5 mg/day	Clearance reduced by 50% in ESRD		No clear role for TDM	34
Trazodone (Desyrel)	Metachlorophenylpiperazine	Hypomania Dizziness Confusion Somnolence Headache Priapism	150–400 mg/day (50 mg in PM for insomnia)	4–11 hr	Few data	No data	H: moderate	Predialysis levels of 50 mg: 85–89 ng/mL; postdialysis level 29–40 ng/mL. No clear role for TDM. Parkinsonism: case report	36,109, 110
Venlafaxine (Effexor)	O-Desmethylvenlafaxine (ODV)	Asthenia Disturbed sleep Dizziness	37.5–225 mg/day XR	4 hr ODV 4 hr	37.5–112.5 mg/day XR	6–11 hr ODV 9 hr	H: no	No clear role for TDM. Half usual dose in dialysis patient, withhold until post-dialysis	37

Continued

Table 73-1 Neuropsychiatric Drugs with Comments on Likely Effects for Patients with Renal Failure—cont'd

Drugs	Active Metabolites	Neurologic/ Psychiatric Adverse Reaction	Typical Adult Dose	$t_{1/2}$	Adult Dose in ESRD	$t_{1/2}$ in ESRD	Removed by Dialysis?	Comment	Ref.
Antimanic Agents									
Lithium (Eskalith, Lithobid, Lithonate)	None	Multiple	900–1200 mg/day	14–28 hr	200–600 mg/day	40 hr	H: considerable CAPD: variable reports	Single dose after dialysis. Titrate dose to level/response 25%–50% standard dose in ESRD	38,111
Lamotrigine (Lamictil)	Inactive metabolites	Dizziness Headache Ataxia	Dose dependent on indications/concurrent interacting drugs	13–30 hr	Conflicting reports. Reduced dose recommended by manufacturer	43–58 hr	H: moderate		145,146
Valproic acid/divalproex (Depakene, Depakote)	Unclear whether active metabolites	Somnolence Dizziness Headache	15–60 mg/kg/day	6–17 hr	15–60 mg/kg/day		H: modest	? Increased risk of pancreatitis with ESRD. Increased free levels in ESRD. Use free VPA levels with TDM	39,112
Antipsychotics (Typical)									
Chlorpromazine (Thorazine)	Chlorpromazine-N-oxide CPA sulfate 7-OH-CPZ Nor-1-CPZ Nor-2-CPZ Nor-2-CPZ sulf 3-OH-CPZ	EPSs Somnolence Dizziness	50–400 mg/day	11–42 hr	Few data. No longer in common use	Few data	H: no	Accumulation in ESRD in case report. No longer in common use among psychiatrists	40,110, 113, 114
Haloperidol (Haldol)	Hydroxyhaloperidol plus other metabolites (activity not clear)	Dizziness EPSs ↑QT interval	1–2 mg q8–12h	14–26 hr	1–2 mg q8–12h	Similar	H: no	<1% excreted in urine	41,115

Antipsychotics (Atypical)

Aripiprazole (Abilify)	Dehydroaripiprazole (DHA)	Headache Insomnia Somnolence	10–15 mg	75–146 hr DHA: 94 hr	10–15 mg	Unknown	H: unknown	Few data	117
Clozapine (Clozaril)	N-Desmethylclozapine (NDC)	Dizziness Somnolence Vertigo Delirium and psychosis on withdrawal	12.5–450 mg slowly titrated. Monitoring ANC weekly per manufacture's guidelines	8–12 hr NDC 13.2 hr	Titrate to response and use TDM	Large interindividual variation	H: probably minimal	Best left to psychiatrists TDM may assist dosing in unclear circumstances. Avoid levels > 400 µg/L. Risks are multiple, including seizures, agranulocytosis, thromboembolic events, cardiomyopathy	42,116
Olanzapine (Zyprexa)	N-Desmethylolanzapine Olanzapine-10-N-glucuronide (activity may be minimal)	Somnolence Dizziness Abnormal gait	5–20 mg/day	32–38 hr	5–20 mg	32–38 hr	H: no CAPD: no	Dose adjustment not necessary in renal failure per manufacturer	43
Quetiapine (Seroquel)	7-Hydroxyquetiapine N-Dealkylated quetiapine	Dizziness Somnolence	50–800 mg/day in divided dose	6 hr	50–800 mg/day in divided dose		H: no CAPD: no	Dose adjustment not necessary in renal failure per manufacturer	118
Risperidone (Risperdal)	9-Hydroxyrisperidone (9ROH)	EPSs Dizziness Somnolence	1–3 mg bid	3–30 hr 9ROH 19 hr	0.5–1.5 mg bid	9ROH: 25 hr	H: no CAPD: no	Wide variation in clearance noted between poor and extensive metabolizers. Clearance of risperidone and 9ROH are reduced by 60% in renal failure	44, 119

Continued

Table 73-1 Neuropsychiatric Drugs with Comments on Likely Effects for Patients with Renal Failure—cont'd

Drugs	Active Metabolites	Neurologic/ Psychiatric Adverse Reaction	Typical Adult Dose	$t_{1/2}$	Adult Dose in ESRD	$t_{1/2}$ in ESRD	Removed by Dialysis?	Comment	Ref.
Ziprasidone (Geodon)	Inactive metabolites	Somnolence Dizziness ↑QT	20–80 mg bid	7 hr	10–80 mg bid			No adjustment required for CrCl 10–60 mL/min per manufacturer. Some clinicians recommend avoiding in ESRD due to prolonged QT interval and risk of life-threatening arrhythmias that may be higher with electrolyte shift	45
Anxiolytics/Hypnotics									
Alprazolam (Xanax)	α-Hydroxyalprazolam 4-Hydroxyalprazolam	Hallucinations Somnolence Memory impairment Interdose rebound anxiety	0.25–6 mg/day (tid dosing)	9–19 hr	0.25–3.0 mg (tid dosing)	9–19 hr	H: minimal	Increased free fraction in ESRD. Minimal kinetic differences in dialysis-dependent patients, but increased potential for psychomotor and memory impairment	28,46, 120

Medication	Active metabolites	Side effects	Dose	Half-life	Dose	Half-life	Dialyzability	Comments	References
Buspirone (Buspar)	1-Pyrimidinylpiperazine (1-PP)	Dizziness Nervousness	5 mg bid–20 mg tid	0.5–2.5 hr 1-PP 6.3 hr	2.5–5.0 mg q8h	1–5 hr 1-PP 9 hr	H: no	Considerable inter-individual and intraindividual variability in kinetics in ESRD. Patients with renal failure may benefit from a 25%–50% dose reduction. Manufacturer does not recommend in severe renal failure	47, 121
Clorazepate (Tranxene)	Desmethyldiazepam (DMD)	Somnolence Dizziness	15–60 mg/day PO	DMD 57.3 hr	15–60 mg/day PO	DMD 36.1 hr	H: no	Increased free fraction DMD resulting in similar free levels in normal and renal insufficiency	48
Clonazepam (Klonopin)	No active metabolites	Dizziness Impaired cognition	0.5 mg tid	18–80 hr	0.5 mg tid	? Same	H: no	Useful in restless legs syndrome	49, 122
Diazepam (Valium)	DMD Oxazepam	Delusions Hallucinations Ataxia Sedation Somnolence Memory impairment	5–40 mg/day	92 hr DMD 57.3 hr	5–15 mg/day	37 hr DMD 36.1 hr	H: no	Elevated free levels of diazepam in ESRD. Increased free fraction DMD resulting in similar free levels in normal and renal insufficiency	28, 50
Lorazepam (Ativan)	No active metabolites	Sedation Unsteady gait	1–2 mg bid or tid	9–16 hr	0.5–2 mg bid	32–70 hr	H: reports vary CVVH: no		28, 123
Midazolam (Versed)	α-Hydroxymidazolam conjugate (AHM-C)	Prolonged sedation	1.25 mg IV titrate to response	1.2–12.3 hr AHM-C: 1 hr	1.25 mg IV titrate to response	1.2–12.3 hr AHM-C: 50.4–76.8 hr	H: CVVH: no	? Increased effect due to altered protein binding. Accumulation of AHM-C	28, 51, 123

Continued

Table 73-1 Neuropsychiatric Drugs with Comments on Likely Effects for Patients with Renal Failure—cont'd

Drugs	Active Metabolites	Neurologic/Psychiatric Adverse Reaction	Typical Adult Dose	$t_{1/2}$	Adult Dose in ESRD	$t_{1/2}$ in ESRD	Removed by Dialysis?	Comment	Ref.
Oxazepam (Serax)	No active metabolites	Dizziness Somnolence	30–120 mg/day usually in divided dose	6–25 hr	30–120 mg/day usually in divided dose	25–90 hr	H: no		28
Temazepam (Restoril)	No active metabolites	Dizziness Somnolence	7.5–30 mg hs prn	4–10 hr	15–30 mg hs prn		H: no CAPD: no		28
Eszopiclone (Lunesta)	N-Desmethylzopiclone (NDZ)	Confusion Dizziness	2–3 mg hs prn	5–6 hr	2 mg hs prn				124
Zaleplon (Sonata)	No active metabolites	Dizziness Incoordination	5–20 mg hs prn	1 hr	? 5–10 mg hs prn			No dose adjustment needed per manufacturer for mild to moderate renal impairment. Not studied in ESRD	125
Zolpidem (Ambien)	No active metabolites	Somnolence Dizziness	10 mg hs prn	2–3 hr	May decrease dose by 50%	4–6 hr		Increased free fraction	126
Ramelteon (Rozerem)	M-II	Somnolence Dizziness	8 mg hs prn	1–2.5 hr M-II: 2–5 hr	8 mg hs prn		H: no	No dose adjustment required per manufacturer	127
Anticonvulsants									
Carbamazepine (Tegretol)	Carbamazepine-10-11-epoxide 9-Hydroxymethyl-10-carbamoylacridan	Dizziness Confusion Nystagmus Diplopia	100 mg bid to 400 mg qid	12–17 hr (chronic dosing)	100 mg bid to 400 mg qid	Similar to normal renal function	H: moderate CAPD: minimal		28, 128

Drug	Active Metabolite	Adverse Effects	Dose	Half-Life	Dose in ESRD	Half-Life in ESRD	Dialyzability	Comments	References
Gabapentin (Neurontin)		Confusion Lethargy Hypoxia Coma Myoclonus Hypoglycemia	300–600 mg tid	5–7 hr	300 mg every other day or 200–300 mg after each 4-hr hemodialysis	132 hr	H: yes CAPD: partial	Significant accumulation has occurred with typical dosing or interruption in hemodialysis. May be helpful for uremic pruritus and restless legs syndrome (RLS). Dose-related mental status changes. ? Increase myoclonus, hypoglycemia	52, 58, 129–137
Phenytoin (Dilantin)	Conjugated and unconjugated 5-(4-hydroxyphenyl)-5-phenylhydantoin: 4-OH-DPH (? activity)	Loose associations Psychosis Ataxia	200–400 mg/day	24 hr (at low to moderate levels)	200–300 mg/day	24 hr (at low to moderate levels) 4-OH-DPH levels (? significance)	H: no CAPD: no CVVH: moderate if high ultrafiltration rate	Increased free levels secondary to uremia. Monitor free phenytoin levels 1–2 mg/L. Hyperphosphatemia with fosphenytoin use.	28, 53, 138, 139
Phenobarbital (Luminal)	Inactive metabolite	Dizziness Somnolence Irritability	60–250 mg/day	1.5–4.9 days	Unknown	Unknown	H: yes CAPD: conflicting reports	Partial renal clearance 15% for patients with normal renal function. Generally avoid long-term long-acting barbiturates in severe renal failure.	59, 140
Pregabalin (Lyrica)	N-methyl-pregabalin (probably not clinically significant)	Dizziness Somnolence Ataxia	50–100 mg tid	5–6.5 hr	25–75 mg once daily	Increased and correlated with CrCl	H: yes	Supplemental dose after hemodialysis of 100%–150% of daily renal dose	141, 142

Continued

Table 73-1 Neuropsychiatric Drugs with Comments on Likely Effects for Patients with Renal Failure—cont'd

Drugs	Active Metabolites	Neurologic/ Psychiatric Adverse Reaction	Typical Adult Dose	$t_{1/2}$	Adult Dose in ESRD	$t_{1/2}$ in ESRD	Removed by Dialysis?	Comment	Ref.
Antiparkinsonian									
Amantadine (Symmetrel)		Hallucinations Agitation	100 mg q8–12h	12 hr	100 mg q7d	500 hr	H: variable reports	Accumulation in renal failure	28,54
Carbidopa/ levodopa (Sinemet)	Active metabolites	Hallucinations Agitation	25/100 mg tid RLS: 25/100 mg at HS, MRxl	Carbidopa 2 hr L-dopa 0.8–1.6 hr	Conflicting data	Unknown	H: no		28,144
Ropinirole (Requip)	Inactive metabolites	Dizziness Somnolence Dyskinesias	RLS: 0.25–4.0 mg hs		RLS: 0.25– 2 mg hs	Unknown	H: no		143
Analgesics									
Ibuprofen (Motrin, Advil)	Metabolites ? activity	Aseptic meningitis with lethargy Coma	200–800 mg tid	2.0–3.2 hr	200–800 mg tid	2.0–3.2 hr	H: no CAPD: no	Prostaglandin inhibition may result in renal dysfunction, uremic and gastrointestinal bleeding, nephrotic syndrome, interstitial nephritis, hyperkalemia	28,56
Indomethacin (Indocin)	Inactive metabolites	Visual hallucinations Paranoid delusions	25–50 mg tid	4–12 hr	25–50 mg tid	4–12 hr	H: no CAPD: no	Prostaglandin inhibition may result in renal dysfunction, uremic and gastrointestinal bleeding	28

AUC, area under the curve; CAPD, continuous ambulatory peritoneal dialysis; CPZ, chlorpromazine; CrCl, creatinine clearance; CVVH; continuous venovenous hemofiltration; EPSs, extrapyramidal symptoms; ESRD, end-stage renal disease; hs, at bedtime; MRX1, may repeat once; SSRI, selective serotonin reuptake inhibitor; VPA, valproic acid; XR, extended release.

pressure fluctuations; derangement of calcium, magnesium, sodium, and glucose; intradialytic air emboli fever; hypoxia; and occult alcohol or sedative withdrawal may all participate in precipitating seizures.[10] Seizures may be induced by toxic accumulations of drugs (e.g., penicillins, cephalosporins, amantadine, intravenous contrast agents, acyclovir) or their metabolites (e.g., normeperidine). Lacerda and colleagues[9] have reviewed the clinical literature describing convulsive and nonconvulsive status epilepticus in renal failure patients on β-lactam penicillins, cephalosporins quinolone antibiotics, and carbapenems. Even intended drug effects can have epileptiform consequences, for example, a rapid increase in hematocrit with epoetin alfa. Seizure treatment and prophylaxis are made more difficult by altered anticonvulsant pharmacokinetics. Drug levels can be decreased by dialysis, whereas interdialytic accumulation of unexcreted waste products and hypoalbuminemia can lead to unintended accumulation of anticonvulsants, including valproic acid, gabapentin, vigabatrin, levatiracetam, topiramate, and phenytoin.[9] The risk of metabolic and hemodynamically related seizures with the first dialysis treatment can be decreased by a gradual decrease in blood urea nitrogen by low blood flows (200 mL/min) and by short dialysis (2–3 hours), a small surface area dialyzer, and lower dialysate flow rates. Dialysis disequilibrium with its attendant seizure risk can be prevented by phenytoin prophylaxis early in dialysis by administering intravenous mannitol (12.5 g of 25% solution) midway through sessions and by careful infusion of hypertonic saline if symptoms emerge.[3] The theoretical effects of idiogenic osmoles on intracranial pressure can be countered by gradually adjusting the dialysate sodium concentration from hypernatremic early in the session to normal levels as the session finishes. Hypertension should be controlled, and epoetin doses should initially be low to prevent a rapid increase in hematocrit (see Chapters 60 and 67).

Management of intradialytic seizures should be standardized; dialysis must be halted and the airway secured, intravenous glucose is given as indicated, and then a series of anticonvulsant medications is used if the seizure has not promptly resolved. Intravenous lorazepam 4 mg over 2 minutes is a first step in ending seizure activity; a repeat dose can be given after 10 to 15 minutes if required. Phenytoin is then loaded via a large-bore intravenous catheter, at no more than 50 mg/minute to avoid hypotension; then a total dose should be 10 mg/kg rather than the standard 18 mg/kg loading dose for adults with intact kidney function Once the seizure has ended, maintenance anticonvulsants may not be necessary, particularly if the seizure is thought to have been triggered by uremia or the dialysis procedure. Abou Khaled and Hirsch[10] have published a generic, polydrug treatment protocol for status epilepticus in the critically ill patient, along with remarks particularly relevant to seizure management in renal failure. Where feasible, free serum levels of anticonvulsants should be monitored in patients with epilepsy. On maintenance anticonvulsant treatment with phenytoin, free serum levels of 1.0 to 2.5 mg/L should be maintained. Consideration should be given to using lower doses of renally eliminated anticonvulsants (specifically topiramate), whereas carbonic anhydrase inhibitors require caution because of enhanced risk of nephrolithiasis. Dialyzable agents, including gabapentin, phenobarbital, topiramate, levetiracetam, ethosuximide, pregabalin, and (to a lesser extent) lamotrigine can require postdialysis supplementation.[10] This is less likely to be required for highly protein-bound agents such as carbamazepine and valproic acid.[9]

Insomnia

Sleep disruption is present in 50% to 90% of patients,[12,13] and primary sleep disorders are common, including restless legs syndrome (RLS), periodic leg movements in sleep, and sleep apnea.[1,14–16] Studies of nonpharmacologic and pharmacologic treatments of this problem are limited, and much of the treatment is by inference from the non-ESRD population.[17]

RLS is found in more than half of patients treated with long-term dialysis and manifests itself with predominantly nocturnal lower extremity "jitteriness," necessitating frequent leg movement and, often, pacing. Periodic leg movements in sleep are found in most patients with RLS, whereas RLS is found in a minority of patients with periodic leg movements in sleep. Nonpharmacologic treatment with heat packs and exercise can be effective. Dopaminergics are first-line pharmacologic agents for both conditions, with carbidopa/levodopa, pramipexole, and ropinirole among the most commonly used agents; the ergot dopamine agonists are problematic because they can induce cardiac valve regurgitation.[18] Narcotics, benzodiazepines, and gabapentin follow dopaminergics as RLS/periodic leg movements in sleep treatments. Although dopaminergics, gabapentin, clonidine, and (subsequently) opioids are used in uremia-associated RLS,[1,19,20] the efficacy of these standard treatments in uremic patients is not yet clear.[21,22] Uremic patients are vulnerable to neuropsychiatric respiratory and gastrointestinal side effects with medications, and tachyphylaxis may necessitate dose escalation and drug class rotation. Sloand and colleagues[23] reported double-blind, placebo-controlled data on the successful use of intravenous iron dextran in uremic RLS. Sleep apnea also occurs in patients with ESRD and is likely underdiagnosed and potentially precipitated by hypocarbia, metabolic acidosis, and uremic toxins in the bloodstream.[16,24] There are reports of intensive dialysis, nocturnal dialysis, and renal transplantation reversing sleep apnea.[25–28] Optimal dialysis, modification of the usual risk factors and continuous positive airway pressure and biphasic positive airway pressure are used in uremia-associated sleep apnea. Sleep hygiene methods, including avoidance of caffeine and nicotine, are recommended for sleep disorders, and relaxation therapy, biofeedback, stimulus control therapy, and cognitive-behavioral therapy can also be considered.[17] Pharmacotherapy with sedative hypnotics can be considered in patients without sleep apnea, including newer generation benzodiazepine-receptor agonists (e.g., zolpidem), benzodiazepines, and sedating antidepressants. Of these, the benzodiazepine-receptor agonists seem promising, with good tolerability and low liability to cause residual sedation, withdrawal, dependence, or tolerance.[17] Antihistamines should be avoided, as they are likely to aggravate problems such as xerostomia and to contribute to cognitive impairment. Nocturnal melatonin levels are decreased in dialysis patients, but melatonin and the melatonin agonist ramelteon have yet to be investigated as primary hypnotics in ESRD.[17,29]

Sleep-onset insomnia may be best addressed with short-acting agents such as benzodiazepine-receptor agonists and triazolam. Triazolam's potential for inducing rebound insomnia, anterograde amnesia, and behavioral disinhibition at low doses is likely no greater than that of other benzodiazepines,[30,31] but its potential for inducing delirium is a concern. Zaleplon is more rapidly eliminated than zolpidem and zolpiclone, and there is evidence that adverse effects may be shorter or milder than those found in benzodiazepines and the other benzodiazepine-receptor agonists.[17,32] There is a small, randomized, double-blind crossover study available on zaleplon's use in hemodialysis patients with insomnia, in which it was well tolerated and performed well, with improved sleep quality and reduced sleep latency.[33] Zaleplon does have significant renal elimination and although there is no recommended dose adjustment for mild to moderate renal impairment, caution is indicated in severe renal disease. Difficulty in maintaining sleep may be best dealt with by using medium half-life agents like temazepam or lorazepam, although the longer pharmacokinetics of zolpidem and zolpiclone may also make them appropriate for maintaining sleep.[17,30] Longer acting hypnotics like flurazepam present a potential problem with residual daytime effects. Antidepressants are commonly pressed into service as sedatives and agents such as amitriptyline, trazodone, and mirtazepine may be of some use. However, tricyclics have significant drawbacks, as noted in the subsequent section on treatment of depression, whereas the use of trazodone in dialysis patients may be limited by its tendency to cause hypotension and by the risk of trazodone-associated arrhythmias in patients with comorbid cardiac disease.[17,34]

Delirium

Delirium implies one or more identifiable etiologies and should prompt a vigorous search for reversible causes, including dyspnea related to volume overload, adverse medication reactions, inadequately treated pain, and fever. There is some evidence implicating older age and longer term therapy as risk factors for delirium in hemodialysis patients.[35] As always, medications are frequent offenders, and there are some common, potentially neurotoxic agents that require monitoring in this respect (see Box 73-1). Acyclovir can cause delirium as can meperidine's excitotoxic normeperidine metabolite.[36,37] Clarithromycin has precipitated visual hallucinations in peritoneal dialysis.[38] Many patients have multifactorial causes.

Delirium can be accompanied by agitation when waste products accumulate,[39] and treatment of agitation in uremic delirium follows the general delirium approach, with considerations attendant to renal failure. Antipsychotics are the usual "platform" upon which regimens for the treatment of agitation are built. There are 14 prospective studies and various case reports to support the use of haloperidol, chlorpromazine, olanzapine, risperidone, ziprasidone, quetiapine, and aripiprazole in delirious patients. However, there are limited prospective studies to go on; there are no randomized, double blind, placebo-controlled data for any of the antipsychotics in delirium. At this point, haloperidol remains the mainstay psychotropic for agitated delirium.[40] The drug is documented to be effective and metabolized in the liver, and its metabolites are not active. It is often used at initial doses of 0.5 to 1 mg PO/SC/IM/IV hourly, titrating to effect.[38] There are several more aggressive haloperidol regimens for severe agitation; a recent guideline lists the episodic use of 5 to 10 mg haloperidol,[41] whereas another protocol calls for a starting dose of 5 mg, doubling the dose every 20 minutes until the patient is tranquilized, but arousable.[38] Although commonly used, intravenous haloperidol is not

formally approved by the FDA, and there have been rare cases in which torsade de pointes developed, as noted later. Haloperidol-induced akathisia, dystonia, and parkinsonism can be dealt with by using diphenhydramine 25 to 50 mg IV every 4 to 6 hours in the usual manner, although the use of this agent will likely worsen cognitive decline. Psychiatric units often medicate severely agitated patients using alternating doses of haloperidol and a benzodiazepine (e.g., lorazepam 1 or 2 mg) every 30 minutes to 1 hour, but the treating nephrologist should be alert for paradoxical disinhibition and accelerated confusion when using benzodiazepines in the neuropsychiatrically compromised patient. Olanzapine, ziprasidone, and aripiprazole are now available in intramuscular form and in the future may come into more common use in agitated delirium.

Dementia

Dementia is common in the ESRD population and may be the result of uremia with associated metabolic and physiologic disturbances or comorbid neurodegenerative or cerebrovascular disorders. A single study available did not find a significant difference in the prevalence of dementia between patients on hemodialysis and those on peritoneal dialysis.[42] Dialysis dementia is accompanied by facial grimacing, myoclonus, asterixis dyspraxia, and convulsions.[3] It has been divided into three categories: an epidemic form that is often associated with aluminum, a sporadic form, and a type that is associated with congenital or early childhood renal disease. Dialysis dementia related to aluminum toxicity has decreased with the use of aluminum-free dialysate. It can be treated with deferoxamine, large surface area dialyzers, or charcoal hemoperfusion. Dialysis patients can become thiamine deficient, and this should be suspected in patients presenting with cognitive impairment. Thiamine deficiency can present as a cryptogenic delirium or rapidly progressive dementia, accompanied by chorea, loss of vision, myoclonus, convulsions, and coma; it is potentially reversible with intravenous supplementation.[43] Other sporadic causes of dialysis-associated dementia include vascular lesions, such as cerebrovascular accidents precipitated by ultrafiltration-related hypotension, hemorrhagic stroke, and subdural hematoma.[44,45] There is at least one case report involving the use of donepezil in a patient with comorbid renal failure and Alzheimer's disease, but the use of acetylcholinesterase inhibitors as a treatment for uremic or dialysis dementia is not substantiated.[46] It should be noted that the most commonly employed acetylcholinesterase inhibitor, donepezil, is predominantly excreted in the urine. The manufacturer's information does not indicate a decrease in its clearance in patients with moderate to severe renal impairment. It may be administered safely at the 5-mg dose to Alzheimer's patients with mild to moderate renal impairment.[47]

PRIMARY PSYCHIATRIC PROBLEMS AND THEIR MANAGEMENT

Adjustment Disorders

All renal replacement therapies and procedures place patients in a position of forced passivity and unaccustomed dependence.[14] Loss of autonomy is stressful, and prolonged dependence can promote regression; dependency issues are particularly brought out in hemodialysis patients. Personality and the patient's ability to withstand the dependent position should be considered in making choices between treatment options. Decisions must be flexible and the staff must be aware of the possibility of a poor fit for the chosen dialysis method and be willing to shift to a different modality.

Most chronic illnesses afford at least some periods of respite. This is not the case in ESRD. Its victims are continually involved in the management of their disease and its symptoms. Multiple medications, fluid and dietary restrictions, dialysis schedules, and vascular procedures all ensure that the patient has very little opportunity to escape a continual dialogue with the disease. Treatment alters the individual's appearance with skin discoloration, surgical scars, and fistula sites. Peritoneal dialysis distorts the patient's body shape and may be punctuated by episodes of peritonitis. Work, normally a source of identity and self-esteem, is no longer possible for many patients because of age or illness. Financial stress increases in this context, and increased expenditures for care, diet, and transport are often unmet by social resources and available insurance coverage. The strain on the family of the ESRD patient may be accentuated by the patient's increased caretaking needs and by role reversal required for spouse and/or children.[48]

Subjective adequacy of social supports has been reported to be a significant factor in the survival of dialysis patients. Discrepancy between a patient's expectations and available levels of support has been found in a recent study to be associated with increased mortality in both peritoneal dialysis and hemodialysis populations.[49] The connection does not appear to be mediated by clinical depression and may reflect the effects of stress and anxiety attendant to dialysis, particularly when inadequately buffered by significant human attachments.

Short-term, reversible changes in emotional state due to proximal stressors are defined as adjustment disorders and can be characterized by predominant depression, anxiety, disturbances in behavior, or any combination thereof. Treatment of an adjustment disorder involves supportive, cognitive, and psychoeducational therapy, along with group and individual peer support and family intervention as indicated. Most psychotherapy is provided by renal social workers, with referral to the local mental health resources or consultants as needed. Pastoral counseling may also be beneficial. Advance preparation, appropriate support, and judicious treatment can, along with time, help the patient's recovery. If the patient's symptoms are protracted, disabling, or complicated by mania, psychosis, or lethal ideation, the diagnosis of adjustment disorder is no longer appropriate.

Anxiety Disorders

Anxiety is commonly encountered in ESRD patients and may present in multiple forms. Fears can center on prognosis, the ability to adjust to the demands of the disease and its treatment, or sexual performance or may be fueled by anticipated effects of the disease on the family and the patient's place within it.[50] Anxiety may be triggered by the dialysis experience, with its attendant fluid shifts, electrolyte disturbances, and gastrointestinal upset and cramping. Needles and blood can provoke phobic reactions, and the methodical draining of

the patient's blood from the body can be subjectively terrifying.[1] Panic attacks can be the vector result of psychological, physiologic, and familial stress.

Pharmacologic management is symptomatic and can be directed at persistent generalized anxiety, acute panic episodes, or a combination of the two (see Table 73-1). Because benzodiazepines are metabolized in the liver, a decrease in dose is generally not necessary in ESRD, with the exceptions of midazolam and chlordiazepoxide. Diazepam, lorazepam, alprazolam, and clonazepam can be used as needed before or during dialysis sessions. In recent years, antidepressants have become first-line treatments for most anxiety disorders. Selective serotonin reuptake inhibitors (SSRIs) are used increasingly to treat panic and generalized anxiety disorders in the general population and are also helpful in CKD patients. Venlafaxine, a serotonin-norepinephrine reuptake inhibitor and its metabolite O-desmethylvenlafaxine are subject to decreased clearance and elimination in renal disease; the manufacturer recommends decreasing the dose by 25% to 50% in patients with renal impairment and 50% in hemodialysis-dependent patients (dose is withheld until 4 hours post-dialysis). Mirtazepine, another dual neurotransmitter antidepressant, may also need to have its dose adjusted downward for decreased clearance and elimination in ESRD.

Depression and Manic Depression

Depression is quite common in the dialysis population. The 1997 review of O'Donnell and Chung[51] found major depression in 5% to 22% of ESRD patients and subclinical depression in an additional 25%. Major depression may be driven by losses of autonomy, productivity and sexual function. Depression in dialysis patients often goes unrecognized and untreated,[52] and suicide rates are elevated.[53,54] The traditionally quoted 500-fold increase in suicide among dialysis patients is a gross overestimate,[1] but dialysis-dependent patients can, with unconscious intent, take their own lives by missing treatments or not complying with dietary and fluid restrictions. Depression and mortality in ESRD have been associated in several studies but not in all.[55,56] In one study,[56] low scores on the Beck Depression Inventory were associated with 85% 2 year survival rate, whereas high depression scores were associated with a 25% survival rate. A 2000 study by Kimmel and colleagues[55] found that depressive indices predicted survival at 1 year and that higher levels of depressive affect were associated with increased mortality. Diagnosis of depression begins with suspecting it. The diagnostic inquiry starts with a simple question about mood (though patients may be unable to recognize changes in their emotional state). It makes sense to follow the initial mood question by additional questions about psychiatric symptoms. Characteristics used to classify major depression can be found in the *Diagnostic and Statistical Manual of Mental Disorders, 4th Edition* (DSM-IV) (http://psyweb.com/Mdisord/DSM_IV/jsp/dsm_iv.jsp). If patient and clinician then believe that "the shoe fits," additional relevant history can be explored, including personal and family history of depression, history of substance abuse, and (especially important) past suicide attempts.[53]

Treatment of depression involves both psychotherapy and pharmacotherapy. Most psychotherapy in the ESRD/dialysis setting is provided by renal social workers; there also should be access to more specialized psychotherapists in the community for patients with particularly complicated or intensive needs. Pharmacotherapy relies on antidepressants, often in combination with or augmented by other agents such as thyroid hormone, buspirone, or stimulants. The nephrologist should refer for psychiatric consultation those depressed patients for whom antidepressant monotherapy is ineffective.

Double-blind, placebo-controlled trials of pharmacotherapy in ESRD depression are needed, but the available data consistently support the use of both SSRIs and tricyclic antidepressants in this population.[57,58] As the oldest generation of antidepressants, tricyclics have accumulated the most data and experience. They are prone to cause anticholinergic and antihistaminic side effects, can precipitate or aggravate postural hypotension, will lower seizure threshold, and lengthen cardiac conduction intervals. Nortriptyline, a secondary amine tricyclic, is particularly useful because of a meaningful therapeutic window in its serum levels and a relatively lower side effect burden, at least in terms of anticholinergic effects and sedation. Imipramine and amitriptyline, tertiary amines, have hydroxylated metabolites that contribute to both therapeutic and toxic effects. Tricyclics can be used adjunctively in the treatment of neuropathic pain, commonly found in ESRD. Although useful and well established, tricyclics are cumbersome, with a low therapeutic index and potential lethality in overdose. At this point, they have been superseded as the first-line of treatment by newer agents and are best reserved for treatment-resistant depression in ESRD.

SSRIs are the first-line treatment of depression in the general population. They are also beneficial in ESRD-related depression, although they are not as well researched as tricyclics. Fluoxetine is the best studied SSRI and appears to be both effective and well tolerated.[59] Fluoxetine is metabolized hepatically; the kinetic profile of single doses of fluoxetine is unchanged in renal failure, even in anephric patients. Renal function does not significantly alter either fluoxetine or norfluoxetine serum levels. Sertraline is also widely used as it too is metabolized hepatically, and urinary excretion of the unchanged drug is insignificant. Subjects with mild to severe renal impairment and matched controls show no significant differences in pharmacokinetics. As noted, sertraline can be used to help prevent sudden hemodialysis-related hypotension.[60] Citalopram kinetics follows the SSRI pattern and is minimally changed in patients with ESRD; dose adjustment is probably not necessary.[61] Paroxetine is unusual among SSRIs in that its blood level is sensitive to renal impairment; in patients with severe renal insufficiency, it should be started at 10 mg or half the usual starting dose.[62]

There are several non-SSRI new-generation antidepressant medications that should be used with caution or avoided in ESRD patients. Careful dose adjustment for patients with renal impairment is necessary with venlafaxine, as noted.[63] With this drug, hypertension can be a risk, and regular blood pressure monitoring on venlafaxine is indicated. Bupropion is contraindicated in patients with seizure disorders and must be used with caution in patients with lower seizure thresholds. In ESRD patients, proconvulsive metabolites may accumulate and predispose to seizures, along with the electrolyte disturbances caused by the disorder. Duloxetine, another nontricyclic serotonin-norepinephrine reuptake inhibitor, has been used as a treatment for diabetic neuropathy as well as for depression and anxiety. It is, however, eliminated by the kidneys, and its use is contraindicated in patients with renal failure. Mirtazepine is an atypical noradrenergic/serotonergic antidepressant often used for depression with prominent insomnia, anorexia, and anxiety. Single-dose oral clearance of mirtazepine is decreased by 33% in moderate and by 50% in severe renal failure. There is inadequate documentation of its use in patients with renal failure.[64,65] Little is known about the use of nefazodone for depression in the ESRD population; its potential hepatotoxicity and cytochrome P-450 3A4 inhibition argue against its use.[66] As a rule, care must be taken when prescribing antidepressants to patients on cytochrome-dependent drugs, as many of the antidepressants, particularly the SSRIs, will inhibit selected isoenzymes of the P-450 system. 3A4 inhibition can be particularly common and problematic, affecting multiple drugs used in the renal failure/transplant population (e.g., tacrolimus, cyclosporine, sildenafil). Inhibitors of the 3A4 subsystem include nefazodone, fluoxetine/norfluoxetine, fluvoxamine, paroxetine (weakly), sertraline, and valproic acid (weakly). In patients with unexplained toxicities, including delirium, careful examination of the use of antidepressant drugs and their interactions with other drugs is critical.[67,68] The pharmacologic management of mania and of depression in the context of a bipolar disorder is considerably more difficult than the management of unipolar depression. Use of polypharmacy by psychiatrists is the rule, and combinations of mood stabilizers, antipsychotics, antidepressants, and other agents are commonly used. In addition, the risk of switching a bipolar patient from a depressed state to mania when antidepressant therapy is required complicates the treatment of bipolar depression. Lithium has traditionally been the primary mood stabilizer used in bipolar disorder. There are many years of experience with the use of lithium, and it has demonstrated efficacy in acute episodes and in prevention of relapses. In the past decade or two, it has been gradually displaced by anticonvulsant medications, particularly valproic acid, carbamazepine, and, more recently, lamotrigine. These drugs are effective, and lamotrigine has particular efficacy in patients with bipolar depression. These useful anticonvulsants can have drug interactions with each other, with antidepressants, and with nonpsychiatric medications, and they are eliminated by the kidneys. The latter property requires dosing adjustment for lamotrigine alone. Titration of the lamotrigine dose is slow and must be carefully monitored to minimize the risk of rapid increase in drug level precipitating Stevens-Johnson syndrome or toxic epidermal necrolysis. For those bipolar disorder patients with ESRD who require lithium, treatment involves administration of a single dose (usually 600 mg) after each dialysis. Lithium is removed by dialysis and a single dose should result in a steady serum level,[69] but serum lithium levels obtained before and after dialysis sessions can help adjust the dose. Lithium levels should be obtained immediately before dialysis and 2 hours after its completion; the immediate level after dialysis is misleadingly low and will increase with subsequent redistribution.

Lithium can be nephrotoxic, and other mood stabilizers are preferable in patients with renal insufficiency. A long-term follow-up study found that when the drug is discontinued, renal function may improve.[70]

Electroconvulsive therapy can also be used as an antidepressant strategy in patients with renal failure. Individual case reports in the literature document successful treatment of bipolar depression in ESRD patients with electroconvulsive therapy.[71,72] Salient issues include renal osteodystrophy with attendant increased fracture risk, hyperkalemia with potential cardiotoxicity when using succinylcholine in the uremic patient, altered pharmacokinetics of anesthetic induction agents, and adverse effects of metabolic acidosis and of changes in volume status complicate the treatment. Careful attention to both muscle relaxation and potassium level is necessary; the use of a nondepolarizing paralytic rather than succinylcholine may also be a consideration.

Schizophrenia and Psychotic Disorders

Pharmacologic treatment of schizophrenia has been shifted away from the reliance on traditional neuroleptics with the advent of the atypical antipsychotics, including clozapine, risperidone, ziprasidone, aripiprazole, and olanzapine. Unlike traditional neuroleptics, this new generation of antipsychotics does not rely primarily on D_2 receptor blockade for efficacy and so is less prone to aggravate negative symptoms of the disease, such as emotional blunting and apathy. Before the Clinical Antipsychotic Trials of Intervention Effectiveness (CATIE) in 2005, atypical antipsychotics were largely uncontested as the standard of care for the treatment of psychotic disorders. In CATIE, the atypical antipsychotics did not seem as a class to show improved tolerance or better results than a standard neuroleptic (perphenazine), but there was much greater cost. CATIE has left the field in doubt as to any reflexive preference for atypical agents and may reshuffle existing treatment guidelines in the coming years. For example, there may be a renewed appreciation for traditional neuroleptics like haloperidol.[73]

There are few data concerning the use of atypical agents in the ESRD population and peer-reviewed data to guide their use in psychotic patients with comorbid renal failure is scanty. There has been a re-emergence of tics in an adolescent treated with risperidone when the patient was switched from peritoneal to hemodialysis; this may have been due to altered gut absorption, as the level of the water-soluble 9-OH metabolite was unaffected by dialysis.[74] In a study of healthy young and elderly subjects compared with patients with cirrhosis or moderate and severe renal insufficiency, the elimination and clearance of risperidone and 9-OH risperidone were decreased in patients with renal disease. This implies there should be a reduced dose and slower titration of risperidone in patients with renal failure.[75] Ziprasidone pharmacokinetics have been studied; mild to moderate renal insufficiency did not alter pharmacokinetics of ziprasidone and hemodialysis did not significantly alter ziprasidone pharmacokinetics.[76] Single-dose data for quetiapine showed no pharmacokinetic difference between nonpsychotic healthy subjects and subjects with renal impairment.[77] There is a case study describing the development of protracted hypothermia in a hemodialysis patient after a single dose of olanzapine, possibly due to an enhanced hypothalamic effect. However, product information for olanzapine indicates no change in pharmacokinetics with severe renal insufficiency, leaving the issue unresolved.[78] Finally, there have been cases of acute renal failure associated with clozapine treatment, including a documented case of acute renal failure due to interstitial nephritis.[79] These reports leave the prescribing physician somewhat at sea in dosing these agents, and caution is warranted. The traditional neuroleptics are still used in the management of schizophrenia and other psychotic disorders and may see a resurgence in future use.

Emerging data show a significant increase in mortality among the demented elderly treated with atypical antipsychotics. Initially recognized and quantified with Risperdal (risperidone) results, the association appears to be a class effect. An increase in stroke risk was also postulated, but this has not been borne out in larger meta-analyses of randomized, controlled trials. Development of the metabolic syndrome is another growing concern with the use of atypical antipsychotics. Clozapine and olanzapine appear to be the worst offenders in this regard, whereas aripiprazole has a more favorable profile in terms of diabetes and hyperlipidemia. Regardless, hemoglobin A1c, weight, blood pressure, and lipids should be monitored when any atypical agent is prescribed.

In vulnerable CKD patients, dopamine-blocking drugs, especially higher potency neuroleptics and risperidone, can cause hyperprolactinemia, affecting gonadotropin levels and bone metabolism.

Cardiac conduction effects and the potential for lethal arrhythmias have become a prominent source of concern in the treatment of medically ill patients with both typical and atypical antipsychotics. In CKD patients and especially ESRD patients who are subjected to disturbances in electrolytes, this is of particular concern. Antipsychotics can cause QTc prolongation, presumed to be related to drug antagonism of the Ikr delayed rectifier current. There are reports of the development of torsade de pointes with haloperidol, pimozide, droperidol, sertindole, thioridazine, chlorpromazine, ziprasidone, risperidone, and quetiapine. In terms of QTc prolongation, ziprasidone and thioridazine are the most problematic, with ziprasidone midway between thioridazine and a number of other, more modestly prolonging antipsychotics, including haloperidol, risperidone, quetiapine, and olanzapine.[80] Aripiprazole may be preferable in this regard, with a low propensity for QTc prolongation.[81] After a U.S. Food and Drug Administration review, thioridazine was found to be contraindicated when other drugs that prolong QTc or that interfere with thioridazine's metabolism or elimination are used. The potentially offending drugs include fluvoxamine, propranolol, paroxetine, and fluoxetine. Thioridazine is no longer a widely used agent, but the consideration of increased cardiac risk with pharmacodynamic or pharmacokinetic drug interactions should be reflexive on the part of the prescribing clinician. On general principles, alternatives to thioridazine (other low-potency neuroleptics such as chlorpromazine) should be preferred for the patient with renal impairment.[82]

Sexual Disorders

Sexual dysfunction in CKD patients has multiple causes, including vascular disease, malnutrition, anemia, hormonal abnormalities, iatrogenic drug effects, and psychiatric disorders. It is found in both men and women, is significantly distressing, and can precipitate lapses in treatment compliance. A recent study has demonstrated an independent association between sexual dysfunction and depression in male hemodialysis patients; the association may be bidirectional.[83]

A majority of patients on dialysis experience a decrease in sexual interest or frequency. Levy and Cohen[57] state that approximately 70% of men have partial or total impotence, that the majority of women are amenorrheic or infertile, and that even successful kidney transplantation does not always restore a patient's sexual function. Dialysis also does not seem to ameliorate sexual dysfunction.[84] SSRIs and other psychiatric medications can be significant offenders. Treatment addresses underlying causes (e.g., correction of anemia and secondary hyperparathyroidism, hormone replacement therapy).[85] Behavioral psychotherapies may be helpful and treatment of clinical depression is indicated, with recognition that antidepressants have side effects that impair sexual performance. Sildenafil is highly effective in the treatment of many cases of erectile dysfunction found in CKD patients,[86] but is contraindicated in people taking nitrates for coronary artery disease (these drugs can cause fatal hypotension). They may not be as effective in diabetic dialysis patients[87]; apomorphine was far less effective than sildenafil in a study comparing the two drugs in the treatment of erectile dysfunction in dialysis patients.[88]

For patients with ESRD who have not developed significant hypotension during dialysis and are not receiving cytochrome P-450 3A4-inhibiting drugs, a low dose of sildenafil (25 mg) may be considered. Men may need surgical intervention to preserve sexual function (see Chapter 71).

INITIAL NEUROPSYCHIATRIC ALGORITHM

Making sense of an array of neuropsychiatric symptoms can be a confusing and unsettling task for the nephrologist. Diagnostic categories and treatments frequently overlap, and comorbidities are routine. This chapter's algorithm should be taken with an "osmole of sodium"—it is simplified and generalized and will apply in some cases far better than in others. An algorithm must not be substituted for informed clinical judgment, and the threshold for referring patients for psychiatric consultation should be low, particularly if problems are persistent, severe, or refractory to initial attempts at management. It should also be emphasized that suicidal or homicidal ideation or threats represent emergent situations requiring an immediate response from the treating physician. If the safety of the patient or others is in doubt, prompt assessment, rapid psychiatric consultation, and careful consideration of inpatient treatment are indicated. Local crisis resources should be identified and emergency contact numbers easily accessed by all clinical personnel.

In more routine situations, a good starting point is to ask whether neuropsychiatric problems involve the mental status of the patient and whether they have an impact on awareness, cognition, mood, thought, or perception.

References

1. USRDS: Excerpts from the United States Renal Data System 2000 Annual Report. National Institutes of Health NIDDK/DKUHD. Am J Kidney Dis 2000;36(Suppl 2):S1–S239.
2. Fraser CL, Arieff AI: Neuropsychiatric complications of renal failure. In Brady HR, Wilcox CS (eds): Therapy in Nephrology and Hypertension: A Companion to Brenner and Rector's The Kidney. Philadelphia: WB Saunders, 2001, pp 488–490.
3. Tzamaloukas AH, Agaba ET: Neurological manifestations of uraemia and chronic dialysis. Niger J Med 2004;13:98–105.
4. Fraser CL, Arieff AI: Metabolic encephalopathy as a complication of renal failure: Mechanisms and mediators. New Horiz 1994;2:518–526.
5. Palmer BF, Henrich WL: Uremic mononeuropathy. In Rose BD (ed): UpToDate. Wellesley, MA: UpToDate, 2001. Available at: http//www.uptodate.com.
6. Krishnan AV, Phoon RK, Pussell BA, et al: Sensory nerve excitability and neuropathy in end stage kidney disease. J Neurol Neurosurg Psychiatry 2006;77:548–551.
7. Krishnan AV, Kiernan MC: Uremic neuropathy: Clinical features and new pathophysiological insights. Muscle Nerve 2007;35:273–290.
8. Barri YM, Golper TA: Seizures in patients undergoing hemodialysis polyneuropathy. In Rose BD (ed): UpToDate. Wellesley, MA: UpToDate, 2001. Available at: http//www.uptodate.com.
9. Lacerda G, Krummel T, Sabourdy C, et al: Optimizing therapy of seizures in patients with renal or hepatic dysfunction. Neurology 2006;67(Suppl 4):S28–S33.
10. Abou Khaled KJ, Hirsch LJ: Advances in the management of seizures and status epilepticus in critically ill patients. Crit Care Clin 2006;22:637–659.
11. Arieff AI: Dialysis disequilibrium syndrome: Current concepts on pathogenesis and prevention. Kidney Int 1994;45:629–635.
12. Walker S, Fine A, Kruger MH: Sleep complaints are common in a dialysis unit. Am J Kidney Dis 1995;26:751–756.
13. Kimmel PL, Gavin C, Miller G, et al: Disordered sleep and noncompliance in a patient with end-stage renal disease. Adv Ren Replace Ther 1997;4:55–67.
14. Levy NB: Psychiatric consideration in the primary medical care of the patient with renal failure. Adv Ren Replace Ther 2000;7:231–238.
15. Noda A, Nakai S, Soga T, et al: Factors contributing to sleep disturbance and hypnotic drug use in hemodialysis patients. Intern Med 2006;45:1273–1278.
16. Jurado-Gamez B, Martin-Malo A, Alvarez-Lara MA, et al: Sleep disorders are underdiagnosed in patients on maintenance dialysis. Nephron Clin Pract 2007;105:c35–c42.
17. Novak M, Shapiro CM, Mendelssohn D, Istvan M: Diagnosis and management of insomnia in dialysis patients. Semin Dial 2006;199:25–31.
18. Schade R, Andersohn F, Suissa S, et al: Dopamine agonists and the risk of cardiac-valve regurgitation. N Engl J Med 2007;356:29–38.
19. Thorp ML, Morris CD, Bagby SP: A crossover study of gabapentin in treatment of restless legs syndrome among hemodialysis patients. Am J Kidney Dis 2001;38:104–108.
20. Wagner ML, Walters AS, Coleman RG, et al: Randomized, double-blind, placebo-controlled study of clonidine in restless legs syndrome. Sleep 1996;19:52–58.
21. Pieta J, Millar T, Zacharias J, et al: Effect of pergolide on restless legs and leg movements in sleep in uremic patients. Sleep 1998;21:617–622.
22. Molnar MZ, Novak M, Musci I: Management of restless legs syndrome in patients on dialysis. Drugs 2006;66:607–624.
23. Sloand JA, Shelly MA, Feigin A, et al: A double-blind, placebo-controlled trial of intravenous iron dextran therapy in patients with ESRD and restless legs syndrome. Am J Kidney Dis 2004;43:663–670.
24. Fletcher EC: Obstructive sleep apnea and the kidney. J Am Soc Nephrol 1993;4:1111–1121.
25. Fein AM, Niederman MS, Imbriano L, Rosen H: Reversal of sleep apnea in uremia by dialysis. Arch Intern Med 1987l;147:1355–1356.
26. Langevin B, Fouque D, Leger P, Robert D: Sleep apnea syndrome and end-stage renal disease. Cure after renal transplantation. Chest 1993;103:1330–1335.
27. Shayamsunder AK, Patel SS, Jain V, et al: Sleepiness, sleeplessness, and pain in end-stage renal disease: Distressing symptoms for patients. Semin Dial 2005;18:109–118.
28. Hanly PJ, Pierratos A: Improvement of sleep apnea in patients with chronic renal failure who undergo nocturnal hemodialysis. N Engl J Med 2001;344:102–107.
29. Karasek M, Szuflet A, Chrzanowski W, et al: Decreased melatonin nocturnal concentrations in hemodialyzed patients. Neurol Endocrinol Lett 2005;26:653–656.

30. Rothschild AJ: Disinhibition, amnestic reactions, and other adverse reactions secondary to triazolam: A review of the literature. J Clin Psychiatry 1992;53(Suppl):69–79.

31. Mendelson WB, Jain B: An assessment of short-acting hypnotics. Drug Saf 1995;3:257–270.

32. Drover DR: Comparative pharmacokinetics and pharmacodynamics of short-acting hypnosedatives: Zaleplon, zolpidem and zopiclone. Clin Pharmacokinet 2004;43:227–238.

33. Sabbatini M, Crispo A, Ragosta A, et al: Zaleplon improves sleep quality in maintenance hemodialysis patients. Nephron Clin Pract 2003;94:c99–c103.

34. James SP, Mendelson WB: The use of trazodone as a hypnotic: A critical review. J Clin Psychiatry 2004;65:752–755.

35. Fukunishi I, Kitaoka T, Shirai T, et al: Delirium in patients on hemodialysis therapy. Nephron 2002;90:236.

36. Revenkar SG, Applegate AL, Markovitz DM: Delirium associated with acyclovir treatment in a patient with renal failure. Clin Infect Dis 1995;21:435–436.

37. Stock SL, Catalono G, Catallano MC: Meperidine associated mental status changes in a patient with chronic renal failure. J Fla Med Assoc 1996;83:315–319.

38. Steinman MA, Steinman TI: Clarithromycin-associated visual hallucinations in a patient with chronic renal failure on continuous ambulatory peritoneal dialysis. Am J Kidney Dis 1996;27:143–146.

39. Neely KJ, Roxe DM: Palliative care/hospice and the withdrawal of dialysis. J Palliat Med 2000;3:57–67.

40. Cassem NH, Hackett TP: The setting of intensive care. In Hackett TP, Cassem NH (eds): Massachusetts General Hospital Handbook of General Hospital Psychiatry. St. Louis: CV Mosby, 1978, pp 326–327.

41. Schmidt RJ, Holley JL: Psychiatric illness in dialysis patients. In Rose BL (ed): UpToDate. Wellesley, MA: UpToDate, 2001. Available at: http://www.uptodate.com

42. Sithinamsuwan P, Niyasom S, Nidhinandana S, Supasyndh O: Dementia and depression in end stage renal disease: Comparison between hemodialysis and continuous ambulatory peritoneal dialysis. J Med Assoc Thai 2005;88(Suppl 3):S141–S147.

43. Hung SC, Hung SH, Tarng DC, et al: Thiamine deficiency and unexplained encephalopathy in hemodialysis and peritoneal dialysis patients. Am J Kidney Dis 2001;38:941–947.

44. Brouns R, De Deyn PP: Neurological complications in renal failure: A review. Clin Neurol Neurosurg 2004;107:1–16.

45. Sengul G, Tuzun Y, Kadioglu HH, Aydin IH: Acute interhemispheric subdural hematoma due to hemodialysis: Case report. Surg Neurol 2005;64(Suppl 2):S113–S114.

46. Suwata J, Kamata K, Nishijima T, et al: New acetylcholinesterase inhibitor (donepezil) treatment for Alzheimer's disease in chronic dialysis patient. Nephron 2002;91:330–332.

47. Seltzer B: Donepezil: A review. Expert Opin Drug Metab Toxicol 2005;1:527–536.

48. Reiss D: Patient, family and staff responses to end-stage renal disease. Am J Kidney Dis 1990;15:194–200.

49. Thong MSY, Adrian A, Kapstein R, et al: Social support predicts survival in dialysis patients. Nephrol Dial Transplant 2007;22:845–850.

50. Levy NB: Sexual dysfunctions of hemodialysis patients. Clin Exp Dial Apheresis 1983;7:275–288.

51. O'Donnell K, Chung Y: The diagnosis of major depression in end-stage renal disease. Psychosomatics 1997;66:38–43.

52. Finkelstein FO, Finkelstein SH: Depression in chronic dialysis patients: Assessment and treatment. Nephrol Dial Transplant 2000;15:191–192.

53. Haenel T, Brunner F, Battegay R: Renal dialysis and suicide: Occurrence in Switzerland and Europe. Compr Psychiatry 1980;21:140–145.

54. Cohen LM, Steinberg MD, Hails KC, et al: The psychiatric evaluation of death-hastening requests: Lessons from dialysis discontinuation. Psychosomatics 2000;41:195–203.

55. Kimmel PL, Peterson RA, Weihs KL, et al: Multiple measurements of depression predict mortality in a longitudinal study of chronic hemodialysis outpatients. Kidney Int 2000;57:2093–2098.

56. Shulman R, Price JD, Spinelli J: Biopsychosocial aspects of long-term survival on end-stage renal failure therapy. Psychol Med 1989;19:945–954.

57. Levy NB, Cohen LM: Central and peripheral nervous systems in uremia. In Massry SG, Glassock R (eds): Textbook of Nephrology, 4 ed. Philadelphia: Williams & Wilkins, 2001, pp 1279–1282.

58. Wuerth D, Finkelstein SH, Finkelstein FO: The identification and treatment of depression in patients maintained on dialysis. Semin Dial 2005;18:142–146.

59. Blumenfeld, M, Levy NB, Spinowitz B, et al: Fluoxetine in depressed patients on dialysis. Int J Psychiatry Med 1997;27:71–80.

60. Dheenan S, Venketesan J, Grubb BP, Henrich WL: Effect of sertraline hydrochloride on dialysis hypotension. Am J Kidney Dis 1998;31:624–630.

61. Joffe P, Larsen FS, Pedersen V, et al: Single-dose pharmacokinetics of citalopram in patients with moderate renal insufficiency or hepatic cirrhosis compared with health subjects. Eur J Clin Pharmacol 1998;54:237–242.

62. Doyle CD, Laher M, Kelly JG, et al: The pharmacokinetics of paroxetine in renal impairment. Acta Psychiatr Scand 1989;80 (Suppl 350):89–90.

63. Troy SM, Schultz RW, Parker VD, et al: The effect of renal disease on the disposition of venlafaxine. Clin Pharmacol Ther 1994;56:14-21.

64. Crone CC, Gabriel GM: Treatment of anxiety and depression in transplant patients: Pharmacokinetic considerations. Clin Pharmacokinet 2004;43:361–394.

65. Timmer CJ, Ad Sitsen JM, Delbressine LP: Clinical pharmacokinetics of mirtazepine. Clin Pharmacokinet 2000;38:461–474.

66. Seabolt JL, DeLeon OA: Response to nefzaodone in a depressed patient with end-stage renal disease. Gen Hosp Psychiatr 2001:23:45–46.

67. Aronoff GR, Berns JS, Brier ME, et al: Drug Prescribing in Renal Failure. Dosing Guidelines for Adults, 4th ed. Philadelphia: American College of Physicians–American Society for Internal Medicine, 1999.

68. Brater DC: Drug Dosing in Renal Failure in Therapy in Nephrology and Hypertension. A Companion to Brenner and Rector's The Kidney. Philadelphia: WB Saunders, 2001, pp 641–653.

69. Port FK, Kroll PD, Rosenzweig J: Lithium therapy during maintenance hemodialysis. Psychosomatics 1979;20:130–132.

70. Braden GL: Lithium-induced renal disease. In Greenberg A, Coffman TM, Cheung AK, et al (eds): Primer on Kidney Disease, 3rd ed., San Diego, CA: Academic Press, 2001, pp 322–324.

71. Williams S, Ostroff R: Chronic renal failure, hemodialysis, and electroconvulsive therapy: A case report. J ECT, 2005;21:41–42.

72. Varghese ST, Sagar R, Jhanjee S: Chronic renal failure and electroconvulsive therapy. Indian J Med Sci 2006;60:114–115.

73. Lieberman JA, Stroup TS, McAvoy JP, et al: Clinical Antipsychotic Trials of Intervention Effectiveness (CATIE) investigators. N Engl J Med 2005;353:1209–1223.

74. Railton CJ, Kapur B, Koren G: Subtherapeutic risperidone serum concentrations in an adolescent during hemodialysis: A pharmacological puzzle. Ther Drug Monit 2005;27:558–561.

75. Snoeck E, Van Peer A, Sack M, et al: Influence of age, renal and liver impairment on the pharmacokinetics of risperidone in man. Psychopharmacology (Berl) 1995;122:223–229.

76. Aweeka F, Jayesekara D, Horton M, et al: The pharmacokinetics of ziprasidone in subjects with normal and impaired renal function. Br J Clin Pharmacol 2000;49(Suppl 1):27S–33S.

77. Thyrum PT, Wong YW, Yeh C: Single-dose pharmacokinetics of quetiapine in subjects with renal or hepatic impairment. Prog Neuropsychopharmacol Biol Psychiatry 2000;24:521–533.

78. Fukunishi I, Sato Y, Kino K, et al: Hypothermia in a hemodialysis patient treated with olanzapine monotherapy. J Clin Psychopharmacol 2003;23:314.

79. Fraser D, Jibani M: An unexpected and serious complication of treatment with the atypical antipsychotic drug clozapine. Clin Nephrol 2000;54:78–80.

80. Haddad PM, Anderson IM: Antipsychotic-related QTc prolongation, torsade de pointes and sudden death. Drugs 2002;62: 1649–1671.

81. Swainston HT, Perry CM: Aripiprazole: A review of its use in schizophrenia and schizoaffective disorder. Drugs 2004;64: 1715–1736.

82. Hoehns JD, Stanford RH, Geraets DR, et al: Torsades de pointes associated with chlorpromazine: Case report and review of associated ventricular arrhythmias. Pharmacotherapy 2001;21:871–883.

83. Peng Y-S, Chiang C-K, Hung K-Y, et al: The association of higher depressive symptoms and sexual dysfunction in male haemodialysis patients. Nephrol Dial Transplant 2007;22: 857–861.

84. Soykan A, Boztas H, Kutlay S, et al: Do sexual dysfunctions get better during dialysis? Results of a six-month prospective follow-up study from Turkey. Int J Impot Res 2005;17:359–363.

85. Palmer BF: Sexual dysfunction in men and women with chronic kidney disease and end-stage kidney disease. Adv Ren Replace Ther 2003;10:48–60.

86. Turk S, Karalezli G, Tonbul HZ, et al: Erectile dysfunction and the effects of sildenafil treatment in patients on haemodialysis and continuous ambulatory peritoneal dialysis. Nephrol Dial Transplant 2001;16:1818–1822.

87. Hyodo T, Ishida H, Masui N, et al: Kidney disease quality of life of Japanese dialysis patients who desire administration of sildenafil and the treatment of erectile dysfunction using sildenafil. Ther Apher Dial 2004;8:340–346.

88. Dachille G, Pagliarulo V, Ludovico GM, et al: Sexual dysfunction in patients under dialytic treatment. Minerva Urol Nephrol 2006;58:195–200.

89. Spigset O, Hagg S, Stegmayr B, Dahlqvist R: Citalopram pharmacokinetics in patients with chronic renal failure and the effect of haemodialysis. Eur J Clin Pharmacol 2000;56:699–703.

90. Drewes P, Thijssen I, Mengel H, et al: A single-dose cross-over pharmacokinetic study comparing racemic citalopram (40 mg) with the S-enantiomer of citalopram (escitalopram, 20 mg) in healthy male subjects. Presented at the Annual Meeting of New Clinical Drug Evaluation Unit, Phoenix, AZ, 2001.

91. Momen MN, Sebastian CS, Buckley PF: Paradoxical reaction to fluoxetine. Psychosomatics 2003;44:259–260.

92. Kamo T, Horikawa N, Tsuruta Y, et al: Efficacy and pharmacokinetics of fluvoxamine maleate in patients with mild depression undergoing hemodialysis. Psychiatry Clin Neurosci 2004;58:133–137.

93. Koo JR, Yoon JY, Joo MH, et al: Treatment of depression and effect of antidepression treatment on nutritional status in chronic hemodialysis patients. Am J Med Sci 2005;329:1–5.

94. Brewster UC, Ciampi MA, Abu-Alfa AK, Perazella MA: Addition of sertraline to other therapies to reduce dialysis-associated hypotension. Nephrology 2003;8:296–301.

95. Yalcin AU, Kudaiberdieva G, Sahin G, et al: Effect of sertraline hydrochloride on cardiac autonomic dysfunction in patients with hemodialysis-induced hypotension. Nephron Physiol 2003;93:21–28.

96. Yalcin AU, Sahin G, Erol M, Bal C: Sertraline hydrochloride treatment for patients with hemodialysis hypotension. Blood Purif 2002;20:150–153.

97. Perazella MA: Pharmacologic options available to treat symptomatic intradialytic hypotension. Am J Kidney Dis 2001;38 (4 Suppl 4):S26–S36t.

98. Degen J, Wolke E, Seiberling M, et al: [Comparative study of the pharmacokinetics of amitriptyline oxide and trimipramine after single administration in healthy male probands and patients with renal failure]. Med Klin 1993;88:129–133.

99. Lieberman JA, Cooper TB, Suckow RF, et al: Tricyclic antidepressant and metabolite levels in chronic renal failure. Clin Pharmacol Ther 1985;37:301–307.

100. Kennedy SH, Craven JL, Rodin GM: Major depression in renal dialysis patients: An open trial of antidepressant therapy [erratum appears in J Clin Psychiatry 1989;50:148]. J Clin Psychiatry 1989;50:60–63.

101. Sunderrajan S, Brooks CS, Sunderrajan EV: Nortriptyline-induced severe hyperventilation. Arch Intern Med 1985;145: 746–747.

102. Sandoz M, Vandel S, Vandel B, et al: Metabolism of amitriptyline in patients with chronic renal failure. Eur J Clin Pharmacol 1984;26:227–232.

103. Dawlilng S, Lynn K, Rosser R, Braithwaite R: The pharmacokinetics of nortriptyline in patients with chronic renal failure. Br J Clin Pharmacol 1981;12:39–45.

104. Worrall SP, Almond MK, Dhillon S: Pharmacokinetics of bupropion and its metabolites in haemodialysis patients who smoke. A single dose study. Nephron 2004;97:c83–c89.

105. Product information. Cymbalta capsules, duloxetine hydrochloride capsules. Eli Lilly and Company, Indianapolis, IN, 2004, 2007.

106. Bymaster FP, Lee TC, Knadler MP, et al: The dual transporter inhibitor duloxetine: A review of its preclinical pharmacology, pharmacokinetic profile, and clinical results in depression. Curr Pharm Des 2005;11:1475–1493.

107. Bennett WM, Aronoff GR, Golper TA, et al: Drug Prescribing in Renal Failure, 3rd ed. Philadelphia: American College of Physicians, 1994.

108. Fukunishi I, Kitaoka T, Shirai T, Watanabe S: Cardiac arrest caused by maprotiline in an elderly hemodialysis patient. Nephron 1998;78:225.

109. Fukunishi I, Kitaoka T, Shirai T, et al: A hemodialysis patient with trazodone-induced parkinsonism. Nephron 2002;90: 222–223.

110. Catanese B, Dionisio A, Barillari G: A comparative study of trazodone serum concentration in patients with normal or impaired renal function. Boll Chim Farm 1978;117:424–427.

111. Walcher J, Schoecklmann H, Renders L: Lithium acetate therapy in a maintenance hemodialysis patient. Kidney Blood Pressure Res 2004;27:200–202.

112. Moreiras Plaza M, Rodriguez Goyanes G, Cuina L, Alonso R: On the toxicity of valproic-acid. Clin Nephrol 1999;51: 187–189.

113. Dorson PG, Crismon ML: Chlorpromazine accumulation and sudden death in a patient with renal insufficiency. Drug Intell Clin Pharm 1988;22:776–778.

114. McAllister CJ, Scowden EB, Stone WJ: Toxic psychosis induced by phenothiazine administration in patients with chronic renal failure. Clin Nephrol 1978;10:191–195.

115. Sanga M, Shigemura J: Pharmacokinetics of haloperidol in patients on hemodialysis. Nihon Shinkei Seishin Yakurigaku Zasshi 1998;18:45–47.

116. Schaber G, Stevens I, Gaertner HJ, et al: Pharmacokinetics of clozapine and its metabolites in psychiatric patients: Plasma protein binding and renal clearance. Br J Clin Pharmacol 1998;46:453–459.

117. Product information. Abilify oral tablets, disintegrating tablets, solution, aripiprazole oral tablets, disintegrating tablets, solution. Bristol-Myers Squibb Company, Princeton, NJ, 2006.

118. Product information. Seroquel oral tablets, quetiapine fumarate oral tablets. AstraZeneca Pharmaceuticals, LP, Wilmington, DE, 2006.

119. Railton CJ, Kapur B, Koren G: Subtherapeutic risperidone serum concentrations in an adolescent during hemodialysis: A pharmacological puzzle. Ther Drug Monit 2005;27:558–561.

120. Schmith VD, Piraino B, Smith RB, Kroboth PD: Alprazolam in end-stage renal disease. II. Pharmacodynamics. Clin Pharmacol Ther 1992;51:533–540.

121. Mahmood I, Sahajwalla C: Clinical pharmacokinetics and pharmacodynamics of buspirone, an anxiolytic drug. Clin Pharmacokinet 1999;36:277–287.

122. Joy MS: Clonazepam: Benzodiazepine therapy for the restless legs syndrome. ANNA J 1997;24:686–689.

123. Swart EL, de Jongh J, Zuideveld KP, et al: Population pharmacokinetics of lorazepam and midazolam and their metabolites in intensive care patients on continuous venovenous hemofiltration. Am J Kidney Dis 2005;45:360–371.

124. Product information. Lunesta, eszopiclone. Sepracor, Marlborough, MA, 2005.

125. Product information. Sonata oral capsules, zaleplon oral capsules. King Pharmaceuticals, Inc, Bristol, TN, 2004.

126. Product information. Ambien oral tablets, zolpidem tartrate oral tablets. Sanofi-Aventis US, LLC, Bridgewater, NJ, 2007.

127. Product information. Rozerem tablets, ramelteon tablets. Takeda Pharmaceuticals America, Inc., Lincolnshire, IL, 2005.

128. Kandrotas RJ, Oles KS, Gal P, Love JM: Carbamazepine clearance in hemodialysis and hemoperfusion. DICP 1989;23:137–140.

129. Dogukan A, Aygen B, Berilgen MS, et al: Gabapentin-induced coma in a patient with renal failure. Hemodial Int 2006;10:168–169.

130. Manenti L, Vaglio A, Costantino E, et al: Gabapentin in the treatment of uremic itch: An index case and a pilot evaluation. J Nephrol 2005;18:86–91.

131. Zhang C, Glenn DG, Bell WL, O'Donovan CA: Gabapentin-induced myoclonus in end-stage renal disease. Epilepsia 2005;46:156–158.

132 Gunal AI, Ozalp G, Yoldas TK, et al: Gabapentin therapy for pruritus in haemodialysis patients: A randomized, placebo-controlled, double-blind trial. Nephrol Dial Transplant 2004;19:3137–3139.

133. Micozkadioglu H, Ozdemir FN, Kut A, et al: Gabapentin versus levodopa for the treatment of restless legs syndrome in hemodialysis patients: An open-label study. Ren Fail 2004;26:393–397.

134. Penumalee S, Kissner PZ, Migdal SD: Gabapentin-induced hypoglycemia in a long-term peritoneal dialysis patient. Am J Kidney Dis 2003;42:E3–E5.

135. Jones H, Aguila E, Farber HW: Gabapentin toxicity requiring intubation in a patient receiving long-term hemodialysis. Ann Intern Med 2002;137:74.

136. Bassilios N, Launay-Vacher V, Khoury N, et al: Gabapentin neurotoxicity in a chronic haemodialysis patient. Nephrol Dial Transplant 2001;16:2112–2113.

137. Blum RA, Comstock TJ, Sica DA, et al: Pharmacokinetics of gabapentin in subjects with various degrees of renal function. Clin Pharmacol Ther 19994;56:154–159.

138. McBryde KD, Wilcox J, Kher KK: Hyperphosphatemia due to fosphenytoin in a pediatric ESRD patient. Pediatr Nephrol 2005;20:1182–1185.

139. Lau AH, Kronfol NO: Effect of continuous hemofiltration on phenytoin elimination. Ther Drug Monit 1994;16:53–57.

140. Porto I, John EG, Heilliczer J: Removal of phenobarbital during continuous cycling peritoneal dialysis in a child. Pharmacotherapy 1997;17:832–835.

141. Product information: Lyrica, pregabalin. Pfizer, New York, NY, 2005.

142. Randinitis EJ, Posvar EL, Alvey CW, et al: Pharmacokinetics of pregabalin in subjects with various degrees of renal function. J Clin Pharmacol 2003;43:277–283.

143. Pellecchia MT, Vitale C, Sabatini M, et al: Ropinirole as a treatment of restless legs syndrome in patients on chronic hemodialysis: An open randomized crossover trial versus levodopa sustained release. Clin Neuropharmacol 2004;27:178–181.

144. Janzen L, Rich JA, Vercaigne LM: An overview of levodopa in the management of restless legs syndrome in a dialysis population: Pharmacokinetics, clinical trials, and complications of therapy. Ann Pharmacother 1999;33:86–92.

145. Wootton R, Soul-Lawton J, Rolan PE, et al: Comparison of the pharmacokinetics of lamotrigine in patients with chronic renal failure and healthy volunteers. Br J Clin Pharmacol 1997;43:23–27.

146. Product information: Lamictal, lamotrigine. GlaxoSmithKline, Research Triangle Park, NC, 2004.

Further Reading

Cohen LM, Levy NB, Tessier E, Germain M: Renal disease. In Levenson JL (ed): Textbook of Psychosomatic Medicine. Washington, DC: American Psychiatric Publishing, 2005, pp 483–493.

Finkelstein FO, Finkelstein SH: Depression in chronic dialysis patients: Assessment and treatment. Nephrol Dial Transplant 2000;15:191–192.

Kimmel PL, Tharner M, Richard CM, et al: Psychiatric illness in patients with end-stage renal disease. Am J Med 1998;105:214–221.

Levy NB: Psychiatric considerations in the primary medical care of the patient with renal failure. Adv Ren Replace Ther 2000;7:231–238.

Novak M, Shapiro CM, Mendelssohn D, Istvan M: Diagnosis and management of insomnia in dialysis patients. Semin Dial 2006;199:25–31.

Chapter 74

Measures to Improve Quality of Life in End-Stage Renal Disease Patients

Catherine Blake and William D. Plant

BACKGROUND

Health outcomes in end-stage renal disease (ESRD) have traditionally been measured in terms of morbidity and mortality. The focus has broadened in recent years to an increase in emphasis on patient-reported outcomes. In addition to sustaining life, the success of renal replacement therapy may now be considered in terms of maintenance and improvement of health status and quality of life (QOL).[1–3] The change in emphasis is based on the principle that health is "a state of complete physical, mental and social well-being and not merely the absence of disease and infirmity."[4]

Health is, therefore, a personal and abstract concept, influenced by both medical and nonmedical factors.[5] It can neither be measured directly nor can its essence be captured using single variables such as physiologic measures of organ function.[6–8] Multidimensional assessment of health is required, and the patient's own perception of well-being and QOL is a vital component.[6,9,10]

DEFINING QUALITY OF LIFE

QOL is a difficult concept to describe, with no single operational definition. This causes difficulties when interpreting results and comparing studies.[7,11] The terms functional status, health status, and QOL are often used interchangeably and are (incorrectly) considered by many sources to define similar constructs.[12] Measures of functional status are largely concerned with physical health, based on measurement of disability. Health status and QOL are far broader concepts, encompassing both the physical, psychological, and social dimensions of health.[13,14] QOL includes the personal beliefs, values, perceptions, and responses that are exclusive to each individual within the context of his or her unique social environment.[7]

The term health-related QOL is used to refer specifically to the physical, psychological, and social dimensions of health.[15] For the purpose of this text, QOL is defined as a concept that takes account of the multidimensional nature of a person's well-being, reflecting the physical, psychological, and social dimensions of health, which is influenced by personal beliefs, experiences, and expectations as well as socioeconomic and cultural factors. This definition is consistent with the World Health Organization's International Classification of Functioning, Disability and Health.[16]

MEASURING QUALITY OF LIFE

Personal subjective perceptions are key to QOL assessments, which should evaluate daily-life performance in physical, psychological, and social dimensions.[9,15,17–19] Numerous QOL scales exist. Selection (generic vs. disease specific, self-report vs. interview, single item vs. battery, preference-based or utility indices) should reflect the purpose of measurement and the target patient group, and the validity, reliability, and responsiveness of the instrument should be established. Disease-specific instruments are generally more sensitive to changes in the target population and may be more useful for sequential monitoring of individual patients or in clinical trials; generic instruments are of greater value when comparing groups of patients with different conditions and when relating results from patients to characteristics of the general population.[14] Single-index, preference-based, and utility scores are useful for multivariate and economic analyses,[20–24] but multi-item profiles emphasize the diverse aspects of QOL and allow a broader personal and clinical perspective.[8,14,23]

QOL instruments are thus useful for characterizing patient groups, discriminating between groups at one point in time, monitoring change over time, predicting outcomes, and economic analysis.[6]

QUALITY OF LIFE IN END-STAGE RENAL DISEASE

Studies reporting QOL in renal patients were first published in the 1980s,[25–27] and interest in QOL outcome measurement for predialysis, dialysis, and transplant groups has grown dramatically since then.[17,28–36] PubMed searches for "Dialysis AND Quality of Life" and "Renal Transplant AND Quality of

Life" currently produce 1997 and 926 citations, respectively. The variation in the type and number of instruments used is notable; some studies have focused on one dimension only, whereas others consider global QOL.[29] Commonly reported multidimensional measures include the Short Form 36 health survey,[37] and the Kidney Disease Quality of Life Questionnaire.[38,39] The Kidney Disease Quality of Life Questionnaire is an increasingly widely used instrument; in particular, it has been rendered into 24 language/cultural translations and been validated in a range of countries.

There is unequivocal evidence that QOL is impaired in dialysis patients compared with the general population.[40–48] Transplant recipients also demonstrate impaired QOL, although this is not as marked as in dialysis groups.[34,35,49–52] Limitations are most marked in the physical and social dimensions, whereas mental health scores tend to remain comparable with those in healthy individuals.[46,53,54] The maintenance of high psychological well-being in the majority of ESRD patients may result from an alteration in health values and expectations with chronic disease.[54–56] However between 20% and 30% of ESRD patients report significant psychological distress and depression.[43,57]

FACTORS ASSOCIATED WITH DIFFERENCES IN QUALITY OF LIFE IN END-STAGE RENAL DISEASE

Factors associated with differences in QOL in ESRD have been identified mainly by cross-sectional studies, which allow comparisons between groups based on existing clinical and sociodemographic characteristics. Many of these report univariate relationships only, whereas others have used multivariate analysis to identify independent associations with QOL. Several prospective single-group and case-control studies using QOL indices as outcome measures have been conducted, and the number of randomized, controlled trials is growing. Problems arise when comparing studies because of the considerable diversity in methodology, definition of QOL, choice of measurement instrument, and sample characteristics. Direct relationships between measures of clinical status and QOL may not always exist, and variables affecting QOL are often interrelated. Broadly speaking, these may be divided into sociodemographic variables, clinical variables, and comorbid medical variables.

Relationships between these characteristics and the multidimensional Short Form 36, and Kidney Disease Quality of Life questionnaires are summarized in Table 74-1, and a sample of randomized, controlled clinical trials reporting QOL outcomes in predialysis and ESRD groups is presented in Table 74-2.

The main sociodemographic factors associated with QOL are age, gender, socioeconomic status, income, employment, and educational level, whereas the relationship with ethnicity is variable. Aging of the ESRD population is a worldwide trend, and this phenomenon brings older patients with greater comorbidity to renal replacement therapy.[58] In general, older age is associated with declining physical function, but when combined with the physical sequelae of chronic renal insufficiency (cardiovascular, neurologic, myopathic, and skeletal), the physical dimension of QOL is especially compromised in this older ESRD group.[40,59] Physical limitations are, however, universally reported in ESRD patients of all ages, to varying degrees. There is now a significant body of evidence that

strongly supports exercise as an effective therapy to ameliorate the physical impact of ESRD and improve QOL for dialysis and transplant cohorts.[60,61]

Renal transplantation is associated with improved QOL, but this in part reflects patient selection. There are conflicting reports regarding the benefit of peritoneal dialysis over hemodialysis. A 2004 Cochrane review concluded that there was not enough evidence to indicate significant differences in QOL between dialysis modalities.[62] Early referral for specialist treatment, adequacy of dialysis, maintenance of nutritional indices, correction of anemia, management of symptoms, and prescription of exercise are the main clinical factors associated with better QOL. Severity of comorbid illness is a strong predictor of poorer QOL. Other factors affecting QOL are perceived burden of illness and the degree of social support.

RECOMMENDATIONS

QOL measurement is a valuable adjunct to objective clinical assessment in ESRD and recent Cochrane reviews have highlighted the need to include QOL outcomes in clinical trial design.[62–64] Close relationships exist between self-reported QOL and morbidity and mortality outcomes,[65–73] and these subjective measures may even be better predictors of outcome than clinical parameters.[43,74] There is also growing evidence that self-assessed physical and psychosocial well-being influences compliance and survival.[64,73,75,76]

The inclusion of QOL assessment in the routine management of ESRD patients offers several advantages. Specific patient problems may be identified, thus directing clinical intervention to alleviate the symptom burden affecting the patient's life. For example, older patients and those reporting specific physical problems will benefit from referral for physical therapy and targeted physical rehabilitation.

Through formal QOL assessment, nonmedical factors such as patient satisfaction, personal beliefs, and social and environmental issues affecting QOL may be highlighted and ways of improving quality of care identified. QOL assessment fosters more patient-centered treatment, enhancing communication between the patient and the health care team, and there is evidence that patient empowerment results in better outcomes.[77] Serial QOL measurement is valuable for patient surveillance over time, and QOL assessment may direct health care planning and quality assurance initiatives.

Factors to consider when attempting to improve QOL are summarized in Figure 74-1, and these reflect the five Es of renal rehabilitation identified by the Life Options Rehabilitation Council: education, encouragement, employment, exercise, and evaluation.[78] Evaluation and regular reassessment are central to any initiative aimed at improving QOL, and early referral to specialist multidisciplinary nephrology services is crucial. Adequacy of dialysis, correction of anemia, careful management of comorbidity, maintenance of nutritional status, and exercise programs designed to enhance physical fitness are key factors in physical management. Exercise prescription is a routine part of patient management in some centers, aimed at improving physical function and QOL in addition to reducing cardiovascular risk,[79–81] and exercise counseling of patients by nephrologists should be promoted.[60,81–83] There is ongoing research on the optimal dose, duration, and setting for exercise, but the current consensus is that individually tailored,

Table 74-1   Factors Affecting Quality of Life in End-Stage Renal Disease

Sociodemographic Variables

Age of patient

Older	↓ Physical health scores[45,46,56]
Younger	↓ Mental health scores[45,46,48,65,96]

Sex: female	↓ Global QOL scores[65,97–99]
Lower educational level	↓ global QOL scores[45,50,65,66,96]
Lower socioeconomic group	↓ Global QOL scores[65,96,97]
Employment: unemployed	↓ Global QOL scores[46,66,100]
Higher income/health insurance	↑ Global QOL scores[66,100,101]

Social Support

Living alone	↓ Mental health scores[48]
Married	↑ Social function scores[52]
Supportive relationship	↑ Global QOL scores[5]

Race

UK: Asian vs. European UK dialysis patients	↓ Global QOL scores[97]
US: African American vs. white	↑ Global QOL scores[102–106]
International: Japan vs. Europe and US	↑ Physical QOL scores[105] ↑ Disease burden
US: Native American vs. white	↑ Physical health scores[106] ↓ Mental health scores
US: Hispanic vs. white	↑ Physical health scores[106] ↓ Mental health scores

Clinical Variables

Treatment modality

Transplant vs. dialysis	↑ Global QOL scores[41,44,51,52,96,98,99,107,108]
Home HD and PD vs. in-center HD	↑ Global QOL scores[42,44]
HD vs. PD	Same global QOL scores[109,110]
PD vs. HD	↑ Mental health status[42,111]
APD vs. CAPD	Same QOL scores[112,113]
	Cochrane review
	APD ↑ psychosocial benefit[63]

CAPD vs. home or in-center HD	Cochrane review: same[62]
Preparation for dialysis: early referral	Better global QOL scores[100,114,115]
Time since transplantation: longer duration	↓ Global QOL scores[51]
Low serum albumin	↓ Global QOL scores[45,48,65,66,116]
Nutritional status: low	↓ Physical health scores[117–119]
Anemia: low hemoglobin/hematocrit	↓ Global QOL scores[42,51]
Dialysis dose and efficacy: better Kt/V/higher dose	↑ Global QOL scores[48,120–122]
Low serum creatinine	↑ Global QOL scores[107]

Table 74-1 Factors Affecting Quality of Life in End-Stage Renal Desease—cont'd

Comorbidity	
Complex comorbidity	↓ Global QOL scores[41,42,44,51,96,97]
Diabetes mellitus	↓ Global QOL scores[45]
Cardiovascular disease	↓ Global QOL scores[48,65]
COPD	↓ Global QOL scores[48]
Musculoskeletal disease	↓ Physical status scores[46]
Erectile dysfunction	↓ Global QOL scores[123,124]
Other	
Severe physical symptoms	↓ Global QOL scores[74]
Pain	↓ Global QOL scores[125,126]
Restless legs syndrome	↓ Global QOL scores[127–129]
Sleep disturbance	↓ Global QOL scores[47,127,128,130,131]
Dialysis symptoms	↓ Global QOL scores[47]
High burden of disease	↓ Global QOL scores[47]

APD, automated peritoneal dialysis; CAPD, continuous ambulatory peritoneal dialysis; COPD, chronic obstructive pulmonary disease; HD, hemodialysis; PD, peritoneal dialysis.

Table 74-2 Randomized Controlled Trials of Interventions to Improve Quality of Life

Intervention	Sample	Outcome in Intervention Group	Ref.
Erythropoietin			
EPO vs. placebo	Predialysis (N = 603)	↑ Physical function ↑ General health	Drueke et al[132]
EPO doses to achieve normal vs. subnormal Hgb	HD, PD, and predialysis (N = 416)	Dialysis patients ↓ Physical symptoms, fatigue, depression, and frustration in normal Hgb group	Furuland et al[133]
EPO doses to achieve high target Hgb vs. low target Hgb	Predialysis (N = 1432)	Same change in QOL both groups Higher risk of adverse events with high target Hgb	Singh et al[134]
EPO doses to achieve normal Hgb vs. low target Hgb	HD (N = 14)	↑ QOL normal target Hgb group	McMahon et al[135]
EPO vs. placebo	PD (N = 152)	↑ QOL EPO group	Nissenson et al[136]
EPO vs. control	Predialysis (N = 83)	↑ QOL in physical and vitality domains in EPO group	Revicki et al[137]
EPO doses to achieve normal vs. subnormal Hgb	HD: placebo (N = 40) Normalized Hgb (N = 40) Subnormal Hgb (N = 38)	↑ QOL both EPO groups vs. placebo	Canadian Erythropoietin Study[138]

Continued

Table 74-2 Randomized Controlled Trials of Interventions to Improve Quality of Life—cont'd

Intervention	Sample	Outcome in Intervention Group	Ref.
Carnitine			
Carnitine vs. placebo	HD (N = 50)	↑ QOL scores in physical domains in carnitine group	Steiner et al[139]
Carnitine vs. placebo	HD (N = 20)	↑ QOL scores in carnitine group	Rathod et al[140]
Gabapentin vs. Levodopa Restless Legs Syndrome	HD (N = 15)	↑ QOL scores in gabapeatin group	Micozkadioglu et al[141]
Glucose in Dialysis Fluid vs. Usual Care	HD (N = 34)	No change in QOL; decreased blood pressure decreased variability in blood glucose levels	Sangill and Pedersen[142]
Predilution Online Hemofiltration vs. Low-Flux HD	Dialysis (N = 40)	↑ QOL scores: hemofiltration	Beerenhout et al[143]
High-Dose HD	HD	High-dose HD: ↑ Physical QOL scores and ↓ pain	Unruh et al[121]
Exercise Training			
Resistance exercise ± nandrolone decanoate	HD (N = 79)	↑ QOL scores in physical domains with exercise	Johansen et al[144]
Moderate conditioning exercise + counseling vs. control	HD (N = 96)	↑ QOL scores	van Vilsteren et al[145]
Outpatient vs. intradialytic exercise	HD (N = 48)	↑ QOL in both exercise groups	Kouidi et al[146]
Intradialytic exercise vs. control	HD (N = 13)	8-wk exercise program in high function patients: no effect on QOL	Parsons et al[147]
Exercise vs. control	HD (N = 33)	Exercise group ↑ QOL scores in physical domains	Molsted et al[148]
Progressive exercise vs. nonprogressive exercise	HD	12-wk exercise program high function patients: no effect on QOL	DePaul et al[149]
Exercise vs. usual care	Transplant recipients (N = 167)	Exercise group ↑ QOL scores in physical domains	Painter et al[150]
Exercise ± normalize hematocrit	HD (N = 65) 4 groups, 2 exercise	Exercise groups ↑ QOL scores in physical domains	Painter et al[151]
Physical rehabilitation vs. control	HD (N = 82)	Exercise group ↑ QOL scores	Tawney et al[152]
Exercise coaching and counseling vs. control	Predialysis (N = 18) HD (N = 18)	Exercise group ↑ QOL scores Greater effect in predialysis	Fitts et al[153]
Exercise vs. control	HD (N = 31)	Exercise group ↑ QOL and depression scores	Kouidi et al[154]

EPO, erythropoietin; HD, hemodialysis; Hgb, hemoglobin; PD, peritoneal dialysis; QOL, quality of life.

submaximal exercise prescribed by a qualified health professional is safe, effective, and feasible for all ESRD patients and can be carried out both during dialysis as an outpatient and in the community.[84–89] Sustained benefits require long-term commitment to exercise, so motivation through regular monitoring is necessary, and supervised settings generally demonstrate

greater improvement. There are, however, barriers to exercise for the patient and resource issues for the health care provider.[61]

The importance of diagnosis and management of depression is increasingly emphasized in the literature, and the role that that patient's own coping mechanisms and psychosocial status play is recognized.[74,90–93] In this regard, education,

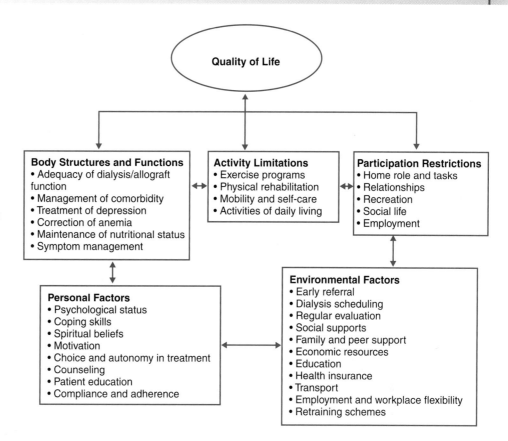

Figure 74-1 Considerations for improving quality of life in end-stage renal disease patients: International Classification of Functioning Disability and Health (ICF) framework.

patient involvement in decision making, counseling, motivation, and the promotion of a positive ethos of rehabilitation are necessary components in psychological management and in ensuring compliance. Vocational rehabilitation is an important consideration in social well-being, and every effort should be made to keep patients employed or allow them to return to work. Efforts to enhance QOL therefore require a multidimensional and multidisciplinary approach, and this process should be started in the predialysis phase of CKD.[94,95]

References

1. Apolone G, Mosconi P: Review of the concept of quality of life assessment and discussion of the present trend in clinical research. Nephrol Dial Transplant 1998;13(Suppl 1):65–69.
2. Reitig RA, Sadler JH, Mayer KB, et al: Assessing health and quality of life outcomes in dialysis: A report on an Institute of Medicine workshop. Am J Kidney Dis 1997;30:140–155.
3. Schrier RW, Burrows-Hudson S, Diamond L, et al: Measuring, managing and improving quality in the end-stage renal disease treatment setting: Committee statement. Am J Kidney Dis 1994;24:383–388.
4. World Health Organization: The First Ten Years of the World Health Organization. Geneva: WHO, 1958, p 459.
5. Rosenberger J, Van Dijk JP, Nagyova I, et al: Do dialysis and transplantation-related medical factors affect perceived health status? Nephrol Dial Transplant 2005;20:2153–2158.
6. Guyatt GH, Feeney DH, Patrick DL: Measuring quality of life. Ann Intern Med 1993;118:622–629.
7. Leplege A, Hunt S: The problem of quality of life in medicine. JAMA 1997;278:47–50.
8. Woodend AK, Nair RC, Tang AS: Definition of quality from a patient versus health care professional perspective. Int J Rehabil Res 1997;20:71–80.
9. Muldoon MF, Barger SD, Flory JD, Manuck SB: What are quality of life measurements measuring? Br Med J 1998;316:542–545.
10. Slevin ML, Plant H, Lynch D, et al: Who should measure quality of life, the doctor or the patient? Br J Cancer 1988;57:109–112.
11. Gill TM, Feinstein AR: A critical appraisal of the quality of life measures. JAMA 1994;272:619–626.
12. Dijkers MPJM, Whiteneck G, El-Jaroudi R: Measures of social outcomes in disability research. Arch Phys Med Rehabil 2000;81 (Suppl 2):S46–S52.
13. Keith RA: Functional status and health status. Arch Phys Med Rehabil 1994;75:478–483.
14. McDowell I, Newell C: Measuring Health: A Guide to Rating Scales and Questionnaires, 2nd ed. New York: Oxford University Press, 1996, pp 381–383.
15. Testa MA, Simonson DC: Assessment of quality of life outcomes. N Engl J Med 1996;334:835–840.
16. World Health Organization: International Classification of Functioning, Disability and Health. Geneva: WHO, 2001.
17. Bergner M: Quality of life, health status, and clinical research. Med Care 1989;27(Suppl 3):S148–S156.
18. Gokal R: Quality of life in patients undergoing renal replacement therapy. Kidney Int 1993;40(Suppl 1):S23–S27.
19. Kimmel PL: Just whose quality of life is it anyway? Controversies and consistencies in measurement of quality of life. Kidney Int 2000;57(Suppl 74):S113–S120.
20. Sennfalt K, Magnusson M, Carlsson P: Comparison of hemodialysis and peritoneal dialysis—a cost-utility analysis. Perit Dial Int 2002;22:39–47.
21. McFarlane PA, Bayoumi AM, Pierratos A, Redelmeier DA: The impact of home nocturnal hemodialysis on end-stage renal disease therapies: A decision analysis. Kidney Int 2006;69:798–805.
22. Brazier JE, Roberts J: The estimation of a preference-based measure of health from the SF-12. Med Care 2004;42:851–859.

23. Coons SJ, Rao S, Keininger DL, Hays RD: A comparative review of generic quality-of-life instruments. Pharmacoeconomics 2000;17:13–35.

24. Gorodetskaya I, Zenios S, McCulloch CE, et al: Health-related quality of life and estimates of utility in chronic kidney disease. Kidney Int 2005;68:2801–2808.

25. Simmons RG, Anderson C, Kamstra L: Comparison of quality of life of patients on continuous ambulatory peritoneal dialysis, hemodialysis, and after transplantation. Am J Kidney Dis 1984;4:253–255.

26. Evans RW, Manninen DL, Garrison LP Jr, et al: The quality of life of patients with end stage renal disease. N Engl J Med 1985;312:553–559.

27. Kutner NG, Brogan D, Kutner MH: End-stage renal disease treatment modality and patients' quality of life. Longitudinal assessment. Am J Nephrol 1986;6:396–402.

28. Edgell ET, Coons SJ, Carter WB, et al: A review of health-related quality-of-life measures used in end-stage renal disease. Clin Ther 1996;18:887–938.

29. Cagney KA, Wu AW, Fink NE, et al: Formal literature review of quality-of-life instruments used in end-stage renal disease. Am J Kidney Dis 2000;36:327–336.

30. Fukahara S, Yamazaki S, Marumo F, et al: Health related quality-of-life of predialysis patients with chronic renal failure. Nephron Clin Pract 2007;105:c1–c8.

31. Perlman RL, Finkelstein FO, Roys E, et al: Quality of life in chronic kidney disease (CKD): A cross-sectional analysis in the Renal Research Institute-CKD study. Am J Kidney Dis 2005;45:658–666.

32. Kutner NG, Zhang R, Barnhart H, et al: Health status and quality of life reported by incident patients after 1 year on hemodialysis or peritoneal dialysis. Nephrol Dial Transplant 2005;20:2159–3267.

33. Kimmel PL, Patel SS: Quality of life in patients with chronic kidney disease; focus on end-stage renal disease treated with hemodialysis. Semin Nephrol 2006;26:68–79.

34. Wu AW, Fink ME, Marsh-Manzi JV, et al: Changes in quality of life during hemodialysis and peritoneal dialysis treatment: Generic and disease-specific measures. J Am Soc Nephrol 2004;15:743–753.

35. Fiebiger W, Mitterbauer C, Oberbauer R: Health related quality of life outcomes after kidney transplantation. Health Qual Outcomes 2004;2:2.

36. Neipp M, Karavul B, Jackobs S, et al: Quality of life in adult transplant recipients more than 15 years after kidney transplantation. Transplantation 2006;81:1640–1644.

37. Ware JE, Snow KK, Kosinski M, Gandek B: SF-36 Health Survey Manual and Interpretation Guide. Boston: Nimrod Press, 1993.

38. Hays RD, Kallich JD, Mapes DL, et al: Development of the kidney disease quality of life (KDQOL) instrument. Qual Life Res 1994;3:329–338.

39. Bartofi S, Molnar MZ, Almasi C, et al: Validation of the Kidney Disease Quality of Life-Short Form questionnaire in kidney transplant patients. J Psychosom Res 2006;60:495–504.

40. Altintepe L, Levendoglu F, Okudan N, et al: Physical disability, psychological status and health-related quality of life in older hemodialysis patients with age-matched controls. Hemodial Int 2006;10:260–266.

41. Khan IH, Garratt AM, Kumar A, et al: Patients' perception of health on renal replacement therapy: Evaluation using a new instrument. Nephrol Dial Transplant 1995;10:684–689.

42. Merkus MP, Jager KJ, Dekker FW, et al: Quality of life in patients on chronic dialysis: Self-assessment 3 months after the start of treatment. The Necosad Study Group. Am J Kidney Dis 1997;29:584–592.

43. DeOreo PB: Hemodialysis patients assessed functional health status predicts continued survival, hospitalisation and dialysis attendance compliance. Am J Kidney Dis 1997;30:204–212.

44. Merkus MP, Jager KJ, Dekker FW, et al: Quality of life over time in dialysis: The Netherlands Cooperative Study on the Adequacy of Dialysis. NECOSAD Study Group. Kidney Int 1999;56:720–728.

45. Mingardi G, Cornalba L, Cortinovis E, et al: Health-related quality of life in dialysis patients. A report from an Italian study using the SF-36 Health Survey. DIA-QOL Group. Nephrol Dial Transplant 1999;14:1503–1510.

46. Blake C, Codd MB, Cassidy A, et al: Physical function, employment and quality of life in end-stage renal disease. J Nephrol 2000;13:142–149.

47. Carmichael P, Popoola J, John I, et al: Assessment of quality of life in a single centre dialysis population using the KDQOL-SF questionnaire. Qual Life Res 2000;9:195–205.

48. Mittal SK, Ahern L, Flaster E, et al: Self-assessed physical and mental function of haemodialysis patients. Nephrol Dial Transplant 2001;16:1387–1394.

49. Shield CF III, McGrath MM, Goss TF: Assessment of health-related quality of life in kidney transplant patients receiving tacrolimus (FK560)-based versus cyclosporine-base immunosuppression. FK560 Kidney Transplant Study Group. Transplantation 1997;64:1738–1743.

50. Tsuji-Hayashi Y, Fukuhara S, Green J, et al: Health-related quality of life among renal-transplant recipients in Japan. Transplantation 1999;68:1331–1335.

51. Rebollo P, Ortega F, Baltar JM, et al: Health related quality of life (HRQOL) of kidney transplant patients: Variables that influence it. Clin Transpl 2000;14:199–207.

52. Chisholm MA, Spivey CA, Nus AV: Influence of economic and demographic factors on quality of life in renal transplant recipients. Clin Transplant 2007;21:285–293.

53. Kutner NG: Renal rehabilitation: Where are the data? A progress report. Semin Dial 1996;9:387–389.

54. Lamping DL, Constantinovici N, Roderick P, et al: Clinical outcomes, quality of life, and costs in the North Thames Dialysis Study of elderly people on dialysis: A prospective cohort study. Lancet 2000;356:1543–1550.

55. Dolan P: The effect of experience of illness on health status valuations. J Clin Epidemiol 1996;49:551–564.

56. Singer MA, Hopman WA, MacKenzie TA: Physical functioning and mental health in patients with chronic medical conditions. Qual Life Res 1999;8:687–691.

57. Wuerth D, Finkelstein SH, Finkelstein FO: The identification and treatment of depression in patients maintained on dialysis. Semin Dial 2005;18:142–146.

58. Apostolou T: Quality of life in the elderly patients on dialysis. Int Urol Nephrol 2007;39:679–683.

59. Sterky E, Stegmayr BG: Elderly patients on haemodialysis have 50% less functional capacity than gender and age-matched healthy subjects. Scand J Urol Nephrol 2005;39:423–430.

60. Cheema BS, Singh MA: Exercise training in patients receiving maintenance hemodialysis: A systematic review of clinical trials. Am J Nephrol 2005;25:352–364.

61. Johansen KL: Exercise and chronic kidney disease: Current recommendations. Sports Med 2005;35:485–499.

62. Vale L, Cody J, Wallace S, et al: Continuous ambulatory peritoneal dialysis (CAPD) versus hospital or home haemodialysis for end-stage renal disease in adults. Cochrane Database Syst Rev 2004;4:CD003963.

63. Rabindranath K, Adams J, Ali T, et al: Continuous ambulatory peritoneal dialysis versus automated peritoneal dialysis for end-stage renal disease. Cochrane Database Syst Rev 2007;2:CD006515.

64. Macleod AM, Campbell M, Cody JD, et al: Cellulose, modified cellulose and synthetic membranes in the haemodialysis of patients with end-stage renal disease. Cochrane Database Syst Rev 2005;3:CD003234.

65. Harris LE, Luft FC, Rudy DW, et al: Clinical correlates of functional status in patients with chronic renal insufficiency. Am J Kidney Dis 1993;21:161–166.

66. Lopes AA, Bragg-Gresham JL, Goodkin DA, et al: Factors associated with health-related quality of life among hemodialysis patients in the DOPPS. Qual Life Res 2007;16:545–557.

67. Ifudu O, Paul HR, Homel P, et al: Predictive value of functional status for mortality in patients on maintenance hemodialysis. Am J Nephrol 1998;18:109–116.

68. Lopez Revuelta K, Garcia Lopez FJ, de Alvaro Moreno F, Alonso J: Perceived mental health at the start of dialysis as a predictor of morbidity and mortality in patients with end-stage renal disease (CALVIDIA Study). Nephrol Dial Transplant 2004;19:2347–2353.

69. McClellan WM, Anson C, Birkeli K, et al: Functional status and quality of life: Predictors of early mortality among patients entering treatment for end stage renal disease. J Clin Epidemiol 1991;44:83–89.

70. Morsh CM, Goncalves LF, Barros E: Health-related quality of life among haemodialysis patients—relationship with clinical indicators, morbidity and mortality. J Clin Nurs 2006;15:498–504.

71. Mapes DL, Lopes AA, Satayathum S, et al: Health-related quality of life as a predictor of mortality and hospitalization: The Dialysis Outcomes and Practice Patterns Study (DOPPS). Kidney Int 2003;64:339–349.

72. Knight EL, Ofsthun N, Teng M, et al: The association between mental health, physical function, and hemodialysis mortality. Kidney Int 2003;63:1843–1851.

73. Kimmel PL, Peterson RA, Weihs KL, et al: Multiple measures of depression predict mortality in a longitudinal study of chronic hemodialysis outpatients. Kidney Int 2000;57:2093–2098.

74. Merkus MP, Jager KJ, Dekker FW, et al: Predictors of poor outcome in chronic dialysis patients: The Netherlands Cooperative Study on the Adequacy of Dialysis. The NECOSAD Study Group. Am J Kidney Dis 2000;35:69–79.

75. DiMatteo MR, Lepper HS, Croghan TW: Depression is a risk factor for non-compliance with medical treatment: Meta-analysis of the effects of anxiety and depression on patient adherence. Arch Intern Med 2000;160:2101–2107.

76. Akman B, Uyar M, Afsar B, et al: Adherence, depression and quality of life in patients on a renal transplantation waiting list. Transpl Int 2007;20:682–687.

77. Tsay SL, Hung LO: Empowerment of patients with end-stage renal disease—a randomized controlled trial. Int J Nurs Stud 2004;41:59–65.

78. Life Options Rehabilitation Advisory Council: Renal Rehabilitation: Building Quality of Life. Madison, WI: Medical Education Institute, 1997.

79. Deligiannis A, Kouidi E, Tassoulas E, et al: Cardiac effects of exercise rehabilitation in hemodialysis patients. Int J Cardiol 2000;72:299–300.

80. Storer TW, Casaburi R, Sawelson S, Kopple JD: Endurance exercise training during haemodialysis improves strength, power, fatigability and physical performance in maintenance haemodialysis patients. Nephrol Dial Transplant 2005;20:1429–1437.

81. Painter P: Physical functioning in end-stage renal disease patients: Update 2005. Hemodial Int 2005;9:218–235.

82. Johansen KL, Sakkaa GK, Doyle J, et al: Exercise counseling practices among nephrologists caring for patients on dialysis. Am J Kidney Dis 2003;41:171–178.

83. Krause R, WGRR-European Working Group on Renal Rehabilitation and Exercise Physiology: Nephrologists' view on exercise training on chronic kidney disease. Clin Nephrol 2004;61(Suppl 1):S2–S4.

84. Cheema BS, O'Sullivan AJ, Chan M, et al: Progressive resistance training during hemodialysis: Rationale and method of a randomized-controlled trial. Hemodial Int 2006;10:303–310.

85. Parsons TL, Toffelmire EB, King-VanVlack CE: Exercise training during hemodialysis improves dialysis efficacy and physical performance. Arch Phys Med Rehabil 2006;87:680–687.

86. Daul AE, Schafers RF, Daul K, et al: Exercise during hemodialysis. Clin Nephrol 2004;61(Suppl 1):S26–S30.

87. Cheema BS, Smith BC, Singh MA: A rationale for intradialytic exercise training as standard clinical practice in ESRD. Am J Kidney Dis 2005;45:912–916.

88. Fuhrmann I, Krause R: Principles of exercising in patients with chronic kidney disease, on dialysis and for kidney transplant recipients. Clin Nephrol 2004;61(Suppl 1):S14–S25.

89. Johansen KL: Exercise in the end-stage-renal disease population. J Am Soc Nephrol 2007;18:1845–1854.

90. Svebak S, Kristoffersen B, Aasarod K: Sense of humor and survival among a county cohort of patients with end-stage renal failure: A two-year prospective study. Int J Psychiatry Med 2006;36:269–281.

91. Kimmel PL, Emont SL, Newmann JM, et al. ESRD patient quality of life: Symptoms, spiritual beliefs, psychosocial factors, and ethnicity. Am J Kidney Dis 2003;42:713–721.

92. Kutner NG, Zhang R, McClellan WM, et al: Psychosocial predictors of non-compliance in haemodialysis and peritoneal dialysis patients. Nephrol Dial Transplant 2002;17:93–99.

93. Patel SS, Shah VS, Peterson RA, et al: Psychosocial variables, quality of life, and religious beliefs in ESRD patients treated with hemodialysis. Am J Kidney Dis 2002;40:1013–1022.

94. Clyne N: The importance of exercise training in predialysis patients with chronic kidney disease. Clin Nephrol 2004;61(Suppl 1):S10–S13.

95. Horl WH: A need for an individualized approach to end-stage renal disease patients. Nephrol Dial Transplant 2002;17(Suppl 6):17–21.

96. Rebollo P, Ortega F, Baltar JM, et al: Health-related quality of life (HRQOL) in end stage renal disease (ESRD) patients over 65 years. Geriatr Nephrol Urol 1998;8:85–94.

97. Bakewell AB, Higgins RM, Edmunds ME: Does ethnicity influence perceived quality of life of patients on dialysis and following renal transplant? Nephrol Dial Transplant 2001;16:1395–1401.

98. Jofre R, Lopez-Gomez JM, Moreno F, et al: Changes in quality of life after renal transplantation. Am J Kidney Dis 1998;32:93–100.

99. Wight JP, Edwards L, Brazier J, et al: The SF-36 as an outcome measure of services for end stage renal failure. Qual Health Care 1998;7:209–221.

100. Caskey FJ, Wordsworth S, Ben T, et al: Early referral and planned initiation of dialysis: What impact on quality of life? Nephrol Dial Transplant 2003;18:1330–1338.

101. Chisholm MA, Spivey CA, Nus AV: Influence of economic and demographic factors on quality of life in renal transplant recipients. Clin Transplant 2007;21:285–293.

102. Unruh M, Miskulin D, Yan G, et al, HEMO Study Group: Racial differences in health-related quality of life among hemodialysis patients. Kidney Int 2004;65:1482–1491.

103. Hicks LS, Cleary PD, Epstein AM, et al: Differences in health related quality of life and treatment preferences among black and white patients with end-stage renal disease. Qual Life Res 2004;13:1129–1137.

104. Kutner NG, Devins GM: A comparison of the quality of life reported by elderly whites and elderly blacks on dialysis. Geriatr Nephrol Urol 1998;8:77–83

105. Mapes DL, Bragg-Gresham JL, Bommer J, et al: Health related quality of life in the Dialysis Outcomes and Practice Patterns Study (DOPPS). Am J Kidney Dis 2004;44(5 Suppl 2):54–60.

106. Lopes AA, Bragg-Gresham JL, Satayathum S, et al: Health-related quality of life and associated outcomes among hemodialysis patients of different ethnicities in the United States: The Dialysis Outcomes and Practice Patterns Study (DOPPS). Am J Kidney Dis 2003;41:605–615.

107. Fujisawa M, Ichikawa Y, Yoshiya K, et al: Assessment of health-related quality of life in renal transplant and hemodialysis patients using the SF-36 health survey. Urology 2000;56:201–206.

108. Gross CR, Limwattananon C, Matthees B, et al: Impact of transplantation on quality of life in patients with diabetes and renal dysfunction. Transplantation 2000;70:1736–1746.

109. Gokal R, Figueras M, Ollé A, et al: Outcomes in peritoneal dialysis and haemodialysis—a comparative assessment of survival and quality of life. Nephrol Dial Transplant 1999; 14(Suppl 6):S24–S30.

110. Manns B, Johnson JA, Taub K, et al: Quality of life in patients treated with hemodialysis or peritoneal dialysis: What are the important determinants? Clin Nephrol 2003;60:341–351.

111. Diaz-Buxo JA, Lowrie EG, Lew NL, et al: Quality of life evaluation using short form 36: Comparison of hemodialysis and peritoneal dialysis patients. Am J Kidney Dis 2000;35: 293–300.

112. Bro S, Bjorner JB, Tofte-Jensen P, et al: A prospective randomized multicenter study comparing APD and CAPD treatment. Perit Dial Int 1999;19:526–533.

113. De Wit GA, Merkus MP, Krediet RT, et al: A comparison of quality of life of patients on automated and continuous peritoneal dialysis. Perit Dial Int 2001;21:306–312.

114. Sesso R, Yoshihiro MM: Time of diagnosis of chronic renal failure and assessment of quality of life in hemodialysis patients. Nephrol Dial Transplant 1997;12:2111–2116.

115. Frimat L, Loos-Ayav C, Panescu V, et al: Early referral to a nephrologist is associated with better outcomes in type 2 diabetes patients with end-stage renal disease. Diabetes Metab 2004;30: 67–74.

116. Allen KL, Miskulin D, Yan G, et al: Association of nutritional markers with physical and mental health status in prevalent hemodialysis patients form the HEMO study. J Ren Nutr 2002;12: 160–169.

117. Kalender B, Ozdemir AC, Dervisoglu E, Ozdemir O: Quality of life in chronic kidney disease: Effects of treatment modality, depression, malnutrition and inflammation. Int J Clin Pract 2007;61:569–576.

118. Raimundo P, Ravasco P, Proenca V, et al: Does nutrition play a role in the quality of life of patients under chronic haemodialysis? Nutr Hosp 2006;21:139–144.

119. Dwyer JT, Larive B, Leung J, et al: Nutritional status affects quality of life in hemodialysis (HEMO) study patients at baseline. J Ren Nutr 2002;12:213–223.

120. Chen YC, Hung KY, Kao TW, et al: Relationship between dialysis adequacy and quality of life in long-term peritoneal dialysis patients. Perit Dial Int 2000;20:534–540.

121. Unruh M, Benz R, Greene T, et al: Effects of hemodialysis dose and membrane flux on health-related quality of life in the HEMO Study. Kidney Int 2004;66:355–366.

122. Martin CR, Thompson DR: Prediction of quality of life in patients with end-stage renal disease. Br J Health Psychol 2000;5:41–55.

123. Turk S, Guney I, Altintepe L, et al: Quality of life in male hemodialysis patients. Role of erectile dysfunction. Nephron Clin Pract 2004;96:c21–c27.

124. Rosas SE, Joffe M, Franklin E, et al: Association of decreased quality of life and erectile dysfunction in hemodialysis patients. Kidney Int 2003;64:232–238.

125. Nourbala MH, Hollisaaz MT, Nasiri M, et al: Pain affects health-related quality of life in kidney transplant recipients. Transplant Proc 2007;39:1126–1129.

126. Wasserfallen JB, Halabi G, Saudan P, et al: Quality of life on chronic dialysis: Comparison between haemodialysis and peritoneal dialysis. Nephrol Dial Transplant 2004;19:1594–1599.

127. Kawauchi A, Inoue Y, Hashimoto T, et al: Restless legs syndrome in hemodialysis patients: Health-related quality of life and laboratory data analysis. Clin Nephrol 2006;66:440–446.

128. Mucsi I, Molnar MZ, Ambrus C, et al: Restless legs syndrome, insomnia and quality of life in patients on maintenance dialysis. Nephrol Dial Transplant 2005;20:571–577.

129. Unruh ML, Levey AS, D'Ambrosio C, et al., Choices for Healthy Outcomes in Caring for End-Stage Renal Disease (CHOICE) Study: Restless legs symptoms among incident dialysis patients: Association with lower quality of life and shorter survival. Am J Kidney Dis 2004;43:900–909.

130. Walker S, Fine A, Kryger MH: Sleep complaints are common in a dialysis unit. Am J Kidney Dis 1995;26:751–756.

131. Erylimaz MM, Ozdemir C, Yurtman F, et al: Quality of sleep and quality of life in renal transplant patients. Transplant Proc 2005;37:2072–2076.

132. Drueke TB, Locatelli F, Clyne N, et al: Normalization of hemoglobin level in patients with chronic kidney disease and anemia. N Engl J Med 2006;355:2071–2084.

133. Furuland H, Linde T, Ahlmen J, et al: A randomized controlled trial of haemoglobin normalization with epoetin alfa in pre-dialysis and dialysis patients. Nephrol Dial Transplant 2003;18:353–361.

134. Singh AK, Szczech L, Tang KL, et al: CHOIR Investigators. Correction of anemia with epoetin alfa in chronic kidney disease. N Engl J Med 2006;16;355:2085–2098.

135. McMahon LP, Mason K, Skinner SL, et al: Effects of haemoglobin normalisation on quality of life and cardiovascular parameters in end-stage renal failure. Nephrol Dial Transplant 2000;15:1425–1430.

136. Nissenson AR, Korbet S, Faber M, et al: Multicentre trial of erythropoietin on peritoneal dialysis. J Am Soc Nephrol 1995; 5:1517–1519.

137. Revicki DA, Brown RE, Feeny DH, et al: Health-related quality of life associated with recombinant human erythropoietin therapy for predialysis chronic renal disease patients. Am J Kidney Dis 1995;25:548–554.

138. Canadian Erythropoietin Study: Association between recombinant erythropoietin and quality of life and exercise capacity of patients receiving haemodialysis. Br Med J 1990;300: 573–578.

139. Steiner AL, Davis AT, Spry L, et al: Carnitine treatment improved quality-of-life measure in a sample of Midwestern hemodialysis patients. J Parenter Enteral Nutr 2006;30:10–15.

140. Rathod R, Baig MS, Khandelwal PN, et al: Results of a single blind, randomized, placebo-controlled clinical trial to study the effect of intravenous L-carnitine supplementation on health-related quality of life in Indian patients on maintenance hemodialysis. Indian J Med Sci 2006;60:143–153.

141. Micozkadioglu H, Ozdemir FN, Kut A, et al: Gabapentin versus levodopa for the treatment of restless legs syndrome in hemodialysis patients: An open-label study. Ren Fail 2004;26:393–397.

142. Sangill M, Pedersen EB: The effect of glucose added to the dialysis fluid on blood pressure, blood glucose, and quality of life in hemodialysis patients: A placebo-controlled crossover study. Am J Kidney Dis 2006;47:636–643.

143. Beerenhout CH, Luik AJ, Jeuken-Mertens SG, et al: Pre-dilution on-line haemofiltration vs low-flux haemodialysis: A randomized prospective study. Nephrol Dial Transplant 2005;20:1155–1163.

144. Johansen KL, Painter PL, Sakkas GK, et al: Effects of resistance exercise training and nandrolone decanoate on body composition and muscle function among patients who receive hemodialysis: A randomized, controlled trial. J Am Soc Nephrol 2006;17:2307–2314.

145. van Vilsteren MC, de Greef MH, Huisman RM: The effects of a low-to-moderate intensity pre-conditioning exercise programme linked with exercise counselling for sedentary haemodialysis patients in The Netherlands: Results of a randomized clinical trial. Nephrol Dial Transplant 2005;20:141–146.

146. Kouidi E, Grekas D, Deligiannis A, Tourkantonis A: Outcomes of long-term exercise training in dialysis patients: Comparison

of two training programs. Clin Nephrol 2004;61(Suppl 1): S31–S38.

147. Parsons TL, Toffelmire EB, King-VanVlack CE: The effect of an exercise program during hemodialysis on dialysis efficacy, blood pressure and quality of life in end-stage renal disease (ESRD) patients. Clin Nephrol 2004;61:261–274.

148. Molsted S, Eidemak I, Sorensen HT, et al: Five months of physical exercise in hemodialysis patients: Effects on aerobic capacity, physical function and self-rated health. Nephron Clin Pract 2004;96:c76–c81.

149. DePaul V, Moreland J, Eager T, et al: The effectiveness of aerobic and muscle strength training in patients receiving hemodialysis and EPO: A randomized controlled trial. Am J Kidney Dis 2002;40:1219–1229.

150. Painter PL, Hector L, Ray K, et al: A randomized trial of exercise training after renal transplantation. Transplantation 2002;15:74: 42–48.

151. Painter P, Moore G, Carlson L, et al: Effects of exercise training plus normalization of hematocrit on exercise capacity and health-related quality of life. Am J Kidney Dis 2002;39: 257–265.

152. Tawney KW, Tawney PJW, Hladik G, et al: The Life Readiness Program: A physical rehabilitation program for patients on hemodialysis. Am J Kidney Dis 2000;36:581–591.

153. Fitts SS, Guthrie MR, Blagg CR: Exercise coaching and rehabilitation counseling improve quality of life for predialysis and dialysis patients. Nephron 1999;82:115–121.

154. Kouidi E, Iacovides A, Iordanidis P, et al: Exercise renal rehabilitation program: Psychosocial effects. Nephron 1997;77:152–158.

Further Reading

Cagney KA, Wu AW, Fink NE, et al: Formal literature review of quality-of-life instruments used in end-stage renal disease. Am J Kidney Dis 2000;36:327–336.

Cheema BS, Singh MA: Exercise training in patients receiving maintenance hemodialysis: A systematic review of clinical trials. Am J Nephrol 2005;25:352–364.

Johansen KL: Exercise in the end-stage renal disease population. J Am Soc Nephrol 2007; 18:1845–1854.

Kalantar-Zadeh K, Unruh M: Health related quality of life in patients with chronic kidney disease. Int Urol Nephrol 2005;37:367–378.

Kimmel PL: Just whose quality of life is it anyway? Controversies and consistencies in measurement of quality of life. Kidney Int 2000;57(Suppl 74):S113–S120.

Kimmel PL, Patel SS: Quality of life in patients with chronic kidney disease: Focus on end-stage renal disease treated with hemodialysis. Semin Nephrol 2006;26:68–79.

Kutner NG, Jassal SV: Quality of life and rehabilitation of elderly dialysis patients. Semin Dial 2002;15:107–112.

Life Options Rehabilitation Advisory Council: Renal Rehabilitation: Building Quality of Life. Madison, WI: Medical Education Institute, Inc, 1997.

Painter P: Physical functioning in end-stage renal disease patients: Update 2005. Hemodial Int 2005;9:218–235.

Chapter 75

Palliative and Supportive Care

Sara N. Davison, Lewis M. Cohen, and Michael J. Germain

BACKGROUND

Despite technological advancements, more than 80,000 dialysis patients die each year in the United States with an unadjusted mortality rate of 22% to 25%.[1] The age- and sex-matched life expectancy is only 16% to 37% that of the general population. Cardiovascular complications account for at least half of the deaths, and the risk of death for a 45-year-old patient is 20 times that of a person of the same age not receiving dialysis. On average, a 50-year-old dialysis patient will live 5.2 additional years and a 75-year-old could expect to live 2.4 more years.[1] Symptom burdens are very high in this population,[2–6] and the dying experience for patients with end-stage renal disease (ESRD) is less than optimal.[7–10] For these reasons, the integration of modern palliative care principles into the care of patients with ESRD is essential to the practice of nephrology.[11]

The World Health Organization defines palliative care as an approach that improves the quality of life of patients and their families faced with a life-limiting illness through the prevention and relief of suffering by means of early identification and impeccable assessment and treatment of pain and other problems—physical, psychosocial, and spiritual. As the dialysis population ages and experiences multiple comorbidities, it is becoming increasingly difficult to maintain a reasonable health-related quality of life (HRQOL) for these patients. Patients with diabetes represent more than one third of the ESRD population, and many of these patients experience amputations, neuropathies, blindness, and other complications. Other common comorbid disorders of incident patients include congestive heart failure (34%), coronary artery disease (25%), peripheral vascular disease (15%), and cerebrovascular disease (10%). Although dialysis supports life, it may not provide what many people consider to be an adequate HRQOL.

A systematic approach to palliative care in dialysis units, emphasizing shared decision making and advance care planning, is discussed in Chapter 84. This chapter focuses on symptom management and the logistics of end-of-life care for patients who withdraw from dialysis or who choose to not initiate dialysis.

SYMPTOM PREVALENCE AND IMPACT

Given the aging population and the increasing incidence of comorbidities, it is not surprising that dialysis patients experience multiple symptoms.[12] Until recently, little attention was paid to the prevalence of symptoms in ESRD and consequently, symptoms are frequently underrecognized and inadequately treated. The overall symptom burden in ESRD is extensive and matches or exceeds that reported by patients hospitalized in palliative care settings with cancer.[13,14] For the following symptoms, the reported mean prevalence rates are fatigue/tiredness, 71%; pruritus, 55%; constipation, 53%; anorexia, 49%; pain, 47%; sleep disturbance, 44%; anxiety, 38%; dyspnea, 35%; nausea, 33%; restless legs syndrome, 30%; and depression, 27%.[14] Chronic pain in this population is typically severe, with 82% experiencing moderate to severe pain.[2] The cause of pain is often multifactorial and may be due to comorbidity, the primary renal disease, or the dialysis procedure itself. There are also painful syndromes associated with chronic kidney disease such as renal osteodystrophy, calcific uremic arteriolopathy, and dialysis-related amyloidosis. Symptoms, both physical and psychological, are highly relevant patient outcomes in evaluating HRQOL. In fact, recent research suggests that dialysis patients' perceptions of symptom burden are more important than objective clinical assessments in determining HRQOL.[4,15–19] A recent study showed that symptom burden in dialysis patients accounted for 29% of the impairment in physical HRQOL and 39% of the impairment in mental HRQOL.[13] Moreover, a change in symptom burden accounted for 46% of the change in mental HRQOL and 34% of the change in physical HRQOL.[20] These results suggest that a palliative care focus on symptom assessment and management would greatly enhance the HRQOL of ESRD patients.

If there is a subgroup of ESRD patients who ought to receive quality palliative care, it is those whose dialysis has been withdrawn and who consequently have a mean of 8 days to live.[21] Data are limited, but recent studies demonstrate an unacceptable degree of suffering of these patients in their last days of life.[8,10] The most common terminal symptoms following withdrawal of dialysis are confusion/agitation (70%), pain (55%), and dyspnea (48%): 24% of patients continued to have unrelieved symptoms at the time of death.[10]

There are patients with stage 5 chronic kidney disease (glomerular filtration rate < 15 mL/min) who are managed without dialysis, either through their own preference or because dialysis is unlikely to benefit them. This group of patients also has extensive palliative care needs. Although data on symptom prevalence in this population are limited, it appears that their overall symptom burden may approach that of dialysis patients.[22]

SYMPTOM ASSESSMENT

Until now, laboratory tests have played a primary role in the assessment and care of patients with chronic kidney disease. However, it is increasingly becoming clear that the patient's symptoms should be the first priority. Regular comprehensive assessment of physical and emotional symptoms, together with proactive management of identified symptoms, is essential if efforts to improve HRQOL are to be successful. Although the most commonly used HRQOL instruments in dialysis patients, the Medical Outcomes Study 36-Item Short-Form Health Survey[23] and the Kidney Disease Quality of Life questionnaire,[24] have items pertaining to physical and psychological symptoms, they do not directly assess patient self-report of troublesome symptoms. In addition, these tools are time-consuming and difficult for patients to complete. Tools used to evaluate symptom burden must be simple and easily understood and take little time to complete. They must also be reliable, valid, sensitive, and responsive to change; yield useful information; and be self-reported because outcomes are dependent on the perceptions and lived experience of individual patients.

The Edmonton Symptom Assessment System is a simple, short, and self-completed measurement tool that was developed for symptom assessment in cancer patients and has been used extensively in palliative care settings. More recently, it has been modified and validated to assess physical and psychological symptoms in ESRD.[3,13,20] The respondent burden is low, and the instrument can even be successfully completed by patients close to death (Fig. 75-1). In contrast to the use of HRQOL instruments, the resources required for data collection, analysis, and reporting of the Edmonton Symptom Assessment System are minimal.

SYMPTOM MANAGEMENT

Management of Pain

It has only recently been recognized that chronic pain is one of the most common and distressing symptoms for patients with ESRD. Medical management is complicated by the high incidence of comorbidity, polypharmacy, and advanced age. However, the greatest barrier to effective pharmacologic management of chronic pain is the altered pharmacokinetics and pharmacodynamics of analgesics in renal failure. More than 90% of most opioids are excreted by the kidneys, and many have active metabolites that accumulate

in chronic kidney disease, causing opioid toxicity. This difficult situation is worsened by a paucity of data on the use of analgesics in ESRD. Drug dosing is covered in greater detail in Chapter 91.

Given the lack of pharmacokinetic and pharmacodynamic data and systematically tested symptom treatment protocols, it is difficult to advocate specific pain management algorithms, but the basic principles of pain assessment and management can be adapted and integrated into the care of ESRD patients (summarized in Box 75-1). Research is needed to test the effectiveness of various interventions.[25] The World Health Organization analgesic ladder is advocated for the pharmacologic management of malignant and nonmalignant pain (Fig. 75-2) and relies on a stepwise approach with analgesics. There is limited evidence to support its use in ESRD patients,[26] and not all analgesics are recommended for patients with ESRD (Table 75-1). Although morphine is the mainstay of pain control for most palliative care programs,[27] active metabolites accumulate in ESRD. The metabolite morphine-6-glucuronide equilibrates very slowly across the blood-brain barrier, and patients may remain sedated for days after the drug is stopped. This may be beneficial if the patient is agitated or in intractable pain after the withdrawal of dialysis, but it could also deny an individual the level of alertness necessary to achieve spiritual and interpersonal goals. For these reasons, morphine is not recommended.

The essentials of opioid dosing are reviewed in Box 75-2. Adverse effects of opioids should be aggressively treated and ideally prevented with a prophylactic bowel regimen and a gradual titration of dose. When titrated slowly, most patients will develop tolerance to the adverse effects of opioids, allowing the higher dose often required for adequate analgesia. Patient and health care professional fears about opioid addiction remain a major barrier to the effective use of opioids. Fortunately, opioid addiction is extremely rare in patients being treated for chronic pain (Box 75-3). Adjuvant therapies are important components of an effective pain management strategy and often permit the use of lower doses of opioids. Tricyclic antidepressants and anticonvulsants are particularly beneficial in controlling neuropathic pain (Table 75-2). Future strategies will likely include cannabinoids.

Management of Other Symptoms Common in End-Stage Renal Disease

Table 75-3 lists some common ESRD symptoms and our suggested guidelines based on the available literature. We caution that these particular protocols have not been validated or tested with sufficient numbers of patients. They should be considered only as rough guidelines and may not be appropriate for those patients who withdraw from dialysis.

Withholding and Withdrawing Dialysis

Increasing numbers and percentages of patients are dying after dialysis withdrawal: 24% of patient deaths were due to discontinuation of dialysis in 2004.[1] Given that withdrawal from dialysis is an accepted and increasingly common treatment option, one might hope that ongoing discussions about terminal care preferences would be routinely occurring with staff, patients, and the families.[28] Instead, research has found that such communications are rare and that written advance directives are completed by only 7% to 35% of long-term

Modified Edmonton Symptom Assessment System:
Numerical Scale
Northern Alberta Renal Program

Please circle the number that best describes:

No pain	0	1	2	3	4	5	6	7	8	9	10	Worst possible pain
Not tired	0	1	2	3	4	5	6	7	8	9	10	Worst possible tiredness
Not nauseated	0	1	2	3	4	5	6	7	8	9	10	Worst possible nausea
Not depressed	0	1	2	3	4	5	6	7	8	9	10	Worst possible depression
Not anxious	0	1	2	3	4	5	6	7	8	9	10	Worst possible anxiety
Not drowsy	0	1	2	3	4	5	6	7	8	9	10	Worst possible drowsiness
Best appetite	0	1	2	3	4	5	6	7	8	9	10	Worst possible appetite
Best feeling of well-being	0	1	2	3	4	5	6	7	8	9	10	Worst possible feeling of well-being
No itching	0	1	2	3	4	5	6	7	8	9	10	Worst possible itching
No shortness of breath	0	1	2	3	4	5	6	7	8	9	10	Worst possible shortness of breath
No insomnia	0	1	2	3	4	5	6	7	8	9	10	Worst possible insomnia

Patient's Name —————————————————————

Date —————————————————— Time ——————————

Completed by (*check one*)
☐ Patient
☐ Caregiver
☐ Caregiver assisted

Figure 75-1 Modified Edmonton Symptom Assessment System.

Please mark on these pictures where it is you hurt.

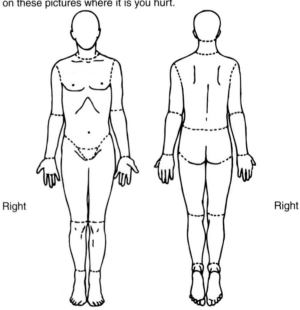

Right   Right

Box 75-1   The Essentials of Pain Management

1. Regular, systematic pain assessment
   a. Believe the patient's report of pain
   b. Assess pain in its site, character, intensity, extent, relieving and aggravating factors, and temporal relationships.
   c. Use a simple assessment tool such as a numerical scale of 0–10, e.g., the Modified Edmonton Symptom Assessment System
   d. Educate patients or their caregivers at home on pain assessment and charting
2. Patients may have more than one kind of pain; each pain syndrome must be independently diagnosed and treated.
3. Aim to achieve control at a level acceptable to the patient. It may not be necessary or possible to make the patient completely pain free.
4. Refer for nonpharmacologic interventions such as physical therapy (e.g., transcutaneous nerve stimulation, hot and cold therapy, exercise, and neuromuscular massage) where appropriate.
5. Educate patients and their caregivers on the goals of therapy, management plan, and potential complications. This will help minimize noncompliance.
   a. Distress at and confusion about previous treatment has a powerful influence on patients' reactions to pain and disability.
6. Early and aggressive treatment of pain is important in minimizing progression to chronicity.

Concurrent Psychosocial Issues
1. Pain may be associated with and aggravated by concurrent psychological symptoms. The psychological state of the patient must be assessed and treated appropriately with equal concern.
2. Use an interdisciplinary team to manage total pain. Total pain refers to any unmet need of the patient that may aggravate pain (e.g., financial, spiritual). Pain may not be controlled unless these needs are addressed. This may require a consultation to a palliative care team.
3. Psychological factors typically have a stronger influence on outcome than do biomedical factors.
   a. Psychological response to acute pain is predictive of chronic incapacity.
   b. Better management of psychological reactions at early stages of treatment has the potential for preventing unnecessary chronicity.

Guidelines to Be Followed When Using Opioids
1. Before initiating opioids, screen for risk factors for addiction using tools such as the Opioid Risk Tool (ORT) or the Screening Instrument for Substance Abuse Potential (SISAP).
2. Use a specific opioid for a specific type of pain.
3. Use adjuvants judiciously.
   a. Adjuvants may be used with opioids to control side effects.
   b. Adjuvants may be used for specific pains not responding well to opioids.
   c. Adjuvants may be used as an opioid-sparing agent to decrease the dose of opioid when side effects of opioids become troublesome.

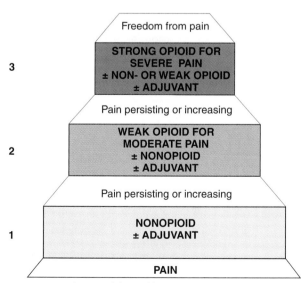

Figure 75-2   The World Health Organization analgesic ladder.

dialysis patients.[29,30] Patients often do not know that they have the option of withdrawing from dialysis, and they frequently believe that their physicians would not support such a choice.[31] Even the relatively simpler discussion around cardiopulmonary resuscitation is not consistently done well in dialysis units. Six months following cardiopulmonary resuscitation, only 3% of ESRD patients are alive: approximately 78% of successfully resuscitated dialysis patients die a mean of 4.4 days later, and 95% of these patients are on mechanical ventilation at the time of death.[32] Despite the extremely poor chance of survival after cardiopulmonary resuscitation, relatively few dialysis patients choose do not resuscitate orders.[33] Issues around advanced care planning are discussed further in Chapter 84.

Less is known about the numbers of patients who choose not to initiate dialysis. In the United States, it is estimated that less than 5% of patients who present to a nephrologist elect to forgo dialysis. In Canada and Great Britain, as many as 15% to 20% of patients may choose to not start dialysis. For each patient, the decision to commence dialysis or have conservative management (without dialysis) is complex and involves discussions on prognosis, anticipated quality of life (with and without dialysis), treatment burden, and patient preferences. A recent retrospective analysis of the survival of all patients older than 75 years with chronic kidney disease

Table 75-1 Analgesic Use in End-Stage renal Disease

WHO Ladder	Analgesic	Recommendation	Comments
Step 1	Acetaminophen	Recommended	No dose adjustment required
	Nonsteroidal anti-inflammatories	Use with caution	Increased incidence of bleeding in CKD. More appropriate for acute pain management
Step 2	Tramadol	Use with caution	Maximum dose 50 mg q12h; associated with a lower seizure threshold
	Codeine	Avoid	Several case reports of profound toxicity, which can be delayed and unexpected
	Dextropropoxyphene	Avoid	Levels of parent compound and active metabolites increase in CKD and are associated with CNS and cardiac toxicity
Step 3	Fentanyl/alfentanil	Recommended	Should only be prescribed by a clinician experienced in its use
	Methadone	Recommended	Should only be prescribed by a clinician experienced in its use
	Hydromorphone	Recommended	Appears well tolerated in dialysis patients, but toxic metabolites rapidly accumulate in patients with stage 5 CKD being managed conservatively and should probably be avoided in this situation
	Oxycodone	Insufficient evidence	
	Buprenorphine	Insufficient evidence	
	Morphine/diamorphine	Avoid	Accumulation of metabolites; metabolite morphine-6-glucuronide is a more potent analgesic than morphine itself and accumulates in ESRD. It equilibrates very slowly across the blood-brain barrier. Thus, patients may remain sedated for days after the drug is stopped
	Meperidine	Avoid	Accumulation of normeperidine, which is only half as potent an analgesic as the parent compound, but is 2–3 times more likely to cause CNS toxicity (agitation, myoclonus, and seizures)

CNS, central nervous system.

stage 5 attending dedicated multidisciplinary predialysis care clinics showed that the survival advantage of dialysis may be lost in patients with high comorbidity scores, especially when the comorbidity includes ischemic heart disease.[34] Because dialysis is a demanding treatment associated with a tremendous symptom burden, data of this sort should help inform discussions for dialysis options including no dialysis.

Box 75-2 The Five Essentials of Analgesic Dosing

By mouth:	Whenever possible, drugs should be given orally.
By the clock:	For continuous pain, schedule doses over 24 hours on a regular basis. Additional breakthrough medication should be available on an as-needed basis.
By the ladder:	Use analgesics stepwise according to the World Health Organization analgesic ladder.
For the individual:	There is no standard dose for strong opioids. The right dose is the dose that relieves pain without causing unacceptable side effects.
Attention to detail:	Pain changes over time: thus, there is the need for constant reassessment.

INTEGRATING PALLIATIVE CARE

Palliative care can best be thought of as supportive care initiated at the time of diagnosis of a life-limiting illness and occurring throughout the illness, depending on the needs of individual patients (Fig. 75-3). All elements of a successful palliative care program require good patient-doctor communication. Specific

Box 75-3 Facts about Opioid Addiction

1. The incidence of addiction in patients receiving opioid therapy for acute pain relief is less than 1%. The incidence of addiction in patients receiving opioid therapy for chronic pain is less clear but is felt to be less than 5%.
2. Patients will become physically dependent when treated with opioids for a time and therefore will have effects of withdrawal if the opioid is stopped suddenly.
3. Physical dependency is easily managed by a slow taper of the opioid when pain has resolved.
4. Physical dependency is not synonymous with addiction.
5. Addiction is a psychological problem rather than a physical one and is characterized by patients engaging in manipulative behaviors to secure the drug.
6. Individuals who are addicted use opioids for reasons other than pain. Taking drugs for pain management is different from taking them for pleasure.

Table 75-2 Adjuvant Use for Neuropathic Pain in Stage 5 Chronic Kidney Disease

Class of Drug	Dose	Comments
Tricyclic Antidepressant		
Amitriptyline	10–100 mg od	Dose alteration not usually necessary in ESRD, although may be poorly tolerated due to common anticholinergic adverse effects; lowers seizure threshold
Desipramine	10–150 mg od	Less sedating and fewer anticholinergic adverse effects than amitriptyline
Anticonvulsants		
Carbamazepine	200 mg od, titrate weekly to effectiveness Maximum dose 1600 mg	No dose adjustment in ESRD
Gabapentin	100–300 mg od	Cases of neurotoxicity reported when using >300 mg od
Benzodiazepines		No dose adjustment required for most benzodiazepines

ESRD, end-stage renal disease; od, once daily.

Table 75-3 Symptom Guidelines

Symptom	Treatment	Dose	Comment
Cramps	Quinine	260–325 mg PO prn	Give before symptoms; limit to 3 doses/day
	Carnitine	1000–2000 mg IV during dialysis	Also used for myopathy, cardiomyopathy, refractory anemia
Restless legs syndrome	Clonazepam	0.5–2.0 mg hs prn	
	Carbidopa-levodopa	25/100 mg hs prn	
	Pergolide	0.05–0.2 mg qd	
	Pramipexole	0.3 mg qd	
Pruritus	Skin moisturizer		Limited effectiveness
	Hydrourea cream		
	Capsaicin	0.025% cream qid	Burning sensation may be problematic; expensive, therefore, not practical for generalized pruritus
	Antihistamines Clemastine Ketotifen	 1–3 mg bid prn 2 mg bid prn	Trial any H_1 antagonist; inexpensive, safe, but often poor clinical response
	UVB light	2–3 times/wk	Effective but potentially noxious in the long term, impractical, and often not available
	Ondansetron	2–4 mg bid	High cost, constipating
	IV lidocaine	100 mg IV during dialysis	Potential seizures
	Activated charcoal	6 g qd × 8 wk	Impractical, poorly tolerated
	Plasmapheresis	3–4 exchanges	Impractical

Continued

Table 75-3   Symptom Guidelines—cont'd

Symptom	Treatment	Dose	Comment
Hypotension, intradialytic or persistent	Alterations to the dialysis bath, temperature, sodium, ultrafiltration		
	Midadrine	1–10 mg tid prn or pre-dialysis	Oral α-adrenergic agonist
	Sertraline	25–50 mg pre-dialysis	
Anorexia	Megestrol	40–400 mg	Has been used in ESRD
	Dronabinol	2.5–5.0 mg bid/tid	Cannabinoid
Lethargy, fatigue	Methylphenidate	5–10 mg AM and noon	Psychostimulant, limited use and effectiveness in ESRD

ESRD, end-stage renal disease.

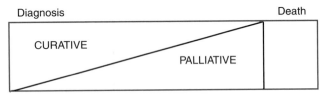

Figure 75-3   The World Health Organization model of cancer management.

Box 75-4   Principles of a Good Death

Anticipate death and know what to expect
Retain control of choices and have those wishes respected (advance care planning)
Maintain dignity
Control of pain and other troublesome symptoms
Choose where death occurs
Easy access to needed care and expertise (palliative care)
Spiritual and emotional support as needed
Access to hospice at all locations (home, hospital, nursing home)
To have those present at death that one chooses
To have time to say goodbye and choose the time of death (withdrawal from dialysis if appropriate)
Bereavement services for those left behind

key elements of a renal palliative care program would include regular symptom assessment and treatment protocols or guidelines available at clinics and dialysis units, advance care planning, enhanced referrals to hospice, morbidity and mortality conferences to review the deaths of recently deceased patients, and annual bereavement services for families, loved ones, and staff who wish to celebrate the memories of patients who died in the previous year. Memorial services, in particular, have been rated very highly by attendees and have been shown to markedly influence the culture in renal centers, making it more open to end-of-life care issues.[35] Hospice can also significantly enhance end-of-life care for patients with ESRD,[36] but United States Renal Data System data indicate that current hospice use is fivefold lower in dying dialysis patients when compared with nondialysis patients.[1] When death becomes imminent, end-of-life care should become the focus of our treatment. Principles of a good death can be seen in Box 75-4. However, achieving these goals takes time. Because death occurs quickly after withdrawal from dialysis, palliative care must be initiated well in advance. The key to end-of-life symptom management is aggressive symptom management before death is imminent. Early pain management is particularly beneficial in reducing the adverse effects of narcotics during the final days of life. Patients in pain who have not been exposed to opioids for some time are at a greater risk of depression, whereas respiratory depression is rare in most terminally ill patients receiving long-term treatment with opioids as long as the dose does not exceed the dose needed for pain relief. Although there remains great concern among health care professionals about using opioids in patients with ESRD or any dying patient for fear of hastening death, the most common form of narcotic abuse in the care of the dying is undertreatment of pain.[37] Although most symptoms associated with dying with ESRD can be managed before death is imminent, some symptoms such as agitation, twitching, nausea, and shortness of breath due to the accumulation of toxins may become more troublesome in the final days of life after withdrawal of dialysis and need to be anticipated and aggressively treated. Table 75-4 lists the treatment of the most troubling terminal symptoms.

SUMMARY

Expertise in pain and symptom management, psychological and spiritual support, and dealing with issues surrounding end-of-life care defines the specialty of palliative care. As tools for measuring patient symptoms and quality of dying are validated in ESRD, and treatment algorithms are developed and tested, the nephrology community will have the opportunity to incorporate these elements of modern palliative/supportive care into their facilities. Collaboration between renal and palliative specialists will likely help identify ways to achieve best care for these patients in the final phase of life.

Table 75-4 Symptoms at the End of Life

Symptom	Treatment
Retained secretions	Scopolamine
Shortness of breath	Fan, oxygen, patient position (upright), opioids
Agitation (includes involuntary twitching)	Ensure that pain and psychosocial issues addressed, haloperidol, methotrimeprazine (effective for anxiety, restlessness, nausea, and pain), and benzodiazepines
Nausea and vomiting	Metaclopramide, prochlorproperazine, ondansetron
Hiccups	Chlorpromazine, haloperidol, metoclopramide

References

1. 2004 Annual Data Report: Atlas of end-stage renal disease in the United States. Am J Kidney Dis 2007;49(Suppl):S1–S235.
2. Davison SN: Pain in hemodialysis patients: Prevalence, cause, severity, and management. Am J Kidney Dis 2003;42:1239–2347.
3. Fainsinger RL, Davison SN, Brenneis C: A supportive care model for dialysis patients. Palliat Med 2003;17:81–82.
4. Kimmel PL, Emont SL, Newmann JM, et al: ESRD patient quality of life: Symptoms, spiritual beliefs, psychosocial factors, and ethnicity. Am J Kidney Dis 2003;42:713–721.
5. Weisbord SD, Carmody SS, Bruns FJ, et al: Symptom burden, quality of life, advance care planning and the potential value of palliative care in severely ill haemodialysis patients. Nephrol Dial Transplant 2003;18:1345–1352.
6. Weisbord SD, Fried LF, Arnold RM, et al: Development of a symptom assessment instrument for chronic hemodialysis patients: The Dialysis Symptom Index. J Pain Symptom Manage 2004;27:226–240.
7. Chambers, EJ, Germain, M, Brown E: Supportive Care for the Renal Patient. New York: Oxford University Press, 2004.
8. Cohen LM, Germain MJ, Poppel DM, et al: Dying well after discontinuing the life-support treatment of dialysis. Arch Intern Med 2000;160:2513–2518.
9. Cohen LM, Germain M, Poppel DM, et al: Dialysis discontinuation and palliative care. Am J Kidney Dis 2000;36:140–144.
10. Chater S, Davison SN, Germain MJ, Cohen LM: Withdrawal from dialysis: A palliative care perspective. Clin Nephrol 2006;66:364–372.
11. Davison SN: Quality end-of-life care in dialysis units. Semin Dial 2002;15:41–44.
12. Weisbord SD, Fried LF, Mor MK, et al: Renal provider recognition of symptoms in patients on maintenance hemodialysis. Clin J Am Soc Nephrol 2007;2:960–967.
13. Davison SN, Jhangri GS, Johnson JA: Cross-sectional validity of a modified Edmonton symptom assessment system in dialysis patients: A simple assessment of symptom burden. Kidney Int 2006;69:1621–1625.
14. Murtagh FE, Addington-Hall JM, Higginson IJ: The prevalence of symptoms in end-stage renal disease: A systematic review. Adv Chron Kidney Dis 2007;14:82–99.
15. Cameron JI, Whiteside C, Katz J, Devins GM: Differences in quality of life across renal replacement therapies: A meta-analytic comparison. Am J Kidney Dis 2000;35:629–637.
16. Davison SN, Jhangri GS: The impact of chronic pain on depression, sleep, and the desire to withdraw from dialysis in hemodialysis patients. J Pain Symptom Manage 2005;30:46–73.
17. Kimmel PL, Peterson RA, Weihs KL, et al: Aspects of quality of life in hemodialysis patients. J Am Soc Nephrol 1995;6:1418–1426.
18. Valderrabano F, Jofre R, Lopez-Gomez JM: Quality of life in end-stage renal disease patients. Am J Kidney Dis 2001;38:443–464.
19. Patel SS, Shah VS, Peterson RA, Kimmel PL: Psychosocial variables, quality of life, and religious beliefs in ESRD patients treated with hemodialysis. Am J Kidney Dis 2002;40:1013–1022.
20. Davison SN, Jhangri GS, Johnson JA: Longitudinal validation of a modified Edmonton Symptom Assessment Dystem (ESAS) in haemodialysis patients. Nephrol Dial Transplant 2006;21:3189–3195.
21. Neu S, Kjellstrand CM: Stopping long-term dialysis. An empirical study of withdrawal of life-supporting treatment. N Engl J Med 1986;314:14–20.
22. Murtagh FE, Addington-Hall JM, Donohoe P, Higginson IJ: Symptom management in patients with established renal failure managed without dialysis. EDTNA ERCA J 2006;32:93–98.
23. Hays RD: RAND-36 Health Status Inventory. Lincoln, RI: Harcourt Brace, 1998.
24. Hays RD, Kallich JD, Mapes DL, et al: Kidney Disease Quality of Life Short Form (KDQOL-SF), Version 1.3: A manual for use and scoring. Qual Life Res 1994;3:329–338.
25. Davison SN: Chronic pain in end-stage renal disease. Adv Chronic Kidney Dis 2005;12:326–334.
26. Barakzoy AS, Moss AH: Efficacy of the World Health Organization analgesic ladder to treat pain in end-stage renal disease. J Am Soc Nephrol 2006;17:3198–3203.
27. Levy MH: Pharmacologic treatment of cancer pain. N Engl J Med 1996;335:1124–2232.
28. Singer PA, MacDonald N: Bioethics for clinicians: 15. Quality end-of-life care. CMAJ 1998;159:159–162.
29. Holley JL, Nespor S, Rault R: Chronic in-center hemodialysis patients' attitudes, knowledge, and behavior towards advance directives. J Am Soc Nephrol 1993;3:1405–1408.
30. Cohen LM, McCue JD, Germain M, Woods A: Denying the dying. Advance directives and dialysis discontinuation. Psychosomatics 1997;38:27–34.
31. Cohen LM, Germain M, Woods A, et al: Patient attitudes and psychological considerations in dialysis discontinuation. Psychosomatics 1993;34:395–401.
32. Moss AH, Holley JL, Upton MB: Outcomes of cardiopulmonary resuscitation in dialysis patients. J Am Soc Nephrol 1992;3:1238–1243.
33. Moss AH, Hozayen O, King K, et al: Attitudes of patients toward cardiopulmonary resuscitation in the dialysis unit. Am J Kidney Dis 2001;38:847–852.
34. Murtagh FE, Marsh JE, Donohoe P, et al: Dialysis or not? A comparative survival study of patients over 75 years with chronic kidney disease stage 5. Nephrol Dial Transplant 2007;3:480–481.
35. Poppel DM, Cohen LM, Germain MJ: The renal palliative care initiative. J Palliat Med 2003;6:321–326.
36. Murray AM, Arko C, Chen S-C, et al: Use of hospice in the United States dialysis population. Clin J Am Soc Nephrol 2006;1:1248–1255.
37. Buchan ML, Tolle SW: Pain relief for dying persons: Dealing with physicians' fears and concerns. J Clin Ethics 1995;6:53–61.

Further Reading

Chambers E, Germain M, Brown E: Supportive Care for the Renal Patient. New York: Oxford University Press, 2004.
Davison SN: Chronic pain in end-stage renal disease. Adv Chronic Kidney Dis 2005;12:326–334.

Chapter 76

Health Economics of End-Stage Renal Disease Treatment

Robert J. Rubin

In 2004, nearly $32.5 billion was spent on end-stage renal disease (ESRD) care in the United States.[1] The U.S. government, under the Medicare program, paid approximately 62% ($20.1 billion), and private insurers and patients paid the rest. Medicare beneficiaries receiving treatment for ESRD represent less than 1% of the Medicare population, but in 2004, they accounted for nearly 7% of the Medicare outlays. Thus, a strikingly disproportionate share of Medicare expenditures is spent annually on Medicare ESRD beneficiaries: ESRD beneficiaries cost an average of at least five times more than beneficiaries in other categories (Fig. 76-1). This disproportionate spending will keep the economics of ESRD treatment under the close scrutiny of legislators and regulators.

The Medicare ESRD program has continued to grow in absolute terms (slightly more than 11.7% in 2003–2004).[1] There is a belief that care can be delivered for a lower cost while offering higher quality care to ESRD patients. In the United States, physicians are paid a monthly fee to care for dialysis patients (monthly capitation payment), and dialysis providers are paid a fixed amount per dialysis treatment per month (composite rate). As this amount has remained relatively stable over time, its value has decreased relative to inflation. Physicians and dialysis providers have had to find ways to increase their productivity by delivering the same or better quality care at a lower cost. To evaluate various measures to improve patient care as well as maintain the economic viability of a practice or dialysis unit, it is useful to understand the economic tools available and how they can be used.

METHODOLOGIES

There are several ways to evaluate the economic and clinical effects of changes in the treatment of ESRD patients.

Cost-Benefit Analysis

This technique compares the costs of an intervention or treatment protocol with the benefits, identified in terms of monetary units. The benefits are typically measured as the change in medical expenditure and productivity. By converting the outcome to a monetary unit, interventions with a variety of outcomes can be compared. There are drawbacks to these types of analyses. They do not reflect changes in quality of life, and determining the impact on productivity among non-working people, such as the very old or young, is problematic. Although it is difficult to assign a value to a year of life that is free of disease, a standard benchmark is $100,000.[2] Multiple interventions can be ranked by their cost-to-benefit ratios. Clearly, as the cost-to-benefit ratio approaches a value of 1, the intervention becomes less desirable.

Cost-Effectiveness Analysis

This technique compares the costs of an intervention or treatment protocol with a measure of effectiveness. It identifies the trade-offs involved in making decisions about care. The costs are monetary, and the effectiveness measure is reported in outcomes (life-years gained or episodes averted) that are adjusted to reflect a measure of quality of life. The results are reported as cost per quality-adjusted life years, or QALYs. The advantage is that it avoids placing a value on a year of life. A recent example is the cost-effectiveness of retransplantation, which was determined as $9656 per QALY saved.[3] Table 76-1 shows the cost per QALY of some treatments for ESRD.

Cost-Minimization Analysis

This technique analyzes two or more interventions or treatment protocols that are believed to be equal clinically, such that the only difference is the economic cost. An example of this type of study would be the cost consequences of using generic versus branded drugs.

Cost-Identification Analysis

This technique identifies and totals all the costs of a particular intervention or treatment protocol. It is useful when comparing a new treatment protocol with an existing one. An example would be the effect of increasing Kt/V (K is the clearance time,

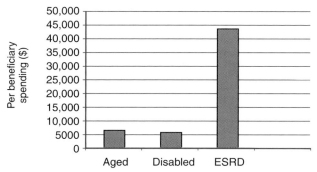

Figure 76-1 Medicare spending by type of beneficiary, 2003. ESRD, end-stage renal disease. (From the Medicare Payment Advisory Commission: A Data Book: Health Care Spending and the Medicare Program. Washington, DC: Medicare Payment Advisory Commission, 2006.)

t is the dialysis time, and V is the volume of distribution) to 1.2 for all Medicare dialysis patients who have a Kt/V of less than 1. This intervention would increase dialysis costs by approximately $2340 per patient-year at risk, but would decrease nondialysis spending by approximately $4670, a savings per patient-year at risk of $2330.[4] Patient-year at risk is a technique used to standardize reporting of data on patients with varying follow-up times. The expenditures for all patients are summed, and all patients receiving therapy during a given year contribute to the denominator based on the days during that year that they were in the program; thus, a patient who was alive and on hemodialysis (HD) for 30 days in 1999 contributes to the cost (numerator) and the time (denominator) for those 30 days. These economic studies are frequently lumped together under the heading of cost-effectiveness. However, it is important to understand a few methodologic characteristics of these studies.

Perspective

Economic studies consider one or more perspectives, such as patient, provider, and payer. For example, per-patient spending for a transplantation in 1996 was $148,959, but Medicare

Table 76-1 Estimated Cost per Quality-Adjusted Life Year Gained by Investing in Different Treatments

Treatment	Cost per QALY (US$)
Kidney transplantation	9099
Home hemodialysis	33,345
Continuous ambulatory peritoneal dialysis	38,387
Hospital hemodialysis	42,444
Erythropoietin for dialysis anemia (with 10% reduction in mortality)	105,057
Erythropoietin for dialysis anemia (with no increase in survival)	243,978

Adapted from Maynard A: Developing the health-care market. The Economic Journal 1991;101:1277–1286 with permission from the publisher.

spending per patient was $141,968. The difference between Medicare spending and total spending is relatively small for transplantation (5%), and substantially larger for HD (17%).[4] The difference is accounted for by payments that patients make, such as those relating to Part A (deductible) and Part B (copayments). Therefore, an analysis that ignores these costs would be appropriate from the perspective of the government, but not from the perspective of the patient.

In the example of cost identification cited previously, increasing Kt/V to 1.2 would increase costs to the providers of dialysis care, but would decrease total costs from the government's perspective. Therefore, it would be cost-effective for Medicare, but not for providers. However, if providers were responsible for all the costs (as they would be under a capitated system), then it would become cost-effective for the provider as well.

The societal perspective measures the net effect of all these perspectives. Generally, health economic studies analyze interventions for their effect on the health care system and the benefits to patients. A truly societal view should also value the effect of interventions on the non–health-related aspects of society, referred to as indirect costs. For example, if daily HD enabled patients to continue to work and be productive members of society, then from a societal perspective, the increased productivity of those patients might well offset any increased costs.

To better understand how these economic tools can be used, we describe the economics of renal replacement therapies.

HEMODIALYSIS

Hemodialysis (HD) is the renal replacement treatment of choice for the majority of ESRD patients in the United States, as 91% of patients receiving renal replacement treatment use this modality compared with 6% for peritoneal dialysis (PD) and 2% for those who go directly to transplantation. Direct comparison of cost-effectiveness between HD and PD is not possible as no prospective study has satisfactorily determined differences in effectiveness between the two modalities. Differences in costs, as determined by Medicare payments, between the two modalities are well documented. In 2004, Medicare paid $67,733 per patient-year at risk for HD patients and $48,796 per patient-year at risk for PD patients.[1]

Currently, routine payment for HD patients is composed of two main components: the monthly capitation payment made to physicians on a per-patient basis and the dialysis facility reimbursement, which consists of the composite rate payment plus separately billable items such as drugs and biologics.

The monthly capitation payment includes physician services related to all routine dialysis treatment in a given month. Services not covered include surgical services, interpretation of tests, training of patients to encourage self-treatment, services not related to patients' renal disease, evaluation for renal transplantation, and physician services covered during a hospital stay as an inpatient. The monthly capitation payment was revised in 2004 to encourage physicians to see their patients more frequently and since that time has been based on the number of times that a physician visits a patient while on dialysis during a month. The rates for 2007 were published in the Federal Register on December 1, 2006, and are displayed in Table 76-2. It is clear from this table that a physician is paid the same whether a patient is seen two or three times per month. It is not yet clear whether this change has resulted in physicians seeing patients two, three, or four times per month on average.

The dialysis facility reimbursement also changed in 2004 as a result of enactment of the Medicare Modernization Act in 2003. Previously, there was a composite rate payment for all necessary dialysis services, equipment, and supplies established in 1981 and effective in 1983. The composite rate has declined substantially on an inflation-adjusted basis. There was no increase in the composite rate between 1983 and 1991. In fact, there were decreases. Subsequent increases in 2000, 2001, 2005, and 2006 were less than half the inflation rate. Dialysis providers point out that the ESRD program is the only payment program in Medicare that does not have an annual inflation adjustment mechanism.

Some dialysis-related pharmaceuticals and supplies are paid as an add-on to the composite rate. These include erythropoietin, vitamin D injections, intravenous iron, and antibiotics. Payments for these ancillary services are an important component of dialysis facility revenues. For example, erythropoietin, iron, and vitamin D account for almost 90% of incremental payments above the composite rate. The Medicare Modernization Act changed the drug reimbursement to an average sales price methodology and added the estimated historical average wholesale price margins to the composite rate, such that the payment rate for most dialysis drugs decreased while the composite rate increased.

There is widespread expectation that some or all of ESRD care will move toward capitation in the near future. There are two ways to achieve this and both are under active consideration in the United States. The first method would capitate the entire cost of care for Medicare beneficiaries with ESRD. This methodology is currently being tested by several organizations, but the results are not expected for a number of years. The second method would only capitate the costs related to the dialysis procedure. It was the intent of the U.S. Congress that the latter would also be tested shortly after passage of the Medicare Modernization Act; however, constructing the test has proven to be difficult. A major concern is that patients require different levels of resources to provide optimal care, and the capitation amount therefore needs to be adjusted to reflect that variation from the average patient. This is called "case-mix adjustment and is an important analytical tool that is used to ensure that the variation (in dollars) that is attributable to patients' needs is accounted for. For example, erythropoietin, iron, and vitamin D account for almost 90% of the incremental cost to the composite rate, yet there is wide variability in the drug utilization from patient to patient and for a single patient over time. Constructing a case-mix adjustment

Table 76-2 The Monthly Capitation Payment: 2007

Visits/Month	Code	2007 Reimbursement Rate (National Average)
1	G-0319	$184.94
2-3	G-0318	$233.83
4	G-0317	$283.09

Table 76-3 Estimated Increase in Dialysis Spending to Achieve 1.2 Kt/V Threshold for All Patients Based on 1997 Levels

	Kt/V VALUE			
	≤1.0	1.0–1.1	≥1.2	Total
Percentage of adult hemodialysis patients	7%	15%	78%	100%
Increase in monthly capitation payment spending	$34	$0	$0	$2
Increase in dialysis facility/supplier spending	$393	$0	$0	$28
Total increase in dialysis-related spending	$427	$0	$0	$30

K, dialyzer clearance of urea; t, dialysis time; V, patient's total body water.
With permission from The Lewin Group: Capitation Models for ESRD. Methodology and Results. Renal Physicians Association, and American Society of Nephrology. Rockville, MD, and Washington, DC: RPA-ASN, 2000.

system with no inherent incentives for overutilization has proven to be difficult. This is true not only in dialysis, but in all capitated systems. Ideally, in a capitated system, patients are provided optimal care and providers are rewarded for delivering optimal care.

Under the current payment scheme, the incentives to decrease use of high-cost health care may not rest with the individuals who have the greatest opportunity to affect change. For example, approximately 40% of total ESRD payments were for hospitalizations.[1] Decreasing hospitalizations would benefit both the Medicare program and the individual patient, but the cost of providing additional services to the patient would likely be borne by the facility. Dialysis adequacy provides a useful illustration of such costs. Increasing Kt/V from 0.82 to 1.33 is associated with a 32% decrease in hospital days, which translates to an average savings of $5400 per patient.[5] A recent study found that a 0.1 lower Kt/V was associated with an 11% increase in hospitalizations and $940 more for Medicare inpatient reimbursement.[6]

Thus, a strategy to deliver an improved level of dialysis should decrease costs. This would require increasing treatment times or increasing the size of the dialyzer used.[7] At present, however, most ESRD providers have little incentive to do so. An increase in spending by the dialysis facility or supplier of $393 should increase the Kt/V value of all patients from less than 1.0 to 1.2 (Table 76-3).[7] An increase in dialysis treatment time is a much less expensive means to increase Kt/V than a change in dialysis membrane (Table 76-4).

VASCULAR ACCESS

There are three types of vascular access used today: arteriovenous fistulas, arteriovenous grafts, and catheters. In 2004, 38% of patients had arteriovenous grafts, 36% had arteriovenous fistulas, and 26% had catheters. Although catheter use has

Table 76-4 Cost Estimates Using Three Methods of Increasing Dialysis Dose Based on 1997 Data

	Increase in Kt/V	Increase in Cost (%)
Increase in dialysis time (10 min)	0.05	1.4
Switch to synthetic membrane	0.05	5.3
Switch to modified cellulose membrane	0.05	20.7

With permission from The Lewin Group: Capitation Models for ESRD. Methodology and Results. Renal Physicians Association, and American Society of Nephrology. Rockville, MD and Washington, DC: RPA-ASN, 2000.

remained relatively constant in this century, graft use has fallen by 30% and fistula use has grown by a third. Medicare has instituted an initiative called Fistula First with a goal of 66% of patients having their vascular access by arteriovenous fistula. A recent article used economic modeling to determine the effect of reaching this goal.[8]

If we reached the 66% goal, and the relative proportions of grafts and catheters remained constant, it is estimated that the shift would provide an additional 35,000 years of survival for the 2003 incident patient cohort, resulting in $2.25 billion in additional Medicare expenditures. This is offset by the $840 million savings in vascular access–attributed costs, yielding Medicare's net additional expenditure of $1.4 billion over the cohort's lifetime. Relative to the current mix of access options, the shift to 66% fistula would be achieved at a cost-effectiveness ratio of $40,000 per year of life gained ($1.4 billion/35,000 years gained).[8]

It is believed that the current payment rate for creating a fistula discourages surgeons from performing the procedure, yet Schon and colleagues[8] demonstrate that trebling the payment from approximately $610 to $1830 while achieving the 66% goal would only decrease Medicare savings from $840 million to $765 million over the life of the cohort and increase the cost-effectiveness ratio by only $2000 per year of life gained.

PERITONEAL DIALYSIS

PD is the choice of only 8% of dialysis patients in the United States.[1] In the past 10 years, PD has declined by nearly 54% in some parts of the country; however, the highest prevalence of PD tends to be in areas with low population densities, suggesting that people choose PD if going to a facility poses a travel burden. Interestingly, its use has declined in recent years despite evidence that outcomes are generally similar and costs are lower than those of HD.[9,10] However, there are no prospective, randomized trials that conclusively determine whether equivalent outcomes exist for morbidity and mortality.

Even if we assume equivalent efficacy between the two modalities and thus propose that PD is the least expensive (cost minimization) modality, it may still lag behind HD as the modality of choice. Traditional cost-effectiveness analysis reflects patient preferences and the perceived impact on quality of life. For PD patients, it is possible that the impact of assuming responsibility for one's treatment reduces quality of life and thus diminishes the benefits of the lower cost therapy.

TRANSPLANTATION

Transplantation is the most cost-effective renal replacement therapy (see Table 76-1). The high cost of surgery is offset by a "long" period in which the patient requires little medical care. It is the only therapy that, if successful, is curative. However, the number of people eligible for receiving a kidney transplant far exceeds the current supply of donor kidneys. In the prevalent population, the number of patients waiting to receive a kidney has grown at an annual rate of 7% to 12% over the past 3 years, and in 2004 numbered more than 60,000. In the same year, there were only slightly more than 10,000 deceased donor transplants as demand clearly outstripped supply. One way to increase the supply of available kidneys is to use expanded criteria donor kidneys. These kidneys are offered to those on the waiting list who have agreed, in advance, to accept them. In 2004, almost one in five deceased donor kidney transplants used an expanded criteria donor kidney.[1] The use of these donors is significantly more expensive than either cadaver or living-related transplants, although graft survival is similar.[11] Are the costs of expanded criteria donor transplants greater than, less than, or equal to alternate renal replacement therapies, assuming roughly similar clinical outcomes? Modeling data show that HD costs would be expected to exceed expanded criteria donor transplant costs after 6.6 years.[12] Therefore, it would be reasonable to proceed with the use of expanded criteria donor transplants, assuming a graft survival, on average, of at least 6.6 years, while collecting economic data to verify the modeling results.

Given the scarcity of kidneys available for transplantation, it is useful to understand the cost-effectiveness of offering re-transplantation to patients with failed grafts. The question to be answered is whether improvement in QALYs from a second transplant is greater than the loss of QALYs from someone else having to wait longer for their first transplant. The answer is that this policy has a cost per QALY of $9656.[3] The policy is, not unexpectedly, better for younger patients, lowering costs while increasing QALYs; however, it remains cost-effective for older patients. Costs are lower because the patients would be on dialysis less often and, on average, would be healthier after receiving a transplant.

All payers would like to be able to predict, and therefore manage, their financial risks. A risk (or case-mix) adjustor model allows the payer to measure the degree to which its patient population may differ from a reference population. The risk adjustor may use demographic information, typically age or gender, or clinical information such as cause of renal failure. In patients receiving a transplant, one can construct a risk adjustor model using both demographic and clinical data (Table 76-5).[4] The base or reference case is a 20- to 34-year-old white woman who has had ESRD as a result of diabetes for less than 1 year who lives in an average-cost city in the Midwestern United States and who will receive a living-related donor kidney for her first transplant. As can be seen in Table 76-4, various demographic factors can dramatically affect the

Table 76-5 Risk Adjuster Model Results for Within-Year Transplant Recipients

	Estimated Coefficient (Spending per Years of Age US$)	Patients in Sample with Characteristic (%)		Estimated Coefficient (Spending per Years of Age US$)	Patients in Sample with Characteristic (%)
Demographic Factors			**Demographic Factors–cont'd**		
Years of age (reference cases 20–34)			Geographic region (reference case midwest)		
0–1	13,939	0	Northeast	10,273‡	20
2–6	9517	1	West	–342	20
7–12	14,050	1	South	–2717	36
13–15	3940	1	U.S. Territories	7876	0.4
16–19	–3622	2			
35–44	7668†	23	**Disease-Specific Factors**		
45–54	6243†	24	Diagnosis causing ESRD (reference case diabetes)		
55–64	13,280‡	17			
65+	21,191‡	7	Cystic kidney disease	–12,053‡	7
Race (reference case white)			Other causes	–11,569‡	14
Black	13,106‡	25	Hypertension	–13,685‡	20
Sex (reference case female)			Glomerulonephritis	–14,548‡	26
Male	–3168	60	Other urological	–8902	2
Years since onset of ESRD (reference case <1)			No. of transplants (reference case 1 Tx)		
1–2	–17,215‡	40	Two transplants	–85,624‡	1
3–4	–21,965‡	18	Transplant donor (reference case living-related donor)		
5+	–22,768‡	20	Cadaver transplant	–10,333‡	81
Wage index (reference case mid 85 < index < 1.10)			Intercept‡		
High index >1.10	6042*	27		–152,268	
Low index <0.85	–3793	23			

*P < .1
†P < .05
‡P < .01
Variables indicating missing or unknown data were included in the regression analysis, but are not given here.
ESRD, end-stage renal disease.
Reproduced with permission from The Lewin Group: Capitation Models for ESRD. Methodology and Results. Renal Physicians Association, and American Society of Nephrology, Rockville, MD, and Washington, DC: RPA–ASN, 2000.

cost. For example, if she were 45 to 54 years old, as are almost one fourth of transplant recipients, costs would be expected to increase by $6243. The cost would increase by an additional $10,333 if she received a cadaver transplant rather than a living-related donor transplant.

It is necessary to understand how good the model is in predicting actual costs. Table 76-6 shows that the model's ability to predict cost is a function of the number of patients or sample size. Thus, for groups of 100 patients, the model would be ±4% to 5% of actual spending 90% of the time and 6% to 8% for 98% of the time. These models are generally useful for predicting costs for larger groups of patients, but they are based on historical costs and treatment protocols. When new treatment protocols are used, both costs and outcomes change and the old paradigms are no longer valid. Newer immunosuppressive agents demonstrate this well.

The cost of immunosuppressive drugs is an important posttransplantation cost. In the United States, patients who are not at least 65 years of age or disabled have to pay for these drugs beginning 3 years after receiving their transplant. The U.S. Food and Drug Administration approved mycophenolate mofetil in 1995, 12 years after the approval of cyclosporine. Tacrolimus and sirolimus have also been approved. Economic analyses will be important in determining whether

Table 76-6 Percentage of Difference between Actual and Predicted Spending-within-Year Transplant Recipients

Group Size	Mean Predicted as % of Actual Spending*	90% of the Time, Predicted $ Are within (of Actual Spending)	98% of the Time, Predicted $ Are within (of Actual Spending)
10 patients	101%	16% to −13%	29% to −16%
20 patients	100%	11% to −9%	17% to −11%
40 patients	100%	7% to −7%	11% to −8%
60 patients	100%	6% to −5%	9% to −7%
100 patients	100%	5% to −4%	8% to −6%
500 patients	100%	2% to −2%	3% to −3%
600 patients	100%	2% to −2%	3% to −3%

*Rounded to nearest whole number.
Reproduced with permission from The Lewin Group: Capitation Models for ESRD. Methodology and Results. Renal Physicians Association, and American Society of Nephrology. Rockville, MD, and Washington, DC: RPA-ASN, 2000.

these newer drugs alone or in combination with older therapies provide better clinical outcomes at equal or lower cost.[13] In performing the analyses, the perspective will be especially important as outpatient drug costs 3 years after a successful transplant place a real burden on patients.

CONCLUSION

Applying the tools of economics to ESRD enhances the decision-making powers of patients, providers, and payers. This chapter has identified a variety of analyses and health care scenarios that show that proper use of economic analysis can result in changes in practice and policy that might achieve more efficient use of resources as well as better patient outcomes.

References

1. USRDS: U.S. Renal Data System: Excerpts from the USRDS 2006 annual data report. Am J Kidney Dis 2006;49(Suppl 1):S1–S296.
2. Cutler DM, McClellan M: Is technological change in medicine worth it? Health Affairs 2001;20:11–29.
3. Hornberger JC, Best JH, Garrison LP Jr: Cost-effectiveness of repeat medical procedures: Kidney transplantation as an example. Med Decis Making 1997;17:363–372.
4. The Lewin Group: Capitation Models for ESRD. Methodology and Results. Renal Physicians Association, and American Society of Nephrology. Rockville, MD, and Washington, DC: RPA-ASN, 2000.
5. Hakim RM, Breyer J, Ismail N, et al: Effects of dose of dialysis on morbidity and mortality. Am J Kidney Dis 1996;23:661–669.
6. Sehgal AR, Dor A, Tsai AC: Morbidity and cost implications of inadequate hemodialysis. Am J Kidney Dis 2001;37:1223–1231.
7. Daugridas JT, Ing T: Handbook of Dialysis. Boston: Little, Brown, 1994.
8. Schon D, Blume SW, Niebauer K, et al: Increasing the use of arteriovenous fistula in hemodialysis: Economic benefits and economic barriers. Clin J Am Soc Nephrol 2007;2:268–276.
9. Held PJ, Port FK, Turenne MN, et al: Continuous ambulatory peritoneal dialysis and hemodialysis: Comparison of patient mortality with adjustment for comorbid conditions. Kidney Int 1994;45:1163–1169.
10. Goeree R, Manalich J, Grootendorst P, et al: Cost analysis of dialysis treatments for end-stage renal disease. Clin Invest Med 1995; 18:455–464.
11. Whiting JF, Golconda M, Smith R, et al: Economic costs of expanded criteria donors in renal transplantation. Transplantation 1998;65:204–207.
12. Whiting, JF, Zavala, JW: The cost-effectiveness of transplantation with expanded donor kidneys. Transplant Proc 1999;31: 1320–1321.
13. Gonin JM: Maintenance immunosuppression: New agents and persistent dilemmas. Adv Renal Replace Ther 2000;7:95–116.

Further Reading

USRDS: U.S. Renal Data System: Excerpts from theUSRDS 2006 annual data report Am J Kidney Dis 49(Suppl 1):S1–S296.
Medicare Payment Advisory Commission: A Data Book: Healthcare Spending and the Medicare Program. Washington, DC: Medicare Payment Advisory Commission, 2006.
Smith MD (ed): Health Care Cost, Quality and Outcomes: ISPOR Book of Terms. Princeton, NJ: International Society for Pharmacoeconomics and Outcomes Research, 2007.

PART XIII

Maintenance Dialysis

CONTENTS

Chapter 77

Technical Aspects of Hemodialysis

Bryan N. Becker and Gerald Schulman

GENERAL PRINCIPLES

Hemodialysis is a complex process performed with apparent simplicity. By attaching an extracorporeal circuit to a patient, the procedure of hemodialysis effectively removes uremic toxins and corrects acid-base disturbances in a manner approximating some of the functions of a natural kidney. This chapter presents a discussion of dialyzers, dialysate composition, water treatment systems, and some of the technical aspects of hemodialysis.

THE HEMODIALYSIS PROCEDURE

Blood Circuit

Blood in the extracorporeal circuit is contained within tubing that is connected to the venous and arterial sides of a patient's access (Fig. 77-1). Needles are inserted into the patient's blood access, and blood tubing is connected to the needle hubs. Blood is withdrawn from the arterial segment by the blood pump and pumped through the dialyzer back to the patient via the venous segment of tubing. Inadvertent entry of air into the dialysis circuit, *air embolism,* is a potentially lethal complication and is most likely to occur between the vascular access site and the blood pump. Air can enter the dialysis circuit from areas around the arterial needle, through leaky or broken tubing or tubing connections, and through the saline infusion set. Air traps are located in the blood tubing to trap air and prevent it from entering the patient's circulation. Air detectors are linked to a relay switch that automatically clamps the venous blood line and shuts off the blood pump if air is detected.

Blood pumps used for hemodialysis (HD) are roller pumps that use the principles of peristaltic pumping to move blood through tubing. A compressible part of the tubing (the *pump segment*) is occluded between rollers and a curved rigid track. Elastic recoil refills the pump tubing after the roller has passed over it. The flow rate of the blood pump is dependent on the stroke volume, the speed of rotation of the rollers, and the volume of the pump segment. The blood flow rate displayed on the dialysis machine is based on these three parameters, rather than an actual value from a blood flow probe. This can lead to significantly higher values for the displayed blood flow compared to the true blood flow rate. Incomplete occlusion of the pump segment due to a pump maladjustment leads to a reduced volume of blood with each pump rotation. This is a common cause of overestimation of blood flow and hence clearance. Careful maintenance of the pump is essential to ensure that the prescribed dialysis dose is actually delivered to the patient.

Pressure monitors are usually located proximal to the blood pump and immediately distal to the dialyzer. The proximal monitor, the *arterial monitor,* guards against excessive suction on the vascular access site by the blood pump; the distal monitor, the *venous monitor,* gauges the resistance to blood return to the venous side of the vascular access. Some machines place the arterial monitor distal to the blood pump and proximal to the dialyzer to detect clotting in the dialyzer and more precisely estimate pressure in the dialyzer blood compartment. To prevent blood clotting in the dialyzer, an anticoagulant such as heparin is often infused into the circuit. A peristaltic pump or syringe pump delivers the anticoagulant into blood in the circuit via a T-tube or T-fitting usually located between the blood pump and the dialyzer.

A blood leak detector is usually placed in the dialysis circuit in the dialysate outflow line. If a blood leak develops through

Figure 77-1 Components of a water treatment system. Deionizers are optional if reverse osmosis (RO) produces water of adequate quality. Granular-activated carbon filters are always placed before the RO system to reduce water hardness and prevent scaling of the RO membranes. Deionization does not remove bacteria or endotoxins and should always be followed by ultrafiltration or submicron filters. (From Ismail N, Becker BN, Hakim RM: Water treatment for hemodialysis. Am J Nephrol 1996;16:60–72. Reproduced with permission of S Karger AG, Basel.)

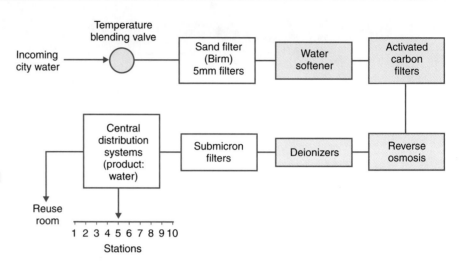

the dialysis membrane, the blood leaking into the dialysate is sensed by the blood leak detector and the appropriate alarm is activated.

Dialysis Solution Circuit

Two properties of the dialysis solution that require constant monitoring are conductivity and temperature. A proportioning system dilutes a concentrated dialysis solution with water. If this system malfunctions, patient blood can be exposed to a hyperosmolar dialysis solution, resulting in hypernatremia, or a hypo-osmolar dialysis solution, leading to hyponatremia and hemolysis. The primary solutes in the dialysis solution are electrolytes. Therefore, the concentration of the dialysis solution is reflected by the concentration of electrolytes and their electrical conductivity. Appropriate proportioning of water and the dialysis solution is monitored by a meter measuring conductivity of the dialysis solution fed into the dialyzer.

A temperature monitor prevents complications related to warm dialysis solution. In most situations, the dialysate temperature is higher than that of the patient, resulting in the transfer of thermal energy into the patient. The energy transfer may prevent a rise in total peripheral resistance as fluid is removed by ultrafiltration (UF), resulting in hypotension during hemodialysis. A cool dialysis solution (i.e., 35°C) can be uncomfortable for the patient and may be dangerous when the patient is unconscious. However, the use of cool dialysate otherwise may have therapeutic value in preventing hypotension. Overheated dialysis solution (>42°C), however, can lead to hemolysis. If the conductivity or the temperature is outside the normal range, a bypass valve diverts the dialysis solution around the dialyzer and directly to a drain.

On-line Monitoring

Dialysis machines function as more than just dialysis delivery systems. Built-in monitors assess the physical characteristics of the dialysis solution, as noted above, and accrue data ranging from patient blood pressure and heart rate to treatment parameters, medication data, measures of delivered dialysis dose, plasma volume, thermal energy loss, and even dialysis access recirculation. Computerized medical information systems have been linked with dialysis delivery systems to provide information networks that can control treatments at individual patient stations while maintaining information and treatment records for future use. Some of these systems include the Smart Connection from Baxter Healthcare, RenalSoft, and a similar system designed by Fresenius Medical Care. Real-time information regarding treatment parameters and patient information also can be visualized during dialysis treatments with the Cobe Centry System 3, the Althin Drake Willock System 1000, and the Fresenius 2008H system. It is now possible to integrate data, such as comparing present and past dialysis treatments, into a real-time display to help gauge therapy, change prescription and ultrafiltration goals, and generate better immediate assessment of a patient's and unit's overall status.[1,2] Such on-line monitoring that allows sensors from the machine to change treatment parameters has been termed a *biofeedback system* (Fig. 77-2). Automatic biofeedback systems have the potential to reduce adverse events such as hypotension, to monitor the state of the hemodialysis access, and to increase the efficiency of the hemodialysis treatment (Table 77-1).

Other monitoring systems have been developed and are used to monitor access flow and function during dialysis and to make accurate determinations of circulating blood volume during the dialytic procedure. Single- and dual-sensor systems using saline injections and sound velocity dilution calibration have been investigated as a method for accurately determining access flow during hemodialysis.[3] Similar efforts have led to noninvasive optical hematocrit monitoring that continually measure hematocrit during dialysis to better determine circulating blood volume.[4] As blood volume deceases, hematocrit increases. It is often possible to define a hematocrit above which hypotension is likely to occur in a patient. A critical hematocrit can be determined with these devices above which hypotension can be reliably predicted in up to 75% of patients.[5]

The measurement of on-line blood volume with these devices can identify patients who are not near their estimated dry weight. In 18% of hemodialysis patients, a less than 5% decrease in blood volume was noted during routine hemodialysis sessions. In subsequent treatments, increased volume was successfully removed without hypotensive episodes.[6] The patients were able to have intradialytic fluid removal intentionally increased by 47% (average, 0.8 L). The change in blood volume can be determined noninvasively during hemodialysis with these devices.[7] Thus, these devices provide an added on-line safety measure to the treatment.

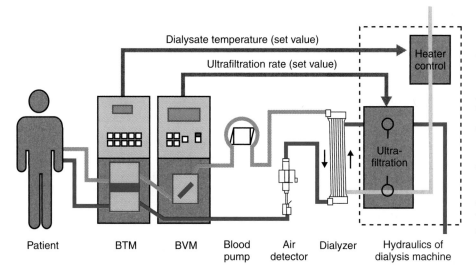

Patient · BTM · BVM · Blood pump · Air detector · Dialyzer · Hydraulics of dialysis machine

Figure 77-2 Elements of a hemodialysis biofeedback system. Patient input variables include blood pressure, plasma volume, sodium concentration, and plasma temperature. These inputs are measured by an on-line blood pressure monitor, a blood volume monitor (BVM), and a blood temperature monitor (BTM). The inputs lead to automatic adjustments by the hemodialysis machine of the ultrafiltration rate, dialysate temperature, and dialysate sodium concentration.

Table 77-1 On-line Features of the Hemodialysis Machine

Parameter	Consequence
Blood pressure	Changes in ultrafiltration rate, sodium modeling
Plasma volume by hemoglobin	Changes in ultrafiltration rate, sodium modeling
Thermal energy loss/gain	Change in dialysate temperature
Transient change in dialysate	Measurement of Kt/V sodium
Transient change in hemoglobin	Access blood flow, recirculation, cardiac output
Transient change in temperature	Access recirculation

CHARACTERISTICS OF DIALYZERS

The classical view of membranes as inert structures providing solely fluid, ion, and molecular transport is now obsolete. Modern dialysis membranes display numerous physical and adsorptive properties that contribute to the degree to which blood components are activated by them. Membranes that produce little interaction with blood components such as white blood cells and the humoral components of plasma are described as being *biocompatible*. The structural compounds comprising the dialysis membranes may be their simplest distinguishing feature, dividing dialyzers into cellulosic, semisynthetic, and synthetic membranes. Cellulose extracted from cotton lint is dissolved in sodium hydroxide and regenerated, and the membrane is then formed in an acid bath. Cuprophane is generated with an ammonium solution of copper hydroxide. Copper-ammonia-cellulose complexes are extruded into an acid bath, producing a membrane with cuprammonium radicals. This modification yields greater diffusion and UF capabilities for cuprophane membranes compared to straight cellulose. Increasing glycerine content in membranes (average content for cuprophane = 5%) also affects these

characteristics, as does membrane acetylation, yielding greater solute and flux capacities to the membrane.

Synthetic membranes differ from cellulose-based dialyzers in several ways. All cellulose membranes have hydroxyl radicals at the surface, which increase their hydrophilicity (membrane wettability). Techniques that mask hydroxyl radicals enhance hydrophobicity and increase protein adsorption.[8] Most synthetic membranes are thicker than less permeable cellulosic membranes. Membrane permeability is inversely proportional to membrane thickness and directly proportional to the membrane's intrinsic diffusion coefficient. However, synthetic membranes also display greater intrinsic diffusion coefficients and maintain their thickness when wet. Cuprophane and cellulose acetate membranes swell when wet.[9,10] A number of synthetic membranes also strongly bind blood proteins, causing decreases in their filtration efficiency.

Membranes can be symmetric or asymmetric. The smooth "skin" side of asymmetric membranes interacts with blood. Asymmetry, obtained by altering membrane precipitation during manufacturing,[11] allows for greater diffusive permeability. Hence, asymmetric membranes are very useful for hemofiltration. Polyacrylonitrile (PAN) and polysulfone (PS) membranes are commonly used asymmetric membranes. Polymethylmethacrylate (PMMA) membranes also manifest many of these characteristics. PAN, polyamide (PA), and PMMA membranes have low hydrophilicity and appreciable protein adsorption. Cellulose-based membranes have greater hydrophilicity and less adsorptive capacity.[11] Surface charge of the membranes also differs, which affects the sieving of charged solutes.[12]

Types of Dialyzers

Three forms of dialyzers have been used for hemodialysis. Plate dialyzers, used in the early days of dialysis, consist of sheets of membranes separated by a spacer in rectangular compartments that are placed in parallel. This arrangement allows for low blood flow resistance and controlled UF.

Coil dialyzers are constructed from one or several pieces of membrane tubing wound around a central core. A support screen maintains the tubing in position. Blood flows through the tubing while dialysate flows through the supporting screen.

Coil dialyzers are of historical interest only because they are rarely used today. They are highly compliant with high blood flow resistance and variable UF rates.

Hollow-fiber dialyzers are the most common dialyzers in use today (Table 77-2). They consist of 10,000 to 15,000 hollow fibers wrapped in a bundle inside a plastic jacket. Each fiber has a diameter of 200 to 300 μm. Blood flows through the fibers while dialysate flows outside the fibers, typically in a countercurrent fashion. Hollow-fiber dialyzers are easy to use and provide low blood flow resistance, excellent mass transfer, low compliance, and controllable UF. Thus, the extracorporeal blood volume is constant and remains independent of transmembrane pressures. They require low (100–200 mL) priming volumes and are easier to reuse than the other types of dialyzers. Problems associated with early hollow-fiber dialyzers include increased blood clotting, blood loss, and residual ethylene oxide or formaldehyde in the potting compound that anchors the fibers to the dialyzer. These problems have largely been overcome with newer dialyzers.[13]

Dialyzers are classified as conventional, high efficiency, or high flux, but with some imprecision surrounding these definitions. The blood flow and the length of treatment employed when using these dialyzers should not be part of the definition. Nor should urea clearance be used in the definition because clearance, or *dialysance*, varies with blood flow. Instead, the dialyzer is defined by the urea mass transfer coefficient (KoA_{urea}) of its membrane, its ultrafiltration coefficient (K_{uf}), and its degree of hydrophobicity or hydrophilicity (Table 77-3). The latter parameter governs the permeability of the membrane to high-molecular-weight substances, its degree of biocompatibility, and its ability to adsorb plasma proteins and peptides to its surface.

The conventional dialyzer has a homogenous membrane that permits effective small-sized solute clearance, but its clearance of medium-sized solute is relatively low. Urea clearance at a blood flow of 300 mL/min is less than 200 mL/min. The relatively low hydraulic permeability of the membrane usually permits treatment with a dialysis machine that does not have an ultrafiltration controller. These membranes are cellulose-based and contain nucleophilic groups that permit complement activation unless they have been chemically modified. The blood flow and membrane structural limitations on urea mass transfer preclude their use in high-efficiency hemodialysis.

Both high-efficiency and high-flux dialyzers have membranes with a KoA_{urea} greater than 450 mL/min. Under standard operating conditions (blood flow of 400 mL/min), the urea clearance is more than 250 mL/min. The high-flux membranes are semisynthetic or synthetic thermoplastics that permit some passage of molecules exceeding 10,000 daltons with a clearance as high as 40 mL/min. In addition, significant adsorption of protein and peptides from the blood onto the membrane may occur with these membranes. When the high-flux membrane is chemically modified such that the hydraulic permeability and the permeability to high-molecular-weight substances is reduced, a high-efficiency membrane is created.

Table 77-2 Representative List of Commonly Used Hollow-Fiber Dialyzers

Model	Membrane	K_{uf}	KoA_{urea}	Surface Area (m²)	Urea Clearance (mL/min) $Q_b = 200$	Vitamin B_{12} Clearance (mL/min) $Q_b = 200$
Cobe 400-HG	Hemophan	5.3	570	0.9	177	57
Terumo C-101	Cellulose	3.5	520	1.0	171	54
Fresenius F-50	PS	30	700	0.9	176	95
Fresenius F-80	PS	60	945	1.8	192	139
Toray B1-1.6-H	PMMA	12	720	1.6	186	94
Gambro polyflux 160	PA	55	690	1.6	183	122
Gambro/Hospal	AN-69	25	400	0.8	161	62

PA, polyamide; PMMA, polymethylmethacrylate; PS, polysulfone.
For a more extensive list of commonly used dialyzers and their specications, refer to Sigdell JE: Operating characteristics of hollow-fiber dialyzers. In Nissenson AR, Fine RN, Gentile DE (eds): Clinical Dialysis, 2nd ed. San Mateo, CA: Appleton & Lange, 1990, pp 106–107.
From Daugirdas JT, Blake PG, Ing TS: Handbook of Dialysis, 2nd ed. Boston: Little Brown, 1994, pp 30–52.

Table 77-3 Comparison of Different Dialyzers

Dialyzer	KoA_{urea} (mL/min)	Ultrafiltration Coefficient	Hydrophobic/Hydrophilic	Membrane Structure
Conventional	<450	<10 mL/mm Hg/hr	Hydrophilic	Symmetrical
High efficiency	>450	10–19 mL/mm Hg/hr	Intermediate	Intermediate
High flux	>450	>15 mL/mm Hg/hr	Hydrophobic	Asymmetrical

Thus, with respect to these low-molecular-weight substances, high-flux and high-efficiency dialyzers have similar performance characteristics. They differ in their respective clearance rates of high molecular substances.

Several reasons suggest use of high-efficiency and high-flux dialyzers. Each of these dialyzer types has a low-molecular-weight solute clearance rate far greater than that of conventional dialyzers. They are useful in large patients with high urea volumes to ensure delivery of an adequate level of therapy. In addition, high-flux dialyzers also clear higher-molecular-weight substances, including substances proven to produce toxicity, such as β_2-microglobulin (MW 11,800 daltons). The surfaces of these membranes are more biocompatible; they cause less activation of complement, less neutropenia, and less immune cell dysfunction during dialysis. Several studies have suggested that biocompatible membranes have a favorable impact on morbidity and mortality in hemodialysis patients. However, the primary motivation behind the use of efficient dialyzers is often the facilitation of shorter dialysis times.

Each dialyzer includes a specification sheet that gives operating information for the dialyzer. The K_{uf} is a function of the hydraulic permeability of the membrane and is expressed as the number of milliliters per hour ultrafiltration achieved for every mm Hg of transmembrane pressure. For example, if the K_{uf} is 4.0, the transmembrane pressure required to remove 1000 mL/hr is 250 mm Hg. This pressure is assessed at the midpoint of the fibers. The values for K_{uf} supplied by manufacturers are derived from in vitro data and usually underestimate the actual clinical K_{uf} by 5% to 30%.[14] Because most hollow-fiber dialyzers have pressure drops across the fibers, because blood is pushed by the blood pump at high pressures (generally 300–350 mm Hg) and exits the dialyzers at lower pressures (generally 100 mm Hg), a "natural" transmembrane pressure of 100 to 150 mm Hg is possible. Thus, with a K_{uf} exceeding 5 mL/mm Hg/hr there is an obligate loss of 500 mL/hr. Patients on these dialyzers may require fluid replacement if their UF requirements are less than 500 mL/hr. Because of this, with most synthetic membranes that have a K_{uf} of more than 6.0, monitoring is necessary to prevent hemodynamically significant errors in UF.

Solute clearance values for urea, creatinine, and vitamin B_{12} are also often supplied on the specification sheet. Clearance of these substances varies directly with hydraulic permeability, and the normal K_{uf} of many synthetic dialyzers can be altered by the manufacturer without requiring relabeling of the dialyzer. Dialyzer urea clearance is usually reported at various blood flow rates (e.g., 200, 300, and 400 mL/min) but at a specific dialysate flow rate (e.g., 500 mL/min). Creatinine clearance approximates 80% of urea clearance. Vitamin B_{12} clearance denotes the ability of the membrane to allow passage of solutes of larger molecular weight. High-flux and high-efficiency dialyzers significantly increase vitamin B_{12} clearance (>100 mL/min at 200 mL/min blood flow) compared to conventional dialyzers (30–60 mL/min at 200 mL/min blood flow). For most dialyzers, in vivo clearance is 20% to 25% less than in vitro clearance.

Dialyzer Reuse

Dialyzer reprocessing for reuse of disposable dialyzers has been widely practiced in the United States, largely due to financial constraints. Dialyzer reuse may be performed manually or with an automated rinsing device. Sterility during reprocessing is maintained either by the use of a chemical disinfectant (such as paracetic acid, glutaraldehyde, or formaldehyde) or via heat sterilization. After reprocessing, dialyzer adequacy is assessed indirectly by measuring the volume of the dialysis fiber bundle in the blood compartment (*fiber bundle volume*) and by pressurizing the dialyzer to evaluate the structural integrity of the fibers (*pressure test*). For a dialyzer to have acceptable reuse parameters, the fiber bundle volume must be greater than 80% of the initial value, the in vitro ultrafiltration rate must be greater than 20% of the manufacturer's stated value, and the dialyzer should not leak at a pressure that is within 20% of the maximal operating pressure.

Reuse of dialyzer can impose its own direct effects on reactions during hemodialysis treatment as well as indirectly via alterations in membrane biocompatibility. During repetitive use, plasma proteins can coat dialysis membranes. The use of formaldehyde or glutaraldehyde without a bleach cycle fixes protein to the surface. This attenuates cuprophane-induced complement activation. However, many reuse procedures with these sterilants also include a bleach-containing cleansing cycle. This tends to restore the original surface of the membrane. Reuse with a mixture of peracetic acid and hydrogen peroxide also allows the surface of the membrane to become coated with protein, improving biocompatibility after reuse.

The increasing use of the newer synthetic membranes raises new issues with respect to reuse. Dialyzers manufactured with synthetic membranes have a favorable biocompatibility profile, even on first use. Therefore, there is no direct clinical benefit associated with reuse. However, the substantial cost of these dialyzers often means that reusing them saves costs. Reuse in this setting permits the introduction of these membranes into situations in which the cost would otherwise be prohibitive. A second issue relating to reuse of high-flux synthetic membranes involves changes to the fundamental characteristics of the membrane induced by the reuse procedure. A procedure using bleach increases porosity and makes the membrane more permeable to substances of larger molecular weight. This is obviously advantageous for removing injurious substances such as β_2-microglobulin. However, if the membrane opens too much, losses of albumin can be substantial. If hydrogen peroxide or peracetic acid is used as the sterilant, an opposite phenomenon occurs, and the permeability of the membrane declines. This is clearly disadvantageous if removal of high-molecular-weight substances is deemed important.

The safety of dialyzer reuse practices has been closely scrutinized, and data concerning the practice have been controversial. Recent data suggest that overall, facilities that reuse dialyzers have a similar risk-adjusted mortality to facilities that do not reuse dialyzers. Most nephrologists believe that patients are not placed at increased risk if strict infection control precautions and quality assurance measures are implemented in dialyzer reprocessing. However, data compiled from the practice of a large dialysis organization suggest that outcome may be improved if dialyzer reuse is discontinued.

Permeability and Porosity

Synthetic high-flux membranes are being increasingly used in the United States. Advantages (or disadvantages) related to their use may result from improved biocompatibility, enhanced clearance or adsorption of large-molecular-weight substances, or both of these features. Even cellulose-triacetate membranes, cellulose-based high-efficiency membranes, have a relatively good biocompatibility profile. The majority of membranes used for conventional or high-efficiency hemodialysis are cellulose or PMMA based. Polysulfone membranes, when configured as low-flux membranes for use without UF control (i.e., "biocompatibility" dissociated from "flux"), cause intermediate degrees of neutropenia and complement activation. The use of polyvinylpyrrolidone to accomplish this dissociation restores some hydrophilicity to the membrane and, thus, a tendency for complement activation.[15]

No large prospective long-term studies have attempted to differentiate effects related to high flux and effects related to biocompatibility. Potential benefits of high flux include enhanced middle-molecule clearance, removal of activated substances such as complement, clearance of β_2-microglobulin, and better lipid control due to the removal of a circulating inhibitor of lipoprotein lipase.[16] Potential disadvantages include albumin loss into the dialysate and the risk of introducing endotoxins or similar substances into the blood.

It is also apparent that reuse procedures may affect membrane properties. As mentioned, bleach may increase high-flux membrane permeability to substances with large molecular weights, whereas hydrogen peroxide or peracetic acid may decrease the permeability of the membrane. This alteration in permeability affects the membrane only when the membrane is configured as a high-flux membrane (e.g., polysulfone or PMMA), but it is unimportant when the membrane is configured as a low-flux membrane. Reuse procedures may also alter the surface charge, potentially resulting in elaboration of bradykinin.

Membrane Choice for Optimal Dialysis

In recent years, there has been a major shift away from the use of celluosic membranes in favor of synthetic membranes. This is clearly due to the multiple lines of evidence describing the adverse blood-membrane interactions associated with cellulosic membranes. Membrane selection influences the frequency and number of adverse events related to hemodialysis therapy (Box 77-1). The membrane may also influence the response to vaccines or erythropoietin and injury to various organs, which may be mediated by inflammatory substances generated during blood-membrane interactions. Some recommendations have been suggested regarding membrane choice for optimal dialysis:

1. Newer synthetic membranes offer established and theoretical advantages over cellulosic membranes.
2. Synthetic membranes are beneficial when used in acute renal failure.

Box 77-1 Factors Influencing Membrane Choice

Biocompatibility of the membrane structure
 Composition and format
 Blood-membrane interactions
 Adsorptive properties
 Effect of reuse
Porosity/permeability
Diffusive and convective clearance

From Schulman G, Levin NW: Membranes for hemodialysis. Semin Dialysis 1994;7:251–256.

3. There is not enough information about the superiority of one synthetic membrane over another (one reasonable approach is to use the specific membrane found in a given study to ameliorate the particular adverse reaction of concern to the nephrologist); currently, the expense of the membrane should also factor in the decision.
4. Avoid the use of angiotensin-converting enzyme inhibitors when PAN membranes (specifically AN-69) are selected. Caution must also be applied with reused membranes.
5. In most cases, the absence of complement activation and of neutropenia is a useful marker of biocompatibility.

Future Developments in Dialyzers

Advances in membrane manufacturing techniques are likely to yield dialyzers better able to remove substances of larger molecular weight (*middle molecules*). Advances have been seen in techniques for regulating pore-size dimensions, distribution, and geometry; these advances have allowed for increased sieving coefficients for molecules such as β_2-microglobulin but not larger substances such as albumin.[17,18] Reducing the inner diameter of the hollow fibers has been shown to increase resistance in the blood compartment, which permits greater filtration of substances in the middle-molecule range.[19] A sorbent system is being developed that also enhances the removal of larger substances; it will be placed in series with the dialyzer in the extracorporeal circuit.[20]

DIALYSATE COMPOSITION

One of the major aims of hemodialysis is the restoration of normal ion concentrations. As such, the levels of individual ions in the dialysate can be set to their desired plasma levels; however, in some instances dialysate levels are set for the diffusible fraction of the ion found in plasma. Dialysis solutions have undergone substantial changes since the inception of hemodialysis.

Dialysate Glucose

In the early 1960s, high glucose concentrations in dialysis fluid were used to provide osmotic pressure for water removal. However, advances in hydraulic UF and the demonstration that high dialysate glucose (>320 mg/dL) increased the risk for hyperosmolar syndrome, postdialysis hyperglycemia, and hyponatremia[21] rendered the use of high dialysate glucose obsolete. Contemporary dialysis fluids range from glucose-free to slightly hyperglycemic (up to 200 mg/dL).[22] Most noninsulin-dependent diabetic patients tolerate dialysis with glucose-free dialysate well, despite losing 25 to 30 g of glucose across the dialyzer. However, this glucose loss may potentiate hypoglycemia[23–25] and adversely affect hemodialysis catabolism, raising levels of free amino acids during dialysis[26] and increasing the intradialytic protein catabolic rate.[27] Ketogenesis and gluconeogenesis are usually sufficient to maintain serum glucose in the physiologic range despite reductions in plasma insulin, lactate, and pyruvate. By contrast, physiologic dialysate glucose (200 mg/dL) has few adverse effects,[28] aside from aggravating hypertriglyceridemia. Dialysate glucose can affect potassium removal, the risk of dialysis disequilibrium syndrome, and postdialysis fatigue. In general, an optimal dialysate glucose concentration is 100 to 200 mg/dL. However, in diabetic patients, insulin doses may require adjustment to account for this dialysis-imposed *glucose clamp,* in which levels of plasma glucose may be kept constant during dialysis as a result of the concentration in the dialysate.

Dialysate Sodium

Investigators comparing hemodynamic changes induced by conventional dialysis, ultrafiltration, and sequential ultrafiltration dialysis found that plasma osmolality plays a pivotal role in maintaining hemodynamic stability during hemodialysis.[29-31] Iso-osmolar fluid removal improved hemodynamic stability. During hemodialysis, the fall in extracellular osmolality is more rapid than corresponding changes in intracellular osmolality, resulting in extracellular to intracellular (ECF–ICF) fluid shifts, exacerbating volume depletion. This decline in plasma osmolality (P_{osm}) is more apparent with rapid solute removal that is not counteracted by sodium diffusing from dialysate into the blood. A low-sodium dialysate (<135 mEq/L) favors this ICF shift because plasma becomes more hypo-osmolar after sodium movement from plasma to dialysate.

The reduction in plasma volume with UF and HD also increases plasma oncotic pressure and decreases capillary hydrostatic pressure. Both forces mobilize extravascular fluid. The degree to which plasma volume decreases depends on the UF rate, fluid shifts, and the plasma refilling rate from the ICF and interstitial fluid compartments. By maintaining a constant P_{osm}, a high-sodium dialysate minimizes intracellular water movement during dialysis, preserving plasma volume.[29,30] A stable P_{osm} during dialysis enhances blood pressure stability,[31,32] especially when the dialysate sodium concentration is increased to at least 135 mEq/L.[33-35] Hypo-osmolality impairs peripheral vasoconstriction during volume removal and exacerbates autonomic insufficiency. Hence, high-sodium dialysate, by maintaining stable P_{osm}, favorably influences compensatory mechanisms during volume removal.[27,36] Improved hemodynamic stability is paralleled by a reduction in cramping, nausea, vomiting, and headache during dialysis.[35-37] Furthermore, patients given higher dialysate sodium concentrations (144 mEq/L) appear to have fewer hypotensive episodes.[37] Thus, a dialysate sodium concentration of 140 to 145 mEq/L is reasonable, gauging the optimal concentration to the patient's blood pressure, weight gain, and symptoms on dialysis.

The use of dialysates with higher sodium concentrations may lead to higher interdialytic weight gain because of increased thirst stimulated by an elevated serum tonicity. In addition, higher dialysate sodium concentrations are associated with a net increase in total sodium shift into the patient. There was concern that hypertension or volume overload would be a consequence of this practice. Although higher dialysate sodium concentration is associated with increased interdialytic weight gain, the excess volume is able to be removed successfully by carefully and frequently assessing the patients' estimated dry weight and increasing the ultrafiltration rate as needed. Adverse symptoms such as hypotension are mitigated by the greater hemodynamic stability associated with the higher sodium concentration. Indeed, it can be argued that of all the changes in dialysate composition, the greatest improvement in intradialytic symptoms such as hypotension has been the result of the introduction of dialysate with a higher sodium concentration.

Sodium Modeling

A strategy combining high and low levels of dialysate sodium is known as *sodium-gradient hemodialysis.* A high-sodium dialysate of 150 mEq/L is used initially and is then reduced automatically and progressively toward isotonic levels in one of three patterns. A linear, ramp pattern lowers sodium concentration at a constant rate throughout the treatment. A step pattern maintains the high sodium level for three quarters of the treatment time and decreases it to 135 to 140 mEq/L for the rest. Finally, sodium is reduced from 150 to 140 mEq/L in an exponential pattern. Sodium modeling can be incorporated into the biofeedback system described in this chapter. Sodium modeling allows the greatest sodium influx to the patient when urea and solute flux from the body is greatest. Theoretically, this technique is associated with fewer symptomatic hypotensive episodes, although in reality it may not be any more advantageous than fixed high-sodium dialysate.[38-41] However, a recent prospective, crossover study in hypotension-prone hemodialysis patients (used as their own controls) compared standard dialysis (138 mEq/L sodium) to step-sodium modeling, isolated ultrafiltration, cool dialysate, and constant high-sodium dialysate (144 mEq/L). The volume removed was similar throughout the study. Sodium modeling and cool dialysate were found to be of greatest benefit in reducing hypotensive events and preserving postdialysis blood pressure. High-sodium dialysate was also shown to reduce hypotensive events. The authors conclude that sodium modeling should be the first approach in patients with intradialytic hypotension.[42] Sodium-gradient dialysis may be beneficial in the initial dialysis of patients with advanced renal insufficiency and urea concentrations higher than 200 mg/dL to decrease the risk of dialysis disequilibrium syndrome. Modeling may also be useful in patients with a low KoA_{urea}, who have delayed urea equilibration between ICF and ECF.[29,43,44] Although sodium modeling has been of unquestionable benefit in selected patients with intradialytic hypotension, it should not be used indiscriminately because of the risk of volume overload and hypertension. The patient must be carefully monitored for symptoms of volume overload.

The concepts of sodium modeling can also be applied to UF, resulting in volume to be removed early in the dialytic session when the patient's intravascular volume is greatest. The UF rate can be gauged to decrease during dialysis as the intravascular volume declines: 50% UF during the first hour, 25% UF during the second hour, 15% UF during the third hour, and 10% UF during the fourth hour. Such a protocol, especially in combination with concurrent sodium modeling, may minimize cramping and symptomatic hypotension in patients prone to these complications.[45]

Dialysate Buffer

Bicarbonate dialysis is the dialytic treatment of choice, conferring benefits over acetate dialysis, including a lower incidence of hypotension and hypoxemia and improved left ventricular stroke work.[46-50] Metabolism of acetate occurs predominantly in skeletal muscle. Healthy people can metabolize acetate at a rate of up to 300 mM/hr, whereas for elderly people and those on chronic hemodialysis, who often have decreased muscle mass, the rate is approximately 3 to 3.5 mM/hr.[51,52] If acetate accumulates due to its reduced rate of metabolism to bicarbonate, reduced myocardial contractility and lowered systemic vascular resistance may occur. In addition, the low P_{CO_2} of the acetate buffered dialysate results in the net transfer of carbon dioxide (CO_2) from the blood to the dialysate, leading to hypoventilation and hypoxia. Thus, older patients, especially those with underlying myocardial dysfunction and low muscle mass, may benefit from bicarbonate dialysate. Dialyzers with a large surface area and increased blood flow rates enhance acetate transfer to the patient, thereby increasing the acetate load for patients to metabolize.[48]

The hemodynamic instability associated with acetate dialysate buffer may be related to a number of factors, including adenosine production,[29] interleukin-1 release,[53] and hypoxemia as a result of myocardial hypoperfusion and dysfunction.[54–57] Dialysate delivery systems also may play a role, because a change from a single-pass system to recirculation with cellulosic membranes can reduce hypoxemia during acetate dialysis.[58] In acetate dialysis, the transfer of CO_2 from blood to dialysate results in reflex hypoventilation and hypoxemia with a decrease in the respiratory quotient (CO_2 produced)/(O_2 consumed), producing hypocapnia and hypoventilation. Bicarbonate dialysate solutions with elevated P_{CO_2} levels reduce reflex hypoventilation and hypoxemia. However, when the dialysate bicarbonate concentration is more than 35 mEq/L, hypoventilation may result from metabolic alkalosis.

Higher dialysate sodium concentrations may improve hemodynamic instability related to acetate dialysis.[33,57–59] Nonetheless, bicarbonate is the dialysate buffer of choice in critically ill patients. In chronic hemodialysis patients, bicarbonate buffer may not offer added hemodynamic benefit when the sodium dialysate is higher than 140 mEq/L. However, patients who metabolize acetate poorly tolerate bicarbonate dialysate better.[60]

Dialysate Calcium

Because dialysate calcium equilibrates with the diffusible (ionized) fraction of plasma calcium, a dialysate calcium concentration of 2.5 mEq/L is equivalent to a serum calcium level of 10 mg/dL. High dialysate calcium (3.5 mEq/L) or low dialysate calcium (<2.5 mEq/L) has certain risks and advantages. Serum calcium level is often reduced in advanced renal failure as a result of reduced sun exposure, depressed production of 1,25-dihydroxyvitamin D_3, and decreased absorption of calcium from the gastrointestinal tract. High dialysate calcium concentration can improve indices of metabolic bone disease and reduce parathyroid hormone levels.[61,62] High dialysate calcium concentration can also improve hemodynamic stability during dialysis[63–65] as well as echocardiographic measures of left ventricular function.[66,67]

The main disadvantage of high dialysate calcium concentration is hypercalcemia. Calcium-based phosphate binders, used preferentially over aluminum-containing antacids and oral or intravenous 1,25-dihydroxyvitamin D_3, are presently used in the management of hyperphosphatemia and to prevent uncontrolled secondary hyperparathyroidism.[68–70] High dialysate calcium concentration can limit the effectiveness of this therapy by inducing hypercalcemia. To obviate hypercalcemia, lower dialysate calcium concentrations (2.5 mEq/L) have been combined with high doses of oral calcium-containing phosphate binders and vitamin D sterols to control hyperphosphatemia[71] and secondary hyperparathyroidism.[72] Mild hypotension was the only major adverse effect associated with such dialysate calcium

concentrations.[66,71] Thus, a dialysate calcium concentration of 2.5 to 2.7 mEq/L is recommended for hemodynamically stable patients, particularly for those prone to hypercalcemia during treatment with vitamin D and calcium salts.

Dialysate Potassium

Dialysis is the primary route of potassium elimination for hemodialysis patients[73,74] although the gastrointestinal tract also contributes to potassium excretion in individuals with end-stage renal disease. Typically, 50 to 80 mEq of potassium are removed with each dialysis treatment.[75] The rate of potassium removal during dialysis is largely a function of the concentration gradient between blood and dialysate. Blood and dialysate flow rates, dialyzer efficiency, and factors affecting transcellular potassium distribution, such as pH, insulin, and catecholamines, are also important.

The majority of dialyzed potassium originates intracellularly and must cross cell membranes before crossing the dialyzer membrane. Plasma potassium concentrations tend to rebound 4 to 5 hours after dialysis, averaging 30% greater potassium values than immediately postdialysis.[76–78] This postdialysis rebound is important because an immediate postdialysis potassium value of more than 5.5 mEq/L is not considered safe, and supplementation for postdialysis hypokalemia is not warranted.

The potassium rebound after hemodialysis reflects a two-compartment model. Potassium transit across cell membranes is believed to be the limiting factor in its removal during dialysis. As a result, potassium dysequilibrium is established, with transfer from ICF to ECF compartments during dialysis failing to replenish external potassium transfer to the dialysate. Net internal transfer continues after the termination of dialysis until a new steady-state potassium gradient is established. Potassium transfer is affected by many factors. Acidosis promotes potassium efflux from cells, and alkalosis causes cellular potassium uptake; this is particularly important in hypokalemic patients with metabolic acidosis. Dialyzing patients with depletion of total body potassium can worsen hypokalemia when concurrent metabolic acidosis is corrected with parenteral bicarbonate during dialysis. Also, plasma tonicity can affect potassium distribution because tonicity favors movement of potassium into extracellular spaces and consequently its removal during dialysis. Hypertonic saline solution or mannitol, used to treat hypotension or muscle cramps during dialysis, thus favors potassium removal during dialysis. Glucose-free dialysate also promotes the dialytic removal of potassium by lowering plasma insulin concentrations.

Low dialysate potassium concentrations can precipitate atrial and venticular ectopic beats, especially in patients with left ventricular hypertrophy or impaired left ventricular function or in patients taking digoxin.[79] The frequency of arrhythmias is greatest during the first 2 hours of dialysis, when potassium flux is greatest. Therefore, in some arrhythmia-prone patients, a "sequential" reduction in dialysate potassium level may be safer for potassium removal.

WATER TREATMENT

Hemodialysis patients are exposed to as much as 600 liters of dialysis water a week, and to all its potential contaminants. Although water treatment systems (WTS) used by dialysis centers produce high-quality water for safe dialysis, WTS are susceptible to malfunction or to user error. Technical advances, such as high-flux and high-efficiency dialysis, reuse, and bicarbonate dialysate, have heightened awareness about water safety.

Hazards Associated with Dialysis Water

Numerous reports of patient injury or death have been linked to improperly treated or inadequately monitored water used for hemodialysis. High levels of aluminum sulfate in dialysate water have been linked to bone disease (osteomalacia and aplastic bone disease) and dialysis-associated encephalopathy (dialysis dementia).[80–82] Limiting aluminum levels in dialysate water to 10 μg/L has resulted in a continued decline in the incidence and case fatality rate of dialysis dementia.[83,84]

Chloramines, used as bactericidal agents in treatment of municipal water, denature hemoglobin by oxidation and inhibition of the hexose monophosphate shunt. Chloramine exposure during dialysis has been associated with hemolysis, Heinz body hemolytic anemia, and methemoglobinemia.[85–87] Other compounds also have adverse effects in dialysis patients. Sodium azide, used frequently with glycerine as a preservative for WTS ultrafilters, has been associated with hypotension.[88] Fluoride, even at the recommended level of 1 mg/L, can cause osteomalacia and bone disease[89] as well as cardiac death.[90] Excess calcium and magnesium in dialysate water have been linked to the *hard water syndrome*, a constellation of symptoms that includes nausea, vomiting, weakness, flushing, and fluctuations in blood pressure.[91,92] Untoward effects have also been reported with nitrates (methemoglobinemia with cyanosis and hypertension),[93] copper (hemolytic anemia),[94,95] and zinc[96] in excess concentrations in dialysate water. Formaldehyde toxicity, secondary to improper disinfectant use and leaching from sediment filters, has caused hemolytic anemia and death.[97,98]

Essential Components of Water Purification

The efficiency of a WTS depends on the capacity of the system, the nature of the water supply, variations in quality of municipal water, and the quality of product water. Figure 77-1 represents a WTS with temperature-blending valves, filters, water softening, carbon filters, reverse osmosis (RO), and deionizing stations. Temperature-blending valves mix incoming hot and cold water to provide an optimum water temperature for downstream components. Most RO membranes work with greatest efficacy at 77°F (26°C). Water temperature lower than 77°F reduces the flow rate of the RO system; water warmer than 100°F (38°C) may damage RO membranes. Filters remove particulate matter from the water. Sand filters remove particles of 25 to 100 μm, cartridge filters extract particles of 1 to 100 μm, and submicron filters remove particles as small as 0.25 μm. In general, 5-μm filters are accepted as adequate protection for equipment and water treatment.

Water softeners, often sodium-containing cation-exchange resins, can remove calcium, magnesium, and other polyvalent cations from the feedwater. Because calcium and magnesium are removed from water in exchange for sodium, the amount of sodium released can be problematic. Removing calcium and magnesium prevents these ions from depositing on the

RO system with resulting malfunction. Granular activated-carbon filters absorb chlorine, chloramines, and other organic substances from the water. Carbon filters are porous, with a high affinity for organic material. Granular activated-carbon filters can be contaminated with bacteria if they are not serviced properly or exchanged frequently. The size of the activated carbon bed depends on the empty bed contact time (EBCT). The EBCT calculation is:

$$EBCT = V \times 7.48 \text{ (gallons/cu. ft.)}/Q$$

where V = carbon volume required in cubic feet and Q = water flow rate in gallons/min. EBCT differs for different substances. Recommended EBCT values are 6 minutes for chlorine removal and 10 minutes for chloramine removal. The Food and Drug Administration recommends that two granular activated-carbon filter-filled tanks are used in series, with each tank having an EBCT of 3 to 5 minutes.

Reverse osmosis applies high hydrostatic pressure to a solution across a semipermeable membrane to prepare a purified solvent. RO rejects 90% to 99% of monovalent and divalent ions and microbiologic contaminants, producing water safe for dialysis. An RO device is often used as pretreatment to deionization, as an economic measure to provide longer service life for the deionization system. Subsequent deionization of permeate (product) RO water is usually unnecessary. Deionization removes all types of cations and anions. The cation-exchange resin exchanges hydrogen ions (H^+) for other cations; the anion-exchange resin exchanges hydroxyl ions (OH^-) for other anions. Deionizing efficacy is determined by measuring the resistivity of the effluent. Resistivity varies with temperature; therefore, resistivity monitors must be temperature-compensated. When the deionization system is exhausted, previously adsorbed ions can elute into the effluent, causing ion-related toxicities.[94,99]

MICROBIOLOGY OF HEMODIALYSIS SYSTEMS

Water used by HD centers is usually obtained from the community water supply. Community water treatment can reduce bacteria and the concentration of endotoxins in the water, yet the dialysis WTS (apart from ultraviolet light) can still become contaminated with bacteria and endotoxins.[100,101] The primary microbial contaminants in dialysis fluids are water bacteria, gram-negative bacteria, and nontuberculous mycobacteria (Box 77-2). Nontuberculous mycobacteria in particular are problematic. They do not produce endotoxins, but they are more resistant to germicides than gram-negative bacteria and are infectious, especially in the setting of inadequately disinfected dialyzers.[102–105] They can survive and multiply in RO-treated water or deionization water that contains little organic matter.[100] Indeed, the Centers for Disease Control documented the presence of nontuberculous mycobacteria in the water of 83% of dialysis centers surveyed in 1984.[102]

Sterilization destroys microorganisms, including highly resistant bacterial spores. Disinfection, in contrast, eliminates all but the highly resistant microorganisms.[106,107] Disinfection can be high level, intermediate, or low level, depending on the germicidal activity. High-level disinfection inactivates all microorganisms except bacterial spores. Low-level disinfection

Box 77-2 Naturally Occurring Water Bacteria Commonly Found in Hemodialysis Systems

Gram-negative Bacteria
Pseudomonas
Flavobacterium
Actinobacillus
Alcaligenes
Xanthomonas
Serratia
Achromobacter
Aeromonas

Nontuberculous Mycobacteria
Mycobacterium chelonae
M. fortuitum
M. gordonae
M. scrofulaceum
M. avium
M. abscessus
M. intracellulare

From Ismail N, Becker BN, Hakin RM: Water treatment for hemodialysis. Am J Nephrol 1996;16:60–72. Reproduced with permission of S. Karger AG, Basel.

reduces the bacterial population to a "safe" level. WTS disinfection generally utilizes low-level disinfection. High-level disinfection is more often used for dialyzer reprocessing.

PYROGENIC REACTIONS DURING HEMODIALYSIS

Pyrogenic reactions (PRs) often develop during or after dialysis treatment, with an incident rate of 0.5% to 12%.[107,108] A *pyrogenic reaction* can be defined as chills (or rigors) and/or fever (oral temperature > 37.8°C[100°F]) in a previously afebrile patient with no recorded signs or symptoms of infection before dialysis.[107,108] Hypotension is sometimes also included in the definition. Other signs of a PR are headache, myalgia, nausea, and vomiting. The symptoms usually begin 30 to 60 minutes into the dialysis treatment and stop shortly after, unless they are extreme. There appears to be little difference in rates of PRs between different hemodialysis modalities.[108]

Three lines of evidence implicate endotoxin in the pathogenesis of PR: (1) antiendotoxin antibodies in dialysis patients,[109,110] (2) *Limulus* lysate reactivity in plasma from patients experiencing PRs,[111,112] and (3) an association of PRs with fluids contaminated with gram-negative bacteria.[112,113] It is unlikely that microorganisms cross intact dialyzer membranes because of the diameter of their pores. Rather, it is endotoxins and other pyrogenic substances that probably gain access to the patient's bloodstream across the dialysis membrane.[112,114] Some of these substances are bacterial pyrogens released by gram-negative bacteria (see Box 77-2),[115] including lipopolysaccharides (LPS), the A-layer LPS subunit, other LPS fragments, peptidoglycans, muramylpeptides, exotoxins, and exotoxin fragments.

Assays for determining the permeability of pyrogens include the *Limulus* amoebocyte lysate assay, the mononuclear cell (MNC) assay, radiolabeled LPS fragments, and neutrophil activation. Many bacterial substances, such as endotoxin fragments, are small enough to penetrate tight cellulosic membranes. These fragments go undetected in the *Limulus* amoebocyte lysate assay. Thus, measuring in vitro cytokine production by MNCs may be more sensitive and specific, allowing detection of these low-molecular-weight substances.[116–118]

The inability to detect passage of endotoxin across intact dialyzer membranes during conventional or high-flux dialysis[119–121] suggests that additional factors are probably involved in PRs. Bacterial products such as endotoxins induce human MNC production of interleukin-1 and tumor necrosis factor alpha.[115] Experimental data suggest that cultured MNCs increase interleukin-1 production in response to LPS, LPS fragments, or plasma proteins in the dialysate.[118,121,122] Moreover, LPS-like fragments can cross dialyzer membranes.[122] Interestingly, plasma must be present on the blood side for cytokine induction. LPS-binding proteins, complement, and other plasma proteins can be activated by regenerated cellulosic membranes[122] and amplify MNC cytokine production.[122–125] Evidence also suggests that endotoxin fragments can cross intact hemodialysis membranes and induce MNC cytokine production, particularly in the presence of plasma.

Additionally, severe PRs in hemodialysis patients appear to correlate with the extent of bacterial contamination in the dialysate.[113] Recent studies have suggested that up to 35% of all water samples and 19% of all dialysate samples in the United States do not comply with AAMI (Association for the Advancement of Medical Instrumentation) standards (<200 colony-forming units [CFU]/mL in water, 2000 CFU/mL in dialysate). Presumably, bacteria adhere to and grow in the dialysis tubing, releasing endotoxin and endotoxin fragments into the dialysate.

Changing dialysis practices have had an impact on PRs, which have been reported with higher frequency in association with dialyzer reuse. Theoretically, use of RO and membrane integrity monitoring should lead to a decrease in the incidence of PRs.[126] The use of bicarbonate and high-flux dialysis have been linked with a higher risk of PRs.[84] In dialysis units that used bicarbonate dialysis, a higher frequency of PRs occurred only in centers that also performed high-flux dialysis. Centers that prepared their own bicarbonate dialysate also were more likely to report pyrogenic reactions than centers that used commercially prepared bicarbonate dialysate. The method for preparing bicarbonate dialysate entails potential contamination.[125] Acetate dialysate is prepared from a single concentrate at a concentration that prohibits bacterial growth (4.8 mol/L). However, bicarbonate dialysate must be prepared from two concentrates: an acid concentrate with a pH of 2.8 that is not conducive to bacterial growth and a 1.2 mol/L bicarbonate concentrate with a neutral pH. Bicarbonate concentrates can support halotolerant endotoxin-producing, gram-negative organisms. As many as 10^5–10^6 CFU/mL can develop in liquid bicarbonate in as few as 10 days after dialysate preparation. Because of this, active quality assurance should be exercised to use liquid bicarbonate concentrate as soon as possible after manufacture or receipt by the dialysis center. Tanks and distribution lines containing stored liquid bicarbonate concentrate should be disinfected at least twice weekly.

Finally, dialyzer reuse practices have been associated with PRs independent of high-flux dialyzer use.[84] Manual dialyzer reprocessing has been associated with a higher incidence of PRs compared to automated reprocessing.[106] Manual reprocessing can allow defects in dialyzer membranes to go undetected because testing for integrity of the membrane is generally not performed with this technique.

Several outbreaks of patient infection and PRs have been reported in HD patients.[127-130] Many of these involved substandard reprocessing or poor water quality.[107] Inadequate mixing of germicide or the use of a new germicide (e.g., chlorine dioxide) have been implicated in several of these outbreaks.[108,131,132] Errors in the design and maintenance of a WTS were responsible for PRs and gram-negative bacteremia in another center.[132] Damage to RO membranes contributed to this outbreak, leading to the recommendation of a thorough inspection for RO damage whenever the RO system removes less than 90% to 95% of total dissolved solids. Finally, although HD has been safely conducted outside the hospital or dialysis center setting, fatal endotoxemia has occurred in dialysis patients at summer camp,[133] illustrating the importance of dialysis WTS in different environmental conditions.

The formaldehyde content used for disinfection also may be important for PRs. Formaldehyde 2% does not effectively or reproducibly eradicate mycobacterial organisms within 36 hours.[104,128] If the concentration of formaldehyde is increased to 4%, mycobacteria cannot survive at room temperature beyond 24 hours.[134] However, there is increasing evidence that lower concentrations of formaldehyde (e.g., 1%) can be effective if the dialyzers are kept at a temperature of 37° to 40°C.[135]

References

1. Ronco C, Brendolan A, Milan M, et al: Impact of biofeedback-induced cardiovascular stability on hemodialysis tolerance and efficiency. Kidney Int 2000;58:800–808.
2. Ronco C, Ghezzi PM, La Greca G: The role of technology in hemodialysis. J Nephrol 1999;12(Suppl 2):S68–S81.
3. Krivitski NM: Theory and validation of access flow measurement by dilution technique during hemodialysis. Kidney Int 1995;48:245–250.
4. Leypoldt JK, Cheung AK, Steuer RR, et al: Determination of circulating blood volume by continuously monitoring hematocrit during hemodialysis. J Am Soc Nephrol 1995;6:214–219.
5. Steuer RR, Leypoldt JK, Cheung AK, et al: Hematocrit as an indicator of blood volume and a predictor of intradialytic morbid events. ASAIO J 1994;40:M691–M696.
6. Steuer RR, Germain MJ, Leypoldt JK, Cheung AK: Enhanced fluid removal guided by blood volume monitoring during chronic hemodialysis. Artif Organ 1998;22:627–632.
7. Steuer RR, Leypoldt JK, Cheung AK, et al: Reducing symptoms during hemodialysis by continuously monitoring the hematocrit. Am J Kidney Dis 1996;27:525–532.
8. Mujais S, Schmidt B: Operating characteristics of hollow-fiber dialyzers. In Nissenson AR, Fine RN, Gentile DE (eds): Clinical Dialysis, 3rd ed. Norwalk, CT: Appleton & Lange, 1995, p 82.
9. Konstantin P, Bailey RM: Polycarbonate-polyether (PC-PE) flat sheet membrane: Manufacture, structure and performance. Blood Purif 1985;4:6–12.
10. Gohl H, Raff M, Harttig D, et al: PC-PE hollow-fiber membrane. Structure, performance characteristics, and manufacturing. Blood Purif 1985;4:23–31.
11. Gohl H, Konstantin P: Membrane and filters for hemofiltration. In Henderson LW, Quellhorst EA, Baldamus CA, Lysaght MJ (eds): Hemofiltration. Berlin: Springer-Verlag, 1986, p 41.
12. Leypoldt JK, Frigon RP, Henderson LW: Macromolecular charge affects hemofilter solute sieving. Trans Am Soc Artif Intern Organs 1986;32:384–387.
13. Kaufman AM, Frinak S, Godmere RO, Levin NW: Clinical experience with heat sterilization for reprocessing dialyzers. ASAIO J 1992;38:M338–M340.
14. Sigdell JE: Operating characteristics of hollow-fiber dialyzers. In Nissenson AR, Fine RN, Gentile DE (eds): Clinical Dialysis, 2nd ed. San Mateo, CA: Appleton & Lange, 1990, pp 106–107.
15. Deppisch R, Betz M, Hansch GM, et al: Biocompatibility of the polyamide membranes in polyamide—the evaluation of a synthetic membrane for renal therapy. In Shaldon S, Koch KM (eds): Contribution to Nephrology. Basel: Karger, 1992, pp 26–46.
16. Seres DS, Strain GW, Hashim SA, et al: Improvement of plasma lipoprotein profiles during high-flux dialysis. J Am Soc Nephrol 1993;3:1409–1415.
17. Bowry SK, Ronco C: Surface topography and surface elemental composition analysis of Helixone, new high-flux polysulfone dialysis membrane. Int J Artif Organs 2001 24:757–764.
18. Ronco C, Brendolan A, Crepaldi C, et al: Blood and dialysate flow distributions in hollow-fiber hemodialyzers analyzed by computerized helical scanning technique. J Am Soc Nephrol 2002;13(Suppl l):S53–S61.
19. Ronco C, Brendolan A, Lupi A, et al: Effects of a reduced inner diameter of hollow fibers in hemodialyzers. Kidney Int 2000;58:809–817.
20. Winchester JF, Ronco C, Brady JA, et al: The next step from high-flux dialysis: Application of sorbent technology. Blood Purif 2002;20:81–86.
21. Mendelssohn S, Swartz CD, Yudis M, et al: High glucose concentration dialysate in chronic hemodialysis. ASAIO J 1967;13:249–253.
22. Rosborough DC, Van Stone JC: Dialysate glucose. Semin Dialysis 1993;6:260–263.
23. Ward RA, Wathen RL, Williams TE, et al: Hemodialysate composition and intradialytic metabolic, acid-base, and potassium changes. Kidney Int 1987;32:129–135.
24. Wathen RA, Keshaviah P, Hommeyer P, et al: The metabolic effects of hemodialysis with and without glucose in the dialysate. Am J Clin Nutr 1978;31:1870–1875.
25. Grajower MM, Walter L, Albin J: Hypoglycemia in chronic hemodialysis patients: Association with propranolol use. Nephron 1980;26:126–129.
26. Kopple JD, Swendseid ME, Shinaberger JH, et al: The free and bound amino acids removed by hemodialysis. ASAIO J 1973;19:309–303.
27. Ward RA, Shirlow MJ, Hayes JM, et al: Protein catabolism during hemodialysis. Am J Clin Nutr 1979;32:2443–2449.
28. Ramirez G, Butcher DE, Morrison AO: Glucose concentration in the dialysate and lipid abnormalities in chronic hemodialysis patients. Int J Artif Organs 1987;10:31–36.
29. Daugirdas JT: Dialysis hypotension: A hemodynamic analysis. Kidney Int 1991;39:233–246.
30. de Vries PMJM: Plasma volume changes during hemodialysis. Semin Dialysis 1992;5:42–47.
31. Palmer BF: The effect of dialysate composition on systemic hemodynamics. Semin Dialysis 1992;5:54–60.
32. Rosansky SJ, Rhinehart R, Shade R: Effect of osmolar changes on plasma arginine vasopressin (PAVP) in dialysis patients. Clin Nephrol 1991;35:158–164.
33. Wehle B, Asaba H, Castenfors J, et al: Hemodynamic changes during sequential ultrafiltration and dialysis. Kidney Int 1979;15:411–418.
34. Baldamus CA, Ernst W, Frei U, et al: Sympathetic and hemodynamic response to volume removal during different forms of renal replacement therapy. Nephron 1982;31:324–332.
35. Petitclerc T, Drueke T, Man N, Funck-Brentano JL: Cardiovascular stability on hemodialysis. Adv Nephrol 1987;16:351–370.

36. Raja R, Henriquez M, Kramer M, et al: Intradialytic hypotension—role of osmolar changes and acetate influx. Artif Organs 1985;9:17–21.

37. Henrich WL, Woodard TD, Blachley JD, et al: Role of osmolality in blood pressure stability after dialysis and ultrafiltration. Kidney Int 1980;18:480–488.

38. Dumler F, Grondin G, Levin NW: Sequential high/low sodium hemodialysis: An alternative to ultrafiltration. ASAIO J 1979;25:351–353.

39. Daugirdas JT, Al-Kudsi RR, Ing TS, et al: A double-blind evaluation of sodium gradient hemodialysis. Am J Nephrol 1985;5:163–168.

40. Raja R, Kramer M, Barber K, et al: Sequential changes in dialysate sodium (D_{Na}) during hemodialysis. ASAIO J 1983;24:649–651.

41. Bedichek E, Kirschbaum B, Sica D: Comparison of the hemodynamic and hormonal effects of hemodialysis using programmable vs. constant sodium dialysate (abstract). J Am Soc Nephrol 1992;3:354.

42. Dheenan S, Henrich WL: Preventing dialysis hypotension: A comparison of usual protective maneuvers. Kidney Int 2001;59:1175–1181.

43. Heineken FS, Evans MC, Keen ML: Intercompartmental fluid shifts in hemodialysis patients. Biotech Prog 1987;3:69.

44. Star RA, Hootkins R, Thompson JR, et al: Variability and stability of two pool urea mass transfer coefficient (abstract). J Am Soc Nephrol 1992;3:395.

45. Prospert FL, Ruffenach P: Ramped sodium dialysis (RSD) versus combined ramped sodium and ultrafiltration dialysis (RSD + RUD) compared to standard sodium dialysis (SD) (abstract). J Am Soc Nephrol 1996;7:1524.

46. Leunissen KML, Hoorntje SJ, Fiers HA, et al: Acetate versus bicarbonate hemodialysis in critically ill patients. Nephron 1986;42:146–151.

47. Graefe U, Milutenovich J, Follette WC, et al: Less dialysis induced morbidity and vascular instability with bicarbonate in dialysate. Ann Intern Med 1978;88:332–336.

48. Vincent JL, Vanherweghem JL, Degante JP, et al: Acetate induced myocardial depression during hemodialysis for acute renal failure. Kidney Int 1982;22:653–657.

49. Novello A, Kelsch RC, Easterling RE: Acetate intolerance during hemodialysis. Clin Nephrol 1976;5:29–32.

50. Hakim RM, Ponzer M-A, Tilton D, et al: Effects of acetate and bicarbonate dialysate in stable chronic dialysis patients. Kidney Int 1985;28:535–540.

51. Tolchin N, Roberts JL, Hayashi J, et al: Metabolic consequences of high mass-transfer hemodialysis. Kidney Int 1977;11:306.

52. Henrich WL: Hemodynamic instability during hemodialysis. Kidney Int 1986;30:605–612.

53. Lonnemann G, Bingel M, Koch KM, et al: Plasma interleukin-1 activity in humans undergoing hemodialysis with regenerated cellulosic membranes. Lymph Res 1987;6:63–70.

54. Garella S, Chang BS: Hemodialysis-associated hypoxemia. Am J Nephrol 1984;4:273–279.

55. Ross EA, Nissenson AR: Dialysis-associated hypoxemia: Insights into pathophysiology and prevention. Semin Dialysis 1988;1:33–39.

56. Wolff J, Pendersen T, Rossen M, et al: Effects of acetate and bicarbonate dialysis on cardiac performance, transmural myocardial perfusion and acid-base balance. Int J Artif Organs 1986;9:105–110.

57. Henrich WL, Woodard TD, Meyer BD, et al: High sodium bicarbonate and acetate hemodialysis: Double-blind crossover comparison of hemodynamic and ventilatory effects. Kidney Int 1983;24:240–245.

58. Vaziri ND, Wilson A, Mukai D, et al: Dialysis hypoxemia—role for dialyzer membrane and dialysate delivery system. Am J Med 1984;77:828–834.

59. Mehta BR, Fischer D, Ahmad M, et al: Effects of acetate and bicarbonate hemodialysis on cardiac function in chronic dialysis patients. Kidney Int 1983;24:782–787.

60. Vinay P, Prud'homme M, Vinet B: Acetate metabolism and bicarbonate generation during hemodialysis: 10 years of observation. Kidney Int 1987;31:1194–1204.

61. Wing AJ: Optimum calcium concentration of dialysis fluid for maintenance haemodialysis. BMJ 1968;4:145–149.

62. Johnson WJ, Goldsmith RS, Beabout JW: Prevention and reversal of secondary hyperparathyroidism in patients maintained by hemodialysis. Am J Med 1974;56:827–833.

63. Maynard JC, Cruz C, Kleerekoper M, et al: Blood pressure response to changes in serum ionized calcium during hemodialysis. Ann Intern Med 1986;104:358–361.

64. Sherman RA, Bialy GB, Gazinski B, et al: The effect of dialysate calcium levels on blood pressure during hemodialysis. Am J Kidney Dis 1986;8:244–247.

65. Fellner SK, Lang RM, Neumann A, et al: Physiological mechanisms for calcium-induced changes in systemic arterial pressure in stable dialysis patients. Hypertension 1989;13:213–218.

66. Henrich WL, Hunt JM, Nixon JV: Increased ionized calcium and left ventricular contractility during hemodialysis. N Engl J Med 1984;310:19–23.

67. Lang RB, Fellner SK, Neuman A, et al: Left ventricular contractility varies directly with blood ionized calcium. Ann Intern Med 1988;108:524–529.

68. Morton AR, Hercz G, Coburn JW: Control of hyperphosphatemia in chronic renal failure. Semin Dialysis 1990;3:219–223.

69. Mai ML, Emmett M, Shelkh MS, et al: Calcium acetate, an effective phosphorus binder in patients with renal failure. Kidney Int 1989;36:690–695.

70. Coburn JW: Use of oral and parenteral calcitriol in the treatment of renal osteodystrophy. Kidney Int 1990;38(Suppl 29):S54–S61.

71. Slatopolsky E, Weerts C, Norwood K, et al: Long-term effects of calcium carbonate and 2.5 mEq/L calcium dialysate on mineral metabolism. Kidney Int 1989;36:897–903.

72. Van der Merwe WM, Rodger RSC, Grant AC: Low calcium dialysate and high-dose oral calcetriol in the treatment of secondary hyperparathyroidism in haemodialysis patients. Nephrol Dial Transpl 1990;5:874–877.

73. Ketchersid TL, Van Stone JC: Dialysate potassium. Semin Dialysis 1991;4:46–51.

74. Spital A, Sterns RH: Potassium homeostasis in dialysis patients. Semin Dialysis 1988;1:14–20.

75. Sherman RA, Hwang ER, Bernholc AS, et al: Variability in potassium removal by hemodialysis. Am J Nephrol 1986;6:284–288.

76. Feig PU, Shook A, Sterns RH: Effect of potassium removal during hemodialysis on the plasma potassium concentration. Nephron 1981;27:25–30.

77. Hou S, McElroy PA, Nootens J, et al: Safety and efficacy of low-potassium dialysate. Am J Kidney Dis 1989;13:137–143.

78. Morgan AG, Burkinshaw L, Robinson PJA, et al: Potassium balance and acid-base changes in patients undergoing regular hemodialysis therapy. BMJ 1970;I:779–783.

79. Morrison G, Michelson EL, Brown S, et al: Mechanism and prevention of cardiac arrhythmias in chronic hemodialysis patients. Kidney Int 1980;17:811–819.

80. Dunea G, Mahurkar SD, Mamdani B, Smith EC: Role of aluminum in dialysis dementia. Ann Intern Med 1978;88:502–504.

81. Coburn JW, Norros KC, Sherrard DJ, et al: Toxic effects of aluminum in end-stage renal disease: Discussion of a case. Am J Kidney Dis 1988;12:171–184.

82. Llach F, Felsenfeld AJ, Coleman MD, et al: The natural course of dialysis osteomalacia. Kidney Int 1986;29(Suppl 18):S74–S79.

83. Tokars JI, Alter MJ, Favero MS, et al: National surveillance of hemodialysis-associated diseases in the United States, 1990. ASAIO J 1993;39:71–80.

84. Alter MJ, Favero MS, Moyer LA, et al: National surveillance of dialysis-associated diseases in the United States, 1989. Trans ASAIO 1991;37:97–109.

85. Topple MA, Bland LA, Favero MS, et al: Investigation of hemolytic anemia after chloramine exposure in a dialysis center (letter). Trans ASAIO 1988;34:1060.

86. Yawata Y, Kjillstrand C, Buselmeier T, et al: Hemolysis in dialyzed patients: Tap water-induced red blood cell metabolic deficiency. Trans ASAIO 1972;18:301–304.

87. Neilan BA, Ehlers SM, Kolpin CF, et al: Prevention of chloramine-induced hemolysis in dialyzed patients. Clin Nephrol 1978;10:105–108.

88. Gordon SM, Drachman J, Bland LA, et al: Epidemic hypotension in a dialysis center caused by sodium azide. Kidney Int 1990;37:110–115.

89. Lough J, Noonan R, Gagnon R, et al: Effects of fluoride on bone in chronic renal failure. Arch Pathol 1975;99:484–487.

90. Dialysis patients in Chicago die from fluoride poisoning; FDA issues safety alert. Contemp Dialysis Nephrol 1993;10:11.

91. Freeman RM, Lawton RL, Chamberlain MA: Hard-water syndrome. N Engl J Med 1967;276:1113–1118.

92. Evans DB, Slapak M: Pancreatitis in the hard water syndrome. BMJ 1975;3:748.

93. Carlson DJ, Shapiro FL: Methemoglobinemia from well water nitrates: A complication of home dialysis. Ann Intern Med 1970;73:757–759.

94. Manzler AD, Schreiner CW: Copper-induced acute hemolytic anemia. A new complication of hemodialysis. Ann Intern Med 1970;73:409–412.

95. Matter BJ, Pederson J, Psimenos G, et al: Lethal copper intoxication in hemodialysis. Trans ASAIO 1969;15:309–315.

96. Gallery ED, Blomfield J, Dixon SR: Acute zinc toxicity in haemodialysis. BMJ 1973;4:331–333.

97. Centers for Disease Control: Formaldehyde intoxication associated with hemodialysis—California. Epidemic Investigation Report EPI 81-73-2, May 7, 1984. Atlanta: Centers for Disease Control, 1984.

98. Orringer EP, Mattern WD: Formaldehyde-induced hemolysis during chronic hemodialysis. N Engl J Med 1976;294:1416–1420.

99. Johnson WJ, Taves DR: Exposure to excessive fluoride during hemodialysis. Kidney Int 1974;5:451–454.

100. Favero MS, Petersen NJ, Carson LA, et al: Gram negative water bacteria in hemodialysis systems. Health Lab Sci 1975;12:321–334.

101. Bland LA, Favero MS: Microbiologic aspects of hemodialysis systems. In Association for the Advancement of Medical Instrumentation (AAMI) Standards and Recommended Practices, Vol. 3: Dialysis. Arlington, VA: American National Standards, 1993, pp 257–265.

102. Carson LA, Bland LA, Cusick LB, et al: Prevalence of nontuberculous mycobacteria in water supplies of hemodialysis centers. Appl Environ Microbiol 1988;54:3122–3125.

103. Lowry P, Beck-Sague CM, Bland LE, et al: *Mycobacterium chelonae* infections among patients receiving high-flux dialysis in a hemodialysis unit in California. J Infect Dis 1990;161:85–90.

104. Bolan G, Reingold AL, Carson LA, et al: Infections with *Mycobacterium chelonae* in patients receiving dialysis and using processed hemodialyzers. J Infect Dis 1985;152:1013–1019.

105. Carson LA, Petersen NJ, Favero MS, et al: Growth characteristics of atypical mycobacteria in water and their comparative resistance to disinfectants. Appl Environ Microbiol 1978;36:839–846.

106. Favero MS: Distinguishing between high-level disinfection, reprocessing, and sterilization. In AAMI Technical Assessment Report No. 6. Reuse of Disposables: Implications for Quality Health Care and Cost Containment. Arlington, VA: American National Standards, 1983, pp 19–20.

107. Favero MS, Bland LA: Microbiologic principles applied to reprocessing hemodialyzers. In Deane N, Wineman RJ, Bemis JA (eds): Guide to Reprocessing of Hemodialyzers. Boston: Martinus Nijhoff, 1986, pp 63–73.

108. Gordon SM, Oettinger CW, Bland LA, et al: Pyrogenic reactions in patients receiving conventional, high-efficiency, or high-flux hemodialysis treatments with bicarbonate dialysate containing high concentrations of bacteria and endotoxin. J Am Soc Nephrol 1992;2:1436–1444.

109. Jones DM, Tobin BM, Harlow GR, et al: Antibody production in patients on regular hemodialysis to organisms present in dialysate. Proc Eur Dial Transpl Assoc 1972;9:575–576.

110. Hindman SH, Favero MS, Carson LA, et al: Pyrogenic reactions during haemodialysis caused by entramural endotoxin. Lancet 1975;2:732–734.

111. Raij L, Shapiro FL, Michael AF: Endotoxemia in febrile reactions during hemodialysis. Kidney Int 1973;4:57–60.

112. Passavanti G, Buongiorno E, De Fino G, et al: The permeability of dialytic membranes to endotoxins: Clinical and experimental findings. Int J Artif Organs 1989;12:505–508.

113. Laurence RA, Lapierre ST: Quality of hemodialysis water: A 7-year multicenter study. Am J Kidney Dis 1995;25:738–750.

114. Dinarello CA: Interleukin-1 and its biologically related cytokines. Adv Immunol 1989;44:153–205.

115. Loppnon H, Brade H, Durbaum I, et al: IL-1 induction-capacity of defined lipopolysaccharide partial structures. J Immunol 1989;142:3229–3238.

116. Duff GW, Atkins E: The detection of endotoxin by in vitro production of endogenous pyrogen: Comparison with limulus amebocyte lysate gelation. J Immunol Methods 1982;52:323–331.

117. Lonnemann G, Bingel M, Floege J, et al: Detection of endotoxin-like interleukin-1-inducing activity during in vitro dialysis. Kidney Int 1988;33:29–35.

118. Evans RC, Holmes CJ: In vitro study of the transfer of cytokine inducing substances across selected high-flux hemodialysis membranes. Blood Purif 1991;9:92–101.

119. Favero MS, Port FK, Bernick JJ: In vivo studies of dialysis related endotoxemia and bacteremia. Nephron 1981;27:307–312.

120. Klinkman H, Falkenhagen D, Smollich BP: Investigation of permeability of highly permeable polysulfone membranes for pyrogens. Contrib Nephrol 1985;46:174–183.

121. Bingel M, Lonnemann G, Sheldon S, et al: Human interleukin-1 production during hemodialysis. Nephron 1986;43:161–163.

122. Hakim RM, Breillat J, Lazarus JM, et al: Complement activation and hypersensitivity reactions to dialysis membranes. N Engl J Med 1984;311:878–882.

123. Cavaillon J-M, Fitting C, Haeffner-Cavaillon N: Recombinant C5a enhances interleukin-1 and tumor necrosis factor release by lipopolysaccharide-stimulated monocytes and macrophages. Eur J Immunol 1990;20:253–257.

124. Schindler R, Gelfand JA, Dinarello CA: Recombinant C5a stimulates transcription rather than translation of interleukin-1 (IL-1) and tumor necrosis factor: Translational signal provided by lipopolysaccharide or IL-1 itself. Blood 1990;76:1631–1638.

125. Urena P, Herbelin A, Zingraff J, et al: Permeability of cellulosic and non-cellulosic membranes to endotoxins subunits and cytokine production during in-vitro haemodialysis. Nephrol Dial Transplant 1992;7:16–28.

126. Gault MH, Duffett AL, Murphy JF, et al: In search of sterile, endotoxin-free dialysate. ASAIO J 1992;38:M431–M435.

127. Centers for Disease Control: Clusters of bacteremia and pyrogenic reactions in hemodialysis patients—Georgia. Epidemic Investigation Report EPI 86-65-2, April 22, 1987. Atlanta: Centers for Disease Control, 1987.

128. Centers for Disease Control: Bacteremia associated with reuse of disposable hollow-fiber hemodialyzers. MMWR 1986;35:417–418.

129. Centers for Disease Control: Pyrogenic reactions in patients undergoing high-flux hemodialysis—California. Epidemic Investigation Report EPI 86-80-2, June 1, 1987. Atlanta: Centers for Disease Control, 1987.

130. Alter MJ, Favero MS, Miller JK, et al: Reuse of hemodialyzers. Results of nationwide surveillance for adverse effects. JAMA 1988;260:2073–2076.

131. Bland LA, Favero MS, Oxborrow GS, et al: Effect of chemical germicides on the integrity of hemodialyzer membranes. Trans ASAIO 1988;34:172–175.

132. Jenkins SR, Lin FUC, Lin RS, et al: Pyrogenic reactions and pseudomonas bacteremias in a hemodialysis center. Dialysis Transplant 1987;16:192–197.

133. Oberle MW, Favero MS, Carson LA, et al: Fatal endotoxemia in dialysis patients at a summer camp. Dialysis Transplant 1980;9:549–550.

134. Bland LA, Favero MS: Microbiologic and endotoxin considerations in hemodialyzer reprocessing. In AAMI Standards and Recommended Practices, Vol. 3: Dialysis. Arlington, VA: American National Standards, 1993, pp 45–52.

135. Gazenfield-Grazit E, Eliabou HE: Endotoxin antibodies in patients on maintenance hemodialysis. Israel J Med Sci 1969;5:1032–1035.

Further Reading

Dheenan S, Henrich WL: Preventing dialysis hypotension: A comparison of usual protective maneuvers. Kidney Int 2001;59:1175–1181.

Eknoyan G, Beck G, Cheung A, et al: Dialyzer best practice: Single use or reuse. Semin Dial 2006;19:120–128.

Locatelli F, Buoncristiani U, Canaud B, et al: Haemodialysis with on-line monitoring equipment: Tools or toys? Nephrol Dial Transplant 2005;20:22–33.

Rocco M, Schulman G, Schwab S, for the HEMO Study investigators: Effect of dialysis dose and membrane flux on morbidity and mortality in chronic hemodialysis patients: Primary results of the HEMO Study. N Engl J Med 2002;347:2010–2019.

Wystrychowski G, Levin N: Dry weight: Sine qua non of adequate dialysis. Adv Chronic Kidney Dis 2007;14:e10–e16.

Chapter 78

Choice and Maintenance of the Vascular Access

Bradley S. Dixon

Hemodialysis may be performed acutely to treat complications of acute kidney injury or remove dialyzable toxins or chronically to treat end-stage renal disease (ESRD). In either situation, to be effective hemodialysis requires a well-functioning access to the bloodstream. To serve this role, significant demands are placed on the vascular access. It must be easy to connect to the external hemodialysis blood circuit, capable of delivering the blood flows of up to 400 to 500 mL/min required for high-efficiency hemodialysis, and must remain patent and free of infection despite frequent, repetitive use—particularly in long-term maintenance hemodialysis. For acute hemodialysis the focus is on ease of creation and rapid access to the circulation. For chronic maintenance hemodialysis the access must be convenient to use and have a low incidence of long-term complications despite repetitive use.

The National Kidney Foundation/Kidney Disease Outcomes Quality Initiative (K/DOQI) established clinical practice guidelines for vascular access in 1997. The guidelines were updated and revised in 2006.[1,2] These guidelines, based on published evidence and expert opinion, represent an excellent resource and an authoritative guide to direct clinicians in the choice and maintenance of the vascular access. They also serve as a source for clinical performance measures being developed by the Centers for Medicare & Medicaid Services (CMS) ESRD Quality Initiative. This chapter endorses most of the K/DOQI guidelines; the reader is referred to published recommendations for more discussion on the background and rationale for those guidelines.[1,2]

VASCULAR ACCESS FOR ACUTE HEMODIALYSIS

Dual-lumen, noncuffed temporary catheters are best used for acute hemodialysis.[3] These catheters are rigid at room temperature, thus aiding insertion, but become pliable when they achieve body temperature after insertion. Acute dialysis catheters may be placed in one of three anatomic locations: the femoral, jugular, or subclavian vein.

In most patients, the femoral vein is the easiest site to insert a catheter; it is associated with the lowest risk of life-threatening complications. The major disadvantage of use of the femoral vein is that the patient generally must lie down while the catheter is in place, and there is a high rate of infection if the catheter is left in place for more than 5 days.[4] Thrombosis is also a concern with femoral vein catheterization. A femoral catheter is particularly useful for short-term treatment of acute renal failure, emergent stabilization of a critically ill patient with a coagulopathy, or acute toxin removal when the patient will only need a few dialysis treatments. It is preferable to use femoral catheters 19 to 20 cm long, because recirculation in the femoral position is considerably lower than when shorter catheters (13–15 cm) are used.[5]

For patients who require longer periods of hemodialysis, the jugular approach is preferable.[3] Catheters placed under aseptic conditions in either jugular vein may be left in place for up to 3 weeks. The complication rate associated with insertion into the jugular is higher than that associated with femoral-line insertion; complications include pneumothorax and arterial or great vein puncture with associated mediastinal, pleural, or pericardial hemorrhage.[3,6] There is also the risk of introducing an air embolism when inserting these catheters, and patients should be maintained in the Trendelenburg position while the catheter is being inserted until the caps have been placed on the end of the catheter. The risk of perforation of the great vein is probably greatest in patients who have previously had many line insertions and have developed central vein stenosis. A chest radiograph is imperative after a jugular or subclavian line is inserted and before initiation of hemodialysis, both to exclude the development of a pneumothorax and to confirm that the catheter is positioned appropriately. If there is any doubt that the tip of the catheter is not within the great vessels, a vascular study should be performed by injecting a small amount of contrast into the catheter under fluoroscopic control.

Subclavian vein catheterization can also be performed, with a rate of immediate complications and catheter-life similar to that seen with jugular vein insertions. However, central vein stenosis—a late complication—occurs more commonly with subclavian than with jugular insertions.[7–9] Thus, subclavian vein catheterization for hemodialysis should be avoided in patients with chronic renal failure who will need future arteriovenous access placement.

Use of ultrasound guidance for catheter insertion can decrease the rate of complications and is strongly recommended.[3,10,11] Ultrasound is used before the procedure to localize the position of the vein and artery and exclude intramural thrombus. Use of real-time ultrasound while cannulating the vein can further enhance successful catheterization and reduce the incidence of inadvertent arterial catheterizations.

All temporary catheters carry the risk of bacterial infection due to contamination of the insertion tract or lumen.[3,6] Strict adherence to aseptic technique in placement and care of the catheter is crucial (for details see www.cdc.gov/mmwr/preview/mmwrhtml/rr5110a1.htm and Posa and colleagues[12]). At the first sign of systemic infection or the development of fever, the catheter should be removed. The most common offending organism with jugular lines is *Staphylococcus aureus* or *S. epidermidis*.[13–15] Any signs of systemic infection should be treated with antibiotics after appropriate cultures. Typically vancomycin (10–20 mg/kg, up to a maximum dose of 2 g) is given initially, pending bacteriologic identification of the organism and sensitivities. Patients with femoral catheters are also likely to become bacteremic from gram-negative organisms and should be treated with vancomycin and either a third-generation cephalosporin, quinolone, or an aminoglycoside, pending the results of blood cultures. The culture results should guide antibiotic therapy after the initial dose. Combinations of vancomycin and an aminoglycoside must be used with caution because of the risk of ototoxicity. These patients must be treated for 2 to 3 weeks when cultures are positive and to confirm adequate antibiotic levels. The trough level of vancomycin is 10 to 15 mg/mL. Patients with some residual renal function or those receiving continuous venovenous hemofiltration will have increased vancomycin clearance and require more frequent dosing.

Uremic patients who develop *S. aureus* bacteremia have a relatively high incidence of metastatic complications; these patients may develop infectious endocarditis, septic arthritis, or epidural abscess.[15] Patients who develop a metastatic focus of infection should have any accumulation of pus drained and should be treated for up to 6 weeks with parenteral antibiotics.

VASCULAR ACCESS FOR MAINTENANCE HEMODIALYSIS

Three main classes of vascular access are currently used for maintenance hemodialysis: the autogenous arteriovenous fistula (AVF), arteriovenous bridge graft (AVG), and central venous catheter (CVC).[16] Common types of AVFs include the radiocephalic fistula, brachiocephalic fistula, and basilic vein transposition to the brachial artery.[17–19] Most current AVGs are composed of expanded polyfluorotetraethylene (ePTFE)

and are placed either in a loop configuration in the forearm (brachial artery to cephalic or basilic vein), straight configuration in the upper arm (brachial artery to axillary vein), or a loop configuration in the upper thigh (femoral artery to vein).[20] Compared to ePTFE, biografts have a lower infection rate but tend to degenerate quicker.[21–23] Autogenous vessels also have other uses (e.g., coronary artery bypass), so they generally are not favored for AVGs over ePTFE. Tunneled central venous catheters (TCCs) are most commonly placed in the internal jugular vein but can be placed in the subclavian vein, femoral vein or, in exceptional circumstances, directly into the inferior vena cava via a transhepatic or translumbar approach.[24]

Selection of a Permanent Vascular Access

An algorithm for the selection of a vascular access is shown in Figure 78-1. Each type of vascular access has advantages and disadvantages. An AVF placed in the most distal location possible in the arm is the preferred access.[1,25] In our practice an AVF is preferred not only for the first, but also subsequent accesses even if the patient is already on dialysis.[26] Once mature, an AVF has the longest cumulative patency, lowest incidence of thrombosis or infection, lowest per patient per year cost, and is associated with prolonged patient survival (though reported differences in survival are admittedly confounded by indication).[14,27–36] The main disadvantages of an AVF are a slower rate of maturation and a higher rate of primary access failure, leading to the increased need for CVCs and subsequent surgery for new access creation.[37–43] Hence, early referral for access creation about 6 months before the expected need for hemodialysis is important to avoid the need for a central venous catheter.[34,44,45] For patients already on hemodialysis, placement of an AVF can lead to longer CVC use with its attendant risks. In this setting, whether the long-term benefits of an AVF outweigh the short-term increased risks compared to an AVG has not been completely resolved.[42] However, we prefer to use an AVF whenever possible and try to be proactive about assessing and facilitating AVF maturation and early catheter removal. The choice between using a basilic vein transposition fistula versus an AVG is debated, but we generally prefer to create the basilic vein transposition fistula before an AVG.[46–53] An additional problem for AVFs is that they can be more difficult to cannulate, particularly when they are deep or not fully developed. The "graftula," created by placing a piece of ePFTE around the adventitial side of the fistula, is a novel approach to the problem of a deep fistula that can be used in selected instances to provide an easier target to cannulate.

An AVG is preferred over a central venous catheter.[30,35,36,54–56] In our practice an AVG is primarily a salvage procedure, reserved for situations in which adjacent vessels are not available to create a suitable AVF.[26] An AVG can typically be cannulated and used for dialysis within 3 to 6 weeks after creation and is often easier than a new AVF to cannulate.[57–60] Grafts can also be used to create heroic types of vascular accesses, such as axilloaxillary arteriovenous grafts or arterioarterial grafts.[61–63] However, AVGs have a significantly increased frequency of stenosis, thrombosis, and infections, leading to an increase in per patient per year costs and morbidity compared to an AVF.[29,30,35,36,54–56,64] Frequent access

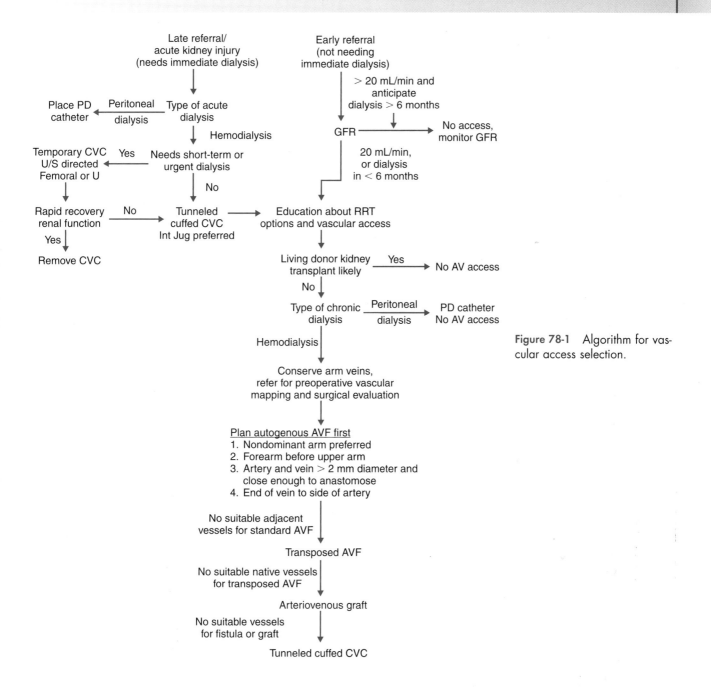

Figure 78-1 Algorithm for vascular access selection.

monitoring is also needed to detect and treat AVG stenosis before it leads to thrombosis.[1,65]

Central venous catheters are discouraged. They should be reserved only for short-term bridging to a permanent AVF or AVG and in situations in which an AVF or AVG is contraindicated (e.g., severe congestive heart failure) or cannot be constructed.[24,66] CVCs are appealing because of the ease and rapidity of creation, the absence of repetitive needle sticks, and lack of problems with postdialysis hemostasis.[24] These advantages are more than offset by the higher risk of infection, leading to increased hospitalizations, higher mortality, and the highest per patient per year costs of any access.[29,34–36,41,44,54,67] Problems with catheter clotting and slow blood flow rates with CVCs also can limit adequate dialysis.[24,55,68] CVCs carry the additional risk of developing central venous stenosis (particularly with subclavian catheters) that is difficult to treat and may prevent subsequent creation of an AVF or AVG in that arm.[7,9]

Preoperative Evaluation and Vascular Mapping

Creation of a successful AVF is enhanced by careful preoperative evaluation.[69] In most cases this should include preoperative arterial and venous imaging.[70–76] The preoperative history includes a review of any prior arteriovenous access surgeries, the location of any current or past CVCs or peripherally inserted central catheters, the presence of a transvenous pacemaker or other significant operations involving the extremities, and the presence of symptomatic organic heart disease. Symptoms and signs, such as swelling, atrophy, ulcers, skin lesions, surgical scars, catheters, pacemakers, and pain or ischemia of the extremity or central vessels, are noted.[1] Arterial pulses in the extremity should be palpated and an Allen's test performed to assess hand perfusion by the radial and ulnar artery.[75] Venous anatomy in the extremity is assessed using a tourniquet. However, given the age and underlying vascular disease in the current ESRD population, the history and physical examination are usually not sufficient to determine the optimal site for AVF creation.[70,77] Preoperative vascular mapping has been shown to increase the percentage of successful AVFs created.[72–74,77] At this time no cross-center standardized protocol exists. Duplex ultrasonography is the current procedure of choice to look at the arterial and venous anatomy for significant stenoses, thrombosis, an atypical vascular pattern, and vessel size. It has a reported sensitivity of 80% to 90% and specificity of 90% to 100% for significant arterial and venous stenosis (>50% luminal narrowing) and other lesions in the distal extremity.[70,78,79] However, duplex ultrasonography is less sensitive in detecting central arterial or venous stenosis.[70,78] If this is suspected on clinical grounds or the patient has had a current or prior CVC (especially a subclavian catheter), further imaging by contrast-enhanced digital subtraction angiography or magnetic resonance angiography is recommended.[78] Both of these techniques have some risks, including contrast-induced nephropathy and nephrogenic systemic fibrosis, respectively.[80–82] The risks need to be discussed with the patient before the procedure.

Vessel size is an important determinant of successful fistula creation.[38,74] This appears to be a threshold effect: below a critical size the likelihood of a successful outcome is negligible, but above that threshold, size does not appear to be strongly predictive of outcome.[83–86] The exact threshold has not been established and may vary with surgical expertise and measurement technique but is probably approximately 2 to 2.5 mm for both arteries and veins.[69,74,85] Venous size should be measured using compression of 30 to 40 mm Hg. Some surgeons favor performing the examination themselves in the operating room just before access creation because vessel size may vary from preoperative assessment due to changes in ambient temperature or sympathetic activity. Studies have also reported that endothelial function, as measured by brachial artery flow-mediated dilation, or venous compliance, as measured by venous plethysmography, are predictive of AVF success.[86,87] However, these are not routinely measured.

Unique Considerations

A number of unique situations influence the timing and choice of vascular access placement. Patients under consideration for kidney transplantation pose a challenge as to when to place a vascular access. Because deceased donor transplantation is unpredictable and may require that the patient wait for several years on dialysis, I recommend placement of an AVF in such patients. However, for patients with a high likelihood of receiving a living donor kidney before starting dialysis, it seems an acceptable risk to delay vascular access placement until that workup is completed. Patients with severe heart failure from organic heart disease are unique because they may decompensate after vascular access placement due to their inability to increase cardiac output sufficient to meet the demands of an arteriovenous shunt.[88,89] A tapered AVG may be considered in such cases to limit the volume flow through the fistula, but most of these patients will likely need a CVC for dialysis. No well-defined parameters exist to predict this outcome. However, patients with organic heart disease who have significant dyspnea at rest or minimal exertion should probably start hemodialysis with a CVC rather than

an arteriovenous shunt. If their symptoms improve on dialysis, conversion to an AVF should be reconsidered. Similarly, patients whose remaining lifespan from comorbidities apart from ESRD is predicted to be very short (i.e., a few months) that nonetheless choose to go on hemodialysis may be suitable candidates for a CVC rather than AVF. However, given the uncertainty in predicting survival in any given person, it seems prudent to recommend placement of an AVF for most patients who are deemed suitable candidates for maintenance hemodialysis. Age, race, and gender should not deter placement of an AVF.[18,69,90,91] With appropriate preoperative vascular mapping, an AVF can be constructed; it remains the first access of choice.

Process Improvement: Achieving Increased Fistula Prevalence

Whereas surgeons and radiologists are responsible for placement of most permanent hemodialysis accesses in the United States, the referring nephrologist plays a critical role in choosing the surgeon, educating the patient and primary care physicians, timing the referral, and communicating with the interventionalist and dialysis staff the type of access that he or she wants in their patients.[38,69,92,93] The nephrologist, in concert with the access surgeon and dialysis staff, should establish access practice goals for the unit.[25,94] Clinical practice guidelines for vascular access established by K/DOQI are a good source for these goals.[1] The CMS ESRD Quality Initiative has currently established three clinical performance measures for vascular access: (1) number of hemodialysis patients with an AVF, (2) number of hemodialysis patients with a catheter, and (3) monitoring of AVGs for stenosis.[95] Current targets are for at least 50% incident patients and 40% prevalent patients to have an AVF. The future goal of the CMS Fistula First Breakthrough Initiative is a 65% prevalence of AVFs by 2009. K/DOQI recommends that less than 10% of hemodialysis accesses should be permanent CVCs (those not used as a bridge to AVF).[1] These targets are challenging but achievable.[91,96–99]

The Fistula First National Vascular Access Improvement Initiative has established 11 core strategies to increase fistula placements. These strategies are listed in Box 78-1. Additional information and resources for implementing these strategies can be found at the Fistula First website (www.fistulafirst.org/index.htm). Central to achieving these goals is the creation and maintenance of a vascular access database.[69,100] At a minimum the database should contain the date, location, and type of each access placement; the surgeon who placed the access; and the date and reason the access was abandoned. Optimally, the database should also record the date of first use for hemodialysis and the date and description of each access study, complication, and intervention, along with the person who performed the intervention. (An electronic database program is available on request from the author.) A vascular access coordinator needs to be assigned to input the data into the database in a timely manner. The database then allows for ongoing continuous quality improvement to monitor progress toward achieving the clinical vascular access practice goals established by the unit. Periodic meetings with the surgeon and vascular access management group are needed to review the data and implement changes to achieve the established goals or to set new goals if prior targets have been attained.

Box 78-1 Core Strategies to Increase AVF Placements (Fistula First Initiative)

1. Routine CQI review of vascular access
2. Timely referral to nephrologist
3. Early referral to surgeon for "AVF only" evaluation and placement
4. Surgeon selection based on best outcomes, willingness, and ability to provide access surgeries
5. Full range of appropriate surgical approaches to AVF evaluation and placement
6. Secondary AVF placement in patients with AVGs
7. AVF placement in patients with catheters where indicated
8. Cannulation training for AVFs
9. Monitoring and maintenance to ensure adequate access function
10. Education for caregivers and patients
11. Outcomes feedback to guide practice

Most of the strategies listed in Box 78-1 to increase AVF prevalence are self-explanatory. Further details can be found at the Fistula First website, as well as in recent reviews.[38,69,93,101] Early identification of patients with stage 4 chronic kidney disease when glomerular filtration rate is approximately 30 mL/min allows for timely education about types of dialysis and vascular access.[69] Preservation of vessels by avoiding intravenous or arterial catheters, particularly in the nondominant upper extremity, is important but admittedly often difficult to enforce. Choice of a surgeon with an interest in vascular access, who is willing to participate in continuous quality improvement and has expertise in creating all types of AVFs (as well as AVGs if needed), is critical. Early referral to the surgeon about 6 months before the expected time of starting hemodialysis is crucial to allow time for AVF maturation, particularly if a radiocephalic AVF is placed.[45,97,102,103] Recommendation of arm exercises for 4 to 6 weeks before and after AVF placement may assist maturation, but this has not been conclusively proven.[104–106] Most AVFs should be mature and safe to cannulate by 4 to 8 weeks after surgery.[57,107,108] Re-evaluation of the AVF at this time allows earlier detection and intervention, if necessary, for AVFs that are slow to mature. If primary AVF failure occurs, there is time to create a second AVF before hemodialysis is needed (or minimize catheter use if already on dialysis). Utilizing the services of a nurse coordinator who assists in education and coordinating care for patients with stage 4 chronic kidney disease is an invaluable asset to help with vascular access education and referrals.[69,100] Patients already dialyzing with CVCs should be routinely identified and considered for AVF (or AVG) placement. Patients with an AVG that fails should be evaluated by vascular mapping for conversion to an AVF.[109] We have had experience with converting failed AVGs to an upper arm AVF; the AVF survival in these cases is the same as in primary upper arm AVF placements.[110] Finally, ongoing education and training of patients and hemodialysis staff in proper techniques of AVF cannulation and the benefits of an AVF for the patient and healthcare system is important to achieve acceptance of the change.[111]

Fistula Maturation

Fistula maturation is the process of arterial and venous dilation that permits an increase in access blood flow sufficient to allow repetitive cannulation with two needles to support maintenance hemodialysis. It is the principal problem associated with AVFs.[112,113] Primary failure due to impaired maturation occurs in approximately 25% to 50% of new AVFs.[38] However, maturation as currently defined in terms of clinical usability is an unsatisfactory criteria and leads to delays in detecting and treating the failing AVF. To promote earlier detection and salvage of a failing fistula, K/DOQI proposed the Rule of 6's (>600 mL/min flow rate, 0.6 cm vein diameter, and no more than 0.6 cm below the skin as measured by duplex ultrasonography by 6 weeks after access creation) as a working biologic definition of fistula maturation.[1] Failure to reach this goal should prompt a search for reversible etiologies. The goal is laudable, but the definition has not been validated and may be too aggressive, potentially leading to unnecessary investigations and intervention. More work is needed to establish the optimal criteria.[114] Importantly, examination of the access by an experienced observer looking for how far the palpable thrill and bruit extend up the arm, as well as the diameter, depth, and length of usable vein, and a pulse augmentation test may be nearly as accurate at predicting maturation.[113,114] However, the specific criteria to use have not been validated across centers.

The etiologies of impaired maturation include stenosis, impaired arterial and/or venous dilation, thrombosis, and the presence of accessory veins.[112,113] Failure to mature as defined above should prompt a search for reversible etiologies. The physical examination (Table 78-1) and a duplex ultrasound can help to assess the likely etiology, but contrast angiography will be needed for any intervention.[113,115,116] The most common etiology for impaired maturation is a focal venous stenosis,

Table 78-1 Physical Examination Characteristics of a Normal and Stenotic Access

Parameter	Normal	Stenosis*
Thrill	Present at arterial anastomosis and decreases along vein	Present at site of stenotic lesion (decreased at arterial anastomosis)
Pulse	Soft, easily compressible throughout access	Water-hammer upstream of stenosis
		Falls off after stenosis
Bruit	Low-pitched	High-pitched
	Continuous	Discontinuous
	Diastolic and systolic	Systolic only

*Abnormalities listed are for the two extremes: completely normal and severe stenosis. With lesser degrees of stenosis the findings will be between these two extremes.

From Beathard GA: Physical examination of the dialysis vascular access. Semin Dial 1998;11:231–236.

typically at or just downstream of the juxta-arterial anastomosis.[40,117–119] This lesion can be treated successfully with angioplasty, although the lesion often recurs, requiring additional angioplasty.[117,119–121] If angioplasty fails to correct the stenosis and improve maturation, consideration should be given to using the downstream good vein to create a new arteriovenous anastomosis at a more proximal site on the artery.[122] Another cause of impaired maturation is accessory veins that divide the flow and limit maturation of a single superficial target vein. This has been treated successfully by ligating the accessory veins to increase flow through a single superficial vein.[117,123] Finally, early thrombosis or a generalized impairment of arterial and venous dilation are reportedly less common but are difficult to treat and typically require creation of a new access. Careful attention should be paid to whether an upstream arterial stenosis is also present that is limiting access blood flow and fistula maturation.[124] An aggressive interventional approach to impaired fistula maturation has led to excellent results in some reports but more modest success in others.[117,119–121] The important message is to not wait too long for a fistula to mature before identifying an etiology and working on a solution.

No pharmacologic strategies have been proved to improve AVF maturation. Several small studies have suggested that using an antiplatelet agent at the time of surgical creation may prevent early thrombosis and allow an AVF to mature.[125] Recently a large multicenter randomized controlled trial demonstrated that administration of clopidogrel for 6 weeks starting at the time of fistula creation decreased early thrombosis from 19.5% to 12.2% at 6 weeks. However, despite the impressive decrease in thrombosis, fistula suitability for hemodialysis, which was only 40% in the placebo group, was not improved by treatment with clopidogrel.[125] Small trials studying allogeneic endothelial cells or human elastase placed on the adventitial side of the vein and arteriovenous anastomosis are currently underway as possible novel therapies to improve fistula maturation.[112]

MAINTENANCE OF THE VASCULAR ACCESS

Stenosis and Thrombosis

Stenosis leading to impaired access flow and thrombosis is the most common etiology of arteriovenous shunt failure.[126] Median primary patency of an AVG is less than 1 year; and median secondary patency is about 2 years.[27,47,64,110,127,128] In the absence of routine monitoring, approximately 70% to 95% of AVG failure is due to thrombosis (0.6–1.4 thromboses/access-year).[64,129–131] Stenosis is found to underlie the thrombosis in approximately 85% of cases.[126,132] Stenosis and thrombosis occur much less frequently in an AVF.[27,64,110,127,128,130] Whereas median primary patency of a lower arm AVF is similar to an AVG (due to failed maturation), median secondary patency, particularly for an upper arm AVF, is typically longer and can exceed 3 to 4 years.[110] Overall, the thrombosis rate in an AVF is approximately 0.25 per fistula-year when the initial maturation phase is included, but drops to approximately 0.1 per fistula-year in a mature AVF.[130,133,134] Stenosis in an AVG typically occurs at the vein-graft anastomosis or downstream vein; stenosis in an AVF typically occurs at the arteriovenous anastomosis or in the immediate downstream vein.[117,132] Importantly, stenosis

may also occur in the feeding artery, the graft itself, or the central veins.[124,132]

Access Surveillance and Prophylactic Angioplasty

Observational studies have demonstrated that a regular vascular access surveillance program can detect stenosis and that early intervention with angioplasty can decrease the rate of subsequent thrombosis in grafts and fistulas.[129,130,134–136] A recent small, randomized study has also reported that prophylactic angioplasty of hemodynamically significant stenosis increases survival in fistulas.[137] However, several recent small, randomized, controlled trials in AVGs found mixed results for preventing thrombosis; only one study found evidence for prolonging AVG survival.[138–143] Nevertheless, routine surveillance and prophylactic angioplasty of hemodynamically significant stenoses is currently recommended to decrease thrombosis and prevent the resulting disruption of dialysis unit function and missed dialysis sessions that otherwise occur.[65]

Development of access stenosis can be detected by various techniques (Box 78-2). Broadly, these techniques include a physical examination (Table 78-1); measurement of access recirculation, intra-access pressure (IAP), and access flow rate (Qa); and imaging studies for direct visualization of the stenosis.[1] The optimal approach would have a high sensitivity and specificity for the detection of access stenosis, be easy to perform on a frequent basis, and be inexpensive. Currently no surveillance technique has been shown to meet all of these criteria. A key principle of access surveillance, however, is that due to biologic and technical variability a single measurement of access flow or pressure has limited usefulness.[144–148] Performing repetitive measurements over time, as well as trend analysis, can improve sensitivity and specificity.[148,149] For AVGs, in which the risk for thrombosis is high, reliance simply on the physical examination and measurement of access recirculation is not sufficient; additional surveillance tools are needed.[65,150] However, for AVFs the risk of thrombosis even at low flow rates is much lower. For AVFs, careful attention on a regular basis to the physical examination, measures of access recirculation (including adequacy of dialysis), and the ability to achieve the target blood flow rate may be sufficient to detect and correct stenosis before thrombosis.[133,150] Regular measurements of IAP, Qa, or duplex ultrasonography (stenosis detection) have all been validated as surveillance tools with modest accuracy to detect stenosis.[148,151–156] Measurement of IAP is better suited for detecting stenosis in an AVG, where the stenosis is typically downstream of the needles, than in an AVF, where the stenosis is typically upstream of the needles.[157,158] Measurement of Qa or use of duplex ultrasonography is equally suited for surveillance of an AVF or AVG.

For measurement of IAP, the blood pump flow rate is set at zero and the blood line clamped proximal to the venous drip chamber.[159] IAP is then determined from the drip chamber pressure after correcting for the decreased hydrostatic pressure due to the height of the drip chamber above the access. The IAP is normalized for the mean arterial pressure (MAP) taken in the contralateral arm (IAP/MAP). An IAP/MAP ratio in an AVG consistently greater than 0.5 (venous drip chamber) or 0.75 (arterial chamber) is an indication to investigate for a downstream venous stenosis.[95] Alternatively, an equivalent IAP can be calculated from the drip chamber pressures measured at a fixed low blood pump flow rate. This is done using a computer algorithm

Box 78-2 Arteriovenous Access Surveillance Techniques and Criteria for Fistulogram

---

A. Clinical Criteria
Recommended for both fistulae and grafts. Use of additional monitoring technique recommended for grafts (see below). Trend analysis more specific than isolated measurement or event.

  Examine access each dialysis (see Table 78-1)
  Arm swelling (if persistent)
  Inability to cannulate access
  Aspiration of clot from access
  Prolonged postdialysis bleeding at cannulation sites
  Increased recirculation (trend data over time, measured at least monthly)
  Indicator dilution techniques (e.g., UDT, GIT, K dilution) >0% is abnormal (if persistent)
  Urea-based recirculation test not recommended, >10% abnormal if persistent or increasing
  Inability to maintain target blood flow (trend Qb over time)
  Inadequate dialysis (trend monthly Kt/V or URR)
  Increasing DVP or decreasing DAP (trend over time; *not* a substitute for IAP)

B. Additional Monitoring[1,2]
Recommend using at least one of these three techniques for monitoring grafts; optional for fistulae.

1. IAP Monitoring (at least monthly; perform trend analysis)
Measurement:
  IAP (mm Hg) = static drip chamber pressure at 0 pump speed with ultrafiltration off or line between dialyzer and drip chamber clamped (mm Hg) + height of drip chamber above access (cm) × 0.74
  Mean arterial pressure (MAP) = DBP + 1/3(SBP − DBP) measured in contralateral arm
  Arterial pressure ratio (APR) = arterial IAP/MAP
  Venous pressure ratio (VPR) = venous IAP/MAP
Criteria for AVG
  Venous stenosis: APR > 0.75 *or* VPR > 0.5
  Intra-access stenosis: APR ≥ 0.65 *and* VPR < 0.5
  Arterial inflow stenosis: APR < 0.3 and clinical criteria

Criteria for AVF (less sensitive for detecting upstream lesions most common in fistulae)
  Venous stenosis: APR > 0.43 *or* VPR > 0.35
  Intra-access stenosis: ARP ≥ 0.65 *and* VPR < 0.35
  Arterial inflow stenosis: APR < 0.13 and clinical criteria

2. Access Flow (Qa) Monitoring (at least monthly; perform trend analysis)
Measurement:
Various techniques.[162] UDT using saline infusion in the reversed dialysis flow configuration is standard (e.g., HD01, Transonics Systems)

Criteria for AVG
  Qa < 600 mL/min *or*
  Qa < 1000 mL/min and ≥ 25% decrease in Qa over 4 months

Criteria for AVF
  Qa < 400 mL/min *or*
  Qa < 1000 mL/min and ≥ 25% decrease in Qa over 4 months

3. Stenosis Monitoring (duplex ultrasound; quarterly)
Measurement:
Requires experienced technician and appropriate ultrasound equipment. Evaluate entire arterial, graft, and venous limbs of access circuit,
Criteria (AVG or AVF)
  Evidence of stenosis by B mode and color Doppler
  Peak systolic velocity ratio ≥ 2.0 (compared to upstream vessel)

DAP, dynamic arterial pressure; DVP, dynamic venous pressure; GIT, glucose infusion technique[239,240]; UDT, ultrasound dilution technique[239]; URR, urea reduction ratio.

based on hematocrit, flow rate, and needle size to correct for the pressure drop in the needle.[160] A company (Vasc-Alert, W. Lafayette, Ind.) has been established that uses on-line machine data to calculate equivalent IAP and notifies the clinic when the threshold for investigation has been exceeded.

Access blood flow is typically measured using an indicator-dilution technique.[161] In most cases this is done with the arterial and venous blood lines reversed in the "recirculation" configuration. Multiple techniques are available for Qa, but the gold standard is the ultrasound dilution technique (UDT).[162,163] In this technique, an ultrasound probe placed on the dialysis tube withdrawing blood from the downstream needle detects the dilution of saline injected upstream into blood flowing through the access. Typical threshold values used for detecting stenosis by UDT are 600 mL/min in an AVG or 400 to 500 mL/min in an AVF, or a drop of 25% in Qa from baseline when Qa is below 1000 mL/min for both an AVG and AVF.[1,2] The main disadvantages of Qa measurements are the need to reverse the blood lines and the need for an experienced technician to make the measurements. Newer technologies may obviate these problems in the future.

Use of duplex ultrasonography can provide both anatomic and flow data to assess the presence of stenosis.[153–155] Unfortunately, it requires a skilled technician, is time intensive, and cannot be done effectively during dialysis, so it is not a practical screening tool for most dialysis units.

At this time the choice of which surveillance techniques to use should be based on considerations of cost, availability of equipment, efficiency, and type of accesses currently used in the unit. At a minimum, all accesses should be regularly monitored by clinical criteria as shown in Box 78-2. For AVFs this may be sufficient without resorting to additional techniques.[133,150] For AVGs, it is recommended that an additional technique, such as IAP, Qa, or duplex ultrasonography surveillance, be used.

K/DOQI recommends that with monitoring and surveillance the incidence of AVG thrombosis should be less than 0.5 episodes per patient-year at risk; the median AVG patency should exceed 2 years.[1,2] It is important to note that a significant fraction of AVGs (15%) will thrombose with a high flow rate above 600 mL/min and no definitive stenosis.[158] This may be due to volume depletion, hypotension, or access compression. Thrombosis in this situation will not be prevented by active surveillance for stenoses. For an AVF, K/DOQI recommends a thrombosis rate of less than 0.25 episodes per patient-year at risk and median patency of more than 3 years.

A stenosis in which the lumen diameter is ≤50% of the reference diameter of the normal upstream or downstream vessel is considered hemodynamically significant and is an indication for intervention.[164,165] Either angioplasty or surgical revision can be used to treat hemodynamically significant access stenosis in an AVG or forearm AVF.[166–172] However, angioplasty is generally the first choice. Stenosis in an upper arm AVF is treated with angioplasty. Central venous stenosis is difficult to treat and often requires stenting in addition to repeated angioplasty or occasionally surgical bypass grafting.[7,173–178] Median patency is typically no more than 6 months after angioplasty of an AVG but greater than 6 months in an AVF, particularly in a forearm AVF.[132,166,172,179,180] Thrombosis of an AVG or AVF can be treated by either percutaneous thrombolysis (mechanical or pharmacomechanical) or surgical thrombectomy with satisfactory results.[181–189] However, survival after access thrombosis in most reports is decreased compared to angioplasty of a nonthrombosed access.[138,166,168,190] Salvage of a thrombosed AVF should be performed as soon as possible after recognizing the thrombosis.[181] Routine stenting after angioplasty does not improve access survival but may be necessary to prevent elastic recoil, treat complications of venous rupture, and obtain a satisfactory result in central venous lesions.[191–195]

There is no proven pharmacologic therapy to prevent access thrombosis or stenosis. Randomized, placebo-controlled trials have examined the use of low-dose warfarin as well as the combination of aspirin and clopidogrel; neither has proven successful in prolonging AVG survival.[196,197] The trial of aspirin plus clopidogrel was closed early due to excessive bleeding.[197] Small trials have suggested a benefit of dipyridamole or fish oil to prevent AVG thrombosis.[198,199] A large multicenter trial is testing whether Aggrenox extended-release dipyridamole/aspirin will prevent AVG stenosis and thereby prolong AVG survival.[200]

Infection

Infection occurs in approximately 5% to 15% of AVGs and no more than 1% of AVFs over the duration of patency.[33,64,127,201,202] Most infections are due to *Staphylococcus aureus* and *S. epidermidis*.[33,203] Less commonly encountered organisms include Enterococcus, gram-negative bacteria, and occasionally candida or other fungal species.[33,203] Infection or abscess around the access may present with localized erythema and tenderness over the site, but AVG infection can also present with fever and systemic symptoms without localized evidence of infection.[204] An indium-tagged white blood cell scan has been used to detect occult AVG infections.[13,204–206] Serious complications of access infection include thrombosis, metastatic seeding leading to endocarditis, osteomyelitis, or murantic abscess, as well as sepsis and death. Careful attention to bactericidal cleansing of the skin and infection control practices at the time of needle insertion in the dialysis unit are important quality control measures.[1,2] The use of preoperative vancomycin before access surgery has been recommended to decrease the frequency of subsequent postoperative graft infections.[207]

Management of AVG infection typically requires excision of the infected graft material and treatment with antibiotics.[13,203] AVFs can usually be treated with 6 weeks of appropriate antibiotics without resection unless thrombosis is present. Vancomycin, with addition of gram-negative coverage if the patient is septic, is appropriate. However, indiscriminant use of vancomycin has led to an emerging epidemic of vancomycin-resistant organisms. Hence, long-term use of vancomycin should be avoided, and alternative antibiotics chosen as soon as results of antibiotic sensitivity testing are known. An alternative strategy being studied recently for infected AVGs is to replace the infected graft with a biograft that is more resistant to infection.[22] If an endovascular source of infection is present, it should be treated for 6 weeks with appropriate intravenous antibiotics to reduce the risk for late sequelae from metastatic seeding.

Vascular Steal

Vascular steal results from retrograde flow from the distal artery into the access and occurs in approximately 75% of AVFs.[208] Symptoms such as vague neurosensory changes, mild swelling, stiffness, or decreased temperature distal to the access may occur after access creation, usually improving or resolving with time. In more severe cases the ischemia may progress to produce painful paresthesias, numbness, ischemic ulcers, trophic changes, or dry gangrene in the extremity. These more severe complications requiring intervention have been reported to occur in 1.6% to 8% of accesses and can occur rapidly after the surgery or arise months or years after access placement.[201,209] The diagnosis can often be made clinically by noting the decrease in symptoms and return of the radial pulse with compression of the fistula.[210] In difficult cases, digital plethysmography can be performed, looking for a digital pressure lower than 50 mm Hg or a digital-brachial index of less than 0.47.[210] In severe cases, the digital pulse waveform contours are monophasic or flat, and occlusion of the fistula leads to augmentation of the pulse wave and normalization of the waveform contour.[211]

If symptomatic steal occurs, it is important to look for and correct any arterial stenosis in the artery proximal to the access.[124] If the symptoms persist, the options include banding the access, ligating the distal artery, ligating the access itself, or performing a distal revascularization with interval ligation procedure. Banding the access or ligating the distal artery is frequently unsuccessful either due to persistent steal, insufficient flow, or thrombosis of the access. Ligating the access solves the problem but leaves the patient without an access. The distal revascularization with interval ligation procedure is often successful at salvaging the distal extremity while maintaining function of the access.[212] However, it carries the risk of putting the distal extremity at the mercy of an autogenous vein bypass graft.

Heart Failure and Pulmonary Hypertension

Heart failure after arteriovenous shunt placement can develop in the setting of underlying organic heart disease, in which the heart is not able to increase its cardiac output to compensate for the increased flow through the shunt.[88,89] In addition, many patients with an arteriovenous shunt also demonstrate an increase in pulmonary artery pressure. In the presence of underlying lung disease or primary pulmonary hypertension, this could exacerbate right heart failure.[213] An access blood flow to cardiac output ratio above 0.3 has been suggested as a risk factor for heart failure, but there is currently no well-validated tool to predict who will develop symptomatic heart failure after access placement; this remains a clinical judgment.[214] Development of symptomatic heart failure after access placement can be treated with banding or placing a tapered AVG to reduce flow but usually requires ligation of the access.

Aneurysms and Pseudoaneurysms

Aneurysms and pseudoaneurysms typically result when regional cannulation of one site is used repetitively, leading to weakening of the wall of the vein or graft.[19] Vessel trauma with extravasation of fluid can also lead to pseudoaneurysm formation. Avoidance of this complication involves employing either the ladder approach to needle placement, in which the entire length of the access is used for cannulation, or the buttonhole technique, in which the same hole is repetitively cannulated with a blunt needle.[215] If an aneurysm develops, it may be corrected surgically. The presence of a stenosis just downstream of the aneurysm should be investigated and corrected if present.

Chronic Catheter Maintenance

Current tunneled cuffed catheters (TCC, typical size approximately 15F) used for maintenance hemodialysis can deliver blood flows of 400 mL/min or more at arterial and venous pressures approximately −100 mmHg and +100 mmHg, respectively. Impaired catheter flow may lead to insufficient dialysis. Catheters should be monitored each dialysis session, looking for evidence of impaired function. Criteria for catheter dysfunction include an inability to achieve 300 mL/min blood pump flow rate (BPFR), a prepump arterial pressure (PPAP) no more than 250 mm Hg or venous pressure higher than 250 mm Hg, a conductance ratio (i.e., BPFR/PPAP) lower than 1.2, progressive decrease in urea reduction ratio below 65% (or Kt/V < 1.2), or trouble aspirating and returning blood in the catheter.[1,2] A trend indicating impaired function should be investigated. Catheter dysfunction occurring within the first 1 to 2 weeks after placement that cannot be resolved by repositioning the patient and flushing the catheter lumens suggests a technical or mechanical problem, such as failure to place the catheter tip in the right atrium, kinked catheter, improperly placed suture, or catheter leak. If persistent or severe this requires evaluation by interventional radiology.

Catheter dysfunction that occurs later is most often due to the presence of thrombus or an external fibrin sheath that impairs catheter flow. This can be treated by intracatheter thrombolysis.[216] The most convenient agent currently available in the United States for catheters is recombinant tissue plasminogen activator (t-PA; e.g., alteplase, Cathflo Activase). A variety of approaches have been used; currently there is no standardized approach to therapy.[216] Typically 1 to 2 mg of t-PA (1 mg/mL) is infused into each lumen and allowed to dwell for 30 to 60 minutes before assessing catheter function.[217] If flow is not restored with the first dose, it can be replaced by a second dose; if necessary this dose may be allowed to dwell longer or until the next dialysis session. Complications have been reported to be low. Restoration of function is expected in 70% to 90% of cases, but recurrence is frequent.[218] Failure to relieve the obstruction or frequent repeated need for thrombolysis requires evaluation by interventional radiology and probable catheter replacement. If dialysis is needed urgently, it can be attempted with the lines reversed while waiting for catheter revision.[219] A fibrin sheath may be the source of dysfunction in a substantial number of patients.[220] It can be diagnosed by injecting a small dose of contrast into the catheter, looking for contrast tracking up the sheath.[221] If present, balloon dilation of the catheter track can be used to disrupt any external fibrin sheath before reinsertion of the new TCC.[222]

The major complications of CVCs are thrombosis, infection, and central venous stenosis.[6] Median TCC survival is approximately 1 year, with thrombosis accounting for the majority of failures.[223] Monitoring as above and prevention are the keys to dealing with catheter thrombosis. Currently, unfractionated heparin (5,000 U/mL) is the standard catheter lock solution used to prevent thrombosis. Low fixed-dose (1 mg) oral warfarin did not improve TCC survival.[224] Higher doses of warfarin or use of oral antiplatelet agents has not been studied. A study is ongoing to determine whether substituting t-PA instead of heparin once a week for intracatheter lock solution will improve outcomes.[225] Various citrate solutions (4% to 47%) have been studied as an alternative to heparin as a catheter lock[226,227]; 4% citrate appears to be equivalent to heparin but potentially less expensive. The U.S. Food and Drug Administration has not approved the use of higher concentrations of citrate in the United States.[228]

Infections associated with TCCs can involve the exit site, the subcutaneous tunnel, or the bloodstream.[229] Catheter-related bloodstream infection (BSI) is the most feared complication of TCCs, carrying the potential for endocarditis, metastatic infection, and septic shock.[229] The reported risk of catheter-related bacteremia ranges from about 1 to 6.5 episodes/1000 catheter-days and rises with duration of use.[14] K/DOQI recommends a goal of less than 1.5 episodes/1000 catheter-days.[1,2] Staphylococcal species account for over 60% of all BSIs, but enterococcus and gram-negative organisms are also frequent.[67,229]

Exit site infections can typically be treated with topical and oral antibiotics without the need for catheter replacement.[229,230] Development of fever, chills, or unexplained hypotension in a patient with a CVC suggests a BSI.[67,229] Blood cultures should be drawn both from the catheter and a peripheral site if possible. For a probable BSI, treatment is begun with empiric intravenous antibiotics, typically vancomycin until appropriate therapy can be refined by the culture results. Empiric gram-negative coverage (e.g., aminoglycoside or third-generation cephalosporin) may be added, particularly if the patient appears ill or hemodynamically unstable. If the patient is hemodynamically stable and there is no exit site or tunnel infection, the BSI can be treated with either catheter exchange over a guidewire or catheter removal, followed in several days by catheter replacement.[67,229,231,232] In either case, 3 weeks of appropriate intravenous antibiotics are recommended followed by surveillance blood cultures 1 to 2 weeks after antibiotics are completed. Catheter exchange over a guidewire has been reported to be more cost-effective than either catheter salvage or catheter removal and replacement.[233] Catheter salvage using systemic antibiotics in conjunction with a concentrated antibiotic/anticoagulant intracatheter lock solution has also been reported to be an acceptable alternative.[234] However, if the fever persists or blood cultures remain positive, the catheter must be replaced. In all cases, follow-up surveillance cultures are critical. Given the difficulty of eradicating *S. aureus* from indwelling catheters and the devastating consequences that can occur, we prefer to treat most BSIs with this organism by catheter removal and replacement after 48 hours when the patient is afebrile and follow-up cultures are negative. Patients who are septic or have a tunnel infection require immediate catheter removal and subsequent replacement. Use of a team approach with an access infection control manager may improve patient outcomes.[235]

Attention to good infection control practices when working with CVCs is critical to preventing infections.[12] This includes hand washing and wearing gloves before working with the catheter, using a sterile drape, carefully disinfecting the caps and hub of the catheter, and using a face mask for both patient and dialysis technician during catheter connection and disconnection. Regular attention to cleaning the exit site and changing the catheter dressing is important to reduce the incidence of exit site infections. Numerous studies have shown that combined antibiotic plus anticoagulant lock solutions can decrease the rate of infection compared to heparin.[234,236,237] In addition, application of mupirocin ointment or "medihoney" to the exit site may also decrease catheter infections.[238] However, these strategies are not recommended until the long-term effect of these approaches on antibiotic resistance is known.

References

1. Besarab A, Work J, Brouwer D, et al: Clinical practice guidelines for vascular access. Am J Kidney Dis 2006;48(Suppl 1): S176–S247.
2. Besarab A, Work , Brouwer D, et al: Clinical practice guidelines for vascular access. Am J Kidney Dis 2006;48(Suppl 1): S248–S273.
3. Oliver MJ: Acute dialysis catheters. Semin Dial 2001;14:432–435.
4. Oliver MJ, Callery SM, Thorpe KE, et al: Risk of bacteremia from temporary hemodialysis catheters by site of insertion and duration of use: A prospective study. Kidney Int 2000;58:2543–2545.
5. Leblanc M, Fedak S, Mokris G, Paganini EP: Blood recirculation in temporary central catheters for acute hemodialysis. Clin Nephrol 1996;45:315–319.
6. Bagul A, Brook NR, Kaushik M, Nicholson ML: Tunnelled catheters for the haemodialysis patient. Eur J Vasc Endovasc Surg 2007;33:105–112.
7. Agarwal AK, Patel BM, Haddad NJ: Central vein stenosis: A nephrologist's perspective. Semin Dial 2007;20:53–62.
8. Barrett N, Spencer S, McIvor J, Brown EA: Subclavian stenosis: A major complication of subclavian dialysis catheters. Nephrol Dial Transplant 1988;3:423–425.
9. Schwab SJ, Quarles LD, Middleton JP, et al: Hemodialysis-associated subclavian vein stenosis. Kidney Int 1988;33: 1156–1159.
10. Work J: Chronic catheter placement. Semin Dial 2001;14: 436–440.
11. Forauer AR, Glockner JF: Importance of US findings in access planning during jugular vein hemodialysis catheter placements. J Vasc Interv Radiol 2000;11:233–238.
12. Posa PJ, Harrison D, Vollman KM: Elimination of central line-associated bloodstream infections: Application of the evidence. AACN 2006;17: 446–454.
13. Lew SQ, Kaveh K: Dialysis access related infections. ASAIO J 2000;46:S6–S12.
14. Nassar GM, Ayus JC: Infectious complications of the hemodialysis access. Kidney Int 2001;60:1–13.
15. Sexton DJ: Vascular access infections in patients undergoing dialysis with special emphasis on the role and treatment of *Staphylococcus aureus*. Infect Dis Clin North Am 2001;15: 731–742.
16. Himmelfarb J, Dember LM, Dixon BS: Vascular access. In Pereira BJG, Sayegh MH, Blake PG (eds): Chronic Kidney Disease, Dialysis and Transplantation, 2nd ed. Philadelphia: Elsevier, 2005, pp 341–362.
17. Konner K: The initial creation of native arteriovenous fistulas: Surgical aspects and their impact on the practice of nephrology. Semin Dial 2003;16:291–298.
18. Konner K, Hulbert-Shearon TE, Roys EC, Port FK: Tailoring the initial vascular access for dialysis patients. Kidney Int 2002; 62:329–338.
19. Konner K, Nonnast-Daniel B, Ritz E: The arteriovenous fistula. J AmSoc Nephrol 2003;14:1669–1680.

20. Warnock DG, Tolwani AJ, Gallichio M, Allon M: Vascular grafts for hemodialysis: Types, sites and techniques. Contrib Nephrol 2004;142:73–93.

21. Matsuura JH, Johansen KH, Rosenthal D, et al: Cryopreserved femoral vein grafts for difficult hemodialysis access. Ann Vasc Surg 2000;14:50–55.

22. Lin PH, Brinkman WT, Terramani TT, Lumsden AB: Management of infected hemodialysis access grafts using cryopreserved human vein allografts. Am J Surg 2002;184:31–36.

23. Bosman PJ, Blankestijn PJ, van der Graaf Y, et al: A comparison between PTFE and denatured homologous vein grafts for haemodialysis access: A prospective randomised multicentre trial. The SMASH Study Group. Study of Graft Materials in Access for Haemodialysis. Eur J Vasc Endovasc Surg 1998;16:126–132.

24. Schwab SJ, Beathard G: The hemodialysis catheter conundrum: Hate living with them, but can't live without them. Kidney Int 1999;56:1–17.

25. Harland RC: Placement of permanent vascular access devices: Surgical considerations. Adv Ren Replace Ther 1994;1:99–106.

26. Huber TS, Seeger JM: Approach to patients with "complex" hemodialysis access problems. Semin Dial 2003;16:22–29.

27. Huber TS, Carter JW, Carter RL, Seeger JM: Patency of autogenous and polytetrafluoroethylene upper extremity arteriovenous hemodialysis accesses: A systematic review. J Vasc Surg 2003;38:1005–1011.

28. Perera GB, Mueller MP, Kubaska SM, et al: Superiority of autogenous arteriovenous hemodialysis access: Maintenance of function with fewer secondary interventions. Ann Vasc Surg 2004;18:66–73.

29. U.S. Renal Data System: Excerpts from the USRDS 2005 Annual Data Report. Am J Kidney Dis 2006;47:S1–S286.

30. Dhingra RK, Young EW, Hulbert-Shearon TE, et al: Type of vascular access and mortality in U.S. hemodialysis patients. Kidney Int 2001;60:1443–1451.

31. Woods JD, Turenne MN, Strawderman RL, et al: Vascular access survival among incident hemodialysis patients in the United States. Am J Kidney Dis 1997;30:50–57.

32. Xue JL, Dahl D, Ebben JP, Collins AJ: The association of initial hemodialysis access type with mortality outcomes in elderly Medicare ESRD patients. Am J Kidney Dis 2003;42:1013–1019.

33. Colville LA, Lee AH: Retrospective analysis of catheter-related infections in a hemodialysis unit. Infect Control Hosp Epidemiol 2006;27:969–973.

34. Ortega T, Ortega F, Diaz-Corte C, et al: The timely construction of arteriovenous fistulae: A key to reducing morbidity and mortality and to improving cost management. Nephrol Dial Transplant 2005;20:598–603.

35. Astor BC, Eustace JA, Powe NR, et al: Type of vascular access and survival among incident hemodialysis patients: The Choices for Healthy Outcomes in Caring for ESRD (CHOICE) Study. J Am Soc Nephrol 2005;16:1449–1455.

36. Polkinghorne KR, McDonald SP, Atkins RC, Kerr PG: Vascular access and all-cause mortality: A propensity score analysis. J Am Soc Nephrol 2004;15:477–486.

37. Miller PE, Tolwani A, Luscy CP, et al: Predictors of adequacy of arteriovenous fistulas in hemodialysis patients. Kidney Int 1999;56:275–280.

38. Allon M, Robbin ML: Increasing arteriovenous fistulas in hemodialysis patients: Problems and solutions. Kidney Int 2002;62:1109–1124.

39. Patel ST, Hughes J, Mills JL Sr: Failure of arteriovenous fistula maturation: An unintended consequence of exceeding Dialysis Outcome Quality Initiative guidelines for hemodialysis access. J Vasc Surg 2003;38:439–445.

40. Tordoir JH, Rooyens P, Dammers R, et al: Prospective evaluation of failure modes in autogenous radiocephalic wrist access for haemodialysis. Nephrol Dial Transplant 2003;18:378–383.

41. Rayner HC, Besarab A, Brown WW, et al: Vascular access results from the Dialysis Outcomes and Practice Patterns Study (DOPPS): Performance against Kidney Disease Outcomes Quality Initiative (K/DOQI) Clinical Practice Guidelines. Am J Kidney Dis 2004;44:22–26.

42. Lee T, Barker J, Allon M: Comparison of survival of upper arm arteriovenous fistulas and grafts after failed forearm fistula. J Am Soc Nephrol 2007;18:1936–1941.

43. Lee T, Barker J, Allon M: Tunneled catheters in hemodialysis patients: Reasons and subsequent outcomes. Am J Kidney Dis 2005;46:501–508.

44. Oliver MJ, Rothwell DM, Fung K, et al: Late creation of vascular access for hemodialysis and increased risk of sepsis. J Am Soc Nephrol 2004;15:1936–1942.

45. Arora P, Obrador GT, Ruthazer R, et al: Prevalence, predictors, and consequences of late nephrology referral at a tertiary care center. J Am Soc Nephrol 1999;10: 1281–1286.

46. Hossny A: Brachiobasilic arteriovenous fistula: Different surgical techniques and their effects on fistula patency and dialysis-related complications. J Vasc Surg 2003;37:821–826.

47. Gibson KD, Gillen DL, Caps MT, et al: Vascular access survival and incidence of revisions: A comparison of prosthetic grafts, simple autogenous fistulas, and venous transposition fistulas from the United States Renal Data System Dialysis Morbidity and Mortality Study. J Vasc Surg 2001;34:694–700.

48. Woo K, Farber A, Doros G, et al: Evaluation of the efficacy of the transposed upper arm arteriovenous fistula: A single institutional review of 190 basilic and cephalic vein transposition procedures. J Vasc Surg 2007;46:94–99.

49. Yilmaz M, Senkaya I, Saba D, Bicer M: Long-term outcomes of basilic vein transposition fistula for hemodialysis. Vasa 2007;36: 29–32.

50. Rao RK, Azin GD, Hood DB, et al: Basilic vein transposition fistula: A good option for maintaining hemodialysis access site options? J Vasc Surg 2004;39:1043–1047.

51. El Sayed HF, Mendoza B, Meier GH, et al: Utility of basilic vein transposition for dialysis access. Vascular 2005;13:268–274.

52. Wolford HY, Hsu J, Rhodes JM, et al: Outcome after autogenous brachial-basilic upper arm transpositions in the post-National Kidney Foundation Dialysis Outcomes Quality Initiative era. J Vasc Surg 2005;42:951–956.

53. Dix FP, Khan Y, Al-Khaffaf H: The brachial artery-basilic vein arterio-venous fistula in vascular access for haemodialysis—a review paper. Eur J Vasc Endovasc Surg 2006;31:70–79.

54. Allon M, Daugirdas J, Depner TA, et al: Effect of change in vascular access on patient mortality in hemodialysis patients. Am J Kidney Dis 2006;47:469–477.

55. Cortez AJ, Paulson WD, Schwab SJ: Vascular access as a determinant of adequacy of dialysis. Semin Nephrol 2005;25:96–101.

56. Taylor G, Gravel D, Johnston L, et al: Prospective surveillance for primary bloodstream infections occurring in Canadian hemodialysis units. Infect Control Hosp Epidemiol 2002;23: 716–720.

57. Saran R, Dykstra DM, Pisoni RL, et al: Timing of first cannulation and vascular access failure in haemodialysis: An analysis of practice patterns at dialysis facilities in the DOPPS. Nephrol Dial Transplant 2004;19:2334–2340.

58. Fan PY, Schwab SJ: Vascular access: Concepts for the 1990s. J Am Soc Nephrol 1992;3:1–11.

59. Bartlett ST, Schweitzer EJ, Roberts JE, et al: Early experience with a new ePTFE vascular prosthesis for hemodialysis. Am J Surg 1995;170:118–122.

60. Bay WH, Van Cleef S, Owens M: The hemodialysis access: Preferences and concerns of patients, dialysis nurses and technicians, and physicians. Am J Nephrol 1998;18:379–383.

61. Zanow J, Kruger U, Petzold M, et al: Arterioarterial prosthetic loop: A new approach for hemodialysis access. J Vasc Surg 2005;41:1007–1012.

62. Rizzuti RP, Hale JC, Burkart TE: Extended patency of expanded polytetrafluoroethylene grafts for vascular access using optimal configuration and revisions. Surg Gynecol Obstet 1988;166: 23–27.

63. Chemla ES, Morsy M, Anderson L, Makanjuola D: Complex bypasses and fistulas for difficult hemodialysis access: A prospective, single-center experience. Semin Dial 2006;19:246–250.

64. Hodges TC, Fillinger MF, Zwolak RM, et al: Longitudinal comparison of dialysis access methods: Risk factors for failure. J Vasc Surg 1997;26:1009–1019.

65. Besarab A: Access monitoring is worthwhile and valuable. Blood Purif 2006;24:77–89.

66. Quarello F, Forneris G, Borca M, Pozzato M: Do central venous catheters have advantages over arteriovenous fistulas or grafts? J Nephrol 2006;19:265–279.

67. Allon M: Dialysis catheter-related bacteremia: Treatment and prophylaxis. Am J Kidney Dis 2004;44:779–791.

68. Atherikul K, Schwab SJ, Conlon PJ: Adequacy of haemodialysis with cuffed central-vein catheters. Nephrol Dial Transplant 1998;13:745–749.

69. Lok CE, Oliver MJ: Overcoming barriers to arteriovenous fistula creation and use. Semin Dial 2003;16:189–196.

70. Planken RN, Tordoir JH, Duijm LE, et al: Current techniques for assessment of upper extremity vasculature prior to hemodialysis vascular access creation. Eur Radiol 2007;17:3001–3011.

71. Asif A, Ravani P, Roy-Chaudhury P, et al: Vascular mapping techniques: Advantages and disadvantages. J Nephrol 2007;20: 299–303.

72. Allon M, Lockhart ME, Lilly RZ, et al: Effect of preoperative sonographic mapping on vascular access outcomes in hemodialysis patients. Kidney Int 2001;60:2013–2020.

73. Robbin ML, Gallichio MH, Deierhoi MH, et al: US vascular mapping before hemodialysis access placement. Radiology 2000; 217:83–88.

74. Silva MB Jr, Hobson RW 2nd, Pappas PJ, et al: A strategy for increasing use of autogenous hemodialysis access procedures: Impact of preoperative noninvasive evaluation. J Vasc Surg 1998;27:302–308.

75. Rutherford RB: The value of noninvasive testing before and after hemodialysis access in the prevention and management of complications. Semin Vasc Surg 1997;10:157–161.

76. Nursal TZ, Oguzkurt L, Tercan F, et al: Is routine preoperative ultrasonographic mapping for arteriovenous fistula creation necessary in patients with favorable physical examination findings? Results of a randomized controlled trial. World J Surg 2006;30:1100–1107.

77. Mihmanli I, Besirli K, Kurugoglu S, et al: Cephalic vein and hemodialysis fistula: Surgeon's observation versus color Doppler ultrasonographic findings. J Ultrasound Med 2001;20: 217–222.

78. Doelman C, Duijm LE, Liem YS, et al: Stenosis detection in failing hemodialysis access fistulas and grafts: Comparison of color Doppler ultrasonography, contrast-enhanced magnetic resonance angiography, and digital subtraction angiography. J Vasc Surg 2005;42:739–746.

79. Grogan J, Castilla M, Lozanski L, et al: Frequency of critical stenosis in primary arteriovenous fistulae before hemodialysis access: Should duplex ultrasound surveillance be the standard of care? J Vasc Surg 2005;41:1000–1006.

80. Kian K, Wyatt C, Schon D, et al: Safety of low-dose radiocontrast for interventional AV fistula salvage in stage 4 chronic kidney disease patients. Kidney Int 2006;69:1444–1449.

81. Asif A, Cherla G, Merrill D, et al: Venous mapping using venography and the risk of radiocontrast-induced nephropathy. Semin Dial 2005;18:239–242.

82. Perazella MA, Rodby RA: Gadolinium use in patients with kidney disease: A cause for concern. Semin Dial 2007;20: 179–185.

83. Lockhart ME, Robbin ML, Allon M: Preoperative sonographic radial artery evaluation and correlation with subsequent radiocephalic fistula outcome. J Ultrasound Med 2004;23:161–168.

84. Wong V, Ward R, Taylor J, et al: Factors associated with early failure of arteriovenous fistulae for haemodialysis access. Eur J Vasc Endovasc Surg 1996;12:207–213.

85. Mendes RR, Farber MA, Marston WA, et al: Prediction of wrist arteriovenous fistula maturation with preoperative vein mapping with ultrasonography. J Vasc Surg 2002;36:460–463.

86. Malovrh M: Native arteriovenous fistula: preoperative evaluation. Am J Kidney Dis 2002;39:1218–1225.

87. van der Linden J, Lameris TW, van den Meiracker AH, et al: Forearm venous distensibility predicts successful arteriovenous fistula. Am J Kidney Dis 2006;47:1013–1019.

88. Engelberts I, Tordoir JH, Boon ES, Schreij G: High-output cardiac failure due to excessive shunting in a hemodialysis access fistula: An easily overlooked diagnosis. Am J Nephrol 1995;15: 323–326.

89. Young PR Jr, Rohr MS, Marterre WF Jr: High-output cardiac failure secondary to a brachiocephalic arteriovenous hemodialysis fistula: Two cases. Am Surg 1998;64:239–241.

90. Weyde W, Letachowicz W, Kusztal M, et al: Outcome of autogenous fistula construction in hemodialyzed patients over 75 years of age. Blood Purif 2006;24:190–195.

91. McGill RL, Marcus RJ, Healy DA, et al: AV fistula rates: Changing the culture of vascular access. J Vasc Access 2005;6:13–17.

92. Young EW, Dykstra DM, Goodkin DA, et al: Hemodialysis vascular access preferences and outcomes in the Dialysis Outcomes and Practice Patterns Study (DOPPS). Kidney Int 2002;61:2266–2271.

93. Nguyen VD, Griffith C, Treat L: A multidisciplinary team approach to increasing AV fistula creation. Nephrol News Issues 2003;17:54–60.

94. Elsharawy MA, Moghazy KM: Pre-operative evaluation of hemodialysis access fistula. A multidisciplinary approach. Acta Chir Belg 2005;105:355–358.

95. Besarab A: Preventing vascular access dysfunction: Which policy to follow. Blood Purif 2002;20:26–35.

96. Kizilisik AT, Kim SB, Nylander WA, Shaffer D: Improvements in dialysis access survival with increasing use of arteriovenous fistulas in a Veterans Administration medical center. Am J Surg 2004;188:614–616.

97. Pisoni RL, Young EW, Dykstra DM, et al: Vascular access use in Europe and the United States: Results from the DOPPS. Kidney Int 2002;61:305–316.

98. Glazer S, Diesto J, Crooks P, et al: Going beyond the kidney disease outcomes quality initiative: hemodialysis access experience at Kaiser Permanente Southern California. Ann Vasc Surg 2006;20:75–82.

99. Nguyen VD, Lawson L, Ledeen M, et al: Successful multidisciplinary interventions for arterio-venous fistula creation by the Pacific Northwest Renal Network 16 vascular access quality improvement program. J Vasc Access 2007;8:3–11.

100. Allon M, Bailey R, Ballard R, et al: A multidisciplinary approach to hemodialysis access: Prospective evaluation. Kidney Int 1998;53:473–479.

101. Hemphill H, Allon M, Konner K, et al: How can the use of arteriovenous fistulas be increased? Semin Dial 2003;16: 214–223.

102. Lee T, Barker J, Allon M: Associations with predialysis vascular access management. Am J Kidney Dis 2004;43:1008–1013.

103. Goncalves EA, Andreoli MC, Watanabe R, et al: Effect of temporary catheter and late referral on hospitalization and mortality during the first year of hemodialysis treatment. Artif Organs 2004;28:1043–1049.

104. Leaf DA, MacRae HS, Grant E, Kraut J: Isometric exercise increases the size of forearm veins in patients with chronic renal failure. Am J Med Sci 2003;325:115–119.

105. Oder TF, Teodorescu V, Uribarri J: Effect of exercise on the diameter of arteriovenous fistulae in hemodialysis patients. ASAIO J 2003;49:554–555.

106. Rus RR, Ponikvar R, Kenda RB, Buturovic-Ponikvar J: Effect of local physical training on the forearm arteries and veins in patients with end-stage renal disease. Blood Purif 2003;21:389–394.

107. Rayner HC, Pisoni RL, Gillespie BW, et al: Creation, cannulation and survival of arteriovenous fistulae: Data from the Dialysis Outcomes and Practice Patterns Study. Kidney Int 2003;63:323–330.

108. Basile C, Casucci F, Lomonte C: Timing of first cannulation of arteriovenous fistula: Time matters, but there is also something else. Nephrol Dial Transplant 2005;20:1519–1520.

109. Asif A, Unger SW, Briones P, et al: Creation of secondary arteriovenous fistulas: Maximizing fistulas in prevalent hemodialysis patients. Semin Dial 2005;18:420–424.

110. Dixon BS, Novak L, Fangman J: Hemodialysis vascular access survival: Upper-arm native arteriovenous fistula. Am J Kidney Dis 2002;39:92–101.

111. Ball LK: Improving arteriovenous fistula cannulation skills. Nephrol Nurs J 2005;32:611–617.

112. Dixon BS: Why don't fistulas mature? Kidney Int 2006;70:1413–1422.

113. Asif A, Roy–Chaudhury P, Beathard GA: Early arteriovenous fistula failure: A logical proposal for when and how to intervene. Clin J Am Soc Nephrol 2006;1:332–339.

114. Robbin ML, Chamberlain NE, Lockhart ME, et al: Hemodialysis arteriovenous fistula maturity: US evaluation. Radiology 2002;225:59–64.

115. Beathard GA: An algorithm for the physical examination of early fistula failure. Semin Dial 2005;18:331–335.

116. Kian K, Vassalotti JA: The new arteriovenous fistula: The need for earlier evaluation and intervention. Semin Dial 2005;18:3–7.

117. Beathard GA, Arnold P, Jackson J, Litchfield T: Aggressive treatment of early fistula failure. Kidney Int 2003;64:1487–1494.

118. Sivanesan S, How TV, Bakran A: Sites of stenosis in AV fistulae for haemodialysis access. Nephrol Dial Transplant 1999;14:118–120.

119. Turmel-Rodrigues L, Mouton A, Birmele B, et al: Salvage of immature forearm fistulas for haemodialysis by interventional radiology. Nephrol Dial Transplant 2001;16:2365–2371.

120. Clark TW, Cohen RA, Kwak A, et al: Salvage of nonmaturing native fistulas by using angioplasty. Radiology 2007;242:286–292.

121. Falk A: Maintenance and salvage of arteriovenous fistulas. J Vasc Interv Radiol 2006. 17:807–813.

122. Berman SS, Gentile AT: Impact of secondary procedures in autogenous arteriovenous fistula maturation and maintenance. J Vasc Surg 2001;34:866–871.

123. Faiyaz R, Abreo K, Zaman F, et al: Salvage of poorly developed arteriovenous fistulae with percutaneous ligation of accessory veins. Am J Kidney Dis 2002;39:824–827.

124. Asif A, Gadalean FN, Merrill D, et al: Inflow stenosis in arteriovenous fistulas and grafts: A multicenter, prospective study. Kidney Int 2005;67:1986–1992.

125. Dember LM, Beck JG, Allon M, et al: Effect of clopidogrel on early failure of arteriovenous fistulas for hemodialysis. JAMA 2008, in press.

126. Schwab SJ, Harrington JT, Singh A, et al: Vascular access for hemodialysis [clinical conference]. Kidney Int 1999;55:2078–2090.

127. Miller PE, Carlton D, Deierhoi MH, et al: Natural history of arteriovenous grafts in hemodialysis patients. Am J Kidney Dis 2000;36:68–74.

128. Glickman MH, Stokes GK, Ross JR, et al: Multicenter evaluation of a polytetrafluoroethylene vascular access graft as compared with the expanded polytetrafluoroethylene vascular access graft in hemodialysis applications. J Vasc Surg 2001;34:465–472.

129. Besarab A, Sullivan KL, Ross RP, Moritz MJ: Utility of intra-access pressure monitoring in detecting and correcting venous outlet stenoses prior to thrombosis. Kidney Int 1995;47:1364–1373.

130. Sands JJ: Vascular access monitoring improves outcomes. Blood Purif 2005;23:45–49.

131. Sullivan KL, Besarab A, Bonn J, et al: Hemodynamics of failing dialysis grafts. Radiology 1993;186:867–872.

132. Kanterman RY, Vesely TM, Pilgram TK, et al: Dialysis access grafts: Anatomic location of venous stenosis and results of angioplasty. Radiology 1995;195:135–139.

133. Shahin H, Reddy G, Sharafuddin M, et al: Monthly access flow monitoring with increased prophylactic angioplasty did not improve fistula patency. Kidney Int 2005;68:2352–2361.

134. McCarley P, Wingard RL, Shyr Y, et al: Vascular access blood flow monitoring reduces access morbidity and costs. Kidney Int 2001;60:1164–1172.

135. Schwab SJ, Oliver MJ, Suhocki P, McCann R: Hemodialysis arteriovenous access: Detection of stenosis and response to treatment by vascular access blood flow. Kidney Int 2001;59:358–362.

136. Safa AA, Valji K, Roberts AC, et al: Detection and treatment of dysfunctional hemodialysis access grafts: Effect of a surveillance program on graft patency and the incidence of thrombosis. Radiology 1996;199:653–657.

137. Tessitore N, Mansueto G, Bedogna V, et al: A prospective controlled trial on effect of percutaneous transluminal angioplasty on functioning arteriovenous fistulae survival. J Am Soc Nephrol 2003;14:1623–1627.

138. Dember LM, Holmberg EF, Kaufman JS: Randomized controlled trial of prophylactic repair of hemodialysis arteriovenous graft stenosis. Kidney Int 2004;66:390–398.

139. Moist LM, Churchill DN, House AA, et al: Regular monitoring of access flow compared with monitoring of venous pressure fails to improve graft survival. J Am Soc Nephrol 2003;14:2645–2653.

140. Ram SJ, Work J, Caldito GC, et al: A randomized controlled trial of blood flow and stenosis surveillance of hemodialysis grafts. Kidney Int 2003;64:272–280.

141. Robbin ML, Oser RF, Lee JY, et al: Randomized comparison of ultrasound surveillance and clinical monitoring on arteriovenous graft outcomes. Kidney Int 2006;69:730–735.

142. Malik J, Slavikova M, Svobodova J, Tuka V: Regular ultrasonographic screening significantly prolongs patency of PTFE grafts. Kidney Int 2005;67:1554–1558.

143. Martin LG, MacDonald MJ, Kikeri D, et al: Prophylactic angioplasty reduces thrombosis in virgin ePTFE arteriovenous dialysis grafts with greater than 50% stenosis: Subset analysis of a prospectively randomized study. J Vasc Interv Radiol 1999;10:389–396.

144. McDougal G, Agarwal R: Clinical performance characteristics of hemodialysis graft monitoring. Kidney Int 2001;60:762–766.

145. Paulson WD: Blood flow surveillance of hemodialysis grafts and the dysfunction hypothesis. Semin Dial 2001;14:175–180.

146. Ram SJ, Nassar R, Sharaf R, et al: Thresholds for significant decrease in hemodialysis access blood flow. Semin Dial 2005;18:558–564.

147. Besarab A, Lubkowski T, Vu A, et al: Effects of systemic hemodynamics on flow within vascular accesses used for hemodialysis. ASAIO J 2001;47:501–506.

148. Paulson WD, Ram SJ, Birk CG, Work J: Does blood flow accurately predict thrombosis or failure of hemodialysis synthetic grafts? A meta-analysis. Am J Kidney Dis 1999;34:478–485.

149. Neyra NR, Ikizler TA, May RE, et al: Change in access blood flow over time predicts vascular access thrombosis. Kidney Int 1998;54:1714–1719.

150. Wijnen E, Planken N, Keuter X, et al: Impact of a quality improvement programme based on vascular access flow monitoring

on costs, access occlusion and access failure. Nephrol Dial Transplant 2006;21:3514–3519.

151. Bosman PJ, Boereboom FT, Smits HF, et al: Pressure or flow recordings for the surveillance of hemodialysis grafts. Kidney Int 1997;52:1084–1088.

152. May RE, Himmelfarb J, Yenicesu M, et al: Predictive measures of vascular access thrombosis: a prospective study. Kidney Int 1997;52:1656–1662.

153. Gadallah MF, Paulson WD, Vickers B, Work J: Accuracy of Doppler ultrasound in diagnosing anatomic stenosis of hemodialysis arteriovenous access as compared with fistulography. Am J Kidney Dis 1998;32:273–277.

154. Robbin ML, Oser RF, Allon M, et al: Hemodialysis access graft stenosis: US detection. Radiology 1998;208:655–661.

155. Schwarz C, Mitterbauer C, Boczula M, et al: Flow monitoring: performance characteristics of ultrasound dilution versus color Doppler ultrasound compared with fistulography. Am J Kidney Dis 2003;42:539–545.

156. Tessitore N, Bedogna V, Gammaro L, et al: Diagnostic accuracy of ultrasound dilution access blood flow measurement in detecting stenosis and predicting thrombosis in native forearm arteriovenous fistulae for hemodialysis. Am J Kidney Dis 2003;42:331–341.

157. Besarab A, Lubkowski T, Frinak S, et al: Detection of access strictures and outlet stenoses in vascular accesses. Which test is best? ASAIO J 1997;43:M543–M547.

158. Besarab A, Lubkowski T, Frinak S, et al: Detecting vascular access dysfunction. ASAIO J 1997;43:M539–M543.

159. Besarab A, al-Saghir F, Alnabhan N, et al: Simplified measurement of intra-access pressure. ASAIO J 1996;42:M682–M687.

160. Frinak S, Zasuwa G, Dunfee T, et al: Dynamic venous access pressure ratio test for hemodialysis access monitoring. Am J Kidney Dis 2002;40:760–768.

161. Krivitski NM: Theory and validation of access flow measurement by dilution technique during hemodialysis. Kidney Int 1995;48:244–250.

162. Lopot F, Nejedly B, Sulkova S, Blaha J: Comparison of different techniques of hemodialysis vascular access flow evaluation. Int J Artif Organs 2003;26:1056–1063.

163. Lindsay RM, Rothera C, Blake PG: A comparison of methods for the measurement of hemodialysis access recirculation: An update. ASAIO J 1998;44:191–193.

164. Berguer R, Hwang NH: Critical arterial stenosis: A theoretical and experimental solution. Ann Surg 1974;180:39–50.

165. May AG, Van De Berg L, Deweese JA, Rob CG: Critical arterial stenosis. Surgery 1963;54:250–259.

166. Turmel-Rodrigues L, Pengloan J, Baudin S, et al: Treatment of stenosis and thrombosis in haemodialysis fistulas and grafts by interventional radiology. Nephrol Dial Transplant 2000;15:2029–2036.

167. Beathard GA: Angioplasty for arteriovenous grafts and fistulae. Semin Nephrol 2002;22:202–210.

168. Lilly RZ, Carlton D, Barker J, et al: Predictors of arteriovenous graft patency after radiologic intervention in hemodialysis patients. Am J Kidney Dis 2001;37:945–953.

169. Dapunt O, Feurstein M, Rendl KH, Prenner K: Transluminal angioplasty versus conventional operation in the treatment of haemodialysis fistula stenosis: Results from a 5-year study. Br J Surg 1987;74:1004–1005.

170. Mori Y, Horikawa K, Sato K, et al: Stenotic lesions in vascular access: Treatment with transluminal angioplasty using high-pressure balloons. Intern Med 1994;33:284–287.

171. Tessitore N, Lipari G, Poli A, et al: Can blood flow surveillance and pre-emptive repair of subclinical stenosis prolong the useful life of arteriovenous fistulae? A randomized controlled study. Nephrol Dial Transplant 2004;19:2325–2333.

172. Asif A, Lenz O, Merrill D, et al: Percutaneous management of perianastomotic stenosis in arteriovenous fistulae: Results of a prospective study. Kidney Int 2006;69:1904–1909.

173. Kwok PC, Wong KM, Ngan RK, et al: Prevention of recurrent central venous stenosis using endovascular irradiation following stent placement in hemodialysis patients. Cardiovasc Intervent Radiol 2001;24:400–406.

174. Maskova J, Komarkova J, Kivanek J, et al: Endovascular treatment of central vein stenoses and/or occlusions in hemodialysis patients. Cardiovasc Intervent Radiol 2003;26:27–30.

175. Maya ID, Saddekni S, Allon M: Treatment of refractory central vein stenosis in hemodialysis patients with stents. Semin Dial 2007;20:78–82.

176. Mickley V, Gorich J, Rilinger N, et al: Stenting of central venous stenoses in hemodialysis patients: Long-term results. Kidney Int 1997;51:277–280.

177. Bhatia DS, Money SR, Ochsner JL, et al: Comparison of surgical bypass and percutaneous balloon dilatation with primary stent placement in the treatment of central venous obstruction in the dialysis patient: One-year follow-up. Ann Vasc Surg 1996;10:452–455.

178. Shoenfeld R, Hermans H, Novick A, et al: Stenting of proximal venous obstructions to maintain hemodialysis access. J Vasc Surg 1994;19:532–538.

179. Beathard GA: Percutaneous transvenous angioplasty in the treatment of vascular access stenosis. Kidney Int 1992;42:1390–1397.

180. Maya ID, Oser R, Saddekni S, et al: Vascular access stenosis: Comparison of arteriovenous grafts and fistulas. Am J Kidney Dis 2004;44:859–865.

181. Diskin CJ, Stokes TJ, Panus LW, et al: The importance of timing of surgery for hemodialysis vascular access thrombectomy. Nephron 1997;75:233–237.

182. Sands JJ, Patel S, Plaviak DJ, Miranda CL: Pharmacomechanical thrombolysis with urokinase for treatment of thrombosed hemodialysis access grafts. A comparison with surgical thrombectomy. ASAIO J 1994;40:M886–M888.

183. Beathard GA: Thrombolysis versus surgery for the treatment of thrombosed dialysis access grafts. J Am Soc Nephrol 1995;6:1619–1624.

184. Palmer RM, Cull DL, Kalbaugh C, et al: Is surgical thrombectomy to salvage failed autogenous arteriovenous fistulae worthwhile? Am Surg 2006;72:1231–1233.

185. Green LD, Lee DS, Kucey DS: A meta-analysis comparing surgical thrombectomy, mechanical thrombectomy, and pharmacomechanical thrombolysis for thrombosed dialysis grafts. J Vasc Surg 2002;36:939–945.

186. Haage P, Vorwerk D, Wildberger JE, et al: Percutaneous treatment of thrombosed primary arteriovenous hemodialysis access fistulae. Kidney Int 2000;57:1169–1175.

187. Turmel-Rodrigues L, Pengloan J, Rodrigue H, et al: Treatment of failed native arteriovenous fistulae for hemodialysis by interventional radiology. Kidney Int 2000;57:1124–1140.

188. Trerotola SO, Lund GB, Scheel PJ Jr, et al: Thrombosed dialysis access grafts: percutaneous mechanical declotting without urokinase. Radiology 1994;191: 721–726.

189. Ponikvar R: Surgical salvage of thrombosed arteriovenous fistulas and grafts. Ther Apher Dial 2005;9:245–249.

190. Sands JJ, Miranda CL: Prolongation of hemodialysis access survival with elective revision. Clin Nephrol 1995;44:329–333.

191. Beathard GA: Gianturco self-expanding stent in the treatment of stenosis in dialysis access grafts. Kidney Int 1993;43:872–877.

192. Hoffer EK, Sultan S, Herskowitz MM, et al: Prospective randomized trial of a metallic intravascular stent in hemodialysis graft maintenance. J Vasc Interv Radiol 1997;8:965–973.

193. Turmel-Rodrigues LA, Blanchard D, Pengloan J, et al: Wallstents and Craggstents in hemodialysis grafts and fistulas: Results for selective indications. J Vasc Intervent Radiol 1997;8:975–982.

194. Patel RI, Peck SH, Cooper SG, et al: Patency of Wallstents placed across the venous anastomosis of hemodialysis grafts after percutaneous recanalization. Radiology 1998;209:365–370.

195. Funaki B, Szymski GX, Leef JA, et al: Wallstent deployment to salvage dialysis graft thrombolysis complicated by venous rupture: early and intermediate results. Am J Roentgenol 1997;169:1435–1437.

196. Crowther MA, Clase CM, Margetts PJ, et al: Low-intensity warfarin is ineffective for the prevention of PTFE graft failure in patients on hemodialysis: A randomized controlled trial. J Am Soc Nephrol 2002;13: 2331–2337.

197. Kaufman JS, O'Connor TZ, Zhang JH, et al: Randomized controlled trial of clopidogrel plus aspirin to prevent hemodialysis access graft thrombosis. J Am Soc Nephrol 2003;14: 2313–2321.

198. Sreedhara R, Himmelfarb J, Lazarus JM, Hakim RM: Antiplatelet therapy in graft thrombosis: Results of a prospective, randomized, double-blind study. Kidney Int 1994;45:1477–1483.

199. Schmitz PG, McCloud LK, Reikes ST, et al: Prophylaxis of hemodialysis graft thrombosis with fish oil: Double-blind, randomized, prospective trial. J Am Soc Nephrol 2002;13:184–190.

200. Dixon BS, Beck GJ, Dember LM, et al: Design of the Dialysis Access Consortium (DAC) Aggrenox Prevention Of Access Stenosis Trial. Clin 2005;2:400–412.

201. Zibari GB, Rohr MS, Landreneau MD, et al: Complications from permanent hemodialysis vascular access. Surgery 1988; 104:681–686.

202. Taylor G, Gravel D, Johnston L, et al: Incidence of bloodstream infection in multicenter inception cohorts of hemodialysis patients. Am J Infect Control 2004;32:155–160.

203. Anderson JE, Chang AS, Anstadt MP: Polytetrafluoroethylene hemoaccess site infections. ASAIO J 2000;46:S18–S21.

204. Ayus JC, Sheikh-Hamad D: Silent infection in clotted hemodialysis access grafts. J Am Soc Nephrol 1998;9:1314–1317.

205. Palestro CJ, Vega A, Kim CK, et al: Indium-111-labeled leukocyte scintigraphy in hemodialysis access-site infection. J Nuclear Med 1990;31:319–324.

206. Lawrence PF, Dries DJ, Alazraki N, Albo D Jr: Indium 111-labeled leukocyte scanning for detection of prosthetic vascular graft infection. J Vasc Surg 1985;2:165–173.

207. Zibari GB, Gadallah MF, Landreneau M, et al: Preoperative vancomycin prophylaxis decreases incidence of postoperative hemodialysis vascular access infections. Am J Kidney Dis 1997; 30:343–348.

208. Sivanesan S, How TV, Bakran A: Characterizing flow distributions in AV fistulae for haemodialysis access. Nephrol Dial Transplant 1998;13:3108–3110.

209. DeCaprio JD, Valentine RJ, Kakish HB, et al: Steal syndrome complicating hemodialysis access. Cardiovasc Surg 1997; 5:648–653.

210. Miles AM: Vascular steal syndrome and ischaemic monomelic neuropathy: Two variants of upper limb ischaemia after haemodialysis vascular access surgery. Nephrol Dial Transplant 1999;14:297–300.

211. Wixon CL, Hughes JD, Mills JL: Understanding strategies for the treatment of ischemic steal syndrome after hemodialysis access. J Am Coll Surg 2000;191:301–310.

212. Knox RC, Berman SS, Hughes JD, et al: Distal revascularization-interval ligation: A durable and effective treatment for ischemic steal syndrome after hemodialysis access. J Vasc Surg 2002;36:250–255.

213. Nakhoul F, Yigla M, Gilman R, et al: The pathogenesis of pulmonary hypertension in haemodialysis patients via arterio-venous access. Nephrol Dial Transplant 2005;20: 1686–1692.

214. Wijnen E, Keuter XH, Planken NR, et al: The relation between vascular access flow and different types of vascular access with systemic hemodynamics in hemodialysis patients. Artif Organs 2005;29:960–964.

215. Ball LK: The buttonhole technique for arteriovenous fistula cannulation. Nephrol Nurs J 2006;33:299–304.

216. Lok CE, Thomas A, Vercaigne L: A patient-focused approach to thrombolytic use in the management of catheter malfunction. Semin Dial 2006;19:381–390.

217. Haymond J, Shalansky K, Jastrzebski J: Efficacy of low-dose alteplase for treatment of hemodialysis catheter occlusions. J Vasc Access 2005;6:76–82.

218. Little MA, Walshe JJ: A longitudinal study of the repeated use of alteplase as therapy for tunneled hemodialysis catheter dysfunction. Am J Kidney Dis 2002;39:86–91.

219. Carson RC, Kiaii M, MacRae JM: Urea clearance in dysfunctional catheters is improved by reversing the line position despite increased access recirculation. Am J Kidney Dis 2005;45:883–890.

220. Suhocki PV, Conlon PJ Jr, Knelson MH, et al: Silastic cuffed catheters for hemodialysis vascular access: Thrombolytic and mechanical correction of malfunction. Am J Kidney Dis 1996; 28:379–386.

221. Crain MR, Mewissen MW, Ostrowski GJ, et al: Fibrin sleeve stripping for salvage of failing hemodialysis catheters: Technique and initial results. Radiology 1996;198:41–44.

222. Merport M, Murphy TP, Egglin TK, Dubel GJ: Fibrin sheath stripping versus catheter exchange for the treatment of failed tunneled hemodialysis catheters: Randomized clinical trial. J Vasc Interv Radiol 2000;11:1115–1120.

223. Develter W, De Cubber A, Van Biesen W, et al: Survival and complications of indwelling venous catheters for permanent use in hemodialysis patients. Artif Organs 2005;29: 399–405.

224. Mokrzycki MH, Jean-Jerome K, Rush H, et al: A randomized trial of minidose warfarin for the prevention of late malfunction in tunneled, cuffed hemodialysis catheters. Kidney Int 2001;59:1935–1942.

225. Hemmelgarn BR, Moist L, Pilkey RM, et al: Prevention of catheter lumen occlusion with rT-PA versus heparin (Pre-CLOT): Study protocol of a randomized trial [ISRCTN35253449]. BMC Nephrol 2006;7:8.

226. Grudzinski L, Quinan P, Kwok S, Pierratos A: Sodium citrate 4% locking solution for central venous dialysis catheters—an effective, more cost-efficient alternative to heparin. Nephrol Dial Transplant 2007;22:471–476.

227. Weijmer MC, van den Dorpel MA, Van de Ven PJ, et al: Randomized, clinical trial comparison of trisodium citrate 30% and heparin as catheter-locking solution in hemodialysis patients. J Am Soc Nephrol 2005;16:2769–2777.

228. Doorenbos CJ, Van den Elsen-Hutten M, Heuven MJ, Hessels J: Estimation of trisodium citrate (Citra-Lock) remaining in central venous catheters after the interdialytic interval. Nephrol Dial Transplant 2006;21:543–545.

229. Saad TF: Central venous dialysis catheters: Catheter-associated infection. Semin Dial 2001;14:446–451.

230. Mermel LA, Farr BM, Sherertz RJ, et al: Guidelines for the management of intravascular catheter-related infections. J Intraven Nurs 2001;24:180–205.

231. Shaffer D: Catheter-related sepsis complicating long-term, tunnelled central venous dialysis catheters: Management by guidewire exchange. Am J Kidney Dis 1995;25:593–596.

232. Lok CE: Avoiding trouble down the line: The management and prevention of hemodialysis catheter-related infections. Adv Chronic Kidney Dis 2006;13:225–244.

233. Mokrzycki MH, Singhal A: Cost-effectiveness of three strategies of managing tunnelled, cuffed haemodialysis catheters in clinically mild or asymptomatic bacteraemias. Nephrol Dial Transplant 2002;17:2196–2203.

234. Allon M: Saving infected catheters: Why and how. Blood Purif 2005;23:23–28.

235. Mokrzycki MH, Zhang M, Golestaneh L, et al: An interventional controlled trial comparing 2 management models for the treatment of tunneled cuffed catheter bacteremia: A collaborative

team model versus usual physician-managed care. Am J Kidney Dis 2006;48:587–595.

236. Saxena AK, Panhotra BR, Sundaram DS, et al: Enhancing the survival of tunneled haemodialysis catheters using an antibiotic lock in the elderly: A randomised, double-blind clinical trial. Nephrology (Carlton) 2006;11:299–305.

237. Manierski C, Besarab A: Antimicrobial locks: Putting the lock on catheter infections. Adv Chronic Kidney Dis 2006;13:245–258.

238. Johnson DW, van Eps C, Mudge DW, et al: Randomized, controlled trial of topical exit-site application of honey (Medihoney) versus mupirocin for the prevention of catheter-associated infections in hemodialysis patients. J Am Soc Nephrol 2005;16:1456–1462.

239. Magnasco A, Bacchini G, Cappello A, et al: Clinical validation of glucose pump test (GPT) compared with ultrasound dilution technology in arteriovenous graft surveillance. Nephrol Dial Transplant 2004;19:1835–1841.

240. Brancaccio D, Tessitore N, Carpani P, et al: Potassium-based dilutional method to measure hemodialysis access recirculation. Int J Artif Organs 2001;24:606–613.

Further Reading

Allon M: Saving infected catheters: Why and how. Blood Purif 2005;23:23–28.

Asif A, Roy-Chaudhury P, Beathard GA: Early arteriovenous fistula failure: A logical proposal for when and how to intervene. Clin J Am Soc Nephrol 2006;1:332–339.

Besarab A, Work J: Clinical practice guidelines for vascular access. Am J Kidney Dis 2006;48(Suppl 1):S176–S247.

Besarab A, Work J: Clinical practice guidelines for vascular access. Am J Kidney Dis 2006;48(Suppl 1):S248–S273.

Bagul A, Brook NR, Kaushik M, Nicholson ML: Tunnelled catheters for the haemodialysis patient. Eur J Vasc Endovasc Surg 2007;33:105–112.

Besarab A: Access monitoring is worthwhile and valuable. Blood Purif 2006;24:77–89.

Dixon BS: Why don't fistulas mature? Kidney Int 2006;70:1413–1422.

Lok CE: Avoiding trouble down the line: The management and prevention of hemodialysis catheter-related infections. Adv Chronic Kidney Dis 2006;13:225–244.

Paulson WD: Access monitoring does not really improve outcomes. Blood Purif 2005;23:50–56.

Ravani P, Spergel LM, Asif A, et al: Clinical epidemiology of arteriovenous fistula in 2007. J Nephrol 2007;20:141–149.

Roy-Chaudhury P, Sukhatme VP, Cheung AK: Hemodialysis vascular access dysfunction: A cellular and molecular viewpoint. J Am Soc Nephrol 2006;17:1112–1127.

Spergel LM, Ravani P, Asif A, et al: Autogenous arteriovenous fistula options. J Nephrol 2007;20:288–298.

Weijmer MC, ter Wee PM: Temporary vascular access for hemodialysis treatment. Current guidelines and future directions. Contrib Nephrol 2004;142:94–111.

White JJ, Bander SJ, Schwab SJ, et al: Is percutaneous transluminal angioplasty an effective intervention for arteriovenous graft stenosis? Semin Dial 2005;18:190–202.

Chapter 79

Hemodialysis Adequacy

Jane Y. Yeun and Thomas A. Depner

CHAPTER CONTENTS

Hemodialysis currently sustains life for more than a million patients throughout the world, with a projected growth of 7% per year.[1] At this growth rate, the projected worldwide expenditure for managing dialysis patients will be more than a trillion dollars a year in the next decade.[1] This staggering human endeavor mandates an in-depth understanding of all aspects of hemodialysis and a commitment to reducing morbidity and mortality first and foremost by providing adequate dialysis. Although we now have a better understanding of what constitutes adequate dialysis, our knowledge is still incomplete because we do not yet fully understand its target, the uremic syndrome. This chapter reviews what is known about hemodialysis adequacy and its measurement, starting with a historical perspective, followed by discussions of methods of measurement, including new expressions of adequacy and

quantifying more frequent dialysis, as well as troubleshooting, and ending with some practical clinical scenarios.

HISTORY OF HEMODIALYSIS ADEQUACY MEASUREMENTS

Measurement of hemodialysis adequacy has been steeped in empiricism since the early pioneering days of Kolff, who was the first to apply hemodialysis successfully to patients,[2] and Scribner, who first applied hemodialysis to treatment of chronic kidney disease using a peripheral vascular access.[3] Despite extensive research, the exact identity of the uremic toxin(s) remained elusive. Instead, nonspecific surrogates, such as improvements in the uremic syndrome, severity of anemia, patient activity and performance levels, and nutritional parameters such as appetite and dietary intake, were used to determine the adequacy of dialysis.

The persistently high mortality after patients start dialysis and recognition of the uremic syndrome as a late finding provided the impetus to develop a better way of measuring and optimizing the dialysis dose. Because urea is the most abundant organic substance to accumulate in patients with kidney failure and is readily measured,[4] it became a natural target for measurement of hemodialysis adequacy. Removal of urea as a measure of dialysis adequacy was further fueled by the growing recognition that blood urea levels correlated with morbidity and mortality, but because interpretation of levels is confounded by urea generation, urea clearance became the favorite measure of adequacy.[4]

A prospective interventional study of dialysis adequacy in the late 1970s, the U.S. National Cooperative Dialysis Study (NCDS), provided clear-cut evidence for a level of urea clearance that was inadequate.[5] Hemodialysis patients randomized to the group with a low urea concentration (achieved time-averaged urea concentration, 51–54 mg/dL) had fewer medical complications and fewer hospitalizations than those randomized to the group with a high urea concentration (achieved urea concentration, 88–90 mg/dL).[5] A subsequent mechanistic analysis of the NCDS highlighted the paradox and difficulty of using serum urea concentration as a marker of dialysis adequacy[6]: When urea levels were reduced by dialysis, patient outcome was improved, but when levels were reduced by poor dietary protein intake, outcomes worsened. Because both nutrition and the amount of dialysis contributed to blood urea levels, the focus switched from monitoring absolute urea levels to measuring the relative change in urea concentration during hemodialysis treatments.[5,6] This relative change in urea concentration is the result of both the dialyzer clearance rate (K) and the treatment time (t), expressed mathematically as Kt/V, the *fractional clearance of urea,* or the urea space cleared per dialysis session. The integrated clearance per dialysis (Kt) is normalized to V, the *volume of urea distribution,* which is a measure of patient size. Currently, both the raw urea reduction ratio (URR) and the more precise expression, Kt/V, are widely accepted and used in dialysis clinics to monitor the adequacy of hemodialysis.

Data from the NCDS was used to set a minimum level of dialysis at a Kt/V of 1.0 per dialysis (three treatments per week), below which poorer outcomes were observed.[6] Uncontrolled studies since then have suggested that more dialysis, in the form of more prolonged treatments provided three times per week, was better for the patient.[7–13] Analysis of urea kinetics suggested, however, that providing longer-duration dialysis beyond 3 to 4 hours three times per week provided no additional benefit, because urea concentrations fell logarithmically with time approaching a plateau.[14,15] Extending the treatment time was considered an inconvenience to the patient, worsening the quality of life without providing significant medical benefit.

The National Institutes of Health (NIH)-sponsored Hemodialysis (HEMO) Study confirmed this theoretical construct.[16] This multicenter, prospective clinical trial randomized 1846 patients to receive standard-dose versus high-dose hemodialysis three times per week, at a time when the accepted minimum Kt/V was 1.2 per treatment.[17] The standard-dose group achieved a single pool Kt/V of 1.32 (equivalent to an equilibrated Kt/V of 1.16 and URR of 66%), whereas the high-dose group achieved a single pool Kt/V of 1.71 (equilibrated Kt/V of 1.53 and URR of 75%).[16] The subjects were further randomized to receive dialysis using a high-flux membrane (β_2-microglobulin clearance >20 mL/min) versus a low-flux membrane (clearance <10 mL/min). More dialysis delivered three times per week or the use of a high-flux membrane did not reduce mortality, reduce cardiovascular or infection-related hospitalizations, or maintain higher serum albumin levels. Although subgroup analysis showed a lower mortality and fewer first hospitalizations for cardiac causes in patients treated with high-flux membranes[16] and lower overall mortality in women receiving high-dose dialysis,[18] these findings were of borderline significance and must be confirmed by other studies. As with any randomized study, the power of the study diminishes and the probability of error increases exponentially with subgroup analysis.

Current Target for Hemodialysis Adequacy

Based on current available data and the results of the HEMO Study, all hemodialysis patients should receive a minimum single pool Kt/V of 1.2 per dialysis three times weekly. A higher urea clearance should be considered in women if symptoms or signs suggest inadequate dialysis, but this is not routinely recommended. Providing more frequent dialysis in the form of daily short-duration hemodialysis or daily nocturnal hemodialysis may reduce mortality and morbidity further, based on solute kinetics that assume that the more toxic uremic solutes are more secluded than urea and not as available to the dialyzer because of their resistance to diffusion across cell membranes or protein binding.[14,15,19–22]

SOLUTE ACCUMULATION AND UREMIC TOXICITY

Reversing uremia and the uremic syndrome is the purpose of hemodialysis. To better understand the current methods of determining hemodialysis adequacy and dosing of hemodialysis, one must first understand the uremic syndrome. A full discussion of uremia and the candidates for uremic toxins is beyond the scope of this chapter but is presented in Section IV, Chapter 48, Pathophysiology of Uremia, in Brenner and Rector's The Kidney, 7th edition. The salient points are reviewed here.

Uremia: The Target of Hemodialysis

All patients with uremia accumulate fluid and solutes, collectively known as *uremic toxins,* which act in concert to create the uremic syndrome.[4,23–28] Removal of these toxins and fluid is the goal of hemodialysis. Monitoring patients and determining the adequacy of their dialysis is made more difficult because the exact nature or identity of the uremic toxins is not known. Like urine solutes, most of the solutes known to accumulate in uremic patients are low in molecular weight and water soluble, rendering them easily removed with dialysis. The most abundant solute of this type is urea.[4] However, some solutes are larger, some are lipid soluble or significantly protein bound, and some are relatively sequestered because of a higher resistance to diffusion across cell membranes than urea.[4,20,23,28,29]

Although urea is a poor marker of native kidney function and demonstrates little toxicity when added to the dialysate to prevent its removal,[30,31] it has become a surrogate marker for uremic toxins and dialysis adequacy because it is easily measured, the most abundant molecule to accumulate in patients with kidney failure, a marker for protein catabolism and hence nutritional status, and its level correlates with survival on dialysis.[5,17,32–34] However, the dual effect of urea generation and removal by dialysis makes interpretation of any measured level difficult unless the relative contributions from kidney failure and protein catabolism are separately identified. Mathematical models of urea kinetics using serum urea concentrations measured before and after dialysis treatments allow such a separation and a better quantification of hemodialysis.

Although the HEMO Study confirmed the validity of using urea kinetics to determine dialysis adequacy, it also highlighted the inherent inefficiency of thrice-weekly dialysis. The logarithmic reduction of urea levels during a short-duration hemodialysis,[14,15] magnified further for the uremic toxins that are not as easily removed as urea,[4,19–23,28,29] markedly reduces the efficiency of intermittent dialysis. Although thrice-weekly dialysis sustains life, it leaves patients with the *residual syndrome,* consisting of a below-average quality of life and significant morbidity, including increased risk of infection, renal osteodystrophy, and cardiovascular disease. The effectiveness of increasing the frequency of dialysis to eliminate the residual syndrome remains to be proven,[35,36] although accumulating data suggest that daily dialysis improves removal of sequestered and protein-bound solutes,[19,21,22] improves blood pressure control, improves anemia and cytokine profiles, and enhances the quality of life.[35,37–39]

Dialysis versus Filtration

Only pertinent points on the physics of dialysis are discussed here; a more detailed analysis of the physical laws that govern dialysis is available in formal texts dealing with kinetic modeling.[40–42]

Dialysis removes solutes by molecular diffusion across a semipermeable membrane. The rate of diffusion varies inversely with the membrane thickness and directly with the solute concentration gradient, the membrane surface area, and the *coefficient of diffusion,* a constant that describes the permeability of a particular membrane material to a particular solute. Solutes with higher molecular weight move more slowly and collide with the membrane less frequently, resulting in a lower coefficient of diffusion. Protein-bound or lipid-soluble substances are even less likely to diffuse across the dialyzer membrane.

An alternative to hemodialysis is hemofiltration, which removes solutes by convection across similar semipermeable membranes. Unlike diffusive clearance, convective clearance is governed mainly by the hydrostatic pressure gradient across the membrane. As long as the solute is small enough to easily traverse the pores in the membrane, larger molecules will be removed at the same rate as smaller molecules. When diffusion and convection occur simultaneously across the same membrane, they can interfere with each other even if solute movement is in the same direction.

When to Start Dialysis

Delaying the initiation of dialysis until frank uremic symptoms are present is clearly deleterious.[43] Based on theoretical grounds, the National Kidney Foundation clinical practice guidelines (K/DOQI)[44,45] suggested starting hemodialysis when the patient's glomerular filtration rate falls below 10 mL/min/1.73 m². Studies that examine the timing of dialysis initiation have yielded conflicting results, some showing a benefit and others equivalence.[46–53] A randomized, controlled trial, the IDEAL (Initiating Dialysis Early And Late) Study, is underway to better answer this question.[54] For now, patients with an estimated glomerular filtration rate near or below 10 mL/min/1.73 m² should be considered for initiation of dialysis, weighing the risks and benefits of vascular access type, quality of life, nutritional status, and comorbidities. If the patient is symptomatic from uremia or volume overload or has significant comorbid conditions,[33] he or she may require initiation of dialysis at a glomerular filtration rate above 10 mL/min/1.73 m².

METHODS FOR MEASURING THE DOSE OF HEMODIALYSIS

Why and How Clearance Substitutes for Toxin Levels

A mechanistic analysis of the NCDS highlighted the difficulty of using urea concentration as a marker of dialysis adequacy[6] and shifted the focus from monitoring absolute urea levels to the relative change in urea concentration during dialysis (i.e., clearance).[5,6] By measuring solute clearance instead of an absolute solute level, the focus shifts to dialyzer function, so the measured marker substance need not be toxic.[55] Because urea is a small molecule that diffuses readily across the dialysis membrane, accumulates in abundance in patients with kidney failure, and is easily measured, it is an excellent solute for monitoring clearance despite its low toxicity. The K/DOQI guidelines recommend using formal urea kinetic modeling to calculate Kt/V to monitor urea clearance and dialysis adequacy, although the URR is acceptable if formal urea kinetic modeling is not possible.[33]

Clearance versus Dialysance

Dialyzer clearance can be defined as the removal rate of a substance (urea) relative to its blood concentration (C):

$$\text{Clearance} = \text{removal rate}/C \qquad \text{(Eq. 79-1)}$$

For single-pass dialysis, in which the dialysate is continually replenished with fresh solution, the clearance of urea is a reasonable measure of dialyzer function. However, if the measured solute is also present in the dialysate, then *dialysance* becomes a more robust term to describe dialyzer function. *Dialysance* is the removal rate of a substance relative to the concentration gradient from blood (C) to dialysate (D):

$$\text{Dialysance} = \text{removal rate}/(C - D) \qquad \text{(Eq. 79-2)}$$

When changes in sodium concentration are used to measure dialyzer "clearance" on-line (see Ionic Dialysance in this chapter), *dialysance* is the more proper term because sodium is also present in the dialysate.

Dialyzer Mass Transfer Area Coefficient (K_OA)

The *mass transfer area coefficient* (K_OA) describes the maximum clearance of a solute across the dialyzer when blood (QB) and dialysate (QD) flow rates are infinite. It is the product of the solute's membrane permeability, or *mass transfer coefficient* (K_O), and the membrane area (A). K_OA is a property of the solute and the dialyzer, including the membrane's pore size and thickness, but is independent of solute concentrations and flow rates. Like clearance or dialysance, it has units of mL/min; it is also known as the *intrinsic clearance of the dialyzer* for the measured solute. K_OA is the most specific constant describing the efficiency of a particular dialyzer for removing a particular solute, with higher values indicating more efficient solute removal. K_OA is used clinically to compare dialyzers and to predict the prescribed dialysis dose.

When QB and QD are finite, dialyzer clearance is lower than K_OA because both flow rates govern diffusion. As QB increases, the inflow concentration is unchanged, but the dialyzer clearance increases logarithmically and approaches K_OA because of a flow-dependent increase in the mean concentration gradient across the membrane, driving more solute into the dialysate. The relationship among dialyzer clearance (K_d), K_OA, QB, and QD can be described mathematically by the following two equations[40–42]:

$$K_OA = \frac{QB \cdot QD}{QB - QD} \ln\left(\frac{QD\,(QB - K_d)}{QB\,(QD - K_d)}\right) \quad \text{(Eq. 79-3)}$$

Equation 79-3 is a practical equation for calculating K_OA from an instantaneous measurement of solute clearance, QB, and QD when flow is countercurrent. This equation is useful clinically to measure in vivo K_OA, which is usually lower than the manufacturer-published in vitro K_OA.

$$K_d = QB\left[\frac{e^{K_OA\left(\frac{QD - QB}{QD\,QB}\right)} - 1}{e^{K_OA\left(\frac{QD - QB}{QD\,QB}\right)} - \frac{QB}{QD}}\right] \quad \text{(Eq. 79-4)}$$

Equation 79-4, which is a rearrangement of Equation 79-3, provides a practical method for calculating expected clearance from QB, QD, and K_OA. This equation is used to calculate a patient's prescribed or predicted Kt/V using the prescribed QB and QD. It also aids in adjusting the patient's dialysis prescription and eliminates the need to measure blood solute concentrations to predict the effect of changes in flow on clearance. It is often used to compare the prescribed with the achieved or predicted Kt/V; the latter is determined primarily from predialysis and postdialysis urea concentrations. A full discussion of the derivation of these formulas is available in formal texts on kinetic modeling.[40–42]

Previously, K_OA was thought to be a constant that did not vary with either blood or dialysate flow rates. More recent studies suggest that QB does not influence K_OA,[58,60] but that at high dialysate flow rates, in vitro K_OA can increase by as

much as 14%.[58] Subsequent data demonstrated a smaller effect of high dialysate flow rates on in vitro[60] and in vivo[56] K_OA values ($\approx$5% higher); they also demonstrated that low dialysate flow rates, such as those used in daily dialysis, resulted in lower K_OA values.[61] That K_OA varies with dialysate flow rates has implications for prescribing dialysis, because predicted clearance calculated from Equation 79-4 may overestimate or underestimate actual clearance, depending on the value for K_OA used. This variation in K_OA renders even more important the use of formal urea kinetics to measure delivered Kt/V using blood urea concentrations that do not depend on K_OA.

Formal Urea Modeling to Measure Clearance

Dialysis in vitro is a simple procedure, but it becomes much more complicated when applied in vivo. Many factors influence the delivery of dialysis; these include the access device, the patient's compliance with the dialysis prescription and dietary restrictions, and solute disequilibrium. Because the precise uremic toxins are not known, measures of dialysis adequacy have been tested using surrogate endpoints, such as mortality, morbidity, serum albumin concentration, and health-related quality of life.[5–13,16,24,28,32,34,62–73] To determine that the observed effect is due to dialysis, detailed studies of large populations with careful attention paid to the many variables that affect outcome are required, preferably by randomizing subjects to different doses of dialysis. To date, only two such randomized studies are available.[5,6,16] Because of the diversity of parameters required for the measurements, such as patient size, ultrafiltration rate, and solute generation rate, complex mathematical models with multiple variables are required even when a simple solute such as urea is used to monitor clearance. These factors add complexity to the relatively simple laws of diffusion and flow, so that the results of solute clearance calculations in patients are often approximations.

Why Kt/V_{urea}?

The simplest measure of clearance is the *instantaneous cross-dialyzer clearance* (K_d), which can be measured by sampling blood on both sides of the dialyzer while simultaneously recording QB using the following equation:

$$K_d = QB(C_{in} - C_{out})/C_{in} \quad \text{(Eq. 79-5)}$$

C_{in} is the inflow solute concentration, and C_{out} is the outflow concentration. Care must be taken to account for ultrafiltration during the measurement and for blood water content because clearances may differ for substances that do not distribute in red cells or are significantly protein bound.[40–42,55] Lastly, loss of surface area from clotting or changes in QB or QD during dialysis may reduce the dialyzer clearance later in the treatment, rendering instantaneous dialyzer clearance less useful.

The *effective clearance,* or integrated dialyzer clearance, accounts for these differences and changes by linking the clearance measurement to the predialysis and postdialysis blood urea nitrogen (BUN) concentration. This clearance, also known as the *delivered clearance,* is the average urea clearance required to reduce the BUN from the measured predialysis value to the postdialysis value. The formal mathematical solution for effective clearance using predialysis and postdialysis BUN values requires a computer-dependent iterative process known as *urea modeling*. Urea modeling can take into account all of the contributing and confounding variables discussed here. Both single- and two-compartment mathematical models have been applied. The single-compartment model requires a predialysis and immediate postdialysis BUN, and the two-compartment model requires intradialysis or postdialysis BUN measurements as well. The most widely accepted expression of the hemodialysis dose, both prescribed and delivered, is Kt/V_{urea}, validated by the NCDS and the HEMO Study[5,6,16] and recommended by the K/DOQI.[17,33]

The Delivered Dose: Mathematical Model of Single Pool Urea Kinetics

The molecular properties of urea that allow it to distribute in aqueous environments and the presence of membrane transporters allow it to diffuse rapidly among the various body water compartments so that a single space of distribution (total body water) can be assumed for most approximations of urea clearance. If urea generation and volume changes during hemodialysis are ignored, fractional urea removal (dC/C) is constant.

$$\left(dC/C\right)/dt = -k = -K/V \qquad \text{(Eq. 79-6)}$$

where k is the fractional removal rate, K the average clearance, and V the volume of urea distribution. Because the fractional removal rate is constant, the absolute removal rate is proportional to the concentration.

Integration and log transformation of Equation 79-6 yields a powerful expression for the normalized clearance (Kt/V):

$$Kt/V = \ln\left(C_0/C\right) \qquad \text{(Eq. 79-7)}$$

Equation 79-7 shows that the effective delivered clearance, integrated over an entire dialysis session and factored for patient size (V), can be determined simply by measuring a predialysis BUN (C_0) and a postdialysis BUN (C), eliminating the need to measure the dialyzer clearance, K_0A, the native kidney clearance during dialysis, the patient's urea volume, or even the duration of each dialysis. However, the simplified Equation 79-7 ignores the change in volume that occurs during dialysis from ultrafiltration (dV) and the contribution of ultrafiltration to clearance (together up to 30% more clearance), as well as the small amount of urea generation that occurs during dialysis (G).

A consideration of urea mass balance requires that the opposing contributions of ultrafiltration and urea generation be added to Equation 79-6. After its synthesis in the liver, urea enters the blood, is quickly distributed in total body water, and is eliminated by the patient's native kidneys (K_r) and by the dialyzer (K_d). Hence, the rate of change of urea content in the pool [d(CV_{urea})/dt] is the difference between the generation rate (G) and the elimination rate [($K_d + K_r$) C]:

$$d\left(CV_{urea}\right)/dt = G - \left(K_d + K_r\right)C = G - KC \qquad \text{(Eq. 79-8)}$$

where C is the concentration of urea and K is the total clearance or the sum of K_r and K_d. Equation 79-8 is the mathematical foundation of the single pool urea model; integration

yields a more complicated equation than Equation 79-7, with four variables that cannot be resolved directly but can be determined using computer iteration, or *modeling*, considering BUN changes during and between dialyses:

$$C = C_0 \left[\frac{V - B{\cdot}t}{V}\right]^{\left(\frac{K_r + K_d + B}{B}\right)} + \frac{G}{K_r + K_d + B}\left[1 - \left[\frac{V - B{\cdot}t}{V}\right]^{\left(\frac{K_r + K_d + B}{B}\right)}\right]$$

$$\text{(Eq. 79-9)}$$

where V is total body water after dialysis (mL) and B is the rate of change in V (mL/min), which is usually negative during dialysis and positive between dialyses. The model allows calculation of the delivered or effective dose of hemodialysis as a single-pool (sp)Kt/V_{urea} from the measured predialysis BUN (C_0), postdialysis BUN (C), and the change in weight during dialysis (B). It gives a more accurate measure of delivered Kt/V, and it also provides a method for calculating G and V.

Simplified Methods

Because the complexity of urea modeling requires a computer program to model spKt/V_{urea} and modeling is not implemented in all dialysis facilities, simplified methods for estimating urea clearance have been developed and are available to clinicians.

Urea Reduction Ratio

The most commonly available and easy to use method is the URR,[74] recommended as the alternative if calculation of Kt/V_{urea} is not available.[33] It is simply the fraction of urea removed during dialysis [($C_0 - C$)/C_0] expressed as a percentage:

$$URR = \left[1 - \left(C/C_0\right)\right] \times 100 \qquad \text{(Eq. 79-10)}$$

where C_0 is the predialysis BUN and C the postdialysis BUN. Several retrospective clinical studies have validated use of URR as an indicator of mortality in hemodialysis patients.[10,75,76] However, URR does not take into account convective clearance provided by ultrafiltration during dialysis, because ultrafiltration does not alter the BUN level. URR also does not allow calculation of V, residual kidney function, urea generation rate, and normalized protein catabolic rate (PCR_n) and is therefore less useful in rooting out the causes of errors in the delivered dose of dialysis (see the section Pitfalls and Troubleshooting in this chapter). Also, it cannot be applied to continuous dialysis or account for continuous native kidney function.

Simplified Equations for spKt/V_{urea}

Alternatives to URR that take into account ultrafiltration and convective clearance, yet do not require computer iteration, are available as simplified explicit equations that approximate spKt/V_{urea}.[77,78] The most widely used equation, proposed by Daugirdas in 1993, is also known as the second-generation logarithm formula.[79,80] This equation was formulated to approximate results from the single pool urea model, including urea generation and volume changes during dialysis, and provides reasonably accurate estimates of Kt/V in the range of 0.7 to 2.1.[79]

$$Kt/V = -\ln\left[(C/C_0) - 0.008 \cdot t\right] +$$
$$\left[4 - 3.5 \cdot (C/C_0)\right] \cdot \Delta BW/BW$$

$$(Eq. 79\text{-}11)$$

where C_0 is predialysis BUN, C is postdialysis BUN, t is treatment time in hours, and BW is body weight.

Equation 79-11 has been compared with other empiric equations and is one of the most accurate.[78,81,82] Like URR, it does not provide a value for G and PCR_n, and it does not permit a rigorous and quantitative analysis of the dialysis prescription to detect sources of errors. However, once $spKt/V_{urea}$ is determined, PCR_n can be estimated using similar empirical equations based on the predialysis BUN.[79,80,83]

Solute Sequestration and Disequilibrium

When solutes are sequestered in a remote body compartment during hemodialysis, the efficiency of dialysis is reduced. The lower BUN levels during dialysis and the BUN rebound after dialysis, compared with levels predicted by the single-compartment model (Figs. 79-1 and 79-2), provide evidence for solute disequilibrium, even for a very diffusible solute like urea. Hemodialysis-induced solute disequilibrium has two forms: (1) diffusion-dependent

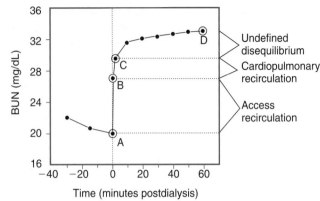

Figure 79-2   Postdialysis blood urea levels. Because of the rapid changes that occur in the postdialysis blood urea nitrogen (BUN) level, timing of blood sampling is critical to ensure consistent and accurate measurements of the urea kinetics value and normalized protein catabolic rate. Sampling blood at Point A may yield a falsely low BUN due to a dilution artifact from access recirculation. Obtaining a blood sample at Point B from the arterial or inflow port 10 to 20 seconds after slowing the blood pump at the end of dialysis eliminates this artifact. Drawing the blood sample 2 minutes postdialysis at Point C eliminates the effects of cardiopulmonary recirculation on urea disequilibrium. Urea equilibration is complete 1 hour after dialysis (Point D). (From Depner TA: Assessing adequacy of hemodialysis: Urea modeling. Kidney Int 1994;45:1522–1535. Used with permission of Kidney International.)

disequilibrium caused by resistance to diffusion across cell membranes, and (2) flow-dependent disequilibrium due to varying blood flow rates among vascular beds.

Two-Compartment Kinetics: Diffusion Model

Urea is unique because it diffuses rapidly across cell membranes, especially the red cell membrane, where its diffusion is facilitated by urea transporters.[84,85] Therefore, the single-compartment model assumption that urea distributes rapidly through all body fluid compartments, including plasma, interstitial fluid, and intracellular water, is reasonable in the interval between dialyses when urea accumulates slowly and urea concentrations change slowly. However, during hemodialysis, when blood concentrations change quickly, urea gradients appear (see Figs. 79-1 and 79-2). To better explain these discrepancies, more complicated mathematical models assuming more than one body fluid compartment were developed.[40–42]

The two-compartment model assumes that total body water is divided into two pools and that solutes must diffuse from one pool into another through a barrier to reach the dialyzer. Typically, for urea, the two pools are thought to be intracellular and extracellular water, and the cell membrane is the semipermeable barrier. The resistance to diffusion is inversely proportional to the intercompartment mass transfer coefficient, K_C. This solute-specific constant is analogous to K_OA and, like K_OA, has units of mL/min. The higher the resistance to diffusion, the lower the K_C, and the slower the solute equilibrates between the fluid compartments. Because solutes are removed rapidly during

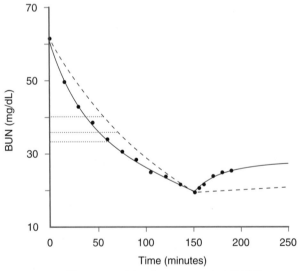

Figure 79-1   Changes in blood urea nitrogen (BUN) concentrations during and after dialysis. BUN levels measured during and immediately after dialysis best fit a two-compartment variable-volume mathematical model (*solid line*). The single-compartment variable-volume model (*dashed line*) overestimates BUN levels during dialysis and does not predict the rebound. The upper horizontal line is the simple arithmetic mean of the predialysis and postdialysis BUN (40 mg/dL). The middle horizontal line depicts the log mean BUN during the treatment (36 mg/dL), as predicted by the single-compartment model. The lower horizontal line is the true mean BUN (34 mg/dL), obtained from multiple measurements throughout dialysis.

hemodialysis, resistance to diffusion between compartments sets up intercompartment solute gradients that subsequently cause a rebound in solute concentration after completion of dialysis.

Solute disequilibrium is more pronounced for solutes other than urea, presumably due to lower rates of diffusion among body compartments, as reflected in their lower K_C values. Most solutes require a multicompartment model to explain their behavior during dialysis.

Recirculation: Flow Model

The two-compartment model described above accounts for solute disequilibrium on the basis of a finite resistance to diffusion among body compartments. The model assumes that the concentration is uniform throughout the blood compartment. More recent data show that blood concentrations are not uniform and that flow-dependent mechanisms contribute to solute disequilibrium.[86–92] Mathematical models developed to describe pure flow-dependent disequilibrium assume that diffusion among compartments is instantaneous and that solute gradients are caused solely by differing blood flow rates to various vascular beds.[90] Regardless, both types of solute disequilibrium lead to lower intradialysis solute concentrations than predicted by the single-pool model, followed by a postdialysis rebound in solute concentration, thereby reducing the efficiency of dialysis (see Fig. 79-1). The largest contributors to flow-dependent disequilibrium are vascular access recirculation[87,93–95] and cardiopulmonary recirculation.[89]

When dialyzer blood flow is higher than vascular access blood flow (as occurs in venous outflow or central venous stenosis), the dialysis needles are too close together, or the arterial and venous needle placements are reversed, blood that has just been dialyzed can return immediately to the dialyzer, creating access recirculation. Because the dialyzer is functioning properly, dialyzer clearance is not reduced, but the recirculated venous blood dilutes the concentration of solute in the dialyzer inflow (arterial blood), lowering the solute concentration gradient across the dialyzer membrane, which decreases total solute removal. Although access recirculation is uncommon (≈5% of dialyses), when it is present, the timing of blood sampling for the postdialysis BUN is critical for accurate measurement of the delivered Kt/V. Sampling arterial (inflow) blood immediately at the end of dialysis without slowing the blood pump (Point A in Fig. 79-2) yields an artificially low BUN and inflates Kt/V. Instead, arterial (inflow) blood should be sampled 10 to 20 seconds after slowing the blood pump at the end of dialysis to eliminate the dilution effect of access recirculation (Point B in Fig. 79-2).

In dialysis patients with peripheral arteriovenous shunts and fistulas, cardiopulmonary recirculation is always present.[89] The circulatory system can be represented as blood flowing from the heart, essentially through various parallel vascular circuits before returning back to the heart. The shunt or fistula has a lower resistance to flow and diverts blood directly from the arterial to the venous circulation, bypassing all capillary beds and returning more quickly to the heart. Because the blood in this circuit has a lower solute concentration, it dilutes the solute concentration of blood returning from other vascular circuits to other parts of the body. Dialyzer clearance is preserved, but the concentration gradient across the dialyzer

membrane is reduced, thus reducing total solute removal and dialysis efficiency. Cardiopulmonary recirculation contributes to the early phases of rebound in urea concentration (and other solutes) seen after completion of dialysis when the various vascular circuits equilibrate (see Fig. 79-2). Patients with central venous catheters as their dialysis access do not have cardiopulmonary recirculation because blood is obtained from and returned to the central blood pool in these patients. This has implications for simplified methods for calculating eKt/V (see Rate Equations in this chapter).

Cardiopulmonary recirculation is a special instance of flow-dependent solute disequilibrium. Differential blood flow rates through other vascular circuits also contribute to solute disequilibrium,[86] such as slower blood flow through dermal vascular beds when the patient is cold or increased gastrointestinal blood flow in the patient who ate before undergoing dialysis. This type of flow-dependent solute disequilibrium invalidated the previous practice of peripheral venous blood sampling for calculating vascular access recirculation.[88,91,92]

Rate Equations

Two-compartment urea kinetic models have been developed to explain the more complex behavior of urea as well as most other solutes, such as creatinine, phosphate, and β_2-microglobulin, during dialysis. Such models allow calculation of whole body or patient clearance that is always lower than the delivered dialyzer clearance calculated from single-pool models. This effective or equilibrated clearance can also be calculated using the single-compartment model but obtaining the postdialysis BUN after re-equilibration among the fluid compartments (Point D in Fig. 79-2). For urea, measuring the equilibrated postdialysis concentration requires delayed blood sampling, at least 30 minutes after the treatment, which is not practical clinically. Fortunately, simple mathematical equations have been derived that predict the equilibrated, or eKt/V_{urea}, from $spKt/V_{urea}$ and either the intensity (K/V) or the duration of dialysis (t).[76,96–100]

For arteriovenous fistulas:

$$eKt/V = spKt/V - 0.6\,(K/V) + 0.03 \qquad \text{(Eq. 79-12)}$$
$$= spKt/V\,(1 - 0.6/t) + 0.03$$

For venous catheters:

$$eKt/V = spKt/V - 0.47\,(K/V) + 0.02 \qquad \text{(Eq. 79-13)}$$
$$= spKt/V\,(1 - 0.47/t) + 0.02$$

where K/V is spKt/V divided by t in hours. The equilibrated eKt/V is lower when the vascular access device is an arteriovenous fistula because of the added presence of cardiopulmonary recirculation. Equation 79-12 has been validated by other investigators and was the basis for prescribing doses of hemodialysis in the HEMO Study.[101,102] The targeted dose of dialysis for the control arm of the HEMO Study[16] was an eKt/V of 1.05, but the achieved eKt/V was 1.16 ± 0.08.

Impact of Treatment Time

Equations 79-12 and 79-13 predict that for the same spKt/V, eKt/V varies with treatment time. In other words, even though dialyzer clearance, expressed in mL/min, remains constant, patient or whole body clearance improves with longer dialysis treatment times, likely due to reducing the effects of solute disequilibrium on the efficiency of dialysis. This effect of time on patient clearance is even more pronounced for solutes that are less diffusible than urea (lower K_C).

The NCDS, which was the first controlled study of dialysis dose versus outcome, reported a borderline significant effect of treatment time on outcome.[5,6] This effect was attributed to larger molecules that are removed more slowly by diffusion. Kinetic studies assessing rebound after short and conventional hemodialysis treatments found that urea concentrations rebounded more after short treatments,[103] as would be expected. However, the postdialysis rebound of β_2-microglobulin was similar for both short and conventional dialysis, suggesting that sequestration may play a more important role than the molecular weight of the solute.

An extreme example of solute disequilibrium is exhibited by phosphate. Phosphate removal varies directly with the serum phosphate concentration and dialyzer clearance, and is greatest during the first hour of dialysis.[37,104,105] After the first hour, phosphate removal falls to half of its initial rate, and the serum level does not decrease further, suggesting that initial phosphate removal is from the blood compartment, and subsequent removal is from sequestered compartments with low K_C values.[37,105,106] From the previous discussion, increasing dialysis treatment time should enhance phosphate removal. Clinical studies have shown that although postdialysis phosphate rebound is greatest when phosphate removal is greatest during dialysis, increasing the duration of each dialysis session eventually reduces predialysis serum phosphate concentrations.[37,104,107] Increasing the dialysis frequency may also increase phosphate removal and lower blood levels. Short daily treatments may improve removal,[107] but long-duration nocturnal hemodialysis has the greatest impact,[37,107] confirming the importance of treatment time for removing sequestered solutes.

Using Other Solutes to Monitor Adequacy

Measuring dialysis adequacy using urea clearance, whether in simple equations or formal urea kinetic modeling, requires careful and precisely timed blood sampling to minimize the effects of solute disequilibrium. Because of these challenges, adequacy is usually measured once a month, which may not be frequent enough to detect vascular access dysfunction or other factors that may reduce the effectiveness of dialysis. Previous advances in on-line monitoring of urea clearance made it possible to monitor urea removal and dialysis adequacy during each dialysis treatment.[108–114] However, urea monitoring devices are cumbersome and expensive to use and therefore are not used widely in clinical practice.[106,113] More recently, on-line monitoring of conductivity has become increasingly available in routine dialysis practice as a reliable surrogate marker for urea clearance.

Ionic Dialysance

The electrical conductivity of dialysate is influenced mainly by the concentration of sodium and its anions. To determine ionic dialysance (Dt/V), which is equivalent essentially to sodium dialysance, conductivity is measured at the dialysate inlet and outlet at baseline and after pulsing the dialysate sodium concentration.[106,113,115,116] Because the out-

let conductivity is determined by the inlet conductivity, the patient's plasma conductivity, and the ionic dialysance, two separate measures of outlet conductivity allow calculations of both plasma conductivity and ionic dialysance.[116,117] This calculation rests on the assumption that the plasma conductivity remains constant between the two sets of conductivity measurements. Therefore, the time elapsed between the dialysate sodium pulse and the second measure of outlet conductivity is critical. If the time period is too long, plasma conductivity may change due to ongoing solute removal. If the elapsed time is too short, there may be insufficient time for the outlet conductivity to stabilize. Currently, most methods allow an elapsed time of 2 minutes before obtaining the second set of inlet and outlet conductivity measurements.

Several studies have validated the use of ionic or sodium dialysance in place of urea clearance.[106,113,115,116,118–120] The correlation with both urea clearance and Kt/V derived from formal urea kinetic modeling is excellent, achieving R values greater than 0.9 in most studies. The main sources of discrepancies between ionic dialysance and urea clearance are: (1) not correcting urea clearance for access and cardiopulmonary recirculation, because ionic dialysance is an effective or patient dialysance by virtue of Dt/V being derived from conductivity measured in the dialysate,[106,113,116,118] and (2) using an anthropometrically derived V to calculate Dt/V instead of a V derived from formal urea kinetic modeling.[106,118,120] If the latter is used as the denominator, values for Dt/V are virtually identical to eKt/V values derived from either formal urea kinetic modeling using a 30-minute postdialysis BUN or from simplified rate equations (Equations 79-12 and 79-18).[106,116,120]

MEASURES AND APPLICATION OF UREA GENERATION

As is evident from the NCDS and other studies, poor protein intake leading to a low urea generation rate (G) and low BUN is associated with a poor outcome.[121,122] Therefore, to assess prognosis and allow intervention, measuring urea generation and its derivative, the patient's protein catabolic rate (PCR), is clinically useful.

Two-BUN Method

As can be seen from Equation 79-9, formal urea kinetic modeling allows calculation of G. Only two BUN values are required if the computer iterative method is used.[41] Once G (mg/min) is available, PCR (g/day) can be calculated from the following equation[123,124]:

$$PCR = 9.35 \cdot G + 11 \qquad (Eq. 79-14)$$

Equation 79-14 illustrates that, under steady state conditions, most of the nitrogen released from net catabolism of endogenous and dietary protein is converted to urea. Only about 11 grams ($\approx$10%) are converted each day to nonurea nitrogenous compounds, such as creatinine, hippurate, and uric acid.[123,124] Urea generation varies directly with protein intake, whereas generation of the other nitrogenous products varies with patient size but not with protein intake. During steady states of protein balance, PCR approximates protein intake, so PCR is a useful marker of protein nutrition.

Clinically, PCR is normalized by ideal body size based on total body water or V_{urea} to yield PCR_n (g/kg/day), allowing comparison among patients of varying size:

$$PCR_n = 5420\,(G/V) + 0.17 \qquad \text{(Eq. 79-15)}$$

ADDITION OF RESIDUAL NATIVE KIDNEY CLEARANCE

When significant residual native kidney function is present, it may contribute significantly to clearance and, therefore, reduce the clearance required from dialysis. However, because residual native kidney clearance (K_r) is continuous and exerts most of its effect between dialysis treatments, it cannot be directly added to dialyzer clearance.

The intermittent clearance obtained with thrice-weekly hemodialysis is less efficient than the continuous clearance provided by native kidneys. The reduced efficiency is due to inherent limitations of intermittent dialysis, which are enhanced by the effects of solute disequilibrium. First, although dialyzer clearance remains constant throughout each dialysis session, the amount of solute removed declines with time as blood solute concentrations decrease logarithmically.[41,125,126] Even if each hemodialysis session were able to remove all of the solute, accumulation between dialysis sessions would result in time-averaged concentration (TAC) and average predialysis concentration that are higher than would be seen in the absence of kidney failure. Solute disequilibrium accentuates this inefficiency by lowering the blood concentration sooner, thereby limiting access of the solute to the dialyzer. For continuous modalities, solute concentrations are stable at a lower level, and the amount of solute removed each hour remains constant. In addition, solute disequilibrium is minimal or absent with continuous modalities.

Because residual kidney clearance is continuous, adding it directly to the intermittent dialyzer clearance would grossly underestimate the contribution of K_r to total clearance. To allow a direct comparison of the relative clearances from the dialyzer and the native kidney and to report a total clearance, two approaches have been proposed. The first, which is used more commonly, involves converting the continuous native clearance to an equivalent intermittent clearance to allow direct addition[41,42]:

$$Kt/V_T = (K_d \cdot t_d + K_r \cdot t_r)\,/\,V_{urea} \qquad \text{(Eq. 79-16)}$$

where Kt/V_T is total Kt/V, K_d is dialyzer clearance, K_r is residual kidney function, and V_{urea} is the volume of distribution of urea or total body water. T_d is the duration of each dialysis session, and t_r is the mean time interval between dialysis sessions. Because continuous clearance is more efficient than intermittent clearance, t_r must be inflated to account for the effect of K_r. The magnitude of the upward adjustment varies with the frequency of dialysis, such that as dialysis becomes more frequent, the adjustment is smaller[41,42] (Table 79-1).

The second, less commonly used, method involves reducing the intermittent dialyzer clearance to a continuous equivalent clearance and then simply adding the residual clearance

Table 79-1 Adjustment to Residual Kidney Function (Values for T_r) to Allow Direct Addition of K_r to K_d Using Equation 79-16

Treatments/ wk (N)	No Adjustment	Adjust to Mean BUN	Adjust to Predialysis BUN
2	5040	6500	9500
3	3360	4000	5500
4	2520	2850	3700
5	2016	2200	2700
6	1680	1780	2100
7	1440	1500	1700

BUN, blood urea nitrogen

without adjustment. Methods for calculating a continuous equivalent clearance are discussed here.

SOLUTE DISTRIBUTION VOLUME

To ensure that patients of varying sizes receive the same dose of dialysis, clearances are adjusted for body size. This adjustment is analogous to the practice of adjusting creatinine clearance to body surface area. For mathematical convenience, dialysis clearance is typically normalized to total body water, which is equal to the volume of distribution of urea (V), an intrinsic element in the term Kt/V. Various methods can be used to calculate V, including indicator dilution,[41] bioimpedance,[127] anthropometric methods,[128–130] and formal urea kinetic modeling.[41] The most common methods used in clinical practice are anthropometry and formal urea kinetic modeling.

Anthropometric V

Anthropometric formulas using the patient's height in centimeters, weight in kilograms, gender, and age in years are the easiest methods to estimate V. Although other formulas are available,[127,128] the most commonly used is the Watson formula[130]:

Males: V (liters) = $2.447 - 0.09516 \cdot$ age $+$

$0.1074 \cdot$ height $+ 0.3362 \cdot$ weight

$$\text{(Eq. 79-17)}$$

Females: V (liters) = $-2.097 + 0.1069 \cdot$ height $+$

$0.2466 \cdot$ weight

$$\text{(Eq. 79-18)}$$

These equations were designed for a wide range of anatomy, but the coefficient of variation is large[130] because variables other than height and weight can influence V.[128]

Modeled V

Urea kinetic modeling yields a more accurate measure of V in individuals because the model makes no anthropometric assumptions and because V is obtained from an average of repeated modeling sessions in the same patient. This method is analogous to the use of indicator dilution methods to measure V, with urea as the indicator. In the HEMO Study, modeled V was 13% to 19% lower than anthropometrically derived V,[131] and lower in whites than in blacks. The difference between modeled and anthropometric V was least for the Watson formula. The etiology for this discrepancy is debated; it may be due to measurement errors in anthropometry, a contracted total body water space in dialysis patients, or differences between the urea distribution volume and total body water.

FREQUENCY OF DIALYSIS

The HEMO Study finding that a higher delivered dose of dialysis did not improve survival[16] has stimulated renewed interest in daily hemodialysis. Observational data suggest that daily hemodialysis improves blood pressure control and may reduce the need for erythropoietin, improve nutrition, regress cardiac hypertrophy, improve phosphate control, reduce inflammation, and improve both quality of life and survival.[35–39,132–139] Currently, daily dialysis is provided either as short daily sessions lasting 1.5 to 3 hours or as nocturnal sessions lasting at least 6 hours while the patient is asleep. Because treatments occur daily, the effects of solute disequilibrium and solute sequestration are minimized, effectively increasing dialysis efficiency while improving its tolerance. In particular, nocturnal dialysis given 6 to 7 nights weekly is expected to control levels of sequestered, protein-bound, and larger molecular weight solutes more effectively.

Available data to date on daily dialysis are observational and frequently retrospective.[36] Two randomized, multicenter studies are currently underway to evaluate the safety and efficacy of more frequent hemodialysis.[140] The Frequent Hemodialysis Network (FHN) Trial Group is conducting two linked studies comparing both short in-center daily hemodialysis and home daily nocturnal hemodialysis with conventional thrice-weekly hemodialysis. Primary outcomes are left ventricular mass index, quality of life, and mortality; secondary endpoints consist of cognitive function, depression index, serum albumin, serum phosphate, blood pressure control, anemia, and hospitalization rates. Complications and the economics of daily dialysis are also monitored. Results of the FHN Trial are not yet available, but mathematical models of solute kinetics suggest that approximately 50% of the benefit derived from daily dialysis can be achieved by increasing the frequency from three to four treatments per week.[15]

RECENT MODIFICATIONS OF UREA MODELING

As discussed, intermittent hemodialysis has inherent inefficiencies because of the effects of solute disequilibrium, solute sequestration, logarithmic decline in solute concentration during dialysis, and the obvious lack of clearance between dialysis sessions. These inefficiencies are attenuated by more frequent or more prolonged treatments, but the improvement is not reflected in currently used measurements of spKt/V and even equilibrated eKt/V.[15,141,142] Several modifications to formal urea kinetic modeling have been proposed to allow improved assessment of dialysis adequacy for more frequent dialysis: equivalent continuous clearance, standard Kt/V, and normalized Kt/V.

Equivalent Continuous Clearance (EKR)

One method, as mentioned in the Addition of Residual Native Kidney Clearance section in this chapter, converts the intermittent hemodialysis component to an equivalent continuous clearance[143]:

$$EKR = G/TAC \qquad \text{(Eq. 79-19)}$$

where EKR is the continuous equivalent of intermittent clearance, has units of mL/min, and includes both the dialyzer and residual kidney clearance. G is the urea generation rate, and TAC the mean concentration (time averaged concentration) of urea; both are obtained from formal urea kinetic modeling.

EKR is the equivalent continuous urea clearance required to maintain the BUN at a level equal to the measured mean level, assuming a steady state of urea nitrogen balance. An example of the clinical application of EKR is its use to explain the discrepancy between the targeted dialysis dose in hemodialysis versus peritoneal dialysis. The minimum spKt/V per hemodialysis treatment is 1.2, giving a weekly Kt/V of 3.6, which results in a hemodialysis mortality rate comparable to that for peritoneal dialysis at a weekly Kt/V of 2.0. Using Equation 79-19, the quantity of dialysis needed to keep a patient's time-averaged BUN constant decreases from 3.6/week to an EKRt/V of approximately 3/week.[141] Converting an intermittent hemodialysis urea clearance to a continuous equivalent brings weekly urea clearance closer to the targeted weekly peritoneal clearance, but there remains a significant difference. This logic suggests that simply maintaining an equivalent mean BUN is not sufficient to explain the discrepancy between hemodialysis and peritoneal dialysis targets.

Standard Kt/V

Substituting average predialysis BUN (average peak BUN) for TAC in Equation 79-19 yields standard clearance (stdKt/V)[15,55,141,144]:

$$stdK = G/(\text{average predialysis BUN}) \qquad \text{(Eq. 79-20)}$$

G and average peak BUN are derived from formal urea kinetic modeling. An alternative mathematical calculation for stdKt/V from eKt/V is also available and has been validated against the computer-based modeling.[145]

Because the predialysis BUN is always higher than the mean BUN, standard clearance is always lower than EKR. Although stdKt/V more closely approximates the peritoneal dialysis weekly Kt/V target, it is unlikely that peak urea levels mediate uremic toxicity because urea itself is not very toxic.[30,125] Rather, the more potent uremic toxins probably are more sequestered than urea, so levels correlate better with the peak urea levels.

Normalized Kt/V

A third new expression for continuous equivalent clearance is the normalized fractional clearance (nKt/V).[55,141] Unlike the previous Kt/V expressions, in which the urea removal rate (equal to the generation rate when in steady state) is divided by a urea concentration, the normalized clearance (nK) is redefined as the urea removal rate divided by the mean concentration of a sequestered solute:

$$nKt/V = G/(\text{mean concentration of sequestered solute})$$

(Eq. 79-21)

This theoretical solute behaves like urea in being easily dialyzed, but is more sequestered than urea in other solute compartments, leading to more solute disequilibrium during dialysis and larger rebound after dialysis. Preliminary estimates suggest that a solute with K_C of approximately 100 mL/min and dialyzer clearance similar to urea would provide an excellent model.[146]

Scaling by Surface Area Instead of V

Use of V to adjust urea clearance for body size and to allow direct comparison of urea clearance among patients and populations is debated for several reasons.[33,147–149] First, V itself is associated independently and inversely with mortality and may confound analyses of dialysis dose versus mortality. Second, factoring urea clearance for V may lead to underdialysis of women and small patients, especially if the assumption that smaller patients need proportionally less dialysis is incorrect. Third, true uremic toxins may not behave like urea and therefore may not distribute only in total body water or V.

Instead, some authors have proposed using Kt alone as a measure of dialysis adequacy.[150] Others suggest factoring clearance (Kt) by body surface area as an adjustment for body size. Factoring for body surface area augments the adjusted dialysis dose for smaller patients (i.e., relatively higher clearance) and reduces the adjusted dialysis dose for larger patients (i.e., relatively lower clearances). This adjustment is straightforward for on-line monitoring of adequacy, which yields Kt. However, if adequacy is obtained using predialysis and postdialysis BUN levels and urea kinetic modeling, the expression for adequacy already includes V. Multiplying Kt/V obtained from kinetic modeling by $3.27 \times V/V^{0.667}$ effectively converts the denominator from total body water to body surface area.[33] Applying this correction to the modeled Kt/V yields the same dialysis dose when V is 35 L, augments the dose if V is less than 35 L, and reduces the dose if V is higher, similar to the effect described above for factoring Kt by body surface area.

REQUIREMENTS FOR DIALYSIS AMONG PATIENT SUBPOPULATIONS

As discussed, the NCDS showed that both high and low blood urea concentrations were associated with increased mortality, due to insufficient dialysis in the former and to poor nutrition in the latter.[6,121] This ambiguity in interpreting the blood urea concentration led to the adoption of urea clearance as the determinant of dose. A mechanistic analysis of the NCDS data demonstrated improved outcomes when spKt/V was 1.0 or greater per dialysis performed three times weekly.[121] Subsequently, data from observational studies suggested that increasing Kt/V to 1.2 or greater yielded additional benefit.[7–13]

Recommendations from the Renal Physicians Association, the National Kidney Foundation, and the National Institutes of Health adopted a Kt/V of 1.2 per dialysis as the minimum dose. Findings from the HEMO Study confirmed the above minimum, showing that increasing the single pool Kt/V from 1.3 to 1.7 did not further reduce morbidity or mortality in patients dialyzed three times weekly.[16]

Factors other than dialysis dose also influence mortality. Several studies have demonstrated that a larger body size, whether assessed by body weight, body mass index, or total body water (as determined by the Watson formula), was associated with a lower mortality.[18,150–155] Black race also confers a survival advantage for patients on hemodialysis.[152] Whether increasing the dialysis dose has a further impact on the effects of body size and race on mortality is controversial.[150,152,154,155] A secondary analysis of the HEMO Study confirmed that a larger body size is associated with a lower mortality, but a higher dialysis dose had no further effect.[18] However, even after adjusting for the effect of body size (smaller in women), women benefited from a higher dose of dialysis, with a 19% lower mortality risk.[18] Men did not appear to benefit from a higher dialysis dose. Analysis of two large databases (Dialysis Outcomes and Practice Patterns Study and Centers for Medicare and Medicaid Services) also showed that women may benefit from a higher dose of dialysis, whereas men did not.[156] Because of the potential errors seen with secondary analysis and with retrospective studies, current recommendations are to provide women with the same dose of dialysis as men, unless symptoms suggestive of uremia are present.

PITFALLS AND TROUBLESHOOTING

Discrepancies in the Delivered versus Prescribed Dialysis Dose

Formal urea kinetic modeling provides a measurement of the delivered dose of dialysis, allowing a comparison with the prescribed dose. A discrepancy between the two may result from large difference between total body water calculated from anthropometric formulas (V_{Calc}) such as the Watson formula (see Equations 79-17 and 79-18) and the modeled V derived from formal urea kinetics (V_{UKM}). Assuming that V_{Calc} is accurate, when V_{UKM} is larger than V_{Calc}, the delivered Kt/V is lower than that prescribed (Box 79-1). The converse is true when V_{UKM} is smaller than V_{Calc}. Various common causes of differences between V_{UKM} and V_{Calc} are listed in Box 79-1.

Alternatively, if the urea kinetic modeling program only reports Kt/V, both prescribed and delivered, a significant difference between the two should prompt an evaluation to detect errors in the delivery or monitoring of dialysis (Boxes 79-2 and 79-3; see also Box 79-1). When delivered Kt/V is greater than prescribed Kt/V or V_{Calc} is greater than V_{UKM}, the cause is usually an error in sampling the postdialysis urea level (see Box 79-1), and not from an erroneous dialysis prescription.

Blood sampling errors can also lead to an artificially low delivered Kt/V when the prescribed Kt/V is appropriate (see Boxes 79-1 to 79-3). In addition, other problems can lead to a real reduction in delivered Kt/V despite an adequate prescribed Kt/V (see Boxes 79-1 to 79-3). These problems include a poorly functioning vascular access, inadequate

Box 79-1 Causes of a Discrepant Volume of Urea Distribution Obtained from Formal Urea Kinetic Modeling (V_{UKM}) Versus that Obtained from Anthropometry (V_{calc})

$V_{UKM} > V_{Calc}$*	**$V_{Calc} > V_{UKM}$**
Delivered Kt/V $<$ Prescribed Kt/V	**Delivered Kt/V $>$ Prescribed Kt/V**
Low blood flow in vascular access	Postdialysis urea level drawn from venous line
Inadequate dialyzer performance	Postdialysis urea level drawn with recirculation present
Low dialysate flow during dialysis	Postdialysis urea level drawn after very efficient dialysis in small patient → urea disequilibrium
Prescription entered incorrectly	
Early termination of dialysis	Postdialysis urea level diluted with normal saline
Predialysis urea level drawn too late	

*assuming that V_{Calc} is accurate

Box 79-2 Common Causes for a Lower Delivered Dose of Hemodialysis than the Prescribed Dose*

Compromised Urea Clearance
Access recirculation
Poor dialyzer function
- Overestimation of dialyzer performance
- Inadequate dialyzer reprocessing
- Dialyzer clotting during hemodialysis
- Dialyzer leaks

Actual QB $<$ prescribed QB
- Poor vascular access function
- Blood pump malfunction

Actual QD $<$ prescribed QD
- Dialysate flow miscalibration

Reduced Treatment Time
Delay in starting dialysis
Failure to account for interruptions
Premature discontinuation of dialysis
- Staff convenience or error
- Patient request

Laboratory or Blood Sampling Errors
Predialysis blood sample diluted with saline
Predialysis blood sample drawn after dialysis initiated
Postdialysis blood sample drawn before dialysis ended
Postdialysis blood sample drawn >5 minutes after dialysis ended
Laboratory measurement error

*An expanded analysis is presented in Box 79-3.

dialyzer performance, lower than prescribed dialysate flow, and shortened dialysis treatment time, all of which compromise urea clearance directly (see Box 79-2). Clinical events, such as hypotension, muscle cramping, chest pain, problems with needle placement, and hemodialyzer blood leaks, also contribute to reduced urea clearance, either by shortening the dialysis treatment time or by lowered QB below that prescribed (see Box 79-3).

Most troubleshooting focuses on causes of a reduced delivered Kt/V, because interventions to improve the dialysis treatment itself are necessary to correct the underlying problem and because the delivered Kt/V is actually low in most cases, not artificially low due to blood sampling errors. A discussion of some specific clinical problems that can affect delivered Kt/V follows.

Measurement Errors

Because of the nonlinear removal of urea at the beginning of hemodialysis and the rapid rebound in BUN at the end of dialysis, timing of blood sampling is critical for accurate determination of the delivered dialysis dose. Drawing the predialysis blood sample for urea measurement after dialysis has begun or contaminating the predialysis blood sample with saline solution or with the catheter lock solution will falsely lower the predialysis urea level and result in a falsely lower delivered Kt/V (see Boxes 79-1 to 79-3). Similarly, poor technique in blood sampling at the end of dialysis can result in erroneously high or low urea levels and a spuriously inaccurate delivered Kt/V (see Boxes 79-1 to 79-3). Falsely low postdialysis urea levels will result if blood is sampled from the venous instead of arterial line, without flushing the blood tubing and needle to eliminate recirculated blood, or while saline solution or blood is infused. These errors all lead to an artificially high delivered Kt/V. Sampling blood too late after discontinuation of dialysis will result in a falsely low delivered spKt/V because of the effects of urea rebound (Point C and beyond in Fig. 79-2). These causes of a spuriously low delivered spKt/V must be distinguished from causes of a true reduction in delivered Kt/V.

Guidelines from The Kidney Disease Outcomes Quality Initiative (K/DOQI) on hemodialysis adequacy provide evidence-based recommendations for sampling of blood both predialysis (Box 79-4) and postdialysis (Box 79-5).[33] Accurate laboratory processing of the blood sample to measure BUN is also important to yield a true measure of the delivered dialysis dose.

Procedure for Sampling Blood Postdialysis

At the completion of hemodialysis, if access recirculation is present, the arterial blood entering the dialyzer may be contaminated with just-dialyzed blood from the venous return. The urea concentration is lower in this recirculated blood, diluting the urea concentration of the arterial blood and leading to an artificially high delivered Kt/V. Hence, postdialysis blood samples will yield an appropriate BUN value only if the effect of access recirculation is eliminated. Two methods exist to reduce the effect of access recirculation: the slow-blood-flow method[33,157] and the stop-dialysate-flow method[33,158,159] (see Box 79-5).

Box 79-3 Error Analysis Algorithm to Detect One of Several Potential Common Problems in Hemodialysis Delivery That Is Responsible for a Lower Delivered Dose of Hemodialysis Than the Prescribed Dose

Actual Dialyzer Clearance < Assumed Dialyzer Clearance
Elements of the hemodialysis procedure affecting solute clearance include dialyzer permeability (K_OA), effective dialyzer surface area, blood flow rate (QB), and dialysate flow rate (QD).
1. Assess fistula for recirculation
   - Review arterial and venous needle placement, proximity, and orientation
   - Verify direction of blood flow through the vascular access device
2. Review record of hemodialysis treatment on the date of measured dialysis adequacy
   - Hemodialyzer reuse log to evaluate total cell volume of dialyzer
   - Maintenance log for dialysis machine for last calibration date and results
   - Hemodialysis treatment log to determine whether prescribed treatment parameters for the following were followed: blood flow rate (QB), dialysate flow rate (QD), and type of hemodialyzer
   - Hemodialysis treatment log to assess for the presence of clinical events that may have altered QB: hypotension, muscle cramp, chest pain, and problems with needle placement
3. Assess for episodes of dialyzer clotting
   - Review anticoagulation regimen for hemodialysis
4. To determine whether hemodialyzer clearance is overestimated, review results of formal urea kinetic modeling of other patients using the same dialyzer

Effective Hemodialysis Treatment Time < Prescribed Treatment Time
Hemodialysis treatment time is the total time at the prescribed blood and dialysate flow rates with the prescribed dialyzer. If the hemodialysis treatment is interrupted, the total dialysis time must be extended by an equivalent amount to ensure the same solute clearance.
1. Review the hemodialysis treatment log to determine the total effective treatment time

2. Review the treatment log for the following:
   - Patient arrival time in the clinic
   - Late hemodialysis start time without compensatory extension at the end
   - Patient request for early termination of treatment
   - Clinical events that may have interrupted or caused premature termination of treatment: hypotension, muscle cramps, chest pain, dialyzer clotting, hemodialyzer blood leak, problems with needle placement that required recannulation of the vascular access, pressures in the extracorporeal circuit close to alarm limits

Errors in Sampling or Processing Blood Specimen
Blood samples that provide predialysis and postdialysis urea levels to allow calculation of delivered dialysis dose with formal urea kinetic modeling must be obtained consistently to avoid: (a) dilution with saline or heparin, (b) contamination by recirculated blood, or (c) confounding by urea disequilibrium
1. Causes of falsely low predialysis BUN concentration
   - Dialysis needle was filled with saline
   - Heparin or locking agent was incompletely removed from the hemodialysis catheter
   - Blood sample was drawn after initiation of hemodialysis
   - Laboratory error in assaying blood sample
2. Causes of falsely high postdialysis BUN concentration
   - Blood sample was drawn too late after the discontinuation of hemodialysis
   - Laboratory error in assaying blood sample
3. Causes of falsely low postdialysis BUN concentration
   - Blood sample was drawn from the venous line
   - Blood sample was drawn without flushing the blood tubing and needle to eliminate recirculated blood
   - Blood sample was contaminated with infused saline
   - Laboratory error in assaying blood sample

Box 79-4 Blood Sampling Techniques for Determination of Predialysis BUN

Arteriovenous Fistula or Graft
Obtain the blood sample from the arterial needle immediately after insertion and before flushing the needle with heparin or connecting to blood tubing
Ensure no saline or heparin is in the arterial needle
Do not draw blood specimen if dialysis has begun

Venous Catheter
Using sterile technique, withdraw any heparin or saline, along with blood, from the arterial port to a total volume of 5 mL; discard
Using a new syringe, draw the blood sample for BUN measurement
Start hemodialysis per clinic protocol

The slow-blood-flow method is by far the most popular and has been in use longer[33,157] (see Box 79-5). Reducing the blood flow rate to 100 mL/min eliminates or greatly reduces access recirculation. Waiting for 15 seconds at the lower QB before obtaining a blood sample allows nonrecirculated blood from the vascular access to replace any potentially recirculated blood. Because 100 mL/min is about 1.6 mL/sec, waiting for 15 seconds at this blood flow rate will allow 24 mL of nonrecirculated blood to displace an equivalent amount of potentially recirculated blood. If the blood tubing volume from the arterial needle tip to the arterial sampling port approaches 24 mL, the waiting period must be longer than 15 seconds. This volume in most blood tubing/needle sets is closer to 8 mL. An alternative site for blood sampling is the arterial needle hub, which eliminates the use of additional needles but requires a sterile disconnect (see Box 79-5). Although the slow-blood-flow method eliminates the error from access recirculation, which resolves immediately

Box 79-5   Blood Sampling Techniques for Determination of Postdialysis BUN

Slow-Blood-Flow Method
Drawing the sample from the blood line sampling port
1. At completion of hemodialysis, turn off QD, or decrease to its minimum setting.
2. Turn off ultrafiltration or decrease it to the lowest setting.
3. Decrease QB to 100 mL/min for 15 seconds (longer if bloodline volume from needle tip to sampling port > 15 mL).
4. Obtain the sample, either with QB at 100 mL/min or off.
5. After sampling, stop the blood pump if not already done, and complete dialysis takeoff.

Stop-Dialysate-Flow Method
1. At completion of hemodialysis, turn off QD.
2. Turn off ultrafiltration or reduce it to the lowest setting.
3. Wait 3 minutes; do *not* reduce QB.
4. Obtain the blood sample from the arterial sampling port, the arterial needle hub, or the arterial port of the dialysis catheter. Stopping QB during blood sampling is optional.
5. After sampling, complete dialysis takeoff.

after stopping dialysis (Point A to B in Fig. 79-2), it does not account for the effect of cardiopulmonary recirculation (Point B to C in Fig. 79-2), which takes about 2 to 3 minutes to resolve.

The stop-dialysate-flow method offers an alternative to the above[158,159] (see Box 79-5). To apply this method, the dialysate flow is stopped for 3 to 5 minutes before the postdialysis arterial blood sample is drawn. By stopping dialysate flow and thus eliminating urea removal, the urea concentration in the dialyzer outlet and venous blood tubing approaches that in the dialyzer inlet and arterial blood tubing.

Errors from Access Recirculation

Not only does access recirculation interfere with accurate measurement of the postdialysis BUN, but it also reduces the efficiency of hemodialysis by diluting the arterial solute concentrations, effectively decreasing delivery of solutes to the dialyzer. Causes of access recirculation are myriad. If the venous needle is placed incorrectly and abuts the venous wall, turbulence results and slows the egress of blood from the access, promoting recirculation. Placing the arterial and venous needles too closely together promotes recirculation, especially at high QB. Vascular access malfunctions, such as venous outflow stenosis, arterial insufficiency either from atherosclerotic disease in the supplying artery or inflow anastomotic stenosis, or a fibrin sheath around the dialysis catheter, may also cause access recirculation. Vascular access dysfunction can be detected through a combination of physical examination, measuring vascular access blood flow and recirculation, direct imaging of the access, and venous pressure monitoring.[160]

Dialyzer Clotting

Clotting of the hemodialyzer during a dialysis session reduces the surface area available for solute removal and compromises the efficiency of dialysis. If reuse is practiced, some of the thrombosed hollow fibers may not respond to cleaning and may continue to adversely affect dialyzer clearance. Adequate anticoagulation is therefore important to maintain dialyzer clearance throughout treatment.

Blood Pump Malfunction

Because dialyzer clearance is a function of dialyzer blood flow (QB) (see Equations 79-4 and 79-5), errors in QB due to blood pump malfunction can reduce the delivered dialysis dose or patient clearance. The blood pump in most dialysis machines is a peristaltic roller pump with two or three rollers that move blood through the tubing by sequentially compressing the tubing pump segment against a curved rigid track. The elastic tubing then recoils and refills with blood after one roller arm has passed and before the next one arrives.

QB displayed on the dialysis machine flowmeter is calculated only from the speed of rotation of the roller pump, but true QB is the product of the rotation speed and the volume of blood forced from the tubing during each cycle. If the pre-pump pressure is too low or the blood tubing is too pliable, the pump segment may not re-expand fully between the roller excursions, leading to a lower QB than indicated by the flowmeter. The lower QB reduces the actual dialyzer clearance. This error is more likely to occur at the higher QB used for high-efficiency and high-flux dialysis, or if the vascular access cannot support the prescribed blood flow.[161]

PRACTICAL EXAMPLES

Four Dialysis Treatments per Week

Many patients receive dialysis four times weekly to help manage refractory anemia, to improve solute clearance in larger patients, to control volume in those with excessive weight gain, and to improve blood pressure control. The challenge is how to measure the delivered dialysis accurately. Ideally, formal kinetic modeling to calculate standard Kt/V (stdKt/V) (see Equation 79-20) or normalized Kt/V (see Equation 79-21) expressed as a weekly dialysis dose would allow comparisons among different dialysis schedules. Alternatively, stdKt/V may be approximated using the following equation[145]:

$$\text{stdKt/V} = \left\{100803\left[(1-e^{-eKt/V})/t\right]\right\} \div$$
$$\left\{\left[(1-e^{-eKt/V})/\text{spKt/V}\right]+(10080/Nt)-1\right\}$$

(Eq. 79-22)

where N is the number of treatments per week. Single pool Kt/V (spKt/V) must be available and converted to equilibrated Kt/V (eKt/V) using Equations 79-12 and 79-13. Derivation of Equation 79-22 is based on a symmetric weekly schedule, no residual kidney function, and a fixed urea volume, but the result is approximately accurate in most patients. Also, the minimal goal has not been firmly established for these newer expressions of clearance.

A simple but practical way to determine the solute clearance needed for four treatments per week is to take the minimum total weekly spKt/V of 3.6 for three treatments per week and divide by 4 to yield a minimum spKt/V of 0.9 for each dialysis session.[33] This simple calculation does not take into account the gain in efficiency with more frequent dialysis and therefore overestimates the dialysis dose needed, but protects the patient from underdialysis.

Phosphate Removal

Because phosphate is a secluded solute with significant resistance to diffusion across cell membranes, standard thrice-weekly hemodialysis has little effect on controlling its level despite its ready diffusion from plasma into the dialysate.[29,105] Even short daily hemodialysis fails to improve control of hyperphosphatemia in most studies.[36,37,107] For patients with persistent symptomatic hyperphosphatemia uncontrolled by dietary restriction and phosphate binders, daily long-duration hemodialysis may provide the solution.[36,37]

Shortening versus Extending Treatment Time

Near-universal use of high-efficiency dialyzers has reduced the treatment time in many dialysis clinics, especially those in the United States. However, Equations 79-12 and 79-13 show that effective dialyzer clearance (eKt/V) is time dependent and that shortening the treatment reduces its efficiency. Shortening the treatment accentuates the effects of intermittence and exacerbates solute rebound.[41,98,162,163] Additional problems with shortening the treatment include reduced removal of larger molecules, which is more time dependent,[164,165] and an obligatory increase in the filtration rate above the maximum 0.35 mL/min/kg (1.5 L/hr in a 70-kg patient) that is tolerated.[164,166,167] Also, any time lost during dialysis due to technical problems, late arrival, or access recirculation is magnified with shorter treatments.

Patients with large interdialysis weight gains will benefit from a longer treatment time because more time is available for fluid removal. However, beyond 4 hours or so of treatment, removal of small solutes is greatly reduced. Larger size patients would benefit more from increasing the frequency than the duration of thrice-weekly dialysis.

SUMMARY

It would be a mistake to consider preservation of life the only goal of hemodialysis. The quality of the life preserved must be linked to the adequacy of dialysis in ways that are not yet fully understood, but without question, removal of small solutes, analogous to removal of the same solutes by the native kidney, must be a major target of treatment. This chapter focuses on methods for ensuring adequate control of small solute concentrations in the patient using a variety of monitoring and measuring techniques. The successful dialysis caregiver must be aware of these methods and how they can be applied, including their pitfalls and recent modifications that will hopefully continue to improve patient outcomes.

References

1. Lysaght MJ: Maintenance dialysis population dynamics: Current trends and long-term implications. J Am Soc Nephrol 2002; 13(Suppl 1):S37–S40.
2. Kolff WJ, Berk HT, ter Welle M, et al: The artificial kidney: A dialyser with a great area. 1944 [classic article]. J Am Soc Nephrol 1997;8:1959–1965.
3. Quinton W, Dillard D, Scribner BH: Cannulation of blood vessels for prolonged hemodialysis. ASAIO Trans 1960;6:104–113.
4. Depner TA: Uremic toxicity: Urea and beyond. Semin Dial 2001;14:246–251.
5. Lowrie EG, Laird NM, Parker TF, et al: Effect of the hemodialysis prescription of patient morbidity: Report from the National Cooperative Dialysis Study. N Engl J Med 1981;305: 1176–1181.
6. Gotch FA, Sargent JA: A mechanistic analysis of the National Cooperative Dialysis Study (NCDS). Kidney Int 1985;28: 526–534.
7. Charra B, Calemard E, Ruffet M, et al: Survival as an index of adequacy of dialysis. Kidney Int 1992;41:1286–1291.
8. Collins AJ, Ma JZ, Umen A, et al: Urea index and other predictors of hemodialysis patient survival. Am J Kidney Dis 1994;23: 272–282.
9. Hakim RM, Breyer J, Ismail N, et al: Effects of dose of dialysis on morbidity and mortality. Am J Kidney Dis 1994;23:661–669.
10. Held PJ, Port FK, Wolfe RA, et al: The dose of hemodialysis and patient mortality. Kidney Int 1996;50:550–556.
11. Owen WF Jr, Lew NL, Liu Y, et al: The urea reduction ratio and serum albumin concentration as predictors of mortality in patients undergoing hemodialysis. N Engl J Med 1993;329: 1001–1006.
12. Parker TF, Husni L, Huang W, et al: Survival of hemodialysis patients in the United States is improved with a greater quantity of dialysis. Am J Kidney Dis 1994;23:670–680.
13. Yang CS, Chen SW, Chiang CH, et al: Effects of increasing dialysis dose on serum albumin and mortality in hemodialysis patients. Am J Kidney Dis 1996;27:380–386.
14. Depner TA: Benefits of more frequent dialysis: lower TAC at the same Kt/V. Nephrol Dial Transplant 1998;13(Suppl 6):20–24.
15. Depner TA, Bhat A: Quantifying daily hemodialysis. Semin Dial 2004;17:79–84.
16. Eknoyan G, Beck GJ, Cheung AK, et al: Effect of dialysis dose and membrane flux in maintenance hemodialysis. N Engl J Med 2002;347:2010–2019.
17. National Kidney Foundation: K/DOQI Clinical Practice Guidelines for Hemodialysis Adequacy: Update 2000. Am J Kidney Dis 2001;37(1 Suppl 1):S7–S64.
18. Depner TA, Daugirdas JT, Greene T, et al: Dialysis dose and the effect of gender and body size on outcome in the HEMO study. Kidney Int 2004;65:1386–1394.
19. Clark WR, Henderson LW: Renal versus continuous versus intermittent therapies for removal of uremic toxins. Kidney Int 2001;78(Suppl):S298–S303.
20. Eloot S, Torremans A, De Smet R, et al: Complex compartmental behavior of small water-soluble uremic retention solutes: Evaluation by direct measurements in plasma and erythrocytes. Am J Kidney Dis 2007;50:279–288.
21. Fagugli RM, De Smet R, Buoncristiani U, et al: Behavior of non-protein-bound and protein-bound uremic solutes during daily hemodialysis. Am J Kidney Dis 2002;40:339–347.
22. Maduell F, Navarro V, Torregrosa E, et al: Change from three times a week on-line hemodiafiltration to short daily on-line hemodiafiltration. Kidney Int 2003;64:305–313.
23. Dhondt A, Vanholder R, Van Biesen W, et al: The removal of uremic toxins. Kidney Int 2000;76(Suppl):S47–S59.
24. Mason M, Resnik H, Mino A, et al: Mechanism of experimental uremia. Arch Intern Med 1993;60:312.

25. Niwa T: Organic acids and the uremic syndrome: Protein metabolite hypothesis in the progression of chronic renal failure. Semin Nephrol 1996;16:167–182.

26. Vanholder R, Argiles A, Baurmeister U, et al: Uremic toxicity: Present state of the art. Int J Artif Organs 2001;24:695–725.

27. Vanholder R, De Smet R: Pathophysiologic effects of uremic retention solutes. J Am Soc Nephrol 1999;10:1815–1823.

28. Vanholder R, Smet RD, Glorieux G, et al: Survival of hemodialysis patients and uremic toxin removal. Artif Organs 2003;27:218–223.

29. Spalding EM, Chamney PW, Farrington K: Phosphate kinetics during hemodialysis: Evidence for biphasic regulation. Kidney Int 2002;61:655–667.

30. Johnson WJ, Hagge WW, Wagoner RD, et al: Effects of urea loading in patients with far-advanced renal failure. Mayo Clin Proc 1972;47:21–29.

31. Merrill J, Legrain, Hoigne R: Observations on the role of urea in uremia. Am J Med 1953;14:519–520.

32. Consensus Development Conference Panel: Morbidity and mortality of renal dialysis: An NIH consensus conference statement. Ann Intern Med 1994;121:62–70.

33. National Kidney Foundation: K/DOQI Clinical Practice Guidelines for Hemodialysis Adequacy 2006. Am J Kidney Dis 2006;48(1 Suppl 1):S2–S90.

34. Renal Physicians Association: Clinical Practice Guideline on Adequacy of Hemodialysis. Washington, DC: Renal Physicians Association, 1993.

35. Pierratos A, McFarlane P, Chan CT, et al: Daily hemodialysis 2006. State of the art. Minverva Urol Nefro 2006;58:99–115.

36. Suri RS, Nesrallah GE, Mainra R, et al: Daily hemodialysis: A systematic review. Clin J Am Soc Nephrol 2006;1:33–42.

37. Achinger SG, Ayus JC: The role of daily dialysis in the control of hyperphosphatemia. Kidney Int 2005;95(Suppl):S28–S32.

38. Heidenheim AP, Muirhead N, Moist L, Lindsay RM: Patient quality of life on quotidian hemodialysis. Am J Kidney Dis 2003;42(1 Suppl):36–41.

39. Yuen D, Richardson RM, Fenton SS, et al: Quotidian nocturnal hemodialysis improves cytokine profile and enhances erythropoietin responsiveness. ASAIO J 2005;51:236–241.

40. Colton CK, Lowrie EG: Hemodialysis: Physical principles and technical considerations. In Brenner BM, Rector FC Jr (eds): The Kidney. Philadelphia: Saunders, 1981, pp 2425–2489.

41. Depner TA: Prescribing Hemodialysis: A Guide to Urea Modeling. Boston, Kluwer Academic Publishers, 1991.

42. Gotch FA: Kinetic modeling in hemodialysis. In Nissenson AR, Fine RN, Gentile DE, Norwalk CT (eds): Clinical Dialysis. Norwalk, CT: Appleton and Lange, 1995, pp 156–188.

43. Hakim RM, Lazarus JM: Initiation of dialysis. J Am Soc Nephrol 1995;6:1319–1328.

44. Keshaviah PR, Emerson PF, Nolph KD: Timely initiation of dialysis: A urea kinetic approach. Am J Kidney Dis 1999;33:344–348.

45. Levey AS, Coresh J, Balk E, et al: National Kidney Foundation practice guidelines for chronic kidney disease: Evaluation, classification, and stratification. Ann Intern Med 2003;139:137–147.

46. Ellis PA, Reddy V, Bari N, Cairns HS: Late referral of end-stage renal failure. QJM 1998;91:727–732.

47. Fink JC, Burdick RA, Kurth SJ, et al: Significance of serum creatinine values in new end-stage renal disease patients. Am J Kidney Dis 1999;34:694–701.

48. Ifudu O, Dawood M, Homel P, Friedman EA: Timing of initiation of uremia therapy and survival in patients with progressive renal disease. Am J Nephrol 1998;18:193–198.

49. Korevaar JC, Jansen MA, Dekker FW, et al: When to initiate dialysis: Effect of proposed US guidelines on survival. Lancet 2001;358:1046–1050.

50. Roubicek C, Brunet P, Huiart L, et al: Timing of nephrology referral: Influence on mortality and morbidity. Am J Kidney Dis 2000;36:35–41.

51. Sesso R, Belasco AG: Late diagnosis of chronic renal failure and mortality on maintenance dialysis. Nephrol Dial Transplant 1996;11:2417–2420.

52. Tattersall J, Greenwood R, Farrington K: Urea kinetics and when to commence dialysis. Am J Nephrol 1995;15:283–289.

53. Traynor JP, Simpson K, Geddes CC, et al: Early initiation of dialysis fails to prolong survival in patients with end-stage renal failure. J Am Soc Nephrol 2002;13:2125–2132.

54. Cooper BA, Branley P, Bulfone L, et al: The Initiating Dialysis Early and Late (IDEAL) Study: Study rationale and design. Perit Dial Int 2004;24:176–181.

55. Depner TA: Hemodialysis adequacy: Basic essentials and practical points for the nephrologist in training. Hemodial Int 2005;9:241–254.

56. Depner TA, Greene T, Daugirdas JT, et al: Dialyzer performance in the HEMO Study: In vivo K_0A and true blood flow determined from a model of cross-dialyzer urea extraction. ASAIO J 2004;50:85–93.

57. Langsdorf LJ, Krankel LG, Zydney AL: Effect of blood-membrane interactions on solute clearance during hemodialysis. ASAIO J 1993;39:M767–M772.

58. Leypoldt JK, Cheung AK, Agodoa LY, et al: Hemodialyzer mass transfer-area coefficients for urea increase at high dialysate flow rates. The Hemodialysis (HEMO) Study. Kidney Int 1997;51:2013–2017.

59. Saha LK, Van Stone JC: Differences between Kt/V measured during dialysis and Kt/V predicted from manufacturer clearance data. Int J Artif Organs 1992;15:465–469.

60. Ouseph R, Ward RA: Increasing dialysate flow rate increases dialyzer urea mass transfer-area coefficients during clinical use. Am J Kidney Dis 2001;37:316–320.

61. Leypoldt JK, Kamerath CD, Gilson JF, Friederichs G: Dialyzer clearances and mass transfer-area coefficients for small solutes at low dialysate flow rates. ASAIO J 2006;52:404–409.

62. Allen KL, Miskulin D, Yan G, et al: Association of nutritional markers with physical and mental health status in prevalent hemodialysis patients from the HEMO study. J Ren Nutr 2002;12:160–169.

63. Arora P, Kausz AT, Obrador GT, et al: Hospital utilization among chronic dialysis patients. J Am Soc Nephrol 2000;11:740–746.

64. Bergstrom J, Heimburger O, Lindholm B, et al: Elevated serum CRP is a strong predictor of increased mortality and low serum albumin in hemodialysis (HD) patients. J Am Soc Nephrol 1995;6:573 Abstract.

65. Bologa RM, Levine DM, Parker TS, et al: Interleukin-6 predicts hypoalbuminemia, hypocholesterolemia, and mortality in hemodialysis patients. Am J Kidney Dis 1998;32:107–114.

66. Fukuhara S, Lopes AA, Bragg-Gresham JL, et al: Health-related quality of life among dialysis patients on three continents: The Dialysis Outcomes and Practice Patterns Study. Kidney Int 2003;64:1903–1910.

67. Hull A, Parker T: Proceedings from the Morbidity, Mortality and Prescription of Dialysis Symposium: Dallas, TX, September 15–17, 1989. Am J Kidney Dis 1990;15:375–383.

68. Iliescu EA, Coo H, McMurray MH, et al: Quality of sleep and health-related quality of life in haemodialysis patients. Nephrol Dial Transplant 2003;18:126–132.

69. Knight EL, Ofsthun N, Teng M, et al: The association between mental health, physical function, and hemodialysis mortality. Kidney Int 2003;63:1843–1851.

70. Lowrie EG, Curtin RB, LePain N, et al: Medical outcomes study short form-36: A consistent and powerful predictor of morbidity and mortality in dialysis patients. Am J Kidney Dis 2003;41:1286–1292.

71. Metcalfe W, Khan IH, Prescott GJ, et al: Can we improve early mortality in patients receiving renal replacement therapy? Kidney Int 2000;57:2539–2545.

72. U.S. Renal Data System: The USRDS dialysis morbidity and mortality study (Wave 1). Am J Kidney Dis 1996;28(3 Suppl 2): S58–S78.

73. Valderrabano F, Jofre R, Lopez-Gomez JM: Quality of life in end-stage renal disease patients. Am J Kidney Dis 2001;38:443–464.

74. Lowrie EG, Lew NL: The urea reduction ratio (URR): A simple method for evaluating hemodialysis treatment. Contemp Dial Nephrol 1991;12:11–20.

75. Shaldon S: Unanswered questions pertaining to dialysis adequacy in 1992. Kidney Int 1993. 41:S274–S277.

76. Szczech LA, Lowrie EG, Li Z, et al: Changing hemodialysis thresholds for optimal survival. Kidney Int 2001;59:738–745.

77. Movilli E: Simplified approaches to calculate Kt/V. It's time for agreement. Nephrol Dial Transplant 1996;11:24–27.

78. Prado M, Roa LM, Palma A, Milan JA: Double target comparison of blood-side methods for measuring the hemodialysis dose. Kidney Int 2005;68:2863–2876.

79. Daugirdas JT: Second generation logarithmic estimates of single-pool variable volume Kt/V: An analysis of error. J Am Soc Nephrol 1993;4:1205–1213.

80. Daugirdas JT: Simplified equations for monitoring Kt/V, PCRn, eKt/V, and ePCRn. Adv Ren Replace Ther 1995;2:295–304.

81. Daugirdas JT: Rapid methods of estimating Kt/V: Three formulas compared. Trans ASAIO 1990;36:M362–M364.

82. Flanigan MJ, Fangman J, Lim VS: Quantitating hemodialysis: A comparison of three kinetic models. Am J Kidney Dis 1991;17:295–302.

83. Depner TA, Daugirdas JT: Equations for normalized protein catabolic rate based on two-point modeling of hemodialysis urea kinetics. J Am Soc Nephrol 1996;7:780–785.

84. Kaplan MA, Hays L, Hays RM: Evolution of a facilitated diffusion pathway for amides in the erythrocyte. Am J Physiol 1974;226:1327–1332.

85. Macey RI, Yousef LW: Osmotic stability of red cells in renal circulation requires rapid urea transport. Am J Physiol 1988;254 (5 Pt 1):C669–C674.

86. Depner T, Rizwan S, Cheer A, et al: Peripheral urea disequilibrium during hemodialysis is temperature-dependent. J Am Soc Nephrol 1991;2:321.

87. Depner TA: Assessing adequacy of hemodialysis: Urea modeling. Kidney Int 1994;45:1522–1535.

88. Depner TA, Rizwan S, Cheer AY, et al: High venous urea concentrations in the opposite arm. A consequence of hemodialysis-induced compartment disequilibrium. ASAIO Trans 1991;37: M141–M143.

89. Schneditz D, Kaufman AM, Polaschegg HD, et al: Cardiopulmonary recirculation during hemodialysis. Kidney Int 1992; 42:1450–1456.

90. Schneditz D, Van Stone JC, Daugirdas JT: A regional blood circulation alternative to in-series two compartment urea kinetic modeling. ASAIO J 1993;39:M573–M577.

91. Tattersall JE, Farrington K, Raniga PD, et al: Haemodialysis re-circulation detected by the three-sample method is an artefact. Nephrol Dial Transplant 1993;8:60–63.

92. Van Stone J, Jones M: Peripheral venous blood is not the appropriate specimen to determine recirculation rate. J Am Soc Nephrol 1991;2:354.

93. Collins DM, Lambert MB, Middleton JP, et al: Fistula dysfunction: Effect on rapid hemodialysis. Kidney Int 1992;41: 1292–1296.

94. Levy SS, Sherman RA, Nosher JL: Value of clinical screening for detection of asymptomatic hemodialysis vascular access stenoses. Angiology 1992;43:421–424.

95. Windus DW, Audrain J, Vanderson R, et al: Optimization of high-efficiency hemodialysis by detection and correction of fistula dysfunction. Kidney Int 1990;38:337–341.

96. Daugirdas JT: Estimation of the equilibrated Kt/V using the un-equilibrated post dialysis BUN. Semin Dial 1995;8:283–284.

97. Daugirdas JT, Schneditz D: Overestimation of hemodialysis dose depends on dialysis efficiency by regional blood flow but not by conventional two pool urea kinetic analysis. ASAIO J 1995;41:M719–M724.

98. Smye SW, Dunderdale E, Brownridge G, et al: Estimation of treatment dose in high-efficiency haemodialysis. Nephron 1994;67:24–29.

99. Smye SW, Evans JH, Will E, Brocklebank JT: Paediatric haemo-dialysis: Estimation of treatment efficiency in the presence of urea rebound. Clin Phys Physiol Meas 1992;13:51–62.

100. Tattersall JE, DeTakats D, Chimney P, et al: The post-hemodialysis rebound. Predicting and quantifying its effect on Kt/V. Kidney Int 1996;50:2094–2102.

101. Daugirdas JT, Depner TA, Gotch FA, et al: Comparison of methods to predict equilibrated Kt/V in the HEMO Pilot Study. Kidney Int 1997;52:1395–1405.

102. Leblanc M, Charbonneau R, Lalumiere G, et al: Post-dialysis urea rebound: Determinants and influence on dialysis delivery in chronic hemodialysis patients. Am J Kidney Dis 1996;27: 253–261.

103. Leypoldt JK, Cheung AK, Deeter RB, et al: Kinetics of urea and β_2-microglobulin during and after short hemodialysis treatments. Kidney Int 2004;66:1669–1679.

104. Giannattasio P, Minutoo R, Bellizzi V, et al: Effects of efficiency and length of acetate-free biofiltration session on postdialysis solute rebound. Am J Kidney Dis 2006;47:1045–1054.

105. Minutolo R, Bellizzi V, Cioffi M, et al: Postdialytic rebound of serum phosphorus: Pathogenetic and clinical insights. J Am Soc Nephrol 2002;13:1046–1054.

106. Locatelli F, Buoncristiani U, Canaud B, et al: Haemodialysis with on-line monitoring equipment: Tools or toys? Nephrol Dial Transplant 2005;20:22–33.

107. Lindsay RM, Alhejaili F, Nesrallah G, et al: Calcium and phosphate balance with quotidian hemodialysis. Am J Kidney Dis 2003;42(Suppl 1):S24–S29.

108. Argiles A, Ficheux A, Thomas M, et al: Precise quantification of dialysis using continuous sampling of spent dialysate and total dialysate volume measurement. Kidney Int 1997;52: 530–537.

109. Calzavara P, Calconi G, Da Rin G, et al: A new biosensor for continuous monitoring of the spent dialysate urea level in standard hemodialysis. Int J Artif Organs 1998;21: 147–150.

110. Chauveau P, Naret C, Puget J, et al: Adequacy of haemodialysis and nutrition in maintenance haemodialysis patients: Clinical evaluation of a new on-line urea monitor. Nephrol Dial Transplant 1996;11:1568–1573.

111. Depner TA, Keshaviah PR, Ebben JP, et al: Multicenter clinical validation of an on-line monitor of dialysis adequacy. J Am Soc Nephrol 1996;7:464–471.

112. Gotch FA: On-line clearance: Advanced methodology to monitor adequacy of dialysis at no cost. Contrib Nephrol 2002;137: 268–271.

113. Lindsay RM, Sternby J: Future directions in dialysis quantification. Semin Dial 2001;14:300–307.

114. Rahmati MA, Rahmati S, Hoenich N, et al: On-line clearance: A useful tool for monitoring the effectiveness of the reuse procedure. ASAIO J 2003;49:543–546.

115. Del Vecchio L, Di Filippo S, Andrulli S, et al: Conductivity: On-line monitoring of dialysis adequacy. Int J Artif Organs 1998;21:521–525.

116. Mercadal L, Ridel C, Petitclerc T: Ionic dialysance: Principle and review of its clinical relevance for quantification of hemodialysis efficiency. Hemodial Int 2005;9:111–119.

117. Petitclerc T, Goux N, Reynier AL, Bene B: A model for non-invasive estimation of in vivo dialyzer performances and patient's conductivity during hemodialysis. Int J Artif Organs 1993;16: 585–591.

118. Lindsay RM, Bene B, Goux N, et al: Relationship between effective ionic dialysance and in vivo urea clearance during hemodialysis. Am J Kidney Dis 2001;38:565–574.

119. McIntyre CW, Lambie SH, Taal MW, Fluck RJ: Assessment of haemodialysis adequacy by ionic dialysance: Intra-patient variability of delivered treatment. Nephrol Dial Transplant 2003;18:559–562.

120. Moret K, Beerenhout CH, van den Wall Bake AW, et al: Ionic dialysance and the assessment of Kt/V: The influence of different estimates of V on method agreement. Nephrol Dial Transplant 2007;22:2276–2282.

121. Laird NM, Berkey CS, Lowrie EG: Modeling success or failure of dialysis therapy: The National Cooperative Dialysis Study. Kidney Int 1983;(13):S101–S106.

122. Lowrie EG, Lew NL: Death risk in hemodialysis patients: The predictive value of commonly measured variables and an evaluation of death rate differences between facilities. Am J Kidney Dis 1990;15:458–482.

123. Borah MF, Schoenfeld PY, Gotch FA, et al: Nitrogen balance during intermittent dialysis therapy of uremia. Kidney Int 1978;14:491–500.

124. Cottini EP, Gallina DL, Dominguez JM: Urea excretion in adult humans with varying degrees of kidney malfunction fed milk, egg or an amino acid mixture: Assessment of nitrogen balance. J Nutr 1973;103:11–19.

125. Depner TA: Quantifying hemodialysis and peritoneal dialysis: Examination of the peak concentration hypothesis. Semin Dial 1994;7:315–317.

126. Yeun JY, Depner TA: Complications related to inadequate delivered dose. In Mehta R, Lamiere N (eds): Complications of Dialysis—Recognition and Management. New York: Marcel Dekker, 1999, pp 89–116.

127. Presta E, Segal KR, Gutin B, et al: Comparison in man of total body electrical conductivity and lean body mass derived from body density: Validation of a new body composition method. Metabolism 1983;32:524–527.

128. Chertow GM, Lazarus JM, Lew NL, et al: Development of a population-specific regression equation to estimate total body water in hemodialysis patients. Kidney Int 1997;51:1578–1582.

129. Hume R, Weyers E: Relationship between total body water and surface area in normal and obese subjects. J Clin Pathol 1971;24:234–238.

130. Watson PE, Watson ID, Batt RD: Total body water volumes for adult males and females estimated from simple anthropometric measurements. Am J Clin Nutr 1980;33:27–39.

131. Daugirdas JT, Greene T, Depner TA, et al: Anthropometrically estimated total body water volumes are larger than modeled urea volume in chronic hemodialysis patients: Effects of age, race, and gender. Kidney Int 2003;64:1108–1119.

132. Blagg CR, Kjellstrand CM, Ting GO, Young BA: Comparison of survival between short-daily hemodialysis and conventional hemodialysis using the standardized mortality ratio. Hemodial Int 2006;10:371–374.

133. Buoncristiani U, Fagugli RM, Pinciaroli MR, et al: Reversal of left-ventricular hypertrophy in uremic patients by treatment with daily hemodialysis (DHD). Contrib Nephrol 1996;119:152–156.

134. Kumar VA, Craig M, Depner TA, et al: Extended daily dialysis: A new approach to renal replacement for acute renal failure in the intensive care unit. Am J Kidney Dis 2000;36:294–300.

135. Locatelli F, Buoncristiani U, Canaud B, et al: Dialysis dose and frequency. Nephrol Dial Transplant 2005;20:285–296.

136. Odar-Cederlaif I, Bjellerup P, Williams A, et al: Daily dialyses decrease plasma levels of brain natriuretic peptide (BNP), a biomarker of left ventricular dysfunction. Hemodial Int 2006;10:394–398.

137. Pierratos A: Nocturnal home haemodialysis: An update on a 5-year experience. Nephrol Dial Transplant 1999;14:2835–2840.

138. Pierratos A: Daily hemodialysis: An update. Curr Opin Nephrol Hypertens 2002;11:165–171.

139. Zilch O, Vos PF, Oey PL, et al: Sympathetic hyperactivity in hemodialysis patients is reduced by short daily haemodialysis. J Hypertens 2007;25:1285–1289.

140. Suri RS, Garg AX, Chertow GM, et al for Frequent Hemodialysis Network Trial Group: Frequent Hemodialysis Network (FHN) randomized trials: Study design. Kidney Int 2007;71:349–359.

141. Depner TA: Daily hemodialysis efficiency: An analysis of solute kinetics. Adv Renal Replacement Therapy 2001;8:227–235.

142. Suri R, Depner TA, Blake PG, et al: Adequacy of quotidian hemodialysis. Am J Kidney Dis 2003;42(1 Suppl 1):S42–S48.

143. Casino FG, Lopez T: The equivalent renal urea clearance: A new parameter to assess dialysis dose. Nephrol Dial Transplant 1996;11:1574–1581.

144. Gotch FA: The current place of urea kinetic modeling with respect to different dialysis modalities. Nephrol Dial Transplant 1998;13(Suppl 6):10–14.

145. Leypoldt JK, Jaber BL, Zimmerman DL: Predicting treatment dose for novel therapies using urea standard Kt/V. Semin Dial 2004;17:142–145.

146. Depner TA: Is Kt/V urea a satisfactory measure for dosing the newer dialysis regimens? Semin Dial 2001;14:9–12.

147. Lowrie EG, Li Z, Ofsthun N, Lazarus JM: Body size, dialysis dose and death risk relationships among hemodialysis patients. Kidney Int 2002;62:1891–1897.

148. Lowrie EG, Li Z, Ofsthun N, Lazarus JM: Measurement of dialyzer clearance, dialysis time, and body size: Death risk relationships among patients. Kidney Int 2004;66:2077–2084.

149. Lowrie EG, Li Z, Ofsthun N, Lazarus JM: The online measurement of hemodialysis dose (Kt): Clinical outcome as a function of body surface area. Kidney Int 2005;68:1344–1354.

150. Lowrie EG, Chertow GM, Lew NL, et al: The urea {clearance × dialysis time} product (Kt) as an outcome-based measure of hemodialysis dose. Kidney Int 1999;56:729–737.

151. Chertow GM, Owen WF, Lazarus JM, et al: Exploring the reverse J-shaped curve between urea reduction ratio and mortality. Kidney Int 1999;56:1872–1878.

152. Owen WF Jr, Chertow GM, Lazarus JM, Lowrie EG: Dose of hemodialysis and survival: Differences by race and sex. JAMA 1998;280:1764–1768.

153. Port FK, Ashby VB, Dhingra RK, et al: Dialysis dose and body mass index are strongly associated with survival in hemodialysis patients. J Am Soc Nephrol 2002;13:1061–1066.

154. Port FK, Wolfe RA: Optimizing the dialysis dose with consideration of patient size. Blood Purif 2000;18:295–297.

155. Wolfe RA, Ashby VB, Daugirdas JT, et al: Body size, dose of hemodialysis, and mortality. Am J Kidney Dis 2000;35:80–88.

156. Port FK, Wolfe RA, Hulbert-Shearon TE, et al: High dialysis dose is associated with lower mortality among women but not among men. Am J Kidney Dis 2004;43:1014–1023.

157. Daugirdas JT, Burke MS, Balter P, et al: Screening for extreme post-dialysis urea rebound using the Smye method: Patients with access recirculation identified when a slow flow method is not used to draw the postdialysis blood. Am J Kidney Dis 1996;28:727–731.

158. Geddes CC, Traynor J, Walbaum D, et al: A new method of post-dialysis blood urea sampling: The "stop dialysate flow" method. Nephrol Dial Transplant 2000;15:517–523.

159. Wu MJ, Feng YF, Shu KH, et al: Another simpler bypassing dialysate technique for measuring post-haemodialysis BUN. Nephrol Dial Transplant 1997;12:2124–2127.

160. Allon M: Current management of vascular access. Clin J Am Soc Nephrol 2007;2:786–800.

161. Depner TA, Rizwan S, Stasi TA: Pressure effects on roller pump blood flow during hemodialysis. ASAIO Trans 1990;36:M456–M459.

162. Abramson F, Gibson S, Barlee V, et al: Urea kinetic modeling at high urea clearances: implications for clinical practice. Adv Ren Replace Ther 1994;1:5–14.

163. Spiegel DM, Baker PL, Babcock S, et al: Hemodialysis urea rebound: The effect of increasing dialysis efficiency. Am J Kidney Dis 1995;25:26–29.

164. Locatelli F, Mastrangelo F, Redaelli B, et al: Effects of different membranes and dialysis technologies on patient treatment tolerance and nutritional parameters. The Italian Cooperative Dialysis Study Group. Kidney Int 1996;50:1293–1302.

165. Leypoldt JK, Cheung AK: Removal of high-molecular-weight solutes during high-efficiency and high-flux haemodialysis. Nephrol Dial Transplant 1996;11:329–335.

166. Collins DM, Lambert MB, Tannenbaum JS, et al: Tolerance of hemodialysis: A randomized prospective trial of high-flux versus conventional high-efficiency hemodialysis. J Am Soc Nephrol 1993;4:148–154.

167. Ronco C, Brendolan A, Bragantini L, et al: Technical and clinical evaluation of different short, highly efficient dialysis techniques. Contrib Nephrol 1988;61:46–68.

Further Reading

Achinger SG, Ayus JC: The role of daily dialysis in the control of hyperphosphatemia. Kidney Int Suppl 2005;95:S28–S32.

Allon M: Current management of vascular access. Clin J Am Soc Nephrol 2007;2:786–800.

Daugirdas JT, Greene T, Depner TA, et al: Anthropometrically estimated total body water volumes are larger than modeled urea volume in chronic hemodialysis patients: Effects of age, race, and gender. Kidney Int 2003;64:1108–1119.

Depner TA: Hemodialysis adequacy: Basic essentials and practical points for the nephrologist in training. Hemodial Int 2005;9:241–254.

Depner TA, Bhat A: Quantifying daily hemodialysis. Semin Dial 2004;17:79–84.

Depner TA, Daugirdas JT, Greene T, et al: Dialysis dose and the effect of gender and body size on outcome in the HEMO study. Kidney Int 2004;65:1386–1394.

Eknoyan G, Beck GJ, Cheung AK, et al: Effect of dialysis dose and membrane flux in maintenance hemodialysis. N Engl J Med 2002;347:2010–2019.

Eloot S, Torremans A, De Smet R, et al: Complex compartmental behavior of small water-soluble uremic retention solutes: Evaluation by direct measurements in plasma and erythrocytes. Am J Kidney Dis 2007;50:279–288.

Leypoldt JK, Jaber BL, Zimmerman DL: Predicting treatment dose for novel therapies using urea standard Kt/V. Semin Dial 2004;17:142–145.

Leypoldt JK, Kamerath CD, Gilson JF, Friederichs G: Dialyzer clearances and mass transfer-area coefficients for small solutes at low dialysate flow rates. ASAIO J 2006;52:404–409.

Locatelli F, Buoncristiani U, Canaud B, et al: Dialysis dose and frequency. Nephrol Dial Transplant 2005;20:285–296.

Locatelli F, Buoncristiani U, Canaud B, et al: Haemodialysis with on-line monitoring equipment: Tools or toys? Nephrol Dial Transplant 2005;20:22–33.

Mercadal L, Ridel C, Petitclerc T: Ionic dialysance: Principle and review of its clinical relevance for quantification of hemodialysis efficiency. Hemodial Int 2005;9:111–119.

Moret K, Beerenhout CH, van den Wall Bake AW, et al: Ionic dialysance and the assessment of Kt/V: The influence of different estimates of V on method agreement. Nephrol Dial Transplant 2007;22:2276–2282.

NKF-KDOQI Clinical Practice Guidelines for Hemodialysis Adequacy 2006. Am J Kidney Dis 2006;48(1 Suppl 1):S2–S90.

Prado M, Roa LM, Palma A, Milan JA: Double target comparison of blood-side methods for measuring the hemodialysis dose. Kidney Int 2005;68:2863–2876.

Spalding EM, Chamney PW, Farrington K: Phosphate kinetics during hemodialysis: Evidence for biphasic regulation. Kidney Int 2002;61:655–667.

Suri R, Depner TA, Blake PG, et al: Adequacy of quotidian hemodialysis. Am J Kidney Dis 2003;42(1 Suppl 1):S42–S48.

Suri RS, Garg AX, Chertow GM, et al for Frequent Hemodialysis Network Trial Group: Frequent hemodialysis network (FHN) randomized trials: Study design. Kidney Int 2007;71:349–359.

Suri RS, Nesrallah GE, Mainra R, et al: Daily hemodialysis: A systematic review. Clin J Am Soc Nephrol 2006;1:33–42.

Chapter 80

Complications Associated with Hemodialysis

Ravinder K. Wali, Jay R. Kaluvapalle, and Alfred K. Cheung

CHAPTER CONTENTS

Considering that more than 50 million hemodialysis treatments are performed every year in a single country such as the United States,[1] hemodialysis should be generally regarded as a very safe procedure. This safety is particularly remarkable considering that a large volume of blood is circulated extracorporeally over hours of treatment, with substantial changes in fluid volumes as well as plasma osmolality and chemistry. On one hand, technical advances have been made that make the procedure safer. On the other hand, the older age and higher comorbidities of U.S. dialysis patients predispose to complications. Some of the complications, such as symptomatic hypotension, are expected on a physiologic basis, whereas others, such as erroneous dialysate composition, are technically mishaps. The severity of these reactions ranges from mild and transient to catastrophic and fatal. This chapter covers these spectra, but limits discussion to complications that result from the treatment, rather than those inherent to the patient's underlying uremia and comorbidities.

DIALYSIS REACTIONS

During hemodialysis, large volumes of blood are exposed to components of the extracorporeal circuit, including the dialyzer, tubing, and other foreign substances related to the manufacturing and sterilization processes. This interaction between the patient's blood and the extracorporeal system can lead to various adverse reactions, which manifest as a continuum ranging from subtle to severe and fatal.[2,3] The signs and symptoms are made up of combinations of angioedema, dyspnea, coughing, chest tightness, sneezing, rhinorrhea, lacrimation, skin flushing, pruritus, paresthesia, burning sensation, nausea, vomiting, abdominal cramps, and diarrhea. These reactions are often referred to as *dialysis reactions* or *dialyzer reactions*. The former terminology is preferred because some of these reactions are not caused by the dialyzer per se.

The etiologies of these reactions are diverse and are often difficult to establish in individual cases. In general, they can be classified into two broad categories: anaphylaxis or anaphylactoid reactions and direct toxic effects. Anaphylaxis is caused by degranulation of mast cells or basophils induced by IgE and usually requires prior sensitization by the allergen. *Anaphylactoid reactions* are anaphylaxis-like reactions in response to the direct effectors or mediators, such as complement activation products or histamine, and do not require the release of IgE. *Direct toxic effects* are those induced by other substances, such as ethylene oxide (EtO) or formaldehyde. This classification only provides a general framework to facilitate the understanding and research of these reactions. Neither this nor other classification systems, however, provide definitive clues to the etiology or the management of the individual patient, because there is probably substantial overlap in clinical manifestations between different categories. Some of the etiologies are discussed in the following.

Leachable Substances

Perhaps the best studied leachable substance from the hemodialysis circuit is EtO.[4–6] EtO gas is used to sterilize some dialyzers. The potting compound that anchors the hollow fibers in place has been shown to be a reservoir for EtO, essentially providing sustained release of EtO into the lumen during the functional life of the dialyzer.[6,7] The exposure of chronic dialysis patients to EtO and their immune response to the compound can be demonstrated by the presence of specific IgE antibodies against EtO that has been conjugated to serum albumin in vivo. In some studies, two thirds of patients with apparent reactions to dialyzers have circulating IgE antibodies against EtO.[4] This test is not specific, because 10% of patients with no prior history of dialysis reactions also have circulating levels of anti-EtO IgE.[6,8] Since EtO is a residue in dialyzers and may be important in the pathogenesis of some dialysis reactions, it is not surprising that these reactions are more common when a new, instead of a reprocessed, dialyzer is used. This phenomenon leads to the term *first-use syndrome*.[2,3,9] Accordingly, rinsing the blood compartment of the dialyzer with saline solution can decrease the incidence of these events. Rinsing the dialysate compartment with dialysate is also effective, because the circulating dialysate can also remove the EtO in the blood compartment by diffusion. If EtO allergy is suspected, changing to a dialyzer sterilized by gamma radiation or steam is appropriate.

Dialysis reactions can also be due to residual disinfectants in the dialyzer, such as formaldehyde, glutaraldehyde, and peracetic acid/hydrogen peroxide. Life-threatening reactions have been observed in dialysis patients in whom serum antibody against formaldehyde was detected.[10] Instead of first-use syndrome, these reactions are appropriately called *reuse syndrome*[11,12] because they occur during dialyzer reuse. If the diagnosis is correct, proper reprocessing of the dialyzers and rinsing of the dialyzer before use are also expected to decrease these reactions.

Other leachable substances that have been suspected to cause dialysis reactions include isopropyl myristate, which is used in the spinning process of hollow-fiber fabrication,[4] isocyanates found in the potting compound,[13,14] and nonendotoxin Limulus amebocyte lysate–reactive material.[15,16] The latter is believed to be cellulose in origin and to react to the Limulus amebocyte lysate assay.

Another leachable substance found in the dialysis circuit is the plasticizer, di(2-ethylhexyl)phthalate (DEHP), although this compound has not been incriminated in acute dialysis reactions.[17–19] The flexibility of polyvinylchloride tubing is achieved by the addition of DEHP into the polymer matrix.[20] Although there is no clear evidence to confirm its toxicity, DEHP can bind to plasma lipids and lipoproteins, and significant tissue levels of DEHP have been recovered at autopsy of dialysis patients. Furthermore, hepatitis-like syndrome and necrotizing dermatitis have been reported in association with polyvinylchloride exposure in dialysis patients. The practice of reusing blood tubing may provide a potential clinical advantage by reducing the exposure to plasticizers. Leachability studies of another plasticizer, trimellitate,[21,22] from blood tubing show a lower rate of release compared with DEHP.[20]

Membrane Bioincompatibility

Another causative factor of dialysis reactions is dialysis membrane bioincompatibility; in particular, interactions between the dialysis membrane and plasma proteins. Two cascades of plasma protein activation have been most intensely studied in this regard. Activation of the complement system via the alternative pathway is practically universal for all dialysis membranes, albeit to various degrees.[23,24] Presumably, by virtue of the free hydroxyl moieties on the surface, unsubstituted cellulosic membranes activate complement rigorously. Complement fragments C3a and C5a generated[23–25] from C3 and C5, respectively, are known as *anaphylatoxins*, because of their potential to induce anaphylactoid reactions. The functional activities of these complement fragments are, however, markedly diminished by the action of a serum carboxypeptidase.[26] Thus, despite the high plasma levels of C3a and C5a commonly found during hemodialysis, especially with unsubstituted cellulosic membranes, dialysis reactions are uncommon. The frequency at which complement activation is responsible for dialysis reactions is unknown, but it is likely to be rare. Compared to unsubstituted cellulosic membranes, substituted cellulosic membranes[27,28] (in which some of the hydroxyl moieties are substituted by other moieties) and synthetic membranes[11,23] tend to activate complement less and would therefore be preferable if complement activation is to be minimized.

The second plasma protein cascade that is of particular relevance to hemodialysis is the intrinsic (or contact) pathway of coagulation. Severe anaphylactoid reactions have been reported in patients dialyzed with the AN69 membrane who were also taking angiotensin-converting enzyme (ACE) inhibitors.[29–31] The likely pathogenetic mechanisms are as follows. Binding of Hageman factor (factor XII) to a negatively charged surface leads to its activation and subsequent conversion of kininogen to bradykinin.[29,30] The AN69 membrane is composed of a copolymer of acrylonitrile and methallyl sulfonate. The latter moiety is negatively charged and is therefore an activator of the intrinsic coagulation pathway. Because angiotensin converting enzyme is also a kininase, the catabolism of bradykinin is inhibited in the presence of an ACE inhibitor. The combination of dialysis with the AN69 membrane and use of an ACE inhibitor therefore results in the accumulation of bradykinin in the plasma and consequently anaphylactoid reactions and hypotension.[29] The obvious preventive strategy for this cause of dialysis reaction is the avoidance of this type of dialysis membrane or ACE inhibitors.

Several anaphylactoid reactions have also been reported in patients dialyzed using polysulfone membranes reprocessed with bleach and also treated with ACE inhibitors.[12,32] These reactions ceased once the use of bleach was discontinued. Furthermore, a cluster of anaphylactoid reactions was observed in patients treated with ACE inhibitors and dialyzed with various membranes reprocessed using hydrogen peroxide/peracetic acid. The reactions abated once reprocessing was discontinued, despite continued use of ACE inhibitors.

Other Factors

The use of acetate dialysate has been implicated in dialysis reactions. Potential mechanisms of these reactions include the direct effect of accumulated acetate and the transient loss of bicarbonate in the plasma prior to conversion to bicarbonate,[33] and the stimulation of interleukin-1 production by monocytes.[34] These reactions tend to be mild and are not acutely life-threatening. Acetate dialysate is seldom, if at all, used in the United States currently. Bacterial products, such as endotoxin fragments, present in the dialysate that traverse across the dialysis membranes are also known to induce cytokine release by monocytes and consequently pyrogenic reactions.[35] These pyrogenic reactions tend to be mild. They may occur more frequently with high-flux membranes,[36] especially those reprocessed using bleach, because reprocessing is associated with increased porosity of the membrane,[37,38] thus facilitating the transfer of bacterial products.

Drugs administered during hemodialysis can also cause adverse reactions that are sometimes difficult to distinguish from other causes of dialysis reactions. Intravenous iron dextran is not infrequently associated with adverse reactions, although severe anaphylactoid reactions are rare, occurring in 0.6% to 1% of patients.[39,40] The mechanisms responsible for dextran-induced anaphylactoid reactions are unclear; the dose-dependent release of histamine from basophils may be responsible.[41,42] More frequently, iron dextran administration is associated with various degrees of hypotension, headache, myalgia, arthralgia, and fever.[39,43] Intravenous iron gluconate appears to be associated with fewer adverse reactions.[40,43] Although it is uncommonly used now in dialysis units, deferoxamine therapy for the chelation of aluminum or iron can produce hypotension during dialysis and, rarely, allergic reactions, gastrointestinal disturbances, loss of vision, auditory toxicity, bone pain, or exacerbation of aluminum encephalopathy.[44–46]

Treatment of Dialysis Reactions

Prevention of dialysis reactions depends on identification of the causative factor. Immediate reactions that occur within the first few minutes of the procedure are likely to be due to preformed agents, such as EtO or formaldehyde. Laboratory tests (e.g., assays for plasma EtO antibodies or bradykinins) are not routinely performed in clinical cases. Further, the predictive value of these assays for clinical diagnosis of these reactions has not been established. Most often, the etiology of the reaction is never firmly established and the reaction ceases after the dialyzer is switched empirically to another type (e.g., from an EtO-sterilized dialyzer to a gamma-radiated dialyzer or from an AN69 membrane to a polysulfone membrane). The dialysis reaction may also be caused by the blood tubing[17,18,20,22,47,48] or even medications, such as heparin,[49] that are administered during the hemodialysis procedure. Switching blood tubing and heparin (e.g., from porcine to bovine heparin) should also be considered. Not uncommonly, dialysis reactions cease with extensive rinsing of dialyzers before use or even if the dialysis procedure and the supplies are unchanged.

The immediate treatment of dialysis reactions depends on the severity of the clinical manifestation. If the reaction is severe, and in particular if it occurs early during the treatment, the extracorporeal circulation should be immediately stopped. Under these circumstances, the blood in the circuit should be discarded rather than being returned to the patient, because it likely contains the causative agent. Otherwise, treatment is largely supportive and targets the specific signs and symptoms. Oxygen supplementation, bronchodilators, sympathomimetic agents, and vasoactive medications are used as indicated. Antihistamines and corticosteroids may be helpful. In mild cases, dialysis can be continued with or without other interventions.

CARDIOVASCULAR COMPLICATIONS

Intradialytic Hypotension

The definition of intradialytic hypotension (IDH) has been inconsistent in different reported series.[50–52] Consequently, the reported incidence (<5%–40%) has also varied widely. The incidence of IDH, however, will likely continue to increase despite technological advances,[53] as more patients with advanced age, diabetes mellitus, and underlying cardiovascular diseases will need dialysis therapy in the future. To maintain the consistency of definition and to assess the response to different therapeutic interventions, the K/DOQI guidelines proposed that IDH be defined as a decrease in systolic blood pressure (BP) of at least 20 mm Hg or a decrease in mean arterial pressure by 10 mm Hg in combination with the symptom complex and a need for active therapy.[54]

When evaluating the etiology of hypotension, it is important to consider more ominous events, such as acute coronary syndrome, arrhythmias, pulmonary embolism (blood clots or air embolism), pericardial effusion or constrictive pericarditis, dialysis reactions, and overestimation of dry weight leading to hypotension. At times other nonspecific symptoms, such as sudden onset sensation of dizziness or fainting, nausea, and vomiting with or without diaphoresis, may be indirect predictors of impending hypotension.[55] The symptom complex due to IDH can vary and include generalized lethargy, nausea and vomiting, muscle cramps, restlessness, dizziness, anxiety, diaphoresis, chest pain, acute confusion, presyncope, or syncope.[55] These symptoms may be severe enough to compel termination of the dialysis therapy. Consequently, frequent episodes of IDH can lead to inadequate delivery of the dialysis dose and volume overload.[56,57] Patients at risk of developing IDH are those who have large interdialytic fluid gain due to fluid or salt intake or poorly controlled hyperglycemia that causes osmotic thirst. Other patients at risk for IDH are those with myocardial, valvular, and pericardial diseases.

Healthy people can tolerate a decrease in blood volume of up to 20% before the development of hypotension. In contrast, dialysis patients can develop hypotension with smaller changes in the blood volume (2%–29%).[58,59] The combination of extracorporeal fluid removal and fluid shifts to the intracellular compartment predisposes to acute intravascular hypovolemia, particularly when the rate of fluid loss from the plasma compartment exceeds the plasma refilling rate.[60–62]

The variability in blood volume changes could be explained by the presence of several pathophysiologic conditions, such as (1) the lack of an increase in cardiac output due to the presence of myocardial disease, thus preventing an increase in myocardial contractility in response to changes in intravascular volume[59,60,63,64]; (2) lack of increase in heart rate and peripheral vascular resistance in response to a decrease in blood volume due to the presence of autonomic dysfunction[55,65,66]; (3) paradoxical and sudden withdrawal of sympathetic response, resulting in bradycardia (Bezold-Jarisch reflex) in response to severe ventricular underfilling (defined as bradycardic hypotension)[67,68]; (4) failure of capacitance vessels to constrict in the face of hypovolemia, with impairment in venous return.[69] Impaired reactivity of resistance and capacitance vessels could be secondary to autonomic dysfunction, cytokine release due to exposure to extracorporeal circulation,[70] an increase in core body temperature due to energy transfer from the dialysate, an increased production of nitric oxide,[71] or decreased vasopressin release in the presence of a low-output state.[72] Other patient-related factors are delayed filling of the central blood volume in patients with arteriovenous fistula or graft.[52] Dialysis-related factors that may increase the risk of developing IDH include the use of acetate dialysate[73] or low-calcium dialysate.[74] Occasionally, IDH may develop because the target dry weight has been underestimated[75] or the dialysis machine has been erroneously programmed to remove more than the expected volume.

The management of patients with IDH includes urgent resuscitation to relieve patient discomfort, maintain hemodynamic stability, and monitor for the development of adverse cardiovascular events. Routine measures for the treatment of IDH include placing the patient in Trendelenburg's position to augment venous refilling and administering saline boluses to increase the systolic BP to 100 to 110 mm Hg as appropriate. The amount of saline solution required varies greatly. Some patients are grossly fluid overloaded systemically and should be given as little fluid as possible to temporarily relieve the symptoms related to the acute plasma volume depletion. On the other hand, some patients are systemically volume depleted even before starting dialysis because of a preexisting condition such as diarrhea; fluid resuscitation under these circumstances may require more aggressive intradialytic saline hydration. Hypertonic saline solution (in 5–10 mL bolus of 7.5% concentration) and, less commonly, hypertonic glucose (25–50 mL bolus of 50% concentration) in nondiabetic patients and mannitol (bolus of 12.5–25.0 g) can also be used. All of these agents are readily dialyzable. If mannitol is administered toward the end of the hemodialysis session, however, it may be retained in the plasma and can accumulate in the visceral organs. The long-term consequences of mannitol accumulation are not known. After an episode of severe symptomatic hypotension, the patient should be monitored for the development of cardiovascular events and evaluated for orthostatic hypotension before discharge from the dialysis unit. Strategies to prevent the occurrence of future episodes should be considered if the IDH is recurrent.

Intradialytic hypotension can be prevented by modifying the dialysis prescription based on the individual center experiences and technical skills of the dialysis staff. Hemodialysis therapy using isothermic (same as body temperature) dialysate is invariably associated with an increase in core body temperature despite heat loss by convection in the extracorporeal circuit.[76,77] The increase in core body temperature decreases the reactivity of resistance and capacitance vessels, and venous return may not increase in response to changes in blood volume during ultrafiltration.[61] To avoid these phenomena, dialysate temperature can be adjusted and maintained at 1° to 2°C below the body temperature. This technique is known as *cool-dialysate dialysis*. Dialysis with cool dialysate improves the reactivity of peripheral resistance and capacitance vessels and increases myocardial contractility.[61,78–80] The most common adverse effects are cold sensation and shivering. A lack of response to cool-dialysate hemodialysis could be due to the failure of fluid shifts from the third compartment in the presence of severe vasoconstriction of the capacitance vessels.[61] Urea clearance usually remains unchanged during cool-dialysate hemodialysis.[81] The temperature of the dialysate can be controlled by continuous biofeedback systems,[82,83] but this technology is not widely available.

Another common strategy to prevent IDH is to manipulate dialysate sodium concentrations. High dialysate sodium concentrations increase plasma osmolality, thus enhancing extracellular and plasma refilling rates. Most studies, but not all, found that the use of conventional dialysate sodium (138–144 mmol/L) compared to low sodium (<135 mmol/L) concentration is associated with lower incidence of IDH.[84–88] High sodium (>144 mmol/L) dialysate can further prevent the development of IDH, but may also lead to interdialytic weight gain and hypertension.[89–91] *Sodium profiling* is the technique of varying dialysate sodium concentration during the dialysis session, which is often accomplished automatically by programming the dialysis machine. Dialysate sodium concentration can be increased or decreased linearly or in a stepwise fashion. Less frequently, alternating high and low concentrations of sodium throughout the dialysis session can be employed. The objective of tapering dialysate sodium concentration during dialysis (*sodium ramping*)[86,88] is to avoid high plasma sodium concentrations at the end of the dialysis session. The counterargument to this strategy is that plasma and interstitial fluid volumes and pressure are high at the beginning of the dialysis session, and therefore high dialysate sodium levels are unnecessary. Toward the end of the dialysis session, interstitial fluid pressure has decreased and plasma refilling rate decreases accordingly. At that time, high dialysate sodium levels are more useful in increasing the serum sodium concentration and osmotic pressure that draw fluids from the intracellular compartment. Increasing dialysate sodium levels during the dialysis session is known as reverse sodium modeling.[91] Fine-tuning of sodium concentration during hemodialysis can be guided by the on-line measurement of conductivity of the plasma and ultrafiltrate and on-line measurement of the ionic mass transfer to prevent the salt retention due to sodium ramping.[92–94] Similar to sodium modeling, ultrafiltration profiling can be used to prevent IDH: it allows adjusting ultrafiltration from a high rate at the start to a lower rate at the end of the dialysis session.

Changes in ionized calcium can play an important role in myocardial contractility during hemodialysis therapy, because myocardial contractility decreases in the presence of low dialysate calcium (1.25 mmol/L) compared to normal dialysate calcium (1.75 mmol/L).[50,74,95,96] Very high-calcium dialysate can lead to positive calcium balance, an increase in arterial calcification, and adverse effects on myocardial relaxation.[96,97] One randomized crossover study demonstrated that the combination of dialysate calcium of 1.50 mmol/L and bicarbonate of 32 mmol/L was associated with less significant drop in systolic BP than the combination of calcium and bicarbonate concentrations of 1.25 mmol/L and 26 mmol/L, respectively.[98] Another randomized crossover study compared three different regimens of dialysate calcium levels: constant 1.25 mmol/L versus constant 1.50 mmol/L versus a profiled regimen of 1.25 mmol/L during the first 2 hours and 1.75 mmol/L during the remaining 2 hours.[99] Both the dialysate calcium of 1.50 mmol/L as well as profiled calcium regimens were more effective in reducing the incidence of IDH than the 1.25 mmol/L regimen.[99] Because the impact of dialysate calcium concentration on vascular calcification remains unknown, the K/DOQI working group for Clinical Practice Guidelines for Bone Metabolism and Disease in Chronic Kidney Disease recommends a routine prescription of dialysate calcium of 1.25 mmol/L; higher concentrations of dialysate calcium should be considered for maintaining intradialytic hemodynamic stability.[100,101]

Reducing intradialytic weight gain is the most important strategy for the prevention of IDH in most patients. Careful estimation of the optimal dry weight is useful and can be facilitated by analytic tools, such as inferior vena cava sonogram,[102] bioelectrical impedance,[103] and continuous monitoring of blood volume variations.[104] Serum biomarkers, such as brain natriuretic peptide[105,106] or adrenomedullin,[107] may also be helpful in assessing dry weight.

Short-acting antihypertensive agents should ideally be avoided immediately before the hemodialysis procedure. The avoidance of food intake immediately before and during the dialysis procedure is helpful, because it prevents the diversion of blood flow to the splanchnic circulation.[87] The benefits of vasoactive agents for either treatment or prevention of IDH have been inconsistent. Midodrine is an a_1-adrenergic receptor agonist that constricts the splanchnic circulatory bed, as well as systemic precapillary resistance and capacitance vessels, with an increase in circulatory blood volume. Oral midodrine given at a dose of 2.5 to 10 mg 30 minutes before the dialysis session has been reported to prevent IDH.[108–110] The most frequent adverse effects of midodrine therapy include piloerection, scalp itching or tingling, weakness, paresthesias, flushing, headache, sleep disturbances and, rarely, bradycardia. It is effectively cleared by hemodialysis and its half-life is less than 2 hours in dialysis patients.[110] Sertraline is a selective serotonin reuptake inhibitor; its oral administration in a small number of patients has demonstrated small benefits in the prevention of IDH. Adverse effects of sertraline include dizziness, insomnia, fatigue, somnolence, and headache.[111–113] Recently the use of intravenous vasopressin has been shown to facilitate fluid removal while maintaining hemodynamic stability.[114,115]

Other therapies that have shown inconsistent results for the prevention of IDH include the use of convective therapies such as on-line hemofiltration, hemodiafiltration and acetate-free biofiltration.[61,94,116–118] Although convective therapy compared to standard hemodialysis treatment preserves the reactivity of resistance and capacitance vessels, it is postulated that benefits of convective therapies are mostly due to the cooling effect and therefore vasoconstriction from the infusion of substitution fluids.[119–121] Chronic supplementation with L-carnitine at 20 mg/kg during dialysis therapy has been demonstrated to improve vascular reactivity and prevents IDH in patients with recurrent IDH.[122,123]

Intradialytic Hypertension

Different degrees of increase in blood pressure, even with fluid removal, can develop either during dialysis or immediately after the dialysis session is completed. Repeated episodes of intradialytic hypertension can be an important risk factor for cardiovascular morbidity and mortality. Intradialytic hypertension appears to be less common, and the pathophysiology more elusive, than IDH. Intradialytic hypertension can be precipitated by the use of hypernatremic dialysate during sodium modeling.[90] Other risk factors include the use of erythropoiesis-stimulating agents and hemoglobin levels above 13 g/dL. Increased plasma levels of renin and endothelin-1 and decreased nitric oxide/endothelin-1 ratio[88] result in an increase in peripheral vascular resistance, as is often present in long-term dialysis patients, and may be contributory to intradialytic hypertension The administration of hypertensive medications immediately before dialysis may be useful to minimize intradialytic hypertension in patients who are prone to this phenomenon.

Sudden Death and Cardiac Arrest

Cardiac arrest and cardiac arrhythmias account for more than 50% of all cardiac deaths in chronic hemodialysis patients.[124] Sudden cardiac arrest in dialysis patients is multifactorial and is likely related, at least in part, to fluctuations in fluid and electrolytes during hemodialysis therapy. Survival after cardiac arrest in dialysis patients remains dismal, with 30-day survival of 32% and 1-year survival of less than 15%.[125] K/DOQI guidelines recommend that all dialysis facilities should support on-site availability of an automated external defibrillator.[54] In addition, the K/DOQI recommends performing an echocardiogram in all dialysis patients after achieving the optimal volume control within 30 to 90 days after dialysis initiation and periodically thereafter to detect abnormalities that may predispose to sudden death and other cardiac events.

Dialysis-Associated Steal Syndrome

Diversion of blood flow through the arteriovenous fistula or graft decreases blood flow to the artery that is distal to the arteriovenous or arteriograft anastomosis.[126] The hemodynamics of these shunts that predispose to peripheral ischemia are complex and involve interactions among the high blood flow into a low-resistance vein, reversal of flow away from the higher-resistance distal arterial bed, and competing with distal collateral blood vessels.[127] More than two thirds of these shunts have different degrees of retrograde flow, but only 6% to 10% develop peripheral ischemia (*dialysis-associated steal syndrome*).[128] The symptom complex from the steal syndrome can vary from time to time and can include numbness, weakness, pain, cramps, and cold sensations of the part distal to the fistula or graft. These symptoms may increase in intensity by routine use of the hand, which increases the demand of blood supply, or during dialysis treatment, which may draw more blood from the distal site into the extracorporeal circuit. Physical findings may include cold sensations of the hand, decreased pulse and decreased capillary refilling rate (>3 seconds), acrocyanosis, trophic lesions of nails, hair loss, muscle atrophy, and progression to ischemic ulcers and gangrene.[129–131] Some of these symptoms can also be produced by mononeuritis, carpal tunnel syndrome, ischemic monomelic neuropathy,[132] peripheral neuropathy due to diabetes mellitus, uremia, collagen vascular diseases, and acral calciphylaxis.[133] Doppler ultrasonography, digital blood pressure phlethysmography, and digital-brachial indices (<0.60) can be used as adjunctive tests,[127] although angiography remains the gold standard for the definitive diagnosis of steal syndrome.

The most common conservative treatment is symptomatic relief (e.g., using a mitten to keep the hand warm during hemodialysis). In 1% to 10% of patients with clinical steal symptoms, invasive interventions are required. These interventions include angioplasty of the stenosis that may be present in the inflow artery or ligation of the fistula. Different methods have also been used to decrease the fistula outflow, such as stitching[134] or placement of a cuff[135] around the outflow vessel. These maneuvers, however, often lead to thrombosis of the graft. The most advanced technique for treating dialysis-associated steal syndrome is the distal revascularization-interval ligation procedure, which has a high rate (90%) of relieving symptoms while maintaining graft patency at 1 year in more than 85% of patients.[132,136–138]

Air Embolism

Air embolism is rare nowadays because of technical advances and the keen awareness of most dialysis personnel. Nonetheless, the potential rapid and catastrophic nature of this complication demands particular attention. The prepump tubing segment, arterial needle, and saline infusion tubing are particularly significant points of air entry, because of the high negative pressure that draws the air. The high blood pump speeds used currently also enhance the chance of entry of large volumes of air. Intravenous infusion setups that are attached to, but are not inherent parts of, the dialysis circuit can also be potential points of entry. Yet another point of entry that escapes the safety features of the dialysis circuit is the venous connection of the central venous catheter. The key preventive measure lies in the dialysis machines, which are almost always equipped with a venous air-bubble trap and a foam detector that triggers an alarm and automatically shuts off the blood pump and clamps the venous blood tubing if air is detected.

Clinical manifestations of air embolism depend on the volume of air, the site of entry, and the patient's position.[139] Microbubbles of air introduced at a slow rate dissolve slowly in the blood and may not be associated with clinical sequelae. In the sitting position, air entry through an arm vascular access bypasses the heart, causes venous emboli in the cerebral circulation, and induces central nervous symptoms rapidly. In contrast, a large bubble introduced from the central venous line when the patient is supine will be trapped in the right ventricle and will interfere with cardiac output. Dissemination of microemboli into the pulmonary vasculature under these circumstances induces acute pulmonary symptoms.

The diagnosis of air embolism is based on clinical signs and symptoms and is often triggered by a keen sense of suspicion. The appearance of foam in the tubings and the typical churning sound on cardiac auscultation when the bubble is in the chest facilitate the diagnosis. If the patient lies in the reverse Trendelenburg position, the air emboli actually migrate to the venous circulation, causing ischemia of the lower extremity.[140]

Swift actions are absolutely essential once the diagnosis of air embolism is suspected. The venous blood tubing should be immediately clamped and the blood pump stopped to prevent further air entry.[141] For right heart air emboli, the patient should be placed in a recumbent position on the left side with the chest and head tilted downward. Cardiopulmonary support is then instituted. Aspiration of the air from the ventricle by a percutaneously inserted needle or right atrial dialysis catheter can be attempted. The patient is then transported, in the recumbent position, to an acute care facility for hyperbaric oxygen and other supportive therapies.[142]

NEUROLOGICAL COMPLICATIONS

Dialysis Disequilibrium Syndrome

Although dialysis disequilibrium syndrome (DDS) is no longer a frequent complication of hemodialysis, it is still a potential problem if proper precautions are not taken. DDS can result in central nervous system damage with long-term sequelae. Cerebral edema can be observed on brain imaging studies if DDS is severe.[143,144] An attractive hypothesis for its pathogenesis is that of osmotic disequilibrium between the plasma and cerebrospinal fluid that results from the rapid removal of urea from the former compartment during dialysis, thus causing a shift of water into the brain.[143] Paradoxical acidosis in the cerebrospinal fluid has also been observed.[145,146] Recent studies have shown decreased expression of the urea transporter UT-B1 and increased expression of aquaporins (AQP4 and AQP9) in the brain of uremic rats.[147] These abnormalities would exacerbate the retention of urea in the brain despite the rapid removal of urea in the plasma and the promotion of water entry into the brain cells. The risk factors for DDS include severe azotemia and preexisting neurological disorders, such as recent stroke, head trauma, subdural hematoma, and malignant hypertension.[148–150]

DDS usually occurs toward the end of dialysis and may be delayed up to 24 hours.[151,152] The manifestations are restlessness, headache, nausea, vomiting, blurred vision, muscle twitching, tremor, disorientation, and hypertension.[153] This syndrome is usually self-limited, but full recovery may take several days. Severe symptoms, such as obtundation, seizures, coma, and death, occur occasionally.[154] DDS is usually a clinical diagnosis, although the presence of cerebral edema on brain imaging studies provides supportive evidence. Electroencephalographic findings are nonspecific.

Because DDS occurs during rapid hemodialysis, preventive measures are directed toward slower removal of urea, especially during the first session of hemodialysis for acute kidney injury or end-stage renal disease. This can be accomplished by short and more frequent dialysis for the first few days, initially using small-surface-area dialyzers and slow blood rates.[143] Maintaining plasma osmolality using high-sodium dialysate and infusing sodium bicarbonate or mannitol while plasma urea is being removed would minimize the osmotic disequilibrium between the plasma and the brain. Early initiation of dialysis therapy in both the acute and chronic settings of renal failure, before plasma urea concentrations become very high, can prevent the development of DDS.

Muscle Cramps

Muscle cramps are the most common acute neuromuscular complications; they are observed commonly in the elderly and in hemodialysis-dependent patients,[155] and can occur in 5% to 20% of hemodialysis patients. Cramps usually occur late during dialysis and frequently involve the legs, although muscles in other parts of the body are not spared. Although cramps are transient and are unlikely to result in long-term sequelae per se, they account for premature discontinuation of the dialysis session in some instances. Electromyography performed during hemodialysis has shown tonic electrical activity in the muscles, which steadily increases throughout the session in those who develop cramps, in contrast to a steady decline in electrical activity in those who do not.[156] A subset of patients has elevated predialysis levels of serum creatine kinase during periods of cramps.[157]

The pathogenesis of intradialytic cramps is unknown. Rapid plasma volume contraction is the strongest predisposing factor; changes in osmolality and serum electrolytes, such as potassium and magnesium, induced by hemodialysis, as well as underlying carnitine deficiency, have also been incriminated.[158]

The most important measure to prevent intradialytic muscle cramps is to minimize intradialytic fluid removal, which unfortunately is difficult for some patients. Increasing the duration of the dialysis session or the frequency of dialysis may be necessary. Increasing the dry weight is often useful, if it does not result in significant fluid overload. Low-dose (5 mg) enalapril twice weekly has been shown to be effective in limiting thirst, presumably by inhibiting angiotensin II production. Oral oxazepam (5–10 mg), given 2 hours before, or quinine sulfate (325 mg) given at the initiation of dialysis has been shown to reduce the incidence of muscle cramps.[159] Quinine sulfate is, however, currently considered by the Food and Drug Administration to be both unsafe and ineffective for this purpose. Dialysate sodium modeling, using an exponential, linear, or step-decrease algorithm, was similarly effective in decreasing intradialytic muscle cramping.[160] Finally, stretching exercise of the affected muscle groups or carnitine supplementation has been shown to decrease the frequency of muscle cramps.[161]

The acute management of muscle cramps is directed at restoring plasma volume. Intravenous fluid administration is effective but would defeat the overall goal of dialytic fluid removal. Plasma volume can also be restored by increasing the plasma osmolality, resulting in the recruitment of fluid from the extravascular space.[154] Intravenous infusion of hypertonic (23.5%) saline (15–20 mL), 25% mannitol (50–100 mL), or 50% dextrose (25–50 mL) has been shown to be equally effective in relieving muscle cramps.[162] Both hypertonic saline and mannitol cause transient warmth or flushing during the infusion. In addition, retention of these agents may result in a persistent increase in serum osmolality and hence postdialytic thirst and interdialytic fluid gain. Hypertonic dextrose is preferred, especially in nondiabetic patients, because it is readily catabolized and is inexpensive, but it causes transient hyperglycemia. A sublingual capsule of 10 mg nifedipine has been reported to provide relief of cramps without causing significant hypotension and may be related to the minimization of hypo-osmolality-induced changes in cellular ionized calcium levels.[163]

Headache

Headache during dialysis is common.[163] The pain can be intense, accompanied by nausea or vomiting. It is not typically accompanied by visual disturbances as in migraines. The etiology of intradialytic headache is unknown. It may be a mild manifestation of the dialysis disequilibrium syndrome[153] or may be related to the use of acetate[118,164] or glucose-free dialysate.[165] It can also be due to other common etiologies, such as hypertension and caffeine withdrawal, or, in rare circumstances, intracranial bleeding exacerbated by heparinization for the dialysis procedure. Preventive measures include a reduction in urea clearance, as described in the section on DDS, or a change to dialysate containing bicarbonate and glucose. Treatment of the headache is largely symptomatic with analgesics if no other serious causes are identified.

Restless Legs Syndrome

Restless legs syndrome (RLS) is a common symptom in dialysis patients. The symptoms are deep paresthesias, creeping and crawling sensations or even pain in the calves and legs that occur exclusively when the legs are inactive, such as during hemodialysis.[166] Although the tendency to move can be temporarily suppressed, it is ultimately irresistible; movement of the legs yields prompt relief. Perhaps paradoxically, RLS is encountered in severely uremic patients and is relieved within a few weeks of initiating or intensifying dialysis therapy.[166]

The results of clinical and electromyographic examinations in RLS are generally unremarkable. This disorder is differentiated from peripheral neuropathy, in which the paresthesia is constant and unrelieved by activity. When RLS symptoms develop in an otherwise stable hemodialysis patient, anxiety, progressive lower extremity vascular insufficiency, and inadequate dialysis need to be considered. Benzodiazepines taken before bedtime may mitigate some of the RLS symptoms, but their use may be complicated by drowsiness.[166] Opiates are remarkably effective but are associated with well known adverse effects. Carbamazepine and levodopa have also been advocated, but tolerance to these agents may develop rapidly.[167] A reasonable approach is to alternate these agents with different mechanisms of action on a weekly or biweekly basis. Gabapentin has been used with success in dialysis patients.[167] In the nondialysis population, the dopamine receptor agonists, such as pramipexole and ropinirole, have been shown to markedly ameliorate RLS symptoms.[168] Data on dialysis patients are limited. Nonpharmacologic approaches, such as transcutaneous electrical nerve stimulation, are yet another form of treatment.[166]

HEMATOLOGIC COMPLICATIONS

Blood Loss

Acute blood loss during hemodialysis can be a catastrophic event. The most serious cause is disengagement of the venous needle from the arteriovenous access without initiating remedial action. At a blood pump speed of 400 mL/min drawing blood from the arterial needle, fatal exsanguination within several minutes has been reported. Disconnection of the arterial needle instead leads to entry of air into the dialysis circuit (see the discussion of air embolism in the section Cardiovascular Complications in this chapter). The obvious preventive strategy is proper securement of needles and tubing. A very low venous pressure, resulting from the disconnected circuit and hence low resistance, should trigger an alarm in the dialysis machine, but the sensitivity of this monitoring system depends on the degree of circuit disconnection and the preset venous pressure parameter. In some instances, devices that sense fluids (i.e., enuresis detection devices) can be wrapped around the sites that are more prone to disconnection. These devices are not usually employed in dialysis centers but are sometimes used in home dialysis settings, especially for patients undergoing nocturnal hemodialysis.

Perforation of the vessels and other anatomic structures by femoral or central catheters leads to internal bleeding (e.g., into the pleural sac or retroperitoneum). Inadvertent puncture of the femoral, iliac, or carotid artery can be more troublesome. The clinical sequelae are those related to intravascular volume depletion (e.g., shock) or the presence of the blood in an unintended space (e.g., dyspnea or pain from bleeding into the pleural sac).[169] Perforation of the vessels by the catheter may not always be apparent during the catheter insertion procedure, but may only manifest during the hemodialysis session when the systemic blood is circulated at high pump speeds. Rupture of the dialysis membrane in the dialyzer is a rare occurrence and should be evident by the presence of blood or pink fluid in the dialysate compartment. Creation of local hematoma or false aneurysm of the vascular access can also occur as a result of puncture of the vessel wall. The management of acute blood loss in these settings depends on the circumstances and severity. It may include the immediate discontinuation of hemodialysis, cardiopulmonary support, and detection and management of the extravasated blood as necessary. Attention should also be directed to the assessment and potential reversal of anticoagulation to stop the bleeding.[64]

Chronic blood loss in the dialyzer occurs with the trapping of residual blood in the hollow fiber lumens. Higher heparin doses decrease dialyzer blood loss on one hand, but may enhance bleeding in patients with underlying pathology in the gastrointestinal tract. The amount of blood lost in the dialyzer also depends on patient characteristics (e.g., coagulability) and the rigor of saline rinsing during blood return to the patient. The estimate has been one to several milliliters for each dialysis session. Of course, with the clotting of the whole dialysis circuit, up to 200 mL of blood can be lost. Another source of external blood loss associated with dialysis is the puncture sites remaining after the needles have been removed from the native fistula or graft. In addition to systemic bleeding diathesis as a result of intrinsic clotting defects or heparinization, high hydrostatic pressure in the vascular access as a result of outflow tract stenosis is another cause of prolonged postdialysis bleeding from these sites. This blood loss is difficult to quantify and is often ignored in the estimation of the amount of supplemental iron required on an ongoing basis.

Intradialytic Hemolysis

The survival of red blood cells in the circulation is decreased from the normal of 120 days to 60 days in hemodialysis patients,[170–172] which aggravates the anemia in this population. Certain events during hemodialysis predispose to hemolysis. In the early years of hemodialysis, the roller pump for the dialysis tubing caused traumatic red cell fragmentation,[173] but newer technical designs have effectively eliminated this problem. Other rare mechanical causes of hemolysis include arterial tubing collapse as a result of poor arterial blood inflow generating very high negative pressure, kinking of dialyzer blood tubing, and defective tubing with constricted lumens.

Over a period of 1 year, one dialysis unit reported that 10 patients developed intravascular hemolysis accompanied by severe abdominal pain and back pain. Six of these patients also developed acute pancreatitis; one patient died. After extensive evaluation, a kink was detected in a batch of arterial blood tubings. Further episodes of hemolysis were prevented by changing to a new batch of arterial blood tubing and removing the redundant length of tubing that predisposed to kinking.[48] In another episode, a total of 30 patients from seven dialysis centers in three different states over a period of 15 days experienced intradialytic hemolysis. Five of these patients died. Careful examination of the used dialyzer tubings demonstrated severe narrowing of the aperture at the outlet of the bubble trap through which blood was pumped.[174,175]

Another etiology for the development of hemolysis in dialysis patients can be due to the addition of chloramine to city water supplies to decrease bacterial contamination.[176] Besides public announcements, many municipal offices specifically warn healthcare facilities about such plans. Deionization of the water or neutralization of the chloramine with the addition of ascorbic acid to the dialysate prevents hemolysis from chloramine.[176–178] Nitrate/nitrite intoxication can occur during home hemodialysis in patients who use water from ground wells that is contaminated with urine from domestic animals, causing methemoglobinemia and hemolysis.[173] Clues to methemoglobinemia are nausea, vomiting, hypotension, cyanosis, and the inability of oxygen supplementation to eliminate the black color in the blood in the extracorporeal circuit. Copper from building water pipes also causes oxidative injury to erythrocytes, leading to methemoglobinemia and hemolysis.[173] Copper intoxication is associated with skin flushing, abdominal pain, and diarrhea. Analysis of the water supply confirms the nature of the contamination, such as copper and chloramine.

Residual formaldehyde and hydrogen peroxide from dialyzer reprocessing for reuse has been associated with hemolysis.[173,179] Formaldehyde induces hemolysis via two mechanisms. It is a potent reducing agent that inhibits erythrocyte glycolysis. It may also act as a hapten that induces the formation of anti-N-like cold agglutinins.[173] Other rare causes of hemolysis related to hemodialysis include overheating of dialysate to 42°C, hypotonic dialysate that results from erroneous preparation and defective monitoring of the dialysate conductivity, and hypophosphatemia as a result of dialytic clearance of phosphorus.[173]

The diagnosis of acute severe hemolysis is self-evident when grossly translucent hemolyzed blood is observed in the tubing. More subtle hemolysis can be confirmed by elevated reticulocyte count, serum free hemoglobin, lactate dehydrogenase level, decreased serum haptoglobin, positive Coomb's test, and the presence of schistocytes and Heinz bodies in the peripheral blood smear. Acute hemolysis is a medical emergency, partly because the associated hyperkalemia can be rapidly fatal. Among other diagnostic tests and investigations for the cause of the hemolysis, serum potassium should be immediately determined and an electrocardiogram obtained for hyperkalemic changes, depending on the degree of suspected hemolysis. A safe extracorporeal circuit should be set up for immediate hemodialysis of the patient to correct the hyperkalemia, if the clinical condition (e.g., hemodynamic stability) permits.

Activation of Complement System and Leukocytes

A number of disorders in various types of leukocytes, including neutrophils, lymphocytes and monocytes, and platelets, have been described in hemodialysis patients. The functional defects in these cells are partially attributed to uremia per se, but the extracorporeal circulation during hemodialysis may also be contributory. A general theme of the mechanisms by which extracorporeal circulation impairs cellular functions is the intradialytic activation of the humoral factors and the direct activation of the cells in the blood, as a result of exposure to the dialysis membrane and dialysate constituents. As a consequence of this intradialytic activation, pro-inflammatory and procoagulatory mediators are generated and released, including anaphylatoxins,[11] kinins,[180] reactive oxygen species,[181] proteases,[182,183] and cytokines,[184] leading to tissue injury. In addition, leukocytes[185] and platelets[186] become deactivated and respond suboptimally to stimuli postdialysis. The intradialytic activation of these cellular and noncellular elements has been used as an index of dialysis membrane biocompatibility assessments. Dialysis membranes that are more prone to activate blood constituents are called *bioincompatible membranes*. However, there is no consensus on the criteria by which dialysis membranes are classified as biocompatible or bioincompatible.

Interactions between plasma proteins and dialysis membrane surfaces are known to activate the complement,[25] intrinsic coagulation, and fibrinolytic pathways.[187] The magnitude of complement system activation, usually via the alternative pathway, is often substantial. Therefore, plasma levels of complement activation products, C3a and C5a, and their respective derivatives, $C3a_{desArg}$ and $C5a_{desArg}$, are commonly used as markers of bioincompatibility. The potential acute effects of anaphylatoxins C3a and C5a in mediating dialysis syndromes have been discussed. The desArginine derivatives of anaphylatoxins lack anaphylactic properties, but still have leukocyte-directed properties capable of activating neutrophils and monocytes.[26,188,189] The extent to which these complement fragments are in fact responsible for intradialytic leukocyte activation and postdialysis cell deactivation is unclear.

Unsubstituted cellulosic membranes, which tend to be associated with the highest intradialytic levels of $C3a_{desArg}$,[190] are often classified as bioincompatible. In contrast, substituted cellulosic membranes and synthetic membranes tend to be associated with lower plasma $C3a_{desArg}$ levels[23,190] and are generally considered biocompatible. This schema is unfortunately too simplistic, because it ignores the other factors that determine plasma level of complement activation products (e.g., removal by transport into dialysate and adsorption onto the dialysis membrane) and other cellular and noncellular blood constituents that may be affected.

In addition to C5a, peripheral blood monocytes can be activated by other components of the extracorporeal circuit. Bacterial products, such as endotoxins, are well known to be potent stimulants of monocytes. The degree to which bacterial product contaminants in the dialysate can exert their effects on cells in the blood compartment has been extensively studied.[35,36,191,192] Evidence suggests that, whereas the intact endotoxin molecules are too large to traverse the pores of the dialysis membrane, smaller fragments with molecular weights lower than 5 kDa that are also functionally active would not be restricted by high-flux membranes.[36,191] Thus, some investigators have advocated the use of ultrapure dialysate to minimize the potential transfer of bacterial fragments into the blood compartment.[192] The actetate used in dialysate also activates monocytes,[35] although this type of buffer is not commonly used in the United States nowadays. Regardless of the mechanisms of cell activation, the release of pro-inflammatory cytokines from the monocytes can potentially induce multisystemic complications.

Repeated intradialytic activation of leukocytes and their subsequent deactivation may have subacute or long-term sequelae on dialysis patients. Thus, several reports have suggested that mortality in patients receiving dialysis for either acute kidney injury[193] or end-stage renal disease[194] is influenced by the selection of dialysis membranes, although the results are not uniform. It must be noted that not only were the patient populations, dialysis prescriptions, and study designs different among the various studies, but the types of membranes compared were also highly heterogeneous, making it difficult to conclude if any differences in the observed outcomes were due to differences in certain biocompatibility characteristics or differences in transport or adsorptive properties of the dialysis membranes. Nonetheless, the results of these studies in general suggest that substituted cellulosic membranes and synthetic membranes are associated with better patient survival,[194,195] compared to unsubstituted membranes.

Platelet Abnormalities

By removing urea and other nitrogenous compounds, such as guanidine succinic acid, hemodialysis improves platelet function. On the other hand, the hemodialysis procedure can also acutely predispose the patient to bleeding by several mechanisms. The most obvious one is systemic heparinization. The techniques of regional anticoagulation were devised to avoid systemic anticoagulation. In the regional heparin technique,[196] heparin is infused into the dialyzer arterial tubing, and the heparinization in the extracorporeal circuit is reversed by the infusion of protamine in the dialyzer venous tubing. In the regional citrate technique, citrate is infused into the arterial tubing, and the anticoagulation is reversed by the infusion of calcium in the venous tubing.[197–200] Neither regional technique is widely used in the United States because they are quite cumbersome. Excessive protamine can paradoxically function as an anticoagulant. Citrate infusion involves large fluid volumes and can cause metabolic alkalosis,[199] whereas inaccurate calcium titration induces hypercalcemia or hypocalcemia.[199,200] Decreasing or eliminating the systemic heparin dosages, with periodic flushing of the bubble trap using saline solution,[13,14] is often sufficient to avoid significant systemic anticoagulation and clotting of the extracorporeal circuit.

Heparin-induced thrombocytopenia is often suspected in dialysis patients, although the prevalence is probably lower than the estimated figure of 4%.[201] Transient thrombocytopenia may result from the interaction between blood and the dialysis membrane, with the nadir of the platelet count being lower than $100,000/\mu L$ observed at approximately 1 hour after starting hemodialysis.[186] Impaired aggregation of platelets has also been observed in blood samples obtained after dialysis compared to predialysis samples, despite the removal of plasma uremic toxins during the treatment.[186] This impairment in aggregation is presumably due to intradialytic activation of the platelets by the dialysis membrane and consequent cell deactivation.

PULMONARY COMPLICATIONS

Hypoxemia

Hypoxemia was common during hemodialysis before the 1990s. The arterial oxygen tension usually drops by 5 to 30 mm Hg during dialysis, reaching a nadir between 30 and 60 minutes in some cases and persisting to the end of dialysis in others.[202–204] In either case, the hypoxemia resolves within 60 to 120 minutes after discontinuation of dialysis. The etiology of hemodialysis-induced hypoxemia is probably twofold. First, during dialysis using unsubstituted cellulosic membranes, complement activation and the associated peripheral leukopenia occur intensely during the initial 15 minutes. Experiments in animals and limited data in patients showed that the peripheral leukopenia was due to the accumulation of leukocytes in the pulmonary arterioles, in essence resulting in diffuse leukocyte thromboembolism. This leukocyte-based pulmonary embolism causes a ventilation/perfusion mismatch and complement-induced extravasation of vascular fluids; both of these events result in impairment in gas diffusion.[203] This mechanism is responsible for the early and transient type of hypoxemia that can develop during the early stages of hemodialysis therapy regardless of the use of different types of hemodialysis membranes.

The more significant cause of dialysis-induced hypoxemia is the loss of carbon dioxide into the dialysate when acetate-containing dialysate is employed.[202] This leads to central hypoventilation and hypoxemia. This type of hypoxemia tends to be more persistent during the hemodialysis session, especially in patients with slow metabolism of acetate, and can be prevented by the use of bicarbonate-containing dialysate.[205,206]

In the modern era of hemodialysis, unsubstituted cellulosic membranes and acetate dialysate are not commonly employed. The most important cause of dialysis-associated hypoxemia nowadays is probably related to hypoventilation as a result of intentional or unintentional sedation or perhaps mild disequilibrium syndrome. Transient dialysis-associated hypoxemia is usually of no clinical significance unless underlying cardiopulmonary diseases are present. Oxygen supplementation should be provided as necessary.

METABOLIC DISTURBANCES

Potassium

The most important danger of potassium removal during hemodialysis is the genesis of cardiac arrhythmia. Potassium removal during hemodialysis does not conform to single-pool kinetics.[207,208] The rate of removal of potassium from the extracellular space exceeds its rate of removal from the intracellular space. The transfer of potassium from the intracellular to extracellular compartment occurs at a relatively slow rate and is modulated by many factors, including pH, insulin, catecholamines, and membrane-bound Na^+/K^+-ATPase. Serum potassium levels rebound rapidly within 5 hours of completing dialysis and may be 30% higher than immediate postdialysis values.[207,208] Therefore, potassium supplementation based solely on the immediate postdialysis values should be largely avoided.

The use of potassium modeling (changing dialysate potassium concentration during treatment) and longer hemodialysis sessions have been advocated to avoid severe rebound.[208] The use of potassium-free dialysate is usually unnecessary and can induce arrhythmias.[209] Even in the presence of severe hyperkalemia, for example, with a serum potassium of 8 mEq/L, dialysate potassium of 2 to 3 mEq/L would provide a steep gradient for potassium diffusion.[210] The pace of hyperkalemia correction is also influenced by the simultaneous correction of metabolic acidosis during hemodialysis, which shifts potassium into cells. Thus, the correction of hyperkalemia may occur faster than the scenario in which acidosis is absent. Although a dialysate potassium concentration of 2 mEq/L is quite safe for most chronic dialysis patients, it should be tailored to the specific patient's need. A dialysate potassium concentration of 3 mEq/L may be necessary for patients with underlying cardiac arrhythmias or those receiving digitalis therapy.

Sodium

Both hyponatremia and hypernatremia can occur during hemodialysis, depending on the sodium concentration in the dialysate employed. Dysnatremias resulting from technical errors in the dialysate are discussed under "Intradialytic Hypotension." Although sodium concentrations usually do not equilibrate between the serum and dialysate compartments during a regular 4-hour hemodialysis session, prescribed dialysate sodium levels that are higher than 145 mEq/L will tend to increase serum sodium concentration and induce thirst during the interdialytic period. Low dialysate sodium concentrations promote hypotension by enhancing the shifting of serum water into the extravascular space to achieve osmolar equilibrium.[211] In the presence of severe predialysis hypernatremia or hyponatremia, extra precautions should be exercised in the prescription of dialysate sodium concentrations to avoid rapid correction of the dysnatremic state and central nervous system symptoms.

Calcium, Phosphorus, and Magnesium

Similarly, hypercalcemia and hypocalcemia can also occur during hemodialysis, with or without technical errors. High dialysate calcium concentration (e.g., 3 mEq/L) allows the transfer of calcium to plasma and may promote vascular calcification. In contrast, low dialysate calcium (e.g., 2 mEq/L) often enhances calcium loss from the plasma, thereby impairing myocardial contractility and inducing hyperparathyroidism, unless supplemental calcium or vitamin D is provided. Very low dialysate calcium is sometimes used to remove body calcium for the treatment of hypercalcemia, tumoral calcinosis, calciphylaxis, or vascular calcification.[212] For these purposes, dialysate calcium of 1 to 1.5 mEq/L can be used judiciously,[213] preferably with cardiac monitoring. The use of calcium-free dialysate is generally discouraged, except under extreme circumstances or experimental conditions, because of the high potential for cardiac arrhythmias.[214] Correction of acidosis during dialysis can also decrease the plasma ionized calcium; this should be taken into consideration for patients with significant predialysis acidemia.

All commercial dialysates are free of phosphorus. Hypophosphatemia is not usually a concern in dialysis patients. In patients with poor dietary intake, total parenteral nutrition supplementation without phosphorus, excessive phosphate-binder administration, or intensive hemodialysis such as nocturnal dialysis[215] can induce hypophosphatemia. If severe, hypophosphatemia can cause muscular weakness and respiratory arrest. Although dialysate enriched with phosphorus has been used,[216] oral or intravenous phosphorus supplementation is simpler and usually sufficient.

Because commercial dialysates do not contain magnesium, hypomagnesemia can also develop with hemodialysis. Oral or intravenous magnesium supplementation can be used as indicated.

Dyslipidemia

Although a variety of lipid and lipoprotein abnormalities are observed in chronic dialysis patients,[217] they are primarily the results of uremia rather than the hemodialysis procedure. Hypertriglyceridemia is a hallmark of chronic kidney disease and is a manifestation of the accumulation of triglyceride-containing lipoprotein remnant particles. A decrease in plasma lipase activity, with consequent impairment in lipoprotein catabolism, appears to be an important mechanism by which these remnant particles accumulate in the plasma. The repeated administration of heparin for hemodialysis has been postulated to be a cause of lipase depletion.[218,219] To what extent dialysis-associated heparinization actually contributes to the hypertriglyceridemia in dialysis patients is unclear.

The intradialytic activation of neutrophils by unsubstituted cellulosic membranes results in the release of reactive oxygen species and oxidation of proteins.[220] Vitamin E coating of cellulosic membranes has been developed to provide antioxidative properties.[221] In spite of this potential sequence of events, the association of intradialytic release of reactive oxygen species with atherosclerosis remains speculative.

Protein Catabolism

Hypoalbuminemia is a strong predictor of mortality in chronic dialysis patients. The etiology of this disorder is multifactorial, with chronic inflammation and poor dietary intake likely to be the two major causes. The hemodialysis procedure may be contributory by several mechanisms. First, the loss of plasma amino acids into the dialysate has been well documented.[222] The magnitude of this loss is substantial, regardless of the use of low-flux or high-flux dialyzers,[223] because of the low molecular weights of these molecules. An average of 1.5 to 3 g[223] are often lost per session of dialysis; that is equivalent to approximately 4% to 8% of the weekly dietary intake of amino acids in proteins. The loss of glucose into the dialysate would exacerbate the catabolic state, but commercial dialysates nowadays usually contain 200 mg/dL of glucose, thus minimizing or eliminating the glucose loss. Second, plasma albumin can also be lost directly into the dialysate.[38,223] Albumin has a molecular weight of 60 kDa and does not usually traverse even high-flux dialysis membranes. Large amounts of plasma protein loss—as high as 20 g in a single hemodialysis session—have been reported during treatment using high-flux polysulfone dialyzers reprocessed with bleach.[38] Presumably, the pore size increases as a result of the action of the bleach on the copolymer of the dialysis membrane. Subsequent changes in the fabrication of these membranes have apparently markedly diminished the permeability of the polysulfone membranes to albumin, even when bleach is included in the reprocessing.[224] Finally, protein catabolism has been reported during sham hemodialysis using unsubstituted cellulosic membranes, apparently mediated by the generation of prostaglandin E_2 after interactions between blood and the dialysis membrane.[225] Although the transmembrane loss of amino acids and albumin and the protein catabolism induced by membrane bioincompatibility contribute to the hypoalbuminemia, it is unclear if hypoalbuminemia from these mechanisms carries the same prognostic value as hypoalbuminemia associated with uremic inflammation or poor dietary intake.

Vitamins

Similar to most other hydrophilic small molecules, water-soluble vitamins, including folate, ascorbate, and vitamin B, are readily diffusible through low-flux and high-flux dialysis membranes. Daily supplementation of these vitamins is therefore recommended. In contrast, the fat-soluble vitamins—vitamins A, D, E, and K—are not dialyzable. Commercially available multivitamins specifically designed for dialysis patients usually contain 1 mg of folate, 1.5 mg of thiamine (vitamin B_1), 1.2 mg of riboflavin (vitamin B_2), 10 mg of pantothenic acid (vitamin B_5), 10 mg of pyridoxine (vitamin B_6), 6 μg of cyanocobalamin (vitamin B_{12}), and 300 μg of biotin. Vitamin B_{12} is of particular interest in hemodialysis because this molecule (13.5 kDa) had been commonly used as a middle-molecule marker.[226] Although low-flux dialyzers are also permeable to vitamin B_{12}, clearance of this molecule is higher with high-flux dialyzers. Vitamin doses higher than those that are necessary to replace dialytic losses are sometimes used for pharmacologic purposes. For example, high doses of folate and pyridoxine have been used to lower serum homocysteine levels, but did not improve survival and did not reduce vascular events in these patients.[227,228]

DIALYSATE CONTAMINATION

Dialysate contamination occurs when either the dialysate concentrates or the water supply is contaminated. Dialysate concentrates are stored in each dialysis facility. The "acid" dialysate concentrates (without bicarbonate) and the bicarbonate concentrates are usually mixed to produce the final dialysate. Bicarbonate concentrates are particularly prone to bacterial growth. The chronic dialysis patient is exposed to 2000 to 3000 L of water in the dialysate during each month of therapy. The water in the dialysate is usually tap water from municipal sources, which has undergone purification using reverse osmosis or carbon filter treatment before it reaches the dialysis machine. Although the majority of dialysis units use reverse osmosis, which has reduced the clinical occurrence of water contamination, serious accidents due to chemical contamination of dialysis water can still occur.[229] In addition, microbial contaminants can be detected in the water system, including bacteria and their cell wall degradation products, such as endotoxins and peptidoglycans. Fungi, viruses, and protozoa may also be present in the dialysis water treatment system. Microbial contamination of the dialysate can lead to intradialytic pyrogenic reactions and hypotension. Exposure to bacterial contaminants over a prolonged period potentially leads to the chronic inflammatory state, which initiates or aggravates dialysis-related amyloidosis, atherosclerosis, and malnutrition.[230]

The Association for the Advancement of Medical Instrumentation's (AAMI) Renal Disease and Detoxification Committee in 2006 revised its standards for water treatment; the new standards include alternative and supplementary methods of removing toxic chloramines from water, because water supply quality and municipal water treatment practices vary substantially. The revised standards should be applied to the water used for the preparation of concentrates from dialysis powder, the preparation of bicarbonate solution, and the reprocessing of dialyzers for multiple uses. It covers all devices, piping, and fittings between the point at which potable water is delivered to the water treatment system and the point-of-use of the treated water. Disinfection must involve all the pipes in the distribution system of either water or dialysate solution and connectors to the dialysis machine to prevent the development of *biofilm,* a layer of polymeric organic matrix in which bacteria and fungi can grow. Once developed, biofilms are resistant to disinfecting techniques.[231,232]

Both AAMI as well as the European Pharmacopoeia have established standards for chemical and microbial quality. The AAMI recommends that tryptic soy agar at 37°C for 48 hours should be used for the detection of microbial contamination and endotoxin levels. The European Pharmacopoeia, however, does not make any prespecified recommendations as to the type of medium to be used for such testing. The use of other specialized mediums, such as Reasoner's agar and tryptone glucose extract agar, along with extended incubation for 5 to 7 days at 20° to 25°C, are more sensitive techniques to detect contamination.[233] AAMI recommends that microbial contamination should not exceed the upper limit of 22 cfu (colony forming units) per mL and endotoxin levels should not exceed 2 IU/mL. Bacterial growth of more than 50 cfu/mL and endotoxin concentration of more than 1 IU/mL should be followed by a corrective action plan that includes a new cycle of disinfection and retesting. The European Pharmacopoeia recommends that bacterial growth at any time should not exceed 100 cfu/mL and endotoxin level should remain less than 0.25 IU/mL.[234,235] These standards for water treatment should be applied to chronic dialysis facilities, acute hospital dialysis units, and homes for patients undergoing home hemodialysis therapy. During the past decade, several studies have demonstrated that more than 35% of water samples from different dialysis centers did not fulfill the expected standards specified by AAMI.[229,236] The medical directors of dialysis units should participate in the quality assurance process for water treatment.[192]

Ultrapure dialysate is defined as a dialysate in which the microbial contamination is less than 0.1 cfu/mL and endotoxin level is less than 0.03 IU/mL.[237] A relatively convenient method of achieving this level of water purity is by techniques of on-line purification of the dialysate.[238,239] Only France has put forth a national directive regarding the use of on-line dialysate production and the achievement of ultrapure dialysate in dialysis units. The use of ultrapure dialysates has been reported to decrease peripheral blood cytokine production during dialysis therapy,[240,241] improve the chronic inflammatory state and nutritional status,[242–244] prevent the development of amyloidosis,[245,246] decrease serum pentosidine levels (a marker of systemic oxidation),[246,247] decrease the dose requirement of erythropoietin,[248,249] and preserve the residual kidney function.[250]

These reports notwithstanding, the effects of ultrapure water in the prevention of long-term dialysis complications remain controversial.[251–254]

HEPATITIS IN HEMODIALYSIS UNITS

Hepatitis C

Chronic dialysis patients are at risk for nosocomial infections due to regular exposure to extracorporeal circulation.[255,256] The environment of dialysis facilities also directly increases the risk for person-to-person transmission of infectious agents and indirectly through the transmission to equipment and supplies.[257] When the Centers for Disease Control and Prevention investigated three different outbreaks of hepatitis C virus (HCV) infection in chronic hemodialysis centers, seroconversions were found to be associated with (1) lack of disinfection of the dialysis machines between patient use, (2) sharing of multiple-dose medication vials, (3) use of common medication carts to prepare and distribute medications at patients' station, (4) blood spills that were not cleaned up immediately, and (5) potential contamination by blood of the pressure-sensing port of the machine, which is not easily accessible to routine disinfection. Multiple blood groups have been found in pressure transducers of the dialysis machine, which are most difficult to disinfect, suggesting cross-contamination by multiple patients.[257,258] Blood transfusions and frequent surgical procedures for various indications, such as the placement and revision of dialysis vascular access, pose additional risks.

The prevalence of HCV infection among patients receiving dialysis varies between countries[259] and between different centers within a given country, ranging from 3% to more than 70%.[260,261] The risk of HCV transmission to patients on maintenance dialysis has not been eliminated despite a significant reduction in blood transfusion as a result of the availability of erythropoiesis-stimulating agents and the introduction of a blood-donor screening program for the detection of anti-HCV antibodies. Among the risk factors associated with HCV seroconversion are the history of blood transfusion and number of years on dialysis. The prevalence increased from an average of 12% in patients with less than 5 years on dialysis to 37% in those receiving dialysis for more than 5 years.

To prevent transmission of HCV and other blood-borne viruses from both recognized and unrecognized sources of infection, the hemodialysis staff requires training and education, with strict adherence to infection control precautions. Patients who are anti-HCV positive or HCV RNA-positive do not need to be isolated from other patients or dialyzed separately on dedicated machines. Such patients can even participate in dialyzer reuse programs, because reprocessing of such dialyzers does not appear to increase the risk for infection to either dialysis staff members or other dialysis patients.

Hepatitis G

Similar to HCV infection, hepatitis G virus (HGV) or GB-virus type C (GBV-C) is a blood-borne virus, a member of the family Flaviviridae. HGV is distributed globally; nearly 1.7% of volunteer blood donors are positive for HGV. An epidemiologic study demonstrated that among new cases of non-A, non-B hepatitis in the United States, 80% were due to HCV infection and the other 20% were due to HGV infection.[262] Also, among patients with HCV infection, more than 20% can have HGV-RNA present in the blood.[263]

The prevalence of HGV infection in hemodialysis patients has been reported to be variable among countries and in different regions within a country. HGV has been reported in 20% of hemodialysis patients in the United States and Europe,[264-267] less than 4% in the Japanese dialysis population,[268] 58% of those in France,[269,270] but in more than 55% of those in Indonesia.[271] It is known that HGV follows the patterns of blood-borne transmission and that HGV viremia can persist for years. Whether HGV will cause liver damage or remains an innocent bystander in the long term is, however, unclear.[263,272]

PREGNANCY AND HEMODIALYSIS

Women of childbearing age seldom become pregnant while on chronic dialysis due to disturbances in the hypothalamic-pituitary-ovarian axis and other associated psychological factors.[273-275] The incidence of pregnancy, defined by a gestational age of 3 months or more, was only 0.3 per 100 patient-years over a period of 20 years even in women of reproductive age; the successful live birth rate is less than 60%.[276] The risk of intrauterine growth retardation, polyhydramnios, and premature rupture of membranes is increased. Most living babies are born prematurely. The likelihood of a successful pregnancy is higher in patients with kidney transplants compared to patients on dialysis therapy. These differences are most likely due to the lesser degree of uremia in the transplant patient, although complications of the hemodialysis procedure cannot be ruled out.

During pregnancy, it is recommended that the predialysis blood urea nitrogen be maintained at less than 50 mg/dL, which may require increasing the dose of dialysis therapy.[276,277] It is particularly important to frequently and carefully estimate and adjust the dry weight to minimize maternal hypotension and fetoplacental circulatory compromise. The dry weight adjustments should take into consideration that there is a 30% increase in plasma volume during pregnancy and almost a linear physiologic weight gain of approximately 1 pound per week after the first 12 weeks of gestation. In addition, pregnant women on dialysis will need to maintain 1.8 g/kg/day of protein intake.[278-280] The dialysate bicarbonate concentration may need to be adjusted because pregnancy is associated with respiratory alkalosis.[279,281] The dialysate calcium concentration and vitamin D supplement should be reassessed to account for the placental production of 1,25-dihydroxyvitamin D_3.[279,281] The dose of folate supplement should be increased to 2 mg/day to account for the increased requirement during the pregnancy to prevent neural tube defects.[280,282] In addition, the dose of erythropoeisis-stimulating agent needs to be increased to maintain hemoglobin levels at 10 to 11 g/dL as the demand for erythropoiesis increases with gestational age. Iron stores should be frequently monitored.[276,277,283] Although definitive evidence is lacking, there appears to be an increased incidence of congenital anomalies associated with the exposure to formaldehyde and ethylene oxide; thus, these agents should be avoided during the gestational period.

References

1. National Kidney and Urologic Diseases Information Clearinghouse. Available at http://kidney.niddk.nih.gov/kudiseases/pubs/kustats/index.htm. Accessed March 23, 2008.
2. Key J, Nahmias M, Acchiardo S: Hypersensitivity reaction on first-time exposure to cuprophan hollow fiber dialyzer. Am J Kidney Dis 1983;2:664–666.
3. Popli S, Ing TS, Daugirdas JT, et al: Severe reactions to Cuprophan capillary dialyzers. Artif Organs 1982;6:312–315.
4. Lemke HD: Mediation of hypersensitivity reactions during hemodialysis by IgE antibodies against ethylene oxide. Artif Organs 1987;11:104–110.
5. Poothullil J, Shimizu A, Day RP, Dolovich J: Anaphylaxis from the product(s) of ethylene oxide gas. Ann Intern Med 1975;82:58–60.
6. Rumpf KW, Seubert S, Seubert A, et al: Association of ethylene-oxide-induced IgE antibodies with symptoms in dialysis patients. Lancet 1985;2:1385–1387.
7. Gotch FA: Mass transport in reused dialyzers. Proc Clin Dial Transplant Forum 1980;10:81–85.
8. Grammer LC, Roberts M, Nicholls AJ, et al: IgE against ethylene oxide-altered human serum albumin in patients who have had acute dialysis reactions. J Allergy Clin Immunol 1984;74 (4 Pt 1):544–546.
9. Lemke HD, Heidland A, Schaefer RM: Hypersensitivity reactions during hemodialysis: Role of the complement fragments and ethylene oxide antibodies. Nephrol Dial Transplant 1990;5:264–269.
10. Maurice F, Rivory JP, Larsson PH, et al: Anaphylactic shock caused by formaldehyde in a patient undergoing long-term hemodialysis. J Allergy Clin Immunol 1986;77:594–597.
11. Chenoweth DE, Cheung AK, Ward DM, Henderson LW: Anaphylatoxin formation during hemodialysis: Comparison of new and reused dialyzers. Kidney Int 1983;24:770–774.
12. Parnes EL, Shapiro WB: Anaphylactoid reactions in hemodialysis patients treated with the AN69 dialyzer. Kidney Int 1991;40:1148–1152.
13. Sanders PW, Taylor H, Curtis JJ: Hemodialysis without anticoagulation. Am J Kidney Dis 1985;5:32–35.
14. Schwab SJ, Onorato JJ, Sharar LR, Dennis PA: Hemodialysis without anticoagulation. One-year prospective trial in hospitalized patients at risk for bleeding. Am J Med 1987. 83:405–410.
15. Henne W, Schulze H, Pelger M, et al: Hollow-fiber dialyzers and their pyrogenicity testing by Limulus amebocyte lysate. Artif Organs 1984;8:299–305.
16. Moss AH, Hamrick RM III, Shen SH: Limulus amebocyte lysate reactivity, complement activation, and patients' symptoms. Comparison of dialyzer membranes. ASAIO Trans 1989. 35:812–815.
17. Faouzi MA, Dine T, Gressier B, et al: Exposure of hemodialysis patients to di-2-ethylhexyl phthalate. Int J Pharm 1999;180:113–121.
18. Mettang T, Thomas S, Kiefer T, et al: Uraemic pruritus and exposure to di(2-ethylhexyl) phthalate (DEHP) in haemodialysis patients. Nephrol Dial Transplant 1996;11:2439–2443.
19. Wahl HG, Hong Q, Hildenbrand S, et al: 4-Heptanone is a metabolite of the plasticizer di(2-ethylhexyl) phthalate (DEHP) in haemodialysis patients. Nephrol Dial Transplant 2004;19:2576–2583.
20. Hoenich NA, Thompson J, Varini E, et al: Particle spallation and plasticiser (DEHP) release from extracorporeal circuit tubing materials. Int J Artif Organs 1990;13:55–62.
21. Flaminio LM, De Angelis L, Ferazza M, et al: Leachability of a new plasticizer tri-(2-ethylhexyl)-trimellitate from haemodialysis tubing. Int J Artif Organs 1988;11:435–439.
22. Kambia K, Dine T, Azar R, et al: Comparative study of the leachability of di(2-ethylhexyl) phthalate and tri(2-ethylhexyl) trimellitate from haemodialysis tubing. Int J Pharm 2001;229:139–146.

23. Chenoweth DE, Cheung AK, Henderson LW: Anaphylatoxin formation during hemodialysis: Effects of different dialyzer membranes. Kidney Int 1983;24:764–769.

24. Cheung AK, Chenoweth DE, Otsuka D, Henderson LW: Compartmental distribution of complement activation products in artificial kidneys. Kidney Int 1986;30:74–80.

25. Chenoweth DE, Cooper SW, Hugli TE, et al: Complement activation during cardiopulmonary bypass: Evidence for generation of C3a and C5a anaphylatoxins. N Engl J Med 1981;304:497–503.

26. Bokisch VA, Muller-Eberhard HJ: Anaphylatoxin inactivator of human plasma: Its isolation and characterization as a carboxypeptidase. J Clin Invest 1970;49:2427–2436.

27. Spencer PC, Schmidt B, Samtleben W, et al: Ex vivo model of hemodialysis membrane biocompatibility. Trans Am Soc Artif Intern Organs 1985;31:495–498.

28. Henne W, Duenweg G, Bandel W: A new cellulose membrane generation for hemodialysis and hemofiltration. Artif Organs 1979;3(Suppl):466–469.

29. Verresen L, Fink E, Lemke HD, Vanrenterghem Y: Bradykinin is a mediator of anaphylactoid reactions during hemodialysis with AN69 membranes. Kidney Int 1994;45:1497–1503.

30. Schulman G, Hakim R, Arias R, et al: Bradykinin generation by dialysis membranes: Possible role in anaphylactic reaction. J Am Soc Nephrol 1993;3:1563–1569.

31. Fink E, Lemke HD, Verresen L, Shimamoto K: Kinin generation by hemodialysis membranes as a possible cause of anaphylactoid reactions. Braz J Med Biol Res 1994;27:1975–1983.

32. Pegues DA, Beck-Sague CM, Woollen SW, et al: Anaphylactoid reactions associated with reuse of hollow-fiber hemodialyzers and ACE inhibitors. Kidney Int 1992;42:1232–1237.

33. Graefe U, Milutinovich J, Follette WC, et al: Less dialysis-induced morbidity and vascular instability with bicarbonate in dialysate. Ann Intern Med 1978;88:332–336.

34. Henderson LW, Koch KM, Dinarello CA, Shaldon S: Hemodialysis hypotension: The interleukin hypothesis. Blood Purif 1983;1:3–8.

35. Weber V, Linsberger I, Rossmanith E, et al: Pyrogen transfer across high-and low-flux hemodialysis membranes. Artif Organs 2004;28:210–217.

36. Bommer J, Becker KP, Urbaschek R: Potential transfer of enotoxin across high-flux membranes. J Am Soc Nephrol 1996;7:883–888.

37. Tokars JI, Alter MJ, Miller E, et al: National surveillance of dialysis associated diseases in the United States—1994. ASAIO J 1997;43:108–119.

38. Kaplan AA, Halley SE, Lapkin RA, Graeber CW: Dialysate protein losses with bleach processed polysulphone dialyzers. Kidney Int 1995;47:573–578.

39. McCarthy JT, Regnier CE, Loebertmann CL, Bergstralh EJ: Adverse events in chronic hemodialysis patients receiving intravenous iron dextran—a comparison of two products. Am J Nephrol 2000;20:455–462.

40. Chertow GM, Mason PD, Vaage-Nilsen O, Ahlmen J: Update on adverse drug events associated with parenteral iron. Nephrol Dial Transplant 2006;21:378–382.

41. Novey HS, Pahl M, Haydik I, Vaziri ND: Immunologic studies of anaphylaxis to iron dextran in patients on renal dialysis. Ann Allergy 1994;72:224–228.

42. Hedin H, Richter W, Ring J: Dextran-induced anaphylactoid reactions in man: Role of dextran reactive antibodies. Int Arch Allergy Appl Immunol 1976;52:145–159.

43. Fishbane S, Kowalski EA: The comparative safety of intravenous iron dextran, iron saccharate, and sodium ferric gluconate. Semin Dial 2000;13:381–384.

44. Baker LR, Barnett MD, Brozovic B, et al: Hemosiderosis in a patient on regular hemodialysis: treatment by desferrioxamine. Clin Nephrol 1976;6:326–328.

45. Ciancioni C, Poignet JL, Mauras Y, et al: Plasma aluminum and iron kinetics in hemodialyzed patients after I.V. infusion of desferrioxamine. Trans Am Soc Artif Intern Organs 1984;30:479–482.

46. McCarthy JT, Milliner DS, Johnson WJ: Clinical experience with desferrioxamine in dialysis patients with aluminium toxicity. Q J Med 1990;74:257–276.

47. Hoenich NA: Spallation and plasticizer release from hemodialysis blood tubing: A cause of concern? Semin Dial 1991;4:227–230.

48. Sweet SJ, McCarthy S, Steingart R, Callahan T: Hemolytic reactions mechanically induced by kinked hemodialysis lines. Am J Kidney Dis 1996;27:262–266.

49. Berkun Y, Havis YS, Schwartz LB, Shalit M: Heparin-induced recurrent anaphylaxis. Clin Exp Allergy 2004;34;1916–1918.

50. Daugirdas JT: Pathophysiology of dialysis hypotension: an update. Am J Kidney Dis 2001;38(4 Suppl 4):S11–S17.

51. Daugiridas JT: Clinical dilemmas in dialysis: Managing the hypotensive patient. Am J Kidney Dis 2001;38:S1–S10.

52. Davenport A: Intradialytic complications during hemodialysis. Hemodial Int 2006;10:162–167.

53. Donauer J: Hemodialysis-induced hypotension: Impact of technologic advances. Semin Dial 2004;17:333–335.

54. National Kidney Foundation: K/DOQI clinical practice guidelines for cardiovascular disease in dialysis patients. Am J Kidney Dis 2005;45(4 Suppl 3):S76–S80.

55. Tisler A, Akocsi K, Harshegyi I, et al: Comparison of dialysis and clinical characteristics of patients with frequent and occasional hemodialysis-associated hypotension. Kidney Blood Press Res 2002;25:97–102.

56. Ronco C, Brendolan A, Milan M, et al: Impact of biofeedback-induced cardiovascular stability on hemodialysis tolerance and efficiency. Kidney Int 2000;58:800–808.

57. Schreiber M Jr: Clinical dilemmas in dialysis: Managing the hypotensive patient. Am J Kidney Dis 2001;38(4 Suppl 4):S1–S10.

58. Barth C, Boer W, Garzoni D, et al: Characteristics of hypotension-prone haemodialysis patients: Is there a critical relative blood volume? Nephrol Dial Transplant 2003;18:1353–1360.

59. Krepel HP, Nette RW, Akcahuseyin E, et al: Variability of relative blood volume during haemodialysis. Nephrol Dial Transplant 2000;15:673–679.

60. Maggiore Q, Dattolo P, Piacenti M, et al: A pathophysiological overview of dialysis hypotension. Contrib Nephrol 1996;119:182–188.

61. Maggiore Q, Pizzarelli F, Dattolo P, et al: Cardiovascular stability during haemodialysis, haemofiltration and haemodiafiltration. Nephrol Dial Transplant 2000;15(Suppl 1):68–73.

62. Santoro A, Mancini E: Clinical significance of intradialytic blood volume monitoring. Int J Artif Organs 1997;20:1–6.

63. Movilli E, Camerini C, Viola BF, et al: Blood volume changes during three different profiles of dialysate sodium variation with similar intradialytic sodium balances in chronic hemodialyzed patients. Am J Kidney Dis 1997;30:58–63.

64. Van der Sande F, Kooman JP, Leunissen KML: Intradialytic hypotension—new concepts on an old problem. Nephrol Dial Transplant2000;15:1746–1748.

65. Stojceva-Taneva O, Masin G, Polenakovic M, et al: Autonomic nervous system dysfunction and volume nonresponsive hypotension in hemodialysis patients. Am J Nephrol 1991;11:123–126.

66. Sulowicz W, Radziszewski A: Pathogenesis and treatment of dialysis hypotension. Kidney Int 2006;Suppl(104):S36–S39.

67. Converse RL Jr, Jacobsen TN, Jost CM, et al: Paradoxical withdrawal of reflex vasoconstriction as a cause of hemodialysis-induced hypotension. J Clin Invest 1992;90:1657–1665.

68. Heber ME, Lahiri A, Thompson D, Raftery EB: Baroreceptor, not left ventricular, dysfunction is the cause of hemodialysis hypotension. Clin Nephrol 1989;32:79–86.

69. Nette RW, van den Dorpel MA, Krepel HP, et al: Hypotension during hemodialysis results from an impairment of arteriolar tone and left ventricular function. Clin Nephrol 2005;63:276–283.

70. Pomianek MJ, Colton CK, Dinarello CA, Miller LC: Synthesis of tumor necrosis factor alpha and interleukin-1 receptor antagonist, but not interleukin-1, by human mononuclear cells is

enhanced by exposure of whole blood to shear stress. ASAIO J 1996;42:52–59.

71. Nishimura M, Takahashi H, Maruyama K, et al: Enhanced production of nitric oxide may be involved in acute hypotension during maintenance hemodialysis. Am J Kidney Dis 1998;31:809–817.

72. Friess U, Rascher W, Ritz E, Gross P: Failure of arginine-vasopressin and other pressor hormones to increase in severe recurrent dialysis hypotension. Nephrol Dial Transplant 1995;10:1421–1427.

73. Leunissen KM, Cheriex EC, Janssen J, et al: Influence of left ventricular function on changes in plasma volume during acetate and bicarbonate dialysis. Nephrol Dial Transplant 1987;2:99–103.

74. Henrich WL, Hunt J, Nixon JV: Increased ionized calcium and left ventricular contractility during hemodialysis. N Engl J Med 1984;310:19–23.

75. Wizemann V, Schilling M: Dilemma of assessing volume state—the use and the limitations of a clinical score. Nephrol Dial Transplant 1995;10:2114–2117.

76. Schneditz D, Martin K, Kramer M, et al: Effect of controlled extracorporeal blood cooling on ultrafiltration-induced blood volume changes during hemodialysis. J Am Soc Nephrol 1997;8:956–964.

77. Van der Sande F, Kooman JP, Burema J, et al: Effect of dialysate temperature on energy balance during hemodialysis: Quantification of extracorporeal energy transfer. Am J Kidney Dis 1999;33:1115–1121.

78. Ayoub A, Finlayson M: Effect of cool temperature dialysate on the quality and patients' perception of haemodialysis. Nephrol Dial Transplant 2004;19:190–194.

79. Levy FL, Grayburn PA, Foulks CJ, et al: Improved left ventricular contractility with cool temperature hemodialysis. Kidney Int 1992;41:961–965.

80. Selby NM, McIntyre CW: A systematic review of the clinical effects of reducing dialysate fluid temperature. Nephrol Dial Transplant 2006;21:1883–1898.

81. Kaufman AM, Morris AT, Lavarias VA, et al: Effects of controlled blood cooling on hemodynamic stability and urea kinetics during high-efficiency hemodialysis. J Am Soc Nephrol 1998;9:877–883.

82. Maggiore Q: Isothermic dialysis for hypotension-prone patients. Semin Dial 2002;15:187–190.

83. Rosales LM, Schneditz D, Morris AT, et al: Isothermic hemodialysis and ultrafiltration. Am J Kidney Dis 2000;36:353–361.

84. de Paula FM, Peixoto AJ, Pinto LV, et al: Clinical consequences of an individualized dialysate sodium prescription in hemodialysis patients. Kidney Int 2004;66:1232–1238.

85. Flanigan MJ: Role of sodium in hemodialysis. Kidney Int 2000;76 (Suppl):S72–S78.

86. Song JH, Park GH, Lee SY, et al: Effect of sodium balance and the combination of ultrafiltration profile during sodium profiling hemodialysis on the maintenance of the quality of dialysis and sodium and fluid balances. J Am Soc Nephrol 2005;16:237–246.

87. Straver B, de Vries PM, Donker AJ, ter Wee PM: The effect of profiled hemodialysis on intradialytic hemodynamics when a proper sodium balance is applied. Blood Purif 2002;20:364–369.

88. Zhou YL, Liu HL, Duan XF, et al: Impact of sodium and ultrafiltration profiling on haemodialysis-related hypotension. Nephrol Dial Transplant 2006;21:3231–3237.

89. Flanigan MJ, Khairullah QT, Lim VS: Dialysate sodium delivery can alter chronic blood pressure management. Am J Kidney Dis 1997;29:383–391.

90. Sang GL, Kovithavongs C, Ulan R, Kjellstrand CM: Sodium ramping in hemodialysis: A study of beneficial and adverse effects. Am J Kidney Dis 1997;29:669–677.

91. Song JH, Lee S, Suh C-K, Kim M-J: Time-averaged concentration of dialysate sodium relates with sodium load and interdialytic weight gain during sodium-profiling HD. Am J Kidney Dis 2002;40:291–301.

92. Begin V, Deziel C, Madore F: Biofeedback regulation of ultrafiltration and dialysate conductivity for the prevention of hypotension during hemodialysis. ASAIO J 2002;48:312–315.

93. Locatelli F, Buoncristiani U, Canaud B, et al: Haemodialysis with on-line monitoring equipment: Tools or toys? Nephrol Dial Transplant 2005;20:22–33.

94. Moret K, Aalten J, van den Wall BW, et al: The effect of sodium profiling and feedback technologies on plasma conductivity and ionic mass balance: A study in hypotension-prone dialysis patients. Nephrol Dial Transplant 2006;21:138–144.

95. Lang RM, Fellner SK, Neumann A: LV contractility varies directly with blood ionized calcium. Ann Intern Med 1988;108:524–529.

96. Van Kuijk WHM, Mulder AW, Peels CH, et al: Influence of changes in ionized calcium on CV reactivity during HD. Clin Nephrol 1997;47:190–196.

97. Nappi SE, Saha HH, Virtanen VK, et al: Hemodialysis with high-calcium dialysate impairs cardiac relaxation. Kidney Int 1999;55:1091–1096.

98. Gabutti L, Ross V, Duchini F, et al: Does bicarbonate transfer have relevant hemodynamic consequences in standard hemodialysis? Blood Purif 2005;23:365–372.

99. Kyriazis J, Glotsos J, Bilirakis L, F et al: Dialysate calcium profiling during hemodialysis: Use and clinical implications. Kidney Int 2002;61:276–287.

100. National Kidney Foundation: K/DOQI clinical practice guidelines for bone metabolism and disease in CKD. Am J Kidney Dis 2003;42(Suppl 3):S1–S201.

101. Fujimori A, Yorifuji M, Sakai M, et al: Low-calcium dialysate improves mineral metabolism in hemodialysis patients. Clin Nephrol 2007;67:20–24.

102. Chang ST, Chen CL, Chen CC, Hung KC: Clinical events occurrence and the changes of quality of life in chronic haemodialysis patients with dry weight determined by echocardiographic method. Int J Clin Pract 2004;58:1101–1107.

103. Kraemer M, Rode C, Wizemann V: Detection limit of methods to assess fluid status changes in dialysis patients. Kidney Int 2006;69(9):1609–1620.

104. Reddan DN, Szczech LA, Hasselblad V, et al: Intradialytic blood volume monitoring in ambulatory hemodialysis patients: A randomized trial. J Am Soc Nephrol 2005;16:2162–2169.

105. Sheen V, Bhalla V, Tulua-Tata A, Bhalla MA, Weiss D, Chiu A et al: The use of β-type natriuretic peptide to assess volume status in patients with end-stage renal disease. Am Heart J 2007;153:244–245.

106. van de Pol AC, Frenken LA, Moret K, et al: An evaluation of blood volume changes during ultrafiltration pulses and natriuretic peptides in the assessment of dry weight in hemodialysis patients. Hemodial Int 2007;11:51–61.

107. Yoshihara F, Horio T, Nakamura S, et al: Adrenomedullin reflects cardiac dysfunction, excessive blood volume, and inflammation in hemodialysis patients. Kidney Int 2005;68:1355–1363.

108. Cruz D: Midodrine: a selective alpha-adrenergic agonist for orthostatic hypotension and dialysis hypotension. Exp Opin Pharmacother 2000;1(4):835–840.

109. Perazella MA: Pharmacologic options available to treat symptomatic intradialytic hypotension. Am J Kidney Dis 2001;38 (4 Suppl 4):S26–S36.

110. Prakash S, Garg AX, Heidenheim AP, House AA: Midodrine appears to be safe and effective for dialysis-induced hypotension: a systematic review. Nephrol Dial Transplant 2004;19:2553–2558.

111. Dheenan S, Venkatesan J, Grubb BP, Henrich WL: Effect of sertraline hydrochloride on dialysis hypotension. Am J Kidney Dis 1998;31:624–630.

112. Yalcin AU, Sahin G, Erol M, Bal C: Sertraline hydrochloride treatment for patients with hemodialysis hypotension. Blood Purif 2002;20:150–153.

113. Yalcin AU, Kudaiberdieva G, Sahin G, et al: Effect of sertraline hydrochloride on cardiac autonomic dysfunction in patients with hemodialysis-induced hypotension. Nephron Physiol 2003;93:21–28.

114. van der Zee S, Thompson A, Zimmerman R, et al: Vasopressin administration facilitates fluid removal during hemodialysis. Kidney Int 2007;71:318–324.

115. Flanigan MJ: Vasopressin: A look at dialysis hypertension and autonomic dysfunction. Kidney Int 2007;71:285–287.

116. Maggiore Q, Pizzarelli F, Santoro A: The effects of control of thermal balance on vascular stability in HD patients: Results of the European randomized clinical trial. Am J Kidney Dis 2002;40:280–290.

117. van der Sande FM, Kooman JP, Konings CJ, Leunissen KM: Thermal effects and blood pressure response during postdilution hemodiafiltration and hemodialysis: The effect of amount of replacement fluid and dialysate temperature. J Am Soc Nephrol 2001;12:1916–1920.

118. Movilli E, Camerini C, Zein H, et al: A prospective comparison of bicarbonate dialysis, hemodiafiltration, and acetate-free biofiltration in the elderly. Am J Kidney Dis 1996;27:541–547.

119. Beerenhout C, Dejagere T, van der Sande FM, et al: Haemodynamics and electrolyte balance: A comparison between on-line pre-dilution haemofiltration and haemodialysis. Nephrol Dial Transplant 2004;19:2354–2359.

120. Karamperis N, Sloth E, Jensen JD: Predilution hemodiafiltration displays no hemodynamic advantage over low-flux hemodialysis under matched conditions. Kidney Int 2005;67:1601–1608.

121. Van der Sande F, Gladziwa U, Kooman JP: Energy transfer is the most important factor for the divergent vascular response between isolated UF and HD at different dialysis temperatures. J Am Soc Nephrol 1999;Abstract 1559:307A.

122. Eknoyan G, Latos DL, Lindberg J: Practice recommendations for the use of L-carnitine in dialysis-related carnitine disorder. National Kidney Foundation Carnitine Consensus Conference. Am J Kidney Dis 2003;41:868–876.

123. Riley S, Rutherford S, Rutherford PA: Low carnitine levels in HD patients: Relationship with functional activity status and intra-dialytic hypotension. Clin Nephrol 1997;48:392–393.

124. U.S. Renal Data System: USRDS 2003 Annual Data Report. Am J Kidney Dis 2003;42(6 Suppl 5):1–230.

125. Karnik JA, Young BS, Lew NL, et al: Cardiac arrest and sudden death in dialysis units. Kidney Int 2001;60:350–357.

126. Gibson KD, Gillen DL, Caps MT, et al: Vascular access survival and incidence of revisions: A comparison of prosthetic grafts, simple autogenous fistulas, and venous transposition fistulas from the United States Renal Data System Dialysis Morbidity and Mortality Study. J Vasc Surg 2001;34:694–700.

127. Goff CD, Sato DT, Bloch PH, et al: Steal syndrome complicating hemodialysis access procedures: Can it be predicted? Ann Vasc Surg 2000;14:138–144.

128. Wong V, Ward R, Taylor J, et al: Factors associated with early failure of arteriovenous fistulae for haemodialysis access. Eur J Vasc Endovasc Surg 1996;12:207–213.

129. Mattson WJ: Recognition and treatment of vascular steal secondary to hemodialysis prostheses. Am J Surg 1987;154:198–201.

130. Morsy AH, Kulbaski M, Chen C, et al: Incidence and characteristics of patients with hand ischemia after a hemodialysis access procedure. J Surg Res 1998;74:8–10.

131. Valji K, Hye RJ, Roberts AC, et al: Hand ischemia in patients with hemodialysis access grafts: Angiographic diagnosis and treatment. Radiology 1995;196:697–701.

132. Brennan AM, McNamara B, Plant WD, O'Halloran DJ: An atypical case of acute ischaemic monomelic neuropathy post vascular access surgery in a patient with Type 1 diabetes mellitus. Diabet Med 2005;22:813–814.

133. Miles AM: Upper limb ischemia after vascular access surgery: Differential diagnosis and management. Semin Dial 2000;13:312–315.

134. Shemesh D, Mabjeesh NJ, Abramowitz HB: Management of dialysis access-associated steal syndrome: Use of intraoperative duplex ultrasound scanning for optimal flow reduction. J Vasc Surg 1999;30:193–195.

135. Stary D, Thaow CP: Banding of the venous limb of surgically created arteriovenous fistula in the treatment of ischaemic steal syndrome. Aust N Z J Surg 2002;72:367–368.

136. Katz S, Kohl RD: The treatment of hand ischemia by arterial ligation and upper extremity bypass after angioaccess surgery. J Am Coll Surg 1996;183:239–242.

137. Knox RC, Berman SS, Hughes JD, et al: Distal revascularization-interval ligation: A durable and effective treatment for ischemic steal syndrome after hemodialysis access. J Vasc Surg 2002;36:250–255.

138. Schanzer H, Schwartz M, Harrington E, Haimov M: Treatment of ischemia due to "steal" by arteriovenous fistula with distal artery ligation and revascularization. J Vasc Surg 1988;7:770–773.

139. O'Quin RJ, Lakshminarayan S: Venous air embolism. Arch Intern Med 1982;142:2173–2176.

140. Bregman H, Daugirdas JT, Ing TS: Complications during hemodialysis. In Daugirdas JT, Ing TS (eds): Handbook of Dialysis. New York: Little, Brown, 1994, p 149.

141. Butler BD: Biophysical aspects of gas bubbles in blood. Med Instrum 1985;19:59–62.

142. Baskin SE, Wozniak RF: Hyperbaric oxygenation in the treatment of hemodialysis-associated air embolism. N Engl J Med 1975;293:184-185.

143. Arieff AI, Lazarowitz VC, Guisado R: Experimental dialysis disequilibrium syndrome: Prevention with glycerol. Kidney Int 1978;14:270–278.

144. Chen CL, Lai PH, Chou KJ, et al: A preliminary report of brain edema in patients with uremia at first hemodialysis: Evaluation by diffusion-weighted MR imaging. Am J Neuroradiol 2007;28:68–71.

145. Kishimoto T, Yamagami S, Tanaka H, et al: Superiority of hemofiltration to hemodialysis for treatment of chronic renal failure: Comparative studies between hemofiltration and hemodialysis on dialysis disequilibrium syndrome. Artif Organs 1980;4:86–93.

146. Posner JB, Plum F: Spinal-fluid pH and neurologic symptoms in systemic acidosis. N Engl J Med 1967;277:605–613.

147. Trinh-Trang-Tan MM, Cartron JP, Bankir L: Molecular basis for the dialysis disequilibrium syndrome: Altered aquaporin and urea transporter expression in the brain. Nephrol Dial Transplant 2005;20:1984–1988.

148. Basile C, Miller JD, Koles ZJ, et al: The effects of dialysis on brain water and EEG in stable chronic uremia. Am J Kidney Dis 1987;9:462–469.

149. Platts MM, Anastassiades E: Dialysis encephalopathy: Precipitating factors and improvement in prognosis. Clin Nephrol 1981;15:223–228.

150. Uysal S, Renda Y, Saatci U, Yalaz K: Neurologic complications in chronic renal failure: A retrospective study. Clin Pediatr (Phila) 1990;29:510–514.

151. Ali II, Pirzada NA: Neurologic complications associated with dialysis and chronic renal insufficiency. In Henrich WL (ed.): Principles and Practice of Dialysis. Philadelphia: Lippincott, Williams and Wilkins, 2004, p 507.

152. Arieff AI: Dialysis disequilibrium syndrome: Current concepts on pathogenesis and prevention. Kidney Int 1994;45:629–635.

153. Mahoney CA, Arieff AI: Uremic encephalopathies: Clinical, biochemical, and experimental features. Am J Kidney Dis 1982;2:324–336.

154. Port FK, Johnson WJ, Klass DW: Prevention of dialysis disequilibrium syndrome by use of high sodium concentration in the dialysate. Kidney Int 1973;3:327–333.

155. Riley JD, Antony SJ: Leg cramps: Differential diagnosis and management. Am Fam Physician 1995;52:1794–1798.

156. Caress JB, Walker FO: The spectrum of ectopic motor nerve behavior: From fasciculations to neuromyotonia. Neurologist 2002;8:41–46.

157. Feinfeld DA, Kurian P, Cheng JT, et al: Effect of oral l-carnitine on serum myoglobin in hemodialysis patients. Ren Fail 1996;18: 91–96.

158. Ahmad S: l-Carnitine in dialysis patients. Semin Dial 2001;14: 209–217.

159. Roy L, Bannon P, Villeneuve JP: Quinine pharmacokinetics in chronic haemodialysis patients. Br J Clin Pharmacol 2002;54: 604–609.

160. Sadowski RH, Allred EN, Jabs K: Sodium modeling ameliorates intradialytic and interdialytic symptoms in young hemodialysis patients. J Am Soc Nephrol 1993;4:1192–1198.

161. Rathod R, Baig MS, Khandelwal PN, et al: Results of a single blind, randomized, placebo-controlled clinical trial to study the effect of intravenous L-carnitine supplementation on health-related quality of life in Indian patients on maintenance hemodialysis. Indian J Med Sci 2006;60:143–153.

162. Canzanello VJ, Hylander-Rossner B, Sands RE, et al: Comparison of 50% dextrose water, 25% mannitol, and 23.5% saline for the treatment of hemodialysis-associated muscle cramps. ASAIO Trans 1991;37:649–652.

163. Bana DS, Yap AU, Graham JR: Headache during hemodialysis. Headache 1972;12:1–14.

164. Goksan B, Karaali-Savrun F, Ertan S, Savrun M: Haemodialysis-related headache. Cephalalgia 2004;24:284–287.

165. Ramirez G, Bercaw BL, Butcher DE, et al: The role of glucose in hemodialysis: The effects of glucose-free dialysate. Am J Kidney Dis 1986;7:413–420.

166. Kruger BR: Restless leg syndrome and periodic movements of sleep. Mayo Clin Proc 1990;65:999–1006.

167. Molnar MZ, Novak M, Mucsi I: Management of restless legs syndrome in patients on dialysis. Drugs 2006;66:607–624.

168. Montplaisir J, Nicolas A, Denesle R, Gomez–Mancilla B: Restless legs syndrome improved by pramipexole: A double-blind randomized trial. Neurology 1999;52:938–943.

169. McGee DC, Gould MK: Preventing complications of central venous catheterization. N Engl J Med 2003;348:1123–1133.

170. Eschbach JW, Adamson JW: Anemia of end-stage renal disease (ESRD). Kidney Int 1985;28:1–5.

171. Eschbach JW, Adamson JW: Modern aspects of the pathophysiology of renal anemia. Contrib Nephrol 1988;66:63–70.

172. Eschbach JW, Haley NR, Adamson JW: The anemia of chronic renal failure: Pathophysiology and effects of recombinant erythropoietin. Contrib Nephrol 1990;78:24–36.

173. Eaton JW, Leida MN: Hemolysis in chronic renal failure. Semin Nephrol 1985;5:133–139.

174. Centers for Disease Control and Prevention: Multistate outbreak of hemolysis in hemodialysis patients—Nebraska and Maryland, 1998. JAMA 1998;280:1299–1300.

175. Duffy R, Tomashek K, Spangenberg M, et al: Multistate outbreak of hemolysis in hemodialysis patients traced to faulty blood tubing sets. Kidney Int 2000;57:1668–1674.

176. Fluck S, McKane W, Cairns T, et al: Chloramine-induced haemolysis presenting as erythropoietin resistance. Nephrol Dial Transplant 1999;14:1687–1691.

177. Fenves AZ, Gipson JS, Pancorvo C: Chloramine-induced methemoglobinemia in a hemodialysis patient. Semin Dial 2000;13: 327–329.

178. Perez-Garcia R, Verde E, Sanz A, Valderrabano F: r-HuEPO resistance and dialysate chloramine contamination in patients on hemodialysis. Nephron 2000;86:222–223.

179. Gordon SM, Bland LA, Alexander SR, et al: Hemolysis associated with hydrogen peroxide at a pediatric dialysis center. Am J Nephrol 1990;10:123–127.

180. Van der Niepen P, Sennesael JJ, Verbeelen DL: Kinin kinetics during different dialysis protocols with AN69 dialyser in ACEI-treated patients. Nephrol Dial Transplant 1995;10:1689–1695.

181. Samouilidou E, Grapsa E, Karpouza A, Lagouranis A: Reactive oxygen metabolites: A link between oxidative stress and inflammation in patients on hemodialysis. Blood Purif 2007; 25:175–178.

182. Coskun C, Kural A, Doventas Y, et al: Hemodialysis and protein oxidation products. Ann N Y Acad Sci 2007;1100:404–408.

183. Horl WH, Schaefer RM, Heidland A: Effect of different dialyzers on proteinases and proteinase inhibitors during hemodialysis. Am J Nephrol 1985;5:320–326.

184. Pereira BJ, Dinarello CA: Role of cytokines in patients on dialysis. Int J Artif Organs 1995;18:293–304.

185. Vanholder R, Ringoir S, Dhondt A, Hakim RM: Phagocytosis in uremic an hemodialysis patients: A prospective and cross sectional study. Kidney Int 1991;39:320–327.

186. Sreedhara R, Itagaki I, Lynn B, Hakim RM: Defective platelet aggregation in uremia in transiently worsened by hemodialysis. Am J Kidney Disease 1995;25:555–563.

187. Speiser W, Wojta J, Korninger C, et al: Enhanced fibrinolysis caused by tissue plasminogen activator release in hemodialysis. Kidney Int 1987;32:280–283.

188. Gerard C, Hugli TE: Identification of classical anaphylatoxin as the des-Arg form of the C5a molecule: Evidence for a modulator role for the oligosaccharide unit in human des-Arg74-C5a. Proc Natl Acad Sci U S A 1981;78:1833–1837.

189. Hugli TE: The structural basis for anaphylatoxin and chemotactic functions of C3a, C4a, and C5a. Crit Rev Immunol 1981;1: 321–366.

190. Ivanovich P, Chenoweth DE, Schmidt R, et al: Symptoms and activation of granulocytes and complement with two dialysis membranes. Kidney Int 1983;24:758–763.

191. Laude-Sharp M, Caroff M, Simard L, et al: Induction of IL-1 during hemodialysis: Transmembrane passage of intact endotoxin (LPS). Kidney Int 1990;38:1089–1094.

192. Lonnemann G: The quality of dialysate: An integrated approach. Kidney Int 2000;76(Suppl):S112–S119.

193. Hakim RM, Wingard RL, Parker RA: Effect of the dialysis membrane in the treatment of patients with acure renal failure. N Engl J Med 1994;331:1338–1342.

194. Hakim RM: Influence of the dialysis membrane on outcome of ESRD patients. Am J Kidney Dis 1998;32(6 Suppl 4):S71–S75.

195. Bloembergen WE, Hakim RM, Stannard DC, et al: Relationship of dialysis membrane and cause-specific mortality. Am J Kidney Dis 1999;33:1–10.

196. Lindholm DD, Murray JS: A simplified method of regional heparinization during hemodialysis according to a predetermined dosage formula. Trans Am Soc Artif Intern Organs 1964; 10:92–97.

197. Lohr JW, Slusher S, Diederich DA: Regional citrate anticoagulation for hemodialysis following cardiovascular surgery. Am J Nephrol 1988;8:368–372.

198. Lohr JW, Slusher S, Diederich D: Safety of regional citrate hemodialysis in acute renal failure. Am J Kidney Dis 1989;13:104–107.

199. Kelleher SP, Schulman G: Severe metabolic alkalosis complicating regional citrate hemodialysis. Am J Kidney Dis 1987;9:235–236.

200. Hocken AG, Hurst PL: Citrate regional anticoagulation in haemodialysis. Nephron 1987;46:7–10.

201. Yamamoto S, Koide M, Matsuo M, et al: Heparin-induced thrombocytopenia in hemodialysis patients. Am J Kidney Dis 1996;28:82–85.

202. Aurigemma NM, Feldman NT, Gottlieb M, et al: Arterial oxygenation during hemodialysis. N Engl J Med 1977;297:871–873.

203. Craddock PR, Fehr J, Brigham KL, et al: Complement and leukocyte-mediated pulmonary dysfunction in hemodialysis. N Engl J Med 1977;296:769–774.

204. De Backer WA, Verpooten GA, Borgonjon DJ, et al: Hypoxemia during hemodialysis: Effects of different membranes and dialysate compositions. Kidney Int 1983;23:738–743.

205. bu-Hamdan DK, Desai SG, Mahajan SK, et al: Hypoxemia during hemodialysis using acetate versus bicarbonate dialysate. Am J Nephrol 1984;4:248–253.

206. Fawcett S, Hoenich NA, Laker MF, et al: Haemodialysis-induced respiratory changes. Nephrol Dial Transplant 1987;2:161–168.

207. Feig PU, Shook A, Sterns RH: Effect of potassium removal during hemodialysis on the plasma potassium concentration. Nephron 1981;27:25–30.

208. Spital A, Sterns RH: Potassium homeostasis in dialysis patients. Semin Dial 1988;1:14–20.

209. Redaelli B, Sturzini S, Bonoldi L: Potassium removal as a factor limiting the correction of acidosis during dialysis. Proc EDTA 1982;19:366–371.

210. Redaelli B, Locatelli F, Limido D, et al: Effect of a new model of hemodialysis potassium removal on the control of ventricular arrhythmias. Kidney Int 1996;50:609–617.

211. Kimura G, Van Stone JC, Bauer JH, Keshaviah PR: A simulation study on transcellular fluid shifts induced by hemodialysis. Kidney Int 1983;24:542–548.

212. Joki N, Nikolov IG, Drueke TB: Optimal dialysate calcium concentration and vascular calcification. Nephrol Dial Transplant 2007;22:3354–3355.

213. Carney SL, Gillies AH: Effect of an optimum dialysis fluid calcium concentration on calcium mass transfer during maintenance hemodialysis. Clin Nephrol 1985;24:28–30.

214. Morrison G, Michelson EL, Brown S, Morganroth J: Mechanism and prevention of cardiac arrhythmias in chronic hemodialysis patients. Kidney Int 1980;17:811–819.

215. Uldall R, Ouwendyk M, Francoeur R, et al: Slow nocturnal home hemodialysis at the Wellesley Hospital. Adv Ren Replace Ther 1996;3:133–136.

216. Yu AW, Soundararajan R, Nawab ZM, et al: Raising plasma phosphorus levels by phosphorus-enriched, bicarbonate-containing dialysate in hemodialysis patients. Artif Organs 1992;16:414–416.

217. Kwan BC, Kronenberg F, Beddhu S, Cheung AK: Lipoprotein metabolism and lipid management in chronic kidney disease. J Am Soc Nephrol 2007;18:1246–1261.

218. Ibels SL, Reardon MF, Nestel PJ: Plasma post-heparin lipolytic activity and triglyceride clearance in uremic and hemodialysis patients and renal allograft recipients. J Lab Clin Med 1976;87:648–658.

219. Nasstrom B, Stegmayr B, Gupta J, et al: A single bolus of a low molecular weight heparin to patients on haemodialysis depletes lipoprotein lipase stores and retards triglyceride clearing. Nephrol Dial Transplant 2005;20:1172–1179.

220. Himmelfarb J, McMonagle E, McMenamin E: Plasma protein thiol oxidation and carbonyl formation in chronic renal failure. Kidney Int 2000;58:2571–2578.

221. Triolo L, Malaguti M, Ansali F, et al: Vitamin E-bonded cellulose membrane, lipoperoxidation, and anemia in hemodialysis patients. Artif Cells Blood Substit Immobil Biotechnol 2003;31:185–191.

222. Tepper T, van der Hem GK, Tuma GJ, et al: Loss of amino acids during hemodialysis: Quantitative and qualitative investigations. Clin Nephrol 1978;10:16–20.

223. Ikizler TA, Flakoll PJ, Parker RA, Hakim RM: Amino acid and albumin losses during hemodialysis. Kidney Int 1994;46:830–837.

224. Cheung AK, Agodoa LY, Daugirdas JT, et al, for the Hemodialysis (HEMO) Study Group: Effects of hemodialyzer reuse on clearances of urea and β_2-microglobulin. J Am Soc Nephrol 1999;10:117–127.

225. Gutierrez A, Alvestrand A, Wahren J, Bergöstrom J: Effect of in vivo contact between blood and dialysis membranes on protein catabolism in humans. Kidney Int 1990;38:487–494.

226. Leypoldt JK, Cheung AK, Carroll CE, et al: Effect of dialysis membranes and middle molecule removal on chronic hemodialysis patient survival. Am J Kidney Dis 1999;33:349–355.

227. Wrone EM, Hornberger JM, Zehnder JL, et al: Randomized trial of folic acid for prevention of cardiovascular events in end-stage renal disease. J Am Soc Nephrol 2004;15:420–426.

228. Jamison RL, Hartigan P, Kaufman JS, et al, for the Veterans Affairs Site Investigators: Effect of homocysteine lowering on mortality and vascular disease in advanced chronic kidney disease and end-stage renal disease: A randomized controlled trial. JAMA 2007;298:1163–1170.

229. Canaud B, Bosc JY, Leray H, et al: Microbiologic purity of dialysate: Rationale and technical aspects. Blood Purif 2000;18:200–213.

230. Terrier N, Senecal L, Dupuy AM, et al: Association between novel indices of malnutrition-inflammation complex syndrome and cardiovascular disease in hemodialysis patients. Hemodial Int 2005;9:159–168.

231. Marion K, Pasmore M, Freney J, et al: A new procedure allowing the complete removal and prevention of hemodialysis biofilms. Blood Purif 2005;23:339–348.

232. Tapia G, Yee J: Biofilm: Its relevance in kidney disease. Adv Chronic Kidney Dis 2006;13:215–224.

233. van der Linde K, Lim BT, Rondeel JM, et al: Improved bacteriological surveillance of haemodialysis fluids: A comparison between Tryptic soy agar and Reasoner's 2A media. Nephrol Dial Transplant 1999;14:2433–2437.

234. Lonnemann G: Chronic inflammation in hemodialysis: The role of contaminated dialysate. Blood Purif 2000;18:214–223.

235. Lonnemann G: Should ultra-pure dialysate be mandatory? Nephrol Dial Transplant 2000;15(Suppl 1):55–59.

236. Laurence RA, Lapierre ST: Quality of hemodialysis water: A 7-year multicenter study. Am J Kidney Dis 1995;25:738–750.

237. Ledebo I, Nystrand R: Defining the microbiological quality of dialysis fluid. Artif Organs 1999;23:37–43.

238. Ouseph R, Ward RA: Ultrapure dialysate for home hemodialysis? Adv Chronic Kidney Dis 2007;14:256–262.

239. Tetta C, David S, Marcelli D, et al: Clinical effects of online dialysate and infusion fluids. Hemodial Int 2006;10(Suppl 1):S60–S66.

240. Schindler R, Lonnemann G, Schaffer J, et al: The effect of ultrafiltered dialysate on the cellular content of interleukin-1 receptor antagonist in patients on chronic hemodialysis. Nephron 1994;68:229–233.

241. Sitter T, Bergner A, Schiffl H: Dialysate related cytokine induction and response to recombinant human erythropoietin in haemodialysis patients. Nephrol Dial Transplant 2000;15:1207–1211.

242. Arizono K, Nomura K, Motoyama T, et al: Use of ultrapure dialysate in reduction of chronic inflammation during hemodialysis. Blood Purif 2004;22(Suppl 2):26–29.

243. Kleophas W, Haastert B, Backus G, et al: Long-term experience with an ultrapure individual dialysis fluid with a batch type machine. Nephrol Dial Transplant 1998;13:3118–3125.

244. Schiffl H, Lang SM, Stratakis D, Fischer R: Effects of ultrapure dialysis fluid on nutritional status and inflammatory parameters. Nephrol Dial Transplant 2001;16:1863–1869.

245. Baz M, Durand C, Ragon A, et al: Using ultrapure water in hemodialysis delays carpal tunnel syndrome. Int J Artif Organs 1991;14:681–685.

246. Furuya R, Kumagai H, Takahashi M, et al: Ultrapure dialysate reduces plasma levels of β_2-microglobulin and pentosidine in hemodialysis patients. Blood Purif 2005;23:311–316.

247. Izuhara Y, Miyata T, Saito K, et al: Ultrapure dialysate decreases plasma pentosidine, a marker of "carbonyl stress." Am J Kidney Dis 2004;43:1024–1029.

248. Hsu PY, Lin CL, Yu CC, et al: Ultrapure dialysate improves iron utilization and erythropoietin response in chronic hemodialysis patients—a prospective cross-over study. J Nephrol 2004;17:693–700.

249. Schiffl H, Lang SM, Bergner A: Ultrapure dialysate reduces dose of recombinant human erythropoietin. Nephron 1999;83:278–279.

250. Schiffl H, Lang SM, Fischer R: Ultrapure dialysis fluid slows loss of residual renal function in new dialysis patients. Nephrol Dial Transplant 2002;17:1814–1818.

251. Bommer J, Jaber BL: Ultrapure dialysate: Facts and myths. Semin Dial 2006;19:115–119.

252. Lamas JM, Alonso M, Sastre F, et al: Ultrapure dialysate and inflammatory response in haemodialysis evaluated by darbepoetin requirements—a randomized study. Nephrol Dial Transplant 2006;21:2851–2858.

253. Tielemans C, Hoenich NA, Levin NW, et al: Are standards for dialysate purity in hemodialysis insufficiently strict? Semin Dial 2001;14:328–336.

254. Ward RA: Ultrapure dialysate. Semin Dial 2004;17:489–497.

255. Delarocque-Astagneau E, Baffoy N, Thiers V, et al: Outbreak of hepatitis C virus infection in a hemodialysis unit: Potential transmission by the hemodialysis machine? Infect Control Hosp Epidemiol 2002;23(6):328–334.

256. Olmer M, Bouchouareb D, Zandotti C, et al: Transmission of the hepatitis C virus in an hemodialysis unit: Evidence for nosocomial infection. Clin Nephrol 1997;47:263–270.

257. Hardy NM, Chiao J, Arora N, et al: Hepatitis C virus in the hemodialysis setting: Detecting viral RNA from blood port caps by reverse transcription-polymerase chain reaction. Clin Nephrol 2000;54:143–146.

258. Marmion BP, Burrell CJ, Tonkin RW, Dickson J: Dialysis-associated hepatitis in Edinburgh; 1969–1978. Rev Infect Dis 1982;4:619–637.

259. Fissell RB, Bragg-Gresham JL, Woods JD, et al: Patterns of hepatitis C prevalence and seroconversion in hemodialysis units from three continents: The DOPPS. Kidney Int 2004;65:2335–2342.

260. Hinrichsen H, Leimenstoll G, Stegen G, et al: Prevalence and risk factors of hepatitis C virus infection in haemodialysis patients: A multicentre study in 2796 patients. Gut 2002;51:429–433.

261. Petrosillo N, Gilli P, Serraino D, et al: Prevalence of infected patients and understaffing have a role in hepatitis C virus transmission in dialysis. Am J Kidney Dis 2001;37:1004–1010.

262. Di Bisceglie AM: Hepatitis G virus infection: A work in progress. Ann Intern Med 1996;125:772–773.

263. Tanaka E, Alter HJ, Nakatsuji Y, et al: Effect of hepatitis G virus infection on chronic hepatitis C. Ann Intern Med 1996;125:740–743.

264. Alter HJ: The cloning and clinical implications of HGV and HGBV-C. N Engl J Med 1996;334:1536–1537.

265. de Medina M, Ashby M, Schluter V, et al: Prevalence of hepatitis C and G virus infection in chronic hemodialysis patients. Am J Kidney Dis 1998;31:224–226.

266. Hinrichsen H, Leimenstoll G, Stegen G, et al: Prevalence of and risk factors for hepatitis G (HGV) infection in haemodialysis patients: A multicentre study. Nephrol Dial Transplant 2002;17:271–275.

267. Sampietro M, Badalamenti S, Graziani G, et al: Hepatitis G virus infection in hemodialysis patients. Kidney Int 1997;51:348–352.

268. Masuko K, Mitsui T, Iwano K, et al: Infection with hepatitis GB virus C in patients on maintenance hemodialysis. N Engl J Med 1996. 334:1485–1490.

269. de Lamballerie X, Charrel RN, Dussol B: Hepatitis GB virus C in patients on hemodialysis. N Engl J Med 1996;334:1549.

270. Sampietro M, Badalamenti S, Lunghi G: Hepatitis GB virus C. N Engl J Med 1996;335:1392.

271. Tsuda F, Hadiwandowo S, Sawada N, et al: Infection with GB virus C (GBV-C) in patients with chronic liver disease or on maintenance hemodialysis in Indonesia. J Med Virol 1996;49:248–252.

272. Yu ML, Chuang WL, Dai CY, et al: GB virus C/hepatitis G virus infection in chronic hepatitis C patients with and without interferon-alpha therapy. Antiviral Res 2001;52:241–249.

273. Espersen T, Schmitz O, Hansen HE, et al: Ovulation in uremic women: The reproductive cycle in women on chronic hemodialysis. Int J Fertil 1988. 33:103–106.

274. Toorians AW, Janssen E, Laan E, et al: Chronic renal failure and sexual functioning: Clinical status versus objectively assessed sexual response. Nephrol Dial Transplant 1997;12:2654–2663.

275. Diemont WL, Vruggink PA, Meuleman EJ, et al: Sexual dysfunction after renal replacement therapy. Am J Kidney Dis 2000;35:845–851.

276. Bagon JA, Vernaeve H, De Muylder X, et al: Pregnancy and dialysis. Am J Kidney Dis 1998;31:756–765.

277. Okundaye I, Abrinko P, Hou S: Registry of pregnancy in dialysis patients. Am J Kidney Dis 1998;31:766–773.

278. Brookhyser J, Wiggins K: Medical nutrition therapy in pregnancy and kidney disease. Adv Ren Replace Ther 1998;5:53–63.

279. Hou S: Pregnancy in chronic renal insufficiency and end-stage renal disease. Am J Kidney Dis 1999;33:235–252.

280. Hull AR: More dialysis appears beneficial for pregnant ESRD patients (at least in Belgium). Am J Kidney Dis 1998;31:863–864.

281. Giatras I, Levy DP, Malone FD, et al: Pregnancy during dialysis: Case report and management guidelines. Nephrol Dial Transplant 1998;13:3266–3272.

282. Toma H, Tanabe K, Tokumoto T, et al: Pregnancy in women receiving renal dialysis or transplantation in Japan: A nationwide survey. Nephrol Dial Transplant 1999;14:1511–1516.

283. Maruyama H, Shimada H, Obayashi H, et al: Requiring higher doses of erythropoietin suggests pregnancy in hemodialysis patients. Nephron 1998;79:413–419.

Further Reading

Herzog CA: Can we prevent sudden cardiac death in dialysis patients? Clin J Am Soc Nephrol 2007;2:410–412.

Pun PH, Lehrich RW, Smith SR, Middleton JP: Predictors of survival after cardiac arrest in outpatient hemodialysis clinics. Clin J Am Soc Nephrol 2007;2:491–500.

Reddy SS, Holley JL: Management of the pregnant chronic dialysis patient. Adv Chronic Kidney Dis 2007;14:146–155.

Sun CY, Wu MS: Renal transplantation reversed intractable hypotension in a diabetic patient. Diabetes Care 2007;30:e65.

Veldt BJ, Heathcote EJ, Wedemeyer H, et al: Sustained virologic response and clinical outcomes in patients with chronic hepatitis C and advanced fibrosis. Ann Intern Med 2007;147:677–684.

Chapter 81

Techniques in Peritoneal Dialysis

John Burkart

In 2004, there were 335,963 patients on dialysis in the United States. Of these, 91.4% were on in-center hemodialysis, 0.6% on home hemodialysis, 3.2% on continuous ambulatory peritoneal dialysis (CAPD), and 4.4% on automated peritoneal dialysis (APD).[1] There were 6686 incident peritoneal dialysis (PD) patients that year, 40% of whom had diabetes mellitus as their primary cause of end-stage renal disease, 31% of whom were older than age 65 years, and 59% of whom were male. Where PD is an accepted practice, in 2004 the reported percentages of dialysis patients on PD varied from lows of 3.6% in Japan and 5.1% in Germany to 42.6% in New Zealand and a high of 69.9% in Mexico, suggesting that there may not be medical reasons for the modality distribution between PD and hemodialysis (HD) seen in the United States.[1] It appears there are other, nonmedical reasons for modality distribution that are multifactorial in origin and include but are not limited to access to PD, physician comfort/expertise with the therapy, and government reimbursement policies.[2,3]

Potential benefits of PD include simplicity of use, lower cost, relatively less restricted diet, easier availability to travel, and potential survival advantage for certain subgroups of patients compared to hemodialysis. The principal components of the therapy are rather simple and have been reviewed elsewhere.[4] As with hemodialysis, the dialysate and blood compartments in PD are separated by a semipermeable membrane, which serves as a selective barrier for the diffusive clearance of retained solutes and osmotic-driven removal of excess water from the peritoneal capillaries to the peritoneal dialysis fluids.

Unlike hemodialysis, in which the blood is brought to the dialysate so that the blood circuit and dialysis fluids are extracorporeal, in PD, the dialysis fluids are intraperitoneal and therefore sterile, and the blood supply is that of the peritoneal organs and abdominal wall. Peritoneal fluid is instilled into the peritoneal cavity and allowed to "dwell" therein while diffusion and ultrafiltration takes place. The fluid is then drained at specified intervals so new fluid can be instilled and the processes of diffusion and ultrafiltration renewed. Patients can either do all these dialysis fluid "exchanges" manually (i.e., CAPD) or one can use an automated device (i.e., APD) to assist in these exchanges while the patient sleeps.

To understand the nuances between these techniques and how to individualize a patient's prescription, it is important to have a basic understanding of peritoneal physiology and the physics of peritoneal ultrafiltration. This physiology and types of PD solutions available are briefly reviewed in this chapter. As with any form of dialysis, it is important to have access to the blood system, so PD catheters are also reviewed.

COMPONENTS OF THE PERITONEAL DIALYSIS SYSTEM

Renal replacement therapies require three key components: (1) access to the bloodstream so that blood and dialysate compartments are separated by a semipermeable membrane, (2) dialysis solutions, and (3) the semipermeable membrane.

In the case of PD, this semipermeable membrane is the peritoneal membrane itself and its associated vascular supply. Each of these components has some distinct differences from its counterpart in hemodialysis. First, the optimal chronic PD access must traverse both a sterile (intraperitoneal portion) and a nonsterile (extraperitoneal portion) environment as opposed to the sterile, subcutaneous placement of the optimal accesses in use for chronic hemodialysis (the subcutaneous fistula or synthetic graft). The access is for delivery of the PD solutions in PD, whereas it is used to access the blood supply and establish an extracorporeal circuit in HD. Second, PD solutions must be sterile, easily stored, and easily transported to the patient's home. Third, PD patients are "born" with their dialyzer membrane. However, just as with HD, PD patients have different membrane types (in terms of diffusion of small solutes). The physician must learn how to tailor the therapy for each patient's peritoneal membrane type by adjusting dwell time and dialysis solutions.

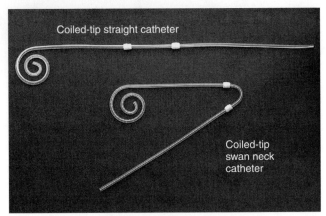

Figure 81-1   Standard peritoneal dialysis catheters.

CATHETERS

Catheter Design

The sole purpose of the PD catheter is to provide quick and easy access for the dialysis fluids to the intraperitoneal space in a way that minimizes risk for bacterial or fungal contamination and resultant infection.

Acute Use Catheters

Acute use PD catheters were a historical approach to access the peritoneum. Introduced by Westin and Roberts[5] in 1965, they were straight, relatively rigid conduits about 3 mm in diameter and 25 to 30 mm in length that could be placed at the bedside. This catheter design was associated with a high risk for peritonitis, malfunction, and bowel perforation. Therefore, their use has largely been abandoned; if PD is contemplated for acute renal failure, even in an intensive care unit setting, the safer, more current chronic use catheter is recommended.

Chronic Use Catheters

Standard chronic indwelling peritoneal catheters are constructed of soft materials, such as silicone rubber or polyurethane. The most frequently used material is silicone rubber, a polymer of methylsilicate. It is relatively biocompatible and inert, has no leachable plasticizers, and is not traumatic to surrounding tissues. Polyurethane catheters have better wall strength and, therefore, can be manufactured with a smaller catheter wall thickness, larger internal lumen, and increased flow rates with the same external diameter catheter.[6] However, cracking of the polyurethane catheter has been reported, especially after prolonged exit site care with polyethylene glycol, alcohol, or topical mupirocin. This catheter material is therefore not likely to be reliable for long-term use.

Design Modifications

Historical chronic use PD catheters were a straight tube with multiple side holes at the intraperitoneal end for dispersion of PD fluid. Straight PD catheters were associated with a high rate of pain on inflow, external cuff extrusion, and catheter migration (often resulting in failure to drain). These complications led to design modifications to both the subcutaneous and intraperitoneal portions of the catheter. The intraperitoneal portion of chronic use catheters usually contains many 1-mm side holes for passage of fluids, but it may also have modifications to facilitate fluid movement, alleviate symptoms associated with inflow or drainage, decrease catheter migration, and prevent trapping by omentum. These modifications include a curled tip, two perpendicular discs (Oreopoulos-Zellerman), and a column disc (Lifecath). Extraperitoneal modifications include various means of external fixation and preformed angles in the subcutaneous portion designed to prevent catheter infections, migrations, and dialysate leaks. Some of these are shown schematically in Figure 81-1.

Design modifications to the subcutaneous portion of the catheter include alterations in location and number of subcutaneous Dacron cuffs and the use of disc-bubble cuffs. Other alterations of the subcutaneous portion of the catheter include a pail-handle design (Cruz catheter), a 90-degree turn (Lifecath), and a fixed bend, or swan neck in the catheter.[7] Catheters with two cuffs allow the fixation of both the deep preperitoneal and subcutaneous portions of the catheter. If the superficial subcutaneous cuff is infected, one can shave it off and the deep cuff still serves as an anchor. Swan neck catheters have two cuffs, but they also have a permanent bend in the subcutaneous portion of the catheter. This results in an arcuate tunnel that is convex upward so that both the internal (peritoneal) and external (skin) exits point downward. This is designed to decrease the likelihood of cuff extrusion and exit site infections. A description of the insertion technique has been reported elsewhere.[8] These catheters are reported to have a longer 3-year survival probability, lower peritonitis rates, and fewer problems with cuff extrusion or catheter migration in small cohort studies; these studies, however, do not mention patient selection criteria, and that caveat must be remembered. A further modification of this catheter type has the exit site in the presternal area.[8] This modification is based on the theory that presternal exit sites would be subject to less trauma and therefore less infection. Another advantage to the presternal exit location is that it allows patients to "immerse" in water (i.e., to use hot tubs and baths without immersing the exit site). Conventional wisdom suggests that obese patients should all have this type of catheter because it allows for better exit site location and care.

Catheter Implantation Techniques

PD catheter implantation and postoperative care have a significant influence on long-term catheter outcome. Sterile conditions are essential, and an experienced catheter insertion team is needed. A panel of experts has agreed on five general standards for catheter placement: (1) the deep cuff should be in the anterior abdominal musculature; (2) the subcutaneous cuff should be near the skin surface and not less than 2 cm from the exit site to allow for drainage and provide a firm anchorage that prevents pistonlike movements of the catheter[9]; (3) the catheter exit should be positioned laterally; (4) the exit site should be directed downward or laterally; and (5) the intra-abdominal portion of the catheter should be placed between the visceral and parietal peritoneum and should not be placed in the middle of loops of bowel.[10]

The techniques for catheter insertion include the following. Surgical insertion of catheters (placement by dissection) is the most commonly used placement procedure in clinical practice today. After surgical dissection through the rectus muscle, the catheter is placed in the pelvis under direct visualization.[11] Peritoneoscopic insertion, which allows direct visualization of the course of the catheter, has results similar to those seen with surgical insertion in experienced hands.[12,13] Blind placement does not allow direct visualization of the catheter or peritoneum. This procedure should not be used in markedly obese patients and in those who have had previous abdominal surgery because of the higher risk of complications, such as bowel perforation, in patients with unsuspected adhesions. In the Moncrief-Popovich technique, at the time of implantation, the entire extraperitoneal portion of the catheter is placed subcutaneously, theoretically allowing the cuff to heal in a sterile environment and preventing any bacterial colonization. At a subsequent date (typically 4–6 weeks after implantation), the external portion of the catheter is exteriorized, and dialysis can be initiated immediately.[14]

Historical review of these techniques suggests that in appropriate patients, outcome does not depend on the technique used for implantation as much as on the person who inserts the catheter. The most important requirement may be to have a trained, knowledgeable, and dedicated catheter insertion team.[10] A recent modification of these techniques, coined the advanced laproscopic insertion technique, which includes rectus sheath tunneling (to prevent catheter tip migration), prophylactic omentopexy in appropriate patients (to prevent omental entrapment), selective resection of epiploic appendages (to prevent catheter obstruction), and adhesiolysis to eliminate compartmentalization,[15] has been reported to even further reduce complication rates. With this technique, reported risk of pericatheter dialysate leaks was 2% compared to published reports of 1% to 27%.[16]

Catheter Break-in

It is normal to flush the peritoneal cavity with between 500 and 1500 mL of dialysis fluid until clear immediately after placement. Heparin (500–1000 U/L) can be added in cases where fibrin is present. Optimally, PD should not be initiated until 10 to 14 days after catheter placement to allow wound healing and cuff maturation and to minimize the risk of leaks or infection. However, the PD catheter *can be used immediately* after placement if clinically indicated. In these cases, low-volume (if possible starting with as little as 500 mL/exchange, aiming for < 1500 mL/exchange), supine PD should be prescribed. Often the patient has some residual renal function, so "full doses" of PD are not needed. Furthermore, the risk of leak and peritonitis during these urgent PD starts should be less than the risk of bacteremia from a tunneled HD catheter in experienced hands. Experience from using the Moncrief-Popovich insertion technique suggests that the catheter does not need to be flushed during the postoperative period. Nevertheless, some authors recommend periodic flushing; if done, a once-weekly approach seems reasonable. After catheter implantation, the exit site should be covered by sterile gauze and a nonocclusive dressing. The dressing should not be changed for several days unless there is evidence of excessive bleeding. To ensure optimal tissue healing during this period, the catheter should be immobilized to prevent trauma to the exit site.[17] Sutures at the exit site should be avoided. During this time, patients should avoid submerging the exit site in water. Once the catheter exit site has "matured," daily exit site care is initiated. This includes cleansing agents and prophylactic antibiotics.

Catheter Survival

Transfer from PD to HD is often precipitated by catheter-related problems; in a recent review of cohorts that started dialysis in 2000, 2001, 2002, and 2003, catheter-related problems were responsible for 17% of transfers.[18] Transfer is usually due to an issue related to catheter infection, but occasionally due to catheter migration or dialysate leaks. Early CAPD registry data (based on patients who were undergoing dialysis between January 1981 and August 1987) showed that the cumulative probability of a CAPD patient's experiencing at least one catheter replacement was 32% at 2 years and 42% at 3 years.[19] These data were collected before widespread use of swan neck type catheters, which have improved catheter survival, and laparoscopic insertion techniques. Catheter survival has been shown to correlate with the patient's weight, and weight at initiation of dialysis was predictive of catheter loss due to infectious complications.[20] Outcomes of 213 curled catheters placed either surgically or percutaneously (63%) were analyzed over a 4-year period.[21] Actuarial catheter survival was 61% at 3 years and did not differ with the implantation technique used. Kaplan-Meier survival of 138 surgically placed straight double-cuff catheters at one center was 87%, 69%, and 65%, at 1, 2, and 3 years, respectively.[22] Others[23] report a 90% 3-year survival with swan neck catheters versus 80% with the straight PD catheter. Using the advanced laparoscopic placement approach, the initial catheter success rate was 99%.[16] Once placed, catheters usually function well although occasionally there is failure to fill or drain due to malposition, kinking, or omental wrapping. This can be treated surgically or with laparoscopic intervention.[24,25]

Indications for Catheter Removal

Indications for catheter removal include malfunction, relapsing or recurrent peritonitis, peritonitis that fails to resolve, chronic exit site or tunnel infection, fungal peritonitis, *Pseudomonas*-related peritonitis that is slow to respond to therapy, perforated viscus, multiorganism-related peritonitis, recovery of kidney function, and permanent transfer to hemodialysis.[26]

DIALYSIS SOLUTIONS

The history of PD fluid development and currently available PD solutions has been reviewed elsewhere.[4] Typical peritoneal dialysis fluid solute concentrations are found in Table 81-1. These solutions have historically used lactate as the buffer (although bicarbonate-based solutions are now approved), are sterile, are easily shipped, and come in various volumes (such as 1.5-, 2-, 2.5-, and 3-L volumes for manual or automated exchanges and 5- and 6-L bags for automated exchanges). The typical osmotic agent is glucose-based (although others are available), and the ultrafiltration profile is varied by choice of osmotic agent instilled and the percent glucose concentration for glucose-containing solutions. Peritoneal dialysis solutions have an unphysiologic pH, a high osmolality, use lactate for the buffer, and contain aldehydes or glucose degradation products (GDPs) that form during the sterilization process or during storage. These GDPs can be absorbed and may cause local and systemic inflammation. Recent development and modification of these fluids has made them more *biocompatible* (lower GDP content, more physiological pH), with a more sustained ultrafiltration profile (polyglucose-icodextrin-containing solutions).

Electrolytes

Sodium

Sodium (Na^+) has been added to the dialysate in concentrations ranging from 120 to 140 mEq/L. The lower the dialysate sodium, the greater the potential for diffusion-related sodium removal.

Early during a dwell with glucose-containing fluids and crystalloid-induced ultrafiltration, some water is transported from the blood to the dialysate compartments via aquaporin channels, which allow for movement of water only and do not allow for the passage of any solutes, such as Na^+. This portion of the ultrafiltrate volume is sodium free or, in other words, *free water*. The physiologic phenomenon is called *sodium sieving*. As a result, early during a dextrose dwell, dialysate sodium decreases. This decrease is most pronounced in patients who are slow transporters and when hypertonic dialysis fluids are used. The clinical consequence is that, after multiple rapid exchanges with hypertonic glucose, systemic hypernatremia can occur.[27] During long dwells, after transcellular water movement ceases, sodium is transported from the blood to the dialysate and dialysate sodium concentrations are eventually equilibrated.

Potassium

Potassium (K^+) is not typically added to PD dialysis fluids. During a dwell, dialysate K^+ approaches equilibrium with that of plasma. Therefore, if one were to do four 2-L exchanges a day with an ultrafiltrate volume of an additional 2 L using dialysis fluid with no added K^+, the patient would tend to lose approximately 35 to 40 mEq/day in the dialysate while maintaining a serum K^+ concentration of approximately 4 mEq/L.[28] Net ultrafiltration increases K^+ removal. However, as with Na^+, ultrafiltrate concentrations are less than that in serum because of potassium sieving across transcellular aquaporins. With rapid cycling, K^+ losses are augmented, but maximal rates are approximately 8 mEq/hr.[29] If needed, K^+ removal can be slowed by adding K^+ to the dialysate. As a result of this daily removal of K^+, most PD patients do not need a potassium-restricted diet.

Calcium

It is now recognized that the calcium (Ca^{2+}) concentration of PD fluids needs to be tailored to different clinical situations.[30,31] During the late 1970s and early 1980s, the standard of care was to use calcium- or aluminum-containing binders along with dietary phosphate restriction to control serum phosphate levels. It was also common practice to treat the tendency for hypocalcemia by using a relatively high dialysate Ca^{2+} concentration (3.5 mEq/L) that would facilitate mass transfer of Ca^{2+} from the dialysis fluids to the blood. When calcium salts are used as the phosphate binder in patients also using dialysis fluids containing Ca^{2+} concentrations of 3.5 mEq/L, hypercalcemia (in 35%–56% of patients) and metastatic calcification have been frequent complications.[32–36] Because of these complications, dialysis fluids were developed with a lower, more nearly physiologic Ca^{2+} concentration (2.5 mEq/L).[37,38] Clinical trials have shown that use of dialysis fluids with a lower Ca^{2+} concentration (2.5 mEq/L) is associated with a net Ca^{2+} flux from the blood to the dialysate under most physiological conditions.[39,40] However, there is a risk of net Ca^{2+} loss in some patients, resulting in negative Ca^{2+} balance and an increase in parathyroid hormone levels.[40,41] Estimated Ca^{2+} loss with 2.5 mEq/L Ca^{2+} solutions is approximately 100 mg/dL of ultrafiltrate or 45 g/year of Ca^{2+} ($\approx$3%–4% of total bone mineral content per year). As has been noted for Na^+ and K^+, the greater the ultrafiltration volume, the greater the potential dialysate calcium loss. Although individualization is needed, it seems reasonable to use low-calcium fluids as the standard peritoneal dialysis solution for most patients. This allows the use of higher doses of Ca^{2+}-containing oral phosphate binders with

Table 81-1 Typical Peritoneal Dialysis Fluids

Components	Dextrose Fluid	Icodextrin Fluid
Dextrose (g/dL)	1.5, 2.5, 4.25	—
Icodextrin (g/dL)	—	7.5
Sodium (mEq/L)	132.0	132.0
Chloride (mEq/L)	96.0	96.0
Calcium (mEq/L)	3.5/2.5	3.5
Magnesium (mEq/L)	0.5	0.5
Lactate (mEq/L)	40.0	40.0
Osmolality (mOsm/kg)	346–485	282
pH	5.2	5.2

a lower risk of hypercalcemia or a progressive positive Ca^{2+} balance.

Buffers

Most PD fluids have a racemic mixture of both D- and L-lactate as the buffer. The normal physiologic form of lactic acid is the L-form,[42] and the normal blood level of this isomer is about 300 times that of the D-form.[43] Nolph and coworkers[44] have shown that despite the high concentration of both isomers in standard dialysis preparations (35–40 mmol/L), even with rapid cycling such as with tidal peritoneal dialysis (TPD), D-lactate levels are only minimally elevated. One significant drawback of lactate-based solutions is that the fluids have an unphysiologically low pH. This may impair cellular functions of resident peritoneal cells and cause pain on inflow in some patients. This pain can be mitigated by using TPD therapies, using bicarbonate-based solutions when available, or adding $NaHCO_3$ to the dialysate.

A bicarbonate-based buffer system would be preferable for dialysis fluids, but if stored in a single chamber precipitation of Ca^{2+} and Mg^{2+} carbonates would occur. Furthermore, a low pH is favored when heat-sterilizing glucose-containing fluids to prevent formation of aldehydes (i.e., GDPs) during sterilization and storage.[45] Use of a two-chamber bag, in which the two solutions are combined at the time of use, has been shown to be a safe and easy way to minimize GDP exposure and pain on inflow.[46,47] Long-term studies using a lactate/bicarbonate mixture (15 mmol/25 mmol/L) have been well tolerated; when compared with standard solutions, there was no difference in serum HCO_3^- levels at baseline and at the end of the study.[48]

Osmotic Agents

Glucose

Standard dialysis solutions have historically used glucose or its hydrated form, dextrose, as a crystalloid osmotic agent. These fluids have been shown to be safe, effective, readily metabolized, and inexpensive. However, glucose is not an "ideal" osmotic agent because of the following properties or effects: rapid absorption; potential for metabolic derangements, such as hyperglycemia, hyperinsulinemia,[49] hyperlipidemia,[50] and obesity[51]; necessity for an acidic dialysate pH to prevent formation of GDPs; and the potential nonenzymatic glycosylation of peritoneal tissue, especially during periods of mesothelial cell loss.[52] Because of these theoretical and potential downsides to glucose-containing fluids, other osmotic agents (i.e., polyglucose and amino acids) are also used in clinical practice. Glucose is a relatively small molecule; as such, it is readily absorbed from the peritoneal cavity by diffusion. Once the osmotic gradient is dissipated, transcapillary ultrafiltration ceases and lymphatic absorption of fluid predominates. The rate of absorption of glucose varies based on transport type, and in many patients who use a low glucose concentration (1.36% glucose = 1.5% dextrose) solution, the osmotic gradient for ultrafiltration is dissipated by 4 to 6 hours of dwell time. To augment the ultrafiltration volume or duration of the ultrafiltration profile, higher instilled concentrations of glucose can be used or alternative osmotic agents, such as the macromolecule icodextrin, which is slowly absorbed from the peritoneal cavity, can be used for the long dwell.

Amino Acids

There is an obligatory daily loss of protein (4–15 g/day) and amino acids (3–4 g/day) into the peritoneal effluent.[53] Amino acid-containing fluids could therefore potentially replace those lost amino acids[54] and provide a caloric source that would be protein-based without the concomitant phosphorus load associated with oral protein sources.[55] Possible complications include the development of metabolic acidosis and increased levels of serum urea nitrogen, at times necessitating an increased dialysis dose. Most,[56,57] but not all,[58] studies have shown a benefit in nutritional parameters with amino acid-containing solutions over the short term. A long-term observational study using 1.1% amino acid solutions in malnourished Korean patients showed a significant improvement in lean body mass (72% of patients) and hand grip strength but no change in serum albumin.[59] Despite data that show that daily absorption of amino acids exceeds daily protein losses and that short-term balance studies suggest a benefit,[54] the long-term usefulness of intraperitoneal amino acids has been controversial. Ultrafiltration rates for 1.1% amino acids are similar to those using 1.5% dextrose solutions. An emerging approach to prescribing PD is to use a *glucose-sparing* PD prescription (i.e., one that minimizes glucose exposure by substituting amino acids, minimizing hypertonic glucose solutions, and using icodextrin for ultrafiltration during the long dwells).[60]

Icodextrin

Traditionally, ultrafiltration in PD is due to *crystalloid* osmotic differences between solutions, but *colloid* osmosis is also possible. In this situation, the direction of the osmotic force is determined by the differences in the number of macromolecules in one solution versus the other, even if both are of similar osmolality. In this case the solvent (water) will move to the solution with the larger number of macromolecules.[61]

Polymers of glucose (polyglucose or icodextrin) can be used to induce colloid-induced ultrafiltration and are currently in clinical use, because there is potentially more sodium and middle molecule removal than seen with some glucose dwells with similar ultrafiltration volumes.[62] Another difference is that ultrafiltration with glucose is rapid and occurs early in the dwell (due to large crystalloid osmotic gradient), decreasing over time as glucose is absorbed, whereas with polyglucose, ultrafiltration is slow but sustained throughout long dwells (up to 16 hours) (see Table 81-1). Furthermore, because removal from the peritoneal cavity is by lymphatic absorption and not by diffusion, the rate of absorption is not influenced by peritoneal transport type, as is the absorption rate of glucose by diffusion. There is a growing indication for polyglucose for the long dwell (nighttime, CAPD; daytime, CCPD) to avoid excessive glucose accumulation and to achieve sustained ultrafiltration without hypertonic glucose. The safety of icodextrin use has been established. Complications include skin rash, which is about twice as likely as with glucose-containing fluids. Although an exfoliative reaction is occasionally seen, there has never been a reported case of Stevens-Johnson syndrome. Sterile peritonitis has been described, and usually resolves with discontinuation of the product.[63,64] The sterile peritonitis was due to an unrecognized peptidoglycan found in some batches of polyglucose that were used in Europe. This has now been identified and the production process revised. There have been no recent documented cases of this complication. Another complication is interference with certain fingerstick glucose estimations (tests that use the dehydrogenase pyrroloquinoline quinone reaction but not those that use glucose oxidation or hexokinase testing) by maltose and or other icodextrin metabolites.[65] Icodextrin and its metabolites may directly interfere with serum amylase determinations, slightly lowering values, suggesting that to make the diagnosis of pancreatitis, one may need to rely more on computed tomography or magnetic resonance imaging or serum lipase levels than serum amylase levels alone.[66]

BIOCOMPATIBILITY

The peritoneal cavity is exposed to new dialysis fluids multiple times a day. These fluids are potentially bioincompatible. They can exert biological and chemical effects locally on the peritoneal membrane, mesothelial cells, and resident leukocytes, macrophages, and fibroblasts and systemically to the absorption of GDPs and glucose itself. Despite these alterations, patients have done well on PD, at times for as long as 20 years. Nevertheless, the concept of biocompatibility is the subject of extensive research. Peritoneal biopsies in patients on long-term PD tend to show ultrastructual changes (e.g., glycosylation of capillary proteins, angioneogenesis, and fibrosis), possibly related to the dialysis solutions themselves.[52] Over time these morphologic alterations seem to be associated with clinically relevant changes in peritoneal transport and ultrafiltration abilities.[67] Occasionally these changes are associated with the development of a debilitating, sclerosing process within the peritoneum. There is concern that this may be due in part to accumulation of advanced glycation end products within the peritoneal membrane structures, precipitation of a local inflammatory state, and alteration of resident cell function.[60,68] Preliminary studies suggest that low-GDP solutions may result in better preserved markers of mesothelial cell function at 1 year of use[69] and, in an observational cohort study, a superior technique and patient survival.[70]

These studies have minor flaws; further long-term data are needed to show that use of these biocompatible solutions will in fact impact positively on patient survival.

CLINICAL USES OF CHRONIC PERITONEAL DIALYSIS

Clinical Observations of Peritoneal Membrane Function

During a typical peritoneal dialysis dwell, the peritoneal effluent drain volume and the concentration of solutes in that drain volume will vary from patient to patient. These differences depend on the individual patients' peritoneal membrane transport characteristics, the infused volume/exchange, the concentration and type of osmotic agent used, rates of lymphatic absorption of fluid, and the dwell time/exchange.[71] Knowledge of individual peritoneal membrane transport characteristics can help efficiently optimize solute and fluid removal.[72]

Multiple tests measure peritoneal membrane transport characteristics; these tests are designed to *define or classify* an individual patients' rate of solute diffusion and potential fluid removal. They do not quantify the actual amount of solute or volume of fluid removed. To perform the test, a patient must bring in a 24-hour collection of dialysate effluent and residual renal volume, which is analyzed for solute clearance. Once an individual patient's peritoneal membrane transport characteristics are defined, such data can be used to *guide* prescription management and *predict* what the delivered solute removal will be with a certain prescription. Multiple tests have been developed to evaluate various aspects of peritoneal membrane function (Table 81-2). No prospective randomized trials have been designed to determine which test is best for prescription management. Each test has its strengths and weaknesses; all are useful. These have been recently reviewed.[67]

In the United States, peritoneal membrane transport/function is typically assessed by the peritoneal equilibration test (PET).[71] This test, based on observations of peritoneal transport,[34,73] is a standardized method used to categorize patients into one of four transport categories using the dialysate-

Table 81-2 Standardized Tests for Evaluating Peritoneal Membrane Transport/Function

Aspect of Peritoneal Function	METHOD OF PERITONEAL FUNCTION TESTING		
	PET	SPA	PDC
Small solute transport	D/P creatinine	MTAC creatinine	Area permeability
Ultrafiltration capacity	Drain volume	Drain volume	Estimated ultrafiltration coefficient
Ultrafiltration via water channels	—	D/P sodium	Model for sodium channel
Fluid absorption	—	Dextran 70	Derived
Permeability to macromolecules	—	Restriction coefficients	Large-pore flow

D/P, dialysate-to-plasma ratio; MTAC, mass transfer area coefficient; PDC, personal dialysis capacity; PET, peritoneal equilibration test; SPA, standard permeability analysis.

to-plasma ratio of creatinine (D/P Cr) at 4 hours: high (D/P Cr ratio > 0.81), high average (D/P Cr ratio 0.81–0.65), low-average (D/P Cr ratio 0.65–0.50), or low (D/P Cr ratio < 0.50). After an overnight dwell the PET is performed, instilling 2 L of 2.5% dextrose dialysis fluid, allowing the dialysate to dwell for 4 hours. Dialysate urea, creatinine, glucose, and Na^+ concentrations are measured at time 0 and after 2 and 4 hours of dwell time. Serum values are determined after 2 hours. In addition, 4-hour drain volume is also obtained. For each for these dwell times, D/P ratios for both urea and creatinine are obtained. The ratios of glucose at time of drain to the initial dialysis fluid glucose (D/D$_o$) are also obtained. On the basis of published data, the membrane type can be identified and prescriptions optimized. Several large retrospective studies have shown that most patients are either high-average or low-average transporters.[34,74]

A modification of the original PET using 1.36% glucose/1.5% dextrose and dextran 70, called the standard peritoneal permeability analysis was developed to better evaluate mass transfer area coefficients of small and middle molecular weight solutes and to better determine residual volume and ultrafiltration kinetics.[75] The 1.36% glucose/1.5% dextrose solutions were chosen so that there would be less of an osmotic gradient for ultrafiltration and therefore one would be better able to determine the true diffusive (i.e., mass transfer area coefficients) characteristics of the membrane under a situation in which there would be less ultrafiltration and its associated convective removal of solutes. This was subsequently modified; 3.86% glucose/4.25% dextrose solutions were substituted to maximize crystalloid osmotic ultrafiltration and optimize one's ability to evaluate pathologic variations in ultrafiltration capacity.[76] This modification allows one to evaluate aquaporin-mediated water transport and the sodium versus water removal characteristics of peritoneal transport. The International Society for Peritoneal Dialysis has recommended that a modified PET (3.86% glucose/4.25% dextrose) dwell be used to optimally evaluate patients with ultrafiltration failure.[18] Most centers use the standardized PET as the baseline test to characterize peritoneal membrane transport. The 1.36% glucose/1.5% dextrose PET and 3.86% glucose/4.25% dextrose PET were compared and no clinical differences between D/P ratios for small solutes such as creatinine were found.[77,78] These data suggest that in common clinical practice, one could compare D/P ratios for small solute transport between tests. If ultrafiltration failure is suspected the 3.86% glucose/4.25% dextrose PET would be most useful even if a 2.27% glucose/2.5% PET was done at baseline.

The initial instillation of dialysate into the peritoneal cavity and the initiation of peritoneal dialysis is associated with mild changes in local cytokine production, peritoneal vascularity, and blood flow.[79] Therefore, it is recommended that the "baseline" peritoneal membrane transport study be obtained after the first 4 to 8 weeks of dialysis.[80] During training one could "estimate" peritoneal membrane transport rate by measuring the drain volume from a 4-hour dwell of 2.5% dextrose and comparing expected D/P Cr ratios to the patient's observed drain volume.

In general, peritoneal transport is stable over time.[81] However, small cohort studies suggest that in some patients peritoneal transport changes.[67] Impaired ultrafiltration is the most common clinically noted abnormality. The prevalence of this change depends on dialysis vintage. One review using a clinical definition for ultrafiltration failure (i.e., need for hypertonic exchanges) suggested that it was present in 3% of patients at 1 year and in 31% after 6 years.[82] In another cross-sectional study of patients on PD a median of 19 months (range, 0.3–178 mo) and using a laboratory definition of ultrafiltration failure (<400 mL after a 4-hour dwell with 4.25% dextrose) impaired ultrafiltration was noted in 23% of patients.[76] The reasons for these changes are unclear. It is thought that continued exposure to nonphysiologic glucose-containing peritoneal dialysis solutions increases the vascularity and thus the "effective" surface area available for transport. Indirect evidence in support of this hypothesis is the observation that increased use of hypertonic glucose solutions preceded the change (increase) in peritoneal transport.[83] In the subgroup in whom there was no clinical need for increased use of hypertonic glucose exchanges, peritoneal transport tended not to change.[84] As a result of the observed stability of peritoneal transport over time in most patients, one does not need to routinely document peritoneal membrane transport characteristics over time with routine laboratory measurement (peritoneal membrane transport testing). However, one should obtain a baseline test to characterize peritoneal transport and then repeat the transport test whenever clinically indicated (such as in patients with unexplained volume overload, decreasing solute removal, or drain volumes).

Choice of Dialysis Modality

Most patients with end-stage renal disease have no contraindication to PD or HD. The patient should be encouraged to learn about dialysis modality choices after a discussion with the physician regarding any potential indications or contraindications to either PD or HD. Potential indications for peritoneal dialysis include patients who have problematic vascular access or who prefer home dialysis but cannot perform home hemodialysis due to a lack of a partner or suitable home environment. Absolute contraindications to peritoneal dialysis include extensive abdominal adhesions that limit dialysate flow or peritoneal surface area; bladder extrophy, gastroschisis or omphalocele and active inflammatory bowel disease because of possible increased infection risk; and physical or mental incapacity to perform peritoneal dialysis. Relative contraindications to peritoneal dialysis include a documented loss of peritoneal function noted during prior use of PD (this may have resolved after a period of peritoneal resting) and patients with recurrent diverticulitis, those with a history of ischemic bowel disease or inflammatory bowel disease, active abdominal wall or skin infections, and those with ostomies (urinary or bowel) because of increased infection risk. Despite the infection risk, PD can be used in patients with ostomies or feeding tubes when clinically indicated, as long as these have been in place for at least 2 months to allow healing at that site to minimize risk of leak.

Obese patients can do well on PD; however, some may not be able to achieve minimal Kt/V goals once anuric, especially low transporters unwilling to do a midday exchange. However, at the start of renal replacement therapy, obese patients often have significant residual kidney function and do not need a "full dose" of PD to achieve the minimal delivered total Kt/V goal. In addition, catheter placement is more challenging in the morbidly obese. Presternal catheters have been advocated to minimize risk of exit-site infections and make daily catheter care easier.

Peritoneal Dialysis Modalities

All PD therapies are based on the same physiologic principles: allow PD fluid to dwell intraperitoneally so that diffusion of solutes from blood to dialysis fluids, ultrafiltration (and convective solute removal), and absorption of wanted solutes from dialysis fluids can occur. These fluids are then drained and replaced at specified intervals to achieve therapeutic goals. Conventional wisdom suggested that patients classified as rapid transporters on PET testing would do best with shorter dwell therapies (i.e., APD, using a cycler); in contrast low transporters would do best with longer dwell therapies (i.e., dwells that are equally spaced out during the day; CAPD). It is now recognized that almost any patient can use either PD therapy at their start of renal replacement therapy; most can still do either once anuric, as long as they are willing to do a midday exchange. For convenience, most patients use a form of APD, and the percentage of patients starting on APD has been increasing yearly.[1]

Continuous Ambulatory Peritoneal Dialysis

Since the original description of CAPD in the 1970s,[85] there have been few changes in the basic therapy. Most patients do four manual exchanges per day—three daytime exchanges of about 5 hours each and one overnight exchange of about 8 or 9 hours. With this type of prescription, one is usually able to achieve adequate daily small-solute clearances due to the continuous nature of the therapy. By adjusting the dwell volumes appropriately or by adding a fourth daytime dwell (see Typical Modifications of the Dialysis Prescription in this chapter), most CAPD patients can achieve an adequate dose of dialysis.

Automated Peritoneal Dialysis or Cycler Peritoneal Dialysis

The technology for APD, prompted by our better understanding of peritoneal physiology, technology development, and attempts to make the therapy more user friendly for the patient, has evolved. The cyclers themselves are smaller and allow the patient to choose more options regarding fill volume, residual volume, and frequency of exchanges. Additionally, they have been altered so that we do not have to rely on gravity for fills and drain. Newer cyclers can interface with the dialysis unit via the internet so that prescriptions can be changed and information about patient usage and troubleshooting can be done at a distance. A typical patient is connected to the cycler for 8 to 10 hours overnight (dwell time usually depends on amount of time the patient would typically sleep).[86]

If dialysis is only done during the nighttime and the patients have a dry peritoneum during the day (*dry day*), this form of APD is called *nightly intermittent peritoneal dialysis* (NIPD). Most patients will also carry dialysate in the peritoneum for part or all of the day; these patients are considered to have a *wet day*; alternatively, they are described as performing *continuous cycling peritoneal dialysis* (CCPD). Patients on CCPD will typically program the cycler machine to perform a last bag fill; that is, the machine will deliver a dialysate exchange at the end of the nighttime cycler dialysis. The patient will disconnect from the cycler with a full abdomen and carry this fluid for part or all of the day. In some cases, the patient will perform one or more manual exchanges during the day in addition to the last bag fill exchange. These additional exchanges are usually performed so that the patient can receive an adequate dose of dialysis (see adequacy of dialysis, below).

Tidal Peritoneal Dialysis

With TPD, after the initial fill, only a portion of the dialysate is drained from the peritoneal cavity, leaving a residual volume, which is then supplemented by the repeated instillation of small tidal volumes of dialysis fluids with the use of an automated cycler.[87] The procedure is usually performed nightly. Variables to be chosen include reserve volume, tidal outflow volume, tidal replacement volume, flow rates, and frequency of the exchanges. Theoretically, maintaining an intraperitoneal reservoir by not attempting to completely drain the peritoneal cavity after each dwell results in more continuous contact of the dialysate with the peritoneal membrane. In addition, the more rapid cycling may increase mixing and prevent formation of stagnant fluid films within the abdomen. In most,[88,89] but not all studies,[90] however, the use of TPD did not result in an increase in urea or creatinine clearances compared to cycler peritoneal dialysis. The differences in results among these studies are likely due to differences in the cycler PD and TPD prescriptions chosen for analysis. Little evidence suggests that TPD can provide clearances superior to those provided by cycler dialysis. It appears that TPD can decrease abdominal discomfort during inflow and outflow due to the continual presence of some dialysate in the peritoneal cavity during the cycling procedure.[91] A major disadvantage of TPD is the cost of the large volume of fluids needed. A recent review of published studies on TPD[92] suggested that there does not appear to be the consistent enhanced clearance over APD with TPD originally suggested by animal studies. However, historical studies may not have "optimized" residual volume and drain time. These parameters and their effect on clearance are being re-examined. Despite the questionable effect on clearance, published data and clinical experience have consistently shown that TPD can improve patient comfort, reducing pain on inflow or drainage, and in some cases may minimize inflow and drainage-related device alarms.

WRITING THE DIALYSIS PRESCRIPTION

Initial Prescription

The peritoneal dialysis prescription can be developed either empirically or through the use of a computer modeling program. To optimize the prescription one should know the patient's weight, residual renal function (i.e., glomerular filtration rate), and peritoneal membrane transport characteristics. At the start of PD, peritoneal transport is not known, so the initial prescription assumes the patient is an average transporter. The prescription can then be adjusted if indicated after a PET (or other test) is performed to determine peritoneal transport and a 24-hour collection of urine and dialysate volumes is obtained to calculate solute clearance/removal (typically Kt/V).[93] To minimize the risk of leak, it is best to let the PD catheter "mature" for 10 to 14 days before starting PD.[94] However, data shows it is safe to start PD the day the catheter is placed if clinically needed. In these cases it is best to use low instilled volumes and keep the patient supine as much as possible to avoid increases in intra-abdominal pressure that could cause leakage at the catheter site. Each center needs to decide if they will use "incremental" dialysis prescriptions (i.e., target total Kt/V—dialysis and residual renal—and only prescribe enough PD so that the combined Kt/V is above the minimal goal, adjusting the PD component as renal function declines.[95] Alternatively, the center's policy may be to ignore the renal component and prescribe a "full dose" of PD no matter how much residual renal function the patient has. Both approaches work equally well as long as one carefully monitors residual renal function (every 2 months) and adjusts the peritoneal component accordingly.

Two to four weeks after initiation of peritoneal dialysis, 24-hour collections of urine and dialysate should be performed, along with serum chemistries and a complete blood count, to determine solute clearances.[93] The initial PET should be performed approximately 1 month after the initiation of dialysis. This waiting period is recommended because PET results can change during the first month of dialysis.[79] The PET is performed to establish baseline transport characteristics, rule out unexpected problems, and identify patients who are either high or low transporters. These patients will need careful attention to their prescription and drain volumes to optimize solute clearance and blood pressure control once they become anuric. If clearances are below target, the prescription should be modified and adequacy testing repeated.

Typical Modifications of the Dialysis Prescription

It is important to remember that solute clearance/exchange equals the drain volume times concentration of solute in that drain volume, and that the daily solute clearance is the sum of the solute clearance for each of the exchanges done that day. Therefore, for patient convenience, a prescription can be written in which the solute removal for one of the dwells may not be the most efficient possible as long as that is "made up" during another dwell. For instance, although diffusion of small solutes would ultimately stop (D/P ratio = 1) some time during the 15-hour daytime dwell of CCPD, one can still obtain minimal Kt/V goals on APD. Similar adjustments can be made to achieve daily ultrafiltration goals.

To increase solute removal in CAPD patients, it is most efficient to increase the instilled volume/exchange. The most common approach is to increase the dwell volume in 500-mL increments, because commercially available fluids come in 500-mL increments. However, one could increase the instilled volume by only 250 mL/exchange if wanted, discarding the remaining dialysis fluids. Alternatively one could increase the number of exchanges/day. However, this is not as user friendly for the patient and typically does not increase solute clearance as much as an increase in instilled volume/exchange does.

For APD patients, the same principles apply as in CAPD; however, one typically has shorter (nighttime) and longer (daytime) dwells to consider. One would typically start by increasing the dwell volume/exchange at night. Other modifications include increasing the time spent overnight on the cycler, increasing the number of exchanges on the cycler, or increasing the number of daytime dwells. Sometimes combinations of the above measures are used in an individual patient. In a review of cycler prescription use in large cohorts of patients on cycler PD during the years 1997, 2000, and 2003,[86] the average instilled volume increased from about 2272 mL to about 2397 mL while number of exchanges on average remained similar (4.5 vs 4.4/day) and percentage of patients with five or more cycles per night decreased from 45% in 1997 to 38% in 2003. These trends are consistent with optimization of therapy based on known peritoneal physiology.

CONCLUSIONS

The goal of renal replacement therapy is not only to keep the patient alive, but at the same time to maintain the patient's previous lifestyle and wellness. Peritoneal dialysis is well suited to do this. The therapy and the solutions used in it have evolved along with the understanding of peritoneal physiology and the development of new technologies. Patients continue to do well on PD with improvement in relative risk of death over past years and outcomes similar to or better than those expected with hemodialysis for most patients.

ACKNOWLEDGMENTS

Many thanks to Sharon Lucas and Laura Harvey for their secretarial assistance.

References

1. U.S. Renal Data System: USRDS 2006 Annual Report. Am J Kidney Dis 2007;49:S1.
2. Lameire N, Biesen WM, Dombros N, et al: The referral pattern of patients with ESRD is a determinant in the choice of dialysis modality. Perit Dial Int 1997;17(Suppl 2):S161.
3. Nissenson AR, Prichard SS, Cheng IKP, et al: Non-medical factors that impact on ESRD modality selection. Kidney Int 1993; 43(Suppl 40):S120–S127.
4. Burkart JM, Daeihagh PD, Rocco MV: Peritoneal dialysis. In Brenner BM (ed): Brenner & Rector's The Kidney, vol 2, 7th ed. 2004, Philadelphia: Elsevier, pp 2625–2695.
5. Westin RE, Roberts M: Clinical use of stylet catheter for peritoneal dialysis. Arch Intern Med 1965;115:659–662.
6. Cruz C: Clinical experience with a new peritoneal access device (the Cruz catheter). In Ota K, Maher J, Winchester JF, et al (eds): Current Concepts in Peritoneal Dialysis. New York, Elsevier Science, 1992, p 164–169.
7. Twardowski ZJ, Nolph KD, Khanna R, et al: The need for a "swan neck" permanently bent, arcuate peritoneal dialysis catheter. Perit Dial Bull 1985;5:219.
8. Twardowski ZJ, Khanna R: Swan neck peritoneal dialysis catheter. In Andreucci VE (ed): Vascular and Peritoneal Access for Dialysis. Dordrecht: Kluwer Academic, 1989, p 271.
9. Twardowski ZJ, Dobbie JW, Moore HL, et al: Morphology of peritoneal dialysis catheter tunnel. Perit Dial Int 1991;11:237–251.
10. Gokal R, Alexander S, Ash S, et al: Peritoneal catheters and exit site practices: toward optimum peritoneal access. Perit Dial Int 1998;18:11–33.
11. Ash SR, Nichols WK: Placement, repair, and removal of chronic peritoneal catheters. In Gokal R, Nolph KD (eds): Textbook of Peritoneal Dialysis. Dordrecht: Kluwer Academic, 1994, p 315.
12. Maffei S, Bonello F, Stramignoni E, et al: Two years experience and 119 peritoneal dialysis catheters placed with peritoneoscopy control and Y-TEC system. Minerva Urol Nefrol 1992;44: 63–67.
13. Nahman NS Jr, Middendorf DF, Bay WH, et al: Modification of the percutaneous approach to peritoneal dialysis catheter placement under peritoneoscopic visualization: Clinical results in 78 patients. J Am Soc Nephrol 1992;3:103–107.
14. Moncrief JW, Popovich RP, Broadrick LJ, et al: The Moncrief-Popovich catheter: A new peritoneal access technique for patients on peritoneal dialysis. ASAIO J 1993;39:62–65.
15. Crabtree JH: Selected best demonstrated practices in peritoneal dialysis access. Kidney Int 2006;70(Suppl 103):S27–S37.
16. Crabtree JH, Fishman A: A laparoscopic method for optimal peritoneal dialysis access. Perit Dial Access Surg 2005;71:135–143.

17. Gokoo CF, Lelah MD, Hauck W, Burkhop KE: External catheter immobilization improves wound healing in micropigs. ASAIO J 1990;35:412–414.

18. Mujias S, Nolph KD, Gokal R, et al: Evaluation and management of ultrafiltration problems in peritoneal dialysis. Perit Dial Int 2000;20(Suppl 4):S5–S21.

19. Lindblad AS, Novak JW, Nolph KD: The USA CAPD registry characteristics of participants and selected outcome measures for the period January 1, 1981 through August 31, 1987. In Nolph KD (ed): Peritoneal Dialysis. Dordrecht: Kluwer Academic Publishers, 1990, p 389.

20. Piraino B, Bernardini J, Centa PK, et al: The effect of body weight on CAPD related infections and catheter loss. Perit Dial Int 1991;11:64–68.

21. Swartz R, Messana JM, Rocher L, et al: The curled catheter: Dependable device for percutaneous access. Perit Dial Int 1990;10:231–235.

22. Weber J, Mettang T, Hübel E, et al: Survival of 138 surgically placed straight double-cuff Tenckhoff catheters in patients on continuous ambulatory peritoneal dialysis. Perit Dial Int 1993;13:224–227.

23. Eklund BH, Honkanen EO, Kala AR, Kyllönen LE: Peritoneal dialysis access: Prospective randomized comparison of the swan neck and Tenckhoff catheters. Perit Dial Int 1995;15:353–356.

24. Guner O: Malfunctioning peritoneal dialysis catheter and accompanying surgical pathology repaired by laparoscopic surgery. Perit Dial Int 2002;22:454–462.

25. Zadronzy D, Niemierko ML, Draczkowski T, et al: Laparoscopic approach for dysfunctional Tenckhoff catheters. Perit Dial Int 1999;19:170–171.

26. Vas SI: Answers to what are the indications for removal of the permanent peritoneal catheter? Perit Dial Bull 1981;1:145.

27. Raja RM, Kramer MS, Rosenbaum JL, et al: Evaluation of hypertonic peritoneal dialysis solutions with low sodium. Nephron 1973;11:342–353.

28. Nolph KD, Twardowski Z, Popovich RP, Rubin J: Equilibration of peritoneal dialysis solutions during long-dwell exchanges. J Lab Clin Med 1979;93:246–256.

29. Brown ST, Ahearn DJ, Nolph KD: Potassium removal with peritoneal dialysis. Kidney Int 1973;4:67–69.

30. Weinreich T, Rambausek M, Ritz E: In control of secondary hyperparathyroidism optimal with the currently used calcium concentration in the CAPD fluid? Nephrol Dial Transplant 1991;6:843–845.

31. Hutchison A, Boulton H, Freemont A, et al: Effective control of phosphate, intact PTH, and osteodystrophy by low calcium dialysate and oral $CaCO_3$ in CAPD. Perit Dial Int 1992;12:S35.

32. Slatopolsky E, Weerts C, Lopez-Hilker S, et al: Calcium carbonate as a phosphate binder in patients with chronic renal failure undergoing dialysis. N Eng J Med 1986;315:157–161.

33. Stein H, Yudis M, Sirota R: Calcium carbonate as a phosphate binder. N Eng J Med 1987;316:109.

34. Slingeneyer A, Laroche B, Loupi G, et al: Calcium concentration in PD dialysate must be lowered. Exclusive use of $CaCO_3$ as a phosphate binder. Perit Dial Int 1992;12(Suppl 2):S161.

35. Cunningham J, Sawyer N, Altmann P, et al: Mineral metabolism in CAPD patients treated with $CaCO_3$ as a phosphate binder. Kidney Int 1992;141:455.

36. Salusky I, Coburn JW, Foley J, et al: Effects of oral calcium carbonate on control of serum phosphorus and changes in plasma albuminium levels after discontinuation of aluminium-containing gels in children receiving dialysis. J Pediatr 1986;108:767–770.

37. Martis L, Serkes KD, Nolph KD: Calcium carbonate as a phosphate binder: Is there a need to adjust peritoneal dialysate calcium concentrations for patients using $CaCO_3$? Perit Dial Int 1989;9:325–328.

38. Brown CB, Hamdy N, Boletis J, et al: Rationale for the use of low calcium solution in CAPD. In La Greca G, Ronco C, Feriani M, et al (eds): Peritoneal Dialysis: Proceedings of the Fourth International Course on Peritoneal Dialysis. Milan: Wichtig Editore, 1991, p 125.

39. Hutchison AJ, Merchant M, Boulton HF, et al: Calcium and magnesium mass transfer in peritoneal dialysis patients using 1.25 mmol/L magnesium dialysis fluid. Perit Dial Int 1993;13:219–223.

40. Weinreich T, Colombi A, Echterhoff HH, et al: Transperitoneal calcium mass transfer using dialysate with a low calcium concentration (1.0 mm). Perit Dial Int 1993;42(Suppl38):S467–S470.

41. Rotellar C, Kinsel V, Goggins M, et al: Does low calcium dialysate accelerate secondary hyperparathyroidism in continuous ambulatory peritoneal dialysis patients? Perit Dial Int 1993;13:S471–S472.

42. Johnson R, Walton J, Krebs H, et al: Metabolic fuels during and after severe exercise in athletes and non-athletes. Lancet 1969;2:452–455.

43. Brandt R, Siegel S, Waters M, et al: Spectroscopic assay for d-lactate in plasma. Anal Biochem 1980;102:39–46.

44. Nolph KD, Twardowski Z, Khanna R, et al: Tidal peritoneal dialysis with racemic or l-lactate solutions. Perit Dial Int 1990;10:161–164.

45. Yatzidis H: A new stable bicarbonate dialysis solution for peritoneal dialysis: Preliminary report. Perit Dial Int 1991;11:224–227.

46. Vaziri N, Ness R, Wellikson L, et al: Bicarbonate buffered peritoneal dialysis. An effective adjunct in the treatment of lactic acidosis. Am J Med 1979;67:392–396.

47. Feriani M, Biasioli S, Borin D, et al: Bicarbonate buffer for CAPD solution. ASAIO J 1985;31:668–672.

48. Coles GA, Gokal R, Ogg C, et al: A randomized controlled trial of a bicarbonate and a bicarbonate/lactate containing dialysis solution in CAPD. Perit Dial Int 1997;17:48–51.

49. Lindholm B, Bergstrom J: Nutritional aspects of CAPD. In Gokal R (ed): Continuous Ambulatory Peritoneal Dialysis. Edinburgh: Churchill Livingstone, 1986, p 228.

50. Gokal R, Ramos J, McGurk J, et al: Hyperlipidemia in patients on continuous ambulatory peritoneal dialysis. In Gahl GM, Kessel M, Nolph KD (eds): Advances in Peritoneal Dialysis. Amsterdam: Excerpta Medica, 1981, p 430.

51. Bouma S, Dwyer JT: Glucose absorption and weight exchange in 18 months of continuous ambulatory peritoneal dialysis. J Am Diet Assoc 1984;84:194–197.

52. Dobbie JW: Pathogenesis of peritoneal fibrosing syndromes (sclerosing peritonitis) in peritoneal dialysis. Perit Dial Int 1992;12:14–27.

53. Blumenkrantz M, Gahl GM, Kopple JD, et al: Protein losses during peritoneal dialysis. Kidney Int 1981;19:593–602.

54. Jones MR, Gehr T, Burkart JM, et al: Replacement of amino acid and protein losses with 1.1% amino acid peritoneal dialysis solution. Perit Dial Int 1998;18:210–216.

55. Oreopoulos DG, Crassweller P, Kartirtzoglou A, et al: Amino acids as an osmotic agent (instead of glucose) in continuous ambulatory peritoneal dialysis. In Legrain M (ed): First International Symposium on CAPD. Paris: Excerpta Medica, 1979, p 335.

56. Williams PF, Marliss E, Anderson GH, et al: Amino acid absorption following intraperitoneal administration in CAPD patients. Perit Dial Bull 1982;2:124.

57. Oren A, Wu G, Anderson GH, et al: Effective use of amino acid dialysate over four weeks in CAPD patients. Perit Dial Bull 1983;3:66.

58. Dombros N, Prutis K, Tong M, et al: Six-month overnight intraperitoneal amino acid infusion in continuous ambulatory peritoneal dialysis patients—no effect on nutritional status. Perit Dial Int 1990;10:79–84.

59. Park MS, Chhoi SR, Song YS, et al: New insight of amino acid-based dialysis solutions. Kidney Int 2006;70(Suppl 103):S110–S114.

60. Holmes C, Mujais S: Glucose sparing in peritoneal dialysis: Implications and metrics. Kidney Int 2006;70(Suppl 103): S104–S109.
61. Krediet RT: Osmotic agents in automated peritoneal dialysis solutions. Contrib Nephrol 1999;50:979–986.
62. Ho-dac-pannekeet MM, Schouten N, Langedijk MJ, et al: Peritoneal transport characteristics with glucose polymer based dialysate. Kidney Int 1996;50:979–986.
63. Pinerolo MC, Porri MT, D'Amico G: Recurrent sterile peritonitis at onset of treatment with icodextrin. Perit Dial Int 1999;19: 491–492.
64. William PF, Foggensteiner L: Sterile/allergic peritonitis with icodextrin in CAPD patients. Perit Dial Int 2002;22:89–90.
65. Wens R, Taminne M, Devriendt J, et al: A previously undescribed side effect of icodextrin, an overestimation of glycemia by glucose analyzer. Perit Dial Int 1998;18:603–609.
66. Schonicke G, Grabensee B, Plum J: Interference of icodextrin with serum amylase activity measurements [abstract]. J Am Soc Nephrol 1999;10:229.
67. Davies SJ, Phillips L, Griffiths AM, et al: What really happens to people on long-term peritoneal dialysis. Kidney Int 1998;54:2207–2217.
68. Honda K, Nitta K, Horita S, et al: Accumulation of advanced glycation end products in the peritoneal vasculature of continuous ambulatory peritoneal dialysis patients with low ultrafiltration. Nephrol Dial Transplant 1999;14:1541–1549.
69. Szeto CC, Chow KM, Lam CW, et al: Clinical biocompatibility of a neutral peritoneal dialysis solution with minimal glucose-degradation products—a 1-year randomized control trial. Nephrol Dial Transplant 2007;22:552–559.
70. Lee HY, Choi HY, Park H, et al: Changing prescribing practice in CAPD patients in Korea: Increased utilization of low GDP solutions improves patient outcome. Nephrol Dial Transplant 2006;21:2684–2686.
71. Twardowski Z, Nolph KD, Khanna R, et al: Peritoneal equilibration test. Perit Dial Bull 1987;7:138–147.
72. Burkart JM, Schreiber M, Korbet SM, et al: Solute clearance approach to adequacy of peritoneal dialysis. Perit Dial Int 1996;16:457–470.
73. Twardowski ZJ: Clinical value of standardized equilibration tests in CAPD patients. Blood Purif 1989;7:95–108.
74. Rodby RA, Firanek CA, Sarpolis AL: Re-evaluation of solute transport groups using the peritoneal equilibration test. Perit Dial Int 1999;19:438–441.
75. Ho-dac pannekeet MM, Imholz ALT, Struijk DG, et al: The standard peritoneal permeability analysis: A tool for the assessment of peritoneal permeability characteristics in CAPD patients. Kidney Int 1995;48:866–875.
76. Ho-dac-pannekeet MM, Atasever B, Struijk DG, Krediet RT: Analysis of ultrafiltration failure in peritoneal dialysis patients by means of the standard peritoneal permeability analysis. Perit Dial Int 1997;17:144–150.
77. Pride ET, Gustafson J, Graham A, et a.: Comparison of a 2.5% and a 4.25% dextrose peritoneal equilibration test. Perit Dial Int 2002;22:365–370.
78. Smit W, van Dijk P, Langedijk MJ, et al: Peritoneal function and assessment of reference values using a 3.86% glucose solution. Perit Dial Int 2003;23:440–449.
79. Rocco MV, Jordan JR, Burkart JM: Changes in peritoneal transport during the first month of peritoneal dialysis. Perit Dial Int 1995;15:12–17.
80. National Kidney Foundation: K/DOQI Clinical Practice Guidelines and Clinical Practice Recommendations for 2006. Updates: Hemodialysis Adequacy, Peritoneal Dialysis Adequacy and Vascular Access. Am J Kidney Dis 2006;48(Suppl 1):S1–S322.
81. Krediet RT, Boeschoten EW, Zuyderhoudt FMJ, et al: Peritoneal transport characteristics of water, low-molecular weight solutes and proteins during long-term continuous ambulatory peritoneal dialysis. Perit Dial Bull 1986;6:61–65.
82. Heimburger O, Waniewski J, Werynski A, et al: Peritoneal transport in CAPD patients with permanent loss of ultrafiltration capacity. Kidney Int 1990;38:495–506.
83. Davies SJ, Phillips L, Naish PF, Gussel GI: Peritoneal glucose exposure and changes in membrane solute transport with time on peritoneal dialysis. J Am Soc Nephrol 2001;12:1046–1051.
84. Davies SJ: Mitigating peritoneal membrane characteristics in modern peritoneal dialysis therapy. Kidney Int 2006;70(Suppl 103):S76–S83.
85. Popovich RP, Moncrief JW, Nolph KD, et al: Continuous ambulatory peritoneal dialysis. Ann Intern Med 1978;88:449–456.
86. Mujais S, Childers RW: Profiles of automated peritoneal dialysis prescriptions in the US 1997–2003. Kidney Int 2006;70(Suppl 103):S84–S90.
87. Twardowski Z, Prowant BF, Nolph KD, et al: Chronic nightly tidal peritoneal dialysis (NTDP). ASAIO J 1990;36:M584–M588.
88. Perez RA, Blake PG, McMurray SD, et al: What is the optimal frequency of cycling in automated peritoneal dialysis? Perit Dial Int 2000;20:548–556.
89. Juergensen PH, Murphy AL, Pherson KA, et al: Tidal peritoneal dialysis: Comparison of different tidal regimens and automated peritoneal dialysis. Kidney Int 2000;57:2603–2607,
90. Fernandez RAM, Vega DN, Palop CL, et al: Adequacy of dialysis in automated peritoneal dialysis: A clinical experience. Perit Dial Int 1997;17:435–439.
91. Juergensen PH, Murphy AL, Pherson KA, et al: Tidal peritoneal dialysis to achieve comfort in chronic peritoneal dialysis patients. Adv Perit Dial 1999;15:125–126.
92. Fernando SK, Finkelstein FO: Tidal PD: Its role in the current practice of peritoneal dialysis. Kidney Int 2006;70:S91–S95.
93. National Kidney Foundation: K/DOQI Clinical Practice Guidelines for Peritoneal Dialysis Adequacy. New York: National Kidney Foundation, 2001.
94. Tzamaloukas AH, Gibel LJ, Eisenberg B, et al: Early and late peritoneal dialysate leaks in patients on CAPD. Adv Perit Dial 1990;6:64–70.
95. Burkart JM, Satko SG: Incremental dialysis: One center's experience over a two-year period. Perit Dial Int 2000;4:418–422.

Further Reading

Clinical practice guidelines and clinical practice recommendations. 2006 Update. Am J Kidney Dis 2006;48:1(Suppl 1): S91–S175.

Mujais S, Holmes C: Modern peritoneal dialysis: Concepts and approaches. Kidney Int 2006;70;S1–S2.

Chapter 82

Complications of Peritoneal Dialysis

John D. Williams and Simon J. Davies

Loss of peritoneal function is a major factor leading to treatment failure in peritoneal dialysis (PD). Although the precise biologic mechanisms responsible for these changes have not been defined, it is widely assumed that alterations in peritoneal function are related to structural changes in the peritoneal membrane. Accumulating, albeit indirect, evidence shows that continuous exposure to components of bioincompatible dialysis solution as well as repeated episodes of bacterial peritonitis play a major role in the long-term changes seen in peritoneal function (i.e., ultrafiltration loss and increased solute clearance). To date, however, the relationship between structure and function has not been fully defined. Although a number of studies have identified various mesothelial, vascular, and interstitial changes in peritoneal morphology during PD, the responsible factors have not been identified. Identified changes include loss or degeneration of mesothelial cells, thickening of the submesothelial compact collagenous zone (variously described as fibrosis or sclerosis), changes in the structure and number of blood vessels, and reduplication of vascular basement membrane.

Recent studies have quantified the changes within the submesothelial collagenous zone and demonstrated a progressive increase in thickness with time on PD (Fig. 82-1). Changes within the peritoneal vascular bed have also been identified. These include progressive changes to the structure of small vessels, ranging from subtle thickening of the subendothelial matrix to complete obliteration of vessels (Fig. 82-2). Thus, evidence is accumulating that changes occur in both the interstitial and vascular compartments of the dialysed peritoneal membrane.[1] The little evidence that is available from matched biopsies also suggests that these changes occur primarily in the parietal membrane, with a lesser degree of involvement of the corresponding visceral membrane.

Although it is likely that these structural changes are related to time on dialysis, episodes of peritonitis, and perhaps to dialysis solution components, the exact relationships are poorly understood, as is the possible contribution of uremia.

Encapsulating peritoneal sclerosis is a rare but serious complication of peritoneal dialysis. It is characterized by a severe fibrotic reaction, frequently inflammatory, that primarily involves the visceral membrane. Encapsulation of the small bowel results in progressive obstruction. Prolonged treatment with PD is the most important risk factor, with an incidence of 5% to 20% after 10 years of continuous therapy.[2] Other risk factors include severe bacterial peritonitis and switching modality (e.g., to hemodialysis or transplant). Cases differ in their severity, some requiring no more than nutritional support; in severe cases surgical intervention, including adhesiolysis and peritonectomy, has proved successful in experienced hands.[2]

INFECTIOUS COMPLICATIONS

Peritonitis

Although the introduction of disconnect systems has reduced the incidence of peritonitis, it remains one of the most important complications of long-term PD. A single episode is rarely life-threatening, but repeated or prolonged infection remains a major cause of treatment failure and results in a forced switch to hemodialysis.

The diagnosis should be suspected in any patient who develops a cloudy bag or abdominal pain. Fever may also be present but is not a universal feature of peritonitis. Patients should be advised to contact their dialysis unit immediately if they have a cloudy bag or persistent abdominal pain. Samples of the dialysate should be analyzed for cell count and undergo microbiologic examination. The diagnosis is confirmed by finding more than 100 white blood cells/μL, of which at least

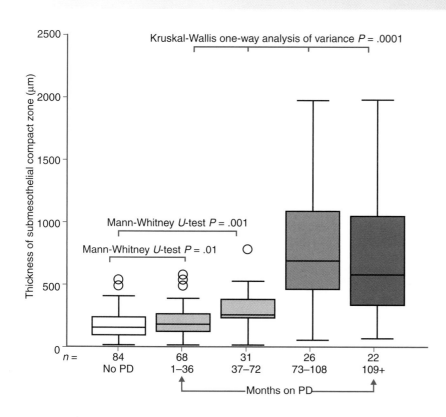

Figure 82-1 Changes in the thickness of the peritoneal membrane with origin of biopsy and time on peritoneal dialysis. The submesothelial compact zone was measured in micrometers in samples taken from normal individuals, uremic predialysis patients, hemodialysis patients, and patients undergoing peritoneal dialysis, grouped according to duration of dialysis. Data are presented as box plots representing interquartile ranges.

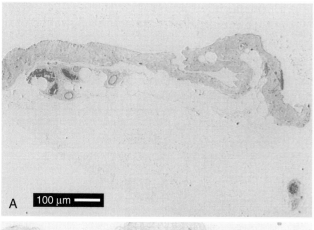

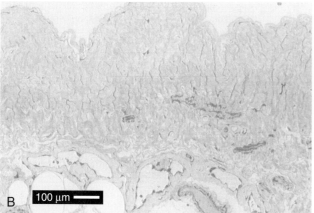

Figure 82-2 Morphologic features of the parietal peritoneum. Biopsies from (**A**) a normal individual and (**B**) a patient who had been on peritoneal dialysis for 7 years. Toluidine blue.

50% are polymorphonuclear leukocytes. A Gram stain should also be performed to help identify the type of causative organism, although this will only reveal the pathogen in a minority of cases. For most patients, treatment will have to be empirical, pending full results of culture and sensitivity tests. Various culture techniques have been proposed, but white cell lysis is often helpful in increasing the yield of a positive growth.

There is no standard treatment for peritonitis in a PD patient. A number of regimens have been found reasonably effective, none of which give a 100% cure rate without relapse. In the few randomized studies that have been conducted, no antibiotic combination or dosing regimen was found to be superior; just one study found that intraperitoneal rather than intravenous administration resulted in a higher cure rate. The emergence of vancomycin-resistant enterococci, methicillin-resistant *Staphylococcus aureus* (MRSA), and other resistant organisms means that local treatment regimens must be developed in consultation with the microbiology services and infection control team.

The Advisory Committee on Peritonitis Management of the International Society of Peritoneal Dialysis (available at ispd.com) has published detailed guidelines and algorithms for the management of this condition.[3,4] The recommended initial empirical therapy is a center-specific regimen, based on known local sensitivities of organisms that frequently cause peritonitis, and must include coverage for both gram-positive and gram-negative organisms. For example, this might be a first-generation cephalosporin, such as cefazolin or cephalothin, combined with an aminoglycoside (paying attention to residual renal function). Both types of antibiotic are administered as a loading dose in the first bag and then as a maintenance dose in subsequent bags. Suggested doses of cephalosporin are 500 mg/L for loading and 125 mg/L for maintenance. Once the culture result is available the regimen should be modified accordingly. If an enterococcus is identified (gram-positive), the cephalosporin should be stopped and ampicillin added at a dose of 125 mg/L. *S. aureus* treatment includes adding oral rifampin 600 mg daily. If the organism is not MRSA, an alternative is to use a specific gram-positive antibiotic such as floxacillin or rifampin. If other gram-positive organisms are identified, the cephalosporin should be continued. Although in vitro tests may suggest resistance of coagulase-negative staphylococci to cephalosporins, the in vivo concentration of the drug is usually sufficient to overcome this potential problem. If, however, clinical improvement is slow or fails to occur, vancomycin may be given at a dose of 30 mg/kg intraperitoneally every 7 days. If the organism is MRSA, vancomycin should be given using the same regimen. For uncomplicated gram-positive infections, an oral cephalosporin can be substituted for the intraperitoneal cephalosporin during the second week of therapy (summarized in Fig. 82-3).

If the culture is negative, combined therapy of cephalosporin and aminoglycoside should be continued for 2 weeks, assuming there is a clinical response (summarized in Fig. 82-4).

If a gram-negative microorganism is identified, subsequent management depends on the sensitivity (summarized in Fig. 82-5). If the bacteria are sensitive to the cephalosporin, it should be continued. On the other hand, isolation of *Pseudomonas* requires withdrawal of the cephalosporin and the addition of an alternative antibiotic with demonstrable activity against the organism, such as a quinolone.

Isolation of multiple organisms, including anaerobes, strongly suggests major bowel pathology, including perforation or a diverticular abscess. Metronidazole should be added

to the regimen intravenously initially (the intravenous dose is 500 mg tid). Bowel pathology should also be considered if a gram-negative peritonitis is associated with severe systemic signs or if the infection proves difficult to bring under control. In these situations, urgent surgical review is required pending a laparotomy.

The identification of yeasts on the Gram stain or isolation of yeasts or fungi on culture is a matter for serious concern. Most clinicians would recommend removing the peritoneal catheter immediately because this type of infection can be difficult to eradicate in the presence of a foreign body. Recent experience suggests that a combination of an imidazole such as fluconazole with flucytosine may be of benefit. The recommendation for adults is daily fluconazole at an oral or intraperitoneal dose of 200 mg, and flucytosine at a loading dose of 2 g orally with a maintenance dose of 1 g/day. Amphotericin B is no longer recommended. Unfortunately, oral flucytosine is not universally available.

The optimum duration of treatment has not been clearly defined by controlled trials. At present it is recommended that for gram-positive organisms therapy should last 14 days, except in the case of *S. aureus,* when 21 days is suggested. For culture-negative episodes 14 days should suffice. The same is true in the case of single-organism gram-negative peritonitis, but 21 days is recommended for *Pseudomonas, Stenotrophomonas,* or multiple organisms. Fungal or yeast infections require 4 to 6 weeks of therapy (or 7 to 10 days of therapy after catheter removal).

A patient who is not systemically ill can be treated successfully on an outpatient basis. It is extremely important, however,

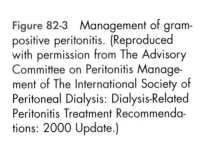

Figure 82-3 Management of gram-positive peritonitis. (Reproduced with permission from The Advisory Committee on Peritonitis Management of The International Society of Peritoneal Dialysis: Dialysis-Related Peritonitis Treatment Recommendations: 2000 Update.)

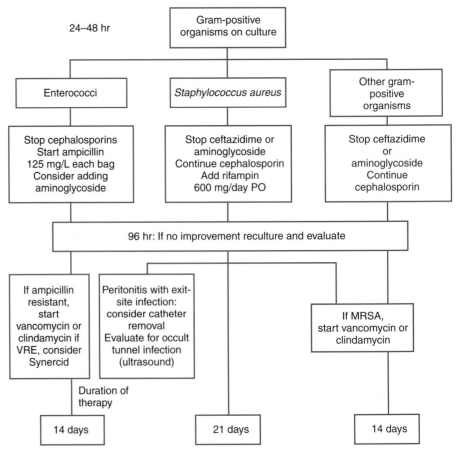

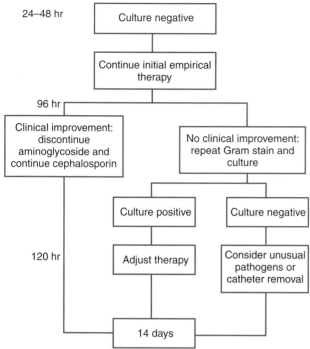

24–48 hr

Culture negative

↓

Continue initial empirical therapy

96 hr

Clinical improvement: discontinue aminoglycoside and continue cephalosporin

No clinical improvement: repeat Gram stain and culture

Culture positive

Culture negative

120 hr

Adjust therapy

Consider unusual pathogens or catheter removal

14 days

Figure 82-4 Management of culture-negative peritonitis. (Reproduced with permission from The Advisory Committee on Peritonitis Management of The International Society of Peritoneal Dialysis: Dialysis-Related Peritonitis Treatment Recommendations: 2000 Update.)

that there is follow-up either in the clinic or by telephone. In the majority of cases, clinical resolution, as judged by clearing of the bags, starts within 48 hours. If there is no improvement within 96 hours despite the correct antibiotic as judged by sensitivity tests, then the fluid must be retested for cell count, Gram stain, and culture. In the case of a persistent *S. aureus* infection, an underlying tunnel infection should be excluded (see Managing Exit-Site and Tunnel Infection in this chapter). In all other situations in which there is failure to improve, serious consideration should be given to removing the catheter. The possibility of intra-abdominal or gynecologic disease, or the presence of unusual organisms such as mycobacterium, should also be considered.

For patients on automated peritoneal dialysis, regimens similar to those outlined above are used, but the dialysis should be modified so that it lasts a full 24 hours, with 3- to 4-hour dwells. Once there is clinical resolution, the usual automated PD regimen can be recommended, but with a daytime bag containing the antibiotics, until completion of the treatment.

Relapsing peritonitis is defined as separate infective episodes caused by the same organism within 4 weeks of finishing the previous course of antibiotics. In gram-positive infections a 4-week course of a cephalosporin together with oral rifampin should be tried. The recurrence of *S. aureus* infection should trigger a search for a pericatheter infection or tunnel. Relapsing MRSA-related peritonitis will require a prolonged course (4 weeks) of vancomycin or clindamycin. If enterococci or gram-negative organisms are the cause, the possibility of intra-abdominal disease or a diverticular abscess should be

considered. Again a repeat course of antibiotics chosen by sensitivity testing should last 4 weeks. As before, in the case of a relapse, removal of the catheter should be considered if there is no improvement within 4 days.

The best regimen for catheter replacement after removal for peritonitis has not been defined. There are theoretical benefits for the withdrawal of PD as replacement renal therapy for a brief period and avoiding the presence of an intraperitoneal foreign body, and altering host defenses by instilling dialysate. Some centers, however, practice removal and replacement of the catheter at the same time under antibiotic cover. Such an approach has met with anecdotal success. Each patient should be judged individually to decide what is in his or her best interests.

Prevention

Because of the high rate of peritonitis experienced during the early years of continuous ambulatory peritoneal dialysis (CAPD), considerable efforts have been made to prevent this serious complication. Approaches that have been shown to reduce infection rates in randomized studies include increased intensity of training,[5] use of flush-before-fill systems,[6] antibiotic prophylaxis to cover catheter insertion,[4] and prevention of exit-site infections.[7,8] There is no evidence that the type of PD catheter used or the approach to insertion (i.e., surgical, medical, or laparoscopic) has any effect on subsequent peritonitis or exit-site infection rates. More important are the experience of the surgical operator and the development of robust preoperative and postoperative care protocols. These should include careful siting of the exit site so that it is visible to the patient and does not lie either on the beltline, where rubbing will occur, or beneath skinfolds. Postoperatively an occlusive dressing should be applied and not removed until healing has occurred. Patients should be trained in exit-site inspection and care; any fresh granulomatous tissue should be removed and kept dry by the careful application of silver nitrate.

Significant advances have been made in the design of delivery systems in an attempt to reduce bacterial entry into the peritoneal cavity and thus reduce peritoneal infection. Buoncristiani and colleagues were the first to show that a Y-set system significantly reduced the rate of infection. This has been confirmed in several randomized, controlled trials.[6] An integrated twin-bag system, one bag for unused fluid and the other for drainage, is connected to a Y-shaped tube, which has a short stem to link it to the catheter. The principle of the system is that the drainage tube is flushed free of contaminating bacteria before fresh fluid is run in. In addition, the number of times that the continuity of the tubing is broken is reduced. These Y-set systems act by greatly reducing the effects of touch contamination, thus reducing the rate of coagulase-negative staphylococcal infection. This system is now the standard for CAPD. The Y set does not, however, affect the incidence of *S. aureus* peritonitis.

In contrast to coagulase-negative staphylococci, carriage of *S. aureus* appears to be confined to 25% to 30% of PD patients who are more likely to acquire exit-site infections and peritonitis. Several studies, using either historical controls or in comparison with oral rifampin, have found that the regular use of mupirocin applied to the nares (e.g., for the first 5 days of each month) or directly to the exit site (on a long-term daily basis) have reduced the frequency of exit-site infections, and in some cases peritonitis, due to *S. aureus*. Recently a

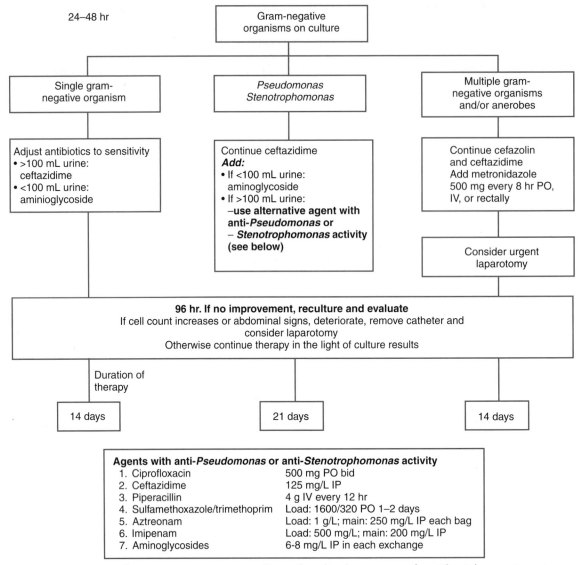

Figure 82-5 Management of gram-negative peritonitis. (Reproduced with permission from The Advisory Committee on Peritonitis Management of The International Society of Peritoneal Dialysis: Dialysis-Related Peritonitis Treatment Recommendations: 2000 Update.)

direct comparison between mupirocin and gentamicin cream applied to the exit site was undertaken; the latter was as effective or even more effective when compared to mupirocin in preventing *S. aureus* infections. It also reduced the frequency of *Pseudomonas* exit-site infection and peritonitis. Concerns remain over the risk of encouraging resistance to gentamicin when used indiscriminately; it is important that any such policy be developed with the local involvement of microbiologists and infection control teams. With the exception of prevention of *Pseudomonas* exit-site infection, there is no proven method of decreasing the incidence of gram-negative infections. Clearly one should avoid PD, if possible, in any patient with a stoma or fistula. Part of the difficulty is that gram-negative organisms often cause problems in the elderly, probably as a result of diverticular disease. Other than keeping the bowels regular by judicious use of fiber, no other measures seem to reduce this type of infection.

Eosinophilic Peritonitis

Eosinophilic peritonitis is diagnosed when the patient presents with a cloudy bag of effluent, which is found to contain eosinophils rather than neutrophils on microscopy. The fluid is culture-negative. It is an uncommon event but tends to occur within the first few weeks of starting PD. The cause is unknown but is assumed to be some form of reaction to the cannula or to the dialysate. It is usually self-limiting, and no treatment is required. Eosinophilic peritonitis has been reported as an allergic response to polyglucose solutions (icodextrin).

Managing Exit-Site and Tunnel Infection

Exit-site infection is an important complication of long-term PD because it influences catheter longevity and increases the risk of peritonitis. The 2005 ISPD guidelines include a simple scoring system that allows standardization of the assessment of inflammatory changes at the exit site. The site is assessed for evidence of swelling, crusting, redness, pain, and exudates; if any of these is present, 1 or 2 points are given according to severity. In the case of the first three, this is determined by extent: less than 0.5 cm from the exit site (1 point) or more than 0.5 cm from the exit site (2 points). An exudate scores 1 point if serous or 2 points if purulent; pain is scored by severity. A total score of 4 or greater indicates infection, unless there is purulent discharge, in which case infection is definite (Table 82-1). Under these circumstances an antibiotic that will cover both *S. aureus* and *Pseudomonas* (e.g., quinolone) should be commenced until sensitivities from culture are available.

Unfortunately, there are no satisfactory trials comparing different therapeutic regimens; thus, the following recommendations are based on anecdotal experiences from a variety of centers in different countries. Consensus guidelines have been published.[3,4] The main treatment options are systemic antibiotics and local therapy. If any discharge or significant associated cellulitis is present, it is essential to start with a systemic antibiotic. Because *S. aureus* is the common organism, an agent effective against this species should be prescribed. Unless there is prior evidence that the patient carries MRSA, dicloxacillin 500 mg two times a day or floxacillin at a dose of 500 mg four times a day is appropriate. Alternatively, a cephalosporin can be used if the patient is allergic to penicillin. In most patients, the drug can be given orally, but if the individual is systemically ill, the antibiotics should be administered intravenously until clinical improvement occurs. Hospitalization is not necessary for most patients unless there is evidence of extension of the infection along the tunnel toward the inner cuff, especially if abscess formation shown by ultrasound is present, necessitating catheter removal. If the infection is resistant to methicillin, an alternative to dicloxacillin or floxacillin should be used. In a few cases, the organism may be sensitive to a cephalosporin. In the majority of resistant cases, however, vancomycin should be given as a 1-g intravenous dose (or intraperitoneally if the dwell time is at least 6 hr). The dose is repeated once a week for up to 4 weeks. Should the culture grow a gram-negative organism, ciprofloxacin in an oral dose of 500 mg twice daily will be effective in most cases. Other antibiotics should be substituted according to the in vitro sensitivity results.

Treatment should continue for a minimum of 2 weeks. In gram-positive infections, if there is no improvement within 7 days, rifampin 600 mg/day should be added. If complete healing does not take place after 4 weeks of therapy, further measures should be considered. A number of centers have recommended exteriorizing and shaving the outer cuff. If this cuff is visible or even close to the exit site, it is likely to be involved in the infection. Under local anesthetic, the cuff is exposed by an incision along the line of the catheter. The cuff is freed by blunt dissection and then carefully shaved off the catheter. Temporary resolution of infection often occurs after this procedure; it may prolong catheter life. If the infection persists or relapses, catheter removal must be considered because there is a high risk that the exit-site infection will lead to peritonitis. It is important that the new exit site be located through a different part of the anterior abdominal wall. If the infection is controlled, and there is no evidence of sepsis along the tunnel, it is possible to insert a new catheter under antibiotic cover at the same time as the old one is removed.

NONINFECTIOUS COMPLICATIONS

Inadequate Ultrafiltration

Insufficient ultrafiltration leading to fluid overload is one of the most common problems associated with long-term PD. The incidence of this problem increases with time on treatment, in part from changes in membrane function, but also from the loss of residual urine volume that contributes to satisfactory fluid balance. One study would suggest that up to 30.9% of patients have this problem by 6 years of treatment.[9]

In defining ultrafiltration failure it is possible to take either a patient- or a membrane-centered approach. The former is a relative definition: it is the inability to achieve sufficient peritoneal fluid removal to maintain adequate fluid balance; it is influenced by many factors, including fluid intake, residual urine volume, and the acceptability of using hypertonic (4.25% dextrose) exchanges. The latter is based on the absolute measurement of the ultrafiltration capacity of the peritoneal membrane, using standardized methods, and is influenced by the intrinsic properties of the membrane, such as characteristics of solute transport and fluid reabsorption rates. The clinician needs to integrate these two approaches to identify and manage fluid balance in the PD patient.

Insufficient ultrafiltration should be suspected if there is clinical evidence of fluid overload (Fig. 82-6). This problem is more difficult to identify in PD patients than in hemodialysis patients, partially because it can develop insidiously, but also because driving the weight down to an appropriate dry weight using sequential ultrafiltration during dialysis sessions is not possible. Edema, hypertension, unexplained low plasma albumin, low daily ultrafiltration volumes in anuric patients (<750 mL), excessive dependence on hypertonic exchanges (≥ 2/day), or increases in weight disproportionate to changes in the midarm circumference all suggest that there is a problem. These findings should lead the clinician to evaluate peritoneal membrane function.

Membrane function should be assessed using a standardized 4-hour dwell as in the peritoneal equilibration test (PET)[10,11] or the simplified standardized permeability analysis (SPA).[12,13] The only important difference between these methods is the

Table 82-1 Classification of Exit-Site Infection

	0 Points	1 Point	2 Points
Swelling	No	Exit only; <0.5 cm	>0.5 and/or tunnel
Crust	No	<0.5 cm	>0.5 cm
Redness	No	<0.5 cm	>0.5 cm
Pain	No	Slight	Severe
Drainage	No	Serous	Purulent

Infection should be assumed with exit-site score of 4 or greater. Purulent drainage, even if alone, is sufficient to indicate infection. A score <4 may or may not represent infection.

Reproduced with permission from Piraino B, Bailie GR, Bernardini J, et al: Peritoneal dialysis-related infections recommendations: 2005 update. Perit Dial Int 2005;25:107–131.

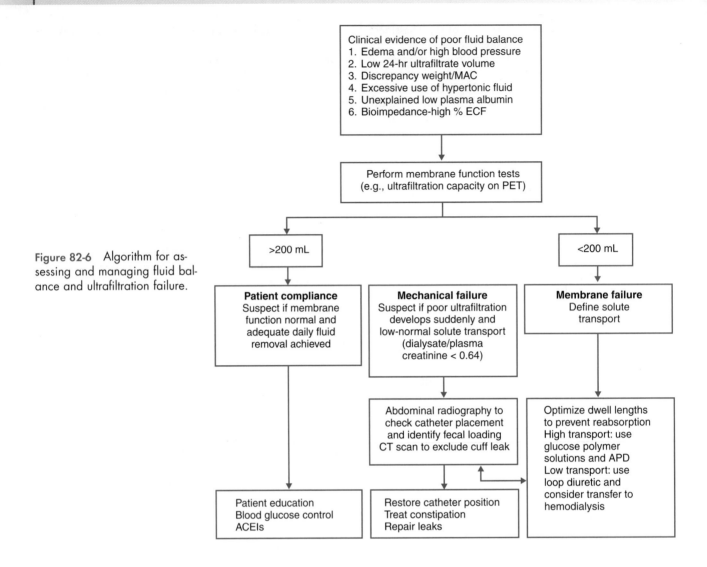

Figure 82-6 Algorithm for assessing and managing fluid balance and ultrafiltration failure.

concentration of dextrose used (2.5% for PET, 4.25% for SPA). Both tests measure two aspects of membrane function, the ultrafiltration capacity and the rate of transfer of creatinine (low-molecular-weight solute transport). The *ultrafiltration capacity* is the net volume of fluid removed during the dwell and is determined by several aspects of membrane function. A value of less than 200 mL (which includes the typical overfill of approximately 150 mL for a 2-L exchange that bypasses the patient in the flush-before-fill procedure) using the PET or less than 400 mL when using the SPA have been taken as indicators of ultrafiltration failure.

If membrane function is normal (Fig. 82-7) and the total achieved ultrafiltration is reasonable (>1000 mL/day minus urine volume), it is likely that fluid balance problems can be addressed through patient education and good glycemic control in diabetics. If the ultrafiltration capacity of the membrane is poor but solute transport normal, it is important to exclude a reversible mechanical cause. This is especially the case if the loss of ultrafiltration appears to have developed rapidly. The reason may be obvious—catheter malposition, constipation (abdominal radiograph), or the development of a scrotal and subcutaneous leak—but deep cuff leaks are more difficult to

identify and require a contrast computed tomography scan. Once mechanical causes are excluded, patients with persistent poor ultrafiltration can be conveniently divided into two groups on the basis of PET or SPA results. In those with high or high average rates of solute transport (4-hr dialysate-to-plasma creatinine ratio [D/P Cr] > 0.64), the cause is early loss of the osmotic gradient during the dwell, leading to a reduced and earlier peak in achieved ultrafiltration combined with a more rapid absorption of fluid in the latter part of the dwell; these problems can both be solved by using shorter exchanges with the aid of automated PD and a glucose polymer (icodextrin) in the long exchange. Increasing evidence demonstrates that the increased mortality and technique failure previously found in high-transport patients[14] can be ameliorated by this approach.[15] More difficult to manage is poor ultrafiltration in the context of a D/P Cr ratio less than 0.64 or a much reduced ultrafiltration capacity of the membrane. This is rare in new PD patients but can develop after prolonged periods on dialysis where it is associated with a reduction in the osmotic conductance (efficiency) of the membrane.[16] This type of ultrafiltration problem usually leads to technique failure and transfer to hemodialysis.

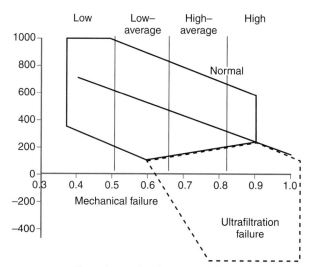

Figure 82-7 The relationship between solute transport (x axis) and ultrafiltration capacity observed in the peritoneal equilibration test. The *bold* regression line reflects the inverse relationship between these measures (see text). This and the areas defined as normal or representing mechanical and ultrafiltration failure were established from 1800 consecutive measurements. (Redrawn from Davies SJ, Brown B, Bryan J, Russell GI: Clinical evaluation of the peritoneal equilibration test: A population-based study. Nephrol Dial Transplant 1993;8(1):64–70.)

Catheter Malfunction

Inflow Failure

A 2-L bag of dialysate should take 15 minutes or less to run into the peritoneal cavity. If inflow is significantly slowed or nonexistent, mechanical causes should first be eliminated. The tubing and catheter should be checked for kinks, all clamps or rollers must be open for the inflow position, and all frangible seals fully broken. In the absence of such problems, the catheter should be flushed vigorously with 20 mL of heparinized saline. If the catheter now becomes patent, it is wise to add heparin at 500 U/L for the next few cycles, because the cause of blockage is usually a fibrin plug. If the catheter remains blocked, a radiograph of the abdomen must be obtained. If the catheter is in a reasonable position in the pelvis, an attempt to restore patency should be made with the use of urokinase; 2 mL containing 25,000 units of urokinase should be infused into the lumen of the catheter and left in situ for 2 to 4 hours. The catheter is then flushed; if inflow is restored, heparin should be added to the dialysate for the next few cycles. Should this procedure not be successful but fibrin is still thought to be the cause, an endoscopy brush may sometimes prove successful in unblocking the catheter.

If the radiographs show the catheter to be malpositioned, an attempt should be made to reposition the catheter tip into the pelvis. This can be done using a sterile semirigid rod, shaped into a curve and slid down the lumen of the catheter under radiographic screening control. The rod is then rotated. Sometimes the catheter will then move easily and slide back into the pelvis. The technique is not practical when the catheter has a swan neck configuration. Alternatively, the catheter

can be repositioned at laparotomy or peritoneoscopy. It will often be found to be wrapped in omentum. Under these circumstances, current practice is to "hitch" the omentum out of the way in the upper abdomen. This avoids an omentectomy (preserving the omentum for future use if necessary) but prevents the omentum from blocking the catheter for a second time. An algorithm for managing inflow failure is shown in Figure 82-8.

Outflow Failure

The reasons for outflow failure are similar to those causing inflow failure. Constipation is another well-recognized cause of outflow problems. Loading of the bowel with fecal material is often obvious on a plain film of the abdomen. If constipation is a likely cause of the problem, it should be treated by oral laxatives or an enema. Sometimes a strong laxative such as sodium picosulfate (Picolax) is necessary to ensure sufficient evacuation for drainage of the dialysate. Subsequently, bowel action should be kept regular by increasing the fiber in the diet and, if necessary, by adding a mild laxative such as lactulose or senna.

Fibrin in Dialysate

In the presence of peritonitis, it is common for fibrin to be present in the dialysate. If there is any restriction of dialysate flow, heparin should be added to the bags to a concentration of 500 units/L. A few patients have fibrin formation in the absence of peritonitis. The bag may appear cloudy immediately on drainage, but the fibrin will aggregate on standing. The first time this happens, a sample must be sent to the microbiology laboratory to exclude infection. If this proves negative, the patient can be reassured. If catheter plugging

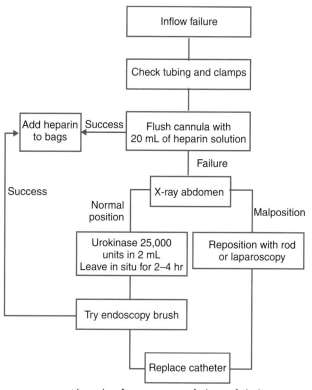

Figure 82-8 Algorithm for managing failure of dialysate inflow.

occurs, regular use of heparin is recommended. This can often be confined to the overnight bag for CAPD or the daytime dwell (if used) for those receiving automated PD.

Fluid Leaks

External

On occasions, fluid may leak from the exit site or even from the incision site where the catheter was inserted into the peritoneal cavity. This problem usually occurs early, particularly if dialysis is started soon after catheter insertion. Whenever possible, elective insertion of the catheter should be performed at least 2 weeks before dialysis is required. In addition, the use of the paramedian approach for the peritoneal entry site is thought to minimize the chances of this complication. If a leak occurs, PD should be withheld for as long as possible. If dialysis is necessary, hemodialysis should be used temporarily for 2 weeks. Alternatively, after at least 48 hours of a "dry" abdomen, PD can be recommenced with the aid of a cycler using a low volume (500 mL for adults) and no dwell. Volumes are then progressively increased over 10 days. Should the leak recur despite either of these regimens, surgical repair of the peritoneal entry site will be required. It may be better to completely remove the first catheter and replace it with a new one at a different site. Once again, if at all possible, the abdomen should be left dry for 2 to 4 weeks to allow full healing with sealing, particularly around the inner cuff.

Internal

Edema of the anterior abdominal wall can occur as part of generalized fluid retention. In this situation there is almost invariably a significant amount of peripheral edema. Treatment involves restricting fluid intake and using more hypertonic bags to improve fluid removal.

Isolated edema of the abdominal wall suggests an internal leak from the peritoneal cavity. This is particularly likely to occur from the catheter insertion site or a previous incision. It also sometimes occurs in association with an overt hernia. The site of the leak can be visualized by computed tomography after the intraperitoneal instillation of contrast media. It may be necessary for the patient to stand or perform other maneuvers to increase intra-abdominal pressure before the leak can be seen. An alternative diagnostic test is to perform scintigraphy after injecting a compound labelled with technetium-99m, such as DTPA. If a major leak is visualized, surgical repair will be required. Often, however, the patient can be managed conservatively by bed rest and using low-volume cycles with little or no dwell. Cessation of PD for 2 weeks with temporary hemodialysis may also allow the leak to seal permanently.

Genital Edema

This symptom can be caused by the same processes as abdominal wall edema; the management is identical. In addition, genital edema can also be caused by a patent processus vaginalis with or without an associated inguinal hernia. As with abdominal wall edema, the leak should be visualized by using computed tomography or scintigraphy. Any hernia requires surgical repair, but once again a small leak may seal off spontaneously if PD is suspended or with continued use of bed rest, low volumes, and a scrotal support for affected men.

Vaginal leakage of dialysate has been described, though relatively rarely. It is not clear whether this phenomenon occurs through the fallopian tubes or by tracking of fluid through fascial planes to the vaginal vault. There is often an associated peritonitis. Diagnosis is confirmed by the presence of fluid in the vagina with a glucose content much higher than the patient's blood glucose level. If the fallopian tubes are the cause, tubal ligation should cure the problem. Otherwise, leaving the abdomen dry for 2 weeks may allow for spontaneous healing. A recurrence may mean that transfer to hemodialysis would be in the patient's best interest.

Hydrothorax

A pleural effusion can occur because of generalized fluid overload or local lung disease, but occasionally it is due to a leak of dialysate through the diaphragm. This more commonly occurs on the right side. A leak is most simply confirmed by aspirating some of the effusion and finding that it has a glucose concentration that is higher than of the patient's blood glucose. Conservative measures should be tried initially. These include stopping PD, aspirating the effusion to dryness, and leaving the abdomen dry for 2 weeks (using hemodialysis if necessary). This regimen is effective in a number of patients. If the condition recurs, pleurodesis should be tried. Various agents have been advocated including tetracycline, talc, autologous blood, and fibrin glue, but there are no comparative studies to indicate the best regimen.

Hernias

Given the inevitable increase in intra-abdominal pressure due to the presence of a large volume of fluid in the abdomen, any weakness in the abdominal wall may give way, creating a hernia. Hernias are relatively common in PD patients. The major risks are incarceration and strangulation of bowel. The most common sites are inguinal, incisional, pericatheter, and periumbilical. Any patient commencing long-term PD with a hernia should have it repaired. This can be done at the same time as catheter insertion. Pericatheter hernias are less likely if the catheter is inserted in a paramedian position and PD is not started for at least 10 days after the procedure. If a hernia subsequently develops during PD treatment, it should be electively repaired. Postoperatively, the patient should be treated by low-volume (500 mL) cycles with no dwell using a cycler. The volume is progressively increased and CAPD can recommence after 10 days. Alternatively, the patient can be treated by temporary hemodialysis. Should hernias become a recurrent problem, a switch to nightly PD should seriously be considered because intra-abdominal pressure is lower in the supine position. The only other option is a transfer to hemodialysis.

Uterine Prolapse

One special form of hernia is uterine prolapse. Once again the increased abdominal pressure, particularly during CAPD, will exacerbate this problem. Though uncommon, it can be difficult to treat. Ring pessaries are sometimes helpful for controlling uterine descent. If these are not successful, a repair should be considered. In the absence of published information, it is suggested that postoperatively the patient should receive low-volume cycles or switch temporarily to hemodialysis (i.e., managed in the same way as for ordinary hernias).

Pain

Inflow Pain

Soon after the commencement of PD, patients may experience pain during inflow of the fluid. This is particularly likely to occur if dialysis commences immediately or within a few days of catheter insertion. It is presumably related to blunt trauma of the peritoneum. This problem usually disappears with time but may require the temporary use of simple analgesics. Slowing the rate of inflow will often reduce the symptoms. Curled-tip catheters are thought to reduce the likelihood of this type of pain. The introduction of air can also produce discomfort. Care with the bag-exchange technique should eliminate this hazard. Pain invariably occurs during peritonitis. The treatment is the same as for any case of peritonitis together with sufficient analgesia if clinically necessary. A small number of individuals have persistent inflow pain. At least some of these can be treated successfully by increasing the pH of the fluid from the usual acidic level of 5.3 to neutral by using neutral pH bicarbonate-based solutions.[17]

Backache

In a minority of patients, particularly those undergoing CAPD or having a daytime dwell in association with automated PD, backache may occur. The presence of a large volume of fluid in the abdomen distorts the normal body balance and posture, exacerbating any tendency to lordosis of the spine. Patients with preexisting back problems are most likely to have an exacerbation of their backache although by no means will they all be affected. It is important to investigate the symptom so as to exclude treatable or serious disease. This includes plain views of the spine and, if necessary, magnetic resonance imaging. Renal osteodystrophy, if present, must be treated appropriately. If, however, the problem appears to be due to degenerative disease of the spine (spondylolisthesis or osteoporosis), adjusting the PD regimen can be beneficial. Reducing the volume of dialysate may help but may adversely affect adequacy. Avoidance of fluid in the abdomen while the patient is upright will often allow considerable improvement. This means transferring those on CAPD to nightly PD and avoiding a daytime dwell. If this is ineffective, a switch to hemodialysis should be tried. In addition to the above, exercises for the back are sometimes useful.

Generalized Pain

If peritonitis occurs, some patients will develop generalized abdominal pain, particularly if treatment is delayed. This symptom usually disappears within a few days of controlling the infection. A fixed or strangulated hernia may also cause persistent abdominal pain. Local pain can occur in association with exit-site or tunnel infections. Specific treatment of the cause will eliminate the symptom.

Outflow Pain

Some patients have discomfort or even pain when the dialysate runs out. This emptying sensation is abolished when the next cycle runs in. This commonly occurs during peritonitis but may be experienced in the absence of infection during the first few weeks of treatment. In the latter situation, the symptom usually disappears with time.

Bleeding

After Catheter Insertion

Immediately after the catheter is placed in the peritoneal cavity, a small amount of bleeding can occur from the operation wounds. If excessive, this will usually respond to firm pressure. Rarely, it may be necessary to reopen the wound and secure the bleeding point.

Exit-Site Bleeding

The exit site can be a source of blood loss at any time while a peritoneal catheter is in place. A common cause is the removal of a crust before actual separation has occurred. The bleeding almost invariably stops with local pressure, but a raw area remains, which is liable to get infected. Regular cleaning of the exit site with povidone-iodine will reduce the chances of this complication. Patients should be instructed not to pull off the crust but await its natural separation. Severe infection of the exit site may, on occasion, be accompanied by secondary hemorrhage. This again will usually respond to firm pressure with gauze dressings. The subsequent management is the same as for any exit-site infection.

Blood-Stained Dialysate

This uncommon event, although rarely serious, can cause considerable alarm to the patient. In some individuals, a clear history of trauma to the abdomen or of unexpected strain is seen. Some women relate the episode to their menstrual cycle at the time of ovulation or menstruation. The treatment is to flush the abdomen with a few cycles of dialysate containing heparin (500 units/L) to minimize the chances of clotting in the catheter. It has been suggested that ice-cold dialysis fluid will stop the bleeding more quickly. There is no controlled trial of this, and the procedure is uncomfortable. The problem usually resolves spontaneously and is often visible in only one outflow. It is unusual for the blood-stained dialysate to be associated with infection, although it is wise to have the fluid cultured. Routine use of antibiotics is not necessary. In the rare event of significant hemorrhage occurring, an urgent laparotomy is required.

Chyloperitoneum

An occasional patient may present with a milky effluent. The initial reaction is to suspect peritonitis, but closer inspection reveals that the fluid is not completely opaque; microscopy does not show excess white cells. This appearance is thought to be due to the presence of chylomicrons in the dialysate. There is no obvious cause in some patients, but malignant neoplasm in the retroperitoneum, including lymphoma, can present this way. Reasonable steps should be taken to exclude such a diagnosis. In the absence of malignant disease there is no specific treatment.

Metabolic Complications

The use of glucose-based hyperosmolar solutions for PD results in a significant increase in the glucose load experienced by the patient. A number of reports have measured the daily glucose absorption, which is estimated as between 100 and 200 g/day.

The resulting metabolic effect is a persistent tendency for patients on CAPD to develop hyperglycemia and hyperinsulinemia. In a number of individuals, frank diabetes may develop. This unused glucose load is also thought to contribute to an increased risk of atherogenesis.

Changes in lipid metabolism peculiar to CAPD are more difficult to define. Triglycerides and cholesterol levels increase during the first year on CAPD. This is due to an increase in very-low-density and low-density lipoproteins. The greater the degree of hyperlipidemia at the start of therapy, the worse will be the changes with time on CAPD. In addition, lipoprotein (a) levels may increase with time on CAPD (although these results are not universally confirmed). On the whole, however, proatherogenic lipid levels are more common in patients on CAPD than those on hemodialysis.

A number of studies have demonstrated the effectiveness of cholesterol-lowering agents in patients on CAPD. Both lovastatin and simvastatin (hydroxymethylglutaryl-coenzyme A reductase inhibitors) have been shown effective in reducing total cholesterol and low-density lipoprotein cholesterol while increasing high-density lipoprotein cholesterol.[18] The long-term effects of such intervention on cardiovascular morbidity and mortality, however, have yet to be established.

References

1. Williams JD, Craig KJ, Topley N, et al: Morphologic changes in the peritoneal membrane of patients with renal disease. J Am Soc Nephrol 2002;13:470–479.
2. Kawanishi H, Watanabe H, Moriishi M, Tsuchiya S: Successful surgical management of encapsulating peritoneal sclerosis. Perit Dial Int 2005;25(Suppl 4):S39–S47.
3. Keane WF, Bailie GR, Boeschoten E, et al: Adult peritoneal dialysis-related peritonitis treatment recommendations: 2000 update. Perit Dial Int 2000;20:396–411.
4. Piraino B, Bailie GR, Bernardini J, et al: Peritoneal dialysis-related infections recommendations: 2005 update. Perit Dial Int 2005;25:107–131.
5. Hall G, Bogan A, Dreis S, et al: New directions in peritoneal dialysis patient training. Nephrol Nurs J 2004;31:149–163.
6. MacLeod A, Grant A, Donaldson C, et al: Effectiveness and efficiency of methods of dialysis therapy for end-stage renal disease: Systematic reviews. Health Technol Assess 1998;2:1–166.
7. Bernardini J, Piraino B, Holley J, et al: A randomized trial of Staphylococcus aureus prophylaxis in peritoneal dialysis patients: Mupirocin calcium ointment 2% applied to the exit site versus cyclic oral rifampin. Am J Kidney Dis 1996;27:695–700.
8. Bernardini J, Bender F, Florio T, et al: Randomized, double-blind trial of antibiotic exit site cream for prevention of exit site infection in peritoneal dialysis patients. J Am Soc Nephrol 2005;16:539–545.
9. Heimbürger O, Waniewski J, Werynski A, et al: Peritoneal transport in CAPD patients with permanent loss of ultrafiltration capacity. Kidney Int 1990;38:495–506.
10. Davies SJ, Brown B, Bryan J, Russell GI: Clinical evaluation of the peritoneal equilibration test: A population-based study. Nephrol Dial Transplant 1993;8:64–70.
11. Davies SJ: Monitoring of long-term peritoneal membrane function. Perit Dial Int 2001;21:225–230.
12. Ho-dac-Pannekeet MM, Atasever B, Struijk DG, Krediet RT: Analysis of ultrafiltration failure in peritoneal dialysis patients by means of standard peritoneal permeability analysis. Perit Dial Int 1997;17:144–150.
13. Smit W, Schouten N, van den Berg N, et al: Analysis of the prevalence and causes of ultrafiltration failure during long-term peritoneal dialysis: A cross-sectional study. Perit Dial Int 2004;24:562–570.
14. Brimble KS, Walker M, Margetts PJ, et al: Meta-analysis: Peritoneal membrane transport, mortality, and technique failure in peritoneal dialysis. J Am Soc Nephrol 2006;17:2591–2598. Epub 2006 Aug 2.
15. Davies SJ: Mitigating peritoneal membrane characteristics in modern PD therapy. Kidney Int 2006;103(Suppl):S76–S83.
16. Parikova A, Smit W, Struijk DG, Krediet RT: Analysis of fluid transport pathways and their determinants in peritoneal dialysis patients with ultrafiltration failure. Kidney Int 2006;70:1988–1994. Epub 2006 Oct 11.
17. Mactier RA, Sprosen TS, Gokal R, et al: Bicarbonate and bicarbonate/lactate peritoneal dialysis solutions for the treatment of infusion pain. Kidney Int 1998;53:1061–1067.
18. Fried L, Hutchison A, Stegmayr B, et al: Recommendations for the treatment of lipid disorders in patients on peritoneal dialysis. International Society for Peritoneal Dialysis guidelines/recommendations. Perit Dial Int 1999;19:7–16.

Further Reading

Feehally J, Floege J, Johnson RJ (eds): Comprehensive Clinical Nephrology. New York: Elsevier, 2007.
International Society for Peritoneal Dialysis. Available at: www.ispd.org. Accessed May 5, 2008.
Renal Association, UK. Available at: www.renal.org. Accessed May 5, 2008.
UpToDate: Putting clinical information into practice. Available at www.uptodate.com. Accessed May 5, 2008.

Adequacy of Peritoneal Dialysis

Peter G. Blake

The term *adequacy of dialysis* has traditionally been used to refer to small solute clearance in both hemodialysis (HD) and peritoneal dialysis (PD). There is, however, an increasing sense, based on recent studies, that the importance of clearances may have been overstated in the past and that an assessment of adequacy should take into account other elements of the dialysis prescription, in particular, control of volume status. In this chapter, emphasis is given to small solute clearance, but attention is also paid to the equally important areas of volume status and nutrition.

The issue of comparative outcomes on PD, relative to HD, is also a key measure of the adequacy of PD as a renal replacement therapy. A controversial topic, it is reviewed here.

SMALL SOLUTE CLEARANCE

In the late 1980s, the first attempts were made to extrapolate to PD the principles of quantification and prescription of dialytic dose established for HD in the aftermath of the National Cooperative Dialysis Study.[1] In the 1990s, numerous studies attempted to show that measurements of fractional urea clearance (Kt/V) and creatinine clearance corrected for body surface area (CrCl) correlated with, or were predictive of, patient well-being and survival; the first clearance guidelines were introduced. In this decade the results of the first major randomized, controlled trials in this area have appeared and have led to a re-evaluation of the importance of clearances and to a revision of clearance guidelines.

Principles of Quantification

Small solute clearance in PD is made up of both a peritoneal and a residual renal component. The latter is particularly important in that it accounts for a greater proportion of overall clearance achieved than is the case in HD and appears to persist longer in PD patients.

The peritoneal component is calculated by collecting dialysate effluent for 24 hours and measuring its urea and creatinine content. These are then divided by the serum urea and creatinine levels, respectively, to give peritoneal urea clearance (Kt$_{urea}$) and creatinine clearance. Dialysate creatinine levels may need to be corrected for the high dialysate glucose content because this interferes with the assay used in some laboratories. The renal component is calculated in the same way, with a 24-hour urine collection. However, in the case of creatinine clearance, an average of residual renal urea and creatinine clearance is typically used, because unmodified creatinine clearance substantially overestimates the true glomerular filtration rate. These clearances are then normalized to total body water (V) to give Kt/V, or to 1.73 m^2 body surface area to give CrCl. The value for V is estimated using anthropometric formulas, such as those of Watson, based on age, sex, height, and weight.[2] These estimates, compared with a standard of measurement such as deuterium oxide dilution, are, on average, reasonably accurate in nonobese patients but tend to give an overestimate of V in those who are overweight.[3] Nevertheless, because most of the clinical literature is based on a V calculated with these equations and because they are relatively simple, they remain the method of choice. Body surface area is estimated by the Du Bois formula.[4] Kt/V and CrCl values are typically expressed as weekly, rather than daily, clearances (Boxes 83-1 and 83-2).

Attempts to estimate Kt/V and CrCl using abbreviated methods based on the peritoneal equilibration test (PET) are not sufficiently accurate for clinical practice. Computer programs that calculate clearances are widely available. These can also be used to "model" patient prescriptions and predict the clearances a given prescription will achieve, but they are not accurate enough to replace the 24-hour collection in clinical practice. Collections are more cumbersome in patients on automated peritoneal dialysis (APD), as compared to continuous ambulatory peritoneal dialysis (CAPD), because of the greater volumes involved, and many units train patients to record or measure cycler effluent volumes and then to take a representative aliquot of dialysate for measurement of urea and creatinine.

Box 83-1   Formulas Required to Calculate Kt/V

Kt/V	$= 7 \times$ (daily peritoneal Kt/V + daily renal Kt/V)
Daily peritoneal Kt	$= \dfrac{\text{24-hr dialysate urea content}}{\text{serum urea}}$
Daily peritoneal Kt	$= \dfrac{\text{24-hr urine urea content}}{\text{serum urea}}$
V (by Watson)	$= 2.447 - 0.09516\ A + 0.1704\ H + 0.3362\ W$ (in males) or
	$= -2.097 - 0.1069\ H + 0.02466\ W$ (in females)

A, age (years); H, height (cm); W, weight (kg).

Box 83-2   Formulas Required to Calculate Creatinine Clearance (CrCl)

Crcl (L/wk)	$= \dfrac{\text{Weekly creatinine clearance (L/wk)} \times \text{body surface area (m}^2)}{1.73\ (\text{m}^2)}$
Weekly creatinine clearance (L/wk)	$= 7 \times$ (daily peritoneal creatinine clearance + daily renal clearance)
Daily peritoneal creatinine clearance	$= \dfrac{\text{24-hr dialysate creatinine content*}}{\text{serum creatinine}}$
Daily renal creatinine clearance	$= \dfrac{\text{24-hr urine creatinine content}}{\text{serum creatinine} \times 2} + \dfrac{\text{24-hr urine urea content}}{\text{serum urea} \times 2}$
Body surface area (by Du Bois):	$\log A\ (\text{cm}^2) = 0.425 \log W + 0.725 \log H + 1.8564$

*Corrected for dialysate glucose by a formula specific to each laboratory.
A, body surface area (m²); H, height (cm); W, weight (kg).

Typically, residual renal function declines gradually towards zero over the first 2 to 3 years on PD; total clearance will also decrease if the dialysis prescription is not modified (Fig. 83-1).[5] The achievement of clearance targets requires such modifications to be made. In general, dialysate and urine collections should be performed shortly after commencing PD, every 4 months subsequently so as to allow timely detection of declines in residual function, and after any alteration in prescription or otherwise unexplained clinical event. Data suggest that daily collections are not very reproducible, particularly due to major variations in the urinary component.[6] A 48-hour urine collection might therefore be preferable in some patients. An unexpected result should be confirmed with a repeat collection.

The urea and protein content of the same 24-hour collections done to calculate clearance can be used to measure normalized protein equivalent of nitrogen appearance (nPNA), which, in a stable patient, is an estimate of dietary protein intake. Numerous formulas are used for calculating nPNA, but evidence suggests that those of Bergstrom are best (Box 83-3).[7,8] Also these collections allow measurement of total

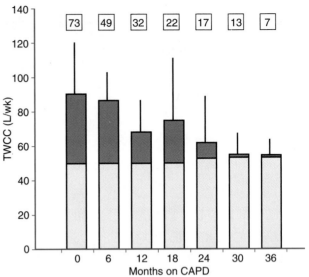

Figure 83-1   Change in creatinine clearance (CrCl) with time and continuous ambulatory peritoneal dialysis (CAPD). *Lighter areas* and *darker areas* indicate the proportions of CrCl accounted for by peritoneal and renal clearance, respectively. Figures in the *boxes* refer to the number of patients at each 6-month interval. (From Blake PG, Balaskas EV, Izatt S, Oreopoulos DG: Is total creatinine clearance a good predictor of clinical outcomes in CAPD? Perit Dial Int 1992;12:353–358.)

creatinine excretion, which can in turn be used to estimate lean body mass (Box 83-4).[9] Similarly, total protein or albumin losses can be helpful in the evaluation of low serum albumin values.

Total Kt/V values achieved with typical PD prescriptions are half to two thirds of those achieved with HD. This might suggest major underdialysis, but it must be remembered that the efficiency, in terms of solute removal, of clearance delivered

Box 83-3   Bergstrom Formulas for Estimating Protein Equivalent of Nitrogen Appearance (PNA) in Patients on Peritoneal Dialysis

PNA (g/day)	$= 20.1 + 7.50$ (daily dialysate + urine urea nitrogen content [g/day])
	or
	$= 15.1 + 6.95$ (daily dialysate + urine urea nitrogen content [g/day]) + daily dialysate + urine protein content (g/day)

The same formulas with urea concentrations expressed in SI units are as follows:

PNA (g/day)	$= 20.1 + 0.209$ (daily dialysate + urine urea content [mmol/day])
	or
	$= 15.1 + 0.195$ (daily dialysate + urine urea content [mmol/day]) + daily dialysate + urine protein content (g/day)

In all cases, normalized PNA (nPNA) = PNA/desirable body weight.
Modified from Bergstrom J, Heimburger O, Lindholm B: Calculation of the protein equivalent of total nitrogen appearance from urea appearance. Which formulas should be used? Perit Dial Int 1998;18:467–473.

Box 83-4 Formulas for Calculating Lean Body Mass by the Method of Keshaviah et al*

Lean body mass (kg)	= 7.38 + 0.029 [creatinine production (mg/day)]
Creatinine production (mg)	= creatinine excretion + creatinine degradation
Creatinine excretion (mg/day) creatinine content (mg)	= 24-hr dialysate creatinine† content (mg) + 24-hr urine
Creatinine degradation	= 0.38 [serum creatinine (mg/day) (mg/dL)] × [body weight (kg)]

*Keshaviah PR, Nolph KD, Moore HL, et al: Lean body mass estimation by creatinine kinetics. J Am Soc Nephrol 1994;4: 1475–1485.
†Corrected for dialysate glucose by a formula specific to each laboratory.

intermittently is much less than that of the same amount of clearance delivered continuously.[10] Also, continuous modalities, in comparison to intermittent modalities, avoid substantial disequilibrium. Furthermore, it has also been suggested that continuous modalities are advantageous because peak levels of uremic toxins are theoretically at a lower level for a given quantity of clearance than is the case with intermittent modalities. It has been proposed that peak rather than mean levels of small solutes are proportional to uremic toxicity.[11]

Clinical Studies on Adequacy of Peritoneal Dialysis

Initial studies correlating small solute clearance and patient outcomes gave varied results and in retrospect have multiple methodologic flaws. The Canada/USA (CANUSA) Study avoided some of these problems in that it was multicenter and prospective, and in that it followed almost 600 incident CAPD patients for up to 3 years, giving it reasonable statistical power.[12] It was, however, a cohort study with no mandated interventions. CANUSA demonstrated a predictive power for both Kt/V and CrCl, such that a 5 L/wk lower CrCl was associated with a 7% greater relative risk of dying, and a 0.1 unit/wk lower Kt/V was associated with a 5% greater relative risk of dying. Patients in CANUSA mainly received standard 4 × 2L per day CAPD with few alterations, so that changes in clearance were mainly due to declines in residual function. CANUSA, on closer analysis, showed a correlation between residual renal clearance and subsequent mortality, but could not show a correlation between peritoneal clearance alone and mortality.[13] However, the design of the study did not really allow this issue to be addressed.

Subsequent to CANUSA, a variety of other prospective and retrospective studies showed similar correlations between small solute clearance and clinical outcomes, but all were similarly confounded by residual renal function.[14–16] None could show an independent effect of peritoneal clearance on outcomes, even when there was significant variation in PD dose.[16] Notwithstanding this, clinical practice guidelines from various bodies proposed target Kt/V and CrCl values in the middle and late 1990s.[17,18] Most notably, the United States National Kidney Foundation's Kidney/Dialysis Outcomes Quality Initiative (K/DOQI) set a weekly Kt/V target of 2.0 for CAPD. For CrCl, the target was set at 60 L/wk, although

this was subsequently modified down to 50 L/wk for low and low-average transporters.[17–19] Slightly higher targets were set for APD, with and without day dwells, on the grounds that these are somewhat more intermittent modalities than is CAPD. These new clearance targets had a major impact on PD prescription and led to increased use of higher dwell volumes in CAPD and of multiple day dwells in APD.[20] The result was a notable increase in delivered clearances.

Randomized, Controlled Trials

The first major randomized, controlled trials addressing the effectiveness of raising peritoneal clearance have appeared since 2000.[21–23]

The best and most definitive was the ADEquacy of Peritoneal Dialysis in MEXico Study (ADEMEX), which involved 960 incident and prevalent CAPD patients recruited from 25 centers in Mexico.[22] Participating patients were randomized to one of two groups. The control group was maintained on a standard 4 × 2L CAPD prescription, and the intervention group had their prescription augmented to achieve a peritoneal creatinine clearance of 60 L/wk. A small number of patients who could achieve a peritoneal creatinine clearance of 60 L/wk on the standard prescription were excluded from the study. The increases in clearance in the intervention group were made using a larger dwell volume or a fifth exchange, delivered with a night exchange device. Follow-up was for an average of 2 years; the primary endpoint was survival. A large variety of secondary endpoints was also examined. Unlike previous studies, ADEMEX had substantial statistical power to detect endpoint differences. The control group achieved, on average, a weekly peritoneal CrCl of 46 L and a weekly peritoneal Kt/V of 1.62; the intervention group had values of 57 L and 2.13, respectively. Corresponding values for total Kt/V were 1.80 and 2.27 and for CrCl were 54 and 63 L/wk, respectively (Table 83-1). There were no significant differences in either primary or secondary outcomes between the two groups. In particular, the relative risk of mortality for a patient included in the intervention group was 1.00 relative to a patient in the control group (Fig. 83-2). This result was surprising to many and, given the high quality of the study, brought into question the appropriateness of the K/DOQI 2000 clearance recommendations.

Concerns have been raised about the ADEMEX findings.[24] These include concerns as to whether the results can be extrapolated to non-Mexican patients, to populations with higher rates of cardiovascular disease, or to patients on APD as distinct from CAPD. In support of the ADEMEX findings, however, are the results of the randomized, controlled trial from Lo and colleagues.[23] This study involved 322 incident

Table 83-1 Peritoneal and Total Clearances Delivered in the ADEMEX Study

	Control	Intervention
Peritoneal Kt/V (per week)	1.62	2.13
Total Kt/V (per week)	1.80	2.27
Peritoneal CrCl (L/week)	46.1	56.9
Total CrCl (L/week)	54.1	62.9

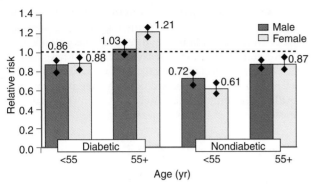

Figure 83-2 Life-table intent-to-treat analysis of patient survival showing no difference in survival between the interventions. (Reproduced from Paniagua R, Amato D, Vonesh E, et al: Effect of increased peritoneal clearances on mortality rates in peritoneal dialysis: ADEMEX, a prospective randomized controlled trial. J Am Soc Nephrol 2002;13:1307–1320.)

CAPD patients recruited from six centers in Hong Kong between 1996 and 1999. These patients were randomized to three different Kt/V targets, 1.5 to 1.7, 1.7 to 2.0, and above 2.0/wk. The three groups achieved the targeted Kt/V levels, and no difference was found in 2-year survival rates. There was, however, a significantly greater study dropout rate for patients in the group with a Kt/V below 1.7/wk; the authors concluded that Kt/V should be maintained above this level. This study was somewhat underpowered to detect mortality differences, but, in the light of the ADEMEX study, its findings are not so surprising.

These studies show that residual renal function is highly predictive of survival but cannot be replaced on a one-to-one basis by peritoneal clearance, which within the usual therapeutic range is not predictive of survival (see Table 83-1). The concept of adding renal and peritoneal clearance together as if they are the same is not justifiable. Given that increasing peritoneal clearance is not a neutral intervention and may have lifestyle implications for the patient in terms of mechanical symptoms, time commitment, and cost, it is important to avoid an unnecessarily aggressive approach to PD prescription. However, these studies do not prove that there is no link between peritoneal clearance and outcome. Clearly there is

some relationship in that zero dialysis guarantees an adverse outcome. There is no evidence that doses below those recorded by the ADEMEX control group, for example, are safe. Furthermore, the Lo study would suggest that total Kt/V values below 1.7 are problematic.

Accordingly, recent revised guidelines produced by K/DOQI have reset the Kt/V target at 1.7/wk.[25] For simplicity and in the absence of evidence to the contrary, the same target is now being used for both CAPD and APD patients, regardless of transport type. Furthermore, K/DOQI suggests that there is no additional benefit from measuring CrCl, although European guidelines still retain this index. This has simplified the prescription of PD and has made the targets easier to achieve.[25]

The reason for the lack of an effect of higher clearance on key outcomes has been debated, especially in the light of analogous findings in HD.[26] One possibility is that substantially higher clearances would be required to improve outcomes, but this is speculative. A plausible alternative is that, once sufficient clearance to control frank uremia has been delivered, outcomes depend much more on critical comorbid conditions such as diabetes and cardiac disease.

PERITONEAL TRANSPORT STATUS

Patients differ in the rapidity with which urea, creatinine, and other solutes equilibrate with dialysis solution across their peritoneal membrane. This is classically measured by the PET, in which dialysate and plasma levels of urea and creatinine are measured during a 4-hour, 2L, 2.5% dextrose dwell, done under standard conditions.[27] Equilibration curves are constructed, and patients are defined as low, low-average, high-average, or high transporters (Fig. 83-3). It is generally believed that PET status is a measure of the effective or vascular surface area of the peritoneal membrane, but interestingly it does not correlate with body size.

Patients who are high transporters equilibrate quickly and so, in that sense, dialyze well but they ultrafilter poorly because the osmotic gradient for glucose dissipates rapidly. They might be expected to do better with short dwell times, as in APD, but they need to avoid prolonged day dwells with glucose-based PD solutions. They also have higher dialysate protein losses and are more prone to marked hypoalbuminemia. Conversely,

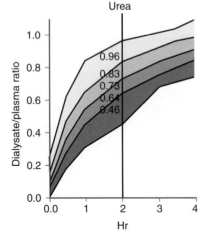
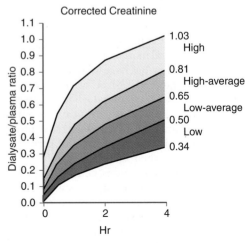

Figure 83-3 Peritoneal equilibration test (PET) results. Ranges of values for dialysate-to-plasma ratios for urea and creatinine (corrected) in standard PET. (From Twardowski ZJ, Nolph KD, Khanna R, et al: Peritoneal equilibration test. Perit Dial Bull 1987;7: 138–147.)

low transporters ultrafilter well, lose less protein in their dialysate, and have higher serum albumin levels, but equilibrate slowly. Thus, large-volume dwells with longer treatment times are best for achieving good clearance. In practice, the choice between CAPD and APD is much more influenced by lifestyle and economic considerations; with the recent reduction in clearance targets, patients of any transporter type can be adequately dialyzed with either modality, although fluid removal can be problematic in high transporters treated with long-duration dwells. Numerous studies suggest that low, rather than high, transporters have substantially superior long-term outcomes on CAPD.[28] This supports the idea that volume status may be more important than clearance. It has led to the suggestion that high transporters might preferentially be directed to APD and to the use of alternative osmotic agents to dextrose, especially when residual renal function is lost.[18] However, there is also evidence to support the alternative suggestion that high transport status may be a marker of older, sicker, more "inflamed" patients; this may be the main driver of the worse outcomes.

INCREASING PERITONEAL DIALYSIS DOSE

Despite the controversy about target clearances in PD, it is important to understand how delivered clearance can be increased in PD patients. In CAPD, the best strategy to raise dialytic dose is to increase dwell volumes to 2.5 L. This is usually well tolerated and minimally disruptive of lifestyle. Larger patients may require and tolerate 3-L volumes. The alternative approach of increasing the frequency of daytime manual exchanges to more than four will tend to lead to inadequate spacing of the exchanges so that equilibration is less complete; this approach also is likely to increase the risk of patient noncompliance.

Automated PD has become increasingly popular in recent years and is the dominant PD modality in the United States. It should not be viewed as a panacea for inadequate PD. If carelessly prescribed, it can lead to clearances that are actually less than those on standard CAPD. Daytime dwells are required to achieve clearance targets in APD patients unless residual renal function is very good, the patient is very small, or the patient is a high transporter. In heavier patients and in low transporters, especially when residual renal function is poor, two day dwells may be required. The cost of this approach can be reduced by using the cycler solutions and tubing to do the daytime exchange. If two daytime exchanges are being done, the number of cycled exchanges at night can be limited to four or even three to minimize cost.

With regard to the actual cycler prescription, 2.5L, and even higher, dwell volumes are usually well tolerated, given that APD is delivered in the supine position. The standard time spent each night on the cycler is 8 to 9 hours. Increasing the frequency of cycler exchanges to more than six or seven over 9 hours gives modest increases in clearance but is generally not cost effective[29,30] because too much of the cycling time is spent on draining and filling, and too little on actual dialysis. Tidal techniques, which maintain a constant residual volume throughout the cycling time, were devised to help with this problem, but they are not effective in increasing clearance and are only useful when the final phase of drainage is slow or painful.

With both CAPD and APD, hypertonic solutions can be used to increase clearance by maximizing ultrafiltration, but this strategy increases the risk of dehydration as well as that of obesity, hyperglycemia, hyperlipidemia and, perhaps, long-term peritoneal membrane damage. With all strategies, patient lifestyle and willingness to comply should be kept in mind. As stated, dialysis dose should be remeasured soon after each prescription alteration.

VOLUME STATUS IN PERITONEAL DIALYSIS

The favorable prognosis associated with low transporter status on PET gives support to the view that volume status is an important determinant of outcome in PD patients.[28] No high-quality data are available that prove that good volume management improves outcome. However, cardiovascular disease is the biggest cause of morbidity and mortality in dialysis patients generally, and hypertension, a crucial risk factor, is common in this population and influenced by volume status. Notwithstanding this, overaggressive volume removal may decrease residual renal function, so a balanced approach is required.

Management of volume status has been the subject of International Society of Peritoneal Dialysis clinical practice guidelines.[31] Key factors that need to be taken into account in managing volume status in PD patients, in addition to PET findings, include salt and water intake, residual renal function, and adherence to the PD prescription. Useful strategies to control volume status include dietary salt and water restriction, when required; the use of high-dose loop diuretics in patients who still have urine output; and education of patients in the significance of fluid overload and hypertension.[32] Randomized trials show that angiotensin receptor blockers and angiotensin-converting enzyme inhibitors help preserve residual renal function and so improve volume control in PD.[32–34]

A number of aspects of the prescription, however, can be modified. These are the dwell time, the tonicity of solution used, and the choice of osmotic agent. Prolonged dwell times are associated with greater peritoneal fluid absorption, which is particularly an issue with the nocturnal dwell in CAPD and with the day dwell in APD. Ultrafiltration can be enhanced, in both short and long dwells, by increasing the tonicity of the glucose solution used. However, this strategy is limited by the adverse effects of increased glucose absorption, including hyperglycemia, hyperlipidemia, obesity, and peritoneal membrane damage. A more attractive approach to avoid fluid absorption from long-duration dwells has become possible with the availability of the osmotic agent icodextrin.[35] This large molecular-weight glucose polymer induces ultrafiltration by colloid osmosis. Because the icodextrin molecule is too large to be absorbed across the peritoneal membrane, the osmotic gradient does not dissipate and there is sustained ultrafiltration throughout the duration of a long dwell. Icodextrin is now frequently used as the long day dwell in APD and as the nocturnal dwell in CAPD. A modest amount of lymphatic absorption of icodextrin occurs, with subsequent metabolism to maltose, but no associated toxicity has been identified after more than 15 years' experience. The disadvantages of icodextrin are its somewhat higher cost and a small rate of exfoliative skin rashes. Evidence from randomized, controlled trials now indicates that icodextrin not only enhances ultrafiltration, but also leads to better control of volume status, as measured by echocardiography, bioimpedance, and other measures of extracellular fluid volume.[36,37] Besides improving ultrafiltration, icodextrin can lead to less weight gain and less hyperglycemia and hypertriglyceridemia due to the reduced exposure to glucose. In general, high and high average transporters should be directed toward APD or icodextrin if problems are arising with volume status.[18] In some countries, icodextrin is now routinely used in the majority of patients.

The growth in APD was initially thought to be a positive development for control of volume status because the shorter dwell times on the cycler would be expected to lead to enhanced ultrafiltration. However, investigators have pointed out that the phenomenon of sodium sieving becomes significant with the typical short dwells of APD, leading to less sodium removal than standard CAPD.[38,39] Sieving of sodium occurs because about half the ultrafiltrate goes through peritoneal aquaporin channels, which transport water only. The longer dwell times in CAPD allow diffusive sodium removal to compensate for sieving, but this is not the case with the short cycles of APD. In practice, studies have not consistently shown worse control of volume or blood pressure in APD, but a randomized trial is required to address this issue. The use of icodextrin in the day dwell can be used to attenuate volume problems in APD.[39]

A problem with volume management in dialysis patients is the lack of a reliable and practical method to measure volume status. Blood pressure and clinical examination may be misleading and bioimpedance has methodologic limitations, as do blood levels of natriuretic peptides.[40] Essentially, volume status is still best optimized by trial and error.

PATIENT COMPLIANCE

Patient compliance with PD exchanges is an important issue for both clearance and volume status. Methodology to detect noncompliance is limited. Ratios between actual and predicted creatinine excretion have not been found to be helpful. Questionnaires are likely to understate the prevalence of noncompliance, and checks on home inventory are probably the nearest to a standard. Using the latter methodology, one U.S. group found a 40% rate of significant noncompliance.[41] A large multicenter questionnaire-based study suggested that the problem was most likely in patients who were young, employed, black, and receiving more than 4 CAPD exchanges daily.[42] There is a need to be aware of this problem.

MALNUTRITION IN PERITONEAL DIALYSIS

Malnutrition is prevalent in dialysis patients generally; one international study found, using subjective nutritional assessment, that 8% of 224 CAPD patients had severe malnutrition and a further 33% had mild to moderate malnutrition.[43]

A number of nutritional indices have been shown to predict adverse outcomes. Lower serum albumin is associated with greater mortality, hospitalization rates, and technique failure.[12] In the CANUSA study, the relative risk of dying decreased 6% for each 1 g/L rise in the serum albumin. In PD patients, however, serum albumin may not primarily be a nutritional marker. A number of studies have shown that high peritoneal transport status and the presence of inflammation, as indicated by a raised serum C-reactive protein level, are the major predictors of a low serum albumin.[44]

Lean body mass, estimated by creatinine excretion, in accordance with the method of Keshaviah,[11] and total body nitrogen, by neutron activation analysis,[45] have also been shown to predict survival, as has the relatively simple clinical tool of Subjective Global Assessment.[12] The predictive data for the nPNA are less consistent. Some of this discrepancy may be related to variation in methods of measurement and normalization. Evidence suggests that the Bergstrom formula, which was specifically derived from PD patients, is most accurate in that it takes full account of the high nonurea, nonprotein nitrogen losses in these patients.[7,46] Normalization to desirable rather than actual weight is preferable. No clear target for nPNA has been validated. On theoretical grounds, 1.2 g/kg/day has been proposed but is rarely achieved and neutral nitrogen balance may be possible at significantly lower values.[7,17] Caloric intake has been relatively poorly studied and, although it has been shown to be as important as protein intake for nitrogen balance, no clear studies correlating it with outcome have been published. The general recommendation is that patients receive 35 kilocalories/kg/day, although this should be reduced for obese patients.[17] In many patients, 20% or more of calories will come from dialysate glucose absorption. Other nutritional indices such as serum prealbumin, insulin-like growth factor-1 levels, anthropometrics, and bioelectric impedance, are not widely used.

Malnutrition in dialysis patients is typically multifactorial. Food intake is often low due to uremia per se, dietary restrictions, socioeconomic issues, possible dialysate-induced compression of viscera and, often most significantly, comorbidity, including gastrointestinal disease, cardiovascular disease, and depression. Patients also have obligatory dialysate nitrogen and protein losses and may be catabolic from inadequate intake as well as from intercurrent illnesses, inflammation, and acidosis. The role of endocrine dysfunction, and in particular of the growth hormone insulin-like growth factor 1 axis in impairing the balance between anabolism and catabolism in uremia, has also been recognized.

Management of Malnutrition

Interventions to treat malnutrition are not well validated. They include increases in dialysis dose, oral protein and carbohydrate supplementation, correction of acidosis, intraperitoneal amino acids, and administration of anabolic hormones, such as androgens, and recombinant growth hormone and insulin-like growth factor-1.

A small number of studies, mostly uncontrolled, have looked at the effect of prospective increases in peritoneal clearance on nutrition.[47] In general, these studies have shown conflicting results with regard to protein intake, with some showing an increase and others no change. The methodology is often confounded by mathematical coupling between indices of dialysis dose and those of nutrition. In studies that have looked at serum albumin, there has been no clear beneficial effect. The ADEMEX study also failed to show a nutritional advantage for the high clearance group.[22]

Numerous studies have examined intraperitoneal amino acids. Initially these were confounded by associated increases in uremia and acidosis, but more recently the amino acid composition of the preparations has been favorably modified and strategies for administering them have improved; they are now given as one exchange in the daytime, in association with oral caloric intake. Recent controlled trials have shown an increase in nitrogen balance and better maintenance of serum albumin over 3 years follow-up.[48] There were additional advantages for women, with better maintenance of lean body mass and body mass index, but the study was too small to detect any survival advantage for treated patients.

Correction of acidosis or even induction of mild alkalosis with oral sodium bicarbonate has been shown to improve nutritional status in PD patients. In one randomized trial of 60 patients followed for 1 year, the bicarbonate-treated patients had superior PNA and Subjective Global Assessment scores and less hospitalization than placebo-treated controls.[49]

One small randomized, controlled trial has shown a benefit for anabolic steroids in increasing lean body mass and functional performance in malnourished HD and PD patients, but concerns about adverse effects have limited their use.[50] Studies on recombinant growth hormone and insulin-like growth factor-1 have been small and short term but have shown impressive anabolic effects.[51] Effects on serum albumin have been less impressive. Cost and toxicity concerns limit the use of these recombinant agents to research studies at present.

The relative ineffectiveness of most of these nutritional interventions in PD patients raises questions about the nature of malnutrition in dialysis patients generally. Although many patients have malnutrition and its presence predicts adverse outcomes, it is not clear that the malnutrition is the proximate cause of those outcomes or that its correction, when possible, will lead to an improvement in those outcomes. It is at least as plausible that the malnutrition is a consequence of the comorbidity or inflammation, which is the true proximate cause of the patients' morbidity and mortality. If the latter is the case, attempts to treat the malnutrition without dealing with underlying causes may be ineffective both in terms of nutritional status and in terms of ultimate clinical outcomes. Recent data linking malnutrition, inflammation, and cardiovascular disease may be pertinent in this regard.[52]

COMPARATIVE OUTCOME STUDIES

Interest in adequacy of dialysis has also focused attention on comparative outcomes between HD and PD. Most data come from national or renal registries; none is from randomized, controlled trials. Patient mortality is the usual endpoint used in these studies. A controversial U.S. Registry study published in 1995 suggested an excess mortality on PD, but the methodology was unusual in that the majority of the first year on dialysis was omitted from the analysis.[53] This leads to a systematic bias against PD because outcomes on the modality are relatively better in the early years on dialysis.

Subsequent and more contemporary studies from the U.S., Canadian, Danish, Dutch, and Lombardy registries all show a similar picture.[54–58] The relative mortality rates of the two modalities change with length of time on dialysis (Fig. 83-4). PD has a survival advantage over HD during the first 1 to 3 years of dialysis. This advantage is most marked in younger

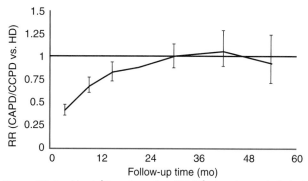

Figure 83-4 Mortality rate ratios (RRs) for peritoneal dialysis relative to hemodialysis (HD) by follow-up interval, adjusted for age, primary renal diagnosis, and comorbid conditions, estimated using Poisson regression. (From Schaubel DE, Blake PG, Fenton SS: Trends in CAPD technique failure: Canada 1981–1997. Perit Dial Int 2001;21:365–371.)

patients and in nondiabetic patients (Fig. 83-5). In the United States, however, no significant early advantage for PD is seen in older diabetic patients, and, indeed, in older female diabetic patients, HD has a significant advantage.[54] After 2 years of dialysis, data are less detailed, but PD appears to lose its advantage and HD is associated with equal or better survival. The reason for the early survival benefit of PD has been debated. One possibility is that it relates to better retention of residual renal function. An alternative is that it simply represents a baseline case mix advantage for PD that cannot be detected in registry studies. This benefit is, however, found in countries with both high and low PD use.[54,55,57]

A particular concern has been raised in the United States by more recent registry studies showing worse outcomes on PD in patients with cardiac disease.[59,60] These findings have not been confirmed in other countries but are a concern; they have heightened interest in glucose-sparing approaches because it is sometimes suggested that systemic glucose absorption may be a particular problem in patients with cardiac disease.

In the absence of randomized trials, a number of prospective but nonrandomized cohort studies have compared HD and PD.

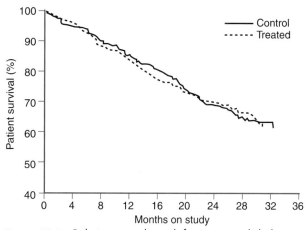

Figure 83-5 Relative mortality risk for peritoneal dialysis compared to hemodialysis in incident in U.S. dialysis patients, 1994–1998. (From Collins AJ, How W, Xia H, et al: Mortality risks of peritoneal dialysis and hemodialysis. Am J Kidney Dis 1999;34:1065–1074.)

A Canadian study of 822 incident patients followed for 2 years found a survival advantage for PD, but this went away after adjustment for the greater comorbidity in HD patients.[61] The Dutch NECOSAD investigators also found some early advantage for PD. There was no overall survival difference in 1222 incident patients over the first 2 years, but there was an advantage for PD in diabetic patients younger than age 60 years. After 2 years, however, a significant benefit for HD was seen in patients age 60 years or older.[62] The CHOICE study, done in the United States, also showed no early difference in survival but reported a worse outcome on PD after the first year and after adjustment for laboratory tests.[63] The methodology used in CHOICE has been questioned, but the high rates of cardiac disease, diabetes, and obesity in the U.S. dialysis population may create particular issues for glucose-based PD.[64] Overall, therefore, prospective studies show a similar pattern of results to the registry-based ones. Technique failure is undoubtedly more common in PD than HD. The most frequent causes are peritonitis, social reasons, and "inadequate dialysis." There is some evidence that technique failure rates in PD are falling, principally due to better prevention and management of peritonitis.[65]

A reasonable conclusion from all this is that modality selection should not be significantly influenced by these comparative studies. Findings are not sufficiently robust to justify making modality decisions based on age, diabetes, or cardiac disease. PD is at least as effective as HD in the early years for patients who choose it. Given its cost advantage in most developed countries, this suggests that PD is a more cost-effective initial therapy. Subsequently, many patients will need to move to HD due to technique failure, and often loss of residual renal function may be associated with this. A dialysis delivery system based on early use of PD but easy availability of HD after 2 to 3 years might be maximally cost effective. This concept has been described as *integrated dialysis care*.[66]

SPECIFIC MANAGEMENT RECOMMENDATIONS

The recent revision of the K/DOQI guidelines on adequacy of dialysis has helped to resolve some of the confusion induced by the results of the ADEMEX study.

A reasonable strategy is to evaluate patients clinically every 1 to 2 months looking for evidence of underdialysis and to monitor both renal and peritoneal Kt/V shortly after the patient initiates PD and routinely at 4- to 6-month intervals with

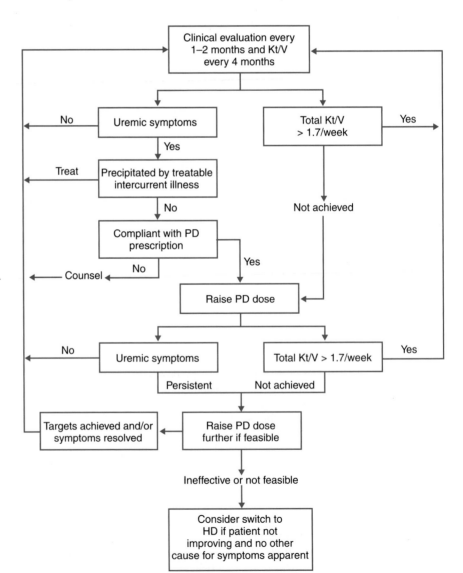

Figure 83-6 Algorithm for the management of clearances in peritoneal dialysis.

a view to keeping the combined value over 1.7/wk (Fig. 83-6). Clearances should also be remeasured soon after any alteration in the prescription and in response to any unexplained clinical changes. Issues such as compliance and the influence of intercurrent illnesses should be kept in mind.

A good approach is to use 4 × 2L daily in CAPD patients and to increase dwell volumes to 2.5 L if the Kt/V target is not reached. Patients with substantial residual renal function may manage for a while with three exchanges daily. With APD, day dry cycling may provide sufficient clearance in those with substantial renal function, but most patients will soon require a day dwell. If icodextrin is easily available, this can be used to minimize glucose absorption and to avoid the need for a daytime drain. Otherwise, glucose-based solution can be used, but consideration should be given to draining it after 4 to 6 hours to minimize absorption and maximize fluid removal. Cycling can be done with 8 to 10 L delivered as 4 or 5 × 2L dwells over 9 hours. Upward adjustments in clearance are best achieved by addition of a day dwell in day dry patients or of a second day dwell if one is already being used. Increasing the volume of cycled fluid is an alternative though less cost-effective option.

Careful attention should be paid to volume status, with the aim of keeping the patient edema free and the blood pressure at or below 130/80 mm Hg while also being aware of the need to avoid volume depletion, with consequent loss of residual renal function, and to limit hypertonic glucose exposure. Long-duration dextrose dwells should be avoided, especially if volume status is a problem. In such settings, the use of APD and icodextrin for long dwells should be considered. PET status should be monitored to identify patients who are at risk for volume overload and who might require these interventions. Loop diuretics and renoprotective agents should be considered.

A multidisciplinary approach to malnutrition is recommended. It should be screened for with a combination of tools, including clinical evaluation; assessment of dietary protein and calorie intake by a renal dietitian; Subjective Global Assessment; measurements of serum urea, creatinine, potassium, and albumin; serial 24-hour creatinine excretion as an index of lean body mass; and nPNA. The limitations of each of these indices should be kept in mind, and no individual one should be emphasized to the exclusion of the others. Warning signs for malnutrition include decreasing body weight, low or declining Subjective Global Assessment status, decreasing lean body mass or blood urea, and nPNA below 0.8 g/kg/day using the Bergstrom formula with normalization to desired or standard weight. Serum albumin below 30 g/L should be investigated, not only with nutrition in mind, but also with regard to PET status and the presence of inflammation, which may frequently not be clinically apparent.

Preventive strategies for malnutrition include a timely start on dialysis, targeting a dietary protein intake above 1 g/kg body weight per day, and a dietary calorie intake above 35 kcal/kg/day, avoidance of acidosis, and an adequate PD prescription.

Therapeutic strategies ideally involve a multidisciplinary approach with dietary counseling, diagnosis and treatment of comorbidity with special attention to upper gastrointestinal disease and depression, correction of poor dentition, awareness of cultural and socioeconomic issues, avoidance of excessive numbers of medications, and correction of acidosis and, where possible, inflammation. If this is unsuccessful, interventions to consider are oral calorie and protein supplementation and the use of intraperitoneal amino acids. Administration of anabolic steroids may sometimes have a role. A trial of HD may be appropriate if the nutritional status is not improving and if no clear cause for this can be identified.

References

1. Teehan BP, Schleifer CR, Sigler MH, et al: A quantitative approach to the CAPD prescription. Perit Dial Bull 1985;5:152–156.
2. Watson PR, Watson ID, Batt RD: Total body water volumes for adult males and females estimated from simple anthropometric measurements. Am J Clin Nutr 1980;23:27–39.
3. Wong K-C, Xiong D-W, Kerr PG, et al: Kt/V in CAPD by different estimations of V. Kidney Int 1995;48:563–569.
4. Du Bois D, Du Bois EF: A formula to estimate the approximate surface area if height and weight be known. Arch Intern Med 1916;17:863–871.
5. Blake PG, Balaskas EV, Izatt S, Oreopoulos DG: Is total creatinine clearance a good predictor of clinical outcomes in CAPD? Perit Dial Int 1992;12:353–358.
6. Rodby RA, Firaneck CA, Cheng YG, et al: Reproducibility of studies of peritoneal dialysis adequacy. Kidney Int 1996;50:267–271.
7. Bergstrom J, Heimburger O, Lindholm B: Calculation of the protein equivalent of total nitrogen appearance from urea appearance. Which formulas should be used? Perit Dial Int 1998;18:467–473.
8. Kopple JD, Gao XL, Qing DP: Dietary protein, urea nitrogen appearance and total nitrogen appearance in chronic renal failure and CAPD patients. Kidney Int 1997;52:486–494.
9. Keshaviah PR, Nolph KD, Moore HL, et al: Lean body mass estimation by creatinine kinetics. J Am Soc Nephrol 1994;4:1475–1485.
10. Depner TA: Quantifying hemodialysis and peritoneal dialysis: Examination of the peak concentration hypothesis. Semin Dial 1994;7:315–317.
11. Keshaviah PR, Nolph KD, VanStone JC: The peak concentration hypothesis: A urea kinetic approach to comparing the adequacy of continuous ambulatory peritoneal dialysis and hemodialysis. Perit Dial Int 1989;9:257–260.
12. Churchill ND, Taylor DW, Keshaviah PR, for the CANUSA Peritoneal Dialysis Study Group: Adequacy of dialysis and nutrition in continuous peritoneal dialysis: Association with clinical outcomes. J Am Soc Nephrol 1996;7:198–207.
13. Bargman JM, Thorpe KE, Churchill DN, for the CANUSA Peritoneal Dialysis Study Group: Relative contribution of residual renal function and peritoneal clearance to adequacy of dialysis: A reanalysis of the CANUSA Study. J Am Soc Nephrol 2001;12:2158–2162.
14. Maiorca R, Brunori G, Zubani R, et al: Predicative value of dialysis adequacy and nutritional indices for mortality and morbidity in CAPD and HD patients: A longitudinal study. Nephrol Dial Transplant 1995;10:2295–2305.
15. Diaz-Buxo JA, Lowrie EG, Lew NL, et al: Associates of mortality among peritoneal dialysis patients with special reference to peritoneal transport states and solute clearance. Am J Kidney Dis 1999;33:523–534.
16. Rocco M, Souci JM, Pastan S, McClellan WM: Peritoneal dialysis adequacy and risk of death. Kidney Int 2000;58:446–457.
17. National Kidney Foundation: NKF–K/DOQI clinical practice guidelines for peritoneal dialysis adequacy. Am J Kidney Dis 1997;30(Suppl 2):S67–S136.
18. Blake PG, Bargman J, Bick J, et al: Clinical practice guidelines of the Canadian Society of Nephrology for peritoneal dialysis adequacy and nutrition. J Am Soc Nephrol 1999;10(Suppl 13):S311–S321.

19. Golper TA, Churchill DN, Blake PG, et al: NKF–K/DOQI clinical practice guidelines for peritoneal dialysis adequacy: Update 2000. Am J Kidney Dis 2001;37(Suppl 1):S65–S136.

20. Perez RA, Blake PG, Jindal KA, et al: Changes in peritoneal dialysis practices in Canada 1996–1999. Perit Dial Int 2003;23:53–57.

21. Mak SK, Wong PN, Lo KT, et al: Randomized perspective study of the effect of increased dialytic dose on nutritional and clinical outcomes in continous ambulatory peritoneal dialysis patients. Am J Kidney Dis 2000;36:105–114.

22. Paniagua R, Amato, D, Vonesh E, et al: Effect of increased peritoneal clearances on mortality rates in peritoneal dialysis: ADEMEX, a prospective randomized controlled trial. J Am Soc Nephrol 2002;13:1307–1320.

23. Lo WK, Ho YW, Li CS, et al: Effect of Kt/V on survival and clinical outcome in CAPD patients in a randomized prospective study. Kidney Int 2003;64:649–656.

24. Churchill DN: The ADEMEX study: Make haste slowly. J Am Soc Nephrol 2002;13:1415–1418.

25. National Kidney Foundation: K/DOQI clinical practice guidelines and clinical practice recommendations for 2006 updates: Peritoneal dialysis adequacy. Am J Kidney Dis 2006;48(Suppl 1):S91–S176.

26. Eknoyan G, Beck GJ, Cheung A: Effect of dialysis dose and membrane flux in maintenance hemodialysis. N Engl J Med 2002;347: 2010–2019.

27. Twardowski ZJ, Nolph KD, Khanna R, et al: Peritoneal equilibration test. Perit Dial Bull 1987;7:138–147.

28. Churchill DN, Thorpe KE, Nolph KD, et al: Increased peritoneal membrane transport is associated with decreased patient and technique survival for continuous peritoneal dialysis patients. J Am Soc Nephrol 1998;9:1285–1292.

29. Perez RA, Blake PG, McMurray S, et al: What is the optimal frequency of cycling in automated peritoneal dialysis? Perit Dial Int 2000;20:548–556.

30. Demetriou D, Habicht A, Schillinger M, et al: Adequacy of automated peritoneal dialysis with and without daytime exchange: A randomized controlled trial. Kidney Int 2006;70:1649–1655.

31. Medcalf JF, Harris KP, Walls M: Role of diuretics in the preservation of residual renal function in patients on continuous ambulatory peritoneal dialysis. Kidney Int 2001;59:1128–1133.

32. Li PK, Chow KM, Wong TY, et al: Effects of an angiotensin-converting enzyme inhibitor on residual renal function in patients receiving peritoneal dialysis. A randomized controlled study. Ann Intern Med 2003;139:105–112.

33. Suzuki H, Kanno Y, Sugahara S, et al: Effects of an angiotensin receptor blocker, Valsartan, in patients on CAPD. Am J Kidney Dis 2004;43:1056–1064.

34. Mujais S, Nolph K, Gokal R, et al: Evaluation and management of ultrafiltration problems in peritoneal dialysis. Perit Dial Int 2000;20(Suppl 4):S5–S21.

35. Mistry CD, Gokal R, Peers E: A randomized multicenter clinical trial comparing isosmolar icodextrin with hyperosmolar glucose solutions in CAPD. Kidney Int 1994;46:496–503.

36. Davies SJ, Woodrow G, Donovan K, et al: Icodextrin improves the fluid status: Results of a double-blind randomized controlled clinical trial. J Am Soc Nephrol 2003;14:2338–2344.

37. Konings CJ, Kooman JP, Schonck M, et al: Effect of icodextrin on volume status, blood pressure and echocardiographic parameters: A randomized study. Kidney Int 2003;63:1556–1563.

38. Rodriguez-Carmona A, Perez-Fontan M: Sodium removal in patients undergoing CAPD and automated peritoneal dialysis. Perit Dial Int 2002;22:705–713.

39. Rodriguez-Carmona A, Perez-Fontan M, Garcia-Naveiro R, et al: Compared time profiles of ultrafiltration, sodium removal and renal function in incident CAPD and automated peritoneal dialysis patients. Am J Kidney Dis 2004;44:132–145.

40. Engel B, Davies SJ: Achieving euvolemia in peritoneal dilaysis. Perit Dial Int 2007;27:514–517.

41. Bernardini J, Piriano B: Compliance in CAPD and CCPD patients as measured by supply inventories during home visits. Am J Kidney Dis 1998;31:101–107.

42. Blake PG, Korbet SM, Blake R, et al: A multicenter study of non-compliance with continuous peritoneal dialysis exchanges in U.S. and Canadian patients. Am J Kidney Dis 2000;35:506–514.

43. Young GA, Kopple J, Lindholm B, et al: Nutritional assessment of CAPD patients: An international study. Am J Kidney Dis 1991;17:462–471.

44. Yeun JY, Kaysen GA: Acute phase proteins in peritoneal dialysate albumin loss are the main determinants of serum albumin in peritoneal dialysis patients. Am J Kidney Dis 1997;30:923–927.

45. Pollock CA, Ibels LS, Allen BJ, et al: Total body nitrogen as a prognostic marker in maintenance dialysis. J Am Soc Nephrol 1995;6:82–88.

46. Mandolfo S, Zucchi A, Cavalieri D'Oro L, et al: Protein nitrogen appearance in CAPD patients: What is the best formula? Nephrol Dial Transplant 1996;11:1592–1596.

47. Davies, SJ, Phillips L, Griffiths AM, et al: Analysis of the effects of increasing delivered dialysis treatment to malnourished peritoneal dialysis patients. Kidney Int 2000;57:1743–1754.

48. Li FK, Chan LYY, Woo JCY, et al: A 3-year, prospective randomized controlled study on amino acid dialysate in patients on CAPD. Am J Kidney Dis 2003;42:173–183.

49. Szeto CC, Wong TY, Chow KM, et al: Oral sodium bicarbonate for the treatment of metabolic acidosis in peritoneal dialysis patients: A randomized placebo-control trial. J Am Soc Nephrol 2003;14:2119–2126.

50. Johansen KL, Mulligan K, Schambelan M: Anabolic effects of nandrolone decanoate in patients receiving dialysis: A randomized controlled trial. JAMA 1999;281:1275–1281.

51. Fouque D, Peng SC, Shamir E, Kopple JD: Recombinant human insulin-like growth factor-one induces an anabolic response in malnourished CAPD patients. Kidney Int 2000;57:646–654.

52. Stenvinkel P, Heimburger O, Lindholm B, et al: Are there two types of malnutrition in chronic renal failure? Evidence for relationships between malnutrition, inflammation, and atherosclerosis. Nephrol Dial Transplant 2000;15:953–960.

53. Bloembergen WE, Port FK, Mauger EA, et al: A comparison of mortality between patients treated with hemodialysis and peritoneal dialysis. J Am Soc Nephrol 1995;6:177–183.

54. Collins AJ, How W, Xia H, et al: Mortality risks of peritoneal dialysis and hemodialysis. Am J Kidney Dis 1999;34:1065–1074.

55. Fenton SSA, Schaubel DE, Desmeules M, et al: Hemodialysis versus peritoneal dialysis: A comparison of adjusted mortality rates. Am J Kidney Dis 1997;30:330–342.

56. Locatelli F, Marcelli D, Conte F, et al: Survival and development of cardiovascular disease by modality of treatment in patients with end-stage renal disease. J Am Soc Nephrol 2001;12:2411–2417.

57. Heaf JG, Lokkegaard H, Madsen M: Initial survival advantage of peritoneal dialysis relative to haemodialysis. Nephrol Dial Transplant 2002;17:112–117.

58. Liem YS, Wong JB, Hunink MG, et al: Comparison of hemodialysis and peritoneal dialysis survival in the Netherlands. Kidney Int 2007;71:153–158.

59. Ganesh SK, Hulbert-Sharon T, Port FK, et al: Mortality differences by dialysis modality among incident ESRD patients with and without coronary artery disease. J Am Soc Nephrol 2003;14:415–424.

60. Stack AG, Molony DA, Rahman NS, et al: Impact of dialysis modality on survival of new ESRD patients with congestive heart failure in the United States. Kidney Int 2003;64:1071–1079.

61. Murphy SW, Foley RN, Barrett BJ, et al: Comparative mortality of hemodialysis and peritoneal dialysis in Canada. Kidney Int 2000;57:1720–1726.

62. Termorshuizen F, Korevaar JC, Dekker FW, et al: Hemodialysis and peritoneal dialysis: Comparison of adjusted mortality rates according to the duration of dialysis: Analysis of the Netherlands Cooperative Study on the Adequacy of Dialysis 2. J Am Soc Nephrol 2003;14:2851–2860.

63. Jaar BG, Coresh J, Plantinga LC, et al: Comparing the risk for death with peritoneal dialysis and hemodialysis in a national cohort of patients with chronic kidney disease. Ann Intern Med 2005;143:174–183.

64. Bargman JM: Worshipping at the altar of St. Cox: Who adjusts the adjustments? Perit Dial Int 2006;26:426–428.

65. Schaubel DE, Blake PG, Fenton SS: Trends in CAPD technique failure: Canada 1981–1997. Perit Dial Int 2001;21:365–371.

66. Van Biesen W, Vanholder RC, Veys N, et al: An evaluation of an integrative care approach for end-stage renal disease patients. J Am Soc Nephrol 2000;11:116–125.

Further Reading

Churchill DN, Thorpe KE, Nolph KD, et al: Increased peritoneal membrane transport is associated with decreased patient and technique survival for continuous peritoneal dialysis patients. J Am Soc Nephrol 1998;9:1285–1292.

National Kidney Foundation: K/DOQI clinical practice guidelines and clinical practice recommendations for 2006 updates: Peritoneal dialysis adequacy. Am J Kidney Dis 2006;48(Suppl 1): S91–S176.

Paniagua R, Amato, D, Vonesh E, et al: Effect of increased peritoneal clearances on mortality rates in peritoneal dialysis: ADEMEX, a prospective randomized controlled trial. J Am Soc Nephrol 2002;13:1307–1320.

Vonesh EF, Snyder JJ, Foley RN, Collins AJ: Mortality studies comparing peritoneal dialysis and hemodialysis: What do they tell us? Kidney Int Suppl 2006;(103): S3–S11.

Chapter 84

Patient Selection for Dialysis and the Decision to Withhold or Withdraw Dialysis

Alvin H. Moss

BACKGROUND

In a span of just 30 years, the process of patient selection for dialysis has been transformed from an intensive one in which each candidate was carefully scrutinized by a multidisciplinary committee for acceptability to one in which almost any patient, or family of a patient, who requests dialysis receives it. Nephrologists, medical ethicists, and health-policy experts have identified many factors to explain this transformation, but most prominent among them are the following: (1) federal legislation that pays for dialysis for all patients with end-stage renal disease (ESRD) who are eligible for Medicare; (2) improvements in medical science and technology that have made it possible to achieve long-term survival for some patients who were previously thought to be too sick to undergo dialysis (for example, the elderly and those with diabetes); (3) a changing ethical and legal environment in which respect for patient autonomy and the right of patient self-determination have become almost decisive in medical decision making to start or stop a life-sustaining treatment such as dialysis; (4) the financial self-interests of nephrologists who stand to increase their incomes by treating larger numbers of dialysis patients; and (5) the absence of any attempt before the issuance of a clinical practice guideline in 2000 by the Renal Physicians Association (RPA) and the American Society of Nephrology (ASN), *Shared Decision-Making in the Appropriate Initiation of and Withdrawal from Dialysis*,[1] to define formally patients who would be inappropriate for dialysis.

The consequences of these factors are twofold: The numbers of patients on long-term dialysis and the cost of the ESRD program to the federal government have exceeded all initial projections several times over and observers of dialysis, including the physicians and nurses actively providing it, have questioned the appropriateness of dialyzing some current patients because of their shortened life expectancy and limited quality of life. Of particular note is the rapid growth in rates of dialysis initiation among octogenarians and nonagenarians with a near doubling of the number of patients with incident ESRD who are older than 80 years of age.[2] These elderly dialysis patients have a survival rate only one sixth that of age-matched patients without kidney disease in the general population and a high prevalence of comorbid conditions including dementia. The controversy about the appropriateness of dialysis initiation inthis older patient population has been particularly strong. This chapter examines the following topics: the reported practices of nephrologists and the preferences of patients regarding dialysis decision making, the recommendations of the RPA and the ASN clinical practice guideline *Shared Decision-Making in the Appropriate Initiation of and Withdrawal from Dialysis*, a process for dialysis decision making in individual cases that is based on ethics and the law, recommendations for caring for a patient who wants to forgo dialysis, and the outcomes of the use of the RPA and ASN clinical practice guideline on nephrologists' end-of-life decision making.

NEPHROLOGISTS' CHANGING PRACTICES REGARDING WITHHOLDING AND WITHDRAWING DIALYSIS

In the 1990s, research studies of nephrologists' dialysis decision-making practices provided insight into which decisions nephrologists would typically make in a variety of circumstances and why they made the decisions that they did. These studies documented that deciding to withhold and withdraw dialysis from patients occurs frequently for the vast majority of nephrologists. Most withhold 1 to 5 patients and withdraw 1 to 10 patients from dialysis each year. These studies showed that most nephrology respondents would honor a competent patient's request to stop dialysis but that there was more variability in starting a permanently unconscious patient on dialysis or stopping dialysis in a permanently demented patient.[3] In one study of nephrologists in New England, 9 out of 10 nephrologists would stop dialysis at the request of a competent patient, but only 6 out of 10 would agree to stop dialysis for an irreversibly incompetent patient at the family's request if the patient's wishes were unknown. In this study, only 1 out of 100 nephrologists would stop dialysis for an irreversibly incompetent patient for whom the nephrologist thought that dialysis should be stopped if the family requested that dialysis be continued and the patient's wishes were unknown. The authors concluded that consensus exists among nephrologists regarding the right of competent patients to determine the course of their care, including stopping dialysis. They also concluded that nephrologists disagree about the management of incompetent patients with unclear previous wishes and that they have difficulty making decisions for such patients.[4]

In a study of medical directors of dialysis units, 9 out of 10 indicated that they would agree to stop dialysis at the request of a competent patient, but only one third would stop dialysis of a permanently and severely demented patient without advance directives. One sixth of the medical directors would start dialysis for a permanently unconscious patient if requested, but the remainder would not. In this study, some respondents indicated that although they thought dialysis was inappropriate for the demented and permanently unconscious patients, they would not withdraw or withhold it unless they could "convince" the families to agree. Other respondents specifically noted that they would be afraid to stop dialysis for the patient with severe dementia if there were the potential for litigation from family members who wanted dialysis continued. In interpreting the results of their study, the authors suggested that some nephrologists may misunderstand the ethical and legal aspects of making decisions for such patients and may feel obligated to provide dialysis to all patients for whom it is requested.[5]

Similarly, in a study of dialysis decision making by nephrologists in Canada, the United Kingdom, and the United States, more than 9 out of 10 nephrologists from all three countries would respect a competent patient's refusal to start dialysis. However, American nephrologists would offer dialysis significantly more often to demented patients, severely disabled diabetic patients, and patients in a persistent vegetative state than would Canadian or British nephrologists. The American nephrologists significantly more often gave "respect for the patient or family request" as the first reason to offer dialysis and ranked "fear of lawsuit" higher as a reason to offer dialysis than their counterparts in the other countries. The British and Canadian nephrologists significantly more often cited "adequate quality of life" as a reason to offer dialysis than the Americans did. Despite these variations, there was never more than a 30% difference in the practice of offering dialysis among the three groups. The greatest agreement on offering dialysis was for the young competent patient with muscular dystrophy (>90% in each group). Less than 10% of each group thought that dialysis should be offered to patients in a persistent vegetative state.[6]

Five years after the introduction of the RPA and ASN clinical practice guideline, a follow-up study of nephrology members of the RPA was conducted to determine whether there had been a change in their attitudes and reported practices with regard to dialysis and end-of-life decision making.[3] In 2005 compared with 1990, there was less variation in nephrologists' responses; nephrologists were significantly more likely to withdraw dialysis from a permanently and severely demented patient (53% vs. 39%) and to withhold dialysis from a permanently unconscious patient (90% vs. 83%). In both time periods, more than 90% of nephrologists would stop dialysis of a competent patient who requests it. Compared with 1990, in 2005 nephrologists reported that the dialysis unit in which they treated most of their patients was significantly more likely to have written policies on cardiopulmonary resuscitation (86% vs. 31%) and withdrawal of dialysis (30% vs. 15%). These dialysis units were also significantly more likely to honor a patient's request for a do-not-resuscitate order in the dialysis unit (83% vs. 66%). The change in clinical decision making by nephrologists in the 15 years between the studies is consistent with the recommendations for dialysis decision making of the RPA and ASN clinical practice guideline. The authors concluded that the development and dissemination of the guideline have been associated with an improvement in nephrologists' end-of-life decision making.[3]

PATIENTS' PREFERENCES FOR DIALYSIS DECISION MAKING

In making decisions about which patients should be selected for dialysis, input from patients is important because they are, as a group, the best to judge under which circumstances dialysis would be viewed as beneficial and when it would be burdensome. Regrettably, there are few studies of patients' preferences regarding dialysis, and only one examined the interaction between health state and treatment modalities. In this study, 25% or less of the patients would want to continue dialysis in three health states: severe stroke, severe dementia, and permanent coma.[7] These findings agree with another study in which 74% of dialysis patients said they would want to stop dialysis if they became permanently and severely demented.[8]

PRACTICE GUIDELINES FOR SELECTION OF DIALYSIS PATIENTS

The idea of practice guidelines for patient selection for dialysis was not new in 2000. In 1978, just 6 years after the passage of the federal legislation creating the Medicare ESRD program, the late Belding Scribner (one of the early nephrologists who pioneered dialysis) was concerned about "how not to dialyze" certain patients with poor prognoses. He recognized even then the need for a "deselection committee."[9] The Institute of Medicine

Committee for the Study of the Medicare End-Stage Renal Disease Program (IOM Committee), which issued its report in 1991, acknowledged that the existence of the public entitlement for treatment of ESRD did not oblige physicians to treat all patients who have kidney failure with dialysis or transplantation.[10] The IOM Committee noted that for some ESRD patients the burdens of dialysis might substantially outweigh the benefits. Specifically, the IOM Committee questioned the appropriateness of providing dialysis to two groups of patients: those with a limited life expectancy despite the use of dialysis and those with severe neurological disease. The first group included patients with kidney failure and other life-threatening illnesses, such as atherosclerotic cardiovascular disease, cancer, chronic pulmonary disease, and acquired immunodeficiency syndrome. The second group included patients whose neurological disease rendered them unable to relate to others, such as those in a persistent vegetative state, those with severe dementia, and those with cerebrovascular disease. The IOM Committee recommended that guidelines be drafted to assist nephrologists in making these decisions so that dialysis could be used appropriately. In 2000, the RPA and the ASN heeded this call for a clinical practice guideline when it published *Shared Decision-Making in the Appropriate Initiation of and Withdrawal from Dialysis*.[1] To draft this guideline, the RPA and ASN organized a working group that included representatives from multiple disciplines and organizations within the dialysis community, kidney patients, internal and family medicine physicians, and experts in bioethics and health policy. The working group developed a priori analytic frameworks regarding decisions to withhold or withdraw dialysis in patients with acute renal failure and ESRD. Systematic literature reviews were conducted to address prespecified questions derived from the frameworks. In most instances, the relevant evidence that was identified was contextual in nature and only provided indirect support for the recommendations. In formulating their nine recommendations, the working group used research evidence, case and statutory law, and ethical principles. They recommended shared decision making as the basis for making decisions about starting and stopping dialysis. Shared decision making is a process by which physicians and patients agree on a specific course of action based on a common understanding of the treatment goals and the risks and benefits of the chosen course compared with the alternative courses. These recommendations appear in Box 84-1. Their recommendations for who should be dialyzed, although more systematically developed and justified, are consistent with those previously recommended.[11] This agreement suggests that there is now a real consensus in the nephrology community on this topic (Box 84-2).

DECIDING TO WITHHOLD OR WITHDRAW DIALYSIS IN INDIVIDUAL CASES

The Process of Informed Consent as the Paradigm for Decision Making

The ethical and legal literature agree that medical decisions for individual patients (such as withholding or withdrawing dialysis) should be made according to the process of informed consent, in which there is active, shared decision making.[12] This agreement formed the basis for the first two recommendations

in the RPA/ASN guideline. Thus, if a physician determines that a patient has decision-making capacity, the patient is informed of his or her medical condition, in this case, ESRD, and all the benefits, risks, and consequences associated with each of the available treatment options, including the option not to undergo dialysis. After determining the patient's values and preferences, the physician recommends what might be best for the patient based on those preferences. Through further conversations, in which there is mutual participation and respect, the patient reaches a decision about dialysis—whether to consent to it or to refuse it. For some patients, the balance of the benefits and the burdens of dialysis may not be clear, and the nephrologist may not know whether to recommend dialysis. In such situations, there is an ethical recommendation for a limited trial of dialysis of approximately 30 days. During this time, the patient's responses to dialysis can be assessed, and afterward, both the patient and physician are in a better position to decide about continuation.

Deciding for the Incompetent Patient

If the patient lacks decision-making capacity, physicians make decisions with the patient's legal agent as designated in the patient's advance directive (e.g., durable power of attorney for health care or health care proxy). If the patient has not completed a written advance directive specifying an agent, physicians need to make decisions with a surrogate who should be appointed according to the provisions of the state law in which the care is being provided. Surrogates should base their decisions on what the patient would choose if he or she were competent to do so; if the patient's views about treatment are unknown, the surrogate's decision should be based on the patient's best interests.

Resolving Conflict between the Surrogate and the Nephrologist

Occasionally, there are conflicts between the patient's legal agent and the nephrologist in which the agent requests dialysis and the nephrologist does not believe that it is appropriate. Based on the studies reviewed in this chapter, many nephrologists report that they would do as the agent requests, even if they thought it was wrong. In yielding to pressure from the agent, nephrologists potentially weaken the integrity of their specialty and shirk their responsibility to be good stewards of the federally funded ESRD program, a program to which every taxpayer, including every nephrologist, contributes. Recommendation 4 of the RPA/ASN guideline provides a systematic approach for resolving these conflicts, and Figure 84-1 presents sequential steps for resolving the conflict.

Withholding or withdrawing dialysis of an incompetent patient, over the objections of the agent, surrogate, or family, may be both ethical and legal.[13] Such decisions should be made openly and should focus clearly on the patient's wishes or best interests. At a minimum, such decisions should be reached only after following Recommendation 4 of the RPA/ASN guideline, which recommends extended conversation with the patient's agent about the diagnosis of ESRD, about options for treatment including palliative care without dialysis, the prognosis, and the reasons for not offering or for stopping dialysis; the agreement of other members of the dialysis team includ-ing at least one other nephrologist; the concurrence of an ethics committee (if available); a detailed note in the patient's medical record

Box 84-1 Renal Physicians Association and the American Society of Nephrology Recommendations for Initiation and Withdrawal of Dialysis

Recommendation No. 1: Shared Decision Making

A patient-physician relationship that promotes shared decision making is recommended for all patients with either acute renal failure or end-stage renal disease. Participants in shared decision making should involve at a minimum the patient and the physician. If a patient lacks the decision-making capacity, decisions should involve the legal agent. With the patient's consent, shared decision making may include family members or friends and other members of the renal care team.

Recommendation No. 2: Informed Consent or Refusal

Physicians should fully inform patients about their diagnosis, prognosis, and all treatment options, including (1) available dialysis modalities, (2) not starting dialysis and continuing conservative management that should include end-of-life care, (3) a time-limited trial of dialysis, and (4) stopping dialysis and receiving end-of-life care. Choices among the options should be made by patients or, if patients lack the decision-making capacity, their designated legal agents. Their decisions should be informed and voluntary. The renal care team, in conjunction with the primary care physician, should ensure that the patient or legal agent understands the consequences of the decision.

Recommendation No. 3: Estimating Prognosis

To facilitate informed decisions about starting dialysis for either acute renal failure or end-stage renal disease, discussions should occur with the patient or legal agent about life expectancy and quality of life. Depending on the circumstances (e.g., availability of nephrologists), a primary care physician or nephrologist who is familiar with prognostic data should conduct these discussions. These discussions should be documented and dated. All patients requiring dialysis should have their chances for survival estimated, with the realization that the ability to predict survival in the individual patient is difficult and imprecise. The estimates should be discussed with the patient or legal agent, the patient's family, and the medical team. For patients with end-stage renal disease, these discussions should occur as early as possible in the course of the patient's renal disease and continue as the renal disease progresses. For patients who experience major complications that may substantially reduce survival or quality of life, it is appropriate to discuss and/or reassess treatment goals, including consideration of withdrawing dialysis.

Recommendation No. 4: Conflict Resolution

A systematic approach for conflict resolution is recommended if there is disagreement regarding the benefits of dialysis between the patient or legal agent (and those supporting the patient's position) and (a) member(s) of the renal care team. Conflicts may also occur within the renal care team or between the renal care team and other health care providers.

This approach should review the shared decision-making process for the following potential sources of conflict: (1) miscommunication or misunderstanding about prognosis, (2) intrapersonal or interpersonal issues, or (3) values. If dialysis is indicated emergently, it should be provided while pursuing conflict resolution, provided the patient or legal agent requests it.

Recommendation No. 5: Advance Directives

The renal care team should attempt to obtain written advance directives from all dialysis patients. These advance directives should be honored.

Recommendation No. 6: Withholding or Withdrawing Dialysis

It is appropriate to withhold or withdraw dialysis for patients with either acute renal failure or end-stage renal disease in the following situations:

- Patients with the decision-making capacity who, being fully informed and making voluntary choices, refuse dialysis or request dialysis be discontinued
- Patients who no longer possess the decision-making capacity who have previously indicated refusal of dialysis in an oral or written advance directive
- Patients who no longer possess the decision-making capacity and whose properly appointed legal agents refuse dialysis or request that it be discontinued
- Patients with irreversible, profound neurological impairment such that they lack signs of thought, sensation, purposeful behavior, and awareness of self and environment.

Recommendation No. 7: Special Patient Groups

It is reasonable to consider not initiating or withdrawing dialysis for patients with acute renal failure or end-stage renal disease who have a terminal illness from a nonrenal cause or whose medical condition precludes the technical process of dialysis.

Recommendation No. 8: Time-Limited Trials

For patients requiring dialysis but who have an uncertain prognosis or for whom a consensus cannot be reached about providing dialysis, nephrologists should consider offering a time-limited trial of dialysis.

Recommendation No. 9: Palliative Care

All patients who decide to forgo dialysis or for whom such a decision is made should be treated with continued palliative care. With the patient's consent, persons with expertise in such care, such as hospice health care professionals, should be involved in managing the medical, psychosocial, and spiritual aspects of end-of-life care for these patients. Patients should be offered the option of dying where they prefer including at home with hospice care. Bereavement support should be offered to patients' families.

Used with permission from the Renal Physicians Association.

Box 84-2 The Consensus on Patients for Whom Dialysis Is Inappropriate

- Patients who refuse dialysis or who have previously indicated they did not want it
- Patients who are terminally ill with a nonrenal disease
- Patients who are permanently unconscious
- Patients who are unable to relate to others
- Patients who are unable to cooperate with the dialysis process

documenting all the factors relevant to the decision; and an attempt to transfer the patient's care if the agent wishes it. If the patient is already receiving dialysis and if (after all the above steps) the agent still requests dialysis and no other nephrologist has been found who is willing to accept the patient in transfer for dialysis, then the agent is given some time (usually 72 hours) to consider other options, including contacting a lawyer, before dialysis is stopped. Such a course of action by the nephrologist is justified for patients who are deemed inappropriate for dialysis (see Box 84-2). In using such an approach, for example, a nephrologist might refuse to dialyze a patient who is permanently unconscious, basing his or her decision on Recommendation 6 of the RPA/ASN guideline. In taking such an approach, nephrologists should indicate that they understand the agent's request and should give an explanation along the lines of "I am sorry, but we do not dialyze patients in your loved one's condition. Our profession is guided by ethical principles that require us to be of benefit and do no harm. In your loved one's case, dialysis cannot help her get better, and it may harm her." Nephrologists say this not because they lack respect or compassion for the agent but because their primary commitment is to the patient.[13]

ETHICAL PRINCIPLES IN DECISION MAKING

In their 1993 annual report, the End-Stage Renal Disease Data Advisory Committee to the U.S. Renal Data System articulated ethical justifications and general and specific principles to be used in making decisions about offering or not offering dialysis. This report included the deliberations of an ad hoc committee gathered to examine bioethical issues related to ESRD; the ad hoc committee was composed of nephrologists, ethicists, and health-policy experts. The Data Advisory Committee endorsed the recommendations of this ad hoc committee. The report described two ethical justifications for withholding or withdrawing dialysis: (1) the right of patients to refuse dialysis based on the ethical principle of respect for autonomy and the legal right of self-determination and (2) a judgment that dialysis does not offer a reasonable expectation of medical benefit based on the ethical principles of beneficence and nonmaleficence.[14]

LEGAL BASIS FOR DECIDING TO WITHHOLD OR WITHDRAW DIALYSIS

The ethical principle of respect for patient autonomy is applied to the treatment of the dialysis patient through the process of obtaining informed consent or refusal. In turn,

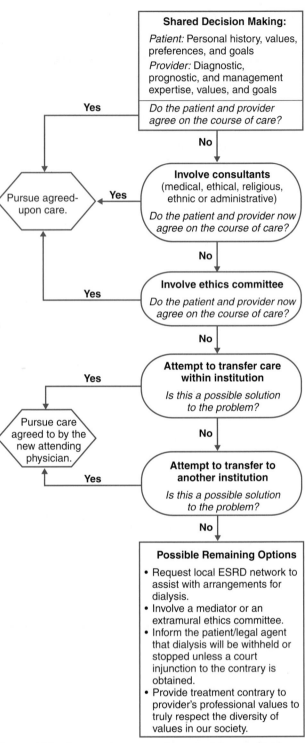

Figure 84-1 Systematic approach to resolving conflict between the patient and the renal care team. (Used with the permission of the Renal Physicians Association.)

the obtaining of consent or refusal is firmly grounded in the law: common law, constitutional law, and federal statute. The right of patients to accept or refuse dialysis is first based on common law dating back to the 1914 case of *Schloendorff v Society of New York Hospital*. In this case, Justice Benjamin Cardozo wrote, "Every human being of adult years and sound mind has a right to determine what shall be done with his body." In the 1990 U.S. Supreme Court case of *Cruzan v*

Director, the legal doctrine of informed consent was determined to be a constitutionally protected right. The Supreme Court justices held that "[t]he doctrine of informed consent arose in recognition of the value society places on a person's autonomy and as the primary vehicle by which a person can protect the integrity of his body. If one can consent to treatment, one can also refuse it. Thus, as a necessary corollary to informed consent, the right to refuse treatment arose."[15] The Patient Self-Determination Act (included in the Congressional Omnibus Reconciliation Act of 1990, Public Law 101-508) became effective on December 1, 1991, and protected by federal statute the right of dialysis patients to consent to or to refuse dialysis. It is important for nephrologists to understand the law because if a nephrologist were to dialyze a competent patient against the patient's will, the nephrologist could be civilly liable for medical battery.

THE ROLE OF ADVANCE CARE PLANNING

Deciding to stop a life-sustaining treatment such as dialysis for an incompetent patient is among the most difficult ethical problems faced by physicians.[16] Because there is a presumption in favor of continued dialysis for patients who cannot and have not expressed their wishes, patients' rights to forgo dialysis in certain situations are usually difficult to achieve unless patients have explicitly stated their preferences in advance or named a legal agent to speak on their behalf. The usual practice of nephrologists in treating patients who have become incompetent and who have provided neither oral nor written advance directives regarding their preferences for stopping dialysis is to continue dialysis. These considerations underscore the importance of advance care planning with patients with chronic kidney disease. Advance care planning is a process in which a patient's preferences for a health care proxy and for future medical care under a variety of circumstances are determined (sometimes in the form of a written advance directive), are updated, and then followed in a manner in which the patient intended once the patient loses decision-making capacity. Advance care planning has been recognized as particularly important for dialysis patients for four reasons[16]: approximately half of the dialysis population is elderly, and the elderly have the shortest life expectancy on dialysis and are the most likely to withdraw or be withdrawn from dialysis; previous discussion of advance directives has been shown to help dialysis patients and their families to approach death in a reconciled fashion[17]; patients who discuss and complete written advance directives are significantly more likely to have their wish to die at home respected; and unless a specific directive to withhold cardiopulmonary resuscitation is obtained—which can be done in the framework of advance care planning—it will be automatically provided, although it rarely leads to extended survival in dialysis patients.[18] For these reasons, nephrologists have been encouraged to discuss the circumstances under which patients would want to discontinue dialysis and forgo cardiopulmonary resuscitation and to urge patients to complete written advance directives.[19]

Despite these benefits, the practice of advance care planning, including the completion of advance directives, has not been optimized for dialysis patients. First, most of these patients do not discuss or complete an advance directive, even though advance directives are particularly important for these chronically ill patients with shortened life expectancy who are dependent on life-sustaining treatment for their daily existence. Dialysis units were not included in the U.S. Patient Self-Determination Act list of health care providers who were required to ask patients about completion of advance directives and also provide them with an opportunity to execute an advance directive. Second, even when patients undergoing dialysis complete written advance directives, only one third have indicated to their family the circumstances under which they may want to stop dialysis.[20] This failure to indicate their preferences is disappointing because, as noted previously, patients undergoing dialysis have strong preferences about stopping dialysis and other life-sustaining treatments in certain health states. Recognizing these deficiencies, the ASN, the National Kidney Foundation, the RPA, and the Robert Wood Johnson Foundation's ESRD Workgroup on End-of-Life Care have all strongly encouraged dialysis units to provide advance care planning to dialysis patients and their families and in the process to include a discussion of health states in which patients would want to stop dialysis and other life-sustaining treatments. Patients undergoing dialysis and their families have been encouraged to view advance care planning as a way to maintain control over present and future health care, relieve burdens on loved ones, strengthen interpersonal relationships, and prepare for death. Research with patients undergoing dialysis and their families shows that patients prefer to center the advance care planning process within the patient-family relationship rather than the patient-physician relationship. Clinicians who treat patients undergoing dialysis should urge them to participate in an advance care planning discussion with their families and should instruct them to tell their families and put in writing under what circumstances they would not want life-sustaining treatment, including dialysis.[21] As part of the advance care planning process, patients should be asked to address where they prefer to die and whether they would like to receive hospice services.

Nephrologist researchers have studied how best to conduct advance care planning with dialysis patients. The nature of advance care planning has changed from a document-driven, decision-focused event in which the goal is completion of a written advance directive to a relational *process* in which the patient's goals for treatment are identified and communicated to those in the patient's support system (Box 84-3).[22]

CARING FOR PATIENTS WHO WANT TO FORGO DIALYSIS

Response to a Patient's Refusal to Start Dialysis

Patients with ESRD may have encephalopathy or depression that renders them incapable of decision making. The first assessment of patients with ESRD who refuse to initiate dialysis is whether they have decision-making capacity. If they have decision-making capacity, then the nephrologist should determine whether the refusal of dialysis is informed and valid. The nephrologist is obligated to determine why the refusal has been made and to ensure that the patient correctly understands the information that has been presented and the consequences of the decision. Patients and families should be informed that

Box 84-3   The Process of Advance Care Planning for Dialysis Patients

Facilitation

Identification and participation of patient's designated proxy decision maker in the planning

Patient and proxy understanding of patient's condition, prognosis, and likely illness course

Elicitation of patient's goals and preferences for treatment in a variety of health states (e.g., permanent coma, advanced dementia, and persistent vegetative state), including those in the likely illness course

Communication between patient and proxy so that proxy/family know and understand patient's goals for future care and are committed to respecting them

Documentation

Patient's designated decision maker and goals and preferences for treatment in the future when incapacitated are recorded in the medical record and on the state-specific advance directive form. Depending on state law, patient may complete a health care proxy form to designate a proxy decision maker and a living will to provide directives for treatment if the patient becomes terminally ill or in a persistent vegetative state.

Completion of a physician order form, called Physician Orders for Life-Sustaining Treatment form in Oregon, specifying the patient's treatment decisions so that they can be honored throughout the health care system[23]; an increasing number of states are using such a form.

Timing

Initial advance care planning discussion is appropriate when the patient is first diagnosed with progressive chronic kidney disease and may include only designation of proxy decision maker and completion of a living will if the patient chooses to execute one.

A more complete discussion of the patient's goals and preferences for treatment is appropriate when the nephrologist answers "no" to the question "Would I be surprised if this patient died in the next year?"[24] At this time in the patient's disease course, complications that are likely to cause the patient's death can be anticipated and the treatments that the patient would and would not want can be identified and documented.

Systems and Processes

Dialysis units need to have a policy and procedure for conducting advance care planning. In most dialysis units, the social workers are assigned primary responsibility for implementing the advance care planning policy.[25]

Quality Improvement

Clinical performance measures can be used to evaluate the advance care planning process and guide further process enhancement.

---

death from uremia is usually a comfortable one in which the patient becomes increasingly somnolent and then dies. Patients also need to be instructed to maintain salt and fluid restrictions so that pulmonary edema does not occur and mar the comfort of the dying process.[26]

If the refusal is judged to be valid, then the patient should be considered terminally ill because a terminal illness is defined as one in which death is expected within 6 months or less. At this point, the RPA and ASN clinical practice guideline and the RPA and ASN statement on Quality Patient Care at the End of Life[27] recommend that the renal care team should refer the patient to a hospice or adopt a hospice-like approach to patient care. Such an approach considers medical, emotional, social, and spiritual needs of the dying patient and the family. If the renal team remains involved in the patient's care after hospice referral—such continuity is desirable—they should, in conjunction with hospice, take the following steps: (1) encourage the patient to participate with them in advance care planning if it has not already been done; (2) issue a do-not-resuscitate order that applies to the outpatient setting; (3) discuss with the patient and family contingencies for the final hours of the patient's life so that the family or caregivers do not panic and call emergency medical services when the patient experiences a cardiopulmonary arrest; and (4) address the needs of the family with regard to grieving while the patient is dying and bereavement after the patient has died.

Response to a Patient's Request to Stop Dialysis

A patient's request to stop dialysis should trigger a systematic response on the part of the dialysis team, including the inquiry in Box 84-4. Such an inquiry might uncover potentially reversible factors responsible for the patient's request, including difficulties with dialysis treatments, concerns about the burdens that the patient is placing on family, undue influence or pressure from outside sources, conflict between the patient and others, and dissatisfaction with the dialysis modality, the time, or the setting. It is usual for most dialysis units to ask a patient who wishes to stop dialysis to be evaluated by a counseling professional, either a psychiatrist, psychologist, or social worker, or someone in pastoral care to be sure that the patient has the decision-making capacity and that reversible factors are identified. Dialysis units also usually try to persuade patients to stay on dialysis for a period of time to see whether patient satisfaction is increased as reversible factors are addressed.

As for ESRD patients who choose not to initiate dialysis, for those who choose to withdraw, nephrologists should assure them and their families that death from uremia is usually a comfortable one as long as patients maintain salt and fluid restrictions so that pulmonary edema does not mar the dying process. Nephrologists are often willing to provide ultrafiltration without

Box 84-4 Questions to Be Answered in Responding to a Patient's Request to Stop Dialysis

1. Does the patient have the decision-making capacity or is the patient's cognitive capacity diminished by depression, encephalopathy, or other disorder?
2. Why does the patient want to stop dialysis?
3. Are the patient's perceptions about the technical or quality-of-life aspects of dialysis accurate?
4. Does the patient really mean what he or she says or is the decision to stop dialysis made to get attention, help, or control?
5. Can any changes be made that might improve life on dialysis for the patient?
6. Would the patient be willing to continue dialysis while the factors responsible for the patient's request are being addressed?
7. Has the patient discussed his or her desire to stop dialysis with significant others such as family, close friends, or spiritual advisors? What do they think about the patient's request?

diffusion dialysis to control symptoms of fluid overload in patients from whom dialysis has been withdrawn. The RPA and ASN recommend that nephrologists refer dialysis patients who stop dialysis to hospice, but research indicates there is room for improvement. Only half as many dialysis patients die with hospice care compared with the general population. Even among dialysis patients who are withdrawn from dialysis and whose death within a month is fairly certain, less than half die with hospice care.[28] Death with hospice care for dialysis patients is associated with lower costs and a much greater percentage of patients dying at home.

NEPHROLOGISTS' PREPAREDNESS FOR END-OF-LIFE DECISION MAKING

The ESRD patient population is increasingly composed of older patients with multiple comorbid conditions, high symptom burden, and a shortened life expectancy. Chapter 75 addresses pain and symptom management for ESRD patients. Because of the changing nature of the ESRD population and the fact that older patients are the most likely to withdraw from dialysis, nephrologists commonly engage in end-of-life decision making with dialysis patients and their families. Researchers have studied how prepared nephrologists report they are for decisions such as withholding or stopping dialysis or initiating it on a time-limited basis. In an online survey of RPA members, 39% identified themselves as being very well prepared for dialysis decision making. Those who reported that they were most prepared had been in practice longer and were knowledgeable of and used the RPA/ASN *Shared Decision-Making* practice guideline more often than those who reported that they were less well prepared.[29] In the preceding year, the very well prepared nephrologists had stopped dialysis of more patients, referred more patients to hospice, and used a time-limited trial of dialysis more often. The benefits of using the guide-

line recommendations prospectively in patient care have also been demonstrated.[30] These findings validate the contribution of the RPA/ASN guideline to nephrology clinical practice and underscore the importance of teaching the guideline recommendations to nephrologists and nephrology fellows.

CONCLUSIONS

Since the inception of dialysis for chronic renal failure in the early 1960s, dialysis decision making has undergone a dramatic transformation. Dialysis selection committees have disappeared, and decisions about whether to start or stop dialysis are made within the confines and privacy of the patient-physician relationship, governed by the process of informed consent.

In the 1990s, the wide range of discretion afforded to patients and nephrologists in making decisions about dialysis had resulted in a large variation in the way in which these decisions were made. Commentators on the ESRD program, including nephrology physicians and nurses, were concerned that some patients receiving dialysis were not appropriate candidates. In 2000, the RPA and ASN published a clinical practice guideline to assist nephrologists in dialysis decision making. Research shows that nephrologists who report that they are most prepared to make dialysis decisions are aware of and use the guideline. Research also shows that nephrologists in 2005 were making dialysis decisions more often in accordance with the guideline recommendations compared with nephrologists in 1990.

Excluding those patients who are identified as inappropriate dialysis candidates by the RPA/ASN guideline, the best approach for patient selection seems to be a liberal policy for accepting patients who might benefit from dialysis, including the use of time-limited trials of dialysis, combined with a readiness to withdraw patients from dialysis when the burdens of treatment outweigh the benefits. Successful implementation of such a policy requires good advance care planning at the start of dialysis and continuing dialogue between the physician, the patient, and the family about the patient's values, wishes, and goals. Patients should be informed that they have the right to stop dialysis. However, the goal of the nephrologist and the dialysis team should be to optimize the care of each patient so that each patient is satisfied with his or her quality of life for as long as possible and chooses to continue dialysis until a catastrophic event or unacceptable disease progression occurs. When it does occur, good advance care planning will prove its worth. Then everyone will know that the patient would no longer wish to receive dialysis, and it may be withdrawn, with the patient, family, and dialysis team all reconciled to the patient's death and knowledgeable about the patient's preferences for terminal care, including the use of hospice, so that those preferences can be honored. Renal palliative care (see Chapter 75) should have been begun at the start of dialysis with pain and symptom management and advance care planning; it will now become especially important to ensure that the patient is comfortable and that the patient and the family receive psychosocial and spiritual support, including bereavement support during and after the patient's death.

References

1. Renal Physicians Association and the American Society of Nephrology: Shared Decision-Making in the Appropriate Initiation of and Withdrawal from Dialysis. Washington, DC: Renal Physicians Association, 2000.
2. Kurella M, Covinsky KE, Collins AJ, Chertow GM: Octagenarians and nonagenarians starting dialysis in the United States. Ann Intern Med 2007;146:177–183.
3. Holley JL, Davison SN, Moss AH: Nephrologists' changing practices in reported end-of-life decision-making. Clin J Am Soc Nephrol 2007;2:107–111.
4. Singer P: The End-State Renal Disease Network of New England: Nephrologists' experience with and attitudes towards decisions to forgo dialysis. J Am Soc Nephrol 1992;2:1235–1240.
5. Moss AH, Stocking CB, Sachs GA, Siegler M: Variations in the attitudes of dialysis unit medical directors toward decisions to withhold and withdraw dialysis. J Am Soc Nephrol 1993;4:229–234.
6. McKenzie JK, Moss AH, Feest TG, et al: Dialysis decision-making in Canada, the United Kingdom, and the United States. Am J Kidney Dis 1998;31:12–18.
7. Singer PA, Thiel EC, Naylor CD, et al: Life-sustaining treatment preferences of hemodialysis patients: Implications for advance directives. J Am Soc Nephrol 1995;6:1410–1417.
8. Kaye M, Lella JW: Discontinuation of dialysis therapy in the demented patient. Am J Nephrol 1986;6:75–79.
9. Fox R, Swazey J: The Courage to Fail: A Social View of Organ Transplants and Dialysis, 2nd ed. Chicago: University of Chicago Press, 1978.
10. Rettig RA, Levinsky NG (eds): Kidney Failure and the Federal Government. Washington, DC: National Academy Press, 1991, pp 51–61.
11. Moss AH: To use dialysis appropriately: the emerging consensus on patient selection guidelines. Adv Renal Replacement Ther 1995;2:175–183.
12. President's Commission for the Study of Ethical Problems in Medicine and Biomedical and Behavioral Research: Making Health Care Decisions. Washington, DC: US Government Printing Office, 1982, pp 27–39.
13. Keating RF, Moss AH, Sorkin MI, Paris JJ: Stopping dialysis of an incompetent patient over the family's objection: Is it ever ethical and legal? J Am Soc Nephrol 1994;4:1879–1883.
14. ESRD Data Advisory Committee: 1993 Annual Report. Washington, DC: U.S. Department of Health and Human Services, 1993, pp 29–33.
15. Meisel A: The Right to Die 1994 Cumulative Supplement 2. New York: John Wiley & Sons, 1994, p 17.
16. Moss AH: Dialysis decisions and the elderly. Clin Geriatr Med 1994;10:463–473.
17. Swartz RD, Perry E: Advance directives are associated with "good deaths" in chronic dialysis patients. J Am Soc Nephrol 1993;3:1623–1630.
18. Lehrich RW, Pun PH, Tanenbaum ND, et al: Automated external defibrillators and survival from cardiac arrest in the outpatient hemodialysis clinic. J Am Soc Nephrol 2007;18:312–320.
19. Moss AH, Hozayen O, King K, et al: Attitudes of patients toward cardiopulmonary resuscitation in the dialysis unit. Am J Kidney Dis 2001;38:847–852.
20. Holley JL, Hines SC, Glover JJ, et al: Failure of advance care planning to elicit patients' preferences for withdrawal from dialysis. Am J Kidney Dis 1999;33:688–693.
21. Hines SC, Glover JJ, Holley JL, et al: Dialysis patients' preferences for advance care planning and end-of-life decision making. Ann Intern Med 1999;130:825–828.
22. Davison SN, Torgunrud C: The creation of an advance care planning process for patients with ESRD. Am J Kidney Dis 2007;49:27–36.
23. Hickman SE, Tolle SW, Brummel-Smith K, Carley MM: Use of the physician orders for life-sustaining treatment program in Oregon nursing facilities: Beyond resuscitation. J Am Geriatr Soc 2004;52:1424–1429.
24. Moss AH, Holley JL, Davison SN, et al: Core curriculum in nephrology: Palliative care. Am J Kidney Dis 2004;43:172–185.
25. Kidney End-of-Life Coalition: Advance Care Planning in Dialysis Facilities. Available at: www.kidneyeol.org/advanced.htm. Accessed May 25, 2007.
26. Neely KJ, Roxe DM: Palliative care/hospice and the withdrawal of dialysis. J Palliat Med 2000;3:57–67.
27. Renal Physicians Association and American Society of Nephrology: RPA/ASN Position on Quality Care at the End of Life, Document 1.02. January 19, 2002. Available at: www.renalmd.org. Accessed May 28, 2007.
28. Murray AM, Arko C, Chen S-C, et al: Utilization of hospice in the United States dialysis population. Clin J Am Soc Nephrol 2006;1:1248–1255.
29. Davison SN, Jhangri GS, Holley JL, Moss AH: Nephrologists' reported preparedness for end-of-life decision-making. Clin J Am Soc Nephrol 2006;1:1256–1262.
30. Cohen LM, Germain MJ, Poppel DM: Practical considerations in dialysis withdrawal: "To have the option is a blessing." JAMA 2003;289:2113–2119.

Further Reading

Cohen LM, Germain MJ, Poppel DM: Practical considerations in dialysis withdrawal: "To have the option is a blessing." JAMA 2003;289:2113–2119.

Chambers EJ, Germain M, Brown E (eds): Supportive Care for the Renal Patient. Oxford: Oxford University Press, 2004.

Davison SN, Torgunrud C: The creation of an advance care planning process for patients with ESRD. Am J Kidney Dis 2007;49:27–36.

Davison SN, Jhangri GS, Holley JL, Moss AH: Nephrologists' reported preparedness for end-of-life decision-making. Clin J Am Soc Nephrol 2006;1:1256–1262.

Moss AH: To use dialysis appropriately: the emerging consensus on patient selection guidelines. Adv Renal Replacement Ther 1995;2:175–183.

Renal Physicians Association and the American Society of Nephrology: Shared Decision-Making in the Appropriate Initiation of and Withdrawal from Dialysis. Washington, DC: RPA, 2000.

PART XIV

Transplantation

CONTENTS

Chapter 85

Evaluation of the Kidney Transplant Recipient and Living Kidney Donor

Connie L. Davis

Kidney transplantation saves lives, especially if performed before a patient with end-stage kidney disease (ESRD) initiates dialysis (Fig. 85-1).[1–3] This survival benefit is seen for the young, the old, and those with diabetes and hepatitis.[1–4] For a full discussion of the outcomes of renal transplantation, see Chapter 87. This chapter focuses on the evaluation of the recipient and donor. These evaluations should be performed within 6 months of the predicted need for recipient dialysis, typically with a glomerular filtration rate (GFR) less than 15 mL/min, especially when a living donor kidney transplant is an option (www.uktransplant.org). If no living donor is available, the average wait for a deceased donor transplant in the United States is 3.3 years for blood group A, more than 5 years for blood group O, and more than 5.6 years for blood group B (www.unos.org). Currently, the time to transplantation is also significantly influenced by geographic location and allosensitization.

RECIPIENT EVALUATION

Guidelines for the evaluation of kidney transplant recipients have been published by the American Society of Transplantation, the European Renal Association-European Dialysis and Transplant Association, and the British Transplantation Society and Renal Association (www .uktransplant.org).[5–7] An overview of the evaluation is shown in Box 85-1.

Blood Type and Histocompatibility

The potential donor and recipient must be ABO blood group compatible to avoid hyperacute rejection; however, Rh factor incompatibility is not a contraindication to transplantation. Likewise, histocompatibility testing is performed to help identify recipient/donor combinations that would result in poor allograft survival. Both donor and recipient HLA-A, HLA-B, and HLA-DR antigens of the major histocompatibility complex are determined. Antigen-specific antidonor profiles are also performed, and unacceptable antigens are determined for the recipient. Histocompatibility testing is discussed in detail in Chapter 87.

Age and Transplantation Success

Older age has been a relative contraindication to transplantation due to concern over decreased survival. From 1988 through 2004 in the United States, 2623 individuals between 71 and 75 years of age underwent transplantation as did 503

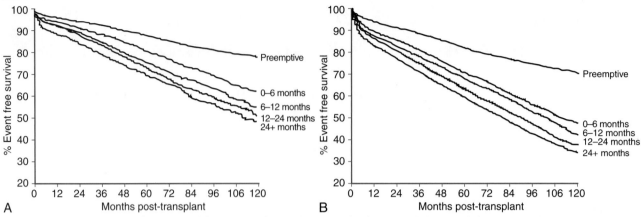

Figure 85-1 Kidney transplant survival by timing of transplantation for living and deceased donor transplants. Patients were evaluated by the timing of transplantation in relation to starting dialysis; preemptive candidates underwent transplantation before starting dialysis. **A,** Graft survival by timing of living donor kidney transplantation. **B,** Graft survival by timing of deceased donor kidney transplantation. (Reprinted from Meier-Kriesche HU, Kaplan B: Waiting time on dialysis as the strongest modifiable risk factor for renal transplant outcomes: A paired donor kidney analysis. Transplantation 2002;74: 1377–1381, with permission.)

Box 85-1   Recipient Evaluation

1. Transplant Specific
   HLA typing
   PRA (panel reactive antibody) determination
   ABO typing
2. General areas of focus
   History
   Cardiovascular: symptoms, smoking, diabetes, exercise tolerance, previous cardiovascular events, hypertension, phosphorus
   Pulmonary: symptoms, limits, treatments, exposures
   Type of renal disease: obtain biopsy report if available
   Family history: malignancy, cardiac disease, renal disease
   Urine output
   Nephrolithiasis
   Infection: residence, travel, work, activity exposure, treatments, transfusions
   Malignancy screening, symptoms
   Surgeries and tolerance
   Medication tolerance
   Gastrointestinal: peptic ulcer disease, bowel habits, bleeding, diverticulitis, cholelithiasis, liver disease
   Neurologic: cerebral ischemia, peripheral neuropathy
   Examination: height, weight, blood pressure; focus on cardiovascular examination; focus on neurological examination; focus on signs of malignancy; focus on signs of infection
   Laboratory
     Complete blood count with platelet count
     Prothrombin time/partial thromboelastin time
     More detailed evaluation if there is a history of coagulation disorders
     Comprehensive panel (electrolytes, transaminase levels, albumin, calcium, phosphorus, alkaline phosphatase, bilirubin)
     Urinalysis if possible, with culture if indicated
     24-Hour urine for volume, protein if possible
3. Cardiovascular
   Electrocardiogram
   Chest radiograph
   As clinically indicated, cardiac stress testing and/or echocardiography
   As clinically indicated, vascular duplex or angiography
4. Malignancy
   PAP test for all adult female candidates
   Mammogram for all women 40 or older, earlier if previous findings or strong family history
   Digital prostate examination and prostate-specific antigen test for all male candidates 40 or older
   Colonoscopy for all candidates older than 50 or younger with increased family risk or positive stool guaiac
5. Infection: screen for
   Cytomegalovirus, Epstein-Barr virus, herpes simplex virus, varicella-zoster virus
   Human immunodeficiency virus types 1 and 2
   Human T-lymphotropic viruses 1 and 2
   Hepatitis B surface antigen
   Hepatitis B core antibody IgM/IgG
   Hepatitis B surface antibody
   Hepatitis C virus
   Rapid plasma reagin
   Tuberculosis
   Toxoplasmosis, depending on exposure risk
   Geographically determined testing: coccidiomycosis, *Strongyloides*, *Trypanosoma cruzi*, malaria, human herpesvirus 8
   Consider human herpesvirus 6 and West Nile virus
6. Recurrent disease
   Review past diagnosis, biopsy results, and clinical course for the risk of diagnoses that frequently recur
7. Psychosocial status: education, support, smoking, recreational drug use, compliance, depression/anxiety

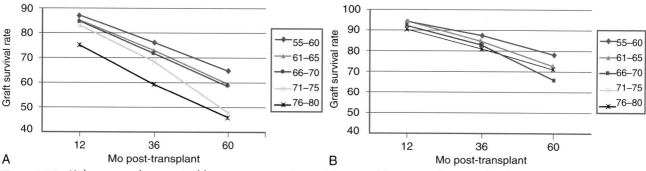

Figure 85-2 Kidney transplant survival by recipient age (over 55 years old) at transplantation for deceased donor and living donor allografts (United Network for Organ Sharing data as of March 2005). **A,** Transplant survival by recipient age for deceased donor transplants. **B,** Transplant survival by recipient age for living donor transplants.

individuals 76 to 80 years old and 48 individuals older than age 80. Although individuals older than 70 must be carefully evaluated, they may successfully undergo transplantation and demonstrate acceptable survival (Fig. 85-2 [www.unos.org; UNOS data as of May 2007]).

Cardiovascular Disease

Cardiovascular disease is a major contributor to the increased premature mortality rate seen in renal transplant recipients. An overview of the work-up algorithm is shown in Box 85-1. There is no general consensus regarding the type or extent of testing.

Ischemic Heart Disease

It is recommended that asymptomatic patients undergo further assessment if they are older than 50 years of age, are diabetic, have smoked cigarettes in the past 5 years, or have a resting electrocardiogram that shows a rhythm disturbance or ST segment abnormalities, although these recommendations are made on underpowered and nonrandomized studies.[8,9] Further assessment begins with a noninvasive test of occult cardiac ischemia, realizing it is not possible to justify one particular test. Exercise tests probably have the most discriminating power but may not be practical, making pharmacologically driven cardiac stress testing more popular. Combined dipyridamole and exercise thallium imaging or dobutamine stress echocardiography are the most commonly used tests.[10] The discovery of significant reversible ischemia requires coronary imaging with subsequent management directed per current protocols. If left ventricular function is adequate and symptoms are controlled, then transplant listing is recommended. Transplantation during treatment with Plavix (clopidogrel) is still without rigorous examination. Coronary calcification testing has not yet predicted posttransplantation outcomes.[11]

Cerebrovascular Disease

There is no evidence to support screening asymptomatic potential renal transplant recipients for cerebrovascular disease, although carotid plaque is positively associated with cardiovascular events.[12,13] Additionally, silent cerebral infarction is not uncommon and not necessarily related to carotid artery disease.[14,15] Patients with a completed stroke or a transient ischemic attack within the past 6 months should be referred for neurological assessment and transplantation reconsidered af-

ter medical and surgical management has been optimized and the patient is free of recurrent transient ischemic attacks for 6 months. Screening in the presence of an asymptomatic carotid bruit is prudent but may not alter the decision for treatment or transplantation.

Peripheral Vascular Disease

If patients are asymptomatic with good femoral pulses, then only a plain radiograph is recommended to rule out extensive vascular calcification.[16] In contrast, patients with claudication or lack of palpable femoral pulses require vascular imaging and a surgical assessment of whether it is technically possible to implant the graft and whether the transplant would be predicted to lead to steal and critical ischemia in the distal leg.[17]

Cancer

Cancer rates are increased in patients with ESRD on dialysis and after transplantation.[18,19] The impact of immunosuppression on recurrence of a previously treated malignancy has not been clarified. However, transplant cancer registries and common sense dictate that potential recipients with an incurable malignancy should not undergo transplantation and those previously successfully treated for cancer should delay transplantation until the time of maximum recurrence of malignancy has passed. Recurrence rates of cancer post-transplantation have been demonstrated to decrease the longer the waiting time, with 53% recurring within 2 years, 34% between years 2 and 5, and the last 13% recurring after 5 years.[20,21] In reality, most programs wait 2 years after successful treatment of most cancers before transplant listing. Exceptions without a recommended delay include asymptomatic incidentally discovered renal cell carcinoma confined to the kidney, in situ cancer of the bladder or cervix, and basal cell and squamous cell carcinomas of the skin. In contrast, cancers with a high risk of recurrence, such as colorectal cancer, malignant melanoma, and cancer of the body of the uterus, should have a 5-year delay. It is difficult to know how best to advise patients with treated breast cancer as the majority of relapses occur after 3 years.[22–25] The safest approach for most cancers due to the heterogeneity of prognosis depending on staging, tumor markers, and treatment advances is to individualize the approach after consultation with an oncologist.

Consensus is nonexistent in the transplant community regarding the necessity of screening for malignancy as the numbers needed to screen to save one life are large and vary from

338 to more than 5000 for colorectal, breast, and prostate cancers.[26] However, to the individual recipient, this may have a huge impact on outcome as well as be a key factor in a possible living donor's decision to donate. Therefore, although some programs will not routinely screen for cervical, prostate, breast, or colon cancer, it is suggested that at least appropriate age, personal history (von Hippel-Lindau disease, analgesic nephropathy), and family history (familial polyposis) screening be performed. Last, renal cell cancer is increased in those with ESRD; some, but not all, recommend that screening start with an ultrasound scan.[27]

Infection

The pretransplantation evaluation for infection should include testing for the infections listed in Box 85-1.[28] Treatable infections must be eradicated before transplantation. Infections of the teeth, sinuses, ears, chest, urinary tract, gastrointestinal tract, and the feet of those with diabetes and patients with peripheral vascular disease must be cleared up before transplantation. Chest radiography should be performed for signs of pulmonary tuberculosis or other pulmonary infection. Controversy exists with regard to patients who are hepatitis B virus surface antigen positive or hepatitis C virus antibody positive because of the risk of immunosuppression leading to enhanced viral replication and promoting progressive liver disease and death from liver failure.[29] However, survival is better with transplantation than with dialysis.[30,31] Patients with active viral infection are recommended to undergo a liver biopsy to stage the disease and to receive antiviral treatment (lamivudine hepatitis B virus or pegylated interferon alfa hepatitis C virus) before transplantation.[31,32] These patients also require monitoring for the development of hepatocellular carcinoma (alpha-fetoprotein and ultrasonography) and progressive liver disease while waiting.[33] If necessary, combined kidney-liver transplantation is an option.

A potential candidate for organ transplantation who is seropositive for human immunodeficiency virus (HIV) antibody but is asymptomatic should be on highly active antiretroviral therapy and compliant and have an undetectable viral load and CD4$^+$ cell counts of at least 200 cells/mm^3.[28,34] In this setting, transplantation success may approach the uninfected population, although rejection remains a significant issue.[34,35] Guidelines have been produced by the British HIV Association and are available via the British Transplantation Society website at www.bts.org.uk/ and information about HIV and transplantation in the United States is available at www.clinicaltrials.gov/ and www.a-s-t.org/.

Testing for fungal or parasitic infections is partially determined by geographic location and travel history (see Box 85-1).[5,28] In regions of the world where herpes hominis virus-8 infection is common, it may be helpful to know the serology of individuals before grafting given the strong association of the virus with Kaposi sarcoma. Recipients who have negative Epstein-Barr virus who receive Epstein-Barr virus–positive renal transplants have a sevenfold increased risk of developing posttransplantation lymphoproliferative disorder. The knowledge of recipient serologies may therefore influence postgraft immunosuppressive strategies. In particular, the cytomegalovirus serology at the time of grafting helps guide antiviral prophylactic strategies.[28]

Tuberculosis may reactivate after transplantation. As such, all patients should undergo chest radiograph to look for inactive disease and have a tuberculin skin (purified protein derivative test) test. Although a positive purified protein derivative test result correlates with past infection, a negative skin test in the uremic patient may represent a false-negative result.[36,37] Patients identified as high risk (history of tuberculosis, positive chest radiograph, positive purified protein derivative test result, or living in an endemic area) and who have not previously received isoniazid should start pretransplantation treatment or receive daily isoniazid for 9 months after transplantation.

Obesity

Obese individuals carry an increased risk of posttransplantation wound infections and perioperative complications.[38] Obesity is also a risk factor for posttransplantation diabetes and allograft dysfunction.[39–41] According to the United States Renal Data System database, a live donor transplant affords an advantage for all obese subjects; however, deceased donors provide survival benefit only for recipients with a body mass index (BMI) of less than 40 kg/m^2.[42] Obese transplantation candidates should be encouraged to lose weight. Many programs have a BMI threshold for acceptance.

Recurrent Disease

Graft loss attributed to recurrent disease has increased in recent years but is still only thought to be responsible for approximately 5% of allograft loss.[43,44] The highest risk of recurrence is seen with membranoproliferative glomerulonephritis type 1 and oxalosis but is also important for hemolytic uremic syndrome, focal segmental glomerulosclerosis, membranoproliferative glomerulonephritis type 1 IgA nephropathy, membranous nephropathy, diabetes, and vasculitis.

Gastrointestinal

The rate of colonic perforation after transplantation is approximately 1% and is most commonly associated with diverticular disease.[45] Although still somewhat controversial, especially in candidates with polycystic kidney disease, screening of asymptomatic patients is not justified as studies have found that patients with significant diverticular disease rarely have symptomatic disease after transplantation.[45–47] Patients with symptomatic disease should undergo imaging and consideration should be given to resection of extensive disease. Screening of asymptomatic individuals for peptic ulcer disease is not recommended because of the low morbidity rate.[48,49] Those with active symptoms or a history of peptic ulcer disease should, however, undergo endoscopic evaluation before transplantation.[50] If an ulcer is present, it should be treated medically for 6 weeks, followed by a repeat endoscopy. If the ulcer has not healed, surgical therapy should be performed before transplantation. Incidentally identified cholelithiasis should be managed expectantly as no advantage has been found to prophylactic cholecystectomy.[51]

Genitourinary

Patients with recurrent urinary tract infections should have a voiding cystourethrogram. If persistent high-grade reflux is demonstrated, bilateral nephrectomy and ureterectomy are indicated. Additionally, native nephrectomy is advised for persistent infection due to nephrolithiasis or infected cysts or uncontrolled hypertension; in patients with polycystic kidney disease and recurrent cystic bleeding, shortness of breath, early satiety; or to make space for the allograft.[52] Consideration of residual renal function is essential. Transplant nephrectomy before retransplantation is indicated if it is the source of infection, there are chronic inflammatory symptoms, or space is needed for the new transplant. Prostate hypertrophy is not a contraindication to transplantation. Treatment depends on the amount of urinary output; less than normal urine output should delay transurethral resection until after transplantation due to the risk of urethral stenosis. Neurogenic bladder or bladder outlet obstruction resulting in high intravesical pressures as suggested by clinical history and examination necessitates evaluation by urology to determine whether urinary diversion, bladder augmentation, or intermittent self-catheterization is the best option.

Failed Allografts

Whether surgical removal of a failed graft minimizes the degree of HLA sensitization is not clear.[53,54] In practice, grafts that fail within 6 months are usually removed. The decision to remove a graft that fails later needs to balance surgical morbidity against the resistance to the effect of erythropoietic agents seen with a failed graft left in situ, the advantage of rapid tapering of immunosuppression, and whether residual urine output contributes meaningfully to fluid balance. Slow tapering of immunosuppression to avoid adrenal insufficiency is usually safe if the graft is not removed.

Bone

Bone fracture rates are increased in patients with ESRD.[55] However, there is important heterogeneity in the association of bone mineral density studies and fractures in this population as well as after transplantation.[56,57] As such, routine bone density measurements are not indicated, but evaluation of the effectiveness of the treatment of hyperparathyroidism, attention to pain medication use, and exercise with fall avoidance is advised.[58]

Pulmonary

Pulmonary function tests are generally performed in the preparation for surgery if the clinical history or examination suggests chronic lung disease. Obstructive lung disease itself is not a contraindication for transplantation. All patients who smoke cigarettes should be advised to quit because active smokers have a 5.5-fold increased risk of pulmonary complications compared with those who do not smoke. Patients with bronchiectasis require careful assessment as they carry significant risk of serious septic complications post-transplantation.

Psychosocial Evaluation

The psychosocial evaluation is critical for the transplantation candidate as psychosocial variables can affect transplantation outcome.[59] The main psychosocial concerns include impaired capacity, treatment adherence and noncompliance, the use of illicit drugs, and lack of social support. Successful postoperative transplant care inevitably requires a supportive environment, frequent hospital attendance, and adherence to a complex drug regimen. Some individuals can be identified before listing for which additional support post-procedure can minimize the risk of premature graft failure due to the inability to comply with management. Other individuals may be at such poor psychosocial risk that transplantation is not in their best interest. It is best

in these circumstances to collate views from several of the health professionals involved in the patient's care as well as from the patient and immediate family members.

Re-evaluation of Patients on the Waiting List

Following placement on the waiting list, patients may wait years before receiving a transplant offer. Due to this wait, candidate medical re-evaluation is a logical step, but there are no data to help decide how often this should be or what tests should be performed. Brief guidelines have been proposed but are not backed by rigorous data. Some assessments are part of regular dialysis care such as monitoring hepatitis and HIV status. Cancer screening should proceed per population guidelines. Cardiovascular assessment, however, is the most controversial; only clinically triggered testing has been shown to be of benefit.[60,61] Even so, it seems prudent to perform cardiac re-evaluation every 2 years on diabetic and every 4 years on nondiabetic wait-listed candidates.[9,62,63]

EVALUATION OF THE LIVING KIDNEY DONOR

Transplant programs have historically used varied evaluation and selection criteria for living donors such that transplant organizations and government transplant agencies have started to devolop guidelines for programs to follow (e.g., UK transplant, the American Society of Transplantation, the American Society of Transplant Surgeons, New York State, and United Network for Organ Sharing [UNOS]).[64–68] The elements necessary in the consenting process are available on the UNOS website, those for the psychological evaluation are shown in Box 85-2 and those for the medical evaluation in Box 85-3.[67,69] Detailed consent is of utmost importance due to the increasing dependence on living donation and because during 2006 in the United States, 21.6% of living donors were unrelated to the recipient (Fig. 85-3) (www.health.state.ny .us/nysdoh/liver_donation/pdf/liver_donor_report_web.pdf).

Optimally, the team evaluating the living kidney donor should include a nephrologist, transplantation surgeon, social worker or psychologist or psychiatrist, dietitian, donor coordinator, and pharmacist. At least one member of the team should be completely independent of the transplantation team taking care of the potential recipient and be able to stop the donation process if discoveries are made that could lead to donor harm.[70] Preferably, the entire donor team would be independent of the team taking care of the recipient with some not being members of the transplantation program at all.

Risk of Living Donation
Death

The risk of death after living donation is reported to be 0.02% to 0.04% within 90 days of donation.[71,72] UNOS initiated tracking of donor deaths in October 1999. From October 1999 through December 2006, 14 (of 43,882 donors, 0.03%) living kidney donor deaths were reported to UNOS or identified by examination of the Social Security Death Master File to have occurred within 30 days of donation. During the same time period, by

Box 85-2   Required Components of the Living Donor Psychosocial Evaluation

To accomplish the goals of the psychosocial evaluation, the following components must be included.[69]

a. *History and current status:* Obtain standard background information regarding such areas as the prospective donor's educational level, living situation, cultural background, religious beliefs and practices, significant relationships, family psychosocial history, employment, lifestyle, community activities, legal offense history, and citizenship.

b. *Capacity:* Ensure that the prospective donor's cognitive status and capacity to comprehend information are not compromised and do not interfere with judgment; determine risk of exploitation.

c. *Psychological status:* Establish the presence or absence of current and previous psychiatric disorders, including but not limited to mood, anxiety, substance use, and personality disorders. Review current or previous therapeutic interventions (counseling, medications); physical, psychological or sexual abuse; current stressors (e.g., relationships, home, work); recent losses; chronic pain management. Assess repertoire of coping skills to manage previous life or health-related stressors. A focus on the extent of anxiety and depression is needed.

d. *Relationship with the transplant candidate:* Review the nature and degree of closeness (if any) to the recipient (e.g., how the relationship developed) and whether the transplant would impose expectations or perceived obligations on the part of either the donor or the recipient.

e. *Motivation:* Explore the rationale and reasoning for volunteering to donate (i.e., the "voluntariness") including whether donation would be consistent with past behaviors and apparent values, beliefs, moral obligations, or lifestyle and whether it would be free of coercion, inducements, ambivalence, impulsivity, or ulterior motives (e.g., to atone or gain approval, to stabilize self-image, to remedy psychological malady).

f. *Donor knowledge, understanding, and preparation:* Explore the prospective donor's awareness of any potential short- and long-term risks of surgical complications and health outcomes, both for the donor and the transplant candidate; recovery and recuperation time; availability of alternative treatments for the transplantation candidate; financial ramifications (including possible insurance risk). Determine that the donor understands that data on long-term donor health and psychosocial outcomes continue to be sparse. Assess the prospective donor's understanding, acceptance, and respect for the specific donor protocol (e.g., willingness to accept potential lack of communication from the recipient, willingness to undergo future donor follow-up).

g. *Social support:* Evaluate significant other, familial, social, and employer support networks available to the prospective donor on an ongoing basis as well as during the donor's recovery from surgery.

h. *Financial suitability:* Determine whether the prospective donor is financially stable and free of financial hardship, has resources available to cover financial obligations for expected and unexpected donation-related expenses, is able to withstand time away from work or established role including unplanned extended recovery time, has disability and health insurance.

i. Discussion with the donor support person.

Box 85-3   Medical Evaluation of the Living Kidney Donor

1. Donor typing to determine the risk of acute transplant failure
   a. ABO blood group typing × 2
   b. HLA typing
   c. Crossmatch
2. General history and physical examination
   a. History specifically includes evaluation of family history of kidney disease, diabetes, hypertension, birth weight if possible, gestational diabetes, birth weight of offspring, clotting disorders or deep venous thrombosis, use of nonsteroidal anti-inflammatory drugs (e.g., ibuprofen, indomethacin), urinary tract infections, nephrolithiasis, chronic infections, cancer and kidney injury; prospective donors should be asked whether they have dental coverage and have had a dental examination recently
   b. Physical examination including blood pressure (done three times at three different times; if possible, it is preferable to perform a 24-hour blood pressure monitor); height; weight; calculated body mass index; waist circumference; a search for evidence of heart, lung, liver, and blood vessel disease; abnormal lymph nodes; and large spleen
   c. Medical psychological evaluation and social history should include questioning about alcohol intake, smoking history, substance use and abuse, history of mental illness and treatment used
3. General laboratory tests: complete blood count with platelet count, prothrombin time/partial thromboelastin time, more detailed evaluation if there is a history of coagulation disorders, comprehensive panel (electrolytes, transaminase levels, albumin, calcium, phosphorus, alkaline phosphatase, bilirubin), human chorionic gonadotropin quantitative pregnancy test if younger than 55 years, urine toxicology screen, serum protein electrophoresis in those older than 60 years
4. Cardiovascular: heart and blood vessel tests
   Chest radiograph
   Electrocardiogram
   Echocardiogram and/or exercise stress test if the prospective donor is more than 50 years old or has risk factors (hypertension, smoking, hyperlipidemia, family history, exercise shortness of breath) or physical findings that demonstrate increased risk of heart disease including, but not limited to, the following: borderline blood pressure, abnormal electrocardiogram, abnormal chest radiograph, murmur
   Pulmonary function tests for smokers

Box 85-3   *Medical Evaluation of the Living Kidney Donor—cont'd*

5. Renal-focused evaluation
Urinalysis, looking for protein and cells in the urine
Urine culture (if symptoms or abnormal urinalysis)
Protein excretion: 24-hour urine for protein and/or microalbumin excretion or protein-to-creatinine ratio and/or albumin-to-creatinine ratio × 2; if one is abnormal, repeat
If protein detected, evaluation for postural proteinuria by split urine collection over 24 hours (8 hours recumbent and 16 hours active)
Serum creatinine
Glomerular filtration rate (GFR) measurement: clearance testing, 24-hour urine for creatinine clearance measurement or preferably a measured clearance using urine or plasma clearance of iothalamate, iohexol, or other suitable marker. GFR should be expressed per 1.73 m². Calculated GFR measurements using the serum creatinine are not felt to be adequate. GFR should be within 2 SD for age or be calculated to be at 40 mL/min/1.73 m² at age 80.
Screen for polycystic kidney disease as indicated by family history, ultrasound scan if older than 30 years, linkage genetic testing if younger than age 30

6. Metabolic-focused evaluation
Fasting blood glucose
Uric acid
Thyroid-stimulating hormone
Fasting lipid profile (cholesterol, triglycerides, high-density lipoprotein cholesterol, low-density lipoprotein cholesterol)
Determine the number of elements of the metabolic syndrome that are present; obtain consent for risk if three or more risk factors
If at increased risk for diabetes (family history of diabetes, gestational diabetes, or elevated triglyceride levels), perform an oral glucose tolerance test and include calculations for insulin secretion/insulin resistance index
Hemoglobin A1C

7. Infection
Cytomegalovirus, Epstein-Barr virus, herpes simplex virus, varicella-zoster virus
Human immunodeficiency virus types 1 and 2
Human T-lymphotropic viruses 1 and 2
Hepatitis B surface antigen

Hepatitis B core antibody IgM/IgG
Hepatitis B surface antibody
Hepatitis C virus
Rapid plasma reagin
Tuberculosis
Toxoplasmosis, depending on exposure risk
Geographically determined testing: coccidiomycosis, *Strongyloides, Trypanosoma cruzi,* malaria, human herpesvirus 8
Consider human herpesvirus 6 and West Nile virus

8. Anatomic evaluation
Determine which kidney is the safest to remove and which kidney (the one with the best function) is to be left with the donor. Additionally, the presence of abnormal liver, nodes, adrenal glands, and spleen can be determined.
a. The test of choice will depend on the local radiological expertise and surgical preference but may include a computed tomography angiogram, magnetic resonance angiogram, or angiogram. It may also be advised to perform an abdominal ultrasound scan to evaluate liver for fatty infiltration and unexpected abnormalities of the liver, pancreas and spleen if a full abdominal computed tomography or magnetic resonance imaging scan is not performed.
b. Renal scan with differential renal function

9. Cancer screening
Determines that the donor does not need both kidneys to help with tolerance of anticancer treatment and that the donor does not have a tumor that would be transferred to the recipient
Testing to be performed depending on gender, age, or family history
a. PAP for all women
b. Mammogram for all women over 40 or according to family risk
c. Prostate-specific antigen test for all men older than 50; for all African American men older than 40, or if from a high-risk family
d. Colonoscopy for all donors older than 50 or younger according to family history
e. Chest computed tomography for those with a history of smoking

12 months post-donation, 37 of 43,882 (0.08%) donors had died. The most common reasons for death at any time were, in descending order of occurrence, unknown (47.2%), cancer (9.4%), cardiovascular disease (7.5%), motor vehicle accident (7.5%), homicide (5.7%), suicide (3.8%), hemorrhage (2.8%), infection (1.9%), and respiratory failure (1.9%).

Morbidity

During the second half of 2006, 14 of 3154 (0.4%) U.S. living kidney donors underwent reoperation before initial discharge.[73] The most common reasons for reoperation were bleeding and bowel obstruction. Readmission after donation was necessary for 47 of 3154 (1.5%) donors.[73] The most common reasons for donor readmission were abdominal problems (nausea, vomiting, abdominal pain, constipation, bowel obstruction) and bleeding. Less frequent reasons included chylous ascites, pancreatitis, pulmonary embolism, subphrenic fluid, and infection (wound, pneumonia, urinary tract). In 2006, 86.9% of donations were performed laparoscopically.[73]

End-Stage Renal Disease

The risk of ESRD varies according to the time after donation, the family history, and donor ethnicity. The impact of access to health care is not known. To date, on average, between 0.1% and 0.5% of living donors have developed ESRD.[74–76]

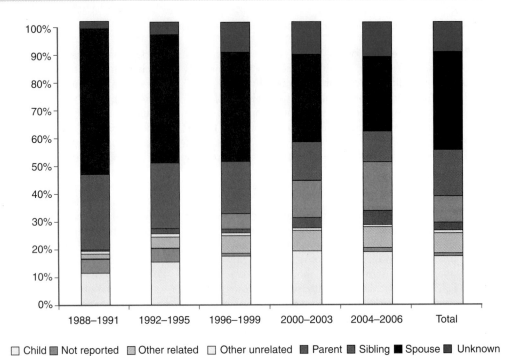

Figure 85-3 United Network for Organ Sharing/ Scientific Registry for Transplant Recipients: Living Kidney Donor Relation. Relationship of living donors to their recipients over time by year (United Network for Organ Sharing data as of December 2006).

☐ Child ■ Not reported ☐ Other related ☐ Other unrelated ■ Parent ■ Sibling ■ Spouse ■ Unknown

From January 1996 through February 2007, UNOS reports that 146 previous living donors have been listed as kidney transplant candidates.[73] Sixty-three percent donated 16 or more years before the onset of ESRD; 8.3% donated 0 to 5 years before listing, 14% between 6 and 10 years, and 14.9% between 11 and 15 years. Donor ethnicity is reported to be white in 42.5%, black in 42.5%, Hispanic in 8.9%, and Asian in 3.4%. The causes of ESRD have been reported as follows: glomerular diseases ($N = 36$, mostly focal segmental glomerulosclerosis), hypertensive nephrosclerosis ($N = 32$), diabetes ($N = 16$), and renovascular and other vascular diseases ($N = 11$). The data reported above do not include those starting dialysis but not wait-listed for a transplant and those dying of ESRD but not receiving renal replacement therapy.

Long-Term Mortality

Most studies have found that long-term mortality after living donation is due to cardiovascular disease and cancer, identical to the general population. Indeed, of donors donating from 1999 onward in the United States, 10 have died of cancer and 8 of cardiovascular causes.[73] Special mention, however, must be made of other causes. Of donors donating from 1999 on in the United States, causes of death were auto accidents in eight, other trauma in four, homicide in six, suicide in four, and drug overdose in one. The last group of causes suggests a renewed focus on the psychosocial evaluation for living donor candidates and that analysis of their support systems is in order.

Evaluation

An outline of the usual donor evaluation is shown in Box 85-3 and includes blood and urine screening tests, chest radiograph, electrocardiogram, an age- and family history–appropriate cardiac stress test and cancer screening, and radiographic assessment of the kidneys and vessels. Accepted contraindications to living donation are listed in Box 85-4.

Box 85-4 Contraindications to Living Kidney Donation

Absolute Exclusion Criteria
1. Age younger than 18 years
2. Hypertension: blood pressure > 130/90 in someone younger than 50, evidence of end-organ damage, nonwhite, on three or more antihypertensive medications
3. Diabetes (diagnosis of diabetes)
4. Abnormal glucose tolerance test: 2-hour oral glucose tolerance test > 140
5. History of thrombosis or embolism
6. Psychiatric contraindications
7. Obesity: body mass index > 35
8. Coronary artery disease, reduced cardiac function
9. Symptomatic valvular disease
10. Chronic lung disease
11. Recent malignancy
12. Urologic abnormalities of donor kidney
13. Creatinine clearance < 80 mL/min or projected glomerular filtration rate with removal of one kidney at 80 years of age of <40 mL/min
14. Peripheral vascular disease
15. Proteinuria > 300 mg/24 hr
16. Human immunodeficiency virus infection
17. Hepatitis C virus infection
18. Hepatitis B virus infection

Relative Contraindications
1. Age 18–21 years, older age relative to the medical condition
2. Obesity (body mass index 30–35)
3. Kidney stones
4. Distant history of cancer
5. History of psychiatric disorder
6. Renovascular disease
7. Thin basement membrane disease

Renal Function and Live Kidney Donation

The threshold of acceptable donor renal function has declined with time. In general, it would appear prudent to require living donors to have a GFR at donation at the average of the age-specific GFR.[77–79] Furthermore, the estimated GFR over time should also fit the average curve for age. Thus, as the GFR decreases with age, a donor's projected GFR at age 80 should be greater than or equal to 40 to 50 mL/min/1.73 m^2 (www.bts.org.uk/).[77,79]

Hypertension

The optimal evaluation of blood pressure for living donors is with 24-hour blood pressure monitoring. This allows detection of white coat hypertension as well as undetected hypertension.[80,81] If elevated blood pressure is detected and the prospective donor is still under consideration, then a chest radiograph, electrocardiogram, echocardiogram, and ophthalmologic evaluation should be obtained to look for secondary consequences of hypertension. Preliminary evidence indicates that donation is acceptable for hypertensive individuals if they are white, blood pressure is controlled, GFR is age appropriate, and protein/albumin excretion is normal.[82] However, more detailed information about these donors and their long-term outcomes is needed before generally accepting hypertensive individuals as donors as donors will on average have a 5-mm Hg increase in blood pressure over 5 to 10 years from donation above that anticipated for normal aging.[83]

Donor Obesity or Family History of Diabetes

Obesity may affect perioperative complications, future renal function, and the cardiovascular health of the living donor. Obesity is a risk factor for the development of nephrolithiasis, renal cell and other cancer, as well as ESRD.[84] For ESRD, the relative risk is 3 for a BMI between 30 and 34.9 kg/m^2 and 4.7 for a BMI of 35 to 39.9 kg/m^2.[85] Obese individuals may be more prone to develop renal disease after donation. In one study, obese (BMI > 30) subjects had an increased rate of proteinuria and renal impairment 10 to 20 years after nephrectomy.[86] Despite these concerns, many programs accept the obese as living donors. Heimbach and colleagues[87] prospectively evaluated obese donors for 12 months. To date, the obese donors have not had lower GFR (by iothalamate clearance) or higher protein excretion rates compared with the normal BMI donors at follow-up. The Swiss donor registry has likewise not noted a change in albuminuria in obese donors over 5 years from donation, although one donor developed diabetes, hypertension, proteinuria, and renal failure.[88] Obesity greatly increases the future risk of diabetes, and as a consequence all obese prospective donors or those nonobese subjects with a first-degree relative with diabetes or with a history of gestational diabetes should be evaluated with an oral glucose tolerance test. This recommendation may change, however, as equations from large population studies are developed to more accurately predict the development of type 2 diabetes.[89–91] Abnormal glucose tolerance is a contraindication to donation.

Nephrolithiasis

Those with a history of bilateral or recurrent stones and those with systemic conditions associated with recurrent stone disease should not donate. An asymptomatic potential donor with a current single stone is suitable if the donor does not have a high risk of recurrence and the stone is less than 1.5 cm in size and is removable during transplantation.[67,92] The evaluation of an asymptomatic donor with a single previous episode of nephrolithiasis should include serum calcium, creatinine, albumin, parathyroid hormone, and spot urine for cystine; a urinalysis and urine culture; a helical computed tomography scan; chemical analysis of the stone if available; and a 24-hour urine for oxalate and creatinine.[93]

History of Malignancy and Infectious Disease

A history of the following malignancies excludes live kidney donation: melanoma, testicular cancer, renal cell carcinoma, choriocarcinoma, hematologic malignancy, bronchial cancer, breast cancer, and monoclonal gammopathy.[67,94,95] A history of malignancy may be acceptable for donation if previous treatment of the malignancy does not decrease renal reserve or place the donor at increased risk of ESRD and does not increase the operative risk of nephrectomy. A history of malignancy may be acceptable if the specific cancer is curable and transmission of the cancer can reasonably be excluded; consultation with an oncologist may be required. Consent to receive a renal transplant must include a discussion with the donor and the recipient that the risk of transmission of malignant disease cannot be completely excluded.

Infection

A living donor should not be accepted if there is a history of active infection that requires nephrotoxic treatments or would put the donor at risk of developing renal disease. These infections include HIV, hepatitis C, hepatitis B, recurrent urinary tract infections, endocarditis, and malaria.[28,67]

Venous Thromboembolism

Unless the history suggests a medical condition that would necessitate a comprehensive coagulation profile, these tests are not likely to yield useful information.[96] Previous thromboembolism is a relative contraindication to live donation and will require an evaluation of the likelihood of recurrence. Oral contraceptives and hormone replacement therapy are commonly used and present an increased risk of postoperative venous thrombosis and thus should be withheld for at least 2 months before elective surgery.[97,98]

Renovascular Disease

Fibromuscular dysplasia is found on average in 2% to 4% of prospective donors.[99,100] Donors with severe and diffuse disease should not be selected for donation. The age of the prospective donor should also be considered with the outcome in donors older than age 50 seemingly more predictable and benign than in younger donors.[101]

Atherosclerotic renal vascular disease is a relative contraindication to living donation. If it is present, the donor should be normotensive, have normal renal function, and have only unilateral disease.[102] Careful evaluation for coronary disease and peripheral vascular disease should be undertaken given the significant correlation with renal artery stenosis.

Isolated Hematuria

Isolated hematuria in a prospective donor necessitates consideration of thin basement membrane nephropathy and IgA nephropathy as well as urinary tract infection, malignancy, and nephrolithiasis. This is a relatively common problem; a mass screening study in Japan found a single test point prevalence of 4% of adult men and 10% of adult women.[103]

Some investigators have reported the development of ESRD in individuals with thin basement membrane disease.[104,105] Currently, one approach to prospective donors with hematuria and thin basement membrane disease would be to limit selection to those older than age 50 who have the least risk and those with predictable family histories of disease and normal functional studies.[106,107]

IgA nephropathy is a contraindication to live donation. The implications of isolated mesangial IgA without other manifestations of nephropathy require further study, and donation should be decided on in the context of family history, absolute renal function, the presence of interstitial disease, and age.[108] If during live donor evaluation, persistent isolated asymptomatic hematuria is detected, the work-up should include a renal biopsy because, in that setting, the biopsy specimen is often abnormal and aids the decision-making process.[109]

Autosomal Dominant Polycystic Kidney Disease

Familial studies have shown the sensitivity of ultrasonography to be 100% in individuals at risk of autosomal dominant polycystic kidney disease who are age 30 or older.[110] Wherever possible, linkage analysis in addition to ultrasound testing should be performed in prospective donors at risk who are younger than age 30.[111,112] Mutation-based molecular diagnostics must still be treated with care in the clinical setting.[112] If linkage studies are not possible, computed tomography and/or magnetic resonance imaging may provide better sensitivity than ultrasonography.[113]

Cardiopulmonary Disease

Cardiac evaluations need to be performed based on the family history, personal history, physical examination, electrocardiogram, and chest radiograph. If the history, examination, and tests suggest ischemia or valvular disease, then an exercise or pharmacologic stress test and/or echocardiogram should be performed. An individual with myocardial dysfunction or coronary ischemia should not donate. Absolute contraindications to donation are symptomatic valvular disease, severe valvular disease even if asymptomatic, and valvular disease with abnormal cardiac function and/or ischemia.[114] The possibility of valvular abnormalities should be particularly considered in family members of those with autosomal dominant polycystic kidney disease. Relative contraindications are the presence of a prosthetic valve and moderate regurgitant valvu-

lar disease with otherwise normal echocardiographic findings. Finally, the donor with valvular disease should be informed of the risk of perioperative endocarditis even with antimicrobial prophylaxis, bleeding in those treated with anticoagulants, and thromboembolism during changes in anticoagulation.

Pulmonary contraindications to donation include chronic lung diseases that significantly increase the risk of anesthesia and hypertension.[115] If indicated by history and examination, pulmonary function testing, echocardiography, and/or sleep studies should be performed. In all cases, donors should cease smoking for at least 4 to 8 weeks before surgery to minimize the risk of pneumonia.[116] Optimally, donors should stop smoking permanently due to the increased risk of vascular disease, renal arteriosclerosis, and cancer.

QUALITY OF LIFE AFTER LIVING DONATION

Physical and psychological function in living donors is higher than the community norm. Physical issues reported by donors after donation frequently include a decrease from baseline in energy, whereas some note a longer time to full recovery (as long as 4 months) than they had anticipated and incision pain that lasted longer than they expected. Psychological factors usually include an improved relationship with the recipient, an improved self-image, and frequently a positive effect on their life. Even though most donors have a very positive experience, a small number do regret the decision to donate (0%–5%).[117,118]

References

1. Meier-Kriesche HU, Kaplan B: Waiting time on dialysis as the strongest modifiable risk factor for renal transplant outcomes: A paired donor kidney analysis. Transplantation 2002;74:1377–1381.
2. Kennedy SE, Mackie FE, Rosenberg AR, McDonald SP: Waiting time and outcome of kidney transplantation in adolescents. Transplantation 2006;82:1046–1050.
3. Ferris ME, Gipson DS, Kimmel PL, Eggers PW: Trends in treatment and outcomes of survival of adolescents initiating end-stage renal disease care in the United States of America. Pediatr Nephrol 2006;21:1020–1026.
4. Gane E, Pilmore H: Management of chronic viral hepatitis before and after renal transplantation. Transplantation 2002;74:427–437.
5. Kasiske BL, Cangro CB, Hariharan S, et al: The evaluation of renal transplantation candidates: Clinical practice guidelines. Am J Transplant 2001;1(Suppl 2):3–95.
6. Steinman TI, Becker BN, Frost AE, et al: Guidelines for the referral and management of patients eligible for solid organ transplantation. Transplantation 2001;71:1189–1204.
7. EBPG, European Renal Association, European Society for Organ Transplantation: European Best Practice Guidelines for Renal Transplantation (part 1). Nephrol Dial Transplant 2000;15(Suppl 7):1–85.
8. Ma IW, Valantine HA, Shibata A, et al: Validation of a screening protocol for identifying low-risk candidates with type 1 diabetes mellitus for kidney with or without pancreas transplantation. Clin Transpl 2006;20:139–146.
9. Gaston RS, Basadonna G, Cosio FG, et al: Transplantation in the diabetic patient with advanced chronic kidney disease: A task force report. Am J Kidney Dis 2004;44:529–542.

10. Kasiske BL, Malik MA, Herzog CA: Risk-stratified screening for ischemic heart disease in kidney transplant candidates. Transplantation 2005;80:815–820.

11. Ferramosca E, De Felice A, Ratti C, et al: Screening for silent ischemia with coronary artery calcium and nuclear stress testing in nondiabetic patients prior to kidney transplant. J Nephrol 2006;19:473–480.

12. Massy ZA, Mamzer-Bruneel MF, Chevalier A, et al: Carotid atherosclerosis in renal transplant recipients. Nephrol Dial Transplant 1998;13:1792–1798.

13. Schwaiger JP, Lamina C, Neyer U, et al: Carotid plaques and their predictive value for cardiovascular disease and all-cause mortality in hemodialysis patients considering renal transplantation: A decade follow-up. Am J Kidney Dis 2006;47:888–897.

14. Anan F, Shimomura T, Imagawa M, et al: Predictors for silent cerebral infarction in patients with chronic renal failure undergoing hemodialysis. Metabolism 2007;56:593–598.

15. Naganuma T, Uchida J, Tsuchida K, et al: Silent cerebral infarction predicts vascular events in hemodialysis patients. Kidney Int 2005;67:2434–2439.

16. Brekke IB, Lien B, Sodal G, et al: Aortoiliac reconstruction in preparation for renal transplantation. Transpl Int 1993;6:161–163.

17. Leskinen Y, Salenius JP, Lehtimaki T, et al: The prevalence of peripheral arterial disease and medial arterial calcification in patients with chronic renal failure: Requirements for diagnostics. Am J Kidney Dis 2002;40:472–479.

18. Maisonneuve P, Agodoa L, Gellert R, et al: Cancer in patients on dialysis for end-stage renal disease: An international collaborative study. Lancet 1999;354:93–99.

19. Vajdic CM, McDonald SP, McCredie MR, et al: Cancer incidence before and after kidney transplantation. JAMA 2006;296:2823–2831.

20. Penn I: Evaluation of transplant candidates with pre-existing malignancies. Ann Transplant 1997;2:14–17.

21. Penn I: The effect of immunosuppression on pre-existing cancers. Transplantation 1993;55:742–747.

22. Brackstone M, Townson JL, Chambers AF: Tumour dormancy in breast cancer: An update. Breast Cancer Res 2007;9:208.

23. Kasiske BL, Snyder JJ, Gilbertson DT, Wang C: Cancer after kidney transplantation in the United States. Am J Transplant 2004;4:905–913.

24. Buell JF, Gross TG, Woodle ES: Malignancy after transplantation. Transplantation 2005;80(2 Suppl):S254–S264.

25. Fischereder M, Jauch KW: Prevalence of cancer history prior to renal transplantation. Transpl Int 2005;18:779–784.

26. Kiberd BA, Keough-Ryan T, Clase CM: Screening for prostate, breast and colorectal cancer in renal transplant recipients. Am J Transplant 2003;3:619–625.

27. Farivar-Mohseni H, Perlmutter AE, Wilson S, et al: Renal cell carcinoma and end stage renal disease. J Urol 2006;175:2018–2020.

28. Screening of donor and recipient prior to solid organ transplantation. Am J Transplant 2004;4(Suppl 10):10–20.

29. Fabrizi F, Martin P, Dixit V, et al: Hepatitis C virus antibody status and survival after renal transplantation: Meta-analysis of observational studies. Am J Transplant 2005;5:1452–1461.

30. Abbott KC, Lentine KL, Bucci JR, et al: The impact of transplantation with deceased donor hepatitis C-positive kidneys on survival in wait-listed long-term dialysis patients. Am J Transplant 2004;4:2032–2037.

31. Maluf DG, Fisher RA, King AL, et al: Hepatitis C virus infection and kidney transplantation: Predictors of patient and graft survival. Transplantation 2007;83:853–857.

32. Kamar N, Toupance O, Buchler M, et al: Evidence that clearance of hepatitis C virus RNA after alpha-interferon therapy in dialysis patients is sustained after renal transplantation. J Am Soc Nephrol 2003;14:2092–2098.

33. Fan WC, King AL, Loong CC, Wu CW: Hepatocellular carcinoma after renal transplantation: The long-term impact of cirrhosis on chronic hepatitis B virus infection. Transplant Proc 2006;38:2080–2083.

34. Abbott KC, Swanson SJ, Agodoa LY, Kimmel PL: Human immunodeficiency virus infection and kidney transplantation in the era of highly active antiretroviral therapy and modern immunosuppression. J Am Soc Nephrol 2004;15:1633–1639.

35. Kumar MS, Sierka DR, Damask AM, et al: Safety and success of kidney transplantation and concomitant immunosuppression in HIV-positive patients. Kidney Int 2005;67:1622–1629.

36. Poduval RD, Hammes MD: Tuberculosis screening in dialysis patients—is the tuberculin test effective? Clin Nephrol 2003;59:436–440.

37. Shankar MS, Aravindan AN, Sohal PM, et al: The prevalence of tuberculin sensitivity and anergy in chronic renal failure in an endemic area: Tuberculin test and the risk of post-transplant tuberculosis. Nephrol Dial Transplant 2005;20:2720–2724.

38. Mehrabi A, Fonouni H, Wente M, et al: Wound complications following kidney and liver transplantation. Clin Transpl 2006;20(Suppl 17):97–110.

39. Gore JL, Pham PT, Danovitch GM, et al: Obesity and outcome following renal transplantation. Am J Transplant 2006;6:357–363.

40. Bosma RJ, Kwakernaak AJ, van der Heide JJ, et al: Body mass index and glomerular hyperfiltration in renal transplant recipients: Cross-sectional analysis and long-term impact. Am J Transplant 2007;7:645–652.

41. Kasiske BL, Snyder JJ, Gilbertson D, Matas AJ: Diabetes mellitus after kidney transplantation in the United States. Am J Transplant 2003;3:178–185.

42. Glanton CW, Kao TC, Cruess D, et al: Impact of renal transplantation on survival in end-stage renal disease patients with elevated body mass index. Kidney Int 2003;63:647–653.

43. Choy BY, Chan TM, Lai KN: Recurrent glomerulonephritis after kidney transplantation. Am J Transplant 2006;6:2535–2542.

44. Hariharan S, Adams MB, Brennan DC, et al: Recurrent and de novo glomerular disease after renal transplantation: A report from Renal Allograft Disease Registry (RADR). Transplantation 1999;68:635–641.

45. Dalla Valle R, Capocasale E, Mazzoni MP, et al: Acute diverticulitis with colon perforation in renal transplantation. Transplant Proc 2005;37:2507–2510.

46. Lederman ED, McCoy G, Conti DJ, Lee EC: Diverticulitis and polycystic kidney disease. Am Surg 2000;66:200–203.

47. McCune TR, Nylander WA, Van Buren DH, et al: Colonic screening prior to renal transplantation and its impact on posttransplant colonic complications. Clin Transpl 1992;6:91–96.

48. Lao A, Bach D: The UGI series in renal transplant candidates. Can Assoc Radiol J 1988;39:195–197.

49. Troppmann C, Papalois BE, Chiou A, et al: Incidence, complications, treatment, and outcome of ulcers of the upper gastrointestinal tract after renal transplantation during the cyclosporine era. J Am Coll Surg 1995;180:433–443.

50. Chen KJ, Chen CH, Cheng CH, et al: Risk factors for peptic ulcer disease in renal transplant patients—11 years of experience from a single center. Clin Nephrol 2004;62:14–20.

51. Kao LS, Flowers C, Flum DR: Prophylactic cholecystectomy in transplant patients: A decision analysis. J Gastrointest Surg 2005;9:965–972.

52. Fuller TF, Brennan TV, Feng S, et al: End stage polycystic kidney disease: Indications and timing of native nephrectomy relative to kidney transplantation. J Urol 2005;174:2284–2288.

53. Abouljoud MS, Deierhoi MH, Hudson SL, Diethelm AG: Risk factors affecting second renal transplant outcome, with special reference to primary allograft nephrectomy. Transplantation 1995;60:138–144.

54. Bennett WM: The failed renal transplant: In or out? Semin Dial 2005;18:188–199.

55. Ball AM, Gillen DL, Sherrard D, et al: Risk of hip fracture among dialysis and renal transplant recipients. JAMA 2002;288:3014–3018.

56. Jamal SA, Hayden JA, Beyene J: Low bone mineral density and fractures in long-term hemodialysis patients: A meta-analysis. Am J Kidney Dis 2007;49:676–681.

57. Grotz WH, Mundinger FA, Gugel B, et al: Bone fracture and osteodensitometry with dual energy X-ray absorptiometry in kidney transplant recipients. Transplantation 1994;58:912–915.

58. Jadoul M, Albert JM, Akiba T, et al: Incidence and risk factors for hip or other bone fractures among hemodialysis patients in the Dialysis Outcomes and Practice Patterns Study. Kidney Int 2006;70:1358–1366.

59. Fisher MS: Psychosocial evaluation interview protocol for pretransplant kidney recipients. Health Soc Work 2006;31:137–144.

60. Zarifian A, O'Rourke M: Managing the kidney waiting list. Prog Transplant 2006;16:242–246.

61. Gill JS, Ma IW, Landsberg DN, et al: Cardiovascular events and investigation in patients who are awaiting cadaveric kidney transplantation. J Am Soc Nephrol 2005;16:808–816.

62. Matas AJ, Kasiske BL, Miller L: Proposed guidelines for re-evaluation of patients on the waiting list for renal cadaver transplantation. Transplantation 2002;73:811–812.

63. Danovitch GM, Hariharan S, Pirsch JD, et al: Management of the waiting list for cadaveric kidney transplants: Report of a survey and recommendations by the Clinical Practice Guidelines Committee of the American Society of Transplantation. J Am Soc Nephrol 2002;13:528–535.

64. Bia MJ, Ramos EL, Danovitch GM, et al: Evaluation of living renal donors. The current practice of US transplant centers. Transplantation 1995;60:322–327.

65. Lumsdaine JA, Wigmore SJ, Forsythe JL: Live kidney donor assessment in the UK and Ireland. Br J Surg 1999;86:877–881.

66. Davis CL, Delmonico FL: Living donor kidney transplantation: A review of current practices for the live donor. J Am Soc Nephrol 2005;16:2098–3110.

67. Delmonico FL: A report of the Amsterdam forum on the care of the live kidney donor: Data and medical guidelines. Transplantation 2005;79(6 Suppl):S53–S66.

68. Kasiske BL, Ravenscraft M, Ramos EL, et al: The evaluation of living renal transplant donors: Clinical practice guidelines. Ad Hoc Clinical Practice Guidelines Subcommittee of the Patient Care and Education Committee of the American Society of Transplant Physicians. J Am Soc Nephrol 1996;7:2288–2313.

69. Dew MA, Jacobs CL, Jowsey SG, et al: Guidelines for the psychosocial evaluation of the living unrelated kidney donors in the United States. Am J Transplant 2007;7:1047–1054.

70. Rudow DL, Brown RS Jr. Role of the independent donor advocacy team in ethical decision making. Prog Transplant 2005;15:298–302.

71. Matas AJ, Bartlett ST, Leichtman AB, Delmonico FL: Morbidity and mortality after living kidney donation, 1999–2001: Survey of United States transplant centers. Am J Transplant 2003;3:830–834.

72. Tooher RL, Rao MM, Scott DF, et al: A systematic review of laparoscopic live-donor nephrectomy. Transplantation 2004;78:404–414.

73. Sharing UNOS. Available at www.unos.org. Accessed May 11, 2007.

74. Ellison MD, McBride MA, Taranto SE, et al: Living kidney donors in need of kidney transplants: A report from the Organ Procurement and Transplantation Network. Transplantation 2002;74:1349–1351.

75. Gracida C, Espinoza R, Cancino J: Can a living kidney donor become a kidney transplant recipient? Transplant Proc 2004;36:1630–1631.

76. Fehrman-Ekholm I, Norden G, Lennerling A, et al: Incidence of end-stage renal disease among live kidney donors. Transplantation 2006;82:1646–1648.

77. Rule AD, Gussak HM, Pond GR, et al: Measured and estimated GFR in healthy potential kidney donors. Am J Kidney Dis 2004;43:112–119.

78. Fehrman-Ekholm I, Skeppholm L: Renal function in the elderly (>70 years old) measured by means of iohexol clearance, serum creatinine, serum urea and estimated clearance. Scand J Urol Nephrol 2004;38:73–77.

79. Garg AX, Muirhead N, Knoll G, et al: Proteinuria and reduced kidney function in living kidney donors: A systematic review, meta-analysis and meta-regression. Kidney Int 2006;70:1801–1810.

80. Textor SC, Taler SJ, Larson TS, et al: Blood pressure evaluation among older living kidney donors. J Am Soc Nephrol 2003;14:2159–2167.

81. Ozdemir N, Guz G, Muderrisoglu H, et al: Ambulatory blood pressure monitoring in potential renal transplant donors. Transplant Proc 1999;31:3369–3370.

82. Textor SC, Taler SJ, Driscoll N, et al: Blood pressure and renal function after kidney donation from hypertensive living donors. Transplantation 2004;78:276–282.

83. Boudville N, Prasad GV, Knoll G, et al: Meta-analysis: Risk for hypertension in living kidney donors. Ann Intern Med 2006;145:185–196.

84. Laber DA:. Risk factors, classification, and staging of renal cell cancer. Med Oncol 2006;23:443–454.

85. Hsu C, McCulloch CE, Iribarren C, et al: Body mass index and risk for end-stage renal disease. Ann Intern Med 2006;144:21–28.

86. Praga M, Hernandez E, Herrero JC, et al: Influence of obesity on the appearance of proteinuria and renal insufficiency after unilateral nephrectomy. Kidney Int 2000;58:2111–2118.

87. Heimbach JK, Taler SJ, Prieto M, et al: Obesity in living kidney donors: Clinical characteristics and outcomes in the era of laparoscopic donor nephrectomy. Am J Transplant 2005;5:1057–1064.

88. Thiel GT, Nolte C, Tsinalis D: Living kidney donors with isolated medical abnormalities: The SOL-DHR experience. In Gaston RS, Wadstrom J (eds): Living Donor Kidney Transplantation. London: Taylor & Francis, 2005, pp 55–73.

89. Abdul-Ghani MA, Williams K, DeFronzo RA, Stern M: What is the best predictor of future type 2 diabetes? Diabetes Care 2007;30:1544–1548.

90. Wilson PW, Meigs JB, Sullivan L, et al: Prediction of incident diabetes mellitus in middle aged adults: The Framingham Offspring Study. Arch Intern Med 2007;167:1068–1074.

91. Norberg M, Eriksson JW, Lindahl B, et al: A combination of HbA1c, fasting glucose and BMI is effective in screening for individuals at risk of future type 2 diabetes: OGTT is not needed. J Intern Med 2006;260:263–271.

92. Worcester E, Parks JH, Evan AP, Coe FL:. Renal function in patients with nephrolithiasis. J Urol 2006;176:600–603.

93. Worcester E, Parks JH, Josephson MA, et al: Causes and consequences of kidney loss in patients with nephrolithiasis. Kidney Int 2003;64:2204–2213.

94. Birkeland SA, Storm HH: Risk for tumor and other disease transmission by transplantation: A population-based study of unrecognized malignancies and other diseases in organ donors. Transplantation 2002;74:1409–1413.

95. Kennecke HF, Olivotto IA, Speers C, et al: Late risk of relapse and mortality among postmenopausal women with estrogen responsive early breast cancer after 5 years of tamoxifen. Ann Oncol 2007;18:45–51.

96. Eckman MH, Erban JK, Singh SK, Kao GS: Screening for the risk for bleeding or thrombosis. Ann Intern Med 2003;138:W15–W24.

97. Ardern DW, Atkinson DR, Fenton AJ: Peri-operative use of oestrogen medications and deep vein thrombosis—a national survey. N Z Med J 2002;115:U26.

98. Grady D, Wenger NK, Herrington D, et al: Postmenopausal hormone therapy increases risk for venous thromboembolic disease. The Heart and Estrogen/Progestin Replacement Study. Ann Intern Med 2000;132:689–696.

99. Andreoni KA, Weeks SM, Gerber DA, et al: Incidence of donor renal fibromuscular dysplasia: Does it justify routine angiography? Transplantation 2002;73:1112–1116.

100. Neymark E, LaBerge JM, Hirose R, et al: Arteriographic detection of renovascular disease in potential renal donors: Incidence and effect on donor surgery. Radiology 2000;214:755–760.

101. Indudhara R, Kenney PJ, Bueschen AJ, Burns JR: Live donor nephrectomy in patients with fibromuscular dysplasia of the renal arteries. J Urol 1999;162:678–681.

102. Zierler RE, Bergelin RO, Davidson RC, et al: A prospective study of disease progression in patients with atherosclerotic renal artery stenosis. Am J Hypertens 1996;9:1055–1061.

103. Iseki K, Ikemiya Y, Iseki C, Takishita S: Proteinuria and the risk of developing end-stage renal disease. Kidney Int 2003;63:1468–1474.

104. Tonna S, Wang YY, MacGregor D, et al: The risks of thin basement membrane nephropathy. Semin Nephrol 2005;25:171–175.

105. Dische FE, Weston MJ, Parsons V: Abnormally thin glomerular basement membranes associated with hematuria, proteinuria or renal failure in adults. Am J Nephrol 1985;5:103–109.

106. Nieuwhof CM, de Heer F, de Leeuw P, van Breda Vriesman PJ: Thin GBM nephropathy: Premature glomerular obsolescence is associated with hypertension and late onset renal failure. Kidney Int 1997;51:1596–1601.

107. Liapis H, Gokden N, Hmiel P, Miner JH: Histopathology, ultrastructure, and clinical phenotypes in thin glomerular basement membrane disease variants. Hum Pathol 2002;33:836–845.

108. Lai KN, Chan LY, Leung JC: Mechanisms of tubulointerstitial injury in IgA nephropathy. Kidney Int Suppl 2005:S110–S115.

109. Koushik R, Garvey C, Manivel JC, et al: Persistent, asymptomatic, microscopic hematuria in prospective kidney donors. Transplantation 2005;80:1425–1429.

110. Nicolau C, Torra R, Badenas C, et al: Autosomal dominant polycystic kidney disease type 1 and 2: Assessment of US sensitivity for diagnosis. Radiology 1999;213:273–276.

111. Garcia-Gonzalez MA, Jones JG, Allen SK, et al: Evaluating the clinical utility of a molecular genetic test for polycystic kidney disease. Mol Genet Metab 2007;92:160–167.

112. Rossetti S, Consugar MB, Chapman AB, et al: Comprehensive molecular diagnostics in autosomal dominant polycystic kidney disease. J Am Soc Nephrol 2007;18:2143–2160.

113. O'Neill WC, Robbin ML, Bae KT, et al: Sonographic assessment of the severity and progression of autosomal dominant polycystic kidney disease: The Consortium of Renal Imaging Studies in Polycystic Kidney Disease (CRISP). Am J Kidney Dis 2005;46:1058–1064.

114. Fox CS, Larson MG, Vasan RS, et al: Cross-sectional association of kidney function with valvular and annular calcification: The Framingham heart study. J Am Soc Nephrol 2006;17:521–527.

115. Krishna J, Shah ZA, Merchant M, et al: Urinary protein expression patterns in children with sleep-disordered breathing: Preliminary findings. Sleep Med 2006;7:221–227.

116. Lawrence VA, Cornell JE, Smetana GW: Strategies to reduce postoperative pulmonary complications after noncardiothoracic surgery: Systematic review for the American College of Physicians. Ann Intern Med 2006;144:596–608.

117. Johnson EM, Anderson JK, Jacobs C, et al: Long-term follow-up of living kidney donors: Quality of life after donation. Transplantation 1999;67:717–721.

118. McCune TR, Armata T, Mendez-Picon G, et al: The living organ donor network: A model registry for living donors. Clin Transpl 2004;18(Suppl 12):33–38.

Further Reading

Barai S, Gambhir S, Prasad N, et al: Levels of GFR and protein-induced hyperfiltration in kidney donors: A single-center experience in India. Am J Kidney Dis 2008;51:407–414.

Giessing M, Fuller F, Tuellmann M, et al: Attitude to nephrolithiasis in the potential living kidney donor: A survey of the German kidney transplant centers and review of the literature. Clin Transplant 2008 Mar 3 [epub ahead of print].

Sung RS, Galloway J, Tuttle-Newhall JE, et al: Organ donation and utilization in the United States, 1997–2006. Am J Transplant 2008;8(4 Pt 2):922–934.

Wright AD, Will TA, Holt DR, et al: Laparoscopic living donor nephrectomy: A look at current trends and practice patterns at major transplant centers across the United States. J Urol 2008; 179:1488–1492.

Chapter 86

Technical Aspects of Renal Transplantation and Surgical Complications

Susan M. Lerner and Jonathan Bromberg

Renal transplantation is regarded by most physicians as the preferred treatment for chronic renal failure.[1] According to the United Network for Organ Sharing, the 1-year graft survival rate for the 15,657 renal allografts (living and cadaveric donor) placed into adult recipients during 2003 to 2004 in the United States was 90%. The recipient mortality in the first year was less than 5%.[2] Rejection and the donor shortage are the major obstacles to the routine application of renal transplantation. As the proportion of grafts lost to rejection decreases and the value of each donor graft increases, the importance of technical perfection is magnified. Surgical skills are best exercised in the context of judicious intra- and perioperative decision making based on a thorough understanding of medicine and biology. It is equally important to evaluate and treat complications as quickly and judiciously as possible to prevent graft loss.

RECIPIENT EVALUATION

- The renal graft is usually transplanted heterotopically in the extraperitoneal iliac fossa of the pelvis. In most cases, the native kidneys are left intact. From the narrow yet important perspective of technical issues, the evaluation of the renal transplant candidate raises several questions:
- Is the domain of either iliac fossa or pelvis adequate?
- Will arterial inflow and venous outflow be sufficient?
- What is the condition of the urine-collecting system and bladder?

Most often, a careful medical history and physical examination of the candidate will provide the answers to these questions and no further anatomical studies are necessary. Examination of the abdomen may reveal surgical scars, masses, organomegaly, or abdominal wall defects that dictate the site of transplantation. In the patient with polycystic kidney disease, physical examination may reveal a large native kidney encroaching on the iliac fossa. Palpation of weak or absent femoral pulses betrays serious vascular disease that may contraindicate renal transplantation or at the very least require further investigation. Previous surgical records should be reviewed to understand any prior vascular reconstruction. If there is any doubt as to the availability of an appropriate vascular site for anastomosis, then additional studies should be obtained (e.g., magnetic resonance angiography, computed tomography angiography, arteriography). If a patient has had multiple previous transplants, then surgical records and imaging studies should be obtained to better understand the anatomy.

Routine cystoscopy or cystography is not indicated. These studies may be of value when there is a history of voiding problems, urinary reflux, recurrent infection, or previous urologic procedures. A cystogram in a patient who has been anuric or oliguric for several years while on dialysis may demonstrate a small-capacity, noncompliant bladder. In the instance of an unsatisfactory urinary reservoir, an ileal loop or bladder augmentation may be needed before transplantation.

Bilateral native nephrectomy is seldom necessary, but indications include symptomatic polycystic kidney disease (e.g., cyst rupture, bleeding), massive vesicoureteral reflux, heavy proteinuria, persistent upper tract infection, severe renovascular hypertension, symptomatic stone disease, and renal cell carcinoma.

DONOR CRITERIA AND PROCUREMENT

Brain death standards for cadaver donors are stringent. There are accepted general donor criteria such as no extracranial malignancy or human immunodeficiency virus infection. However, given the severe donor organ shortage, general criteria are expanding. Currently the United Network for Organ Sharing national waiting list exceeds 103,000 candidates, of whom more than 75,000 are awaiting kidney transplants.[3] The increasing disparity between organ supply and demand challenges the transplantation community to maximize the use of organs from all consented donors. This includes the use of kidneys from older donors, donors with serologies positive for hepatitis C or hepatitis B core antibody, and donors with a history of diabetes and hypertension. United Network for Organ Sharing defined a specific group of these donors, known as extended criteria donors, as all deceased donors older than 60 years of age and deceased donors between the ages of 50 and 59 with any two of the following criteria: history of hypertension, cerebrovascular cause of brain death, or terminal serum creatinine level greater than 1.5 mg/dL.[4] Concerns about the need to assess these kidneys before transplantation have led to initiatives to use ex vivo biopsies and machine-preservation technology. Microscopic analysis is used to determine tubular, interstitial, and vascular changes.

There are other donor kidneys that can be included in this category of extended criteria donors that do not fit the United Network for Organ Sharing definition, but with judicious selection can be transplanted. This includes small pediatric donors (<15 kg) whose renal mass may be considered insufficient—considered extended criteria grafts. The controversy about how to use these grafts centers on whether to transplant them as an en bloc transplant or as single grafts. Using 6-cm length and donor weight of more than 14 kg as basic variables for the ability to split the graft seems to improve the results of these donor grafts.[5] Another large group of donors are non–heart beating organs that are procured as a result of donation after cardiac death. These donors are usually individuals with devastating irreversible neurological injuries who do not meet formal brain death criteria. Despite ethical controversies surrounding this type of organ donation, the contribution of organs from donation after cardiac death has grown rapidly and the organs, when chosen appropriately, function well.[6]

Once a deceased donor kidney is recovered, there are two methods of preservation: simple cold hypothermic storage and pulsatile preservation. Pulsatile perfusion involves an ex vivo hypothermic pulsatile perfusion machine that delivers oxygen and nutrients through a specialized preservation solution to the kidney and removes waste products in an attempt to mimic circulation, thereby preserving endothelial and parenchymal integrity and reducing vasospasm. Some initial data suggest that pumping kidneys decreases the rate of delayed graft function, especially in extended criteria donors. In addition, pump parameters (i.e., flow rates and resistance) can be used in determining the appropriate use of a kidney.[7]

The length of cold ischemia time becomes a factor in organ preservation as well. A time interval up to 24 hours is generally considered to be appropriate, although there are widely differing opinions among centers, with a few centers routinely transplanting organs with 30 to 48 hours of cold time. Most literature suggests that ischemia beyond 24 hours is particularly detrimental, although the increased risk of graft failure associated with this prolonged ischemia is on average only approximately 10%, but with much higher rates of delayed graft function.[8] Kidneys obtained from elderly or extended criteria donors are particularly sensitive to effects of prolonged ischemia. Pulsatile perfusion appears to minimize or ameliorate the delayed graft function observed with longer ischemia time.

The retrieval of cadaver donor kidney grafts is usually one component of a complex multiple organ procurement. A common technique employed is in situ perfusion using iced preservation solution and en bloc removal of both kidneys based on the aorta and inferior vena cava. Multiple arteries are found in approximately 20% of donors. During procurement, care is taken to leave multiple arteries intact. In a cadaver donor, renal arteries can be centered on a Carrel patch of donor aorta to facilitate the arterial anastomosis. The hilum of the renal graft is not disturbed to avoid injuring arterial arborizations. Because the arterial blood supply to the kidney is segmental, inadvertent ligation of a polar artery, for example, creates a discrete infarct. If the vessel supplies the upper pole, a small scar of little consequence may result. Conversely, a lower pole vessel is important because it supplies the ureter. A devascularized ureter will necrose and leak or fibrose and obstruct. To ensure good vascularization of the graft ureter, the procurement surgeon leaves a "fan" of investing periureteral tissue.

With a live donor, the surgeon has the advantage of preoperative imaging of the renal vasculature. Arteriography, computed tomography angiography, or magnetic resonance angiography will identify multiple vessels or an early bifurcation of the renal artery. Gadolinium-enhanced magnetic resonance angiography is an attractive choice because it is minimally invasive, has multiplanar capability, and is able to evaluate the renal parenchyma and the vascular anatomy without using iodinated contrast media and does not expose patients to radiation.[9] If both kidneys have a single artery and vein, the left kidney is preferred because of the longer vein and technical ease of approach. A longer vein facilitates the implantation and the donor nephrectomy, particularly if the surgery is performed laparoscopically. In addition, technical considerations, including the need to retract the liver and the increased number of lumbar veins, make laparoscopic right-side nephrectomy more challenging. At one time, the right side was used as a last resort, but more recently, many groups have endeavored to better define the indications for selecting one kidney over another for donation (e.g., renal vascular abnormalities). Studies show that ischemia time is similar for both sides, and all kidneys had adequate vein length.[10] A guiding principle is that if there is a defect, the live donor is left with the more perfect kidney. In addition, laparoscopic donor nephrectomy is being extended to donors with multiple renal arteries with no difference in warm ischemia time, donor morbidity, or graft outcome.[11]

TRANSPLANTATION

General endotracheal anesthesia is induced with the patient in the supine position on the operating table.[12] A urinary balloon catheter is inserted. The bladder can be filled with antibiotic solution, which is left indwelling, or the Foley catheter can be attached to a Y-connector and irrigation system so the bladder can be filled. Intraoperative monitoring may include a central venous pressure catheter, pulse oximetry, and/or arterial blood pressure line. A curvilinear incision is made in either the right or left lower abdomen. The extraperitoneal iliac fossa is used because of the presence of the iliac vessels and its proximity to the urinary bladder. The transplant is protected by the iliac bone posterolaterally and the abdominal musculature anteriorly, yet the graft is superficial enough for percutaneous biopsy. The right side is generally preferred because the external iliac vessels are more superficial on this side. In theory, the renal graft can be transplanted anywhere that there is a suitable recipient artery, vein, and urine conduit or reservoir.

Three layers of the abdominal wall, the external oblique, internal oblique, and transversus abdominis, are divided to afford access to the iliac fossa. The inferior epigastric vessels are divided, and a long stump of the inferior epigastric artery is preserved in case its use may be necessary in a separate anastomosis to a lower pole renal artery. The spermatic cord is preserved in men, and in women, the round ligament is divided. The diaphanous peritoneal membrane is rolled medially off the external iliac vessels. Lymphatic channels that overlie the iliac vessels are divided to expose the artery and vein. These channels are ligated to prevent lymphatic leaks, lymphocele formation, and subsequent ureteral obstruction or iliac vein compression. It is common practice to anastomose the transplant artery end to side on the external iliac artery. If multiple arteries are present, they can be reconstructed in several ways. They can be syndactylized, the inferior epigastric artery can be used as mentioned earlier, or they can be sewn in on a common aortic patch. The renal vein is routinely sewn to the side of the external iliac vein. The left donor kidney is generally preferred because of its longer vein; however, a short right renal vein of a deceased donor kidney can be extended using the attached inferior vena cava.[13] In the case of multiple draining renal veins, the decision of whether to implant both veins separately, leave them on a common caval patch, or ligate the smaller of the veins must be made. Because venous drainage is not segmental, unlike arterial inflow, it is usually safe to ligate smaller veins.[14] The clamps are then removed and reperfusion begins. The time that transpires between removing the graft from ice and reperfusion with oxygenated blood is known as the warm ischemia time. This period ranges from 20 to 45 minutes. Warm ischemia time longer than 45 minutes is associated with increased incidence of delayed graft function, and longer than 60 minutes may promote primary nonfunction.

Urinary drainage from the renal graft is established by surgically connecting the graft ureter to the bladder. The ureteroneocystostomy is usually accomplished via the extravesical approach, whereby the spatulated end of the transplant ureter is sewn to the bladder, mucosa to mucosa, after incision through the detrusor muscle. The detrusor muscle is then reunited to buttress the anastomosis and create an antireflux valve (an extravesical Lich-Gregoir ureteroneocystostomy.) A double pigtail ureteral stent is sometimes placed to prevent ureteric complications. The stent is then endoscopically removed several weeks later. There are complications associated with stents as well, namely, an increase in the incidence of urinary tract infections, calcification, and stent migration. As a result, studies now support a practice of selective stenting based on the surgeon's judgment (e.g., for anastomoses that are technically difficult, a contracted bladder, or friable mucosa).[15] In addition, stent removal requires a second procedure that not only increases cost, but can also be a source of morbidity. Other techniques of ureteral drainage include tunneling of the graft ureter via cystotomy (Leadbetter-Politano), modifications of the Lich technique using a tunnel but with an extravesical approach, and sewing of the native ureter to the transplant renal pelvis (ureteropyelostomy). After meticulous hemostasis is achieved, the wound is closed in two layers. A drain can be placed if necessary. Depending on the patient's body habitus, the operation lasts for 2 to 4 hours. Postoperatively, the Foley catheter remains in place for 2 to 5 days. If the patient has difficulty voiding spontaneously and bladder urodynamics are markedly abnormal, the bladder may be used as a passive reservoir coupled with intermittent self-catheterization after transplantation.

Some variations on the standard operation deserve special mention. The first is the use of dual-kidney transplantation, where two aged adult kidneys (which were turned down as single transplants) are placed into an adult recipient, as a way to help alleviate the continued organ shortage. The two kidneys are generally implanted as separate transplants on the same side but may be implanted in opposite iliac fossae. Recipients of these transplants have been shown to have acceptable long-term graft survival.[16] It is important to reduce cold storage time when using aged kidneys for dual transplantations to reduce the incidence of delayed graft function.

Patients who have undergone more than one transplantation were once considered to be at higher risk of graft failure than first graft recipients, but retransplantation survival rates have improved substantially as a result of improved pretransplantation screening and posttransplantation management. Recipients of a third or subsequent graft constitute a unique population because of the previous manipulation of two iliac fossae for previous transplants and frequently the removal of earlier grafts. This results in surgical challenges for retransplantation, mainly in vessel and bladder dissection due to scarring from previous surgery.[17]

There are several additional considerations for pediatric recipients. In children, the relative size discrepancy between the graft and the recipient may dictate placement of the renal transplant intraperitoneally with anastomosis to the aorta and inferior vena cava.[18] In particular, children weighing less than 15 kg present a challenging subgroup. The size discrepancy can be troublesome during abdominal closure, and these small patients are at high risk of kinking and obstruction of graft vessels or abdominal compartment syndrome. Even with maximum intravascular volume, an adult kidney transplanted into an infant or small child cannot achieve more than two thirds of the blood flow present in the donor. Therefore, it is imperative to maintain optimum intravascular volume in the intraoperative and postoperative periods.[19] Bladder dysfunction can pose a great challenge in the pediatric population as well. If the pretransplantation evaluation reveals a contracted, noncompliant bladder, a urine reservoir can be established with an ileal loop or bladder augmentation with a segment of intestine. A final consideration in pediatric recipients is the high occurrence of graft loss secondary to vascular thrombosis. Increasingly, centers are now testing for thrombophilias and anticoagulation in patients perioperatively with good results.[20]

SURGICAL COMPLICATIONS

Wound Complications

Wound infection is the most common complication after renal transplantation. Contributory factors include obesity, diabetes, uremia with protein malnutrition, and immunosuppression. Typically, the characteristic findings of fever, local erythema, swelling, and drainage present 4 to 7 days after surgery. However, it is important to remember immunosuppressed patients may not manifest the same signs and symptoms, and one must have a higher level of suspicion for wound and abdominal infections.

For infection confined to the subcutaneous space, treatment consists of opening the skin to allow drainage, followed by local wound care measures such as packing until the wound heals. Antibiotics are usually warranted, and antibiotic selection depends on the culture results. If there is suspicion of a subfascial abscess, an ultrasound study or the removal of fascial sutures will demonstrate deep involvement. Drainage of clear fluid from the wound is common, especially in obese patients. Placement of a collection bag allows the determination of fluid creatinine to distinguish urine (from a urine leak) from serum (lymphatic leak or draining seroma). A seroma, a subcutaneous collection of tissue fluid, can be left alone to resolve with time or can be drained either by repeated needle aspiration or drain placement. The approach depends on the clinical circumstances. Dehiscence of the transplant wound is unusual. However, the inhibition of wound healing from the malnutrition of chronic renal failure, steroids, or sirolimus may contribute to fascial disruption. Dehiscence requires emergent reoperation and reclosure.

Vascular Thrombosis

The prevalence of thrombosis of the transplant artery or vein is 1%. Clinically, acute anuria raises the concern of graft thrombosis. Hyperacute rejection can result in thrombosis, but faulty technique is usually responsible. Technical problems include intimal dissection, especially in recipients with long-standing diabetes or hypertension; kinking of the artery or vein from malpositioning of the graft; torsion of the vessels; and narrowing of the anastomosis. Doppler ultrasonography or radionuclide scanning shows greatly decreased or no flow to the graft. If the index of suspicion for thrombosis is high, for example, an uneventful live donor graft that does not diurese postoperatively, the patient should be taken back to the operating room for immediate exploration. Arteriography is seldom of value and delays surgical exploration. At exploration, arterial thrombosis is suggested by a small, pale kidney; with venous thrombosis, the kidney transplant is blue, swollen, and sometimes bleeding from a fracture. Thrombectomy and graft salvage have been reported, but warm ischemia that lasts more than 45 to 60 minutes results in irreversible injury. When the vascular compromise is incomplete (e.g., venous kinking), the chance of salvage is improved, but a prolonged delay in graft function can be expected. Protracted warm ischemia or primary nonfunction of a graft mandates transplant nephrectomy.

It is imperative to consider risk factors for vascular thrombosis in the recipient evaluation. One must consider and test when appropriate for the presence of an inherited hypercoagulable state such as patients with previous deep vein thrombosis/pulmonary embolism, multiple vascular thromboses, spontaneous abortions, end-stage renal disease due to lupus or hemolytic uremic syndrome. Interventions to decrease the thrombotic risk including heparin, warfarin, and aspirin have been evaluated and appear to decrease the risk of renal allograft thrombosis significantly.[21]

Bleeding

Characteristically, "surgical" bleeding, requiring a return to the operating room, presents in the early postoperative period with tachycardia, hypotension, and, after volume resuscitation, decreasing hematocrit. Bleeding is more likely in renal transplant recipients than in normal patients because of decreased platelet adhesiveness secondary to uremia. Some surgeons fully heparinize renal transplant recipients, and this practice may contribute to bleeding. A decreasing hematocrit in the early postoperative period should not be ascribed to "medical" causes. Correction of clinically significant bleeding is amenable only to re-exploration. A bleed at the vascular anastomosis or a vessel in the graft hilum is often the culprit. Mild hematuria that resolves without intervention is not uncommon.

Urine Leak

The prevalence of urine leak is approximately 2%. A large urine leak at the ureter-to-bladder anastomosis due to a technical flaw results in a rapid decrease in urine output in the early postoperative period. Ureteral necrosis and leak may be due to procurement errors (e.g., degloving) or ischemia from rejection-induced vasculitis and thrombosis of periureteral blood supply. Labial or scrotal edema may occur. Clear fluid from the wound may be distinguished from the more common finding of a draining seroma by creatinine determination. Patients frequently complain of abdominal, pelvic, or rectal discomfort or pain from the inflammation of extravasated urine. A urine leak can be confirmed by a radionuclide scan showing extravasation of "hot" tracer outside the confines of the collecting system.[22] If ultrasonography demonstrates a fluid collection, the collection is tapped and the fluid analyzed for creatinine to make the diagnosis of urinoma. Emergent exploration is the treatment of choice for a urine leak. Treatment of a leak with interventional radiologic techniques such as percutaneous nephrostomy and drain placement is successful only for small leaks at the ureteroneocystostomy. Although these techniques are helpful for diagnosis or as a temporizing measure in patients who are unfit for surgery (e.g., untreated urinary infection), the definitive solution is surgery. Reconstruction of the ureter may involve reimplantation after cutting back to well-vascularized tissue. If the transplant ureter is too short to reach the bladder, the bladder may be extensively mobilized and fixed superiorly to the psoas muscle, a psoas "hitch"; the distal native ureter may be sewn to the transplant pelvis, or a tube can be fashioned from the bladder wall (Boari flap) to bridge the gap. After reconstruction, both a ureteral stent and a drain are placed to allow egress of urine until the urinary mucosa heals watertight. The drain is removed when output ceases, and the stent is cystoscopically removed at approximately 4 to 6 weeks.

Obstruction of the Collecting System

Obstruction occurs in approximately 2% of renal transplants. Blockage of urine flow in the early postoperative period may be the result of technical misadventure in the construction of the ureteroneocystostomy, such as a too-tight antireflux tunnel, or a problem with the graft ureter, such as a twist, entrapment by the spermatic cord, or an extrinsic compression by a hematoma or urinoma. Weeks to months after transplantation, ultrasonographic investigation of an elevated serum creatinine value may reveal a dilated urine collecting system due to ureteral stricture, stone disease (either de novo, retained, or of donor origin), fungus balls, shed tissue from papillary necrosis, or lymphocele. After percutaneous needle biopsy, hemorrhage can fill the pelvis with clot, but the thrombolytic effect of urokinase in urine makes obstruction of the collecting system unusual. Ischemia and acute rejection of the ureter are the most frequent causes of ureteral stricture in adults; however, ureteritis and subsequent ureteral strictures can also be the result of a viral infection. Cytomegalovirus and human polyoma BK virus have both been implicated in the development of stricture formation.

When a dilated transplant ureter with mild to moderate hydronephrosis is seen, the urodynamic significance of the findings may be uncertain. If renal transplant function is only mildly impaired, a furosemide washout radionuclide study may be helpful. An antegrade pyelogram provides the best image and can be converted to a percutaneous nephrostomy to decompress an obstructed system. If there is a clinically significant obstruction, there will be a postobstructive diuresis and decrease in the serum creatinine. In equivocal cases, a Whitaker test or manometric study of urodynamics can be performed by saline infusion through the percutaneous nephrostomy. If there is obstruction, the pressure in the manometer will increase steadily as saline is infused. If ultrasonography reveals the collecting system to be massively dilated, the patient should be scheduled for definitive decompression. Decompression can be accomplished by percutaneous, endourologic, open surgical approaches, or a combination of modalities. Percutaneous decompression with percutaneous nephrostomy is often the first step in relieving obstruction and further defining anatomy and cause for a more definitive and durable repair. Endourologic management of transplant ureteral stenoses with balloon dilatation or Acucise endoureterotomy are used. After either procedure, indwelling stents are left in place and removed cystoscopically at 6 to 8 weeks. These methods, if successful, can avoid the morbidity of open revision.[23] However, disruption of the ureter and recurrent strictures can occur with both methods. Furthermore, stenting introduces a foreign body that may be a nidus for encrustation, stone formation, or infection. Often the best approach is surgical correction. This is usually carried out either by graft ureteral reimplantation into the bladder or by rerouting of urine from the transplant into the native ureter by ureteroureterostomy or pyeloureterostomy. In constructing either bypass, the native kidney does not have to be removed; rather, the proximal native ureter is ligated and residual function is shut down by the resultant hydrostasis.[24]

Vesicoureteral Reflux

Voiding cystography in transplant recipient demonstrates a reflux rate of 2% to 6%. Whether urine reflux per se damages a renal transplant is debatable; what is not debatable is the deleterious effect of reflux when infection is present. Antibiotic suppression of urinary tract infection will decrease the incidence of graft pyelonephritis, but if infections recur, a revision of the ureteroneocystostomy or conversion to transplant-to-native ureteroureterostomy is indicated to eliminate reflux. A newer approach is the endoscopic correction of vesicoureteral reflux with subureteral injections of Deflux (dextranomer microspheres in sodium hyaluronic acid solution.) This substance is biodegradable and has no immunogenic properties and no potential to cause malignant transformation. Most of the available data are in nontransplant pediatric patients with reflux, but show a 69% success rate for endoscopic treatment versus a 38% success rate for antibiotic prophylaxis after 1 year of treatment. Although open surgery achieves a success rate of 92% to 98%, it is an invasive procedure and is not free of complications, especially in transplant recipients. An important advantage of endoscopic treatment is its easy repeatability in cases of failure after the first injection.[25]

Lymphocele

Transected lymphatic channels that course over the iliac vessels may leak lymph and develop into a lymphocele, a cystlike collection of lymph that may impinge on the graft ureter. The standard treatment for lymphocele is surgical fenestration of the peritoneum. A window is created in the lymphocele wall via the laparoscope or open surgery to allow lymph to drain into the peritoneal cavity, where it is absorbed. A lymphocele can also be treated by sclerosis with iodine or caustic antibiotic preparation (e.g., tetracycline) to obliterate the cavity.

Transplant Renal Artery Stenosis

Typically, transplant renal artery stenosis (TRAS) usually occurs months after transplant surgery. The prevalence of this disorder has varied in the literature, ranging from 1% to 23%. This discrepancy has been ascribed to several factors: The definition of hemodynamically significant TRAS has not been standardized, and the ready availability of noninvasive screening modalities, such as color Doppler ultrasonography and magnetic resonance angiography, may lead to increased pursuit of this diagnosis.[26] The diagnosis is suggested by hypertension that is intractable to an escalating regimen of antihypertensive drugs. On physical examination, a bruit may be heard over the transplant, but this finding is nonspecific. The cause of TRAS is multifactorial and includes surgical technique during organ removal and transplantation, acute rejection, delayed graft function, and cytomegalovirus infection.[27] TRAS often has an insidious onset. Angiography is the gold standard in diagnosis, and if TRAS is present, percutaneous transluminal angioplasty can be carried out concurrently. The treatment of TRAS with both surgical and endovascular techniques has been evaluated in multiple studies. Surgical correction has a 66% to 90% initial success rate with a 12% recurrence rate. The reported success rate with percutaneous transluminal angioplasty is lower, but has improved in more recent studies, with a similar recurrence rate. Percutaneous transluminal angioplasty is favored as the first-line treatment because of the technical demand of an open repair with the risks of allograft loss, ureteral injury, and surgical mortality.[26] TRAS is associated with a significant decrease in long-term allograft survival, but it is still unclear as to whether this is due to the stenosis, the repair, or the factors that predisposed to the condition.[27] TRAS can be mimicked by stenosis of the proximal iliac artery ipsilateral to the renal transplant or an arteriovenous fistula after a needle biopsy.[28,29]

MISCELLANEOUS COMPLICATIONS

Leg edema ipsilateral to the graft is common owing to ligation of lymphatics and/or compression of the external iliac vein by the graft. The diagnosis of deep venous thrombosis may be entertained, and a Doppler study or venography may be indicated. Neurapraxia of the femoral nerve is rare and may result from retractor trauma or ischemia. Patients with preexisting diabetic neuropathy are particularly susceptible. Femoral nerve injury is manifested by the inability of the supine patient to lift the leg off the bed. Restoration of function, assisted by physical therapy, takes several weeks.

References

1. Suthanthiran M, Strom TB: Renal transplantation. N Engl J Med 1994;331:365–376.
2. 2004 Annual Report of the U.S. Scientific Registry for Transplant Recipients and the Organ Procurement and Transplantation Network: Transplant Data: 1994–2003 U.S. Department of Health and Human Services, Health Resources and Services Administration, Office of Special Programs, Division of Transplantation, Rockville, MD. Richmond, VA: United Network for Organ Sharing, 2004.
3. United Network for Organ Sharing: National data. Available at: www.unos.org/data. Accessed May 13, 2007.
4. United Network for Organ Sharing: UNOS Policy 3.5.1. Expanded Criteria Donor Definition and Point System. Richmond, VA: United Network for Organ Sharing, 2002.
5. Morgan C, Martin A, Shapiro R, et al: Outcomes after transplantation of deceased-donor kidneys with rising serum creatinine. Am J Transplant 2007;7:1288–1292.
6. Keitel E, Fasolo LR, D'Avila AR, et al: Results of en bloc renal transplants of pediatric deceased donors into adult recipients. Transplant Proc 2007;39:441–442.
7. Cooper JT, Chin LT, Krieger NR, et al: Donation after cardiac death: The University of Wisconsin experience with renal transplantation. Am J Transplant 2004;4:1490–1494.
8. Stratta RJ, Moore PS, Farney AC, et al: Influence of pulsatile perfusion preservation on outcomes in kidney transplantation from expanded criteria donors. J Am Coll Surg 2007;204:873–882.
9. Opelz G, Döhler B: Multicenter analysis of kidney preservation. Transplantation 2007;83:247–253.
10. Lee CM, Carter JT, Randall HB, et al: The effect of age and prolonged cold ischemia times on the national allocation of cadaveric renal allografts. J Surg Res 2000;91:83–88.
11. Kim J, Kim C, Jang M, et al: Can magnetic resonance angiogram be a reliable alternative for donor evaluation for laparoscopic nephrectomy? Clin Transpl 2007;21:126–135.
12. Kieran K, Roberts WW: Laparoscopic donor nephrectomy: An update. Curr Opin Nephrol Hypertens 2005;14:599–603.
13. Desai MR, Ganpule AP, Gupta R, et al: Outcome of renal transplantation with multiple versus single renal arteries after laparoscopic live donor nephrectomy: A comparative study. Urology 2007;69:824–827.
14. Dafoe DC, Alfrey EJ: Urologic aspects of renal transplantation. In Hanno PM, Wein AJ (eds): Clinical Manual of Urology, 2nd ed. New York: McGraw-Hill, 1994.
15. Barry J: Renal transplant-recipient surgery. BJU Int 2007;99:701–717.
16. Gerstenkorn C, Papalois VE, Thomusch O, et al: Surgical management of multiple donor veins in renal transplantation. Int Surg 2006;91:345–347.
17. Dominguez J, Clase C, Mahalati K, et al: Is routine ureteric stenting needed in kidney transplantation? A randomized trial. Transplantation 2000;4:597–601.
18. Alfrey EJ, Boissey AR, Lerner SM: Dual-kidney transplants: Long-term results. Transplantation 2003;75:1232–1236.
19. Loupy A, Anglicheau D, Timsit MO, et al: Impact of surgical procedures and complications on outcomes of third and subsequent kidney transplants. Transplantation 2007;83:385–391.
20. Tejani AH, Fine RN (eds): Pediatric Renal Transplantation. New York: Wiley-Liss, 1994.
21. Mickelson JJ, MacNeily AE, Leblanc J, et al: Renal transplantation in children 15 kg or less: The British Columbia Children's Hospital Experience. J Urol 2006;176:1797–1800.
22. Dick AA, Lerner SM, Boissy AR, et al: Excellent outcome in infants and small children with thrombophilias undergoing kidney transplantation. Pediatr Transplant 2004;9:39–42.
23. Irish A: Hypercoagulability in renal transplant recipients. Identifying patients at risk of renal allograft thrombosis and evaluating strategies for prevention. Am J Cardiovasc Drugs 2004;4:139–149.
24. Becker JA, Choyke PL, Hill M, et al: Imaging the transplanted kidney. In Pollack HM (ed): Clinical Urography. Philadelphia: WB Saunders, 1990.
25. Bhayani SB, Landman J, Slotoroff C, Figenshau RS: Transplant ureter stricture: Acucise endoureterotomy and balloon dilation are effective. J Endourol 2003;17:19–22.
26. Salomon L, Saporta F, Amsellem D, et al: Results of pyeloureterostomy after ureterovesical anastomosis complications in renal transplantation. Urology 1999;53:908–912.
27. Puri P, Pirker M, Mohanan N, et al: Subureteral dextranomer/hyaluronic acid injection as first line treatment in the management of high grade vesicoureteral reflux. J Urol 2006;176:1856–1860.
28. Patel NH, Jindal RM, Wilkin T, et al: Renal arterial stenosis in renal allografts: Retrospective study of predisposing factors and outcome after percutaneous transluminal angioplasty. Radiology 2001;219:663–667.
29. Audard V, Matignon M, Hemery F, et al: Risk factors and long-term outcome of transplant renal artery stenosis in adult recipients after treatment by percutaneous transluminal angioplasty. Am J Transplant 2006;6:95–99.

Further Reading

Kieran K, Roberts WW: Laparoscopic donor nephrectomy: An update. Curr Opin Nephrol Hypertens 2005;14:599–603.

Barry, J: Renal transplant-recipient surgery. BJU Int 2007;99, 701–717.

Opelz G, Döhler B: Multicenter analysis of kidney preservation. Transplantation 2007;83:247–253.

Suthanthiran M, Strom TB: Renal transplantation. N Engl J Med 1994;331:365–376.

Chapter 87

Transplant Immunology and Immunosuppression

Bernd Schröppel and Enver Akalin

CHAPTER CONTENTS

Understanding the basis of transplant immunology is required to comprehend the role of the tissue typing laboratory in managing potential transplant recipients, to understand the mechanisms of immunosuppression, and to be able to appropriately detect and diagnose acute or chronic rejection. The chapter begins with a general overview of the immune response, focusing on those aspects that are important to understand the logic behind the clinical use of immunosuppressive drugs. We then outline clinically relevant characteristics of individual immunosuppressive agents currently used, as well as new immunosuppressive medications, focusing on mechanisms of action, interactions, and toxicities of individual medications. We then provide a rationale for the current immunosuppressive protocols and summarize relevant clinical trials.

BASIC TRANSPLANT IMMUNOLOGY

Components of the Immune System

The human immune system can respond to a nearly infinite range of foreign antigens by generating and maintaining immune responses that are rapid, antigen specific, and protective. The cardinal features of the adaptive system are specificity to antigenic diversity, memory, and tolerance of self.[1,2] The adaptive immune system is composed of cellular (T cells) and humoral (B cells/antibodies) components. T cells are derived from the thymus and play a central role in cellular immunity. They can be divided into subsets of CD4 and CD8 T cells and can recognize antigens presented by the major histocompatibility complex (also called HLA), through T-cell receptors

(TCRs) expressed on their cell surface. B cells express a highly specialized form of antigen receptors, surface immunoglobulins, and are the precursors of plasma cells, which can secrete a soluble form of immunoglobulin, the antibody. In addition to the adaptive system, the mammalian immune system consists of innate components. There are important interactions between the two systems. Innate immunity is composed of a series of nonpolymorphic proteins (e.g., defensins, cytokines, Toll-like receptors, and complement) and cells (e.g., macrophages, dendritic cells, natural killer cells, and neutrophils).

Recognition of Alloantigen

The highly polymorphic HLA loci are the primary targets of the alloimmune response.[3,4] Class I HLA molecules (HLA A, B, and C) are expressed on essentially all somatic cells and are recognized by CD8 T cells. Class II HLA molecules (HLA DR, DP, and DQ) are recognized by CD4 T cells and are found predominantly on a few specialized cell types, including macrophages, dendritic cells, and B cells, which are called professional antigen-presenting cells (APCs).

Humoral Alloimmunity

Alloantibodies are produced by alloreactive B cells specific for HLA molecules and participate in transplant injury. Alloreactive B cells recognize allogenic HLA molecules through surface-bound IgM receptors but require second costimulatory signals (e.g., CD40/CD154) for full activation and differentiation into antibody-secreting plasma cells.[1,2] Donor-specific anti-HLA antibodies (DSAs) can be present in a patient before transplantation due to sensitization through a previously failed allograft, blood transfusion, or pregnancy. In rare circumstances, they may have developed a cross-reactive antibody because of underlying autoimmune disease or an environmental agent mimicking the structure of an HLA molecule. The presence of pretransplant DSAs can predispose kidney transplant recipients to hyperacute rejection of the allograft as well as acute or chronic antibody-mediated rejection. Blood group antigens are other targets for the antidonor humoral immune response. Natural antibodies against these antigens cause complement-mediated hyperacute rejection, generally precluding transplant across ABO differences, but transplantation can be performed in infants, before natural development of the antibodies or after desensitization protocols, which is discussed in the section "Immunosuppression and Sensitization."[5]

Cellular Alloimmunity

Initial recognition of alloantigen predominantly occurs in secondary lymphoid organs as recipient T cells interact with antigens derived from the donor. The primed T cells then migrate back to the allograft where they re-encounter antigen and mediate their effector functions.[6] Alloreactive T cells recognize major histocompatibility complex–peptide complexes via two distinct pathways: the direct and the indirect allorecognition pathways.[7] Direct refers to recipient T cells recognizing donor major histocompatibility complex on donor APCs, and indirect presentation refers to the recognition of the donor alloantigen presented within the groove of recipient major histocompatibility complex on recipient APCs. As donor APCs migrate out of the allograft over time and are replaced by infiltrating recipient APCs, indirect

recognition may be the dominant effector pathway within the allograft.[8] Successful initiation of an adaptive immune response depends on two major signals being delivered to the T cell: (1) antigen-specific recognition via the TCR and (2) a costimulatory signal. The costimulatory signal results from the interaction of a receptor-ligand pair (one on the T cell and the other on the APC) that, in conjunction with TCR ligation, induces T-cell activation, proliferation, and differentiation. Without costimulation, T cells may undergo apoptosis (deletion) or become unresponsive to future encounters with the antigen (anergy). The best characterized costimulatory pathways involve the T cell membrane–bound molecules CD154 (CD40L) and CD28 and their APC-expressed cognate ligands CD40 and CD80/CD86 (B7.1/B7.2).[9,10] A high-affinity variant of cytotoxic T lymphocyte (CTL) A4 immunoglobulin (blocks the CD28 and CD80/CD86 interaction), named LEA29Y (belatacept), is in clinical trials (see "New Immunosuppressive Medications").[11] If a T cell receives a signal through both the TCR and the second costimulatory signal(s), then a number of intracellular activation steps ensue. A calcium flux activates the intracellular molecule calmodulin and allows it to bind to a calcium-binding protein called calcineurin (the target of cyclosporine and tacrolimus). This activates a phosphatase followed by a number of downstream reactions that lead to binding of the transcription activating factor nuclear factor of activated T cells to the interleukin (IL)-2 promoter. As a consequence, up-regulation of IL-2 gene expression occurs followed by synthesis and release of this potent T-cell growth factor. Full T-cell activation leads to up-regulation and expression of the high-affinity α chain of the IL-2 receptor (CD25) on the surface of the T cell (the target of anti-CD25 monoclonal antibodies). The synthesized and released IL-2 acts in an autocrine and paracrine manner and binds to the up-regulated IL-2R. Signaling through the IL-2R then initiates another (kinase-dependent) cascade mediated in part through a protein called mTOR (mammalian target of rapamycin, the therapeutic target of the drug sirolimus). This results in translation of new proteins and allows the cell to progress from the G_1 phase to the S phase of the cell cycle, resulting in proliferation. Azathioprine and mycophenolic acid (MPA) are inhibitors of DNA synthesis and thus inhibit T-cell activation at this stage.

T-cell activation induces differentiation, which can have many manifestations, as reflected by the variety of different T-cell subsets, referred to as T-helper cells (Th)1, Th2, Th17, and T regulatory 1. These phenotypes primarily refer to the pattern of cytokines produced by the activated T cells. In general, Th1 cells secrete interferon-γ and tumor necrosis factor α and Th17 cells secrete IL-17, which lead T-cell traffic to sites of inflammation, facilitate ongoing inflammation at those sites, and promote destructive T-cell immunity, whereas T regulatory 1 phenotypes secrete transforming growth factor β and IL-10 and are associated with T-cell regulation and tolerance. Although such categorizations have utility, the pattern of cytokine production does not necessarily correlate with outcome: Th2 immunity can be associated with rejection, and interferon-γ, the prototypical Th1 cytokine, is required for tolerance in mice.[12]

Effector Mechanisms

In this phase of the immune response, activated effector cells, including T cells, B cells, natural killer cells, and macrophages, migrate to the site of original antigen encounter and use a combination of mechanisms to kill and/or neutralize their targets. In the case of cellular immune responses, the primary mediators are CTLs, macrophages, and selected cytokines produced in the local microenvironment. CTLs, primarily major histocompatibility complex class I–restricted CD8 T cells, kill their targets through direct cell-cell contact by one of two means. The first method uses proteins such as perforin and granzyme B, which are contained in secretory granules of the CTL. These proteins can create pores in the membranes of the target cells and trigger a cascade that results in cell lysis. Once inside the cell, these serine proteinases proceed to cleave the precursors of caspases, activating them to cause the cell to self-destruct by apoptosis (programmed cell death). Fas ligand/Fas provides another means of destroying target cells. Fas ligand is a membrane-bound effector molecule on CD8 T cells and binds to Fas, which is expressed on the graft cells. Activation of Fas, a member of the tumor necrosis factor receptor family, induces apoptosis. In each case, CTLs are antigen specific, meaning that they only kill selected targets after recognition of the antigen and activation through its TCR. Unlike CTLs, macrophages are antigen nonspecific and can kill their target cells by phagocytosis or by soluble factors such as reactive oxygen intermediates, proteases, and tumor necrosis factor. In the case of the humoral immune response, the primary mediators are alloantibodies and complement. Antibody-induced activation of the complement cascade via the classic pathway can induce acute organ damage and intravascular thrombosis. The resultant complement by-products (i.e., C3a and C5a) also act as chemoattractants for additional inflammatory cells. C4d is one split product that is released by the complement activation cascade, and C4d staining of human kidney transplant biopsy specimens has become the primary method for assessing whether antibodies are participating in the antibody-mediated rejection process.

CLINICAL APPLICATION OF TRANSPLANT IMMUNOLOGY

Tissue-Typing Techniques

To define class I and II HLA molecules, the serological microcytotoxicity test has been the standard test for HLA typing since 1964. Currently, DNA-based tests are the method of choice due to their greater accuracy, sensitivity, and specificity. These polymerase chain reaction–based assays use oligonucleotide primers that define a unique HLA locus, allele, or group of alleles.

Detection of Anti-HLA Antibodies

Sera from prospective transplant recipients are routinely screened for the presence of HLA antibodies to determine the extent of HLA alloimmunization. The screening is performed against a panel of 30 to 60 cells, representing most antigens encountered in the general population, using a form of complement-dependent cytotoxicity (CDC) assay. Lymphocytes from a panel of donors are mixed with sera of the recipient, and complement is added to determine whether the recipient has antibodies that bind to donor cells and activate complement and the membrane attack complex leading to cell death. The results are reported as the percentage of panel cells that

are killed by reacting with the HLA antibodies in a patient's serum, thus the term PRA (panel reactive antibody). The CDC method is a nonspecific test, and positive results indicate the existence of antidonor antibodies in the recipient's sera, but depending on the nature of the cells used in the panel, it may be possible to determine the anti-HLA antibody specificity. The solid-phase assays, enzyme-linked immunosorbent assays (ELISA), or flow cytometry bead–based assays (Flow Specific Beads and FlowPRA [Luminex, Canoga Park, CA] which are purified HLA antigens coupled to microparticles) are the most specific and sensitive tests to identify anti-HLA antibodies.[13]

Crossmatch Methods

After Patel and Terasaki[14] reported in 1969 that 80% of the kidneys transplanted into crossmatch-positive patients were lost within 2 days, a CDC assay became obligatory before kidney transplantation. There are two types of CDC crossmatch that depend on the type of donor lymphocytes used (T and B cells). A positive T-cell CDC crossmatch is an absolute contraindication to kidney transplantation. Further modifications have been introduced in the crossmatch technique to increase the sensitivity, such as extending the incubation time to add wash steps to eliminate anticomplementary factors and unbound serum (Amos CDC crossmatch) or to add antihuman globulin (AHG) to detect low-titer anti-HLA antibodies (AHG CDC crossmatch), where antihuman globulin binds to antidonor antibody already bound to lymphocytes.[15] Antihuman globulin CDC assay is now the standard lymphocytotoxicity assay in most tissue-typing centers. IgG-type anti-HLA antibodies are the most detrimental immunoglobulins to the allograft. IgM type antibodies are mostly non–donor-specific antibodies and can be removed by heating or treating the serum with the reducing agent dithiothreitol. However, not all IgM antibodies are benign, and donor-specific IgM anti-HLA antibodies can be detrimental to the allograft.

The flow cytometry crossmatch (FCXM) was introduced in 1983 and detects DSAs independent of complement fixation. Patient sera are incubated with donor lymphocytes and stained with fluorescence-labeled anti-CD3 (T cell) and anti-CD19 (B cell). Flow cytometry may detect very low titers of either complement-fixing DSAs or noncomplement-fixing DSAs as well as non-HLA–related antibodies. It is a sensitive test but lacks specificity. To confirm the specificity of a positive FCXM, specific solid phase assays should be done to determine the specificity of the alloantibody. Another problem with interpreting the results of a positive FCXM on allograft outcome is that the technique does not discriminate between cytotoxic and noncytotoxic antibodies.

The clinical significance of CDC B-cell or flow cytometry T or B cell–positive crossmatches is controversial. A positive CDC or FCXM B-cell may indicate anti–class II, weak anti–class I, or anti-immunoglobulin antibodies, which are abundant on B cells. Most positive B-cell crossmatch results are due to low-affinity and low-titer IgM antibodies, which do not harm the graft, but there are some reports of poor graft outcome in recipients with positive CDC B-cell crossmatches. The main reason for the controversial outcomes in the literature is the lack of studies to confirm DSAs. A recent study using a combination of tests to demonstrate DSAs by CDC, ELISA, and flow cytometry showed that the majority of B cell–positive crossmatches were not due to DSAs. Although B cell–crossmatch positive patients with anti-HLA II antibodies had lower allograft survival, patients without DSAs have a graft survival similar to that of B-cell crossmatch–negative controls.[16] The Fc receptors on B cells bind IgG nonspecifically and may lead to a false-positive crossmatch result. Using pronase to cleave Fc receptors from B-cell surface might decrease those false-positive results.[17]

Most studies have linked T-cell FCXM positivity to increased acute humoral, cellular, or chronic rejection and decreased allograft survival. Gebel and colleagues[15] reviewed the previous studies that investigated the effect of positive FCXM results on allograft survival and reported that although 20% of primary grafts and 60% of regrafts were lost within 3 months if the FCXM was positive, those rates were only 5% and 15%, respectively, with FCXM negative results.

IMMUNOSUPPRESSIVE MEDICATIONS

The mechanisms of actions, dosing, and side effects of immunosuppressive agents used in kidney transplantation are summarized in Figure 87-1 and Table 87-1.

Induction Agents

Induction agents are polyclonal lymphocyte–depleting antibodies (Thymoglobulin), monoclonal lymphocyte–depleting antibodies (alemtuzumab), or monoclonal nondepleting antibodies to IL-2R (basiliximab and daclizumab) that are given during the early peritransplantation period to decrease the risk of delayed graft function (DGF) and acute rejection, which are major factors adversely affecting graft outcome. Induction treatments are given mostly to immunologically high-risk patients (high PRA, crossmatch positive, retransplant, African American, pediatric, combined kidney/pancreas or pancreas transplant recipients), deceased donor recipients, and patients

at higher risk of developing DGF and patients receiving early steroid withdrawal. Some centers use induction treatment in all transplant recipients other than HLA-identical pairs.

Polyclonal Lymphocyte–Depleting Antibodies

Polyclonal antibody preparations are IgG fractions isolated from serum of animals (rabbits or horses) immunized against human lymphocytes. The antigenic preparation used may be human thymocytes (thymoglobulin, lymphocyte immune globulin [Atgam]), or activated human T-cell line (ATG-Fresenius), and the antibodies are directed to a wide variety of T- and B-cell antigens, natural killer cell surface antigens, and adhesion and costimulatory molecules. These antibodies are also used for the treatment of acute rejection.

Mechanism of Action

The exact mechanism of action is not fully understood, but polyclonal lymphocyte–depleting antibodies work by binding to peripheral lymphocytes, blocking their function and targeting them for destruction. Shortly after administration, these preparations lead to lymphocyte depletion via complement-mediated lysis, removal by the reticuloendothelial system, and antibody-dependent cell-mediated cytotoxicity (ADCC).[18] In contrast to other immunosuppressive agents, polyclonal agents do not depend on T-cell activation but can eliminate preactivated noncycling memory lymphocytes, which may be critical in presensitized recipients. The more potent rabbit antithymocyte globulin Thymoglobulin has, for the most part, replaced Atgam.

Dosing and Side Effects

The usual dose of thymoglobulin is 1.5 to 2.0 mg/kg/day and 15 mg/kg/day for Atgam over 4 to 6 hours as an intravenous infusion. Thymoglobulin is recommended to be started during

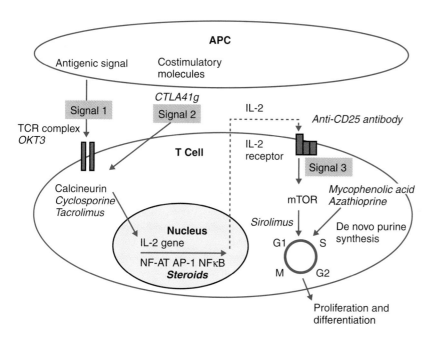

Figure 87-1 Schematic representation of the three signals for T-cell responses and the main mediators in T-cell activation. The major steps involved in T-cell activation are outlined and sites of action of some of the principal immunosuppressive medications are shown in italics. Cyclosporine and tacrolimus prevent the generation of nuclear factor of activated T cells by inhibiting the activity of calcineurin. Sirolimus binds to immunophilin and then combines with mammalian target of rapamycin (mTOR), inhibiting cell-cycle progression. Mycophenolic acid and azathioprine inhibit proliferation by restricting the supply of guanosine available for DNA synthesis. Anti-CD25 antibodies block the interaction between interleukin-2 and CD25. Cytotoxic T-lymphocyte antigen 4 (CTLA4) immunoglobulin blocks the interaction between CD28 on T cells and CD80/CD86 on antigen-presenting cells. OKT3 is directed to the CD3 T-cell receptor (TCR) complex. AP, activator protein; NFκB, nuclear factor κB.

Table 87-1   Immunosuppressive Drugs: Dose Forms, Mechanisms of Action, Adverse Effects, and Dosing Guidelines

Drug	Mechanism of Action	Adverse Effects	Dosing Guidelines
Polyclonal-Depleting Antibodies			
Thymoglobulin: 25-mg/vial Atgam: 50 mg/mL (5 mL)	Causes lymphopenia and impairs T-cell responses. Cell depleting via CDC, removal by the reticuloendothelial system, and ADCC	Fever, chills, arthralgias, serum sickness, anaphylaxis, leukopenia, thrombocytopenia, thrombophlebitis	Given as IV infusion over 4 hr for 3–5 days when used as induction agent, for 5–10 days when used to treat acute allograft rejection. Thymoglobulin 1.5–2.0 mg/kg/day and Atgam 15 mg/kg/day: doses should be titrated according to WBC and platelet counts
Monoclonal-Depleting Antibodies			
Orthoclone (OKT3): 1 mg/mL (5 mL)	Depletes cells by binding to $CD3^+$ T cells and impairs T-cell responses by modulating the TCR–CD3 complex	Cytokine release syndrome: fever, chills, pulmonary edema, hypotension, myalgias, aseptic meningitis	Given as IV infusion for 5–14 days when used as induction agent; standard dose is 5 mg/day
Alemtuzamab (Campath-H1): 30 mg/mL	Directed against the CD52 antigen, which is expressed on all blood mononuclear cells and induces ADCC, CDC, and apoptosis	Fevers, rigors, hypotension, dyspnea, and nausea related to cytokine release	Given as 1 or 2 doses on the day of transplantation and the first postoperative days. The total dose of 30–40 mg is administered as an IV infusion over 2 hours but can be also given subcutaneously
Rituximab (Rituxan): 10 mg/mL	Binds to $CD20^+$ B cells and eliminates B cells in a highly selective fashion directly by CDC, ADCC and indirectly by structural changes and apoptosis	Mainly associated with first dose reactions: hypotension, fever, tachycardia, and arthralgias	Dose depends on indication but usually given as 1 dose of 375 mg/m^2 in desensitization protocols or for treatment of antibody-mediated rejection. Once weekly for up to 4 doses in PTLD
Monoclonal Nondepleting Antibodies			
Basiliximab (Simulect): 10 mg, 20 mg/vial Daclizumab (Zenapax): 5 mg/mL	Targets CD25 of the IL-2 receptor on activated lymphocytes	Uncommon other than hypersensitivity	Basiliximab is given as two 20-mg IV doses, the first on day 0 and the second on day 4 post-transplantation. Daclizumab is given as 1 mg/kg IV infusion (day 0), then every 14 days for four doses. Protocols may vary between centers.
CIs			
Cyclosporine (Sandimmune): 25-, 50-, 100-mg tablets; 100 mg/mL oral solution Cyclosporine microemulsion (Neoral): 25-, 100-mg tablets; 100-mg/mL oral solution (Gengraft): 25-, 100-mg tablets; 100-mg/mL oral solution	Binds to cyclophilin and inhibits calcineurin, leading to impaired T-cell activation	Nephrotoxicity, hypertension, hyperlipidemia, glucose intolerance, hyperkalemia, hyperuricemia, hypomagnesemia, tremor, paresthesias, seizures, thrombotic microangiopathy, hirsutism, gingival hyperplasia, hepatotoxicity	Usually given with antimetabolite/steroid or steroid alone. Initial dose is 6–10 mg/kg/day. For first 3 mo target 12-hr trough levels are 200–350 ng/mL and 80–200 ng/mL beyond 3 mo

Table 87-1   Immunosuppressive Drugs: Dose Forms, Mechanisms of Action, Adverse Effects, and Dosing Guidelines—cont'd

Drug	Mechanism of Action	Adverse Effects	Dosing Guidelines
CIs—cont'd			
Tacrolimus (Prograf): 0.5-, 1-, 5-mg capsules	Binds FK-binding protein, thereby inhibits calcineurin, leading to impaired T-cell activation	Similar as for cyclosporine but compared with cyclosporin A has less common hirsutism, hyperlipidemia, and gingival hyperplasia; more commonly alopecia, neurotoxicity, and glucose intolerance	Initial dose is 0.15–0.3 mg/kg/day. For first 3-mo target 12-hr trough levels are 8–15 ng/mL and 5–10 ng/mL beyond 3 mo
Antimetabolites			
Azathioprine Azasan: 75, 100 mg Imuran: 50 mg	Competitive inhibitor of purine synthesis	Leukopenia, thrombocytopenia, anemia, hepatotoxicity	Oral dose is 1–2 mg/kg/day when combined with a CI and corticosteroids. Dose adjustment with low WBC count
Mycophenolate mofetil (MMF) (CellCept): 250-, 500-mg tablets, 200-mg/mL oral suspension, enteric-coated mycophenolate sodium (EC-MPS) (Myfortic): 180-, 360-mg tablets	Noncompetitive inhibitor of inosine monophosphate dehydrogenase; inhibits purine synthesis. Impairs T-cell responses and decreases B-cell activity and antibody production	Nausea, vomiting, diarrhea, dyspepsia, leukopenia, anemia	When used with tacrolimus 0.5–1.0 g bid, and 1.0–1.5 g bid with Cyclosporin A. Dose adjustment with low WBC count; 500 mg of MMF corresponds to 360 mg EC-MPS
TOR Inhibitors			
Sirolimus (Rapamune): 1-, 2-mg tablets, 1-mg/mL oral solution Everolimus (Certican): 250-, 500-, 750-, 1000-µg tablets	Sirolimus–FK binding protein complex inhibits mammalian TOR and blocks cytokine-mediated cellular proliferation at G_1 to S phase	Increased nephrotoxicity when used with CI, proteinuria, hypokalemia, hypomagnesemia, thrombotic microangiopathy, thrombocytopenia, anemia, hyperlipidemia, lymphocele, impaired wound healing, oral ulcers, interstitial pneumonitis	Used with CI or antimetabolite. For sirolimus, starting dose is 2–5 mg/day. Target trough levels 5–10 ng/mL with CI, 12–20 ng/mL with MMF, and 15–25 ng/mL if CI is withdrawn. Everolimus is given twice daily (not available in U.S.)
Corticosteroids			
Prednisone, prednisolone, methylprednisolone (Solu-Medrol)	Inhibition of genes encoding proinflammatory cytokines	Glucose intolerance, hypercholesterolemia, hypertension, impaired wound healing, skin fragility, growth retardation, osteoporosis, central obesity, suppression of pituitary-hypothalamic axis, cataracts, glaucoma, psychosis	Initiated intraoperatively at 250–1000 mg of methylprednisolone followed by an oral taper to a maintenance dose, usually 5–10 mg/day by 2–6 mo after transplantation. Pulse steroids (250–500 mg/day for 3 days) are used to treat acute rejection.

Suggested target levels depend on use of concomitantly administered drugs, immunologic risk, transplanted organs, and assay used (range based on immunoassay).

ADCC, antibody-dependent cellular cytotoxicity; CDC, complement-dependent cytotoxicity; CI, calcineurin inhibitor; IL, interleukin; PTLD, posttransplantation lymphoproliferative disease; TCR, T-cell receptor; TOR, target of rapamycin; WBC, white blood cell.

the transplantation before reperfusion due to a decreased incidence of DGF rather than administered postoperatively.[19] The duration is usually 3 to 5 days for induction treatment and 5 to 10 days for treatment of rejection. Polyclonal antibody preparations are foreign proteins and may cause a variety of ad-verse effects. Most common are fever, chills, and arthralgias. Allergic reactions can be avoided with premedication consisting of methylprednisolone, diphenhydramine, and acetaminophen. Anaphylaxis and serum sickness occur rarely. Leukopenia and thrombocytopenia are common and need dose adjustment. Patients with white blood cell counts between 2000 and 3000 or platelet counts between 50,000 and 75,000 require half-dose Thymoglobulin, and it should be held if the white blood cell count is less than 2000 or the platelet count is less than 50,000.[18]

Monoclonal Lymphocyte–Depleting Antibodies

Anti-CD3 Monoclonal Antibodies

Muromonab-CD3 (Orthoclone OKT3) was the first monoclonal antibody approved for human use by the U.S. Food and Drug Administration in 1986. A humanized anti-CD3 monoclonal antibody, hOKT3γ1(Ala-Ala) was developed to eliminate some of the toxicities of OKT3. The current use of OKT3 as an induction agent is extremely rare (<1%) in the United States. OKT3 can be used for the treatment of acute rejection.

Mechanism of Action

OKT3 is a xenogeneic murine IgG$_2$ antibody directed against the ε chain of the human CD3 complex, which is a protein linked to the TCR. Within minutes after administration, CD3$^+$ cells (T cells) disappear from the circulation, returning only after several days. This is a result of complement-mediated lysis and opsonization for clearance by phagocytic cells. OKT3 can also modulate the TCR-CD3 complex off the T-cell surface, thereby rendering T cells, even if present, incapable of antigen recognition.[18]

Dosing and Side Effects

The standard dose of OKT3 is 5 mg/day given as 7 to 14 single daily doses. Approximately 50% of patients develop anti-mouse antibodies and 20% of these have high titers (>1:1000) that may make a second course of OKT3 ineffective.[20] During an effective course, the percentage of CD3$^+$ cells decreased from 60% to less than 5% within 24 to 48 hours. The most dangerous adverse effect of OKT3 administration is a cytokine release syndrome usually seen during the first few doses and characterized by high fever, chills, headache, arthralgias, nausea, diarrhea, and pulmonary edema. These reactions are due to the binding of OKT3 to proteins in the TCR complex leading to transient T-cell activation and cytokine release.[18] The severity of these reactions may decrease by premedication with high doses of corticosteroids and antihistamines.[21] To avoid the occurrence of life-threatening pulmonary edema, it is important to ensure that the patient is euvolemic before administration. OKT3 is associated with an increased incidence of posttransplantation lymphoproliferative disorders

and opportunistic infections, most commonly cytomegalovirus infection.[22,23]

Alemtuzumab (Campath-1H)

Alemtuzumab (Campath-1H) is a monoclonal humanized rat monoclonal antibody (rat IgG2b) directed against the CD52 antigen, which is expressed on all blood mononuclear cells, including T and B lymphocytes, monocytes, macrophages, and eosinophils, as well as on the lining of the male reproductive system. It has been used to treat chronic B-cell lymphocytic leukemia since 1988, but was first used in organ transplantation in 1998. Due to its strong cytolytic activity, alemtuzumab has been mainly used in minimization of immunosuppressive protocols (rapid steroid withdrawal, calcineurin inhibitor (CI) free or reduced-dose CI).[24]

Mechanism of Action

Alemtuzumab's proposed mechanism of action includes ADCC, CDC, and induction of apoptosis.[24] It causes profound and long-lasting lymphopenia and may take months to years for the depressed lymphocyte levels to return to normal levels.

Dosing and Side Effects

The protocol usually consists of one or two doses (total dose 30–40 mg) on the day of transplantation and the first postoperative days. Alemtuzumab traditionally has been administered intravenously over 2 hours but can be also given subcutaneously.[25] In theory, alemtuzumab should leave patients seriously immunocompromised due to profound and long-lasting CD4 T-cell depletion, but surprisingly few serious infections were encountered in all studies reported. Infusion-related toxicities are common and include fevers, rigors, hypotension, dyspnea, and nausea. These reactions are related to cytokine release during administration and can be minimized by premedication regimens.

Rituximab (Rituxan)

Rituximab is a chimeric anti-CD20 (B-cell) monoclonal antibody, approved for the therapy of B-cell lymphomas including posttransplantation lymphoproliferative disorders. It has not been evaluated in a rigorous fashion in kidney transplantation but has been employed in desensitization protocols of crossmatch-positive or ABO-incompatibile kidney transplant recipients. Rituximab is also used in the treatment of acute antibody-mediated rejection.[26]

Mechanism of Action

Rituximab eliminates B cells in a highly selective fashion via multiple mechanisms: directly by CDC and ADCC and indirectly by structural changes and apoptosis. B-cell recovery takes 6 to 12 months after the completion of the treatment.

Dosing and Side Effects

Rituximab has been used in kidney transplant recipients during desensitization protocols or for the treatment of acute antibody-mediated rejection as a single dose (325 mg/m^2) and infused over 6 hours. For the treatment of posttransplantation lymphoproliferative disorders, it is given the same dose but for four consecutive weeks. The reactions include transient hypotension that responds to intravenous fluids, low-grade fever, mild tachycardia, and arthralgias.[27] Persistent hypogammaglobulinemia has been shown in patients with autoimmune hemolytic anemia and bone marrow transplant recipients.

Monoclonal Nondepleting Antibodies (Anti-CD25)

The humanized antibody daclizumab (Zenapax) and the chimeric antibody basiliximab (Simulect) are two similar compounds that became available in 1998. They are not used for the treatment of acute rejection but rather to prevent rejection when used as an induction agent. These agents have been shown clinically to result in a lower incidence of acute rejection compared with standard three-drug therapy in renal transplantation and may allow for steroid sparing.

Mechanism of Action

IL-2 receptor antibodies target the α chain (CD25) of the IL-2 receptor, blocking the autocrine and paracrine survival and growth effects of IL-2, which play a central role in antigen-induced proliferation of T cells.[28]

Dosing and Side Effects

Both drugs have a half-life of more than 7 days, which permits a long dose interval and results in diminished T-cell responses for at least 4 to 6 weeks. Basiliximab is given as two intravenous doses of 20 mg (days 0 and 4). Daclizumab is given as IV doses of 1 mg/kg starting on day 0 and then four times every other week.[28] Some recent studies demonstrated the efficacy of using two-dose courses of daclizumab. Neither IL-2 receptor antibody has significant serious adverse effects or first-dose reactions. There is no increased risk of posttransplantation infections or malignancy.

Calcineurin Inhibitors (Cyclosporine and Tacrolimus)

The introduction of CIs in kidney transplantation, first cyclosporin A (CsA) in 1983 and later tacrolimus (Prograf) in 1994, has significantly improved the 1-year graft survival, and they became the main immunosuppressive agents. The original formulation Sandimmune (cyclosporine) has been largely replaced by Neoral, the microemulsion formulation, due to improved gastrointestinal absorption and bioavailability. The generic formulations of cyclosporine microemulsion, Gengraf and cyclosporine USP, have been used widely in the United States. Tacrolimus is now the predominantly used CI in the United States (85% tacrolimus vs. 15% CsA).

Mechanism of Action

CsA and tacrolimus inhibit the expression of multiple genes involved in T-cell activation and proliferation, including IL-2 and other lymphokines. CsA and tacrolimus bind respectively to cytoplasmic immunophilins called cyclophilin and FK-binding protein, thereby producing a complex that inhibits the calcium-sensitive phosphatase calcineurin.[29] Calcineurin normally dephosphorylates transcription factors including nuclear factor of activated T cells, allowing their translocation into the nucleus where they are responsible for induction of gene transcription.[30]

Dosing and Side Effects

The optimal maintenance doses of CIs are still not fully stratified. CsA is usually administered orally in doses of 6 to 10 mg/kg/day and tacrolimus in doses of 0.15 to 0.3 mg/kg/day, in two divided doses. Monitoring blood levels is important because of variation in interpatient and intrapatient metabolism and a narrow therapeutic index. In patients receiving triple immunosuppressive therapy, the target 12-hour trough level (C0) for CsA and tacrolimus are 200 to 350 ng/mL and 8 to 15 ng/mL up to 3 months, 100 to 200 ng/mL and 5 to 10 ng/mL within 3 to 12 months, and 80 to 150 ng/mL and 4 to 8 ng/mL thereafter, respectively. There are several assays currently available to measure the CsA and tacrolimus levels, and physicians should know the type of method used at their center due to differences in results between the methods. Immunoassays using monoclonal antibodies against CsA and tacrolimus are the most common methods used. Recent attention has been given to 2-hour peak CsA levels (C2), which may predict clinical events such as acute rejection and nephrotoxicity better than 12-hour trough levels. Suggested target C2 levels are 1200 to 2000 ng/mL for the first 3 months, 800 to 1000 ng/mL months 4 through 6, and 800 ng/mL thereafter.[31] However, there are no large, multicenter, randomized trials to compare the long-term effects of C2 with C0 trough levels on allograft outcome. After significant dose adjustment, levels of CsA and tacrolimus should be rechecked within 2 to 4 days.

Both CIs are associated with numerous adverse effects. Although there are minor differences in the incidence of individual adverse effects, the spectrum is essentially similar for both agents. Both CIs are nephrotoxic and cause acute and chronic renal insufficiency. Acute renal insufficiency may be related to renal vasoconstriction as well as tubular toxicity. The vasoconstriction can be marked, involving both the afferent and efferent glomerular arterioles and persisting with time. Long-term use of CIs leads to renal insufficiency due to chronic tubulointerstitial disease, which may be characterized by "striped" interstitial fibrosis or multinodular arteriolar hyalinosis. However, none of the pathologic changes are specific for CIs.[32] CsA is associated with hypertension that appears to be salt sensitive and associated with low renin levels.[33] It also causes hyperlipidemia and glucose intolerance. Tacrolimus causes the same problems, but there seems to be a greater tendency to diabetogenicity with a slightly lower incidence of hypertension and hyperlipidemia. Posttransplantation diabetes mellitus was reported in 5% to 10% of CsA-treated and 10% to 20% of tacrolimus-treated patients. The mechanisms underlying the development of these adverse defects are not fully clear. Hyperkalemia is common, seen with both agents, and often associated with mild hyperchloremic acidosis (type 4 renal tubular acidosis). Hyperuricemia is more common with CsA. Both drugs lead to magnesium wasting and hypomagnesemia. Neurotoxicity may occur with both agents and manifests as paresthesias, tremors, convulsions, and encephalopathy. Thrombotic microangiopathy may develop secondary to CIs that may manifest with or without systemic features. Thrombotic microangiopathy mostly develops early after the introduction of a CI, but can be seen at later stages as well. At high drug levels, hepatotoxicity manifested by hyperbilirubinemia and elevated transaminases may occur with both agents. Hirsutism, coarse facies, and gingival hyperplasia are troubling adverse effects that appear to occur only with cyclosporine, and patients may respond to a switch to tacrolimus. In contrast, tacrolimus may cause hair loss.

Antimetabolites

Azathioprine (Imuran, Azasan)

Azathioprine (Imuran, Azasan) was first synthesized in the late 1950s as a prodrug of 6-mercaptopurine and has been the most commonly used immunosuppressive agent first with steroids and later with CsA and steroids until the introduction of mycophenolate mofetil (MMF). Currently less than 1% of de novo renal transplant recipients are started on azathioprine. However, given the costs and clinical efficacy, it remains a reasonable alternative to MMF in immunologically low-risk recipients, pregnancy, and recipients unable to tolerate MMF due to side effects.[34]

Mechanism of Action

Azathioprine is a prodrug, whose active metabolite, 6-mercaptopurine, competitively inhibits the formation of phosphoribosyl pyrophosphate, a key intermediate in purine synthesis. Lymphocytes are relatively unique in their dependence on de novo purine synthesis. Other cells are able to use a "salvage pathway" for recycling of purines. Thus azathioprine and related compounds are relatively selective for lymphocytes.

Dosing and Side Effects

The daily oral dose is 1.0 to 2.0 mg/kg/day when combined with a CI. Therapeutic drug monitoring is usually not necessary but possible by measuring 6-thioguanine levels in red blood cells. Myelosuppression is the most serious adverse effect leading to leukopenia, megaloblastic anemia, and thrombocytopenia in that order of frequency. It is important to be aware of a significant drug interaction between azathioprine and allopurinol. The latter drug impairs the degradation of the active metabolites of azathioprine, with the risk of profound and long-lasting neutropenia. Azathioprine should be switched to MMF in patients requiring allopurinol. Hepatotoxicity, reflected by a cholestatic picture, is another serious side effect.

Mycophenolate Mofetil (CellCept) and Enteric-Coated Mycophenolate Sodium (Myfortic)

MMF (CellCept) was introduced in clinical transplantation in 1995 and has almost completely replaced azathioprine in the United States.[35] Enteric-coated mycophenolate sodium (Myfortic) is an advanced formulation of mycophenolic acid characterized by a delayed release at the level of the small bowel and became available in 2004.[36]

Mechanism of Action

MMF is metabolized to MPA, which causes noncompetitive inhibition of inosine monophosphate dehydrogenase, a key enzyme in the de novo synthesis of guanine nucleotides.[37] Due to their significant dependence on this pathway, in addition to salvage mechanisms for purine synthesis, proliferating lymphocytes are especially susceptible to inhibition of inosine monophosphate dehydrogenase. Consequently, exposure to MPA impairs T-cell proliferation in response to antigen stimulation, decreases B-cell activity and antibody production, inhibits generation of cytotoxic T cells, and also decreases adhesion molecule function.[38]

Dosing and Side Effects

The standard dose is 1.0 g twice daily for CellCept and 720 mg twice daily for Myfortic. Blacks require higher doses of CellCept (1.5 g twice daily) when used with CsA. Trough levels of MPA are not routinely measured in kidney transplant recipients. Pharmacokinetic studies demonstrated that the area under the curve 0-12 for MPA correlates with its clinical efficacy and side effect profile. This relationship with random or 12-hour trough levels is less consistent.[39] Trough levels of MMF seem to be lowered by concurrent administration of cyclosporine but not tacrolimus.[40] The optimal dose of MMF in long-term stable kidney transplant recipients (>1 year) on CsA or tacrolimus is not certain. MMF causes significant gastrointestinal adverse effects that may manifest as severe nausea, vomiting, and persistent diarrhea (infectious or noninfectious Crohn's disease–like enterocolitis).[41] The only effective therapy for the noninfectious enterocolitis is to decrease the dose or even discontinue the drug, which is, however, associated with an increased risk of rejection. It is therefore important to reintroduce or increase the drug dose as soon as clinically possible. Enteric-coated mycophenolate sodium was developed as an alternative way to deliver MPA with the goal of reducing gastrointestinal adverse effects, but most clinical trials demonstrated a similar gastrointestinal side effect profile compared with MMF. The gastrointestinal side effects are due to systemic MPA and occur even when the drug is given intravenously. Other causes of diarrhea, such as infections, should be investigated before attribution to MMF or enteric-coated mycophenolate sodium and dose reduction of these agents. In clinical trials of MMF, leukopenia was found to occur at a frequency similar to that seen with the use of azathioprine, and may require dose adjustment.[42] However, other causes of leukopenia, such as viral infections, or other drugs (ganciclovir, valganciclovir) should be considered before dose reduction due to increased risk of acute rejection in patients whose MMF dose was reduced due to leukopenia.[43] Those patients on a reduced dose of MMF require closer monitoring. Nephrotoxicity, neurotoxicity, and hepatotoxicity have not been observed with MMF.

The Target of Rapamycin Inhibitors: Sirolimus (Rapamune) and Everolimus (Certican)

Sirolimus, formerly known as rapamycin, was introduced to transplantation in 1999[44] and its derivate with a shorter half-life, everolimus, is approved for use in Europe but is not currently available in the United States.[45–47] Since the approval of sirolimus by the U.S. Food and Drug Administration, this drug has been used in combination with CIs or MMF.

Mechanism of Action

Although TOR inhibitors bind to the same immunophilin FK binding protein as FK506 tacrolimus, they act through an entirely different mechanism. The resulting TOR inhibitor–FK binding protein complex does not bind to calcineurin phosphatase, but rather to cytosolic protein kinases known as TOR that are centrally involved in the regulation of cell proliferation and differentiation. Binding to this target results in inhibition of signal transduction through several growth factor receptors (such as the IL-2 receptor), thus preventing cell-cycle progression and immune activation.[48] The net result of these actions is potent antiproliferative activity against T cells and smooth muscle cells. Due to actions at a later stage in the immune response, TOR inhibitors can prevent cell proliferation even after immune stimulation and may function synergistically with a CI.

Dosing and Side Effects

Sirolimus is given once daily due to its long half-life (62 hours). It is rapidly absorbed from the gastrointestinal tract, reaching peak concentrations within 1 to 2 hours. It is usually given as a loading dose (6–15 mg/day), which is three times the maintenance dose (2–5 mg/day). Therapeutic drug level monitoring is an important part of its use and provides a good reflection of drug exposure. The doses and the target levels for sirolimus depend on the concomitant immunosuppressive agent, whether it is a CI or MMF. CIs augment the blood concentrations of sirolimus and vice versa, potentiating the nephrotoxicity of the CIs when these two drugs are used in combination.[44] Sirolimus should be administered 4 hours after the morning CI dose. Current recommendations are sirolimus trough levels of 5 to 10 ng/mL, CsA levels 50 to 100 ng/mL, or tacrolimus levels 3 to 6 ng/mL, if used together. Sirolimus trough levels should be 15 to 25 ng/mL if the CI is withdrawn after 3 months or 12 to 20 ng/mL if used with MMF. Sirolimus has direct adverse effects on the kidney even in the absence of CI use, causing proteinuria,[49] hypokalemia, and hypomagnesemia as a result of kaliuresis, and magnesuria. Everolimus has a shorter half-life (23 hours) and is given twice daily. The adverse effect profile of sirolimus is better established than that of everolimus, although preliminary data suggest that they are similar. The major adverse effects of sirolimus appear to be related to higher concentrations of drug in the blood. In the early posttransplantation period, impaired wound healing and an increased tendency for lymphocele formation have been noted.[50] It may cause myelosuppression, especially anemia and thrombocytopenia. Hyperlipidemia, particularly with hypertriglyceridemia, is a common complication of TOR inhibitors.[51] Other important complications described with sirolimus use include pulmonary toxicity (bronchiolitis obliterans organizing pneumonia) and painful oral ulcers.[52]

Glucocorticoids

Glucocorticoids are potent anti-inflammatory and immunosuppressive agents and have been used for several decades. Rapid steroid withdrawal protocols have gained popularity and are discussed under "Immunosuppressive Protocols." Pulse steroids are used to treat acute cellular rejection.

Mechanism of Action

Glucocorticoids bind to a cytosolic receptor that translocates to the nucleus, where the complex binds to DNA regulatory sequences, called glucocorticoid-responsive elements.[53] Glucocorticoids decrease the transcription of key cytokines, where glucocorticoid-responsive element sequences have been found in the critical promoter regions of several cytokine genes, or may also affect the transcription of genes that do not contain glucocorticoid-responsive elements.[54] As evidenced by the large number of target genes for glucocorticoids, their effects are exerted on a variety of cells, including lymphocytes and macrophages. Despite our understanding of the molecular mechanisms of these drugs, it is not certain which mecha-

nisms predominate in vivo, and this may depend on the drug dose. It is likely that for low doses used for daily maintenance therapy for prophylaxis of rejection, the nonspecific anti-inflammatory effects are most important. At higher doses, glucocorticoids are directly lympholytic, that is, they kill T and B cells, and this action may explain the rapid and potent immunosuppressive effects of pulse steroids.

Dosing and Side Effects

Steroids are given at high doses intravenously (250–1000 mg) starting before the transplantation surgery and gradually tapered over a few weeks, reaching maintenance doses of 5 to 10 mg/day at 2 to 3 months after transplantation. For rapid steroid withdrawal protocols, steroids are given for only 3 to 7 days after transplantation in a rapid taper. Glucocorticoids have multiple adverse effects that depend on the dose and duration of use, with the majority of effects becoming a serious problem only after prolonged use. These include impaired glucose tolerance, hyperlipidemia, and hypertension. These adverse effects can significantly enhance progression of atherosclerosis and cardiovascular morbidity and mortality. Glucocorticoids have devastating effects on connective tissues, causing poor wound healing, skin fragility, growth retardation in children, accelerated bone loss leading to osteoporosis, avascular necrosis of bones, cataracts, and proximal myopathy. Corticosteroid-induced osteoporosis may be diminished by the use of calcium and vitamin D supplements as well as agents to decrease bone resorption, including bisphosphonates and calcitonin.[55]

Drug Interactions of Immunosuppressive Drugs

Cyclosporine, tacrolimus, and sirolimus are catabolized by the same hepatic cytochrome P-450 systems (CYP3A4/5) that are involved in the degradation of other commonly used drugs. CYP3A4/5 is also present in the intestinal wall,[56] and oral absorption is decreased by the multidrug resistance gene *MDR-1*. This gene produces a transmembrane protein, P-glycoprotein[57] that actively transports a large number of molecules (including cyclosporine, tacrolimus, and sirolimus) back into the intestinal lumen. Due to genetic and/or environmental factors, the activity of both of these systems varies greatly from individual to individual. Box 87-1 lists some of the more common drugs that are particularly prone to produce changes in blood levels. In any immunosuppressed patient who has developed impaired renal function or toxic drug side effects, it is important to ascertain whether there have been any changes in medications, including over-the-counter medications such as herbal and antioxidant supplements.

Intravenous Immunoglobulins

Intravenous immunoglobulin (IVIG) products have immunomodulatory effects and have been used in the treatment of inflammatory and autoimmune disease.[58] IVIG products are prepared from IgG derived from thousands of donors. IVIG has been used in the field of transplantation since the 1990s, after in vitro studies demonstrated the inhibition of anti-HLA lymphocytotoxicity of sera from highly sensitized patients, and later in vivo studies showing decreased titers of anti-HLA antibodies.[59] A randomized, double-blind, placebo-controlled, multicenter National Institutes of Health–sponsored trial

Box 87-1   Common Drugs That Alter Blood Levels of Cyclosporine, Tacrolimus, and Sirolimus

Increase Levels	Decrease Levels
Diltiazem, nicardipine, verapamil	Phenobarbital, phenytoin, carbamazepine
Clarithromycin, erythromycin	Rifampin, rifabutin
Fluconazole, itraconazole, ketoconazole, voriconazole	St. John's wort *(Hypericum perforatum)*
Danazol, estradiol	Cholestyramine
Amiodarone, carvedilol	
Metoclopramide	
Antiretroviral treatment, HAART, particularly protease inhibitors (ritonavir)	
Grapefruit juice	

HAART, highly active antiretroviral therapy.

involving 101 end-stage renal disease patients with PRA levels greater than 50% and on the transplant waiting list for more than 5 years have shown decreased PRA levels and an increased transplantation rate in patients receiving IVIG (2 g/kg monthly for 4 months).[60] IVIG is currently used in desensitization protocols of crossmatch-positive or ABO-incompatible kidney transplant recipients. IVIG is also used in the treatment of acute antibody-mediated rejection.

Mechanisms of Action

There are many proposed mechanisms of IVIG, involving different parts of the immune response, including inhibition of the activation and effector functions of complement, cytokine cascades, and T- and B-lymphocyte function, and modulation of dendritic cells. Anti-idiotypic antibodies binding to anti-HLA antibodies might be the immediate mechanism of IVIG, but the immunomodulatory effects of IVIG treatment persist well beyond its half-life, indicating ongoing active inhibitory mechanisms. IVIG interacts with Fcγ receptor IIB, which is a negative signaling receptor on B cells and inhibits the expression of CD19 on activated B cells.[61,62]

Dosing and Side Effects

The dose of IVIG ranges from 100 to 2000 mg/kg depending on the type of protocol used. Desensitization protocols combining IVIG with plasmapheresis used lower doses of IVIG or 2.0 g/kg if used alone (maximum 140 g in a single administration). There are many IVIG products with different osmolality, pH, sodium, and sugar components, which results in specific side effect profiles. Adverse reactions to IVIG occur in less than 5% of patients. These side effects include headache, chills, nausea, myalgia, arthralgia, back pain, and increased blood pressure. Premedication with acetaminophen and diphenhydramine is required before infusion. A rare side effect is acute aseptic meningitis, which occurs 48 to 72 hours after the administration of IVIG and resolves spontaneously or can be prevented with nonsteroidal anti-inflammatory drugs. Renal failure secondary to osmotic injury to proximal tubular epithelium may occur due to sucrose or sorbitol components in some IVIG preparations. IVIG preparations that do not include sucrose or sorbitol are preferred to avoid renal failure (such as Gamimune-N, Gammagard, and Polygam). IVIG should be given during hemodialysis in end-stage renal disease patients or as a 6- to 8-hour infusion in nondialysis patients. Very rarely, serious anaphylactoid reactions occur within the first hour of administration of IVIG. In this situa-

tion, the infusion should be stopped and patients be treated with intravenous glucocorticoids.

New Immunosuppressive Medications

LEA29Y (belatacept) is a second-generation CTL-associated antigen 4 (CTLA4) immunoglobulin, a fusion protein combining CTLA4 with the Fc portion of IgG, which blocks costimulation (signal 2) of T cells by binding to CD80 and CD86. A phase II, randomized, multicenter trial comparing belatacept, mycophenolate mofetil, and prednisone to cyclosporine microemulsion, mycophenolate mofetil, and prednisone treatment showed similar rates of acute rejection but a better glomerular filtration rate and less chronic allograft nephropathy at 12-month protocol biopsies in the belatacept group.[11] All patients received basiliximab induction treatment, and belatacept was administered as a 30-minute intravenous infusion and divided into two groups, intensive and less intensive regimen, depending on the frequency of dosing. Efalizumab is a humanized IgG$_1$ monoclonal antibody that prevents LFA1–intracellular adhesions molecule interaction by binding to CD11a chain of leukocyte function antigen 1 (LFA1). In a phase I/II open-label, multidose, multicenter trial involving 38 patients, efalizumab was administered weekly for 12 weeks (0.5 or 2.0 mg/kg subcutaneously) after renal transplantation along with full-dose CsA, MMF, and prednisone or half-dose CsA, sirolimus, and prednisone.[63] The overall acute rejection rate at 6 months was 11%. However, three patients receiving high-dose efalizumab with full-dose CsA developed posttransplantation lymphoproliferative disease. Leflunomide (Arava) is metabolized to its active metabolite, A77 1726, which inhibits dihydroorotic acid dehydrogenase, an enzyme required for de novo pyrimidine synthesis in lymphocytes. It also inhibits selected tyrosine kinases involved in T- and B-cell activation. In addition, leflunomide seems to have antiviral activity against herpesviruses and polyomaviruses and has been used in the treatment of polyoma nephropathy.[64] FK778 is an analogue of A77 1726 with a shorter plasma half-life. It was used in a phase II multicenter trial in renal transplant recipients in combination with tacrolimus and steroids.[65] Anemia was the most frequently reported side effect of FK778 in this trial. Another phase II study comparing FK778 with MMF, along with tacrolimus and steroids, did not show efficacy of FK778 over MMF, and the manufacturer decided not to pursue the use of FK778 in renal transplantation. FTY720 is a novel immunomodulator agent with unique mechanisms of action. It is a sphingosine-

1-phosphate receptor agonist that modulates lymphocyte trafficking by reducing the recirculation of lymphocytes from lymph nodes to blood and peripheral tissues, including inflammatory lesions and graft sites. A phase II, multicenter, open-label study compared four different doses of FTY720 with MMF, in combination with cyclosporine and steroids.[66] Reversible bradycardia during the first doses of FTY720 raised concerns about the safety of the drug. Higher doses of FTY720 were found to be as effective as MMF, but the manufacturer decided not to pursue clinical use of FTY720 in renal transplant recipients. Janus kinase 3 is a tyrosine kinase associated with the cytokine receptor γ chain, which participates in the signaling of many cytokine receptors (IL-2, 4, 7, 9, 15, and 21). The Janus kinase 3 inhibitor CP-690,550 has been used in kidney transplant patients in a multicenter, randomized, phase II clinical trial comparing it with MMF in combination with tacrolimus and steroids. AEB071 is a highly potent and reversible inhibitor of all classic and novel protein kinase C isoforms. Protein kinase C isoforms are important mediators of intracellular signaling of T and B cells. AEB071 has completed phase I trials and is now in phase II trials in kidney transplant recipients. A modified extended-release tacrolimus formulation (Prograf XL, previously referred to as MR4) for once-daily administration has been shown to be safe in renal transplant patients converted from tacrolimus standard twice-daily dosing.[67] A large randomized, multicenter, phase III trial involving 638 de novo kidney transplant recipients comparing Prograf XL with twice-daily tacrolimus and cyclosporine microemulsion, along with MMF, steroids, and basiliximab induction has shown a similar patient and graft survival and safety profile.[68]

IMMUNOSUPPRESSIVE PROTOCOLS

Conventional immunosuppressive protocols consist of a CI (tacrolimus or cyclosporine), an adjuvant agent (MMF, azathioprine, or sirolimus), and corticosteroids with or without an induction agent. Immunosuppressive regimens have significantly changed over the past decade in the United States (Table 87-2). Although 76.5% of patients undergoing transplantation in 1997 received cyclosporine and 12.5% received tacrolimus, this ratio was reversed in 2005 such that 78.7% received tacrolimus and 14.9% received cyclosporine. As an adjuvant agent, 81.8% of 2005 kidney transplant recipients received MMF, 9.1% sirolimus, 5.1% Myfortic (mycophenolate sodium), 0.6% azathioprine, and 0.3% everolimus. The tacrolimus/MMF regimen was the most common combination (80.4%), followed by CsA/MMF (9.4%). The remaining 10% of the recipients received sirolimus with tacrolimus (4.5%), CsA (2.8%), or MMF (3.0%). The induction regimen has also been changed over the past decade such that while 65.7% of transplant recipients in 1997 did not receive any induction treatment; this rate was only 26.4% for patients receiving a transplant in 2005. Thymoglobulin was the most commonly used induction agent in 2007 (38.6%), followed by basiliximab (16.4%), daclizumab (11.5%), and alemtuzumab (8.8%). The use of Atgam and OKT3 was extremely rare, 1.6% and 0.4%, respectively. The use of rapid steroid withdrawal protocol has also increased recently so that although 97.4% of transplant recipients in 1997 were discharged with steroids, this rate decreased to 73.5% in 2007, indicating that 26.5% of the patients underwent rapid steroid withdrawal or steroid avoidance protocol.

Table 87-2 Immunosupressive Treatment of Kidney Transplant Recipients in 2005 (United States)

Agent	%
Induction	
Thymoglobulin	38.6
Basiliximab	16.4
Daclizumab	11.5
Alemtuzumab	8.8
Atgam	1.6
OKT3	0.4
No induction	26.4
Calcineurin Inhibitors	
Tac	78.7
Cyclosporine	14.9
Adjuvant Treatment (Antimetabolite)	
MMF	81.8
SRL	9.1
Myfortic (enteric-coated mycophenolate sodium)	5.1
Azathioprine	0.6
Everolimus	0.3
Steroids	73.5
Immunosupressive Treatment Combinations	
Tac/MMF	80.4
CsA/MMF	9.4
Tac/SRL	4.5
SRL/MMF	3.0
CsA/SRL	2.8

CsA, cyclosporine; MMF, mycophenolate mofetil; SRL, sirolimus; Tac, tacrolimus.

What Type of Calcineurin Inhibitor? (Tacrolimus vs. Cyclosporine)

Both CsA and tacrolimus have similar efficacy but different side effect profiles. Randomized, controlled studies or large database analyses comparing tacrolimus with CsA revealed conflicting results.[69,70] Initial randomized, multicenter, controlled trials showed decreased acute rejection rates in tacrolimus-treated patients compared with CsA-treated patients, but patients received Sandimmune (cyclosporine oral solution) instead of microemulsion CsA.[69] Follow-up studies comparing tacrolimus with Neoral showed similar patient and graft survival rates, but some advantages of tacrolimus in subgroups of patients, such as patients with DGF and black patients. Retrospective data analysis of patients undergoing transplantation between 1996 and 2000 in the United States has showed a similar graft survival rate in tacrolimus- and CsA-treated patients.[71] Another study analyzed deceased donor pairs between 1995 and 2002, in which one kidney was allocated to a patient receiving Neoral and the other kidney to a patient receiving tacrolimus to minimize the donor variability and selection bias.[72] Multivariate analyses could not demonstrate a difference in 5-year patient survival or graft loss. More recent studies analyzing patients receiving a transplant between 2000 and 2005 using the Scientific Registry of Transplant Recipients database demonstrated a slight but statistically significant increase in risk for 6-month acute rejection rate and decreased graft survival in CsA/MMF-treated patients compared with tacrolimus/MMF-treated patients (relative risk, 1.16 for both parameters, $P < .01$).[73] Initial studies demonstrated a higher rate of posttransplantation diabetes mellitus in tacrolimus-treated patients compared with CsA-treated patients, especially in African American and Hispanic patients, but more recent studies targeting lower tacrolimus levels revealed a decreased incidence of posttransplantation diabetes mellitus. Although CsA decreases MPA levels, tacro-limus does not have any significant effect; thus, patients on tacrolimus/MMF may receive more overall immunosuppression that may affect allograft outcome. Tacrolimus is preferred in immunologic high-risk kidney transplant recipients, pancreas transplant recipients, and in patients receiving minimization of immunosuppressive protocols (rapid steroid withdrawal).

What Type of Adjuvant Agent? (Mycophenolate Mofetil vs. Sirolimus)

Sirolimus use peaked in 2001; 9.7% of kidney transplant recipients were treated with sirolimus with tacrolimus, 4.1% with CsA, and 4.2% with MMF. Despite a decrease in acute rejection rates in patients treated with the sirolimus and CI combination, the studies also demonstrated a significant decrease in the glomerular filtration rate, indicating increased nephrotoxicity with this combination. This synergistic nephrotoxicity was attributed to impaired tubular recovery from CIs and/or ischemia/reperfusion injury by sirolimus. A meta-analysis of the studies using lower dose sirolimus with standard dose CI or higher dose sirolimus with lower dose CI still demonstrated a lower glomerular filtration rate compared with patients receiving a CI and MMF.[44] This analysis also showed that patients on sirolimus and a CI developed more thrombocytopenia, anemia, hypercholesterolemia, hypertriglyceridemia, and lymphocele. Due to these adverse effects, later studies were designed to withdraw the CI from the sirolimus/CI combination after 3 months or use sirolimus with MMF without using a CI.[74] A meta-analysis analyzed six randomized, controlled trials that involved initial immunosuppression with CI and sirolimus, followed by CI withdrawal in stable patients at 3 months after transplantation. The results demonstrated an increased risk of acute rejection (6%), but a higher glomerular filtration rate at 1 year in patients with CI withdrawal compared with patients remaining on sirolimus/CI.[75] There was no difference in patient and graft survival. A single-center study using sirolimus and MMF with basiliximab induction found excellent patient and graft survival,

kidney function, and low acute rejection rates (<10%).[76] The protocol biopsy specimens at 2 years also had significantly fewer chronicity findings in sirolimus/MMF-treated patients compared with patients treated with CI/MMF.[77] Another single-center study demonstrated similar acute rejection rates and graft function in sirolimus/MMF-treated patients compared with tacrolimus/MMF patients.[78] However, two multicenter, controlled, randomized trials were halted due to higher than expected acute rejection rates in patients receiving sirolimus/MMF. Analysis of patients receiving transplants between 2000 and 2005 using Scientific Registry of Transplant Recipients data showed the lowest 5-year graft survival in sirolimus/MMF-treated patients (57.7%) compared with patients treated with tacrolimus/MMF (73.8%), CsA/MMF (71.8%), CsA/sirolimus (68.9%), and tacrolimus/sirolimus (67.6%).[73] The risk of acute rejection was also the highest (relative risk = 1.53) compared with other combinations. Sirolimus is probably a more potent but also more toxic immunosuppressant compared with MMF. These studies raised questions regarding the safety of using sirolimus in kidney transplantation as a de novo agent with CIs or MMF. Use of sirolimus as a secondary agent in stable patients on a CI and MMF, in whom the CI will be switched to sirolimus after 3 months, in a multicenter trial is currently ongoing. However, another concern about sirolimus is proteinuria, and some studies found increased proteinuria in patients who were switched to sirolimus from a CI.

Sirolimus and everolimus have antiangiogenic and antiproliferative actions leading to inhibition of tumor growth in animal models. Maintenance immunosuppression with the TOR inhibitors is associated with a decreased risk of developing any posttransplantation de novo malignancy, using a large database analysis of kidney transplant recipients.[79] Conversion from CIs to sirolimus has been shown to cause regression of Kaposi's sarcoma.[80] These results indicate a potential use of sirolimus in transplant recipients with de novo malignancy.[81]

What Type of Induction Treatment?

A prospective, randomized trial comparing Thymoglobulin with Simulect in deceased donor recipients at high risk of acute rejection or DGF showed higher acute rejection rates in Simulect-treated patients (25.5% vs. 15.6%) but a similar incidence of DGF (44.5% vs. 40.4%).[82] Another prospective, randomized trial demonstrated a significant decrease in DGF incidence in patients treated with intraoperative Thymoglobulin induction treatment compared with postoperative thymoglobulin administration.[19] The main concerns using polyclonal or monoclonal lymphocyte-depleting agents are increased risk of developing opportunistic infections and malignancy after transplantation.[83] A meta-analysis of randomized trials using anti–IL-2R antibodies compared with placebo showed decreased acute rejection rates but no improvement in patient or graft survival at 1 year.[84] Using the Scientific Registry of Transplant Recipients database of patients receiving a transplant between 1998 and 2003, analysis demonstrated that anti–IL-2R antibodies decreased acute rejection at 6 months and decreased graft failure over a follow-up of 1059 days compared with no induction.[85] The benefit of anti-IL-2R antibodies in reducing acute rejection increased significantly with greater HLA mismatch. However, despite a statistically significant decrease in acute rejection rate (10.2% vs. 8.1%) and graft failure (11.8% vs. 10.4%) due to the large number of the patients analyzed,[49,50] the clinical meaning of these small differences is questionable. Anti–IL-2R antibodies were not found to increase the risk of cytomegalovirus infection or malignancy in this meta-analysis. The use of OKT3 as an induction agent has almost been completely eliminated due to cytokine-release syndrome as well as increased risk of infection and posttransplantation lymphoproliferative disorders. Alemtuzumab is a powerful cytolytic agent and has been used mainly for minimization of immunosuppressive treatment.[24] The first single-center study using alemtuzumab induction treatment with CsA monotherapy showed similar patient and graft survival and acute rejection rates compared with patients receiving triple immunosuppression.[86] Sirolimus monotherapy with alemtuzumab induction treatment showed increased acute antibody-mediated rejection.[87] A number of nonrandomized, retrospective, single-center studies with large patient numbers using alemtuzumab with rapid steroid withdrawal and low-dose tacrolimus and MMF found good patient and graft survival and acute rejection rates without increases in the incidence of infection and malignancy. However, there is a need for large, prospective, randomized, controlled studies with long-term follow-up of patients to determine the safety of alemtuzumab treatment as well as the advantages over the other induction agents.

Induction treatment has also been used to delay the initiation of CIs, but a recent randomized trial comparing early versus delayed CsA in renal transplant recipients with anti–IL-R2 antibody showed similar DGF, graft function, and graft loss in both groups.[88] Patients receiving delayed CsA had higher rate of acute rejection (26.5% vs. 15.5%), but the difference was not statistically significant.

Steroid Withdrawal

The widely known adverse effects of long-term steroid treatment have stimulated interest in using lower doses of steroid in kidney transplant recipients. Although most recent transplant patients decrease their maintenance dose of steroids to 5 mg once daily at 3 months after transplantation, an increasing number of transplant recipients have been receiving rapid steroid withdrawal before discharge. Steroid-free protocols using CsA and azathioprine in kidney transplant recipients from the 1980s and early 1990s showed increased risks of acute rejection.[89] In the past decade, the paradigm for timing of steroid withdrawal has shifted from late withdrawal to early withdrawal, eliminating steroids within 7 days after transplantation, and using more potent immunosuppressive treatment along with induction treatment. Two retrospective studies using rapid steroid withdrawal with induction treatment have shown low acute rejection rates and good patient and graft survival and graft function up to 5 years in immunologically low-risk patients.[90,91] However, randomized, controlled trials have shown increased acute rejection rates in steroid withdrawal groups.[89] Data on the beneficial effects of steroid withdrawal on posttransplantation diabetes mellitus, hyperlipidemia, osteopenia, weight gain, and blood pressure control have been mixed and could not be demonstrated in all studies. Some investigators raised the question of whether low-dose maintenance steroid treatment can achieve similar outcomes in prevention of side effects without increasing the risk of acute rejection. Due to a lack of protocol allograft biopsy specimens and long-term follow-up, it is not clear whether steroid withdrawal may increase the risk of developing chronic allograft nephropathy. Despite the increased popularity of using steroid-free protocols and the good short-term outcome, there is still a need for additional research to investigate the safety of those protocols, which induction agent to use (Thymoglobulin, Campath-1H, or anti–IL-2R antibodies), and what patient population to use (immunologically high versus low risk) in multicenter, randomized, controlled trials incorporating protocol biopsies and bone densitometry compared with patients treated with a low maintenance dose of steroids.

Calcineurin Inhibitor Withdrawal

CIs have been the cornerstone of immunosuppressive treatment and primarily responsible for increased 1-year graft survival rates of more than 90% in the past decade. However, CI-induced nephrotoxicity is still a hurdle to achieving better long-term graft survival. Other CI-related cardiovascular side effects, including posttransplantation diabetes, hyperlipidemia, and hypertension may decrease patient survival. CI withdrawal or dose reduction in patients receiving a transplant before 1996 and receiving CsA, azathioprine, and steroids have resulted in increased acute rejection.[92,93] In a prospective, multicenter trial involving 212 stable kidney transplant recipients receiv-ing CsA/MMF/steroids randomized at 6 months post-transplantation to either CsA withdrawal or to continue their triple-drug therapy,[94] the CsA withdrawal group had 22% and 11% biopsy-proven acute and chronic rejection compared with 1.4% and 0% in controls, respectively. CsA withdrawal or complete avoidance using sirolimus also increases the risk of acute rejection. Current ongoing trials using new immunosuppressive medications, such as LEA29Y (belatacept), Janus kinase 3 inhibitor (CP-690,550), and protein kinase C inhibitor (AEB071), along with MMF and steroids, compared with standard treatment with CI/MMF/steroids may show the safety of CI avoidance in the future.

Immunosuppression and Sensitization

Unsensitized recipients of HLA-identical living donor or zero antigen mismatched deceased donor kidney transplant recipients have a lower risk of acute rejection and much longer graft survival. Those patients need less immunosuppressive treatment with lower dose CIs and MMF and are also good candidates for rapid steroid withdrawal or CI avoidance protocols with anti–IL-2R antibodies. However, immunosuppressive management of sensitized recipients of HLA-identical living donor or 0-mismatched deceased donor kidney transplant recipients may require more immunosuppression. Recent findings by Opelz[95] suggest that the long-term outcome in kidney recipients from HLA-identical siblings depends on the degree of sensitization before transplantation. Although unsensitized HLA-identical siblings showed a 72% ten-year survival rate, recipients with

1% to 50% and more than 50% PRA had 63% and 55% graft survival rates after a decade, respectively. Whether PRA indicates a higher responsiveness or a reaction against a non-HLA antigen remains to be elucidated. In general, unsensitized living donor kidney transplant recipients usually receive standard triple immunosuppressive treatment with or without an induction agent per transplantation center preference. Unsensitized deceased donor kidney transplant recipients may require induction treatment along with standard triple immunosuppressive treatment, especially in patients at higher risk of developing DGF. Immunosuppressive management of the sensitized patients depends on the type of crossmatch result and the specificity of anti-HLA antibodies (i.e., whether it is donor specific). CDC T-cell crossmatch positivity is an absolute contraindication to transplantation and requires pretransplantation desensitization. Therapeutic strategies for desensitization protocols include combinations of plasmapheresis or immunoadsorption, IVIG, rituximab (anti-CD20), and splenectomy.

Currently, there are no randomized, controlled, prospective studies that compare different desensitization protocols, and all published studies are retrospective, single-center studies using high-dose IVIG or immunoadsorption alone or plasmapheresis with low- or high-dose IVIG.[96] The selection of the desensitization protocol also depends on the strength of the DSA, so that patients with high titers probably require pretransplantation plasmapheresis.[97] Patients with low DSA titers (<1:8) may require two to three sessions of plasmapheresis, whereas patients with high DSA titers (>1:128) may require six to 10 sessions to decrease the antibody titers. Patients undergo transplantation if the crossmatch becomes negative with an induction agent (anti–IL-2R antibody, Thymoglobulin, or alemtuzumab), IVIG, and continuation of posttransplantation plasmapheresis for two to five sessions depending on the titers of the DSA. Rituximab has been added to some desensitization protocols as a single dose (375 mg/m^2) before or at the time of transplantation. However, early acute antibody-mediated rejection is an important obstacle seen in 30% to 40% of the recipients, despite the type of desensitization, whether they receive high-dose IVIG or low-dose IVIG/plasmapheresis protocol or rituximab is added to the protocol.

CDC B-cell or FC T-or B cell–positive crossmatch patients are at higher risk of developing acute antibody-mediated or cellular rejection as well as chronic rejection leading to decreased graft survival. Those patients also require desensitization protocols with IVIG and pre- and/or peritransplantation plasmapheresis depending on the titers of the DSAs.[98] All sensitized patients require induction agents along with triple immunosuppressive treatment and the CI levels should be kept at higher target levels plus standard doses of MMF and steroids. Those patients should be closely followed after transplantation with monitoring DSAs and probably with protocol allograft biopsies to diagnose acute or chronic antibody-mediated rejection. Future prospective, randomized, multicenter studies are required to define the most appropriate desensitization protocol for highly sensitized kidney transplant recipients.

References

1. Delves PJ, Roitt IM: The immune system. Second of two parts. N Engl J Med 2000;343:108–117.
2. Delves PJ, Roitt IM: The immune system. First of two parts. N Engl J Med 2000;343:37–49.
3. Klein J, Sato A: The HLA system. First of two parts. N Engl J Med 2000;343:702–709.
4. Klein J, Sato A: The HLA system. Second of two parts. N Engl J Med 2000;343:782–786.
5. West LJ: B-cell tolerance following ABO-incompatible infant heart transplantation. Transplantation 2006;81:301–307.
6. Lakkis FG, Arakelov A, Konieczny BT, Inoue Y: Immunologic 'ignorance' of vascularized organ transplants in the absence of secondary lymphoid tissue. Nat Med 2000;6:686–688.
7. Gould DS, Auchincloss H Jr: Direct and indirect recognition: The role of MHC antigens in graft rejection. Immunol Today 1999;20:77–82.
8. Saiki T, Ezaki T, Ogawa M, et al: In vivo roles of donor and host dendritic cells in allogeneic immune response: Cluster formation with host proliferating T cells. J Leukoc Biol 2001;69:705–712.
9. Clarkson MR, Sayegh MH: T-cell costimulatory pathways in allograft rejection and tolerance. Transplantation 2005;80:555–563.
10. Sayegh MH, Turka LA: The role of T-cell costimulatory activation pathways in transplant rejection. N Engl J Med 1998;338:1813–1821.
11. Vincenti F, Larsen C, Durrbach A, et al: Costimulation blockade with belatacept in renal transplantation. N Engl J Med 2005;353:770–781.
12. Lakkis FG: Role of cytokines in transplantation tolerance: Lessons learned from gene-knockout mice. J Am Soc Nephrol 1998;9:2361–2367.
13. Bray RA, Nickerson PW, Kerman RH, Gebel HM: Evolution of HLA antibody detection: Technology emulating biology. Immunol Res 2004;29:41–54.
14. Patel R, Terasaki PI: Significance of the positive crossmatch test in kidney transplantation. N Engl J Med 1969;280:735–739.
15. Gebel HM, Bray RA, Nickerson P: Pre-transplant assessment of donor-reactive, HLA-specific antibodies in renal transplantation: Contraindication vs. risk. Am J Transplant 2003;3:1488–1500.
16. Le Bas-Bernardet S, Hourmant M, Valentin N, et al: Identification of the antibodies involved in B-cell crossmatch positivity in renal transplantation. Transplantation 2003;75:477–482.
17. Vaidya S, Cooper TY, Avandsalehi J, et al: Improved flow cytometric detection of HLA alloantibodies using pronase: Potential implications in renal transplantation. Transplantation 2001;71:422–428.
18. Norman DJ: Antilymphocyte antibodies in the treatment of allograft rejection: Targets, mechanisms of action, monitoring, and efficacy. Semin Nephrol 12:315–324, 199.
19. Goggins WC, Pascual MA, Powelson JA, et al: A prospective, randomized, clinical trial of intraoperative versus postoperative thymoglobulin in adult cadaveric renal transplant recipients. Transplantation 2003;76:798–802.
20. Schroeder TJ, First MR, Mansour ME, et al: Antimurine antibody formation following OKT3 therapy. Transplantation 1990;49:48–51.
21. Chatenoud L, Ferran C, Legendre C, et al: In vivo cell activation following OKT3 administration. Systemic cytokine release and modulation by corticosteroids. Transplantation 1990;49:697–702.
22. Swinnen LJ, Costanzo-Nordin MR, Fisher SG, et al: Increased incidence of lymphoproliferative disorder after immunosuppression with the monoclonal antibody OKT3 in cardiac-transplant recipients. N Engl J Med 1990;323:1723–1728.
23. Penn I: Cancers complicating organ transplantation. N Engl J Med 1990;323:1767–1769.

24. Morris PJ, Russell NK: Alemtuzumab (Campath-1H): A systematic review in organ transplantation. Transplantation 2006;81: 1361–1367.

25. Magliocca JF, Knechtle SJ: The evolving role of alemtuzumab (Campath-1H) for immunosuppressive therapy in organ transplantation. Transpl Int 2006;19:705–714.

26. Becker YT, Samaniego-Picota M, Sollinger HW: The emerging role of rituximab in organ transplantation. Transpl Int 2006;19:621–628.

27. Vieira CA, Agarwal A, Book BK, et al: Rituximab for reduction of anti-HLA antibodies in patients awaiting renal transplantation: 1. Safety, pharmacodynamics, and pharmacokinetics. Transplantation 2004;77:542–548.

28. Waldmann TA: Anti-Tac (daclizumab, Zenapax) in the treatment of leukemia, autoimmune diseases, and in the prevention of allograft rejection: A 25-year personal odyssey. J Clin Immunol 2007;27:1–18.

29. O'Keefe SJ, Tamura J, Kincaid RL, et al: FK-506- and CsA-sensitive activation of the interleukin-2 promoter by calcineurin. Nature 1992;357:692–694.

30. Liu J, Farmer JD Jr, Lane WS, et al: Calcineurin is a common target of cyclophilin-cyclosporin A and FKBP-FK506 complexes. Cell 1991;66:807–815.

31. Schiff J, Cole E, Cantarovich, M: Therapeutic monitoring of calcineurin inhibitors for the nephrologist. Clin J Am Nephrol 2007;2:374–384.

32. Remuzzi G, Perico N: Cyclosporine-induced renal dysfunction in experimental animals and humans. Kidney Int Suppl 1995;52:S70–S74.

33. Curtis JJ: Hypertension following kidney transplantation. Am J Kidney Dis 1994;23:471–475.

34. Remuzzi G, Lesti M, Gotti E, et al: Mycophenolate mofetil versus azathioprine for prevention of acute rejection in renal transplantation (MYSS): A randomised trial. Lancet 2004;364:503–512.

35. Ciancio G, Miller J, Gonwa TA: Review of major clinical trials with mycophenolate mofetil in renal transplantation. Transplantation 2005;80:S191–S200.

36. Gabardi S, Tran JL, Clarkson MR: Enteric-coated mycophenolate sodium. Ann Pharmacother 2003;37:1685–1693.

37. Sollinger HW: Mycophenolate mofetil for the prevention of acute rejection in primary cadaveric renal allograft recipients. U.S. Renal Transplant Mycophenolate Mofetil Study Group. Transplantation 1995;60:225–232.

38. Allison AC, Eugui EM: Immunosuppressive and other effects of mycophenolic acid and an ester prodrug, mycophenolate mofetil. Immunol Rev 1993;136:5–28.

39. van Gelder T, Le Meur Y, Shaw LM, et al: Therapeutic drug monitoring of mycophenolate mofetil in transplantation. Ther Drug Monit 2006;28:145–154.

40. van Hest RM, Mathot RA, Pescovitz MD, et al: Explaining variability in mycophenolic acid exposure to optimize mycophenolate mofetil dosing: A population pharmacokinetic meta-analysis of mycophenolic acid in renal transplant recipients. J Am Soc Nephrol 2006;17:871–880.

41. Maes BD, Dalle I, Geboes K, et al: Erosive enterocolitis in mycophenolate mofetil-treated renal-transplant recipients with persistent afebrile diarrhea. Transplantation 2003;75:665–672.

42. Placebo-controlled study of mycophenolate mofetil combined with cyclosporin and corticosteroids for prevention of acute rejection. European Mycophenolate Mofetil Cooperative Study Group. Lancet 1995;345:1321–1325.

43. Knoll GA, MacDonald I, Khan A, Van Walraven C: Mycophenolate mofetil dose reduction and the risk of acute rejection after renal transplantation. J Am Soc Nephrol 2003;14:2381–2386.

44. Webster AC, Lee VW, Chapman JR, Craig JC: Target of rapamycin inhibitors (sirolimus and everolimus) for primary immunosuppression of kidney transplant recipients: A systematic review and meta-analysis of randomized trials. Transplantation 2006;81:1234–1248.

45. Vitko S, Margreiter R, Weimar W, et al: Everolimus (Certican) 12-month safety and efficacy versus mycophenolate mofetil in de novo renal transplant recipients. Transplantation 2004;78: 1532–1540.

46. Vitko S, Tedesco H, Eris J, et al: Everolimus with optimized cyclosporine dosing in renal transplant recipients: 6-month safety and efficacy results of two randomized studies. Am J Transplant 2004;4:626–635.

47. Nashan B, Curtis J, Ponticelli C, et al: Everolimus and reduced-exposure cyclosporine in de novo renal-transplant recipients: A three-year phase II, randomized, multicenter, open-label study. Transplantation 2004;78:1332–1340.

48. Chung J, Kuo CJ, Crabtree GR, Blenis J: Rapamycin-FKBP specifically blocks growth-dependent activation of and signaling by the 70 kd S6 protein kinases. Cell 1992;69:1227–1236.

49. Letavernier E, Peraldi MN, Pariente A, et al: Proteinuria following a switch from calcineurin inhibitors to sirolimus. Transplantation 2005;80:1198–1203.

50. Dean PG, Lund WJ, Larson TS, et al: Wound-healing complications after kidney transplantation: A prospective, randomized comparison of sirolimus and tacrolimus. Transplantation 2004; 77:1555–1561.

51. Murgia MG, Jordan S, Kahan BD: The side effect profile of sirolimus: A phase I study in quiescent cyclosporine-prednisone-treated renal transplant patients. Kidney Int 1996;49:209–216.

52. Morelon E, Stern M, Israel-Biet D, et al: Characteristics of sirolimus-associated interstitial pneumonitis in renal transplant patients. Transplantation 2001;72:787–790.

53. Beato M: Gene regulation by steroid hormones. Cell 1989;56: 335–344.

54. Auphan N, DiDonato JA, Rosette C, et al: Immunosuppression by glucocorticoids: Inhibition of NF-kappa B activity through induction of I kappa B synthesis. Science 1995;270: 286–290.

55. Sambrook P, Birmingham J, Kelly P, et al: Prevention of corticosteroid osteoporosis. A comparison of calcium, calcitriol, and calcitonin. N Engl J Med 1993;328:1747–1752.

56. Lin YS, Dowling AL, Quigley SD, et al: Co-regulation of CYP3A4 and CYP3A5 and contribution to hepatic and intestinal midazolam metabolism. Mol Pharmacol 2002;62:162–172.

57. Hochman JH, Chiba M, Yamazaki M, et al: P-glycoprotein-mediated efflux of indinavir metabolites in Caco-2 cells expressing cytochrome P450 3A4. J Pharmacol Exp Ther 2010;298:323–330.

58. Kazatchkine MD, Kaveri SV: Immunomodulation of autoimmune and inflammatory diseases with intravenous immune globulin. N Engl J Med 2001;345:747–755.

59. Jordan SC, Vo AA, Peng A, et al: Intravenous gammaglobulin (IVIG): A novel approach to improve transplant rates and outcomes in highly HLA-sensitized patients. Am J Transplant 2006;6:459–466.

60. Jordan SC, Tyan D, Stablein D, et al: Evaluation of intravenous immunoglobulin as an agent to lower allosensitization and improve transplantation in highly sensitized adult patients with end-stage renal disease: Report of the NIH IG02 trial. J Am Soc Nephrol 2004;15:3256–3262.

61. Samuelsson A, Towers TL, Ravetch JV: Anti-inflammatory activity of IVIG mediated through the inhibitory Fc receptor. Science 2001;291:484–486.

62. Toyoda M, Pao A, Petrosian A, Jordan SC: Pooled human gammaglobulin modulates surface molecule expression and induces apoptosis in human B cells. Am J Transplant 2003;3:156–166.

63. Vincenti F, Mendez R, Pescovitz M, et al: A phase I/II randomized open-label multicenter trial of efalizumab, a humanized anti-CD11a, anti-LFA-1 in renal transplantation. Am J Transplant 2007;7:1770–1777.

64. Josephson MA, Gillen D, Javaid B, et al: Treatment of renal allograft polyoma BK virus infection with leflunomide. Transplantation 2006;81:704–710.

65. Vanrenterghem Y, van Hooff JP, Klinger M, et al: The effects of FK778 in combination with tacrolimus and steroids: A phase II multicenter study in renal transplant patients. Transplantation 2004;78:9–14.

66. Tedesco-Silva H, Mourad G, Kahan BD, et al: FTY720, a novel immunomodulator: Efficacy and safety results from the first phase 2A study in de novo renal transplantation. Transplantation 2004;77:1826–1833.

67. Alloway R, Steinberg S, Khalil K, et al: Two years postconversion from a Prograf-based regimen to a once-daily tacrolimus extended-release formulation in stable kidney transplant recipients. Transplantation 2007;83:1648–1651.

68. Silva HT Jr, Yang HC, Abouljoud M, et al: One-year results with extended-release tacrolimus/MMF, tacrolimus/MMF and cyclosporine/MMF in de novo kidney transplant recipients. Am J Transplant 2007;7:595–608.

69. Vincenti F, Jensik SC, Filo RS, et al: A long-term comparison of tacrolimus (FK506) and cyclosporine in kidney transplantation: Evidence for improved allograft survival at five years. Transplantation 2002;73:775–782.

70. Gonwa T, Johnson C, Ahsan N, et al: Randomized trial of tacrolimus + mycophenolate mofetil or azathioprine versus cyclosporine + mycophenolate mofetil after cadaveric kidney transplantation: Results at three years. Transplantation 2003;75:2048–2053.

71. Woodward RS, Kutinova A, Schnitzler MA, Brennan DC: Renal graft survival and calcineurin inhibitor. Transplantation 2005;80:629–633.

72. Kaplan B, Schold JD, Meier-Kriesche HU: Long-term graft survival with Neoral and tacrolimus: A paired kidney analysis. J Am Soc Nephrol 2003;14:2980–2984.

73. Srinivas TR, Schold JD, Guerra G, et al: Mycophenolate mofetil/sirolimus compared to other common immunosuppressive regimens in kidney transplantation. Am J Transplant 2007;7:586–594.

74. Mota A, Arias M, Taskinen EI, et al: Sirolimus-based therapy following early cyclosporine withdrawal provides significantly improved renal histology and function at 3 years. Am J Transplant 2004;4:953–961.

75. Mulay AV, Hussain N, Fergusson D, Knoll GA: Calcineurin inhibitor withdrawal from sirolimus-based therapy in kidney transplantation: A systematic review of randomized trials. Am J Transplant 2005;5:1748–1756.

76. Flechner SM, Goldfarb D, Modlin C, et al: Kidney transplantation without calcineurin inhibitor drugs: A prospective, randomized trial of sirolimus versus cyclosporine. Transplantation 2002;74:1070–1076.

77. Flechner SM, Kurian SM, Solez K, et al: De novo kidney transplantation without use of calcineurin inhibitors preserves renal structure and function at two years. Am J Transplant 2004;4:1776–1785.

78. Larson TS, Dean PG, Stegall MD, et al: Complete avoidance of calcineurin inhibitors in renal transplantation: A randomized trial comparing sirolimus and tacrolimus. Am J Transplant 2006;6:514–522.

79. Kauffman HM, Cherikh WS, Cheng Y, et al: Maintenance immunosuppression with target-of-rapamycin inhibitors is associated with a reduced incidence of de novo malignancies. Transplantation 2005;80:883–889.

80. Stallone G, Schena A, Infante B, et al: Sirolimus for Kaposi's sarcoma in renal-transplant recipients. N Engl J Med 2005;352:1317–1323.

81. Campistol JM, Albanell J, Arns W, et al: Use of proliferation signal inhibitors in the management of post-transplant malignancies—clinical guidance. Nephrol Dial Transplant 2007;22 (Suppl 1):i36–i41.

82. Brennan DC, Daller JA, Lake KD, et al: Rabbit antithymocyte globulin versus basiliximab in renal transplantation. N Engl J Med 2006;355:1967–1977.

83. Meier-Kriesche HU, Arndorfer JA, Kaplan B: Association of antibody induction with short- and long-term cause-specific mortality in renal transplant recipients. J Am Soc Nephrol 2002;13:769–772.

84. Webster AC, Playford EG, Higgins G, et al: Interleukin 2 receptor antagonists for renal transplant recipients: A meta-analysis of randomized trials. Transplantation 2004;77:166–176.

85. Patlolla V, Zhong X, Reed GW, Mandelbrot DA: Efficacy of anti-IL-2 receptor antibodies compared to no induction and to antilymphocyte antibodies in renal transplantation. Am J Transplant 2007;7:1832–1842.

86. Watson CJ, Bradley JA, Friend PJ, et al: Alemtuzumab (CAMPATH 1H) induction therapy in cadaveric kidney transplantation—efficacy and safety at five years. Am J Transplant 2005;5:1347–1353.

87. Knechtle SJ, Pirsch JD, H Fechner JJ Jr, et al: Campath-1H induction plus rapamycin monotherapy for renal transplantation: Results of a pilot study. Am J Transplant 2003;3:722–730.

88. Kamar N, Garrigue V, Karras A, et al: Impact of early or delayed cyclosporine on delayed graft function in renal transplant recipients: A randomized, multicenter study. Am J Transplant 2006;6:1042–1048.

89. Augustine J, Hricik DE: Steroids sparing in kidney transplantation: Changing paradigms, improving outcomes, and remaining questions. Clin J Am Nephrol 2006;1:1080–1089.

90. Matas AJ, Kandaswamy R, Gillingham KJ, et al: Prednisone-free maintenance immunosuppression—a 5-year experience. Am J Transplant 2005;5:2473–2478.

91. Kaufman DB, Leventhal JR, Axelrod D, et al: Alemtuzumab induction and prednisone-free maintenance immunotherapy in kidney transplantation: Comparison with basiliximab induction—long-term results. Am J Transplant 2005;5:2539–2548.

92. Wong W, Venetz JP, Tolkoff-Rubin N, Pascual M: 2005 immunosuppressive strategies in kidney transplantation: Which role for the calcineurin inhibitors? Transplantation 2005;80:289–296.

93. Kasiske BL, Chakkera HA, Louis TA, Ma JZ: A meta-analysis of immunosuppression withdrawal trials in renal transplantation. J Am Soc Nephrol 2000;11:1910–1917.

94. Smak Gregoor PJ, de Sevaux RG, Ligtenberg G, et al: Withdrawal of cyclosporine or prednisone six months after kidney transplantation in patients on triple drug therapy: A randomized, prospective, multicenter study. J Am Soc Nephrol 2002;13:1365–1373.

95. Opelz G: Non-HLA transplantation immunity revealed by lymphocytotoxic antibodies. Lancet 2005;365:1570–1576.

96. Akalin E, Bromberg JS: Kidney transplantation in highly-sensitized recipients. Acta Nephrol 2007;21:1–8.

97. Montgomery RA, Zachary AA: Transplanting patients with a positive donor-specific crossmatch: A single center's perspective. Pediatr Transplant 2004;8:535–542.

98. Akalin E, Bromberg JS: Intravenous immunoglobulin induction treatment in flow cytometry cross-match-positive kidney transplant recipients. Hum Immunol 2005;66:359–363.

Further Reading

Akalin E, Watschinger B: Antibody-mediated rejection. Semin Nephrol 2007;27:393–407.

Augustine J, Hricik, DE: Steroids sparing in kidney transplantation: changing paradigms, improving outcomes, and remaining questions. Clin J Am Nephrol 2006;1:1080–1089.

Bray RA, Nickerson PW, Kerman RH, Gebel HM: Evolution of HLA antibody detection: technology emulating biology. Immunol Res 2004;29:41–54.

Gebel HM, Bray RA, Nickerson P: Pre-transplant assessment of donor-reactive, HLA-specific antibodies in renal transplantation: contraindication vs. risk. Am J Transplant 2003;3:1488–1500.

Halloran PF: Immunosuppressive drugs for kidney transplantation. N Engl J Med 2004;351:2715–2729.

Morris PJ, Russell NK: Alemtuzumab (Campath-1H): A systematic review in organ transplantation. Transplantation 2006;81:1361–1367.

Srinivas TR, Schold JD, Guerra G, et al: Mycophenolate mofetil/sirolimus compared to other common immunosuppressive regimens in kidney transplantation. Am J Transplant 2007;7:586–594.

Webster AC, Lee VW, Chapman JR, Craig JC: Target of rapamycin inhibitors (sirolimus and everolimus) for primary immunosuppression of kidney transplant recipients: A systematic review and meta-analysis of randomized trials. Transplantation 2006;81:1234–1248.

Chapter 88

Diagnosis and Management of Renal Allograft Dysfunction

John P. Vella and Mohamed H. Sayegh

IMMEDIATELY POST-TRANSPLANTATION

Delayed graft function (DGF) is defined as the requirement for dialysis within the first week after transplantation or as less than 25% decrease in creatinine within the first 24 hours after surgery.[1,2] The term *primary nonfunction* describes the outcome of approximately 5% of kidneys that never work. The dominant cause of DGF is acute tubular necrosis consequent to ischemia and the events surrounding organ procurement.[2,3] Acute tubular necrosis rarely occurs in living donor kidney recipients, although the incidence may be higher if the kidney is procured laparoscopically.[4] The incidence of DGF increases when the cold ischemia time exceeds 24 hours and when calcineurin inhibitors (CIs) are included in the induction regimen.[5,6]

The organ donor shortage has spawned several previously underused and innovative strategies to increase the donor pool from nontraditional sources. Over the past 10 years, there has been a marked increase in the number of donors whose death was defined by cardiac standstill (donation after cardiac death).[7–9] Wider use of donation after cardiac death organs has the potential to greatly increase the number of organ transplants. Cooper and colleagues[9] reported on the experience of the University of Wisconsin of 382 donation after cardiac death organ donors over a 16-year period starting in 1984 and compared the function of these kidneys to more than 1000 brain-dead donors over the same time period. They found that there was no statistical difference in cold ischemia time, rate of primary nonfunction, and short- or long-term graft loss. However, the incidence of delayed graft function (DGF) was significantly higher in donation after cardiac death organ recipients compared with standard criteria recipients.

The United Network for Organ Sharing recently defined a class of deceased donor kidney grafts for special allocation procedures to enhance use of such organs. The criteria defining these expanded-criteria donor kidneys (ECDs) are donor age older than 60 years or donor age between 50 and 59 years plus two of the following characteristics: donor history of cerebrovascular accident, donor history of hypertension, and elevated creatinine (1.5 mg/dL) at any time during donor management.[10] The risk of DGF is higher in expanded-criteria donor recipients, although the risk may be mitigated by pulsatile perfusion of the graft before transplantation.[11] Recipients older than the age of 60 years who receive an expanded-criteria donor kidney and experience DGF have a higher risk of death compared with other patient groups,[12] although overall survival is improved compared with dialysis.

Diagnosis

Renal ultrasonography should always be performed to exclude a vascular catastrophe such as thrombosis of the transplant renal artery or vein. Isotope renography may also detect functionally significant obstruction or a urine leak and exclude kidney infarction. The diagnosis of allograft rejection in patients with DGF who are maintained on dialysis can be made only histologically.

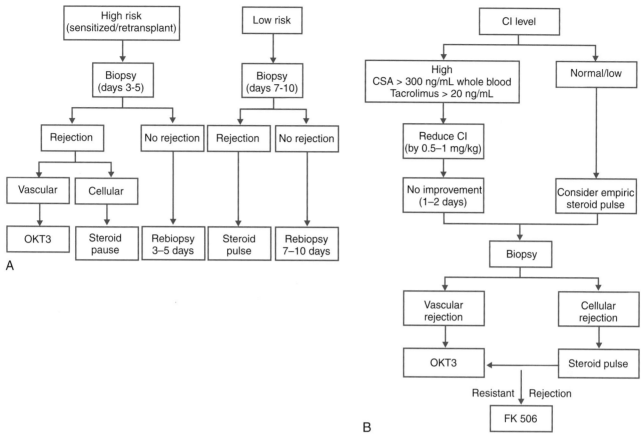

Figure 88-1 **A,** The approach to patients with delayed graft function. **B,** The approach to patients with rising creatinine levels after immediate graft function. The causes and approach to the management of renal allograft dysfunction vary with time after transplantation. Therefore, the differential diagnosis is best approached by considering the time periods separately. The surgical complications leading to allograft dysfunction that include obstruction and vascular thromboses are addressed in Chapter 86. The attention of the reader is directed to a recently published update of the Banff diagnostic categories for renal allograft biopsies that is discussed in detail in the text[1] (Table 88-1).

The approach to DGF varies with patient risk (Fig. 88-1). Factors indicating high-risk include sensitization, retransplantation, and cold ischemia time exceeding 24 hours. Such patients should have a renal biopsy performed on days 3 to 5 to rule out acute rejection. A repeat biopsy should be performed in 3 to 5 days if rejection is not seen and DGF persists. In the absence of antibody induction therapy, low-risk patients should have a biopsy performed on days 7 to 10, which can be repeated should DGF persist. For those patients receiving potent antilymphocyte antibody induction therapy, it may be reasonable to defer the biopsy as the risk of early rejection is low.[13]

Management

Prolongation of DGF by concurrent calcineurin inhibitor (CI) therapy has led to the use of sequential induction regimens with antilymphocyte antibody therapies. Provision of adequate immunosuppression while avoiding CI therapy is desirable during DGF as there is evidence to suggest that the incidence of acute rejection is increased by DGF.[13,14] Initial studies suggested that DGF is associated with poorer long-term graft survival.[15] More recent reports indicate that graft survival is not significantly different when comparing DGF versus no DGF for patients without rejection.[16,17] Immunologic injury may play a role in some cases of DGF.[18] Evidence to support this is provided by the ob-

servation that the incidence of DGF is increased in presensitized, retransplant patients.[15] Therapy of DGF includes supportive care[19] and minimizing nephrotoxins (notably CIs and some antibiotics). The use of vasodilators such as dopamine in the recipient with DGF has been largely discredited. However, a recent report of dopamine use in the donor before organ procurement suggests that such an approach may have a favorable impact on DGF rates after implantation.[20] Reports that rabbit antithymocyte globulin (thymoglobulin) may reduce the incidence of DGF[21] have not been universally reproduced.[13,22]

Hyperacute rejection is a rare and generally preventable cause of primary nonfunction.[23] It is caused by unrecognized ABO incompatibility or donor-specific antibody, both of which have long been deemed to be contraindications to kidney transplantation.[24] More recently, successful transplantation across such immunologic barriers has been described in which a pretransplantation conditioning regimen involving plasmapheresis and intravenous immunoglobulin is used.[20] Other causes of hyperacute rejection include anti-HLA class II antibodies and antidonor endothelial/monocyte antibodies, which may cause a delayed-onset hyperacute rejection-like syndrome in HLA-identical grafts.[19,25,26] The diagnosis of hyperacute rejection is usually made by the surgeon in the operating room. The initially pink kidney becomes mottled and cyanotic. There is little or no urine output, and the renal biopsy specimen shows intrarenal coagulopathy and cortical necrosis. The differential diagnosis includes pulsatile perfusion–induced endothelial injury, cryoglobulinemia, disseminated intravascular coagulation, fat embolization, and antiglomerular basement membrane disease.[27,28] There is no effective therapy, and graft nephrectomy is necessary.

Accelerated rejection can occur in patients with or without DGF; it refers to rejection episodes occurring 2 to 5 days after transplantation.[23] It is caused by previous sensitization to donor antigens (occult T-cell crossmatch), a positive B-cell crossmatch, or a positive flow cytometry crossmatch in patients who underwent a repeat transplantation.[29] The differential diagnosis includes CI toxicity, thrombotic angiopathy, and urinary tract obstruction. The diagnosis of accelerated rejection is usually established by renal biopsy. The biopsy specimen may show predominantly either cellular rejection or vascular rejection. It is important to make this pathologic distinction because the approach to therapy is different.

EARLY POST-TRANSPLANTATION

The major causes of a decrease in graft function early after transplantation include acute rejection, which is most common, polyoma virus allograft nephropathy (PVAN) CI nephrotoxicity, thrombotic microangiopathy, and urinary tract obstruction or decreased renal perfusion due to effective circulating volume depletion, infection, and recurrent or de novo renal disease.

Approach to Diagnosis

Early allograft dysfunction is typically characterized by a blood creatinine concentration that is stable at an elevated level or is increasing. Unfortunately, the blood creatinine is a rather crude marker of allograft health, lacking sensitivity and specificity for rejection, especially in children.[30] Indeed, there is the growing realization that subclinical rejection exists as an entity that is treatable that affects long-term graft survival.[31] Unless there is evidence suggestive of infection or recurrent disease, the evaluation of such patients is commenced by measuring the plasma CI concentrations (see Fig. 88-1). If the drug level is elevated, the cyclosporine or tacrolimus dose may be decreased. A renal biopsy is performed if no improvement is noted within 1 to 2 days or if the creatinine continues to increase. If, conversely, the CI level is normal or low, a biopsy is performed or empirical pulse steroid therapy may be given with the CI dose adjusted until the level is within the therapeutic range.

Acute Renal Allograft Rejection

Acute renal allograft rejection is defined as an acute deterioration in allograft function associated with specific pathologic changes in the transplant that have been categorized by the Banff consortium described in Figure 88-1.[1,32] The incidence of acute rejection and the time at which it occurs vary with the induction and maintenance therapy protocol used for immunosuppression. Registry data indicate that the incidence of acute rejection has greatly decreased over the past decade and is now consistently less than 20% depending on donor and recipient characteristics and the immunosuppressive protocol.[33] Kidneys that recover function still have a 10% decrease in 1-year survival compared with rejection-free kidneys.[34]

Acute rejection episodes also have a negative impact on long-term graft survival, being a major clinical predictor of chronic allograft nephropathy.[35]

Diagnosis

The presence of acute renal allograft rejection should be suspected in every transplant recipient in whom the creatinine fails to settle or is increasing. Most patients are asymptomatic. Fever and graft pain are rarely encountered unless immunosuppression has been discontinued. Most episodes of acute rejection occur within the first 3 months post-transplantation. Only 8% of patients with functioning grafts have a first episode of rejection after 1 year,[36] often associated with noncompliance with medical therapy or low drug levels.[37] The differential diagnosis includes ongoing acute tubular necrosis, CI nephrotoxicity, and urinary tract obstruction. Obstruction can usually be ruled out by renal ultrasonography. Duplex Doppler ultrasonography, although noninvasive, is not sufficiently sensitive or specific for the diagnosis of acute rejection.[38]

Percutaneous renal allograft biopsy is frequently necessary and may be complicated by macroscopic hematuria, transient anuria due to obstructing blood clots, perirenal hematoma, retroperitoneal hematoma, and rarely traumatic intrarenal arteriovenous fistula or bowel injury.[39] Fine-needle aspiration biopsy[40] has not been widely accepted as a replacement for core biopsy techniques.

Pathology

The 8th Banff Conference on Allograft Pathology held in 2005 represented the latest iteration of the international consensus meeting that develops standards for interpretation of allograft biopsy results.[1] The meeting is generally perceived to be an important force behind the standardization of slide interpretation for use in clinical trials. The current classification of renal allograft biopsy pathology is summarized in Box 88-1.[41–43] The characteristic pathologic changes that occur during acute cellular rejection include interstitial infiltration with mononuclear cells and disruption of the tubular basement membranes.[44] The presence of patchy mononuclear cell infiltrates without tubulitis is not uncommon in normally functioning renal allografts and is not sufficient to make the diagnosis of acute rejection. The presence of neutrophils is uncommon and should suggest the diagnosis of infection. Immunohistologic evaluation of rejecting renal allografts shows an increased number of infiltrating major histocompatibility complex (MHC) class II–positive and interleukin-2 receptor–positive mononuclear cells.[45] Acute vascular rejection, conversely, is characterized pathologically by capillary endothelial swelling, arteriolar fibrinoid necrosis, fibrin thrombi in glomerular capillaries, and frank cortical necrosis in severe cases. Glomerular involvement is associated with a worse prognosis.[44,46]

Antibody-mediated rejection (AMR) has now been incorporated into the Banff schema and is summarized in Table 88-1. To satisfy current diagnostic criteria, three of the four parameters must be present[41]: allograft dysfunction, histology, positive immunofluorescence for C4d, and demonstration of donor-specific antibody. It should be noted that the histology in type 1 AMR is not typically thought of as being associated with rejection (minimal inflammatory infiltrate with microscopic evidence of tubular necrosis). Consequently, all allograft biopsy material should be processed for C4d with an additional search for donor-specific antibody performed as necessary.

Box 88-1 Banff 97 Diagnostic Categories for Renal Allograft Biopsies (2005 Revision)

1. Normal
2. Antibody-mediated rejection
Acute antibody-mediated rejection (C4d$^+$) type
    I. Acute tubular necrosis–like
    II. Capillary margination and/or thrombosis
    III. Arterial

Chronic Active Antibody-Mediated Rejection*
Glomerular double contours, peritubular capillary basement membrane multilayering, interstitial fibrosis, tubular atrophy, fibrous intimal thickening
3. Borderline changes
4. T cell–mediated rejection
Acute
    IA. Significant interstitial infiltration (>25% of parenchyma) and moderate tubulitis
    IB. Significant interstitial infiltration (>25% of parenchyma) and severe tubulitis
    IIA. Mild to moderate intimal arteritis
    IIB. Cases with severe intimal arteritis comprising >25% of the luminal area
    III. Transmural arteritis

Chronic Active T Cell–Mediated Rejection
5. Interstitial fibrosis and tubular atrophy, no evidence of any specific etiology
Grade
    I. Mild (<25% of cortex)
    II. Moderate (26%–50% of cortex)
    III. Severe (>50% of cortex)
6. Other: Categories not considered to be due to rejection; may coincide with categories 2–5.

---

*Changes in the updated Banff 2005 schema
Adapted from Solez K, Colvin RB, Racusen LC, et al: Banff '05 Meeting Report: Differential diagnosis of chronic allograft injury and elimination of chronic allograft nephropathy ('CAN'). Am J Transplant 2007;7:518–526.

Unusual Rejection Variants

Colovai and colleagues[47] reported three cases of hyperacute rejection and AMR of renal allografts in recipients who had received rabbit antithymocyte globulin (thymoglobulin) as induction therapy. A variety of studies failed to reveal either antilymphocytic or antiendothelial cell antibodies either pre- or post-transplantation. However, xenoantibodies that strongly bound to human lymphocytes to activated endothelial cells were identified in the sera obtained at the time of rejection. Campath-1H (alemtuzumab) is a humanized monoclonal antibody against CD52 that is being studied as an induction agent in transplantation. Although rejection rates with alemtuzumab treatment are low, a number of reports describe acute rejection dominated by monocytes.[48–50] Such rejections tend to be steroid sensitive.

Management of Renal Allograft Rejection

Treatment of rejection should be started when the diagnosis is suspected and should not be unduly delayed until the results of the allograft biopsy are available. There are several thera-peutic options available for rejection. The intensity of therapy will largely be dictated by the severity of the rejection episode as well as response to initial therapy (see Table 88-1). In this age of greatly reduced rejection risk, it is useful to investigate the root cause of a rejection episode (Box 88-2). Certainly, from a continuous quality improvement process viewpoint, every rejection should be evaluated to ascertain whether there was a program or patient failure that led to rejection.

Corticosteroids remain one of the cornerstones of most induction, maintenance, and rescue immunosuppressive regimens.[51,52] Steroids are lympholytic when given in high doses (e.g., methylprednisolone 0.5–1g/day given over 3–5 days) and can reverse acute rejection in as many as 75% of cases.[51] After completing the steroid pulse, oral steroids are restarted using the same dose that the patient had been taking. The urine output increases, and the serum creatinine starts decreasing within 3 to 5 days after initiating therapy. The major complication of pulse steroids is increased susceptibility to infection, especially oral candidiasis. Other potential problems include acute hyperglycemia, hypertension, peptic ulcer disease, and psychiatric disturbances including euphoria and depression. Prophylactic antacids/H$_2$ blockers as well as oral antifungal therapy are generally recommended.[53] Steroid resistance is defined as a lack of improvement in urine output or the plasma creatinine concentration within 5 days. In this setting, second-line therapy consists of the administration of tacrolimus and antilymphocyte antibodies, either as rabbit antithymocyte globulin (thymoglobulin) or OKT3.[54–56]

Polyclonal Anti–T Cell Antibodies

Rabbit antithymocyte globulin (thymoglobulin) is prepared by immunizing rabbits with human lymphoid cells derived from cultured B-cell lines. Antithymocyte globulin, a preparation commonly used in Europe, is an equine hyperimmune globulin. Such agents have been used for prophylaxis and first- and second-line therapy of acute rejection. A typical recommended dose for acute rejection is 10 to 15 mg/kg/day for 7 to 10 days. The reversal rate has been between 75% and 100% in different series,[57,58] with the plasma creatinine concentration returning to baseline several days after initiating therapy. Fever and chills develop in a majority of patients during the initial infusion. Anaphylactic reactions, including respiratory distress and hypotension, are rare. To minimize the allergic manifestations, patients are usually pretreated with corticosteroids, antihistamines, and acetaminophen.

OKT3 was the first murine monoclonal antibody licensed for use in humans.[59,60] It is directed against the CD3 antigen causing complex, which is closely associated with the T-cell receptor modulation or clearing of CD3$^+$ T cells.[61] OKT3 has been used as the primary treatment of acute rejection and also as rescue therapy for resistant rejection.[62] The usual dose of OKT3 is 5 mg/day intravenously for 10 to 14 days. As many as 94% of steroid- or ALS-resistant rejections can be expected to reverse with OKT3 treatment.[59] The plasma creatinine concentration typically increases for the first 2 to 3 days of OKT3 therapy and then decreases. OKT3 is also used as primary therapy in patients who have vascular rejection, a process that is generally resistant to steroids.[59] In vitro, OKT3 acts as a T-cell mitogen, and many of the first dose reactions commonly seen are generally thought to be due to initial binding to the CD3 complex, mediating T-cell release of cytokines. These reactions include fever, rigors, nausea, vomiting, diarrhea, hypotension,

Table 88-1   Rejection Rescue Protocol

Rejection (Banff 1997 Classification)		Treatment Options
Borderline Change		Optimize immunosuppressive drug levels
Grade IA	Moderate tubulitis (>4 mononuclear cells in >25% of biopsy sample)	1. Optimize immunosuppressive drug levels
Grade IB	Severe tubulitis (>10 mononuclear cells in >25% of biopsy sample)	2. Consider switch to tacrolimus or myco-phenolate mofetil or sirolimus 3. Adjunctive therapy (statin)
Grade IIA	Mild to moderate arteritis in at least one blood vessel	4. Recycle oral steroids or pulse intravenous steroids
Grade IIB	Severe arteritis (>25% loss of luminal area)	5. If unresponsive: Polyclonal anti–T cell antibody therapy or OKT3
Grade III	Transmural arteritis with fibrinoid necrosis and perivascular inflammation	Optimize immunosuppressive drug levels Switch to tacrolimus OKT3
Antibody-mediated rejection		Optimize immunosuppressive drug levels Switch to tacrolimus OKT3 Therapeutic plasma exchange until donor-specific antibody is removed

chest pain, dyspnea and wheezing, and occasionally frank pulmonary edema.[63] This latter complication is rarely seen unless the patient is volume overloaded, and, thus, patients should be dialyzed or diuresed before OKT3 therapy. Dyspnea may also be related to complement activation and subsequent pulmonary vascular neutrophil sequestration.[64] Antihistamines, acetaminophen, and steroids are usually given before OKT3 to minimize adverse effects, all of which should decrease with repeated exposure. Higher steroid doses should be avoided to prevent a potential increase in the procoagulant effect of OKT3.[65] Other serious complications that can occur after the administration of OKT3 include graft thrombosis[66] and thrombotic microangiopathy.[66] OKT3 can predispose to potentially life-threatening infections, especially those due to cytomegalovirus.[67] Total exposure is an important determinant of risk, with almost 100% of patients experiencing an episode of infection after three courses.[63] There is also evidence that OKT3 may be associated with an increased risk of certain malignancies such as Epstein-Barr virus–related lymphoproliferative disorders.[60] Aseptic meningitis characterized by lymphocytosis and elevated cerebrospinal fluid protein occurs in as many as 5% of patients who receive OKT3 and is usually self-limiting, although differentiation from other causes of infectious meningitis is essential.

Box 88-2   Preventable Causes of Rejection

Inadequate drug: azathioprine
Inadequate dose: failure to aggressively optimize CI or SRL levels in the early post-transplantation period
Noncompliance: failure to take medication
  Youth
  Side effects (especially cosmetic such as weight gain, acne, and hirsutism)
  Drug or alcohol abuse
  Financial
Drug interaction: various drugs can reduce CI and SRL drug levels
  Dilantin
  Phenobarbital
  Rifampin
  St. John's wort

CI, calcineurin inhibitor; SRL, sirolimus.

Recurrent Rejection

Approximately 15% to 20% of transplant patients have recurrent episodes of acute rejection. The success rate of retreatment with OKT3 in this setting is related to its ability to modulate/clear CD3+ T cells.[68] This in turn is determined by two important factors: circulating anti-mouse antibody titers and timing of the rejection episode. Approximately 50% to 60% of patients who receive OKT3 will produce human anti-mouse antibodies,[69] generally in low titers (<1:100). Low antibody titers do not affect the response to retreatment (reversal rate almost 100%) if the rejection episode occurs within 90 days after transplantation. Conversely, titers of more than 1:100 or recurrent rejection beyond 90 days is associated with a reversal rate of less than 25%. The reversal rate is essentially zero when both high human anti-mouse antibodies titers and late rejection are present. OKT3 is also indicated in primarily vascular rejection.[59] It is important to confirm the diagnosis of rejection by renal biopsy before starting antilymphocyte therapy.

Recent uncontrolled trials suggest that tacrolimus may be effective as rescue therapy for refractory rejection. One report, for example, switched 77 patients with biopsy-proven ongoing acute rejection from cyclosporine to tacrolimus.[70] The overall response rate was 74%, with responders having a mean plasma creatinine concentration of 2.35 mg/dL (207 μmol/L) at 14 months. Even dialysis-dependent patients had a 50% response rate. Preliminary data on the role of mycophenolic acid as rescue therapy for biopsy-proven acute rejection revealed a response rate of 69% in patients who failed standard pulse steroid or OKT3. Tacrolimus is currently the dominant CI at the time of discharge from hospital in the United States.[52]

Antibody-Mediated Rejection Therapy

The optimal therapy for antibody-mediated rejection remains to be defined, although an aggressive approach with plasmapheresis and intravenous immunoglobulin to remove donor-specific antibodies is gaining support. In a retrospective study of nine patients with AMR, White and colleagues[71] reported that eight grafts were successfully rescued with mean serum creatinine levels at 3 and 12 months of 1.9 and 1.8 mg/dL, respectively. Another group described a series of seven patients with AMR who received approximately seven plasmapheresis treatments combined with rabbit antithymocyte globulin (thymoglobulin).[72] One graft was lost to rejection. Renal function improved to baseline in the remaining six patients. Lehrich and colleagues[73] described a retrospective analysis of 23 patients with AMR treated with plasmapheresis and intravenous immunoglobulin. Two-year graft survival was numerically worse in patients with AMR versus acute cellular rejection (ACR) (78% vs. 85%), but the difference was not statistically significant.

LATE ACUTE DYSFUNCTION

When acute allograft dysfunction develops more than 3 months after transplantation, the differential diagnosis should include prerenal azotemia due to volume depletion, CI nephrotoxicity, urinary tract infection or obstruction, acute rejection—possibly due to reduction in immunosuppression or noncompliance, recurrent or de novo renal disease, and renal artery stenosis.[74] The risk of late acute rejection is increased in patients who are tapered off cyclosporine[37] or steroids.[75] Bearing in mind that renal transplant recipients rarely achieve a glomerular filtration rate (GFR) exceeding 55/60 mL/min, a creatinine level less than 2 mg/dL represents good, although certainly not normal, renal function. Thus, under circumstances of volume depletion or infection, the creatinine can increase alarmingly quickly and still reflect small decreases in the GFR. Dehydration secondary to diarrhea can occur rapidly on exposure to enteropathogens in immunosuppressed transplant recipients. The principal aim of therapy under these circumstances is to ensure adequate volume and electrolyte replacement and maintain drug levels to prevent intercurrent rejection. Long-term transplant patients who miss several doses of steroids risk adrenal insufficiency.

Polyomavirus Nephropathy

The polyomaviruses that are known to cause disease in humans include BK, JC, and, much less commonly, SV40.[76] It is known that as many as 85% of adults in the general population are seropositive for BK and JC viruses as a consequence of exposure during childhood.[77] By themselves, polyomaviruses tend not to be overtly pathogenic. However, in the setting of immunosuppression, malignancy, or acquired immunodeficiency syndrome, BK virus can cause nephropathy and hemorrhagic cystitis and JC virus can cause progressive multifocal leukoencephalopathy.

BK virus is the dominant pathogen causing polyomavirus nephropathy (PVN), although occasional cases have been reported due to JC and SV40. BK virus generally remains latent in kidney tissue and can induce inflammatory changes when the immune system is suppressed after transplantation. It has generally been assumed that PVN is due to reactivation of recipient disease. More recent data cast doubt on this premise. In a longitudinal study of almost 200 transplant recipients, pretransplant donor and recipient samples were analyzed for BK virus antibody titer and HLA alleles.[78] The donor antibody titer was found to be inversely proportional to onset of viruria, directly proportional to duration of viruria, and directly proportional to peak urine viral titer. Recipient pairs receiving kidneys from the same donor were concordant for BK virus infection and had matched sequences of segments of the defined genes that tend to vary among recipients of kidneys from different donors. All 11 recipients with sustained BK viremia received kidneys from donors lacking HLA C7, and 10 recipients also lacked C7.

The incidence of polyomavirus infection may differ among different organ recipients. For example, in a study of 263 heart, kidney, liver, and pancreas transplant patients, BK virus and JC virus DNAemia were observed most commonly in kidney and/or pancreas transplant patients (26%), although they were also observed, to a lesser extent, in heart (7%) and liver (4%) transplant patients.[79] As many as 8% of kidney transplant recipients will develop PVN with a concomitant risk of graft loss at 1 year ranging from 35% to 65%.[80] PVN has been described rarely in recipients of nonkidney transplants and can cause nephrosis and end-stage renal disease.[76,81,82]

The incidence of PVN seems to be increasing, although it remains unclear whether this observation is related to enhanced recognition or more potent immunosuppression. Currently recognized risk factors include length of time after transplantation, rejection rescue therapy, type of immunosuppression, and co-infection with cytomegalovirus.[83–85] Brennan and colleagues[83] examined 200 adult renal transplant recipients who were randomized to either tacrolimus or CsA. Urine and blood samples were collected at defined intervals for BK polymerase chain reaction. At 1 year, 35% had developed viruria and 11.5% viremia. Viral replication was not affected independently by tacrolimus, cyclosporin A (CsA), mycophenolate mofetil (MMF), or azathioprine, although viruria was highest with tacrolimus/MMF (46%) and lowest with cyclosporin/MMF (13%). After reduction of immunosuppression, viremia resolved in 95%, without increased acute rejection, allograft dysfunction, or graft loss. No BK nephropathy was observed. More recently, a significant association between BK virus nephropathy and HLA mismatching has been suggested.[86] This study also showed that BK virus nephritis was associated with a greater number of rejection episodes and a higher incidence of steroid-resistant rejection requiring antilymphocyte treatment. There was no association between BK virus nephropathy and any specific HLA allele. Active infection starts typically within the first 3 months in 80% of patients.[84] Cold ischemia time that exceeded 24 hours and the administration of tacrolimus were identified as significant risk factors for viruria. The risk of viremia was greatest in patients with viruria (especially when the viral load exceeded 4 log/mL) and those treated with tacrolimus. No relationship was found between the development of nephropathy and genetic variability in the viral sequence.

Diagnosis

Many transplantation programs now routinely screen allograft recipients for polyomavirus infection either by urinary cytology or, more frequently, the more sensitive polymerase chain reaction assay in which viral DNA can be quantified in urine and blood.[78,87,88] A consensus conference was recently held, and the report recommended that all renal transplant recipients should have their urine screened for BK virus replication[89] every 3 months during the first 2 years post-transplantation, when allograft dysfunction is noted, and when an allograft biopsy is performed. It should be noted that polyoma viruria is demonstrable as early as 4 weeks post-transplantation, and some programs initiate screening earlier than 12 weeks post-transplantation. They also recommended that positive screening results should be confirmed and assessed by quantitative assays and that a definitive diagnosis of PVAN requires allograft biopsy. In a simulation model in which patients positive for blood DNA polymerase chain reaction had their immunosuppression reduced, screening saved $1912 and produced 0.02 more quality-adjusted life years than not screening.[88]

The impact of the histologic features on the diagnosis and outcome of PVN was described in 90 patients.[90] Viral cytopathic changes, tubular atrophy (TA) and interstitial fibrosis (IF) as well as inflammation were scored and classified into defined histologic patterns. The histologic findings were correlated with viruria, viremia, and graft survival. PVAN lesions were found to be random and multifocal and affected both cortex and medulla. Areas with PVAN coexisted with areas of unaffected parenchyma. In 36.5% of biopsies with multiple tissue cores, discordant findings with PVAN-positive and -negative cores were observed. However, all patients with PVAN had decoy cells in urine as well as significant viruria and viremia. Biopsy specimens showing lesser degrees of renal scarring at the time of diagnosis were associated with, more likely, resolution of the infection, in response to decrease of immunosuppression. More advanced tubulointerstitial atrophy, active inflammation, and higher creatinine level at diagnosis correlated with a significantly worse graft outcome. Due to the focal nature of PVAN, correlation of biopsy results with viruria and viremia is required for diagnosis.

Treatment

Therapeutic options for established PVN include reducing immunotherapy, conversion to leflunomide, treatment of intercurrent infection, if present, with cidofovir, and retransplantation. It is generally agreed that decreasing immunosuppression is the primary therapy for PVN and alone is effective in reducing viremia and viruria in most cases.[83,91] Leflunomide is an antimetabolite immunosuppressive agent that inhibits pyrimidine synthesis. The drug is licensed for the treatment of rheumatoid arthritis and is known to have antiviral and immunosuppressive properties. Williams and colleagues[80] provided a brief, nonrandomized report of 17 patients with biopsy-proven PVN in whom MMF was stopped and leflunomide commenced initially with a loading dose of 100 mg/day for 5 days

followed by a maintenance dose of 20 to 60 mg/day. Treatment was monitored by serial measurements of viral load as well as that of an active metabolite of leflunomide, A77 1726. This is an important point because leflunomide is P-450 metabolized and has an extremely long half-life All patients who achieved a drug level in excess of 40 μg/mL either cleared or reduced their viral load. Two patients also required cidofovir.

Cidofovir is a monophosphate nucleotide analogue of deoxycycytidine that competitively inhibits viral DNA polymerase. In vitro activity against a number of DNA viruses, including adenovirus, polyomavirus, papillomavirus, and herpesviruses has been demonstrated. Cidofovir also retains activity against thymidine kinase–negative herpes simplex virus and cytomegalovirus that are resistant to acyclovir and ganciclovir. Eighty percent of the drug is excreted unchanged in the urine within 24 hours. However, cidofovir diphosphate is an active metabolite that is eliminated more slowly with first- and second-phase intracellular half-lives of 24 and 65 hours, respectively, permitting the drug to be dosed every 2 weeks. Kuypers and colleagues[92] reported a nonrandomized study of 8 of 21 patients who were treated with weekly adjuvant low-dose cidofovir in addition to reduction of immunosuppressive therapy. PVN caused irreversible deterioration of graft function in all patients, but renal function stabilized after antiviral treatment and no graft loss occurred in cidofovir-treated recipients during 25 months of follow-up. No cidofovir-related renal toxicity occurred. In contrast, 9 of 13 patients who received no adjuvant cidofovir therapy lost their graft after approximately 8 months.

The outcomes of 10 patients from 5 transplantation centers who had lost their primary renal allografts to PVN who underwent retransplantation were described.[93] Repeat transplantation occurred approximately 13 months after failure of the first graft. Allograft nephrectomy had been performed in 7 of the 10 patients. PVAN recurred in one patient 8 months after retransplantation, but stabilization of graft function was achieved with a decrease in immunosuppression and treatment with low-dose cidofovir. After a mean follow-up of 34 months, all patients were found to have good graft function with a mean creatinine level of 1.5 mg/dL. The authors concluded that patients with graft loss caused by PVN can safely undergo retransplantation. Initial results suggesting that ciprofloxacin may be useful in treating PVAN have not been confirmed.

LATE CHRONIC DYSFUNCTION

Many patients have slowly progressive azotemia over a period of years after kidney transplantation. The major etiologic considerations in this setting include chronic rejection, chronic CI nephrotoxicity, hypertensive nephrosclerosis, chronic urinary tract obstruction, and recurrent or de novo renal disease. The use of the nonspecific term chronic allograft nephropathy has now been formally abandoned by the Banff consortium due to concerns that this term "undermines recognition of morphologic features enabling diagnosis of specific causes of chronic graft dysfunction."[1]

Interstitial Fibrosis and Tubular Atrophy

IF/TA, previously referred to as chronic allograft nephropathy, is one of the most common causes of end-stage renal disease, accounting for 20% of kidney transplantations performed in the United States and as many as 30% of patients awaiting renal transplantation.[94] Various terms have been used to describe this condition over time, although the acronym IF/TA is that chosen by the most recent iteration of the Banff consortium. The syndrome is clinically associated with progressive loss of graft function and hypertension with variable degrees of proteinuria. Approximately 2.6% of kidney grafts are lost yearly due to IF/TA.[94,95]

Pathogenesis

The exact mechanisms responsible for the pathogenesis of IF/TA are varied and are summarized in Table 88-2. It has been postulated, however, that chronic graft dysfunction is mediated by both alloantigen-dependent and alloantigen-independent factors.[96,97] Data from experimental models indicate a role for all elements of the immune system, including cell-mediated immune responses (delayed-type hypersensitivity responses mediated by macrophages and CD4$^+$ T cells), humoral alloantibody responses against donor antigens, inflammatory cytokines, fibrogenic growth factors (such as platelet-derived growth factor and transforming growth factor β), and possibly the vasoactive and mitogenic peptide endothelin.

T-cell recognition of alloantigen in the presence of the appropriate costimulatory signal is the central and primary event that initiates the immunologic component of the rejection process that ultimately leads to chronic allograft loss. Such antigen is recognized either directly in the form of intact allo–major histocompatibility complex (MHC) on the surface of donor cells or indirectly in the form of processed peptide(s) that is itself derived from donor MHC presented by recipient antigen-presenting cells. There is increasing interest in this indirect pathway as peptide antigens are relatively simple structures that are readily synthesized.[98] This novel experimental approach permits the investigation of the molecular mechanisms of allograft rejection. Recent evidence indicates that allopeptide-primed T cells are present during both acute and chronic rejection.[99] Although primary immune responses are characterized by T-cell proliferative responses to a limited number of immunogenic MHC allo-

peptides under experimental circumstances, secondary responses, such as those that occur in chronic or late acute rejection, are associated with T-cell proliferative responses to a more variable repertoire.[100] This repertoire includes responses to peptides that were previously immunologically silent. Such a change in the pattern of T-cell responses has been termed epitope switching or spreading and can occur to peptides representing alternative regions within a given MHC β chain hypervariable region (intramolecular spreading) or, alternatively, peptides representing different MHC chains (intermolecular spreading). The precursor frequency of such MHC allopeptide reactive T cells is typically low, as evidenced by studies in humans with chronic renal allograft rejection. However, such a finding is not unexpected given the indolent nature of chronic rejection. Recent studies have provided a link between MHC allopeptide primed T cells and the development of acute vascular type rejection mediated in part by accelerating the production of alloantibodies. Such studies suggest that chronic allograft vasculopathy, the sine qua non of experimental chronic rejection, may also be mediated by T cells primed by the indirect pathway. Additional evidence of the importance of T-cell activation in chronic rejection is provided by experimental observations that inhibiting costimulatory signals such as the CD28:B7 pathway using cytotoxic T lymphocyte antigen 4 immunoglobulin or blockade of the CD40:CD40L pathway can prevent or even interrupt progression of chronic rejection in experimental models of cardiac and renal allograft rejection.[98] The development of the C4d assay in which the complement component gets covalently bound to endothelial structures in response to antibody activity has also cast a new light on immunopathogenesis. For example, glomerular C4d deposits were found in a cohort of 10 of 11 biopsies with IF/TA and in only 2 of 13 controls.[101]

Therapeutic Options for Interstitial Fibrosis and Tubular Atrophy

Despite the frequency of IF/TA as a cause of premature graft failure and the frequency with which clinical research papers are published annually, therapeutic options are limited. Treatment strategies include prevention and management of established disease and are summarized in Box 88-3.

Prevention

Most programs strive to minimize acute rejection rates based on the understanding that either clinical or subclinical rejection is a major risk factor for the development of IF/TA.[35] Data are accumulating that some of the newer immunosuppressive medications currently in clinical practice are associated with a lower incidence of IF/TA compared with older regimens. For example, in a small single-center study, the incidence of biopsy-confirmed IF/TA was 31% in patients treated with MMF compared with 63% in those treated with azathioprine when both groups also received prednisone and cyclosporine.[102] Meier-Kriesche and colleagues[103] performed an analysis of registry data and found that continued therapy with MMF compared with azathioprine was associated with a protective effect against declining renal function at 1 year. Continued therapy with MMF at 2 years was associated with a further reduction in the risk of decreased renal function.

Protocols that avoid the deleterious effects of CI continue to be pursued. Renal function, structure, and gene expression were studied in a prospective, randomized trial that compared a CI-free to CI-based immunosuppressive regimen.[104] Kidney

Table 88-2 Interstitial Fibrosis and Tubular Atrophy: Morphology and Causes of Specific Chronic Renal Allograft Diseases

Etiology	Morphology
Chronic hypertension	Arterial thickening with reduplication of elastica and hyaline arteriosclerosis
Calcineurin inhibitor toxicity	Arteriolar hyalinosis and tubular cell injury with vacuolization
Chronic obstruction	Marked tubular dilatation
Bacterial pyelonephritis	Intratubular neutrophils
Viral infection	Viral inclusions on histology, immunohistochemistry, and electron microscopy

Adapted from Solez K, Colvin RB, Racusen LC, et al: Banff '05 Meeting Report: Differential diagnosis of chronic allograft injury and elimination of chronic allograft nephropathy ('CAN'). Am J Transplant 2007;7:518–526.

Box 88-3 Interstitial Fibrosis and Tubular Atrophy Therapeutic Strategies

Prophylactic Interventions
A. Alloantigen-dependent mechanisms
  Optimize HLA match
  Long term benefit greatest with matching for HLA-A>
    HLA-B>HLA-DR
  Avoidance of sensitization to HLA
  As much as 6% differential in 3-year graft survival in
    patients who are highly sensitized versus nonsensi-
    tized (treated with cyclosporin A)
  Blood transfusion effect
    1-DR matching
    Donor-specific transfusion
  As much as 10% improvement in 3-year graft survival
    in those who did not become sensitized to HLA
  Avoidance of acute rejection
    Mycophenolate mofetil
    Neoral versus cyclosporin A (?)
    Tacrolimus
    Antibody induction therapy
  Impact of newer immunosuppressive agents and anti-
    body induction protocols on chronic graft loss re-
    mains unproven. Tacrolimus can negate impact of
    sensitization on long-term graft loss.
B. Alloantigen-independent mechanisms
  Nephron undersupply
    Donor-recipient age matching
    Donor-recipient weight matching
    Double kidney transplants
  Theoretical benefits from providing adequate nephron
    dose. Optimizing this variable may conflict with
    organ procurement.
  Renal Injury
    Minimize cold ischemia time
    Preservation solution
  Risk of ATN is greatly increased when cold ischemia
    exceeds 24 hours. Risk of CAD increases if ATN is
    complicated by acute rejection.

Therapeutic Interventions
Cytomegalovirus
Potential benefits of antiviral chemotherapy
Hyperfiltration
Potential benefits of preventing/treating hyperfiltration
Hypertension
Calcium channel blockers probably of maximal benefit in
  early posttransplantation period when calcineurin in-
  hibitor dose is highest
Proteinuria
Potential benefit of reducing proteinuria (unproven)
Hyperhomocysteinemia
Potential benefit of reducing homocysteine levels (un-
  proven)
Hyperlipidemia
3-Hydroxy-3-methylglutaryl coenzyme A reductase inhibi-
  tors reduce risk of acute rejection. Unproven benefit in
  preventing coronary artery disease

recipients were treated with basiliximab, MMF, and predni-sone and were randomly assigned to either sirolimus (SRL) or cyclosporine. Renal function as measured by iothalamate GFR was 60 mL/min in the SRL group compared with almost 50 mL/min in the CsA group. Regression analysis of calculated GFRs yielded a positive slope for SRL of 3.36 mL/min per year and a negative slope for CsA of −1.58 mL/min per year. Gene expression profiles from kidneys with higher Banff IF/TA scores confirmed significant up-regulation of the genes responsible for inflammation, fibrosis, and tissue remodeling.

Vincenti and colleagues[105] reported a study in which patients were randomized to either cyclosporine-based immunotherapy or a novel costimulatory blockade molecule, belatacept (LEA29Y). Various animal studies have previously indicated that such a strategy can effectively prevent allograft rejection and in some cases induce tolerance.[98] In this protocol, patients received conventional immunosuppression with basiliximab, MMF, and steroid along with either cyclosporine or two different dosing regimens of belatacept. At 6 months, the incidence of acute rejection was similar among the groups and at 12 months, the GFR was significantly higher in both belatacept groups compared with cyclosporine. Biopsy-confirmed IF/TA was less common in both belatacept groups compared with the cyclosporine group. Lipid levels and blood pressure values were similar or slightly lower in the belatacept groups, despite the greater use of lipid-lowering and antihypertensive medications in the cyclosporine group.

Treatment of Established Interstitial Fibrosis and Tubular Atrophy

The limited therapeutic options for established chronic allograft nephropathy include inhibition of the renin-angiotensin system and altering the immunosuppressive drug strategy. One retrospective European study found that renal allograft outcome was influenced by the relative change in renal function over time, urinary protein excretion, hypertension, and renin-angiotensin system blockade.[106] In this nonrandomized cohort, renal allograft survival after treatment with renin-angiotensin system blockade was significantly longer at 6.3 years as opposed to 1.8 years in untreated patients. It has also been suggested that 3-hydroxy-3-methylglutaryl coenzyme A reductase inhibitor therapy may have an impact on renal allograft survival. Unfortunately, the null hypothesis was supported in a post hoc analysis of the ALERT (Assessment of Lescol in Renal Transplantation) study.[95] More than 2000 renal transplant recipients were randomized to receive either fluvastatin or placebo and followed for as long as 6 years. Although fluvastatin treatment significantly lowered cholesterol, no significant effect on the incidence of renal graft loss or GFR was seen. It should be noted that fluvastatin had no impact on total mortality or graft loss.[107] However, fluvastatin was a safe and effective agent for reducing low-density lipoprotein cholesterol and was associated with a reduced risk of major adverse cardiac events in kidney transplant recipients.

A variety of immunosuppressive strategies for treatment of established IF/TA have been studied over time. Such approaches have included the addition of MMF, withdrawal of CIs, and the addition of SRL.

Most transplantation centers routinely use MMF as part of their standard induction and maintenance immunosuppressive protocol. Nevertheless, a limited number of patients continue to take azathioprine as the antimetabolite component of their immunosuppressive regimen. It has been suggested that such patients may benefit from switching to MMF. In a non-randomized study of renal allograft recipients with biopsy-proven chronic allograft nephropathy, MMF was substituted for azathioprine.[108] At inclusion, each group received 2 g/day of MMF and azathioprine was stopped. Before the introduction of MMF, renal function had been deteriorating progressively. After the introduction of MMF, renal function stabilized and a significant change in the slope of the GFR was observed.

The long-term nephrotoxic potential of both CIs has been well characterized. Although tacrolimus may be less nephrotoxic than cyclosporine, elimination of either drug remains an attractive strategy in patients with established IF/TA who are losing graft function. The withdrawal of a nephrotoxin must be balanced against the risk of rejection and, consequently, CI withdrawal strategies usually employ the introduction of a potent, nonnephrotoxic agent such as MMF or SRL. A prospective, randomized study compared the introduction of MMF with or without CI withdrawal in long-term transplant recipients with histologically proven IF/TA and deteriorating renal function.[109] An interim analysis found a greater than expected difference between groups in terms of renal function deterioration, and the study was stopped prematurely. There were 20 patients in the MMF/CI continuation and 19 patients in the MMF/CI withdrawal groups. Renal function and blood pressure control improved in the dual-therapy compared with the triple-therapy group, and no acute rejections occurred. In a controlled, multicenter study, CsA-treated renal allograft recipients with IF/TA were randomized to have their CsA discontinued with the concomitant addition of MMF to their regimen or to continue treatment with CsA.[110] Fifty-eight percent of patients who had the CsA withdrawn achieved the primary endpoint defined as a stabilization or reduction of serum creatinine, as evidenced by an improvement in slope of the 1/SCr plot and no graft loss compared with 32% of patients who continued CsA. There were no acute rejections in CsA withdrawal group during the study period.

Various studies have indicated that SRL is equally effective as cyclosporine in preventing early allograft rejection. Adverse effects of SRL include edema, thrombocytopenia, hyperlipidemia, and delayed wound healing. The pivotal trials that studied SRL in place of CsA indicated that SRL-treated patients had a significantly higher GFR at the end of the first posttransplantation year. It is now also recognized that SRL is associated with at least some nephrotoxicity as evidenced by prolongation of DGF immediately post-transplantation and the development of long-term proteinuria in some patients. In an analysis of pretransplantation and 1-year renal allograft biopsies of patients enrolled in a multicenter trial, patients who received cyclosporine and SRL during the first 3 months post-transplantation were randomly assigned to continue cyclosporine or have it withdrawn.[111] The proportion of patients in whom chronic pathologic lesions progressed was lower in the cyclosporine elimination group. There was significantly less chronic interstitial and tubular disease, whereas no differences were observed in rejection. In a study of 59 renal transplant patients with IF/TA who were converted to SRL, renal function improved in 54% and deteriorated in 46%.[112] Patient and graft survival rates were 100% and 92%, respectively, at 1 year. In a multivariate analysis, proteinuria less than 800 mg/day was the only independent variable that predicted a favorable outcome.

Calcineurin Inhibitor Nephrotoxicity

The toxic effects of CI therapy can be divided temporally and pathogenically into two discrete categories. Acute nephrotoxicity manifests as azotemia, which is largely reversible after dose reduction and is due predominantly to vasoconstriction. Chronic CI toxicity manifests as irreversibly progressive renal disease and hypertension and is due to fibrogenesis. Most of the literature devoted to the mechanisms of CI nephrotoxicity examines the effects of cyclosporine as opposed to the newer agent tacrolimus. Although it is now generally agreed that tacrolimus is less nephrotoxic compared with cyclosporine, this drug can have a significant impact on kidney function in both the short and long term via mechanisms that are largely presumed to be the same as those of cyclosporine.

Acute Toxicity

Renal transplant patients treated with cyclosporine may develop nephrotoxicity that can manifest in many ways. In addition to azotemia, other renal effects of cyclosporine include tubular dysfunction with concomitant electrolyte and acid base disturbances and rarely thrombotic microangiopathy. A similar pattern of renal injury associated with the use of tacrolimus may be less severe.[113,114] Attention must also be paid to drug dose and to drug interactions to minimize toxicity and maximize efficacy. In the earliest clinical renal transplantation trials using cyclosporine, a high incidence of oliguric acute tubular necrosis and primary nonfunction was observed; the risk was greatest with prolonged ischemia time of the donated kidney before transplantation. Subsequent trials using lower doses of cyclosporine showed that these problems were dose related. Studies in experimental animals have demonstrated that cyclosporine causes vasoconstriction of the afferent and efferent glomerular arterioles and decreases in renal blood flow and GFR. Cyclosporine is not a direct vasoconstrictor, however, and the exact mechanism of vasoconstriction is unclear, but there appears to be substantial impairment of endothelial cell function, leading to decreased production of vasodilators (prostaglandins and nitric oxide) and enhanced release of vasoconstrictors (endothelin and thromboxane).[115–118] Increased sympathetic tone also may be present, although renal vasoconstriction occurs even in denervated kidneys.[119] The increase in renal vascular tone induced by cyclosporine does not attenuate with time. Maintenance cyclosporine therapy is associated with transient reductions in renal plasma flow and GFR, which correlate with both dose and peak cyclosporine levels reached 2 to 4 hours after the oral dose and reverse when reasonable drug levels are attained. Administration of a calcium channel blocker can prevent the renal vasoconstriction.[120,121] This observation constitutes part of the rationale for the use of calcium channel blockers to treat hypertension in cyclosporine-treated transplant recipients. The increase in vascular resistance may be reflected clinically by an elevated plasma creatinine concentration and hypertension. Acute cyclosporine nephrotoxicity is usually reversible with cessation of therapy, as both the plasma creatinine concentration and systemic blood pressure decrease toward baseline values for that patient. The important clinical problem is to differentiate cyclosporine-induced renal dysfunction from acute rejection. The only definitive diagnostic test is biopsy of the renal allograft. Although there are no specific pathologic changes induced acutely by cyclosporine, the absence of cellular or vascular rejection, coupled with tubular damage including vacuolization of the tubular epithelial cells, strongly suggests cyclosporine nephrotoxicity. In addition, the presence of rejection does not exclude concomitant cyclosporine toxicity. Rarely, vascular lesions similar to those seen in the thrombotic microangiopathies are seen. This lesion is idiosyncratic and presumably initiated by cyclosporine-induced injury to the vascular endothelial cells.

Chronic cyclosporine nephrotoxicity manifests as renal insufficiency due to glomerular and vascular disease, abnormalities in tubular function, and an increase in blood pressure. The biopsy specimen reveals an obliterative arteriolopathy, ischemic collapse or scarring of the glomeruli, vacuolization of the tubules, and focal areas of IF/TA.[122] These changes are typically seen with high-dose cyclosporine therapy (>6 mg/kg/day). The factors responsible for chronic cyclosporine nephrotoxicity are not well understood. It has been proposed that the arterial lesions are the primary abnormality, with ischemia being responsible for the tubular and interstitial lesions. However, animal studies have shown that the vascular and interstitial findings can be dissociated. It is now accepted that transforming growth factor β, a cytokine with both potent immunosuppressive and fibrogenic properties, is up-regulated by cyclosporine in an experimental model of chronic cyclosporine nephropathy.[123-125] The development of IF is also associated with increased expression of osteopontin, a potent macrophage chemoattractant, by the tubular epithelial cells.[126] Other evidence that supports an alternative mechanism for cyclosporine toxicity is the observation that administration of either an endothelin A receptor antagonist or calcium channel blocker can prevent hypertension and decreases in renal plasma flow and yet have no impact on the development of arteriolopathy.[127]

Perhaps the best information available to support the hypothesis of chronic cyclosporine nephrotoxicity comes from nonkidney solid organ transplant patients in whom the nephrotoxic potential of cyclosporine can be evaluated in the absence of coexisting acute or chronic renal allograft rejection.[128] During a median follow-up of 36 months, chronic kidney disease developed in 16.5% of almost 70,000 recipients of (nonkidney) solid organ transplants.[128] Almost 30% required maintenance dialysis or renal transplantation. The 5-year risk of chronic renal failure varied according to the type of organ transplanted, from 7% among recipients of heart-lung transplants to 21% among recipients of intestine transplants. Factors associated with an increased risk of chronic kidney disease included increasing age, female sex, hepatitis C infection, hypertension, diabetes mellitus, and postoperative acute kidney injury. The applicability of these findings to renal allografts is uncertain; it has been suggested, for example, that the denervated kidney may be less susceptible to cyclosporine-induced renal injury.[129]

Calcineurin Inhibitor Dosing

There are few studies that clearly define the optimal dose of cyclosporine in renal transplantation. More recently, a number of investigators have focused on tailoring cyclosporine to a 2-hour peak (C2) level as against the traditional 12-hour trough (C0) level.[130-134] Some such studies have indicated that targeting higher peak levels may be associated with delivery of higher doses of cyclosporine in the early posttransplantation period and lower early rejection rates.[130,134] However, C2 monitoring has not been shown to have an impact on patient or

graft survival, and the whole endeavor has been eclipsed by the emergence of tacrolimus as the dominant CI over the past few years.[52] It should also be noted that the introduction of cyclosporine microemulsion preparations in the mid-1990s has had no appreciable impact on patient or graft survival rates.

Tacrolimus is 100 times more potent than cyclosporine on a milligram-per-milligram basis. As such, the starting dose is generally in the range of 0.05 to 0.1 mg/kg twice daily. As the bioavailability of tacrolimus is more predictable than cyclosporine, 12-hour trough levels are deemed sufficient for monitoring.[135] The desired target level within the first 3 months is generally 8 to 15 ng/mL.[136] Thereafter, levels are allowed to run at a lower level.

In view of the utility of calcineurin inhibition in transplantation and autoimmune diseases, there has been a great deal of interest in developing novel therapeutic strategies to minimize their nephrotoxic potential. Animal data and preliminary observations in humans that suggested that fish oil may be beneficial were never confirmed.[137,138] Animal and human data also suggest that concurrent administration of calcium channel blockers may be protective against cyclosporine nephrotoxicity, at least in part by minimizing renal vasoconstriction.[120,121] However, there is at present no proof that these agents increase graft survival. The likely explanation for the inability to demonstrate a long-term benefit with calcium channel blockers in patients treated with cyclosporine is that reversal of renal vasoconstriction, although beneficial, does not affect the concurrent up-regulation of transforming growth factor β, and, therefore, fibrosis can proceed uninterrupted.

RECURRENT AND DE NOVO RENAL DISEASE POST-TRANSPLANTATION

Virtually all primary renal diseases can recur in a kidney transplant with the exception of polycystic kidney disease, hereditary nephritis, and chronic tubulointerstitial nephritis.[139-141] The diagnosis of recurrent glomerular disease post-transplantation depends on an initial complete and accurate histologic evaluation of the primary nephropathy leading to renal failure and the documentation of the same disease in the transplanted kidney. Although disease recurrence is relatively common post-transplantation, the precise incidence is unknown and recurrence accounts for only 2% to 5% of all graft failures.[139,142,143] Clearly, recurrent primary and secondary glomerulonephritides are a cause of concern for patients and their physicians, and there is some evidence to suggest that recipients of living related donor transplants[144] and pediatric recipients are at greater risk. Recurrent glomerular disease in the allograft is the third most common cause of premature graft failure after death with function and chronic allograft nephropathy.[141]

The presence of focal glomerulosclerosis on the transplant biopsy specimen must be distinguished from recurrent disease in those patients in whom primary focal glomerulosclerosis was responsible for the initial renal failure.[139] The onset of proteinuria typically occurs within hours or days in recurrent focal glomerulosclerosis, whereas in the chronic de novo disease, protein excretion does not begin to increase until 3 or more months after transplantation and then increases slowly. Early data indicated that staphylococcal protein A immunoabsorption can induce partial or complete remission in such patients with recurrent disease. More recent reports have focused on the use of plasmapheresis for recurrent focal segmental glomerulosclerosis post-transplantation.[145]

Patients with Alport syndrome can develop antiglomerular basement membrane nephritis post-transplantation.[146,147] These patients lack the α5 chain of type IV collagen and presumably mount a humoral response on receiving an allograft that contains the offending collagen structure. Interestingly, the antibodies produced are directed against the α-3 chain, the reason for which is not known.[148] The frequency with which this complication arises is unclear due to variable reporting; however, it appears to be uncommon. It is more often associated with graft failure in patients who have undergone retransplantation, probably due to previous sensitization to the glomerular basement membrane antigen.

Metabolic diseases that recur include diabetes mellitus, oxalosis, amyloidosis, and, to a lesser extent, cystinosis. There is in these patients clearly a milieu that is not altered per se by renal transplantation. When a patient with diabetes receives a kidney, typical histologic changes generally can be seen within 2 years. The clinical course is variable, however, and progression does not correlate with donor age, human leukocyte antigen match, recipient age, or chronic rejection.[149] Simultaneous pancreas-kidney transplantation may prevent such complications.[150]

Pessimism resulted from early reports of rapid recurrence of oxalosis after renal transplantation alone. However, better results have been achieved more recently.[151] Combined liver and kidney transplantation in this setting, however, may be curative.

References

1. Solez K, Colvin RB, Racusen LC, et al: Banff '05 Meeting Report: Differential diagnosis of chronic allograft injury and elimination of chronic allograft nephropathy ('CAN'). Am J Transplant 2007; 7:518–526.
2. Perico N, Cattaneo D, Sayegh MH, Remuzzi G: Delayed graft function in kidney transplantation. Lancet 2004;364:1814–1827.
3. Lim EC, Terasaki PI (eds): Early Graft Function. Los Angeles: UCLA Tissue Typing Laboratory, 1991.
4. Troppmann C, McBride MA, Baker TJ, Perez RV: Laparoscopic live donor nephrectomy: A risk factor for delayed function and rejection in pediatric kidney recipients? A UNOS analysis. Am J Transplant 2005;5:175–182.
5. Matas AJ, Tellis VA, Quinn TA, et al: Timing of cyclosporine administration in patients with delayed graft function. J Surg Res 1987;43:489–494.
6. Asderakis A, Dyer P, Augustine T, et al: Effect of cold ischemic time and HLA matching in kidneys coming from "young" and "old" donors: Do not leave for tomorrow what you can do tonight. Transplantation 2001;72:674–678.
7. Johnson SR: Donors after cardiac death: Opportunity missed. Transplantation 2005;80:569–570.
8. Howard RJ, Schold JD, Cornell DL: A 10-year analysis of organ donation after cardiac death in the United States. Transplantation 2005;80:564–568.
9. Cooper JT, Chin LT, Krieger NR, et al: Donation after cardiac death: The University of Wisconsin experience with renal transplantation. Am J Transplant 2004;4:1490–1494.
10. Johnston TD, Thacker LR, Jeon H, et al: Sensitivity of expanded-criteria donor kidneys to cold ischaemia time. Clin Transpl 2004;18(Suppl 12):28–32.
11. Matsuoka L, Shah T, Aswad S, et al: Pulsatile perfusion reduces the incidence of delayed graft function in expanded criteria donor kidney transplantation. Am J Transplant 2006;6:1473–1478.
12. Kauffman HM, McBride MA, Cors CS, et al: Early mortality rates in older kidney recipients with comorbid risk factors. Transplantation 2007;83:404–410.
13. Brennan DC, Daller JA, Lake KD, et al: Rabbit antithymocyte globulin versus basiliximab in renal transplantation. N Engl J Med 2006;355:1967–1977.
14. Yokoyama I, Uchida K, Kobayashi T, et al: Effect of prolonged delayed graft function on long-term graft outcome in cadaveric kidney transplantation. Clin Transpl 1994;8:101–106.
15. Sanfilippo F, Vaughn WK, Spees EK, Lucas BA: The detrimental effects of delayed graft function in cadaver donor renal transplantation. Transplantation 1984;38:643–648.
16. Troppmann C, Gillingham KJ, Gruessner RW, et al: Delayed graft function in the absence of rejection has no long-term impact. A study of cadaver kidney recipients with good graft function at 1 year after transplantation. Transplantation 1996;61:1331–1337.
17. Kamar N, Garrigue V, Karras A, et al: Impact of early or delayed cyclosporine on delayed graft function in renal transplant recipients: A randomized, multicenter study. Am J Transplant 2006;6:1042–1048.
18. Quiroga I, Salio M, Koo DD, et al: Expression of MHC class I-related chain B (MICB) molecules on renal transplant biopsies. Transplantation 2006;81:1196–1203.
19. Halloran PF, Schlaut J, Solez K, Srinivasa NS: The significance of the anti-class I response. II. Clinical and pathologic features of renal transplants with anti-class I-like antibody. Transplantation 1992;53:550–555.
20. Schnuelle P, Yard BA, Braun C, et al: Impact of donor dopamine on immediate graft function after kidney transplantation. Am J Transplant 2004;4:419–426.
21. Goggins WC, Pascual MA, Powelson JA, et al: A prospective, randomized, clinical trial of intraoperative versus postoperative thymoglobulin in adult cadaveric renal transplant recipients. Transplantation 2003;76:798–802.
22. Lebranchu Y, Bridoux F, Buchler M, et al: Immunoprophylaxis with basiliximab compared with antithymocyte globulin in renal transplant patients receiving MMF-containing triple therapy. Am J Transplant 2002;2:48–56.
23. Braun WE: The immunobiology of different types of renal allograft rejection. In Milford EL (ed): Renal Transplantation: Contemporary Issues in Nephrology. New York: Churchill Livingstone, 1989, pp 45–64.
24. Carpenter CB, Winn HJ: Hyperacute rejection. N Engl J Med 1969;280:47–48.
25. Kissmeyer-Nielsen F, Olsen S, Petersen VP, Fjeldborg O: Hyperacute rejection of kidney allografts, associated with pre-existing humoral antibodies against donor cells. Lancet 1966;2:662–665.
26. Jordan SC, Yap HK, Sakai RS, et al: Hyperacute allograft rejection mediated by anti-vascular endothelial cell antibodies with a negative monocyte crossmatch. Transplantation 1988;46:585–587.
27. Cross DE, Whittier FC, Cuppage FE, et al: Hyperacute rejection of renal allografts following pulsatile perfusion with a perfusate containing specific antibody (letter). Transplantation 1974;17:626–629.
28. Light JA, Annable C, Perloff LJ, et al: Immune injury from organ preservation. A potential cause of hyperacute rejection in human cadaver kidney transplantation. Transplantation 1975;19:511–516.
29. Scornik JC, LeFor WM, Cicciarelli JC, et al: Hyperacute and acute kidney graft rejection due to antibodies against B cells. Transplantation 1992;54:61–64.
30. Seikku P, Krogerus L, Jalanko H, Holmberg C: Better renal function with enhanced immunosuppression and protocol

biopsies after kidney transplantation in children. Pediatr Transplant 2005;9:754–762.

31. Nickerson P, Jeffery J, Rush D: Long-term allograft surveillance: The role of protocol biopsies. Curr Opin Urol 2001;11:133–137.

32. Racusen LC, Solez K, Colvin RB, et al: The Banff 97 working classification of renal allograft pathology. Kidney Int 1999;55: 713–723.

33. Cecka JM: The UNOS Scientific Renal Transplant Registry. Clin Transpl 1999:1–21.

34. Cecka JM, Terasaki PI: Early rejection episodes. In Terasaki PE (ed): Clinical Transplants. Los Angeles: UCLA Tissue Typing Laboratory, 1989, p 425.

35. Nankivell BJ, Borrows RJ, Fung CL, et al: Natural history, risk factors, and impact of subclinical rejection in kidney transplantation. Transplantation 2004;78:242–249.

36. Burke JF, Pirsch JD, Ramos EL, et al: Long-term efficacy and safety of cyclosporine in renal-transplant recipients. N Engl J Med 1994;331:358–363.

37. Sanders CE, Curtis JJ, Julian BA, et al: Tapering or discontinuing cyclosporine for financial reasons—a single center experience. Am J Kidney Dis 1993;21:9–15.

38. Meyer M, Paushter D, Steinmuller DR: The use of duplex Doppler to evaluate renal allograft dysfunction. Transplantation 1990;50:974–978.

39. Huraib S, Goldberg H, Katz A, et al: Percutaneous needle biopsy of the transplanted kidney: Technique and complications. Am J Kidney Dis 1989;14:13–17.

40. Helderman JH, Hernandez J, Sagalowski A, et al: Confirmation of the utility of fine needle biopsy of the renal allograft. Kidney Int 1988;34:376–381.

41. Racusen LC, Colvin RB, Solez K, et al: Antibody-mediated rejection criteria—an addition to the Banff 97 classification of renal allograft rejection. Am J Transplant 2003;3:708–714.

42. Racusen LC, Halloran PF, Solez K: Banff 2003 meeting report: New diagnostic insights and standards. Am J Transplant 2004;4:1562–1566.

43. Racusen LC: The Banff schema and differential diagnosis of allograft dysfunction. Transplant Proc 2004;36:753–754.

44. Solez K, Axelsen RA, Benediktsson H, et al: International standardization of criteria for the histologic diagnosis of renal allograft rejection: The Banff working classification on renal transplant pathology. Kidney Int 1993;44:411–422.

45. Hancock WW: Analysis of intragraft effector mechanisms associated with human renal allograft rejection: Immunohistological studies using monoclonal antibodies. Immunol Rev 1984;77: 61–84.

46. Salmela KT, von Willebrand EO, Kyllonen LEJ, et al: Acute vascular rejection in kidney transplantation—Diagnosis and outcome. Transplantation 1992;54:858–862.

47. Colovai AI, Vasilescu ER, Foca-Rodi A, et al: Acute and hyperacute humoral rejection in kidney allograft recipients treated with anti-human thymocyte antibodies. Hum Immunol 2005;66: 501–512.

48. Bartosh SM, Knechtle SJ, Sollinger HW: Campath-1H use in pediatric renal transplantation. Am J Transplant 2005;5: 1569–1573.

49. Zhang PL, Malek SK, Prichard JW, et al: Acute cellular rejection predominated by monocytes is a severe form of rejection in human renal recipients with or without Campath-1H (alemtuzumab) induction therapy. Am J Transplant 2005;5: 604–607.

50. Zhang PL, Malek SK, Prichard JW, et al: Monocyte-mediated acute renal rejection after combined treatment with preoperative Campath-1H (alemtuzumab) and postoperative immunosuppression. Ann Clin Lab Sci 2004;34:209–213.

51. Bell PR, Briggs JD, Calman KC, et al: Reversal of acute clinical and experimental organ rejection using large doses of intravenous prednisolone. Lancet 1971;1:876–880.

52. Meier-Kriesche HU, Li S, Gruessner RW, et al: Immunosuppression: Evolution in practice and trends, 1994–2004. Am J Transplant 2006;6:1111–1131.

53. Delmonico FL, Tolkoff-Rubin N: Treatment of acute rejection. In Milford EL (ed): Renal Transplantation: Contemporary Issues in Nephrology. New York: Churchill Livingstone, 1989. pp 129–138.

54. Luke PP, Scantlebury VP, Jordan ML, et al: Reversal of steroid- and anti-lymphocyte antibody-resistant rejection using intravenous immunoglobulin (IVIG) in renal transplant recipients. Transplantation 2001;72:419–422.

55. Midtvedt K, Tafjord AB, Hartmann A, et al: Half dose of OKT3 is efficient in treatment of steroid-resistant renal allograft rejection. Transplantation 1996;62:38–42.

56. Mathew A, Talbot D, Minford EJ, et al: Reversal of steroid-resistant rejection in renal allograft recipients using FK506. Transplantation 1995;60:1182–1184.

57. Gaber LW, Moore LW, Gaber AO, et al: Correlation of histology to clinical rejection reversal: A thymoglobulin multicenter trial report. Kidney Int 1999;55:2415–2422.

58. Khositseth S, Matas A, Cook ME, et al: Thymoglobulin versus ATGAM induction therapy in pediatric kidney transplant recipients: A single-center report. Transplantation 2005;79:958–963.

59. Ortho Multicenter Transplant Study Group: A randomized trial of OKT3 monoclonal antibody for acute rejection of cadaveric renal transplants. N Engl J Med 1985;313:337–342.

60. Swinnen LJ, Costanza-Nordin MR, Fisher SG: Increased incidence of lymphoproliferative disorders after immunosuppression with the monoclonal antibody OKT3 in cardiac transplant recipients. N Engl J Med 1990;323:1723–1728.

61. Schroeder TJ, First MR: Monoclonal antibodies in organ transplantation. Am J Kidney Dis 1994;23:138–147.

62. Norman DJ, Barry JM, Bennett WM, et al: The use of OKT3 in cadaveric renal transplantation for rejection that is unresponsive to conventional anti-rejection therapy. Am J Kidney Dis 1988;11:90–93.

63. Thistlethwaite JRJ, Stuart JK, Mayes JT: Complications and monitoring of OKT3 therapy. Am J Kidney Dis 1988;11:112–119.

64. Raasvekt MHM, Bemelman FJ, Schellekens P, et al: Complement activation during OKT3 treatment: A possible explanation for respiratory side effects. Kidney Int 1993;43:1140–1149.

65. Abramowicz D, Pradier O, De Pauw L, et al: High dose glucocorticoids increase the procoagulant effects of OKT3. Kidney Int 1994;46:1596–1602.

66. Abramowicz D, Pradier O, Marchant A, et al: Induction of thromboses within renal grafts by high-dose prophylactic OKT3. Lancet 1992;339:777–778.

67. Oh CS, Stratta J, Fox RJ: Increased infections associated with the use of OKT3 for the treatment of steroid resistant rejection in renal transplantation. Transplantation 1988;45:68–73.

68. Norman DJ, Shield CF, Henell KR, et al: Effectiveness of a second course of OKT3 monoclonal anti-T cell antibody for treatment of renal allograft rejection. Transplantation. 1988;46: 523–529.

69. Hu H, Aizenstein BD, Puchalski A, et al: Elevation of CXCR3-binding chemokines in urine indicates acute renal-allograft dysfunction. Am J Transplant 2004;4:432–437.

70. Jordan ML, Shapiro R, Vivas SA, et al: FK506 "rescue" for resistant rejection of renal allografts under primary cyclosporine immunosuppression. Transplantation 1994;57:860–865.

71. White NB, Greenstein SM, Cantafio AW, et al: Successful rescue therapy with plasmapheresis and intravenous immunoglobulin for acute humoral renal transplant rejection. Transplantation 2004;78:772–774.

72. Shah A, Nadasdy T, Arend L, et al: Treatment of C4d-positive acute humoral rejection with plasmapheresis and rabbit polyclonal antithymocyte globulin. Transplantation 2004;77: 1399–1405.

73. Lehrich RW, Rocha PN, Reinsmoen N, et al: Intravenous immunoglobulin and plasmapheresis in acute humoral rejection: Experience in renal allograft transplantation. Hum Immunol 2005;66:350–358.

74. Frem GJ, Rennke HG, Sayegh MH: Late renal allograft failure secondary to thrombotic microangiopathy-human immunodeficiency virus nephropathy. J Am Soc Nephrol 1994;4:1643–1648.

75. Hricik DE, Whalen CC, Lautman J, et al: Withdrawal of steroids after renal transplantation—clinical predictors of outcome. Transplantation 1992;53:41–45.

76. Milstone A, Vilchez RA, Geiger X, et al: Polyomavirus simian virus 40 infection associated with nephropathy in a lung-transplant recipient. Transplantation 2004;77:1019–1024.

77. Greene M, Avery R, Preiksaitis JE: BK virus. Am J Transplant 2004;4(Suppl 10):89–91.

78. Bohl DL, Storch GA, Ryschkewitsch C, et al: Donor origin of BK virus in renal transplantation and role of HLA C7 in susceptibility to sustained BK viremia. Am J Transplant 2005;5:2213–2221.

79. Razonable RR, Brown RA, Humar A, et al: A longitudinal molecular surveillance study of human polyomavirus viremia in heart, kidney, liver, and pancreas transplant patients. J Infect Dis 2005;192:1349–1354.

80. Williams JW, Javaid B, Kadambi PV, et al: Leflunomide for polyomavirus type BK nephropathy. N Engl J Med 2005;352:1157–1158.

81. Schmid H, Burg M, Kretzler M, et al: BK virus associated nephropathy in native kidneys of a heart allograft recipient. Am J Transplant 2005;5:1562–1568.

82. Limaye AP, Smith KD, Cook L, et al: Polyomavirus nephropathy in native kidneys of non-renal transplant recipients. Am J Transplant 2005;5:614–620.

83. Brennan DC, Agha I, Bohl DL, et al: Incidence of BK with tacrolimus versus cyclosporine and impact of preemptive immunosuppression reduction. Am J Transplant 2005;5:582–594.

84. Bressollette-Bodin C, Coste-Burel M, Hourmant M, et al: A prospective longitudinal study of BK virus infection in 104 renal transplant recipients. Am J Transplant 2005;5:1926–1933.

85. Toyoda M, Puliyanda DP, Amet N, et al: Co-infection of polyomavirus-BK and cytomegalovirus in renal transplant recipients. Transplantation 2005;80:198–205.

86. Awadalla Y, Randhawa P, Ruppert K, et al: HLA mismatching increases the risk of BK virus nephropathy in renal transplant recipients. Am J Transplant 2004;4:1691–1696.

87. Gai M, Piccoli GB, Motta D, et al: Detecting 'decoy cells' by phase-contrast microscopy. Nephrol Dial Transplant 2004;19:1015–1016.

88. Kiberd BA: Screening to prevent polyoma virus nephropathy: A medical decision analysis. Am J Transplant 2005;5:2410–2416.

89. Hirsch HH, Brennan DC, Drachenberg CB, et al: Polyomavirus-associated nephropathy in renal transplantation: Interdisciplinary analyses and recommendations. Transplantation 2005;79:1277–1286.

90. Drachenberg CB, Papadimitriou JC, Hirsch HH, et al: Histological patterns of polyomavirus nephropathy: Correlation with graft outcome and viral load. Am J Transplant 2004;4:2082–2092.

91. Mannon RB: Polyomavirus nephropathy: What have we learned? Transplantation 2004;77:1313–1318.

92. Kuypers DR, Vandooren AK, Lerut E, et al: Adjuvant low-dose cidofovir therapy for BK polyomavirus interstitial nephritis in renal transplant recipients. Am J Transplant 2005;5:1997–2004.

93. Ramos E, Vincenti F, Lu WX, et al: Retransplantation in patients with graft loss caused by polyoma virus nephropathy. Transplantation 2004;77:131–133.

94. Cecka JM: The UNOS Renal Transplant Registry. Clin Transpl 2002;16:1–20.

95. Fellstrom B, Holdaas H, Jardine AG, et al: Effect of fluvastatin on renal end points in the Assessment of Lescol in Renal Transplant (ALERT) trial. Kidney Int 2004;66:1549–1555.

96. Carpenter CB: Long term failure of renal transplants: Adding insult to injury. Kidney Int 1995;48:S40–S44.

97. Tullius SG, Hancock WW, Heeman U, et al: Reversibility of chronic renal allograft rejection. Critical effects of time after transplantation suggest both host immune dependent and independent phases of progressive injury. Transplantation 1994;58:93–99.

98. Sayegh MH, Turka LA: The role of T-cell costimulatory activation pathways in transplant rejection. N Engl J Med 1998;338:1813–1821.

99. Vella JP, Spadafora-Ferreira M, Murphy B, et al: Indirect allorecognition of major histocompatibility complex allopeptides in human renal transplant recipients with chronic graft dysfunction. Transplantation 1997;64:795–800.

100. Vella JP, Vos L, Carpenter CB, Sayegh MH: Role of indirect allorecognition in experimental late acute rejection. Transplantation 1997;64:1823–1828.

101. Sijpkens YW, Joosten SA, Wong MC, et al: Immunologic risk factors and glomerular C4d deposits in chronic transplant glomerulopathy. Kidney Int 2004;65:2409–2418.

102. Merville P, Berge F, Deminiere C, et al: Lower incidence of chronic allograft nephropathy at 1 year post-transplantation in patients treated with mycophenolate mofetil. Am J Transplant 2004;4:1769–1775.

103. Meier-Kriesche HU, Steffen BJ, Hochberg AM, et al: Mycophenolate mofetil versus azathioprine therapy is associated with a significant protection against long-term renal allograft function deterioration. Transplantation 2003;75:1341–1346.

104. Flechner SM, Kurian SM, Solez K, et al: De novo kidney transplantation without use of calcineurin inhibitors preserves renal structure and function at two years. Am J Transplant 2004;4:1776–1785.

105. Vincenti F, Larsen C, Durrbach A, et al: Costimulation blockade with belatacept in renal transplantation. N Engl J Med 2005;353:770–781.

106. Artz MA, Hilbrands LB, Borm G, et al: Blockade of the renin-angiotensin system increases graft survival in patients with chronic allograft nephropathy. Nephrol Dial Transplant 2004;19:2852–2857.

107. Holdaas H, Fellstrom B, Cole E, et al: Long-term cardiac outcomes in renal transplant recipients receiving fluvastatin: The ALERT extension study. Am J Transplant 2005;5:2929–2936.

108. Gonzalez Molina M, Seron D, Garcia del Moral R, et al: Mycophenolate mofetil reduces deterioration of renal function in patients with chronic allograft nephropathy. A follow-up study by the Spanish Cooperative Study Group of Chronic Allograft Nephropathy. Transplantation 2004;77:215–220.

109. Suwelack B, Gerhardt U, Hohage H: Withdrawal of cyclosporine or tacrolimus after addition of mycophenolate mofetil in patients with chronic allograft nephropathy. Am J Transplant 2004;4:655–662.

110. Dudley C, Pohanka E, Riad H, et al: Mycophenolate mofetil substitution for cyclosporine A in renal transplant recipients with chronic progressive allograft dysfunction: The "creeping creatinine" study. Transplantation 2005;79:466–475.

111. Ruiz JC, Campistol JM, Grinyo JM, et al: Early cyclosporine A withdrawal in kidney-transplant recipients receiving sirolimus prevents progression of chronic pathologic allograft lesions. Transplantation 2004;78:1312–1318.

112. Diekmann F, Budde K, Oppenheimer F, et al: Predictors of success in conversion from calcineurin inhibitor to sirolimus in chronic allograft dysfunction. Am J Transplant 2004;4:1869–1875.

113. Cantarovich D, Renou M, Megnigbeto A, et al: Switching from cyclosporine to tacrolimus in patients with chronic transplant dysfunction or cyclosporine-induced adverse events. Transplantation 2005;79:72–78.

114. Artz MA, Boots JM, Ligtenberg G, et al: Conversion from cyclosporine to tacrolimus improves quality-of-life indices, renal

graft function and cardiovascular risk profile. Am J Transplant 2004;4:937–945.

115. Bunchman TE, Brookshire CA: Cyclosporine-induced synthesis of endothelin by cultured human endothelial cells. J Clin Invest 1991;88:310–314.

116. Fogo A, Hakim RC, Sugiura M, et al: Severe endothelial injury in a renal transplant patient receiving cyclosporine. Transplantation 1990;49:1190–1192.

117. Smith JR, Kubacki VB, Rakhit A, et al: Chronic thromboxane synthesis inhibition with CGS 12970 in human cyclosporine nephrotoxicity. Transplantation 1993;56:1422.

118. Lanese DM, Falk SA, Conger JD: Sequential agonist activation and site-specific mediation of acute cyclosporine constriction in rat renal arterioles. Transplantation 1994;58:1371–1378.

119. Scherrer U, Vissing SF, Morgan BJ, et al: Cyclosporine-induced sympathetic activation and hypertension after heart transplantation. N Engl J Med 1990;323:693–699.

120. Ruggenenti P, Perico N, Mosconi L, et al: Calcium channel blockers protect transplant patients from cyclosporine-induced daily renal hypoperfusion. Kidney Int 1993;43:706–711.

121. Palmer BF, Davidson I, Sagalowsky A, et al: Improved outcome of cadaveric renal transplantation due to calcium channel blockers. Transplantation 1991;52:640–645.

122. Solez K: International standardization of criteria for histologic diagnosis of chronic rejection in renal allografts. Clin Transpl 1994;8:345–350.

123. Shihab FS, Andoh TF, Tanner AM, et al: Role of transforming growth factor-beta 1 in experimental chronic cyclosporine nephropathy. Kidney Int 1996;50:45–53.

124. Shehata M, Cope GH, Johnson TS, et al: Cyclosporine enhances the expression of TGF-beta in the juxtaglomerular cells of the rat kidney. Kidney Int 1996;49:1141–1151.

125. Khanna A, Li B, Stenzel KH, Suthanthiran M: Regulation of new DNA synthesis in mammalian cells by cyclosporine. Demonstration of a transforming growth factor beta-dependent mechanism of inhibition of cell growth. Transplantation 1994;57:1727–1731.

126. Pichler RH, Franceschini N, Young BA, et al: Pathogenesis of cyclosporine nephropathy: Roles of angiotensin II and osteopontin. J Am Soc Nephrol 1995;6:1186–1196.

127. Lanese DM, Conger JD: Effects of endothelin receptor antagonist on cyclosporine-induced vasoconstriction in isolated rat renal arterioles. J Clin Invest 1993;91:2144–2149.

128. Ojo AO, Held PJ, Port FK, et al: Chronic renal failure after transplantation of a nonrenal organ. N Engl J Med 2003;349:931–940.

129. Elzinga LW, Rosen S, Burdmann EA, et al: The role of renal sympathetic nerves in experimental chronic cyclosporine nephropathy. Transplantation 2000;69:2149–2153.

130. Thervet E, Pfeffer P, Scolari MP, et al: Clinical outcomes during the first three months posttransplant in renal allograft recipients managed by C2 monitoring of cyclosporine microemulsion. Transplantation 2003;76:903–908.

131. Levy G, Villamil F, Samuel D, et al: Results of lis2t, a multicenter, randomized study comparing cyclosporine microemulsion with C2 monitoring and tacrolimus with C0 monitoring in de novo liver transplantation. Transplantation 2004;77:1632–1638.

132. Holt DW: Cyclosporin monitoring based on C2 sampling. Transplantation 2002;73:840–841.

133. Hardinger KL, Schnitzler MA, Koch MJ, et al: Cyclosporine minimization and cost reduction in renal transplant recipients receiving a C2-monitored, cyclosporine-based quadruple immunosuppressive regimen. Transplantation 2004;78:1198–1203.

134. Birsan T, Loinig C, Bodingbauer M, et al: Comparison between C0 and C2 monitoring in de novo renal transplant recipients: Retrospective analysis of a single-center experience. Transplantation 2004;78:1787–1791.

135. Gruessner RW, Burke GW, Stratta R, et al: A multicenter analysis of the first experience with FK506 for induction and rescue therapy after pancreas transplantation. Transplantation 1996;61:261–273.

136. Ciancio G, Burke GW, Gaynor JJ, et al: A randomized trial of three renal transplant induction antibodies: Early comparison of tacrolimus, mycophenolate mofetil, and steroid dosing, and newer immune-monitoring. Transplantation 2005;80:457–465.

137. Homan van der Heide JJ, Bilo HJ, Donker JM, et al: Effects of dietary fish oil on renal function and rejection in cyclosporine-treated recipients of renal transplants. N Engl J Med 1993;329:769–773.

138. Kooijmans-Coutinho MF, Rischen-Vos J, Hermans J, et al: Dietary fish oil in renal transplant recipients treated with cyclosporin-A: No beneficial effects shown. J Am Soc Nephrol 1996;7:513–518.

139. Ramos EL, Tisher CC: Recurrent diseases in the renal transplant. Am J Kidney Dis 1994;24:142–154.

140. Hariharan S, Johnson CP, Bresnahan BA, et al: Improved graft survival after renal transplantation in the United States, 1988 to 1996. N Engl J Med 2000;342:605–612.

141. Briganti EM, Russ GR, McNeil JJ, et al: Risk of renal allograft loss from recurrent glomerulonephritis. N Engl J Med 2002;347:103–109.

142. Mathew TH: Recurrence of disease following renal transplantation. Am J Kidney Dis 1988;12:85–96.

143. Dantal J, Giral M, Hoormant M, Soulillou JP: Glomerulonephritis recurrence after kidney transplantation. Curr Opin Nephrol Hypertens 1995;4:146–154.

144. Michielsen P: Recurrence of the original disease. Does it influence renal graft failure. Kidney Int 1995;52(Suppl):S79–S84.

145. Ohta T, Kawaguchi H, Hattori M, et al: Effect of pre-and postoperative plasmapheresis on posttransplant recurrence of focal segmental glomerulosclerosis in children. Transplantation 2001;71:628–633.

146. Kalluri R, Weber M, Netzer KO, et al: COL4A5 gene deletion and production of post-transplant anti-alpha 3(IV) collagen alloantibodies in Alport syndrome. Kidney Int 1994;45:721–726.

147. Brainwood D, Kashtan C, Gubler MC, Turner AN: Targets of alloantibodies in Alport anti-glomerular basement membrane disease after renal transplantation. Kidney Int 1998;53:762–766.

148. Kalluri R, van den Heuvel LP, Smeets HJ, et al: A COL4A3 gene mutation and post-transplant anti-alpha 3(IV) collagen alloantibodies in Alport syndrome. Kidney Int 1995;47:1199–1204.

149. Mauer SM, Goetz FC, McHugh LE, et al: Long-term study of normal kidneys transplanted into patients with type I diabetes. Diabetes 1989;38:516–523.

150. Bilous RW, Mauer SM, Sutherland DE, et al: The effects of pancreas transplantation on the glomerular structure of renal allografts in patients with insulin-dependent diabetes. N Engl J Med 1989;321:80–85.

151. Broyer M, Brunner FP, Brynger H, et al: Kidney transplantation in primary oxalosis: Data from the EDTA registry. Nephrol Dial Transplant 1990;5:332–336.

Further Reading

Bennett W, Vella JP: NephSAP transplantation. J Am Soc Nephrol 2005;44(1).

Koch MJ, Brennan DC. Acute renal allograft rejection: Treatment. Waltham, MA: UpToDate.

Vella JP, Danovitch GD: NephSAP transplantation. J Am Soc Nephrol 2008;7.

Vella JP, Danovitch GD: NephSAP transplantation. J Am Soc Nephrol 2006;5.

Vella JP, Koch MJ, Brennan DC: Acute renal allograft rejection: Diagnosis. Waltham, MA: UpToDate.

Chapter 89

Cardiovascular and Other Noninfectious Complications after Renal Transplantation in Adults

William E. Braun

CHAPTER CONTENTS

Recommendations for outpatient surveillance of renal transplant recipients have been provided by the Clinical Practice Guidelines Committee of the American Society of Transplantation.[1] Three useful points should be kept in mind when prescribing medications for renal transplant recipients. First, because most renal transplant recipients have renal function at stage 3 chronic kidney disease (CKD) (i.e., glomerular filtration rate [GFR] 30–59 mL/min), dosage adjustments will be necessary for many medications (see Chapter 91). Second, because cyclosporine, tacrolimus, and sirolimus are metabolized by the cytochrome P450 3A4 (CYP3A4) pathway, and many other drugs share this pathway, their various drug interactions need to be considered[2] (see the section on Hyperlipidemia in this chapter). Third, tablet splitting should not be used for special formulations such as enteric-coated and unscored extended release tablets, nor for certain combination tablets (e.g., amoxicillin/clavulanicacid, irbesartan/hydrochorthiazide, ezetimibe/simvastatin).[3]

CARDIOVASCULAR DISEASE

Cardiovascular disease (CVD; see also Chapter 70) remains the leading cause of mortality in recipients of renal allografts, and its proportion of total deaths in these patients has increased. Moreover, CVD accounts for 36% of patients dying with a functioning graft in the first 10 years after transplantation. By 15 years after renal transplantation, approximately 23% of patients develop coronary heart disease (CHD), 15% develop cerebrovascular disease, and 15% develop peripheral arterial disease.[1] "The annual risk of a fatal or nonfatal CVD event of 3.5% to 5% in renal transplant recipients is 50-fold higher than in the general population."[4]

Coronary Heart Disease

The annual mortality from CHD in renal transplant recipients age 25 to 34 years is equivalent to mortality from CHD in those age 45 to 54 years in the general population; CHD mortality for renal transplant recipients age 45 to 54 years is comparable to that of those age 55 to 64 years in the general population, with mortality rates converging at age 75 to 84 years.[5] When compared with CHD in renal transplant recipients before 1986, the relative risk of CHD decreased to 0.60 between 1986 and 1992, and even further, to 0.27, after 1992.[6] Moreover, in patients who suffered an acute myocardial infarction (MI) between 1990 and 1996, compared with those who suffered an acute MI between 1977 and 1984, there has been a 51% reduction in the risk of cardiac mortality.[7]

Three important new themes in CHD have recently emerged. (1) Patients in high-risk and very high-risk categories for CHD (this could apply to many renal transplant recipients) had a low-density lipoprotein cholesterol (LDL-C) goal set at less than 70 mg/dL as a therapeutic option (Treating to New Targets, TNT study)[8,9]; based on a meta-analysis of studies in nontransplant patients with either stable CHD or acute coronary syndrome, a 16% to 22% event reduction can be expected.[8,10] (2) In patients with stable CHD, percutaneous coronary intervention, when added to optimal medical therapy, did not reduce the risk of death, MI, or other major cardiovascular events.[11] (3) In 40,450 patients with established CHD, those who had not undergone either percutaneous coronary intervention or coronary artery bypass graft (CABG) and were dependent on medical therapy only, were the *least* likely to be receiving evidence-based therapies.[12]

The management of CHD can be directed at two levels: medical treatment of CHD risk factors and diagnosis of CHD, and medical and interventional treatment of established CHD.

Level I: Medical Treatment of CHD Risk Factors and Diagnosis of CHD

Posttransplantation risk factors for CHD may be classified as not modifiable, difficult-to-modify, in transition, and modifiable (Box 89-1).[6] In one major study, hypertension and LDL-C could no longer be identified as CHD risk factors, apparently because of intensive treatment.[13] Applying the Framingham Heart Study CHD Risk Score (Framingham Risk Score) to renal transplant recipients tends to underestimate the risks, especially for diabetics.[6,14] CHD risk factors in renal transplant recipients, when compared with those in the nontransplant population, include risks specific to transplantation (e.g., acute rejection, use of certain immunosuppressants [see Box 89-1], pretransplant splenectomy), risks disproportionately accentuated by transplantation (e.g., diabetes mellitus, age, cigarette smoking),[6] risks of similar magnitude (e.g., male gender, hypertension, decreased high-density lipoprotein cholesterol [HDL-C] and high LDL-C), risks related to CKD and proteinuria, and risks that may reflect another process (e.g., hypoalbu-minemia reflecting increased interleukin-1 and interleukin-6 inflammatory activity).[6,13,15–19] A recent study of 643 patients with a bone mineral density (BMD) T-score of −1.0 or less quantitated the known risk that created for CHD.[20] Overall, patients with a BMD T-score of −1.0 or lower had a 43% greater hazard of CHD compared to those with normal BMD (see Box 89-1).

Risk Assessment

The first step in risk management is risk assessment. The 10-year risk for developing CHD can be assessed by a risk scoring system that expands the original three major risk categories for CHD— high risk (10-year risk > 20% mortality); moderately high risk (10-year risk 10%–20%); moderate risk (<10% risk)—by adding two new groups: *very high risk* and *lower risk*.[9, 21] The new designation of a *very* high-risk patient includes the following criteria: the presence of established CVD plus (1) multiple major risk factors (especially diabetes mellitus); (2) severe and poorly controlled risk factors (especially cigarette smoking); (3) multiple risk factors of the metabolic syndrome (especially high triglycerides ≥ 200 mg/dL plus non-HDL-C ≥130 mg/dL with low HDL-C < 40 mg/dL); and (4) patients with acute coronary syndrome.[9]

Box 89-1   Posttransplantation Risk Factors* for Coronary Heart Disease

Not Modifiable	**In Transition**[†]
Increasing age[‡,§]	Each acute rejection[‡,§] (↓)
Male gender[‡,§]	Prednisone dose[‡,"] (↓)
Pretransplantation CHD	Cyclosporine dose[‖] (↓)
Atherosclerotic disease	Tacrolimus dose[‖] (↑)
• In carotid arteries[‡,§]	Sirolimus dose[‖] (↑)
• In peripheral vessels[‡,§]	Hyperuricemia** (↑)
Plaque burden in coronary arteries	Hyperparathyroidism (↑)
Pretransplantation diabetes mellitus[‡,§]	Osteoporosis[††] (↑)
Family history of premature CHD	Hyperhomocysteinemia[‡‡] (↓)
Pretransplantation splenectomy[‡]	
	Modifiable
Difficult-to-Modify	Hypertension[¶]
Smoking[‡]	Elevated total cholesterol[§]
Excess weight	LDL-C ≥ 130 mg/dL[¶]
Sedentary lifestyle	Left ventricular hypertrophy
HDL-C (each 10 mg/dL)[‡]	
Lipoprotein (a)	
Stages 3–5 CKD proteinuria	

*Not all risk factors have been subjected to analysis.
[†]Arrow indicates direction of change based on frequency of occurrence (acute rejection), trends to treatment minimization or avoidance (prednisone, cyclosporine), trends to increased use (tacrolimus, sirolimus), and evolving evidence that hyperuricemia, hyperparathyroidism, and osteoporosis are, and hyperhomocysteinemia is not, likely to be significant coronary risk factors.
[‡]Independent risk factor for post-transplantation CHD identified by multivariate analysis.
[§]Risk factor for posttransplantation CHD identified by discriminate analysis. (Kasiske BL, Chakkera HA, Roel J: Explained and unexplained ischemic heart disease risk after renal transplantation. J Am Soc Nephrol 2000;11:1735–1743.)
[¶]These traditional risk factors did not appear in some analyses presumably because they were aggressively treated.
["]Although each of these immunosuppressants has not been subjected to specific analysis as a coronary risk factor, they may be considered risk factors because each has potential significant risk(s) for provoking known coronary risk factors: prednisone (hypertension, hypercholesterolemia, diabetes); cyclosporine (hypertension, hypercholesterolemia, diabetes); tacrolimus (hypertension, diabetes); sirolimus (hypercholesterolemia and more frequent rejection).
**From Nakagawa T, Kang DH, Feig D, et al: Unearthing uric acid: An ancient factor with recently found significance in renal and cardiovascular disease. Kidney Int 2006;69:1722–1725.
[††]From From AM, Hyder JA, Kearns AM, et al: Relationship between low bone mineral density and exercise-induced myocardial ischemia. Mayo Clin Proc 2007;82:679–685.
[‡‡]From Winkelmayer WC, Kramar R, Curhan GC, et al. Fasting plasma total homocysteine levels and mortality and allograft loss in kidney transplant recipients: A prospective study. J Am Soc Nephrol 2005;16:255–260 and Winkelmayer WC: Cardiovascular risk in adult kidney transplant patients. Nephrol Rounds 2007;5:1–6.

The diagnosis of CHD is usually based on a description of angina pectoris or MI, but many patients have atypical pain; those with diabetes mellitus often are asymptomatic. Clinical suspicion and use of the expanded Framingham Risk Score will often lead the clinician to consider stress imaging. Imaging stress testing is usually either nuclear-based (assessing perfusion) or echo-based (assessing myocardial contractility); each of these may use either exercise or pharmacologic stressors (i.e., dipyridamole, adenosine, or dobutamine). From a practical point of view, dipyridamole and adenosine stress tests are not heart-rate dependent. Screening for CHD by electron beam computed tomography and coronary calcium scoring remains unproved.[22, 23] Although plaque burden is a coronary risk factor[24] and coronary calcium scoring reflects plaque,[25] calcified plaques are relatively stable.[26] The threshold for performing coronary arteriography rests with the interventional cardiologist, but generally it is based on the presence of ischemic symptoms or evocable ischemia.

Hypertension

Hypertension is a well-established risk factor for CHD (see Chapters 58 and 59).

Hyperlipidemia

Hyperlipidemia occurs in 50% to 80% of renal transplant recipients treated with prednisone and calcineurin inhibitors. It usually consists of elevated LDL-C, apolipoprotein B, triglycerides (particularly when sirolimus is used), and very low-density lipoproteins; and low, normal, or even slightly elevated serum HDL-C levels.[27–29] Elevated LDL-C levels have been identified as a risk factor for cardiovascular disease in several, but not all, studies, probably because of treatment effects.[13,30] Glucocorticoids, cyclosporine, and sirolimus promote hyperlipidemia.[28,31] Severe hypercholesterolemia and hypertriglyceridemia were 3 to 4 times more frequent with sirolimus than with cyclosporine and were maximal after approximately 2 months of therapy.[32] The Framingham Risk Score has been used to estimate that sirolimus in doses of 2 or 5 mg/day would cause an increased incidence of two or three new cases of CHD per thousand renal transplant recipients per year, respectively.[32,33] Hypercholesterolemia tends to improve within the first 6 to 12 months after transplantation, when prednisone and cyclosporine, sirolimus, or tacrolimus doses are being tapered, as may hypertriglyceridemia when sirolimus and prednisone doses are decreased. Nevertheless, significant persistent hyperlipidemia warrants treatment (Table 89-1).

It is important to consider secondary causes of dyslipidemias: for hypercholesterolemia these include hypothyroidism, nephrotic syndrome, obstructive liver disease, and use of prednisone, cyclosporine, and sirolimus; for hypertriglyceridemia these include diabetes mellitus, chronic excessive alcohol consumption, prednisone, and sirolimus. Other drugs that can cause dyslipidemias include anticonvulsants, isotretinoin, β-blockers, diuretics, androgens/anabolic steroids, oral contraceptives, and highly active antiretroviral agents.[31]

Lowering LDL-C is achieved by therapeutic lifestyle changes and drug therapy (see also Chapter 63).[31]

Drug therapy includes statins, ezetimibe, bile acid sequestrants, nicotinic acid, fibric acid derivatives, and omega-3-acid ethyl esters. A complete description of lipid-lowering agents, their mechanisms of action, and side effects is given in Chapter 63. However, their use in renal transplant recipients often requires modification because of impaired renal func-

tion and the use of certain immunosuppressants. Cyclosporine can cause significant blood level elevations of those statins metabolized by the CYP3A4 pathway (i.e., atorvastatin, lovastatin, and simvastatin), as well as pravastatin, metabolized in the liver by sulfation, and rosuvastatin, metabolized by the CYP2C9 pathway.[31,34] Cyclosporine may not raise the level of fluvastatin, which has multiple metabolic pathways, including CYP2C9.[31,34,35] Ingestion of food increases the bioavailability of lovastatin.[36] Cyclosporine levels can be increased by pravastatin, simvastatin and, to a minor degree, by atorvastatin.[34,36] Recommended daily statin doses need to be adjusted for the level of renal function and certain immunosuppressants (Table 89-2).[31] "It is recommended that the maximum doses of statins be reduced in patients receiving either cyclosporine or tacrolimus. The effects of sirolimus on statins are unknown."[31] It has not been established that the addition of coenzyme Q10 to statin treatment reduces its potential for causing myopathy.[37] The phosphate binder sevelamer binds bile acids and can lower LDL-C.[38]

The only prospective, randomized, controlled trial of statin therapy in renal transplant recipients is the Assessment of LEscol in Renal Transplantation (ALERT) study, which compared 40 to 80 mg/day of fluvastatin with placebo in 2102 cyclosporine-treated stable recipients followed for 5 to 6 years.[39] The primary endpoint of a composite of cardiac death, definite or probable MI, and coronary revascularization was reduced 17% by fluvastatin.[39] Although the difference in this endpoint did not achieve statistical significance, a post hoc analysis using cardiac death or definite nonfatal MI did show a significant decrease with fluvastatin from 104 to 70 events ($P = .005$).[40] In a study of 12 cyclosporine-treated patients with elevated LDL-C levels, atorvastatin was more effective in reducing LDL-C than was a change from cyclosporine to tacrolimus, although a combination of atorvastatin and a change to tacrolimus had the greatest effect.[41] Reviews of 13 statin trials in renal transplant recipients, including the ALERT study, confirmed in 6 of 7 studies their benefit in reducing cardiac events, but in 3 of the largest and most recent studies, there was no evidence that they reduced acute rejection.[42–44] Additional benefits of statins include a reduction in the level of circulating endothelin 1; decreases in systolic, diastolic, and pulse pressure[45]; reduced CRP and reduction of acute primary coronary events[46]; and antiproliferative[47,48] and immunomodulatory effects.[42]

Patients should be monitored every 3 to 6 months, or as clinically indicated, with alanine aminotransferase (ALT) levels for hepatic toxicity and creatine kinase (CK) enzymes for muscle toxicity (although dose-related myopathy can occur with or without CK elevation),[49] and at more frequent intervals with serum creatinine and blood levels of the immunosuppressants that can be affected by statins.[31,34] Proteinuria was associated with the use of 80 mg of rosuvastatin, a dose no longer marketed.[50] The possibility that proteinuria is actually a statin-class effect with a renal tubular mechanism involving blocked endocytosis by megalin and cubilin has been analyzed in meta-analyses[51,52] and will be further elucidated in ongoing trials.[53]

Ezetimibe was used as additional therapy for 18 renal transplant patients receiving cyclosporine ($N = 11$), tacrolimus ($N = 6$), or sirolimus ($N = 1$) plus 7.5 prednisone, and whose LDL-C levels were uncontrolled by high-dose statin therapy (80 mg fluvastatin in 14, 40 mg fluvastatin in 1, 40 mg pravastatin in 2, 80 mg simvastatin in 1).[54] LDL-C levels were reduced from 178 ± 41 mg/dL to 117 ± 40 mg/dL after 3 months of additional ezetimibe 10 mg daily. There were no significant changes

Table 89-1   Adult Treatment Panel III Low-density Lipoprotein Cholesterol (LDL-C) Goals and Cutpoints for Therapeutic Lifestyle Changes (TLC) and Drug Therapy in Different Risk Categories and Proposed Modifications Based on Recent Clinical Trial Evidence

Risk Category	LDL-C Goal	Initiate TLC	Consider Drug Therapy*
Very high risk: (10-yr risk >20% plus other features) (see text)	<100 mg/dL (optional goal: <70 mg/dL[†])	≥70 mg/dL	≥70 mg/dL
High risk: CHD[‡,¶] or CHD risk equivalents[§] (10-yr risk > 20%)	<100 mg/dL (optional goal: <70 mg/dL)[†,§]	≥100 mg/dL[¶]	>100 mg/dL[‖] (<100 mg/dL: consider drug options)*
Moderately high risk: 2+ risk factors** (10-yr risk 10%–20%)[††]	<130 mg/dL[‡‡]	≥130 mg/dL[¶]	≥130 mg/dl (100–129 mg/dL: consider drug options)[§§]
Moderate risk: 2+ risk factors** (10-yr risk < 10%)[‡‡]	<130 mg/dL	≥130 mg/dL	≥160 mg/dL
Lower risk: 0–1 risk factors[¶¶]	<160 mg/dL	≥160 mg/dL	≥190 mg/dL (160–189 mg/dL: LDL-lowering drug optional)

*When LDL-lowering drug therapy is employed, it is advised that intensity of therapy be sufficient to achieve at least a 30%–40% reduction in LDL-C levels.

†Very high risk favors the optional LDL-C goal of < 70 mg/dL, and in patients with high triglycerides, non-HDL-C < 100 mg/dL (see Risk Assessment in this chapter). However, there are increased risks with this approach, which is not universally accepted (Hayward RA, Hofer TP, Vijan S: Narrative review: Lack of evidence for recommended low-density lipoprotein treatment targets: A solvable problem. Ann Intern Med 2006;145:520–530; Grundy SM: Promise of low-density lipoprotein-lowering therapy for primary and secondary prevention. Circulation 2008;117:569–573.

‡CHD includes history of myocardial infarction, unstable or stable angina, coronary artery procedures (angioplasty, stenting, or bypass surgery), or evidence of clinically significant myocardial ischemia.

§CHD risk-equivalents include clinical manifestations of noncoronary forms of atherosclerotic disease (peripheral arterial disease, abdominal aortic aneurysm, and carotid artery disease [transient ischemic attacks or stroke of carotid origin or > 50% obstruction of a carotid artery]), diabetes, and 2+ risk factors with 10-year risk for hard CHD > 20%.

¶Any person at high risk or moderately high risk who has a lifestyle-related risk factor (e.g., obesity, physical inactivity, elevated triglyceride levels, low HDL-C, or metabolic syndrome) is a candidate for TLC to modify these risk factors regardless of LDL-C level.

‖If baseline LDL-C is < 100 mg/dL, institution of an LDL-lowering drug is a therapeutic option on the basis of available clinical trial results. If a high-risk person has high triglycerides or low HDL-C, combining a fibrate or nicotinic acid with an LDL-lowering drug can be considered.

**Risk factors include cigarette smoking, hypertension (BP ≥ 140/90 mm Hg or on antihypertensive medication), low HDL-C (<40 mg/dL), family history of premature CHD (CHD in male first-degree relative < 55 years of age; CHD in female first-degree relative < 65 years of age), and age (men ≥ 45 years; women ≥ 55 years).

††Electronic 10-year risk calculators are available at www.nhlbi.nih.gov/guidelines/cholesterol.

‡‡Optional LDL-C goal is < 100 mg/dL.

§§For moderately high-risk persons, when LDL-C level is 100–129 mg/dL, at baseline or on TLC, initiation of an LDL-lowering drug to achieve an LDL-C level < 100 mg/dL is a therapeutic option on the basis of available clinical trial results.

¶¶Almost all people with 0 or 1 risk factor have a 10-year risk < 10%, and 10-year risk assessment in people with 0 or 1 risk factor is thus not necessary.

Modified from Grundy SM, Cleeman JI, Merz CN, et al: Implications of recent clinical trials for the National Cholesterol Education Program Adult Treatment Panel III guidelines. Circulation 2004;110:227–239.

in cyclosporine or tacrolimus blood levels or in liver or muscle enzymes, although two patients stopped treatment because of nausea and muscle pain without CK enzyme elevation.[54] In the Canadian experience with nontransplant patients, some taking ezetimibe without a statin did develop rhabdomyolysis.[55] The use of the combination drug ezetimibe/simvastatin has been reported in nontransplant patients, and there are indications of a higher frequency of adverse effects.[56]

Hypertriglyceridemia, when associated with sirolimus, may diminish as the dosage of sirolimus declines, but treatment may be necessary for severe elevations (see Chapter 63). The use of fibric acid analogs (e.g., gemfibrozil, bezafibrate, fenofibrate, and ciprofibrate) or nicotinic acid may be indicated. Bezafibrate, fenofibrate, and ciprofibrate may increase serum creatinine in cyclosporine-treated patients, and fenofi-

brate and bezafibrate may increase plasma homocysteine.[27,57] Fibric acid analogs should be avoided in those with severe renal disease or severe hepatic disease, and the dose should be reduced in patients with impaired renal function.[27,31] The use of omega-3-acid ethyl esters has not been tested in renal transplant recipients, but in nontransplant patients loses of 3 to 12 g daily can decrease fasting triglycerides by 20% to 50% and do not interact with statins to cause rhabdomyolysis.[58,59]

Combined lipid abnormalities characterized by both high LDL-C and triglyceride levels are more difficult and riskier to treat. Statins can reduce triglycerides modestly,[59] but the addition of a second agent may be necessary. Under such circumstances, very close clinical and laboratory follow-up are warranted. Pharmacologic approaches to raising HDL-C as a means to reduce cardiovascular risk and disease are just emerging.[60]

Table 89-2 Modification of Statin Doses According to Glomerular Filtration Rate (GFR) and Cyclosporine Use

Statin	LEVEL OF GFR (mL/min/1.73 m²)		
	≥30	<30 or Dialysis	With Cyclosporine
Atorvastatin	10–80 mg	10–80 mg	10–40 mg
Fluvastatin	20–80 mg	10–40 mg	10–40 mg
Lovastatin	20–80 mg	10–40 mg	10–40 mg
Pravastatin	20–40 mg	20–40 mg	20–40 mg
Simvastatin	20–80 mg	10–40 mg	10–40 mg

Most manufacturers recommend once-daily dosing, but consider giving 50% of the maximum dose twice daily.
Adapted from Executive summary of the third report of the National Cholesterol Education Program (NCEP) Expert Panel on Detection, Evaluation, and Treatment of High Blood Cholesterol in Adults (Adult Treatment Panel III). JAMA 2001;285:2486–2497, and Kasiske B, Cosio FG, Beto J, et al: Clinical practice guidelines for managing dyslipidemias in kidney transplant patients: A report from the Managing Dyslipidemias in Chronic Kidney Disease Work Group of the National Kidney Foundation Kidney Disease Outcomes Quality Initiative. Am J Transplant 2004;4(Suppl 7):13–53.

Transplant-Associated Hyperglycemia: New-Onset Diabetes Mellitus and Prediabetic Conditions

Current criteria from the American Diabetes Association (ADA) classify patients with a fasting plasma glucose of ≥126 mg/dL as having diabetes, and those with values between 100 and 125 mg/dL as having impaired fasting glucose.[61] When a 2-hour 75-g oral glucose tolerance test is used, a 2-hour plasma glucose level greater than 200 mg/dL represents diabetes, and a 2-hour level between 140 and 200 mg/dL defines impaired glucose tolerance.[61] Because varying criteria were used for the diagnosis of new-onset diabetes mellitus (NDOM), its frequency within the first year after transplantation was reported to be from 4% to 20%.[62] In subsequent studies diabetes occurred at a 6% annual rate while patients were on the waiting list for a deceased donor kidney transplant, increased to 14% to 16% as NODM in the first year after transplant, and then settled at an annual incidence of 4% to 6%, so that the cumulative incidence of NODM 3 years after transplantation was 24%.[63-65] In addition to patients with overt NODM, approximately a third to a half of the others have either impaired fasting glucose or impaired glucose tolerance 1 year after transplantation.[65-67] Impaired fasting glucose and insulin resistance are components of a cluster of CVD risk factors designated the *metabolic syndrome* that also includes triglycerides greater than 150 mg/dL, HDL-C less than 40 mg/dL, blood pressure greater than 130/80 mm Hg, and obesity.[21]

Risk factors for NODM include most of the major immunosuppressants (glucocorticoids, tacrolimus, cyclosporine, and sirolimus, but not mycophenolate mofetil or azathioprine), excess weight, age older than 45 years, male gender, African-American and Hispanic race, family history of diabetes mellitus, hepatitis C, possibly cytomegalovirus, and autosomal dominant polycystic kidney disease (ADPKD).[63,65,68-70] Acute rejection episodes, which are often treated with high-dose IV

methylprednisolone and conversion to tacrolimus, also raise the risk of NODM.[65]

Complications of NODM are essentially the same as those seen in patients with pretransplant diabetes mellitus.[71] At least 10 cases of de novo diabetic nephropathy evolving from NODM have been reported, with a time from onset to histologic diabetic nephropathy of approximately 6 years, similar to that with recurrent diabetic nephropathy.[72,73]

A recent expert opinion recommends that "a 75-g 2-hour oral glucose tolerance be performed at 3 to 6 months after transplantation and annually thereafter in all kidney recipients without diabetes. Testing should be repeated in all patients who meet diabetic criteria to confirm a diagnosis of NODM. NODM should be treated with medical nutrition therapy and, as required, by drug therapy to target American Diabetes Association–defined glycemic goals for patients with diabetes: fasting plasma glucose 90 to 130 mg/dL, 2-hour postprandial glucose less than 180 mg/dL, and glycosylated hemoglobin (HbA$_{1C}$ less than 7%."[61,65,74]

Patients with new-onset diabetes mellitus require diabetes education and diet instruction. They should monitor their glycemic control with a home glucose diary; have their HbA$_{1C}$ levels checked every 3 months; have annual ophthalmologic evaluations, regular foot care, and regular evaluation of complications from a variety of neuropathies (i.e., autonomic neuropathy with orthostatic hypotension, peripheral neuropathy, gastroenteropathy, bladder dysfunction, neuropathic bone disease); and receive appropriate periodic cardiovascular evaluation of the coronary arteries, carotid arteries, and peripheral vascular system.[61,71]

Because of the dramatic increase in new drugs with new mechanisms of action that now constitute nine classes of antidiabetes medications for treating diabetes, patients with NODM are usually best managed by collaborative care with an endocrinologist or diabetologist.[75] However, lifestyle changes can achieve a 58% risk reduction for diabetes in patients at high risk for the disease.[76,77] The nine classes of antidiabetes classes are insulin, sulfonylureas (oral), biguanides/metformin (oral), alpha-glycosidase inhibitors (oral), thiazolidinediones (TZDs; rosiglitazone and pioglitazone; oral), meglitinides/glinides (nateglinide, repaglinide; oral), glucagon-like peptides (GLP analogs; exenatide; parenteral), amylin analogs (pramlintide; parenteral), and dipeptidyl peptidase-IV (DPP-IV) inhibitors (sitagliptin; oral).[75] Selection of NODM treatment and dosing will be influenced by the level of renal function, which may fluctuate; intermittent courses of IV methylprednisolone; use of drugs, including immunosuppressants, that share metabolism by the CYP3A4 pathway; and compromised cardiopulmonary situations that may not permit the fluid retention often seen with TZDs. The four commonly used groups of oral agents have been sulfonylureas (glipizide and glyburide), biguanides (metformin), TZDs (pioglitazone and rosiglitazone), and meglitinides/glinides (repaglinide and nateglinide).[75] A consensus algorithm for initiation and adjustment of therapy has recently been published, but it was developed before the availability of DPP-IV inhibitors.[78] Various combinations of these drugs also are available, and dose modification or avoidance is required according to the more hazardous component. Sulfonylureas, which act by stimulating insulin, cannot be used for type 1 diabetes mellitus; they are renally excreted and should generally be avoided with significant allograft dysfunction because of the risk of protracted hypoglycemia. Biguanides act by decreasing hepatic glucose production and increasing muscle glucose uptake and utilization, may aid in avoiding further weight gain, and are usually titrated from doses of 500 mg up to a maximum of 2000 mg; they are contraindicated with either transient renal insufficiency or fixed elevations of the serum creatinine or impaired liver function. TZDs are agonists for peroxisome proliferator-activated receptor-gamma receptors in target tissues for insulin action, such as adipose tissue, skeletal muscle, and liver, an effect that translates into enhanced sensitivity to insulin. An interim analysis of 4437 nontransplant type 2 diabetic patients (RECORD study) confirmed rosiglitazone's risk for congestive heart failure and had insufficient data to determine whether there was an increased risk of MI,[79] a provocative finding reported in a recent meta-analysis.[80] Durability of therapy is an important consideration in medication selection. In A Diabetes Outcome Progression Trial (ADOPT), which evaluated rosiglitazone, metformin, and glyburide as initial treatment for recently diagnosed type 2 diabetes mellitus in 4360 patients treated for a median of 4 years, the cumulative incidence of monotherapy failure at 5 years was 34% with glyburide, 21% with metformin, and only 15% with rosiglitazone.[81] In studies done before concerns were raised about an increased risk of myocardial infarction,[80] rosiglitazone had been used with apparent safety and efficacy for NODM after renal transplantation and did not appear to have any significant effect on calcineurin dosing.[65,82] However, concerns do exist about its risk for MI based on a recent meta-analysis.[80,83] Meglitinides/glinides that act by stimulating insulin secretion cannot be used for type 1 diabetic patients, are dosed 15 minutes before each meal, and appear to have less of a hypoglycemic potential than sulfonylureas. Nateglinide is metabolized by several pathways, including CYP3A4, which is involved in the metabolism of cyclosporine, tacrolimus, and sirolimus. Because approximately 75% of the administered dose appears in the urine within 6 hours, the dose effect should be monitored in patients with impaired renal function. In a single study of NODM after renal transplantation, repaglinide was reported to be safe and efficacious.[84] The newest drugs that either mimic, and thereby compensate for deficient production of the incretin hormone glucagon-like peptide-1 (GLP-1) in type 2 diabetic patients (e.g., the GLP analog exenatide), or limit proteolysis of native GLP-1 (e.g., the DPP-IV inhibitor sitagliptin) have not been evaluated in renal transplant recipients.[75,85–87] A recent review of oral medications for type 2 diabetes in nontransplant patients concluded, "Compared with newer, more expensive agents (thiazolidinediones, α-glucosidase inhibitors, and meglitinides), older agents (second-generation sulfonylureas and metformin) have similar or superior effects on glycemic control, lipids, and other intermediate endpoints.[88] Insulin therapy is an alterative for treating NODM. Insulin analogues in both long-acting (glargine, detemir) and short-acting (lispro, aspart, and glulisine) forms have a reduced risk for hypoglycemia compared to older formulations.

The transplant nephrologist needs to carefully evaluate the medications being used because of the potential for adverse effects that include edema and congestive heart failure (the TZD derivatives pioglitazone and rosiglitazone), possible risk for MI[80] and fractures in women[81] (rosiglitazone), higher blood levels of drugs because of decreased renal function (insulin, metformin, sulfonylurea derivatives, exenatide, and sitagliptin), lactic acidosis (metformin), competitive metabolism by CYP3A4 (the meglitinides repaglinide and nateglinide to a lesser extent and the DPP-IV inhibitor sitagliptin), and the effect of hepatic insufficiency on drug metabolism. Control of the edema associated with TZDs has been more effectively accomplished with spironolactone or thiazide diuretics than it has with furosemide.[89]

In 1994, a 5-year, randomized, controlled clinical trial of kidney transplant recipients who had type 1 diabetes mellitus as their original disease compared standard insulin therapy with optimized glycemic control.[90] The standard therapy group had more than a twofold increase in the volume of the mesangial matrix per glomerulus, a threefold increase in arteriolar hyalinosis, and greater thickening of the glomerular basement membrane. In this early study that did not have currently available insulin formulations, severe hypoglycemic episodes were more frequent in the optimized group. Very recently, it has been shown that "in at-risk patients with type 2 diabetes, intensive intervention with multiple drug combinations and behavior modification has sustained beneficial effects with respect to vascular complications and on rates of death from any cause and from cardiovascular causes."[94]

Ancillary but possibly important contributors to glucose control are statins and drugs that block the renin-angiotensin system, both angiotensin-converting enzyme (ACE) inhibitors and angiotensin receptor blockers. Statins increase insulin sensitivity; in a retrospective study of 300 Canadian renal transplant recipients, statins were associated with a 70% decrease in the occurrence of NODM.[65,91] There is suggestive evidence from studies in nontransplant patients that blockade of the renin-angiotensin system may be associated with a reduction in the occurrence of diabetes.[65,92–94] The avoidance or withdrawal of diabetogenic immunosuppressants is discussed in Chapter 87. It is worthwhile to note that "trials that reduce one drug often improve the effects of that drug, but not graft and patient survival."[95]

Cigarette Smoking

In a study of 1334 transplant recipients, 24.7% of whom smoked, the relative risk for a major cardiovascular event was 1.56 for those smoking 11 to 25 pack-years at transplant and 2.14 for those smoking for more than 25 pack-years ($P < .001$).[96] For smokers, the relative risk of invasive malignancy was 1.91 and of death with a functioning graft 1.42. Adverse renal hemodynamic effects, coagulation alterations, and endothelial injury result from smoking and are particularly injurious in diabetic patients.[97,98] Cigarette smoking is also an independent risk factor for type 2 diabetes mellitus.[99]

There are basically three ways in which smoking cessation may be achieved: self-motivated spontaneous cessation, counseling and behavioral therapies, and pharmacotherapies.[100] One or more of these should be offered to every smoker. It has been estimated that approximately 50 million Americans have stopped smoking, 95% of whom have stopped of their own accord.[100,101] Individuals who stop smoking typically experience physical withdrawal symptoms, which peak in 2 to 4 days and generally disappear in 10 to 14 days. Even years later, many individuals will continue to experience the periodic desire to smoke. Smoking even a single cigarette in response to these urges can frequently lead to an extended relapse. When conducted by a psychologist or physician experienced in smoking cessation therapy the next most effective methods after spontaneous cessation are behavior-oriented programs.[100]

Pharmacologic aids to smoking cessation include nicotine replacement therapy (gum, lozenge, transdermal patch, nasal spray, and inhaler), bupropion, and varenicline.[100–112] Recommended dosage schedules for transdermal nicotine patches are widely available. If patients continue to smoke while using nicotine replacement therapy, there is an increased risk of adverse effects and higher peak nicotine levels. Up to 23% of patients using nicotine replacement therapy complain of sleep disturbances; nausea is also common, as is skin irritation with transdermal patches.

Bupropion's mechanism for smoking cessation is unknown. Under the brand name Zyban, bupropion is approved by the U.S. Food and Drug Administration (FDA) for smoking cessation with a prescription, but under the brand name Wellbutrin, bupropion is FDA-approved for the management of depression. Because bupropion takes 5 to 8 days to reach steady-state concentrations, patients must select a quit date for smoking.[105] The initial dose of bupropion is usually 150 mg orally for several days that may be followed by an increase to 150 mg twice daily for a total treatment period of 7 to 12 weeks. Bupropion 150 mg each morning for 9 weeks, when compared with a nicotine patch alone, a combination of the nicotine patch and bupropion, or placebo, resulted in abstinence rates after 1 year of 30.3%, 16.4%, 35.5%, and 15.6%, respectively, clearly indicating greater success with combination therapy that included bupropion or bupropion alone.[103] Sustained-release bupropion reduced the relapse rate and weight gain after smoking cessation.[104] Bupropion appears to be metabolized in the liver by enzyme systems other than CYP3A4 (which is involved in the metabolism of cyclosporine, tacrolimus, and sirolimus). Bupropion has not been studied in patients with renal insufficiency, but dose reduction may be needed in these patients. Adverse effects of bupropion include seizure and other neurological symptoms (insomnia [21%], headache, abnormal dreams, dizziness, disturbed concentration), dry mouth, and nausea. Contraindications include seizure disorder, prior or current bulimia or anorexia nervosa, and monoamine oxidase inhibitor use.

Varenicline has a dual effect in smoking cessation because it binds to the $\alpha_4\beta_2$ neuronal nicotinic acetylcholine receptors and acts as an agonist to enhance dopamine release and curb nicotine withdrawal; it also prevents the binding of nicotine to these receptors.[105–110] Because varenicline does not reach steady state for 4 days, patients must have a quit date, just as with bupropion. Varenicline doses begin with 0.5 mg once daily on days 1 to 3, 0.5 mg twice daily on days 4 to 7, and 1 mg twice daily from day 8 to the end of treatment, which is usually 12 weeks. In a randomized, double-blind, parallel-group, placebo-controlled trial that compared varenicline titrated to 1 mg bid ($N = 352$), sustained-release bupropion titrated to 150 mg bid ($N = 329$), or placebo ($N = 344$) orally for 12 weeks, continuous abstinence rates from weeks 9 to 12 (the primary endpoint) were 44%, 29.5%, and 17.7%, respectively.[108] However, continuous abstinence rates for these same three groups for weeks 9 to 52 fell to 29.9%, 16.1%, and 8.4%, respectively. At 1 year varenicline was not superior to sustained-release bupropion.[106,108] However, in a study of relapse after quitting, addition of another 12 weeks of varenicline versus placebo in those who were abstinent at week 12 in-

creased the continuous abstinence rates to 43.6% versus 36.9% at week 52, respectively ($P = 0.02$). Weight gain in the two groups was comparable.[110] Serious neuropsychiatric symptoms including agitation, depression, and suicidal behavior have been reported with varenicline. Other adverse effects from varenicline with greater than 5% frequency include nausea (28%), sleep disturbance, constipation, vomiting, frequent arthralgia, diarrhea, chest pain, edema, polyuria, psychiatric disturbances, flushing, and abnormal liver function tests. Varenicline must be used with caution in patients with impaired renal function and creatinine clearances less than 50 mL/min because blood levels increase by 1.5- to 2.1-fold. Varenicline's place in therapy is still evolving, but "it might prove to be particularly appropriate for those in whom other therapies have failed."[106] Multicomponent behavior-oriented programs can improve the long-term cessation rates of pharmacologic therapies.[102,111]

Level II: Medical and Interventional Treatment of Established CHD

Four evidence-based medical therapies have been proven to decrease morbidity and mortality in nonrenal transplant patients with documented CHD.[12,113] These are antiplatelet agents (aspirin, adenosine diphosphate receptor antagonists, or dipyridamole), β-blockers, inhibitors of the renin-angiotensin system, and statins or certain other lipid-lowering agents. Compliance with recommendations for medical therapy was evaluated in 40,450 patients from the REduction of Atherothrombosis for Continued Health (REACH) International Registry who had documented CHD (previous MI, percutaneous coronary intervention, CABG, or angina pectoris), approximately 33% having had previous CABG, 33% percutaneous coronary intervention, and 33% no revascularization.[12] When compared to those who had no intervention and were medically managed, the groups who had previous CABG (usually older, male, and diabetic) or percutaneous coronary intervention (usually younger) were significantly more likely to be receiving antiplatelet therapy (79% vs. 86% and 91%, respectively), a lipid-lowering agent (70% vs. 86% and 86%, respectively), or a β-blocker (55% vs. 64% and 66%, respectively). The use of ACE inhibitors and angiotensin II receptor blockers was comparable in the three groups (50% vs. 48% and 46%, respectively, for ACE inhibitors; and 19% vs. 21% and 21%, respectively, for angiotensin receptor blockers). These data clearly indicate that "those patients with CHD managed only with medications appear to be receiving the *fewest* evidence-based pharmacologic treatments."[12] To paraphrase Shakespeare, "the fault, . . . is not in our stars, but in ourselves. . ." (Julius Caesar, Act I, Scene II). In the TNT study of 10,001 patients with clinically evident CHD and LDL-C less than 130 mg/dL who were randomly assigned to receive either 80 mg or 10 mg of atorvastatin, a primary event (CHD death, nonfatal nonprocedure-related MI, resuscitation after cardiac arrest, or fatal or nonfatal stroke) occurred in 8.7% of those receiving the 80-mg dose vs. 10.9% of those given a 10-mg dose, a 22% relative reduction in risk ($P < .001$).[8] Persistent elevation of liver enzymes was seen in 0.2% of those receiving 10 mg atorvastatin versus 1.2% of those on 80 mg atorvastatin.[8] Among 15,603 nontransplant patients in the Clopidogrel for High Atheroembolic Risk and Ischemia Stabilization, Management and Avoidance (CHARISMA) study) who had either clinically evident CVD or multiple risk factors and received either 75 mg clopidogrel plus low-dose aspirin (75–162 mg) daily or placebo plus low-dose aspirin, there was no significantly greater effect with clopidogrel plus aspirin than with aspirin alone in reducing MI, stroke, or death from CVD over 28 months.[114] However, in the CREDO study of 2116 higher-risk cardiac patients, long-term (1 year) clopidogrel plus aspirin versus placebo plus aspirin was associated with a 26.9% relative reduction in the combined risk of death, MI, or stroke ($P = .02$).[115]

Experimental and clinical data suggest that at least part of the benefit of renin-angiotensin-aldosterone system blockers and statins is related to their additional secondary antiproliferative or antifibrotic effects. ACE inhibitors block transforming growth factor-β-mediated extracellular matrix protein synthesis by fibroblasts,[116] and angiotensin receptor blockers shunt angiotensin II to binding sites on AT_2 receptors that inhibit endothelial cell proliferation.[117] Spironolactone (25 mg/day) reduced morbidity and mortality in patients with severe congestive heart failure who were also receiving ACE inhibitors, probably because it reduced myocardial and vascular fibrosis.[118] Careful attention to spironolactone dosing, concurrent medications, and level of renal function should permit its safe use in some patients without serious hyperkalemia.[119] Statins can block the proliferative effect of epidermal growth factor,[48] have an antihypertensive effect,[120] and have no clearly defined benefit for osteoporosis.[121]

Coronary artery stenting (CAS) using drug-eluting stents (DES) (sirolimus or paclitaxel) has decreased restenosis from approximately 15% to 6% (9 events per 100 patients) whereas the risk of thrombosis has increased from 0.2% to 0.4% (2 events per 1000 patients).[122–125] Prolonged use of clopidogrel has improved the outlook.[126] In an observational study from the Duke Heart Center, patients with DES who were event-free at 6 months and received clopidogrel ($N = 637$), when compared to those not receiving clopidogrel ($N = 579$), had significantly lower death rates (2.0% vs. 5.3%) and death or MI (3.1% vs. 7.2%) at 24 months.[126] Among patients who had bare metal stents, clopidogrel was beneficial for the first 3 to 6 months but not beyond.

In a 25-year single-institution experience examining outcome after CABG among 2989 renal transplant recipients, 83 required myocardial revascularization (percutaneous transluminal coronary angioplasty [PTCA] or CABG) before or after renal transplantation.[127] None of the 45 patients revascularized after transplantation experienced allograft loss or significant change in renal function. Survival rates of the 45 patients were 93%, 78%, and 60% at 1, 3, and 5 years, respectively.[127] Early-phase risk factors for death included hypertension and revascularization carried out before 1989. Late-phase risk factors for death included diabetes mellitus, a greater number of pre-CABG myocardial infarctions, renal transplantation before 1984, older age, and unstable angina before CABG. These authors concluded that coronary angiography, PTCA, and CABG are safe in patients with functioning renal allografts.[127] In another series of 31 patients who received CABG after renal transplantation, there was one early postoperative death and two episodes of renal transplant dysfunction.[128] A retrospective U.S. Renal Data System (USRDS) database search from 1995 to 1998 identified 912 patients who were hospitalized for CABG, 613 hospitalized for PTCA, and 626 for PTCA/CAS.[129] In-hospital deaths were 4.9% for CABG, 4.2% for PTCA, and 2.2% for CAS. At 3 years, event-free survival from combined cardiac endpoints (cardiac death and acute MI) was 88.9% for

CABG, 84.8% for CAS, and 80.2% for PTCA.[129] After comorbidity adjustment, renal transplant patients in the United States have similar 3-year survival after PTCA, CAS, and CABG (75.8%, 78.9%, and 77.0%, respectively), but fewer serious cardiac events after CABG.

Cerebrovascular Disease

A duplex ultrasound or imaging study of the carotid arteries should be performed if a decreased carotid arterial pulse, a bruit over the carotid artery, or a neurological syndrome consistent with carotid artery disease is present. A systematic review and meta-analysis involving more than 90,000 nontransplant patients that examined the effect of statins on incident strokes concluded that statin use was associated with a 21% reduction for stroke and no increase in hemorrhagic stroke; for every 10% reduction in LDL-C a 15.6% decrease in all strokes and 0.73% decrease in carotid intima-media thickness was seen.[130] However, in 69 nontransplant patients (CKD $N = 38$; CHD $N = 31$) there was no significant reduction in carotid intima-media thickness after 2 years in the CKD group despite lowering LDL-C to 70 ± 27 mg/dL with atorvastatin 80 mg/day.[131] Recently a randomized, double-blind, placebo-controlled study (Measuring Effects on intimal-media Thickness: an Evaluation Of Rosuvastatin [METEOR]) of 984 nontransplant patients with an average age of 57 years and Framingham Risk Score less than 10% demonstrated that rosuvastatin 40 mg, when compared to placebo, significantly reduced carotid intima-media thickness over 2 years.[132]

If carotid artery stenosis 80% or larger (but not total occlusion) is detected in asymptomatic patients, intervention should be considered.[133] In the Asymptomatic Carotid Atherosclerosis Study (ACAS), the estimated incidence of ipsilateral strokes within 5 years and perioperative strokes or death within 30 to 42 days of randomization was reduced with surgical intervention by 66% in men and by 17% in women.[133]

As secondary prevention, in the Stroke Prevention by Aggressive Reduction in Cholesterol Levels (SPARCL) study of 4731 nontransplant patients, 80 mg of atorvastatin, initiated within 6 months of a stroke or transient ischemic episode, significantly reduced recurrent stroke by 16% and fatal stroke by 43% when compared to placebo.[134] Although atorvastatin decreased ischemic strokes significantly more than placebo (218 vs. 274), with a 5-year 3.5% absolute reduction in risk of a major cardiovascular event, atorvastatin was associated with a nonsignificant increased frequency of hemorrhagic strokes (55 vs. 33). Overall mortality rate was similar in the two groups, but elevated liver enzyme values were more common in those taking atorvastatin. The SPARCL results differed somewhat from those of the Heart Protection Study (HPS), in which 40 mg of simvastatin or placebo was used.[135] Patients with preexisting cerebrovascular disease in the HPS study ($N = 3280$ adults) had no significant reduction in stroke rate. A major protocol difference in the HPS study was that patients were enrolled an average of 4.3 years after the index event, a period well after the highest risk of stroke recurrence.[136] However, in the HPS study there was a significant reduction in the first event rate for stroke, from 5.7% to 4.3%, a 28% reduction in presumed ischemic strokes with no apparent difference in hemorrhagic strokes.[135] Data are conflicting as to whether low cholesterol levels represent a risk for hemorrhagic stroke.[137–140] The combined use of intensive LDL-C-lowering and antiplatelet drugs has not been specifically studied for either primary or secondary prevention, and not in transplant recipients. The combination of these two treatment modalities might be hazardous because of the suggestion of an increase in hemorrhagic strokes in one study with high-dose statin therapy.[134]

The choice of endarterectomy over stenting has become clearer.[141–143] Both a review of five randomized trials that compared stenting to endarterectomy[141] and a recent Endarterectomy Vs. Angioplasty in Patients with Symptomatic Severe Carotid Stenosis (EVA-3S) study support using carotid endarterectomy as the standard treatment because of lower rates of death and stroke at 1 and 6 months when compared to stenting: 3.9% versus 9.6%, and 6.1% versus 11.7%, respectively.[142] Expert commentary on these findings stated: "the only widely accepted indication for carotid artery stenting remains its use in symptomatic patients who have stenosis of the internal carotid artery exceeding 70% and who also have a high surgical risk. All other patients should be treated medically, undergoing carotid endarterectomy if indicated, or should be placed in a clinical trial."[144]

Patients with ADPKD require special attention for CVD because the overall prevalence of an asymptomatic intracranial aneurysm as determined by magnetic resonance angiography is approximately 12% and increases to about 20% in those with a positive family history of an intracranial aneurysm or subarachnoid hemorrhage in conjunction with ADPKD.[145,146] Magnetic resonance angiography with gadolinium has recently been associated with the risk of nephrogenic systemic fibrosis in some patients with severely impaired renal function, but cerebral MRA can be done without it.[147–149] For those patients with ADPKD and a family history of intracranial aneurysm or subarachnoid hemorrhage, or who have neurological symptoms suggestive of an intracranial aneurysm, magnetic resonance angiography is usually the initial study. Repeat scanning for those with a history of intracranial aneurysm has been recommended every 5 to 10 years.[150,151] These patients should know the significance of for those with a history of intro crarial aneurysm a "sentinel" headache relating to the initial intracranial bleed and the need to seek immediate medical/surgical treatment. Control of hypertension and timely neurosurgical judgment and skill are the main elements of treatment.

Peripheral Arterial Disease

A report based on data from the Atherosclerosis Risk In Communities (ARIC) study in 14,280 middle-aged adults with either normal kidney function, mildly decreased kidney function, or stages 3 to 4 CKD indicated by multivariate analysis, that CKD created a 1.56 relative risk for peripheral arterial disease (PAD).[152] Among 43,427 adult renal transplant recipients and 53,309 adults on the renal transplant waiting list, the 3-year cumulative incidence of de novo PAD in diabetics was 24% for those on the waiting list versus 20% after transplantation, and for those without diabetes mellitus, 9% on the waiting list versus 5% after transplantation.[153] For both diabetic and nondiabetic patients a diagnosis of PAD on the waiting list was associated with approximately a threefold increase in the relative risk for death. After transplantation in both groups the development of de novo PAD increased the relative risk

for death approximately twofold. Nondiabetic patients with renal allografts functioning for longer than 20 years also can have vascular calcification and lower limb ischemia requiring amputation.[154]

Diminished femoral and/or pedal pulses; iliofemoral bruits; the presence of coronary, carotid, or renal arterial disease; a high-risk CHD profile, and claudication are indications to measure the ankle-brachial index ratios. An ankle-brachial index value less than 0.90 at rest, or more than 0.90 at rest but that decreases by 20% after exercise, represents the earliest diagnostic assessment of PAD.[155] The presence of vascular calcification prevents the interpretation of the ankle-brachial index but at times may be circumvented by using a toe-brachial index rather than the ankle-brachial index.[155,156] About one third of patients with PAD in the general population have typical claudication, resulting in amputation in 5% of patients within 5 years, and about 5% to 10% of patients have critical leg ischemia with major risk of limb loss. However, more than 50% of patients having PAD on the basis of abnormal ankle-brachial index ratios do not have typical claudication or critical leg ischemia, but they do have reduced ambulatory activity and quality of life.[155]

For patients with PAD in the general population, risk factors should be assessed and treated (e.g., smoking cessation, reduction of LDL-C to less than 100 mg/dL or in very high-risk individuals possibly to less than 70 mg/dL, control of hypertension to less than 130/80 mm Hg, and diabetes control with HbA_{1c} less than 7%).[157] Further treatment includes an exercise program, antiplatelet and other pharmacologic therapy and, when indicated, revascularization that may take the form of open surgical procedures, angioplasty, and stents.[155,157] Currently drug treatment of PAD includes aspirin in daily doses of 75 to 150 mg, which has been shown to be as effective as higher doses and less likely to cause gastrointestinal (GI) bleeding complications.[157–159] Although aspirin has not been shown to improve claudication, it does delay the rate of progression, lessens the need for intervention, and reduces graft failure in patients who have undergone revascularization procedures.[157] Clopidogrel was compared with aspirin in the Clopidogrel versus Aspirin in Patients at Risk of Ischaemic Events (CAPRIE) trial, in which clopidogrel's greatest benefit occurred in the 6452 patients with PAD who had nearly a 24% reduction (4.9%/year with clopidogrel vs. 3.7%/year with aspirin) in the risk of MI, stroke, or cardiovascular death.[160] Clopidogrel is usually given in doses of 75 mg once daily. It is extensively metabolized by the liver. Although there are lower metabolite levels and reduced adenosine diphosphate–induced platelet aggregation in patients with stage 5 CKD, prolongation of bleeding time was similar to that in healthy treated volunteers. Nevertheless, clopidogrel should be used with caution in those with significant liver or kidney disease. Its use is contraindicated in patients with active bleeding or hypersensitivity. Adverse effects include bleeding, thrombotic thrombocytopenic purpura, hypersensitivity reactions, anaphylactoid reactions, serum sickness, neurological symptoms, hepatobiliary disorders, myelotoxicity, and skin lesions, including angioedema, Stevens-Johnson syndrome, and toxic epidermal necrolysis.

Angiographic studies in renal transplant patients, who typically have stage 3 or 4 CKD, are problematic both for the use of intravenous (IV) iodinated contrast agents with their risk of acute kidney injury as well as magnetic resonance angiography employing gadolinium with its risks for nephrogenic systemic fibrosis and possible need for dialysis.[147–149] Because contrast loads are typically larger for the study of PAD, if iodinated contrast agents are to be used, it is still advisable to try to keep the amount of reagent as low as possible, prehydrate patients intravenously according to their cardiopulmonary parameters, and use acetylcysteine before and after the procedure.[161] (See also Chapter 40.)

POSTTRANSPLANTATION ERYTHROCYTOSIS

Posttransplantation erythrocytosis, defined as a persistently elevated hematocrit higher than 51%, used to be seen in about 15% of renal transplant patients (range, 4%–22%), usually within the first 2 years after transplantation.[162] However, in clinical practice since about 2000, it has become an unusual finding. This may be due to the expanding use of sirolimus, with its anemia effect,[28] as well as widespread use of ACE inhibitors or angiotensin receptor blockers. In fact, posttransplant anemia has become a significant issue, initially because it contributed to the risk of CVD, especially in diabetics,[163] and then because its treatment with erythropoietin products after transplantation could create a new risk, as reflected in the CHOIR and CREATE trials in nontransplant patients (see Chapters 67 and 68).[164–166]

The consequences of posttransplantation erythrocytosis (PTE) are primarily thromboembolic events, which may be seen in up to 22% of patients. Remarkably, the development of PTE does not correlate with serum erythropoietin levels.[167] Instead, angiotensin II stimulates the proliferation of normal early erythroid precursors that have increased numbers of AT_1 receptors and correlate with the hematocrit in patients with PTE.[168,169] Consequently, ACE inhibitors and angiotensin receptor blockers are the treatments of choice for PTE, although phlebotomy may be useful at times. Because some patients may have a rapid fall in hematocrit, or less commonly a spontaneous remission, careful monitoring is necessary. Intermittent therapy may be effective in some patients.

MALIGNANT DISEASE

It has been stated that "cancer will surpass cardiovascular complications as a leading cause of death in transplant patients within the next two decades."[170] Skin cancer is the most frequent malignancy seen in renal transplant recipients, and post-transplant lymphoproliferative disease (PTLD) is the second most common, occurring in about 11%.[170] A study of malignancy among 35,765 first-time recipients of deceased or living donor kidney transplants from 1995 to 2001 revealed a twofold increase in common tumors (i.e., colon, lung, prostate, stomach, esophagus, pancreas, ovary, and breast); approximately a fivefold increase in melanoma, leukemia, hepatobiliary tumors, cervical, and vulvovaginal cancers; a threefold increase in testicular and bladder cancers, a 15-fold increase in kidney cancers, and more than a 20-fold increase in Kaposi's sarcoma, non-Hodgkin's lymphoma, and nonmelanoma skin cancers.[171] In data obtained by record linkage between the Australia and New Zealand Dialysis and Transplant Registry and the Australian National Cancer Statistic Clearing-

house, it was noted that among the 18 specific cancers with greater than a threefold increase in risk, five were at sites affected by human papillomavirus (tongue, mouth, vulva, vagina, penis), two were related to Epstein-Barr virus (EBV) (Hodgkin's disease, non-Hodgkin's lymphoma), one was related to hepatitis B and C (hepatocellular carcinoma), and one is universally associated with human herpes virus 8 (HHV-8) (Kaposi's sarcoma).[172] Only five of the high-risk cancers did not have viral infection as a generally accepted primary cause. Azathioprine, cyclosporine, and tacrolimus have been associated with an increased risk of post-transplant malignancies, whereas sirolimus especially, and possibly mycophenolic acid, may lower malignancy frequency.[170,173–180] The full extent of post-transplant malignancies is beyond the scope of this chapter.

When a renal transplant recipient develops a malignancy, the transplant physician/surgeon will need to work closely with the oncologist to develop a plan of therapy that will involve modification of immunosuppressant medication, as well as selection of chemotherapy, radiotherapy, and surgery. The risks of the malignancy itself and each component of therapy must be compared to the morbidity and mortality risks for the patient and stability of renal allograft function. Perhaps the strongest trend in immunosuppression management of post-transplant malignancies has been the use of sirolimus, which followed reports of a reduced incidence of de novo malignancies when it is used.[28,175,178–180] A decreased incidence of both skin and nonskin malignancies 5 years after renal transplant was reported in 430 adult renal transplant recipients randomly assigned to either remain on sirolimus/cyclosporine/ steroids or to have cyclosporine withdrawn at 3 months and sirolimus trough levels increased.[179] It should be noted, however, that the prescribed trough levels for sirolimus are ones that have more frequent and serious adverse effects. Mycophenolic acid appears to have a neutral to possibly beneficial effect on the occurrence of post-transplant de novo malignancies.[175–177] Two major studies of antibody induction therapy and subsequent PTLD are in agreement that PTLD rates were highest with monoclonal OKT3 and polyclonal Atgam and thymoglobulin, with the least risk from interleukin-2 receptor antibodies.[180,181] Somewhat at variance with these results is the SRTR report, which attributes the highest risk for PTLD to rabbit thymoglobulin and then clusters interleukin-2 receptor antibodies, OKT3, and equine antithymocyte globulin in the second tier.[182,183] Thus far, alemtuzumab does not appear to create a higher risk.[184]

Several clinical risk profiles for individuals prone to developing certain malignancies after renal transplantation are: (1) PTLD occurring within the first 12 months after transplantation in a white male (often younger than age 18 years) who is seronegative for EBV, human leukocyte antigen (HLA)–mismatched for both HLA-B locus antigens, lacks HLA-DR7, and receives antithymocyte globulin induction or possibly belatacept[185–189]; (2) Kaposi's sarcoma in a person of Arabic, Jewish, black, or Mediterranean ancestry with evidence of HHV-8 or human immunodeficiency virus infection[174,190]; (3) vulvar and vaginal carcinomas in women with papillomavirus types 16 and 18[191]; (4) hepatocellular carcinoma in those with persistent hepatitis B antigenemia, cirrhosis, or hepatitis C of long duration[192]; (5) carcinomas of the skin in fair-skinned or older individuals with unprotected sun exposure and long-duration use of azathioprine with its metabolite thioguanine[173,193]; (6) recurrent malignant disease in those who before transplantation had a malignant neoplasm with a medium or high rate of recurrence.[194,195] Other nondrug risk factors associated with increased frequency of post-transplantation malignancy are increasing age, a past history of cancer, cigarette smoking, previous splenectomy, and polycystic kidney disease.[175,183]

Recommendations of the American Cancer Society are used for cancer surveillance, but they may need to be applied with increased frequency or with invasive testing in high-risk individuals.[1,195]

Two of the most frequently encountered malignancies after transplantation are PTLD and squamous cell carcinomas of the skin and lip. PTLD occurs within 5 years of renal transplantation in approximately 1.2% of adult renal transplant recipients at a median of 1000 days.[196] Poor prognostic factors include multiple organ involvement at the time of diagnosis, graft organ failure at diagnosis, age greater than 40 years, and lactic dehydrogenase level 2.5 times or more above the upper limit of normal.[197] If none of these risk factors is present, response to treatment can occur in as many as 89% of patients, whereas with two or three factors present, the response rate is essentially zero.[197] Also influencing the prognosis is the clonality of the PTLD. Polyclonal B-cell PTLD has an early onset, is EBV-positive, and offers a better prognosis, whereas monoclonal B-cell PTLD has a late onset, may be EBV-positive or EBV-negative, and is more aggressive. B-cell PTLD constitutes approximately 85% to 90% of PTLD cases, and T-cell PTLD, which carries a worse prognosis, the other 10 to 15%.

Three special characteristics of PTLD after transplantation are its extranodal involvement in 70% of patients, compared with 35% of nontransplant controls, central nervous system involvement in 26% (63% confined to the brain), and microscopic or gross involvement of the allograft in 20% of patients, sometimes simulating rejection. In an early study of 435 patients, total remissions were achieved in 29%, and approximately 25% of the remissions were induced by the decrease or elimination of nonsteroidal immunosuppressants.[174]

Treatment still begins with a reduction in immunosuppression, according to the risks of each noted in this chapter, that will usually involve discontinuation of azathioprine, discontinuation or at least a 50% reduction in cyclosporine or tacrolimus, and often an increase in maintenance prednisone to the 10- to 15-mg range for protection of the allograft. In some cases surgical resection may be indicated.[197] Whether the second step in treatment of B-cell lymphoma should be chemotherapy or rituximab is currently being reassessed.[198] Conventional chemotherapy has a rapid response (days) but significant toxicity, whereas rituximab is slower (weeks) but generally safer.[197,199,200] The usual course had been to proceed with conventional chemotherapy, namely, the CHOP protocol (cyclophosphamide, doxorubicin, vincristine [Oncovin], and prednisone), sometimes with irradiation. However, more recently the anti-CD20 B-cell monoclonal antibody rituximab has been gaining favor for use before chemotherapy.[198,201,202] In a key study, complete remissions were achieved in 13 (59%) of 22 patients who received rituximab and in 13 (57%) of 23 patients who received chemotherapy.[201] No fatalities occurred in the rituximab-treated group, whereas a quarter of those treated with chemotherapy died of treatment-related toxicities. Because failure with one mode of therapy can often be salvaged by the other, the use of rituximab as initial therapy appears to be reasonable.[198–200] Rituximab also has the advantage of being a standardized dose of 375 mg/m^2 usually given weekly for 4 weeks. No adjustment appears to be needed for the level of renal function, although "no formal studies were conducted to examine the effects of either renal or hepatic impairment" on rituximab. Adverse effects of rituximab include fatal infusion reactions, 80% of which occurred with the first dose, tumor lysis syndrome with acute kidney injury and some fatalities seen when treating PTLD, severe mucocutaneous reactions, and severe infection, also with fatalities, reported. One should be thoroughly familiar with the adverse effects before using this agent.

T-cell PTLD is typically aggressive and poorly responsive to conventional therapy centered on reduction of immunosuppression and chemotherapy. However, one case recently reported in a recipient of a combined kidney/pancreas transplant achieved clinical remission after treatment with a novel synthetic retinoid analog, bexarotine.[199]

Although antiviral therapy has been used as adjunctive therapy, it would only be active during the lytic stages of EBV infection. It may well have a more important role in reducing the risk of PTLD in recipients seronegative for EBV.[203]

Newer therapies in limited testing include the use of EBV-specific cytotoxic lymphocytes[204] and arginine butyrate, which may render EBV more susceptible to ganciclovir.[199]

Remarkably, because PTLD is a result of a primary EBV infection, renal retransplantation is acceptable for those who have had a complete remission. The median time from PTLD diagnosis to retransplantation has been 1300 days.[196] Often the same immunosuppressants that were used at the time of the initial PTLD can be used for the next renal transplant.[198]

The second malignancy of particular interest after renal transplant is squamous cell carcinoma (SCC) of the skin and lip, which constitutes about one third of all new malignant neoplasms after renal transplantation. After renal transplantation SCCs tend to be multiple, have a more aggressive course, and are a more common cause of cancer death than in the general population. Transplant recipients developing SCC are about 30 years younger than their counterparts in the general population. Renal transplant recipients at increased risk include those with a history of skin cancer, actinic keratoses, chronic sun exposure or sunburns, or human papillomavirus infection, those who are fair skinned (Fitzpatrick types I to III), older age, those with CD4 lymphocytopenia, and those whose immunosuppression has been either intense or of long duration.[205]

A dermatologist should examine and treat the patient at intervals appropriate to the risks.[205,206] Treatment of SCC may require varying types of surgery. Patient education, guidelines of care, and other aspects of posttransplantation skin cancer are in the process of being placed on the new International Transplant Skin Cancer Collaborative website for AT-RISC Alliance. (After Transplantation Reduce Incidence of Skin Cancer at www.at-risc.org). In addition to information about SCC in allograft recipients, there will also be information about the diagnostic management of basal cell carcinoma, melanoma, and rare carcinomas of the skin.

Skin cancer risk can be lessened by wearing protective clothing, avoiding direct sun exposure, and using appropriate sun block. Sunscreens should have a sun protection factor of at least 15 and be applied 15 to 30 minutes before sun exposure. They do not necessarily avoid all photodamage from prolonged sun exposure even though they prevent erythema.[207]

The first new sunscreen approved by the FDA in 18 years contains ecamsule, which is particularly effective in UVA2 absorption.[207] Medical treatment of recurrent SCC includes cautious decreases in overall immunosuppression, specifically elimination of azathioprine (if being used), careful use of low-dose retinoids, and possible substitution of sirolimus for a calcineurin inhibitor.[179,180,206,208,209] The frequency of SCC of the skin is reported to be reduced by sirolimus.[179,180,208,209] In a series of 23 renal transplant recipients with multiple skin cancers who were treated in 70% of the cases with cyclosporine, azathioprine, and prednisone, 2 mg daily of sirolimus was initiated with rapid withdrawal of cyclosporine or tacrolimus, and azathioprine or mycophenolic acid.[209] With sirolimus levels maintained at 4 to 10 ng/mL and prednisone sustained at 5 to 10 mg/day, the average frequency of skin cancer episodes (predominantly SCC) decreased from 3.2 to 0.7 ($P <$ .001) over mean follow-up of 22.4 months, and 16 patients had no new skin cancers. However, one patient with malignant melanoma and another with Kaposi's sarcoma died within 1 year of conversion. A delay in the onset of the first skin cancer was also seen in a multicenter trial in which 215 renal transplant recipients, who had cyclosporine withdrawn from a cyclosporine/sirolimus/steroid regimen, had the first cancers appearing at an average of 1126 days after transplant compared to 491 days in those who remained on the triple therapy, which included cyclosporine ($P =$ .007).[179]

Other modes of therapy for SCC include topical 5-fluorouracil, and more recently low-dose oral acitretin, whose oral absorption is optimal with food. In collaboration with our dermatologists we have initiated treatment with low doses of 10 mg acitretin daily with careful monitoring for the numerous adverse effects, which include hepatotoxicity, pancreatitis, pseudotumor cerebri, ophthalmologic complications, inflammatory bowel disease, hyperglycemia, hypertriglyceridemia, decreased HDL-C, hyperostosis, osteoporosis, alopecia, mucocutaneous lesions, elevated CK levels, and depression. Postmarketing adverse effects include cardiovascular events, neuropathy, myopathy, and thinning of the skin. Acitretin may require dose adjustment in renal insufficiency and end-stage renal disease. It should not be used in women who are or intend to become pregnant. If this medication is to be used, the manufacturer's drug information should be carefully reviewed.

The treatment of local/regional advanced SCC of the head and neck with a monoclonal antibody against epidermal growth factor receptor (cetuximab) plus radiotherapy significantly lengthened overall survival from approximately 29 months to 49 months.[210]

Sirolimus has demonstrated a remarkable capacity to control Kaposi's sarcoma in renal transplant recipients.[190] Because Kaposi's sarcoma is invariably associated with HHV-8, this implies that sirolimus has activity against HHV-8, as well as against EBV, as noted in the discussion of PTLD.[211] The antineoplastic and antiviral effects of sirolimus, as well as the comprehensive overview of its therapeutic efficacy and tolerability, have recently been reviewed.[28,180] A detailed discussion of malignant melanoma is beyond the scope of this discussion, but a recent comprehensive review is available.[212]

Patients who are hepatitis B carriers or have nonhepatitis B cirrhosis should be monitored at 6- to 12-month intervals for development of hepatocellular carcinoma with liver ultrasound and alpha fetoprotein determinations.[192] Abstinence from alcohol is recommended for those with hepati-tis. Treatment of hepatitis B and C and other infections of the liver are discussed in Chapter 90. Of particular interest are recent studies evaluating cyclosporine as therapy for hepatitis C.[213–215]

GASTROINTESTINAL DISEASE

The primary causes of GI disease after renal transplantation are infections, malignancies, and adverse effects due to immunosuppressant drugs. GI infections, which include tissue-invasive cytomegalovirus, herpes simplex, fungal, bacterial, and parasitic infections, are discussed in Chapter 90 and have been reviewed elsewhere.[216] In addition to creating the susceptibility to infection, use of immunosuppressants produces other complications, including mucosal injury and ulceration associated with atypical chest pain, nausea, vomiting, aphthous ulcers of the mouth and tongue, and diarrhea. Diarrhea has been a major problem with the use of mycophenolate mofetil (MMF), and attempts to avoid it with enteric-coated mycophenolate sodium in two studies showed no significant difference between MMF or enteric-coated mycophenolate sodium in the occurrence of GI symptoms.[217,218] In some patients, changing the MMF dosing schedule from bid to tid dosing may control the diarrhea. Reduction of MMF dose is an option, but it has been reported that when compared to those with no MMF dose reduction or discontinuation, the risk of renal allograft failure increased after MMF dose reduction equal to or greater than 50% (hazard rate, 2.36), and with MMF discontinuation (hazard rate, 2.72).[219] Sirolimus has also been noted to be associated with diarrhea in as high as 38% of renal transplant recipients with elevated trough levels of sirolimus.[220] Other causes of diarrhea include diverticular disease, pancreatitis, unsuspected celiac disease, continued stool softener and laxative use, and other medications such as cinecalcet for hyperparathyroidism, colchicine for gout, and high doses of magnesium supplements.

A nonrandomized multicenter study to identify nonimmunosuppressant factors causing severe diarrhea in renal transplant recipients followed these seven steps: (1) Discontinue or replace any nonimmunosuppressant drug that could cause diarrhea (e.g., antiarrhythmics, antibiotics, antihypertensives, diuretics, diabetic medications, laxatives, proton pump inhibitors, protease inhibitors). (2) Perform a microbiologic stool examination (cultures for pathogenic bacteria, examination for ova and parasites, assays for fungi, and assay for *C. difficile* toxin). (3) Screen for viruses, including CMV, adenovirus, enterovirus, and rotavirus. (4) Test for bacterial overgrowth and treat as indicated. If diarrhea did not resolve after these four steps, (5) adjust the immunosuppressive regimen. If diarrhea persists, (6) perform a colonoscopy. If, after all of the above steps, the diarrhea has not resolved, (7) treat with antidiarrheal drugs, supplemental bacteria, or diets.[221] In this protocol MMF was associated with the largest number of dose reductions or stoppages ($N =$ 34), and the remission rate of diarrhea was 65% in these patients. Tacrolimus was adjusted in 12 patients, with a 42% remission rate; all 3 of the patients who had cyclosporine stopped or reduced had remission of diarrhea; glucocorticoids were reduced in 10 patients, with a 60% remission rate. After the first five steps of this protocol, 67 of the 108 patients had resolution of diarrhea, and 41 patients went on to require colonoscopy and empirical treatment.[221]

Esophagitis and gastritis are most frequently associated with infectious causes, but cyclosporine, tacrolimus, sirolimus, and MMF have been associated with upper GI lesions, and glucocorticoids remain a controversial cause of these lesions.[216] Once again, it is necessary to identify other drugs that might be causing the symptoms, such as nonsteroidal anti-inflammatory drugs (NSAIDs), bisphosphonates, potassium supplements, and alcohol. There should be a low threshold for endoscopy of the upper GI tract. Identification of early malignancy and H. pylori–positive ulcers are obvious benefits of this approach. A search for iron-deficiency anemia and occult blood testing in three or more stool specimens are also indicated. Surprisingly, one still encounters patients who have upper GI symptoms that completely disappear when they stop taking all of their morning medications in a single batch and separate them by about 1 hour into two or three groups. Esophageal reflux disease may be an especially difficult problem for those whose original kidney disease was ADPKD and have very large kidneys and an enlarged liver, provoking reflux symptoms. Setting aside the treatment of H. pylori–positive peptic ulcer disease, which involves triple therapy (2-week course of two antibiotics [e.g., amoxicillin 1000 mg bid and clarithromycin 500 mg bid]), along with lansoprazole 30 mg bid), and other lesions caused by infection, the treatment of esophagitis and gastritis includes the use of proton pump inhibitors, H2 receptor antagonists, and coating agents.[222] The use of clarithromycin for treatment of H. pylori–positive peptic ulcers can increase blood levels of immunosuppressants metabolized by the CYP3A4 pathway. Prolonged use of proton pump inhibitors has been associated with an increased risk of fractures.[223]

When a colonoscopy is to be done, whether for screening purposes over age 50 or for a specific indication, special care needs to be exercised in bowel preparation. Oral phosphate solutions should be avoided to prevent "phosphate nephropathy."[224,225] Nonphosphate-containing preparations should be used.[226]

When a disease process leads to perforation of the colon, it can be managed with low mortality and often maintenance of allograft function, when there is a high clinical index of suspicion leading to prompt treatment with appropriate antibiotics, exteriorization of the perforated colon, and reduction of immunosuppression to minimal levels.[227] In a series of 1000 renal transplant recipients, the incidence of colon perforations was 1.1%. Diverticulitis was the cause in approximately 70%, with smaller contributions from iatrogenic factors, ischemia, impaction, colonic ulcers, and colitis.[227] More than half of the cases of perforation of the colon occurred within 3 months of renal transplantation.

Aphthous ulcers occurring in the course of treatment with sirolimus have been reported to be manageable with clobetasol.[228,229]

Acute pancreatitis and biliary tract diseases are more serious events in renal transplant recipients than in the general population. Cyclosporine has been associated with a higher frequency of cholelithiasis,[230] although this was in an era when higher cyclosporine dosing was common.[231] Some have recommended "eradication of all biliary calculi, electively, before

transplantation and on diagnosis after transplantation before the patients get really sick."[216]

OSTEOPOROSIS

Many renal transplant recipients have unrecognized osteopenia or osteoporosis at transplantation. Compounding that problem is the fact that "as many as 60% of renal transplant recipients treated with corticosteroids may lose sufficient BMD to meet the definition of osteoporosis in the first 18 months after transplantation."[1] Glucocorticoids suppress bone formation (inhibiting synthesis of insulin-like growth factor, transforming growth factor-β action on bone, and osteocalcin) without suppressing, and possibly even stimulating, bone resorption.[232] By 6 months after renal transplant, patients receiving therapy with cyclosporine, azathioprine, and low-dose prednisone had a 2.8% decrease in BMD of the lumbar vertebrae and a 4.2% decrease in BMD of the femoral neck.[233] When the prednisone dose was less than 7.5 mg/day, subsequent decreases in BMD appeared to parallel those for age-matched individuals.[234] However, prednisone doses as low as 5 mg/day have been associated with significant reduction in indices of bone formation in postmenopausal females,[232] and doses of 2.5 to 7.5 mg/day with higher hip and vertebral fracture risks in nontransplant patients.[235,236] Duration of steroid treatment, as well as dose, influence BMD. Moderate use of steroids for 4 months after transplantation when compared to rapid steroid withdrawal had no significant effect on bone mass at 1 year.[237] In a study of 364 renal transplant recipients, all of whom were treated with tacrolimus, MMF, and 3 days of 100 mg/day IV prednisolone, 186 of these patients were randomized to receive either daclizumab and no further steroid, whereas 178 patients had a limited 4-month steroid regimen beginning at 0.3 mg/kg and tapered to zero.[237] Although lumbar BMD decreased significantly in the first 3 months in both the steroid-free (−1.3%) and steroid groups (−2.3%), recovery to baseline occurred at 12 months in both groups. Both regimens prevented accelerated bone loss. In a randomized, controlled study of 92 renal transplant recipients receiving cyclosporine, azathioprine, and prednisone who had stable graft function for at least 1 year (average, 7 years), those who had prednisone withdrawn at a rate of 1 mg/month, when compared to controls maintained at an average of 5.6 mg/day, demonstrated a significant 2.54% per year increase in L1–L4 BMD, a rise in osteocalcin, and no significant change in serum creatinine.[238]

Lumbar spine and hip bone mineral densities should be measured by dual x-ray absorptiometry at the time of transplantation, after 6 months, and then every 12 months if results are abnormal. Bone mineral density measurements are "specific but not necessarily sensitive" and, as a single method, are inadequate for identifying all patients at risk for osteoporosis and in need of treatment.[239] Consequently, a new evaluation scheme is being developed that combines BMD and clinical risk factors to quantitate the absolute probability of risk for hip or clinical fracture over a 10-year period, an approach that resembles estimation of 10-year risk for CHD.[239] Overall, the most important clinical risk factors appear to be patient age, previous fracture, and use of glucocorticoids, although many other risk factors have been described by at least seven sources.[239,240] Disease states relevant to the renal transplant population are diabetes mellitus, hyperparathyroidism, vitamin D deficiency, chronic metabolic acidosis, and hypogonadal states, as well as use of glucocorticoids and possibly other immunosuppressants.[235,240–243] It remains unclear as to whether cyclosporine and tacrolimus, independent of other immunosuppressants, cause osteoporosis.[235] Sirolimus thus far does not appear to significantly affect BMD, but its testosterone-lowering effect may pose a long-term risk for males.[28,235,244,245] Azathioprine, MMF, and cyclophosphamide have not been shown to cause bone loss.[235] There have been recent reports of an increased risk of fractures with prolonged use of proton pump inhibitors,[223] and with pioglitazone in females, but without other indications of osteoporosis.[79,246]

"Multiple current guidelines generally agree that patients with T-scores lower than −2.5 should be treated, and those with T-scores higher than −1.5 should not"; however, glucocorticoid use may modify this statement.[239,240] Treatment of osteoporosis in renal transplant recipients has paralleled that in the general population and is conjoined with adequate calcium (1500 mg daily) and vitamin D (800 IU cholecalciferol) supplementation, after deficiencies have been corrected; blood levels should be monitored. These treatments include bisphosphonates (oral agents: alendronate, ibandronate, and risedronate; IV agents: ibandronate [FDA approved],[247] pamidronate, and zoledronic acid [FDA approved]), calcitonin, estrogen, the selective estrogen receptor modulator raloxifene in postmenopausal females, testosterone in hypogonadal males, and possibly recombinant human parathyroid hormone (teriparatide).[235,248–258] Bisphosphonates have been used in renal transplant recipients because of BMD-documented osteoporosis or glucocorticoid therapy[259,260] and often a plethora of other risk factors. One of the early guidelines for the prevention and treatment of glucocorticoid-induced osteoporosis is given in Box 89-2, and will be updated.[259–261] However, there are reports pointing to the need to reassess both the routine use and duration of bisphosphonate therapy in such renal transplant recipients.[251,262–267] This emerging uncertainty is generated by the diversity of pretransplant bone diseases and their uncharted courses after transplantation even before bisphosphonate use, now further complicated with the use of bisphosphonates.[253,262–269] A meta-analysis[251] of five randomized, controlled trials of bisphosphonates in 180 glucocorticoid-treated renal transplant recipients concluded that bisphosphonates, usually given IV in two to four doses with and soon after transplantation, significantly reduced bone loss by 0.06 g/cm² in the lumbar spine and nonsignificantly in the femoral neck by 0.05 g/cm². Three of the five studies used pamidronate (two IV[264,270] and one orally,[271] one IV ibandronate,[272] and one IV zoledronic acid[273])—all with supplemental calcium and three with supplemental vitamin D. Three of these studies reported the number of fractures, and they were nearly identical in the bisphosphonate-treated versus control patients (4 vs. 3). In a more definitive randomized, prospective, controlled study of 72 renal transplant recipients (21 with bone biopsies at baseline and 14 with 6-month follow-up biopsies) who received glucocorticoids and cyclosporine or tacrolimus, 36 received pamidronate IV within 48 hours after transplantation and at months 1, 2, 3, and 6, as well as oral calcitriol and calcium carbonate, the latter two medications being the ones received by the 36 control patients.[264] Pamidronate-treated

Box 89-2 Guidelines for the Prevention and Treatment of Glucocorticoid-Induced Osteoporosis (see comments in text)

Patient receiving long-term glucocorticoid therapy (prednisone equivalent of ≥ 5 mg/day)
- Modify lifestyle risk factors for osteoporosis
  - Smoking cessation or avoidance
  - Reduction of alcohol consumption if excessive
- Instruct in weight-bearing physical exercise
- Initiate calcium supplementation as needed
- Initiate supplementation with vitamin D (plain or activated form) as needed
- Prescribe treatment to replace gonadal sex hormones if deficient or otherwise clinically indicated
- Measure BMD at lumbar spine and/or hip
- If BMD is not normal (i.e., T-score below −1), then:
  - Prescribe bisphosphonate (use with caution in premenopausal women; avoid in patients with GFR < 30 mL/min/1.73 m² or high-risk condition)
  - Reevaluate at least annually the safety and duration of bisphophonate therapy because of new information on possible adverse effects of these drugs on different underlying pretransplant bone diseases
  - Consider calcitonin as second-line agent if patient has contraindication to or does not tolerate bisphosphonate therapy
- If BMD is normal, followup and repeat BMD measurement either annually or biannually

Modified from the American College of Rheumatology Ad Hoc Committee Guidelines on Glucocorticoid-Induced Osteoporosis– 2001 Update. Arthritis Rheum 2001;44:1496–1503.

patients preserved bone mass at 6 and 12 months whereas the control patients had decreases in vertebral BMD at 6 and 12 months of 4.8% and 6.1%, respectively. However, at baseline 50% of the patients in the subset studied with bone histology had low-turnover bone disease; this increased to 100% at 6 months in all the patients who received IV pamidronate but remained at 50% in control patients.[263] As noted by Cunningham,[235] "These observations are very important, raising the question of whether preservation of BMD, possibly in the face of deteriorating and adynamic bone histology is a reasonable objective in its own right. The overall balance in terms of achieved bone health remains uncertain." These divergent findings of improved BMD and the development of universal adynamic bone histology are unsettling. Furthermore, among 20 renal transplant recipients randomized to receive either two infusions of 4 mg of zoledronic acid or placebo at 2 weeks and 3 months after transplantation, as well as 1000 mg of daily calcium citrate for the first 6 months (also used in the controls), zoledronic acid when compared to placebo showed no sustained benefit at 3 years despite an early decrease in bone loss by the bisphosphonate.[266] The potential use of teriparatide to increase BMD has not been tested in renal transplant recipients in whom preexisting bone disease, probable hyperparathyroidism, and use or nonuse of glucocorticoids and bisphosphonates will create a highly complex picture.[229,255] When nontransplant patients were treated with alendronate the improvement of BMD by teriparatide was blunted, but no interference was exerted by raloxifene.[265] None of the renal transplant studies performed with bisphosphonates have been sufficiently powered to determine the hard endpoint of fracture occurrence. In a long-term retrospective cohort study of 86 renal transplant recipients followed for a median of 10.6 years, the only overall predictors of fracture risk were age and diabetic nephropathy.[267] There were 117 fractures observed in this long-term group with a cumulative incidence of 60% for any fracture at 15 years (compared to the expected 20%), but cumulative corticosteroid dose was remarkably not associated with an increased fracture risk.[267]

No guidelines have been established regarding when to stop bisphosphonate therapy, but a "holiday" period at 5 years is being evaluated in low-risk nontransplant patients.[257,258]

Adverse effects reported with oral bisphosphonates are dysphagia, esophagitis, esophageal and gastric ulcers, decreases in serum calcium and phosphorus, and osteonecrosis of the jaw, most often occurring when bisphosphonates are given IV to patients with cancer, dental disease, or to those undergoing dental surgery.[274] Because bisphosphonates are renally excreted and can accumulate in patients with stages 5 and 4 CKD, their use is avoided under these circumstances because of potential renal and other toxicities. The nephrotoxic effects of bisphosphonates appear to be most closely associated with IV use. Pamidronate given IV has been associated with hypocalcemia, febrile reactions, and collapsing focal segmental glomerulosclerosis reported in seven patients receiving high doses in the course of treatment for malignancy.[275] As noted above, bisphosphonates may aggravate preexisting low-turnover bone disease and hyperparathyroidism.[235,264,276]

A once-yearly infusion of zoledronic acid over a 3-year period in a double-blind, placebo-controlled nontransplant trial of 3889 postmenopausal females with osteoporosis (Health Outcomes and Reduced Incidence with Zoledronic acid ONce yearly [HORIZON]) showed a benefit in terms of a reduction in the risks of vertebral, hip, and other fractures, a similar effect on renal function as in the controls, but significantly more episodes of serious atrial fibrillation more than 30 days later in the zoledronic acid group (50 vs. 20 patients).[255,256]

Calcitonin nasal spray 200 once daily, which reduced new vertebral fractures by 33% in 1255 postmenopausal osteoporotic women,[277] has adverse effects that include allergy and nasal irritation. Raloxifene for postmenopausal women at a dose of 60 mg/day can reduce vertebral fractures by 30%,[278] and it does not interfere with the use of teriparatide.[265] Adverse effects of raloxifene include flushing and hot flashes, leg cramps, and thromboembolic events.

HYPERPARATHYROIDISM

Parathyroid function improves in approximately 50% of patients with pretransplant hyperparathyroidism. However, hyperparathyroidism persists in 17% to 50% of patients if the parathyroid glands have developed nodular hyperplasia or if renal allograft function is impaired; hypercalcemia is present in approximately 10% of recipients at 1 year.[279-281] The majority of functioning renal allografts have a GFR of 30 to 59 mL/min/1.73 m^2 (stage 3 CKD) accompanied by decreasing phosphorus excretion and lower serum calcium and 1,25-dihydroxyvitamin D_3 levels that promote secondary hyperparathyroidism.[282] For interpretation of parathyroid hormone (PTH) function and assays, see Chapter 69.

Hyperparathyroidism can cause osteoporosis (particularly evident as decreased bone density in the forearm), osteitis fibrosa cystica, lytic bone lesions (Brown tumors), pathologic fractures, vascular calcification, ectopic calcification, calciphylaxis, renal stones, and pancreatitis. The K/DOQI guidelines provide a framework for treating renal transplant recipients even though they have not been specifically tested in that population (see Chapter 69).

Treatment of hyperparathyroidism can be medical or surgical. Medical therapy includes vitamin D analogs, the calcimimetic cinacalcet, which suppresses PTH and lowers serum calcium and phosphorus and, if still needed, oral phosphate binders (see Chapter 69).

When secondary hyperparathyroidism is present, typically with hypercalcemia, and 1,25-dihydroxyvitamin D_3 levels are in a normal range with or without vitamin D supplementation, the use of cinacalcet can be considered.[283] Seven small short-term studies totaling 81 kidney-only transplant recipients who received 30 to 180 mg of cinacalcet daily generally demonstrated safety and efficacy, reflected in decreases in serum calcium, elevation of depressed phosphorus levels, and usually decreases in PTH levels.[281,284–289] An extended study of 170 nontransplant patients with secondary hyperparathyroidism who were treated with 30 to 180 mg of cinacalcet daily for 2 years demonstrated control of PTH levels in approximately 60% of patients.[290] Nausea, vomiting, and diarrhea are the most common GI effects and may occur even at the lowest dose. This author has found that dosing on a Monday-Wednesday-Friday schedule can sometimes relieve these symptoms while still retaining partial effectiveness. Diarrhea is a particularly difficult adverse effect because it is also likely to be attributed to mycophenolate mofetil, sirolimus, or colchicine, if one of these drugs is also being used. Cinacalcet is metabolized by multiple enzymes, including CYP3A4. In a recent report cinacalcet reduced the AUC of tacrolimus by 14% and increased formation of the nephrotoxic cyclosporine metabolite AM19.[291] These findings may help to explain the reduced allograft function reported by some when cinacalcet was used. A more complete list of pharmacokinetic interactions with cinacalcet is given in Chapter 69. Those prescribing the drug should read the manufacturer's information thoroughly. Hypocalcemia and excessive reduction of PTH need to be avoided, and monitoring of serum calcium, phosphorus, and PTH is advisable at 3-month intervals. Relapsing hypercalcemia and elevated PTH levels have been reported when cinacalcet is stopped.[281,286,287]

When 1,25-dihydroxyvitamin D_3 was given for various reasons to 26 deceased donor renal allograft recipients with functioning grafts more than 1 year after transplantation, there was evidence of immunosuppressive properties, reflected in deceleration in the loss of graft function and instances of stabilization or slight improvement in function. These clinical results extended findings from animal studies of transplantation in which vitamin D prevented rejection and prolonged graft function.[292,293] The fact that blacks have lower levels of vitamin D than do whites may be relevant to the high risk that blacks have for allograft rejection. Vitamin D has also been reported to have antifibrotic and antirenin effects.[294,295]

Indications for parathyroidectomy have generally been the occurrence of acute hypercalcemia greater than 12.5 mg/dL in the immediate post-transplant period, asymptomatic hypercalcemia greater than 12 mg/dL for more than 1 year after transplantation, and symptomatic hypercalcemia.[296] It should be noted that if cinecalcet was being used in a patient before transplantation and then discontinued, rebound hypercalcemia may occur.[286] The surgical guidelines reported by Kerby were developed before the availability of cinecalcet. The major single center-study by Kerby, extending over a 29-year period, resulted in only 38 of 4344 renal transplant recipients requiring a parathyroidectomy for hyperparathyroidism at a mean of 2.7 years after transplantation. In addition to surgical complications, parathyroidectomy incurs risk for hypocalcemia (*hungry bone syndrome*), hypoparathyroidism that requires resetting "normal" serum calcium levels to 8.0 to 8.5 mg/dL to avoid nephrocalcinosis (because the absence of PTH decreases calcium reabsorption), adynamic bone disease, and a significant decline in renal allograft function.[297] A summary of various forms of vitamin D is given in Chapter 69 and has been reviewed.[298]

ACUTE VASCULAR NECROSIS

When glucocorticoids were the major immunosuppressant, the prevalence of acute vascular necrosis was 3% to 41%, but in the cyclosporine and tocrolimus eras it has generally been less than 5%. Risk factors for acute vascular necrosis include deceased donor transplants, repeat transplants, frequent acute rejections, alcohol consumption, glucocorticoids, severe hypertriglyceridemia, and osteoporosis. However, an analysis of 27,772 solitary renal transplant recipients in the USRDS database indicated that acute vascular necrosis was significantly more common when cyclosporine was used.[299] Unfortunately, the study was unable to determine if the effect was due to differences in the amount of glucocorticoid therapy, hyperlipidemia, or microvascular thrombosis. The weight-bearing long bones are the most frequently affected sites. Diagnosis is confirmed by magnetic resonance imaging, although such imaging now raises concerns for gadolinium toxicity if it has to be used.[147-149]

Initial conservative measures for the hip include avoidance of weight-bearing on the symptomatic side and orthopedic consultation. Orthopedic surgical procedures for acute vascular necrosis include core decompression (with uncertain benefit) before collapse of the femoral head and total hip replacement for more extensive disease. Once the disease has occurred, an abrupt decrease or discontinuation of glucocorticoids does not appear to be helpful and may jeopardize the allograft.

A syndrome of severe, episodic bone pain involving primarily both knees and ankles that is often worse at night and in recumbency has been associated with the use of cyclosporine.[300] The pain often responds to calcium channel blockers, but a small number of patients may develop acute vascular necrosis in the affected knee.

GOUT

Risk factors for the development of gout in the general population include obesity, weight gain, hypertension, and diuretic use, as well as high-purine diets in males.[301] Impaired renal function, treatment with cyclosporine, and the use of diuretics are major contributing factors in renal transplant recipients. In patients receiving cyclosporine, the prevalence of hyperuricemia was 30% to 80%, and 2% to 28% developed symptomatic gout.[302,303] In the era before cyclosporine use, hyperuricemia developed in 19% to 55%, and gout occurred in only 0% to 8% within 10 years of transplantation, although it increased to 23% after 20 years.[241,302,304] The diagnosis of acute gout can be made with a good history, physical examination and, when needed, an examination of the joint fluid for monosodium urate monohydrate crystals during an acute attack. However, gout in transplant patients has differences that include involvement of proximal joints, including the sacroiliac joint[305] a shorter lead time from onset of hyperuricemia to the first gout attack, with a mean time of approximately 1.5 to 2 years; and the more frequent occurrence of tophi.[301] Glucocorticoids may mute the full expression of acute gout.

Treatment of acute gout in renal transplant recipients involves modification of the American College of Rheumatology guidelines used in the general population.[306] These guidelines recommend the use of NSAIDs, colchicine, or corticosteroids for treatment of acute gout in patients who do not have significant renal impairment or peptic ulcer disease. However, in renal transplant recipients both cyclooxygenase-1 and cyclooxygenase-2 NSAIDs are not recommended as first-line treatment for acute gout because of adverse effects on renal hemodynamics, including renal vasoconstriction, with reduced renal blood flow and decreased GFR, sodium and water retention, hyperkalemia, hypertension, and in some cases acute renal failure. Colchicine appears to be a useful medication for acute attacks, but it too must be used with caution and in modified dose (Box 89-3).[307] This author does not recommend titrating colchicine to the point of diarrhea; one of the goals of colchicine therapy should be to avoid diarrhea. Among the adverse effects of colchicine noted in Box 89-3 is myoneuropathy, which can cause elevated serum creatine kinase levels and changes seen on electromyography, particularly when used for long periods of time in patients with impaired renal function or also receiving statins, cyclosporine, or clarithromycin.[301,308-311] Colchicine 0.6 mg may be continued on an every-other-day basis if necessary for a short time with close monitoring for toxicity until acute gouty attacks cease and the serum uric acid has been reduced to a safe level.

An alternative treatment is the use of glucocorticoids at doses of 0.5 to 1.0 mg/kg of prednisone for 3 to 7 days with tapering to a maintenance dose within 14 days.[312] Adrenocorticotropic hormone 40 to 80 IUs given intramuscularly has also been used.[312] A low-purine diet can be a useful adjunct in males.[313,314] In patients receiving cyclosporine, a change to another immunosuppressant not having such adverse renal hemodynamic and hyperuricemic effects may be appropriate. Diuretics should be avoided if possible or used in reduced doses because of their hyperuricemic effects.

According to guidelines for the general population, therapy to lower elevated serum uric acid levels should be undertaken in patients who have hyperuricemia and gouty arthritis with tophi, gouty erosive changes on radiograph, or two or more attacks/year; however, one attack has been deemed sufficient in the transplant population.[301,306] Reduction of serum uric

Box 89-3 A Modified Protocol for Colchicine in the Treatment of Acute Gout in Stable Renal Transplant Recipients

Day 1
Colchicine 0.6 mg orally q1h × 2 maximum, but stop if any dose causes diarrhea

Days 2–8
Colchicine 0.6 mg orally daily, but stop if any dose causes diarrhea

Days 10, 12, 14
Colchicine 0.6 mg orally every other day, but stop if diarrhea occurs

Note: The objective is to terminate the acute painful inflammatory joint symptoms while minimizing the risk of toxicity. One should be thoroughly familiar with each patient's drug sensitivities and with other potential adverse effects, including myopathy, neuropathy, alopecia, myelosuppression and, rarely, fatality, and with drug interactions, especially with immunosuppressants. Lower doses or drug avoidance are necessary for those with a GFR < 50 mL/min/1.73 m^2. The risks and benefits of treatment, alternative treatment, or nontreatment must be carefully evaluated for each patient. Prudent clinical judgment and careful monitoring are essential. Also adjust allopurinol, azathioprine, diuretics, and diet as needed.

Modified from Braun WE: Modification of the treatment of gout in renal transplant recipients. Transplant Proc 2000;32:199.

Box 89-4 A Modified Protocol for Managing Tophaceous Gout in Stable Renal Transplant Recipients

For Patients on Azathioprine
Allopurinol 50 mg/day; azathioprine reduced by 50%–75% (no more than 50 mg/day)
Monitor complete blood count, serum uric acid, and liver and renal function. Leukopenia would be the most likely sign of toxicity and would require discontinuation of both drugs.
Reduce or eliminate diuretic, if possible; diet as needed (males)

For Patients on Mycophenolate Mofetil
Allopurinol 100 mg/day
Monitor complete blood count, serum uric acid, and liver and renal function
Reduce or eliminate diuretic if possible; diet as needed (males)

For All Patients Being Treated for Gout
Ultrasound of renal allograft for obstruction or stones; treat as indicated
Urine alkalinization to pH of ≈6.0–6.5*
Appropriate hydration
If no adverse effects or toxicity are encountered, except for patients on azathioprine, cautiously increase allopurinol toward 200 mg/day if necessary, and continue close monitoring
If GFR is > 50 mL/min/1.73 m^2, probenecid 250 mg bid may be initiated
Addition of losartan for its uricosuric effect can be considered

Note: The objective is to decrease urate deposits while minimizing drug toxicity or damage to the allograft. One should be thoroughly familiar with each patient's drug sensitivities and with the potentially serious adverse effects of each component of treatment, medications, and fluids, including the broad range that may be seen with allopurinol and probenecid. One should also be aware of any potential drug interactions, especially with immunosuppressants. With impaired renal function (GFR < 50 mL/min/1.73 m^2), azathioprine doses are often reduced, and allopurinol and probenecid may need to be avoided entirely. The risks and benefits of treatment, alternative treatment, or nontreatment must be carefully evaluated for each patient. Prudent clinical judgment and careful monitoring are essential.

*Approaches to alkalinizing the urine (and some of their risks) when clinically safe include the use of potassium citrate (hyperkalemia, alkalosis); sodium citrate, sodium bicarbonate (hypertension, fluid retention, possibly nephrocalcinosis and nephrolithiasis), and acetazolamide (paresthesias, renal stones) may be more problematic.

Modified from Braun WE: Modification of the treatment of gout in renal transplant recipients. Transplant Proc 2000;32:199.

acid levels can be achieved through inhibition of uric acid production by means of the xanthine oxidase inhibitor allopurinol or by cautiously employing a uricosuric agent such as probenecid if there is good renal function. Adverse effects of allopurinol, especially the hypersensitivity syndrome, and its interaction with azathioprine, are noted in Box 89-4.

Losartan also has a uricosuric effect that is more pronounced the higher the serum uric acid level.[315-317] Uricosuria could pose a risk for uric acid stone formation, but the solubility of uric acid rises significantly even with a urine pH of 6.0. Renal allografts with impaired function may not be capable of acidifying the urine to a pH of 5.0 where urate stones can form. Nevertheless, urine pH should be kept at 6.0 or above. It has been my experience that the uric acid level does not have to be driven down below 6 mg/dL to suppress acute gouty attacks, and often a reduction from a range of 11 to 13 mg/dL to 8 to 9 mg/dL, which may be achievable with losartan, is sufficient to avoid acute attacks. However, hyperuricemia may still be a cardiovascular risk factor (see the section Coronary Heart Disease in this chapter).[317,318]

Two new agents are under study for the treatment of hyperuricemia: urate oxidase (uricase), which catalyzes the conversion of uric acid to allantoin, and febuxostat, a nonpurine selective inhibitor of xanthine oxidase.[301,311,319] These drugs have not been studied in renal transplant recipients. A single report from Italy in 1997 described the use of urate oxidase in six heart transplant patients receiving cyclosporine, azathioprine, and prednisone; their acute gouty symptoms subsided and plasma uric acid levels normalized with apparently no change in serum creatinine or blood counts.[301,320] Febuxostat has been shown in a randomized, controlled trial of nontransplant patients with gout to reduce serum uric acid levels to 6 mg/dL or lower in 81% of cases, compared to 39% of those receiving 300 mg of allopurinol.[321] Emerging problems with febuxostat include hepatotoxicity, diarrhea, musculoskeletal symptoms, and a high frequency (70%) of gouty flares that developed despite concurrent colchicine or naproxen therapy.[319]

HYPOPHOSPHATEMIA

Hypophosphatemia may be caused by massive diuresis immediately after transplantation, persistence of secondary hyperparathyroidism early post-transplantation, defective proximal tubular phosphate reabsorption because of glucocorticoid therapy or Fanconi-like syndrome, glycosuria, acyclovir (in rat studies),[322] and even the inadvertent use of phosphate binders as antacids. A recent study of the phosphaturic hormone FGF-23, an inhibitor of renal 1-α-hydroxylase activity, in 41 patients at the time of renal transplantation and 3 months after transplant demonstrated that the persistence of FGF-23 after transplant contributed to hypophosphatemia and suboptimal calcitriol levels.[297] Complications of severe hypophosphatemia include rhabdomyolysis, impaired left ventricular function and possibly ventricular arrhythmias, impaired pulmonary function presumably related to respiratory muscle impairment, defects in erythrocyte metabolism with possible hemolysis, insulin resistance, and osteomalacia. Oral supplementation with phosphorus-containing compounds may be needed. Dipyridamole at a dose of 75 mg qid has been reported to increase low Tm PO_4/GFR and improve hypophosphatemia.[323]

HYPOMAGNESEMIA

Cyclosporine, tacrolimus, and sirolimus may cause renal magnesium wasting and hypomagnesemia. Magnesium depletion is associated with intracellular calcium overload, cardiac arrhythmias, and changes in the coronary vasculature similar to those seen in accelerated atherosclerosis, as well as neurological and GI symptoms. The hypomagnesemia caused by cyclosporine is typically not accompanied by hypocalcemia or hypokalemia. Oral magnesium supplements with substantial elemental magnesium content include magnesium oxide, as Mag-Ox 400 (241 mg), Slow-Mag enteric-coated (64 mg), and Uro-Mag (84 mg).

Acknowledgments

I am indebted for helpful suggestions to Dr. Michael Limhoff (Coronary Heart Disease and Medical Interventional Treatment of Established CHD), Dr. Byron Hoogwerf (New-Onset Diabetes Mellitus and Prediabetic Conditions), and Dr. Angelo Licata (Hyperparathyroidism and Osteoporosis).

Mrs. Sandra Bronoff provided excellent editorial assistance.

References

1. Kasiske BL, Vazquez MA, Harmon WE, et al: Recommendations for the outpatient surveillance of renal transplant recipients. American Society of Transplantation. J Am Soc Nephrol 2000; 11(Suppl):S1–S86.
2. CYP3A and drug interactions. Med Lett Drugs Ther 2005;47: 54–55.
3. Tablet splitting. Med Lett Drugs Ther 2004;46:89–91.
4. Ojo AO: Cardiovascular complications after renal transplantation and their prevention. Transplantation 2006;82:603–611.
5. Foley RN, Parfrey PS, Sarnak MJ: Clinical epidemiology of cardiovascular disease in chronic renal disease. Am J Kidney Dis 1998;32:S112–S119.
6. Kasiske BL, Chakkera HA, Roel J: Explained and unexplained ischemic heart disease risk after renal transplantation. J Am Soc Nephrol 2000;11:1735–1743.
7. Herzog CA, Ma JZ, Collins AJ: Long-term survival of renal transplant recipients in the United States after acute myocardial infarction. Am J Kidney Dis 2000;36:145–152.
8. LaRosa JC, Grundy SM, Waters DD, et al: Intensive lipid lowering with atorvastatin in patients with stable coronary disease. N Engl J Med 2005;352:1425–1435.
9. Grundy SM, Cleeman JI, Merz CN, et al: Implications of recent clinical trials for the National Cholesterol Education Program Adult Treatment Panel III guidelines. Circulation 2004;110: 227–239.
10. Cannon CP, Steinberg BA, Murphy SA, et al: Meta-analysis of cardiovascular outcomes trials comparing intensive versus moderate statin therapy. J Am Coll Cardiol 2006;48:438–445.
11. Boden WE, O'Rourke RA, Teo KK, et al: Optimal medical therapy with or without PCI for stable coronary disease. N Engl J Med 2007;356:1503–1516.
12. Steinberg BA, Steg PG, Bhatt DL, et al: Comparisons of guideline-recommended therapies in patients with documented coronary artery disease having percutaneous coronary intervention versus coronary artery bypass grafting versus medical therapy only (from the REACH international registry). Am J Cardiol 2007;99:1212–1215.
13. Kasiske BL, Guijarro C, Massy ZA, et al: Cardiovascular disease after renal transplantation. J Am Soc Nephrol 1996;7:158–165.
14. Greenland P, Smith SC Jr, Grundy SM: Improving coronary heart disease risk assessment in asymptomatic people: Role of traditional risk factors and noninvasive cardiovascular tests. Circulation 2001;104:1863–1867.
15. Kasiske BL: Risk factors for accelerated atherosclerosis in renal transplant recipients. Am J Med 1988;84:985–992.
16. Gerstein HC, Mann JF, Yi Q, et al: Albuminuria and risk of cardiovascular events, death, and heart failure in diabetic and nondiabetic individuals. JAMA 2001;286:421–426.
17. Mann JF, Gerstein HC, Pogue J, et al: Renal insufficiency as a predictor of cardiovascular outcomes and the impact of ramipril: the HOPE randomized trial. Ann Intern Med 2001;134:629–636.
18. Sarnak MJ, Levey AS, Schoolwerth AC, et al: Kidney disease as a risk factor for development of cardiovascular disease: A statement from the American Heart Association Councils on Kidney in Cardiovascular Disease, High Blood Pressure Research, Clinical Cardiology, and Epidemiology and Prevention. Circulation 2003; 108:2154–2169.
19. Wan RK, Mark PB, Jardine AG: Cardiovascular disease management in renal transplant recipients: More or less treatment? Transplantation 2006;82:737–738.
20. From AM, Hyder JA, Kearns AM, et al: Relationship between low bone mineral density and exercise-induced myocardial ischemia. Mayo Clin Proc 2007;82:679–685.
21. Executive summary of the third report of the National Cholesterol Education Program (NCEP) expert panel on detection, evaluation, and treatment of high blood cholesterol in adults (adult treatment panel III). JAMA 2001;285:2486–2497.
22. Detrano RC, Wong ND, Doherty TM, et al: Coronary calcium does not accurately predict near-term future coronary events in high-risk adults. Circulation 1999;99:2633–2638.
23. He ZX, Hedrick TD, Pratt CM, et al: Severity of coronary artery calcification by electron beam computed tomography predicts silent myocardial ischemia. Circulation 2000;101:244–251.
24. Grundy SM: Primary prevention of coronary heart disease: integrating risk assessment with intervention. Circulation 1999; 100:988–998.
25. Block GA, Port FK: Re-evaluation of risks associated with hyperphosphatemia and hyperparathyroidism in dialysis patients: Recommendations for a change in management. Am J Kidney Dis 2000;35:1226–1237.

26. Kullo IJ, Edwards WD, Schwartz RS: Vulnerable plaque: Pathobiology and clinical implications. Ann Intern Med 1998;129:1050–1060.

27. Massy ZA, Kasiske BL: Posttransplant hyperlipidemia: mechanisms and management. J Am Soc Nephrol 1996;7:971–977.

28. Augustine JJ, Bodziak KA, Hricik DE: Use of sirolimus in solid organ transplantation. Drugs 2007;67:369–391.

29. Ligtenberg G, Hene RJ, Blankestijn PJ, Koomans HA: Cardiovascular risk factors in renal transplant patients: Cyclosporin A versus tacrolimus. J Am Soc Nephrol 2001;12:368–373.

30. Rigatto C, Parfrey P: Therapy insight: Management of cardiovascular disease in the renal transplant recipient. Nat Clin Pract Nephrol 2006;2:514–526.

31. Kasiske B, Cosio FG, Beto J, et al: Clinical practice guidelines for managing dyslipidemias in kidney transplant patients: A report from the Managing Dyslipidemias in Chronic Kidney Disease Work Group of the National Kidney Foundation Kidney Disease Outcomes Quality Initiative. Am J Transplant 2004;4(Suppl 7):13–53.

32. Saunders RN, Metcalfe MS, Nicholson ML: Rapamycin in transplantation: A review of the evidence. Kidney Int 2001;59:3–16.

33. Podder H, Stepkowski SM, Napoli KL, et al: Pharmacokinetic interactions augment toxicities of sirolimus/cyclosporine combinations. J Am Soc Nephrol 2001;12:1059–1071.

34. Molitch ME: Management of dyslipidemias in patients with diabetes and chronic kidney disease. Clin J Am Soc Nephrol 2006;1:1090–1099.

35. Neuvonen PJ, Niemi M, Backman JT: Drug interactions with lipid-lowering drugs: Mechanisms and clinical relevance. Clin Pharmacol Ther 2006;80:565–581.

36. Chong PH, Seeger JD, Franklin C: Clinically relevant differences between the statins: Implications for therapeutic selection. Am J Med 2001;111:390–400.

37. Coenzyme Q10. Med Lett Drugs Ther 2006;48:19–20.

38. Phosphate binders. Med Lett Drugs Ther 2006;48:15–16.

39. Holdaas H, Fellstrom B, Jardine AG, et al: Effect of fluvastatin on cardiac outcomes in renal transplant recipients: A multicentre, randomised, placebo-controlled trial. Lancet 2003;361:2024–2031.

40. Jardine AG, Holdaas H, Fellstrom B, et al: Fluvastatin prevents cardiac death and myocardial infarction in renal transplant recipients: Post-hoc subgroup analyses of the ALERT study. Am J Transplant 2004;4:988–995.

41. Wissing KM, Unger P, Ghisdal L, et al: Effect of atorvastatin therapy and conversion to tacrolimus on hypercholesterolemia and endothelial dysfunction after renal transplantation. Transplantation 2006;82:771–778.

42. Steffens S, Mach F: Drug insight: Immunomodulatory effects of statins—potential benefits for renal patients? Nat Clin Pract Nephrol 2006;2:378–387.

43. Lentine KL, Brennan DC: Statin use after renal transplantation: A systematic quality review of trial-based evidence. Nephrol Dial Transplant 2004;19:2378–2386.

44. Kasiske BL, Heim-Duthoy KL, Singer GG, et al: The effects of lipid-lowering agents on acute renal allograft rejection. Transplantation 2001;72:223–227.

45. Glorioso N, Troffa C, Filigheddu F, et al: Effect of the HMG-CoA reductase inhibitors on blood pressure in patients with essential hypertension and primary hypercholesterolemia. Hypertension 1999;34:1281–1286.

46. Ridker PM, Hennekens CH, Buring JE, Rifai N: C-reactive protein and other markers of inflammation in the prediction of cardiovascular disease in women. N Engl J Med 2000;342:836–843.

47. Katznelson S: Immunosuppressive and antiproliferative effects of HMG-CoA reductase inhibitors. Transplant Proc 1999;31:22S–24S.

48. Vrtovsnik F, Couette S, Prie D, et al: Lovastatin-induced inhibition of renal epithelial tubular cell proliferation involves a p21 ras activated, AP-1-dependent pathway. Kidney Int 1997;52:1016–1027.

49. Safety of aggressive statin therapy. Med Lett Drugs Ther 2004;46:95–96.

50. Vidt DG, Cressman MD, Harris S, et al: Rosuvastatin-induced arrest in progression of renal disease. Cardiology 2004;102:52–60.

51. Sandhu S, Wiebe N, Fried LF, Tonelli M: Statins for improving renal outcomes: A meta-analysis. J Am Soc Nephrol 2006;17:2006–2016.

52. Douglas K, O'Malley PG, Jackson JL: Meta-analysis: the effect of statins on albuminuria. Ann Intern Med 2006;145:117–124.

53. Ritz E, Wanner C: Lipid changes and statins in chronic renal insufficiency. J Am Soc Nephrol 2006;17:S226–S230.

54. Kohnle M, Pietruck F, Kribben A, et al: Ezetimibe for the treatment of uncontrolled hypercholesterolemia in patients with high-dose statin therapy after renal transplantation. Am J Transplant 2006;6:205–208.

55. Rhabdomyolosis with ezetimide. Med Lett Drugs Ther 2005;47:17–19.

56. Vytorin: a combination of ezetimibe and simvastatin. Med Lett Drugs Ther 2004;46:73–74.

57. Westphal S, Dierkes J, Luley C: Effects of fenofibrate and gemfibrozil on plasma homocysteine. Lancet 2001;358:39–40.

58. Fish oil supplements. Med Lett Drugs Ther 2006;48:59–60.

59. Omega-3 polyunsaturated fatty acids (Omacor) for hypertriglyceridemia. Med Lett Drugs Ther 2005;47:91.

60. Toth PP: Reducing cardiovascular risk by targeting high-density lipoprotein cholesterol. Curr Atheroscler Rep 2007;9:81–88.

61. American Diabetes Association: Standards of medical care in diabetes—2006. Diabet Care 2006;29:S4–42.

62. Jindal RM: Posttransplant diabetes mellitus—a review. Transplantation 1994;58:1289–1298.

63. Kasiske BL, Snyder JJ, Gilbertson D, Matas AJ: Diabetes mellitus after kidney transplantation in the United States. Am J Transplant 2003;3:178–185.

64. Woodward RS, Schnitzler MA, Baty J, et al: Incidence and cost of new onset diabetes mellitus among U.S. wait-listed and transplanted renal allograft recipients. Am J Transplant 2003;3:590–598.

65. Crutchlow MF, Bloom RD: Transplant-associated hyperglycemia: A new look at an old problem. Clin J Am Soc Nephrol 2007;2:343–355.

66. Cosio FG, Kudva Y, van der Velde M, et al: New onset hyperglycemia and diabetes are associated with increased cardiovascular risk after kidney transplantation. Kidney Int 2005;67:2415–2421.

67. Nam JH, Mun JI, Kim SI, et al: Beta-cell dysfunction rather than insulin resistance is the main contributing factor for the development of postrenal transplantation diabetes mellitus. Transplantation 2001;71:1417–1423.

68. Hamer RA, Chow CL, Ong AC, McKane WS: Polycystic kidney disease is a risk factor for new-onset diabetes after transplantation. Transplantation 2007;83:36–40.

69. Cosio FG, Pesavento TE, Kim S, et al: Patient survival after renal transplantation: IV. impact of post-transplant diabetes. Kidney Int 2002;62:1440–1446.

70. Shah T, Kasravi A, Huang E, et al: Risk factors for development of new-onset diabetes mellitus after kidney transplantation. Transplantation 2006;82:1673–1676.

71. Williams ME: Management of the diabetic transplant recipient. Kidney Int 1995;48:1660–1674.

72. Bhalla V, Nast CC, Stollenwerk N, et al: Recurrent and de novo diabetic nephropathy in renal allografts. Transplantation 2003;75:66–71.

73. Kelly JJ, Walker RG, Kincaid-Smith P: De novo diabetic nodular glomerulosclerosis in a renal allograft. Transplantation 1992;53:688–689.

74. Sharif A, Moore RH, Baboolal K: The use of oral glucose tolerance tests to risk stratify for new-onset diabetes after transplantation: An underdiagnosed phenomenon. Transplantation 2006;82:1667–1672.

75. Nathan DM: Finding new treatments for diabetes—how many, how fast... how good? N Engl J Med 2007;356:437–440.

76. Tuomilehto J, Lindström J, Eriksson JG, for the Finnish Diabetes Prevention Study Group: Prevention of type 2 diabetes mellitus by changes in lifestyle among subjects with impaired glucose tolerance. N Engl J Med 2001;344: 1343–1350.

77. Diabetes Prevention Program Research Group: Reduction in the incidence of type 2 diabetes with lifestyle intervention or metformin. N Engl J Med 2002;346:393–406.

78. Nathan DM, Buse JB, Davidson MB, et al: Management of hyperglycemia in type 2 diabetes: A consensus algorithm for the initiation and adjustment of therapy: A consensus statement from the American Diabetes Association and the European Association for the Study of Diabetes. Diabet Care 2006;29: 1963–1972.

79. Home PD, Pocock SJ, Beck-Nielsen H, et al: Rosiglitazone evaluated for cardiovascular outcomes — an interim analysis. N Engl J Med 2007;357:28–38.

80. Nissen SE, Wolski K: Effect of rosiglitazone on the risk of myocardial infarction and death from cardiovascular causes. N Engl J Med 2007;356:2457–2471.

81. Kahn SE, Haffner SM, Heise MA, et al: Glycemic durability of rosiglitazone, metformin, or glyburide monotherapy. N Engl J Med 2006;355:2427–2443.

82. Pietruck F, Kribben A, Van TN, et al: Rosiglitazone is a safe and effective treatment option of new-onset diabetes mellitus after renal transplantation. Transpl Int 2005;18:483–486.

83. Nathan DM: Rosiglitazone and cardiotoxicity—weighing the evidence. N Engl J Med 2007;357:64–66.

84. Turk T, Pietruck F, Dolff S, et al: Repaglinide in the management of new-onset diabetes mellitus after renal transplantation. Am J Transplant 2006;6:842–846.

85. Kendall DM, Kim D, Maggs D: Incretin mimetics and dipeptidyl peptidase-IV inhibitors: A review of emerging therapies for type 2 diabetes. Diabetes Technol Ther 2006;8:385–396.

86. Sitagliptin (Januvia) for type 2 diabetes. Med Lett Drugs Ther 2007;49:1–3.

87. Exenatide (Byetta) for type 2 diabetes. Med Lett Drugs Ther 2005;47:45–46.

88. Bolen S, Feldman L, Vassy J, et al: Systematic review: Comparative effectiveness and safety of oral medications for type 2 diabetes mellitus. Ann Int Med 2007;147:386–399.

89. Karalliedde J, Buckingham R, Starkie M, et al: Effect of various diuretic treatments on rosiglitazone-induced fluid retention. J Am Soc Nephrol 2006;17:3482–3490.

90. Barbosa J, Steffes MW, Sutherland DE, et al: Effect of glycemic control on early diabetic renal lesions. A 5-year randomized controlled clinical trial of insulin-dependent diabetic kidney transplant recipients. JAMA 1994;272:600–606.

91. Prasad GV, Kim SJ, Huang M, et al: Reduced incidence of new-onset diabetes mellitus after renal transplantation with 3-hydroxy-3-methylglutaryl-coenzyme A reductase inhibitors (statins). Am J Transplant 2004;4:1897–1903.

92. Scheen AJ: Renin-angiotensin system inhibition prevents type 2 diabetes mellitus. Part 2. Overview of physiological and biochemical mechanisms. Diabet Metab 2004;30: 498–505.

93. Bosch J, Yusuf S, Gerstein HC, et al: Effect of ramipril on the incidence of diabetes. N Engl J Med 2006;355:1551–1562.

94. Gaede P, Lund-Andersen H, Parving HH, Pedersen O: Effect of a multifactorial intervention on mortality in type 2 diabetes. N Engl J Med 2008;358:580–591.

95. Kirk AD, Mannon RB, Swanson SJ, Hale DA: Strategies for minimizing immunosuppression in kidney transplantation. Transpl Int 2005;18:2–14.

96. Kasiske BL, Klinger D: Cigarette smoking in renal transplant recipients. J Am Soc Nephrol 2000;11:753–759.

97. Orth SR, Ritz E, Schrier RW: The renal risks of smoking. Kidney Int 1997;51:1669–1677.

98. Ritz E, Benck U, Franek E, et al: Effects of smoking on renal hemodynamics in healthy volunteers and in patients with glomerular disease. J Am Soc Nephrol 1998;9:1798–1804.

99. Manson JE, Ajani UA, Liu S, et al: A prospective study of cigarette smoking and the incidence of diabetes mellitus among US male physicians. Am J Med 2000;109:538–542.

100. Fiore MC, Bailey WC, Cohen SJ, et al: Treating tobacco use and dependence. In Quick Reference Guide for Clinicians. Rockville, MD: U.S. Department of Health and Human Services, Public Health Service, 2000.

101. DeNelsky GY, Bower ME: Smoking cessation in cardiac preventive health. In Robinson K (ed): Preventive Cardiology. Armonk, NY: Futura Publishing, 1998, pp 325–353.

102. Helge TD, Denelsky GY: Pharmacologic aids to smoking cessation. Cleve Clin J Med 2000;67:818,821–824.

103. Jorenby DE, Leischow SJ, Nides MA, et al: A controlled trial of sustained-release bupropion, a nicotine patch, or both for smoking cessation. N Engl J Med 1999;340:685–691.

104. Hays JT, Hurt RD, Rigotti NA, et al: Sustained-release bupropion for pharmacologic relapse prevention after smoking cessation. A randomized, controlled trial. Ann Intern Med 2001; 135:423–433.

105. Leonard M: Medications used for smoking cessation. Pharmacother Update 2006;9:1–5.

106. Schroeder SA, Sox HC: Trials that matter: Varenicline: A designer drug to help smokers quit. Ann Intern Med 2006;145:784–785.

107. Klesges RC, Johnson KC, Somes G: Varenicline for smoking cessation: Definite promise, but no panacea. JAMA 2006;296: 94–95.

108. Gonzales D, Rennard SI, Nides M, et al: Varenicline, an $\alpha_4\beta_2$ nicotinic acetylcholine receptor partial agonist, vs. sustained-release bupropion and placebo for smoking cessation: A randomized controlled trial. JAMA 2006;296:47–55.

109. Jorenby DE, Hays JT, Rigotti NA, et al: Efficacy of varenicline, an $\alpha_4\beta_2$ nicotinic acetylcholine receptor partial agonist, vs. placebo or sustained-release bupropion for smoking cessation: A randomized controlled trial. JAMA 2006;296:56–63.

110. Tonstad S, Tonnesen P, Hajek P, et al: Effect of maintenance therapy with varenicline on smoking cessation: A randomized controlled trial. JAMA 2006;296:64–71.

111. DeNelsky GY: Stop Smoking Now. Cleveland, OH: Cleveland Clinic Press, 2007.

112. Varenicline (Chantix) for tobacco dependence. Med Lett Drugs Ther 2006;48:66–68.

113. Smith SC Jr, Allen J, Blair SN, et al: AHA/ACC guidelines for secondary prevention for patients with coronary and other atherosclerotic vascular disease: 2006 update endorsed by the National Heart, Lung, and Blood Institute. J Am Coll Cardiol 2006;47:2130–2139.

114. Bhatt DL, Fox KA, Hacke W, et al: Clopidogrel and aspirin versus aspirin alone for the prevention of atherothrombotic events. N Engl J Med 2006;354:1706–1717.

115. Steinhubl SR, Berger PB, Mann JT 3rd, et al, for the CREDO Investigators: Early and sustained dual oral antiplatelet therapy following percutaneous coronary intervention: A randomized controlled trial. JAMA 2002;288:2411–2420.

116. Kagami S, Border WA, Miller DE, Noble NA: Angiotensin II stimulates extracellular matrix protein synthesis through induction of transforming growth factor-β expression in rat glomerular mesangial cells. J Clin Invest 1994;93: 2431–2437.

117. Monton M, Castilla MA, Alvarez Arroyo MV, et al: Effects of angiotensin II on endothelial cell growth: Role of AT_1 and AT_2 receptors. J Am Soc Nephrol 1998;9:969–974.

118. Pitt B, Zannad F, Remme WJ, et al, for the Randomized Aldactone Evaluation Study Investigators: The effect of spironolactone

on morbidity and mortality in patients with severe heart failure. N Engl J Med 1999;341:709–717.

119. Schepkens H, Vanholder R, Billiouw JM, Lameire N: Life-threatening hyperkalemia during combined therapy with angiotensin-converting enzyme inhibitors and spironolactone: An analysis of 25 cases. Am J Med 2001;110:438–441.

120. Borghi C, Prandin MG, Costa FV, et al: Use of statins and blood pressure control in treated hypertensive patients with hypercholesterolemia. J Cardiovasc Pharmacol 2000;35:549–555.

121. Rizzo M, Rini GB: Statins, fracture risk, and bone remodeling: What is true? Am J Med Sci 2006;332:55–60.

122. Spaulding C, Henry P, Teiger E, et al: Sirolimus-eluting versus uncoated stents in acute myocardial infarction. N Engl J Med 2006;355:1093–1104.

123. Laarman GJ, Suttorp MJ, Dirksen MT, et al: Paclitaxel-eluting versus uncoated stents in primary percutaneous coronary intervention. N Engl J Med 2006;355:1105–1113.

124. Sousa JE, Costa MA, Abizaid A, et al: Lack of neointimal proliferation after implantation of sirolimus-coated stents in human coronary arteries: A quantitative coronary angiography and three-dimensional intravascular ultrasound study. Circulation 2001;103:192–195.

125. Shuchman M: Trading restenosis for thrombosis? New questions about drug-eluting stents. N Engl J Med 2006;355:1949–1952.

126. Eisenstein EL, Anstrom KJ, Kong DF, et al: Clopidogrel use and long-term clinical outcomes after drug-eluting stent implantation. JAMA 2007;297:159–168.

127. Ferguson ER, Hudson SL, Diethelm AG, et al: Outcome after myocardial revascularization and renal transplantation: A 25-year single-institution experience. Ann Surg 1999;230:232–241.

128. Dresler C, Uthoff K, Wahlers T, et al: Open heart operations after renal transplantation. Ann Thorac Surg 1997;63:143–146.

129. Herzog CA, Ma JZ, Collins A: Three-year survival of renal transplant recipients in the US after coronary artery bypass surgery, coronary angioplasty, and coronary stenting. J Am Soc Nephrol 2001;11:719A.

130. Amarenco P, Labreuche J, Lavallee P, Touboul PJ: Statins in stroke prevention and carotid atherosclerosis: Systematic review and up-to-date meta-analysis. Stroke 2004;35:2902–2909.

131. Fathi R, Isbel N, Short L, et al: The effect of long-term aggressive lipid lowering on ischemic and atherosclerotic burden in patients with chronic kidney disease. Am J Kidney Dis 2004; 43:45–52.

132. Crouse JR III, Raichlen JS, Riley WA, et al: Effect of rosuvastatin on progression of carotid intima-media thickness in low-risk individuals with subclinical atherosclerosis: The METEOR trial. JAMA 2007;297:1344–1353.

133. Executive Committee for the Asymptomatic Carotid Atherosclerosis Study: Endarterectomy for asymptomatic carotid artery stenosis. JAMA 1995;273:1421–1428.

134. Amarenco P, Bogousslavsky J, Callahan A III, et al: High-dose atorvastatin after stroke or transient ischemic attack. N Engl J Med 2006;355:549–559.

135. Collins R, Armitage J, Parish S, et al, for the Heart Protection Study Collaborative Group: Effects of cholesterol-lowering with simvastatin on stroke and other major vascular events in 20536 people with cerebrovascular disease or other high-risk conditions. Lancet 2004;363:757–767.

136. Vickrey BG, Rector TS, Wickstrom SL, et al: Occurrence of secondary ischemic events among persons with atherosclerotic vascular disease. Stroke 2002;33:901–906.

137. Iso H, Jacobs DR Jr , Wentworth D, et al: Serum cholesterol levels and six-year mortality from stroke in 350,977 men screened for the multiple risk factor intervention trial. N Engl J Med 1989;320:904–910.

138. Yano K, Reed DM, MacLean CJ: Serum cholesterol and hemorrhagic stroke in the Honolulu Heart Program. Stroke 1989; 20:1460–1465.

139. Lee SH, Bae HJ, Yoon BW, et al: Low concentration of serum total cholesterol is associated with multifocal signal loss lesions on gradient-echo magnetic resonance imaging: Analysis of risk factors for multifocal signal loss lesions. Stroke 2002;33:2845–2849.

140. Waters DD, Schwartz GG, Olsson AG, et al: Effects of atorvastatin on stroke in patients with unstable angina or non-Q-wave myocardial infarction: A Myocardial Ischemia Reduction with Aggressive Cholesterol Lowering (MIRACL) substudy. Circulation 2002;106:1690–1695.

141. Coward LJ, Featherstone RL, Brown MM: Safety and efficacy of endovascular treatment of carotid artery stenosis compared with carotid endarterectomy: A Cochrane Systematic Review of the randomized evidence. Stroke 2005;36:905–911.

142. Mas JL, Chatellier G, Beyssen B, et al: Endarterectomy versus stenting in patients with symptomatic severe carotid stenosis. N Engl J Med 2006;355:1660–1671.

143. Ringleb PA, Allenberg J, Bruckmann H, et al: 30 day results from the SPACE trial of Stent-Protected Angioplasty versus Carotid Endarterectomy in symptomatic patients: A randomised non-inferiority trial. Lancet 2006;368:1239–1247.

144. Furlan AJ: Carotid-artery stenting—case open or closed? N Engl J Med 2006;355:1726–1729.

145. Ruggieri PM, Poulos N, Masaryk TJ, et al: Occult intracranial aneurysms in polycystic kidney disease: Screening with MR angiography. Radiology 1994;191:33–39.

146. Huston J III, Torres VE, Sulivan PP, et al: Value of magnetic resonance angiography for the detection of intracranial aneurysms in autosomal dominant polycystic kidney disease. J Am Soc Nephrol 1993;3:1871–1877.

147. Marckmann P, Skov L, Rossen K, et al: Nephrogenic systemic fibrosis: Suspected causative role of gadodiamide used for contrast-enhanced magnetic resonance imaging. J Am Soc Nephrol 2006;17:2359–2362.

148. Grobner T, Prischl FC: Gadolinium and nephrogenic systemic fibrosis. Kidney Int 2007;72:260–264.

149. Karlik SJ: Gadodiamide-associated nephrogenic systemic fibrosis. Am J Roentgenol 2007;188:W584.

150. Kasiske BL, Ramos EL, Gaston RS, et al: The evaluation of renal transplant candidates: Clinical practice guidelines. Patient Care and Education Committee of the American Society of Transplant Physicians. J Am Soc Nephrol 1995; 6:1–34.

151. Belz MM, Fick-Brosnahan GM, Hughes RL, et al: Recurrence of intracranial aneurysms in autosomal-dominant polycystic kidney disease. Kidney Int 2003;63:1824–1830.

152. Wattanakit K, Folsom AR, Selvin E, et al: Kidney function and risk of peripheral arterial disease: Results from the Atherosclerosis Risk In Communities (ARIC) study. J Am Soc Nephrol 2007;18:629–636.

153. Snyder JJ, Kasiske BL, Maclean R: Peripheral arterial disease and renal transplantation. J Am Soc Nephrol 2006;17:2056–2068.

154. Braun WE, Avery R, Gifford RW Jr, Straffon RA: Life after 20 years with a kidney transplant: Redefined disease profiles and an emerging nondiabetic vasculopathy. Transplant Proc 1997;29:247–249.

155. Hiatt WR: Medical treatment of peripheral arterial disease and claudication. N Engl J Med 2001;344:1608–1621.

156. Cozzolino M, Brancaccio D, Gallieni M, Slatopolsky E: Pathogenesis of vascular calcification in chronic kidney disease. Kidney Int 2005;68:429–436.

157. Hankey GJ, Norman PE, Eikelboom JW: Medical treatment of peripheral arterial disease. JAMA 2006;295:547–553.

158. Collaborative meta-analysis of randomised trials of antiplatelet therapy for prevention of death, myocardial infarction, and stroke in high risk patients. BMJ 2002;324:71–86.

159. Patrono C, Garcia Rodriguez LA, Landolfi R, Baigent C: Low-dose aspirin for the prevention of atherothrombosis. N Engl J Med 2005;353:2373–2383.

160. CAPRIE Steering Committee: A randomised, blinded, trial of Clopidogrel versus Aspirin in Patients at Risk of Ischaemic Events (CAPRIE). Lancet 1996;348:1329–1339.

161. Tepel M, van der Giet M, Schwarzfeld C, et al: Prevention of radiographic-contrast-agent-induced reductions in renal function by acetylcysteine. N Engl J Med 2000;343:180–184.

162. Gaston RS, Julian BA, Curtis JJ: Posttransplant erythrocytosis: An enigma revisited. Am J Kidney Dis 1994;24:1–11.

163. Djamali A, Becker YT, Simmons WD, et al: Increasing hematocrit reduces early posttransplant cardiovascular risk in diabetic transplant recipients. Transplantation 2003;76:816–820.

164. Singh AK, Szczech L, Tang KL, et al: Correction of anemia with epoetin alfa in chronic kidney disease. N Engl J Med 2006;355:2085–2098.

165. Drueke TB, Locatelli F, Clyne N, et al: Normalization of hemoglobin level in patients with chronic kidney disease and anemia. N Engl J Med 2006;355:2071–2084.

166. Locatelli F, Del Vecchio L, Pozzoni P: Anemia and cardiovascular risk: The lesson of the CREATE trial. J Am Soc Nephrol 2006;17:S262–S266.

167. Danovitch GM, Jamgotchian NJ, Eggena PH, et al: Angiotensin-converting enzyme inhibition in the treatment of renal transplant erythrocytosis: Clinical experience and observation of mechanism. Transplantation 1995;60:132–137.

168. Mrug M, Stopka T, Julian BA, et al: Angiotensin II stimulates proliferation of normal early erythroid progenitors. J Clin Invest 1997;100:2310–2314.

169. Gupta M, Miller BA, Ahsan N, et al: Expression of angiotensin II type I receptor on erythroid progenitors of patients with post transplant erythrocytosis. Transplantation 2000;70:1188–1194.

170. Buell JF, Gross TG, Woodle ES: Malignancy after transplantation. Transplantation 2005;80:S254–S264.

171. Kasiske BL, Snyder JJ, Gilbertson DT, Wang C: Cancer after kidney transplantation in the United States. Am J Transplant 2004;4:905–913.

172. Vajdic CM, McDonald SP, McCredie MR, et al: Cancer incidence before and after kidney transplantation. JAMA 2006;296: 2823–2831.

173. Penn I: Cancers in cyclosporine-treated vs azathioprine-treated patients. Transplant Proc 1996;28:876–878.

174. Penn I: Tumors after renal and cardiac transplantation. Hematol Oncol Clin North Am 1993;7:431–445.

175. Kauffman HM, Cherikh WS, McBride MA, et al: Post-transplant de novo malignancies in renal transplant recipients: The past and present. Transpl Int 2006;19:607–620.

176. Robson R, Cecka JM, Opelz G, et al: Prospective registry-based observational cohort study of the long-term risk of malignancies in renal transplant patients treated with mycophenolate mofetil. Am J Transplant 2005;5:2954–2960.

177. Funch DP, Ko HH, Travasso J, et al: Posttransplant lymphoproliferative disorder among renal transplant patients in relation to the use of mycophenolate mofetil. Transplantation 2005; 80:1174–1180.

178. Andrassy J, Graeb C, Rentsch M, et al: mTOR inhibition and its effect on cancer in transplantation. Transplantation 2005; 80:S171–S174.

179. Campistol JM, Eris J, Oberbauer R, et al: Sirolimus therapy after early cyclosporine withdrawal reduces the risk for cancer in adult renal transplantation. J Am Soc Nephrol 2006;17: 581–589.

180. Gutierrez-Dalmau A, Campistol JM: Immunosuppressive therapy and malignancy in organ transplant recipients: A systematic review. Drugs 2007;67:1167–1198.

181. Cherikh WS, Kauffman HM, McBride MA, et al: Association of the type of induction immunosuppression with posttransplant lymphoproliferative disorder, graft survival, and patient survival after primary kidney transplantation. Transplantation 2003;76:1289–1293.

182. Bustami RT, Ojo AO, Wolfe RA, et al: Immunosuppression and the risk of post-transplant malignancy among cadaveric first kidney transplant recipients. Am J Transplant 2004;4:87–93.

183. Opelz G, Naujokat C, Daniel V, et al: Disassociation between risk of graft loss and risk of non-Hodgkin lymphoma with induction agents in renal transplant recipients. Transplantation 2006;81:1227–1233.

184. Cherikh WS: Updated analysis of dissociation of depletion and PTLD in kidney recipients treated with alemtuzumab induction therapy [abstract]. Am J Transplant 2007;7:233.

185. Smith JM, Rudser K, Gillen D, et al: Risk of lymphoma after renal transplantation varies with time: An analysis of the United States Renal Data System. Transplantation 2006;81:175–180.

186. Subklewe M, Marquis R, Choquet S, et al: Association of human leukocyte antigen haplotypes with posttransplant lymphoproliferative disease after solid organ transplantation. Transplantation 2006;82:1093–1100.

187. Bakker NA, van Imhoff GW, Verschuuren EA, et al: HLA antigens and post renal transplant lymphoproliferative disease: HLA-B matching is critical. Transplantation 2005;80:595–599.

188. Vincenti F, Larsen C, Durrbach A, et al: Costimulation blockade with belatacept in renal transplantation. N Engl J Med 2005;353:770–781.

189. Dharnidharka VR, Tejani AH, Ho PL, Harmon WE: Post-transplant lymphoproliferative disorder in the United States: Young Caucasian males are at highest risk. Am J Transplant 2002;2:993–998.

190. Stallone G, Schena A, Infante B, et al: Sirolimus for Kaposi's sarcoma in renal-transplant recipients. N Engl J Med 2005;352:1317–1323.

191. Joura EA, Leodolter S, Hernandez-Avila M, et al: Efficacy of a quadrivalent prophylactic human papillomavirus (types 6, 11, 16, and 18) L1 virus-like-particle vaccine against high-grade vulval and vaginal lesions: A combined analysis of three randomised clinical trials. Lancet 2007;369:1693–1702.

192. Bruix J, Sherman M: Management of hepatocellular carcinoma. Hepatology 2005;42:1208–1236.

193. Lennard L, Thomas S, Harrington CI, Maddocks JL: Skin cancer in renal transplant recipients is associated with increased concentrations of 6-thioguanine nucleotide in red blood cells. Br J Dermatol 1985;113:723–729.

194. Penn I: The effect of immunosuppression on pre-existing cancers. Transplantation 1993;55:742–747.

195. Penn I: Neoplasia following transplantation. In Turka LA, Norman DJ (eds): Primer on Transplantation. Ames, IA: Blackwell Publishing, 2001, pp 268–275.

196. Johnson SR, Cherikh WS, Kauffman HM, et al: Retransplantation after post-transplant lymphoproliferative disorders: An OPTN/UNOS database analysis. Am J Transplant 2006;6: 2743–2749.

197. Tsai DE, Hardy CL, Tomaszewski JE, et al: Reduction in immunosuppression as initial therapy for posttransplant lymphoproliferative disorder: Analysis of prognostic variables and long-term follow-up of 42 adult patients. Transplantation 2001;71:1076–1088.

198. Tsai D: Advances in management of refractory PTLD. Presentation at the American Transplant Conference: 7th Annual Joint Transplant of the American Society of Transplant Surgeons and American Society of Transplantation 2007.

199. Tsai DE, Aqui NA, Vogl DT, et al: Successful treatment of T-cell post-transplant lymphoproliferative disorder with the retinoid analog bexarotene. Am J Transplant 2005;5:2070–2073.

200. Patel H, Vogl DT, Aqui N, et al: Posttransplant lymphoproliferative disorder in adult liver transplant recipients: A report of 17 cases. Leuk Lymphoma 2007;48:885–891.

201. Elstrom RL, Andreadis C, Aqui NA, et al: Treatment of PTLD with rituximab or chemotherapy. Am J Transplant 2006;6: 569–576.

202. Taylor AL, Bowles KM, Callaghan CJ, et al: Anthracycline-based chemotherapy as first-line treatment in adults with malignant posttransplant lymphoproliferative disorder after solid organ transplantation. Transplantation 2006;82:375–381.

203. Funch DP, Walker AM, Schneider G, et al: Ganciclovir and acyclovir reduce the risk of post-transplant lymphoproliferative disorder in renal transplant recipients. Am J Transplant 2005;5:2894–2900.

204. Comoli P, Basso S, Zecca M, et al: Preemptive therapy of EBV-related lymphoproliferative disease after pediatric haploidentical stem cell transplantation. Am J Transplant 2007;7:1648–1655.

205. Stasko T, Brown MD, Carucci JA, et al: Guidelines for the management of squamous cell carcinoma in organ transplant recipients. Dermatol Surg 2004;30:642–650.

206. Berg D, Otley CC: Skin cancer in organ transplant recipients: Epidemiology, pathogenesis, and management. J Am Acad Dermatol 2002;47:1–17.

207. A new sunscreen agent. Med Lett Drugs Ther 2007;49:41–43.

208. Kauffman HM, Cherikh WS, Cheng Y, et al: Maintenance immunosuppression with target-of-rapamycin inhibitors is associated with a reduced incidence of de novo malignancies. Transplantation 2005;80:883–889.

209. Tessmer CS, Magalhaes LV, Keitel E, et al: Conversion to sirolimus in renal transplant recipients with skin cancer. Transplantation 2006;82:1792–1793.

210. Bonner JA, Harari PM, Giralt J, et al: Radiotherapy plus cetuximab for squamous-cell carcinoma of the head and neck. N Engl J Med 2006;354:567–578.

211. Nepomuceno RR, Balatoni CE, Natkunam Y, et al: Rapamycin inhibits the interleukin 10 signal transduction pathway and the growth of Epstein Barr virus B-cell lymphomas. Cancer Res 2003;63:4472–4480.

212. Markovic SN, Erickson LA, Rao RD, et al: Malignant melanoma in the 21st century, part 1: Epidemiology, risk factors, screening, prevention, and diagnosis. Mayo Clin Proc 2007;82:364–380.

213. Sugawara Y, Kaneko J, Makuuchi M: Cyclosporin A for treatment of hepatitis C virus after liver transplantation. Transplantation 2006;82:579–580.

214. Inoue K, Sekiyama K, Yamada M, et al: Combined interferon alpha2b and cyclosporin A in the treatment of chronic hepatitis C: Controlled trial. J Gastroenterol 2003;38:567–572.

215. Nakagawa M, Sakamoto N, Enomoto N, et al: Specific inhibition of hepatitis C virus replication by cyclosporin A. Biochem Biophys Res Commun 2004;313:42–47.

216. Helderman JH, Goral S: Gastrointestinal complications of transplant immunosuppression. J Am Soc Nephrol 2002;13:277–287.

217. Budde K, Curtis J, Knoll G, et al: Enteric-coated mycophenolate sodium can be safely administered in maintenance renal transplant patients: Results of a 1-year study. Am J Transplant 2004;4:237–243.

218. Salvadori M, Holzer H, de Mattos A, et al: Enteric-coated mycophenolate sodium is therapeutically equivalent to mycophenolate mofetil in de novo renal transplant patients. Am J Transplant 2004;4:231–236.

219. Bunnapradist S, Lentine KL, Burroughs TE, et al: Mycophenolate mofetil dose reductions and discontinuations after gastrointestinal complications are associated with renal transplant graft failure. Transplantation 2006;82:102–107.

220. Kreis H, Cisterne JM, Land W, et al: Sirolimus in association with mycophenolate mofetil induction for the prevention of acute graft rejection in renal allograft recipients. Transplantation 2000;69:1252–1260.

221. Maes B, Hadaya K, de Moor B, et al: Severe diarrhea in renal transplant patients: Results of the DIDACT study. Am J Transplant 2006;6:1466–1472.

222. Helderman JH: Prophylaxis and treatment of gastrointestinal complications following transplantation. Clin Transplant 2001;15 Suppl 4:29–35.

223. Yang YX, Lewis JD, Epstein S, Metz DC: Long-term proton pump inhibitor therapy and risk of hip fracture. JAMA 2006;296:2947–2953.

224. Heher EC, Rennke HG, Humphreys BD: Nephrocalcinosis, oral sodium phosphate solution, and phosphate nephropathy. Nephrol Rounds 2007;5:1–6. Available from www.nephrologyrounds.org.

225. Markowitz GS, Nasr SH, Klein P, et al: Renal failure due to acute nephrocalcinosis following oral sodium phosphate bowel cleansing. Hum Pathol 2004;35:675–684.

226. Colonoscopy preparations. Med Lett Drugs Ther 2005;47:53–54.

227. Church JM, Fazio VW, Braun WE, et al: Perforation of the colon in renal homograft recipients. A report of 11 cases and a review of the literature. Ann Surg 1986;203:69–76.

228. Knechtle SJ, Pirsch JD, Fechner H, et al: Campath-1H induction plus rapamycin monotherapy for renal transplantation: Results of a pilot study. Am J Transplant 2003;3:722–730.

229. Chuang P, Langone AJ: Clobetasol ameliorates aphthous ulceration in renal transplant patients on sirolimus. Am J Transplant 2007;7:714–717.

230. Lorber MI, Van Buren CT, Flechner SM, et al: Hepatobiliary and pancreatic complications of cyclosporine therapy in 466 renal transplant recipients. Transplantation 1987;43:35–40.

231. Soderdahl G, Tyden G, Groth CG: Incidence of gastrointestinal complications following renal transplantation in the cyclosporin era. Transplant Proc 1994;26:1771–1772.

232. Ton FN, Gunawardene SC, Lee H, Neer RM: Effects of low-dose prednisone on bone metabolism. J Bone Miner Res 2005;20:464–470.

233. Kwan JT, Almond MK, Evans K, Cunningham J: Changes in total body bone mineral content and regional bone mineral density in renal patients following renal transplantation. Miner Electrolyte Metab 1992;18:166–168.

234. Grotz WH, Mundinger FA, Gugel B, et al: Bone mineral density after kidney transplantation. A cross-sectional study in 190 graft recipients up to 20 years after transplantation. Transplantation 1995;59:982–986.

235. Cunningham J: Pathogenesis and prevention of bone loss in patients who have kidney disease and receive long-term immunosuppression. J Am Soc Nephrol 2007;18:223–234.

236. Van Staa TP, Leufkens HG, Abenhaim L, et al: Use of oral corticosteroids and risk of fractures. J Bone Miner Res 2000;15:993–1000.

237. ter Meulen CG, van Riemsdijk I, Hene RJ, et al: No important influence of limited steroid exposure on bone mass during the first year after renal transplantation: A prospective, randomized, multicenter study. Transplantation 2004;78:101–106.

238. Farmer CK, Hampson G, Abbs IC, et al: Late low-dose steroid withdrawal in renal transplant recipients increases bone formation and bone mineral density. Am J Transplant 2006;6:2929–2936.

239. Silverman SL: Selecting patients for osteoporosis therapy: A new approach—fracture risk assessment based on clinical risk factors is coming into play. J Musculoskel Med 2007;24:207–218. Available from: find.galegroup.com/itx/infomark.

240. Lewiecki EM: Review of guidelines for bone mineral density testing and treatment of osteoporosis. Curr Osteoporos Rep 2005;3:75–83.

241. Braun WE, Richmond BJ: Osteoporosis and gout before and after 20 years with a functioning renal transplant. Graft Organ Cell Transplant 1999;2:S119.

242. Bushinsky DA: The contribution of acidosis to renal osteodystrophy. Kidney Int 1995;47:1816–1832.

243. Osteoporosis prevention, diagnosis, and therapy. JAMA 2001;285:785–795.

244. Lee S, Coco M, Greenstein SM, et al: The effect of sirolimus on sex hormone levels of male renal transplant recipients. Clin Transplant 2005;19:162–167.

245. Fritsche L, Budde K, Dragun D, et al: Testosterone concentrations and sirolimus in male renal transplant patients. Am J Transplant 2004;4:130–131.

246. Hampton T: Diabetes drugs tied to fractures in women. JAMA 2007;297:1645.

247. Intravenous ibandronate (Boniva). Med Lett Drugs Ther 2006; 48:68–69.

248. Summey BT, Yosipovitch G: Glucocorticoid-induced bone loss in dermatologic patients: An update. Arch Dermatol 2006;142: 82–90.

249. Heffernan MP, Saag KG, Robinson JK, Callen JP: Prevention of osteoporosis associated with chronic glucocorticoid therapy. JAMA 2006;295:1300–1303.

250. Silverman SL, Watts NB, Delmas PD, et al: Effectiveness of bisphosphonates on nonvertebral and hip fractures in the first year of therapy: The risedronate and alendronate (REAL) cohort study. Osteoporos Int 2007;18:25–34.

251. Mitterbauer C, Schwarz C, Haas M, Oberbauer R: Effects of bisphosphonates on bone loss in the first year after renal transplantation—a meta-analysis of randomized controlled trials. Nephrol Dial Transplant 2006;21:2275–2281.

252. de Nijs RN, Jacobs JW, Lems WF, et al: Alendronate or alfacalcidol in glucocorticoid-induced osteoporosis. N Engl J Med 2006;355:675–684.

253. Weisinger JR, Carlini RG, Rojas E, Bellorin-Font E: Bone disease after renal transplantation. Clin J Am Soc Nephrol 2006;1: 1300–1313.

254. Greenspan SL, Bone HG, Ettinger MP, et al: Effect of recombinant human parathyroid hormone (1-84) on vertebral fracture and bone mineral density in postmenopausal women with osteoporosis: A randomized trial. Ann Intern Med 2007;146: 326–339.

255. Black DM, Delmas PD, Eastell R, et al: Once-yearly zoledronic acid for treatment of postmenopausal osteoporosis. N Engl J Med 2007;356:1809–1822.

256. Compston J: Treatments for osteoporosis—looking beyond the HORIZON. N Engl J Med 2007;356:1878–1880.

257. Black DM, Schwartz AV, Ensrud KE, et al: Effects of continuing or stopping alendronate after 5 years of treatment: The Fracture intervention trial Long-term EXtension (FLEX):A randomized trial. JAMA 2006;296:2927–2938.

258. Colon-Emeric CS: Ten vs. five years of bisphosphonate treatment for postmenopausal osteoporosis: Enough of a good thing. JAMA 2006;296:2968–2969.

259. American College of Rheumatology Ad Hoc Committee on Glucocorticoid-Induced Osteoporosis: Recommendations for the prevention and treatment of glucocorticoid-induced osteoporosis: 2001 update. Arthritis Rheum 2001;44:1496–1503.

260. Adler RA, Hochberg MC: Suggested guidelines for evaluation and treatment of glucocorticoid-induced osteoporosis for the Department of Veterans Affairs. Arch Intern Med 2003;163: 2619–2624.

261. Sambrook PN: Anabolic therapy in glucocorticoid-induced osteoporosis. N Engl J Med 2007;357:2084–2086.

262. Westenfeld R, Brandenburg VM, Ketteler M: Bisphosphonates can improve bone mineral density in renal transplant recipients. Nat Clin Pract Nephrol 2006;2:676–677.

263. Kodras K, Haas M: Effect of kidney transplantation on bone. Eur J Clin Invest 2006;36(Suppl 2):63–75.

264. Coco M, Glicklich D, Faugere MC, et al: Prevention of bone loss in renal transplant recipients: A prospective, randomized trial of intravenous pamidronate. J Am Soc Nephrol 2003;14:2669–2676.

265. Ettinger B, San Martin J, Crans G, Pavo I: Differential effects of teriparatide on BMD after treatment with raloxifene or alendronate. J Bone Miner Res 2004;19:745–751.

266. Schwarz C, Mitterbauer C, Heinze G, et al: Nonsustained effect of short-term bisphosphonate therapy on bone turnover three years after renal transplantation. Kidney Int 2004;65: 304–309.

267. Vautour LM, Melton LJ III, Clarke BL, et al: Long-term fracture risk following renal transplantation: A population-based study. Osteoporos Int 2004;15:160–167.

268. Moe S, Drueke T, Cunningham J, et al: Definition, evaluation, and classification of renal osteodystrophy: A position statement from Kidney Disease: Improving Global Outcomes (KDIGO). Kidney Int 2006;69:1945–1953.

269. Rojas E, Carlini RG, Clesca P, et al: The pathogenesis of osteodystrophy after renal transplantation as detected by early alterations in bone remodeling. Kidney Int 2003;63:1915–1923.

270. Fan SL, Almond MK, Ball E, et al: Pamidronate therapy as prevention of bone loss following renal transplantation. Kidney Int 2000;57:684–690.

271. Kovac D, Lindic J, Kandus A, Bren AF: Prevention of bone loss with alendronate in kidney transplant recipients. Transplantation 2000;70:1542–1543.

272. Grotz WH, Mundinger FA, Rasenack J, et al: Bone loss after kidney transplantation: A longitudinal study in 115 graft recipients. Nephrol Dial Transplant 1995;10:2096–2100.

273. Haas M, Leko-Mohr Z, Roschger P, et al: Zoledronic acid to prevent bone loss in the first 6 months after renal transplantation. Kidney Int 2003;63:1130–1136.

274. Bilezikian JP: Osteonecrosis of the jaw—do bisphosphonates pose a risk? N Engl J Med 2006;355:2278–2281.

275. Markowitz GS, Appel GB, Fine PL, et al: Collapsing focal segmental glomerulosclerosis following treatment with high-dose pamidronate. J Am Soc Nephrol 2001;12:1164–1172.

276. Grotz W, Nagel C, Poeschel D, et al: Effect of ibandronate on bone loss and renal function after kidney transplantation. J Am Soc Nephrol 2001;12:1530–1537.

277. Wolpaw T, Deal CL, Fleming-Brooks S, et al: Factors influencing vertebral bone density after renal transplantation. Transplantation 1994;58:1186–1189.

278. Maricic MJ, Gluck OS: Osteoporosis: therapeutic options for prevention and management. J Musculoskel Med 2001;18:415–423.

279. Massari PU: Disorders of bone and mineral metabolism after renal transplantation. Kidney Int 1997;52:1412–1421.

280. Torres A, Lorenzo V, Salido E: Calcium metabolism and skeletal problems after transplantation. J Am Soc Nephrol 2002;13: 551–558.

281. Szwarc I, Argiles A, Garrigue V, et al: Cinacalcet chloride is efficient and safe in renal transplant recipients with posttransplant hyperparathyroidism. Transplantation 2006;82:675–680.

282. Ix JH, Quarles LD, Chertow GM: Guidelines for disorders of mineral metabolism and secondary hyperparathyroidism should not yet be modified. Nat Clin Pract Nephrol 2006;2:337–339.

283. Shahapuni I, Monge M, Oprisiu R, et al: Drug insight: Renal indications of calcimimetics. Nat Clin Pract Nephrol 2006;2: 316–325.

284. Kruse AE, Eisenberger U, Frey FJ, Mohaupt MG: The calcimimetic cinacalcet normalizes serum calcium in renal transplant patients with persistent hyperparathyroidism. Nephrol Dial Transplant 2005;20:1311–1314.

285. Serra AL, Schwarz AA, Wick FH, et al: Successful treatment of hypercalcemia with cinacalcet in renal transplant recipients with persistent hyperparathyroidism. Nephrol Dial Transplant 2005;20:1315–1319.

286. Srinivas TR, Schold JD, Womer KL, et al: Improvement in hypercalcemia with cinacalcet after kidney transplantation. Clin J Am Soc Nephrol 2006;1:323–326.

287. Leca N, Laftavi M, Gundroo A, et al: Early and severe hyperparathyroidism associated with hypercalcemia after renal transplant treated with cinacalcet. Am J Transplant 2006;6: 2391–2395.

288. El Amm JM, Doshi MD, Singh A, et al: Preliminary experience with cinacalcet use in persistent secondary hyperparathyroidism after kidney transplantation. Transplantation 2007;83:546–549.

289. de Francisco AL: New strategies for the treatment of hyperparathyroidism incorporating calcimimetics. Expert Opin Pharmacother 2008;9:795–811.

290. Moe SM, Cunningham J, Bommer J, et al: Long-term treatment of secondary hyperparathyroidism with the calcimimetic cinacalcet HCl. Nephrol Dial Transplant 2005;20:2186–2193.

291. Falck P, Vethe NT, Asber A, et al: Cinacalcet influences the pharmacokinetics of tacrolimus but not cyclosporine A in stable renal transplant recipients. Am Transplant Cong 2007;7:535.

292. Becker BN, Hullett DA, O'Herrin JK, et al: Vitamin D as immunomodulatory therapy for kidney transplantation. Transplantation 2002;74:1204–1206.

293. Aschenbrenner JK, Heisey DM, Sollinger HW: 1,25-dihydroxy vitamin D_3 (1,25-[OH]$^2D_3$) improves renal transplant function. J Am Soc Nephrol 2000;11:677A.

294. Tan X, Li Y, Liu Y: Paricalcitol attenuates renal interstitial fibrosis in obstructive nephropathy. J Am Soc Nephrol 2006;17:3382–3393.

295. Li YC, Kong J, Wei M, et al: 1,25-dihydroxyvitamin D_3 is a negative endocrine regulator of the renin-angiotensin system. J Clin Invest 2002;110:229–238.

296. Kerby JD, Rue LW, Blair H, et al: Operative treatment of tertiary hyperparathyroidism: A single-center experience. Ann Surg 1998;227:878–886.

297. Evenepoel P, Claes K, Kuypers D, et al: Impact of parathyroidectomy on renal graft function, blood pressure and serum lipids in kidney transplant recipients: A single centre study. Nephrol Dial Transplant 2005;20:1714–1720.

298. Andress DL: Vitamin D treatment in chronic kidney disease. Semin Dial 2005;18:315–321.

299. Abbott KC, Koff J, Bohen EM, et al: Maintenance immunosuppression use and the associated risk of avascular necrosis after kidney transplantation in the United States. Transplantation 2005;79:330–336.

300. Barbosa LM, Gauthier VJ, Davis CL: Bone pain that responds to calcium channel blockers. A retrospective and prospective study of transplant recipients. Transplantation 1995;59:541–544.

301. Stamp L, Searle M, O'Donnell J, Chapman P: Gout in solid organ transplantation: A challenging clinical problem. Drugs 2005;65:2593–2611.

302. Gores PF, Fryd DS, Sutherland DE, et al: Hyperuricemia after renal transplantation. Am J Surg 1988;156:397–400.

303. Zurcher RM, Bock HA, Thiel G: Hyperuricaemia in cyclosporin-treated patients: GFR-related effect. Nephrol Dial Transplant 1996;11:153–158.

304. West C, Carpenter BJ, Hakala TR: The incidence of gout in renal transplant recipients. Am J Kidney Dis 1987;10:369–372.

305. Cohen MR: Proximal gout following renal transplantation (letter). Arthritis Rheum 1994;37:1709–1710.

306. Mikuls TR, MacLean CH, Olivieri J, et al: Quality of care indicators for gout management. Arthritis Rheum 2004;50:937–943.

307. Braun WE: The medical management of the renal transplant recipient. In Johnson RJ, Feehally J (eds.): Comprehensive Clinical Nephrology, Vol 1. London: Mosby, 2000, pp 89:1–89:15.

308. Kuncl RW, Duncan G, Watson D, et al: Colchicine myopathy and neuropathy. N Engl J Med 1987;316:1562–1568.

309. Ducloux D, Schuller V, Bresson-Vautrin C, Chalopin JM: Colchicine myopathy in renal transplant recipients on cyclosporin. Nephrol Dial Transplant 1997;12:2389–2392.

310. Simkin PA, Gardner GC: Colchicine use in cyclosporine treated transplant recipients: How little is too much? J Rheumatol 2000;27:1334–1337.

311. Pascual E, Sivera F: Therapeutic advances in gout. Curr Opin Rheumatol 2007;19:122–127.

312. Clive DM: Renal transplant-associated hyperuricemia and gout. J Am Soc Nephrol 2000;11:974–979.

313. Choi HK, Mount DB, Reginato AM: Pathogenesis of gout. Ann Intern Med 2005;143:499–516.

314. Choi HK, Atkinson K, Karlson EW, et al: Purine-rich foods, dairy and protein intake, and the risk of gout in men. N Engl J Med 2004;350:1093–1103.

315. Minghelli G, Seydoux C, Goy JJ, Burnier M: Uricosuric effect of the angiotensin II receptor antagonist losartan in heart transplant recipients. Transplantation 1998;66:268–271.

316. Shahinfar S, Simpson RL, Carides AD, et al: Safety of losartan in hypertensive patients with thiazide-induced hyperuricemia. Kidney Int 1999;56:1879–1885.

317. Schumacher HR Jr, Chen LX: Newer therapeutic approaches: Gout. Rheum Dis Clin North Am 2006;32:235–244.

318. Krishnan E, Baker JF, Furst DE, Schumacher HR: Gout and the risk of acute myocardial infarction. Arthritis Rheum 2006;54:2688–2696.

319. Bruce SP: Febuxostat: a selective xanthine oxidase inhibitor for the treatment of hyperuricemia and gout. Ann Pharmacother 2006;40:2187–2194.

320. Ippoliti G, Negri M, Campana C, Vigano M: Urate oxidase in hyperuricemic heart transplant recipients treated with azathioprine. Transplantation 1997;63:1370–1371.

321. Becker MA, Schumacher HR Jr, Wortmann RL, et al: Febuxostat compared with allopurinol in patients with hyperuricemia and gout. N Engl J Med 2005;353:2450–2461.

322. Monteiro JL, De Castro I, Seguro AC: Hypophosphatemia induced by acyclovir. Transplantation 1993;55:680–682.

323. Prie D, Blanchet FB, Essig M, et al: Dipyridamole decreases renal phosphate leak and augments serum phosphorus in patients with low renal phosphate threshold. J Am Soc Nephrol 1998;9:1264–1269.

Further Reading

Danovich GM: Handbook of Renal Transplantation, 4th ed. Philadelphia, Lippincott Williams & Wilkins, 2004.

DeNelsky GY: Stop Smoking NOW! Cleveland, Ohio: Cleveland Clinic Press, 2007.

Djamali A, Samaniego M, Muth B, et al: Medical care of kidney transplant recipients after the first posttransplant year. Clin J Am Soc Nephrol 2006;1:623–640.

Kasiske BL, Vazquez MA, Harmon WE, et al: Recommendations for the outpatient surveillance of renal transplant recipients. American Society of Transplantation. J Am Soc Nephrol. 2000;11(Suppl):S1–S86.

National Kidney Foundation: K/DOQI clinical practice guidelines for bone metabolism and disease in chronic kidney disease. Am J Kidney Dis 2003;42:S1–S201.

Norman DJ, Turka LA: Primer on Transplantation, 2nd ed. Mt. Laurel, N.J., American Society of Transplantation, 2001.

Chapter 90

Prevention and Treatment of Infection in Kidney Transplant Recipients

Karen D. Sims and Emily A. Blumberg

CHAPTER CONTENTS

Despite advances in immunosuppression, surgical techniques, and donor and recipient screening that have increased the life expectancy of renal transplant recipients, infectious complications remain a significant cause of morbidity and mortality among renal transplant recipients.[1] A recent analysis of the U.S. Renal Data System database found that for patients who received a tranplant between 1991 and 1998, 51% had a hospital discharge diagnosis that included infection during the first year after transplantation.[2] Unfortunately, the incidence of infection in the post-transplant period seems to be increasing; total infection-related hospital discharge diagnoses have increased each year since 1999.[3]

For the clinician, the challenge lies in both the prevention of and the early diagnosis and treatment of infection in this population. This is hampered by the lack of standardized diagnostic testing for many pathogens and the often atypical presentation of infectious diseases in immunocompromised patients. Additionally, many of the more commonly used antimicrobials have significant drug interactions with immunosuppressive medications, putting the patient at risk for allograft rejection or toxic adverse effects.[4] Some drug-drug interactions of importance are listed in Table 90-1; however, the clinician should always check for drug interactions before prescribing any antimicrobial, preferably with the input of a clinical pharmacist, if available.

Although the list of pathogens that may cause disease in the transplant recipient continues to increase, each broad class of infection contains several "typical" organisms with which the practitioner should be familiar. One helpful method of thinking about infection in the transplant patient is to consider how much time has elapsed since the transplant occurred, because some infections tend to manifest during certain time windows after surgery. This finding has been summarized in chart form by Fishman[5] (Fig. 90-1). In the first month post-transplant, nosocomial infections tend to predominate, including wound and catheter-related bacterial and fungal infections, and flares of prior latent or allograft-transmitted viruses if no prophylaxis is given (i.e., herpes simplex virus [HSV], hepatitis B, hepatitis C). During the following 5 months, viral infections predominate, including reactivation or primary infection with varicella-zoster virus (VZV), Epstein-Barr virus (EBV), or cytomegalovirus (CMV), although if the patient is receiving antiviral prophylaxis, disease may be delayed until prophylaxis is discontinued. Patients are also increasingly susceptible to community-acquired respiratory viruses, environmental fungi, and parasites as they begin to travel and congregate with others outside the healthcare setting. After 6 months, the risk of opportunistic infections declines as the period of maximum immunosuppression passes, and community-acquired pathogens and post-transplant lymphoproliferative disease (PTLD) tend to be more common.

The use of vaccines before transplantation and selected prophylaxis regimens after transplantation, along with good infection control practices and common sense guidelines for the recipient to minimize high-risk exposures after discharge, will greatly reduce the risk of infectious complications.[6,7] However, there are still many pathogens for which there are no vaccines or effective prevention strategies. This chapter discusses the more common infections encountered in the transplant setting; however, an exhaustive review of infectious diseases is beyond the scope of this chapter. An excellent resource containing comprehensive guidelines for the majority of infectious diseases encountered by the clinician is available in a recent supplement to the *American Journal of Transplantation.*[8]

Table 90-1   Important Drug-Drug Interactions

	Drugs By Class	Cyclosporine Interaction	Tacrolimus Interaction	Nephrotoxic?
Antifungals	Amphotericin B/lipid amphotericin B	—	—	Yes
	Caspofungin	*	↓	
	Fluconazole/itraconazole	↑↑	↑↑	
	Ketoconazole	↑↑↑	↑↑↑↑†	
	Voriconazole	↑↑↑	↑↑↑↑†	
Antibacterials	Erythromycin/clarithromycin	↑↑↑	↑↑↑	
	Nafcillin	↓↓	—	Yes
	Aminoglycosides	—	—	Yes
	Rifampin	↓↓↓	↓↓↓	
	Trimethoprim/sulfamethoxazole	—	—	Yes
	Dapsone	—	↑	
	Chloramphenicol	↑↑	↑↑	
	Quinupristin/dalfopristin	↑↑	—	
	Metronidazole	↑↑	↑↑	
Antivirals	Foscarnet	—	—	Yes
	Cidofovir	—	—	Yes
	Protease inhibitors	↑↑	↑↑	
	Tenofovir	—	—	Yes

*Combination may increase caspofungin levels and induce hepatotoxicity.
†Use with sirolimus contraindicated.
Adapted from Immunosuppressive drug interactions with anti-infective agents. Am J Transplant 2004;4(Suppl 10):164–166.

VIRAL INFECTIONS

Cytomegalovirus

Cytomegalovirus is the most important viral infection that develops after solid organ transplant and is associated with significant morbidity and mortality.[9] CMV is a member of the Betaherpesvirus family; its seroprevalence in the general adult population ranges from 50% to 80% by age 40, and the virus establishes lifelong latency in the host.[10] Primary infection with CMV in the immunocompetent host may be asymptomatic or may manifest as fever, malaise, and a mononucleosis-type syndrome. After primary infection, the virus typically remains latent with no systemic signs or symptoms of reactivation. However, in the transplant recipient, the effects of CMV are myriad, including a *viral syndrome* with fever, leukopenia, and thrombocytopenia that may be compounded by immunosuppressive medications, and also tissue-invasive disease, potentially involving the transplanted organ as well as the lungs, liver, gastrointestinal tract and, rarely, the retina.[11] CMV also has been associated with several indirect effects in solid organ tranplant patients, including increased risk of rejection, reduced long-term survival, increased risk of other opportunistic infections, bacterial infections, and allograft dysfunction.[12]

Prior to the widespread use of antiviral prophylaxis, most CMV disease occurred in the first 3 months after solid organ

transplantation, with donor-seropositive/recipient-seronegative patients at the highest risk for disease. In addition to donor seropositivity, other major risk factors for CMV infection and disease include the degree of immunosuppression, including the use of antilymphocyte and OKT3 monoclonal antibody therapy for induction or treatment of rejection, rejection itself, and other concurrent viral infections (e.g., human herpesvirus 6 [HHV-6] infection).[9] Primary CMV infection via the transplanted organ in the seronegative recipient, reactivation of latent disease in the seropositive recipient, and superinfection of donor virus in the seropositive recipient can all cause symptomatic disease. Two strategies have been used for CMV prevention in at-risk patients: universal prophylaxis and preemptive therapy.

Universal CMV prophylaxis involves giving antiviral therapy to all "at-risk" patients (i.e., those with either a CMV-seropositive donor or recipient) at the time of transplantation or immediately afterward for a specified period with the goal of preventing CMV disease during the period of maximum immunosuppression. This approach may be preferable in patients in whom close monitoring for CMV disease is not possible or practical. Although numerous approaches (including acyclovir, valacyclovir, and CMV immunoglobulin) have been associated with a reduction in CMV disease, ganciclovir has been the mainstay of both CMV treatment and prophylaxis in solid organ transplant recipients after studies showed improved efficacy over acyclovir in this population.[13–15] The

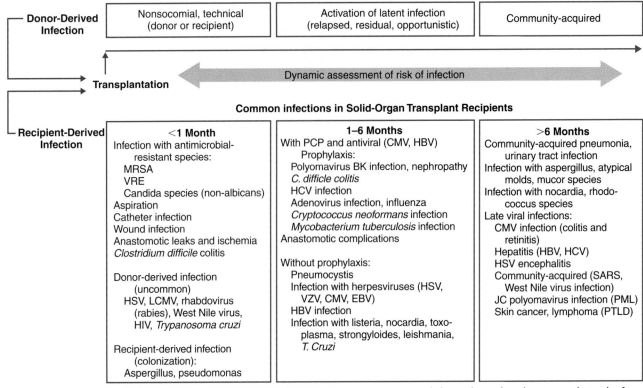

Figure 90-1 Timeline of infection after solid organ transplantation, summarizing typical donor-derived and recipient-derived infections. CMV, cytomegalovirus; EBV, Epstein-Barr virus; HBV, hepatitis B virus; HCV, hepatitis C virus; HIV, human immunodeficiency virus; HSV, herpes simplex virus; LCMV, lymphocytic choriomeningitis virus; MRSA, methicillin-resistant *Staphylococcus aureus*; PCP, *Pneumocystis carinii* pneumonia; PML, progressive multifocal leukoencephalopathy; PTLD, post-transplant lymphoproliferative disorder; SARS, severe acute respiratory syndrome; VRE, vancomycin-resistant *Enterococcus faecalis*; VZV, varicella-zoster virus. (From Fishman JA: Infection in solid-organ transplant recipients. N Engl J Med 2007;357:2601–2614.)

intravenous form of ganciclovir has given way to oral formulations at many centers due to ease of administration. Oral ganciclovir has a significantly lower bioavailability than the intravenous form, but at doses of 1 gram three times a day it has proven efficacy in reducing the incidence of CMV disease.[16] The valine ester prodrug of ganciclovir, valganciclovir, has improved bioavailability compared to oral ganciclovir, and at doses of 900 mg daily has been shown to be equally efficacious in renal transplant patients,[17] with a slightly increased incidence of neutropenia compared to ganciclovir (8.2% vs. 3.2%). Valganciclovir is not indicated for patients undergoing combined liver and kidney transplantation due to reports of breakthrough CMV disease in liver transplant recipients receiving valganciclovir prophylaxis.[18]

Preemptive therapy requires close monitoring of patients for signs of CMV reactivation or primary infection, with prompt initiation of anti-CMV therapy to prevent progression to CMV disease. Blood CMV DNA or RNA levels or CMV antigenemia assays can be utilized at weekly intervals for the initial post-transplantation phase, and then at longer intervals as immunosuppression is reduced. Culture techniques, including shell vials, have fallen out of favor due to long turnaround times or poor sensitivity. A randomized trial of prophylactic or preemptive oral valganciclovir was published in 2006, comparing prophyloctic valganciclavir 900 mg daily for 100 days posttransplant and preemptive valganciclovir 900 mg twice a day for 21 days; the trial measured whether

CMV DNA levels rose above 2000 copies/mL in blood samples assessed weekly for the first 16 weeks and then at 5, 6, 9, and 12 months post-transplant. There were no significant differences in efficacy in the prevention of CMV disease, and a cost-sensitivity analysis was similar for both approaches.[19]

The optimal duration of CMV prophylaxis remains unclear. Now that many centers use prophylaxis for the first 3 months after transplant, CMV disease typically occurs later after transplantation, most often at a median of 5 months post-transplant in donor-seropositive/recipient-seronegative patients.[20,21] Unfortunately, extension of prophylaxis beyond 3 months raises concerns of drug toxicity or the development of drug resistance, although a study of 301 high-risk solid organ transplant patients who received 100 days of valganciclovir prophylaxis failed to show the development of drug resistance.[22] Monitoring immune markers of CMV also does not appear to be predictive of the development of CMV disease, as a recent study by LaRosa and colleagues[23] suggests. This study examined interferon gamma release from T cells at biweekly intervals between 4 and 6 months after transplant. No association was found between presence or absence of T-cell response and development of CMV disease.[23] However, the failure to develop IgG antibodies at 6 months' post-transplant in patients seronegative at the time of transplant may be predictive of late-onset CMV disease (10% developed disease vs. 1.3% of patients with CMV IgG by 6 months).[24]

Standard treatment of CMV disease uses intravenous ganciclovir, 5 mg/kg twice daily (with dose adjustments for renal insufficiency) and reduction of immunosuppression until resolution of symptoms and CMV viremia. Unfortunately, ganciclovir-resistant CMV has emerged as an uncommon but growing problem in the solid organ transplant population, perhaps due to prolonged use of oral ganciclovir prophylaxis and more potent immunosuppression regimens.[25] Although this has not been commonly reported in recipients of kidney transplants alone, it may occur more frequently in pancreas transplant recipients; a major risk factor for this is prolonged exposure to low-dose ganciclovir during periods of asymptomatic infection. Resistance can be detected via phenotypic or genotypic testing, but usually requires additional time. Failure to respond to adequate dosing of ganciclovir should raise a suspicion of ganciclovir resistance, and substitution of another antiviral agent may be warranted. Options for the treatment of resistant CMV include foscarnet with or without ganciclovir and cidofovir, both of which may be highly nephrotoxic, especially when used in the context of calcineurin inhibitors. Adjunctive intravenous immunoglobulin (CMV specific or nonspecific) has been used for treatment of refractory CMV disease, although there are no large-scale trials or specific guidelines for its use.[11]

Epstein-Barr Virus

Similar to CMV, EBV is a ubiquitous herpesvirus that also establishes latent infection in the host. EBV is a member of the Gammaherpesvirus family along with human herpesvirus 8 (HHV-8)/Kaposi's sarcoma-associated herpesvirus (KSHV). EBV infection in the immunocompetent host may be asymptomatic if acquired during childhood or may result in infectious mononucleosis in young adults. More than 90% of the population is seropositive by adulthood. In the transplant recipient, EBV is associated with PTLD, a group of disorders involving varying degrees of abnormal B-cell and T-cell proliferation. Patients at highest risk for PTLD are seronegative recipients who acquire primary infection after transplantation, making pediatric patients especially vulnerable. The virus is efficiently transmitted via saliva and other body fluids, but may also be transmitted by lymphocytes in the transplanted allograft. The risk of PTLD varies by the organ transplanted, with small-bowel transplant recipients at highest risk; lung, heart, pancreas, and liver patients at moderate risk; and renal transplant recipients at lowest risk (approximately 1%).[26–28] Other risk factors include the type and duration of immunosuppression, including OKT3 and polyclonal antibody use. A recent analysis of the French Registry of PTLD in renal transplant recipients demonstrated an incidence of 1.18% after 5 years, with a 61% survival rate at 5 years after diagnosis.[29] Infection with hepatitis B or C was also noted to be a risk factor for patient death, in addition to the more commonly recognized risk factors.

The diagnosis of PTLD initially requires clinical suspicion, because the presentation may be variable, ranging from an infectious mononucleosis-like syndrome to localized or diffuse lymphatic tissue involvement or even isolated allograft involvement. The standard test for diagnosis is biopsy of the involved site with examination of cellular phenotype and clonality, as well as examination for the presence of EBV gene products, such as EBER, via in situ hybridization. Staging should be performed with special attention paid to allograft involvement, the presence of multifocal disease, including

involvement of the central nervous system, and the category of PTLD (i.e., monomorphic vs. polymorphic, B cell vs. T cell). EBV viral load testing has not yet been established as an accepted diagnostic test for PTLD because viremia is variable and does not correlate specifically with the presence or absence of PTLD. A low viral load has good negative predictive value, but a high viral load is nonspecific, and certain subtypes of PTLD are EBV-negative.[30,31] Studies are currently underway examining different EBV antigens as markers for patients at risk for developing PTLD and possibly also as surrogate markers for global immunosuppression levels.

Prevention strategies for PTLD are limited, because systematic study of various modalities is lacking. Identification of high-risk recipients is recommended, specifically EBV-seronegative recipients and those at risk for CMV disease. Avoidance of overzealous immunosuppression should be encouraged as well, because this has been shown to be a risk factor for development of PTLD. The benefit of antiviral prophylaxis specifically targeted toward EBV has not been established, but CMV prophylaxis regimens may have some benefit in reducing the risk for PTLD. The use of prophylactic CMV intravenous immunoglobulin (IVIG) did not prove efficacious in a small clinical trial.[32]

Treatment of early PTLD begins with reduction of immunosuppression, which may result in spontaneous regression in 23% to 50% of cases. In renal transplant patients, confirmed PTLD should prompt cessation of immunosuppression, even at the expense of rejection of the allograft. Retransplantation after recovery from PTLD is possible, with a recent OPTN/UNOS database study showing retransplantation patient survival of 100% and graft survival of 88.9% at a mean follow-up of 742 ± 107 days.[33] Other treatment modalities include surgical debulking of the tumor or explant of the allograft, if involved; referral to an oncologist for monoclonal B-cell antibody therapy (rituximab) if the tumor cells are CD20+; and cytotoxic chemotherapy for refractory disease. A variety of other treatment modalities are under investigation, including anti-interleukin-6, interferon alfa, and adoptive immunotherapy using the patient's own lymphocytes activated ex vivo.[27] Late-onset or EBV-negative PTLD typically does not respond as well to reduction of immunosuppression and thus requires more aggressive therapeutic measures, so early consultation with an oncologist is prudent in these patients.

Herpes Simplex Viruses 1 and 2 and Varicella-Zoster Virus

Herpes simplex virus-1, HSV-2, and VZV are members of the Alphaherpesvirus family and, like other herpesviruses, establish lifelong latency after primary infection. Seroprevalence of HSV-1, the common etiological agent for orolabial lesions, is >60% in the United States, whereas seroprevalence of HSV-2 (genital ulcer disease) exceeds 20%.[34] Antibodies to VZV, the cause of chickenpox and zoster/shingles, are present in more than 90% of adults, although the epidemiology of this virus may change in the future due to the adoption of universal vaccination of children in the United States in 1995. Most disease caused by these viruses is secondary to reactivation of latent infection; however, in seronegative patients primary infection may be acquired rarely via transmission from the allograft or more commonly from community spread, usually early in the post-transplant course if prophylaxis is not given.

Reactivation of HSV-1 and HSV-2 may present as localized orolabial or genital ulcers, but disseminated disease may occur, causing pneumonitis and hepatitis. Similarly, VZV may reactivate as dermatomal zoster, but can also cause more generalized skin disease as well as invasive disease involving the lungs, gastrointestinal tract, and central nervous system.

Most centers use oral acyclovir 400 to 800 mg orally bid to tid[35] or valacylovir 500 mg daily as prophylaxis against HSV-1, HSV-2, and VZV in patients who are not receiving prophylaxis for CMV; regimens for CMV prophylaxis using ganciclovir or valganciclovir are also effective.[34] The VZV serostatus of prospective transplant recipients should be assessed early in the evaluation process so the live, attenuated varicella vaccine can be administered well before transplantation occurs. In the previously infected, immunocompetent host, varicella vaccine has been shown to reduce the incidence of zoster.[36] Whether varicella vaccine is safe and effective for the prevention of zoster after transplantation is unknown.

Human Herpesviruses 6 and 7

The Betaherpesviruses HHV-6 and HHV-7 were identified in 1986 and 1990, respectively. Both tend to cause primary infection in childhood, such as roseola infantum, exanthema subitum, or other nonspecific febrile illnesses, and then establish latency in adults, with 90% of adults demonstrating seropositivity for the viruses.[34] The role of reactivation of these viruses in the post-transplantation period is still under investigation, but it appears that they may have immunomodulatory effects either independently or in combination, especially in that reactivation of HHV-6 and HHV-7 is often found in the context of CMV disease. Primary disease caused by HHV-6 has been reported to include bone marrow suppression, encephalitis, hepatitis, colitis, pneumonitis, and fatal hemophagocytic syndromes,[34,37–39] whereas primary HHV-7 syndromes have been less well-described. In a prospective study of Betaherpesvirus viremia after renal transplantation, CMV was the most commonly detected virus, occurring in 58% of patients; HHV-7 occurred earliest (in 47%) of patients, and HHV-6 occurred in 23% of patients.[40] Interestingly, the authors found a correlation between HHV-7 viremia and increased number of rejection episodes in an analysis restricted only to patients with rejection (overall there was no association between presence of Betaherpesvirus viremia and occurrence of rejection), and there was an increased incidence of CMV disease in patients who demonstrated infection with both CMV and HHV-7.[40]

Detection of HHV-6 and HHV-7 can be accomplished by nucleic acid testing, but prevention strategies remain undefined. Ganciclovir may be effective for HHV-6 prophylaxis, but variability of susceptibility to this agent may exist between the A and B variants of the virus. HHV-7 does not appear to be affected by ganciclovir prophylaxis,[41] and both viruses appear to be resistant to acyclovir. Optimal treatment of these viruses is clouded by frequent coinfection with CMV. Ganciclovir, foscarnet, and cidofovir appear to reduce HHV-6 and HHV-7 viremia when used for coincident CMV disease, but it is unclear if this reduction is due to clearance of CMV and resolution of its immunomodulatory effects, or direct antiviral effects on HHV-6 or HHV-7. Individual case reports of reduction of immunosuppression and ganciclovir treatment for HHV-6 infection have been published.[37]

Human Herpesvirus 8/Kaposi's Sarcoma–Associated Herpesvirus

Human herpesvirus 8 is a Gammaherpesvirus related to EBV that similarly establishes latency after primary infection, and is the cause of Kaposi's sarcoma (KS), primary effusion lymphoma, and some forms of multicentric Castleman's disease. Seropositivity for HHV-8 is more geographically restricted than for other herpesviruses, with highest prevalence rates in Africa and the Middle East. In the United States, seroprevalence is estimated to be less than 5%, although in certain populations (i.e., men who have sex with men) the rates may be higher.[42] Seroconversion post-transplant appears to depend on the donor status and perhaps the geographical location of the recipient, although a study of 100 solid organ transplant recipients in Pittsburgh showed seropositivity rose from 5.3% to 15.8% after transplantation with presumed donor-negative organs (90% documented as negative via serum sample), regardless of patient age or type of organ received.[43] Incidence of KS has been estimated to be up to 500 times higher in solid organ transplant recipients as compared to the general population,[44] and rates in the United States have been reported to be from 0.5% to 6%. Most U.S. patients present with cutaneous KS, and disease occurs a median of 30 months after transplantation.[34]

Detection of HHV-8 antibodies is useful for establishing seroconversion, and an assay for the detection of serum nucleic acid is available for detection of viremia. No guidelines exist for prevention of disease, although the replicating virus appears to be susceptible in vitro to ganciclovir, foscarnet, and cidofovir.[34] Treatment of post-transplantation KS depends on the extent of disease (i.e., cutaneous or visceral involvement), but typically begins with reduction of immunosuppression; if necessary radiotherapy and chemotherapy may be added for more extensive disease. Recently a series of 15 renal transplant recipients with post-transplantation KS were successfully treated with discontinuation of cyclosporine and mycophenolate mofetil and addition of sirolimus.[45] Sirolimus, an immunosuppressive medication that targets mTOR and prevents interleukin-2-induced proliferation of T cells, inhibits the growth of several tumor cell lines in vitro, and inhibits Akt, a protein kinase in the mTOR signaling pathway that has been implicated in KS pathogenesis. Sirolimus trough levels were maintained between 6 and 10 ng/mL, and no episodes of rejection occurred in any of the patients.[45]

Respiratory Viruses (Adenovirus, Respiratory Syncytial Virus, Influenza, Parainfluenza)

Recipients of renal transplants are at risk of contracting common community-acquired respiratory viruses from household contacts and others. In many cases, these viruses may be seasonal (e.g., respiratory syncytial virus [RSV], parainfluenza, and influenza), and the impact on the patient varies with the proximity to the transplant and the degree of immunosuppression of the recipient. Polymerase chain reaction (PCR) techniques have made the rapid diagnosis of most of these pathogens possible (fluorescent antibody detection is also available in many centers), but prevention strategies and treatment are limited for many of these viruses. Infection control practices to prevent nosocomial spread and hand hygiene in and outside of the hospital are the primary means of prevention of these viruses, along with yearly influenza vaccination for all transplant recipients, household contacts, and healthcare workers.

Adenovirus can cause symptomatic and invasive disease (i.e., hemorrhagic cystitis, gastroenteritis, pneumonitis) that can occasionally be fatal in transplant recipients, more commonly in pediatric patients. No vaccine or prophylaxis is currently available against adenovirus, and definitive treatment recommendations have not been established. Several case reports suggest that cidofovir may be efficacious in treating hematopoetic stem cell transplant patients, although dosing recommendations are unclear.[46] Dosing of cidofovir at 5 mg/kg every 1 to 2 weeks may cause nephrotoxicity, but dosing at 1 mg/kg three times per week may cause breakthrough CMV or HSV infections.[46,47] Ribavirin has also been used for treatment of tissue-invasive adenoviral disease, but its antiviral activity is limited to certain serotypes of adenovirus, there are significant toxicities associated with its use, and convincing efficacy data has not been shown to warrant recommendation of its use.[46,47] Ganciclovir has in vitro activity against adenovirus, but there is no definitive data supporting its use for treatment of adenoviral disease, and conflicting data exist regarding prophylactic benefits. Insufficient evidence exists for the use of other agents, such as zalcitabine and vidarabine, for treatment.[47] Reduction of immunosuppression should be attempted in all cases along with supportive care.

RSV is a common pediatric pathogen that causes seasonal disease in the winter months, usually among children age 2 and younger. It appears that immunity to the virus is not lifelong, and transplant recipients may manifest more severe disease than immunocompetent hosts. Manifestations are typically pulmonary, and the development of lower respiratory tract disease portends a worse prognosis.[48] The benefit of prophylaxis with palivizumab or RSV-IVIG in adult transplant recipients has not been proven. Data are limited for treatment of established RSV disease in solid organ transplant patients, but some benefit may exist for the use of aerosolized ribavirin in combination with palivizumab or RSV-IVIG early in lower tract disease.[48]

The mainstay of prevention of influenza A and B is the yearly vaccination of the transplant recipient and their close contacts.[6,49] The preferred vaccine is a combination of inactivated antigens from strains of influenza A and B that are predicted via epidemiological studies to circulate for a given year; thus, the composition may change on a yearly basis. Although the response of transplant patients is lower than that of healthy immunocompetent individuals, sufficient levels of protection are likely to occur in most individuals. Early concerns about an increased risk of graft rejection as a result of the immune response to vaccination have not been supported by the literature, and a recent multicenter retrospective analysis of rejection in more than 3000 heart transplant recipients found no association between influenza vaccination and episodes of rejection.[50] If infection is suspected, rapid treatment should be initiated within 48 hours of symptom development concurrently with a diagnostic test such as nucleic acid detection. Neuraminidase inhibitors (oseltamivir, zanamivir) have become the mainstay of therapy because they are efficacious against both A and B strains of influenza; however, studies specifically evaluating their efficacy in transplant recipients have yet to be conducted.[48] Treatment dosing of oseltamivir is 75 mg orally twice a day for 5 days (zanamivir is only available as an inhaled agent). Prophylaxis with oseltamivir may also be beneficial within 48 hours in cases of known or suspected exposure to influenza at a dose of 75 mg orally once a day for a minimum of 10 days. The use of amantidine or rimantidine has fallen out of favor due to the lack of efficacy against influenza B and the recent reports of resistance of influenza A during the 2006 influenza season.[51]

Parainfluenza viruses 1 and 2 tend to circulate in the fall and winter months, and typically produce nonspecific upper respiratory tract symptoms. There is currently no vaccine, prophylaxis, or accepted treatment regimens for these viruses.[48]

Hepatitis B

The incidence of new acquisition of hepatitis B during the hemodialysis period has been markedly reduced since the adoption of improved infection control practices in 1977. Widespread use of the hepatitis B vaccine was adopted in 1982, further reducing the incidence of hepatitis B acquisition.[52] Vaccination of all patients with compensated renal disease well in advance of dialysis dependence should be encouraged using a four-dose vaccine schedule (0, 1, 2, and 6 months), and yearly monitoring of HBsAb titers should be conducted, with booster vaccination given as needed.[53] Currently the prevalence among hemodialysis patients is approximately 1.6%. Among dialysis patients who seroconvert, 80% may develop chronic hepatitis B, and a subset of patients who undergo transplantation after becoming HBsAg-negative will reactivate after the transplant.[54] Patients who receive a transplant when HBsAg-positive have a poorer prognosis with high rates of chronic hepatitis by 10 years (85%) and also an increased likelihood of sepsis and hepatocellular carcinoma in the posttransplant period.[54] A high risk of HBV transmission exists when grafting an HBsAg-positive organ into a seronegative recipient, so this circumstance should be avoided. Transplantation of a hepatitis BsAg-negative/cAb-positive kidney may be undertaken in a seronegative recipient if the recipient is fully vaccinated and the donor is HBV DNA-negative; although the recipient may seroconvert based on the presence of new HBcAb, this did not affect patient survival or graft function.[55] Close follow-up of these recipients with monitoring for transmission of hepatitis B is important; the use of hepatitis B immunoglobulin and pharmacotherapy may be warranted in this situation.

For recipients with hepatitis B, close monitoring of viral load and HBeAg is warranted, and a liver biopsy before transplantation to assess the extent of hepatitis or cirrhosis should be performed, because the more extensive the liver disease present before transplantation, the higher the liver-associated mortality after transplantation.[54] Treatment of these patients may include use of the nucleoside analogs lamivudine, adefovir, entecavir, and telbivudine, and nucleotide analogs such as tenofovir. Treatment with lamivudine typically results in a large reduction in HBV DNA, but resistance may develop with prolonged use of the drug (>1 to 2 years).[56] This approach is advocated before transplantation to suppress the viral load and should be continued after transplantation in nonhepatic recipients with chronic hepatitis B. Tenofovir and adefovir have both been associated with nephrotoxicity in patients who are not transplant recipients, raising concerns about their safety in renal transplant recipients. Recent data regarding the use of long-term (up to 5 years) adefovir in chronic hepatitis B patients was recently published, suggesting that this agent is well tolerated, with a small risk of renal insufficiency at 1 to 3 years and a low risk of development of resistance after 5 years.[57] A smaller analysis of renal transplant recipients with chronic hepatitis B resistant to lamivudine was reported that showed a significant reduction in hepatitis B DNA with no evidence of adefovir-related renal toxicity after a median of 15 months of treatment, although several patients required phosphorus supplementation.[58] Pretransplant treatment with interferon-alfa to reduce viral load and promote seroconversion has been investigated in renal transplant recipients, but specific guidelines regarding its use have not been published; this approach is not currently recommended.

Hepatitis C

Infection with hepatitis C leads to chronic infection in 85% of exposed individuals, and cirrhosis develops after approximately 20 years in 10% to 30% of these individuals.[54] Fortunately, the rates of HCV infection in the hemodialysis population have declined due to improved infection control measures and screening of blood products.[52] However, de novo infection still occurs in the dialysis setting, with a seroconversion rate of 2.5% per 100 person-years in a recent prevalence study.[59] Screening of potential renal transplant recipients and donors is critical, because discovery of chronic infection with HCV has implications for treatment and surveillance.

Hepatitis C can be efficiently transferred via the transplanted organ, with seroconversion occurring in 67% of recipients of an HCV-positive organ and detection of HCV RNA in 96% of recipients.[60] This result underscores the difficulty of relying solely on serological testing in transplant recipients, and nucleic acid testing for HCV is required for the immunocompromised host, including both dialysis patients and transplant recipients. Because transmission of the virus occurs frequently, HCV-seropositive donors now are considered extended-criteria donors and are typically reserved for HCV-positive recipients or other special circumstances. Nucleic acid testing for hepatitis C RNA in antibody-positive renal donors can help identify those donors who are viremic and therefore likely to transmit hepatitis C.[61]

The effects of HCV positivity on graft and patient survival have been variable. In a cohort of patients on a renal transplant waiting list, HCV-positive patients had a higher risk of death compared to HCV-negative patients regardless of whether they remained on dialysis or underwent transplantation.[62] However, HCV-positive recipients who underwent transplantation or seronegative recipients who received a HCV-positive kidney had improved long-term survival compared to patients who remained on dialysis after 6 months.[60,63-65] HCV infection in the post-transplant period is associated with increased chance of new-onset diabetes mellitus, sepsis, and HCV-related glomerulonephropathy; long-term mortality; and graft failure.[54,66-69] Recent studies have suggested that hepatitis C infection in renal transplant patients may not necessarily predispose recipients to rapid progression of liver disease.[70] Increased variability of the hypervariable region (HVR-1) of HCV E_2 glycoprotein may be a predictor of lack of progression of fibrosis.[70,71]

Because of the implications of chronic hepatitis C infection in the post-transplant period, efforts should be made to stage the extent of disease in transplant candidates. Serum transaminases do not reflect the extent of liver fibrosis or cirrhosis, so a liver biopsy should be performed during the transplant evaluation to determine the extent of liver damage. Treatment of hepatitis C in the pretransplant period should also be considered in an effort to eradicate the virus.[66] Ribavirin and PEG-interferon-alfa combinations are the treatments of choice, but adverse effects such as anemia prevent the use of ribavirin in this population. After transplantation, interferon-alfa has been associated with an increased risk of renal failure and possible graft rejection, so it is generally not recommended for use after renal transplantation.[54,72,73]

BK Virus

The BK virus is a double-stranded DNA polyoma virus that infects up to 90% of the adult population and appears to be primarily asymptomatic in the immunocompetent host, although upper respiratory symptoms and cystitis have been reported.[74] In the renal transplant recipient, BK virus can be transmitted by the transplanted organ or can reactivate from latency in seropositive recipients. Typically the virus causes asymptomatic viruria in this population, but in some patients nephropathy with allograft dysfunction or ureteral stenosis or stricture develops as a result of BK disease. The risk factors for development of BK viremia or viruria are unclear, but the extent of immunosuppression appears critical, as does antirejection treatment.[75]

The methods and screening intervals used for the diagnosis of BK virus infection are not well-defined, but include frequent urine cytological examination looking for abnormal epithelial *decoy cells* and more sensitive PCR methods of detection of both urine and blood specimens.[76] Nucleic acid techniques also can provide a quantitative assessment of viral load and are able to differentiate between BK virus infection and other viruses that may produce a similar cytological appearance of epithelial cells (i.e., JC virus). Plasma viral loads greater than 10^4 copies/mL and urine viral loads greater than 10^7 copies/mL are suggestive of underlying BK virus nephropathy (BKVN).[77] The diagnosis and staging of BKVN requires renal biopsy, and the incidence of BKVN appears to range between 1% and 10% of renal transplant recipients. Recent research has examined the utility of nucleic acid-based detection techniques as screening tools for the development of BK viruria, viremia, and nephropathy.[78] Both the level of BK viremia and the presence of recurrent viremia have been correlated with the presence of BKVN.[75,79]

Treatment and prevention of BK virus is still evolving. Reduction of immunosuppression remains the mainstay of prevention and therapy of BK viruria, viremia, and nephropathy. Antiviral agents have not been uniformly efficacious in the prevention or treatment of BK viruria, but several have been anecdotally reported, including cidofovir and leflunomide. Unfortunately, no randomized, controlled clinical trials have been performed with either of these agents, but their use may be warranted in patients who have severe BKVN with concurrent rejection that may limit reduction of immunosuppresion.[80] Cidofovir has activity against polyoma viruses in vitro, but its nephrotoxicity has led to reduced dosing in renal transplant patients for treatment of BK virus infection (0.25–1 mg/kg given intravenously every 1–3 weeks), and clinical results remain mixed.[80] Of 26 patients with BKVN treated with cidofovir at the University of Pittsburgh, viremia cleared in 25 patients, and 15% lost the graft, compared to a historical graft loss rate of 45% without cidofovir.[81]

Leflunomide, a drug used for the treatment of rheumatoid arthritis, also has antiviral activity against BK virus in vitro, and a limited amount of data is available regarding its clinical utility.

A series of 17 patients with biopsy-proven BKVN was treated with leflunomide at a loading dose of 100 mg/day for 5 days and then 20 to 60 mg per day titrated to maintain blood levels higher than 40 µg/mL.[82] Those patients who achieved blood levels greater than 40 µg/mL had reduction or clearance of the virus in the urine and blood by 6 months, with persistence of response beyond that time.[78] However, the pharmacokinetics of leflunomide are unpredictable, making uniform dosing recommendations difficult and serum drug level monitoring necessary.

Quinolones and IVIG have also been explored for the treatment of BK virus infection, but limited clinical data is available on efficacy, and no recommendations can be made about these agents until further studies are performed.[80,81]

Retransplantation after BKVN is feasible, with a low risk of recurrence of BKVN, regardless of transplant nephrectomy before retransplantation or the presence of active BKVN and viremia.[83,84]

FUNGAL INFECTIONS

The morbidity and mortality of fungal infections in transplant recipients remains high despite recent advances in antifungal medications and diagnostic testing. Compared with other transplant recipients, renal transplant patients are at lower risk for fungal infections unless they are receiving a simultaneous pancreas transplant.[85] Despite this reduced risk, clinicians need to remain vigilant for unexplained fever, respiratory symptoms, or skin lesions as possible manifestations of fungal disease. The unpredictability of the clinical signs and symptoms of fungal infections, the difficulty of interpreting radiological studies and biopsies, and the limited number of laboratory-based markers of fungal infection often result in the dissemination and invasion of fungal disease before proper treatment can be initiated. The added difficulties of managing the interactions between immunosuppressive medications and many antifungal medications increase the complexity of treating these infections.

Fungal infections in the early transplant period (<1 month) typically involve *Candida* species or, in rare instances, nosocomial transmission of other environmental fungal pathogens, such as *Cryptococcus neoformans* or *Aspergillus* species.[9,85] A variety of risk factors have been associated with early invasive fungal infections after transplant, including simultaneous pancreas transplant or pancreas transplant after kidney transplant, enteric or bladder drainage procedures, primary allograft dysfunction, prolonged transplantation surgery, high intraoperative blood loss, prolonged intensive care unit stay, chronic graft dysfunction/rejection, presence of immunomodulating viruses, prolonged use of antibiotics, artificial stents, donor fungemia, and prior or concurrent fungal infection in the recipient.[85] Care must be taken to identify the species of *Candida* isolated for therapeutic reasons, because *Candida albicans* remains susceptible to fluconazole, but other *Candida* species are becoming more frequent pathogens and are not uniformly susceptible to fluconazole (i.e., *Candida glabrata* may be resistant or have dose-dependent susceptibility, *Candida kruseii* is intrinsically resistant). The choice of empirical therapy for life-threatening candidal infections depends on the epidemiology of isolates at an individual institution and may include high-dose fluconazole, voriconazole or an echinocandin.

In the later post-transplant period, patients are at risk for environmental pathogens and endemic mycoses, both via primary exposure and reactivation of latent disease.[9,85] *Aspergillus* and *Cryptococcus neoformans* infections are the most commonly encountered fungal pathogens during this period. Risk factors for fungal infection include diabetes, prolonged pre-transplant dialysis, use of tacrolimus, and treatment for rejection.[86] A careful history, including travel, workplace and home exposures (i.e., construction or remodeling, pets), and hobbies such as gardening or spelunking should be elicited, and a careful review of systems performed. Radiological studies may be warranted, and any suspicious skin lesions should be biopsied. Suggested diagnostic testing and treatment regimens for *Candida*, *Aspergillus*, and *Cryptococcus* are summarized in Table 90-2.

PNEUMOCYSTIS JIROVECI INFECTIONS

Pneumocystis jiroveci (formerly *Pneumocystis carinii*) remains an important cause of respiratory disease in transplant recipients despite excellent prophylaxis regimens. The use of more potent immunosuppression and the ultimate cessation of prophylaxis at approximately 6 months post-transplant require the physician to consider *Pneumocystis* infection in any transplant recipient with flulike symptoms and persistent respiratory complaints, including dry cough and dyspnea. Radiographic findings may be atypical in transplant recipients and can manifest as diffuse ground-glass infiltrates, more focal consolidation, or pneumothorax.[87]

Prophylaxis with trimethoprim-sulfamethoxazole for the first 6 months after transplant is strongly recommended, because it also reduces the risk of other opportunistic infections, such as toxoplasmosis, listeriosis, and nocardiosis, as well as bacterial urinary tract infections (UTIs). If the patient cannot tolerate trimethoprim-sulfamethoxazole, other agents can be used, such as aerosolized pentamidine, atovaquone, and dapsone, but care must be taken to monitor for compliance and adverse effects of the medications.[87] Treatment of *Pneumocystis* disease should be with trimethoprim-sulfamethoxazole 15 to 20 mg/kg daily in four divided doses, with corticosteroids given if hypoxia with a PO_2 lower than 70 mm Hg by arterial blood gas is documented. A minimum 14-day course of trimethoprim-sulfamethoxazole is often sufficient if immunosuppression can be reduced, and 40 to 60 mg of prednisone for 5 to 7 days followed by a taper is recommended for concomitant hypoxemia.

BACTERIAL URINARY TRACT INFECTIONS

Urinary tract infections, especially involving the transplanted kidney, are the most commonly encountered bacterial infections in renal transplant recipients. The incidence of UTI in this population has been estimated to be between 35% and 79%, and this infection is the most common source of gram-negative bacteremias.[88] The high rate of infection is likely due to several factors, including surgical factors (e.g., refluxing vs. nonrefluxing anastomosis of the ureters, ureteral stent placement, impaired bladder emptying), presence and duration of bladder catheters, and immunosuppression.[88,89] Of increasing concern is the number of highly resistant gram-negative

Table 90-2 Suggested Diagnostic Testing and Treatment Regimens for *Candida*, *Aspergillus*, and *Cryptococcus*

Pathogen	Prophylaxis	Diagnosis	Treatment of Invasive Disease	Special Considerations
Candida species	Candiduria: fluconazole 400 mg/day until eradication SPK: fluconazole 400 mg/day or liposomal amphotericin B 3–5 mg/kg/day for ≥4 wks until risk factors resolved	Smear/culture of blood or sterile site Nucleic acid detection (not universally accepted) Radiology: CT of viscera, MRI of brain Histopathology	Fluconazole 200–800 mg/day depending on site and isolate MIC, renal function Amphotericin B lipid formulations: 1–5 mg/kg/day Amphotericin B: 0.5–1.5 mg/kg/day Echinocandins: caspofungin 75 mg × 1 loading dose then 50 mg/day, dose reduction for liver disease Anidulafungin 200 mg × 1 loading dose, then 100 mg/day Triazoles: voriconazole 6 mg/kg IV q12h × 2 doses, then 4 mg/kg q12h; 400 mg PO q12h × 2 doses, then 200 mg q12h for patients >40 kg; dose reduction for liver disease; itraconazole 200 mg PO or IV q12–24h Other options not yet FDA approved for this indication: micafungin, posaconazole	*C. glabrata* MICs/resistance increasing to fluconazole, *C. kruseii* intrinsically resistant *C. lusitaniae* intrinsically resistant; monitor renal function and electrolytes Monitor renal function and electrolytes May be hepatotoxic if given with cyclosporine; may decrease tacrolimus levels IV form not recommended if renal impairment, significant drug interactions, including contraindication of voriconazole use with sirolimus; reduce dose of tacrolimus by two thirds and reduce cyclosporine by one half; monitor levels
Aspergillus species	None recommended	Culture of sterile site Antigen detection: galactomannin assay not universally accepted, false positives with concurrent piperacillin use Radiology: CT of viscera with nodules, cavities; halo sign, crescent sign may be seen/MRI of brain Histopathology	Voriconazole: dosed as above Liposomal amphotericin B: 5 mg/kg/day Amphotericin B: 1–1.5 mg/kg/day Caspofungin: dosed as above Role of combination therapy unclear Other options not yet FDA approved for this indication: micafungin, posaconazole	As above As above As above As above
Cryptococcus neoformans	None recommended (fluconazole may provide some protection)	Smear/culture of blood, CSF, sterile site (transplant patients *must* have CSF evaluation, may have elevated opening pressure) India ink preparation of CSF Antigen detection in CSF, blood (false-negatives if nonencapsulated strain, prozone effect) Nucleic acid detection (not universally accepted) Radiology: CT of viscera, MRI of brain Histopathology	Liposomal amphotericin B: 5 mg/kg/day OR Amphotericin B: 0.5–1 mg/kg/day PLUS 5-flucytosine 100 mg/kg/day divided q6h; renal dosing required × 14 days THEN Fluconazole 400 mg/day, duration unknown	As above As above Monitoring serum creatinine and 5-flucytosine levels suggested, goal 30–80 µg/mL 2 hr after dose

CSF, cerebrospinal fluid; CT, computed tomography; FDA, Food and Drug Administration; MRI, magnetic resonance imaging; SPK, simultaneous pancreas-kidney transplantation.

Adapted from Fungal infections. Am J Transplant 2004;4(Suppl 10):110–134, Tables 3 and 4.

organisms isolated from these patients and the limited number of antimicrobial options for treatment.

The impact of early UTI in renal transplant recipients has been associated with pyelonephritis, bacteremia/septicemia, and increased mortality compared to the general population[88–91]; late UTI may also be associated with increased mortality,[92] although most tend to mimic UTIs in the immunocompetent host. Most centers provide prophylaxis against early UTI using either trimethoprim-sulfamethoxazole or a quinolone for the first 6 to 12 months after transplant.[93–95] Use of trimethoprim-sulfamethoxazole is not only inexpensive, but also provides prophylaxis against *Pneumocystis*, toxoplasmosis, listeriosis, and nocardiosis, although quinolones may be better tolerated.[93] Most centers use low-dose trimethoprim-sulfamethoxazole daily, but some studies have suggested that higher doses (320 mg/1600 mg) may be more efficacious in the prevention of UTI during the first month after transplant.[95,96] Whether higher doses may be associated with increased toxicity is unknown.

Treatment of UTI in this population requires that close attention be paid to the susceptibilities of the isolate, because rates of highly resistant gram-negative pathogens appear to be increasing.[97,98] Most centers use a longer duration of treatment in transplant recipients, typically 14 days.[88] Candidal UTIs in this population are also problematic because they may lead to the formation of fungal balls and resultant urinary obstruction, so the finding of yeast in a sterile urine specimen should prompt further investigation.

TUBERCULOSIS AND NONTUBERCULOUS MYCOBACTERIA

Although tuberculosis (TB) remains a relatively rare disease after renal transplantation, the complexities of treatment and high associated mortality require vigilance of the provider during both the pretransplant and posttransplant periods. The incidence of TB after renal transplantation in the United States is estimated to be less than 1%, but the mortality rate in these patients approaches 25% to 30%.[99,100] Most patients develop symptomatic disease within the first year after transplantation.

Evaluation of the transplant recipient should include a detailed history of prior TB, possible exposure to the disease, or travel to endemic areas. Tuberculin skin testing is recommended for all potential recipients, and should be interpreted as positive if greater than 5 mm of induration is detected.[101] If no prior prophylaxis has been given, or if the patient's response to the test has recently converted to positive, the patient should be treated as having latent TB infection. Unfortunately many patients with severe renal disease may be anergic, rendering the test unreliable if negative. The recent release of a blood test for interferon-gamma release from patient's sensitized lymphocytes after exposure to purified protein derivative (QuantiFERON test) is promising, but as yet is not indicated for use in immunosuppressed individuals.[102] Chest radiographs may be useful for finding evidence of prior or active disease that would warrant further evaluation, especially if no prior treatment or prophylaxis was given. In patients in whom latent TB infection is suggested, treatment with 300 mg of isoniazid daily for 9 months is recommended after evaluation for underlying liver disease. Ideally, prophylaxis should be completed before transplantation and the

onset of more severe immunosuppression; however, if the donor had risk factors for latent TB infection, the recipient should receive prophylaxis after transplantation to reduce the risk of transmission of disease.[101] Liver function tests should be monitored every 2 weeks for the first 6 weeks of therapy, then monthly, looking for elevations of transaminases greater than 4 times normal.

Diagnosis and treatment of active tuberculosis after transplantation is complex; the involvement of an infectious diseases specialist is recommended, as well as involvement of local public health departments. Patients are likely to present in the first year after transplantation and are more likely to present with disseminated disease than immunocompetent patients, although pulmonary disease remains the most common manifestation.[99,100] Diagnosis may require extensive imaging and multiple specimens from suspicious areas for microbiological culture and susceptibility testing. The use of the QuantiFERON test has not been validated for diagnosis of active infection in immunosuppressed patients.[103] The standard four-drug regimen typically initiated at diagnosis of TB (isoniazid, rifampin, pyrazinamide, and ethambutol) is problematic in the transplant recipient due to the interaction between rifampin and calcineurin inhibitors that induces the metabolism of these agents. Substitution with rifabutin or a quinolone such as levofloxacin is a common approach to eliminate this problem, although rifabutin is still associated with significant drug interactions.[101] Once susceptibility of the isolate to isoniazid and rifampin is confirmed, therapy should continue for a minimum of 6 months, if isoniazid and rifampin or rifabutin are used, and longer with other regimens or more severe disease.

Nontuberculous mycobacterial infections in transplant recipients are rare and not well-studied. Many of these organisms are environmental contaminants and can cause disease as a result of nosocomial transmission or exposure in the community. Again, a high index of suspicion must be maintained, and early involvement of an infectious diseases specialist is helpful, because many of these organisms require special growth conditions in the microbiology laboratory and do not have uniform susceptibilities to antimicrobial agents. More detailed recommendations can be found in recently published guidelines.[104,105]

HUMAN IMMUNODEFICIENCY VIRUS AND RENAL TRANSPLANTATION

The widespread use of highly active antiretroviral therapy (HAART) has changed the prognosis for patients with human immunodeficiency virus (HIV) infection, allowing these patients to be considered for renal transplantation.[106] Prior to the widespread use of HAART, a retrospective analysis of HIV-positive renal transplant recipients suggested a slightly worse 3-year survival compared to HIV-negative patients during the same 10-year period (83% vs. 88%).[107] More recently, several case series have reported encouraging results after renal transplantation in HIV-positive patients, showing similar graft survival and mortality at 1 year compared to controls from the UNOS database.[108,109] Unfortunately, graft rejection rates appear to be higher in the HIV-positive groups. Currently a prospective, multicenter trial is underway to study HIV-positive renal and liver transplant recipients to study the effects of immunosuppressive medications on patient survival and how HIV infection and HAART affect graft survival.

Ideally, HIV-positive patients being considered for transplantation should have $CD4^+$ cell counts greater than 200 cells/μL and an undetectable viral load for 3 months on stable antiretroviral therapy.[110] Comorbid conditions should be assessed, including the presence of other viral infections (i.e., HBV, HCV) that may have accelerated courses in the presence of both HIV and immunosuppression, and history of opportunistic infections that may reactivate post-transplantation. After transplantation, these patients require close monitoring, because the pharmacokinetics and drug interactions of antiretroviral medications and immunosuppressive medications may be complex; notably, there are significant drug interactions between calcineurin inhibitors and antiretroviral agents, including both protease inhibitors and nonnucleoside reverse transcriptase inhibitors.[108,111] Frequent assessment of serum drug levels of the calcineurin inhibitors is therefore mandatory for patients on protease inhibitor-based HAART. More comprehensive guidelines have been established by the Cooperative Clinical Trials in Adult Transplantation group and include specific recommendations regarding inclusion and exclusion criteria and pharmacological considerations for HAART, immunosuppression, and prophylaxis regimens.[111]

Management of infectious disease complications continues to pose a challenge for physicians treating transplant recipients. As the use of newer, more potent immunosuppressive regimens becomes more common, the risk for opportunistic pathogens and more severe manifestations of both community-acquired and nosocomial pathogens increases. Continued attention to improved preventive, diagnostic, and treatment strategies to minimize the impact of infections on outcomes is required.

References

1. Scientific Registry of Transplant Recipients. 2007.
2. Dharnidharka VR, Caillard S, Agodoa LY, Abbott KC: Infection frequency and profile in different age groups of kidney transplant recipients. Transplantation 2006;81:1662–1667.
3. U.S. Renal Data System: USRDS 2006 Annual Data Report: Atlas of End-Stage Renal Disease in the United States. Bethesda, Md: National Institutes of Health, National Institute of Diabetes and Digestive and Kidney Diseases, 2006
4. Immunosuppressive drug interactions with anti-infective agents. Am J Transplant 2004;4(Suppl 10):164–166.
5. Fishman JA: Infection in solid-organ transplant recipients. N Engl J Med 2007;357:2601–2614.
6. Guidelines for vaccination of solid organ transplant candidates and recipients. Am J Transplant 2004;4(Suppl 10):160–163.
7. Strategies for safe living following solid organ transplantation. Am J Transplant 2004;4 (Suppl 10):156–159.
8. Guidelines for the prevention and management of infectious complications of solid organ transplantation. Am J Transplant 2004;4(Suppl 10):1–166.
9. Fishman JA, Rubin RH: Infection in organ-transplant recipients. N Engl J Med 1998;338:1741–1751.
10. Staras SA, Dollard SC, Radford KW, et al: Seroprevalence of cytomegalovirus infection in the United States, 1988–1994. Clin Infect Dis 2006;43:1143–1151.
11. Cytomegalovirus. Am J Transplant 2004;4(Suppl 10):51–58.
12. Rubin RH:. Cytomegalovirus in solid organ transplantation. Transpl Infect Dis 2001;3(Suppl 2):1–5.
13. Rubin RH, Kemmerly SA, Conti D, et al: Prevention of primary cytomegalovirus disease in organ transplant recipients with oral ganciclovir or oral acyclovir prophylaxis. Transpl Infect Dis 2000;2:112–117.
14. Winston DJ, Wirin D, Shaked A, Busuttil RW: Randomised comparison of ganciclovir and high-dose acyclovir for long-term cytomegalovirus prophylaxis in liver-transplant recipients. Lancet 1995;346:69–74.
15. Turgeon N, Fishman JA, Doran M, et al: Prevention of recurrent cytomegalovirus disease in renal and liver transplant recipients: Effect of oral ganciclovir. Transpl Infect Dis 2000;2:2–10.
16. Gane E, Saliba F, Valdecasas GJ, et al, for The Oral Ganciclovir International Transplantation Study Group: Randomised trial of efficacy and safety of oral ganciclovir in the prevention of cytomegalovirus disease in liver-transplant recipients [corrected]. Lancet 1997;350:1729–1733.
17. Paya C, Humar A, Dominguez E, et al: Efficacy and safety of valganciclovir vs. oral ganciclovir for prevention of cytomegalovirus disease in solid organ transplant recipients. Am J Transplant 2004;4:611–620.
18. Jain A, Orloff M, Kashyap R: Does valganciclovir hydrochloride (Valcyte) provide effective prophylaxis against cytomegalovirus infection in liver transplant recipients? Transplant Proc 2005;37:3182–3186.
19. Khoury JA, Storch GA, Bohl DL: Prophylactic versus preemptive oral valganciclovir for the management of cytomegalovirus infection in adult renal transplant recipients. Am J Transplant 2006;6:2134–2143.
20. Boeckh M, Riddell SR: Immunologic predictors of late cytomegalovirus disease after solid organ transplantation—an elusive goal? J Infect Dis 2007;195:615–617.
21. Limaye AP, Bakthavatsalam R, Kim HW, et al: Late-onset cytomegalovirus disease in liver transplant recipients despite antiviral prophylaxis. Transplantation 2004;78:1390–1396.
22. Boivin G, Goyette N, Gilbert C, et al: Absence of cytomegalovirus-resistance mutations after valganciclovir prophylaxis, in a prospective multicenter study of solid-organ transplant recipients. J Infect Dis 2004;189:1615–1618.
23. La Rosa C, Limaye AP, Krishnan A: Longitudinal assessment of cytomegalovirus (CMV)-specific immune responses in liver transplant recipients at high risk for late CMV disease. J Infect Dis 2007;195:633–644.
24. Humar A, Mazzulli T, Moussa G, Clinical utility of cytomegalovirus (CMV) serology testing in high-risk CMV D+/R− transplant recipients. Am J Transplant 2005;5:1065–1070.
25. Limaye AP, Corey L, Koelle DM, et al: Emergence of ganciclovir-resistant cytomegalovirus disease among recipients of solid-organ transplants. Lancet 2000;356:645–649.
26. Epstein-Barr virus and lymphoproliferative disorders after transplantation. Am J Transplant 2004;4(Suppl 10):59–65.
27. Lim WH, Russ GR, Coates PT: Review of Epstein-Barr virus and post-transplant lymphoproliferative disorder post-solid organ transplantation. Nephrology (Carlton) 2006;11: 355–366.
28. Caillard S, Dharnidharka V, Agodoa L, et al: Posttransplant lymphoproliferative disorders after renal transplantation in the United States in era of modern immunosuppression. Transplantation 2005;80:1233–1243.
29. Caillard S, Lelong C, Pessione F, Moulin B: Post-transplant lymphoproliferative disorders occurring after renal transplantation in adults: Report of 230 cases from the French Registry. Am J Transplant 2006;6:2735–2742.
30. Rowe DT, Webber S, Schauer EM, et al: Epstein-Barr virus load monitoring: Its role in the prevention and management of post-transplant lymphoproliferative disease. Transpl Infect Dis 2001;3:79–87.
31. Tsai DE, Nearey M, Hardy CL, et al: Use of EBV PCR for the diagnosis and monitoring of post-transplant lymphoproliferative

disorder in adult solid organ transplant patients. Am J Transplant 2002;2:946–954.

32. Green M, Michaels MG, Katz BZ, et al: CMV-IVIG for prevention of Epstein Barr virus disease and posttransplant lymphoproliferative disease in pediatric liver transplant recipients. Am J Transplant 2006;6:1906–1912.

33. Johnson SR, Cherikh WS, Kauffman HM, et al: Retransplantation after post-transplant lymphoproliferative disorders: An OPTN/UNOS database analysis. Am J Transplant 2006;6:2743–2749.

34. Other herpesviruses: HHV-6, HHV-7, HHV-8, HSV-1 and -2, VZV. Am J Transplant 2004;4(Suppl 10):66–71.

35. Seale L, Jones CJ, Kathpalia S, et al: Prevention of herpesvirus infections in renal allograft recipients by low-dose oral acyclovir. JAMA 1985;254:3435–3438.

36. Oxman MN, Levin MJ, Johnson GR, et al: A vaccine to prevent herpes zoster and postherpetic neuralgia in older adults. N Engl J Med 2005;352:2271–2284.

37. Delbridge MS, Karim MS, Shrestha BM, McKane W: Colitis in a renal transplant patient with human herpesvirus-6 infection. Transpl Infect Dis 2006;8:226–228.

38. Karras A, Thervet E, Legendre C: Hemophagocytic syndrome in renal transplant recipients: Report of 17 cases and review of literature. Transplantation 2004;77:238–243.

39. Rossi C, Delforge ML, Jacobs F, et al: Fatal primary infection due to human herpesvirus 6 variant A in a renal transplant recipient. Transplantation 2001;71:288–292.

40. Kidd IM, Clark DA, Sabin CA, et al: Prospective study of human Betaherpesviruses after renal transplantation: Association of human herpesvirus 7 and cytomegalovirus co-infection with cytomegalovirus disease and increased rejection. Transplantation 2000;69:2400–2404.

41. Galarraga MC, Gomez E, de Ona M, et al: Influence of ganciclovir prophylaxis on citomegalovirus, human herpesvirus 6, and human herpesvirus 7 viremia in renal transplant recipients. Transplant Proc 2005;37:2124–2126.

42. Lennette ET, Blackbourn DJ, Levy JA: Antibodies to human herpesvirus type 8 in the general population and in Kaposi's sarcoma patients. Lancet 1996;348:858–861.

43. Jenkins FJ, Hoffman LJ, Liegey-Dougall A: Reactivation of and primary infection with human herpesvirus 8 among solid-organ transplant recipients. J Infect Dis 2002;185:1238–1243.

44. Hayward GS: Initiation of angiogenic Kaposi's sarcoma lesions. Cancer Cell 2003;3:1–3.

45. Stallone G, Schena A, Infante B, et al: Sirolimus for Kaposi's sarcoma in renal-transplant recipients. N Engl J Med 2005;352:1317–1323.

46. Adenovirus. Am J Transplant 2004;4(Suppl 10):101–104.

47. Ison MG: Adenovirus infections in transplant recipients. Clin Infect Dis 2006;43:331–339.

48. Community-acquired respiratory viruses. Am J Transplant 2004;4(Suppl 10):105–109.

49. Grekas D, Alivanis P, Kiriazopoulou V, et al: Influenza vaccination on renal transplant patients is safe and serologically effective. Int J Clin Pharmacol Ther Toxicol 1993;31:553–556.

50. White-Williams C, Brown R, Kirklin J, et al: Improving clinical practice: Should we give influenza vaccinations to heart transplant patients? J Heart Lung Transplant 2006;25:320–323.

51. Smith NM, Bresee JS, Shay DK, et al: Prevention and control of influenza: Recommendations of the Advisory Committee on Immunization Practices (ACIP). MMWR Recomm Rep 2006;55(RR-10):1–42.

52. Recommendations for preventing transmission of infections among chronic hemodialysis patients. MMWR Recomm Rep 2001;50(RR-5):1–43.

53. Kotton CN, Fishman JA: Viral infection in the renal transplant recipient. J Am Soc Nephrol 2005;16:1758–1774.

54. Viral hepatitis guidelines in hemodialysis and transplantation. Am J Transplant 2004;4(Suppl 10):72–82.

55. Fong TL, Bunnapradist S, Jordan SC, Cho YW: Impact of hepatitis B core antibody status on outcomes of cadaveric renal transplantation: Analysis of United Network of Organ Sharing database between 1994 and 1999. Transplantation 2002;73:85–89.

56. Gane E, Pilmore H: Management of chronic viral hepatitis before and after renal transplantation. Transplantation 2002;74:427–437.

57. Delaney WE: Progress in the treatment of chronic hepatitis B: Long-term experience with adefovir dipivoxil. J Antimicrob Chemother 2007;59:827–832.

58. Fontaine H, Vallet-Pichard A, et al: Efficacy and safety of adefovir dipivoxil in kidney recipients, hemodialysis patients, and patients with renal insufficiency. Transplantation 2005;80:1086–1092.

59. Fissell RB, Bragg-Gresham JL, et al: Patterns of hepatitis C prevalence and seroconversion in hemodialysis units from three continents: The DOPPS. Kidney Int 2004;65:2335–2342.

60. Pereira BJ, Wright TL, Schmid CH, Levey AS for the New England Organ Bank Hepatitis C Study Group: A controlled study of hepatitis C transmission by organ transplantation. Lancet 1995;345:484–487.

61. Schweitzer EJ, Perencevich EN, Philosophe B, Bartlett ST: Estimated benefits of transplantation of kidneys from donors at increased risk for HIV or hepatitis C infection. Am J Transplant 2007;7:1515–1525.

62. Batty DS Jr., Swanson SJ, Kirk AD, et al: Hepatitis C virus seropositivity at the time of renal transplantation in the United States: Associated factors and patient survival. Am J Transplant 2001;1:179–184.

63. Bloom RD, Sayer G, Fa K, et al: Outcome of hepatitis C virus-infected kidney transplant candidates who remain on the waiting list. Am J Transplant 2005;5:139–144.

64. Pereira BJ, Natov SN, Bouthot BA, et al, for the New England Organ Bank Hepatitis C Study Group: Effects of hepatitis C infection and renal transplantation on survival in end-stage renal disease. Kidney Int 1998;53:1374–1381.

65. Abbott KC, Lentine KL, Bucci JR, et al:. The impact of transplantation with deceased donor hepatitis C-positive kidneys on survival in wait-listed long-term dialysis patients. Am J Transplant 2004;4:2032–2037.

66. Kamar N, Ribes D, Izopet J, Rostaing L: Treatment of hepatitis C virus infection (HCV) after renal transplantation: Implications for HCV-positive dialysis patients awaiting a kidney transplant. Transplantation 2006;82:853–856.

67. Bloom RD, Lake JR: Emerging issues in hepatitis C virus-positive liver and kidney transplant recipients. Am J Transplant 2006;6:2232–2237.

68. Wells JT, Lucey MR, Said A: Hepatitis C in transplant recipients of solid organs, other than liver. Clin Liver Dis 2006;10:901–917.

69. Hanafusa T, Ichikawa Y, Kishikawa H, et al: Retrospective study on the impact of hepatitis C virus infection on kidney transplant patients over 20 years. Transplantation 1998;66:471–476.

70. Izopet J, Rostaing L, Sandres K, et al: Longitudinal analysis of hepatitis C virus replication and liver fibrosis progression in renal transplant recipients. J Infect Dis 2000;181:852–858.

71. Kamar N, Rostaing L, Selves J, et al: Natural history of hepatitis C virus-related liver fibrosis after renal transplantation. Am J Transplant 2005;5:1704–1712.

72. Rostaing L, Modesto A, Baron E, et al: Acute renal failure in kidney transplant patients treated with interferon alpha 2b for chronic hepatitis C. Nephron 1996;74:512–516.

73. Fabrizi F, Martin P, Ponticelli C: Hepatitis C virus infection and renal transplantation. Am J Kidney Dis 2001;38:919–934.

74. BK virus. Am J Transplant 2004;4(Suppl 10):89–91.

75. Hirsch HH, Knowles W, Dickenmann M, et al: Prospective study of polyomavirus type BK replication and nephropathy in renal-transplant recipients. N Engl J Med 2002;347:488–496.

76. Randhawa P, Brennan DC: BK virus infection in transplant recipients: An overview and update. Am J Transplant 2006;6:2000–2005.
77. Drachenberg CB, Papadimitriou JC: Polyomavirus-associated nephropathy: Update in diagnosis. Transpl Infect Dis 2006;8:68–75.
78. Vera-Sempere FJ, Rubio L, Felipe-Ponce V, et al: PCR assays for the early detection of BKV infection in 125 Spanish kidney transplant patients. Clin Transplant 2006;20:706–711.
79. Basse G, Mengelle C, Kamar N, et al: Prospective evaluation of BK virus DNAemia in renal transplant patients and their transplant outcome. Transplant Proc 2007;39:84–87.
80. Trofe J, Hirsch HH, Ramos E: Polyomavirus-associated nephropathy: Update of clinical management in kidney transplant patients. Transpl Infect Dis 2006;8:76–85.
81. Josephson MA, Williams JW, Chandraker A, Randhawa PS: Polyomavirus-associated nephropathy: Update on antiviral strategies. Transpl Infect Dis 2006;8:95–101.
82. Williams JW, Javaid B, Kadambi PV, et al: Leflunomide for polyomavirus type BK nephropathy. N Engl J Med 2005;352:1157–1158.
83. Ramos E, Vincenti F, Lu WX, et al: Retransplantation in patients with graft loss caused by polyoma virus nephropathy. Transplantation 2004;77:131–133.
84. Womer KL, Meier-Kriesche HU, Patton PR, et al: Preemptive retransplantation for BK virus nephropathy: Successful outcome despite active viremia. Am J Transplant 2006;6:209–213.
85. Fungal infections. Am J Transplant 2004;4(Suppl 10):110–134.
86. Abbott KC, Hypolite I, Poropatich RK, et al: Hospitalizations for fungal infections after renal transplantation in the United States. Transpl Infect Dis 2001;3:203–211.
87. *Pneumocystis jiroveci* (formerly *Pneumocystis carinii*). Am J Transplant 2004;4(Suppl 10):135–141.
88. Tolkoff-Rubin NE, Rubin RH: Urinary tract infection in the immunocompromised host. Lessons from kidney transplantation and the AIDS epidemic. Infect Dis Clin North Am 1997;11:707–717.
89. Chuang P, Parikh CR, Langone A: Urinary tract infections after renal transplantation: A retrospective review at two US transplant centers. Clin Transplant 2005;19:230–235.
90. Dharnidharka VR, Agodoa LY, Abbott KC: Risk factors for hospitalization for bacterial or viral infection in renal transplant recipients—an analysis of USRDS data. Am J Transplant 2007;7:653–661.
91. Abbott KC, Oliver JD 3rd, Hypolite I, et al: Hospitalizations for bacterial septicemia after renal transplantation in the United States. Am J Nephrol 2001;21:120–127.
92. Abbott KC, Swanson SJ, Richter ER, et al: Late urinary tract infection after renal transplantation in the United States. Am J Kidney Dis 2004;44:353–362.
93. Hibberd PL, Tolkoff-Rubin NE, Doran M, et al: Trimethoprim-sulfamethoxazole compared with ciprofloxacin for the prevention of urinary tract infection in renal transplant recipients. A double-blind, randomized controlled trial. Online J Curr Clin Trials 11 August 1992 (Doc No. 15).
94. Tolkoff-Rubin NE, Cosimi AB, Russell PS, Rubin RH: A controlled study of trimethoprim-sulfamethoxazole prophylaxis of urinary tract infection in renal transplant recipients. Rev Infect Dis 1982;4:614–618.
95. Fox BC, Sollinger HW, Belzer FO, Maki DG: A prospective, randomized, double-blind study of trimethoprim-sulfamethoxazole for prophylaxis of infection in renal transplantation: Clinical efficacy, absorption of trimethoprim-sulfamethoxazole, effects on the microflora, and the cost-benefit of prophylaxis. Am J Med 1990;89:255–274.
96. Khosroshahi HT, Mogaddam AN, Shoja MM: Efficacy of high-dose trimethoprim-sulfamethoxazol prophylaxis on early urinary tract infection after renal transplantation. Transplant Proc 2006;38:2062–2064.
97. Valera B, Gentil MA, Cabello V et al: Epidemiology of urinary infections in renal transplant recipients. Transplant Proc 2006;38:2414–2415.
98. Dantas SR, Kuboyama RH, Mazzali M, Moretti ML: Nosocomial infections in renal transplant patients: Risk factors and treatment implications associated with urinary tract and surgical site infections. J Hosp Infect 2006;63:117–123.
99. Singh N, Paterson DL: Mycobacterium tuberculosis infection in solid-organ transplant recipients: Impact and implications for management. Clin Infect Dis 1998. 27:1266–1277.
100. Klote MM, Agodoa LY, Abbott K: Mycobacterium tuberculosis infection incidence in hospitalized renal transplant patients in the United States, 1998–2000. Am J Transplant 2004;4:1523–1528.
101. Mycobacterium tuberculosis. Am J Transplant 2004;4(Suppl 10):37–41.
102. Mazurek GH, Villarino ME: Guidelines for using the QuantiFERON-TB test for diagnosing latent Mycobacterium tuberculosis infection. Centers for Disease Control and Prevention. MMWR Recomm Rep 2003;52(RR-2):15–18.
103. Mazurek GH, Jereb J, Lobue P, et al: Guidelines for using the QuantiFERON-TB Gold test for detecting Mycobacterium tuberculosis infection, United States. MMWR Recomm Rep 2005;54(RR-15):49–55.
104. Nontuberculous mycobacteria. Am J Transplant 2004;4(Suppl 10):42–46.
105. Griffith DE, Aksamit T, Brown-Elliott BA, et al: An official ATS/IDSA statement: Diagnosis, treatment, and prevention of nontuberculous mycobacterial diseases. Am J Respir Crit Care Med 2007;175:367–416.
106. Stock PG, Roland ME, Carlson L, et al: Kidney and liver transplantation in human immunodeficiency virus-infected patients: A pilot safety and efficacy study. Transplantation 2003;76:370–375.
107. Swanson SJ, Kirk AD, Ko CW, et al: Impact of HIV seropositivity on graft and patient survival after cadaveric renal transplantation in the United States in the pre highly active antiretroviral therapy (HAART) era: An historical cohort analysis of the United States Renal Data System. Transpl Infect Dis 2002;4:144–147.
108. Roland ME: Solid-organ transplantation in HIV-infected patients in the potent antiretroviral therapy era. Top HIV Med 2004;12:73–76.
109. Abbott KC, Swanson SJ, Agodoa LY, Kimmel PL: Human immunodeficiency virus infection and kidney transplantation in the era of highly active antiretroviral therapy and modern immunosuppression. J Am Soc Nephrol 2004;15:1633–1639.
110. Wyatt CM, Murphy B: Kidney transplantation in HIV-infected patients. Semin Dial 2005;18:495–498.
111. Solid organ transplantation in the HIV-infected patient. Am J Transplant 2004;4(Suppl 10):83–88.

Further Reading

Abbott KC, Swanson SJ, Richter ER, et al: Late urinary tract infection after renal transplantation in the United States. Am J Kidney Dis 2004;44:353–362.

Dharnidharka VR, Agodoa LY, Abbott KC: Risk factors for hospitalization for bacterial or viral infection in renal transplant recipients—an analysis of USRDS data. Am J Transplant 2007;7:653–661.

Guidelines for the prevention and management of infectious complications of solid organ transplantation. Am J Transplant 2004;4(Suppl 10):1–166.

Recommendations for preventing transmission of infections among chronic hemodialysis patients. MMWR Recomm Rep 2001;50(RR-5):1–43.

Trofe J, Hirsch HH, Ramos E: Polyomavirus-associated nephropathy: Update of clinical management in kidney transplant patients. Transpl Infect Dis 2006;8:76–85.

Drugs and the Kidney

CONTENTS

Chapter 91

Drug Dosing in Renal Failure

D. Craig Brater

Many drugs are eliminated by the kidney and therefore require dose adjustment in patients with renal insufficiency.[1-4] Other drugs that themselves are not dependent on the kidney for excretion are converted in the liver to active metabolites that accumulate in patients with diminished renal function.[5,6] Thus, to avoid toxicity doses of many drugs must be diminished in patients with decreased renal function. The precision required depends on the therapeutic index of individual drugs. For example, penicillins and cephalosporin antibiotics have wide margins of safety. Dosing does not require the same precision as with drugs having narrow therapeutic indices, such as aminoglycoside antibiotics or digoxin, in which, in some instances, serum concentrations are measured to assure attainment of therapeutic, yet nontoxic, levels.

Patients treated with hemodialysis, hemofiltration, or peritoneal dialysis present an additional challenge. Drug may be removed by the procedure itself, thereby requiring compensatory dose supplementation, the extent of which is a function of the amount of drug removed.[1] The ability of dialysis to remove drugs is influenced by the binding of the drug to protein, which limits dialyzability, and molecular size, for example. These factors are highly variable among drugs, even those in the same chemical class, rendering a priori predictions impossible. Published data from appropriate patient populations guide therapy, which should be complemented with measurements of serum drug concentrations when assays are available.

This chapter discusses principles of drug dosing as a framework for adjustment in dosing regimens in patients with renal insufficiency. Dosing guidelines for patients with renal dysfunction, including dialysis, are offered in the appendix (Tables A91-1 to A91-3).

It is possible to anticipate some of the effects that renal disease and dialysis will have on drug disposition. Renal insufficiency will cause drugs eliminated by the kidney to accumulate. In general, accumulation sufficient to be of clinical concern occurs if 30% or more of the drug is eliminated in the urine unchanged. A characteristic of renal insufficiency is accumulation of endogenous organic acids in plasma, which compete with acidic xenobiotics for binding to albumin and thereby diminish protein binding. Hypoalbuminemia results in diminished binding of drugs bound to albumin. Thus, changes in protein binding influence the concentration of unbound, pharmacologically active drug in plasma.

All forms of dialysis require passage of the removed substance across a membrane. Certain characteristics of a drug predict its removal by dialysis. Avid binding to circulating proteins prevents dialytic removal. Theoretically, large size also restricts removal, but most xenobiotics are sufficiently small that this is only rarely important. A drug that is widely distributed in tissues, with only a small component of the total body burden circulating in plasma, may readily cross a dialysis membrane. However, the amount removed during dialysis will be clinically unimportant.

Understanding the pharmacokinetic characteristics of a drug is the framework on which the following discussion is based. This allows predictions that can be helpful in clinical situations in which insufficient dosing information is available.

PRINCIPLES OF DOSE ADJUSTMENT

Loading Dose

Use of some drugs entails administration of a loading dose to rapidly attain therapeutic drug concentrations.[7-9] This approach is usually employed when an effective drug concentration is needed quickly. Whether to give a loading dose depends on the urgency to achieve a pharmacologic effect compared to the half-life of the drug. If a loading dose is not given, the time needed to reach plateau drug concentrations is 4 times the half-life. If this time is long relative to the clinical need, a loading dose strategy should be employed. The loading dose needed is a function of the *volume of distribution* (V_d) of the drug and its *initial blood concentration* ($C_{initial}$):

$$\text{Loading dose} = (C_{initial})\,(V_d)$$

For example, if the V_d for a drug such as an aminoglycoside antibiotic is 0.25 L/kg and the desired peak serum concentration is 8 mg/L, the necessary loading dose can be calculated as follows:

$$\text{Loading dose} = (8\ \text{mg/L})\,(0.25\ \text{L/kg}) = 2\ \text{mg/kg}$$

It is customary for clinicians to consider a standard loading dose rather than calculating it from V_d and the desired concentration. This can be hazardous in settings in which the patient's disease may influence V_d and thereby mandate a change in the loading dose. For example, if the V_d of a drug in a patient with renal insufficiency is one-half that in a patient with normal renal function, and the patient with renal disease received a "standard" loading dose, the resulting initial concentration would be twice that expected, with a consequent risk of toxicity. To illustrate this from the previous example, if the "normal" loading dose of 2 mg/kg were administered to a patient whose V_d was 0.125 L/kg (i.e., one-half the usual value), a concentration of 16 mg/L would result:

$$2 \text{ mg/kg} = (C_{initial}) (0.125 \text{ L/kg})$$

$$C_{initial} = 2 \text{ mg/kg} \div 0.125 \text{ L/kg} = 16 \text{ mg/L}$$

It should be clear that clinicians need to be alert to changes in the V_d of drugs. Such data are provided in the appendix (see Table A91-1) for patients with renal disorders. The loading dose can be calculated as shown above. Alternatively, if the clinician knows the usual loading dose, the data in Table A91-1 can be used to calculate a modified dose:

Usual loading dose/Modified loading dose =
$$\text{Normal } V_d/\text{Patient's } V_d$$

or,

Modified loading dose = (Patient's V_d/Normal V_d) ×
$$\text{Usual loading dose}$$

The direct proportionality between loading dose and V_d makes such dose adjustments quite easy. A caution is the influence of changes in drug protein binding, which in many drugs is decreased in patients with renal insufficiency,[10,11] particularly for acidic drugs bound to serum albumin, wherein accumulated endogenous organic acids can displace drug from albumin binding sites.[12]

For highly protein-bound drugs, such as phenytoin, valproate, and warfarin, a decrease in binding to albumin might be expected to cause an increase in the unbound concentration, thereby resulting in increased drug effect. However, the increased free drug is also readily available for metabolism by the liver, such that the unbound concentration is no different from that in patients with normal renal function.[10,11,13,14] As an example, in a patient with normal renal function, a total serum concentration of phenytoin of 10 mg/L yields 1 mg/L of free drug. In contrast, in a patient with end-stage renal disease, the same dose results in a lower total concentration of 5 mg/L but the same free, pharmacologically active phenytoin concentration (Table 91-1).

The lesson is that for phenytoin (and valproate) the same pharmacologically active unbound serum concentration occurs at a lower total concentration. Clinical laboratories usually measure total drug concentration. Hence, in a patient with renal insufficiency or hypoalbuminemia, the "therapeutic" serum concentration, expressed as total drug, is less than in patients with normal renal function. This may prompt the physician to administer inappropriately larger doses to increase the total drug concentration. The result is a concomitant increase in the unbound concentration to potentially toxic levels. Although there is a similar scenario for warfarin,

Table 91-1 Phenytoin Concentration in Patients with Normal Renal Function and Those with End-stage Renal Disease

Concentration	Bound	+	Free	=	Total	Percentage Bound
Normal renal function	9	+	1	=	10 mg/L	90
ESRD	4	+	1	=	5 mg/L	80

ESRD, end-stage renal disease.

physicians normally monitor this drug's effect using the International Normalized Ratio as opposed to measuring the drug concentration. This spares the need to contemplate the role of protein binding with this agent.

Maintenance Dose

A maintenance dose maintains the desired steady-state drug concentrations,[7-9] as determined by the target *average drug concentration*, $C_{average}$, and the *clearance* (Cl) of the drug from the body:

$$\text{Maintenance dose} = (C_{average}) (Cl)$$

If a drug is administered as a continuous intravenous infusion, the maintenance dosing rate is the infusion rate of the drug. If a drug is administered as separate, intermittent intravenous doses, the dosing rate is expressed as:

$$\text{Dosing rate} = \text{Individual dose/Dosing interval}$$

If a drug is administered by mouth, a term to account for incomplete bioavailability must be incorporated, with the *fraction of the dose absorbed* (F). The maintenance dosing rate becomes:

$$\text{Dosing rate} = (F) (\text{Individual dose})/\text{Dosing interval}$$

Hence, depending on the route of administration, any of the following relationships may apply:

$$\text{Infusion rate} = (C_{average}) (Cl)$$

$$\text{Dose/Dosing interval} = (C_{average}) (Cl)$$

$$F \times \text{Dose/Dosing interval} = (C_{average}) (Cl)$$

Thus, a change in clearance mandates a proportional change in the rate of drug administration to maintain a constant average drug concentration. The clearance of drugs or their metabolite(s) in patients with renal insufficiency is often diminished; consequently, maintenance doses must be adjusted. Guidelines for doing so are offered in the appendix (see Table A91-3).

Half-life

The *half-life* ($t_{1/2}$) of a drug refers to the time required for the serum concentration to decrease by 50%. The rate of elimination of most drugs (exceptions being phenytoin and salicylate) is linear and independent of the drug serum concentration. This implies that the $t_{1/2}$ is independent of the serum concentration. Therefore, the time for a drug's concentration to decrease from 100 to 50 units of concentration is the same as for a decrease from 10 to 5 units.

Many clinicians use $t_{1/2}$ synonymously with clearance of a drug. This presumes that an increase in $t_{1/2}$ indicates a proportional decrease in clearance, which thereby requires a compensatory and proportional decrease in the maintenance dose. This misconception can lead to errors in dose adjustment in patients with renal insufficiency because $t_{1/2}$ is a function of both V_d and Cl and does not solely reflect the clearance of a drug:

$$t_{1/2} = 0.693 \, V_d/Cl$$

A change in $t_{1/2}$ can reflect a change in V_d, a change in Cl, or both. The correct dosing regimen adjustment depends on whether an alteration in V_d or in Cl is responsible for the change in $t_{1/2}$. If $t_{1/2}$ increases solely because of an increase in V_d, the loading dose should be increased, while the maintenance dose should remain unchanged. If it is assumed that the $t_{1/2}$ increased because Cl decreased, a "normal" loading dose and a diminished maintenance dose would be administered. This would result in a loading dose that is too small, which would fail to attain the desired initial concentration, and an inappropriately diminished maintenance dose, which would maintain a lower drug concentration than desired. The result could be lack of efficacy.

A good example of this is the use of digoxin in patients with renal insufficiency. In patients with mild to moderate renal insufficiency, the V_d of digoxin is little changed, whereas Cl may be reduced to about one-half to two-thirds normal.[15] In such patients, the $t_{1/2}$ rises in proportion to the diminished Cl. However, in patients with severe renal insufficiency, the V_d is decreased to one-half to two-thirds normal, and Cl is decreased further to about one-third normal.[15,16] In this setting, the $t_{1/2}$ is influenced by both parameters. Although the half-life is prolonged in severe renal dysfunction, it is little different from that in the patient with mild to moderate renal insufficiency. If the change in $t_{1/2}$ in the patient with severe renal insufficiency compared to normal subjects was erroneously presumed to reflect only the decrease in digoxin clearance and thereby to affect only the maintenance dose, a serious dosing error would occur. Because no downward adjustment in loading dose would be made, the initial concentration would be higher than desired. The decrease in maintenance dose would be underestimated so that the patient's steady-state serum concentration would be maintained at a higher concentration than desired. The hazards of such an error are obvious.

A realization of the limitations of using $t_{1/2}$ to predict dosing adjustments mandates the need to dissect it into its component parts of V_d and Cl. Of what use, then, is $t_{1/2}$? Knowing $t_{1/2}$ allows one to determine the time necessary for serum drug concentrations to reach a steady state. Steady state is reached after administering the drug for 4 to 5 times the $t_{1/2}$. This delay in attaining plateau drug concentrations can be avoided by giving a loading dose designed to attain the desired drug concentration quickly.

The attainment of steady state applies to a change in dose. For example, if a maintenance dose is doubled, 4 to 5 times the $t_{1/2}$ is required for the serum concentration to reach the new plateau. Similarly, if the maintenance dose is decreased, 4 to

5 times the $t_{1/2}$ must elapse for the new, lower steady-state concentration to be reached. Lastly, if a drug is stopped, 4 to 5 times the $t_{1/2}$ is needed for concentrations to become negligible.

In summary, the half-life should be used to predict the time for a drug to reach steady-state concentrations. It is a hybrid value influenced by both V_d and Cl and provides no direct information about loading or maintenance dose.

Dosing Regimens

Changes in loading dose entail giving a larger or smaller dose depending on whether V_d is increased or decreased. The need to modify a loading dose may be unclear, in which case a decision must be made concerning whether a loading dose strategy is necessary. In such cases it is wise to err on the side of caution and administer a smaller loading dose. If monitoring of clinical endpoints or serum drug concentrations shows the dose to have been too low, a supplementary dose can be given. In contrast, too large a loading dose can lead to iatrogenic drug toxicity.

Several strategies can be employed for adjusting maintenance doses of a drug. The primary objective is to maintain the same average drug concentration in a patient without renal disease. Because the majority of drugs obey linear or first-order elimination kinetics, change in clearance can be compensated for by a proportional change in the dosing rate:

Usual maintenance dose/Modified maintenance dose =
Usual clearance/Patient's clearance

or,

Modified maintenance dose =
(Patient's clearance/Usual clearance) × Usual maintenance dose

Hence, if the clearance of a drug in a patient with renal insufficiency is one-half the "normal" value, the patient's maintenance dose should be one-half that usually administered. Such dose modifications will maintain a normal average steady-state drug concentration.

If a patient is receiving a drug by continuous intravenous infusion, maintenance dose modification simply requires a modified infusion rate. If the patient is receiving intermittent doses, reduction of the total dose administered can be accomplished in three ways:

1. Decreasing each individual dose and maintaining the same dosing frequency. This is referred to as the *variable dose method.*
2. Maintaining the same individual dose but administering each dose less frequently. This is referred to as the *variable frequency method.*
3. Modifying both individual doses and the frequency of their administration, which is a combination method.

All three methods attain the same average drug concentration. For example, if 2400 mg of a drug is administered to a patient with normal renal function as 600 mg every 6 hours, and one wished to administer one half as much total drug to a patient with renal insufficiency, options include the following:

- 300 mg every 6 hr (variable dose)
- 600 mg every 12 hr (variable frequency)
- 400 mg every 8 hr (combination)

The total drug administered with each of these regimens is the same (1200 mg). It is half that administered to a patient with normal renal function. These regimens differ in the profile of serum drug concentrations. Regimens with closer dosing frequencies and smaller individual doses result in less difference between peak and trough drug concentrations. Determining which option is best is a function of the drug and the disease being treated. For example, having low serum concentrations for a considerable period of time with an antibiotic with a long postantibiotic effect may not be worrisome. In contrast, for a drug that must be maintained within a narrow concentration range to maximize efficacy (e.g., an antiarrhythmic or anticonvulsant), a regimen would be needed that minimizes fluctuations in serum concentrations.

No general rule can be applied to the maximum length of a dosing interval; 24 hours seems a reasonable rule of thumb and would likely be helpful for patient adherence. If a patient is not responding to a drug, the clinician should anticipate a possible inappropriate dosing regimen. Signs of toxicity shortly after administration of an individual dose may indicate a need to give the drug more frequently in smaller doses to optimize the dosing regimen.

Dialysis

Patients with endstage renal disease treated with dialysis (including hemofiltration) have an additional mechanism by which drugs can be eliminated.[17–20] If substantial elimination by these routes occurs, supplemental dosing must be given. This is most easily accomplished by administering a supplemental dose of drug at the completion of dialysis. The dose given is the amount of drug removed during the procedure.

With continuous ambulatory peritoneal dialysis (CAPD), drug removal is continuous. The patient's total clearance of a drug is the sum of the clearance by residual renal function and clearance via CAPD. The dosing regimen (individual dose, dosing interval, or both) should be adjusted upward in proportion to the added increment in clearance from CAPD.

Where information on dialytic removal of the agent is lacking, insight into the dialyzability of a drug may be appreciated from its pharmacokinetic parameters. If a drug such as vancomycin or amphotericin is too large to pass across the dialysis membrane (including the peritoneum), it will not be removed by dialysis. If a drug is bound in excess of 90% to plasma proteins, it is unlikely that dialysis will contribute appreciably to its elimination. Drugs that are water soluble are more readily dialyzed. A clue that a drug is water soluble is that these drugs are usually eliminated predominantly by the kidney as unchanged drug. Lastly, drugs with large volumes of distribution have minimal dialyzability because, of the total amount of drug in the body, only a small portion resides in the vascular space where it can be removed. Once dialysis ends, the large amount of drug in the tissues can refill the vascular compartment. The dialysis procedure therefore removes only an insignificant quantity of the total amount of drug in the body.

Specific examples can be used to illustrate these principles. Aminoglycoside antibiotics are water soluble, eliminated primarily by the kidney (100% of the dose is normally excreted unchanged in the urine), have negligible protein binding, have a small volume of distribution (0.25 L/kg), and are removed by dialysis procedures sufficiently to require dose supplementation. In contrast, cefonicid also has a small V_d (0.10 L/kg), but is highly bound to serum proteins (98%) and therefore is not removed by hemodialysis or CAPD. Cefadroxil, on the other hand, despite having a somewhat larger V_d than cefonicid (0.30 L/kg) is only 16% bound to serum proteins. Dialytic removal is sufficient with this cephalosporin to require supplemental dosing. Last, drugs such as phenothiazines and tricyclic antidepressants that have large V_d values (>10 L/kg) are not eliminated by dialysis even if they are negligibly bound to serum proteins.

Table A91-2 in the appendix lists the amount of a drug removed by dialysis (as a percentage of a "normal" dose in a patient with normal renal function). This value allows calculation of the increment in dosing that must be given to compensate for removal by dialysis. The table does not include removal of drugs by hemoperfusion, hemofiltration, or hemodiafiltration. Hemoperfusion is applicable to toxicologic settings and is discussed in Chapter 92.

Hemofiltration removes unbound drug in the serum. The amount removed (and thereby the dose increment needed) can be calculated as:

$$\text{Amount removed (mg)} = \text{Serum concentration (mg/L)} \times \text{Unbound fraction} \times \text{Ultrafiltration rate (L/min)} \times \text{Time of procedure (min)}$$

The ultrafiltration rate and the duration of hemofiltration are known. The unbound fraction can be found in the published literature.[1] Serum concentration can be directly measured for many drugs. Alternatively, the average concentration at steady state can be reasonably estimated as:

$$\text{Average concentration (mg/L)} = \text{Dosing rate (mg/min)}/\text{Clearance (mL/min)}$$

Active Metabolites

Although many drugs are not themselves eliminated by renal routes, they are converted by the liver to active metabolites that depend on the kidney for excretion. Hence, in patients with renal disease, the metabolite can accumulate, causing its own pharmacologic effect(s).[5,6] For example, meperidine is converted to normeperidine, which unlike the parent drug is not an analgesic but rather a central nervous system stimulant. The metabolite is excreted by the kidney and accumulates in patients with renal insufficiency. Even in elderly patients with mild decrements in renal function, this metabolite can reach sufficient concentrations to cause seizures. Its use in patients with renal compromise requires lower doses of meperidine (which may limit its efficacy). A better alternative is to use another analgesic such as morphine for which the parent drug and metabolite(s) do not depend on the kidney for elimination. For many drugs, it is not known whether there are active metabolites or if these accumulate in renal disease. Unanticipated responses to drugs should raise the consideration of active metabolites and may prompt discontinuation of a drug in the hope that an adverse response dissipates.

DOSING RECOMMENDATIONS

When renal insufficiency affects the volume of distribution of a drug (see Table A91-3 in the appendix), the loading dose must be modified. More commonly, one needs to compensate for decreased clearance of drugs by adjusting the maintenance dose. Principles for doing so have been discussed previously, the most important of which is the proportionality that exists between clearance, dose, and steady-state serum drug concentration. Hence, a clearance that is one-half that of normal can be compensated for by decreasing the dose to one-half normal. Different strategies for dose adjustment have also been discussed. The clinician can change each individual dose, the interval between them, or both. Which strategy to use depends on the drug and the individual patient, but a reasonable starting point for most drugs is to first lengthen the interval until a maximum of 24 hours is reached, after which further modification of the individual dose is appropriate.

Table A91-3 in the appendix offers recommendations for modification of the maintenance dose in patients with various degrees of renal insufficiency. These guidelines should serve only as starting points of therapy. Subsequent dosing requires tailoring the regimen to each individual patient, which in turn must be based on clinical endpoints or measurement of serum concentrations of drugs.

References

1. UpToDate, Wellesley, MA: 2007.
2. Brater DC: The pharmacological role of the kidney. Drugs 1980; 19:31–48.
3. Clinical Drug Use. Available at: www.clinicaldruguse.com. Accessed May 6, 2008.
4. Swan SK, Bennett WM: Drug dosing guidelines in patients with renal failure. West J Med 1992;156:633–638.
5. Drayer DE: Pharmacologically active drug metabolites: Therapeutic and toxic activities, plasma and urine data in man, accumulation in renal failure. Clin Pharmacokinet 1976;1:426–443.
6. Verbeeck RK, Branch RA, Wilkinson GR: Drug metabolites in renal failure: Pharmacokinetic and clinical implications. Clin Pharmacokinet 1981;6:329–345.
7. Holford NHG, Sheiner LB: Kinetics of pharmacologic response. Pharm Ther 1982;16:143–166.
8. Gibaldi M, Levy G: Pharmacokinetics in clinical practice. I. Concepts. JAMA 1976;235:1864–1867.
9. Gibaldi M, Levy G: Pharmacokinetics in clinical practice. 2. Applications. JAMA 1976;235:1987–1992.
10. Oie S: Drug distribution and binding. J Clin Pharmacol 1986; 26:583–586.
11. Reidenberg MM, Drayer DE: Alteration of drug-protein binding in renal disease. Clin Pharmacokinet 1984;9:18–26.
12. Gulyassy PF, Bottini AT, Stanfel IA, et al: Isolation and chemical identification of inhibitors of plasma ligand binding. Kidney Int 1986;30:391–398.
13. Benet LZ, Hoener B-A: Changes in plasma protein binding have little clinical relevance. Clin Pharmacol Ther 2002;71:115–121.
14. Greenblatt DJ, Sellers EM, Koch-Weser J: Importance of protein binding for the interpretation of serum or plasma drug concentrations. J Clin Pharmacol 1982;22:259–263.
15. Sheiner LB, Rosenberg BG, Marathe VV: Estimation of population characteristics of pharmacokinetic parameters from routine clinical data. J Pharmacokinet Biopharm 1977;5:445–479.
16. Gault MH, Churchill DN, Kalra J: Loading dose of digoxin in renal failure. Br J Clin Pharmacol 1980;9:593–597.
17. Gibson TP, Nelson HA: Drug kinetics and artificial kidneys. Clin Pharmacokinet 1977;2:403–426.
18. Keller E, Reetz P, Schollmeyer P: Drug therapy in patients undergoing continuous ambulatory peritoneal dialysis. Clinical pharmacokinetic considerations. Clin Pharmacokinet 1990;18:104–117.
19. Reetz-Bonorden P, Böhler J, Keller E: Drug dosage in patients during continuous renal replacement therapy. Pharmacokinetic and therapeutic considerations. Clin Pharmacokinet 1993;24:362–379.
20. Bressolle F, Kinowski J-M, de la Coussaye JE, et al: Clinical pharmacokinetics during continuous haemofiltration. Clin Pharmacokinet 1994;26:457–471.

Further Reading

Gibaldi M, Levy G: Pharmacokinetics in clinical practice. I. Concepts. JAMA 1976;235:1864–1867.
Gibaldi M, Levy G: Pharmacokinetics in clinical practice. 2. Applications. JAMA 1976;235:1987–1992

APPENDIX

Table A91-1   Effect of Renal Disease on Volume of Distribution

Drug	V_d (L/kg) Normal Renal Function	ESRD
Analgesics		
Codeine	3.5–6.0	7.3
Nalmefene	8.2	17.1
Salicylate	0.15	Increase (no change)*
Anesthetics and Drugs Used during Anesthesia		
Thiopental	1.9 (12)	3.0 (12)
Antianxiety Agents		
Abecarnil	14	19 (no change)
Oxazepam	0.6–2.0	Increase (no change)
Anticonvulsants		
Phenytoin	0.5–1.0	Increase (no change)
Valproate	0.2–0.4	Increase (no change)
Antihistamines		
Roxatidine	3.2	2.0
Anti-inflammatory Agents		
Anakinra	0.11	0.17
Azapropazone	0.15–0.25	No change (decrease)
Diflunisal	0.10–0.13	0.27 (no change)
Oxaprozin	0.07–0.25	(Decrease)
Antifungals		
Miconazole	2–3	Decrease
Antimicrobial Agents/Antibacterials		
Cephalosporins		
Cefazolin	0.11–0.14	0.17
Cefoxitin	0.27	Increase
Macrolide Antibiotics		
Erythromycin	0.6–0.8	1.2
Penicillins		
Azlocillin	0.18	0.3
Quinolones		
Norfloxacin	3.2	1.7

Table A91-1 Effect of Renal Disease on Volume of Distribution—cont'd

Drug	V_d (L/kg)	
	Normal Renal Function	ESRD
Bronchodilators		
Albuterol	2.0–2.5	0.8
Cardiovascular Agents		
Blood Lipid-Lowering Agents		
Acifran	0.5	(Decrease to 1/3 normal)
Cardiac Inotropes		
Digitoxin	0.73	Increase (no change)
Digoxin	$V_d = 3.84 + 0.0446$ CrCl	
Hormonal Agents		
Insulin-like growth factor	0.15	0.07–0.09

V_d, volume of distribution; ESRD, end-stage renal disease; CrCl, creatinine clearance.
*Values in parentheses indicate data for unbound drug.

Table A91-2 Percentage of a Dose Removed by One Session of Hemodialysis or 24 Hours of Continuous Ambulatory Peritoneal Dialysis

Drug	Hemodialysis	CAPD
Analgesics		
Meperidine	Negligible	Negligible
Methadone	Negligible (1%)	Negligible (1%)
Nalmefene	Negligible (3.3%)	
Propoxyphene	Negligible	Negligible
Salicylates	Negligible	Negligible
Tilidine	Negligible (<1%)	
Tramadol	Negligible (7%)	
Anesthetics and Drugs Used during Anesthesia		
Gallamine	Considerable	Considerable
Antianxiety Agents, Sedatives, and Hypnotics		
Buspirone	Negligible	
Chloral hydrate	Negligible	
Ethchlorvynol	Negligible	
Glutethimide	Negligible	
Meprobamate	Negligible	
Methaqualone	Negligible	
Oxazepam	Negligible	

Continued

Table A91-2 Percentage of a Dose Removed by One Session of Hemodialysis or 24 Hours of Continuous Ambulatory Peritoneal Dialysis—cont'd

Drug	Hemodialysis	CAPD
Phenobarbital	Negligible	
Zopiclone	Negligible	
Anticholinergics and Cholinergics		
Cisapride	Negligible	
Metoclopramide	Negligible	
Pirenzipine	11%–15%	
Anticoagulants, Antifibrinolytics, and Antiplatelet Agents		
Warfarin	Negligible	Negligible
Low-molecular-weight heparins	Negligible	
Anticonvulsants		
Gabapentin	50%	
Ethosuximide	45%	
Levetiracetam	25%–50%	
Phenytoin	Negligible	Negligible
Pregabalin	50%	
Primidone	30%	
Topiramate	50%	
Valproic acid	Negligible (1%)	Negligible
Antihistamines		
Cetirizine		Negligible (9%)
Cimetidine	10%–20%	Negligible (1.6%)
Famotidine	Negligible (6%–16%)	Negligible (4.5%)
Fexofenadine	Negligible (<1.7%)	
Levocabastine	Negligible (11%)	
Loratadine	Negligible	
Nizatidine	Negligible (10%)	
Ranitidine	50%–60%	Negligible (<1%)
Anti-inflammatory Agents		
Anakinra	Negligible	
Azapropazone	Negligible	Negligible
Bromfenac	Negligible	
Leflunomide	Negligible	Negligible
Lornoxicam	Negligible	
Nabumetone	Negligible	
Oxaprozin	Negligible	Negligible

Table A91-2 Percentage of a Dose Removed by One Session of Hemodialysis or 24 Hours of Continuous Ambulatory Peritoneal Dialysis—cont'd

Drug	Hemodialysis	CAPD
Penicillamine	30%	
Sulindac	Negligible	
Antimicrobial Agents		
Aminoglycosides		
Aminoglycosides	50%	20%–25%
Spectinomycin	50%	
Carbapenems		
Biapenem	90%	
Imipenem	80%–90%	Negligible
Meropenem	50%–70%	
Cephalosporins		
Cefaclor	33%	
Cefadroxil	50%	
Cefamandole	50%	Negligible (5%)
Cefazolin	50%	20%
Cefdinir		Negligible (1.4%–7.2%)
Cefipime	40%–70%	26%
Cefixime	Negligible (1.6%)	Negligible
Cefmenoxime	16%–51%	Negligible (<10%)
Cefmetazole	60%	
Cefodizime	50%	Negligible (15%)
Cefonicid	Negligible	Negligible (6.5%)
Cefoperazone	Negligible	Negligible
Ceforanide	20%–50%	
Cefotaxime	60%	Negligible (5%)
Cefotetan	Negligible (5%–9%)	
Cefotiam	30%–40%	
Cefoxitin	50%	Negligible
Cefpirome	32%–48%	Negligible (12%)
Cefpodoxime	50%	
Cefprozil	55%	
Cefroxadine	50%	
Cefsulodin	60%	
Ceftazidime	50%	Negligible
Ceftibuten	39%	
Ceftizoxime	50%	Negligible (16%)
Ceftriaxone	40%	Negligible (4.5%)

Continued

Table A91-2 Percentage of a Dose Removed by One Session of Hemodialysis or 24 Hours of Continuous Ambulatory Peritoneal Dialysis—cont'd

Drug	Hemodialysis	CAPD
Cefuroxime		20%
Cephacetrile	50%	
Cephalexin	50%–75%	30%
Cephalothin	50%	
Cephapirin	20%	
Glycopeptides		
Vancomycin	Negligible	Negligible (15–20%)
Teicoplanin	Negligible	Negligible (5%)
Macrolide Antibiotics		
Clindamycin	Negligible	Negligible
Dirithromycin	Negligible	
Lincomycin	Negligible	Negligible
Monobactams		
Aztreonam	40%	Negligible
Carumonam	51%	
Moxalactam	30%–50%	Negligible (15%–20%)
Nitroimidazoles		
Metronidazole	45%	Negligible (10%)
Ornidazole	42%	Negligible (6%)
Tinidazole	40%	
Oxazolidinones		
Linezolid	33%	
Penicillins		
Amdinocillin	32%–70%	Negligible (<4%)
Amoxicillin	30%	
Ampicillin	40%	
Azlocillin	30%–45%	
Carbenicillin	50%	
Cloxacillin	Negligible	
Dicloxacillin	Negligible	
Methicillin	Negligible	
Mezlocillin	20%–25%	24%
Nafcillin	Negligible	
Oxacillin	Negligible	
Penicillin	50%	
Piperacillin	30%–50%	Negligible (6%)

Table A91-2 Percentage of a Dose Removed by One Session of Hemodialysis or 24 Hours of Continuous Ambulatory Peritoneal Dialysis—cont'd

Drug	Hemodialysis	CAPD
Temocillin	50%	Negligible
Ticarcillin	50%	Negligible
Polymyxins		
Colistin	Negligible	Negligible
Quinolones		
Ciprofloxacin	Negligible (2%)	Negligible (0.4%–1.6%)
Enoxacin	Negligible	
Fleroxacin	Negligible (3%–7%)	Negligible (<10%)
Gatifloxacin	Negligible (14%)	Negligible (11%)
Levofloxacin	Negligible	Negligible
Lomefloxacin	Negligible	
Norfloxacin	Negligible	
Ofloxacin	Negligible (15%–25%)	Negligible (4%–6%)
Pefloxacin	Negligible	
Temafloxacin	Negligible (9.4%)	
Streptogramins		
Quinupristin/dalfopristin		Negligible
Sulfonamides		
Sulfamethoxazole	50%	Negligible (8%)
Trimethoprim	50%	Negligible (7%)
Tetracyclines		
Doxycycline	Negligible	Negligible
Minocycline	Negligible	Negligible
Antifungals		
Amphotericin B	Negligible	
Fluconazole	40%	Negligible (18%)
Flucytosine	50%	
Itraconazole	Negligible	Negligible
Ketoconazole	Negligible	Negligible
Miconazole	Negligible	Negligible
Antimalarials		
Chloroquine	Negligible	
Mefloquine	Negligible	
Quinine	Negligible	

Continued

Table A91-2 Percentage of a Dose Removed by One Session of Hemodialysis or 24 Hours of Continuous Ambulatory Peritoneal Dialysis—cont'd

Drug	Hemodialysis	CAPD
Antineoplastics and Antimetabolites		
Cyclophosphamide	30%–60%	
Etoposide	Negligible	
Methotrexate	Negligible	
Paclitaxel	Negligible	
Antituberculous Agents		
Para-aminosalicylic acid	50%	
Ethambutol	Negligible (12%)	
Isoniazid	75%	
Antiulcer Agents		
Lansoprazole	Negligible	
Omeprazole	Negligible	
Pantoprazole	Negligible	
Rabeprazole	Negligible	
Antiviral Agents		
Abacavir	24%	
Acyclovir	60%	Negligible (<10%)
Amantadine	Negligible	
Cidofovir	50%	Negligible
Didanosine	20%–67%	Negligible
Foscarnet	27%–58%	
Ganciclovir	Negligible	
Lamivudine	Negligible	
Ribavirin	Negligible (8%)	
Vidarabine	50%	
Zidovudine	Negligible	Negligible
Bronchodilators		
Dyphylline	28%	
Theophylline	40%	
Zileuton	Negligible (0.5%)	
Cardiovascular Agents		
Antianginal Agents		
Amlodipine	Negligible	Negligible
Bepridil	Negligible	
Diltiazem		Negligible (<0.1%)

Table A91-2 Percentage of a Dose Removed by One Session of Hemodialysis or 24 Hours of Continuous Ambulatory Peritoneal Dialysis—cont'd

Drug	Hemodialysis	CAPD
Felodipine	Negligible	
Isradipine	Negligible	
Nifedipine	Negligible (<1%)	Negligible
Antiarrhythmics		
N-Acetylprocainamide	50%	Negligible
Amiodarone	Negligible	
Bretylium	Negligible	
Cibenzoline	Negligible	
Disopyramide	Negligible (2%–4%)	
Flecainide	Negligible (1%)	Negligible
Lorcainide	Negligible (8%–12%)	
Mexiletine	Negligible	Negligible
Procainamide	Negligible	Negligible (<5%)
Propafenone	Negligible	
Quinidine	Negligible (<1%)	
Recainam	Negligible (9%)	
Sematilide	20%–25%	
Sotalol	40%–57%	
Tocainide	25%	Negligible (2%)
Antihypertensives		
α₁-Adrenergic Antagonists		
Doxazosin	Negligible	
Urapadil	Negligible (6.5%)	
Angiotensin Receptor Antagonists		
Candesartan	Negligible (0.2%)	
Erbesartan	Negligible	
Irbesartan	Negligible	
Losartan	Negligible	Negligible
β-Adrenergic Antagonists		
Acebutolol	Negligible	
Atenolol	50%	
Carvedilol	Negligible	
Esmolol	Negligible	Negligible
Labetalol	Negligible (2%–5%)	Negligible (0.14%)
Metoprolol	Negligible	
Nadolol	50%	

Continued

Table A91-2 Percentage of a Dose Removed by One Session of Hemodialysis or 24 Hours of Continuous Ambulatory Peritoneal Dialysis—cont'd

Drug	Hemodialysis	CAPD
Centrally Acting α_2-Stimulants		
Clonidine	Negligible	
Guanfacine	Negligible	
Angiotensin-Converting Enzyme Inhibitors		
Captopril	35%–40%	Negligible (<1%)
Cilazapril	Negligible (14%)	
Enalapril	50%	
Fosinopril		Negligible (2%)
Lisinopril	50%–60%	
Omapatrilat	Negligible	
Perindopril	55%	
Quinapril		Negligible (2.6%)
Ramipril	Negligible	
Blood Lipid-Lowering Agents		
Bezafibrate	Negligible	Negligible (1.6%)
Clofibrate	Negligible	
Fenofibrate	Negligible	
Gemfibrozil	Negligible	
Pravastatin	Negligible	
Cardiac Inotropes		
Digoxin	Negligible	Negligible (8%)
Fab	Negligible	Negligible
Vasodilators		
Buflomedil	Negligible (3.4%–6.7%)	
Diazoxide	Negligible	
Ketanserin	Negligible	
Minoxidil	24%–43%	
Hormonal Agents		
Epoetin		Negligible (2.3%)
Hypoglycemic Agents		
Repaglinide	Negligible	
Rosiglitazone	Negligible	
Hypouricemic Agents		
Allopurinol	40%	

Table A91-2 Percentage of a Dose Removed by One Session of Hemodialysis or 24 Hours of Continuous Ambulatory Peritoneal Dialysis—cont'd

Drug	Hemodialysis	CAPD
Immunologic Agents		
Cyclosporine	Negligible	
Mycophenolate	Negligible	
Psychotherapeutic Agents		
Citalopram	Negligible (<1%)	
Lithium	Considerable	Considerable
Olanzapine	Negligible	
Sertindole	Negligible (<0.1%)	
Sertraline	Negligible	
Tianeptine	Negligible	
Steroids		
Prednisone	Negligible	
Miscellaneous		
Sulbactam		Negligible
Tazobactam	30%–50%	Negligible (11%–13%)

Table A91-3 Dosing Recommendations in Patients with Renal Insufficiency (Relative to Normal Dose)

Drug	CREATININE CLEARANCE (mL/min)		
	>50	20–50	<20
Analgesics			
Butorphanol			1/2
Codeine			1/2
Meperidine		Avoid	
Metamizol			1/3
Nalmefene			1/2
Propoxyphene		Avoid	
Tramadol			1/2
Anesthetics and Drugs Used during Anesthesia			
Alcuronium			1/3
Doxacurium			1/2
Gallamine		Avoid	
Metocurine			1/2
Pancuronium		Avoid	
Pipecuronium			1/2

Continued

Table A91-3 Dosing Recommendations in Patients with Renal Insufficiency (Relative to Normal Dose)—cont'd

Drug	CREATININE CLEARANCE (mL/min)		
	>50	20–50	<20
Rapacuronium			2/3
D-Tubocurarine			1/2
Vecuronium		Avoid	
Anthelmintics			
Diethylcarbamazine		Decrease	
Antianxiety Agents			
Acamprosate			1/3
Buspirone		1/2	1/4
Anticholinergics and Cholinergics			
Metoclopramide		1/2	1/4
Neostigmine		1/2	1/3
Pirenzipine			1/2
Pyridostigmine	1/2	1/3	1/5
Anticoagulants, Antifibrinolytics, and Antiplatelet Agents			
Bivalirudin			1/4
Desirudin		1/3	1/6
Iloprost			1/2
Lamifiban		Avoid	
Lotrafiban			1/2
Low-molecular-weight heparins			1/2
Sulotroban	1/2	1/5	1/20
Tirofiban			1/2
Tranexamic acid	1/2	1/4	1/8
Anticonvulsants			
Gabapentin	1/2	1/4	1/8
Levetiracetam		1/2	1/3
Oxcarbazepine			1/2
Pregabalin	1/2	1/3	1/6
Topiramate			1/2
Vigabatrin		1/2	1/4
Antihistamines			
Cetirizine			1/3
Cimetidine		1/2	1/6
Ebastine			1/2
Emedastine			2/3

Table A91-3 Dosing Recommendations in Patients with Renal Insufficiency (Relative to Normal Dose)—cont'd

Drug	CREATININE CLEARANCE (mL/min)		
	>50	20–50	<20
Famotidine	1/2	1/3	1/5
Fexofenadine			1/2
Levocabastine			1/3
Nizatidine	1/2	1/4	1/4
Ranitidine	1/2	1/3	1/4
Roxatidine	3/4	1/2	1/4
Anti-inflammatory agents			
Anakinra			1/5
Azapropazone	1/2	1/5	1/10
Diacerein			1/2
Diflunisal			1/2
Indobufen		1/2	1/3
Ketoprofen			1/2
Ketorolac		Avoid	
Oxaprozin			1/2
Penicillamine		Avoid	
Tiaprofenic acid			1/2
Ximoprofen			1/3
Antimicrobial Agents/Antibacterials			
Aminoglycosides	1/3	1/2	1/4
Carbapenems			
Biapenem			1/5
Imipenem		1/2	1/4
Meropenem	2/3	1/3	1/6
Cephalosporins			
Cefaclor		1/2	1/4
Cefadroxil	1/2	1/4	1/8
Cefamandole	1/2	1/3	1/4
Cefazolin	1/2	1/4	1/6
Cefdinir			1/10
Cefditoren pivoxil			1/3
Cefepime	2/3	1/5	1/8
Cefetamet	1/2	1/4	1/8
Cefixime		1/2	1/3
Cefmenoxime	1/2	1/4	1/6
Cefmetazole	2/3	1/2	1/3
Cefodizime			1/2

Continued

Table A91-3 Dosing Recommendations in Patients with Renal Insufficiency (Relative to Normal Dose)—cont'd

Drug	CREATININE CLEARANCE (mL/min)		
	>50	20–50	<20
Cefonicid	1/2	1/5	1/10
Ceforanide	1/2	1/3	1/5
Cefotaxime		1/2	1/4
Cefotetan	1/2	1/4	1/10
Cefotiam		3/4	1/2
Cefoxitin	1/2	1/4	1/6
Cefpirome		1/2	1/4
Cefpodoxime		1/4	1/8
Cefprodoxime	1/2	1/3	1/5
Cefprozil			1/2
Cefroxadine		1/2	1/4
Cefsulodin	1/2	1/4	1/10
Ceftazidime	1/2	1/5	1/10
Ceftibuten		1/2	1/6
Ceftizoxime	1/2	1/4	1/10
Cefuroxime		1/2	1/4
Cephacetrile	1/2	1/4	1/10
Cephalexin		1/3	1/10
Cephalothin	2/3	1/2	1/6
Cephapirin		1/2	1/3
Cephradine		1/3	1/10
Loracarbef	1/2	1/4	1/10
Chloramphenicol and Thiamphenicol			
Thiamphenicol	1/2	1/3	1/10
Glycopeptides			
Teicoplanin		1/2	1/3
Vancomycin	2/3	1/2	1/10
Macrolide Antibiotics			
Clarithromycin			1/3
Lincomycin		1/2	1/3
Roxithromycin			1/2
Telithromycin			1/2
Monobactams			
Aztreonam	1/2	1/3	1/4
Carumonam	2/3	1/3	1/6
Moxalactam	1/2	1/3	1/10

Table A91-3   Dosing Recommendations in Patients with Renal Insufficiency (Relative to Normal Dose)—cont'd

Drug	CREATININE CLEARANCE (mL/min)		
	>50	20–50	<20
Penicillins			
Amdinocillin		1/2	1/4
Amoxicillin		1/2	1/6
Ampicillin	1/2	1/4	1/10
Azlocillin		1/2	1/4
Carbenicillin	1/3	1/5	1/10
Methicilin		1/2	1/4
Mezlocillin	1/2	1/4	1/8
Penicillin		1/5	1/8
Piperacillin		1/2	1/3
Ticarcillin	1/2	1/3	1/4
Timocillin		1/2	1/4
Polymyxins			
Colistin		Avoid	
Polymyxin B		Avoid	
Quinolones			
Ciprofloxacin			1/2
Fleroxacin	3/4	1/2	1/3
Gatifloxacin			1/4
Gemifloxacin			1/2
Levofloxacin		1/4	Avoid
Lomefloxacin			1/6
Norfloxacin			1/2
Ofloxacin			1/2
Rufloxacin			2/3
Sparfloxacin			1/2
Sulfonamides			
Sulfamethoxazole			1/2
Sulfisoxazole	3/4	1/2	1/4
Trimethoprim			1/2
Tetracyclines			
Tetracycline		Avoid	
Urinary Bacteriostatics			
Cinoxacin			1/10
Fosfomycin			1/4

Continued

Table A91-3 Dosing Recommendations in Patients with Renal Insufficiency (Relative to Normal Dose)—cont'd

Drug	CREATININE CLEARANCE (mL/min)		
	>50	20–50	<20
Nalidixic acid		Avoid	
Nitrofurantoin		Avoid	
Antifungals			
Fluconazole		1/2	1/3
Flucytosine	1/2	1/3	1/4
Miconazole			1/3
Terbinafine			1/2
Antimalarials			
Chloroquine	1/2	1/5	1/10
Quinine		1/2	1/3
Antineoplastic Agents			
Bleomycin			1/2
Capecitabine		Avoid	
Carboplatin		1/2	1/3
Etoposide		1/2	1/3
Exemestane			1/3
Methotrexate		Undefined	
Oxaliplatin			1/2
Pentostatin			1/2
Raltitrexed		1/2	Avoid
Topotecan			1/4
Antiparasitics			
Pentamidine		Avoid	
Antispasticity Agents			
Baclofen		Decrease	
Tizanidine			1/4
Antituberculous Agents			
Ethambutol		1/2	1/3
Isoniazid			1/2
Antiulcer Agents			
Colloidal bismuth subcitrate		Avoid	
Antiviral Agents			
Acyclovir		1/2	1/5

Table A91-3 Dosing Recommendations in Patients with Renal Insufficiency (Relative to Normal Dose)—cont'd

Drug	CREATININE CLEARANCE (mL/min)		
	>50	20–50	<20
Amantadine	1/2	1/5	1/10
Cidofovir	1/2	1/5	1/10
Didanosine			1/3
Emtricitabine	1/2	1/3	1/4
Entecavir	1/2	1/4	1/10
Foscarnet		Decrease	
Ganciclovir	1/2	1/5	1/10
Lamivudine		1/3	1/10
Oseltamivir		Avoid	
Penciclovir		1/2	1/4
Ribavirin			1/3
Rimantadine			1/2
Stavudine		1/5	1/10
Vidarabine		Decrease	
Zalcitabine		1/2	1/4
Zanamivir		1/5	1/10
Zidovudine			1/2
Bisphosphonates		Avoid	
Bronchodilators			
Albuterol			1/3
Dyphylline		Avoid	
Enprofylline		Avoid	
Prenalterol		Decrease	
Terbutaline		Decrease	
Tiotropium	1/2	1/5	1/10
Cardiovascular Agents			
Antianginal Agents			
Isradipine			1/4
Lercanidipine			1/2
Ranolazine			1/2
Antiarrhythmics			
Acecainide (N-acetyl-procainamide; NAPA)		1/2	1/4
Bretylium			1/5
Cibenzoline		1/2	1/3

Continued

Table A91-3 Dosing Recommendations in Patients with Renal Insufficiency (Relative to Normal Dose)—cont'd

Drug	CREATININE CLEARANCE (mL/min)		
	>50	20–50	<20
Disopyramide		1/2	1/5
Dofetilide		1/2	Avoid
Flecainide			1/3
Procainamide (see NAPA)			
Recainam		1/2	1/4
Sematilide	1/2	1/4	1/4
Sotalol		1/3	1/8
Tocainide		3/4	1/2
Antihypertensives			
Acebutolol		1/2	1/3
Atenolol		1/2	1/4
Betaxolol			1/2
Benazepril			1/4
Bisoprolol		1/2	1/3
Bosentan			1/2
Buflomedil			1/2
Candesartan			1/2
Captopril	1/2	1/6	1/12
Carteolol		1/2	1/4
Celiprolol		Decrease	
Cetamolol			1/3
Cilazapril	3/4	1/2	1/4
Clonidine		1/2	1/3
Delapril			1/3
Diazoxide		2/3	1/2
Enalapril		1/3	1/5
Eposartan			2/3
Fosinopril			1/2
Guanadrel	1/2	1/5	1/10
Imidapril			1/2
Lisinopril		1/2	1/4
Methyldopa			1/2
Metoprolol			1/2
Minoxidil			1/2
Moexipril			1/4
Moxonidine			1/3
Nadolol	3/4	1/2	1/4

Table A91-3 Dosing Recommendations in Patients with Renal Insufficiency (Relative to Normal Dose)—cont'd

Drug	CREATININE CLEARANCE (mL/min)		
	>50	20–50	<20
Nebivolol			1/2
Olmesartan			1/3
Pentopril		Avoid	
Perindopril			1/10
Pinacidil			1/2
Quinapril	1/2	1/4	1/8
Ramipril		2/3	1/3
Rilmenidine	2/3	1/3	1/5
Spirapril			1/3
Temocapril			1/2
Trandolapril			1/3
Valsartan			1/2
Blood Lipid-Lowering Agents			
Acifran		1/4	Avoid
Bezafibrate	2/3	1/3	1/6
Cerivastatin			2/3
Ciprofibrate			1/2
Clofibrate		Avoid	
Fenofibrate			1/6
Lovastatin			1/2
Cardiac Inotropes			
Digoxin	1/2	1/3	1/5
Flosequinan			1/3
Milrinone	1/3	1/4	1/10
Piroximone			1/2
Cognitive Impairment			
Memantine			1/2
Diuretics			
Acetazolamide (for glaucoma)	1/2	1/2	1/3
Eplerenone		Avoid	
Mannitol		Avoid	
Triamterene	1/2	1/3	1/4
Erectile Dysfunction			
Sildenafil			1/2
Tadalafil		1/2	1/4

Continued

Table A91-3 Dosing Recommendations in Patients with Renal Insufficiency (Relative to Normal Dose)—cont'd

Drug	CREATININE CLEARANCE (mL/min)		
	>50	20–50	<20
Hormonal Agents			
Goserelin			1/4
Lanreotide			1/2
Octreotide			1/2
Triptorelin			1/2
Hypoglycemic Agents			
Acetoheximide		Avoid	
Chlorpropamide		Avoid	
Metformin		Avoid	
Repaglinide			1/3
Tolrestat			1/2
Hypouricemic Agents			
Allopurinol	2/3	1/3	1/6
Colchicine			1/2
Psychotherapeutic Agents			
Acamprosate		Avoid	
Amisulpride			1/2
Milnacipran		1/2	1/4
Mirtazapine			2/3
Quetiapine			3/4
Reboxetine			2/3
Remoxipride			1/2
Risperidone			2/3
Sulpiride	2/3	1/2	1/4
Venlafaxine			1/2
Sympathomimetics			
Almotriptan			1/2
Dolasetron			1/2
Pramipexole			1/4
Selegiline		Avoid	
Miscellaneous			
Dextran 40		Avoid	
Sulbactam			1/5
Tazobactam			1/4

"Decrease" indicates a need to decrease the dose in patients with renal insufficiency, but data are not sufficient to offer quantitative guidelines.

Chapter 92

Dialysis and Hemoperfusion in the Treatment of Poisoning and Drug Overdose

Nikolas B. Harbord, Zachary Z. Brener, Donald A. Feinfeld, and James F. Winchester

In 2004, the American Association of Poison Control Centers (AAPCC) reported approximately 2.43 million human poison exposures.[1] Although incidence far exceeds mortality, fatal ingestions occurred in 1183 patients.

The nephrologist is often consulted in poisoning cases for assistance in drug removal. The 2004 AAPCC data show that 8654 patients were treated with urine alkalinization, 1726 received hemodialysis, and 62 received either hemoperfusion or another extracorporeal intervention.

This chapter outlines the approach to the poisoned subject. It covers initial management, enteric decontamination, enhanced drug elimination, and principles and application of dialysis and related procedures. Emphasis is given to clinical criteria for use of dialysis and extracorporeal techniques, decision making among available modalities, and recent advances.

INITIAL APPROACH

The algorithm in Figure 92-1 provides a reasonable approach to the treatment of all poisoned patients, in combination with appropriate triage and disposition. Initial assessment should include evaluation of the airway and breathing status, with administration of supplemental oxygen, intubation, and mechanical ventilation as necessary. Impaired circulatory status requires hemodynamic support with intravenous fluids or pressor agents. Core temperature should be frequently assessed, because autonomic dysfunction is possible. Hyperthermia or hypothermia should be corrected by passive external cooling or warming or peritoneal lavage. Hypoglycemia should also be assessed and corrected if present.

Although all patients require a complete neurological examination, comatose patients and those with seizures need immediate intervention. With coma or altered consciousness, dextrose (25 g) should be administered empirically in combination with thiamine (100 mg) given before the dextrose in alcoholics and malnourished patients.[2,3] Empiric administration of naloxone should be reserved for patients with signs of opiate intoxication, such as respiratory depression and pupillary miosis. Empirical flumazenil can precipitate seizure. It should be used only for reversal of conscious sedation and not for presumed benzodiazepine overdose.[2] Treatment of seizures after poisoning is similar to treatment of seizures from other causes. If intravenous access is difficult, intranasal midazolam or rectal administration of diazepam is an effective treatment for acute seizures, particularly in children.[4] Seizures and coma after acute overdose of isoniazid are typically unresponsive to conventional antiepileptics and should be treated with pyridoxine (vitamin B_6) in doses equivalent to ingested isoniazid.[5,6] Physostigmine should be used to treat anticholinergic poisonings even without seizures. It may be safer and more effective than benzodiazepines.[7]

Subsequent evaluation should include an investigation of the offending or suspected drug or chemical. This should include the route, estimated dose, quantity, and timing of ingestion. Multiple drugs should be considered, especially with intentional or suicidal ingestions. Further information might be obtained from physician and pharmacy records, family members, paramedics, and medication containers. An accurate and thorough medical history with regard to chronic illness or organ dysfunction, medications, and allergies should be attempted. A complete physical examination with attention to pupillary size, breath odors, skin changes, unusual vital signs, and respiratory pattern should be performed.

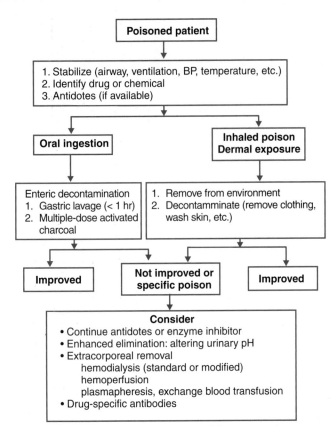

Figure 92-1 Simplified management of the poisoned patient.

Finally, laboratory studies should include toxicology panels with serial blood levels of identified ingestions. Metabolic panels with electrolytes and an arterial blood gas should be obtained to determine acid-base status and identify an increased anion gap or electrolyte disturbance. Calculation of the serum osmolal gap and examination of urine for crystals may further aid in the identification and treatment of ingestion. Additional laboratory tests should include calcium, magnesium, liver function tests, ketones, lactate level and, if applicable, a urine pregnancy test.

ENTERIC DECONTAMINATION: GASTRIC LAVAGE, EMETICS, WHOLE BOWEL IRRIGATION, AND ORAL SORBENTS/CATHARTICS

Use of lavage, induction of emesis, bowel irrigation, and oral sorbents should be preceded in unconscious patients by airway intubation with a cuffed tube to prevent aspiration of gastric contents. Enteric decontamination is contraindicated in petroleum distillate ingestions and caustic ingestions because of the risk of hydrocarbon aspiration pneumonitis and gastrointestinal rupture, respectively. Gastric lavage is recommended only up to 1 hour after ingestion. Lavage provides limited total drug removal and may increase the risk of aspiration or hasten the passage of drug into the small bowel.[8–10] Syrup of ipecac is not recommended for routine use for induced emesis of ingestions.[11] Gastric lavage and ipecac may, however, be useful for drugs that delay gastric emptying, such as tricyclic antidepressants and large quantities of aspirin or barbiturates.[12] Whole-bowel irrigation with large volumes of polyethylene glycol is an effective method for clearing the bowel of poisons, particularly if the in-

gestion is an enteric-coated drug (e.g., aspirin), a slow-release preparation (e.g., lithium, theophylline, verapamil), iron tablets, foreign bodies, or ingested packets of illicit drugs.[13–15] Multiple-dose activated charcoal is the most effective method of enteric decontamination. It is recommended for a wide variety of ingestions.[16] Oral charcoal (50 g q2–6h) reduces oral bioavailabilty by preventing drug absorption and also significantly shortens drug half-life through interruption of the enterohepatic circulation of some agents (e.g., barbiturates, digitalis preparations, and theophylline). The cation exchange resin kayexalate is an oral sorbent that may be effective in the prevention of gastrointestinal absorption of ingested lithium.[17] The addition of the cathartic sorbitol to oral sorbents prevents constipation and increases passage of the charcoal–poison complex.

ENHANCED ELIMINATION: ALTERING URINE PH

Elimination is the irreversible removal of a drug from the body. It refers principally to excretion and biotransformation. In patients with renal function, excretion involves drug concentration movement in (and out of) the urine through three processes: glomerular filtration, tubular secretion, and tubular reabsorption. With an understanding of drug properties, clinicians can increase renal excretion of drugs through modulation of urine pH.

Drugs that are weak acids or bases exist in solution as mixtures of ionized and nonionized species. The dissociation of a weak acid or base is determined by its *dissociation constant* (pKa). At a pKa equal to the pH, the concentrations of nonionized drug and ionized drug are equivalent. In the renal tubule, the nonionized molecules are generally lipid soluble, readily diffuse across cell membranes, and are reabsorbed. In contrast, the ionized form is reflected from cell membranes and excreted. Because the dissociation constant is a logarithmic function, small alterations of the pH of tubular fluid increase ionization greatly and have a disproportionately larger effect on drug clearance. In short, excretion of weak acid drugs with pKa in the range of 3.0 to 7.5 can be increased with urinary alkalinization. Conversely, excretion of weak bases with pKa 7.5 to 10.5 can be increased with urinary acidification. Drugs that will respond to urine pH manipulation are renally excreted, with pKa in the weakly acidic and basic range, confined to the extracellular fluid compartment, and minimally protein bound. For example, phenobarbital (pKa 7.2) and thiopental (pKa 7.6) have similar dissociation constants, but, due to differences in distribution, 25% to 50% of phenobarbital is excreted unmetabolized in the urine compared with less than 1% of thiopental. In this case, alkalinization of the urine will clearly not increase the excretion of the weak acid thiopental.

The administration of alkali to raise urine pH above 7.5 increases the urinary excretion of chlorpropamide, 2,4-dichlorophenoxyacetic acid, diflunisal, fluoride, mecoprop, methotrexate, phenobarbital, and salicylate.[18] Urinary alkalinization is recommended for salicylate poisoning when the plasma level exceeds 50 mg/dL, even when alkalemia is initially present. In salicylate poisoning, estimating the severity of poisoning with the assistance of serum levels and a nomogram will help in the decision to use alkalinization. However, clinical deterioration, pulmonary edema, development of renal failure or severe acid-base disorders, and salicylate levels greater than 100 mg/dL should prompt a change to hemodialysis to remove salicylate and correct acid-base status. Urinary alkalinization remains first-line therapy for treatment of salicylate intoxication when hemodialysis is not appropriate.[18] Acetazolamide is not recommended as the method of urinary alkalinization due to competitive inhibition of protein binding and risk of increase in salicylate levels.[19] Urinary alkalinization for drug removal in phenobarbital poisonings is not likely to be as effective as multiple-dose activated charcoal.[18,20] Intravenous bicarbonate solutions should be administered as a bolus followed by a constant infusion. Urine pH should be maintained within the range of 7.5 to 8.5. Urinary modulation is the objective of treatment.

"Forced" diuresis or alkaline diuresis with large quantities of intravenous fluids is recommended for chlorophenoxy herbicides, 2,4-dichlorophenoxyacetic acid, and mecoprop.[18] Furthermore, forced diuresis (achieving urine outputs of 300–500 mL/hr) may be complicated by the development of hyponatremia and water intoxication, pulmonary edema, and cerebral edema. Salicylate excretion has been found to be similar after urinary alkalinization without forced diuresis.[21] Although alkalinization is well tolerated, hypokalemia after potassium shifts is frequent. Severe alkalemia with tetany and hypocalemia may occur.[18] Urine pH, serum pH, and electrolytes should be measured frequently in the initial period of treatment.

Urinary acidification, to pH less than 5.5, has been attempted to increase the excretion of weakly basic drugs such as amphetamines, fenfluramine, phencyclidine (PCP), and quinine. However, acidification is not recommended in the management of poisoning with these agents because most patients recover with supportive care.[22] Furthermore, lowering urine pH increases PCP excretion only modestly and is only of benefit for deeply comatose patients.[22] Acidification has been performed using arginine- or lysine-hydrochloride, ammonium chloride, or ascorbic acid. There is a risk of acidemia and hyperkalemia. Serum potassium should be monitored closely and urine pH measured at least hourly. Bromide intoxication, often with high serum chloride levels and negative anion gap at presentation, may follow ingestion of dextromethorphan bromide, bromide salts in sleeping draughts, and colas.[23–25] Chloride loading with ammonium chloride increases the elimination of bromide, which can be increased further with the administration of mannitol, loop diuretics, or dialysis.[25]

INDICATIONS FOR EXTRACORPOREAL TECHNIQUES IN POISONING

Extracorporeal techniques deserve special consideration for removal of agents with delayed toxicity, such as mushrooms, paraquat, methanol, and ethylene glycol; when endogenous clearance is impaired (e.g., cardiac, renal, or hepatic failure); or when the agent can be removed at a rate exceeding endogenous elimination.

The decision to use dialysis modalities for drug removal is made on clinical criteria. Symptoms to consider include abnormalities in vital signs suggesting hemodynamic instability, deterioration despite adequate supportive treatment, mental status alteration (including confusion, lethargy, stupor, and coma), pneumonia due to coma, and midbrain dysfunction (i.e., hypothermia, hypotension, and bradycardia). Dialysis may not only remove the offending agent, but also improve electrolyte abnormalities and correct concomitant acid-base disorders.

Hypotensive patients requiring hemodynamic support with an indication for extracorporeal drug removal should receive an infusion of pressors distal to the dialyzer or sorbent cartridge. Careful monitoring of circulatory status is essential as dialysis may enhance the clearance of the pressor agents.

DIALYSIS TECHNIQUES FOR REMOVING POISONS

Many substances can be removed from the body by hemodialysis, peritoneal dialysis, hemofiltration, hemoperfusion, and combined modalities.[26] The underlying principles of dialysis for drug removal, and the potential problems associated with it, are reviewed first.

Principles of Dialysis

Hemodialysis is the most commonly used method of extracorporeal drug removal for the treatment of poisoning.[1] In conventional practice, the apparatus consists of a blood circuit (arteriovenous or venovenous), electronic and mechanical devices (blood pump, pressure monitors and alarms, and transmembrane pressure controller), a dialyzer cartridge containing the synthetic (or semisynthetic) membrane, and a countercurrent dialysate circuit of purified water and added electrolytes. In dialysis, solutes and poisons are removed from blood by diffusion across the porous membrane and into the dialysate.

Hemofiltration is a related procedure that does not employ dialysate but removes drugs and poisons by convective clearance. Blood within the filtration cartridge is subject to pressure across the porous membrane, creating an ultrafiltrate of plasma and solutes. Hemofiltration requires both anticoagulation of the blood circuit and continuous replacement of fluid and electrolytes lost into the ultrafiltrate. Ultrafiltration dialysis provides efficient clearance of large-molecular-weight intoxicants. It requires lower rates of blood and dialysate flow but a prolonged or continuous treatment protocol.

Hemodiafiltration combines ultrafiltration across a high-flux (large-pore) dialysis membrane with countercurrent flow of dialysate for combined diffusive and convective clearance.

Factors Governing Drug Removal with Dialysis

Drug characteristics that increase removal by dialysis are small molecular size (molecular weight < 500 Da), high water solubility, low protein binding, small volume of distribution (<1 L/kg), and rapid equilibration of plasma and tissue to maintain a concentration gradient.[27,28] Characteristics that limit dialysis clearance include high lipid-solubility, tight tissue binding, large volume of distribution, and slow plasma equilibration with other body compartments. For example, amitriptyline is tightly bound to albumin and muscle protein, resulting in a large apparent volume of distribution (8.3 L/kg of body weight). Consequently, it is poorly dialyzable. In contrast, lithium distributes in whole body water and is not protein bound. Consequently, it is eminently dialyzable. Although protein binding is an important factor, some drugs, such as salicylates, are reversibly protein bound and are highly dialyzable. Dialysis factors that determine drug removal include access type, blood and dialysate flow rates, and dialyzer properties (i.e., material, surface area, and pore size). Low blood flow may prevent hemodynamic instability but necessitates longer or continuous treatments for adequate clearance. Although higher flow rates increase diffusive clearance, this plateaus above a blood flow rate of 200 to 300 mL/min and a dialysate flow rate above 1.5 times that of blood. For drugs of high molecular weight, removal can be increased by increasing the dialyzer surface area, pore size, and length of the treatment.

As the molecular weight of a drug increases, its removal becomes less dependent on diffusion and more on *convection* (the creation of an ultrafiltrate).[26] Therefore, the efficient clearance of large-molecular-weight intoxicants is best accomplished with hemofiltration and hemodiafiltration. Depending on the pore size of the dialyzer, these modalities can remove drugs with molecular weight up to 50,000 Da. The degree of protein binding also limits drug clearance with ultrafiltration. The *sieving coefficient* (SC) is a measure of the ability of a molecule to pass convectively across a membrane. The drug clearance is the product of the sieving coefficient and the ultrafiltration rate. For molecules that pass completely (an SC of 1), the clearance is equal to the ultrafiltration rate. Increasing the ultrafiltration rate will thus increase clearance of any intoxicant with an SC greater than 0.

The complications of extracorporeal elimination include hypotension, blood loss, metabolic disequilibrium, catheter problems such as hematomas, and mechanical problems such as air embolism. Dialysis is most frequently employed to remove alcohols, lithium, and salicylate. Prolonged (or repeat) dialysis may be required to remove lithium, ethchlorvynol, glutethimide, and midazolam to avoid rebounds in drug concentration and relapse of intoxication. Box 92-1 lists drugs and chemicals that are removed by dialysis.

Sorbent Hemoperfusion and Complications of Hemoperfusion

Although first introduced in the 1940s[29] and adopted for clinical use in the 1970s and 1980s,[30–32] hemoperfusion is used infrequently to treat acute intoxications.[1] The apparatus consists of a blood circuit identical to that of hemodialysis, including blood pumps and pressure monitors, but with a cartridge containing a large surface area column of charcoal or resin. The column is primed with saline solution. Anticoagulated blood is pumped through the cartridge, where drugs with molecular weight between 100 and 40,000 Da are removed by adsorption. Table 92-1 lists several available hemoperfusion devices.

Available columns include activated charcoal and resin columns, and antibody- or antigen-coated columns for specific states (e.g., lupus erythematosus,[33] cytotoxic antibody removal before renal transplantation,[34] or endotoxin binding[35]). Activated charcoal has greater affinity for water-soluble molecules, whereas resins (e.g., XAD-4) have greater affinity for lipid-soluble molecules (e.g., glutethimide and methaqualone).[36] The sorbent column may become saturated during use, leading

to a progressive decline in extraction ratios. The use of short, intermittent treatments provides several advantages: less clinical "rebound" effect as the drug redistributes from tissues into plasma, reduction in hematologic side effects, and improved drug clearance.

Drug clearance with hemoperfusion exceeds that seen with dialysis for lipid-soluble drugs, cardiac glycosides, barbiturates, and other types of hypnotics, sedatives, and tranquilizers. For example, the extraction ratio of theophylline is 99%, as compared to 50% with hemodialysis. If there is near-equivalent clearance, dialysis is preferred because it is less expensive and can address any superimposed metabolic disorder (e.g., those that complicate salicylate poisoning).[37] Box 92-2 lists drugs that have been reported to be removed by various types of hemoperfusion.

The specific complications of hemoperfusion include thrombocytopenia, leukopenia, hypocalcemia, and hypoglycemia. Transient platelet depletion (average loss 30%) occurs with both coated and uncoated charcoal and resin sorbent columns. More severe thrombocytopenia, flushing, and dyspnea were reported with the original resin columns, but changes to preparatory methods and coatings have made resins more biocompatible.[38] A transient reduction in body temperature of several degrees can be expected. However, hypotension is less likely with hemoperfusion than with dialysis modalities.

Plasma Exchange and Exchange Blood Transfusion

Plasma exchange and exchange blood transfusion are used infrequently in the treatment of poisoning[39] but can remove highly protein-bound drugs. With a 3- to 4-L plasma exchange, the maximal quantity of drug removed is the plasma concentration multiplied by the volume of plasma removed. Attempts to use plasma exchange to treat chromic acid and chromate poisoning have not been fully successful,[40] whereas treatment of acute cyclosporine[41] and cisplatin[42] intoxications have been more successful. Exchange blood transfusion is employed with hemolysis when methemoglobinemia complicates the poisoning (e.g., sodium chlorate poisoning).

Hemoperfusion and Hemodialysis with Chelation

Intoxication with aluminum in dialysis patients can be treated with desferoxamine (DFO) chelation combined with hemodialysis or hemoperfusion to remove the DFO–aluminum complex. Dialysis with high-flux membranes and charcoal hemoperfusion are superior to cuprophane membranes in removing the DFO–aluminum complexes.[43] Recently, in an aluminum-intoxicated patient, we demonstrated higher clearances with a 1.8 m² high-flux dialyzer than with a 300-g charcoal sorbent column. Steady clearance was observed throughout a 4-hour treatment with the dialyzer; the sorbent saturated by 2 hours.[44] Clinical improvement of osteomalacia, encephalopathy, and anemia have also been reported in aluminum-intoxicated dialysis patients treated with DFO chelation combined with extracorporeal elimination.[45]

Desferoxamine chelation and hemoperfusion or hemodialysis also effectively clears iron from acutely intoxicated and overloaded patients.[46] Heavy metals and their salts are not removed efficiently by dialysis or hemoperfusion alone. During

Box 92-1 Drugs and Chemicals Removed with Dialysis

Antimicrobials/Anticancer
Cefaclor
Cefadroxil
Cefamandole
Cefazolin
Cefixime
Cefmenoxime
Cefmetazole
(Cefonicid)
(Cefoperazone)
Ceforamide
(Cefotaxime)
Cefotetan
Cefotiam
Cefoxitin
Cefpirome
Cefroxadine
Cefsulodin
Ceftazidime
(Ceftriaxone)
Cefuroxime
Cephacetrile
Cephalexin
Cephalothin
(Cephapirin)
Cephradine
Moxalactam
Amikacin
Dibekacin
Fosfomycin
Gentamicin
Kanamycin
Neomycin
Netilmicin
Sisomicin
Streptomycin
Tobramycin
Bacitracin
Colistin
Amoxicillin
Ampicillin
Azlocillin
Carbenicillin
Clavulinic acid
(Cloxacillin)
(Dicloxacillin)
(Floxacillin)
Mecillinam
(Mezlocillin)
(Methicillin)
(Nafcillin)
Penicillin
Piperacillin
Temocillin
Ticarcillin
(Clindamycin)
(Erythromycin)
(Azithromycin)
(Clarithromycin)

Metronidazole
Nitrofurantoin
Ornidazole
Sulfisoxazole
Sulfonamides
Tetracycline
(Doxycycline)
(Minocycline)
Tinidazole
Trimethoprim
Aztreonam
Cilastatin
Imipenem
(Chloramphenicol)
(Amphotericin)
Ciprofloxacin
(Enoxacin)
Fleroxacin
(Norfloxacin)
Ofloxacin
Isoniazid
(Vancomycin)
Capreomycin
PAS
Pyrizinamide
(Rifampin)
(Cycloserine)
Ethambutol
5-Fluorocytosine
Acyclovir
(Amantadine)
Didanosine
Foscarnet
Ganciclovir
(Ribavirin)
Vidarabine
Zidovudine
(Pentamidine)
(Praziquantel)
(Fluconazole)
(Itraconazole)
(Ketoconazole)
(Miconazole)
(Chloroquine)
(Quinine)
(Azathioprine)
Bredinin
Busulfan
Cyclophosphamide
5-Fluorouracil
(Methotrexate)

Barbiturates
Amobarbital
Aprobarbital
Barbital
Butabarbital
Cyclobarbital
Pentobarbital

Phenobarbital
Quinalbital
(Secobarbital)

**Nonbarbiturate Hypnotics,
Sedatives, Tranquilizers,
and Anticonvulsants**
Carbamazepine
Atenolol
Betaxolol
(Bretylium)
Clonidine
(Calcium channel blockers)
Captopril
(Diazoxide)
Carbromal
Chloral Hydrate
(Chlordiazepoxide)
(Diazepam)
(Diphenylhydantoin)
(Diphenylhydramine)
Ethiamate
Ethchlorvynol
Ethosuximide
Gallamine
Glutethimide
(Heroin)
Meprobamate
(Methaqualone)
Methsuximide
Methyprylon
Paraldehyde
Primidone
Valproic acid

Cardiovascular Agents
Acebutolol
(Amiodarone)
Amrinone
(Digoxin)
Enalapril
Fosinopril
Lisinopril
Quinapril
Ramipril
(Encainide)
(Flecainide)
(Lidocaine)
Metoprolol
Methyldopa
(Ouabain)
N-Acetylprocainamide
Nadolol
(Pindolol)
Practolol
Procainamide
Propranolol
(Quinidine)
(Timolol)
Sotatol

Tocainide

Alcohols
Ethanol
Ethylene glycol
Isopropanol
Methanol

**Analgesics and
Antirheumatics**
Acetaminophen
Aspirin
Colchicine
Methylsalicylate
Phenacetin
(D-Propoxyphene)
Salicylic acid

Antidepressants
(Amitriptyline)
Amphetamines
(Imipramine)
Isocarboxazid
MAO inhibitors
Moclobemide
(Pargyline)
(Phenelzine)
Tranylcypromine
(Tricyclic antidepressants)

Solvents and Gases
Acetone
Camphor
Carbon monoxide
(Carbon tetrachloride)
(Eucalyptus oil)
Thiols
Toluene
Trichloroethylene

**Plant and Animal Toxins,
Herbicides, and Insecticides**
Alkyl phosphate
Amanitin
Demeton sulfoxide
Dimethoate
Diquat
Glufosinate
Methylmercury complex
(Organophosphates)
Paraquat
Snake bite
Sodium chlorate
Potassium chlorate

Miscellaneous
Acipimox
Allopurinol
Aminophylline
Aniline
Borates
Boric acid

Continued

Box 92-1 Drugs and Chemicals Removed with Dialysis—cont'd

Miscellaneous—cont'd	4-Methylpyrazole	Barium	Potassium
(Chlorpropamide)	Sodium citrate	Bromide	(Potassium dichromate)*
Chromic acid	Theophylline	(Copper)*	Phosphate
(Cimetidine)	Thiocyanate	(Iron)*	Sodium
Dinitro-O-cresol	Ranitidine	(Lead)*	Strontium
Folic acid		Lithium	(Thallium)*
Mannitol	**Metals and Inorganics**	(Magnesium)	(Tin)
Methylprednisolone	(Aluminum)*	(Mercury)*	(Zinc)
	Arsenic		

( ), poor removal; ( )*, removed with chelating agent.
From Watson WA, Litovitz TL, Rodgers Jr GC, et al: 2004 Annual report of the American Association of Poison Control Centers Toxic Exposure Surveillance System. Am J Emerg Med 2005;23:589–666.

Table 92-1 Some Available Hemoperfusion Devices

Manufacturer	Device	Sorbent Type	Amount of Sorbent	Polymer Coating
Clark*	Biocompatible system	Carbon	50, 100, 250 mL	Heparinized polymer
Gambro*	Adsorba	Norit carbon	100 or 300 g	Cellulose acetate
Nextron Medical	Hemosorba Ch-350	Petroleum bead carbon	170 g	PolHema

*Smaller devices for use in children.

Box 92-2 Drugs and Chemicals Removed with Hemoperfusion

Antimicrobials/Anticancer	**Nonbarbiturate Hypnotics,**	Metoprolol	Demeton sulfoxide
Ampicillin	**Sedatives, Tranquilizers, and**	N-Acetylprocainamide	Dimethoate
Carmustine	**Anticonvulsants**	Procainamide	Diquat
Chloramphenicol	Carbamazepine	Quinidine	Endosulfan
Chloroquine	Carbromal		Glufosinate
Clindamycin	Chloral hydrate	**Analgesics and**	Methylparathion
Dapsone	Chlorpromazine	**Antirheumatics**	Nitrostigmine
Doxorubicin	(Diazepam)	Acetaminophen	(Organophosphates)
Gentamicin	Diphenhydramine	Aspirin	Phalloidin
Ifosfamide	Ethchlorvynol	Colchicine	Polychlorinated biphenyls
Isoniazid	Glutethimide	D-Propoxyphyene	Paraquat
(Methotrexate)	Meprobamate	Methylsalicylate	Parathion
Pentamidine	Methaqualone	Phenylbutazone	
Thiabendazole	Methsuximide	Salicylic acid	**Miscellaneous**
(5-Fluorouracil)	Methyprylon		Aminophylline
Vancomycin	Phenytoin	**Antidepressants**	Cimetidine
	Promazine	(Amitryptiline)	(Fluoroacetamide)
Barbiturates	Promethazine	(Imipramine)	(Phencyclidine)
Amobarbital	Valproic acid	(Tricyclic antidepressants)	Phenols
Butabarbital			(Podophyllin)
Hexabarbital	**Cardiovascular Agents**	**Solvents and Gases**	Theophylline
Pentobarbital	Atenolol	Carbon tetrachloride	
Phenobarbital	Cibenzoline succinate	Ethylene oxide	**Metals**
Quinalbital	Clonidine	Trichloroethane	(Aluminum)*
Secobarbital	Digoxin	Xylene	(Iron)*
Thiopental	(Diltiazem)		Thallium
Vinalbital	(Disopyramide)	**Plant and Animal Toxins,**	
	Flecainide	**Herbicides, and Insecticides**	
		Amanitin	
		Chlordane	

( ), poor removal; ( )*, removed with chelating agent.
From Muran PJ: Mercury elimination with oral DMPS, DMSA, vitamin C, and glutathione: An observational clinical review. Altern Ther Health Med 2006;12:70–75.

hemodialysis, metal removal may be enhanced with certain antioxidants (N-acetylcysteine, cysteine, zinc, or methionine) when used in conjunction with chelating agents.[47] In contrast, the modest removal of mercury and thallium by hemoperfusion can be enhanced with high-dose vitamin C and intravenous glutathione.[48,49]

IMMUNOPHARMACOLOGY

Immunopharmacologic treatment of poisonings is limited to digoxin toxicity,[50] scorpion sting,[51] and snakebite.[52] Fab (fragments of antibodies to drugs or venom) fragment preparations for treating acute colchicine and tricyclic antidepressant poisonings have been developed but are not available commercially.[53] When injected, Fabs combine specifically with their antigenic targets. Digoxin Fabs are effective in the treatment of toad venom poisoning[54] and after ingestion of yellow oleander, which is a frequent source of natural cardiac glycoside poisoning in South Asia.[55]

When given in potentially fatal cases of cardiac glycoside poisoning, digoxin Fabs can improve outcomes.[56] Digoxin Fabs should not be dosed differently in patients with renal impairment,[57] although renal failure delays clearance of both Fab and total digoxin.[58] Digoxin poisoning can relapse in patients with renal failure 24 to 48 hours after receiving Fab antibodies. This may relate to dissociation of Fab from the glycoside (C. Ronco, personal communication). The risk of rebound toxicity necessitates prolonged monitoring in patients with renal failure. Although immobilized antibody on hemoperfusion devices is logical,[59] successful treatment of digoxin toxicity with hemoperfusion and hemofiltration has not been well substantiated. Newer resin hemoperfusion devices (BetaSorb) have been shown to remove digoxin in vitro.[60]

References

1. Watson WA, Litovitz TL, Rodgers Jr. GC, et al: 2004 Annual report of the American Association of Poison Control Centers Toxic Exposure Surveillance System. Am J Emerg Med 2005;23:589–666.
2. Hoffman RS, Goldfrank LR: The poisoned patient with altered consciousness. Controversies in the use of a "coma cocktail." JAMA 1995;274:562–569.
3. Doyon S, Roberts JR: Reappraisal of the "coma cocktail." Dextrose, flumazenil, naloxone and thiamine. Emerg Med Clin North Am 1994;12:301–306.
4. Pang T, Hirsch LJ: Treatment of convulsive and nonconvulsive status epilepticus. Curr Treat Options Neurol 2005;7:247–259.
5. Morrow LE, Wear RE, Schuller D: Acute isoniazid toxicity and the need for adequate pyridoxine supplies. Pharmacotherapy. 2006 Oct;26:1529–32.
6. Topcu I, Yentur EA, Ekici NZ, et al: Seizures, metabolic acidosis and coma resulting from acute isoniazid intoxication. Anaesth Intensive Care 2005;33:518–520.
7. Burns MJ, Linden CH: A comparison of physostigmine and benzodiazepines for the treatment of anticholinergic poisoning. Ann Emerg Med 2000;35:374–381.
8. Vale JA, Kulig K: Position paper: Gastric lavage. J Toxicol Clin Toxicol 2004;42:933–943.
9. Comstock EG, Faulkner TP, Boisaubin EV, et al: Studies on the efficacy of gastric lavage as practiced in a large metropolitan hospital. Clin Toxicol 1981;18:581–597.
10. Saetta JP, March S, Gaunt ME, Quinton DN: Gastric emptying procedures in the self-poisoned patient: Are we forcing gastric content beyond the pylorus? J R Soc Med 1991;84:274–276.
11. Position paper: Ipecac syrup. J Toxicol Clin Toxicol 2004;42:133–143.
12. Kulig K: Initial management of ingestions of toxic substances. N Engl J Med 1992;326:1677–1681.
13. Position paper: Whole bowel irrigation. J Toxicol Clin Toxicol 2004;42:843–854.
14. Smith SW, Ling LJ: Whole-bowel irrigation as a treatment for acute lithium overdose. Ann Emerg Med 1991;20:536–539.
15. Rosenberg PJ, Livingstone DJ, McLellan BA: Effect of whole-bowel irrigation on the antidotal efficacy of oral activated charcoal. Ann Emerg Med 1988;17:681–683.
16. Chyka PA, Seger D: Position statement: Single-dose activated charcoal. American Academy of Clinical Toxicology; European Association of Poisons Centres and Clinical Toxicologists. J Toxicol Clin Toxicol 1997;35:721–741.
17. Belanger DR, Tierneg MG, Dickinson G: Effect of sodium polystyrene sulfonate on lithium bioavailability. Ann Emerg Med 1992;21:1312–1315.
18. Proudfoot AT, Krenzelok EP, Brent J, Vale JA: Position paper on urine alkalinization. J Toxicol Clin Toxicol 2004;42:1–26.
19. Sweeney KR, Chapron DJ, Brandt JL, et al: Toxic interaction between acetazolamide and salicylate: Case reports and a pharmacokinetic explanation. Clin Pharmacol Ther 1986;40:518–524.
20. Frenia ML, Schauben JL, Wears RL, et al: Multiple-dose activated charcoal compared to urinary alkalinization for the enhancement of phenobarbital elimination. J Toxicol Clin Toxicol 1996;34:169–175.
21. Prescott LF, Balali-Mood M, Crithley JA, et al: Diuresis or urinary alkalinization in salicylate poisoning? BMJ 1982;285:1383–1386.
22. Garrettson LK, Geller RJ: Acid and alkaline diuresis. When are they of value in the treatment of poisoning? Drug Saf 1990;5:220–232.
23. Hung YM: Bromide intoxication by the combination of bromide-containing over-the-counter drug and dextromethorphan hydrobromide. Hum Exp Toxicol 2003;22:459–461.
24. Steinhoff BJ, Paulus W: Chronic bromide intoxication caused by bromide-containing combination drugs. Dtsch Med Wochenschr 1992;117:1061–1064.
25. Horowitz BZ: Bromism from excessive cola consumption. J Toxicol Clin Toxicol 1997;35:315–320.
26. Depner T, Garred L: Solute transport mechanisms in dialysis. In Horl W, Koch KM, Lindsay RM, et al (eds): Replacement of Renal Function by Dialysis, 5th ed. Dordrecht, Kluwer Academic Publishers, 2004, pp 73–93.
27. Maher JF: Principles of dialysis and dialysis of drugs. Am J Med 1977;62:475–481.
28. Gibson TP, Atkinson AJ JR: Effect of changes in intercompartment rate constants on drug removal during hemoperfusion. J Pharm Sci 1978;67:1178–1179.
29. Muirhead EE, Reid AF: Resin artificial kidney. J Lab Clin Med 1948;33:841–844.
30. Hampel G, Crome P, Widdop B, Goulding R: Experience with fixed-bed charcoal haemoperfusion in the treatment of severe drug intoxication. Arch Toxicol 1980;45:133–141.
31. Gelfand MC, Winchester JF, Knepshield JH, et al: Charcoal hemoperfusion in severe drug overdosage. Trans Am Soc Artif Intern Organs 1977;23:599–605.
32. Verpooten GA, De Broe ME: Combined hemoperfusion–hemodialysis in severe poisoning: Kinetics of drug extraction. Resuscitation 1984;11:275–289.
33. Terman DS, Buffaloe G, Mattioli C, et al: Extracorporeal immunoadsorption: Initial experience in human systemic lupus erythematosis. Lancet 1979;2:824–827.

34. Jacobsen D, Hakim RM, Milford E, et al: Extracorporeal removal of anti-HLA antibodies in transplant candidates. Am J Kidney Dis 1990;16:423–431.

35. Ronco C, Brendolan A, Scabardi M, et al: Blood flow distribution in a polymyxin coated fibrous bed for endotoxin removal. Effect of a new blood path design. Int J Artif Organs 2001;24:167–172.

36. Rosenbaum JL, Kramer MS, Raja R: Resin hemoperfusion for acute drug intoxication. Arch Intern Med 1976;136:263–266.

37. Jacobsen D, Wiik-Larsen E, Bredersen J, et al: Haemodialysis or haemoperfusion in severe salicylate poisoning? Hum Toxicol 1988;7:161–163.

38. Ronco C, Brendolan A, Winchester JF, et al: First clinical experience with an adjunctive hemoperfusion device designed specifically to remove β_2-microglobulin in hemodialysis. Contrib Nephrol 2001;133:166–173.

39. Gurland HJ, Samtleben W, Lysaght MJ, Winchester JF: Extracorporeal blood purification techniques: plasmapheresis and hemoperfusion. In Jacobs C, Kjellstrand CM, Koch KM, Winchester JF (eds): Replacement of Renal Function by Dialysis, Fourth Edition, Dordrecht: Kluwer Academic Publishers, 1996, p 472.

40. Meert KL, Ellis J, Aronow R, Perrin E: Acute ammonium dichromate poisoning. Ann Emerg Med 1994;24:748–750.

41. Kwon SU, Lim SH, Rhee I, et al: Successful whole blood exchange by apheresis in a patient with acute cyclosporine intoxication without long-term sequelae. J Heart Lung Transplant 2006;25:483–485.

42. Choi JH, Oh JC, Kim KH, et al: Successful treatment of cisplatin overdose with plasma exchange. Yonsey Med J 2002;43:128–132.

43. National Kidney Foundation: K/DOQI clinical practice guidelines for bone metabolism and disease in chronic kidney disease. Am J Kidney Dis 2003;42(Suppl 3):S1–S201.

44. Bouchard NC, Malostovsker I, Harbord N, et al: Acute encephalopathy: Aluminum extraction with high-flux dialysis is superior to charcoal hemoperfusion. Clin Toxicol 2005;43:677–678.

45. Chang TM, Barre P: Effect of desferrioxamine on removal of aluminum and iron by coated charcoal haemoperfusion and haemodialysis. Lancet 1983;2:1051–1053.

46. Winchester JF: Management of iron overload. Semin Nephrol 1986;4(Suppl 1):22–26.

47. Patrick L: Toxic metals and antioxidants: Part II. The role of antioxidants in arsenic and cadmium toxicity. Altern Med Rev 2003;8:106–128.

48. Patrick L: Mercury toxicity and antioxidants: Part 1: Role of glutathione and alpha-lipoic acid in the treatment of mercury toxicity. Altern Med Rev 2002;7:456–471.

49. Muran PJ: Mercury elimination with oral DMPS, DMSA, vitamin C, and glutathione: An observational clinical review. Altern Ther Health Med 2006;12:70–75.

50. Bateman DN: Digoxin-specific antibody fragments: How much and when? Toxicol Rev 2004;23:135–143.

51. Muzard J, Billiald P, Goyffon M, et al: Recombinant antibodies: A new application in scorpion envenomation? Bull Soc Pathol Exot 2005;98:383–385.

52. Dart RC, Seifert SA, Boyer LV, et al: A randomized multicenter trial of crotalinae polyvalent immune Fab (ovine) antivenom for the treatment for crotaline snakebite in the United States. Arch Intern Med 2001;161:2030–2036.

53. Flanagan RJ, Jones AL: Fab antibody fragments: Some applications in clinical toxicology. Drug Saf 2004;27:1115–1133.

54. Gowda RM, Cohen RA: Toad venom poisoning: Resemblance to digoxin toxicity and therapeutic implications. Heart 2003;89:e14.

55. Roberts DM, Buckley NA: Antidotes for acute cardenolide (cardiac glycoside) poisoning. Cochrane Database Syst Rev 2006(4):CD005490.

56. Smith TW: Review of clinical experience with digoxin immune Fab (ovine). Am J Emerg Med 1991;9(2 Suppl 1):1–6.

57. Renard C, Grene-Lerouge N, Beau N, et al: Pharmacokinetics of digoxin-specific Fab: Effects of decreased renal function and age. Br J Clin Pharmacol 1997;44:135–138.

58. Ujhelyi MR, Robert S, Cummings DM, et al: Disposition of digoxin immune Fab in patients with kidney failure. Clin Pharmacol Ther 1993;54:388–394.

59. Savin H, Marcus L, Margel S, et al: Treatment of adverse digitalis effects by hemoperfusion through columns containing antidigoxin antibodies bound to agarose polyacrolein microsphere beads. Am Heart J 1987;113:1078–1084.

60. Reiter K, Bordoni V, Dall'Olio G, et al: In vitro removal of therapeutic drugs with a novel adsorbant system. Blood Purif 2002;20:380–388.

Further Reading

Feinfeld DA, Harbord N: Renal principles. In Goldfrank LR, Flomenbaum NE, Lewin NA, et al (eds): Goldfrank's Toxicologic Emergencies, 8th ed. New York, McGraw-Hill, in press.

Shannon MS, Borron SW, Burns MJ (eds): Haddad and Winchester's Clinical Management of Poisoning and Drug Overdose, 4th ed. Philadelphia, Elsevier, 2007.

Winchester JF, Harbord N: Extracorporeal removal of drugs and toxins. In Jörres A, Ronco C, Kellum J (eds): Management of Acute Kidney Problems. New York, Springer, in press.

Winchester JF, Harbord N, Feinfeld DA: Use of dialytic therapies for poisoning in clinical nephrotoxins. In De Broe ME, Porter GA, Bennett WM, Deray G (eds): Renal Injury from Drugs and Chemicals, 3rd ed. Heidelberg, Springer, in press.

PART XVI

Use of the Internet

CONTENTS

Chapter 93

Internet Resources for Nephrologists

Stephen Z. Fadem

Computers have a mystique that either attracts or repels prospective users. Regardless, they have become a necessity for the health profession. This chapter will deal with the practical aspects of applying the Internet to problems clinicians commonly encounter.

The history of computing and the Internet, though beyond the scope of this chapter, is fascinating.[1-3] What started as a tabulating machine to enable a burgeoning nation to compute the 1890 census grew into a mammoth device that provided a military advantage during World War II. After the invention of the transistor and solid-state circuitry, the computer shrank in size and cost, resulting in the digital transformation that erupted in the last part of the 20th century. Modern users carry computers in their pocket that have the computing power of the most sophisticated machines of 50 years ago.

BASICS

It is impossible to understand the Internet without a brief introduction to computer basics. One can easily become confused by the terminology and jargon used in this industry, and getting started may be difficult because of the learning curve required to master computer skills. Keeping in mind that the software of today is engineered to create ease of use and that skills gained are cumulative may alleviate the reader's trepidation.

The general principle of computing is the same regardless of use and can be divided in terms of hardware, software, or location. With respect to *hardware* (machinery), there must always be input devices (i.e., the keyboard and mouse), a processor with storage devices such as the server or workstation, and output devices, such as the monitor or printer. The *software* is divided into the operating system, a specific application, and data management. Regarding *location*, processing may be done by a stand-alone machine, connected within an office to a network, or extended off-site via the Internet. Details of how each of these components work are discussed elsewhere.[4,5]

The Internet is a worldwide network of computers communicating with each other through standard protocols. It became popular in 1990 when scientists at CERN, the European Organization for Nuclear Research, conceptualized and developed the World Wide Web. Several books are available to give the reader an in-depth view of how the Internet developed and information about the technical side of its management.[6]

INTEGRATING THE INTERNET WITH THE WORD PROCESSOR

Word processing replaced the typewriter; the only remnant left is the QWERTY keyboard developed in the 1860s.[7] Word processing programs also feature a toolbar menu, enabling users to change and adapt styles, layouts, and font size easily. They also allow the nephrologist to generate manuscripts in the format required by the publisher, saving time and costs.

Specifically, users can add pictures, charts, tables, or diagrams into text by using the Insert dropdown menu.

Microsoft Word integrates with EndNote and Reference Manager, applications that allow users to create a library of bibliographic data downloaded from the Internet sources such as the National Library of Medicine's (NLM) PubMed. The author simply drags a selected reference from the End-Note or Reference Manager library, which consists of references the user has entered into the program, onto the document. It is automatically formatted in the selected style required by the publisher.[8] Chickenfoot, a Mozilla Firefox Browser extension, enables users to automate web browsing functions on their personal computers. A script to automate EndNote use with PubMed can be found at http://szf.com.[9]

SPREADSHEETS: FROM LIST MANAGEMENT TO FORECASTING

Soon after the advent of personal computing in the late 1970s, software emerged that could modify data stored in the cells of computer-generated tables. This advance is known as the *spreadsheet.* Today, Microsoft Excel, the most heavily used spreadsheet application, enables users to add values to a cell, specify mathematical arguments for each value, and relate the results of the manipulation to any other cell or to an entire row or column of cells. Consequently, large bodies of data can be summed or averaged, and projections and regression analyses can be modified within milliseconds. With very little learning time, complex statistical manipulations of data can be performed by physicians as well as researchers. Changing one value in the spreadsheet will change all values that depend on it, giving users the power to design prediction and simulation templates. For instance, a practice that projects a 20% increase in patient services per year can simulate future requirements for employees, supplies, office space, and other expenses. Likewise, data transferred between large databases can be manipulated, reformatted, and shared with other applications.[10]

Useful accounting tools are also available; in Microsoft Excel, the *net present value* (NPV) formula enables users to predict whether it is more advantageous to place capital in an interest-bearing account than to invest it in a new enterprise; this can be used for clinical purposes. Take, for example, a nephrology practice that is trying to determine whether it will be economical to purchase a new electronic health record system. The system being investigated will allow the group to examine additional patients, eliminate dictation services and, when the practice becomes paperless, eliminate the chart room. They also will be able to reduce the time staff spends filing reports, laboratory reports, and imaging studies. The group carefully calculates how much they will reduce expenses and what revenue and additional services can be incorporated. But the application has fixed costs: purchasing the basic software application, the required computers and server, and the operating system licensing fee. In addition, there also is a hefty monthly service charge. With a spreadsheet containing all expenses and projected revenue, the practice can use the NPV formula, taking into account the current prime interest rate for investments, to ascertain if it would be more feasible just to place the money in the bank or to purchase the new electronic health record. A positive NPV means that the profits from capitalizing a system are greater than placing funds in an interest-bearing account, giving the practice solid data on which to base their decision.[9,11]

Patient List Management

By placing dates into spreadsheet columns and patient names in rows, a nephrologist can track which of his or her list of dialysis patients has been visited. A PDA (*personal digital assistant*) spreadsheet can be synchronized over the Internet to the main computer used by the billing and coding department to generate bills.

The spreadsheet can also keep track of laboratory information. The physician can refer to the spreadsheet during future visits to seek trends in patient care, as in this example: A patient with chronic kidney disease (CKD) is prescribed a 0.6 g/kg protein-restricted diet. Every 3 months the physician measures the 24-hour urine nitrogen, tracks the urine nitrogen, and uses it to calculate the patient's protein intake. The urine protein-to-creatinine ratio is also entered in the spreadsheet so the physician can determine if the patient is following the dietary restriction and if there are changes in proteinuria.

In clinics with large numbers of patients, this activity would be impractical, and other physicians would want to share this information. In addition, the visit needs to be tied to billing. In such clinics, the database, a large repository of structured information, should be useful for patient management.

CREATING PRESENTATIONS

Although most nephrologists use Microsoft PowerPoint for creating slide presentations, a few "tricks" can make any user appear professional. For example, a photograph of a saddle-nose deformity can be downloaded from the web to a desktop computer. This image is taken from the screen by pressing the "alt" and "PrtSc" buttons simultaneously, allowing the photograph to be immediately pasted into Microsoft PowerPoint. The "crop" tool on the "picture" toolbar can then be used to tailor-fit the photograph perfectly into a slide.[12,13] In addition, highly complex tables created in Microsoft Excel can be converted to charts or graphs and imported into PowerPoint. Mastering a few simple keystrokes can allow one to create complex diagrams and figures because the PowerPoint program uses a technology that enables the embedding of practically any kind of binary data. Consequently, movies, charts, and photographs can be portrayed with equal ease.[11]

THE OFFICE SYSTEM

The use of the computer as a practice management tool and electronic health record is gaining in popularity, but still only one in four physicians uses computers in this manner.[14] Although computer systems are expensive and require sophisticated programming and upkeep, they can be an invaluable tool to increase the quality of health care delivered.[15] Without computers, 30 minutes of care requires on average 1 hour of paperwork.[16] Multiple benefits of using a computer include a reduction in redundant data entry; once entered, data is permanently available for future use.[17] Next, a well-designed system can provide checkpoints for patient safety. An example is the medication list: Should two agents have the potential to interact, the physician can be warned to make necessary changes. If a computer is at the point of service, whether a hospital room or a dialysis station, the physician will have instant access to data, and patient entries can be made on site. This reduces reliance on faulty physician memory. Once entered, other physicians and health personnel will have access to the information.

The computer is an Internet-based, patient-centered tool. Some health care providers, such as the Palo Alto Medical Foundation, allow patients to review their medications and laboratory values online.[18] Patient organizations such as the American Association of Kidney Patients (AAKP) have developed patient health records that enable a patient to enter medical information, check definitions, and share data with their physician. Based on these advances, it is obvious that physician use of computers will decrease inequities in medical care and reduce administrative costs (presently 31 cents of each dollar[19]) while helping to make medical care accessible to the growing number of uninsured patients.

A well-designed health information system takes into account the need to protect patient confidentiality. Data must be sent from computer to computer over a secure network (a so-called *virtual private network*), which must be established on the physician's workstation or laptop computer. By using strong encryption algorithms when storing data on the server and allowing Internet access only directly to that server's address, the private network is not needed, so information can be securely viewed from any website. Physician passwords must be designed so that hackers cannot easily guess them; security is compounded by each letter or number added to the password, and when numbers and shifted numbers (characters and capitals) are added. Other security items, such as no repudiation, and digital signatures must be in place to prevent the record from being nefariously altered. Data security is beyond the scope of this chapter, but the Health Insurance Portability and Accountability Act (HIPAA) spells out specific requirements for using a computer online to share information. Information about a patient's health records must also follow these rules.

Selection of an office system should never be a decision made in haste. It requires time and energy and is often accompanied by periods of frustration; a purchase should be preceded by understanding the workflow of the office and by determining how a computer can speed each step, as in the following example: A group practice with offices at several locations is trying to decide whether to own or lease a computer system. If owned, it will reside on a local server, offering heightened security, but if leased, it will reside on the vendor's server and will be Internet-based. This offers the advantage of data access from remote sites. The group approaches the choice systematically, comparing costs, benefits, risks, and tradeoffs to make an ideal choice. Several outstanding resources, including the Hartley book,[20] can help clinicians select office systems.[21–24]

PRACTICE ANALYSIS

Well-designed software enables the physician to gather and manipulate data. The physician can analyze growth patterns, define demographic and geographic centers where patients live, and give attention to areas for new recruits to practice. For example, a practice group can sort its end-stage renal disease patients by ZIP code and rank them according to the first date of dialysis. Using a commercially available software package, Microsoft MapPoint, they can visualize their patients' homes by ZIP code. In one practice, it was noted that over the past 3 years there had been a steady growth of patients from the northwest side of the city, yet there were no dialysis centers in that area and patients were driving long distances for dialysis care. It became obvious that placing a dialysis facility near the heaviest density of patients would yield a financial "break-even" point in 2 years and would enhance the ability of the practice to deliver care. When presented with these data, the group decided to build a facility to accommodate patients based on the patterns recognized during their analysis.

THE COMPUTER AND CLINICAL RESEARCH

With expansive technology, particularly as we utilize knowledge of the human genome to create better therapies, there will be a greater demand for clinical trials. The office computer is an ideal analytic tool to help detect, recruit, and screen study subjects,[25] as in this example: The opportunity to screen patients with stage 4 CKD and diabetic nephropathy arose; one nephrology practice group promised to enroll 30 patients over a 12-month period to study a more aggressive lipid-lowering regimen. The inclusion criteria were patients over age 18 years with an estimated glomerular filtration rate (GFR) value of less than 30 mL/min, serum cholesterol levels lower than 200 mg/dL, and a negative history of myocardial infarction. The practice queried its database using these variables and notified patients of the possibility of participating in screening for enrollment or exclusion. Meanwhile, the physician group generated a list of referring physicians likely to send patients meeting these criteria, and in cooperation with the study sponsor, arranged educational seminars to help recruit additional patients. This computer-driven exercise allowed them to fulfill the recruitment goal.

INTERNET TOOLS FOR NEPHROLOGISTS

In the United States, 70.8% of the population uses the Internet.[26] The advent of mobile telephones and PDAs allow Internet access without carrying a large device. Technology adds dimension to effectiveness, knowledge, and confidence[27] to the physician's decision-making powers through instant access and sharing of patient data, guidelines, clinical trials results, and publications.

The Nephron Information Center

Nephron.org has embedded formulas for calculating the Modification of Diet in Renal Disease study (MDRD) GFR (eGFR) and has text boxes to link to PubMed, Google, and Wikipedia in its header. It receives 17,000 unique visits each day because users are searching for news or literature pertinent to patients with kidney disease. Newsdesk, a technology built for Nephron.org, aggregates and syndicates resources about kidney disease that are published on the Internet each day. The information is organized and displayed on the front page of the site as "news."

The site also has calculators for body mass index, mean arterial pressure, and conversions for laboratory values as well as direct access to the National Kidney Foundation's K/DOQI guidelines (also available at http://kidney.org).

Finding Drug Reactions from a PDA

The site epocrates.com enables physicians to look up medication dosing, indication, drug interactions, and adverse events using a PDA. The package also includes several handy calculators. This information is available at http://www.epocrates.com.

Calculating Protein Intake

An online protein intake calculator (http://nephron.org/protein_intake) allows a nephrologist to advise a patient. It can be used as in this example: A mechanical engineer was prescribed a 0.6 g/kg protein-restricted diet in an effort to help preserve kidney function. The patient collected a 24-hour urine, and the urea nitrogen content in the collection was 4.5 g/day; his weight was 70 kg. The calculator converted these data into a protein intake of 41.69 g/day, which is on target with the prescribed diet.[28,29]

Tracking Dialysis Units during a Catastrophe

The site dialysisunits.com enables users to search for dialysis facilities and details. Based on the Centers for Medicare & Medicaid Services (CMS) national provider list, it is updated monthly. Search can be made by name, city, ESRD Network, state, ZIP code, or dialysis modality. After Hurricane Katrina, the program informed dialysis patients which dialysis units were operating when they returned to Louisiana. CMS and the ESRD Networks control portions of the site to track facility closures during emergencies.

How to Calculate the MDRD GFR

The four-variable MDRD study equation is a popular method of predicting the GFR from serum creatinine, age, race, and gender. It is based on stepwise multiple linear regression analyses of the demographic and laboratory data from the Modification of Diet in Renal Disease clinical trial.[30–33] To correct for the variation in the calibration of laboratory instruments that leads to a variation in performance of the equation at higher levels of GFR, serum creatinine levels measured using the original laboratory equipment were recalibrated to a Roche/Hitache enzymatic assay traceable to serum samples analyzed at the National Institute of Standards and Technology (NIST) using isotope-dilution mass spectrometry. The original GFR equation is used when laboratory creatinine values have not been standardized. The formula, which gives users the option to choose which creatinine methodology was used, is available online at http://mdrd.com and is used by both the National Kidney Foundation (http://www.kidney.org) and the Nephron Information Center (http://nephron.org). A third site, that of the National Kidney Disease Education Program (http://nkdep.nih.

gov), also gives users this option. The formula can be used as in this example: A 55-year-old Hispanic female with a creatinine of 2 mg/dL 4 months ago now has a creatinine of 2.1, both traceable to diabetic nephropathy. Her GFR has declined from 26 to 24 mL/min/1.73 m^2, indicating that she has stage 4 CKD.

Wikikidney

Wikikidney.org is a collaborative nephrology encyclopedia patterned after Wikipedia. Information is not copyrighted and is reviewed or edited by other volunteer professionals. The *wiki concept*[34] is that placing information in open view facilitates peer review, editing, and upgrading until contributors are satisfied with the content. Wiki etiquette dictates that all articles uploaded must have references. The wikis allow for broad dissemination but lack the structured peer review of conventional publications. This source can serve as a first-line resources for medical information.

Search Articles on PubMed, HighWire, and HubMed

The NLM's PubMed enables searching for publications by keyword, author, date, or medical subject heading. It is also available for PDAs or phones at http://pubmedhh.nlm.nih.gov. One can enter keywords into a text field on a cell phone, for instance, and scroll through the same database of references and abstracts used with conventional computers. PubMed is invaluable during rounds, conferences, and in the midst of patient care. Many other features are listed on the ncbi.nlm.nih.gov website.

HighWire Press, a large repository of peer-reviewed content, hosts more than 4.2 million full-text articles, of which nearly 1.7 million are free. Surprisingly, it receives the overwhelming majority of its referrals from Google, not from PubMed.[35] HubMed.org also uses the NLM database, but it allows direct transfer to reference managers such as EndNote. In addition, it takes advantage of a standardized Web format that syndicates published articles that can be viewed on an individual's website. This new format, RSS (Really Simple Syndication[36]), is becoming highly popular in the news publishing industry and is widely used by CNN and the *New York Times*. In the past special software was required to read files sent in this format, but lately this functionality is available on freely accessible web browsers such as Mozilla Firefox (http://firefox.com).

An example will serve to illustrate how these searches work: A new faculty member was interested in learning more about CKD. By searching for "chronic kidney disease" on hubmed.org and then clicking the "feeds" button, all NLM articles on CKD were fed to her Firefox browser. Each time a new article appears on PubMed or HubMed, the feed distributes the reference to her computer, and it is available for viewing.

SHIFTS: Tracking Dialysis Patients between Center, Hospital, and Office

Tracking a visit to a patient in a dialysis unit is possible using a spreadsheet format, but there are disadvantages; it is not secure and may be difficult to send across the Internet. Using online programs enables users to log in and track their visits. A well-designed computer program should automatically stamp the date, place, and physician's initials and generate a report for billing. The program should be encrypted so that the data are secure. To see an example of the SHIFTS program, go to http://interoperablesoftware.com.

NEPHROL: The Nephrology Discussion Group

NEPHROL, sponsored by the National Kidney Foundation, is an e-mail listserv, or discussion group, that comprises 2000 nephrologists from around the world. Subjects vary, and discussions can be lively. Many of the participants are experts in their field, and erudite discussions enable physicians in practice to get answers to difficult clinical problems from colleagues. This group can be found at http://kidney.org/professionals/cyber.cfm.

How to Look Up a Lecture from HDCN

The site hdcn.com (Hypertension, Dialysis and Clinical Nephrology) publishes key lectures from national meetings, offering streaming video as well as a PDF handout. Lectures can be downloaded and "burned" on a CD-ROM. The site requires a subscription.

USRDS

The USRDS (U.S. Renal Data System) is a database of information on every dialysis patient in the Medicare program. As patients become eligible for enrollment, their facilities must complete a Federal 2728 form. Using this and claims data, the registry makes available statistics about the incidence, prevalence, morbidity, and economics of end-stage renal disease (http://usrds.org).

Google

This popular search engine also accesses 3 billion medical articles. In a recent study of 26 *New England Journal of Medicine* weekly clinical pathologic conferences, three to five keyword Google searches had a 58% success rate of making the correct diagnosis.[37] Google Scholar is a refined version of Google that, by allowing a more selective search of scientific articles, filters out extraneous information. An additional feature of Google is the ability to automatically find images for keywords. This comprehensive tool is indispensable when trying to find charts and diagrams.

For example, a renal fellow was asked to give a talk on WNT signaling. She was working on a set of MS PowerPoint slides and needed another image. By going to http://google.com, typing "wnt signaling" into the textbox, and clicking the "images" menu item above the logo, she retrieved 3800 images in 0.02 seconds. She double-clicked on one of them, saved it to the desktop, and imported it into her PowerPoint presentation using the Insert:picture menu.

PHYSICIAN QUALITY REPORTING INITIATIVE (PRQI)

As part of the Tax Relief and Health Care Act of 2006, CMS has created the Physician Quality Reporting Initiative as the initial step toward a shift in payment strategy to value or performance-based payments. This phase enabled providers to earn bonus payments of up to 1.5% of total allowed Medicare charges by voluntarily reporting codes that reflect quality of care with their claims. These "zero dollar quality-data codes" are specific for measures pertinent to one's practice.

This scheme forced physicians to review how they capture data related to clinical events, generate appropriate codes and include them with billing information. It is the first step toward tying claims processing to an outcomes-based reimbursement model.

Figure 93-1 is an algorithm for high blood pressure control in patients with diabetes. This algorithm can be converted into a simple software applet that, when integrated into one's electronic health system, simplifies the capture and analysis of relevant information and, after being reviewed by the provider, passes it along to the billing department.

A PRACTICAL TIP ON INTERNET SECURITY

Standard e-mail uses nonencrypted protocols. For example, secure e-mail used within a university only assures privacy when the sender and user are in the same institution. Consequently, an email that is sent unencrypted is not secure for patient communication.[38,39] Patients should be advised of this fact, and physicians should use caution when sending sensitive laboratory data to their patients.

The Health Insurance Portability and Accountability Act of 1996 specifies that patient health information sent over the Internet must be secure and encrypted. The CMS has authority over HIPAA and has created guidance documents on their website, http://cms.hhs.gov/SecurityStandard. They have pointed out risks and vulnerabilities associated with the use of laptops, backup devices, flash drives, and e-mails. These include the potential for stolen passwords, malicious stealing of sensitive data off a server, inappropriate access by an employee, workstations being left unattended, and corruption of a system due to a virus. Rules are complex, but in principle, specify that practices must have sound security policies and ongoing risk management initiatives and that electronic personal health information should always be protected from access by nonauthorized users through the use of strong encryption. CMS points out the risk of not using a strong encryption system when sending or receiving e-mails containing sensitive patient information.

CONCLUSIONS

A complete discussion of the resources and applications available to nephrologists would require much more space, but this chapter should serve as an introduction and review of some of the more practical web and computer applications, and as a starting point for those in the field to discover other available sites. Tables 93-1 to 93-3 list several sites useful to nephrologists.

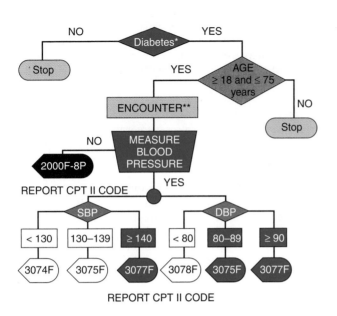

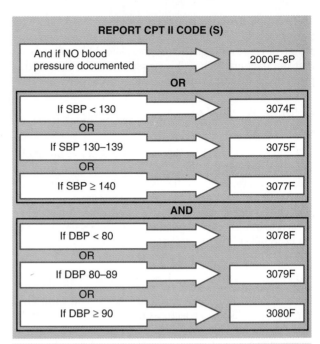

REPORT CPT II CODE (S)

PERFORMANCE IS MET IF 3074F, 3075F, 3078F
PERFORMANCE IS NOT MET IF 3079F, 3080F, 3077F, 2000F–8P

Both a systolic and diastolic code are required
SBP—systolic blood pressure in mm Hg
DBP—diastolic blood pressure in mm Hg

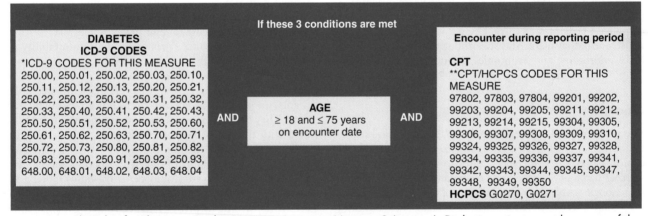

Figure 93-1 Algorithm for Physician Quality Reporting Initiative, Measure 3 (see text). Diabetic patients must have one of the listed ICD-9 codes, meet age criteria, and have a recent encounter during the reporting period that meets the listed CPT or HCPCS codes. If no documented blood pressure, use CPT II code 2000F-8P. Both a systolic and diastolic code are required. Performance is met if CPT II codes are 3074F or 3075F and 3078F. Performance is not met if code is 3079F or 3080F or 3077F. CPT, Current Procedural Terminology; DBP, diastolic blood pressure in mm Hg; HCPCS, Healthcare Common Procedure Coding System; ICD-9, International Statistical Classification of Diseases; SBP, systolic blood pressure in mm Hg.

Table 93-1   Information Sites

Site Name	Site Address
AAKP My Health	http://aakp.org/my-health/
Dialysis & Transplantation	http://eneph.com
Dialysis Units in the USA	http://dialysisunits.com
Epocrates	http://epocrates.com
Fistula First	http://fistulafirst.org
Hypertension Dialysis & Clinical Nephrology (HDCN)	http://hdcn.com/
Kidney Community Emergency Response Coalition	http://kcercoalition.com
Kidney Disaster Page	http://kidneydisasters.com
Kidney Times	http://ikidney.com
NEPHROL	http://www.kidney.org/professionals/cyber.cfm
Nephron Information Center	http://nephron.org
Nephronline	http://www.nephronline.org/
National Kidney Foundation KDOQI	http://kdoqi.org
HighWire Press	http://highwire.stanford.edu
PubMed	http://ncbi.nlm.nih.gov/pubmed
HubMed	http://hubmed.org
Recent Journals	http://journals.nephron.org
Renal Business Today	http://renalbusiness.com
UK Renal Association	http://www.renal.org/
UpToDate	http://uptodate.com
USRDS	http://usrds.org/
wikikidney	http://wikikidney.org

From Wikikidney, http://wikikidney.org. Accessed May 1, 2008. AAKP, American Association of Kidney Patients; KDOQI, Kidney Disease Oucomes Quality Initiative; USRDS, U.S. Renal Data System.

Table 93-2   Renal Organizations

Organization	Website
American Association of Kidney Patients (AAKP)	http://aakp.org
American Kidney Fund (AKF)	http://kidneyfund.org
American Nephrology Nurses Association (ANNA)	http://annanurse.org
American Society for Bone & Mineral Research (ASBMR)	http://asbmr.org
American Society of Nephrology (ASN)	http://asn-online.org
American Society of Transplant Surgeons (ASTS)	http://asts.org
American Society of Transplantation (AST)	http://a-s-t.org/
European Renal Association (ERA-EDTA)	http://era-edta.org
International Federation of Kidney Foundations (IFKF)	http://ifkf.net
International Society for Hemodialysis (ISHD)	http://ishd.net
International Society of Nephrology (ISN)	http://nature.com/isn
International Society for Peritoneal Dialysis (ISPD)	http://ispd.org
Kidney Care Partners (KCP)	http://kidneycarepartners.org/
National Kidney Foundation (NKF)	http://www.kidney.org
National Renal Administrators Association (NRAA)	http://nraa.org
Renal Physicians Association (RPA)	http://renalmd.org
UK Renal Registry (UKRR)	http://renalreg.com/
United Network for Organ Sharing (UNOS)	http://unos.org/
USRDS	http://usrds.org
Vascular Access Society (VAS)	http://www.vascularaccesssociety.com/

From: Wikikidney, http://wikikidney.org. Accessed May 1, 2008.

Table 93-3 Government Organizations

Organization	Web site
Agency for Healthcare Research and Quality (AHRQ)	http://ahrq.gov
Center for Medicare & Medicaid Services (CMS)	http://cms.hhs.gov
Centers for Disease Control and Prevention (CDC)	http://cdc.gov
Clinical Trials	http://clinicaltrials.gov
FirstGov	http://firstgov.gov
Forum of ESRD Networks	http://esrdnetworks.org/
U.S. Department of Health and Human Services (HHS)	http://hhs.gov
Institute of Medicine (IOM)	http://iom.edu
Library of Congress (THOMAS)	http://thomas.loc.gov/
National Kidney Disease Education Program (NKDEP)	http://nkdep.nih.gov
National Heart, Lung, and Blood Institute (NHLBI)	http://nhlbi.nih.gov
National Institute of Diabetes and Digestive and Kidney Diseases (NIDDK)	http://niddk.nih.gov
National Institutes of Health (NIH)	http://nih.gov
National Kidney and Urologic Diseases Information Clearinghouse (NKUDIC)	http://kidney.niddk.nih.gov

From: Wikikidney. http://wikikidney.org. Accessed May 1, 2008.

References

1. Cringley RX: Accidental Empires. New York: HarperCollins, 1996.
2. Chandler AD Jr: Inventing the Electronic Century. Cambridge, Mass.: Harvard University Press, 2005.
3. Manes S, Andrews P: Gates. New York: Doubleday, 1993.
4. Cannon DL, Luecke G: Understanding Microprocessors. Dallas: Texas Instruments Learning Center, 1979.
5. Gralla P: How the Internet Works. Indianapolis: Que, 2002.
6. Winston B: Media Technology & Society. London: Routledge, 2004.
7. The Typewriter. Toronto: Dover Publications, 2000.
8. Edhlung BM: Pubmed and Endnote: A User's Guide that Helps You Organize Bibliographic Information. Stallarholmen, Sweden: Form & Kunskap, 2005, AB.
9. Bott E, Leonard W: Microsoft Office XP, T.F. Hayes (ed). Indianapolis: Que, 2001.
10. Hefferin L: Learning Microsoft Office XP Advanced Skills: An Integrated Approach. New York: DDC Publishing, 2002.
11. Cornell P: Accessing and Analyzing Data with Microsoft Excel. Redmond, Wash.: Microsoft Press, 2003.
12. Maran R: Maran Illustrated Windows XP 101 Hot Tips. Boston: Thomsen Course Technology PTR, 2005.
13. Kinkoph SW: Teach Yourself Visually Microsoft Office 2003. Hoboken, N.J.: Wiley, 2006.
14. Jha AK, Ferris TG, Donelan K, et al: How common are electronic health records in the United States? A summary of the evidence. Health Affairs 2006;256: w496–w507.
15. Adler KG, Edsall RL: Electronic health records: A user-satisfaction survey. Fam Pract Manag 2005;12:47–51.
16. Gingrich N, Pavey D, Woodbury A: Saving Lives and Saving Money. Washington, D.C.: Alexis de Tocqueville Institution, 2003.
17. Laflamme MR, Dexter PR, Graham MF, et al: Efficiency, comprehensiveness and cost-effectiveness when comparing dictation and electronic templates for operative reports. Proc AMIA Symp 2005:425–429.
18. Palo Alto Medical Foundation. Available at: http://mychart.sutterhealth.org/pamf/default.asp. Accessed May 1, 2008.
19. Woolhandler S, Campbell T, Himmelstein DU: Costs of health care administration in the United States and Canada. N Engl J Med 2003;349:768–775.
20. Hartley CP, Jones EP: EHR Implementation: A Step-by-Step Guide for the Medical Practice. Chicago: AMA, 1996.
21. Kim E, Mayani A, Modi S, et al: Evaluation of patient-centered electronic health record to overcome digital divide. Conf Proc IEEE Eng Med Biol Soc 2005;2:1091–1094.
22. Orlova AO, Dunnagan M, Finitzo T, et al: Electronic health record–public health (EHR–PH) system prototype for interoperability in 21st century healthcare systems. Proc AMIA Symp 2005;575–579.
23. Walker JM, Buckley S, Richards F, Bieber EJ: Implementing an Electronic Health Record System. London: Springer-Verlag, 2006.
24. Bruun-Rasmussen M, Bernstein K, Vingtoft S, et al: Quality labelling and certification of electronic health record systems. Stud Health Technol Inform 2005;116:47–52.
25. Zoccali C: Clinical databases in nephrology: Research and clinical practice goals and challenges. J Nephrol 2006;19:551–555.
26. Internet World Stats. Accessed 31 March 2007. Available from http://internetworldstats.com/stats2.htm.
27. Fogg BJ: Persuasive Technology. San Francisco: Morgan Kaufmann, 2003.
28. Maroni BJ, Steinman TI, Mitch WE: A method for estimating nitrogen intake of patients with chronic renal failure. Kidney Int 1985;27:58–65.
29. Masud T, Manatunga A, Cotsonis G, Mitch WE: The precision of estimating protein intake of patients with chronic renal failure. Kidney Int 2002;62:1750–1756.
30. Hebert LA, Kusek JW, Greene T, et al, for the Modification of Diet in Renal Disease Study Group: Effects of blood pressure control on progressive renal disease in blacks and whites. Hypertension 1997;30(3 Pt 1):428–435.
31. Levey AS, Bosch LP, Lewis JB, et al, for the Modification of Diet in Renal Disease Study Group: A more accurate method to estimate glomerular filtration rate from serum creatinine: A new prediction equation. Ann Intern Med 1999;130:461–470.
32. Levey AS, Coresh J, Greene T, et al, for the Chronic Kidney Disease Epidemiology Collaboration: Using standardized serum creatinine values in the Modification of Diet in Renal Disease study equation for estimating glomerular filtration rate. Ann Intern Med 2006;145:247–254.
33. Levey AS, Coresh J, Greene T, et al, for the Chronic Kidney Disease Epidemiology Collaboration: Expressing the Modification of Diet in Renal Disease Study equation for estimating glomerular filtration rate with standardized serum creatinine values. Clin Chem 2007;53:766–772.
34. Leuf B, Cunningham W: The Wiki Way: Quick Collaboration on the Web. Boston: Addison-Wesley Professional, 2001.
35. Steinbrook R: Searching for the right search—reaching the medical literature. N Engl J Med 2006;354:4–7.
36. Hammersley B: Content Syndication with RSS. Sebastopol, Calif.: O'Reilly Media, 2003.
37. Tang H, Ng JHK: Googling for a diagnosis—use of Google as a diagnostic aid: Internet based study. BMJ 2006;333:1143–1145.

38. Ali Pabrai UO: Getting Started with HIPAA. Boston: Premier Press, 2003.
39. Garfinkel SL, Margrave D, Schiller JI, et al: How to make secure email easier to use. Conference on Human Factors in Computing Systems 2005;701–710.

Further Reading

Ali Pabrai UO: Getting Started with HIPAA. Boston: Premier Press, 2003.

Chandler AD: Inventing the Electronic Century. Cambridge, MA: Harvard University Press, 2005.

Gralla P: How the Internet Works. Indianapolis: Que, 2002.

Hammersley B: Content Syndication with RSS. Sebastopol, CA: O'Reilly Media, 2003.

Hartley CP Jones, EP: EHR Implementation: A Step-by-Step Guide for the Medical Practice. Chicago: AMA, 1996.

Kinkoph SW: Teach Yourself Visually Microsoft Office 2003. Hoboken, N.J.: Wiley Publishing, 2006.

Leuf B, Cunningham W: The Wiki Way: Quick Collaboration on the Web. Boston: Addison-Wesley Professional, 2001.

Walker JM, Buckley S, Richards F, Bieber EJ: Implementing an Electronic Health Record System. London: Springer-Verlag, 2006.

Winston B: Media Technology & Society. London: Routledge, 2004.

Index

Erectile dysfunction (ED) *(Continued)*
    improvement after renal transplantation, 788–789
    incidence of, 783
    medication-induced, 785, 786b
    due to neurogenic alterations, 784, 784b, 785f
    due to physiologic alterations, 783–785, 784b
    treatment of, 786–788, 787b
    due to vascular compromise, 784b, 785
Ergocalciferol
    for chronic kidney disease, 744, 768
    for hypocalcemia, 418
Erythropoiesis-stimulating agents (EPAs)
    for anemia in chronic kidney disease, 751–752, 751t,
        753, 757–758, 761b
    complications of treatment with, 752, 758, 759
    suboptimal responses to, 752–753, 758–759
Erythrocytosis, posttransplantation, 1018
Erythromycin, in renal failure, 1054t
Erythropoietin (EPO)
    for acute kidney injury, 95–96
    for anemia in childhood and adolescence, 525
    in chronic kidney disease, 749, 756
    human recombinant, 757, 760t
    physiology of, 749, 756
    and quality of life in end-stage renal disease, 821t
Erythropoietin (EPO) gene therapy for renal anemia,
    561–562
Escherichia coli, urinary tract infection with, 447–448
Escherichia coli O157:H7
    hemolytic-uremic syndrome due to, 509, 510
    Shiga toxin due to, 295, 309
Escitalopram (Lexapro), in renal failure, 798t
Eskalith. *See* Lithium.
Esmolol
    for hypertensive urgencies, 629
    in renal failure, 1061t
Esophagitis, posttransplantation, 1021
ESRD. *See* End-stage renal disease.
Essential fatty acid (EFA) deficiency, 116–117
Estrogens, conjugated, for uremic bleeding, 760t, 761,
    762t
Eszopiclone (Lunesta), in renal failure, 806t
ET_A (endothelin type A) receptor antagonists, for
    prevention of progressive renal failure, 709
Etanercept, for focal segmental glomerulosclerosis, 230t
Ethacrynic acid
    for acute kidney injury, 37t
    dosage of, 390t
Ethambutol, in renal failure, 1060t, 1068t
Ethanol, for ethylene glycol intoxication, 374
Ethchlorvynol, in renal failure, 1055t
Ethics, of withholding or withdrawal of dialysis, 950
Ethosuximide, in renal failure, 1056t
Ethylene glycol, acidosis due to, 373–374
Ethylene glycol intoxication, hemodialysis for, 62t
Ethylene oxide (EtO), dialysis reactions due to, 894–895,
    896
Etidronate
    for calciphylaxis, 771
    for hypercalcemia, 415
Etoposide, in renal failure, 1060t, 1068t
European Society of Hypertension, 570–571, 571t
EVA-3S (Endarterectomy vs. Angioplasty in Patient with
    Symptomatic Severe Carotid Stenosis) study, 1017
Everolimus (Certican), for renal transplantation, 981t,
    984–985
Excel spreadsheet, 1084
Exchange blood transfusion, for poisoning, 1076
Exemestane, in renal failure, 1068t
Exercise
    for end-stage renal disease, 774, 775t
    for hypertension, 576t, 577–578, 639–640
    and quality of life in end-stage renal disease, 819–823,
        822t
Exit-site infections
    with hemodialysis vascular access, 868
    with peritoneal dialysis, 928–929, 929t
EXP-3174, pharmacology of, 603, 603t
Expenditures, in end-stage renal disease, 836–841
    for hemodialysis, 837–838, 838t, 839t
    Medicare spending in, 836, 837, 837f
    methodologies for evaluating, 836–837, 837t
    for peritoneal dialysis, 839
    for transplantation, 839–840, 840t, 841t
    for vascular access, 838–839

Experimental strategies, for acute kidney injury, 92–96,
    95b
Extended daily dialysis (EDD), 58, 59, 61t, 78
Extended daily dialysis with filtration (EDDf), 78
Extended dialysis, 78
Extracellular fluid (ECF), potassium ions in, 353–354,
    354f
Extracellular fluid (ECF) volume depletion, due to
    diuretics, 398
Extracorporeal albumin dialysis for hepatorenal
    syndrome, 48t, 51–52
Extracorporeal circuit, for hemodialysis, 845–846, 846f
Extracorporeal shock wave lithotripsy, 430, 437
    antibiotics and, 442
    for cystine stones, 548
    efficacy of, 438–439
    indications for, 471
    for renal calculi, 440, 441, 441f
    technique of, 470–471
    for ureteral calculi, 441–442
Extracorporeal therapy. *See also* Renal replacement
    therapy (RRT).
    metabolic impact of, 84, 84b
    for poisoning, 1075–1079, 1077b–1078b, 1078t
Ezetimibe
    for lipid management, 719t
    for posttransplant hyperlipidemia, 1011–1012

F

FA(s). *See* Fatty acids (FAs).
Fab(s)
    for poisoning, 1079
    in renal failure, 1062t
Fabry's disease, 554–555, 554t
FACET (Fosinopril versus Amlodipine Cardiovascular
    Events Randomized Trial), 612, 612t
Falciparum malaria, glomerulonephritis due to,
    146–147
Familial hypocalciuric hypercalcemia (FHH), 413
Familial Mediterranean fever (FMF), 553–554, 554t
Familial rickets, 548–550, 549t
Famotidine, in renal failure, 1056t, 1065t
Fanconi syndrome, 550–552, 551t
Fasudil, for focal segmental glomerulosclerosis, 230t
Fat emulsions, in parenteral nutrition for acute renal
    failure, 88, 88t
Fat intake
    with chronic kidney disease, 742t
    and hypertension, 575–576, 576t
Fatigue in end-stage renal disease, 834t
Fatty acids (FAs)
    dietary manipulation of intake of, 117
    essential, deficiency of, 116–117
    n-3, 112
        biologic properties and effects of, 113–116,
            113f–115f
        dietary supplementation with, 117
    n-6, deficiency of, 116–117
FAVORIT study, 725
FCXM (flow cytometry crossmatch), 978–979
Febuxostat for posttransplant gout, 1025
Felodipine (Plendil)
    cardiovascular effects of, 612, 612t, 613
    with dialysis, 684t, 1061t
    pharmacology of, 610, 611t
Femoral catheter, for hemodialysis, 61–62, 859
Fenofibrate
    for lipid management, 719t
    in renal failure, 1062t, 1071t
Fenoldopam mesylate
    for acute renal failure, 22–23, 24t–27t
    for contrast-induced nephropathy, 23, 24t–25t
    for hypertensive emergencies, 627t, 629
Fentanyl, for pain management in end-stage renal
    disease, 832t
Ferric gluconate, for chronic kidney disease, 752, 753t,
    758
Ferritin, serum, in chronic kidney disease, 752, 753f, 758
Fetal effects, of renal transplant, 492t, 493
Fetus, obstructive uropathy in, 474
Fexofenadine, in renal failure, 1056t, 1065t
FFP (fresh frozen plasma)
    for plasmapheresis, 128
    for thrombotic microangiopathy, 297t, 306t

FGF-23 (fibroblast growth factor 23), and posttrans-
    plant hypophosphatemia, 1026
FHH (familial hypocalciuric hypercalcemia), 413
FHN (Frequent Hemodialysis Network) Trial Group,
    884
Fiber bundle volume, of dialyzer, 849
Fibric acid analogues, for posttransplant hypertriglyc-
    eridemia, 1012
Fibric acid derivatives
    for lipid management, 719t
    for nephrotic syndrome, 286
Fibrillary glomerulonephritis, 258t, 268–269
Fibrillary kidney disease, 257, 258t
    amyloidosis as, 257–264, 258t, 259t
    fibrillary glomerulonephritis and immunotactoid
        glomerulopathy as, 258t, 268–269
Fibrin, in dialysate, 931–932
Fibrinogen Aα amyloidosis, 259t, 263
Fibroblast growth factor 23 (FGF-23), and
    posttransplant hypophosphatemia, 1026
Fibromuscular dysplasia
    in living kidney donor, 965
    renal artery stenosis due to, 647–648, 666, 666f, 667t
Filariasis, glomerulonephritis due to, 147
Filtration, extended daily dialysis with, 78
Finasteride, for benign prostatic hypertrophy, 472
Finnish-type congenital nephrotic syndrome (CNF),
    502
First-use syndrome, 895
Fish oil(s), 112
    biologic properties and effects of, 113–116,
        113f–115f
    for IgA nephropathy, 179, 182t, 507
Fistula First Initiative, 862, 863, 863b
Fistula maturation, for hemodialysis vascular access,
    863–864, 863t
FK506. *See* Tacrolimus.
FK778, for renal transplantation, 986
Flecainide, in renal failure, 1061t, 1070t
Fleet Enema (phosphate enema), for
    hypophosphatemia, 422
Fleroxacin, in renal failure, 1059t, 1067t
Flosequinan, in renal failure, 1071t
Flow cytometry crossmatch (FCXM), 978–979
Flow model, for hemodialysis, 881
Floxacillin, for exit-site infections, 929
Fluconazole
    for candidal UTI, 452
    for peritonitis, 926
    for posttransplant infections, 1042t
    in renal failure, 1059t, 1068t
Flucytosine
    for candidal UTI, 452
    for peritonitis, 926
    for posttransplant infections, 1042t
    in renal failure, 1059t, 1068t
Fludrocortisone acetate
    for hyperkalemia, 364, 365
    for renal tubular acidosis, 378
Fluid administration, for contrast-induced nephropathy,
    42, 42t
Fluid challenge, 7, 7f
Fluid intake
    with chronic kidney disease, 742t
    for end-stage renal disease in childhood and adoles-
        cence, 523
    for prevention of nephrolithiasis, 431, 470
Fluid overload, with peritoneal dialysis, 929–930, 930f,
    931f
Fluid removal, in continuous renal replacement therapy,
    76
Fluid restriction, for hyponatremia, 345
Fluid resuscitation
    monitoring and administration of, 6–7
    selection of, 5–6
Fluid retention, in end-stage renal disease, 681–682
Flumazenil, for poisoning, 1073
Fluoride, in dialysate fluid, 853
Fluoroquinolone, for UTI, 450, 451
Fluoxetine (Prozac, Sarafem), in renal failure, 798t, 812
Fluvastatin
    for lipid management, 719t
    for posttransplant hyperlipidemia, 1011, 1013t
Fluvoxamine (Luvox), in renal failure, 798t
FMF (familial Mediterranean fever), 553–554, 554t